VASCULAR DIAGNOSIS

VASCULAR DIAGNOSIS

EDITED BY

Eugene F. Bernstein, M.D., Ph.D.

Division of Vascular and Thoracic Surgery
Scripps Clinic and Research Foundation;
Clinical Professor of Surgery
University of California, San Diego
La Jolla, California

FOURTH EDITION

with 960 illustrations

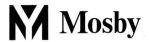 Mosby

St. Louis Baltimore Boston Chicago London Madrid Philadelphia Sydney Toronto

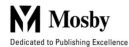

Publisher: George Stamathis
Editor: Susie Baxter
Assistant Developmental Editor: Anne Gunter
Project Manager: Carol Sullivan Wiseman
Senior Production Editor: Linda McKinley
Senior Designer: Jeanne Wolfgeher
Manufacturing Supervisor: Kathy Grone

FOURTH EDITION

Printed in the United States of America

Mosby–Year Book, Inc.
11830 Westline Industrial Drive
St. Louis, Missouri 63146

Library of Congress Cataloging in Publication Data

Vascular diagnosis / edited by Eugene F. Bernstein.—4th ed.
    p. cm.
    Rev. ed. of: Noninvasive diagnostic techniques in vascular
disease. 3rd ed. 1985.
    Includes bibliographical references and index.
    ISBN 0-8016-6557-4
    1. Blood-vessels—Diseases—Diagnosis. 2. Blood-vessels—Imaging.
3. Diagnosis, Noninvasive. I. Bernstein, Eugene F., 1930–
II. Noninvasive diagnostic techniques in vascular disease.
    [DNLM: 1. Vascular Diseases—diagnosis. WG 500 V3312 1993]
RC691.6.N65N66 1993
616.1′3075—dc20
DNLM/DLC
for Library of Congress   93-4086
                                       CIP

93 94 95 96 97 GW/WA 9 8 7 6 5 4 3 2 1

CONTRIBUTORS

ROB G.A. ACKERSTAFF, M.D., Ph.D.

Chairman, Department of Clinical Neurophysiology,
St. Antonius Hospital, Koekoekslaan 1, Nieuwegein,
The Netherlands

FREDERICK A. ANDERSON, Jr., Ph.D.

Research Associate Professor, Department of Surgery,
University of Massachusetts Medical Center, Worcester,
Massachusetts

JEFFREY L. BALLARD, M.D.

Vascular Surgery Fellow, Department of Vascular Surgery,
Loma Linda University Medical Center, Loma Linda, California

DENNIS F. BANDYK, M.D.

Professor of Surgery, Director, Division of Vascular Surgery,
University of South Florida, Tampa, Florida

ROBERT W. BARNES, M.D.

Professor and Chairman, Department of Surgery, University
Hospital of Arkansas, Veterans Administration Medical Center,
University of Arkansas for Medical Sciences, Little Rock,
Arkansas

KIRK W. BEACH, Ph.D., M.D.

Research Associate Professor, Department of Surgery, RF-25,
University of Washington, Seattle, Washington

GIANNI BELCARO, M.D.

Professor, Medicine and Surgery, General Surgery, Thoracic
Surgery, Institute of Cardiovascular Clinic, Microcirculation
Laboratory, ACV (Angiologia, Chirurgia Vascolare, Pierangeli
Clinic, Pescara); G.D'Annunzio University, Chieti, Italy

EUGENE F. BERNSTEIN, M.D.

Division of Vascular and Thoracic Surgery, Scripps Clinic
Medical Group; Clinical Professor of Surgery, University of
California, San Diego, La Jolla, California

HENRI BISMUTH, F.A.C.S.

Professor of Surgery, Hepato-Biliary Surgery and Liver
Transplantation Department, Hopital Paul Brousse, Villejuif,
France

M. GENE BOND, Ph.D.

Director, Division of Vascular Ultrasound Research, Department
of Neurobiology and Anatomy, Bowman Gray School of
Medicine, Winston-Salem, North Carolina

EDWIN C. BROCKENBROUGH, M.D., F.A.C.S.

Past Chief of Staff, Northwest Hospital; Clinical Professor of
Surgery, University of Washington, Seattle, Washington

NORMAN L. BROWSE, M.D., P.R.C.S.

President, Royal College of Surgeons,
Professor, Department of Surgery, St. Thomas Hospital,
London, England

CYNTHIA B. BURNHAM, B.S.N., R.N., R.V.T.

Technical Director, Peripheral Vascular Laboratory, UNC
Hospitals; Clinical Assistant Professor, Department of Surgery,
University of North Carolina School of Medicine, Chapel Hill,
North Carolina

PETER N. BURNS, M.D.

Senior Scientist, Sunnybrook Health Science Centre; Professor
of Medical Biophysics and Radiology, University of Toronto,
Ontario, Canada

STEFAN A. CARTER, M.D., B.Sc. (Med), M.Sc., F.R.C.P.(C)

Director, Vascular Laboratory, Department of Medicine, St.
Boniface General Hospital; Professor, Department of Physiology
and Medicine, University of Manitoba, Winnipeg, Manitoba,
Canada

DOUGLAS M. CAVAYE, M.D., B.S., F.R.A.C.S.

Vascular Surgeon, Division of Vascular Surgery, Department of
Surgery, Harbor-UCLA Medical Center, Torrance, California;
Visiting Vascular Surgeon, Wadsworth Veterans Administration
Medical Center; Instructor in Surgery, UCLA School of
Medicine, Los Angeles, California

BENJAMIN B. CHANG, M.D.

Department of Surgery, Albany Medical College, Albany,
New York

DIMITRIS CHRISTOPOULOS, M.D., Ph.D.

Senior Lecturer in General and Vascular Surgery, B2 Surgical Unit, Hippokrateion Hospital, University of Salonica, Greece

ROBERT COURBIER, M.D.

Professor, Vascular Surgery, Chief, Department of Cardiovascular Surgery, St. Joseph Hospital, Marseille, France

JOHN J. CRANLEY, M.D.

Director of Surgery Emeritus, Director Emeritus, The John J. Cranley Vascular Laboratory, Good Samaritan Hospital, Cincinnati, Ohio; Director, Kachelmacher Memorial Clinic, Logan, Ohio; Chairman, The Cranley Surgical Associates, Inc., Cincinnati, Ohio

DAVID L. DAWSON, M.D.

Staff Surgeon, Vascular Laboratory Director, Vascular Surgery Service, Wilford Hall USAF Medical Center, Lackland AFB, Texas; Assistant Professor of Surgery, Uniformed Services University of the Health Sciences, F. Edward Hèbert School of Medicine, Bethesda, Maryland

RALPH B. DILLEY, M.D.

Head, Division of Vascular Surgery, Director, Heart, Lung, and Vascular Center, Scripps Clinic and Research Foundation; Clinical Professor, Department of Surgery, University of California Medical School, San Diego, La Jolla, California

JAMES M. EDWARDS, M.D.

Assistant Professor, Division of Vascular Surgery, Department of Surgery, Oregon Health Sciences University; Staff Surgeon, Department of Surgery, Portland Veterans Administration Medical Center, Portland, Oregon

BERT C. EIKELBOOM, M.D.

Professor of Vascular Surgery, Department of Surgery, University Hospital Utrecht, The Netherlands

MICHEL FERDANI, M.D.

Cardiovascular Surgery, St. Joseph Hospital, Marseille, France

PETER J. FITZGERALD, M.D., Ph.D.

Senior Cardiology Fellow, Department of Cardiology, University of California, San Francisco, California

WILLIAM R. FLINN, M.D.

Associate Professor of Surgery, Department of Vascular Surgery, Northwestern University Medical School, Northwestern Memorial Hospital; Director, Center for Vascular Disease, Columbus Hospital, Chicago, Illinois

ARNOST FRONEK, M.D., Ph.D.

Professor, Department of Surgery and Bioengineering, University of California, San Diego, La Jolla, California

DON P. GIDDENS, Ph.D.

Dean, G.W.C. Whiting School of Engineering, Johns Hopkins University, Baltimore, Maryland

ROBERT R.M. GIFFORD, M.D.

Professor of Surgery, Department of Surgery, The Pennsylvania State University College of Medicine, Hershey, Pennsylvania

EDWARD G. GRANT, M.D.

Professor and Vice Chairman, Department of Radiological Sciences, UCLA School of Medicine; Chief, Radiology Service, Veterans Affairs Medical Center—West Los Angeles, Los Angeles, California

LAZAR J. GREENFIELD, M.D.

Frederick A. Coller Professor and Chairman, Department of Surgery, Surgeon-in-Chief, University of Michigan Hospitals, Ann Arbor, Michigan

DEAN A. HEALY, M.D.

Assistant Professor, Vascular Surgery Center, Department of Surgery, Pennsylvania State University College of Medicine, Hershey, Pennsylvania

CHARLES B. HIGGINS, M.D.

Professor and Vice Chairman of Radiology, Chief, Magnetic Resonance Imaging, University of California, San Francisco, California

JACK HIRSH, M.D.

Director, Hamilton Civic Hospitals Research Center; Professor, Department of Medicine, McMaster University, Hamilton, Ontario, Canada

ROBERT W. HOBSON II, M.D.

Professor of Surgery, Chief, Section of Vascular Surgery, Department of Surgery, University of Medicine of New Jersey, New Jersey Medical School, Newark, New Jersey

TIMOTHY C. HODGES, M.D.

Vascular Research Fellow, Division of Vascular Surgery, Department of Surgery, University of Washington School of Medicine, Seattle, Washington

RUSSELL D. HULL, M.B.B.S.

Professor of Medicine, Head, Division of General Internal Medicine, University of Calgary, Foothills Hospital; Head, Division of General Internal Medicine, Department of Medicine, University of Calgary—Faculty of Medicine, Calgary, Alberta, Canada

E. MEREDITH JAMES, M.D.

Associate Professor of Radiology, Department of Diagnostic Radiology, Mayo Clinic, Rochester, Minnesota

CESS JANSEN, M.D.

Department of Clinical Neurophysiology, St. Antonius Hospital, Koekoekslaan 1, Nieuwegein, The Netherlands

KAJ JOHANSEN, M.D., Ph.D.

Director, Surgical Education, Providence Medical Center; Professor of Surgery, University of Washington School of Medicine, Seattle, Washington

K. WAYNE JOHNSTON, M.D., F.R.C.S.(C)

Professor of Surgery and Associate Chair, Department of Surgery, University of Toronto, Ontario, Canada

ANNE M. JONES, R.N., B.S.N., R.V.T. (RDMS)

Co-Director, Vascular Laboratory, Department of Surgery, Montefiore Medical Center, Albert Einstein College of Medicine, Bronx, New York

EVI KALODIKI, M.D., B.A.

Surgeon, Vascular Department, Academic Surgical Unit, St. Mary's Hospital, Paddington; Senior Vascular Research Fellow, Vascular Department Academic Surgical Unit, St. Mary's Hospital Medical School and Imperial College, London, England

RICHARD F. KEMPCZINSKI, M.D.

Professor, Department of Surgery, Chief, Division of Vascular Surgery, University of Cincinnati Medical Center, Cincinnati, Ohio

THOMAS M. KERR, M.D.

Assistant Professor of Surgery and Anesthesiology, University of South Florida College of Medicine; Chief, Section of Vascular Surgery, Director, Surgical Intensive Care Unit, Director, Noninvasive Vascular Laboratory, Veterans Administration Medical Center, Bay Pines, Florida

PROFESSOR RICHARD I. KITNEY

Director, Centre for Biological and Medical Systems and the Department of Electrical Engineering, Imperial College of Science, Technology and Medicine, London, England

TED R. KOHLER, M.D.

Chief, Vascular Surgery, Seattle Veterans Affairs Medical Center; Associate Professor, Department of Surgery, University of Washington, Seattle, Washington

GEORGE E. KOPCHOK, B.S.

Biomedical Engineer, Division of Vascular Surgery, Harbor-UCLA Medical Center, Torrance, California

FREDERICK W. KREMKAU, Ph.D.

Professor and Director, Center for Medical Ultrasound, Bowman Gray School of Medicine, Wake Forest University, Winston-Salem, North Carolina

ANN MARIE KUPINSKI, M.S.

Department of Surgery, Albany Medical College, Albany, New York

NIKOS LABROPOULOS, B.Sc.

St. Mary's Hospital, London, England

ROBERT P. LEATHER, M.D.

Professor of Surgery and Head Division of Vascular Surgery, Department of Surgery, Albany Medical College, Albany, New York

TREVOR LEESE, M.D., F.R.C.S.

Consultant Surgeon, Department of Surgery, Royal Lancaster Infirmary, Lancaster, England

ANTHONIE W.A. LENSING, M.D., Ph.D.

Assistant Professor, Department of Neurology, Academic Medical Center, University of Amsterdam, The Netherlands

MIGUEL LEON, M.D.

Vascular Surgeon, Irvine Laboratory Academic Surgical Unit, St. Mary's Hospital, Central University-Quito-Ecuador, London, England

MICHAEL P. LILLY, M.D.

Assistant Professor of Surgery, Director, Noninvasive Vascular Laboratory, Department of Surgery, University of Maryland Hospital; Assistant Professor, Department of Surgery, University of Maryland, Baltimore, Maryland

JOANN M. LOHR, M.D.

Director, John J. Cranley Vascular Laboratory, Good Samaritan Hospital, Cincinnati, Ohio; Co-Director, Kachelmacher Clinic, Logan, Ohio

THOMAS G. LYNCH, M.D.

Associate Professor and Chief, Section of Vascular Surgery, Department of Surgery, University of Nebraska Medical Center, Omaha, Nebraska

JAMES M. MALONE, M.D.

Chairman, Department of Surgery, Maricopa Medical Center; Clinical Professor, Department of Surgery, University of Arizona, Phoenix, Arizona

MARK A. MATTOS, M.D.

Assistant Professor of Surgery, Section of Peripheral Vascular Surgery, Southern Illinois University, Springfield, Illinois

ROBERT F. MATTREY, M.D.

Professor, Department of Radiology, UCSD Medical Center, San Diego, California

MARK H. MEISSNER, M.D.

Senior Vascular Fellow, Department of Surgery, University of Washington School of Medicine, Seattle, Washington

MICHELE MERCURI, M.D., Ph.D.

Research Assistant Professor Deputy Director Division of Vascular Ultrasound Research, Department of Neurobiology and Anatomy, Bowman Gray School of Medicine, Wake Forest University, Winston-Salem, North Carolina

CHRISTOPHER R.B. MERRITT, M.D.

Chairman, Department of Radiology, Ochsner Clinic and Alton Ochsner Medical Foundation, New Orleans, Louisiana

JOSEPH M. MESSICK, Jr., M.D.

Professor of Anesthesiology, Mayo Medical School, Department of Anesthesiology, Mayo Clinic, Mayo Foundation, Rochester, Minnesota

LOUIS M. MESSINA, M.D.

Assistant Professor of Surgery, Director, Diagnostic Vascular Laboratory, Section of Vascular Surgery, University of Michigan Medical Center, Ann Arbor, Michigan

MARSHA M. NEUMYER, B.S., R.V.T.

Instructor of Surgery, Department of Surgery, The Pennsylvania State University College of Medicine, Hershey, Pennsylvania

ANDREW N. NICOLAIDES

Professor of Vascular Surgery, Director, Academic Vascular Surgery Unit, St. Mary's Hospital, London, England

M. LEE NIX, B.S.N., R.N., R.V.T.

Director of Vascular Laboratory, University Hospital; Instructor, Department of Surgery, University of Arkansas for Medical Sciences, Little Rock, Arkansas

JOHN W. NORRIS, M.D., F.R.C.P.

Professor of Neurology, University of Toronto, Ontario, Canada

STEVEN P. OKUHN, M.D.

Assistant Clinical Professor of Surgery, Department of Surgery, Division of Vascular Surgery, University of California, San Francisco Medical Center; Staff Surgeon, Kaiser Hospital, San Francisco, California

SHIRLEY M. OTIS, M.D.

Senior Consultant, Division of Neurology, Medical Director, Vascular Laboratories, Division of Neurology, Scripps Clinic and Research Foundation, La Jolla, California

BILL C. PENNEY, Ph.D.

Associate Professor, Departments of Nuclear Medicine and Surgery, University of Massachusetts, Worcester, Massachusetts

JOHN M. PORTER, M.D.

Professor, Department of Surgery, Head, Division of Vascular Surgery, Oregon Health Sciences University, Portland, Oregon

THOMAS A. PORTS, M.D.

Director, Cardiac Catheterization Laboratories, Adult Cardiology Services, University of California San Francisco Medical Center, San Francisco, California

JEFFREY K. RAINES, M.D.

Associate Professor, Department of Epidemiology, University of Miami School of Medicine, Miami, Florida

GARY E. RASKOB, M.Sc.

Assistant Professor, Department of Biostatistics and Epidemiology, College of Public Health, Department of Medicine, College of Medicine, University of Oklahoma, Oklahoma City, Oklahoma

MICHEL REGGI, M.D.

Chief, Angiology Department, St. Joseph Hospital, Marseille, France

LINDA M. REILLY, M.D.

Associate Professor of Surgery, University of California, San Francisco, California

WILLIAM G. REISS, PHARM. D.

Department of Pharmacy Practice, University of Wisconsin, Madison, Wisconsin

FERNAND RIES, M.D.

Privatdozent (Associate Professor of Neurology), Department of Neurology, University Clinic Bonn, F.R. Germany

E. BERND RINGELSTEIN, M.D.

Professor and Chairman, Department of Neurology, University Hospital, Westfalische Wilhelms-University, Domagkstr. 5, Munster, Germany

ROBERT J. RIZZO, M.D.

Vascular Surgery Fellow, Northwestern University Medical School, Chicago, Illinois

ROBERT B. RUTHERFORD, M.D.

Professor and Chief, Vascular Surgery Section, University of Colorado Health Services Center, Denver, Colorado

GAIL P. SANDAGER, R.N., R.V.T.

Technical Director, Vascular Laboratory, Columbus Hospital, Chicago, Illinois

MICHAEL J. SCHINA, Jr., M.D.

Resident in Vascular Surgery, Department of Surgery, The Pennsylvania State University College of Medicine, Hershey, Pennsylvania

TORBEN V. SCHROEDER, M.D., Ph.D.

Consultant Vascular Surgeon, Department of Vascular Surgery, Rigshospitalet; Professor of Surgery, University of Copenhagen, Denmark

DHIRAJ M. SHAH, M.D.

Department of Surgery, Albany Medical College, Albany, New York

PRAVIN M. SHAH, M.D.

Professor of Medicine, Director, Academic Program, Section of Cardiology, Loma Linda University Medical Center, Loma Linda, California

FRANK W. SHARBROUGH, M.D.

Department of Neurologic Surgery, Mayo Clinic, Rochester, Minnesota

RONALD J. STONEY, M.D.

Professor, Department of Surgery, Division of Vascular Surgery, University of California, San Francisco Medical Center, San Francisco, California

D. EUGENE STRANDNESS, Jr., M.D.

Attending Vascular Surgeon, Department of Surgery, University of Washington Medical Center; Professor of Surgery and Chief, Division of Vascular Surgery, Department of Surgery, University of Washington School of Medicine, Seattle, Washington

KRISHNANKUTTY SUDHIR, M.D., Ph.D.

Senior Cardiology Research Fellow, Cardiology Division Moffit Hospital, Clinical Research Fellow; Cardiovascular Research Institute, University of California, San Francisco, California

DAVID S. SUMNER, M.D.

Distinguished Professor, Department of Surgery, Chief, Section of Peripheral Vascular Surgery, Southern Illinois University School of Medicine, Springfield, Illinois

†THORALF M. SUNDT, Jr., M.D.

Professor, Department of Neurologic Surgery, Mayo Clinic, Rochester, Minnesota

RONG TANG, M.D.

Research Associate, Division of Vascular Ultrasound Research, Department of Neurobiology and Anatomy, Bowman Gray School of Medicine, Wake Forest University, Winston-Salem, North Carolina

KENNETH J.W. TAYLOR, M.D., Ph.D., F.A.C.P.

Professor, Department of Diagnostic Radiology, Yale New Haven Hospital; Director, Vascular Laboratory, Director of Experimental Laboratory, Academic Research Director, Department of Diagnostic Radiology, Yale University School of Medicine, New Haven, Connecticut

PETER TAYLOR, M.D.

Consultant Vascular Surgeon, Guy's Hospital, London, England

BRIAN L. THIELE, M.D.

Professor of Surgery, Department of Surgery, The Pennsylvania State University College of Medicine, Hershey, Pennsylvania

OLAV THULESIUS, M.D., Ph.D.

Professor, Department of Clinical Physiology, University Hospital, Linköping, Linköping, Sweden

JAN H.M. TORDOIR, M.D., Ph.D.

Vascular Surgeon, Department of Surgery, University Hospital Maastricht, The Netherlands

PAUL S. van BEMMELEN, M.D., Ph.D.

Clinical Vascular Fellow, Section of Peripheral Vascular Surgery, St. John's Hospital, Southern Illinois University, Springfield, Illinois

TREVOR M. Van WAGENEN, B.A.

Vascular Technologist, John J. Cranley Vascular Laboratory, Good Samaritan Hospital, Cincinnati, Ohio

SPIROS N. VASDEKIS, M.D.

Vascular Surgeon, Pireus General Hospital, Athens, Greece

NICOS VOLTEAS, M.D.

St. Mary's Hospital, London, England

H. BROWNELL WHEELER, M.D.

Harry M. Haidak Distinguished Professor of Surgery, Professor and Chairman, Department of Surgery, University of Massachusetts Medical Center, Worcester, Massachusetts

RODNEY A. WHITE, M.D.

Chief, Vascular Surgery, Harbor-UCLA Medical Center, Torrance, California; Professor of Surgery, Department of Surgery, UCLA School of Medicine, Los Angeles, California

YEHUDA G. WOLF, M.D.

Attending Surgeon, Department of Surgery, Veterans Administration Hospital, La Jolla, California; Assistant Clinical Professor, Department of Surgery, University of California School of Medicine, San Diego, California

HAROLD C. YANG, M.D., Ph.D.

Associate Professor of Surgery, The Pennsylvania State University College of Medicine, Hershey, Pennsylvania

JAMES S.T. YAO, M.D., Ph.D.

Attending Surgeon, Department of Surgery, Northwestern Memorial Hospital; Magerstadt Professor of Surgery, Chief, Division of Vascular Surgery, Department of Surgery, Northwestern University Medical School, Chicago, Illinois

PAUL G. YOCK, M.D.

Associate Professor, Department of Medicine and Cardiovascular Research Institute, University of California, San Francisco, California

BRENDA K. ZIERLER, B.S.N., R.V.T.

Department of Surgery, University of Washington, Seattle, Washington

R. EUGENE ZIERLER, M.D.

Associate Professor of Surgery, Division of Vascular Surgery, University of Washington School of Medicine, Seattle, Washington

---

†Deceased.

PREFACE

The first edition of this work was published in 1978 when it was apparent that a new technology of vascular investigation had emerged from the research laboratory and was rapidly spreading throughout the clinical world. Subsequent editions were published to update and supplement the original material in 1982 and 1985 under the title, *Noninvasive Diagnostic Techniques in Vascular Disease*. Although the field continued to expand, a full fourth edition was not undertaken until now because the basic methods and underlying principles had not changed significantly, and therefore an interim update, *Recent Advances in Noninvasive Diagnostic Techniques in Vascular Disease,* was considered adequate and was published in 1990. Further rapid advances in technology have propelled this field forward during the last few years and now justify a complete and full revision of the volume to comprehensively cover this growing field.

As an indication of the magnitude of the changes that have occurred, the title has been altered to *Vascular Diagnosis* to reflect the fact that not all of the instruments are still completely noninvasive. Some powerful advances with ultrasound applicable to the diagnosis of vascular conditions include the transvaginal visualization of the pelvic vessels as well as the use of "semiinvasive" devices such as the endovascular ultrasound probes and subsequent three-dimensional reconstructions. Thus the older *Noninvasive* title no longer seemed appropriate. The vast majority of this book is new, and the few continuing chapters have been completely revised and updated.

In this volume, we have attempted to continue to provide the reader with a complete source of information, which includes the basic science underlying the development of each of the diagnostic instruments. In addition, all of the currently useful approaches to a given problem are presented by their originator or by another recognized expert in the field. The introductions to each clinical area were written by the section editors to highlight those special advances that follow and those areas in which differences of opinion exist. When a particular conflict regarding the appropriate device or approach to a specific problem has continued without resolution, we have attempted to present all sides of the discussion, with current information and arguments, so that the reader may be up-to-date and make a choice based on the latest information rather than one editor's opinion.

Another area of this book differing from some others in the field is the inclusion of "derived information" that has been obtained with vascular diagnostic testing over the years and that may influence clinical judgments regarding the appropriate use of the vascular laboratory. In addition, the expanded range of application of vascular technology to the diagnosis of diseases of the parenchyma of the visceral and pelvic organs, including questions of malignancy and transplant rejection, has been covered in this volume, since they employ the same technology and are often supervised by the same physicians.

The continuing maturation of the field of vascular diagnosis is evidenced by the concurrent evolution of training programs, testing, and certification of both the personnel and the facilities involved. Detailed information regarding this evolving process is included because of its increasing importance in ensuring a basic level of quality performance, which is correctly demanded by both our patients and the payment systems.

Fortunately, most of the editors of the original volumes, including Drs. Ralph B. Dilley, Arnost Fronek, D. Eugene Strandness, Jr., and James S.T. Yao, have continued to participate in the planning and preparation of this edition. We have been joined by a number of distinguished colleagues, including Drs. Dennis F. Bandyk, Bernardus C. Eikelboom, Edward G. Grant, Christopher R.B. Merritt, Andrew N. Nicolaides, Brian S. Thiele, and R. Eugene Zierler. Together, the editorial group represents the entire spectrum of vascular diagnosis with an international, multispecialty background. Without their contributions and those of the many experts whose chapters are the heart of this volume, the full and authoritative coverage we have aimed for would not be possible.

The editorial and production staff of Mosby–Year Book has been ably directed by Anne Gunter, who was heavily involved in the preparation of the third edition, and by Susie Baxter, the surgery editor, and Linda McKinley, the production editor. The authors would also like to express their profound appreciation to Mrs. Gita Braude for her expert work as the San Diego medical editor of this volume.

Eugene F. Bernstein

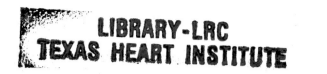

TABLE OF CONTENTS

Introduction

EUGENE F. BERNSTEIN

Rapid and profound strides have been made in vascular diagnosis since the first edition of this book was published in 1978.[1] That volume marked the beginning of an era of widespread clinical application of noninvasive instrumentation, which permitted identifying the site and quantifying the degree of vascular disease in many locations in the body. Before that, the history and physical examination and a few devices such as the blood pressure cuff and the plethysmograph were the limits of our diagnostic armamentarium, short of formal contrast angiography. Vascular laboratories were confined to a few research centers, and most vascular diagnosis was performed by the vascular surgeon, who offered the only effective methods of therapy.

Most important in the development of our contemporary ability to characterize vascular conditions has been the development of ultrasound techniques. Devices employing the Doppler effect to detect the presence and velocity of moving particles in the blood stream became clinically available in the late 1960s, and the early A-mode and B-mode imaging modalities first were available to clinicians around 1970. The concept of obtaining blood pressures at several segmental levels in the lower extremities, both at rest and with stress, and the development of carotid bruit analysis and two forms of oculoplethysmography to indirectly assess the presence of carotid stenosis provided enough additional insight into vascular conditions to justify the formation of independent vascular laboratories in a number of clinical centers in the United States and Europe in the early 1970s.

The original plan for the first edition of this book was to provide a single source of information about "noninvasive" vascular diagnosis, which included a solid foundation in the basic principles underlying the various instruments, considerations of the selection of diagnostic approaches for a given clinical situation, details of device operation, methods of data analysis and interpretation, and a repository of useful data. Our goal was to provide guidance to the physician planning to initiate and direct a vascular laboratory, the practitioner with a clinical problem to analyze, and the researcher who needed to know the state of the art to improve upon it. In the subsequent two editions and the supplementary volume, *Recent Advances,* published in 1990, we have endeavored to continue to fulfill these objectives by attempting to remain up-to-date in a rapidly evolving and improving field.

In the current edition, we deleted the word *noninvasive* from the title because the field of vascular diagnosis has become so broad and now involves the vascular laboratory, conventional radiology, new imaging modalities (CT and MRI), and a variety of percutaneous invasive radiologic and surgical methods. Thus *noninvasive* becomes too limiting a definition of the choices currently available to the clinician (box). The role of the vascular laboratory continues to be the detection and documentation of vascular disease, characterization of arterial and venous obstruction and venous valvular incompetence and their functional significance, localization of anatomic site, and evaluation of the results of

---

CURRENT ROLE OF THE VASCULAR LABORATORY

Structure

Pressure (screening and detection)
Localization (number, extent)
Characterization (composition, age)

Function

Doppler velocity ($\times$ A = flow)
Pressure (at rest/with stress)
Volume = plethysmography (impedance, strain gauge, air, liquid)
  With inflow or outflow occlusion or respiration
Cutaneous circulation
  Microscopy
  Photoplethysmography
  Laser Doppler
  Transcutaneous oxygen and carbon dioxide
  Temperature

SPECTRUM OF VASCULAR DIAGNOSIS

Noninvasive   *Invasive*

(Vascular lab ⟷ Radiology)   (Radiology ⟷ Surgery)

STRUCTURE

B-mode ultrasound   Angioscopy
CT/MRI   Angiography
                                       Endovascular ultrasound

FUNCTION

Doppler ultrasound
Pressure
Volume
Temperature
Gas tension
Microscopy

---

treatment. In addition to this structural information, however, there is an obligation to provide more functional information than was available in the past by using many measurement modalities (box).

Newer technology is often so expensive and so multipotent that it must be shared or duplicated in the medical center or hospital setting. Nevertheless, these more sensitive and sophisticated devices provide so much information that methods of data reduction have become principal requirements for their clinical usefulness. Placing such technology in appropriate perspective is another important role for this edition. In a parallel effort, we have attempted to gracefully "retire" those techniques that now seem archaic while retaining others for which significant applications still appear to exist.

This volume updates descriptions of all the basic methodology previously published in the third edition in 1985 and, in addition, adds the developments of the past 3 years to the material covered in *Recent Advances* in 1990.[2,3] The focus of the newest information must be the real-time color flow Doppler systems, which have rapidly become a standard, not only for many vascular laboratories but also for many other specialties, such as obstetrics and radiology, with interests in pregnancy, pelvic and abdominal tumors, the breast, the neck, and the extremity. We have attempted to cover only those applications that are fundamentally vascular, but the basic principles of these instruments, the differences among them, and the basis for selection and application of a specific system are all within the range of this effort. Because many vascular laboratories are currently in radiology departments, we have added additional material relevant to vascular problems in areas not usually included under the traditional definition of vascular disease. These areas, such as the pancreas and female pelvis, are currently studied by similar ultrasound methods, and information regarding the techniques and results of such studies appears relevant and valuable to anyone concerned with vascular diagnosis.

Newer, low-frequency probes have expanded the areas that may be examined by our ultrasound systems. We now expect to obtain information about the great vessels of the aortic arch, the vertebral arteries, and the intracranial circulation in any patient sent to the vascular laboratory for cerebrovascular evaluation. Endovaginal and endorectal probes permit examination of the iliac veins deep within the pelvis. Several new chapters deal with the role of transcranial Doppler, both as a diagnostic and as a monitoring method. Real-time color flow transcranial Doppler also has become available and will increase our ease in obtaining three-dimensional information.

Other significant advances in vascular laboratory capability, particularly in obtaining quantitative information, are those systems directed at measuring cutaneous functions, including laser Doppler and transcutaneous oxygen tension. Characterization of the cutaneous circulation is becoming progressively more important in our understanding of both arterial and venous disease and in evaluating specific ischemic lesions for potential healing, the need for reconstructive surgery, or amputation.

Applications of vascular laboratory methodology have brought us a great deal of new information about the natural history of atherogenesis and those interventions that may affect it. Arterial wall thickness, particularly of the carotid arteries, appears to be a useful index of atherosclerosis elsewhere in the body. Additional data regarding the role of surgery in cerebrovascular disease and the proper place of intraoperative and postoperative monitoring have been accumulated, placing our knowledge of both these areas on a sounder footing.

In the peripheral arterial tree, increasing therapeutic applications of invasive radiologic techniques have emphasized the need for screening those patients with less extensive disease than would warrant surgery as potential candidates for angioplasty, atherectomy, and stent placement. Duplex and real-time color devices are particularly valuable for this function. In addition, low-frequency transducers now permit scanning the abdominal aorta for both aneurysms and occlusive disease and evaluation of the renal and mesenteric circulations for significant stenoses. In many situations in the periphery, as at the carotid bifurcation, vascular laboratory information has reached such a high level of reliability that formal contrast angiography may not be necessary as a diagnostic technique. These include postoperative monitoring of both renal and hepatic transplants as well as renal and visceral artery reconstructions.

In the venous system, increased sensitivity has moved the emphasis from the detection of acute venous thrombosis in the larger vessels of the thigh to the detection of very small clots in the gastrocnemius and soleus muscles. Often these lesions do not produce symptoms, and controversy regarding their management has become an important clinical problem. The significance of a negative scan for DVT and of a free-floating venous thrombus is also recognized as important, and significant new information has been generated. Additional interest has focused on the diseased venous valve, both congenital and postthrombotic. Identification of the location and degree of reflux in the critical valves protecting the veins of the thigh and calf, when coupled with better surgical methods of repair and/or replacement, may open a wide area of therapy for many people who are seriously handicapped with chronic venous insufficiency. Current approaches, which must be placed on trial for their clinical usefulness, include several concepts for evaluating and quantitating valve insufficiency.

Finally, the frontier of vascular diagnosis, which includes magnetic resonance angiography, endovascular Doppler, three-dimensional representations, and Doppler contrast agents, will provide us with even better methods within the next several years and a promise to change this entire area once again. We are looking forward to these exciting advances, which will add to our ability to provide our patients and their doctors with more precise, safe, and appropriate diagnostic information.

REFERENCES

1. Bernstein EF, ed: *Noninvasive diagnostic techniques in vascular disease,* St Louis, 1978, Mosby.
2. Bernstein EF, ed: *Noninvasive diagnostic techniques in vascular disease,* ed 3, St Louis, 1985, Mosby.
3. Bernstein EF, ed: *Recent advances in noninvasive diagnostic techniques in vascular disease,* St Louis, 1990, Mosby.

PART ONE

GENERAL ASPECTS OF VASCULAR DIAGNOSIS

CHAPTER 1

The history and physical examination in vascular disease

RALPH B. DILLEY

Although this book deals predominately with methods of vascular diagnosis that are noninvasive or minimally invasive, many conditions encountered by vascular specialists may be accurately diagnosed by obtaining a careful history and performing a detailed physical examination. Consequently, the experienced clinician should be able to predict the status of the circulation to the lower extremities, often before the physical examination, if a careful history is obtained. Physical findings add certainty to the diagnosis in most cases, and the techniques described in this book provide confirmation of the clinical impression, quantitate the severity of the problem, and provide follow-up information after therapeutic interventions.

In some areas the history and physical findings are not as specific, such as in occlusive peripheral vascular disease. For example, the history in patients with neurologic syndromes associated with carotid artery disease is suggestive, the physical findings are nonspecific, and these diagnoses almost always require confirmation by other techniques. Similarly, the symptoms and physical findings in patients with mesenteric artery stenosis and renal artery stenosis are frequently nonspecific and always require investigation by other techniques. Finally, the symptoms and signs associated with the leg pain of acute venous disease are not as characteristic as arterial pain syndromes, and they too require evaluation by noninvasive testing for an accurate diagnosis.

In this chapter, important aspects of the history and physical findings are reviewed as they relate to arterial and venous obstructions in various vascular beds.

EXTRACRANIAL CAROTID OCCLUSIVE DISEASE

The history is important in patients with carotid artery stenosis or occlusion. The symptoms include a spectrum of neurologic complaints and may range from a minor problem, such as blurring of vision in one eye, to profound obtundation, aphasia, and hemiparesis. Because a majority of patients with hemispheric neurologic symptoms have significant related carotid artery disease, which is amenable to surgical repair, recognizing the various neurologic symptom complexes that may occur is important.

Amaurosis fugax

Amaurosis fugax, or fleeting blindness, is a common symptom most often caused by emboli that originate from an atherosclerotic plaque in the ipsilateral internal carotid artery and migrate to the ophthalmic artery and its branches. The patient complains of temporary loss of vision in one eye caused by transient interference of its arterial blood supply. In general, the attacks occur without a precipitating factor and commonly involve the entire monocular visual field. Vision becomes hazy, beginning in the upper visual field and extending downward, like a window shade being pulled down. Occasionally, patients describe patchy loss of vision. The attacks last from a few seconds to a few minutes, after which vision returns to normal. Careful attention must be paid to whether the symptoms are monocular or binocular. If both eyes are involved, the cause is rarely carotid artery disease.

Because visual disturbances are common symptoms, other causes of transient visual loss must be considered. These include emboli from the great vessels or heart, primary ocular pathology, neurologic diseases (e.g., optic neuritis, optic nerve compression), blood disorders (e.g., polycythemia), and systemic conditions (e.g., migraine, arteritis).[1]

Transient ischemic attacks

Transient ischemic attacks (TIAs) are brief episodes of neurologic dysfunction most frequently caused by embolic showers from an atheromatous carotid artery to the ipsilateral cerebral hemisphere. Patients may complain of paresthesia or anesthesia in an arm or leg. When a motor abnormality is prominent, weakness, paralysis, or incoordination on the involved side of the body may be present. Brief aphasic or dysphasic symptoms may occur with involvement of the dominant hemisphere. The attacks are quite brief, lasting from a few seconds to minutes and only rarely extending beyond 3 hours. TIAs are the result of focal neurologic deficits and occur on the side opposite the involved area of the brain and carotid artery. If patients complain of global symptoms such as dizziness or vertigo, the diagnosis becomes complex because these symptoms generally are not caused by carotid artery stenosis.

Reversible ischemic neurologic deficit

Reversible ischemic neurologic deficits (RINDs) persist for longer than 24 hours and ultimately disappear completely. When the symptoms of RINDs occur and are identical with TIAs, the patient may have sustained a small area of cerebral infarction, which is often not visible on a computerized tomographic scan. Finally, neurologic symptoms that persist for long periods are generally related to cerebral infarction and are diagnosed as a completed stroke.

Stroke in evolution and crescendo TIAs

These two clinical syndromes have recently been recognized more frequently. A patient with a stroke in evolution complains of an acute neurologic deficit, which progresses over a period of hours or days and ultimately results in a fixed deficit caused by cerebral infarction. Occasionally, exacerbations of the neurologic deficit or a waxing and waning pattern with incomplete recovery between episodes may be seen. This pattern is clearly different from a TIA in which recovery is complete after each episode. Crescendo carotid territory TIAs define a syndrome in which multiple TIAs occur within a short time, but each attack is followed by complete recovery. These two clinical syndromes generally indicate high-grade carotid artery stenosis with embolization and are an urgent indication for further evaluation.[2,3]

Vertebrobasilar disease

Symptoms of vertebrobasilar insufficiency are numerous and difficult to relate to specific areas in the brain. They arise from transient ischemia to the areas of the brain supplied by the vertebrobasilar arteries or the more proximal subclavian and innominate vessels. Because of the anatomic pattern, symptoms rarely arise when the vertebral system on one side is involved; both vertebrals must be obstructed for symptoms to develop. If no carotid disease is present and the posterior communicating arteries are patent, the patient may remain free of symptoms in the presence of significant bilateral vertebrobasilar disease; thus progression of carotid artery occlusion may imitate symptoms of vertebrobasilar insufficiency.

One group of symptoms associated with cranial nerve dysfunction consists of facial numbness, vocal cord paralysis, ataxia, and Horner's syndrome. A second symptom complex consists of true subjective or objective vertigo (not just light-headedness), vomiting, lack of coordination, alternating hemiparesis or hemisensory symptoms, and a decreased level of consciousness. Finally, patients with vertebral artery disease may suffer from "drop attacks." When this symptom occurs, patients generally state they are unaware of a problem but suddenly find themselves on the floor because of a sudden loss of lower extremity motor function. Many patients complain of dizziness or vertigo, and when these complaints are prominent without other symptoms of posterior circulation insufficiency, ascribing them to vertebrobasilar disease is difficult. Many are the result of intrinsic ear pathology or eighth cranial nerve pathology.

Physical findings in carotid occlusive disease

In patients suspected of having carotid occlusive disease, a thorough physical examination that includes blood pressure measurements in both arms and careful auscultation of the heart should be performed. The presence of a precordial murmur is important because it may radiate to the neck and be confused with bruits in the carotid artery. A cardiac murmur is loudest at the base of the heart (especially if due to aortic stenosis) and becomes less prominent as the vessels are followed up into the neck. If the bruit is much louder at the carotid bifurcation than at the base of the neck, a localized lesion exists at the carotid bifurcation. In the absence of a precordial murmur, a bruit at the carotid bifurcation suggests carotid bifurcation atherosclerosis either in the internal or external artery or both, and no physical finding differentiates which of these sites is involved. In high-grade lesions, the bruit may extend into diastole, and when flow is slowed by a very high-grade carotid artery obstruction, the bruit may disappear. It is important to listen over the supraclavicular region, where a bruit suggests subclavian or innominate artery stenosis. A significant difference in blood pressure between the two extremities confirms the presence of subclavian artery obstruction.

Because the external carotid artery is rarely occluded, a decreased common carotid pulse in the neck is rarely detected. Only with common carotid artery occlusion, a rare condition, will an absent carotid pulse be observed. More often, carotid pulses will be equal even in the presence of significant carotid bifurcation disease.

Examination of the eye grounds (retina) may be highly specific in suggesting carotid bifurcation disease. Embolic material in branches of the retinal artery confirms the diagnosis of amaurosis fugax. Cholesterol emboli appear as bright glistening material within the arterial lumen (Hollenhorst plaque), whereas fibrin and platelet particles tend to be pale. The latter are difficult to visualize because they spontaneously break up and pass into the distal circulation.

In patients with a residual neurologic deficit, a careful neurologic examination is needed to document the degree of disability, particularly when carotid endarterectomy is contemplated. (The details of a careful neurologic evaluation are beyond the scope of this chapter.)

LOWER EXTREMITY PERIPHERAL ARTERIAL OCCLUSIVE DISEASE
Acute arterial occlusion

Classically, the patient with acute arterial occlusion demonstrates the five p's: pain, pallor, pulselessness, paresthesia, and paralysis. The pain of acute arterial occlusion is usually intense. The patient suddenly develops severe lower extremity pain accompanied by weakness and "giving way" of the extremity. Symptoms are most intense immediately and then gradually subside. Improvement depends on the competence of collateral channels and the pain may subside completely or progress to symptoms characteristic of chronic ischemia. The most severe pattern generally occurs with embolic disease and the least severe in patients who thrombose an artery at the site of a high-grade stenosis. In the latter group, collateral vessels may be well established. The most important symptoms that suggest the necessity for rapid intervention include the development of paresthesias and paralysis of the leg and foot. Once this stage is reached, advanced ischemia is present.

Chronic arterial occlusive disease

The most common presenting complaint in patients with chronic arterial occlusion of the lower extremity is intermittent claudication. *Claudication* is derived from the Latin verb "to limp" but has come to mean disabling pain in the lower extremity associated with exercise. The location of the pain depends on the level of arterial obstruction; the most common site is the calf. Pain in the calf with walking results from superficial femoral artery stenosis or occlusion. The patient generally complains of a cramping sensation in the calf that is brought on by a certain amount of exercise. The symptom is generally reproducible with equivalent exercise and is promptly relieved by standing for a few moments. Claudication does not occur at rest and should not be confused with the common complaint of occasional nocturnal calf cramps, which are not caused by vascular obstruction. Patients may "walk through" their calf claudication, which means that once the pain occurs with predictable exercise, they are able to walk farther for a variable distance after resting a few minutes. Careful questioning is important because patients will often limit or adjust walking speed to levels that minimize the onset of claudication.

If the level of arterial obstruction is more proximal (i.e., the aortoiliac segment), the exercised-induced pain may extend into the thigh and buttocks. Buttock and thigh claudication usually does not occur without calf claudication unless significant bilateral aortoiliac occlusive disease is present. Pain in the buttock and thigh is usually not as severe as that in the calf, and patients frequently complain of leg fatigue. As with calf claudication, patients with buttock and thigh claudication report prompt relief of their symptoms with cessation of exercise, and it is not necessary for them to sit down or recline.

In patients with diffuse arterial disease, which often includes the infrapopliteal segments, exercise-induced foot and ankle pain occasionally occurs. This is the rarest form of claudication and may occur in the absence of calf pain. In general, the symptoms are described as a deep aching pain associated with stiffness in the forefoot or ankle, with rest providing prompt relief.

If the lower extremity symptoms are atypical, other causes of a painful extremity must be considered. Important conditions that may confuse the clinician in evaluating the pain of arterial insufficiency include osteoarthritis of the hip or knee, lumbar disk disease with radiculopathy, spinal stenosis with narrowing of the lumbar neurospinal canals, and peripheral neuropathy.

Osteoarthritis of the hip may be associated with complaints similar to those of claudication. Occasionally, symptoms are brought on by exercise; however, the amount of exercise varies from day to day. The symptoms are often more intense in the morning on arising, with gradual improvement during the day. In addition, these symptoms are not relieved as promptly by standing as those caused by vascular claudication, and the patient must often recline to obtain relief. Patients with lumbar disk disease and radiculopathy have characteristic radicular pain associated with nerve root compression. Associated peripheral neurologic changes differentiate this condition from vascular claudication. Symptoms of peripheral neuropathy are usually symmetric and involve the lower aspects of the legs and feet. Patients complain of paresthesias and dysesthesias associated with lancinating, sharp, burning pain in both feet. These symptoms are easily differentiated from those of vascular claudication and most often occur in patients with diabetes mellitus.

The most difficult symptom complex confused with vascular claudication is spinal stenosis or so-called neurogenic claudication. Spinal stenosis is narrowing of the lumbar neurospinal canal. It is usually a slowly progressive acquired degenerative process, which allows the neurologic structures to accommodate. Moreover, many patients may remain free of symptoms. Critical narrowing of the canal produces symptoms of pain, numbness, and weakness in the lower back, buttocks, and lower extremities. The pain is exacerbated by walking and relieved by sitting or lying down. Neurogenic claudication usually starts in the lower back and buttocks, with subsequent involvement of both legs; it may include paresthesias. In addition, this pain requires more time to subside than the pain from arterial insufficiency, and the patient usually must sit down or recline for relief of symptoms. In fact, prolonged standing may initiate symptoms in patients with neurogenic claudication. In spite of these differences, distinguishing the symptoms of spinal stenosis from those caused by vascular occlusion is often difficult. Because both conditions may frequently coexist, which contributes most to the overall symptom complex must be discerned.

A final symptom pattern characteristic of patients with chronic occlusive peripheral arterial disease is ischemic rest pain. Typically, this pain is nocturnal and diffuse in the forefoot, often in the area of an ischemic ulcer or early gangrene. Patients are awakened at night and will often swing the affected foot over the side of the bed or get up and walk around, actions that they learn from experience will relieve the symptoms. In the erect position, gravity improves the perfusion pressure to the lower extremity, which explains the typical occurrence of ischemic rest pain at night when patients are horizontal. In addition, some patients learn to sleep with one foot hanging over the side of the bed or resting on a stool. In some cases, they sleep in a lounge chair with their feet in a dependent position. This pain pattern is characteristic and indicates far advanced peripheral arterial occlusive disease.

Physical findings. In patients with symptoms of occlusive arterial disease of the lower extremity, a complete physical examination should be part of the evaluation. Particular attention should be directed toward blood pressure measurement and examination of upper extremity pulses, including the carotids, brachials, radials, and ulnars. In addition, cardiac abnormalities should be noted, and an examination of the abdomen should focus on the exclusion of an occult abdominal aortic aneurysm or unsuspected abdominal bruits.

Documentation of lower extremity pulses is critical for the evaluation of patients with chronic arterial occlusive disease. Careful pulse examination identifies the distribution and degree of arterial occlusion. If the examination is not performed meticulously, the opportunity to make an accurate diagnosis without additional diagnostic methods may be missed, and a baseline will not be established against which disease progression or treatment can be measured. When peripheral pulses are examined, the abdomen and lower extremities should be exposed and the feet should be supported at the end of the examining table. After the presence of a pulse is established, the pulse should be graded, with *0* assigned to an absent pulse and *4+* assigned to a normal pulse. If the pulse is decreased, the grade of *2+* is recommended. An experienced examiner may recognize a weak pulse (possibly coming from collateral vessels), which may be graded as *1+*, or a slightly decreased pulse, which may be graded as *3+*. However, a 0, 2+, 4+ system of grading is sufficient for most examiners. In addition to grading the femoral, popliteal, dorsalis pedis, and posterior tibial pulses, the presence or absence of bruits in the femoral region and iliac fossa should be noted.

The femoral pulse is generally identified midway between the pubic tubercle and the anterior superior iliac spine. After palpation and grading of the pulses, the presence or absence of a bruit should be recorded. If an iliac fossa bruit is loud and decreases in intensity in the femoral area, iliac artery disease is most likely. On the other hand, if the bruit is loud in the femoral area and softer in the iliac fossa, common femoral artery and/or profunda femoral artery disease should be suspected. A bruit at Hunter's canal, a common site for early obstruction of the superficial femoral artery, is often detected along the course of the superficial femoral artery. If a femoral pulse is weak and no bruits are present, the palpated pulse may be the result of collateral blood flow with a very high-grade or complete proximal obstruction.

The popliteal pulse is the most difficult to palpate, and even experienced clinicians may find assessing this vessel troublesome. The examination is best performed with the patient's knee extended and the examiner placing the hands in the midline of the popliteal fossa while gently lifting the knee to a slightly flexed position. On occasion, the popliteal pulse may be prominent, and it should then be determined whether it is expansile. If so, a popliteal aneurysm may be present. A popliteal pulse that is too easy to feel should make the examiner suspicious.

Pedal pulses are normally present just behind the medial malleolus (posterior tibial) and on the dorsum of the foot between the heads of the first and second metatarsals (dorsalis pedis). The examiner should be certain that the pulse detected is that of the patient and not the examiner's. Simultaneous monitoring of the palpated pulse rate and the patient's radial pulse rate often prevents any confusion.

Physical findings of more advanced ischemia are less specific. Lack of hair growth on the dorsum of the foot, thickening of toenails, and delayed capillary refill are inconstant and less helpful in localizing arterial disease. In patients with rest pain, however, the presence of a chronically edematous, erythematous foot and ankle may reflect the extremity being kept in the dependent position, which aids blood flow and which the patient finds helpful in relieving the symptoms of advanced ischemia.

Ulceration and gangrene of the lower extremity represents the most advanced complication of arterial occlusive disease and is generally associated with diffuse, severe, multilevel arterial obstruction. Although an arterial-to-arterial embolus from an ulcerating atherosclerotic plaque or aneurysm may occasionally result in toe gangrene without significant arterial disease ("blue toe syndrome"), advanced arterial obstruction is usually present. Ischemic ulcers generally occur on the distal portion of the foot, toe, or heel and are particularly painful. The ulcers generally do not bleed and often look necrotic, and the associated pain may be relieved by dependency. In addition, advanced severe arterial occlusive disease with absent pulses is evident, and many patients will have associated diabetes mellitus. The presence of these advanced forms of ischemic vascular disease is an urgent indication for an intervention, since a high percentage of patients will develop extensive gangrene and require amputation unless revascularization is performed.

UPPER EXTREMITY ARTERIAL OCCLUSIVE DISEASE

In patients with symptoms referable to arterial occlusions in the upper extremity, the history is important because lesions of these arterial segments are often the first expression of systemic collagen vascular diseases. In addition, upper extremity arteries are subject to atherosclerosis in both the large vessels and the small vessels of the hand. Patients with arterial obstruction in the upper extremity complain of claudication with exercise, Raynaud's phenomenon, and ischemic ulceration and gangrene of the fingertips.

Claudication in the upper extremity is similar to that in the lower extremity; the major symptom is crampy pain in the muscles of the forearm or arm with exercise. In addition, the patient often complains of weakness or the inability to move the arm after exercise. Holding the arm over the head for long periods frequently initiates the symptoms.

Raynaud's phenomenon is a common symptom complex associated with not only intrinsic vascular occlusions but also generalized collagen vascular disease. The typical complaints are sudden blanching of a finger or fingers in one or both hands after exposure to cold. In addition to blanching, the finger becomes quite painful, and ultimately the blanching is replaced by cyanosis and rubor. Often the fingers feel numb, and there is intense pain. Determination of whether these symptoms occur in only one digit, multiple digits, or in both hands is important. When the process is particularly severe, persistent discolorization and dry gangrene can form at the tips of the fingers, changes that are exquisitely painful and often result in loss of tissue. This advanced condition is usually associated with advanced obstructive disease of the intrinsic arteries of the hand.

Occasionally, patients will present with fingertip gangrene and ulceration without a history of Raynaud's phenomenon. In these cases the symptoms are generally confined to a single hand or digit. This symptom complex may reflect the presence of embolic obstruction of the digital arteries of the finger, for which a source must be determined. Atherosclerosis of the subclavian artery must be suspected.

Physical examination of a patient with upper extremity arterial occlusion should include palpation and grading of carotid pulses as well as the subclavian, brachial, radial, and ulnar pulses. In addition, the presence or absence of bruits in the supraclavicular and infraclavicular areas should be recorded, and an Allen test should be performed to determine the competence of the palmar arch. For the Allen test, the examiner asks the patient to close the fist and then compresses the radial and ulnar arteries. After a minute, the patient opens the hand, revealing a white palm. When radial artery compression is released, flow into the hand and fingers may be noted. The process is then repeated with release of ulnar artery compression. By noting the pattern of palmar refill and the time required, the clinician can diagnose palmar artery obstruction. If a single finger refills slowly, digital artery obstruction or spasm may be present.

MESENTERIC VASCULAR OCCLUSIVE DISEASE
Acute mesenteric ischemia

The symptoms of acute mesenteric ischemia are those of bowel ischemia/infarction, which is an important differential in the patient with an acute abdomen. Mesenteric ischemia may be the cause of acute abdominal pain when the patient complains of severe, generalized, steady pain out of proportion to the physical findings. The pain is intense, and vomiting and bloody diarrhea may be present. However, the findings on the physical examination are often not as significant as might be expected for the severity of symptoms. Early in the development of the disease, the abdomen may be silent to auscultation or hyperactive. In advanced intestinal ischemia and gangrene, diffuse abdominal tenderness and rebound are often prominent.

Chronic mesenteric ischemia

Patients with chronic occlusive disease of the mesenteric circulation complain primarily of abdominal pain, which may occur with or without diarrhea. The pain is located in the midabdomen and is crampy, usually occurring after ingestion of meals. After a period of time this pain syndrome becomes so severe that the patient consciously avoids eating to decrease the expected abdominal pain. Consequently, most patients presenting with this syndrome complain of significant weight loss. The majority of patients with symptoms of chronic mesenteric ischemia are women, and they appear in the physician's office weighing 80 to 90 pounds with typical postprandial pain as their major complaint. In spite of these rather characteristic complaints, the syndrome is similar to many other intraabdominal conditions, and the physician must rule out other causes of abdominal pain, such as carcinoma of the stomach, pancreas, and colon or retroperitoneal tumors.

The most suggestive physical finding is an epigastric bruit, which calls attention to the possibility of visceral artery occlusive disease. However, the bruit is nonspecific, and other tests must be performed to firmly establish the diagnosis.

RENAL ARTERY OCCLUSIVE DISEASE

Hypertension is the major consequence of renal artery occlusion, although renal insufficiency or sudden pulmonary edema may also be the initial presentation. Although hypertension is an extremely common condition, only a small percentage of the cases are the result of renal artery occlusion. Unfortunately, no characteristic is sufficiently discriminating to separate patients with hypertension from renal artery disease from those with essential hypertension, and only general guidelines can be offered. The severity of the hypertension is important in that the more elevated the diastolic pressure (off medication), the more likely a renal vascular cause for the hypertension will be found. In the large population of patients with modest diastolic hypertension (105 mm Hg or less) renal artery disease is an unlikely cause. However, with increasing severity of diastolic hypertension, the chance of significant renal artery stenosis is increased. In addition, younger individuals with severe hypertension are more likely to have renal artery stenosis. In the older age group, when hypertension becomes difficult to manage or worsens on adequate medication or when diastolic pressures increase significantly, the chance of finding renal artery stenosis also increases.

In addition to the measurement of blood pressure, the physical finding of importance is the presence of an abdominal bruit, particularly in the flank. This finding suggests vascular obstruction and, when associated with high blood pressure, indicates possible renal vascular obstruction.

In a few patients, progressively deteriorating renal function suggests renal vascular obstruction. In these instances, both renal arteries are generally involved in the obstructive process (in the absence of parenchymal kidney disease), and appropriate studies should be performed to assess the possibility of renal artery stenosis. These patients almost always have some degree of hypertension associated with their renal failure.

ANEURYSM OF THE AORTA AND ITS BRANCHES
Infrarenal abdominal aortic aneurysm

The most common site for an aneurysm is the infrarenal abdominal aorta, and most patients are free of symptoms. Patients may occasionally notice an abnormal pulsation in the abdomen, which is the only symptom. When the aneurysm expands rapidly or there is disruption of the aortic wall with contained hemorrhage, symptoms may include acute back, hip, and abdominal pain. When bleeding occurs into the vena cava, symptoms of congestive heart failure may be present, or if an aneurysm bleeds into the renal vein, hematuria may occur.

The major physical finding is the presence of a pulsatile mass within the abdomen, which characteristically is in the midabdominal or left epigastric region. The mass is sometimes tender, which suggests the aneurysm may be enlarging.

Peripheral arterial aneurysm

The most common sites for peripheral aneurysms include the femoral and the popliteal regions. Other than the presence of a pulsatile mass, these aneurysms are usually without symptoms, and the diagnosis is confirmed by palpation. When peripheral aneurysms produce symptoms, emboli to the digital arteries with gangrene of the toes ("blue toe syndrome") is the most common manifestation. Acute thrombosis with acute extremity ischemia may occur, but rupture of a peripheral aneurysm is uncommon. The symptoms of acute thrombosis are the same as those of an acutely ischemic extremity with a cold, pallorous foot. This is often an urgent indication for treatment, particularly when the foot is without motor function and sensation.

PERIPHERAL VENOUS DISEASE
Venous disease of the lower extremity

Venous problems of the lower extremity do not present with the characteristic pain syndromes seen in arterial occlusive disease. In patients with primary varicose veins, pain is rarely present. Rather, these patients complain of diffuse aching in the lower extremities, generally at the end of the day after sitting at a desk or standing for long periods. Occasionally, discrete burning pain occurs over a large varicosity, but this is the exception rather than the rule. Mild ankle swelling may occur with primary varicose veins but is unusual, and most symptoms are relieved by wearing compressive stockings and elevating the extremities.

In primary varicose veins, large, tortuous subcutaneous veins, which are tributary to or part of the greater saphenous vein, are the main diagnostic finding when ankle edema or skin changes secondary to chronic venous insufficiency are not seen. Incompetence of the greater saphenous vein at the sapheno-femoral junction may be assessed by the tourniquet test (Fig. 1-1). After application of a thigh tourniquet, the varicose veins below the tourniquet do not fill quickly when the patient stands. Once the tourniquet is removed, prompt filling of varicose veins occurs, confirming the presence of

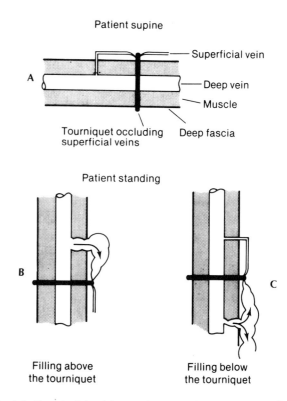

Fig. 1-1. The principle of the tourniquet test. *A,* A tourniquet is placed around the leg to occlude the superficial veins when the patient is supine and the superficial veins empty. The patient is then asked to stand. *B,* Filling of the veins above the tourniquet indicates an incompetent deep-to-superficial communication above the tourniquet. *C,* Filling of the veins below the tourniquet indicates an incompetent connection below the tourniquet. (From Browse NL, Barnard KG, Thomas ML: *Disease of the veins—pathology, diagnosis and treatment,* London, 1988, Hodder and Stoughton [Edward Arnold Division], p 75.)

incompetence of the sapheno-femoral junction. In addition, the examiner can test the competence of perforators by placing the tourniquet at different levels on the leg. In a similar fashion, the competence of the lesser saphenous vein at the sapheno-popliteal junction may be tested.

Acute venous thrombosis of the lower extremity may occur without symptoms or cause severe leg pain. If an inflammatory component is present, as in superficial thrombophlebitis, exquisite pain along the course of the vein (usually the greater saphenous) is the major complaint. Deep vein thrombophlebitis frequently causes calf pain and tenderness associated with swelling, which may be localized in the lower leg or extend into the thigh depending on the level of venous thrombosis. Homans' sign is calf tenderness with foot dorsiflexion. Because the pain pattern in this condition is not specific enough for definitive diagnosis, the clinician must consider noninvasive tests to substantiate the diagnosis. Most examiners agree that the sensitivity of the history and physical findings in diagnosing deep vein thrombophlebitis is only 50%.

In acute superficial thrombophlebitis, the involved saphenous vein feels like a tender cord and is associated with erythema along its course. Occasionally, this type of tenderness is present in deep vein thrombophlebitis, especially in the popliteal fossa.

Chronic venous insufficiency produces symptoms that depend on the degree or level of obstruction and/or degree of valvular insufficiency. Most symptoms occur at the ankle and include ankle swelling, discoloration of the skin, and the development of leg ulcers. In addition, some patients will complain of "bursting" leg pain (venous claudication) brought on by walking. This is a rare condition and usually due to significant venous outflow obstruction.

Chronic venous insufficiency generally produces brawny edema at the ankle with discoloration of the skin, caused by venous stasis and ambulatory venous hypertension. The edema associated with chronic venous disease must be differentiated from other causes of leg swelling, such as lymphatic obstruction or systemic disease (such as cardiac, hepatic, and renal conditions).

Ulcers associated with venous disease usually occur in the area of the medial malleolus. They are caused by sustained ambulatory venous hypertension, are shallow and irregular, and are usually associated with secondary changes of chronic venous insufficiency. These must be differentiated from arterial and neuropathic ulcers (see p. 10). Neuropathic ulcers occur at the sites of pressure points, most often on the plantar aspect of the foot over the first or fifth metatarsal-phalangeal joint or at the heel. They are usually painless and indolent and most commonly are associated with the peripheral neuropathy seen in patients with diabetes mellitus.

Venous disease of the upper extremity

The primary symptoms of acute upper extremity venous obstruction include arm swelling and an aching discomfort secondary to thrombosis of the axillo-subclavian vein. It is common in otherwise healthy individuals and occurs spontaneously, usually after excessive effort, because of partial obstruction of the axillo-subclavian vein at the thoracic outlet. A more indolent form of upper extremity swelling may occur with axillo-subclavian vein thrombosis associated with long-term intravenous cannulation for hyperalimentation, chemotherapy, or measurement of intravascular pressures. Principal physical findings include an asymmetrically swollen upper extremity with an extremely prominent collateral venous pattern involving the upper arm and shoulder girdle.

CONCLUSION

Careful history and physical examination evolution are critical in the clinical judgment required to successfully manage patients with vascular disease. Frequently, the history is the best clue to the diagnosis, such as in distinguishing between leg pain resulting from spinal stenosis and that from arterial insufficiency. In other cases, the physical findings, such as the location or character of a leg ulcer, best discriminate between underlying arterial and venous disease. Use of the other diagnostic modalities described in this text to confirm or disprove the clinical impression will help the physician avoid the dangerous pitfalls of ignoring the patient's complaints and the physical clues to the correct diagnosis.

REFERENCES

1. Gautier JC: *Clinical presentation and differential diagnosis of amaurosis fugax.* In Bernstein EF, ed: *Amaurosis fugax,* New York, 1988, Springer-Verlag.
2. Goldstone J, Moore WS: Emergency carotid artery surgery in neurologically unstable patients, *Arch Surg* 111:1284, 1976.
3. Mentzer RM et al: Emergency carotid endarterectomy for fluctuating neurologic deficits, *Surgery* 89:60, 1981.

CHAPTER 2

What should we measure?

DAVID S. SUMNER

In the rapidly expanding field of noninvasive evaluation of peripheral vascular disease, the question, "What should we measure?" becomes vitally important. With the development of increasingly sophisticated instruments, measurement capabilities far exceed those available only a few years ago.[1,4] No longer are clinicians limited to examination of the extremities and the neck; instruments are now able to probe previously inaccessible areas such as the interior of the skull and the abdominal cavity. No longer are clinicians limited to the basic measurements of pressure, flow, velocity, and pulse contours; the menu now includes velocity profiles, compliance, tissue oxygen tension, vessel and plaque dimensions, and morphologic features such as ulceration and plaque composition. From these, the computer permits the derivation of a host of indices. Some are valuable; others are of dubious significance.

In this state of flux, what to measure is a difficult question. All investigators have their own opinions (perhaps *prejudices* is a better word), and a resolution of their differences must await the acquisition and careful analysis of objective data, a process that is essentially never ending.

WHY MAKE MEASUREMENTS?

According to Lord Kelvin,[2] "When you can measure what you are speaking about and express it in numbers, you know something about it; but when you cannot express it in numbers, your knowledge is of a meager and unsatisfactory kind; it may be the beginning of knowledge, but you have scarcely, in your thoughts, advanced to the edge of science, whatever the matter may be."

A *measurement* is "a figure, extent, or amount obtained by measuring."[3] One definition of the verb *to measure* is "to ascertain the measurements of."[3] "Objective" is among the buzz words most commonly associated with measurements. For a measurement to be objective, it must belong "to the sensible world and be observable or verifiable by scientific methods."[3] It seems doubtful that any "subjective" observation can really be considered a measurement because such an observation belongs "to reality as perceived rather than as independent of mind."[3] With apologies to Lord Kelvin, many noninvasive testing methods depend heavily on subjective assessment—and that includes some of the most successful tests.

Why make measurements? First, they are a means of conveying information from one laboratory to another. Second, they are a way of defining standards: What is meant by normal or abnormal? How severe is a physiologic impairment? How severe is a stenosis? Third, they recognize, document, and quantitate changes in observed parameters. Fourth, only by making measurements can the pathophysiology of a disease process be investigated.

Without measurements, descriptive terms that are open to a variety of interpretations must be used. What exactly is meant by the terms a small or large artery; a thin- or a thick-walled vessel; a compliant or stiff vessel wall; a normal or abnormal pulse contour; a low, normal, or high blood pressure, velocity, or flow; and a slight, small, moderate, large, or great change in some parameter? The use of such nebulous terms leads to confusion.

The use of measurements and the avoidance of purely descriptive terms have facilitated the diagnosis of disease and the evaluation of the resulting physiologic impairment. Measurements permit a more objective assessment of the results of therapy; sometimes allow prediction of the outcome of treatment; are a necessary requirement for conducting studies of the natural history, incidence, and prevalence of disease; and provide concrete data during serial follow-up of patients undergoing medical or surgical therapy that can alert the physician to a deteriorating condition.

REQUIREMENTS

To be meaningful, a measurement should be related in some clearly defined way to physiologic phenomena associated with the disease process. Although numbers convey an aura of accuracy and authority, they may be meaningless. For example, some indices devised to improve diagnostic accuracy failed to do so because they were based on faulty or incomplete assumptions.

Measurements should be accurate, reproducible, and, preferably, simple. Above all, they should provide information that is demonstrably pertinent to clinical evaluation or to scientific studies. Unfortunately, some investigators have ignored this seemingly obvious requirement. Finally, a measurement should not duplicate information that is more readily available by using simpler, more accurate, less invasive, or more cost-effective means.

**INSTRUMENTS FOR NONINVASIVE MEASUREMENT
OF VASCULAR FUNCTIONS**

Ultrasound imagers
  Doppler (continuous wave, pulsed, flow mapping)
  B-mode (sector scanning, linear array)
  Duplex (color-coded flow mapping)
Plethysmographs
  Air (PVR)
  Water (volumeter)
  Strain gauge (SGP)
  Impedance (IPG)
  Photosensitive (PPG)
  Ocular (OPG)
Pressure transducers
Scintillation counters
Thermisters
Clark electrodes (oxygen and carbon dioxide tension)
Laser Doppler flow detection
Electromagnetic flowmeters
Nuclear magnetic resonance imaging and flow detection
Electroencephalogram (EEG)

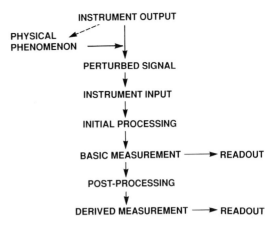

Fig. 2-1. Sequence of processing a measurement.

Currently, a variety of instruments are available, each of which is capable of making a variety of measurements. Even when listed generically, their number is impressive (box). Certainly, the most important and widely used are those that rely on ultrasound, but plethysmographs, which have been in use for many decades, remain firmly entrenched. Because all noninvasive methods of measuring blood pressure are indirect, transducers coupled to intravascular catheters remain essential for the determination of venous pressure and the accurate measurement of systolic and diastolic pressure and pressure waveforms. Oxygen-sensing electrodes and laser Doppler blood flux detection are rapidly finding a place in the vascular laboratory, but the role of nuclear magnetic resonance (NMR) for studying blood flow has yet to be established. Some of the other methods listed in the box are now seldom used.

WHAT CAN BE MEASURED

Despite this imposing and ever-expanding list of instruments, only a few basic measurements can be made. They include pressure, velocity, changes in volume, temperature, dimensions of plaque and vessel walls, uptake and clearance of radionuclides, and tissue oxygen and carbon dioxide tension. Plaque morphology and composition can be characterized to some degree, and perhaps with NMR spectroscopy, metabolic activity can be determined. All other measurements and indices must be derived from these.

To comprehend the meaning of any measurement, the examiner must first recognize what is really being measured. For example, measuring changes in volume with a volumeter is actually the measurement of water displacement; with a pulse volume recorder, changes in air pressure; with a strain gauge, changes in the electrical resistance of a mercury column; with an impedance plethysmograph, the impedance

of the tissues between the electrodes and that of the interface between the electrodes and the skin; and with the photosensitive plethysmograph, light reflected from red cells. Similarly, with a Doppler flow detector, flow velocity is not measured but rather the angle-dependent shifted frequency of the transmitted ultrasound, and with the B-mode image, the position and dimensions of body parts are not measured but rather the transit time of ultrasound reflected from tissue interfaces.

In all cases, the output of the instrument must be modified in some way by the physical phenomenon being measured (Fig. 2-1). The modified signal is then detected and processed by the instrument to provide a basic measurement (e.g., a frequency shift). This may be subjected to further processing to yield derived measurements (e.g., velocity, flow, various indices). Inevitably, each stage in the process increases the chances for error.

The relative inaccuracy and inconsistency of ultrasonic blood flow measurements illustrates how the sequential input of faulty data may confound results. Not only are time-averaged and spatially averaged velocity measurements subject to a variety of errors, but any error in measuring vessel diameter is squared when cross-sectional area (essential for the calculation of total flow) is estimated.

One further problem deserves mention: the instrument itself may actually modify the phenomenon being measured. A simple example of this is shutting off the flow in a vessel by applying a Doppler probe too firmly to the skin; most examples are far more subtle.

DEVELOPMENT OF A MEASUREMENT

Logically, the development of a measurement technique should follow the perception of need for the information that the measurement can convey (Fig. 2-2). Sometimes this sequence is not followed: The measurement appears first as a result of some technologic advance, and then a search is made for a need. Once the measurement is available, it is applied clinically, and criteria are developed on

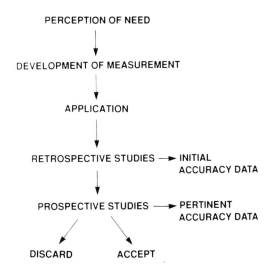

PERCEPTION OF NEED

DEVELOPMENT OF MEASUREMENT

APPLICATION

RETROSPECTIVE STUDIES → INITIAL
ACCURACY DATA

PROSPECTIVE STUDIES → PERTINENT
ACCURACY DATA

DISCARD   ACCEPT

Fig. 2-2. Outline of steps in the development and evaluation of a measurement technique.

the basis of retrospective review of the data generated. Accuracy is estimated at first by applying these criteria to the original data. This always yields splendid figures, which all too often do not hold up when the criteria are applied prospectively. Only after a measurement has been used and critically evaluated by a number of different laboratories can its true value be determined. It then becomes widely accepted or is gradually discarded. Although some techniques continue to be written about and advocated by one or two laboratories, the fact that these techniques have not been generally adopted is usually good evidence that they have proved wanting. Likewise, measurements or instruments that were accurate and useful by the standards prevailing at the time of their introduction tend to be replaced as newer, more accurate, or more versatile technology evolves.

ACCURACY

Just because a measurement has been made and a number obtained, the measurement cannot be assumed to be accurate. Accuracy and reproducibility are affected by biologic variability, the quality of the instrument, the noise that creeps in at all stages of the measurement process, the skill and bias of the observer, and the conditions under which the measurement is made. These sources of error can only be minimized; they cannot be eliminated. Application of statistical techniques (such as analysis of variance) may alert the investigator or clinician to the presence of significant errors. In clinical practice, the precision of the physical sciences can never be achieved, but this does not invalidate the usefulness of many of these measurements. Nevertheless, their limitations must be recognized.

The results of the measurement must be compared with those obtained by using a recognized gold standard to understand the limitations of any measurement. Accuracies are commonly given in terms of sensitivities, specificities, and positive and negative predictive values. Although these

are "hard" numbers, they must be examined skeptically. Among the many things that can affect accuracy are reliability of the gold standard, prevalence of the disease or condition in the population being surveyed, whether the population being studied displays symptoms or is free of symptoms, whether the study is prospective or retrospective, whether any subjects are excluded, whether the sample includes a broad spectrum of disease, and the size of the sample (see Chapter 8).

For some measurements, there are no recognized gold standards; accuracy can be ensured only by compensating for or eliminating all known sources of error. This requires an in-depth understanding of the phenomenon being examined, the physics (or chemistry) involved in the measurement, and the potential errors relating to electronic data processing. Examples are the measurement of velocity profiles or tissue oxygen tension, for which there are no readily available methods for confirming the results.

CLASSIFICATION OF MEASUREMENTS

Measurements can be classified according to their level of sophistication and complexity into three general groups: pattern recognition, basic measurements, and derived measurements. Although pattern recognition is not really a measurement, observations such as the shape of the pulse contour and the extent of spectral broadening are clinically useful and are sometimes as accurate as those to which numbers are applied. Velocity, pressure, and vessel diameter are examples of basic (unadorned) measurements; pulsatility indices, Laplace damping factors, input impedance, principal component analyses, and three-dimensional reconstructions are derived measurements.

No single problem better exposes the vulnerability of these three levels of measurement to close scrutiny than aortoiliac disease. Although total occlusion of this vascular segment can usually be detected by physical examination, the assessment of less severe disease, even by the most experienced clinician, is often grossly inaccurate. Likewise, arteriography frequently underestimates the severity of the occlusive process. These facts have stimulated an immense interest in the development of noninvasive diagnostic techniques capable of grading the degree of aortoiliac stenosis, particularly in limbs with concomitant superficial occlusion of the femoral artery.

Simply stated, none of the methods that depend on Doppler-derived velocity recordings from the femoral artery have stood the test of time. They are all fairly accurate for discriminating between no disease and severe disease, but in between many errors occur. Some investigators maintain that the Laplace transform is better than the computationally less challenging pulsatility index; others find little difference between the two or even the reverse. It is probable that simple pattern recognition is not far inferior. Although the final word is not in, duplex scanning will likely be the most accurate noninvasive method. This method measures "where the action is," the site of the stenosis, not some point farther downstream. A more direct but no longer noninvasive method is intravascular ultrasound imaging—a promising but as yet insufficiently studied technique.

Finally, pressure recorded invasively downstream or directly across the stenosis, an easily comprehended, basic physiologic measurement, remains the gold standard for evaluating aortoiliac disease.

PERIPHERAL ARTERIAL DISEASE

Tests used in the investigation of peripheral arterial disease should identify, locate, and grade the severity of the obstructive process; determine the adequacy of tissue nutrition (both at rest and during exercise); and in some cases, assess the effects of sympathetic activity, limb position, and temperature. A large number of measurements can be used. Of these, measurement of pressure is the most consistently valuable, especially noninvasively at the ankle and invasively in the femoral area. In many cases, measurements of pressure satisfy all the diagnostic requirements. Pulse contours may be helpful in a supplemental role, especially in situations in which the accuracy of the pressure measurements may be doubtful (e.g., calcified vessels). Direct sonographic examination of the artery to detect local flow disturbances and to ascertain degrees of stenosis may be informative in some patients, especially those who have suspected inflow disease, or in the postoperative follow-up of grafts. In both situations, the stenoses may be of insufficient severity to alter the dynamics of blood flow at some distance from the lesion but nevertheless pose a distinct hazard to the survival of an arterial reconstruction. Estimation of tissue oxygen tension and local blood flow in the skin may provide valuable information in cases of ischemia, a situation in which it is necessary to predict the potential for tissue survival or a successful amputation. When symptoms appear only during exercise, it may be necessary to make the measurement under conditions that simulate this form of hemodynamic stress to detect subtle, though important, physiologic effects. Although many other measurements are possible, several are of limited or as yet unproved value.

CEREBROVASCULAR DISEASE

As stated previously, in the investigation of cerebrovascular disease, measurements should identify, locate, and grade the obstructive process. Because the pathophysiology of cerebrovascular problems differs from that of peripheral arterial disease (small emboli assume a much more important role), the potential for embolization should be determined, if possible, by ascertaining plaque morphology and by detecting the presence of local flow disturbances. Evaluating the potential contribution of collateral vessels to cerebral perfusion and how this might influence the susceptibility of the brain to deprivation of flow is also important. In cases of suspected subclavian or innominate arterial occlusion, the direction of blood flow has important diagnostic implications. Direction of intracranial flow may also provide valuable insights into the dynamics of the cerebral blood supply.

Measurements of velocity and flow disturbances, best obtained with duplex Doppler spectroscopy, are used to investigate embolic potential. Real-time, color-coded Doppler flow-mapping devices offer the potential for rapid assessment of two-dimensional flow characteristics at the carotid bifurcation and in other areas of the extracranial circulation where the vascular geometry is conducive to hemodynamic aberrations. B-mode scanning assists in determining plaque dimensions and may contribute to the assessment of plaque morphology. Evaluation of collateral potential has depended on measurements of ocular pressure, but this approach seems likely to be superseded by transcranial Doppler studies. The role of measuring cerebral blood flow by using xenon or other techniques remains uncertain. Pulse-transit times, once popular, are too inaccurate to be of much value and generally have been discarded. Periorbital Doppler or photoplethysmographic studies designed to detect the presence of extracranial collaterals and, by implication, carotid occlusive disease are cumbersome to perform, difficult to interpret, and relatively inaccurate; consequently, these tests are used much less frequently than they were a decade ago.

VENOUS DISEASE

In cases of suspected deep venous thrombosis, measurements should detect and, if possible, locate the clot or clots and should determine the severity of the obstruction and the character of the thrombus, for example, its age (is it acute or chronic) and its adherence to the venous wall. In cases of varicose veins or chronic venous insufficiency, measurements should identify the presence of valvular incompetence, locate incompetent valves, evaluate the severity of venous reflux, and ascertain the efficacy of the venous pump mechanism. When ulcers or other manifestations of venous stasis are present, measurements of local tissue nutrition are highly desirable.

This information can be derived by assessing flow patterns and flow direction with Doppler sonography; by measuring outflow resistance, reflux, and exercise-induced changes in volume with plethysmography; and by visualization of thrombi and incompetent valves with duplex imaging. Real-time, color-coded Doppler flow mapping promises to increase the accuracy of such studies by revealing partial occlusions and by facilitating the examination of veins below the knee.

Measurements of ambulatory venous pressure remain the gold standard for evaluating venous valvular incompetence. The role of measurements of oxygen tension has not been firmly established, and capillaroscopy is likely to remain a research tool for the foreseeable future. Measurement of the uptake of radionuclide-labeled fibrinogen (the ^{125}I-fibrinogen uptake test) as a method for diagnosing clinically suspected deep venous thrombosis has few current advocates. At any rate, this pharmaceutical is no longer commercially available.

MULTIPLE MEASUREMENTS

An eclectic approach that includes all these measurements applicable in any given study is obviously not economical in terms of time, energy, or money—nor is it necessary. Even when the results are incorporated in bayesian analytic systems, multiple overlapping measurements seldom enhance diagnostic accuracy and may actually confuse the diagnostic process (see Chapter 8). Statistical devices, such as multiple linear regression and receiver-operator-characteristic curves, may be necessary to identify those tests that contribute measurably to diagnostic accuracy. The charge, therefore, is to select only those measurements that are pertinent to the solution of a specific problem. In addition, the investigator must weigh the accuracy of each individual test (or combination of tests) in terms of sensitivity, specificity, and predictive values, and these accuracy figures must be shown to pertain to the laboratory making the measurements and to the population on which the measurements are being made.

CONCLUSION

The problem of what to measure is complex. Different measurements are required for evaluating the cerebrovascular, the peripheral arterial, and the venous circulations. Even in these particular areas, the measurement most appropriate for establishing a diagnosis may not be the best for following the patient's condition, for assessing the results of medical or surgical treatment, or for establishing the natural history of the disease process. Only by constantly, carefully, and objectively assessing the results can unnecessary and misleading measurements be eliminated. Ultimately, the decision concerning what to measure is the responsibility of the individual laboratory; the philosophy governing these decisions, however, should incorporate the precepts outlined here.

REFERENCES

1. Sumner DS: Noninvasive testing of vascular disease: fact, fancy, and future, *Surgery* 93:665, 1983.
2. Thomson W: *Popular lectures and addresses,* ed 3, vol 1, *Constitution of matter,* London, 1891, Macmillan.
3. *Webster's new collegiate dictionary,* Springfield, Mass, 1979, G & C Merriam.
4. Yao JST: Precision in vascular surgery, *J Vasc Surg* 5:535, 1987.

CHAPTER 3

Establishing technical competence in the vascular laboratory

CYNTHIA B. BURNHAM and M. LEE NIX

Noninvasive vascular testing has become common in various health care delivery settings, including hospitals, private offices, and mobile services. Although acceptance of this discipline is gratifying, the increase in quantity has not consistently been accompanied by maintenance of quality. Central to the issue of quality assurance is the interrelationship of the physicians, technologists, and instrumentation that forms the foundation of a vascular laboratory.[4-6] Essential to the successful development of the vascular laboratory is the establishment of written procedures, protocols, and policies, as well as implementation of an ongoing method for correlation of noninvasive examination results with angiographic results. This chapter will discuss the role of each variable in the successful development of the technical aspects of the vascular laboratory. (For discussion of quality control of test procedures, see Chapters 5 and 8.)

THE ROLE OF THE PHYSICIAN

The first task in the establishment of the vascular laboratory is selection of the medical director. As in any patient care service, the primary motivation of the physician should be to provide excellent patient care and useful diagnostic information in the evaluation of disease. When a physician makes the decision to become director of a vascular laboratory, a major time commitment is involved. This commitment of time, support, and interest will be concentrated in the developmental phase of the laboratory but must continue on a lesser scale after establishment of the routine procedures. If the physician is inexperienced in noninvasive testing, an even greater investment will be required. In addition to a good understanding of vascular disease, the director must first acquire a working knowledge of noninvasive vascular testing. Formal training is strongly advised. As this knowledge is gained, the physician becomes aware of the interrelationship of physician involvement, technical examiner input, and test modality capabilities and limitations. This will allow the physician to select the appropriate instruments and hire staff capable of fulfilling job expectations. As medical director, the physician is also responsible for correlation of test results with contrast angiography. This initial process of physician input and interaction with the laboratory staff is the foundation of all later laboratory

activity and is important for the survival and success of the operation.

In situations in which the medical director is interested in continuing an active, hands-on, participatory role in the laboratory, the director chooses a supervisory role. The active role includes selection of the appropriate procedures, oversight of each test, interpretation of the results, and communication of the results to the referring physician. This requires a significant time commitment daily, as well as accessibility for consultations with the examiners and referring physicians. A medical director with limited time should choose a collaborative relationship with a capable technical staff rather than a supervisory role that requires constant supervision of patient examinations. A collaborative relationship implies that the physician depends on the technical examiners to make decisions appropriate to each testing situation and requires a high level of confidence in their competence. The wise physician looks beyond the initial role assumed and seeks to hire individuals who will complement the role of the medical director. After the proficiency and competence of the laboratory are established, the physician may choose to continue active participation by overseeing all aspects of the operation or may choose to be involved in a less demanding role by delegating most aspects to examiners. This decision is strongly influenced by the availability of the director for decision making on a patient-by-patient basis. In addition, this delegation of responsibility may occur only if the technical examiners have demonstrated the ability to function independently.

The medical director and other interpreting physicians must have a strong background in the assessment of the patient with vascular disease. Vascular surgery fellowships and radiology residencies may include training in noninvasive vascular studies; however, most interpreting physicians have gained knowledge through continuing education programs, clinical preceptorships, and experience.

THE EXAMINER: TECHNICIAN OR TECHNOLOGIST?

When more than six noninvasive examinations are to be done in a week, the physician will probably choose to hire a technical examiner to perform the procedures. This examiner is either a technician or a technologist. A technician has acquired a specialized skill. A technologist supersedes a technician and is capable of independent work, selecting appropriate tests as dictated by the clinical situation and providing a preliminary interpretation of test results.

A technician should work efficiently and accurately in the performance of objective tests according to strict procedure protocols. In the small hospital or office practice where fewer than five vascular tests are performed daily, a technician can also perform a variety of other tasks. Such an arrangement can be advantageous if the medical director is available to make decisions regarding the performance and interpretation of each procedure in the vascular laboratory. Problems will inevitably follow if either of two situations occurs. If the physician does not maintain a supervisory role, quality will suffer. If technicians are expected to perform subjective testing without direct supervision, quality will be compromised because they are forced to exceed their capabilities.

The technologist is capable of independently performing both objective and subjective tests and must be knowledgeable about vascular disease and test capabilities and limitations. This enables the technologist to evaluate the noninvasive test data obtained during the course of the examination and to modify the procedure to maximize diagnostic accuracy as well as cost effectiveness. This interactive process of using clinical and technical expertise permits the technologist to function independently when the collaborating physician is not present. The technologist is best suited to work in a large community hospital, private laboratory, or medical center where at least five procedures are performed daily. The technologist should be capable of evaluating current technology and educating other health care professionals and patients about vascular disease. This expanded role is essential for the individual with the broad knowledge required for this role and is important for job satisfaction. Physicians play a key role in promoting job satisfaction for technologists by working with them to correlate noninvasive test results with contrast radiographic results, by encouraging review of pertinent periodical information, and by providing the opportunity to participate in vascular conferences and rounds.

Formal education for the technical examiner remains in its infancy and relies primarily on self-initiated study and experience gained during employment. For this reason, the individual hired for a technical position should have a background that includes a knowledge of anatomy, physiology, medical ethics, disease processes, and biophysical principles. In addition, a background in patient care and the scientific method is valuable. Desirable characteristics in a technologist are inquisitiveness, independence, and motivation. Such an individual will seek out answers to physiologic questions and monitor state-of-the-art technology.

Once technologists or technicians have been hired, they should proceed with a course of educational study structured by the physician. This should include a review of pertinent anatomy, physiology, and pathophysiology. Programmed texts afford a simplified review and information about the use of Doppler evaluation of the arterial, venous, and cerebrovascular systems.[1-3] It is helpful to begin learning test procedures by examining normal volunteers. This allows the examiner to become familiar with the variations that occur among normal subjects. Establishing expertise in one area of testing before learning another promotes confidence and reduces frustration.

Good rapport should be established with the vascular radiologists and neuroradiologists because feedback from radiologic procedures is a primary learning tool in identification of problems in technique and in defining limitations of the test method. In the developmental stages of the vascular laboratory, physicians referring patients for invasive radiologic procedures may be approached about the possibility of performing noninvasive tests at no charge to the patient. This provides feedback regarding accuracy for the novice examiner and can also help establish the accuracy of the noninvasive procedure for the particular laboratory.

Once the basic principles of testing are understood, there is no substitute for the experience of working with a knowledgeable preceptor; if the medical director has a working knowledge of noninvasive testing, a valuable resource is provided. Otherwise, the physician and technical examiner will need to seek assistance from an established resource.

TESTING MODALITIES

Equipment selection is a major issue in the organization of the vascular laboratory; the choice between objective and subjective test modalities should be based on the scope of clinical questions to be addressed. Objective tests are those performed according to a rigid protocol and require minimal operator decision making. Although objective tests are restricted in the clinical information they provide, the examiner may be trained within a short time to perform these tests. The use of a stethoscope to obtain blood pressure is an example of an objective test, since it is not necessary to understand Korotkoff's sounds or the physiologic variables that affect pressure changes to obtain accurate blood pressure measurements. The parallel in the vascular laboratory is the measurement of segmental pressures in the limb by Doppler ultrasound.

In general, subjective testing is more versatile, addresses a broader spectrum of clinical questions, and requires maximal operator input to obtain the greatest amount of accurate information. The operator must modify the test protocol during the procedure in accordance with knowledge of anatomy, physiology, pathophysiology, hemodynamics, physics, and instrumentation. An example of such a test is carotid duplex examination. The use of duplex ultrasound to assess the carotid system for stenosis or occlusion requires the examiner to understand cerebrovascular anatomy, hemodynamics and pathophysiology, and Doppler and real-time B-mode ultrasound physics and instrumentation.

Testing modalities that involve the use of plethysmography are generally objective, and those using ultrasound, either Doppler or real-time imaging, are generally subjective. Some instruments can be used for either subjective or objective testing. Duplex ultrasound may be an objective instrument in venous imaging and compression but is subjective in analysis of venous Doppler signals.

Subjective and objective methods rarely assess the same variables. An oculoplethysmograph can provide objective information about the presence of an uncompensated internal carotid lesion, but it cannot provide comprehensive information about the status of the cervical carotid bifurcation. Such information must be obtained with duplex examination of the cervical carotid arteries. An oculoplethysmographic examination may be carried out with little or no understanding of the results, whereas a duplex examination of the carotid bifurcation requires that the technologist have extensive knowledge of anatomy, physiology, and the possible variations in test results.

Another consideration in the choice of subjective or objective test modalities is the availability of contrast arteriographic and venographic studies for validation of noninvasive test results. Without these tests or surgical verification of noninvasive examination results, the logical choices for noninvasive tests are those that allow standardized results and little examiner input or variability. Subjective examinations require ongoing monitoring of results. Correlation of these findings requires the participation of a knowledgeable physician.

Adequate numbers of examinations are required for the examiner to develop proficiency with the subjective tests. A minimum of 6 to 10 studies per week is necessary to attain and maintain an appropriate level of competence with subjective testing modalities. For example, if a review of venograms with a competent interpreter is not possible or if fewer than 6 venous duplex examinations are performed per week, the selection of an objective technique is recommended.

Turnover in technical staff affects the selection of instrumentation. If frequent turnover is anticipated, objective testing modalities should be used. Because of the shorter learning curve involved, these skills are more easily transferred from one individual to another. Conversely, subjective testing modalities require an extended learning curve that may approach a year if the technologist is to perform comprehensive testing in the areas of cerebrovascular, arterial, and venous assessment.

INTERRELATIONSHIP OF PHYSICIAN, TECHNICAL EXAMINER, AND TESTING MODALITIES

The organizational base for the vascular laboratory depends on the interrelationship of the physician, technical examiner, and tests performed (Fig. 3-1). This interrelationship serves effectively if it is structured according to either of the following triads (Fig. 3-2): The inner triad, which addresses a limited clinical role, has a physician in a supervisory role, a vascular technician, and objective testing modalities. The outer triad, which encompasses a more comprehensive range

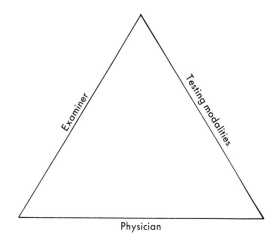

Fig. 3-1. The organizational base for vascular laboratory: physician, examiner, and testing modalities.

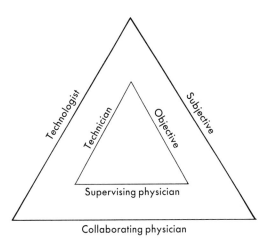

Fig. 3-2. Triads representing appropriate organization of vascular laboratory. The outer triad represents the structure required to address the entire scope of vascular testing. The inner triad represents the structure recommended for laboratories addressing most clinical questions.

of clinical testing, has a physician in a collaborative role, a technologist, and subjective procedures. If factors between the two triads are exchanged, the basic foundation of the laboratory will be weakened, resulting in a sacrifice of quality and personnel conflicts.

In the inner triad the desired clinical information is restricted (see Fig. 3-2). Objective tests are performed competently by a technician under the direction of a physician supervisor. In this pattern the physician is available to communicate with the referring physician and the technician on a patient-by-patient basis. If the physician supervisor is inaccessible, technicians will function beyond their capabilities (Fig. 3-3), and laboratory quality will suffer; in addition, technicians may feel frustrated. Cost-effectiveness and patient safety may be jeopardized if the referring physician, unfamiliar with noninvasive testing or clinical presentation of vascular disease, requests an inappropriate ex-

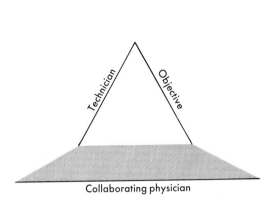

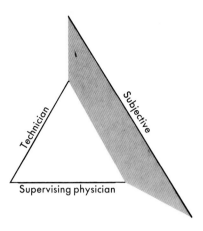

Fig. 3-3. Laboratory credibility decreases because of lack of consistent physician input.

Fig. 3-4. The scope of subjective testing exceeds the capability of the technician.

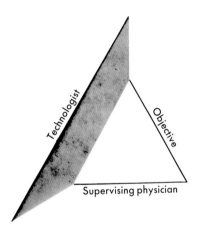

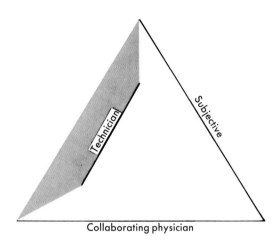

Fig. 3-5. The technologist is underused in the role of technician.

Fig. 3-6. The most dangerous variation of either triad. The technician is expected to function beyond personal capability.

amination. At best, the result is a failure to provide diagnostic information. At worst, the incorrect procedure may result in patient injury. Such a situation may occur if segmental pressures were requested for a patient with confusing clinical signs, such as limb edema and diminished pulses, and the test resulted in dislodgment of thrombotic material from a deep vein thrombosis. Fig. 3-4 illustrates the situation in which subjective testing is performed by a technician who is supervised by the laboratory director. Quality cannot be maintained unless the laboratory director oversees and assumes the responsibility for each subjective testing procedure, and few physicians have the time to participate in each examination. A final variation of the inner triad is to have a technologist fill the role of a technician examiner (Fig. 3-5). Because the technologist is capable of functioning in a more independent role than that of technician examiner, job

dissatisfaction and termination of employment will probably occur.

If maximal efficiency and clinical information are desired, the outer triad should be selected (see Fig. 3-2). Subjective techniques may be used by the technologist in collaboration with the medical director to address a broad scope of clinical questions. This outer triad functions effectively when the physician delegates responsibility to a technologist who is capable of and willing to function independently. The physician should only delegate responsibility if the technologist has demonstrated an appropriate level of knowledge and expertise. The most dangerous variation of either triad is to place the technician in the position of performing subjective tests when the physician performs only a collaborative role (Fig. 3-6). Because a technician is not capable of making independent clinical decisions and

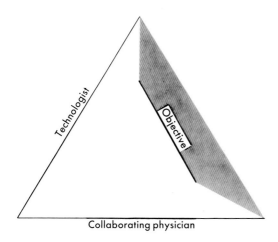

Fig. 3-7. The limited scope of testing modalities underuses the capabilities of personnel.

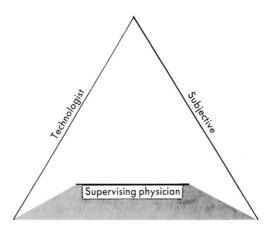

Fig. 3-8. The least dangerous variation of either triad. However, personnel conflicts are likely to occur.

the physician is not present during the examination to make these decisions, the accuracy of the results must suffer. Two other variations of the outer triad are shown in Figs. 3-7 and 3-8. Both of these will result in job dissatisfaction for the technologist. When objective techniques are used, the technologist will become bored. When the physician functions as a supervisor, the technologist will be stifled.

CONCLUSION

During the initial organizational phase of the vascular laboratory, the roles of the physician and examiner in relation to the equipment chosen for the laboratory must be defined precisely. A laboratory planned in accordance with the capability of the medical director and the technical examiner is preferable to one that evolves around premature purchase of instruments. With proper planning, an appropriate relationship may be designed for any given laboratory situation. Attention to this relationship in the planning stage will lead to the development of a harmonious and capable vascular laboratory.

REFERENCES

1. Barnes RW, Wilson MR: *Doppler ultrasonic evaluation of cerebrovascular disease: a programmed instruction,* Iowa City, Iowa, 1975, University of Iowa Audiovisual Center.
2. Barnes RW, Wilson MR: *Doppler ultrasonic evaluation of peripheral arterial disease: a programmed audiovisual instruction,* Iowa City, Iowa, 1976, University of Iowa Press.
3. Barnes RW, Russell HE, Wilson MR: *Doppler ultrasonic evaluation of venous disease: a programmed audiovisual instruction,* ed 2, Iowa City, Iowa, 1975, University of Iowa Press.
4. Essentials and guidelines of an accredited educational program for the cardiovascular technologist, *Joint Review Committee on Education in Cardiovascular Technology,* Bethesda, Md.
5. Essentials and standards for accreditation of noninvasive vascular testing, *Intersocietal Commission for the Accreditation of Vascular Laboratories,* Rockville, Md.
6. Kempczinski RF: *Vascular diagnostic laboratory: organization and operation.* In Kempczinski RL, Yao JST, eds: *Practical noninvasive vascular diagnosis,* Chicago, 1987, Year Book Medical.

CHAPTER 4

Quality control in the vascular laboratory

RICHARD F. KEMPCZINSKI

The term *quality control (QC)* when applied to health care usually means "the objective documentation of institutional results and their comparison against accepted, recognized standards followed by the implementation of appropriate changes in those areas where significant deficiencies are noted." Although the profession has had a well-established commitment to the highest standards of patient care, pressure from local and national regulatory agencies to create formal mechanisms that can objectively monitor and document the quality of the diagnostic services has been growing. Such QC programs have become an essential requirement for hospital accreditation under the auspices of the Joint Commission for the Accreditation of Healthcare Organizations and will almost certainly be expected of vascular diagnostic laboratories seeking accreditation from the newly formed Intersocietal Commission for the Accreditation of Vascular Laboratories.

To ensure the quality of services it provides, the vascular laboratory should be monitored by an internal QC program that audits each of the following elements:

1. Credentialing of the laboratory's professional and technical staff
2. The selection and maintenance of high-quality, state-of-the-art equipment
3. The indications for referral to the laboratory
4. The accuracy of each specific test performed as well as the results for each technologist
5. The availability and the quality of the continuing education provided for the staff

The QC program that has been developed for the vascular diagnostic laboratory at the University of Cincinnati Hospital over the past 12 years is built around a weekly, joint Vascular Surgery/Radiology Indications Conference, a computerized laboratory data base, a monthly Vascular Journal Club, and a weekly, didactic Vascular Conference. This program effectively monitors and hopefully improves the quality of the services provided to patients referred to the laboratory.

CREDENTIALING OF THE STAFF
The laboratory director

The active involvement of a well-trained, knowledgeable medical director is essential to ensuring quality within the laboratory. This individual, irrespective of any formal specialty training, must have a clear understanding of vascular physiology as well as the biomechanics of each of the instruments used in that particular laboratory. Preferably, the laboratory director should have no proprietary or vested interest in the laboratory's financial operations to avoid any semblance of impropriety or conflict of interest. The director should also have first-hand experience with the performance of all tests and must have a sincere, ongoing commitment to the field of vascular medicine and noninvasive testing.

As individuals from diverse clinical backgrounds have become increasingly involved in noninvasive testing, the demand for credentialing of laboratory directors is growing. Some have even suggested that such individuals should sit for a certifying examination to ensure their familiarity with the spectrum of clinical vascular disease and the noninvasive techniques used to diagnose it.[7] Although this may represent an extreme point of view, candidates for the position of director should have clearly documented training in noninvasive vascular diagnosis and should be committed to continuing education to ensure that they remain expert in this field.

If physicians other than the laboratory's director wish to apply for privileges as medical staff in the vascular laboratory, they should have had documented formal training during their residency in the performance and interpretation of the full spectrum of noninvasive techniques. Lacking such training, they can still be considered for vascular laboratory privileges if they have had formal training in any of the clinical disciplines devoted to the diagnosis and/or care of patients with vascular disease and have completed a recognized, didactic course on noninvasive diagnostic techniques.

Initially, these individuals should be granted temporary

privileges for 6 to 12 months. During this time, all their interpretations should be reviewed by the laboratory's medical director. At the end of this trial period, they could be (1) granted full privileges, (2) required to take additional training in the areas where their results fell below the laboratory's standards, or (3) dropped from the panel if they are unwilling to comply with the laboratory's standards. All physicians working in the laboratory must demonstrate a genuine commitment to continuing education in the field of noninvasive diagnosis and must be willing to participate actively in the laboratory's QC efforts.

The technologist

Technologists who perform the tests and are responsible for their preliminary interpretation are equally important in determining the quality of data generated by the laboratory.[8] These individuals have historically come from diverse backgrounds. However, most effective technologists are distinguished by a commitment to quality patient care and a thorough understanding of the vascular physiology and anatomy, tempered with sufficient clinical experience to enable them to select and interpret the test most appropriate to the patient's clinical problem.

Historically, most technologists have learned their craft through a limited period of apprenticeship or observation in an existing laboratory. In the last several years, numerous short-term (3 to 5 day), "hands-on" courses have become available to meet the growing demand for qualified technologists. Until recently, however, no formal guidelines for such training programs existed. In 1985, the Committee on Allied Health Education and Accreditation of the American Medical Association proposed essentials and guidelines for accredited educational programs for "Cardiovascular Technologists."[2] These recommendations gave substantial status to the field and set educational standards that were previously lacking. In brief, the committee stated that "Cardiovascular technology is a multidisciplinary science requiring the student to be suitably trained and educated in the basic and applied science of several diagnostic and/or therapeutic modalities. Upon completion of an educational program, the student must have acquired clinical skills and knowledge consistent with specific clinical performance and objectives in one or more of the following areas of expertise: invasive cardiology, noninvasive cardiology, and noninvasive peripheral vascular studies." In addition, the committee suggests that "for high school graduates without previous postsecondary education, the course of study should normally span a period of 24 months and consist of 1 year of core courses followed by a year of instruction in their area of specialization." For individuals previously qualified in a clinically related health profession, a 1-year course of study was recommended. Obviously, most vascular technologists have not undergone such a rigorous training program. Nevertheless, these standards represent the ideal and should be the goal for prospective vascular technologists.

The Society of Vascular Technology (SVT) has taken a proactive role regarding the training of vascular technologists. Its education committee compiled a list of guidelines for such centers and published a training center directory describing 22 training centers in 14 states.[9] The review of each of the programs listed in the directory, which is available on request from the society, describes its content and objectives in detail.

Once technologists have received appropriate training, they should be encouraged to pursue certification by the American Registry of Diagnostic Medical Sonographers (ARDMS). This registry holds yearly examinations throughout the country and awards successful candidates the title of "Registered Vascular Technologist." Successful completion of the certification process ensures minimum requirements in the field and should be expected of all vascular technologists. It is the only credential currently endorsed by the trustees of the SVT.

All vascular technologists in the laboratory at the University of Cincinnati Hospital are certified by ARDMS and regularly participate in vascular rounds, indications conference, and all other educational activities of the vascular service. This participation enhances their professionalism, helps to stimulate their intellectual growth and curiosity, and may help to avoid complacency and errors.[3]

In addition, technologists' performances are regularly audited, and they are periodically recertified in each specific test area. As new procedures are added to the laboratory's diagnostic armamentarium, technologists may need to obtain additional training from outside laboratories.

EQUIPMENT

The Subcommittee on Peripheral Vascular Disease of the American Heart Association suggests that instruments for the vascular diagnostic laboratory be "simple, reliable, and reproducible; capable of intrinsic standardization; easily used by paramedical personnel; suitable for measurements during and after exercise; and adaptable to current recording devices."[1] With few exceptions, there is no consensus on specific pieces of equipment or on specific manufacturers for that equipment.

The instruments used in each laboratory usually reflect the prejudices and previous training of the laboratory's medical director, the primary purpose for which the laboratory was established (e.g., research versus clinical care), the type of patients being referred to the laboratory, the daily work load, and the skill and training of the technologists working in the laboratory. It is difficult to imagine a modern vascular laboratory that expects to provide the full spectrum of diagnostic services without a high-quality duplex scanner, since this instrument is now generally considered the "standard of care" for the evaluation of extracranial carotid disease, deep venous thrombosis, and the postoperative surveillance of infrainguinal, autologous vascular reconstructions.

Once the appropriate equipment has been purchased and installed and is fully operational, each laboratory must document that its results compare favorably with those that have been published in the medical literature. Furthermore, that information should be made known to all the referring physicians as part of the laboratory's responsibility to educate the hospital's medical staff on appropriate use of its services.

Because most vascular laboratory instruments come with a limited service contract, usually 1 year or less, on-site bioengineering support should be available to help maintain, repair, and modify instruments as needed, or a supplemental service contract should be purchased to provide extended support beyond the warranty period. In addition, a regular, preventive maintenance schedule should be established for all equipment, and adherence to that schedule should be documented. Instruments capable of internal standardization should be standardized daily or weekly depending on need. As appropriate "phantoms" become available, especially for the duplex scanner, they should be used regularly to ensure proper functioning of the equipment.

INDICATIONS CONFERENCE

High-quality patient care mandates that the accuracy of diagnostic procedures be comparable to national/regional standards and that those studies be performed for appropriate indications. In the University of Cincinnati Hospital, all patients being evaluated for interventional therapy of vascular occlusive disease by surgical revascularization or a percutaneous endovascular procedure are initially presented at a weekly Vascular Radiology Indications Conference attended by all members of the vascular staff and the interventional radiologists at the institution. The patient's clinical history and vascular laboratory findings are presented, and the clinical indications for proposed intervention are discussed, along with the propriety of the laboratory studies. Therapeutic options are debated, and an appropriate procedure is chosen after a review of the patient's angiograms and input from all members of the staff.

As they are reviewed, the findings of each angiogram presented at this conference are recorded by a vascular technologist on a standardized data collection form and are subsequently entered into the computerized vascular laboratory registry form containing the data from the study that was performed before the angiogram. This provides essential, objective feedback for the laboratory and is an integral part of its QC program.

In some respects, the vascular laboratory is a victim of its own success. Because the tests are painless and because of the tremendous improvements in accuracy that have resulted from technologic advances in instrumentation and better training of the technologists, there has been enthusiastic acceptance of the vascular laboratory by patients and their referring physicians. This may result in overuse of laboratory services. Because it is difficult for technologists to challenge referring physicians who request what appear to be inappropriate or unnecessary studies, the medical director should educate the physicians who use the laboratory

on appropriate indications for testing and should regularly monitor the indications for each type of testing performed in the laboratory. In addition, the frequency of repeat testing, especially for such conditions as venous thrombosis surveillance and postoperative monitoring of vascular reconstructions, should be carefully audited and performed as infrequently as is consistent with high-quality patient care. In a large, busy laboratory, this can represent a logistic nightmare if indications for referral are not recorded for each study in some type of computerized data base.

DATA STORAGE AND RETRIEVAL

To minimize multiple reentries of the same data, expedite data retrieval, and facilitate comparison of test results with objective standards, all vascular studies performed in the laboratory are entered into a computerized data base as the data are generated.[4] Every examination room, the technologists' office, and the secretarial desks have computer terminals that are linked in a local area network (LAN) that permits new data to be added to each patient's data base from any location within the laboratory. Similarly, all data entered into a patient's file are immediately available at any other location, thus eliminating the need for hard copies of the data or for reentry of duplicate data.

For each patient seen in the laboratory, a unique "Demographic" form is initially created that contains a broad range of demographic and medical data, such as vascular risk factors and previous vascular surgical procedures. This form serves as the common denominator that links each of the specific "Study" forms together and is begun by one of the laboratory's secretaries when the patient is first registered. Information collected by the secretaries is typically limited to factual demographic data. Appropriate clinical information is added by the technologist before beginning the test procedure.

Once the technologist brings the patient into the examination room, the Demographic form is updated and a blank Study form, specific for the type of test that has been requested, is brought up on to the screen. Because these forms are linked electronically, any data required in form Study but already present in form Demographics can be automatically added, thus minimizing the need for retyping data. As each test is performed, the raw data, such as the segmental limb pressures and the peak systolic frequency, are directly entered into the appropriate field on the form. Calculated data, such as the ankle/brachial index, are automatically computed as the raw data are entered. Angiographic data recorded at indications conference are subsequently entered into the corresponding Study form and are readily available for comparison and validation of the laboratory's findings.

All tests are initially interpreted by the technologist and are reviewed later that day by a physician on the laboratory's medical staff. Once the diagnostic impression is approved, the computer automatically generates the final report, which will be inserted into the patient's chart without any additional retyping of data.

All vascular surgical procedures performed in our hospital are entered into a separate computerized vascular registry that contains detailed information on each patient, the indications for the operation, a technical description of the procedure, complications that occurred during the perioperative period, and the status of the repair on the most recent follow-up. These data are regularly updated on the vascular laboratory computer, which allows the technologist to quickly and accurately determine the details of previous vascular reconstructions and to interpret the recent findings more accurately.

INTERNAL AUDITS

Once the appropriate laboratory data and confirmatory angiograms are entered into the computerized data base, periodic audits of specific procedures should be performed to continually monitor the laboratory's diagnostic accuracy. These can be further refined to examine the results for individual technologists or physicians serving on the interpretation panel.

A randomly chosen sample of tests is selected each month for review by a member of the laboratory staff who is unfamiliar with the previous interpretation or the findings of angiography. Specific procedures as well as the performance of each individual technologist within the laboratory are audited, which permits laboratory staff to determine the sensitivity, specificity, and overall accuracy for every procedure and the performance of each technologist.

CONTINUING EDUCATION

The importance of continuing education for the vascular staff cannot be overestimated. At the University of Cincinnati Hospital, a monthly vascular journal club, which is attended by all the members of the staff including the vascular technologists, reviews the current vascular literature, both from the perspective of clinical results and indications as well as technologic advances.[5] This ensures a free exchange of ideas and familiarizes the staff with the latest developments in vascular surgery. In addition, a biweekly vascular conference presents a rotating schedule of didactic lectures covering most topics in vascular disease and basic science over the course of a year. Lunch is served and attendance by all the laboratory staff is required. Finally, regular but well-chosen participation at national meetings and/or noninvasive diagnostic symposia provides regular exposure for all members of the division to current thinking at the regional and national level and helps to stimulate the implementation of new programs within the laboratory.

All vascular technologists should also be encouraged to join the SVT. Participation in this society provides technologists with an important educational resource through its annual meeting and its excellent publication, *The Journal of Vascular Technology*. The society also functions as a forum for the presentation of research and clinical studies that are of interest to vascular technologists.

ACCREDITATION OF THE LABORATORY

Recently, concerns have been voiced about possible financial incentives that may have motivated some of the increased use of the vascular laboratory and about the lack of standardization of instrumentation, testing procedures, and interpretive criteria in these laboratories. Similarly, the growing demand for personnel has raised concerns about their qualifications, training, and supervision.

Overuse of laboratory services, inappropriate testing, self-referral of patients to physician-owned facilities, lack of appropriate quality controls, failure to demonstrate clinical relevance for some forms of testing, and the questionable credentials of some laboratory personnel have been cited as justifications for the recent increased scrutiny by regulatory agencies. Furthermore, those responsible for health care reimbursement have become concerned about the costs of these tests and are increasingly adopting policies aimed at restricting their availability based largely on financial considerations even when these policies appear to be in direct conflict with quality patient care and established clinical data.

In the fall of 1989, two delegates from each of eight sponsoring organizations that represented virtually every professional group historically involved in noninvasive testing began meeting to develop a mechanism for the voluntary accreditation of vascular laboratories (see Chapter 7).[6] However, widespread acceptance and expeditious implementation of the accreditation process may represent the last opportunity to maintain any control over the future of noninvasive vascular testing.

REFERENCES

1. Bergan JJ et al: Report of the Intersociety Commission for Heart Disease Resources: Medical instrumentation in peripheral vascular disease, *Circulation* 54:A-1, 1976.
2. Committee on Allied Health Education and Accreditation (CAHEA): *Proposed essentials and guidelines of an accredited educational program for the cardiovascular technologist,* Chicago, 1985, American Medical Association.
3. Godsey J et al: Quality control in the clinical vascular laboratory, *Bruit* 4:33-34, 1980.
4. Gupta SK et al: System for widespread application of microcomputers to vascular surgery, *J Vasc Surg* 1:601-604, 1984.
5. Kempczinski RF: A microcomputer-based system for the management of vascular surgical references, *J Vasc Surg* 6:542-547, 1987.
6. Kempczinski RF et al: Accreditation of vascular laboratories, *J Vasc Surg* 12:629-630, 1990.
7. Rutherford RB: Qualifications of the physician in charge of the vascular diagnostic laboratory, *J Vasc Surg* 8:732-735, 1988.
8. Strandness DE: The role of the vascular technologist, *Bruit* 4:1-2, 1980.
9. *Training center directory,* Washington, DC, 1983, Society of Vascular Technology.

CHAPTER 5

Education and certification of the vascular technologist

ANNE M. JONES

The vascular technologist is a unique professional whose specialty began in response to the need to accurately evaluate patients with arterial and venous disease. The person performing the evaluations had to be more than a "button pusher" who required constant supervision and direction. The technologist had to function independently, perform multiple examinations, and understand the implications of the results. Despite strong initial affiliations with vascular surgery, the specialty has rapidly expanded to include other specialties. Although vascular laboratories remain largely hospital and university based (58%), the specialty of the physician director now includes vascular and cardiovascular surgery, radiology, cardiology, internal medicine, and neurology.[7] Expansion and diversification are expected to continue, so the need for education, certification, and standardization will become increasingly important.

The Society of Vascular Technology (SVT),* the only professionally allied health organization dedicated to the field of vascular technology, traces its origin to the San Diego symposium on noninvasive diagnostic techniques in vascular disease. At that meeting in 1977, nine vascular technologists created the framework for a society that now has a membership of almost 4000 technologists, scientists, and physicians. The goals and objectives of the society, which are to provide continuing education, maintain a central information source, and facilitate cooperation among health care professionals, remain intact and are perhaps more pertinent today than at the time of inception 15 years ago.

EDUCATION AND INSTRUCTION

As the field of noninvasive vascular technology evolved, much of the early education and training was obtained on the job or by visiting the laboratory of a colleague. Since then, many private and university-based short-term educational programs have emerged in response to the growing demand. Additionally, instrument manufacturers have recognized the importance of proper education and have developed educational programs and on-site instruction tailored to meet the specific needs of the user. Despite sig-

nificant progress in this area, the need for sound, affordable, short-term educational programs remains critical. The challenge is not simple. Because the supply of experienced vascular technologists cannot meet the demand within the field, many inexperienced persons are hired with the expectation that the specialty can be easily learned. Finding an educational program tailored to the specific needs of an individual is difficult. If the course content stresses fundamental principles and appropriate technique, additional technical and interpretive skills can be developed on the job. Courses that provide hands-on instruction are important so that appropriate technique is developed and understood from the onset.

The education committee of the SVT has compiled a list of recommendations and guidelines for training centers. Although the society cannot enforce compliance, the information is published in an effort to provide comparative information for potential trainees. The training center directory,[11] which outlines the available training programs in the United States, is periodically updated by the society to include new programs. Each program is identically reviewed and provides a brief description of the course content and program objectives. (A copy can be obtained by contacting SVT.)

CERTIFICATION

In 1979, the certification committee of the SVT explored the concept of certification. A total of 78% of the membership overwhelmingly endorsed the concept of voluntary certification in 1980. It was generally believed that a national certification process would enhance the professional status of the specialty. In support of the certification process, Beach and Edwards[4] noted that "the purpose of a registry exam in vascular technology is to identify a level of professional achievement which represents the expected practice in the field." The ultimate goal of any certification process is to grant the credentials only to those qualified to practice in the field. Although accreditation is voluntary, compliance is becoming the accepted norm, and the registered vascular technology (RVT) credential is often recognized as the minimum standard for employment. With the introduction of voluntary accreditation of vascular laboratories, the RVT credential may achieve increased stature in the field.

---

*The name was officially changed from Society of Noninvasive Vascular Technology (SNIVT) in 1988.

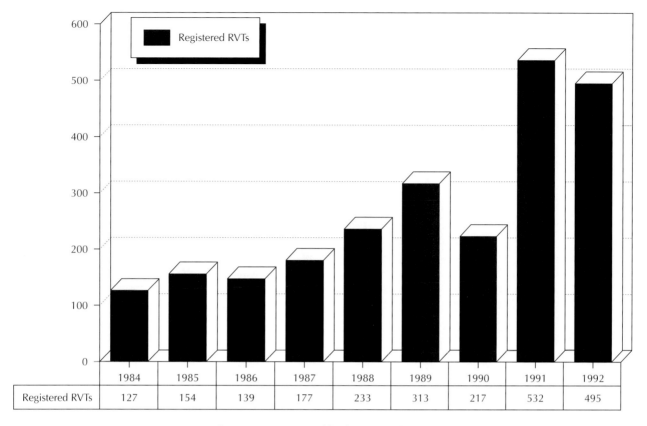

	1984	1985	1986	1987	1988	1989	1990	1991	1992
Registered RVTs	127	154	139	177	233	313	217	532	495

Fig. 5-1. RVTs registered by the ARDMS by year.

The certification committee of the society soon recognized that the testing process should be conducted by a testing organization independent of the society. After considerable research and deliberation, the American Registry of Diagnostic Medical Sonographers (ARDMS) was chosen. The ARDMS is a nonprofit organization incorporated in 1975 for the sole purpose of administering examinations in diagnostic medical sonography. At that time, examinations were offered in all areas of ultrasound, pediatric and adult echocardiography, and peripheral vascular Doppler sonography. As a part of the agreement with the SVT, the examination in peripheral vascular Doppler sonography was discontinued, and an examination in vascular technology was developed. The first vascular technology examination was administered by the ARDMS in 1983. Since then, the RVT credential has been awarded to 2862 technologists, of which 209 are physicians (Fig. 5-1). It is viewed as the accepted standard in noninvasive vascular technology.[3] In 1992, 1100 applicants sat for the vascular technology and vascular physics examinations, a significant increase over the previous year; 495 of the candidates successfully completed both examinations and acquired the RVT credential (Fig. 5-2). The ARDMS has awarded over 22,170 credentials in ultrasound, cardiology, and vascular technology, making it the largest worldwide organization representing vascular technology, ultrasound, and cardiology professionals. Because of the high quality of the program offered by the ARDMS, full membership in the National Commission for Certifying Agencies (NCCA) was awarded in 1985 and renewed in 1990.[2]

Vascular technology examination

The ARDMS board of directors includes physicians, technologists, sonographers, and a consumer representative. Each specialty in represented by a physician or doctor of philosophy and a registered technologist or sonographer who is actively engaged in the practice of clinical or academic ultrasound or vascular technology. The specialty committee members are responsible for development of the examination, and validity studies are conducted to ensure that the examination reflects current practice in the field. The vascular examination is divided into vascular physics and instrumentation and vascular technology; two committee members are assigned to each area. To become an RVT, the candidate must successfully complete both parts of the examination. Before taking the examination, a number of prerequisites must be met.[3] Although the specific requirements can be obtained by contacting the ARDMS, the basic requirement is 2 years of formal education after high school and 24 months of full-time clinical experience in vascular technology. If the candidate has completed college or an educational program accredited by the Committee on Allied Health Education and Accreditation (CAHEA) or the American Medical Association (AMA), the requirement for clinical experience is reduced to 12 months (although the ARDMS executive committee recommends 24 months). An equivalency clause outlines the requirements for persons who do not meet the previously described educational requirements but have extensive on-the-job training in an allied health profession. Candidates preparing to sit for the

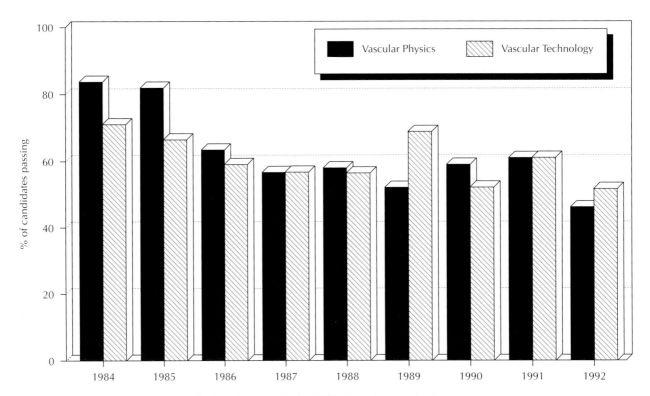

Fig. 5-2. Pass rates for the ARDMS vascular examinations.

vascular technology examination receive a content outline with the application. A study guide that provides relevant references for each topic listed in the content outline can also be obtained from the SVT.[10] The guideline is updated periodically and reflects current and accepted practice in vascular technology.

Continuing education

After the technologist has successfully completed the examination, active status is effective for 1 year. After the first year, a moderate renewal fee is required annually to maintain active status. ARDMS requires proof of continuing education to ensure continued competence in the field. Documentation of 30 hours of continuing education (CME) credit must be submitted every 3 years (triennium). All programs approved for AMA category 1, Society of Diagnostic Medical Sonographers, American Institute of Ultrasound in Medicine, or SVT are accepted. Failure to submit the appropriate documentation verifying CME will result in a provisional rather than active status.

To ease the burden of obtaining CME credits, the SVT has created ARDMS-approved vascular technology credits (VTCs). These credits may apply to regional programs, grant rounds, local educational programs, and small study-group activities, making continuing education more accessible and affordable. Application for VTC credits can be obtained through the education committee of the SVT.

Formal educational programs

In March 1981, the American College of Cardiology (ACC) recognized the profession of cardiovascular technology. In December of the same year, the Council of Medical Education of the AMA formally recognized cardiovascular technology as an allied health profession.[12] Although little impact was felt at the time, the effect of this action has recently created some concern among vascular technologists. This concern is primarily centered on the RVT credential and the position of vascular technology within this recognized allied health profession, which includes invasive and noninvasive cardiovascular technology.

After the recognition of cardiovascular technology as a distinct specialty, an ad hoc committee was formed to develop "Essentials and Guidelines of an Accredited Educational Program for the Cardiovascular Technologist."[1] These guidelines divide the specialty into three distinct parts: invasive cardiology, noninvasive cardiology, and peripheral vascular technology. The ad hoc committee completed the guidelines in 1983, and they were ultimately adopted in 1985 by 12 allied health organizations, including the SVT. Since 1985, a great deal of discussion and confusion about these guidelines and the accreditation process for educational programs has ensued. The guidelines dictate the requirements of a formal educational program in cardiovascular technology. Students enrolled in a CAHEA-accredited program must complete a year of fundamentals and a year of specialized instruction in one or all of the three specialty areas. At this time, only two cardiovascular technology programs have received CAHEA approval. Additional programs should be developed, reviewed, and approved in the near future.

Why is there such confusion about credentialing? It is a complex issue that has not been resolved. After AMA approval of cardiovascular technology as an allied health profession and the development of the guidelines, the issue of who would grant credentials to these specialists emerged. Because the specialty of cardiovascular technology encompasses invasive and noninvasive cardiology as well as peripheral vascular technology, the ACC endorsed the development of one credentialing body offering examinations in all three areas. No such credentialing body currently exists; hence, there is concern and confusion that multiple credentials offered by several credentialing bodies will weaken the current RVT credential. In addition to the ARDMS, two other credentialing bodies exist. These groups provide examinations on entry-level vascular technology and noninvasive cardiology. Despite intermittent negotiations between the three organizations, the problem of multiple or unequal credentials has not been resolved.[6] In an effort to endorse the ARDMS, discourage the development of multiple credentials, and prevent confusion among the membership, the trustees of the SVT endorsed the RVT examination as the only recognized credential in the field of vascular technology. It was believed that the high standards set by the ARDMS would help ensure professionalism in vascular technology.[5]

To meet the needs and address the concerns of the cardiovascular community, the ARDMS developed a cardiovascular principles and instrumentation examination in 1990. This examination is similar in scope to the vascular physical principles and instrumentation examination and is designed to address the unique components of the noninvasive cardiovascular/cardiology specialties. This examination must be successfully completed in conjunction with the pediatric or adult echocardiography examination before the registered diagnostic cardiac sonographer (RDCS) credential is awarded.[9]

Vascular laboratory accreditation

Despite the long-standing efforts designed to accredit the individual technologist, quality assurance and standardization within vascular laboratories have been isolated and variable. To encourage voluntary accreditation of vascular laboratories, a multidisciplinary organization was formed to explore and promote this process. The Intersocietal Commission for the Accreditation of Vascular Laboratories (ICAVL) was officially established in 1990 with the support of 12 sponsoring organizations. These organizations include the American Academy of Neurology, American College of Radiology, American Institute of Ultrasound in Medicine, International Society for Cardiovascular Surgery (North American Chapter), Society for Vascular Medicine and Biology, Society for Vascular Surgery, Society of Diagnostic Medical Sonographers, and SVT. Although each sponsoring organization is represented by two members who sit on the board of directors, the ICAVL is completely independent of the sponsoring organizations' activities. The purpose of the ICAVL is to provide a mechanism for accreditation of facilities that perform comprehensive testing for vascular disease to ensure quality noninvasive vascular testing.[8] A set of standards for arterial, venous, cerebrovascular, and visceral vascular testing has been established through the collaborative efforts of the representatives of the sponsoring organizations. Substantial rather than absolute compliance is required for accreditation, which is voluntary and not designed to be punitive. To date, 230 vascular laboratories have been accredited by ICAVL. Additional information on the voluntary accreditation process can be obtained by contacting the executive offices of the ICAVL (14750 Sweitzer Lane, Laurel, Md, 20707).

CONCLUSION

Although many vascular technologists have little interest in the issues of cardiovascular technology, credentialing, and vascular laboratory accreditation, these issues will ultimately have an effect on the individual as well as the profession. Obtaining the RVT credential is the best way for each technologist to strengthen the credential, the profession, and personal professional credibility. Although the RVT credential does not ensure proficiency in all areas of vascular testing, it assures the employer and the patient that the technologist has demonstrated a minimum level of competence in vascular technology. As technology evolves, the requirement for continuing education credits encourages and promotes competence. The institution of voluntary vascular laboratory accreditation further ensures competency in vascular testing and continuation of the professional goals outlined nearly 15 years ago.

REFERENCES

1. American Medical Association: *Essentials and guidelines of an accredited educational program for the cardiovascular technologist,* Chicago, 1985, The Association.
2. American Registry of Diagnostic Medical Sonographers: ARDMS again meets the standard, *Registry Rep* 8:2, 1990.
3. American Registry of Diagnostic Medical Sonographers: *ARDMS examination and information booklet,* Cincinnati, 1991, American Registry.
4. Beach KW, Edwards CM: Background information for the ARDMS certification examination in vascular technology, *Bruit* 7:42, 1983.
5. Blackburn D: Certification committee report, *Spectrum* 6:5, 1988.
6. Cardullo PA: Support the RVT credential, *J Vasc Tech* 11:164, 1987 (editorial).
7. Fischer PA: SVT membership database, *Spectrum* 6:1, 1988.
8. ICAVL informational booklet: *Who we are and what we do,* Rockville, Md, 1991, Intersocietal commission for the Accreditation of Vascular Laboratories.
9. Skelly AC: A message from the chair, *Registry Rep* 8:2, 1990.
10. Society of Vascular Technology: *Referenced study outline for the registry examination,* Washington, DC, 1991, The Society.
11. Society of Vascular Technology: *Training center directory,* Washington, DC, 1991, Society of Vascular Technology.
12. Waldrup LD: Cardiovascular technology: an informal update, *Registry Rep* 4:1, 1987.

CHAPTER 6

Qualifications of the physician in the vascular diagnostic laboratory

ROBERT B. RUTHERFORD

Now an established entity with rapidly developing technology, the vascular diagnostic laboratory is becoming increasingly concerned with appropriate training, proper job qualifications, need for certification, diagnostic test standards, quality control, and other educational and administrative issues that signal a certain coming of age.

Vascular technologists are now certified by examination, vascular laboratories are soon to be accredited, standards for reports on noninvasive tests have been published, and appropriate indications for test applications have been developed in response to requests by health care agencies and insurers. Will the physicians working in vascular diagnostic laboratories be next?

This discussion focuses on the physicians who direct the laboratory, interpret its tests, supervise its performance, and develop or evaluate new diagnostic methods. What should their training include, what qualifications should they ultimately possess, and how should these be evaluated? Should these physicians be certified and, if so, by whom? Currently there are no accepted answers to these questions, but they deserve serious consideration.

Most areas of physician specialization develop from growing clinical applications and/or expanding technology. Noninvasive vascular diagnosis fits both criteria. Until recently, most physicians who stepped in to fill this void came primarily from one specialty, vascular surgery. The increasing application of duplex scanning and other imaging techniques has now attracted significant numbers of radiologists, neurologists, and cardiologists. It may seem only natural and right that vascular surgeons should continue to harvest the ground they cultivated, but history has taught that it takes continued commitment, involvement, and leadership to protect one's "territory."

Emerging disciplines typically have difficulties in establishing educational and performance standards, approved training programs, and criteria for qualification for examination and certification. Vascular surgeons have recently

gone through the same struggles, and as the primary developers of today's vascular diagnostic laboratories, they may face these issues again, albeit on a smaller scale. Noninvasive vascular diagnosis is not a specialty, but it is a specialized clinical activity that requires a unique background and special skills. Today's vascular diagnostic laboratory is a unique working environment, and some of its characteristics complicate the choice of appropriate qualifications for the physicians who should work there. These characteristics include the following:

1. Noninvasive testing is an adjunct to clinical diagnosis. Ordering appropriate tests and interpreting them require a sound working knowledge of vascular diseases. A request for vascular consultation is often more appropriate than the request for noninvasive testing. Although a combination of tests is often required and normally is considerably more accurate than a single test, clinical judgment helps in determining the most appropriate combination of tests and in interpreting the results of those tests when they disagree with each other or with the presumed clinical diagnosis. *A solid understanding of vascular disease is therefore a prime requisite for the physician working in the vascular diagnostic laboratory.*

2. A wide variety of complaints, presumed or potentially of vascular origin, are evaluated by noninvasive testing: exercise-induced extremity pain, pain occurring at rest, leg swelling, discoloration, ulceration, cold sensitivity, impotence, visual disturbances, syncope, arm weakness, weight loss and postprandial pain, hypertension, pulsatile masses, bruits, birthmarks, and limb asymmetry. All may be caused by arterial or venous occlusive lesions, aneurysms, and arteriovenous fistulas that exist not only in the extremities or neck but also in the chest or abdomen, all of which can be detected, thanks to developments in "deep Doppler" imaging, in today's well-equipped laboratory. *Understanding this breadth of vascular disease and the tests used in its detection requires a vascular specialist.*

3. Today's vascular diagnostic instrumentation is becoming increasingly complex. Where an understanding of the Doppler probe and plethysmography once sufficed, real-

This chapter is based in large part on a presentation made at the San Diego Symposium on Noninvasive Diagnostic Techniques in Vascular Disease in February 1988 and published as an editorial in the *Journal of Vascular Surgery* 8:732-735, 1988.

time B-mode ultrasound imaging, linear-array transducers, and spectral analysis of velocity signals by fast Fourier transform—neatly integrated by microprocessor-based, computer technology—now challenge if not intimidate most clinicians whose formal training in physics, electrical engineering, and computers may be marginal or lacking. An electrical engineering degree need not be a prerequisite for physicians to qualify for work in a vascular diagnostic laboratory. Nevertheless, *they should have a clear understanding of the operating principles behind every instrument used in the laboratory.*

4. Noninvasive tests rarely give yes or no answers. Test results are usually numerical values that are estimates of such variables as intraocular pressure, peak systolic velocity, venous refill time, delay in pulse arrival, ankle systolic pressure, maximal venous outflow rate, and thigh:brachial index. Interpretation is all too often based on ranges of values established in other laboratories for normal subjects and for patients who have certain degrees of categorical levels of disease (e.g., more than 50% stenosis, claudication, "proximal" deep venous thrombosis, vasogenic impotence). Their accuracy is often measured against the dubious gold standard of angiography. Other tests are not as readily quantified and may be given qualitative interpretation. Spectral broadening, a triphasic waveform, vein compressibility, nonhomogenous plaque, and flow augmentation are terms on which considerable reliance may be placed. *The person interpreting these tests results must know not only their accuracy* (in terms of false-negative and false-positive rates and positive and negative predictive values) *but also their true limitations and potential sources of error,* both clinically and because of the manner in which the test was performed.

5. Potential conflicts of interest exist. Revenues from all but the very largest vascular diagnostic laboratories, if interpretive fees only are considered, are rarely enough to support a physician's salary. Therefore almost all physicians who work in these laboratories must pursue other activities (e.g., clinical practice, other diagnostic services, research) to support themselves. This produces potential conflicts of interest and time and may seriously limit the physician's availability for supervision and guidance.

Another potential conflict of interest exists whenever clinicians ordering the tests also run the laboratory or interpret the tests. Even if interpreters do not order the tests, they may end up managing the patient by taking advantage of the opportunity to discuss the findings with the primary physician. This criticism was once leveled against vascular surgeons, but in this era of interventional radiology, it also can be applied to radiologists, and as cardiologists now are invading the field of endovascular surgery, they too may be placed in a similar position.

BACKGROUND AND ACTIVITIES OF THE PHYSICIAN

From just these considerations, it would seem that physicians who direct or work in a vascular diagnostic laboratory must develop major capabilities in areas other than those represented in their original training. That is, the vascular surgeon or physician must master much of the bioengineering behind today's diagnostic instrumentation, and those with backgrounds in radiology, cardiology, clinical psychology, or bioengineering must thoroughly understand the clinical manifestations of peripheral vascular disease. Second, such physicians likely will be obliged to pursue other clinical, diagnostic, or research activities to support themselves but not to the extent that supervision or direction of the laboratory is significantly impaired. Many of the physicians who direct or work in today's vascular diagnostic laboratory are or soon will be unable to satisfy both of these conflicting demands.

Radiologists are adept at imaging methods but often are less familiar with analysis of Doppler velocity signals and plethysmography. They need other diagnostic activities to support themselves, but these can usually be pursued within the same department, so availability is not seriously limited. Detailed knowledge of vascular diseases will likely be lacking initially and may be acquired only with considerable time and interest.

Bioengineers, physicists, and clinical physiologists will probably understand the instrumentation best of all and have the background and time to further its research and development. Their lower salaries are easier to support, but currently, only physicians are able to collect fees for interpretation in the United States. Although this could change, the lack of clinical experience with vascular disease is harder to remedy. However, they have no conflicts of interest between diagnosis and treatment.

Vascular surgeons clearly have the greatest clinical experience in dealing with the broad spectrum of vascular diseases. The same may soon be said for vascular physicians, with their increasing numbers and increasing opportunities for fellowship training. Neurologists and cardiologists normally lack the breadth of clinical experience needed to function in anything but a limited capacity and certainly not in a comprehensive vascular diagnostic laboratory. Instrumentation is likely to be foreign to traditionally trained neurologists; cardiologists are at least familiar with similar instruments used in cardiac diagnosis. Although much of the clinical applications and testing of today's vascular diagnostic instrumentation can be credited to vascular surgeons, newer imaging techniques may place these and the other clinical specialists at an increasing disadvantage compared with radiologists. The demands of clinical practice apply to all these clinicians but particularly to a surgeon.

Limited knowledge of vascular diseases is a criticism that applies to all specialists other than vascular surgeons (or a few vascular internists). An extreme example is podiatrists, but noninvasive testing as an adjunct to their clinical practice cannot be condemned outright any more than it could be for a neurologist or cardiologist or, for that matter, any clinician. Nevertheless, laboratories of limited scope in private offices are vulnerable to the criticism of entrepreneurism and are likely to run into increasing problems with reimbursement from third-party sources and approval by official health care agencies. The same can be said even more emphatically for nonphysician, owner/investors who buy diagnostic equipment and hire technicians to perform tests and physicians to provide interpretation. The mobile vascular diagnostic laboratories that flourished in many states earlier in this decade have created great concern in this regard.

IDEAL QUALIFICATIONS OF THE PHYSICIAN

As a guiding principle, *anyone,* regardless of specialty background, should be considered qualified to run a vascular diagnostic laboratory and/or interpret its findings as long as that person has acquired adequate training and personal experience in both vascular diseases and their noninvasive diagnosis. However, physicians from different backgrounds who do not compensate for the weaknesses of their original specialty will fall short of being well qualified to serve the laboratory.

Therefore total acquired skills are extremely important: (1) What are the ideal qualifications? (2) How can they best be acquired? In formal training programs? (3) How can successful acquisition of the necessary skills be gauged? (4) Who should decide on "appropriate" qualifications and see that they are applied? Currently, there are no recognized formal training, no qualification criteria, and no evaluation or certification, and no medical specialty or society has yet accepted the responsibility for filling these needs.

Ideally, the physician in charge of a vascular diagnostic laboratory should have the following qualifications:

1. Understand the instrumentation (and be able to troubleshoot it)
2. Be able to perform and in turn instruct others in performing all noninvasive tests
3. Have a thorough knowledge of the clinical aspects of the vascular diseases being studied in the laboratory
4. Understand the true meaning, accuracy, and limitations of test results and be able to intrepret them in the light of other tests and the clinical setting
5. Either be completely supported by activities of the laboratory or have other activities that do not interfere seriously with availability to provide direction for the laboratory (e.g., supervise, teach, ensure quality control, consult promptly as needed on problem cases)
6. Have no conflict of interest between the roles of diagnostician and clinician

Few can satisfy these ideal qualifications, and even those who can will need vacations or be absent for illness. Thus these capabilities will often have to be supplied by a group of physicians or a combination of physician(s) and a bioengineer or physicist and/or senior vascular laboratory technologist with advanced training (the last individual handling

instrumentation and day-to-day test performance; the first handling interpretation and overall direction). Although these functions and capabilities are adequately covered in many vascular diagnostic laboratories, they clearly are not in others. Third-party providers and state and federal agencies are already concerned about the indications for noninvasive tests, particularly multiple testing, and who should be compensated for performing and interpreting these tests. It is agreed that standards for noninvasive testing and formal training and qualifications for technologists are necessary. Is it not equally proper that physicians working in these laboratories receive proper training and qualify themselves for their position?

TRAINING AND CERTIFICATION PROGRAMS

A likely and practical direction for this process would be to follow the same developmental steps taken by other emerging specialties. The recent history of vascular surgery provides an example of how to proceed. First, the appropriate educational background and training requirements for physicians must be established. A number of training programs in leading laboratories around the country could be set up and approved by site visit. Physicians already working in the vascular diagnostic laboratory would have to submit a resume of their background in this field as well as some evidence of ongoing activity. Those who are qualified either by approved formal training or by documented acquired experience would then be allowed to take a certification examination. If the example of vascular surgery is followed, only formal training would be accepted as qualification for examination in the future.

It is likely that all vascular diagnostic laboratories eventually will require some official approval to operate, but the ones in which technologists and physicians receive training should satisfy certain requirements, including a formal curriculum and evidence of standardization of procedures, interpretive review, and quality control, all under the direction of an experienced physician who may ultimately need to be certified.

The original background of physicians seeking training will be varied, but so will their training programs. Vascular surgery or angiography fellows could (and should) devote sufficient structured time during their training to vascular diagnosis to qualify them for examination. For example, a vascular surgery fellow could spend a 3-month, full-time elective period devoted to vascular diagnosis, with time spent in both the vascular laboratory and the angiography suite. Currently, daily participation in the end-of-day interpretive sessions is a required activity for up to 1 year in a number of vascular surgery fellowships. Sometimes this is combined with clinical research activities. Radiology residents or angiography fellows who intend to work in the field of vascular diagnosis could, in addition to rotations in angiography, ultrasound, nuclear medicine, and magnetic resonance imaging, spend a period of time on a vascular surgery service, during which they would learn about not only noninvasive testing but also clinical aspects of vascular disease by regularly attending vascular rounds, clinics, and operations. Such educational opportunities probably should be offered during these fellowships even if the recipient did not intend to work on a regular basis in the vascular diagnostic laboratory. In academic centers, at least, vascular surgeons and interventional radiologist angiographers work together closely enough that such "cross-training" arrangements should be possible.

Those who have other backgrounds or who are pursuing other specialty training eventually need to devote a similar amount of structured time studying noninvasive vascular diagnosis and vascular disease. Allowance should be made for those whose other duties prevent them from spending blocks of time in the vascular diagnostic laboratory so that they might acquire the necessary skills and experience more gradually over a longer time. For example, a physician spending 1 day a week for an entire year or, during the same period of time, spending part of each day involved in the vascular diagnostic laboratory (especially in the end-of-day interpretive sessions) might achieve the necessary skills and experience. Somewhere during these periods of training (preferably at the beginning), there should be a series of didactic lectures and hands-on training sessions focused on instrumentation and test performance.

Until formal training programs evolve and gain approval, flexibility regarding the manner in which applying physicians have gained the necessary background and experience to qualify them to take the certifying examination should be allowed, though it should be documented that such experience has been acquired in a deliberate and organized manner. In turn, it will be necessary to emphasize comprehensive examinations. These should test applicants' understanding of the operational principles behind diagnostic instrumentation and test methodology, their appreciation of appropriate indications for testing, and knowledge of the accuracy of the tests and their sources of error. A broad background in the diagnosis and management of vascular diseases should be covered (e.g., vascular physiology and anatomy, the epidemiology and pathophysiology of vascular diseases, their clinical presentation and differential diagnosis). Finally, interpretive skills should be tested by using actual case examples.

The details of this training and certification process deserve more than this or any other single opinion and ultimately must be worked out by appropriate committees of the responsible certifying organizations. However, just who or which organization (specialty board or society) should take the responsibility for the training, qualifications, and certification of such physicians? The first one to take the initiative? The one with the most organizational clout or political power? What if more than one specialty pursues this task simultaneously? Clearly, it would be better if these efforts could be complementary rather than competitive. A multidisciplinary society devoted to vascular diagnosis and organized by directors of leading vascular diagnostic laboratories could achieve this task with the ultimate blessing of their parent specialties.

Finally, does the field of vascular diagnosis deserve or need all this organization and accreditation activity, and if so, how soon? The current laissez-faire approach has spawned many undesirable practices and some laboratories that do not even approach reasonable standards. Patients deserve better than this and so do the technologists working in this field. Just as technologists need good training, certification, and ongoing supervision and direction, physicians responsible for vascular diagnostic laboratories should be expected to live up to similar standards. For noninvasive testing to gain appropriate approval and compensation, standards must be established for the indications, performance, and interpretation of these tests and the training and qualifications for those who perform them. The physicians who interpret the tests and direct and supervise the overall activities of vascular diagnostic laboratories should also meet specific standards.

CHAPTER 7

Accreditation of vascular laboratories

BRIAN L. THIELE

In collaboration with William McKinney, Edward Grant, Philip J. Bendick, Dennis F. Bandyk, John Gocke, J. Dennis Baker, Anne M. Jones, Polly DeCann Wilson, Charles Tegler, Joseph Polak, Christopher R.B. Merritt, Richard Kempczinski, J.R. Young, Marsha M. Neumyer, Cindy Cole Owen, and Sandra Katanick

Noninvasive testing has become an important part of the examination of patients with suspected vascular disease. The application of the various objective testing methods has provided a means of detecting the presence of disease and quantifying the severity of the anatomic lesions and the physiologic disturbances that are related to the patient's signs and symptoms. New equipment has brought a broader application of these tests to virtually all areas of the vascular system and the adoption of these diagnostic procedures by a wide range of health care professionals.

With this expansion of applications has come a need to establish guidelines for testing and a measure of quality control to ensure that these tests are appropriately performed by persons who are adequately trained to conduct the appropriate study and to interpret the results. The Intersocietal Commission for Accreditation of Vascular Laboratories (ICAVL) was formed to deal with this need.

DEVELOPMENT

Initial discussions among members of the Joint Vascular Societies, the American Institute of Ultrasound in Medicine (AIUM), and the Society for Vascular Technology (SVT) commenced in 1989 to address a perceived need to provide a mechanism of accreditation. Increasingly, health care professionals were concerned that if such a mechanism were not in place, governmental agencies would likely impose regulations that might not adequately or appropriately address issues of quality of patient care. To ensure broad acceptance of this approach by the persons involved in providing noninvasive vascular testing, the organization included representatives from the parent organizations: AIUM, the American College of Radiology (ACR), SVT, the Society for Diagnostic Medical Sonography (SDMS), the Society for Vascular Surgery (SVS), the North American chapter of the International Society for Cardiovascular Surgery (ISCVS), the American Academy of Neurology (AAN), and the Society of Vascular Medicine (SVM). Each

of these organizations, termed founding sponsoring organizations, was asked to nominate two representatives to participate in the development and implementation of the new accrediting body.

In 1989 and 1990, these representatives met several times to explore and discuss the feasibility of establishing a mechanism for accreditation, and the formal process of creating an appropriate organization and working guidelines began. This culminated in the incorporation of the ICAVL in Maryland in January 1991. The board of directors consisted of two representatives from each of the sponsoring organizations, and an executive committee was formed by the election of officers, including chairman, secretary, treasurer, and chairman-elect. After incorporation, the commission became financially independent.

An important philosophy of the commission is that the board members, who are elected for terms ranging from 3 to 5 years, report to their respective organizations but are primarily responsible to the commission. In April of 1991, a full-time executive director was appointed, with permanent support staff, and an office was established in Rockville, Maryland. Early discussions and organizational arrangements leading to establishment of the commission were characterized by a unanimous commitment by those involved. This was a unique undertaking by professionals from diverse backgrounds and could serve as a model for professional cooperation in the health care field.

GOALS

The primary goals of the ICAVL are to establish a process of accreditation to recognize facilities performing appropriate quality studies in the field of noninvasive vascular testing, issue certificates as recognition of this function, and maintain a registry of accredited facilities. In this regard, it is important to understand the difference between certification and accreditation. Certification is a process in which applicants' qualifications are reviewed, usually by a certifying agency, to determine if applicants have had appropriate training for performing specific activities. Certification implies that a person has the appropriate qualifications to practice the profession. Accreditation is the process by which applicants' activities are reviewed to determine if the applicants are practicing their certified skills appropriately. Whereas certification is often a legal process, accreditation is an administrative process.

For the accreditation process, the commission compiled a set of standards for each of the four areas of noninvasive testing: cerebrovascular, peripheral arterial, peripheral venous, and abdominal vascular. An additional component of the standards documents was devoted entirely to the organizational characteristics of the testing laboratory, including the qualifications of the personnel working in the facility.

STANDARDS

The standards documents serve as the basis for the accreditation process. They are similar to those used by other accrediting agencies, such as the Joint Commission on Accreditation of Healthcare Organizations, and define the required characteristics of each area to be evaluated. For example, the standards document on the organizational characteristics of the testing laboratory contains statements about the optimal qualifications of the medical director, medical personnel, technical director, and technical staff who work in the facility. The facilities in which studies are performed are evaluated by the commission, and issues such as patients' safety, instrumentation, maintenance of equipment, and quality control policies and procedures are also scrutinized (box).

The standards for the individual areas of testing describe primary instrumentation to be used for certain testing and secondary or complementary examination procedures. The standards for instrumentation use a parallel approach in an attempt to minimize the number of tests performed to arrive at a diagnosis. Anatomic and physiologic tests may be performed in conjunction with one another, but multiple anatomic or physiologic studies are usually considered inappropriate. An important feature of the standards documents is that not all the standards listed are absolute; rather they are defined as being the optimum. Copies of the standards documents can be obtained from the offices of ICAVL in Rockville, Maryland. Each facility should carefully review these standards and, if appropriate, apply for the self-study documents.

SELF-STUDY DOCUMENTS

The process of self-study is the centerpiece of the accreditation process. The self-study documents, which are constructed in parallel with the standards documents, are completed by the facility seeking accreditation. These comprehensive documents require each laboratory to address in detail the various features outlined in the standards. For example, proof of MD certification or certification by the American Registry of Diagnostic Medical Sonographers may be required in the organizational section, as well as information about the quality control measures used. In the various areas of testing, hard-copy results of tests must be submitted, as well as the laboratory's diagnostic criteria and measures taken to confirm the validity of these criteria. The completed self-study documents serve as the objective basis for considering whether the facility should be accredited.

THE ACCREDITATION PROCESS

The permanent staff and board members of the commission carefully review submitted self-study documents for completeness and compliance. Accreditation is awarded if the documents indicate *substantial* compliance with the standards. This is the approach usually adopted by accrediting agencies, particularly when the activity under review is still evolving, so the criteria for substantial compliance are likely to change. The ICAVL accreditation process (Fig. 7-1) is an evolving one, and the quality of laboratory facilities will be gradually upgraded as the discipline matures. Currently, accreditation is valid for 3 years and most likely will be awarded if review indicates the submitted self-study documents are satisfactory. Accreditation can also be denied, but usually a site visit is required before a final decision is made. Random site visits are used to evaluate accredited facilities as a means of assessing the self-study review process. Facilities denied accreditation can appeal the decision, thus ensuring that due process has been followed in all reviews of submitted applications.

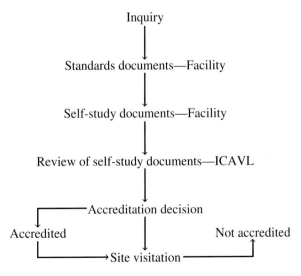

Fig. 7-1. Process for accreditation by ICAVL.

> **COMPONENTS OF THE STANDARDS AND SELF-STUDY DOCUMENTS FOR ACCREDITATION OF VASCULAR LABORATORIES**
>
> | | |
> |---|---|
> | Qualifications of personnel | Quality assurance |
> | Equipment used | Patient safety |
> | Testing protocols | Facilities |
> | Diagnostic criteria | |

THE FUTURE

In an era in which governmental control of practice is increasing, professional organizations should establish appropriate practice standards rather than have legislative agencies dictate these standards. Although the commission recognizes that a vascular laboratory's diagnostic procedures may occasionally be overused, the commission was created primarily to protect the needs of patients. Poor-quality studies, inappropriate studies, and unwarranted studies compromise the quality of services provided to patients. The accreditation process should promote recognition that accredited vascular laboratories provide high-quality, reliable information.

Currently, most vascular laboratories do not completely satisfy all the requirements of the commission as outlined in the standards documents, but most laboratories will be accredited. Although this may sound contradictory, it is important to recognize the principle of evolving sophistication. For example, although many physicians and technologists do not have formal training in noninvasive vascular testing, it will be increasingly important that these people have appropriate training and, if necessary, certification for future accreditation. Because of the comprehensive nature of vascular disease and testing, vascular laboratory investigations constitute a defined area of expertise that requires specific training. It is likely that the accreditation process will stimulate increasing professionalism in the field and will be associated with a significant increase in education.

CHAPTER 8

Evaluation of noninvasive testing procedures: data analysis and interpretation

DAVID S. SUMNER

In clinical practice, many factors influence the choice of a noninvasive test, including availability of the instrument, cost, experience of the technician, convenience, personal prejudices, and accuracy. Of these, accuracy is certainly the most important. Without sufficient accuracy, the results of a test are meaningless and its performance not only constitutes a waste of time but also results in an uncompensated expense for the patient in terms of money, unwarranted concern over a falsely positive diagnosis, or neglect of a lesion that should be treated. Unlike older diagnostic modalities, noninvasive tests came along at a time when investigators were sensitive to the need for demonstrating their accuracy. To the credit of those in the field, earnest efforts have been made to use statistical methods and to be as objective as possible. Despite these efforts, bias invariably creeps in; the multiplicity of instruments, techniques, and methods of analysis has added to the confusion.

This chapter describes some of the statistical methods used to evaluate the accuracy of noninvasive tests, describes how these methods may be used to compare the accuracy of one test with another, examines some of the subtle ways that results may be biased, discusses the advantages and disadvantages of using multiple tests, and points out the way some statistical attributes relate to the practical application of these tests.

BASIC CONSIDERATIONS

The fact that measurements made on one group of patients differ statistically from those made on another group does not mean that these measurements are sufficiently accurate to effectively distinguish between the two groups. For example, the average weight of 50 females on two hospital wards was significantly lower ($p < 0.001$) than that of 50 males on the same wards; yet as shown in Fig. 8-1, the spread of the data was so great in both groups that given a certain weight, it would be impossible to predict with any degree of confidence whether the individual was male or female.

For evaluation of the accuracy of a diagnostic test, the results of the test must be compared with the results obtained on the same patient (or same artery or vein) with a reliable, well-established diagnostic standard (frequently referred to as a "gold standard"). Use of a diagnostic standard is necessary because the true diagnosis is often unknown. In the simplest case, the diagnosis and the test results are considered either positive or negative (Table 8-1). *True negative* (TN) results are those in which both the noninvasive test and the diagnostic standard results are negative; *true positive* (TP) results are those in which both the noninvasive test and the diagnostic standard results are positive. *False negative* (FN) results are those in which the noninvasive test is negative but the definitive test is positive, indicating the presence of disease. *False positive* (FP) results are those in which the noninvasive test is positive but the diagnostic standard is negative, indicating the absence of disease.

From Table 8-1, four useful parameters describing the accuracy of the test can be derived. *Sensitivity,* which is the ability of a test to recognize the presence of disease, is calculated by dividing the number of true positive results by the total number of positive results obtained with the diagnostic standard. *Specificity,* which is the ability to recognize the absence of disease, is calculated by dividing the number of true negative results by the total number of negative results obtained with the diagnostic standard.

$$\text{Sensitivity} = \frac{\text{TP}}{\text{TP} + \text{FN}} \qquad (1)$$

$$\text{Specificity} = \frac{\text{TN}}{\text{TN} + \text{FP}} \qquad (2)$$

Although sensitivity and specificity are the best parameters for comparing the accuracy of one test with that of another, the clinician receiving the results of a test is more concerned with predictive value. *Positive predictive value* (PPV) represents the likelihood that a positive test result actually implies the presence of disease, whereas *negative predictive value* (NPV) is the likelihood that a negative test result actually implies the absence of disease. PPV is the ratio of true positive results to the total number of positive test results, and NPV is the ratio of true negative results to the total number of negative test results.

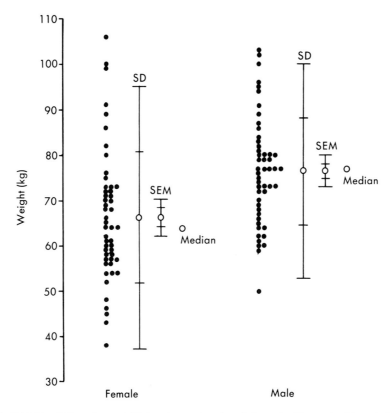

Fig. 8-1. Weights of 50 males and 50 females on two hospital wards. The vertical bars indicate two standard deviations of mean *(SD)* or two standard errors of the mean *(SEM)*. t = 3.866, df = 98, *p*<0.001.

Table 8-1. Matrix for calculating parameters of accuracy

Noninvasive test results	Distribution according to diagnostic standard		Noninvasive test total
	Negative	Positive	
Negative	TN	FN	TN + FN
Positive	FP	TP	
TOTAL FOR DIAGNOSTIC STANDARD	TN + FP	TP + FN	TP + FP

$$PPV = \frac{TP}{TP + FP} \qquad (3)$$

$$NPV = \frac{TN}{TN + FN} \qquad (4)$$

Dividing the sum of the test results that agree with the diagnostic standard results by the total number of tests performed gives the *overall accuracy.*

$$Accuracy = \frac{TN + TP}{TN + FN + TP + FP} \qquad (5)$$

Calculated in this way, accuracy is not very descriptive, since it does not directly reflect the values of the more critical parameters. As shown in Table 8-2, two tests with identical accuracies can have widely different sensitivities, specific-

Table 8-2. Relationship of accuracy to sensitivity and specificity (different tests, same accuracy)

Noninvasive test results	Distribution according to diagnostic standard		Noninvasive test total
	Negative	Positive	
TEST A*			
Negative	84	8	92
Positive	16	92	108
TEST B†			
Negative	98	22	120
Positive	2	78	80

*Accuracy, 88%; sensitivity, 92%; specificity, 84%; PPV, 85%; NPV, 91%.
†Accuracy, 88%; sensitivity, 78%; specificity, 98%; PPV, 98%; NPV, 82%.

ities, PPVs, and NPVs. Except in the unique case when sensitivity and specificity are equal, the prevalence of the disease in the population being studied also affects overall accuracy, despite the same test being used and sensitivity and specificity remaining the same (Table 8-3). Overall accuracy alone, therefore, provides the reader with insufficient information to evaluate the merits of a test.

Prevalence refers to the proportion of the population

Table 8-3. Effect of prevalence on accuracy and predictive values (same test, three different populations)

| Noninvasive test results | Distribution according to diagnostic standard | | Noninvasive test total |
	Negative	Positive	
POPULATION A*—50% PREVALENCE			
Negative	80	10	90
Positive	20	90	110
POPULATION B†—10% PREVALENCE			
Negative	144	2	146
Positive	36	18	54
POPULATION C‡—90% PREVALENCE			
Negative	16	18	34
Positive	4	162	166

*Accuracy, 85%; sensitivity, 90%; specificity, 80%; PPV, 82%; NPV, 89%.
†Accuracy, 81%; sensitivity, 90%; specificity, 80%; PPV, 33%; NPV, 99%.
‡Accuracy, 89%; sensitivity, 90%; specificity, 80%; PPV, 98%; NPV, 47%.

being studied that actually has the disease. In retrospective studies, prevalence can be calculated by dividing the number of positive results as determined by the diagnostic standard (TP + FN) by the total number of tests performed; in actual practice, prevalence is seldom known with certainty.

$$\text{Prevalence} = \frac{\text{TP} + \text{FN}}{\text{TN} + \text{FN} + \text{TP} + \text{FP}} \qquad (6)$$

Table 8-3 illustrates how variations in prevalence can affect predictive values, even when the same test is used. In each of the three examples, sensitivity and specificity are unchanged; however, the PPV increases when prevalence is high and decreases when prevalence is low. Conversely, NPV increases when prevalence is low but decreases when prevalence is high. These relationships are shown in Figs. 8-2 and 8-3.

The important relationships between sensitivity and specificity and predictive values are also illustrated in Figs. 8-2 and 8-3. Given the same specificity, an improvement in sensitivity will have little effect on the PPV (Fig. 8-2) but will have a major effect on the NPV (Fig. 8-3). On the other hand, given the same sensitivity, an improvement in specificity will have little effect on the NPV (Fig. 8-3) but will have a major effect on the PPV (Fig. 8-2). In other words, if the investigation requires a high PPV, a test with a high specificity should be selected—even at the expense of a low sensitivity. If a high NPV is desired, a test with a high sensitivity should be used. How this relates to actual clinical practice is discussed later in this chapter.

Predictive values can be calculated for any disease prevalence if sensitivities and specificities are known. In Table 8-4, the TN, TP, FN, and FP results have been expressed in terms of prevalence, sensitivity, and specificity. This permits the following equations to be derived:

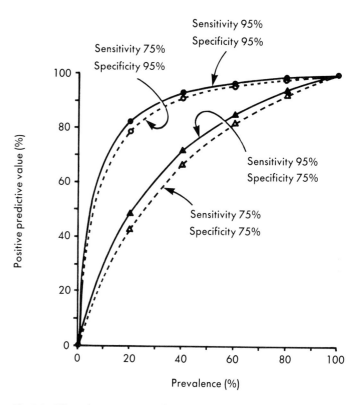

Fig. 8-2. Effect of sensitivity, specificity, and prevalence on the positive predictive value.

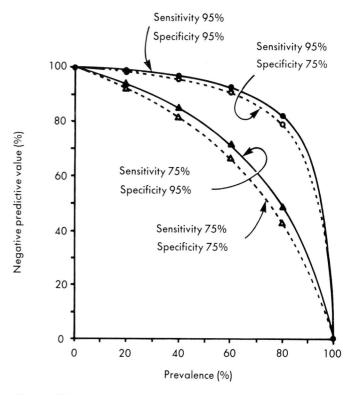

Fig. 8-3. Effect of sensitivity, specificity, and prevalence on the negative predictive value.

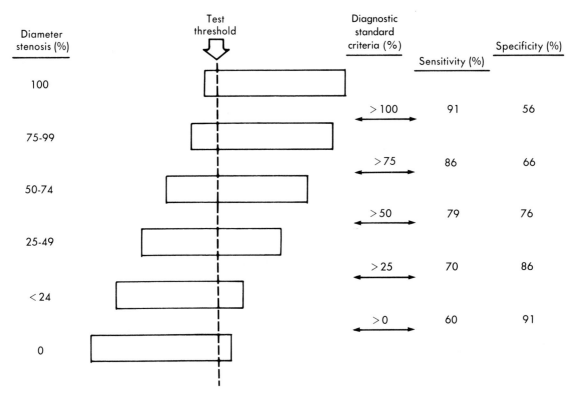

Fig. 8-4. Effect of varying the positive criteria for the presence of disease on the sensitivity and specificity. The test threshold is fixed.

Table 8-4. Matrix for calculating PPV and NPV from sensitivity, specificity, and prevalence

| | Distribution according to diagnostic standard | | |
Noninvasive test results	Negative	Positive	Noninvasive test total
Negative	B (1 − P)	P (1 − A)	B (1 − P) + P (1 − A)
Positive	(1 − P) (1 − B)	PA	(1 − P) (1 − B) + PA
TOTAL FOR DIAGNOSTIC STANDARD	1 − P	P	1

P, Prevalence; *A*, sensitivity; *B*, specificity.

$$PPV = \frac{PA}{(1 - P)(1 - B) + PA} \qquad (7)$$

$$NPV = \frac{B(1 - P)}{B(1 - P) + P(1 - A)} \qquad (8)$$

$$ACC = B + P(A - B) \qquad (9)$$

where P indicates prevalence; A, sensitivity; B, specificity; and ACC, accuracy. P, A, and B are expressed in decimal fractions and are always less than 1. These equations prove very useful in selecting a test to fit a particular study population.

GRADATIONS OF DISEASE

In most conditions to which noninvasive testing is applied, there is a gradation in the severity of the disease process. Arteriosclerosis, for example, can be absent, produce non-

stenotic plaques, cause varying degrees of stenosis, or result in total arterial occlusion. A noninvasive test may be used to detect the presence or absence of any disease regardless of its severity, to distinguish between hemodynamically significant and nonhemodynamically significant stenoses, or to differentiate between stenotic and totally occluded arteries. It is therefore necessary to establish some guidelines to determine what magnitude of disease is to be considered negative and what, positive.

Many noninvasive tests (such as oculoplethysmography and impedance plethysmography) do not become positive unless disease of certain severity is present. Moreover, the percentage of positive test results increases as the severity of the disease process increases. For this reason, the same test applied to the same population will usually appear to be more sensitive and less specific when the criterion for a positive result is set at a high degree of stenosis and less sensitive and more specific when the criterion is set at a lower level of stenosis (Fig. 8-4). A hypothetical population consisting of equal numbers of arteries in each of six categories of stenosis is shown in Fig. 8-4. To the right of the vertical line indicating the *test threshold,* the results of the noninvasive test are positive; to the left, the test results are negative. In the category of no disease (0% diameter stenosis), most of the test results are negative; in the category of total occlusion (100% diameter stenosis), most of the test results are positive. When the degree of stenosis is less severe (for example, 25% to 49% diameter stenosis), the number of positive and negative test results is almost equal. If the criteria for a positive test were set at 50% diameter stenosis, 79% of the arteries with stenoses >50% would have positive studies and 76% of those with stenoses <50% would have negative studies. On the other hand, if the test distinguished between total occlusion and any degree of stenosis (criterion 100%), the sensitivity would rise to 91% and the specificity would fall to 56%. For detecting any stenosis, the sensitivity would drop to 60% and the specificity would increase to 91%.

It is therefore critically important to be aware of the criteria used to distinguish between the presence and absence of disease when comparing the results of two diagnostic tests. Medical literature contains many examples of tests that appear to be highly sensitive merely because the dividing line has been set at a high level of disease (≥70% to 80%). If these same tests had been employed to differentiate between <50% diameter stenosis and >50% or between 0% stenosis and ≥1% stenosis, the results would be considerably less impressive in terms of sensitivity.

DISTRIBUTION OF DISEASE

Because the percentage of positive test results usually increases with the severity of disease, the distribution of disease in a study population affects the various parameters of accuracy. As shown in Table 8-5, a test appears most sensitive and specific when the distribution is skewed toward the more severe and less severe ends of the disease spectrum and least sensitive and specific when the numbers are concentrated in the midportion of the spectrum. When the disease is evenly distributed among the four categories of stenosis, the parameters of accuracy lie between the two extremes. In these three examples, the parameters of accuracy vary even though the same test is used and the apparent disease prevalence remains constant. In Table 8-5, the *percentage* of positive test results from the three populations was the same: 5% positive in the range of 0% to 24% diameter stenosis, 35% positive in the 25% to 49% disease range, 65% positive in the 50% to 74% range, and 95% positive in the 75% to 100% range.

The distribution of disease in the study populations should be carefully examined when test results are compared. *One test may appear better than another merely because the study includes a large number of normal or occluded vessels.*

Table 8-5. Effect of disease distribution on sensitivity and specificity (same test, three different populations; dividing line between positive and negative set at 50% diameter stenosis)

| Noninvasive test results | Distribution according to diagnostic standard (% stenosis) | | | |
| | Negative | | Positive | |
	0-24	25-49	50-74	75-100
EVEN DISTRIBUTION*				
Negative	95	65	35	5
Positive	5	35	65	95
SKEWED TOWARD EXTREMES†				
Negative	171	13	7	9
Positive	9	7	13	171
CONCENTRATED IN MIDPORTION‡				
Negative	19	117	63	1
Positive	1	63	117	19

*Sensitivity, 80%; specificity, 80%; prevalence, 50%.
†Sensitivity, 92%; specificity, 92%; prevalence, 50%.
‡Sensitivity, 68%; specificity, 68%; prevalence, 50%.

RECEIVER OPERATING CHARACTERISTIC CURVES

In the preceding discussion, test results have been considered to be either positive or negative. The results of most noninvasive tests, however, are not so easily classified. For example, carotid Doppler spectra have a wide range of peak frequencies and bandwidths, and the degree of stenosis estimated from B-mode images may vary from none to total occlusion. Other examples of tests in which results vary continuously over a wide range include ankle pressure measurements, venous plethysmography, arterial plethysmography, oculopneumoplethysmography, $TcPO_2$, and laser Doppler flux. To apply these tests, the investigator must decide what level of ankle pressure, rate of venous outflow or venous filling, pulse volume, intraocular/arm pressure ratio, oxygen tension, or millivolts of excursion to consider normal and what to consider abnormal. A threshold or cutoff point must be selected to divide positive from negative results.

Where this threshold is set will have a major effect on the sensitivity and specificity of the test. As shown in Fig. 8-5, if the criterion for a positive test is made very strict (hard reading, indicated by *C*), few lesions that are negative by the diagnostic standard criterion will be called positive, but many positive lesions will be missed. On the other hand, if the criterion for a positive test is made very lenient (soft reading, indicated by *A*), few lesions that are positive by the diagnostic standard criterion will be called negative, but many negative lesions will be wrongly identified as being positive. In other words, when the test reading is hard, specificity increases (few false positives), but sensitivity decreases (many false negatives); when the test reading is

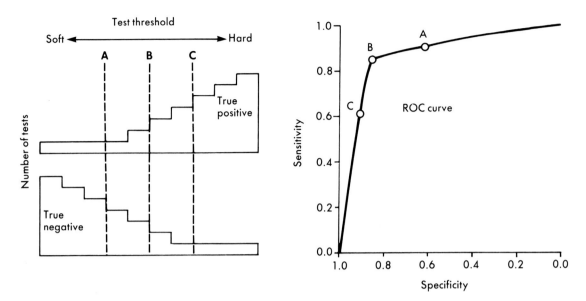

Fig. 8-5. Generation of ROC curve. With varying test threshold, sensitivity and specificity shift in opposite directions. (From Sumner DS: *Noninvasive investigation of the arterial supply to the brain and eye.* In Warlow C, Morris PJ, eds: *Transient ischemic attack,* New York, 1982, Marcel Dekker.)

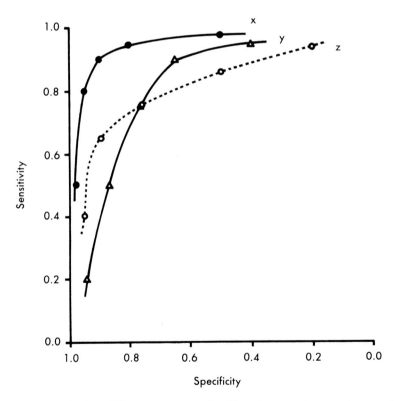

Fig. 8-6. ROC curves for three different tests, *x*, *y*, and *z*. The point on each curve closest to the upper left-hand corner is the best cutoff point in terms of making the fewest mistakes (smallest number of false-positive and false-negative studies). Test *x* is generally more accurate than tests *y* and *z*.

soft, sensitivity increases (few false negatives), but specificity decreases (many false positives).

Receiver operating characteristic (ROC) curves are constructed by plotting the sensitivity of the test versus its specificity at various thresholds. In the example shown in Fig. 8-5, at point *A* (soft threshold) the sensitivity of the test is 92% and its specificity is 62%; at point *C* (hard threshold) the sensitivity is 62% and the specificity is 92%; at point *B* (intermediate threshold) both are 85%. The best compromise would appear to be threshold *B*, but under certain circumstances the purposes of the investigator might be better served by selecting one of the other thresholds.

ROC curves can be used to compare the accuracy of tests at various thresholds. Of the three tests whose ROC curves are illustrated in Fig. 8-6, test *x* is clearly the best. A soft reading of test *y*, however, will provide sensitivities almost as good as those of test *x*, albeit at the expense of specificity. A hard reading of test *z* yields specificities comparable to test *x*, but the sensitivity is reduced. For some purposes, therefore, substitution of test *y* or *z* for test *x* may be justified, especially when *y* or *z* is less expensive, less time consuming, less technically demanding, or more readily available than test *x*.

A family of ROC curves is required to document the accuracy of any given test when different criteria are used to define the presence or absence of disease. Fig. 8-7 illustrates this point. At all test thresholds, sensitivities improve and specificities decline as the definitive criteria for positivity shift toward more significant disease, causing the inflexion of the ROC curve to move upward and to the left. Obviously, the same definitive criterion must be in effect when the ROC curves of two tests are compared.

PRESENTATION OF DATA

Because both the distribution of disease in the study population and the degree of positivity of the test results vary, presentation of data in a 2 × 2 format often obscures differences between studies that may be critical for evaluating the accuracy of a test. Without knowledge of the distribution of disease, the three tests in Table 8-5 would have been interpreted as having widely different accuracies. Without some indication of the threshold criterion used for the test, ROC curves cannot be constructed—again, making it difficult to compare test results. For these reasons, it is preferable to present raw data in tables with enough columns and rows to adequately display categories of increasing disease severity on one axis and categories of increasing test positivity on the other (see Table 14-2).

In some cases there may be multiple disease categories but the test results are either positive or negative; in others, there may be several gradations of test positivity but only two categories of disease. In most cases, more than two rows and columns are required to display the data. The number of cells in such a table will be equal to the product of the number of columns and the number of rows (Fig. 8-8). In the better tests, cells corresponding to high-grade disease and normal or almost normal test results and cells corresponding to low-grade disease and markedly abnormal test results will be empty or nearly so, whereas those in which the disease grade and the test results correlate will be relatively full. Deviations from this ideal pattern are easily perceived, their severity is immediately apparent, and the correlations most responsible for errors are readily identified.

By adjusting the line dividing positive from negative

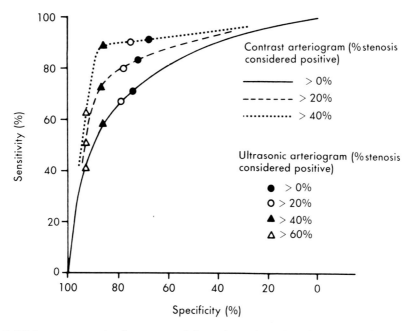

Fig. 8-7. ROC curves comparing the accuracy of ultrasonic arteriography with conventional arteriography. (From Sumner DS, Russell JB, Miles RD: *Surgery* 91:700, 1992.)

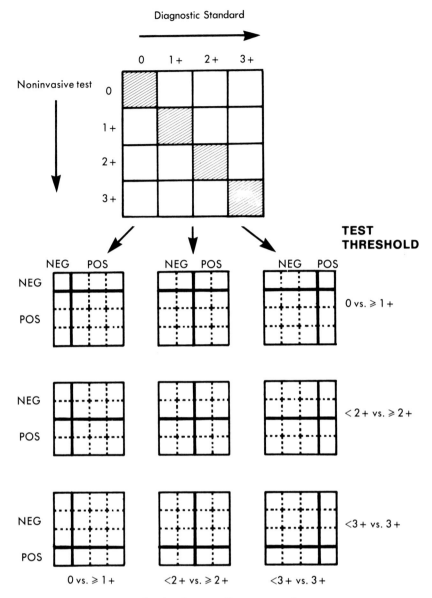

Fig. 8-8. Method for obtaining sensitivities and specificities for different levels of disease and for different test thresholds. Shaded areas in the upper diagram indicate perfect correlation. Dark lines in the lower diagrams indicate dividing lines between positive and negative disease levels or test thresholds.

disease categories and the orthogonal line dividing positive from negative test results, one can calculate the sensitivity and specificity of the test for different disease severities and the ROC curves defining the characteristics of the test for each disease category (Fig. 8-8). From a 4 × 4 matrix, nine sets of sensitivities and specificities can be calculated— the number of sets being equal to the number of columns minus one times the number of rows minus one.

When the data vary continuously, they may be presented with greater precision in a scatter diagram, the coordinates of each point being determined by the test results on one axis and the disease severity (diagnostic standard results) on the other (Fig. 8-9). In some cases, test results vary continuously but disease severity is discontinuous; in others, the opposite occurs. Data from such studies can be presented in columns corresponding to the discontinuous parameter with the vertical position of the points in each column corresponding to the values of the continuous parameter (Fig. 8-1). Continuous data can be analyzed in the same fashion as categorized data by constructing vertical and horizontal dividing lines across the display, thus separating positive from negative disease states and positive from negative test

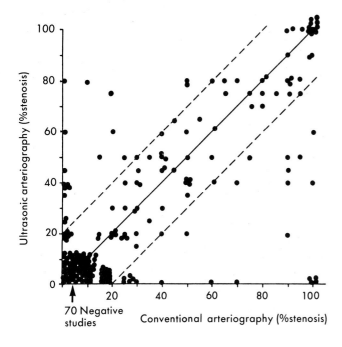

Fig. 8-9. Scatter diagram of continuously varying data comparing ultrasonic arteriography with conventional arteriography in detecting internal carotid artery stenosis in 209 vessels from 122 patients. The results of conventional arteriography are on the abscissa and the results of ultrasonic arteriography are on the ordinate. (From Sumner DS et al: *Arch Surg* 114:1222, 1979.)

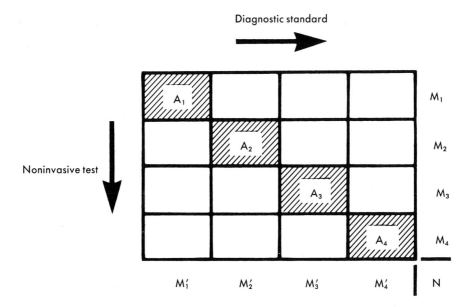

Fig. 8-10. Matrix illustrating the method for calculating κ value. Areas of perfect agreement are indicated by *A*, marginal totals by *M*, and total number of studies by *N*. See text for explanation.

results. Sensitivities and specificities are calculated by counting the number of points in each of the four resulting quadrants and performing the appropriate mathematics.

κ *STATISTIC*

For the most part, the preceding discussions have considered only the ability of noninvasive tests to distinguish disease of lesser severity from that of greater severity. In addition, some noninvasive tests are capable of predicting the actual magnitude of the disease process within certain limits. For example, spectrum analysis, duplex imaging, and B-mode

scans can be used not only to discriminate between hemodynamically and nonhemodynamically significant disease at the carotid bifurcation but also to estimate the degree of stenosis of the internal carotid artery.

To evaluate how well the results of a noninvasive test correlate with the results of the diagnostic standard, a number of investigators have employed the κ statistic, which is a coefficient of agreement for nominal scales. With the data arranged in a matrix with n columns and n rows, there will be n cells in which there are perfect agreement. In Fig. 8-10, there are four columns, four rows, and four cells with perfect agreement (A_1, A_2, A_3, and A_4). The proportion of results that agrees perfectly with the diagnostic standard (P_0) may be obtained by adding the numbers within the A cells and dividing the total by the total number of studies performed (N):

$$P_0 = \frac{\sum_1^n A}{N} \qquad (10)$$

The total number of results in each row is obtained by adding the numbers in each cell of that row. This figure is designated by *M,* or the "marginal" for that row. Similarly, the total number of results in each column is indicated by the marginal, *M'*. The proportion of agreement expected by chance (P_c) is the sum of the products of the marginals of each corresponding row and column divided by the square of the total number of studies performed.

$$P_c = \frac{\sum_1^n MM'}{N^2} \qquad (11)$$

κ is obtained from the observed proportion of agreement (P_0) and that expected by chance (P_c) by means of the following formula:

$$\kappa = \frac{P_0 - P_c}{1 - P_c} \qquad (12)$$

The standard error of κ is given by:

$$\sigma_\kappa = \left(\frac{P_0 (1 - P_0)}{N (1 - P_0)^2} \right)^{1/2} \qquad (13)$$

Table 8-6 demonstrates the use of equations 10 through 13 to calculate κ and its standard error from hypothetical data comparing a noninvasive test having four grades of positivity with a diagnostic standard having four similar grades of positivity. In this example, 84.4% of the results

of the noninvasive test and the diagnostic standard agreed ($P_0 = 0.844$), but 25.4% of the studies could have agreed by chance ($P_c = 0.254$). The difference between the observed agreement and chance agreement divided by the difference between perfect agreement (1.0) and chance gives a κ value of 0.791. The standard error is 0.055; therefore the 95% confidence limits of κ are 0.683 to 0.899 ($0.791 \pm 0.055 \times 1.96 = 0.791 \pm 0.108$).

When the results are "perfectly" randomly distributed, P_0 and P_c are identical and κ equals 0.0, indicating the total lack of correlation (Table 8-7). Perfect correlation, on the other hand, yields a κ value of $+1.0$ (Table 8-7). Reversed

Table 8-6. Calculating κ value

Noninvasive test results	Distribution according to diagnostic standard				Noninvasive test totals
	9	1+	2+	3+	
0	20	2	1	0	23
1+	2	15	1	0	18
2+	0	3	16	2	21
3+	0	0	1	14	15
TOTAL FOR DIAGNOSTIC STANDARD	22	20	19	16	77

$$P_0 = \frac{20 + 15 + 16 + 14}{77} = 0.844.$$

$$P_c = \frac{23(22) + 18(20) + 21(19) + 15(16)}{(77)^2} = 0.254.$$

$$\kappa = \frac{0.844 - 0.254}{1 - 0.254} = 0.791.$$

$$\sigma_\kappa = \left(\frac{0.844(1 - 0.844)}{77(1 - 0.254)^2} \right)^{1/2} = 0.055.$$

Table 8-7. Properties of the κ statistic

Noninvasive test results	Distribution according to diagnostic standard				Noninvasive test total
	0	1+	2+	3+	
*PERFECT RANDOM DISTRIBUTION**					
0	16	12	8	4	40
1+	12	9	6	3	30
2+	8	6	4	2	20
3+	4	3	2	1	10
PERFECT CORRELATION†					
0	40	0	0	0	40
1+	0	30	0	0	30
2+	0	0	20	0	20
3+	0	0	0	10	10

$$*P_0 = \frac{16 + 9 + 4 + 1}{100} = 0.3.$$

$$†P_0 = \frac{40 + 30 + 20 + 10}{100} = 1.0.$$

$$P_c = \frac{(40)^2 + (30)^2 + (20)^2 + (10)^2}{(100)^2} = 0.3.$$

$$P_c = \frac{(40)^2 + (30)^2 + (20)^2 + (10)^2}{(100)^2} = 0.3.$$

$$\kappa = \frac{0.3 - 0.3}{1 - 0.3} = 0.0.$$

$$\kappa = \frac{1.0 - 0.3}{1 - 0.3} = 1.0.$$

Table 8-8. Effect of number of cells on κ value

Noninvasive test results	Distribution according to diagnostic standard						Noninvasive test total
	0	1+	2+	3+	4+	5+	
*6 × 6 MATRIX**							
0	10	5	2	1	0	0	18
1+	5	10	5	2	1	0	23
2+	2	5	10	5	2	1	25
3+	1	2	5	10	5	2	25
4+	0	1	2	5	10	5	23
5+	0	0	1	2	5	10	18
3 × 3 MATRIX†							
	0 to 1+		2+ to 3+		4+ to 5+		
0 to 1+	30		10		1		41
2+ to 3+	10		30		10		50
4+ to 5+	1		10		30		41

*p_0, 0.455; p_c, 0.170; κ, 0.343; standard deviation, 0.052.

†p_0, 0.682; p_c, 0.336; κ, 0.521; standard deviation, 0.061.

correlations are also possible, in which case κ has a negative sign. A perfect negative correlation would have a κ value of -1.0. In other words, κ values may vary from -1.0 through 0.0 to $+1.0$. As κ approaches 1.0, the correlation improves between the noninvasive test and the diagnostic standard.

Even when there is an absolute lack of correlation between the noninvasive test and the diagnostic standard, the results will usually not be as perfectly distributed as they are in the upper part of Table 8-7. For example, the κ values of three 4 × 4 matrices in which the 16 cells were filled with computer-generated random numbers from 1 to 10 were 0.106 ± 0.065, 0.074 ± 0.071, and 0.103 ± 0.061. Thus slight positive or negative correlations are likely to happen by chance. That these three κ values are not statistically significantly different from zero becomes evident when their relatively large standard errors are considered. In each case, the 95% confidence limit extends below 0.

The κ statistic can be used to compare the accuracy of one test with that of another; the test with the higher κ value is expected to be the better predictor of disease severity. The standard errors of the tests must always be considered in determining whether the differences could have occurred by chance. Another pitfall concerns the fact that κ values for the same data are increased when the data are condensed in a matrix with fewer cells (Table 8-8). Therefore the same number of cells should be used when tests are compared.

One further note: Pearson correlation coefficients (r) can also be applied to grouped data. Analyzed in this way, the data in Table 8-6 gives an r value of 0.920, a value that is considerably higher than the κ value for this table, 0.791.

PREDICTING SEVERITY OF DISEASE

The κ statistic measures the overall correlation between the noninvasive test and the diagnostic standard results but does not tell the clinician how reliable a report indicating a specific level of disease is likely to be. To illustrate this point,

Table 8-9. Predictive value (%) of noninvasive test results (derived from Table 8-6)

Noninvasive test results	Distribution of noninvasive percentages according to diagnostic standard			
	0	1+	2+	3+
0	87	9	4	0
1+	11	83	6	0
2+	0	14	76	10
3+	0	0	7	93

the data in each test category of Table 8-6 have been divided by appropriate row totals and are listed as percentages in Table 8-9. Although 87% of the 0 noninvasive tests had 0 disease according to the diagnostic standard, 9% had 1+ disease and 4% had 2+ disease. Similarly, 83% of the 1+, 76% of the 2+, and 93% of the 3+ noninvasive tests were correct. If it were assumed that all future test results from the same laboratory were likely to have a similar distribution, the clinician receiving a report of 2+ disease could predict that this patient has a 76% chance of having a 2+ disease, a 14% chance of having 1+ disease, and a 10% chance of having 3+ disease. The clinician could be reasonably sure, however, that the patient had at least some disease. Likewise, a report of 0 or 1+ would virtually rule out 3+ disease, and a report of 3+ would make 0 or 1+ disease highly unlikely.

An example of this kind of analysis is given in Table 14-2, which summarizes the distribution of degree of internal carotid stenosis according to the color duplex reading. Presenting the data in this way enables the clinician to determine what level of confidence to attach to any given test result.

Calculations of sensitivity and specificity by the method illustrated in Fig. 8-8 may give a distorted impression of the ability of a noninvasive test to discriminate between

Table 8-10. Ability of noninvasive test to discriminate between levels of disease: comparing the results of ultrasonic arteriography and conventional arteriography in 232 internal carotid arteries

Results of ultrasonic arteriography (% stenosis)	Conventional arteriography (% stenosis)					
	Normal	1-24	25-49	50-74	75-99	Total occlusion
Normal	92	14	4	1	0	0
1-24	12	8	7	0	0	0
25-49	10	5	10	2	1	1
50-74	0	1	3	9	9	0
75-99	2	0	1	8	9	1
Total occlusion	3	2	0	2	2	13

	0% vs 1% to 24%	1% to 24% vs 25% to 49%	25% to 49% vs 50% to 74%	50% to 74% vs 75% to 99%	75% to 99% vs 100%
	92 14	22 11	21 3	12 10	19 2
	27 16	8 14	4 19	10 11	2 13
χ^2 (Yates)	9.5174	3.7431	20.4553	0.02221	18.3673
	p = 0.002	p = 0.053	p = 0.000006	p = 0.882	p = 0.00002
	0% vs ≥1%	≤24% vs ≥25%	≤49% vs ≥50%	≤74% vs ≥75%	≤99% vs 100%
Sensitivity	83	86	91	69	87
Specificity	77	85	93	91	96
Accuracy	80	85	93	88	95

levels of disease. As the data in Table 8-10 show, ultrasonic arteriography (UA) has a sensitivity of 86%, a specificity of 85%, and an overall accuracy of 85% for distinguishing internal carotid artery stenoses of <25% from stenoses >25%. Yet χ^2 analysis fails to demonstrate a statistically significant difference between the distribution of UA findings in the 1% to 24% lesions and the 25% to 49% lesions. While this may represent a type II statistical error (too few examples to reach statistical significance), it does show that the test is not very good for discriminating between these disease levels. Similarly, the test cannot reliably discriminate 50% to 74% lesions from 75% to 99% lesions despite a sensitivity of 69%, a specificity of 91%, and an accuracy of 88%. The test does appear to be capable of discriminating between no disease and 1% to 24% stenoses, between 25% to 49% and 50% to 74% stenoses, and between 75% to 99% stenosis and total occlusion. Medical literature contains many examples in which the accuracy implied by sensitivity and specificity data misrepresents the actual capabilities of the noninvasive test.

PROSPECTIVE VERSUS RETROSPECTIVE

After data have been accumulated and compared with the diagnostic standard, the investigator may examine it retrospectively to determine what test threshold provides the optimal combination of sensitivity and specificity. From this retrospective examination, accuracy parameters may (and often are) reported. But when retrospectively determined test thresholds are applied prospectively to new sets of data, the investigator may find that sensitivities and specificities are no longer satisfactory. The data are then reexamined, a

new threshold is selected based on the new data, and sensitivities and specificities are again retrospectively reported. This process ensures that the reported accuracies will always be good. It does not, however, ensure that they will be representative of the capabilities of the test.

To illustrate these points, the data in Table 8-11 were developed using a random number generator programmed to provide 80% negative test results in the 0 range, 6% in the 1+ range, 6% in the 2+ range, and 8% in the 3+ range for an infinite number of trials in which the diagnostic standard is negative. An opposite distribution is assumed for trials in which the standard is positive. Prevalence is assumed to be 50% for all trials. In trial 1 (in which 50 studies were performed), it appears that the optimum threshold would be ≥3+. This would provide a sensitivity and specificity of 92%. Applying this same threshold to 50 more studies in trial 2 gives a sensitivity of only 72%. By readjusting the threshold to ≥1+, the sensitivity is again 92% and the specificity is a respectable 88%. Unfortunately, if this new threshold were reapplied to the data in trial 1, the specificity would fall to 72%. When figures for 23 more trials (1150 studies) are accumulated, it becomes apparent that a ≥2+ threshold provides the best compromise between sensitivity and specificity. With the increasing number of studies, the randomly allocated data approach the infinite distribution, confirming what is already intuitively evident—the larger the study population, the more closely the results approximate truth. Other thresholds could be selected if the investigator wished to optimize sensitivity at the expense of specificity, or vice versa.

As long as the test itself has not been changed (e.g., no

Table 8-11. Variations in accuracy caused by sampling (prevalence, 50%)

Noninvasive test results	Distribution according to standard, infinite trials		Distribution according to standard, trial 1		Distribution according to standard, trial 2		Distribution according to standard, trial 3	
	Negative	Positive	Negative	Positive	Negative	Positive	Negative	Positive
0	80%	8%	18	1	22	2	453	34
1 +	6%	6%	2	0	1	3	44	33
2 +	6%	6%	3	1	1	2	32	42
3 +	8%	80%	2	23	1	18	46	466
Threshold	**Specificity**	**Sensitivity**	**Specificity**	**Sensitivity**	**Specificity**	**Sensitivity**	**Specificity**	**Sensitivity**
≥1 +	80%	92%	72%	96%	88%	92%	79%	94%
≥2 +	86%	86%	80%	96%	92%	80%	86%	88%
≥3 +	92%	80%	92%	92%	96%	72%	92%	81%

new instruments, no new technicians), it is not only valid but quite important to update accuracy figures by a retrospective examination of the data; however, all of the preceding test results should be included in the review and not just those resulting from the most recent trial to minimize errors. Armed with this information, the results of a prospective trial of 50 new studies—such as trial 2—in which sensitivities drop need not be viewed with alarm but could be recognized for what they are, merely the vagaries of chance.

The warning for the student of the medical literature is simply to view accuracy figures derived from retrospective reviews with some skepticism.

CONFIDENCE LIMITS

The previous discussion raises questions regarding the certainty that sensitivities and specificities reported from a limited sample actually represent *true values* (the values expected if the test had been applied to an infinitely large population). Is test A with a reported sensitivity of 80% inferior to test B with a reported sensitivity of 90%, or could the difference be the result of chance? One way of approaching this problem is to calculate the 95% confidence limits of the sensitivity and specificity.

Although confidence limits for means are commonly reported in medical literature (that is, the mean ± the standard of error of the mean), similar data for proportions seldom appear. Sensitivity and specificity are proportions, the former being the proportion of positive noninvasive tests in the sample of tests that are positive according to the diagnostic standard and the latter being the proportion of negative tests in the sample that are negative according to the diagnostic standard.

For example, test A in an infinitely large, well-defined population has a true sensitivity of 80%. Thus the probability (p) that any individual study will correctly identify the presence of disease is 0.80. If an investigator applies the test to a group of patients from this population in which 20 of the diagnostic standard results turn out to be positive, what is the likelihood that exactly 16 (80%) of the test results

will also be positive? The answer, somewhat surprisingly, is that in only about 22% of such samples will exactly 16 studies be positive. Unfortunately, an investigator attempting to estimate the sensitivity of the test from a sample of 20 has a 78% chance of arriving at an erroneous value. In fact, in over 5% of such samples, as few as 13 or as many as 19 positive studies can be expected. In the former case the sensitivity would appear to be 65% and in the latter case, 95%. Table 8-12 lists the probability, f(x), that a certain number of positive test results, x, will be found in samples of n = 20 when p = 0.80. These probabilities are derived from the binomial theorem:

$$f(x) = \frac{n!}{x!(n - x)!} p^x(1 - p)^{n - x} \qquad (14)$$

The calculation for 16 positive studies is as follows:

$$f(16) = \frac{20!}{16!(4)!} 0.8^{16}(0.2)^4 = 0.218$$

Because of the factorials these calculations are cumbersome to do by hand but are easily accomplished with a programmable calculator, a computer, or the aid of tables.

As indicated in Table 8-12, the sum of all the probabilities, $\Sigma f(x)$, from x = 0 to x = 20 is 1.0. Since only 1% of the samples would have 11 or fewer positive results ($\Sigma_0^{11} f(x) = 0.010$), it is unlikely that the investigators would conclude that the sensitivity of the test is 55% or less. It is also unlikely that all 20 studies would be positive (f(x) = 0.012). On the other hand, there is a 21% chance that the sample of 20 would include 18 or more positive studies ($\Sigma_{18}^{20} f(x) = 0.137 + 0.058 + 0.012$), leading to the mistaken conclusion that the sensitivity of the test is 90% or better. There is a 60% chance that the sample of 20 will produce 15 to 17 positive studies, implying a sensitivity of 75% to 85%, which is equal to or within 5% of the true sensitivity of 80%.

To make these observations more intuitively evident, it is helpful to consider an analogous situation. For example, with a sack containing 8000 red marbles and 2000 white marbles, each time a marble is removed blindly from the

Table 8-12. Binomial theorem: probability distribution of positive test results, f(x), in samples of 20 studies

Positive results (%)	No. of positive studies (x)	Test A (p = 0.80)		Test B (p = 0.90)	
		f(x)	$\Sigma_0^x f(x)$	f(x)	$\Sigma_0^x f(x)$
0	0	1×10^{-14}	0.000	1×10^{-20}	0.000
5	1	8×10^{-13}	0.000	2×10^{-18}	0.000
10	2	3×10^{-11}	0.000	2×10^{-16}	0.000
15	3	8×10^{-10}	0.000	8×10^{-15}	0.000
20	4	1×10^{-8}	0.000	3×10^{-13}	0.000
25	5	2×10^{-7}	0.000	9×10^{-12}	0.000
30	6	2×10^{-6}	0.000	2×10^{-10}	0.000
35	7	1×10^{-5}	0.000	4×10^{-9}	0.000
40	8	9×10^{-5}	0.000	5×10^{-8}	0.000
45	9	5×10^{-4}	0.000	7×10^{-7}	0.000
50	10	0.002	0.003	6×10^{-6}	0.000
55	11	0.007	0.010	5×10^{-5}	0.000
60	12	0.022	0.032	4×10^{-4}	0.000
65	13	0.055	0.087	0.002	0.002
70	14	0.109	0.196	0.009	0.011
75	15	0.175	0.370	0.032	0.043
80	16	0.218	0.589	0.090	0.133
85	17	0.205	0.794	0.190	0.323
90	18	0.137	0.931	0.285	0.608
95	19	0.058	0.988	0.270	0.878
100	20	0.012	1.000	0.122	1.000

sack and then replaced, the probability (p) that it will be red is 0.8. If one removes, inspects, and replaces 20 marbles, one would not be surprised to find that the sample of 20 has not produced exactly 16 red marbles but rather, 14, 15, 17, or 18 red marbles. However, one would not expect the sample to contain all red marbles or less than 10 or 11 red marbles.

The probability distribution, f(x), of another test (test B) with a true sensitivity of 90% (p = 0.90) is also shown in Table 8-12. Almost 29% of the samples of 20 studies in which the diagnostic standard is positive would be expected to yield 18 positive test results. In other words, the estimated sensitivity would be correct 29% of the time. But 13% of the samples would indicate a sensitivity of 80% or less ($\Sigma_0^{16} f(x) = 0.133$). Since 21% of the samples from test A might indicate a sensitivity greater than 90%, it would be possible to conclude—given the vagaries of sampling—that test B was inferior to test A. It is interesting that the chances of obtaining exactly 17 positive test results (estimated sensitivity, 85%) are almost the same with either test (A = 0.205; B = 0.190).

These examples emphasize the difficulties involved in making inferences regarding the true sensitivity (or specificity) of a test from a limited number of studies. Inferences could be improved by increasing the sample size. If 100 marbles were withdrawn from the sack instead of 20 marbles, the likelihood that exactly 80% would be red is reduced from 22% to 10%, but the likelihood that 75% to 85% will be red is increased from 60% to 83%. In fact, with a sample size of 100, 62% of the samples should consist of 77% to 83% red marbles. In other words, increasing the sample

size reduces the likelihood that the precise sensitivity of a test would be discovered but permits a more accurate estimation of the range in which the precise sensitivity is likely to occur.

In actual practice, the true sensitivity or specificity of a test is never known. The best that the investigator can do is to estimate the sensitivity or specificity from the proportion of successes (positive results in the case of sensitivity, negative results in the case of specificity) that are found in a sample consisting of positive or negative diagnostic standard results. The estimated probability of success is indicated by $\hat{p}$ to distinguish it from the true probability of success, p. Therefore

$$\hat{p} = x'/n \tag{15}$$

where x' is the number of successes observed in a sample size of n (x' and n are always positive integers).

For any $\hat{p}$, 95% confidence limits can be defined. The lower limit of the true probability (p_a) is that which would be expected to yield x' or more success in only 2.5% of samples of size n; the upper limit of the true probability (p_b) is that which would be expected to yield x' or fewer successes in only 2.5% of samples in size n. Expressed mathematically, the lower limit (p_a) is that which satisfies the following equations:

$$\sum_{x'}^{n} f(x, n, p_a) = 0.025 \tag{16}$$

$$\sum_{0}^{x'-1} f(x, n, p_a) = 0.975 \tag{17}$$

Table 8-13. Finding the 95% confidence limits for $\hat{p} = 0.85$ (n = 20, x' = 17)

p_a	$\sum_{17}^{20} f(x, n, p_a)$	p_b	$\sum_0^{17} f(x, n, p_b)$
0.500	0.0013	0.950	0.0755
0.600	0.0016	0.960	0.0439
0.620	0.0245	0.967	0.0269
0.621	**0.0250**	**0.968**	**0.0249**
0.622	0.0255	0.969	0.0229
0.650	0.0444	0.975	0.0130
0.700	0.1071	0.980	0.0071

and the upper limit is expressed as:

$$\sum_0^{x'} f(x, n, p_b) = 0.025 \tag{18}$$

$$\sum_{x'+1}^{n} f(x, n, p_b) = 0.975 \tag{19}$$

For example, an investigator analyzes data and finds that a noninvasive test is positive in 17 of 20 arteries that had positive results for carotid artery disease according to the diagnostic standard. The number of successes (x') is 17, the sample size (n) is 20, and the estimated sensitivity ($\hat{p}$) is 0.85. To determine the lower limit, p_a, the investigator applies equation 14, uses 17, 18, 19, and 20 for x, and guesses what the p_a value should be. The resulting probabilities are added, as in equation 16, and inspected to see how closely the sum approximates 0.025. If the first estimation of p_a had been 0.5, the resulting sum would be 0.0013 (Table 8-13). Since this value is too low, the estimated p_a must be too low. The process is then repeated, this time using a p_a of 0.7. This gives a sum of 0.1071, indicating that over 10% of the samples taken with a p of 0.7 would yield 17 or more successes. Thus p_a must lie between 0.5 and 0.7. By repeating the process, the p_a can be narrowed down to 0.621, a value that would yield 17 or more successes in only 2.5% of samples having an n of 20.

To determine p_b, the investigator again applies equation 14, this time using all the integers from 0 through 17 for x and totaling the resulting probabilities as in equation 18. If the first guess at a value for p_b had been 0.95, the sum would be too high (0.0755), indicating that almost 8% of the samples would yield 17 or fewer successes (Table 8-13). A p_b of 0.98 would be too high, since the percentage of samples yielding 17 or fewer successes is far less than 2.5%. By process of elimination, 0.968 appears to be the best approximation for p_b.

The investigator can now report that the sensitivity of this test is 85%, with the 95% confidence limits being 62.1% and 96.8%. Clearly, this range would encompass the true p values of test A (0.80) and test B (0.90) in Table 8-12, both of which would frequently yield a $\hat{p}$ of 0.85. As expected, increasing the sample size narrows the confidence limits. If the sample size had been 100 and the apparent

sensitivity had been 85% (x' = 85), the 95% confidence limits would be 76.5% and 91.5%.

Calculating confidence limits in this way can be extremely time consuming and cumbersome, even with the help of a programmable calculator. Computer programs, charts, and tables are available to simplify the task.

Returning to the original question—is test A with a reported sensitivity of 80% inferior to test B with a sensitivity of 90%? If for both tests the positive sample according to the diagnostic standard consisted of 20 arteries, the 95% confidence limits of test A would be 56.3% to 94.3% and that for test B would be 68.3% to 98.8.%. Because of the considerable overlap, it is apparent that the two tests could easily be identical. It is quite possible that test B could be inferior to test A. χ^2 with Yates correction is only 0.196, indicating that differences as large as those observed have a 66% likelihood of occurring by chance. For example, if the sample for test A were increased to 75 and that for test B to 50 and both retained the same sensitivity, the narrowed confidence limits for test A (69.2% to 98.4%) would still overlap those for test B (78.2% to 96.7%). χ^2 with Yates correction (1.550) would still be insufficient to reject the null hypothesis (p = 0.213). It would take sample sizes of about 120 for each of the tests to reject the null hypothesis at the 5.0% level. With these numbers the 95% confidence limits would show little overlap (A $\sim$ 73% to 86% and B $\sim$ 83% to 94%).

Although confidence limits overlap and tests for significant differences between proportions (χ^2 or Fisher's exact test) fail to reject the null hypothesis at the 5.0% levels, the sensitivities (or specificities) of two tests may not be really different. The differences may be less than they appear to be and could have occurred by chance. The cautious investigator may wish to defer judgment on the relative merits of two tests until sufficient data have accumulated to establish with reasonable certainty that one is better than the other. Unfortunately, there is a tendency to accept data at face value, with the result that some tests are discarded prematurely and others accepted too readily. Publications of confidence limits for sensitivity and specificity would do much to dispel this source of confusion.

RELIABILITY OF THE DIAGNOSTIC STANDARD

Ideally, the accuracy of a noninvasive test is evaluated based on concrete knowledge of the presence or absence of disease or its relative severity. Since the truth is seldom known, it is usually necessary to substitute a diagnostic standard. A variety of standards have been used; some are clinical (relief of claudication) and others are physiologic (invasive pressure measurements), but most are anatomic (angiography). Diagnostic standards should be selected to coincide with the objectives of the noninvasive test. For example, it would be more appropriate to compare noninvasive pressure measurements to invasive pressure measurements than to arteriography. Another guideline for selecting the diagnostic standard should be its accuracy. Unfortunately, these guidelines are frequently neglected, and the most readily avail-

Table 8-14. The effect of diagnostic standard errors on the apparent accuracy of a noninvasive test, given the true disease status

DIAGNOSTIC STANDARD VS. TRUE DISTRIBUTION*

Diagnostic standard results	True distribution		Diagnostic standard total
	Negative	Positive	
Negative	285	5	290
Positive	15	95	110

NONINVASIVE TEST VS. TRUE DISTRIBUTION†

Noninvasive test results	True distribution		Noninvasive test total
	Negative	Positive	
Negative	285	5	290
Positive	15	95	110

NONINVASIVE TEST VS. DIAGNOSTIC STANDARD‡

Noninvasive test results	Distribution according to diagnostic standard		Noninvasive test total
	Negative	Positive	
Negative	270	20	290
Positive	20	90	110

SUMMARY

Diagnostic standard results	Noninvasive test results	True distribution	
		Negative	Positive
Negative	Negative	270	0
Negative	Positive	15	5
Positive	Negative	15	5
Positive	Positive	0	90

*Sensitivity, 95%; specificity, 95%; PPV, 86%; NPV, 98%; accuracy, 95%.
†Sensitivity, 95%; specificity, 95%; PPV, 86%; NPV, 98%; accuracy, 95%.
‡Sensitivity, 82%; specificity, 93%; PPV, 82%; NPV, 93%; accuracy, 90%.

able, conventionally used method for diagnosing disease is used.

All too often, the accuracy of a diagnostic standard is unknown. Recently, there have been several reports questioning the reliability of conventional arteriography for assessing disease at the carotid bifurcation. Because most noninvasive tests designed to assess the severity of disease at the carotid bifurcation have been compared to arteriography, one should consider what effect errors made by the diagnostic standard might have on the apparent accuracy of the noninvasive tests.

Table 8-14 illustrates a hypothetical situation in which the truth is known regarding the presence or absence of disease. Based on the true condition, a noninvasive test and its diagnostic standard are both quite accurate, both having sensitivities and specificities of 95%. For the most part, the results coincide; but in a few cases, they disagree. When the test is compared to the diagnostic standard rather than to the true condition, the apparent sensitivity of the test falls

to 82%; the other parameters (specificity, PPV, NPV, and overall accuracy) also suffer. Thus it is possible that the true accuracy of a test may be considerably better than its apparent accuracy. On the other hand, a noninvasive test and its diagnostic standard may be subject to the same errors, in which case the apparent accuracy of the test may exceed its true accuracy.

NONINVASIVE DIAGNOSTIC STANDARDS

In a few reports, one noninvasive test has been employed as the diagnostic standard for another. This practice is perhaps even more likely to yield distorted parameters of accuracy than the use of an independent diagnostic standard, such as conventional arteriography. The accuracy of the noninvasive test being evaluated may appear inferior to that of the test used as the diagnostic standard when its true accuracy may be equally as good or even better. How this can happen is shown in Table 8-15. Test B, with a true sensitivity and specificity of 95%, appears to have a sensitivity and specificity of only 80% when test A, with a true sensitivity and specificity of 85%, serves as the definitive test. Similarly, if test B were selected as the diagnostic standard, test A would appear to have a sensitivity and specificity of 80%. Either way, the parameters of accuracy of the test being evaluated are erroneously low.

If, however, the two tests are basically similar and are likely to make the same errors, the apparent sensitivity and specificity will be deceptively high. Test C in Table 8-15 has a true sensitivity and specificity of 86%, only slightly better than test A, but because they tend to make the same mistakes, test C appears to have a sensitivity and specificity of 97% when compared with test A.

In general, therefore, it seems advisable to avoid using one noninvasive test as the standard for evaluating the accuracy of another. Data derived from studies that use this approach must be viewed with some skepticism.

VARIABILITY OF TEST RESULTS

Like all clinical determinations, the results of noninvasive tests are subject to three main sources of variability: true biologic, temporal, and measurement errors. Intersubject biologic variability includes those differences that relate to the factors distinguishing one individual from another, temporal variability refers to biologic differences occurring within a single individual from one time to the next, and the measurement errors relate to differences attributable to the instruments, test procedures, or interpretation. Since the goals of noninvasive testing are to identify the presence of disease, assess its severity, determine its location, and evaluate disease progression, the clinician must be able to distinguish pathologic changes from normal variation or measurement error. Accomplishing this requires an awareness of the extent to which the test results vary in normal subjects. Ideally, confidence limits should be established so that the likelihood that any result is abnormal (or normal) can be predicted.

Table 8-15. Effect of using noninvasive tests as diagnostic standards

Noninvasive test result	Distribution according to noninvasive test A*		True distribution	
	Negative	Positive	Negative	Positive
TEST B†				
Negative	80	20	95	5
Positive	20	80	5	95
TEST C‡				
Negative	97	3	86	14
Positive	3	97	14	86

SUMMARY

Tests		True distribution		Tests		True distribution	
B vs. A		Negative	Positive	C vs. A		Negative	Positive
Negative	Negative	80	0	Negative	Negative	84	13
Positive	Negative	5	15	Positive	Negative	1	2
Negative	Positive	15	5	Negative	Positive	2	1
Positive	Positive	0	80	Positive	Positive	13	84

*True sensitivity, 85%; true specificity, 85%.
†Apparent sensitivity using Test A as diagnostic standard, 80%; apparent specificity, 80%; true sensitivity, 95%; true specificity, 95%.
‡Apparent sensitivity using Test A as diagnostic standard, 97%; apparent specificity, 97%; true sensitivity, 86%; true specificity, 86%.

Of the three sources of variability, that caused by biologic factors has been the most frequently investigated. Information is available on the range of normal values for many noninvasive tests, including ankle pressure indices, venous outflow, and ophthalmic pressures. Indeed, the calculation of sensitivity and specificity is predicated on knowledge of the spread of normal values (intersubject variability). Less attention, however, has been given to the analysis of temporal variation (intrasubject variability). For some easily repeated tests, such as the determination of ankle pressures, several measurements may be made on the same visit, and the results analyzed to give a single value. But many tests are too difficult, too time consuming, too expensive, or too uncomfortable to be repeated. In such cases, every effort should be made to perform the measurements when the patient has rested long enough to minimize the effects of previous activity or excitement. Variability between visits is usually higher than that observed during any single visit. Between-visits variability may be reduced by careful attention to decreasing the factors implicit in single-visit variability by making the measurements at the same time of day (to standardize the effects of circadian rhythms) and by striving to maintain the same laboratory conditions. Despite all efforts at standardization, there will always be some temporal variation. Unless the extent of this variation is known, the clinician may be uncertain whether a change in the results of a noninvasive test represents a worsening (or improvement) of the patient's condition or merely reflects intrasubject variability. For this reason, serial interpretation of tests that do not lend themselves readily to numerical measurement, such as spectral broadening or Doppler venous surveys, may be difficult.

Measurement errors influence apparent biologic and temporal variability. Although measurement errors cannot be eliminated, they should be sought out, their source identified, their magnitude determined, and—if possible—their cause corrected. Any of the multiple factors that interact to produce the final result of the noninvasive test may be responsible: instruments may be poorly designed, lack stability, or have a tendency to malfunction; technicians may be inadequately trained, careless, fatigued, or distracted; and the patient's physique, mental condition, or physiologic state may preclude an adequate study. Tests that require additional interpretation are conducive to further error—the more subjective the test, the less likely that one interpreter will agree with another or even with earlier results if given the same data at a later date. Finally, the rationale of the test may not be based on sound physiologic principles.

Inaccuracy may represent bias, lack of precision, or both. Since the average results of an unbiased test should approach the true or correct value, bias can usually be recognized by comparing the data derived from the test with the results of a reliable diagnostic standard. The precision of noninvasive tests is less easily determined and consequently is seldom reported. A precise test yields results with little spread. Unfortunately, distinguishing variability resulting from lack of precision from that caused by temporal factors may be difficult. Although the precision of some noninvasive tests can be evaluated by comparing the results to those obtained simultaneously with an accurate invasive test, many noninvasive tests have no readily available invasive counterpart. It is possible, however, to determine the precision with which tests are read by suitably blinding the interpreters. Recent reports concerning the interpretation of carotid arteriograms have called attention to a surprisingly high degree of interobserver and intraobserver variability. The fact that arteriography—which is ordinarily considered to be highly objective—is subject to diverse interpretations should serve as a warning to those who use noninvasive tests.

The message is clear: each laboratory should define the extent of the biologic and temporal variability of the population it serves and should determine the reliabilty and precision of the tests it uses. Only in this way can the significance of aberrant values be determined. Documentation of variability is particularly important when noninvasive tests are used to diagnose disease progression or to define the natural history of a disease.

MULTIPLE TESTS

To improve the accuracy of the overall result, laboratories often use two or more noninvasive tests concurrently. The intuitive rationale for this approach is that if one test is good, two must be better, and three or more should be best. However, each additional test adds to the expense and time required to complete the evaluation. Because of these factors, the premise that a battery of tests will provide superior results should be examined carefully.

Venn diagrams help explain the interaction of multiple noninvasive tests and the study population. In Fig. 8-11, the rectangle represents all the patients included in the study. Patients with disease are represented by the contents of the open circle. Those with no disease are represented by the space between that circle and the rectangle. Positive test results are indicated by the shaded circle and negative results by the space between the shaded circle and the rectangle. If the test were 100% sensitive and specific, the two circles would coincide. As it is, the overlapping areas represent the TP studies, the remaining crescent of the open or "disease" circle represents FN studies, and the shaded crescent outside the disease circle includes all of the FP results. Thus the shaded portion of the disease circle corresponds to the sensitivity of the test. The space within the rectangle not occupied by either of the circles represents TN studies and corresponds to the specificity of the test.

The more the shaded circle overlaps the disease circle, the greater the sensitivity and specificity become, and vice versa—the less the overlap, the poorer the sensitivity and specificity. Although the two circles in Fig. 8-11 are of equal size, they would not necessarily be so. For example, the shaded circle could be smaller or larger than the disease circle, indicating more or less positive studies than the number of patients with disease. In other words, the Venn diagram functions as a graphic representation of Table 8-1.

For example, two similar tests, subject to the same types

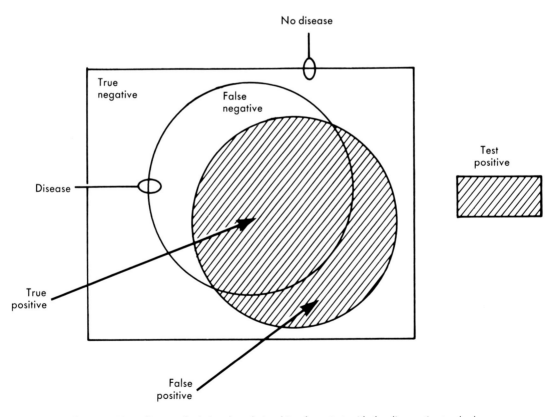

Fig. 8-11. Venn diagram depicting the relationship of one test with the diagnostic standard.

of error, are applied to the same population (e.g., measuring venous refilling times with foot volumetry and air plethysmography). In Fig. 8-12 the test represented by the inner shaded circle (test *A*) is somewhat less sensitive but more specific than the test represented by the outer shaded circle (test *B*). For each battery of two tests there are four possible combinations of results: (1) both tests positive, (2) both tests negative, (3) test *A* positive, test *B* negative, and (4) test *A* negative, test *B* positive. In this particular example, however, there are no tests that fall into the *A* positive, *B* negative category. If the two tests agree, there will be no problem in classifying the overall result, but when *B* is positive and *A* is negative, should the overall result be called positive or negative? If the *B* reading is presumed correct, the overall sensitivity will be greater, but the specificity will be less than if the *A* reading is presumed correct. Either way, the overall result would be the same as if only one test was used, the test whose results were accepted. If, on the other hand, all studies that do not coincide are discarded, a number of studies made in both the disease and no disease categories will be considered uninterpretable and will disappear from the denominator in the sensitivity and specificity calculations. This approach may or may not have a favorable effect on the overall accuracy and is always done at the cost of an increased number of uninterpretable studies. The conclusion that must be drawn is that combining similar tests will not materially affect overall accuracy.

Fig. 8-13 shows a Venn diagram of two dissimilar, totally independent tests. An example of two such tests would be ultrasonic B-mode scanning of the carotid bifurcation and oculopneumoplethysmography. Because the rationales of these tests are different, they would not necessarily make the same errors. Although the two tests depicted in the diagram are equally sensitive and specific, they frequently disagree. All possible combinations of results are pictured: (1) both tests positive; (2) both negative; (3) test *A* (horizontal shading) positive, test *B* (diagonal shading) negative; and (4) test *A* negative, test *B* positive. Both tests can agree and both be falsely positive, falsely negative, truly positive, or truly negative. When the tests disagree, one test will be falsely negative while the other is truly positive or one test will be falsely positive while the other is truly negative. Again when the tests agree, there will be no problem in classifying the overall result. When some of the tests disagree, three options are possible:

1. The tests that disagree can be disregarded and only those that agree considered in formulating the overall result.
2. The overall result can be called positive if one or both tests are positive, and negative if both tests are negative.
3. The overall result can be called positive if both tests are positive, and negative if one or both tests are negative.

As Fig. 8-13 shows, if option 2 is selected, the disease circle is nearly occupied by positive studies, but an increased portion of the area outside the circle (the area corresponding to no disease) is also occupied by positive studies. Thus

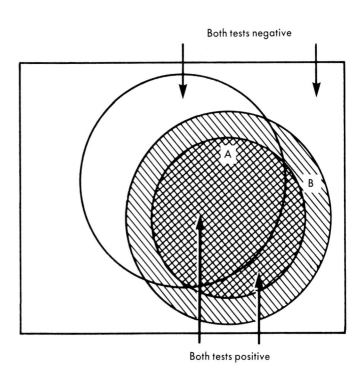

Fig. 8-12. Venn diagram illustrating the relationship between two dependent tests and the diagnostic standard. The tests are convergent: Test *A* is more likely to be positive when test *B* is positive than when test *B* is negative.

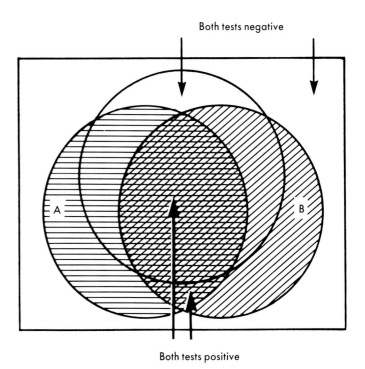

Fig. 8-13. Venn diagram illustrating the relationship between two independent tests and the diagnostic standard. To be completely independent, the positivity rate of test *A* should be the same for patients with positive or negative results of test *B*.

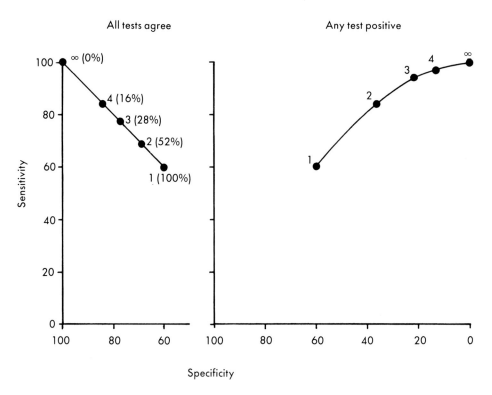

Fig. 8-14. The effect of increasing the number of tests on the sensitivity and specificity. Left panel (option 1): All tests must agree to be positive. Right panel (option 2): Overall result is considered to be positive if one or more test results are positive. The percentages in parentheses (left panel) indicate the percentage of total studies that agree.

calling the result positive when any one or both tests are positive and negative when both are negative always increases sensitivity at the expense of specificity.

The reverse is true when option 3 is selected. In this event, only the areas where the two tests are both positive are considered positive (the crosshatched area in Fig. 8-13). Since this leaves a large portion of the disease circle unoccupied, sensitivity is always decreased. Specificity is always increased because only a small part of the area outside the circle is occupied by the intersection of positive tests.

Overall results are less easily predicted when option 1 is selected. While the elimination of tests that do not agree always increases the number of uninterpretable studies, this undesirable feature may be offset by an increased accuracy. Although the relationships are complicated, sensitivity and specificity both tend to increase when the major portion of the overlapping area of the positive circles of both tests (the crosshatched area in Fig. 8-13) lies in the disease circle with little remaining in the nondiseased area outside. Although it is possible that considering only tests that agree could decrease sensitivity and specificity compared to a single test, this seldom happens in practice.

In summary, in regard to sensitivity, the options rank as follows:
Option 2 > option 1 > option 3
Option 2 > single test > option 3
Option 1 <, =, or > single test

In regard to specificity:
Option 3 > option 1 > option 2
Option 3 > single test > option 2
Option 1 <, =, or > single test

When three or more tests are included in the battery, similar generalizations apply. Fig. 8-14 illustrates the effects on overall sensitivity and specificity that result from the use of multiple tests. All tests are assumed to be totally independent and to have a sensitivity and specificity of 60%. If option 1 is used (all tests must agree to be considered), sensitivity and specificity both increase as more tests are added, but the percentage of tests that agree rapidly declines (Fig. 8-14, *left*). Although the accuracy obtained when four tests agree is much improved over that obtained with a single test, only 16% of the total studies can be used; the remaining 84% would be considered uninterpretable. Eventually, accuracy for agreeing tests would approach 100%, but the percentage that agree would approach 0%.

When option 2 is used (overall result positive if one or more tests are positive, overall result negative only if all tests are negative), increasing the number of tests rapidly improves sensitivity at the expense of rapidly decreasing specificity (Fig. 8-14, *right*). With three or four tests the sensitivity exceeds 90%, but the 20% specificity is unacceptably low. The graph for option 3 (overall result negative if any test is negative) would be identical to that for option 2 except that the labeling of the axes would be reversed.

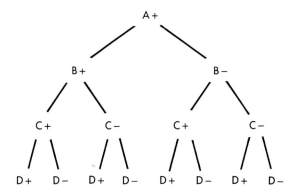

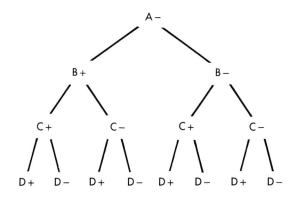

Fig. 8-15. Algorithm illustrating the various possible combinations of results from four diagnostic tests.

Adding tests would increase specificity but decrease sensitivity.

As implied by the graphs in Fig. 8-14, the beneficial effects of adding more tests are offset by the detrimental effects and the incremental increase in accuracy rapidly declines (the sensitivity of four tests is little better than that of three). Thus there appears to be scant justification for using more than two, perhaps three, rarely four tests even if they are totally independent. To illustrate these points, low sensitivities and specificities were deliberately selected for calculating the data in Fig. 8-14. However, the curves would be similar, though less exaggerated, if higher values had been used. The *all tests agree* curve would rotate upward and the *any test positive* curve would shift to left and rotate upward. In other words, increasing the sensitivity and specificity of any or all of the tests used would further decrease the relative benefits of adding more tests.

Bayes theorem

The algorithm in Fig. 8-15 illustrates another approach to combining the results of multiple tests. Because any of the tests must be either positive or negative, the number of combinations is equal to 2^n. Thus three tests yield 8 combinations and four tests yield 16 combinations. By means of a retrospective review of accumulated data, one could determine what percentage of a given combination of test results was actually found to be associated with the presence

of disease when the results were compared with a diagnostic standard. For example, the combination $A+$, $B-$, $C+$, $D+$ might have a PPV of 94%, whereas another combination, $A-$, $B+$, $C-$, $D-$, might have a PPV of only 8% (an NPV of 92%). If enough examples of each combination are available for analysis and if the data are continuously updated, this approach provides a rational method of using multiple tests to predict the likelihood of disease.

Bayes theorem provides a mathematic approach to the same problem. In the following calculations, $p(D+)$ denotes the probability that disease is present, and $p(D-)$ denotes the probability of no disease. These symbols refer to the *prior probability* in that these calculations assume knowledge of the prevalence (prior probability) of the disease in the population being studied. Symbolically, prior probability is:

$$p(D+) = \frac{TP + FN}{TN + FN + TP + FP} = \text{Prevalence} \quad (20)$$

Similarly, the prior probability of no disease is

$$p(D-) = \frac{TN + FP}{TN + FN + TP + FP} = 1 - \text{Prevalence} \quad (21)$$

In equations 22 and 23, $p(T+ \mid D+)$ and $p(T+ \mid D-)$ are the *conditional probabilities* that the test will be positive when disease is either present or absent, respectively, and are expressed symbolically as follows:

$$p(T+ \mid D+) = \frac{TP}{TP + FN} = \text{Sensitivity} \quad (22)$$

$$p(T+ \mid D-) = \frac{FP}{TN + FP} = 1 - \text{Specificity} \quad (23)$$

Bayes theorem calculates the *posterior probability* that disease is present given a positive test result as follows:

$$p(D+ \mid T+) = \quad (24)$$

$$\frac{p(D+) \times p(T+ \mid D+)}{p(D+) \times p(T+ \mid D+) + p(D-) \times p(T+ \mid D-)} =$$

$$\frac{(\text{Prevalence})(\text{Sensitivity})}{(\text{Prevalence})(\text{Sensitivity}) + (1 - \text{Prevalence})(1 - \text{Specificity})} =$$

$$\frac{TP}{FP + TP} = \text{PPV}$$

Thus this formula is merely a complex method of stating the PPV. The conditional probabilities that the test will be negative $(T-)$ when disease is present or absent are expressed as follows:

$$p(T- \mid D+) = \frac{FN}{TP + FN} = 1 - \text{Sensitivity} \quad (25)$$

$$p(T- \mid D-) = \frac{TN}{TN + FP} = \text{Specificity} \quad (26)$$

The posterior probability that disease is present given a negative test result is:

Table 8-16. Probability of disease (prevalence 30%): random number generator vs. Bayes theorem

Test results			Random number generator				Bayes theorem
A*	B†	C‡	Disease present	Disease absent	Total	Probability of disease	Probability of disease
+	+	+	108	0	108	1.000	0.964
+	+	−	44	15	59	0.746	0.743
+	−	+	20	12	32	0.625	0.628
+	−	−	9	97	106	0.085	0.153
−	+	+	14	12	26	0.538	0.429
−	+	−	9	85	94	0.096	0.074
−	−	+	3	37	40	0.075	0.045
−	−	−	3	232	235	0.013	0.005

*Sensitivity, 90%; specificity, 80%.
†Sensitivity, 80%; specificity, 80%.
‡Sensitivity, 70%; specificity, 80%.

$$p(D+ \mid T-) = \tag{27}$$

$$\frac{p(D+) \times p(T- \mid D+)}{p(D+) \times p(T- \mid D+) + p(D-) \times p(T- \mid D-)} =$$

$$\frac{(\text{Prevalence})(1 - \text{Sensitivity})}{(\text{Prevalence})(1 - \text{Sensitivity}) + (1 - \text{Prevalence})(\text{Specificity})} =$$

$$\frac{FN}{FN + TN} = 1 - NPV$$

For any given combination of tests, some of which may be positive (subscript i) and some negative (subscript j), formulas 24 and 27 can be combined to calculate the probability of disease:

$$p(D+ \mid T_{ij}) = \frac{(\text{Prevalence})(\text{Sensitivity}_i)(1 - \text{Sensitivity}_j)}{\begin{array}{c}(\text{Prevalence})(\text{Sensitivity}_i)(1 - \text{Sensitivity}_j) + \\ (1 - \text{Prevalence})(1 - \text{Specificity}_i)(\text{Specificity}_j)\end{array}} \tag{28}$$

Consider three tests, *A* with a sensitivity of 80% and a specificity of 70%, *B* with a sensitivity of 60% and a specificity of 90%, and *C* with a sensitivity of 90% and a specificity of 50%. If tests *A* and *B* were positive and test *C* was negative and if the prevalence were 30%, the calculated disease probability would be as follows:

$$\frac{(0.3)(0.8)(0.6)(1 - 0.9)}{(0.3)(0.8)(0.6)(1 - 0.9) + (1 - 0.3)(1 - 0.7)(1 - 0.9)(0.5)} = 0.578$$

Table 8-16 compares the disease probabilities calculated with Bayes theorem to the disease probabilities obtained with a random number generator programmed to simulate an algorithmic analysis of the results of three totally independent tests. The sample included 700 studies, each consisting of the three tests, and for most of the eight combinations, this sample provided numbers adequate to estimate disease probability. The fact that the results of the two approaches were quite similar supports the validity of Bayes theorem.

Odds and likelihood ratios

Bayes theorem, as stated in equation 28, is somewhat forbidding in its complexity. The use of odds and likelihood ratios simplifies the process of estimating the posterior probability of disease given a combination of positive and negative test results.[9,14]

The odds of an event, *A*, occurring against its not occurring is defined as the probability of *A* divided by the probability of not *A:*

$$\frac{p(A)}{p(\text{not } A)} = \frac{p(A)}{1 - p(A)} \tag{29}$$

For example, the odds for throwing a six when one die of a pair of dice is rolled are 1/5 or 0.2, which is the probability of a six (1/6) divided by the probability of some other number from one to five appearing on the upper face of the cube (5/6).

Reversing the process, starting with the odds, we can calculate the probability of an event *A*, $p(A)$:

$$p(A) = \frac{\text{Odds}}{1 + \text{Odds}} \tag{30}$$

If the prevalence of disease in a population is known or can be estimated, the *prior odds* of disease can be calculated from equations 20, 21, and 29:

$$\text{Prior odds of disease} = \frac{p(D+)}{p(D-)} = \frac{p(D+)}{1 - p(D+)} = \frac{\text{Prevalence}}{1 - \text{Prevalence}} \tag{31}$$

The *likelihood ratio of a positive test (LR+)* is defined as the ratio of the conditional probability of obtaining a positive test result in a patient with disease, $p(T+ \mid D+)$, to that of obtaining a positive result in a patient without disease, $p(T+ \mid D-)$. From equations 22 and 23, it is evident that LR+ equals the sensitivity of the test divided by 1 minus its specificity:

$$LR+ = \frac{p(T+ \mid D+)}{p(T+ \mid D-)} = \frac{\text{Sensitivity}}{1 - \text{Specificity}} \tag{32}$$

Similarly, the *likelihood ratio of a negative test (LR−)* is defined as the ratio of the conditional probability of obtaining a negative test result in a patient with disease, $p(T- \mid D+)$, to that of obtaining a negative result in a patient without disease, $p(T- \mid D-)$. From equations 25 and 26, it is evident that LR− equals 1 minus the sensitivity of the test divided by its specificity:

$$LR- = \frac{p(T- \mid D+)}{p(T- \mid D-)} = \frac{1 - \text{Sensitivity}}{\text{Specificity}} \quad (33)$$

Because likelihood ratios depend only on sensitivity and specificity, they are independent of the prevalence of disease in the population being studied. By multiplying the prior odds of disease by the likelihood ratio (LR + or LR −), one can estimate the *posterior odds* of disease:

$$\text{Posterior odds of disease (Test+)} = \frac{p(D+)}{p(D-)} LR+ \quad (34)$$

which equals:

$$\frac{\text{Prevalence}}{1 - \text{Prevalence}} \times \frac{\text{Sensitivity}}{1 - \text{Specificity}}$$

$$\text{Posterior odds of disease (Test-)} = \frac{p(D+)}{p(D-)} LR- \quad (35)$$

which equals:

$$\frac{\text{Prevalence}}{1 - \text{Prevalence}} \times \frac{1 - \text{Sensitivity}}{\text{Specificity}}$$

By using equation 30, one can calculate the *posterior probability* of disease from the posterior odds of disease. Given a positive test result, the posterior probability of disease is:

$$p(D+ \mid T+) = \frac{\text{Posterior odds (T+)}}{1 + \text{Posterior odds (T+)}} \quad (36)$$

Given a negative test result, the corresponding posterior probability of disease is:

$$p(D+ \mid T-) = \frac{\text{Posterior odds (T-)}}{1 + \text{Posterior odds (T-)}} \quad (37)$$

Equations 36 and 37 give exactly the same result as one would obtain using Bayes theorem (equations 24 and 27, respectively). With Test A in Table 8-16 (which has a sensitivity of 0.9 and a specificity of 0.8) as an example, LR + = 0.9/0.2 = 4.5 (equation 32) and LR − = 0.1/0.8 = 0.125 (equation 33). Since the prevalence of disease in Table 8-16 is 0.3, the prior odds of disease are 0.3/0.7 = 0.429 (equation 31). Therefore the posterior odds for disease given a positive test result are 0.429 × 4.5 = 1.93 (equation 34), and the posterior probability of disease is 1.93 ÷ 2.93 = 0.659 (equation 36), which is identical to the PPV. Similarly, the posterior odds for disease given a negative test result is 0.429 × 0.125 = 0.054 (equation 35), and the posterior probability of disease is 0.054 ÷ 1.054 = 0.051, which is identical to 1 − NPV.

Although these calculations seem cumbersome when one is dealing with a single test, they greatly simplify the task of predicting disease probabilities when multiple tests are considered. This is because the posterior probability obtained after one test becomes the prior probability for the next test applied to the same population, and so on with each subsequent test. Thus the posterior odds for disease given any combination of tests having positive results (tests A, B, and so on) and negative results (tests R, S, and so

Table 8-17. Calculation of likelihood ratios for tests in Table 8-16

Test	Sensitivity	Specificity	LR +	LR −
A	0.9	0.8	0.9/0.2 = 4.5	0.1/0.8 = 0.125
B	0.8	0.8	0.8/0.2 = 4.0	0.2/0.8 = 0.250
C	0.7	0.8	0.7/0.2 = 3.5	0.3/0.8 = 0.375

on) are simply the product of the prior odds for disease and the LR + s for the positive tests and the LR − s for the negative tests:

$$\text{Posterior odds of disease (T+, T-)} = \quad (38)$$

$$\frac{p(D+)}{p(D-)} (LR_A+)(LR_B+)(LR_R-)(LR_S-)$$

Once the posterior odds of disease have been obtained from equation 38, it is quite easy to calculate the posterior probability of disease using equation 30. Mathematically, the combination of equations 30 and 38 is identical to the more complicated equation for Bayes theorem (equation 28).

The data in Table 8-16 may be used to illustrate the relative ease with which these equations can predict the probability of disease given a combination of positive and negative test results. The prior odds of disease (0.429) for a population with a disease prevalence of 0.3 were calculated above. The likelihood ratios of all three tests are listed in Table 8-17. When test A and test C are both positive and test B is negative, the LR + for test A is 4.5, the LR − for test B is 0.25, and the LR + for test C is 3.5. The posterior odds for disease with this combination of test results is (equation 38):

$$\text{Posterior odds (A+, B-, C+)} = 0.429 \times 4.5 \times 0.25 \times 3.5 = 1.69$$

The posterior probability of disease is (equation 30):

$$\text{Posterior probability of disease} = 1.69 \div (1 + 1.69) = 0.628$$

which is identical to the result obtained using Bayes theorem (Table 8-16, last column, third row). Other combinations can be dealt with in a similar manner.

Advantages and limitations of Bayes theorem

The primary advantage of the Bayes approach or the use of odds and likelihood ratios is that it allows prediction of disease probability for any combination of tests based on knowledge of sensitivity, specificity, and estimated prevalence (prior probability) even when the number of studies previously performed by the laboratory is insufficient to use the algorithmic approach. Moreover, in the event that all three tests could not be performed on a given patient, the Bayes approach (or the use of odds and likelihood ratios) would still be applicable. The disadvantage of Bayes theorem—and for that matter, any of the previously discussed schemes for using combinations of tests—is that it is valid only when the tests are totally independent. Obviously, if two tests were similar (as in Fig. 8-11), the results would be fallacious. A further disadvantage is that it presupposes a reasonably accurate estimate of disease prevalence, which varies from time to time in the same laboratory and from one population to the next.

In reality, most tests are not entirely independent. For example, even though the methodologies of toe systolic pressure and pulse volume measurements differ, both depend on arterial perfusion pressure and the contour of the pressure waveform. Furthermore, independence is sacrificed when the result of one test is allowed to influence the reading of another. This is especially likely to happen when both tests are interpreted by the same individual. Consequently, most combinations of tests will fall somewhere between the two extremes of providing little or no benefit (all tests measuring the same parameter, as in Fig. 8-12) and providing maximal benefit (all tests independent, as in Fig. 8-13). This generalization applies to all methods used to combine test results.

Most laboratories using multiple-test batteries probably do not adhere to a strict protocol based on the number of positive or negative tests. The natural tendency of the interpreter is to weigh—either consciously or unconsciously—a personal perception of the relative merits of each test before arriving at a conclusion. No matter how accurate the conclusions, this approach is not particularly satisfying from a scientific viewpoint.

In summary, the use of multiple tests is not without its price. The cost for improving the accuracy of one parameter is borne by the loss of accuracy of another or by an increased incidence of uninterpretable studies. Whether the additional time and expense are justified depends on the goals of the investigator and the demonstration by objective clinical studies that the battery of tests does in fact enhance overall accuracy. Because the point of diminishing returns is rapidly reached as new tests are added, it is usually sufficient to use two, possibly three, but rarely four well-established, independently read tests based on different physiologic principles.

APPLICATION

In general, very sensitive tests (or batteries of tests, such as option 2) should be selected when the goal is to rule out disease. As indicated in Fig. 8-3, the influence of sensitivity on the NPV far outweighs that of specificity. On the other hand, when confirmation of the presence of disease becomes the primary goal, a very specific test (or battery of tests, such as option 3) should be used. In other words, PPV is more dependent on specificity than it is on sensitivity (Fig. 8-2). Thus sensitive tests are used to narrow the range of diagnostic hypotheses, and specific tests are used to increase the level of diagnostic confidence when there is a strong clinical suspicion that a certain disease is present. No test can establish the presence or absence of disease with absolute certainty. The purpose of all noninvasive tests is to reduce the range of uncertainty.

As a rule, tests are most helpful when the prior (pretest) probability of disease is in the 50% range and least helpful when the likelihood of disease is either very low or very high. The figures in Table 8-18 illustrate this point. For example, suppose test B has a sensitivity of 90% and a specificity of 70% and the prior probability of disease was considered to be very small (estimated prevalence = 0.05); the PPV or posterior (posttest) probability of disease given a positive test result (equation 24) would increase to 0.14, which represents a change of only $+0.09$ ($+9\%$) from the prior probability (PPV − Prevalence). Similarly, if the results of test B were negative (equation 27), the posterior probability of disease being present (1-NPV) would diminish to 0.01, a change of only -0.04 (-4%). In other words,

Table 8-18. Effect of prevalence on posterior probability of disease

Test	Sensitivity	Specificity	Prior probability of disease — Prevalence	Posterior probability of disease (positive test) PPV	Posterior probability of disease (positive test) PPV − Prevalence	Posterior probability of disease (negative test) 1 − NPV	Posterior probability of disease (negative test) (1 − NPV) − Prevalence
A	0.70	0.90	0.05	0.27	+0.22	0.02	−0.03
			0.40	0.82	+0.42	0.18	−0.22
			0.70	0.94	+0.24	0.44	−0.26
			0.90	0.98	+0.08	0.75	−0.15
B	0.90	0.70	0.05	0.14	+0.09	0.01	−0.04
			0.40	0.67	+0.27	0.09	−0.31
			0.70	0.88	+0.18	0.25	−0.45
			0.90	0.96	+0.06	0.56	−0.34
C	0.90	0.90	0.05	0.32	+0.27	0.01	−0.04
			0.40	0.86	+0.46	0.07	−0.33
			0.70	0.96	+0.26	0.21	−0.49
			0.90	0.99	+0.09	0.50	−0.40

applying test *B* to a population in which the prevalence of disease is suspected to be very low would not materially affect the likelihood that the individual patient does or does not have the disease. Even if the results were positive, the odds are still 6 to 1 against the disease being present (0.86:0.14).

At the other extreme, applying test *A* with a sensitivity of 70% and a specificity of 90% to a population with a high likelihood of disease (90%) would increase the likelihood by only 8% if the test were positive and would decrease the likelihood by a modest 15% if the test were negative. Even with a negative test, the odds are still 3 to 1 that the patient has the disease (0.75:0.25). Consequently, one would be reluctant to discard the diagnosis based on a negative test result.

If the prior probability were 70% (which approximates the probability that a patient referred to the laboratory with a clinical diagnosis of transient ischemic attack [TIA] will have a lesion in the appropriate carotid artery) and test *C*, with a sensitivity and specificity of 90%, were applied, the posterior probability given a positive result would rise to 0.96—virtually confirming the presence of disease. A negative result would lower the probability of disease significantly to 0.21, stimulating one to consider other diagnoses. In other words, with a negative result the odds against the patient having the disease rise from 0.4:1 to 3.8:1. Of course, the decision to discard a diagnosis will depend not only on the posterior probability of disease but also on one's clinical judgment regarding the potential harm that would ensue if vital treatment were withheld. Therefore if the patient had had a classic TIA, most clinicians would still pursue the diagnosis of carotid disease despite a negative test result. On the other hand, the decision to accept a positive diagnosis will depend on the potential harm that would ensue from a FP diagnosis.

Table 8-18 further confirms what has been mentioned about the relative value of sensitivity and specificity for diagnosing or ruling out disease. A positive result with a very specific test, such as test *A* or *C*, will greatly increase the posterior probability of disease in the middle ranges of

prevalence; whereas a negative result with a very sensitive test, such as test *B* or *C*, will significantly reduce the likelihood that disease is present.

After the first test (or series of tests) has been performed, the clinician may then decide whether further tests are necessary. For the second test, the posterior probability following the first test now becomes the prior probability (estimated prevalence) for the second test. Remembering this fact may influence the decision to select a highly sensitive or highly specific test. The ultimate results of any series of tests follow the precepts of Bayes theorem.

Interpretation of screening tests must be done cautiously. For a population in which the true prevalence of disease is only 5% and a highly sensitive (90%) and specific (90%) test is used to assess the prevalence of disease, the investigator may conclude that the prevalence is much higher, 14% (Table 18-19). This, in fact, was the conclusion of a study in which noninvasive tests with this degree of accuracy were used to ascertain the prevalence of >75% stenosis of the internal carotid artery in a series of patients undergoing cardiovascular and peripheral vascular surgery. Although the use of the test does define two populations—one with a greater likelihood of having the disease than the other—any inferences regarding the true prevalence of disease are likely to be quite inaccurate.

REFERENCES

1. Beyer WH, ed: *Handbook of tables for probability and statistics*, ed 2, Boca Raton, Fla, 1968, CRC Press.
2. Cohen J: A coefficient of agreement for nominal scales, *Educ Psychol Measures* 20:37, 1960.
3. Cohen J: Weighted kappa: nominal scale agreement with provision for scaled disagreement or partial credit, *Psychol Bull* 70:213, 1968.
4. Colton T: *Statistics in medicine*, Boston, 1974, Little, Brown.
5. Griner PF et al: Selection and interpretation of diagnostic tests and procedures: principles and application, *Ann Intern Med* 94:553, 1981.
6. Hall GH: The clinical applications of Bayes' theorem, *Lancet* 2:555, 1967.
7. Haynes RB: Interpretation of diagnostic data. 2. How to do it with a simple table (part A), *Can Med Assoc J* 129:559, 1983.
8. Haynes RB: Interpretation of diagnostic data. 3. How to do it with a simple table (part B), *Can Med Assoc J* 129:705, 1983.
9. Ingelfinger JA et al: *Biostatistics in clinical medicine*, New York, 1983, Macmillan.
10. Lusted LB: *Introduction to medical decision making*, Springfield, Ill, 1968, Charles C Thomas.
11. McNeil BJ, Keeler E, Adelstein SJ: Primer on certain elements of medical decision making, *N Engl J Med* 293:211, 1975.
12. Metz CE: Basic principles of ROC analysis, *Semin Nucl Med* 8:283, 1978.
13. Sackett DL: Interpretation of diagnostic data. 1. How to do it with pictures, *Can Med Assoc J* 129:429, 1983.
14. Sackett DL: Interpretation of diagnostic data. 5. How to do it with simple maths, *Can Med Assoc J* 129:947, 1983.
15. Sumner DS: *Noninvasive investigation of the arterial supply to the brain and eye*. In Warlow C, Morris PJ, eds: *Transient ischemic attack*, New York, 1982, Marcel Dekker.
16. Trout KS: Interpretation of diagnostic data. 6. How to do it with more complex maths, *Can Med Assoc J* 129:1093, 1983.
17. Tugwell PX: Interpretation of diagnostic data. 4. How to do it with a more complex table, *Can Med Assoc J* 129:832, 1983.
18. Vecchio TJ: Predictive value of a single diagnostic test in unselected populations, *N Engl J Med* 274:1171, 1966.

Table 8-19. Apparent prevalence compared with true prevalence of disease

Noninvasive test results	True distribution		Noninvasive test total
	Negative	**Positive**	
Negative	855	5	860
Positive	95	45	140
TRUE TOTAL	950	50	1000

Apparent prevalence, 14%; true prevalence, 5%.

PART TWO

FUNDAMENTALS OF MEASUREMENT
AND CURRENT INSTRUMENTATION

CHAPTER 9

Doppler ultrasonic techniques in vascular disease

D. EUGENE STRANDNESS, JR.

Since publication of the third edition of this book, there has been remarkable progress in the development and application of Doppler methods to the study of vascular disease. Because of this, Doppler, combined with imaging and modern signal processing, will certainly remain the principal method for the study of vascular diseases.[3,4,7,15] Although the technology has become much more sophisticated, there is still a place for the simplest of all Doppler devices—the hand-held units that provide only an audible output.[19,20]

PHYSICAL PRINCIPLES

The basis for the use of Doppler devices is the detection of the frequency shifts that occur when ultrasound encounters moving blood.[11,16] The frequency shift can be amplified to drive a loudspeaker, providing an audible output of the blood flow velocity, or processed by more sophisticated signal methods, such as fast Fourier transform, displaying all the required information in the backscattered Doppler signal.

When ultrasound encounters moving blood, its effect on the transmitted frequency is expressed by the following formula:

$$\Delta F = \frac{2F_0 \times V \times \cos\theta}{C} \qquad (1)$$

where:

F = Frequency shift

2 = Round trip of the ultrasound

C/F_0 = Wavelength of ultrasound

$V \cos\theta$ = Closing speed between the erythrocytes and the Doppler probe

Each factor should be reviewed to understand its application to the study of vascular diseases. For example, doubling the frequency of interrogation (F_0) will double the frequency shift. The particular F_0 that is chosen depends on the intended application. The more superficial vessels can be reached with the higher frequencies (5 to 10 MHz), whereas for deeper vessels such as in the abdomen, lower levels are needed (2 to 5 MHz). For most simple applications such as measurement of systolic blood pressures in the limbs, frequencies in the range of 5 to 10 MHz are often used. This is also true if the device is used to audibly evaluate the type of flow patterns that occur when the arterial and venous system is affected by disease.

Another important factor is the relationship between the frequency of interrogation and its attenuation (power) in tissue. For example, the attenuation is twice as great with a 10 MHz system as it is with a 5 MHz system. However, the red cells—which are the principal reflectors—tend to scatter the higher frequencies better than the lower frequencies. This effect tends to minimize the loss of power that occurs when the higher frequencies are used.

The velocity of ultrasound in tissue determines the travel time between the transducer and the moving red blood cells. With a continuous wave (CV) system the transit time to the vessel of interest is not a concern. Everything in the path of the sound beam is insonated, making it impossible to determine the site or sites from which the flow is being detected. Until the development of pulsed Doppler the source of the backscattered signal could not be identified with certainty. When the sound is transmitted in bursts (pulses), however, the site from which flow is being detected can be determined because the speed of sound in tissue is known. When Doppler is used in this way, an echo must be received for sampling before the next pulse is transmitted, thus limiting the rate at which pulses can be transmitted. For pulsed Doppler, the following relationships are important:

$$\text{PRF (maximum)} = C/2d \qquad (2)$$

where PRF is pulse repetition frequency, C is velocity of sound in tissue, and d is the distance to the reflector.

When the expected peak Doppler frequency shift is greater than twice the PRF, the frequency shift of the detected signal will be lower than expected. The highest frequency shift that can be generated is referred to as the *Nyquist frequency*. For example, if the maximum PRF is 10 kHz, the highest Doppler shift that can be recorded is 5 kHz. Frequencies above this level will not be displayed as expected and will appear as an aliased signal (Fig. 9-1).

The first Doppler method widely used was the zero-crossing detector, which was simple and cheap and provided an analogue display of forward-reverse flow components of arterial and venous velocity patterns (Fig. 9-2).[8,10] However, the zero-crossing detector had several problems.[14] An excellent signal-to-noise ratio was needed for proper functioning. In addition, the output of the backscattered signal

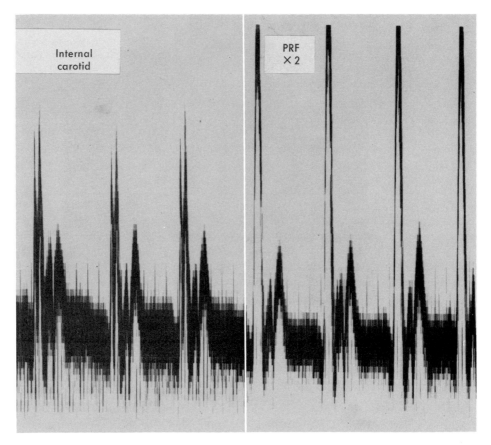

Fig. 9-1. The problem of sharing PRF of the pulsed Doppler with the B-mode system. Left is a velocity spectrum from a normal internal carotid artery when the PRF is shared. Aliasing is seen as the fold-over of the peak velocity information, which is eliminated when the B-mode system is shut off and the PRF is doubled. Now the entire range of the peak systolic velocity is shown.

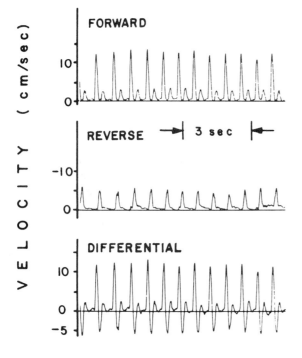

Fig. 9-2. The type of velocity signal that can be recorded when a CW directional Doppler system is used with a zero-crossing detector. The presentation of the Doppler information can be as a differential output with the forward and reverse flow information shown on separate channels. The more conventional method is to display the information in a differential mode *(bottom)*. (From Nippa JH, et al: Phase rotation for separating forward and reverse flow blood velocity signals, *IEEE Trans Ultrasonics* SU-22:340, 1975.)

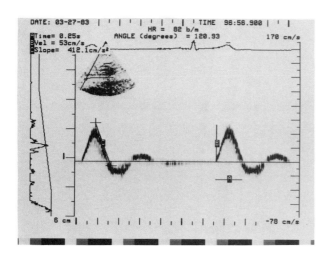

Fig. 9-3. A real-time Doppler spectrum obtained from a peripheral artery and analyzed by an FFT spectrum analyzer. The forward-reverse flow components are displayed. Note that the window beneath the peak systolic peak is clean (no spectral broadening). (From Strandness DE Jr: *Duplex scanning in vascular disorders,* New York, 1990, Raven Press.)

was amplitude dependent and often failed to record high-frequency, low-amplitude signals. In addition, when both an artery and a vein were insonated by a CW Doppler, the flow velocity signals would be mixed together. When this occurred, the recorded waveform would be unintelligible. The disadvantages of the CW Doppler could be avoided by the use of a pulsed system where specific site sampling could be achieved.[1,2]

The best signal-processing method that has been developed is fast Fourier transform spectral analysis. With this method, frequency and intensity of the backscattered signal can be accurately displayed. In addition to velocity data, the temporal relationships of the frequency shifts (special broadening) can also be seen (Fig. 9-3).[3,13,15]

Several aspects of the backscattered Doppler signal are useful. On the arterial side of the circulation, the major components of the velocity signal that can be used for diagnostic purposes include the following:

1. As an artery becomes narrowed, the peak velocity in the narrowest segment of the artery increases.[3,4] If the sampling is done at the same site of narrowing during follow-up visits, the rate of disease progression can be calculated. The end-diastolic velocity reflects the resistance of the vascular bed being supplied by the artery. This can be illustrated by noting the flow patterns in arteries supplying tissues of varying resistance. Low-resistance vascular beds are the brain, liver, and kidneys.[21] The end-diastolic velocity in the arteries supplying these organs is normally well above 0. Flow reversal should not be seen at any time during the pulse cycle. The end-diastolic velocity can also reflect the degree of narrowing. For example, for stenoses of the internal carotid artery that are 80% to 99%, using only the peak systolic velocity as an index of the degree of narrowing is dif-

ficult.[15] The end-diastolic velocity in the carotid artery will not only reflect the degree of narrowing but is also predictive of future clinical events, such as transient ischemic attacks, strokes, and occlusion of the internal carotid artery. For example, if the end-diastolic velocity exceeds 145 cm/sec, this is a useful cut-off point to recognize a stenosis that now exceeds 80% in terms of its reduction in diameter. When this degree of stenosis increases, the end-diastolic velocity will increase to even higher levels.

In other vascular beds, the resistance to flow depends on the metabolic activity of the tissue at the time the measurements are made.[18] Two examples of this are in the small intestine and the limbs. In the small bowel during fasting, there is often a brief period of reverse blood flow in late systole.[9] The end-diastolic velocity is also at or near 0. This changes dramatically after eating. The reverse flow component is lost, and there is a large increase in peak systolic and end-diastolic velocity.

In the normal lower limb, the resting arterial velocity patterns are triphasic, with forward and reverse flow and a second smaller forward flow component in late diastole.[3,4] This can be changed by exercise in which marked vasodilatation and a fall in vascular resistance occur. This results in a loss of the reverse flow component and an increase in the end-diastolic velocity to above the 0 flow level.

For all arterial beds that have a hemodynamically significant stenosis or an occlusion of the inflow vessel, the velocity patterns distal to the area of involvement will become monophasic, with a reduction in the peak systolic velocity and loss of reverse flow. The end-diastolic velocity, however, will be higher than normal as the resistance to flow is reduced to maintain blood flow to the limb in a normal range. This adaptation by the collateral circulation is very efficient.

2. In the normal arterial system, flow tends to both accelerate and decelerate within a fairly narrow range depending on the particular flow laminae that are being examined. If a pulsed Doppler is used to document flow velocity patterns, patterns recorded from the center of the artery will show a narrow bandwidth.[12] This will leave a clear window (absence of data) beneath the systolic peak; however, if a CW Doppler is used, the clear systolic window will be obliterated. Insonation of the entire artery will lead to the recording of all velocities. Filling of the systolic window is referred to as *spectral broadening.* Spectral broadening can be seen even with a pulsed system if the sample volume is placed near the wall of the artery. In this case the velocity gradients are steep, and a spectral display of the signal will reflect the broad band of frequencies (Fig. 9-4).

3. In the posterolateral aspect of the carotid bulb, complex flow patterns involve forward and reverse flow components during each pulse cycle (Fig. 9-5). This is an important phenomenon, since the development of a

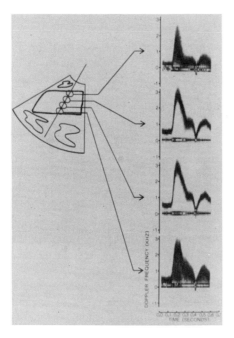

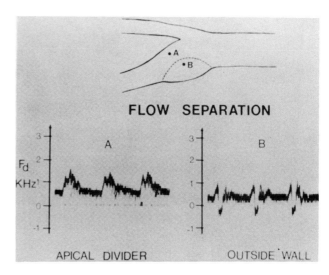

Fig. 9-4. When the sample volume of the pulsed Doppler is placed near the wall of the common carotid artery, the systolic window is filled in (spectral broadening). However, when the sample volume is placed in the center of the artery, the systolic window is clean. If a CW Doppler system were used, the spectrum would be as seen when the samples with the pulsed Doppler were placed against either the near or far wall. (From Strandness DE Jr: *Duplex scanning in vascular disorders,* New York, 1990, Raven Press.)

Fig. 9-5. The sample volume of the pulsed Doppler is moved from the anterior wall of the carotid bulb to the posterolateral wall. As the posterior wall region is encountered, the flow is no longer totally antegrade but has a to and fro motion. This is boundary layer separation. (From Strandness DE Jr: *Duplex scanning in vascular disorders,* New York, 1990, Raven Press.)

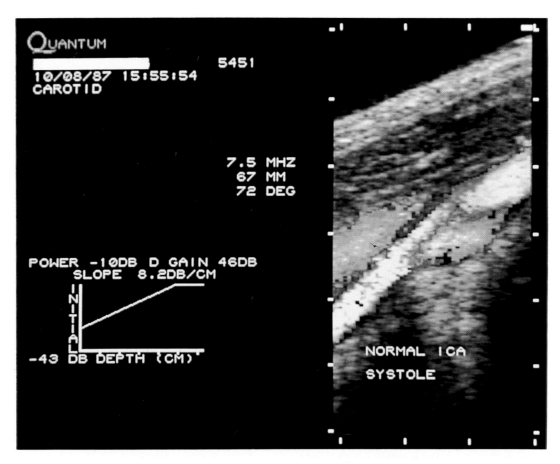

Fig. 9-6. The boundary layer separation shown in Fig. 9-5 can be easily displayed by using color Doppler. The reverse flow component is shown in *blue* during peak systole. (From Strandness DE Jr: *Duplex scanning in vascular disorders,* New York, 1990, Raven Press.)

plaque that fills the bulb will eliminate this from occurring. The normal flow separation noted in this region is easily demonstrated by using color Doppler flow systems (Fig. 9-6).[17] If boundary layer separation is noted in the bulb, atherosclerosis is ruled out in this important arterial segment. However, boundary layer separation can also be seen distal to a plaque.

4. Doppler data can also provide insight into the status of the arterial circulation. With CW Doppler flow must be sampled from areas where the site of insonation is certain, which is where arteries are large; data obtained will provide information about the status of the arterial inflow. The sites where CW Doppler can be used include the common femoral artery, the popliteal artery, and the tibial arteries at the ankle. At these locations, the companion veins can be used as landmarks to identify the adjacent artery. With CW Doppler the angle of incidence of the sound beam with the artery is always unknown. A parameter that is independent of the angle of the sound beam must be used to numerically represent the velocity signal. The indices that have been developed include the pulsatility index (PI) and the Laplace transform damping (LTD) factor (see Chapters 16, 33, and 56). These parameters do not depend on the quantitation of the velocity patterns recorded at the site of study. However, these indirect and "blind" methods have been replaced by the use of duplex scanning. With this method, all arteries from the level of the abdominal aorta to tibial arteries at the level of the ankle can be directly interrogated.[7] It is also possible to examine the arteries with data relative to the angle of insonation. Peripheral arteries can be screened for stenoses and occlusions with a level of accuracy comparable to that found with arteriography.

On the venous side of the circulation the use of velocity data is equally important in documenting the presence of diseases. The pertinent changes in the velocity of flow are as follows:

1. Normally, the velocity of flow in the major proximal veins (popliteal to inferior vena cava) of the lower limb is phasic with respiration. In these large veins, flow will go to 0 during inspiration.[20] This occurs because as the diaphragm descends, the intraabdominal pressure increases, exceeding that in the inferior vena cava. This results in transient cessation of flow from the lower limbs. The reverse occurs with expiration (Fig. 9-7).

2. For veins distal to the knee (toward the foot), the velocity of venous flow is often low and affected by the ambient conditions at the time the study is performed. If the examination room is cool or there is a draft, vasoconstriction often occurs, reducing flow to the skin where it may not be detectable with the CW Doppler system. These units often have a wall filter to remove the frequency shift that occurs with motion of the arterial wall. If venous flow cannot be detected at the level of the ankle, it may be necessary to compress the foot and augment venous flow above this threshold level.

3. In the upper extremity, the intrathoracic pressure decreases during inspiration, which tends to augment venous flow during this phase of the respiratory cycle.

4. When acute venous obstruction is present, there is no flow from the site of occlusion, but the velocity patterns below (toward the foot) lose their phasic component and become continuous.[4,20] This occurs because venous blood flow is diverted through collateral pathways, many of which are not subject to the normal pressure changes that take place with each respiratory cycle. As venous collaterals develop and/or the thrombus begins to lyse, the venous flow patterns may return to a normal state.

5. In chronic venous disease secondary to primary varicose veins or the postthrombotic syndrome, the venous valves no longer function, leading to the development of reverse flow whenever a reverse pressure gradient is created. This occurs with activities such as coughing, sneezing, and the activation of the muscle pump and can be documented by noting the reversal of flow that occurs during maneuvers providing a reversal of the normal pressure gradient. In practice, the maneuver most often used is a Valsalva maneuver. Another simple method for reversing

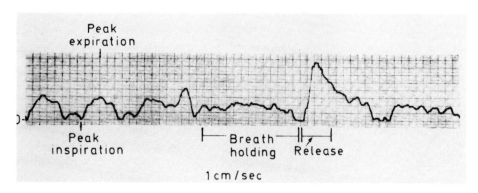

Fig. 9-7. The velocity patterns seen in a normal subject recorded from the common femoral vein. With the patient in a horizontal position, flow will diminish with inspiration. (From Yao JST, Gourmos C, Hobbs JT: Detection of proximal vein thrombosis by Doppler ultrasound flow-detection method, *Lancet* 1:1, 1972.)

the normal antegrade pressure gradient is to forcibly compress the limb proximal (toward the heart) to the transducer. However, neither maneuver always generates sufficient pressures to induce reverse flow at a velocity that is sufficient to result in valve closure.[22]

Testing for venous valvular incompetence is best done with the patient in the upright position.[22] In this position, the veins are maximally dilated as they are during most of the day. With exercise, muscle contraction propels blood toward the heart and the foot only if the valves are incompetent. With muscular relaxation, the empty veins will refill by two mechanisms. The first is by antegrade flow alone if the valves in the area are competent; if not, the veins may also refill secondary to reflux.

Pneumatic cuffs that can be rapidly inflated and deflated are used to simulate normal activity. The cuffs are placed on the thigh, upper and lower calf, ankle, and foot. For each cuff position, the ultrasonic transducer is placed distal to the cuff (less than 5 cm). The pressure used to inflate the cuffs for each limb segment is comparable to that exerted by the force of gravity for the distance from the right heart. When the cuff is rapidly deflated, the veins beneath the cuff can be filled by antegrade or retrograde flow through incompetent venous valves. This method of testing for reflux is done with a duplex scanner. The reverse flow that develops secondary to valvular incompetence is easily and immediately detected. Reflux in both the superficial and deep veins can be tested by using cuffs at different levels of the limb.

COLOR DOPPLER

With the development of ultrasonic duplex scanning, it became possible to take advantage of both imaging and pulsed Doppler. The B-mode image provides the anatomy with the pulsed Doppler, permitting selective sampling of the flow velocity from any point in the scan plane. This method is valuable for examining blood flow wherever a vessel can be imaged. However, for some areas the "black and white" image alone requires considerable skill on the part of the technologist to assess the anatomy of the blood vessels in the region. For example, anatomic variants (coils and kinks) are common in the neck. It can be challenging for ultrasound technologists to unravel these pathways unless they have considerable skill and experience (Fig. 9-8).

The development of color Doppler systems is a major technologic advance.[23] Because this method can be performed in real-time, the local anatomy and the flow patterns for each visualized vascular segment can be examined. In general, red is used for the arterial system and blue for the venous system, resulting in a picture similar to an arteriogram (Fig. 9-9).

Several analytic schemes have been devised to present the color changes. The changes in velocity are usually represented by changes in the hue of the color. For example, lighter shades of red are noted with increasing velocities on the arterial side of the circulation. Attempts have been made

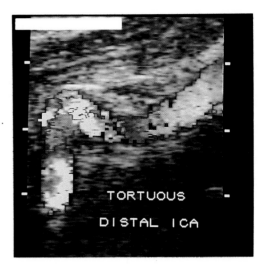

Fig. 9-8. The tortuous carotid artery can easily be displayed with color Doppler. Although the hue and color change throughout this artery, the velocity is not changing. The angle of the incident sound beam is changing as the flow vectors change their direction. (From Strandness DE Jr: *Duplex scanning in vascular disorders,* New York, 1990, Raven Press.)

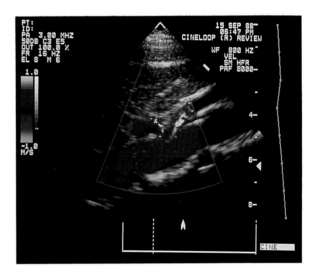

Fig. 9-9. By using color it is often easy to demonstrate the origin and direction of flow in arteries such as the celiac and superior mesenteric arteries. (From Strandness DE Jr: *Duplex scanning in vascular disorders,* New York, 1990, Raven Press.)

to use this information to quantitatively document the degree of stenosis. However, the following must be noted:

1. The angle of incidence with the artery must be known. If the angle of incidence is not constant, the changes seen in the color are not a reflection of a change in velocity. This common problem appears whenever the artery being studied is not parallel to the skin or the face of the transducer.
2. Although aliasing is readily detected with a spectral display whenever the Nyquist limit is exceeded, it may be

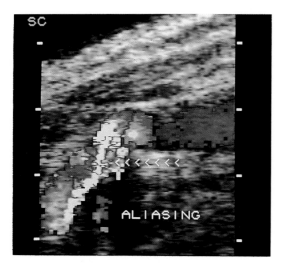

Fig. 9-10. Aliasing can also occur with color Doppler. Blue is seen in the area of narrowing. This is not actual reverse flow but is caused by aliasing. (From Strandness DE Jr: *Duplex scanning in vascular disorders,* New York, 1990, Raven Press.)

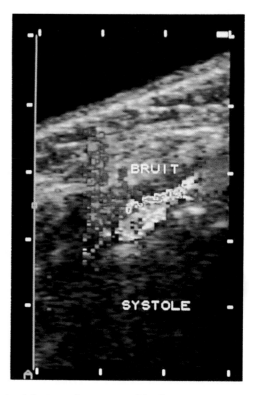

Fig. 9-11. A bruit can be recognized by the appearance of speckles of color outside the artery just beyond an area of stenosis. (From Strandness DE Jr: *Duplex scanning in vascular disorders,* New York, 1990, Raven Press.)

misleading when it occurs with color Doppler systems (Fig. 9-10).

3. Most systems provide frequency and velocity data from the color display alone, but this information must not be used to quantitatively assess the velocity at the point of interest. The single sample volume of the pulsed Doppler must be used to obtain this information.[6] Otherwise, values for the peak systolic and mean velocity will be underestimated.

The flow data can be advantageous if the following are observed:

1. Color Doppler should be used as a "pathfinder." Color makes recognition of the regional anatomy easier and quicker, particularly for the carotid artery and in the abdomen where localization of the origin of the renal and mesenteric vessels may be difficult.
2. In areas where the arteries follow a relatively straight course, the color changes that signify an increase in velocity are quite reliable. In the femoral, popliteal, and tibioperoneal arteries, the color will immediately demonstrate vessel patency as well as its location. Hemodynamically significant stenoses (more than 50% diameter reduction) can be recognized by the appearance of poststenotic turbulence and a bruit in the tissues adjacent to the diseased segment. Because turbulence produces random velocity vectors of differing magnitude, the color changes represent a mixture of colors and hues. Bruits are produced by vibration of the arterial wall at and distal to the stenosis. Since this produces tissue motion, it will produce a color change in the tissues outside the artery (Fig. 9-11).
3. On the venous side of the circulation, color Doppler assists in identifying the major veins of interest to doc-

ument the presence of occlusive and nonocclusive thrombi.

4. One of the most difficult areas to examine is below the knee. The veins are usually paired, and conventional black and white scanning does not easily identify them. Color greatly simplifies this task, making the interrogation of this area quicker and more reliable.

MEASUREMENT OF VOLUME FLOW

Volume flow is the product of mean velocity times the cross-sectional area. Ultrasound appears ideal for measuring volume flow because dimensions (diameter) and the mean velocity of the backscattered Doppler signal can be obtained. However, small errors in the estimation of diameter produce major errors in the volume flow calculation. In addition, information concerning the velocity profile at the site of volume flow measurement is necessary to be certain of the mean velocity calculation—velocity vectors are not always parallel to the arterial wall.[12] The reverse flow component must also be considered.

A single measurement of volume flow is rarely of clinical value. A wide range of normal values exists, and the total volume flow to an organ may be within a normal range even when rather extensive disease is present. However, changes or trends may be valuable in some situations.

REFERENCES

1. Baker DW: Pulsed ultrasonic Doppler blood flow sensing, *IEEE Trans Biomed Engn* 17:170, 1970.
2. Barber FE et al: Ultrasonic duplex echo Doppler scanner, *IEEE Trans Biomed Engn* 21:109, 1974.
3. Jager KA et al: *Noninvasive assessment of lower extremity ischemia.* In Bergan JJ and Yao JST, eds: *Evaluation and treatment of upper and lower extremity circulatory disorders,* New York, 1983, Grune & Stratton.
4. Jager KA et al: Noninvasive mapping of lower limb arterial lesions, *Ultrasound Med Biol* 11:515, 1985.
5. Killewich LA et al: Diagnosis of deep venous thrombosis: a prospective study comparing duplex scanning to contrast venography, *Circulation* 79:810, 1989.
6. Knox RA et al: Empirical findings relating sample volume size to diagnostic accuracy in pulsed Doppler cerebrovascular studies, *J Clin Ultrasound* 10:56, 1982.
7. Kohler TA et al: Duplex scanning for diagnosis of aortoiliac and femoropopliteal disease: a prospective study, *Circulation* 76:1074, 1987.
8. McLeod FD Jr: Progress report, directional Doppler blood flowmeter, NRG 33-010-074, May 1969, Cornell University.
9. Moneta GL et al: Duplex ultrasound measurement of postprandial intestinal blood flow: effect of meal composition, *Gastroenterology* 95:1294, 1988.
10. Nippa JH et al: Phase rotation for separating forward and reverse blood velocity signals, *IEEE Trans Sonic Ultrasonics* 22:340, 1975.
11. Phillips DJ et al: Detection of peripheral vascular disease using the duplex scanner III, *Ultrasound Med Biol* 6:205, 1980.
12. Phillips DJ et al: Flow velocity patterns in the carotid bifurcation of young, presumed normal subjects, *Ultrasound Med Biol* 9:33, 1983.
13. Phillips DJ et al: Should results of ultrasound Doppler studies be reported in units of frequency or velocity? *Ultrasound Med Biol* 15:205, 1989.
14. Reneman RS et al: In vivo comparison of electromagnetic and Doppler flowmeters with special attention to the processing of the analogue Doppler signal, *Cardiovasc Res* 7:557, 1973.
15. Roederer GO et al: *Comprehensive noninvasive evaluation of extracranial cerebrovascular disease.* In Hershey RB, Barnes RW, Sumner DS, eds: *Noninvasive diagnosis of vascular disease,* Pasadena, Calif, 1984, Appleton Davies.
16. Satomura S: Study of flow patterns in peripheral arteries by ultrasonics, *J Acoust Soc Jpn* 15:151, 1959.
17. Strandness DE Jr: *Color.* In *Duplex scanning in vascular disorders,* New York, 1990, Raven Press.
18. Strandness DE Jr, Sumner DS: *Measurement of blood flow.* In *Hemodynamics for surgeons,* New York, 1975, Grune & Stratton.
19. Strandness DE Jr et al: Ultrasonic flow detection: a useful technique in the evaluation of peripheral vascular disease, *Am J Surg* 113:311, 1967.
20. Sumner DS et al: The ultrasonic velocity detector in a clinical study of venous disease, *Arch Surg* 37:75, 1968.
21. Taylor DC et al: Duplex ultrasound in the diagnosis of renal artery stenosis: a prospective study, *J Vasc Surg* 7:363, 1988.
22. van Bemmelen PS et al: Quantitative segmental evaluation of venous valvular reflux with ultrasonic duplex scanning, *J Vasc Surg* 10:425, 1989.
23. Zierler RE et al: Noninvasive assessment of normal carotid bifurcation hemodynamics with color-flow ultrasound imaging, *Ultrasound Med Biol* 13:471, 1987.

CHAPTER 10

Ultrasound bioeffects and safety

CHRISTOPHER R. B. MERRITT

As a diagnostic procedure, ultrasound has established an enviable safety record. The most recent bioeffects statement of the American Institute of Ultrasound in Medicine (AIUM) (box) has concluded that "No confirmed biological effects on patients or instrument operators caused by exposure at intensities typical of present diagnostic ultrasound instruments have ever been reported."[3] In part because of the excellent risk-to-benefit performance reflected in this statement, ultrasound is now the most rapidly growing of all imaging modalities. This growth reflects an increasing acceptance of the clinical value of ultrasound with the dissemination of ultrasound units into the hands of new users, as well as the introduction of new applications such as Doppler. Over 70,000 ultrasound units are currently in operation worldwide, performing up to 90 million examinations each year. Presently, ultrasound equipment sales are growing at an annual rate of 20%, and continued growth at this rate is projected for the next 3 years.

Although experience with ultrasound has shown no hazards, the AIUM bioeffects statement cautions that biologic effects might be identified in the future and notes that "the benefits to patients of prudent use of diagnostic ultrasound outweigh the risk, if any, that may be present." Although reassuring, this statement raises several issues that users of diagnostic ultrasound must consider as knowledge of ultrasound bioeffects increases and new applications of ultrasound are introduced into routine clinical practice. All physicians accept as a fundamental obligation the duty to practice in a way that protects their patients from unnecessary harm. Thus, in interacting with the patient, the physician should attempt to provide maximal benefit with minimal risk. Despite the importance that ultrasound has assumed in medical imaging, these principles have received less attention than they deserve, largely because of the presumed safety of ultrasound at typical diagnostic levels. The continued lack of evidence of harm from diagnostic levels of ultrasound does not remove the obligation of the physician

to consider issues of risk and benefit in performing diagnostic ultrasound examinations and to take all proper measures to ensure maximal benefit with minimal risk. The widespread and growing use of ultrasound makes discussion of safety and benefit both important and timely, particularly when many of the new users of ultrasound are likely to have little or no formal training in sonology.[14]

Most new ultrasound devices will soon be required to display indications of acoustic output related to known bioeffects mechanisms.[2] With this output display, users of ultrasound will be able to implement the common sense principle of as low as reasonably achievable (ALARA).[11] Under this principle, users are encouraged to keep exposure to levels that are as low as reasonably achievable in keeping with diagnostic objectives and economic and social factors. The implementation of ALARA is an important element in the prudent use encouraged by the AIUM safety statement. A few key principles must be understood for the user to apply the information provided in the output display. This chapter will review current concepts regarding the mechanisms by which bioeffects may be produced with ultrasound

---

Adapted with permission from Merritt CRB: *Safety issues in diagnostic US*. In Rifkin MD, Charbonneu JW, Laing FC, eds: *Syllabus: special course in ultrasound 1992*, Oak Brook, Ill, 1991, Radiological Society of North America, pp 73-80.

and the clinical implications of these mechanisms and will suggest ways in which the prudent user of ultrasound can use the display of output information to maximize benefit and minimize risk. The relationship of bioeffects concerns to other issues that affect the risk-to-benefit equation will also be discussed.

ACOUSTIC OUTPUT MEASUREMENT

Familiarity with certain basic concepts and terms used in describing the acoustic power output of an ultrasound device is needed to understand bioeffects.[12] Because most clinical applications involve imaging and Doppler and use pulsed rather than continuous wave ultrasound, only pulsed ultrasound conditions will be discussed. A pulsed ultrasound transducer introduces brief bursts of acoustical energy into the body that are then propagated as waves of alternating compression and rarefaction (Fig. 10-1). The wavelength (λ) is the distance between the pressure waves, and the period (T) is the time between the pressure waves. The reciprocal of the period is the frequency (F). The relationship of ultrasound propagation velocity (C) to wavelength (λ) and frequency (F) is well known to sonographers:

$$C = F\lambda \tag{1}$$

In pulsed operating modes the interval between the initiation of pulses is the pulse repetition period; the reciprocal of this is the pulse repetition frequency (PRF) (Fig. 10-2). The pulse duration or pulse length is the time from the beginning to the end of a pulse. With pulsed ultrasound systems the transducer is energized only a small part of the time. The PRF and pulse duration are related by the duty factor, which is the pulse duration divided by the pulse repetition period. Imaging and Doppler devices differ considerably in pulse duration and PRFs used, and thus duty factors also differ, which has important consequences for bioeffect production.

Each ultrasound pulse results in peak compressional and peak rarefactional pressures (Fig. 10-3). These peak pressure values relate to mechanical mechanisms for bioeffects such as cavitation. Pressure is measured in newtons/meter² (N/m²) or pascals (Pa) or may be displayed in decibels (dB) as a relative measure of amplitude difference.

As pulses of ultrasound are transmitted through tissues, *work* is performed. From a bioeffects viewpoint, the most important result of this work is the heating of tissues. The capacity to perform work is determined by the quantity of acoustic energy produced. *Acoustic power* (expressed in watts or milliwatts) describes the amount of acoustic energy produced in a unit of time. The *time-average acoustic power* is obtained by averaging the energy output from the beginning of one pulse to the beginning of the next pulse. Measures of acoustic power vary depending on the time interval considered. For example, the peak power that occurs during the time interval of a single pulse differs considerably from the average power occurring over a series of pulses (Fig. 10-4). In the case of pulsed ultrasound, the average power is the peak power multiplied by the duty factor.

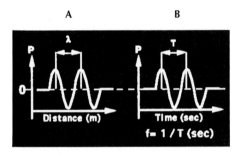

Fig. 10-1. *A,* At a given instant during passage of an ultrasound pulse, acoustic pressure *(P)* varies with distance. *B,* At a given point the acoustic pressure varies in time. The wavelength *(λ)* is the distance between corresponding points of the pressure wave and the period *(T)* is the time interval separating these points. The frequency of the sound *(f)* is the reciprocal of the period.

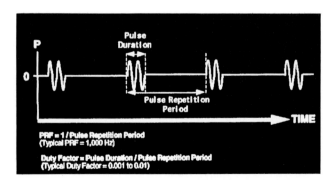

Fig. 10-2. In pulsed operating modes the interval between pulses is the pulse repetition period; the reciprocal of this is the pulse repetition frequency or PRF. The pulse duration or pulse length is the time from the beginning to the end of a pulse. The PRF and pulse duration are related by the duty factor, which is the pulse duration divided by the PRF.

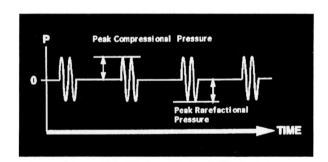

Fig. 10-3. Each ultrasound pulse results in peak compressional and peak rarefactional pressures. These are often not identical. Measurements of peak compressional and rarefactional pressures are measured at a specified point, usually where the value would be maximum. Peak pressure values are of interest with respect to mechanical mechanisms for bioeffects such as cavitation.

Although measurement of power provides an indication of energy as it relates to time, it does not consider the spatial distribution of the energy. A measurement describing the spatial distribution of power is needed to determine bioeffects. This is particularly true in the use of focused transducers where power may be concentrated in small geographic areas. Under these conditions, spatial-peak intensities may be considerably higher than at the transducer face. *Intensity* (I) describes the spatial concentration of power and is used to describe the exposure conditions at the target of the ultrasound beam:

$$I \ (W/cm^2) \ = \ Power \ (W)/Area \ (cm^2) \qquad (2)$$

In pulsed modes of operation, intensity may be calculated in at least six different ways.[8,13] These take into account different power measurements (e.g., peak, average) and the spatial distribution of the power. The *spatial-peak intensity (I$_{SP}$)* is the highest intensity spatially in the ultrasound beam. The *spatial-average intensity (I$_{SA}$)* is the average value of intensity over some specified area. The *spatial-average, temporal-average intensity (I$_{SATA}$)* is obtained by dividing the temporal average power by the area of the transducer face. The *spatial-average, pulse-average intensity (I$_{SAPA}$)* is the spatial average of the intensity during a pulse (I$_{SAPA}$ = I$_{SATA}$/Duty factor). Time-averaged intensity is an indicator of thermal effects and is important in safety considerations.

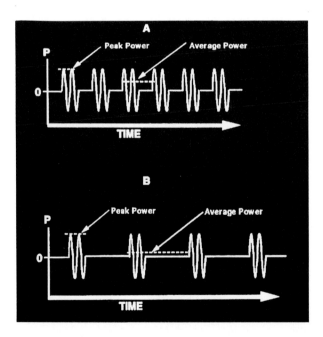

Fig. 10-4. The time average acoustic power is obtained by averaging the energy output from the beginning of one pulse to the beginning of the next pulse. In the case of pulsed ultrasound, the average power is the peak power times the duty factor. *A,* The PRF is high, resulting in a high duty factor and higher average power than in *B,* where a longer pulse repetition period results in a lower duty factor and thus a lower average power.

This is provided in the *spatial-peak, temporal-average intensity (I$_{SPTA}$)*, which is the time-average intensity at the position of the spatial peak (I$_{SPTA}$ = I$_{SATA}$ × I$_{SP/ISA}$). A final measurement is the *spatial-peak, pulse-average intensity (I$_{SPPA}$)*. This is the intensity that exists during a pulse at the position of the spatial peak and is the highest of the four intensities (I$_{SPPA}$ = I$_{SATA}$ × I$_{SP}$/I$_{SA}$/Duty factor). These intensities may be estimated (with limited precision) for typical clinical conditions by using measurements obtained in vitro and applying certain assumptions regarding attenuation of the ultrasound beam.

The measurements most relevant to known bioeffects mechanisms are the I$_{SPTA}$ and the I$_{SPPA}$. The I$_{SPTA}$ is used to estimate thermal bioeffects of ultrasound, whereas the I$_{SPPA}$ is related to the likelihood of mechanical bioeffects such as cavitation. The I$_{SPPA}$ tends to be higher in imaging than in Doppler instruments; the I$_{SPTA}$ is generally higher in Doppler modes. Both intensities are considered in the regulatory process of the FDA.

BIOEFFECTS MECHANISMS

Two potential mechanisms for producing biologic effects with ultrasound are currently understood. These include thermal mechanisms, which result from tissue heating from the absorption of ultrasound as it passes through tissue, and nonthermal (mechanical) effects, such as cavitation and radiation forces. *Cavitation* refers to the formation and collapse of microbubbles around cavitation nuclei. The extent to which these nuclei exist in normal tissue is unclear. Presently, thermal mechanisms are better understood with respect to their relationship to bioeffects than are the nonthermal mechanisms.

Thermal mechanism

Predicting the amount of heating produced by ultrasound in a given clinical situation is difficult and depends on a number of conditions. As previously stated, I$_{SPTA}$ is considered the most appropriate measure of intensity for predicting thermal effects. Local heating is determined not only by the ultrasound intensity at the site to which the ultrasound is directed but also by the rate of removal of heat away from the target by blood flow or conduction, the area of the ultrasound beam, and the duration of exposure. The intensity of ultrasound at the target is affected by the attenuation coefficient of the tissue along the path of the ultrasound beam and the amount of energy removed by the attenuating pathway from the transducer to the site of interest (usually the focal zone of the transducer). Absorption is the part of attenuation responsible for the conversion of ultrasonic energy into heat; tissue heating can thus occur along the entire beam path. As a consequence of increasing attenuation at higher frequencies, transducer frequency is a material factor. Finally, the presence of bone in the ultrasound path is a particularly important factor, since absorption is significantly increased at soft tissue/bone interfaces, resulting in a greater potential for heating than in soft tissues alone.

REPORTED BIOEFFECTS OF ULTRASOUND

Biologic macromolecules

Molecular degradation
Enzyme inactivation
Enhancement of enzyme activity

Cells

Cell disruption
Thrombocyte disruption (clot initiation)
Dislodgment of ribosomes
Release of enzymes from lysosomes
Rupture of nucleolus
Disruption of mitochondrial cristae
Chromosomal anomalies
Mitotic delay
Increase in cell membrane permeability
Intracellular streaming
Abnormal cell division
Cell surface changes

Tissues and organs

Selective heating of peripheral nerves
Reduction of nerve action potentials
Tissue edema
Hemorrhage
Decreased glycogen in muscle and liver
Formation of cataracts
Blood flow stasis
Induction of congenital anomalies
Retardation of fetal growth
Increased rate of tissue regeneration
Lesions

Animals

Fetal weight loss
Hind limb and tail paralysis
Increased heart rate
Retardation of growth
Delayed neuromuscular development
Death

From Safety Code 23: *Guidelines for the safe use of ultrasound. Part I. Medical and paramedical applications,* Pub No 88-EHD-59, Ottawa, Canada, 1989, Environmental Health Directorate, Health Protection Branch, Minister of National Health and Welfare, Canada.

All models for estimating thermal effects of ultrasound make assumptions regarding the attenuating pathway of the ultrasound beam. Conditions of attenuation vary considerably from one ultrasound application to another, and models attempting to predict heating must generalize. One approach is to assume a uniform rate of attenuation by soft tissue. In some obstetric applications, however, the path of the beam through amniotic fluid requires different assumptions. Thus a model based on a uniformly attenuating fluid medium is appropriate for estimating the thermal effects in a first trimester obstetrical evaluation but is inappropriate for an examination of the adult abdomen. On the other hand, in the second and third trimesters the ossification of fetal bone produces soft tissue/bone interfaces where greater absorption is present, resulting in the potential for greater thermal effects under worst-case exposure conditions.

Nonthermal mechanisms

Currently, much less is known about the likelihood of clinically significant bioeffects with nonthermal (mechanical) mechanisms. Cavitation requires the presence of small stabilized gaseous nuclei, but there is some uncertainty about the extent of these nuclei in humans. Ultrasound contrast agents composed of encapsulated microbubbles may increase cavitation potential, which is related to the higher amplitude, short pulses that are typically used with imaging rather than with Doppler modes. Radiation forces are another mechanical mechanism of potential bioeffect significance. Although these effects have not been studied extensively, in certain models, standing pressure waves that can impede flow in small vessels can be created.

Thermal and mechanical mechanisms are each capable of producing biologic effects at high levels. A summary of biologic effects that have been reported in experimental studies is shown in the box. Although these findings are impressive, most are produced under exposure conditions and at exposure levels that are not comparable to those encountered clinically. Nevertheless, these data do serve a useful purpose to remind users that sufficient ultrasound energy under specified conditions is capable of producing quite definite bioeffects.

BIOLOGIC CONSEQUENCES OF HYPERTHERMIA

Because thermal mechanisms for producing ultrasound bioeffects clearly exist, the biologic consequences of heating should be considered. Normal body temperatures may range from slightly less than 36° C to around 40° C, with even greater variation occurring with exercise and in response to disease. In competitive athletic activities, core temperatures as great as 41° C have been recorded.[6] Data show that almost every person experiences at least brief elevations of the body temperature to 4° C above normal as a result of exercise or fever (Fig. 10-5).[9]

Because the fetus is generally regarded as the most sensitive target of ultrasound, information related to teratogenesis is of particular interest. The scientific literature contains a great deal of information describing thermal bioeffects, and teratogenic effects of hyperthermia have been extensively studied in a number of primate and nonprimate animal models.[1,7,9] In general, these studies indicate that for a given biologic defect the exposure time required to produce the defect decreases as the temperature elevation increases.

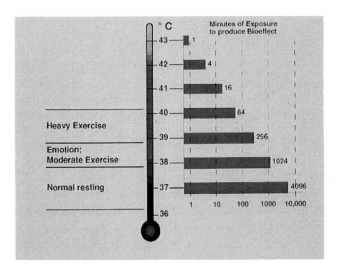

Fig. 10-5. In hyperthermia, examiners should remember that the core temperature of normal individuals varies considerably under different physiologic conditions. Also shown are the results of calculating the expression t = 4$^{(43-T)}$ for temperatures from 37° C to 43° C and the relationship of exposure duration to potential for bioeffect. The length of the bar for each temperature indicates the estimated time of ultrasound exposure that would be necessary to exceed the conditions under which bioeffects due to hyperthermia have been reported.

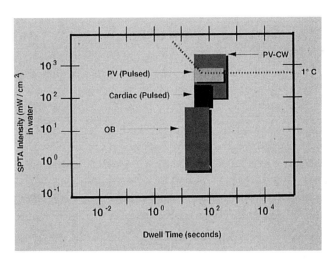

Fig. 10-6. The output (SPTA intensity) of various classes of Doppler instruments is related to the threshold for producing a 1° C temperature rise *(dotted line)* with various dwell times. Most imaging devices fall well below this one degree threshold. Some peripheral vascular Doppler instruments do, however, have the capacity to approach this threshold. (Modified from National Council on Radiation Protection and Measurements: *Biological effects of ultrasound: mechanisms and clinical implications,* NCRP Report No. 74, Bethesda, Md, 1983.)

Bioeffects attributed to hyperthermia include embryonic death (guinea pig, hamster), increased fetal mortality (mice), microcephaly (guinea pigs, sheep, hamster), and exencephaly (sheep).[9] In recording the lowest temperature reported in the literature to produce a given bioeffect and the briefest exposure to that temperature elevation associated with the effect, a boundary is observed below which effects are not reported. This boundary is described by

$$t_{43} = t \times R^{43 - T} = 1 \qquad (3)$$

where t is the exposure time, T is the temperature, and R is a constant with a value of 0.5 for temperatures of 43° C or above and a value of 0.25 for T less than 43° C. For T less than 43° C, the expression is simplified to

$$t = 4^{43 - T} \qquad (4)$$

This equation states the relationship between exposure time in minutes and temperature in degrees Celsius to produce a detectable bioeffect by heating (Fig. 10-5). The boundary line given by this expression might serve as a guide for determining whether a biologic effect due to hyperthermia would be likely.[9] Combinations of temperature elevation and exposure duration falling below the boundary line would be considered unlikely to produce harm, whereas exposure conditions above this line would have a significant possibility of damage. Based on these data, a temperature rise of 1° C to 2° C in an afebrile patient would not be likely to have a damaging effect.[9] For exposures resulting in temperature rises of greater than 2° C, the duration of exposure becomes an important consideration in risk-to-benefit assessment.

Currently available ultrasound devices operate well below this boundary. Fig. 10-6 shows the output of current types of ultrasound instruments and their relationship to the threshold for producing a 1° C temperature rise.[10] Most imaging devices fall well below this 1° C temperature rise. However, some peripheral vascular Doppler instruments do have the capacity to approach this level. The focal zone must be fixed on the target for some time to produce these conditions in vivo, even near a highly absorptive soft tissue/bone interface. In most clinical scanning situations, this is unlikely.

At present, much less is known of the biologic consequences of nonthermal mechanism effects in mammalian systems, at least at levels of intensity likely to be encountered clinically. Tissue damage presumed to be related to cavitation has been noted with lithotriptors at peak pressures of from 2 to 15 MPa, however, these devices operate at much lower frequencies than clinical ultrasound devices. Researchers have failed to identify evidence of hemorrhage in renal tissue with pulsed Doppler devices at peak pressures of up to 10 MPa but have noted a threshold for hemorrhage in aerated mouse lung of the order of 1 MPa for pulsed ultrasound.[4,5] The clinical relevance of these observations remains unclear, and further investigation is warranted.

OPERATING MODES: CLINICAL IMPLICATIONS

Ultrasound devices may operate in several modes, including real-time imaging, color Doppler imaging, spectral Doppler, and M-mode. Pulsed ultrasound is used for real-time imaging, spectral Doppler, and color flow applications. The nature of the ultrasound pulses and the resulting acoustic exposure differ significantly among these operating modes, which results in important bioeffects considerations. Imaging is produced in a scanned mode of operation (Fig. 10-7). In scanned modes, pulses of ultrasound from the transducer are directed down lines of sight that are moved or steered in sequence to generate the image. The number of ultrasound pulses arriving at a given point in the patient

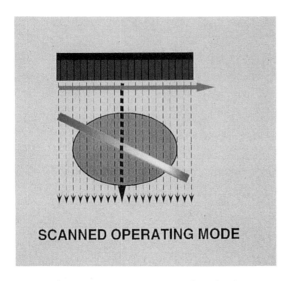

SCANNED OPERATING MODE

Fig. 10-7. Real-time imaging uses a scanned mode of operation. In scanned modes, pulses of ultrasound from the transducer are directed down lines of sight *(dotted lines)* that are moved or steered in sequence to generate the image. The number of ultrasound pulses arriving at a given point in the patient over a given interval of time is relatively few, and relatively little energy is deposited at any given location.

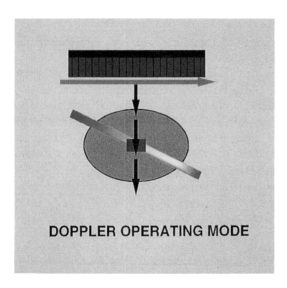

DOPPLER OPERATING MODE

Fig. 10-8. Doppler is an unscanned mode of operation in which multiple ultrasound pulses are sent in repetition along a line to collect the Doppler data. In this mode the beam is stationary, resulting in considerably greater potential for heating than in imaging modes.

over a given interval of time is relatively few, and relatively little energy is deposited at any given location. In contrast, Doppler is an unscanned mode of operation in which multiple ultrasound pulses are sent in repetition along a line to collect the Doppler data (Fig. 10-8). In this mode the beam is stationary, resulting in considerably greater potential for heating than in imaging modes. For imaging, the frequency at which the pulses are emitted (the PRF) is usually in the range of 1000 Hz, with very short pulses. With Doppler, longer pulse durations are often used. In addition, higher PRFs must often be used to avoid aliasing and other artifacts. Longer pulse duration and higher PRF result in higher duty factors for Doppler modes of operation and increase the amount of energy introduced in scanning. Color Doppler, although a scanned mode, produces exposure conditions between those of real-time imaging and Doppler, since color Doppler devices tend to send more pulses down each scan line and may use longer pulse durations than imaging devices. Clearly, users must realize that when they switch from an imaging to a Doppler mode, the exposure conditions and potential for bioeffects change.

With current devices operating in imaging modes, bioeffects concerns are minimal because intensities sufficient to produce measurable heating are seldom used. With Doppler the potential for thermal effects is greater. Preliminary measurements on commercially available instruments suggest that at least some of these are capable of producing temperature rises of greater than 1° C at soft tissue/bone interfaces if the focal zone of the transducer is held stationary for a short time. Care is therefore warranted when Doppler measurements are obtained at or near soft tissue/bone interfaces as may be the case in the second and third trimesters of pregnancy. In these cases, the principle of ALARA is required.

In obstetric ultrasound, Doppler and color Doppler instruments are now being used. As a result, fetuses are now being exposed to different conditions and sometimes higher acoustic output than previously. In obstetric applications the need for prudent use is emphasized. Users should prevent unnecessary exposure and not perform an examination under high-exposure conditions unless the examination is clinically warranted. Examination skill and experience in performing the study are necessary to collect the diagnostic information efficiently and with minimal exposure.

THE FDA AND OUTPUT DISPLAY

Any discussion of issues of ultrasound power output and bioeffects must include the role of the United States Food and Drug Administration. Through its regulation of ultrasound devices, the FDA has been intimately involved with these issues. For over 15 years, the FDA has imposed limits on the acoustic output of diagnostic ultrasound devices intended for various uses (Fig. 10-9). These limits were established as a result of the Medical Devices Amendment enacted by Congress in 1976. Approval of new ultrasound devices for marketing is based on the ability of the manufacturer to demonstrate the substantial equivalence in safety and efficacy of the new device as compared to devices on the market before May 28, 1976. Until recently, the FDA used the production of acoustic output at levels at or below the maximum intensities in use before May, 1976, as its test of equivalent safety. This approach has been criticized because it tends to imply a relationship between ultrasound bioeffects and the output limits used for regulatory purposes. Because the regulatory limits are arbitrary and derived from historical events, this is clearly not the case. A second objection is that the arbitrary limits have the potential for slowing the introduction of promising applications of ultrasound, particularly those involving deep Doppler, in which higher acoustic outputs than are currently available may be necessary for maximal clinical benefit.

The FDA may soon be more flexible. Higher power output levels will be possible when certain user feedback features are incorporated into ultrasound devices with a comprehensive user educational program. Although the range of applications and the benefits of ultrasound may increase, users will have greater responsibility and must understand the possible implications of higher output levels in clinical situations.

Key conditions of the proposed approval process include instrument display features to provide user feedback related to acoustic exposure, low power default output levels, and override controls for certain modes of operation. In proposing this approach, the FDA has accepted the concept that an educated user provided with appropriate exposure feedback and default safeguards is in the best position to make a proper risk-to-benefit assessment. With FDA support, a

voluntary standard for the display of acoustic output information has recently been approved. The premise is that the user should be provided with acoustic output information and use this information to keep exposure as low as possible while keeping with the diagnostic objectives. Since current data indicate that the most relevant mechanisms for production of bioeffects with ultrasound are the thermal and mechanical mechanisms, the output display will provide indices accordingly. As proposed in the output display standard, thermal indices for soft tissue and bone will be displayed in Doppler modes and will indicate a worst-case potential for heating under actual examination conditions. In imaging modes, a mechanical index will be provided as a relative indicator of the potential for nonthermal bioeffects such as cavitation. To use these new feedback features, the user will need a basic understanding of the mechanisms by which ultrasound bioeffects are known to occur and the situations in which the indices are likely to overestimate (and rarely underestimate) exposure conditions in vivo. With this information, the user is adequately prepared to implement the principles of ALARA.

CONCLUSION

Despite the reassurance provided by an excellent safety record to date, there is a growing body of evidence that at sufficiently high intensities, ultrasound can produce biologic effects by thermal and mechanical mechanisms. This provides a basis for concern at clinical levels. Although concerns for current instruments are largely hypothetical, new imaging and Doppler applications providing increased sensitivity may require appreciably higher acoustic output than current instrumentation and thus produce exposures for which the possibility of thermal bioeffects must be considered as part of the risk-to-benefit decision. The knowledge and skill of the user is another major determinant of the risk-to-benefit implications of the use of ultrasound in a specific clinical situation. For example, an unrealistic emphasis on the safety of ultrasound may promote its use when a more invasive examination or one associated with identifiable risks is actually a more appropriate solution to the clinical problem. Conversely, an unrealistic emphasis on risks may discourage appropriate use of ultrasound, resulting in harm to the patient by omission of useful information or by exposure of the patient to another more hazardous examination. The skill and experience of the individual performing and interpreting the examination are likely to have a major effect on the overall benefit of the examination. Because of the rapid growth of ultrasound and its proliferation into the hands of minimally trained clinicians, far more patients are likely to be harmed by misdiagnosis resulting from improper indications, poor examination technique, and errors in interpretation than from biologic effects. The abortion of a normal fetus or the removal of a normal gallbladder on the basis of a faulty ultrasound diagnosis are real dangers, and poorly trained users may turn out to be the greatest current hazard of diagnostic ultrasound.

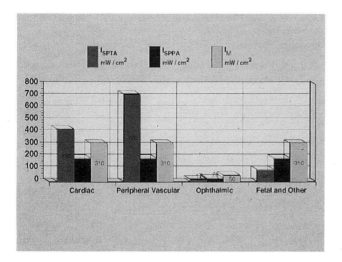

Fig. 10-9. Current FDA limits for acoustic output of various classes of ultrasound devices. These limits are based on historical events and are not derived from any study of their potential for producing bioeffects. A new scheme to display acoustic output indices to users will soon replace the use of these arbitrary limits for regulatory purposes.

REFERENCES

1. Abraham V, Ziskin MC, Heyner S: Temperature elevation in the rat fetus due to ultrasound exposure, *Ultrasound Med Biol* 15:443-449, 1989.
2. AIUM/NEMA: *Standard for the real time display of thermal and mechanical indices,* April 14, 1991.
3. American Institute of Ultrasound in Medicine: Bioeffects considerations for the safety of diagnostic ultrasound, *J Ultrasound Med* (suppl)S4, 1988.
4. Carstensen EL et al: Test for kidney hemorrhage following exposure to intense, pulsed ultrasound, *Ultrasound Med Biol* 16:681-685, 1990.
5. Child SZ et al: Lung damage from exposure to pulsed ultrasound, *Ultrasound Med Biol (England)* 16:817-825, 1990.
6. Clark RP, Edholm OG: *Man and his thermal environment,* London, 1985, Edward Arnold.
7. Edwards MJ: Hyperthermia as a teratogen: a review of experimental studies and their clinical significance, *Teratogenesis Carcinog Mutagen* 6:563-582, 1986.
8. Kremkau FW: Diagnostic ultrasound: principles, instruments, examples, ed 3, Philadelphia, 1989, WB Saunders.
9. Miller MW, Ziskin MC: Biological consequences of hyperthermia, *Ultrasound Med Biol* 15:707-722, 1989.
10. NCRP Report No. 74: *Biological effects of ultrasound: mechanisms and clinical implications,* Bethesda, Md, 1983, National Council on Radiation Protection and Measurements.
11. NCRP Report No 107: *Implementation of the principle of as low as reasonably achievable (ALARA) for medical and dental personnel,* Bethesda, Md, 1990, National Council on Radiation Protection and Measurements.
12. Safety Code 23: *Guidelines for the safe use of ultrasound. Part I. Medical and paramedical applications,* Pub No 88-EHD-59, Ottawa, Canada, 1989, Environmental Health Directorate, Health Protection Branch, Minister of National Health and Welfare, Canada.
13. *Safety considerations for diagnostic ultrasound,* Report of the Bioeffects Committee of the American Institute of Ultrasound in Medicine, Rockville, Md, 1991.
14. Ultrasound imaging, *Health Week* 3(12):19-31, 1989.

CHAPTER 11

Pulsed Doppler ultrasound for blood velocity measurements

KIRK W. BEACH and D. EUGENE STRANDNESS, Jr.

The earliest ultrasonic Doppler instruments were non-directional continuous wave devices that transmitted at an ultrasonic frequency of about 5 MHz. The choice of that frequency was fortunate because it produces the strongest reflected signal from blood at a depth of 2 cm when viewed with ultrasound through muscle. Suppose that the blood velocity is 15.7 cm/sec and the blood is insonated with a 5 MHz ultrasound beam colinear with the blood velocity (a Doppler angle of 0). Because the velocity of sound in blood is 157,000 cm/sec, ultrasound that reflects off the moving erythrocytes would experience a 1/10,000 shift in frequency on reaching the erythrocytes and another 1/10,000 shift on reflecting from them, for a total shift of 2/10,000. A 2/10,000 shift in the frequency of 5,000,000 Hz is equal to 1000 Hz, a frequency that is well within the normal human hearing range. It is only by chance that over the normal range of blood flow velocities, 3 to 150 cm/sec, the Doppler shift produces Doppler signals of 200 Hz to 10,000 kHz with a Doppler angle of 0 degrees, or 100 Hz to 5000 kHz with a Doppler angle of 60 degrees (cos60 = 0.5).

Those relationships, in combination with a simple set of electronics capable of extracting the "beat" (difference) frequency between the transmitted and the received frequencies,[3] made the first Doppler instruments possible. These instruments extended the acoustic examination of patients beyond the stage of the passive stethoscope, but they had limitations. The two major limitations, the inability to separate mixed signals and the need to quantify velocities, could be overcome with the use of technology already developed for radio and radar.

The first limitation appears when two blood vessels are insonated simultaneously by the instrument; the signals appear superimposed in the output and are hard to separate. Although both vessels might be arteries, usually one is an artery and the other a vein. Two strategies were available to separate these signals, one based on the difference in flow direction in arteries and veins and the other on the fact that the two vessels are spatially separated. Flow direction can be identified by the use of methods developed by radio engineers working with single sideband receivers. It was only necessary to recognize the similarity in the two systems and apply the method to Doppler systems. Because flow toward the probe shifts ultrasound to slightly higher frequencies and flow away from the probe shifts ultrasound to slightly lower frequencies, flows in two directions appear as two "sidebands" of the transmitted frequency and can be separated with sideband technology. The bidirectional ultrasonic Doppler system is based on this technology.[5,6] Spatial separation is achieved by focusing the ultrasonic beam to allow the ultrasound to be directed toward one vessel while avoiding the other and by an electronic method of selecting the Doppler-shifted signal from a single depth in tissue while rejecting signals from all other depths. The pulsed Doppler system was devised to accomplish this.

The second limitation is that there is a direct proportional relationship between blood velocity and frequency. The relationship is expressed as the Doppler equation:

$$\Delta F = \frac{2F_0 \times V \times \cos\theta}{C} \qquad (1)$$

where:

ΔF = Frequency shift
2 = Round trip of the ultrasound
C/F_o = Wavelength of ultrasound
$V \cos\theta$ = Closing speed between the erythrocytes and the Doppler transducer

Examiners, aware of this relationship, wanted to quantify blood velocity. Two things were needed: a method of measuring the Doppler angle and a quantitative frequency display. Fortunately, imaging systems are now capable of displaying the Doppler angle, and frequency analyzers are capable of displaying the quantitative spectral waveform.

Of all the advances in ultrasonic Doppler technology, the pulsed Doppler system is the most intriguing. It provides the ability to monitor blood velocity at different depths in tissue: pulsed Doppler systems combine the spatial ability on which ultrasonic imaging is based with the ultrasound phase detection on which Doppler measurement is based.

PHYSICAL BASIS OF PULSED DOPPLER SYSTEM

When a pulse of ultrasound is transmitted into tissue, the echo returned by the tissue consists of a series of radio-frequency oscillations. The strength of the echo depends on the power of the ultrasound pulse and on the attenuation of the tissue. The attenuation in turn depends on the ultrasonic frequency and the tissue type. There is a direct relationship

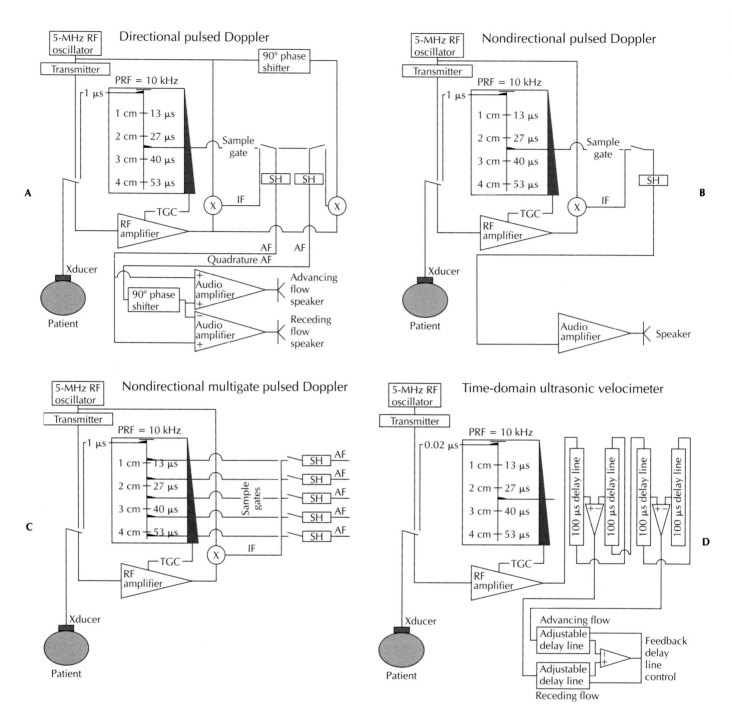

Fig. 11-1. Pulsed Doppler circuit diagrams. At the beginning of the pulse-echo cycle, a transmit pulse is sent from the transmitter via the transmit-receive switch to the transducer. In pulsed Doppler *(A, B, C)* the pulse contains 5 cycles (as in Fig. 11-2, *B*); in time-domain *(D)* the pulse contains 1 cycle (as in Fig. 11-2, *A*). The RF receiver amplifier is on whenever the transmitter is off. The gain (amount that the echo is amplifed) is increased with time by the TGC as deeper and deeper echoes return. *A, B, C,* Pulsed Doppler. *B,* Nondirectional Doppler. *C,* Multigate pulsed Doppler. *D,* Time-domain Doppler. (*Xducer,* ultrasound transducer; *TGC,* time-gain control; *RF,* radiofrequency [5 MHz]; *IF,* intermediate frequency [1 MHz]; *AF,* audio frequency [50 Hz to 5000 Hz]; *S & H,* sample and hold device; *(X),* multipliers; *triangles,* amplifiers; *PRF,* pulse repetition frequency [10 kHz].)

between the duration of a segment of the echo and the depth of tissue involved in that time segment. The relationship is based on the velocity of ultrasound in tissue (154,000 cm/sec) as the pulse travels to and from the reflectors. Each centimeter in tissue depth is displayed as 13 μs in echo duration. Thus to receive an echo from a depth of 3 cm, the operator must wait about 40 μs after the transmission. To accept the signal from a 1 mm slice of tissue at that depth, the operator would have to accept the signal for 1.3 μs after waiting 40 μs for the desired echo.

If the ultrasound frequency is 6 MHz and the sound is passing through muscle, the attenuation rate is 10 dB/cm tissue depth. Inasmuch as the ultrasound must pass through each centimeter twice, once going down and the next time coming back, echoes are attenuated 20 dB, or a factor of 100 in power for each centimeter of tissue depth represented (each 13 μs on the display). Most ultrasonic pulsed echo instruments (imaging and Doppler) are equipped with *time-gain controls* (TGC; sometimes called *depth gain compensation* [DGC]) to compensate for the attenuation. Such a control will amplify echoes from the first 13 μs after pulse transmission (representing the first centimeter) by a factor of 100, echoes from the next 13 μs (second centimeter) by a factor of 10,000, those from the next 13 μs (another centimeter) by 1,000,000, and each successive 13 μs (representing successive centimeters) by successive factors of 100. Thus the intensity of the echoes varies over a wide range, strong from shallow reflectors and weak from deep reflectors. Undesired echoes from beyond the desired depth are ignored because the amplification is inadequate to make these signals visible.

In continuous wave (CW) Doppler systems, two transducers are used, one for transmitting and the other for receiving. In pulsed Doppler systems a single crystal is used for both transmitting and receiving. Voltages required for ultrasound transmission range from 20 to 100 V. Echoes returning from tissue generate voltages in the range of 10 μV (microvolts) to 10 mV (millivolts). It is therefore very important to electrically isolate the receiver from the transmitter. In CW Doppler systems the separation is accomplished by having separate transducers. In pulsed Doppler systems the separation is achieved by switching the same transducer from transmitting to receiving. The beam patterns from the two transducers used in CW Doppler systems do not overlap near the skin. Thus the strong echoes from shallow depths are avoided. CW Doppler systems are therefore able to operate without electronic depth gain compensation; instead the limited overlap of the beam patterns provides automatic depth gain compensation. In pulsed Doppler systems the transmitter beam pattern and the receiver beam pattern are identical, so all of the depth gain compensation must be done by timing. With CW Doppler systems it is not possible to perform depth gain compensation with timing from the transmitted pulse because ultrasound is transmitted continuously and echoes are received from all depths at all times.

An ultrasonic pulsed Doppler instrument consists of a radiofrequency oscillator operating in the range of 1 to 20 MHz, a gate (or switch) to determine the transmission timing and the pulse length, a timing circuit that opens the receiver for the desired echo, an amplifier, a mixer-detector to compare the phase and amplitude of the echo with the reference oscillator, and an audio amplifier to amplify the resultant Doppler signal (Fig. 11-1). The ultrasonic pulse generated by an ultrasonic pulsed Doppler instrument differs from the pulse generated by an ultrasonic pulsed echo imaging instrument. The pulsed echo instrument transmits the shortest possible burst into tissue (Fig. 11-2, A). This is to ensure the best possible depth resolution of the image. The Doppler pulse consists of a series of cycles at the ultrasonic carrier frequency (Fig. 11-2, B). The returned echo contains variations in both amplitude and phase (Fig. 11-2, C). As the echo is received, the portion of the echo from the desired depth is accepted by the receiver gate. That portion, the gated echo, is usually equal in length to the transmitted pulse. The gated echo is multiplied times a reference wave within the instrument. The reference wave is the Doppler carrier frequency. The output voltage of the multiplier depends on the phase relationship between the echo and the

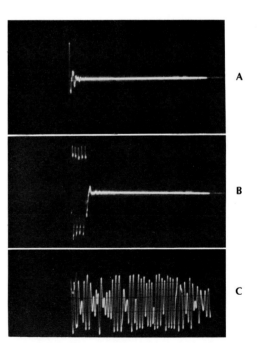

Fig. 11-2. Transmitted and received ultrasonic signals. **A,** Ultrasonic pulsed echo transmission burst. Note the few weak oscillations (ringing) following the single cycle transmitted. In most systems, ringing is suppressed to improve the depth resolution of the system. **B,** Ultrasonic pulsed Doppler transmission pulse. Five cycles of 5 MHz ultrasound are transmitted in a pulse 1μ long. **C,** Radiofrequency A-mode echo. This is an echo recieved at the transducer over the first 8μs after completion of the Doppler pulse transmission. This represents the first 6 mm of tissue depth. An appropriate time gain amplification has been applied to prevent attenuation of the trace from left (skin) to right (deep).

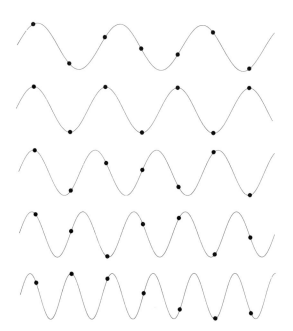

Fig. 11-3. Aliasing of a high-frequency Doppler shift signal. The dots represent ultrasound pulses that sample phase of echo from a particular depth. The horizontal measure represents the timing of pulses; the vertical distance represents the phase alignment measurement from each ultrasonic echo. As the frequency exceeds the Nyquist frequency (equal to half of the PRF), the line connecting the samples would produce erroneously low output frequency rather than the expected frequency drawn. The upper two tracings show the correctly represented frequencies; the lower three tracings represent the signals that would be aliased if the signals were reconstructed from the dot samples. In the lowest tracing, the effect is shown with the greatest clarity. The Doppler shift frequency is nearly equal to the sample frequency.

Table 11-1. Aliasing frequencies for a pulse repetition frequency of 10 kHz

Expected Doppler shift (kHz)	Observed nondirectional Doppler shift (kHz)	Observed directional Doppler shift (kHz)
3	3	+3
4	4	+4
5	5*	±5*
6	4†	−4†
7	3†	−3†
8	2†	−2†
9	1†	−1†
10	0†	0†
11	1†	+1†
12	2†	+2†

*Half of PRF equals aliasing frequency.
†F(observed) = F(expected) − n × (PRF)/2, where n is an integer chosen to locate the result between −(PRF)/2 and +(PRF)/2; the nondirectional result displays only the magnitudes of the aliased frequencies.

reference. If that phase relationship is constant over a period of 100 ms or longer during which 1000 pulse-echo cycles are completed, as with a stationary reflector, the output will be a constant voltage that contains no audio signal. If the phase relationship is changing, as with a moving reflector, the output voltage will vary up and down changing with each pulse-echo cycle, generating the audio output, a sound with frequency proportional to blood velocity. Superimposed on that signal is the pulse repetition frequency (PRF), which is suppressed by a low pass filter set to reject the PRF while preserving the lower frequency audio Doppler signal.

The audio signal generated by the pulsed Doppler unit is similar to the CW Doppler signal. The nondirectional or directional output signals from the pulsed Doppler system can be handled and analyzed just like the CW signals. Pulsed Doppler signals differ from CW Doppler signals in two ways. First, pulsed Doppler signals usually represent velocities in smaller sample volumes than CW Doppler signals. Although CW Doppler units display velocities from the entire vessel cross section, a pulsed Doppler system can obtain Doppler data from a sample volume as small as 3 mm.[3] The small sample volume allows data collection from many adjacent regions in a single artery. This enables the operator to examine the complex nature of the blood flow in detail. Second, because the pulsed Doppler system samples the data rather than collecting data continuously, an artifact of the sampling rate occurs. There is a limit to the Doppler shift frequency that can be displayed by a pulsed Doppler unit.

ALIASING

The output of the pulsed Doppler system is generated by displaying the phase of successive pulse echoes as sound. At least one point must be available for each peak and one for each valley of the output frequency to faithfully create an audible sound of a particular frequency (Fig. 11-3). This means that the audio Doppler output signal will have a frequency that is lower than half of the PRF of the pulsed Doppler instrument. The limiting audio frequency (PRF/2) is called the *Nyquist frequency* (after Harry Nyquist, a Bell Telephone Laboratory scientist). If the PRF is less than half of the expected Doppler frequency, a sound will be generated based on the phase samples available, but the audio output generated is the lowest frequency that satisfies the phase shifts. If the PRF is 10 kHz, the highest magnitude Doppler shift frequencies that can be correctly displayed on the audio channel or the spectral waveform output are ±5 kHz. A tabulation of the effect is helpful for a PRF of 10 kHz (Table 11-1).

Aliasing can be easily recognized on a velocity waveform display (Fig. 11-4). Frequencies that should appear in the forward direction at frequencies higher than the Nyquist frequency are plotted in the reverse direction. The same effect will appear on the audio output channels. Because CW Doppler systems do not sample the phase of the ultra-

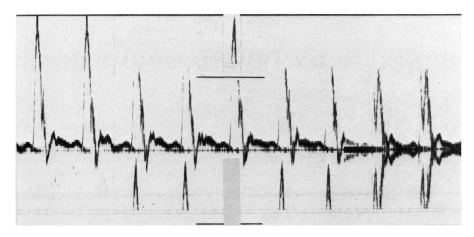

Fig. 11-4. A pulsed Doppler signal with aliasing. First, two cardiac cycles were obtained with a PRF of 19.6 kHz. The range of kHz spectral tracing is $+7$ to -3 kHz. Next, five cardiac cycles were obtained with a directional pulsed Doppler system with a PRF of 7.6 kHz. Aliasing begins at 3.8 kHz. The lines drawn at $+3.8$ kHz allow the aliased signal to be moved to the correct location on the waveform by aligning the two marks. Finally, two cardiac cycles were gathered with a nondirectional pulsed Doppler system at a PRF of 7.6 kHz. Note that the nondirectional aliased signal produces an M-shaped waveform.

sonic echoes but monitor the phase continuously, they do not exhibit aliasing. Digital spectra derived from CW Dopplers may alias because the spectrum analyzer samples the audio output of the Doppler at a frequency equal to twice the maximum frequency of the spectrum analyzer display, and thus if the Doppler frequency is higher than the maximum of the display (half of the spectrum analyzer sample rate), aliasing will result on the display but not on the audio channels.

PULSED DOPPLER SIGNALS

Pulsed Doppler and CW Doppler systems are both subject to the Doppler equation, but the signals obtained from the two instruments are different. Because the pulsed Doppler systems can measure flow velocity in the midstream of a vessel while rejecting signals from near the vessel walls, the width of the frequency spectrum generated by the pulsed Doppler unit is narrower than that from a CW Doppler unit (Fig. 11-5). This difference in spectral width can be heard. The sound from a pulsed Doppler system is a purer tone than that from a CW Doppler system.

A flow profile across the vessel can be generated by stepping the angle of the probe laterally across the vessel or by stepping the Doppler sample volume across the vessel[4] by incrementally increasing the depth (Fig. 11-6). If the steps occur in 1 mm increments, the vessel dimensions can be determined by observing the points at which velocity goes to zero. This is not an ideal way to measure arterial dimensions because the vessel walls move during the cardiac cycle. The motion of the arterial wall will introduce an intense, low-frequency Doppler signal that will make the vessel appear wider. If low-frequency filters are used to suppress these signals, the vessel width will appear incorrectly small, and the width measurement will be velocity dependent.

MULTIGATE PULSED DOPPLER SYSTEMS

The pulsed Doppler system is more difficult to operate than the CW Doppler system. The Doppler probe must be coupled with the skin and directed toward a blood vessel to receive a signal from a CW Doppler unit. This requires that the operator have knowledge of the vascular system as projected in the skin. To obtain a signal with a pulsed Doppler unit, in addition to pointing the probe at the vessel of interest, the operator must adjust the range (depth setting) of the machine so that the Doppler signal will be obtained from within the vessel. This requires that the operator have knowledge of the depth of the blood vessels in addition to their projection on the skin. Recognizing this difficulty, investigators have attempted to develop a convenient pulsed Doppler system that could interrogate multiple depths simultaneously.[2]

As the pulsed Doppler system operates, the echoes from tissue include data from a broad range of depths. The data from all depths of tissue except the depth of the sample gate are discarded. Like the echo from the depth of interest, the data from all other depths can be processed by additional sample gates without degrading the data from the first. Such a system allows the velocity profile across the vessel to be displayed. The operation of such a system requires that the phase of the ultrasound signal from various depths be stored separately. The phase from each depth during successive pulse echoes can be compared with the phase from the preceding pulse to establish the Doppler phase shift. This storage can be accomplished in digital memory devices[1] or in analogue delay lines.[7] In either case, flow profiles across a vessel diameter can be obtained.

Additional insight into the multigate pulsed Doppler system and its nature can be obtained by playing with the operation of a B-mode imaging system. When a B-mode image is viewed, a speckle pattern is apparent in the image.

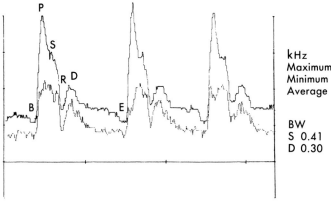

kHz
Maximum 3.98
Minimum 1.07
Average 1.86

BW
S 0.41
D 0.30

Fig. 11-5. Comparing the spectral width of pulsed and CW Doppler systems. The figures show the waveform and spectral width by plotting the 12th and 88th percentile contour lines. The upper curve is from a pulsed Doppler system, and the lower trace is from a CW Doppler system. Both signals were taken at an angle of 45° to the skin. Although the wave shapes are similar, the spectral width of the pulsed Doppler signal is narrower than that of the CW tracing. Note that the peak frequency appears lower on the CW tracing even though the upper envelopes of the signals as viewed on a spectrum analyzer are similar. *S,* Systole; *D,* diastole; *BW,* spectral bandwidth; *B,* automatically selected systolic upslope; *P,* automatically selected peak systole, *B* to *S,* automatically selected systolic period; *R,* automatically selected first zero slope after systole; *S* to *D,* automatically selected diastolic interval; *E,* end-diastolic frequency.

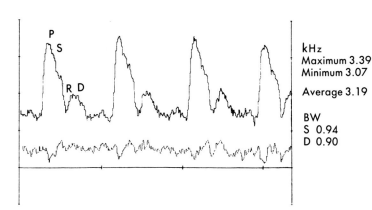

kHz
Maximum 3.39
Minimum 3.07

Average 3.19

BW
S 0.94
D 0.90

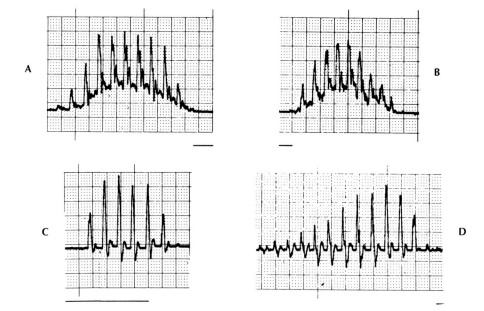

Fig. 11-6. Stepping a pulsed Doppler sample volume across the common carotid artery and external iliac artery. **A,** Stepping the sample volume laterally across the common carotid artery indicates blunt flow in systole and rounded flow in diastole. The probe was handheld without guidance, **B,** Stepping a sample volume in depth at the same point in the common carotid artery indicates more parabolic flow along that diameter of the common carotid artery. **C,** Stepping a sample volume laterally across the external iliac artery shows the profile of both forward and reverse flow. **D,** Stepping a sample volume in depth in the same external iliac artery. The probe is looking into the curve; velocities on the left are on the inside of the arterial bend. The peak velocities show assymetry, whereas the reverse velocities have rounded symmetry.

The size of the speckles in the depth direction depends on the length of the transmission pulse and the response time of the receiver. The speckles do not represent echogenicity fluctuations in the tissue but constructive and destructive interference between the reflections coming from slightly different depths. This is superimposed on the image intensity fluctuations caused by changes in tissue echogenicity.

In normal B-mode imaging the transmission pulse is so short that the speckles may be too small to be apparent. If, however, the B-mode image is generated from a long Doppler transmission pulse, the speckle will be prominent. The speckle associated with stationary regions of tissue will be stationary, but the speckle pattern that represents moving tissues such as blood will fluctuate. This "sparkling" of the image is the visual manifestation of the Doppler effect. If attention is focused on a single spot of the speckle pattern, the fluctuation frequency of the spot is exactly equal to the expected Doppler frequency. Of course, in Doppler signals, the Doppler frequency may vary from a few hundred to thousands of cycles per second (Hertz). It is not possible to follow such frequencies by eye because the flicker fusion rate of the eye is about 20 Hz. By chance, aliasing makes the effect visible.

In a two-dimensional, real-time B-mode imaging system the frame rate is 30 Hz. This means that the PRF for each B-mode line making up the image is 30 Hz. The PRF is much higher, because the pulser is also used to obtain data from many other lines in the image. A pulsed Doppler system that operates at 30 Hz will alias at 15 Hz, which is below the flicker fusion rate of the eye. If one supposes that the velocity in a blood vessel is such that it would create a Doppler shift of 1000 Hz, the pulsed Doppler system operates at a PRF of 30 Hz, and aliasing will occur at 15 Hz. Doppler frequencies that are multiples of 30 Hz will appear stationary because they exhibit an exact integral number of phase shifts between pulses. Thus an expected Doppler shift frequency of 990 Hz would produce a zero Doppler shift in this pulsed system and a stationary speckle pattern. A 1000 Hz shift, 10 Hz higher than 990 Hz, will produce a periodic cycle in the brightness of the speckle pattern at a frequency of 10 Hz. For other frequencies the fluctuation of the speckle pattern will range in frequency between 0 and 15 Hz, well within the range of visibility.

The pattern does not show velocity in an easily understandable manner, but it does show those regions where blood flow is present as a sparkling area of the image and those where it is absent. The pattern was first observed on a wide-aperture B-mode imaging system. The engineers were installing a new transmitter so that the instrument could be used with a pulsed Doppler system. Creating the B-mode image with the Doppler transmitter produced the effect of "worms crawling" within the arteries and veins. The observation was never exploited by the manufacturer.

CONCLUSION

Pulsed Doppler systems are now most popular when used with two-dimensional B-mode imaging systems in the form of duplex scanners. Such systems allow the visualization of a blood vessel in longitudinal section and the location of the Doppler sample volume within the vessel under visual control. The angle between the vessel axis and the Doppler ultrasound can be measured directly, and the location of the measurement with respect to curves and bifurcations can be positively established. In addition, periodic vessel motion with respect to the Doppler sample volume can be observed. Pulsed Doppler signals are usually analyzed with real-time spectrum analyzers that allow the details of the generated frequencies to be displayed. In this context the pulsed Doppler system can be used to display the details of the flow within the vascular system.

Even though many advances have been made in the use of CW and pulsed Doppler systems for the diagnosis of arterial, venous, and cardiac disease, there are still many opportunities to expand the usefulness of the information available from pulsed Doppler systems.

REFERENCES

1. Hoeks APG, Reneman RS, Peronneau PA: A multigate Doppler system with serial data processing, *IEEE Trans Sonics Ultrasonics* SU 28:4, 1981.
2. Hokanson DE, Mozersky DJ, Sumner DS: Ultrasonic arteriography, *Biomed Eng* 6:420, 1971.
3. Jaffe J: Listen to your heart with Doppler ultrasound, *Popular Electronics* 60-63, August 1975.
4. Ku DN et al: Hemodynamics of the normal human carotid bifurcation: in vitro and in vivo studies, *Ultrasound Med Biol* 11:13-26, 1985.
5. McLeod FD: A directional Doppler flowmeter, *Dig Int Conf Med Biol Eng* 7:196-217, 1967.
6. McLeod FD: *A Doppler ultrasonic physiologic flowmeter.* Proceedings of the 17th Annual Conference for Engineering in Medicine and Biology, 1968.
7. Nowicki A, Reid JM: An infinite gate pulsed Doppler, *Ultrasound Med Biol* 7:41-50, 1981.

CHAPTER 12

Principles and pitfalls of real-time color flow imaging

FREDERICK W. KREMKAU

Color flow imaging presents two-dimensional, cross-sectional, blood flow information in real-time in conjunction with two-dimensional, cross-sectional, gray-scale anatomic imaging. Two-dimensional real-time presentations of flow information allow the observer to readily locate regions of abnormal flow for further evaluation. Direction of flow is readily appreciated, and disturbed or turbulent flow is presented in a two-dimensional form quite dramatically. Color flow instruments present pulse-echo, gray-scale anatomic information in the conventional form and include circuitry that allows the rapid detection of Doppler frequency or echo arrival time shifts at several locations along each scan line and presentations of these in color at the appropriate locations in the cross-sectional image.[12] The color flow imaging instrument is therefore a combined pulse-echo gray-scale imaging instrument and pulsed Doppler or time-shift multigate instrument. Conventional continuous-wave and pulsed Doppler spectral analysis[7] capability is commonly included in these instruments.

COLOR FLOW PRINCIPLE

Color flow imaging uses the pulse-echo imaging principle.[3] A pulse of ultrasound is emitted from a transducer that receives the returning echoes from the tissues. Echoes returning from stationary tissues are detected and presented in gray scale in appropriate locations along the scan line. Depth is determined by echo arrival time, and brightness is determined by echo amplitude. If a returning echo has a different frequency from what was emitted, a Doppler shift (frequency change) has occurred because the echo-generating object was moving.[7] If the motion is toward or away from the transducer, the Doppler shift is positive or negative, respectively. At locations along the scan line where Doppler shifts have been detected, the sign, magnitude of the mean, and sometimes the variance are recorded. This information is used to determine the appropriate hue, saturation, and luminance of each color pixel at its location on the display. Doppler-shifted echoes can be recorded and presented at many locations along each scan line (Fig. 12-1). As in all sonography, many scan lines make up one cross-sectional image. Several images are presented each second, yielding what is commonly called *real-time sonography*. Color flow images can also be produced without using the Doppler effect. Instead, the change in echo arrival time as blood cells move closer to or farther away from the transducer is used to determine their speed of motion.

The three components of a color as presented on a display include hue, saturation, and luminance (Fig. 12-2). Hue is the color perceived. It represents the frequency of the light, with the range of frequencies detectable by the human eye ranging from the lowest (red) to the highest (violet), with increasing frequency progression through orange, yellow, green, and blue. Saturation is the amount of hue present in a mix with white (which is a combination of all visible hues). This is similar to mixing a deep color paint with white to produce a pale color (e.g., red mixed with white yields pink). The less white present, the greater the saturation, and the more white present, the less the saturation. Luminance is the brightness of the hue and saturation presented. In conventional gray-scale anatomic imaging, saturation is zero (there is no hue) and luminance represents echo amplitude. This yields gray-scale imaging, ranging from black to white through various shades of gray. In color flow imaging, various combinations of hue, saturation, and luminance are used to indicate the sign, magnitude of the mean, and sometimes the magnitude of the variance (which is a measure of the spread around the mean and therefore an indication of the extent of flow disturbance or turbulence). The mean and variance are encountered because Doppler or time shift representing flow within each sample volume is not the result of a single moving reflector (erythrocyte) but the result of many moving cells that even in normal flow, are not all moving at the same velocity (speed and direction).

This chapter is a combination, expansion, and revision of three earlier articles on the subject.[9-11] They were used as a basis for this chapter with permission. The assistance of Diane Branscome, Marge Cappuccio, Jean Ellison, Marie King, Anne Mansfield, Valerie Perry, Paul Ramsey, Pam Rowland, Dennis Shields, Jackie Sledge, Paul Tesh, and the following companies: Acuson, Advanced Technology Laboratories, Diasonics, Hewlett-Packard, Philips, and Quantum Medical Systems in obtaining scans for figures and of Kim Eldridge in manuscript preparation is gratefully acknowledged.

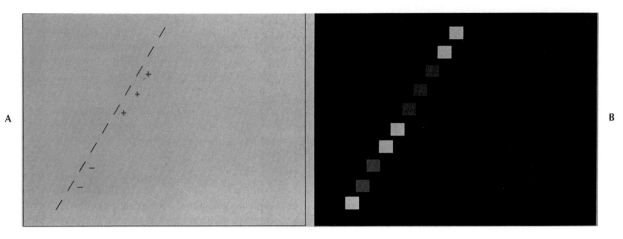

Fig. 12-1. ***A,*** Ten echoes are received as a pulse travels through tissue. Three *(red)* have positive Doppler shifts, and two *(blue)* have negative shifts. ***B,*** Doppler shifts are shown as red and blue pixels, respectively, on this color flow display. (From Kremkau FW: *Doppler ultrasound: principles and instruments,* Philadelphia, 1990, WB Saunders.)

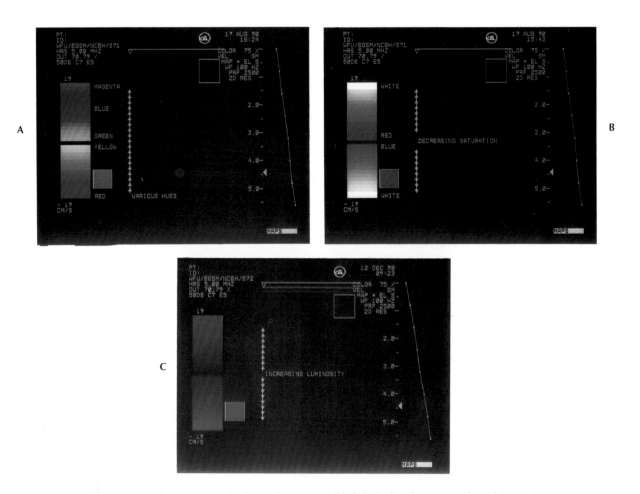

Fig. 12-2. ***A,*** Color map shows the lowest frequency visible light *(red)* and progresses through increasing frequency through yellow, green, and blue to magenta, which is a combination of red and blue. ***B,*** At the center of this bar, red and blue are shown with maximum saturation (no white added). Progressing to the upper and lower ends of the bar, saturation decreases (i.e., less red or blue and more white). ***C,*** Color map shows increasing luminance of red and blue progressing from minimum at the center of the bar to maximum at the ends. (From Kremkau FW: *J Vascular Tech* 15:104, 1991.)

DOPPLER (FREQUENCY-DOMAIN) PRINCIPLE

The *Doppler effect* is a change in frequency or wavelength of sound resulting from motion of the source of sound, the listener or receiver, or a reflector of sound. The changing pitch of an ambulance siren or truck horn as it passes is an example of the Doppler effect resulting from the motion of the sound source. Public building door openers and police radar are examples of devices that make use of the Doppler effect resulting from a moving reflector (approaching person or vehicle, respectively) of sound, infrared light, or microwave. In Doppler ultrasound medical devices, the moving reflector of sound is commonly the erythrocyte in flowing blood. If blood is approaching the transducer, the returning echoes will have a higher frequency than the emitted sound. If the blood is flowing away from the transducer, the returning echoes will have a lower frequency than the emitted sound. The difference between the emitted and received frequencies is called the *Doppler shift*. For physiologic flow speeds (typically less than 5 m/sec) and transducer frequencies (typically 2 to 10 MHz), Doppler shifts normally fall in the audible frequency range. They are consequently applied to loudspeakers or headphones to permit audible evaluation. The Doppler-shifted information is often presented visually in the form of a Doppler spectrum or in two-dimensional coded form for the color-flow instruments.[1,7] The Doppler equation describes the dependence of the Doppler shift ΔF on the speed V of the reflector, the angle θ between the reflector motion and the sound propagation direction (Doppler angle), and the transducer frequency F_0:

$$\Delta F = \frac{2VF_0\cos\theta}{C} \qquad (1)$$

where C is the speed of sound in tissues (1.54 mm/μs). The Doppler shift is proportional to the reflector speed and to the operating frequency. Its dependence on angle is not linear but rather follows the cosine of the angle, which means that for small angles there is a weak dependence on the angle, but for large angles (greater than 60°) there is a strong dependence. For conversion of Dopper shifts (what the instrument detects) to flow velocity (what is usually calibrated on the spectral axis or color bar), the Doppler angle must be known:

$$V \text{ (cm/sec)} = \frac{77 \; \Delta F \text{ (kHz)}}{F_0 \text{ (MHz)} \cos\theta} \qquad (2)$$

As the blood flow speed increases, the Doppler shift increases. The Doppler technique is so valuable because it provides flow speed information for the observer. Because the Doppler shift depends on operating frequency, it is not the same for two different instruments or transducers measuring the same blood flow at different frequencies. The higher frequency will yield a higher Doppler shift. Comparison of Doppler shifts between instruments or laboratories therefore requires a knowledge of operating frequencies. Conversion of Doppler shift information to flow velocity eliminates this difference but also requires incorporation of the operating frequency into the calculation by the instrument.

TIME-DOMAIN PRINCIPLE

Rather than using Doppler shift to identify and quantify the speed of flowing blood, another approach can be used.[18] In Fig. 12-3, a group of blood cells is shown at some location in the vessel at time t_1. At a later time (t_2), this group of cells has moved to a new position, separated from the old position by the distance d. If all the cells move together at the same velocity, the speed (V) is equal to d/T, where T is the difference between the two times ($t_2 - t_1$). When ultrasound pulses are sent into the vessel in a path parallel to the vessel walls from left to right, the echo arrival times for the two times shown in Fig. 12-3 are as illustrated in Fig. 12-4. A longer time is required for the pulse round-trip travel at time t_1 compared with that for time t_2. The difference between the two times is Δt. The instrument measures this difference in echo arrival times (Δt) observed at two different times (t_1 and t_2) to determine flow speed. From this echo arrival time difference, the flow speed is calculated as follows: The average speed of sound in soft tissues is 1.54 mm/μs, yielding the round-trip travel time of 13 μs/cm. When the round-trip

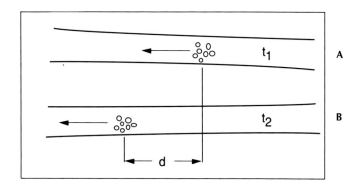

Fig. 12-3. *A,* A group of cells at a location in a vessel at time t_1. *B,* At a later time (t_2), the group has moved a distance d to a new location. (From Tegeler CH, Kremkau FW, Hitchings LP: *J Neuroimaging* 1:85, 1991).

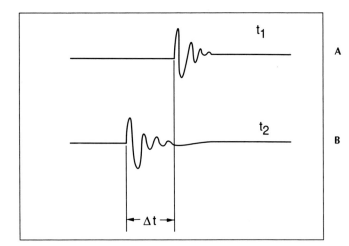

Fig. 12-4. *A,* Echo from the group of cells in Fig. 12-3, *A. B,* Echo from the group of cells in Fig. 12-3, *B,* arrives a time Δt earlier than the echo in *A.* (From Tegeler CH, Kremkau FW, Hitchings LP: *J Neuroimaging* 1:85, 1991.)

travel time is divided by this number, the result is the distance to the group of cells producing the received echo. The difference in echo arrival time (Δt) between the two times, t_1 and t_2, divided by 13 μs/cm yields the distance d, that the group of cells traveled during time T. The time T between two subsequent pulses is equal to the pulse repetition period, which is the reciprocal of the pulse repetition frequency (PRF). Distance d divided by the time difference T yields the speed V of the cell group (i.e., blood flow speed). Combining the mathematical steps described above yields the following expression:

$$V = \frac{\Delta t \times PRF}{13} \qquad (3)$$

where Δt is in μs, PRF in Hz, and V in cm/sec. If the sound beam is not parallel to the flow direction, as is common in clinical practice, the calculated flow speed will be less than the actual flow speed, with the factor being the cosine of the angle between the sound and flow directions. This angular dependence is identical to that in the Doppler equation. Thus, although the two techniques are very different, they have the same angle dependence. Incorporating angle correction yields the following equation:

$$V \,(cm/sec) = \frac{\Delta t \,(\mu s)\, PRF \,(Hz)}{13\cos\theta} \qquad (4)$$

TRANDUCERS

Color flow images are commonly produced by linear and convex sequenced arrays and phased sector arrays. A linear sequenced array is a line of rectangular transducer elements that are operated in groups (sequenced).[3,8] Each group is energized by a voltage from the pulser in the instrument, thus producing an ultrasound pulse that travels through the tissues generating a series of echoes presented as a scan line on the display. Subsequent pulses use different groups of elements shifting across the array, usually shifting by one element for each subsequent pulse. In a conventional linear array, all pulses travel out in the same direction, producing parallel scan lines on a rectangular display. The convex array sends pulses out in various directions to produce a sector display.

A phased array is a small line of rectangular elements that are energized so that the direction of the emitted pulse is determined (by phasing or delays in the voltage applied to each element.)[3,8] With larger delays the pulses are steered farther from center. With no delay the pulse travels out perpendicularly from the face of the array. Electronics in the instrument automatically adjust the delays, so each pulse travels out in a slightly different direction from the previous one. This results in an electronically steered sector image. With phased arrays, curvature can be included in the delays, giving the emitted pulse a curved wave front. This results in focusing at a specific depth that is determined by the amount of curvature. More or less curvature produces shallower or deeper focusing, respectively. This is controllable by the operator. Thus the location of the focus is electronically adjustable.

Linear array presentation of color flow information is sometimes inadequate when the vessel runs parallel to the skin surface.[7,13] The pulses (and scan lines) run perpendicular to the transducer surface (and therefore to the skin surface), resulting in a 90° angle where the pulses intersect the flow in the vessel. This would yield no Doppler or time shift and therefore no color within the vessel if the flow were parallel to the vessel walls. Two approaches have been used to avoid this situation (Fig. 12-5). A standoff wedge

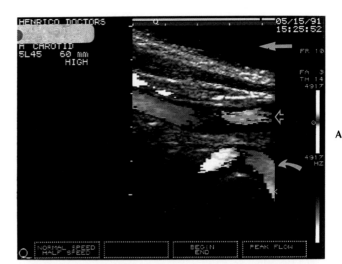

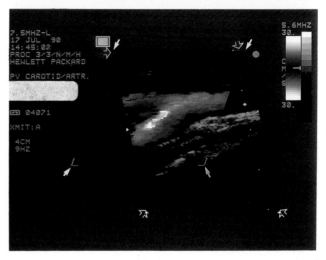

Fig. 12-5. **A,** An anechoic stand-off wedge is located between the face of the transducer and the skin line (straight arrow). This causes the pulse paths (and therefore the scan lines) to be nonperpendicular to the flow of a vessel that runs parallel to the skin. Also shown is the change of the sign of the Doppler shift (and therefore the color) that results from vessel curvature. On the right side of the carotid artery (open arrow), flow is slightly away from the transducer, whereas on the left side it is directed toward the transducer. The opposite situation is seen in the vertebral artery (curved arrow). Flow in both arteries is from right to left. **B,** A perpendicular Doppler angle is avoided by electronically steering the color-producing Doppler pulses to the left of vertical. The corners of the resulting parallelogram in which color can be displayed are shown by the solid arrows. Note that on this instrument the gray-scale anatomic imaging pulses can also be steered (in this case to the right of vertical). The corners of the resulting parallelogram are shown with open arrows.

can be placed between the transducer surface and the skin, causing the emitted pulses to travel at an angle other than perpendicular to the skin and therefore yielding an angle less than 90° for parallel vessels. Another approach is to use phasing to steer each emitted pulse from a linear sequenced array in a given direction (for example, 20° away from perpendicular). All color pulses and color scan lines are steered at this angle, resulting in a parallelogram presentation of color flow information on the display.[8,13]

INSTRUMENTS

The color flow instrument consists of a pulser, a receiver, memory, and the display (Fig. 12-6).[13] The pulser produces the electric voltages that drive the transducer array, providing appropriate sequencing and phasing to electronically scan and focus the sound beam in rectangular or sector format through the tissue cross-section. Control of output intensity, beam steering, and focal depth are accomplished through the pulser. The receiver receives the voltages that represent the echoes returning from tissue as a pulse travels. Non–Doppler-shifted echoes are processed conventionally as in any sonography instrument.[3] This includes amplification, attenuation compensation, dynamic range compression, radiofrequency to video demodulation, and threshold (rejection). The echoes then exit the receiver in the form of voltages representing echo amplitude that are stored in the memory at appropriate locations in digital form with numbers representing amplitudes.

Doppler-shifted echoes are detected in the receiver by using an autocorrelation technique that rapidly determines the mean and variance of the Doppler shift signal at each location along the scan line (at each selected echo arrival time during pulse travel). The autocorrelation technique is a mathematical process that yields the mean Doppler shift and spread around the mean (variance) for each sample time (and corresponding depth) after pulse emission. The Doppler detector yields the mean Doppler shift magnitude, sign (positive or negative), and variance for each location (Fig. 12-7). These three quantities are stored in the memory at appropriate locations corresponding to anatomic sights where Doppler shifts have been found.

The time-domain color flow instrument must determine the echo arrival time shift between subsequent pulses caused by blood flow movement between pulses. This is accomplished by a mathematical technique called *cross-correlation*. In this technique, two wave forms from subsequent pulses (Fig. 12-4) are stored, and the second is delayed a sufficient amount of time so that the two wave forms have maximum correlation (i.e., their overlapping similarity is maximum). At that point, the delay time is equal to Δt. The component of flow velocity parallel to the sound beam can then be calculated and color assignment can be made at the appropriate pixel location on the display. This is done at many locations along each scan line, resulting in a two-dimensional color representation of flow speed on the instrument display.

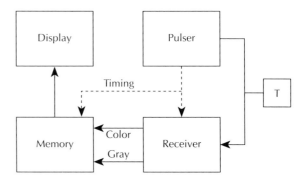

Fig. 12-6. Block diagram of a color Doppler imaging instrument. As for a gray-scale imaging instrument, pulser, receiver, memory, and display are included. However, the receiver can detect Doppler or arrival time shifts throughout the scan field. Information regarding flow is stored in memory through the color line at appropriate locations. The display shows the color flow information superimposed on the gray-scale anatomic image. (*T*, transducer.) (From Kremkau FW: *J Vascular Tech* 15:104, 1991.)

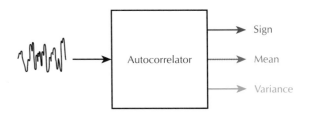

Fig. 12-7. The autocorrelator rapidly performs Doppler demodulation on the complicated echo signal (entering at left). The autocorrelator yields the sign of the mean Doppler shift, the magnitude of the mean Doppler shift, and the magnitude of the Doppler shift variance at each location in the scanned cross section. These three pieces of information are stored in each pixel location in the memory. Color assignments are appropriately made to indicate these three pieces of information two dimensionally on the display. (From Kremkau FW: *J Vascular Tech* 15:104, 1991.)

The display is a color video monitor that includes three electron guns that correspond to triple groups of color phosphor dots (red, green, blue) on the inside face of the tube. At each pixel location on the display, a gray level (brightness) appropriate to the stored number in memory is shown for each non–Doppler-shifted echo stored. Where Doppler-shifted or time-shifted echoes have been stored, a hue, saturation, and luminance appropriate to the shift information are presented according to a choice of schemes shown on the display as a color map or color bar (Fig. 12-8). The map allows the observer to interpret what the hue, saturation, and luminance mean at each location in terms of sign, magnitude, and variance of the Doppler shifts. Hue indicates sign; changes in hue, saturation, or luminance indicate increasing magnitude; and changes in hue indicate increasing variance (Fig. 12-9).

Color controls include rectangle or sector width and depth, steering angle, color inversion, wall filter, priority, baseline shift, velocity range (PRF), color map selection,

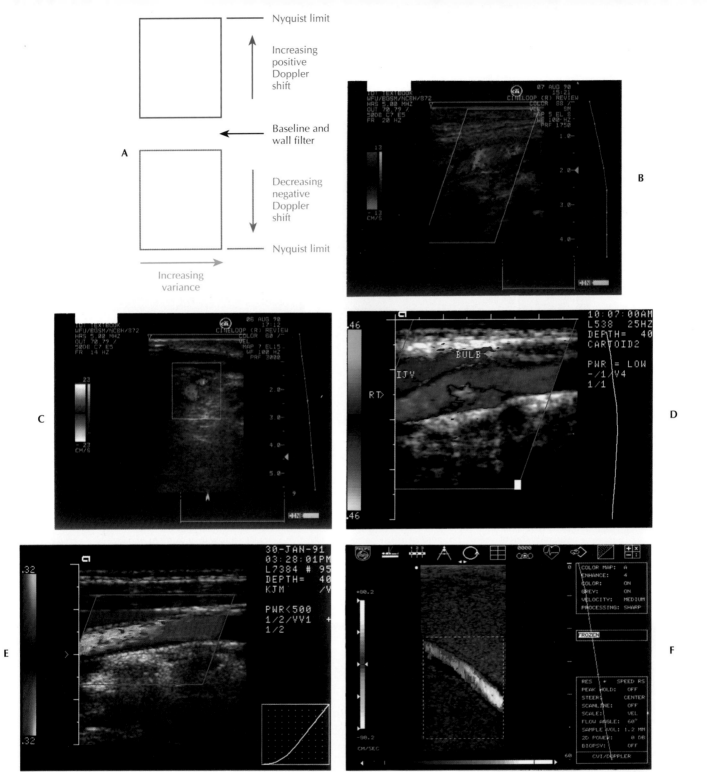

Fig. 12-8. A, The color map (color bar) indicates the color assignments for various values of Doppler shift sign, mean, and variance. Zero Doppler shift is indicated at the baseline. The wall filter eliminates small Doppler shifts in the region of the baseline to avoid clutter due to tissue and wall motion on the display. Increasing positive Doppler shifts are shown progressing upward from the baseline. Negative Doppler shifts are shown downward from the baseline. The limits of these regions are the Nyquist limit beyond which aliasing occurs. Increasing variance is shown as changing color coding from left to right on the color map. **B,** A luminance map. Increasing luminance of red and blue indicates increasing positive or negative mean Doppler shifts, respectively. **C,** A saturation map is used to show cross-sectional flow in two vessels. Flow in the upper vessel is toward the transducer, yielding positive Doppler shifts *(red)*. Flow in the lower vessel is away from the transducer, yielding negative Doppler shifts *(blue)*. Red and blue progress to white with increasing positive and negative Doppler shift means, respectively. **D,** A hue map showing flow in the carotid artery (with reversal in the bulb) and jugular vein. Increasing positive Doppler shifts progress from dark blue to bright cyan (blue and green). Increasing negative Doppler shifts progress from dark red to bright yellow (red and green). **E,** A luminance (dark blue and red to bright blue and red) map with variance included. Increasing variance adds green to red or blue (producing yellow or cyan) from left to right across the map. **F,** A saturation map on an instrument that detects echo arrival time shifts rather than Doppler shifts to generate a color flow display. Red and blue progress toward white as positive and negative time shifts increase. (From Kremkau FW: *J Vascular Tech* 15:104, 1991.)

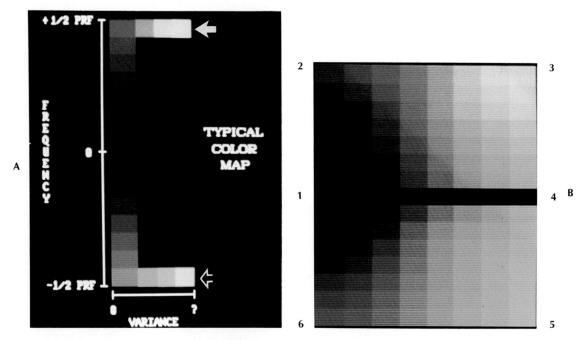

Fig. 12-9. *A,* Increasing positive Doppler shifts progress from black to bright red and negative shifts from black to bright blue (luminance map). Increasing variance for maximum Doppler shift is shown to progress to yellow and cyan for positive and negative Doppler shifts, respectively. Increasing amounts of green are added to red or blue as variance increases. *B,* The various hues and luminances resulting from a combination of red and blue luminance maps for positive and negative increasing means, respectively, and increasing green for increasing variance. (*1,* Zero Doppler shift and variance [black]; *2,* maximum positive Doppler shift with zero variance [bright red]; *3,* maximum positive Doppler shift with maximum variance [bright yellow]; *4,* zero or small positive or negative Doppler shift with maximum variance [green]; *5,* maximum negative Doppler shift with maximum variance [bright cyan]; *6,* maximum negative Doppler shift with zero variance [bright blue].) (From Kremkau FW: *J Vascular Tech* 15:104, 1991.)

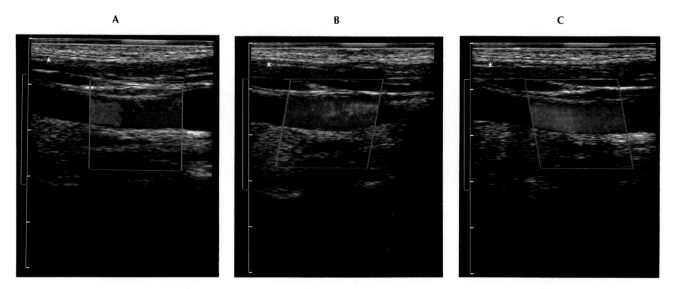

Fig. 12-10. Common carotid arterial flow. Color scan lines are directed, *A,* vertically, *B,* to the left of vertical, and, *C,* to the right of vertical. Flow is from left to right, producing positive and negative Doppler shifts depending on the relationship between scan lines and flow. (From Kremkau FW: *Semin Roentgenol* 27:6, 1992.)

variance, smoothing, and ensemble lengths.[13] Steering angle control avoids 90° angles (Fig. 12-10). Color inversion alternates the color assignments above and below the baseline on the color map (Fig. 12-11). The wall filter eliminates clutter caused by tissue and wall motion (Fig. 12-12). However, care must be taken not to set the wall filter setting too high or slower blood flow signals will be removed. Color

velocity range sets the Nyquist limit at the color bar extremes. Decreasing the value permits observation of slower flows (smaller Doppler shifts) but increases the probability of aliasing for faster flows.[13] Color priority determines the level at which color will be shown instead of gray.[13] Baseline control allows shifting up or down to scroll in a manner similar to that done in spectral displays to eliminate alias-

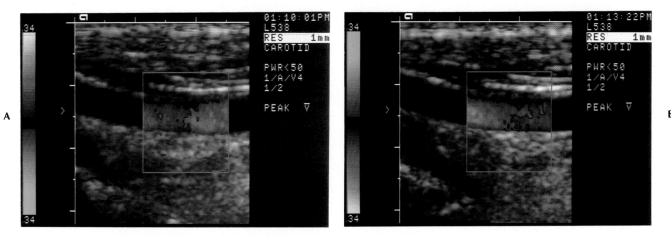

Fig. 12-11. *A,* Red and blue are assigned to positive and negative Doppler shifts, respectively, progressing to yellow and cyan at the Nyquist limits. This is a common color assignment. *B,* The color assignments are reversed.

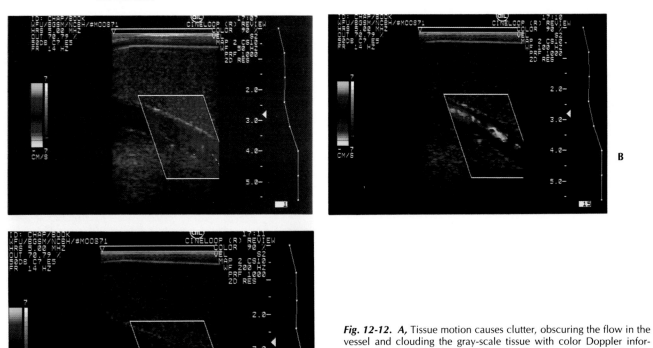

Fig. 12-12. *A,* Tissue motion causes clutter, obscuring the flow in the vessel and clouding the gray-scale tissue with color Doppler information. *B,* Wall filter has been increased to 100 Hz, eliminating the color clutter. *C,* Wall filter has been increased to 200 Hz, eliminating virtually all color flow information in the vessel.

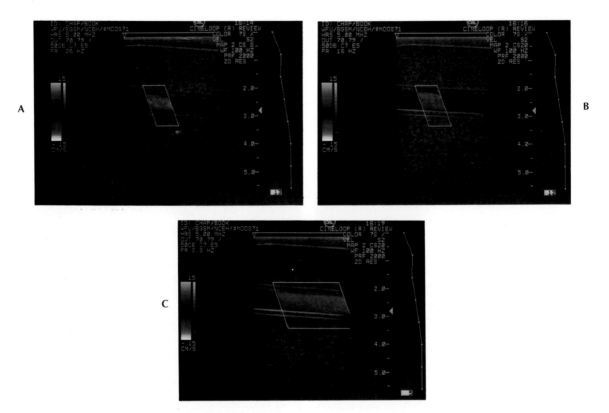

Fig. 12-13. *A,* A relatively high frame rate (26 Hz) is achieved with a small ensemble length and a narrow color box (8 mm). *B,* With ensemble length increased to 20, the frame rate is reduced to 16 Hz. *C,* Maintaining the high ensemble length and increasing the color box width to 25 mm decreases the frame rate to 8.8 Hz.

ing.[13] Smoothing provides frame-to-frame averaging to fill in missing pixels and provide a smoother image.[13] Ensemble length is the number of pulses required for each color scan line. The minimum is 3, with values of 8 to 20 being common. Larger ensemble lengths provide better detection of slow flows and complete representation of flow within a vessel (Fig. 12-13) but at the expense of longer time and therefore lower frame rates. Wider color boxes (viewing areas) also reduce frame rates because more pulses (and scan lines) per frame are required (Fig. 12-13).

PITFALLS

Several aspects of color flow imaging are limiting, including lack of complete spectral information, angle dependence, and lower frame rates. Spectral Doppler presents the entire range of Doppler shift frequencies received as they change over the cardiac cycle (Fig. 12-14). Color Doppler displays can only present statistical representations of the complete spectrum at each pixel location on the display. The sign, mean value, and possibly the variance of the spectrum are color coded into combinations of hue, saturation, and luminance presented at each display pixel location. Some Doppler instruments provide the capability to read out the quantitative digital values for the mean Doppler shift at chosen pixel locations (Fig. 12-15). These mean values are different than the peak systolic values that are commonly used in evaluating spectral displays (Fig. 12-14). Turbu-

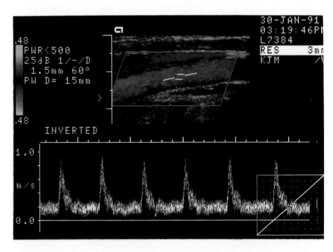

Fig. 12-14. The spectral display shows the complete range of Doppler shift frequencies present at each instant and how it varies over the cardiac cycle. The corresponding color presented at the spectral gate location *(dark red)* can only show a statistical representation of the spectrum (mean and in same cases variance).

lence causes increasing weighting of lower Doppler shifts, thus reducing the mean Doppler shift. The peak is unchanged in the presence of turbulence as observed on a spectral display. However, in the color flow display, the mean is reduced in the presence of turbulence. Time-domain techniques do provide peak and spectral information that can be shown on conventional flow speed versus time plots

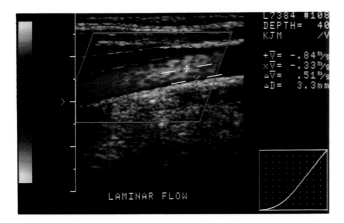

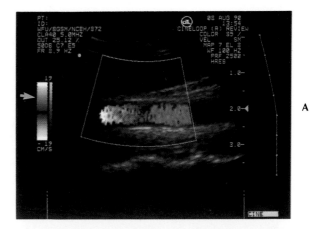

Fig. 12-15. Digital readout of stored mean Doppler shift (converted to mean flow speed) at specific pixel locations. Conversion to speed requires angle correction just as in spectral Doppler techniques. The value at the vessel center (+) is greater than at the edge (x), as expected for laminar flow. (From Kremkau FW: *Semin Roentgenol* 27:6, 1992.

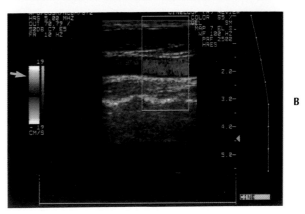

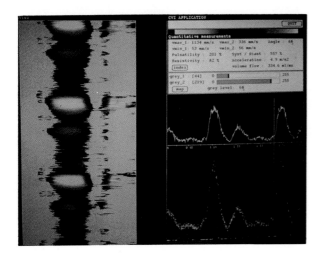

Fig. 12-16. Peak, spectral, and volume flow rate information derived from time-domain color flow information.

Fig. 12-17. *A,* Flow from right to left in the carotid artery experiences a color change because Doppler pulses are sent out in various directions from the convex array transducer. The scan lines on the right are viewing the flow upsteam; those on the left are viewing it downstream. *B,* Flow is from right to left again, but the color change occurred because of slight curvature of the vessel (it is convex up). With this linear array transducer, all pulses and scan lines are directed vertically down.

(Fig. 12-16). These can be converted through calculation to volume flow rate versus time plots (Fig. 12-16).[18]

Color flow techniques have cosine angle dependence just as spectral Doppler techniques do. Thus the colors shown on the display are angle dependent. Fig. 12-17 shows color changes resulting from different pulse vectors (sector image) and different blood flow vectors (curving vessels). In Fig. 12-17, where blood flow is from right to left toward the head in the carotid artery, both show blue on the right and red on the left, seemingly consistent. However, the color bar in *B* is the reverse of that in *A*. How is this apparent contradiction explained? The color change in *A* is caused by the changing Doppler angle resulting from the changing pulse directions across the sector scan. The pulses in the right-hand portion are looking upstream (positive Doppler shifts), whereas those in the left are looking downstream (negative Doppler shifts). In Fig. 12-17, *B*, the pulses all

travel in the same direction (straight down), so the color change is caused by vessel curvature (the vessel is slightly convex up within the color box). Thus on the right-hand side, blood flow is slightly away from the transducer, whereas on the left, it is slightly toward the transducer.

Because color flow techniques require several pulses per scan line (as opposed to one pulse per scan line for single-focus, gray-scale anatomic imaging), frame rates are generally lower than those for comparable depth gray-scale anatomic imaging. If the frame rate is low enough, as in Fig. 12-18, a significant portion of the cardiac cycle is represented across the color image from left to right. In Fig. 12-18 the time across the color box represents about 15% of the cardiac cycle. The bright portion represents the largest Doppler shifts, but these are not a result of a region where the Doppler angle is the smallest (the Doppler angle is approximately constant across the color box in this example) or where there is vessel narrowing (there is none in this example). Here, the bright region represents the largest Doppler shifts at peak systole, with the darker red to the

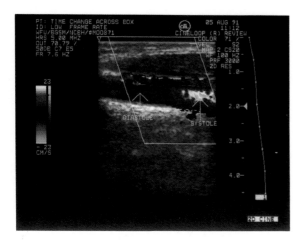

Fig. 12-18. A frame of color flow information generated at a low frame rate (7.6 Hz). A significant portion of the cardiac cycle is represented across this frame from left to right showing late diastole progressing to peak systole.

left representing late diastole and early systole. In such a case, the single frame being viewed is not a representation of the flow at an instant in time. In fact, it is a representation of flow at various instants in time over a significant portion of the cardiac cycle from left to right across the box.

Artifacts that occur with Doppler color flow imaging are color presentations of artifacts traditionally seen in gray-scale imaging and Doppler spectral displays.[7,14] Several artifacts are encountered in Doppler ultrasound. The most common incorrect presentation of Doppler flow information is aliasing.[4-7] However, other artifacts occur, including range ambiguity, anatomic mirror image, spectrum mirror image, Doppler angle effects, grating lobes, shadowing (Fig. 12-19), clutter (Fig. 12-12), and others (Fig. 12-20).[2,7,15-17] Aliasing occurs when the Doppler shift exceeds the Nyquist limit. The result is incorrect flow direction on the color flow image (Fig. 12-21). Increasing the flow speed range (which is actually an increase in PRF) can solve the problem (Fig. 12-22). However, too high a range can cause loss of flow information, particularly if the wall filter is set high (Figs. 12-12, *D*, and 12-22, *D, E*). Too high a range can also cause range ambiguity that places echoes and Doppler gates in incorrect depth locations.[2] Baseline shifting can decrease or eliminate aliasing (Fig. 12-22, *C*) as in spectral displays.

In the mirror artifact (Fig. 12-23), an image of a vessel and source of Doppler-shifted echoes can be duplicated on the opposite side of a strong reflector (e.g., pleura, diaphragm). Array grating lobes[3] can produce Doppler information of incorrect sign and incorrect locations (Fig. 12-24, *A*). Shadowing can weaken or eliminate Doppler-shifted echoes beyond the shadowing object (Fig. 12-24, *B*). Clutter results from tissue, heart, or vessel wall motion (Fig. 12-12) and is eliminated by wall filters. Doppler angle effects include zero Doppler shift when the Doppler angle is 90° and the change of color in a straight vessel viewed with a sector transducer (Fig. 12-25). These artifacts can hinder proper interpretation and diagnosis and must be avoided or properly handled when encountered.

Text continued on p. 105.

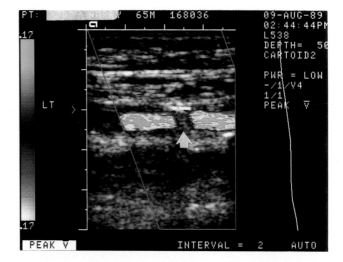

Fig. 12-19. Aliased flow in a vertebral artery. A spinous process shadows part of the flow *(arrow)*.

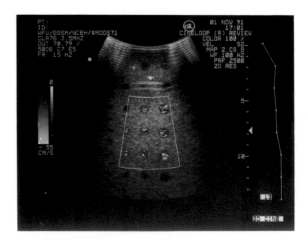

Fig. 12-20. Color flow appears in echo-free (cystic) regions of a tissue-equivalent phantom. The color gain has been increased sufficiently to produce this effect. The instrument tends to write color information preferentially in areas where non-Doppler–shifted echoes are weak or absent.

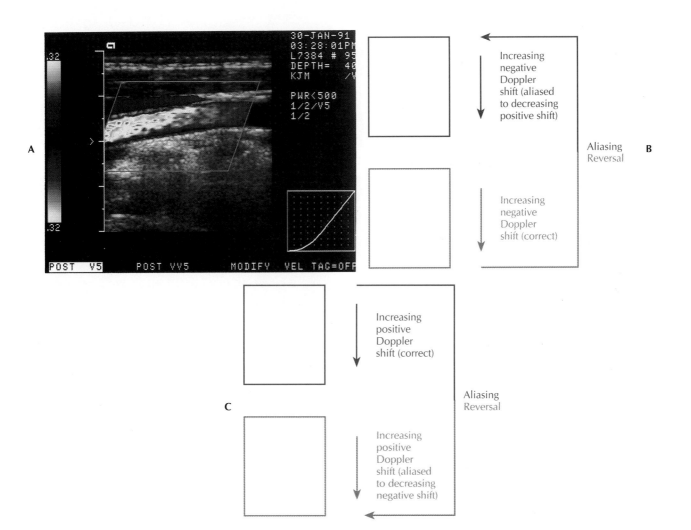

Fig. 12-21. *A,* Positive (blue) Doppler shifts. These are actually negative Doppler shifts that have exceeded the lower Nyquist limit (−0.32 m/sec) and wrapped around to the positive portion of the color bar, *B.* Positive shifts that exceed the +0.32 m/sec limit would alias to the negative side, *C.*

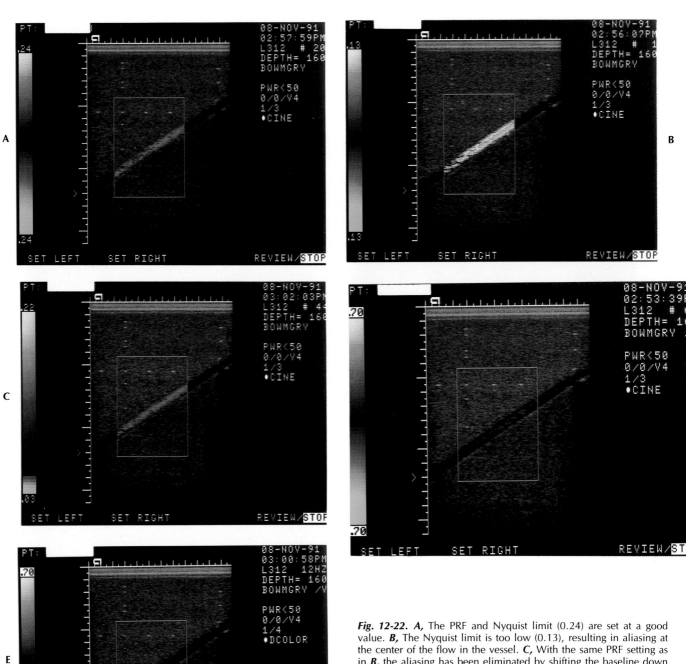

Fig. 12-22. *A,* The PRF and Nyquist limit (0.24) are set at a good value. *B,* The Nyquist limit is too low (0.13), resulting in aliasing at the center of the flow in the vessel. *C,* With the same PRF setting as in *B,* the aliasing has been eliminated by shifting the baseline down 0.10 cm/sec below the center of the color bar. *D,* The Nyquist limit setting (0.70) is too high causing the detected Doppler shifts to be well down the positive scale and producing a dark red appearance. *E,* With the Nyquist limit set as in *D,* an increase in the wall filter setting elimates what little color flow information there was in *D.*

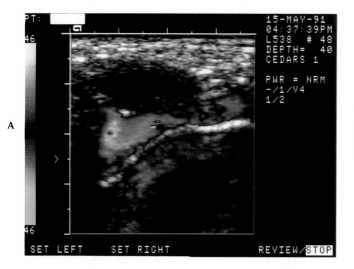
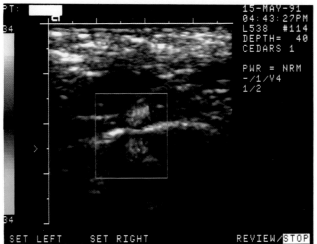
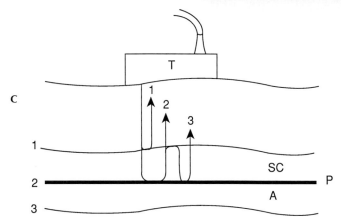

Fig. 12-23. Mirror image of the subclavian artery inferior to the pleura. **A,** Longitudinal view. **B,** Transverse view. **C,** Multiple reflections producing mirror image. Paths 1 and 2 are legitimate, but Path 3 arrives late and produces the artifactual deep arterial wall.

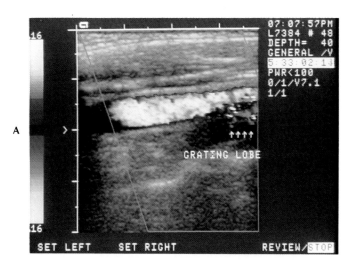
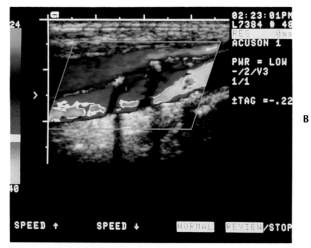

Fig. 12-24. A, Doppler-shifted echoes of different color *(blue)* are a result of grating lobes that are viewing the flow downstream. **B,** Shadowing from calcified plaque follows the gray-scale scan lines straight down while following the angled color scan lines parallel to the sides of the parallelogram. (From Kremkau FW: *Principles and instrumentation.* In Merritt CRB, ed: *Doppler color flow imaging,* New York, 1992, Churchill Livingstone.)

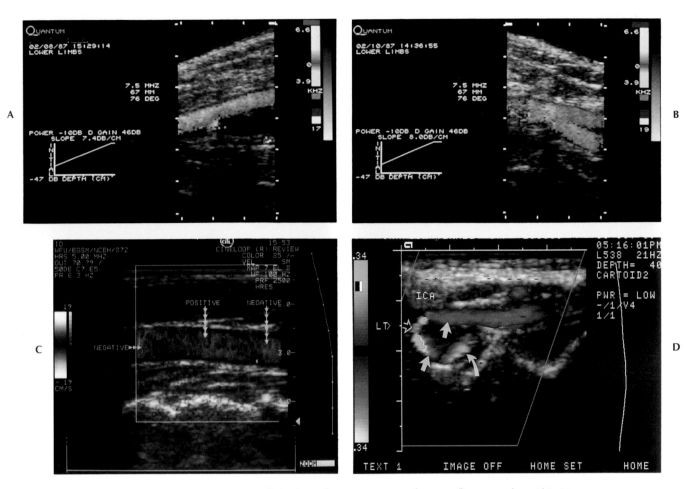

Fig. 12-25. A, Profunda branch off the femoral artery appears to have no flow (no color within it). **B,** This view of the profunda shows color flow within it. The 90° Doppler angle in **A** causes no Doppler shift and lack of color. (**A, B,** From Kremkau FW: *Doppler ultrasound: principles and instruments,* Philadelphia, 1990, WB Saunders.) **C,** All scan lines from this linear array are directed vertically down. Slight curvature of this vessel (concave up on the right and convex up on the left) produces flow slightly away *(blue)* and slightly toward *(red)* in three regions. Positive and negative Doppler shifts are indicated. (From Kremkau FW: *J Vascular Tech* 15:104, 1991.) **D,** In a tortuous internal carotid artery, negative Doppler shifts are indicated in the *red* regions *(solid straight arrows)*. Two regions of positive Doppler shifts *(blue)* are seen *(open arrow* and *curved arrow)*. In the latter, legitimate flow toward the transducer is indicated. In the former, the flow away from the transducer has yielded high Doppler shifts (because of a small Doppler angle, i.e., flow is approximately parallel to scan lines), which produces a color shift to the opposite side of the map due to aliasing. The boundaries from and to normal positive Doppler shifts into and out of the aliased region are *bright yellow* and *cyan* from the ends of the color bars. The transition from unaliased negative Doppler shift into unaliased positive Doppler shift (near the bottom) is *black,* representing the baseline of the color bar. (From Kremkau FW: *J Vascular Tech* 15:265, 1991.)

CONCLUSION

Doppler color flow imaging acquires Doppler-shifted or time-shifted echoes from a cross-section of tissue scanned by an ultrasound beam. These echoes are presented in color and superimposed on the gray-scale anatomic image of non-shifted echoes that were received during the scan. The flow echoes are assigned colors according to the color map chosen. Several pulses (the number is called the *ensemble length*) are needed to generate a color scan line. Linear, convex, and phased arrays are used to acquire the gray-scale and color flow information. Color controls include gain, map selection, variance on/off, persistence, ensemble length, color/gray priority, Nyquist limit (PRF), baseline shift, wall filter, and color window angle, location, and size. Doppler color flow instruments are pulsed Doppler instruments and are subject to the same limitations (e.g., Doppler angle dependence and aliasing) as other Doppler instruments. Time-shift instruments have the same angle dependence. Other artifacts include range ambiguity, mirror image, grating lobes, shadowing, and clutter.

REFERENCES

1. Evans DH et al: Doppler ultrasound physics, instrumentation, and clinical applications, New York, 1989, John Wiley & Sons.
2. Gill RW et al: New class of pulsed Doppler US ambiguity at short ranges, *Radiology* 173:272-275, 1989.
3. Kremkau FW: *Diagnostic ultrasound: principles and instruments,* ed 4, Philadelphia, 1993, WB Saunders.
4. Kremkau FW: Doppler artifacts I, *J Vascular Tech* 14(1):41-142, 1990.
5. Kremkau FW: Doppler artifacts II, *J Vascular Tech* 14(3):123-124, 1990.
6. Kremkau FW: Doppler artifacts III, *J Vascular Tech* 14(5):239-240, 1990.
7. Kremkau FW: *Doppler ultrasound: principles and instruments,* Philadelphia, 1990, WB Saunders.
8. Kremkau FW: Modern transducer terminology, *J Diag Med Sonography* 5:293-295, 1990.
9. Kremkau FW: Color-flow assignments (I), *J Vascular Tech* 15(5):265-266, 1991.
10. Kremkau FW: Color-flow assignments (II), *J Vascular Tech* 15(6):325-326, 1991.
11. Kremkau FW: Principles of color flow imaging, *J Vascular Tech* 15(3):104-111, 1991.
12. Kremkau FW: Doppler principles, *Semin Roentgenol* 27(1):6-16, 1992.
13. Kremkau FW: *Principles and instrumentation.* In Merritt CRB, ed: *Doppler color flow imaging,* New York, 1992, Churchill Livingstone.
14. Kremkau FW, Taylor KJW: Artifacts in ultrasound imaging, *J Ultrasound Med* 5:227-237, 1986.
15. Middleton WD, Erickson S, Melson GL: Perivascular color artifact: pathologic significance and appearance on color Doppler US images, *Radiology* 171:647-652, 1989.
16. Mitchell DG, Burns P, Needleman L: Color Doppler artifact in anechoic regions, *J Ultrasound Med* 9:255-260, 1990.
17. Reading CC et al: Color and spectral Doppler mirror-image artifact of the subclavian artery, *Radiology* 174:41-42, 1990.
18. Tegeler CH, Kremkau FW, Hitchings LP: Color velocity imaging: introduction to a new ultrasound technology, *J Neuroimaging* 1(2):85-90, 1991.

CHAPTER 13

Strategies of color coding

KIRK W. BEACH

A two-dimensional color Doppler image consists of a set of rows and columns of squares. Each square contains either a color or a brightness in the gray scale from black to white. The color in each box represents the blood velocity in a corresponding region of the examination plane in the body. The possible velocities range from 4 to 256. Each range is assigned a color, depending on the speed and direction. Bluish colors have been used to indicate velocities approaching the ultrasound scan head and reddish colors to indicate velocities receding from the ultrasound scan head. The opposite assignment can be used, since the color designation is arbitrary and depends on the preference of the examiner.

Blood velocity can be determined and displayed in several ways with the use of pulsed ultrasound and associated methods. This chapter provides a historical review of display methods and discusses three methods for determining blood velocity: direct Doppler autocorrelation, time domain, and mean spectral fast Fourier transform (FFT) Doppler. Finally, the ultrasound echo signals that are subject to analysis are explored.

SELECTING INFORMATION FOR DISPLAY

Blood velocity information detected by Doppler can be communicated audibly or visually; can be formated to factor, select, or combine information on time in the cardiac cycle; and can be presented in a form that selects or combines locations from a region in space, differentiating the dimension of longitudinal location from the two dimensions of cross section. Blood flow information that is displayed is usually restricted to a particular range of magnitudes and a particular directional component of the velocity vector. Two ways to characterize the Doppler frequency are by indicating the strength of each frequency present (the spectrum of frequencies) and by showing a single characteristic frequency with other descriptive statistics. Most changes in display methods and formats have resulted from changes in technology and not because of striving for the best way to show the aspects of blood flow that are most pertinent to correct diagnosis.

Display methods are shown in Table 13-1. From 1965 to 1990, commercialized Doppler displays have exhibited (1) audio signals, (2) black and white graphs, (3) color

photographs, (4) gray-scale images on printed screens or on paper, and (5) color video that can be moved through time (in a cine-loop). The Doppler information displayed has varied; all, some, and no frequencies have been shown. Display types have also varied. The Doppler waveform shows the cardiac cycle as a graph of time versus one Doppler frequency. The flow mapping systems show two-dimensional images of arteries but report only the highest forward frequencies in the cardiac cycle. The Dopscan and Arteriograph show forward flow as absent in black and present in white. The EchoFlow shows absent forward flow as black, slow flow as red, moderate flow as yellow, and fast flow as blue. The Doppler histogram shows a combined spectrum of all frequencies in the cardiac cycle without regard to time. The color M-mode or displacement M-mode shows a single Doppler frequency at multiple depths as a function of time in the cardiac cycle. Spectral waveforms show all Doppler frequencies at one depth as a function of time in the cardiac cycle. Two-dimensional color Doppler images attempt to show only one characteristic Doppler frequency at one moment in the cardiac cycle. Current two-dimensional color Doppler displays do not show time in the cardiac cycle in an easily understandable form.

REAL-TIME COLOR FLOW IMAGING

A color flow image is formed by moving the ultrasound beam pattern across the region of interest from right to left. Color flow data are displayed as the beam pattern moves. All objects in the region of interest must be stationary to obtain a two-dimensional image without distortion. In a typical image, the color scan line moves across the image at a speed of 45 cm/sec. During image acquisition the pulse may travel through an artery in the region of interest and will move at a speed of 1000 cm/sec in a young, normal patient. Because the entire image width is not acquired simultaneously, the pulse is smeared onto the image. The right edge of the two-dimensional color flow image is often acquired before the onset of systole, and the left edge at peak systole; in this case, the systolic upslope is smeared across the image from right to left.

Although modern color flow imaging systems are said to operate in real time, considerable caution must be used. Faster frame rates make motion appear smooth—an aspect

Table 13-1. Characteristics of Doppler frequency displays

Type	Display	Frequency display	Time character	Spatial character
CW[2,4,6,7]	Audio	All	Temporal*	Region
Pulsed	Audio	All	Temporal*	1 Point
Inst Mean[5]	2-D chart	One	Time waveform†	Region
TIH	2-D chart	All	Time waveform†	1 Point
Flow map[3,8,9]	2-D color	2-4 Level overwrite	Peak overwrite‡	2-D map
Histograph	2-D chart	All	Time average§	Region
Spectral	2-D gray	All	Time waveform†	1 Point
M-color[1]	2-D color	One +	Time waveform†	1-D
2-D color[1]	2-D color	One +	Haphazard-cine‖	2-D map

CW, Continuous wave; *TIH*, time interval histogram.
*Display is shown in real time.
†Time is shown as the horizontal distance on the image.
‡Each pixel is brightened or colored according to the greatest Doppler frequency (or echo intensity) found corresponding to that pixel.
§A spectrum of all frequencies present in the Doppler signal over a period is shown. Systolic and diastolic Doppler frequencies are mixed in the display.
‖Different portions of the image are taken at different times, and relating a particular color region on the image to an event in the cardiac cycle is difficult.

of perception called the *flicker fusion rate of the eye*. Although the observation of motion in real-time color displays is considered a diagnostic advantage, some examiners believe that the flashes of color are confusing. These flashes sometimes move in directions opposite to the direction of blood flow. Usually, color changes from frame to frame are so great that it is not possible to relate the colors in adjacent frames. Because of these factors, the real-time display may not contribute to better diagnosis.

GOALS FOR BLOOD VELOCITY MEASUREMENT

Although there have been many changes in Doppler measurements, the goals of the techniques in vascular diagnosis have not been definitively set. The most modest goal is to establish the presence or absence of flow in blood vessels. To verify the correct diagnosis of an occluded vessel, the examiner must be certain that a vessel (rather than some other structure) is being interrogated and that the Doppler system has sufficient sensitivity under the operating conditions to detect minimal flow. Ensuring that the vessel rather than some other structure is interrogated is easy if the occlusion is caused by a removable blood pressure cuff; the return of flow when the cuff is released verifies the anatomy. A vessel occluded by intraluminal thrombus must be identified by anatomic clues.

A second goal of Doppler blood flow measurements is to determine whether the velocity has changed, and if so, how much. The change may be between systole and diastole as seen in Doppler waveform analysis, or the change may be in systolic Doppler frequency detected by comparing one location with another.

Doppler waveform analysis has also been used to compute pulsatility indices, which can identify high proximal arterial resistance or low distal arterial resistance. A high diastolic/systolic Doppler frequency (velocity) ratio indicates a low distal vascular resistance and possibly high proximal vascular resistance. In carotid and renal arteries, a high diastolic/systolic ratio is a normal pattern; in femoral or

iliac arteries, a high diastolic/systolic ratio indicates a proximal stenosis or distal hyperemia.* Modern two-dimensional color Doppler imaging systems are not set up to show pulsatility conveniently. A measure of pulsatility requires the comparison of the systolic velocity from a Doppler sample volume with the corresponding diastolic velocity available 0.5 seconds later. Because the two measurements are not easily quantified or available simultaneously, any comparison requires a heroic effort.

Doppler systems can be used for venous waveform analysis. In the patient whose legs are supine, venous velocities in the legs are expected to decrease with respiratory inspiration because of the venous obstructive effect of the associated increase in intraabdominal pressure; a constant venous signal is consistent with venous obstruction. Confirmation of these effects is not easily recorded when color flow imaging is used. Such comparison would require a kinetic videotaped image with a physiologic tracing of respiration.

A change in velocity between two locations along the axis of an artery can be shown directly on a color flow image. An increased systolic velocity in one region of an artery compared with an adjacent region often indicates a stenosis near the region of increased velocity. Because measurements are taken in a series and compared within the series, absolute numbers are not required, nor is it necessary to know the relationship between the Doppler frequency shift and the blood velocity. Most vascular Doppler work requires this level of quantitation. This measurement is confounded if the series of measurements in the image represent different time periods in the cardiac cycle.

More difficult goals involve using the Doppler frequency shift to determine quantitative parameters of blood flow.

---

*The diastolic/systolic ratio is preferred over the systolic/diastolic ratio because the former has a value range between -1 and 1. The systolic/diastolic ratio may take the value infinity (if D is 0) before taking the value of negative infinity (if D becomes less than 0).

These include determining the volumetric flow rate, the percentage of area reduction of a stenosis from the prestenotic Doppler frequency and the intrastenotic Doppler frequency (this computation is related to volumetric flow), the kinetic energy of blood and the associated pressure drop in a stenosis, the shape of the blood velocity profile, and the shear rate on the vessel wall.

By using a Doppler angle of 0° to the axis of an aortic stenosis jet and the maximum peak velocity measured on spectral waveform analysis, cardiologists have determined the kinetic energy of blood in the jet and the associated pressure drop across the aortic valve; by using a Doppler angle of 0° to the axis of the aortic outflow tract and the mean velocity integral from a spectral waveform times the cross-sectional area of the tract, cardiologists have determined the volumetric flow rate (cardiac output) through the aortic valve.

VELOCITY INFORMATION FROM ULTRASOUND

The Doppler equation that relates velocity to Doppler frequency has been quoted in almost all material written on the subject. Several methods now exist for extracting velocity data from ultrasound echoes. One new method, time-domain analysis, is considered to be different from Doppler echocardiography. A derivation here identifies the fundamental similarities and differences among the methods in blood velocity measurements.

Speed (S) is the ratio of distance traveled (da) to time of travel (dt):

$$S = \frac{da}{dt} \tag{1}$$

All methods of blood velocity measurement are based on this relationship. The object that is traveling is a cluster of erythrocytes. This unique cluster provides a signature in the radiofrequency echo that can be identified and located on each of a series of pulse-echo cycles, which allows changes in the location of the cluster to be tracked. Most methods in use are limited to measuring the change in location along the ultrasound beam, that is, the change in the distance from the ultrasound transducer to the cluster of erythrocytes. These methods include the time-domain and Doppler methods. One new method, tracking the movement of speckle signature of the cluster on a two-dimensional B-mode image, can measure the complete vector in the plane of the image. The following discussion covers the Doppler and time-domain methods but could be extended to the speckle tracking methods.

S in equation 1 is the speed at which the blood approaches (or recedes from) the ultrasound transducer along the direction of the ultrasound beam. The blood velocity is directed along the velocity vector stream line at some angle to the ultrasound beam. Thus only a fractional component of the velocity magnitude contributes to the Doppler frequency measurement. If a right triangle is formed by using the velocity vector *V* as the hypotenuse, using the line of

the ultrasound beam to form the adjacent side *S*, and using the angle between them as the angle *θ*, *S* is the component of the velocity along the ultrasound beam that contributes to the measurement:

$$\frac{S}{V} = \cos\theta \text{ or } S = V \cos\theta \tag{2}$$

where *θ* is the angle between the ultrasound beam and the velocity vector.

By combining equations 1 and 2, the following equations are obtained:

$$S = \frac{da}{dt} = V \cos\theta \tag{3}$$

or:

$$V = \frac{S}{\cos\theta} = \frac{1}{\cos\theta} \times \frac{da}{dt} \tag{4}$$

The time over which the measurement is made *(dt)* depends on the measurement method but is never shorter than the interval between ultrasound pulse-echo cycles, which may range from 0.02 ms (20 μs) to 1 ms, and is never longer than the period of the lowest audible frequency, 50 ms (20 Hz is the lowest audible frequency). The distance that the cluster of erythrocytes has traveled cannot be determined directly. The signature of the cluster is identified in one pulse-echo cycle at time representing one depth and in another pulse-echo cycle at a slightly different time representing another depth. The distance *(da)* traveled by the cluster in the interval time *(dt)* ranges about from −0.2 mm through 0 to +0.2 mm. If the cluster of erythrocytes has moved to a location in blood that is 0.1 mm (da) farther from the ultrasound transducer between the first pulse-echo cycle and the second, the signature of that cluster arrives 0.1274 μs later (de) after the second transmit pulse than it did after the first.

$$de = \frac{2 \times \text{Depth change}}{\text{Speed of ultrasound in blood}} = \frac{2 \times da}{C} \tag{5}$$

where *C* is 157,000 cm/sec, the speed of ultrasound in blood and *de* is the difference in arrival time of the echo signature.

$$da = \frac{C \times de}{2} \tag{6}$$

Substituting equation 6 into equation 4 provides the equation that is the basis for both time-domain and Doppler blood velocity measurement.

$$V = \frac{1}{\cos\theta} \times \frac{C}{2} \times \frac{de}{dt} \tag{7}$$

In a time-domain system, *de* is measured directly by comparing the echo received from the depth of interest after the initial transmit pulse, with the similar echo received after a subsequent transmit pulse. In signal processing the initial echo is displaced in time until the best alignment with the subsequent echo is achieved; the displacement required is *de*. In a Doppler system *de* is determined by comparing each echo with a reference signal derived from the transmitted ultrasound frequency (F_o). The time relationship between the echo and the reference is called the *phase*. It is a fraction of the period of the transmitted ultrasound wave. The value of *de* is determined by taking the difference between the phase of the initial echo and a subsequent echo and multiplying by the period of the ultrasound frequency. The period of the ultrasound frequency is equal to 1 divided by the frequency.

In Doppler examination:

$$de = \frac{1}{F_0} \times d\phi \qquad (8)$$

Substituting equation 8 into equation 7 yields:

$$V = \frac{1}{\cos\theta} \times \frac{C}{2} \times \frac{1}{F_0} \times \frac{d\phi}{dt} \qquad (9)$$

The Doppler frequency (ΔF) that is heard is equal to $d\phi/dt$. Therefore:

$$V = \frac{1}{\cos\theta} \times \frac{C}{2} \times \frac{\Delta F}{F_0} \qquad (10)$$

which can be rearranged to the conventional Doppler equation:

$$\Delta F = \frac{2F_0 \times V \times \cos\theta}{C} \qquad (11)$$

Blood velocity measurements made by the time-domain method and those made by the Doppler method are similar; the methods differ only in the way that they determine the distance traveled by the echo signature of the erythrocyte cluster. All the methods compute the distance the blood has traveled in the direction of the ultrasound scan lines *(da)* over a time interval *(dt)*. In some systems a fixed change in *da* is detected and *dt* is measured; in other systems a fixed change in *dt* is selected and *da* is measured. (The selected and detected variables are shown in Table 13-2.) The biphasic zero-crossing detector begins the time interval measurement when the erythrocyte cluster passes a predetermined starting depth and ends the time measurement when the erythrocyte cluster passes a depth one-half wavelength greater than the starting depth. Spectrum analyzers monitor the echoes for a fixed period and then determine how many erythrocyte clusters have had depth changes within a set of 64 or 128 predetermined ranges. The result of each test is shown as a spectrum of blood velocities. Most color Doppler velocity instruments use autocorrelation detectors; these measure the distance traveled by an erythrocyte cluster for a fixed short period.

Blood speed varies from a minimum of approximately 1 cm/sec to a maximum of 550 cm/sec. For vessels shallower than 3 cm, the ultrasound pulse interval (1/PRF) is about 50 µs (1/20 KHz). For the deepest vessels (15 cm), the ultrasound pulse interval is 200 µs. Acceleration times at the onset of systole can be as short as 50 ms. Thus the measurement interval for the displacement measurement *dt* ranges between 50 µs and 50 ms. The human hearing range varies from 15,000 Hz (a period of 66 µs) to 20 Hz (a period of 50 ms).

Table 13-3 shows the technical problems associated with

Table 13-2. Methods of speed detection

Method	Benchmark	Variable measured
Audio frequency zero crosser	da = L/2	dt
FFT spectral waveform	dt = 0.01 sec*	P in N × da†
Autocorrelation Doppler	dt = (M−1)/PRF = 0.001 sec*	da†
Time domain	dt = 4/PRF = 0.0004 sec*	da

L, Ultrasound wavelength (C/F_o); C, speed of ultrasound in blood; F, frequency of interrogation; N, integer representing frequencies in the spectrum; M, ensemble length (number of pulse-echo cycles required to complete the measurement); P, number of erythrocyte clusters that match; PRF, pulse repetition frequency; 1/PRF, ultrasound pulse interval.
*Typical value.
†If |da| >L/2, aliasing is present and the value displayed is wrong.

Table 13-3. Distances traveled by erythrocyte clusters and corresponding ultrasound echo phase shifts

	Venous (1 cm/sec)	Arterial (50 cm/sec)	Stenotic (400 cm/sec)
50 µs (shallow pulse interval)	0.0005 mm	0.025 mm	0.2 mm
	0.0033 φ	0.167 φ	1.33 φ*†
200 µs (deep pulse interval)	0.002 mm	0.1 mm	0.8 mm
	0.0133 φ	0.67 φ*	5.33 φ*†
1 ms (instant detectors)	0.01 mm	0.5 mm	4.0 mm
	0.067 φ	3.33 φ	26.7 φ†
10 ms (FFT spectrum)	0.1 mm	5.0 mm	40.0 mm
	0.67 φ	33.3 φ	267.0 φ†
50 ms (lowest audible—20 Hz)	0.5 mm	25.0 mm	200.0 mm
	3.33 φ	166.0 φ	1333.0 φ†

Ultrasound wavelength for 5 MHz ultrasound is 0.3 mm; φ = phase change in echoes (1 φ = 360°).
*Higher than hearing range.
†Aliased because phase shift of the echo is more than 0.5 of a cycle.

measuring blood flow. With phase (Doppler) demodulation, one cycle in phase change is equal to a change in the round trip of the ultrasound travel of one wavelength (L) or a motion of the cluster of the erythrocytes of half a wavelength (L/2). For shallow or deep vessels, the slowest venous flow will change the phase of the echo less than 1% between pulse-echo cycles; over the 1 ms measurement period of the instant methods used in color Doppler imaging, the motion of the erythrocyte cluster changes the phase of the echo by only 6.7%. This phase change is difficult to measure accurately. The minimum phase change detectable by the spectral analysis systems, such as the FFT, is 0.5 cycles, and they use a measurement period of 10 ms. The 1 cm/sec venous blood velocity is barely detected. However, normal hearing can detect a phase change of 100% (or 1) in 50 ms; thus a person can hear a Doppler shift from slow-moving blood that cannot be easily detected by electronic frequency measurement systems. Instrument manufacturers have included "slow flow" options in their instruments, which lengthen the measurement time.

A phase change of more than 0.5 (50%) during a single pulse interval will result in aliasing, the inability to tell the difference between forward and reverse flow. This problem appears whenever phase (Doppler) demodulation is used. Phase changes look the same for:

$$n + p \qquad (12)$$

where n is any integer and p is a fractional phase. Therefore all of the following phase changes look the same:

$$-3.22 = -2.22 = -1.22 = -0.22 = +0.78 = 1.78 = 2.78 \quad (13)$$

Most systems select the one value that lies between -0.5 and $+0.5$ as most likely to be correct. In this case the velocity associated with a phase change of -0.22 is chosen. When aliasing is identified by the examiner (a display showing lower velocity reverse flow where there should be higher velocity forward flow), the examiner may shift the baseline (zero velocity line) on the display to make the velocity waveform look more attractive. Then the velocity associated with a phase change of $+0.78$ is chosen and displayed.

PULSED DOPPLER ULTRASOUND VELOCITY MEASUREMENT

Each pulse of ultrasound transmitted into tissue by a typical 5 MHz-pulsed Doppler instrument comprises 5 cycles of ultrasound, with a pulse duration of 1 μs (Fig. 13-1). At a time corresponding to the depth of interest (33 μs after the transmitted ultrasound pulse for a depth of 2.5 cm), a 1 μs sample of echo is digitized for phase analysis. The portion of the echo that is sampled (*Echo 1* in Fig. 13-2) is compared with two standard waves derived from the transmit pulse: one is a sine wave (*I* in Fig. 13-1) and one is a cosine wave (*Q* in Fig. 13-1). The comparison is made at 20 points along the wave and is marked by dots; the first dot and the last dot each count as half a point. Half of the points have values of 0, one-fourth have values of -1, and one-fourth have

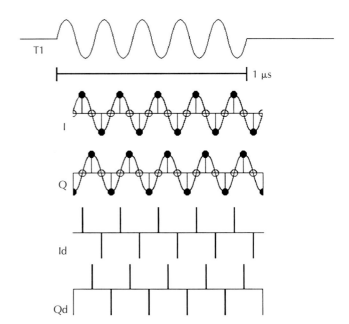

Fig. 13-1. Doppler reference signals. *T1* is a 5 MHz Doppler transmit pulse lasting 1 μs and consisting of 5 cycles. After transmitting the pulse, the instrument receives echoes for 100 μs, including echoes from 1 cm deep at 13 μs and echoes from 7.7 cm at 100 μs. The next pulse will be transmitted 100 μs after this one, a PRF of 10 KHz. *I* & *Q*, A pair of reference signals of the same frequency as the transmit pulse, is sent to the receiver. Q is one quarter cycle delayed behind the I. They are called *quadrature signals*. They are used in the determination of Doppler frequency and direction. *Id* & *Qd* represent digital samples. Modern digital instruments use digital samples of the I and Q waves for comparison. These sampled waves are particularly simple, consisting of the sequence (for I) 0, $+1$, 0, -1, 0, $+1$.

values of $+1$. The sine and cosine waves differ in phase by one-quarter cycle—they are in quadrature. Inside the Doppler instrument, the waves are actually in digital form and look like *Id* and *Qd* in Fig. 13-1. Although the frequency of each wave is 5 MHz, the echo must be digitized at 20 MHz to gather the 20 samples required for the comparison. When the first echo (*Echo 1* in Fig. 13-2) is compared with the I reference, the 20 values of the I reference are multiplied by the corresponding values of the echo (including sign), and the results are added. Only 10 results have to be added because 10 of the results are 0. In this example, the result of the addition is $-20i$ (Fig. 13-3). (The letter i is used for identification.) A corresponding comparison is done with the Q wave to give $+174q$ (Fig. 13-3). After the second pulse is transmitted, similar comparisons are done with Echo 2 × I and Echo 2 × Q to give $-101i$ and $+67q$ (Fig. 13-4).

In a conventional pulsed Doppler system, echoes return from shallow, middle, and deep depths after the first transmit pulse. The "raw" radiofrequency echoes from the first transmit pulse can be shown as a vertical stripe: black marks indicate compressions, and white regions between indicate decompressions. In Fig. 13-5, the echo patterns from 32 pulse-echo cycles are shown as columns: depth is shown in

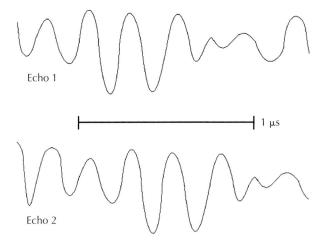

Echo 1

1 μs

Echo 2

Fig. 13-2. Two Doppler echoes from 3 cm deep. Echo 1 is the portion of the echo resulting from the first Doppler transmit pulse received between 39.6 μs and 41.4 μs after transmission. Echo 2 is the portion of the echo resulting from the second Doppler transmit pulse received between 39.6 μs and 41.4 μs after transmission. The central portion (40 μs to 41 μs) is from 3 cm deep. In the time between the first pulse-echo cycle and the second, the echo has displaced, indicating that a group of erythrocytes in the beam has descended.

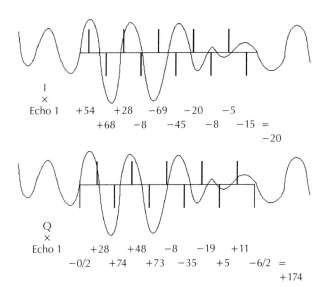

I
×
Echo 1   +54   +28   −69   −20   −5
         +68   −8   −45   −8   −15 =
                                         −20

Q
×
Echo 1   +28   +48   −8   −19   +11
        −0/2   +74   +73   −35   +5   −6/2 =
                                              +174

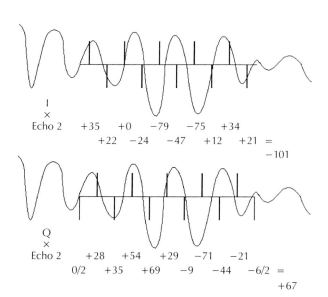

I
×
Echo 2   +35   +0   −79   −75   +34
         +22   −24   −47   +12   +21 =
                                        −101

Q
×
Echo 2   +28   +54   +29   −71   −21
        0/2   +35   +69   −9   −44   −6/2 =
                                             +67

Fig. 13-3. Quadrature Doppler demodulation of the first echo. The value of the transducer voltage is measured at 21 times between 40 μs and 41 μs after ultrasound pulse transmission. The echo is demodulated against *I* by multiplying corresponding values of *I* and the echo. Odd numbered values of I are 0. Even numbered values alternate +1 and −1. By adding the 10 results, the "correlation" between the I reference and the echo is determined. In this case the correlation score is −20i. The echo is demodulated against Q in a similar way by using the odd 11 transducer voltage measurements (the first and last are halved). In this case the correlation score is +174q.

Fig. 13-4. Quadrature Doppler demodulation of the second echo. The I and Q correlation scores obtained as in Fig. 13-3. (The results are used in Fig. 13-7.)

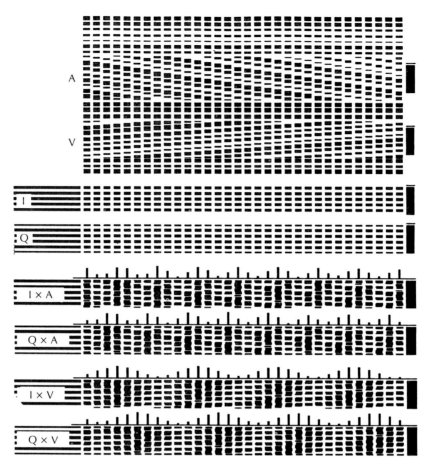

Fig. 13-5. Quadrature demodulation of a series of Doppler echoes. Upper panel, A and V: Each column represents an echo pattern from a transmitted ultrasound pulse. The dark regions represent "compressions," the light "decompressions." Echoes from shallow tissues are depicted near the top of the panel; deeper echoes are near the bottom of the panel. Superficial stationary tissues, flowing arterial blood (A), intermediate stationary tissues, flowing venous blood (V), and deep stationary tissues are represented. The progressive descent of the arterial echoes in succeeding echoes from succeeding transmit pulses and the ascent of the venous echoes indicate arterial flow away from the transducer and venous flow toward the transducer. Second panel, I and Q: these reference signals are used for the directional phase demodulation of A (the arterial signal) and V (the venous signal). Third panel, I X A and Q X A: An overlap comparison of the echo signal from A with either reference signal can be used to visualize the Doppler frequency. A count of the compression regions that fall in the white regions of the reference is shown as a bar above the echo. Together, the 32 bars form a wave with 8 cycles. This is the arterial Doppler frequency. I X A is one quarter cycle displaced from Q X A: the signals are in quadrature. Fourth panel, I X V and Q X V: A similar comparison of the venous can be done. The venous Doppler frequency is half of the arterial Doppler frequency. In the demodulated arterial signal pair, Q X A has peaks one-quarter cycle earlier (to the left) than I X A, representing flow velocities away from the ultrasound transducer; in the venous signal pair, the Q X V is later than I X V, representing flow velocities approaching the ultrasound transducer.

the vertical direction, and time between pulses is shown in the horizontal direction. The time for one set of echoes (from one transmit pulse) to return is about 40 µs (3 cm maximum depth, vertical in Fig. 13-5); the time between pulse transmissions is 100 µs (PRF is 10 KHz), the time for 32 pulse-echo cycles (horizontal in Fig. 13-5) is 3.2 ms. The echo pattern can be divided into five depth regions: static superficial tissues, receding arterial blood "A," static intervening tissues, advancing venous blood "V," and static deep tissues. The quadrature reference signals "I" and "Q" are also shown. One Doppler sample volume is marked by a black box at the arterial depth, and another is marked at the venous depth. By superimposing the I reference signal on the echoes from the arterial sample volume (I × A), a pattern that results from the alignment is seen. All sense of the echoes "moving down" is lost, but an impression of a light-dark oscillation is noted horizontally (in time) along the pattern. A bar graph just above shows the number of spaces in the I pattern filled by the superimposed echo pattern. The 8 cycles in the 3.2 ms period of measurement correspond to a Doppler frequency of 2.5 KHz (2500 c/sec).

The comparison Q × A results in a similar pattern of 8

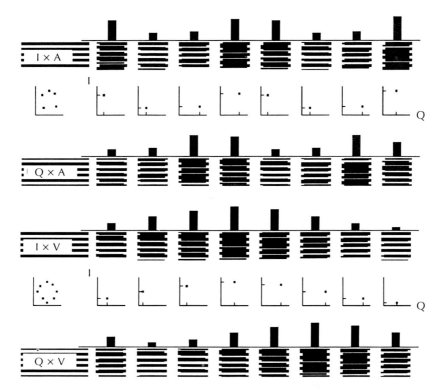

Fig. 13-6. Phase measurement from quadrature signals. The directional demodulation at arterial and venous depth of the first eight echo cycles from Fig. 13-5 are shown. *I* is plotted on the vertical axis, and Q is plotted on the horizontal axis. The eight phase plots are superimposed on a single plot on the left. The points representing the echoes form a circle, which rotates in the counterclockwise direction. The circle indicates that there is a Doppler shift present. Counterclockwise rotation indicates that the flow is away from the transducer. A similar process applied to the venous echoes produces a circle on the phase diagram with clockwise rotation, which is slower than the rotation on the arterial diagram. Slow rotation indicates low velocities; clockwise rotation indicates flow toward the transducer. This method does not result in any negative numbers; therefore the Doppler circle always appears above and to the right of the center of the graph. The multiplication method used in Figs. 13-3, 13-4, and 13-7 does permit negative numbers, so with a pure Doppler signal, the circle will be centered on the center of the graph.

oscillations. Direction is identified by noting that the oscillations of the bar graph in the I × A pattern are delayed for one-quarter cycle from the oscillations in the Q × A pattern. This quadrature delay indicates a flow velocity component away from the ultrasound transducer.

A similar analysis of the venous signals shows a frequency of 1.25 KHz, and I × V one-quarter cycle ahead of Q × V, which indicates flow toward the transducer.

Autocorrelation is one name for direct Doppler frequency analysis. Other names include lambda processing and pulse pair covariance. The differences in these methods are subtle. All are based on the measurement of the phase angle of each echo as an indication of the depth position of a cluster of erythrocytes in the body. The progressive change in depth with time can be determined by monitoring the progressive change in phase in successive echoes taken at regular time intervals.

The phase of the portion of the echo at the sample volume depth is determined by combining the I × A and Q × A results from that echo. If the two values are plotted on a

graph, the I × A on the vertical axis and the Q × A on the horizontal axis, a point on the graph represents the phase of *t*, which is the echo at that depth (Fig. 13-6). The phase at the same depth from the next pulse-echo cycle will be different if the sample volume is in moving blood. An impression of the change of phase can be obtained by plotting the phase values of a series of 8 pulse-echo cycles. When plotted on the same graph, the 8 points, which represent 8 pulse-echo cycles, form a circle that indicates blood flow. The direction of the rotation indicates direction of flow. Clockwise rotation indicates flow toward the ultrasound transducer.

Fig. 13-6 demonstrates the phase measurement effect. Because the ultrasound echo wave, which has many numeric positive and negative values, has been represented as either just positive or just negative, the numeric values for compression and decompression are lost. Counts of 1 and 0 values only were used to make the bar graphs, so no negative values were plotted. In a more realistic phase-plotting method, the numeric values from Figs. 13-3 and

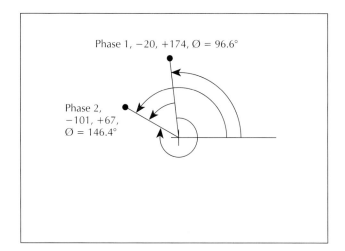

Fig. 13-7. Doppler frequency measurement. The timing or phase of the echo can be determined quantitatively from a phase diagram. Echo 1 (Fig. 13-3) is plotted by measuring −20 mm horizontally (the I value) and +174 mm vertically (the Q value). A line from the center to this point is at an angle of 96.6° to the horizontal. Echo 2 (Fig. 13-4) is plotted by measuring −101 mm horizontally and 67 mm vertically. The line to this point is at angle of 146.4°. The difference between the two angles, 49.8° divided by 360° in a complete circle, is the fraction of a cycle that the phase has changed in the time between pulse-echo cycles. The Doppler frequency is equal to the fractional phase change divided by the time between ultrasound transmit pulses (the pulse period).

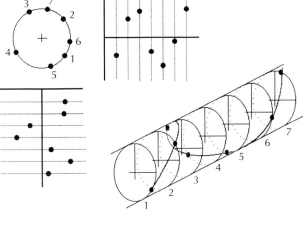

Fig. 13-8. Relating quadrature Doppler frequency and phase. A quadrature Doppler signal can be thought of as a coil spring. Viewed from the axis *(upper left)*, it looks like a circle; viewed from the right side *(upper right)*, it looks like a sine wave; and viewed from the bottom side *(lower left)*, it looks like a cosine wave. The rotational speed indicates the Doppler frequency; the direction of rotation (right-hand or left-hand screw thread) indicates the direction of the flow, toward or away from the transducer. The radius of the helix indicates the strength of the Doppler signal.

13-4 are shown in Fig. 13-7. The −20i and +174q values from the sample volume during the first echo form an angle of 96.6° with a horizontal reference line; the −101i, +67q values from the second echo form the angle of 146.4°. This indicates that the blood has moved enough to change the phase angle by 49.8°. If the wavelength of ultrasound in blood is 0.3 mm, the displacement from the ultrasound transducer is:

$$\text{(14)}$$
$$dS = \tfrac{1}{2} \times d\phi \times L = \tfrac{1}{2} \times (49.8 \times \tfrac{1}{360}) \times 0.3 \text{ mm} = 0.02 \text{ mm}$$

If the pulse interval is 0.0001 second (PRF is 10 KHz), the blood velocity away from the ultrasound transducer is:

$$\text{(15)}$$
$$S = \tfrac{1}{2} \times (49.8 \times \tfrac{1}{360}) \times 0.3 \text{ mm}/0.0001 \text{ sec} = 207.5 \text{ cm/sec}$$

Although two pulse-echo cycles are enough to determine a velocity, most instruments use between 7 and 32 pulse-echo cycles. This is called the *ensemble length, packet length,* or *sensitivity.* The ensemble of phase diagrams can be thought of as a helix in three dimensions (Fig. 13-8). Viewed from the end of the helix, the values form a circle; viewed from the side, the time coordinate can be seen as well as the oscillations of the Doppler frequency. The view from the right side shows the I values of the quadrature pair versus time; the view from the bottom shows the Q values of the quadrature pair versus time. The rotational speed of the points shows the velocity, the direction of rotation shows the direction of flow, and the radius of the circle indicates the strength of the Doppler signal.

The values from 8 echoes are plotted in Fig. 13-9. Although the points form a somewhat circular-type figure, there is some variability among the points in both the echo strength (distance from the origin) and the change in phase angle between successive echoes. Part of the variability is due to electrical noise, and part is due to statistical noise. The velocity is determined from the difference between successive echoes in the phase angle.

The average angle change is 55°. If the differences are listed in order of size from the smallest difference to the greatest (33, 44, 55, 57, 62, 64, 67), five of the seven values lie within 6° of 61. Echo 7 is so close to the center that the angle measurement could contain a large error; therefore the differences computed from that measurement (67° and 64°) should probably be discarded. The average is now only 58°, and three of the remaining five values lie within 4° of 58°. Whichever value is chosen as the characteristic phase angle change, there is a corresponding Doppler frequency, a corresponding velocity, and a corresponding color in hues of red or blue for the color Doppler display.

The echoes from the Doppler sample volume often include strong echoes from the vascular wall mixed with the weak echoes from flowing blood. The stationary echoes from the wall are added to the weak echoes from flowing blood and cause an offset of the center of the Doppler circle (Fig. 13-10); the circle that represents the blood flow forms around the stationary echo. The Doppler circle can be identified by drawing a line from the point that represents sample

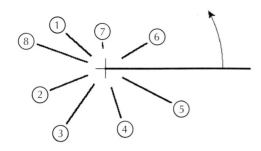

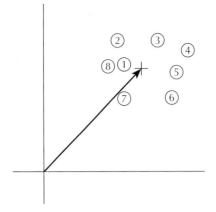

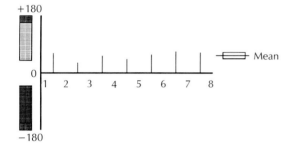

Echo number	Phase angle	Difference
1	139	
		62
2	201	
		33
3	234	
		55
4	289	
		44
5	333	
		57
6	30	
		67
7	97	
		64
8	161	

Fig. 13-10. The effect of stationary echoes. Most echoes from moving blood include echoes from nearby stationary solid tissue. The stationary echoes dominate the signal. The locations of the points on the phase diagram are determined by the combination of two values; the phase of the solid tissues (*arrow* to the center of the Doppler circle) and the rotating vector resulting from the blood flow.

pulse-echo cycles per color line means that creation of each color line requires 0.8 ms. A standard color television creates 30 images per second and thus requires 33 ms per image. At 0.8 ms per line, there is time to create only 41 color Doppler lines per image. Because each B-mode line is created from just 1 pulse-echo cycle, there is time to create 330 B-mode lines during formation of an image. This is why color images have a wider B-mode image than color Doppler box width.

In summary, four types of data are available from each sample volume in the image when the autocorrelation phase diagram showing 8 pulse-echo cycles is used: (1) the Doppler velocity derived from a characteristic angle change between pulse-echo cycles, (2) the strength of the Doppler signal derived from the radius of the Doppler signal, (3) the strength of the stationary echo based on the distance of the center of the Doppler circle from the center of the phase diagram, and (4) the variance of the Doppler signal based on the irregularity of the Doppler circle. Only the Doppler velocity is displayed. By manipulating controls (write priority), the examiner can suppress the color display under certain conditions.

If the stationary echo is large, which indicates that the sample volume is in solid tissue, the Doppler signal may be spurious, perhaps as a result of a reflection. In that case, the Doppler color should be suppressed in favor of the gray-scale solid-tissue brightness. The write priority control permits the operator to make that selection. The manufacturer may program the write priority control to make the selection by Doppler velocity or Doppler echo strength.

If the phase change is greater than 0.5 cycles between pulse-echo cycles, aliasing occurs. For example, two photographs of a clock show the times as 4:00 in one and 9:00 in the other. The time interval between the photographs could be 5 hours, 7 hours, 17 hours, 19 hours, and so on. This uncertainty also occurs with the Doppler system. A

Fig. 13-9. Phase angle measurement. In most instruments, the echo phase angle is determined from 8 pulse-echo cycles. A line connecting the echo points describes the arc of a circle, which represents a Doppler signal. The change in phase angle can be measured between each echo pair. The seven differences are not equal because of noise in the echoes and because of fluctuations in the flow. By taking the average of the seven differences, the mean value can be determined. In this case the phase change between Doppler pulse-echo cycles is 54.6/360 = 0.15. A standard deviation can also be computed. Different manufacturers may compute the characteristic frequency in different ways.

1 to 2 to 3 and so on to 8. If neither noise nor stationary echoes were present, the points would form a perfect circle around the center of the figure and the velocity measurement could be made from just two pulse-echo cycles. In practice, both noise and stationary echoes are present, and seven or eight values are required for a more accurate result. Some systems permit the examiner to increase the number of samples to as many as 32. The greater the *sensitivity* (ensemble length, packet length), the longer it takes to acquire a data set from each sample volume.

It is important to notice the effect of ensemble length on color Doppler images. Long ensemble lengths reduce the statistical noise in the results. However, at a typical pulse interval of 0.1 ms (pulse repetition frequency of 10 KHz, 7 cm maximum Doppler depth), an ensemble length of 8

wheel with a 1 meter circumference is photographed on a cart first with an index arrow pointing up and, 0.28 second later, with the index arrow pointing to the right. The speed of the cart can be computed. The difference in the rotational position of the wheel between the first sample and the second is ¼ rotation. The speed is:

$$\text{Speed} = \frac{\text{Circumference} \times \text{Rotation}}{\text{Time}} \quad \textbf{(16)}$$

Speed = 1 m × ¼ rotation to right ÷ 0.28 sec = 0.9 m/sec to the right

or:

Speed = 1 m × ¾ rotation to left ÷ 0.28 sec = 2.7 m/sec to the left

or:

Speed = 1 m × ⁵⁄₄ rotation to right ÷ 0.28 sec = 3.6 m/sec to the right

The circumference is equivalent to the wavelength of ultrasound or a change in depth of the cluster of erythrocytes of half a wavelength when the round trip for the ultrasound echo is considered. The time between photographs (0.28 sec) is equivalent to the time between pulse-echo cycles, and the possible number of turns of the wheel is equivalent to the phase angle change.

TIME-DOMAIN ULTRASOUND VELOCITY MEASUREMENT

Rather than transmitting long, 1-μs pulses of ultrasound into tissue, the time-domain system uses a short ultrasound pulse like that used in ultrasound B-mode imaging (Fig. 13-11). The echoes that return from the depth of interest after

pulse 1 (Echo 1) and after pulse 2 (Echo 2) are similar to the echoes that return in pulsed Doppler. The echoes do differ in that the waves vary more rapidly with depth than the echoes from the longer transmit pulses. Although the echoes are similar, their processing in the time-domain method is different. A sample of the first echo (E1) is obtained from the depth of interest (Fig. 13-12). A sample from the echo is enclosed in a box window. When the second echo (E2) is returned, the sample from the first echo in the window is compared with the second echo. In the first comparison, the E1 window is placed on E2 at the time corresponding to the depth that the window was captured. The area between the two curves that represents the echoes is an indication of how poorly the two are aligned. If some peaks are aligned and the area between the curves is small, a positive alignment score results. In the second comparison with E2, the window has been displaced 0.12 μs in the direction that represents flow away from the transducer. No

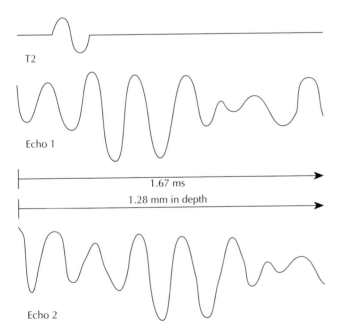

Fig. 13-11. Time-domain transmit pulse and echoes. The ultrasound transmit pulse used for time-domain velocity measurement is short *(T2)* in contrast to the long transmit pulse in Doppler *(T1* in Fig. 13-1). Echo 1 from transmit pulse 1 can be compared to Echo 2 from transmit pulse 2. The portion of the echo displayed begins at 40 μs and ends at 41.67 μs; this duration represents the depths around 3 cm, from a depth of 2.983 cm to a depth of 3.111 cm.

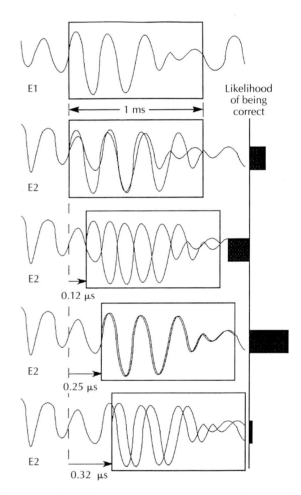

Fig. 13-12. The displacement of the echo signature between ultrasound pulses can be determined by comparing a portion of the echo from the first transmit pulse *(E1)* with a later echo *(E2)* from the same depth. By moving the sample of E1 in the sample box along E2 and assessing the likelihood that the alignment is correct, the most likely echo displacement (0.25 μs) is determined.

peaks align; instead, they all seem to be opposed, and the alignment score is negative. When two other displacements (0.25 μs and 0.32 μs) are tested, the best alignment score is attained at a time displacement of 0.25 μs. Therefore 0.25 μs is the value of *de* in equation 7 on p. 108. A range of negative and positive values of time displacement must be tested to detect velocities toward and away from the transducer. Each alignment score can be plotted at the corresponding time delay. The result is an oscillating curve with peaks and valleys. The highest peak corresponds to the delay *de*. If there is noise in the echoes, other peaks might be enhanced and the expected peak is depressed. In

that case, as in aliasing, the highest peak would not properly represent the blood velocity.

As with Doppler echoes, time-domain echoes often contain stationary phase components superimposed on the shifting phase components that result from blood velocities. When present, these stationary components of the echo dominate the correlation curve, and blood velocity, although present, is not displayed. This problem can be solved by using the echoes from four pulse-echo cycles rather than those from two (Fig. 13-13). If the first pair of echoes is subtracted, the stationary portions disappear completely from the result, but the relative motion (*middle panel,* Fig.

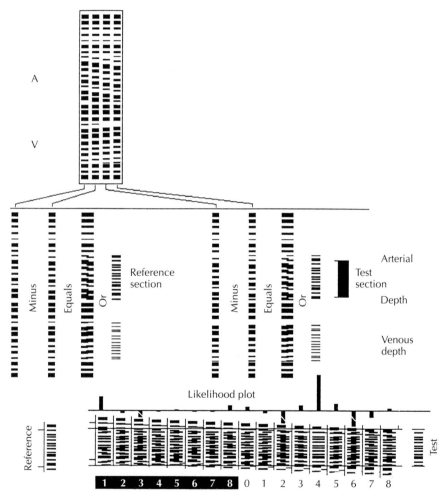

Fig. 13-13. Canceling stationary echoes in time domain. The erythrocyte cluster echo signature is superimposed on strong echoes from solid tissue. By using the echoes from 4 pulses, the effect of stationary echoes can be removed. The difference between the first two echoes removed all effects of stationary echoes; the difference gives zero for all depths where there is no motion. At the arterial depth, a sample depth region (Test Section) is used to select a portion of the difference pattern from the first pair of echoes (Reference Section) for comparison with a similar portion of the difference pattern from the second pair of echoes (Test Section). In the lower panel, the Reference Section is reproduced on the left and the Test Section on the right. Between are 17 comparisons of the reference with the test. In the comparison labeled 0, the Test and the Reference are aligned in time. Those to the left of 0, testing for flow toward the transducer, Reference is displaced to earlier and earlier times for comparison with the Test; to the right of 0, testing for flow away from the transducer, the Reference is displaced to later times. A likelihood bar graph above each comparison adds +1 to the likelihood score for each time segment where both the Reference and Test are the same color (white or black) and −1 for each time segment where the color is different. One value (displacement 4 in the away direction) gives the greatest likelihood.

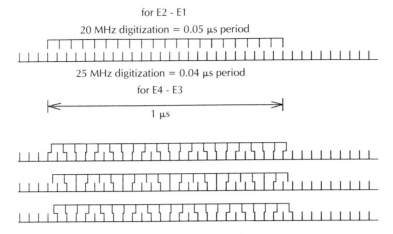

Fig. 13-14. If the radiofrequency digitizing rates of the first and second echo pair are both 20 MHz, the period between samples is 0.05 μs. Therefore the tests for displacement in Fig. 13-13 will be spaced in time at 0.05 μs. With a PRF of 10 KHz (100 μs between ultrasound pulses, 200 μs between pairs of ultrasound pulses), velocity tests can be made at intervals of 0.05 μs/200 μs × 157,000 cm/sec = 39.25 cm/sec. Thus the slowest flow detectable would be about 20 cm/sec, and 65 cm/sec would look the same as 95 cm/sec. By digitizing the first echo pair at one frequency and the second echo pair at a slightly different frequency, the size of the displacement steps can be decreased so that the step size is half the difference between the two periods. Sampling one pair at 20 MHz and the second at 25 MHz permits 8 samples over a 0.5 μs displacement, improving frequency resolution from about 40 cm/sec to about 8 cm/sec.

13-13, at arterial and venous depth) provides unique signatures of the erythrocyte cluster motion. A second subtraction of the second pair of echoes (echoes 3 and 4) provides a similar set of signatures. A time-domain comparison of the differences in signatures at the sample depth results in a likelihood plot (Fig. 13-13, *lower panel*). The peak value corresponds to the best estimate of the time delay *de*.

As with autocorrelation Doppler analysis, the time-domain process does require digitizing the radiofrequency signal. Tests for velocity are made by multiplying corresponding values from the digitized signals, as was done when each echo was compared with the quadrature signal in Doppler.

The rate of digitizing the radiofrequency echo is not restricted to 20 MHz. If a 20 MHz digitizing rate is used, the time-domain method suffers because it is able to test only the few velocities associated with time delays of ($\frac{1}{20}$ MHz) 0.05 μs, ($\frac{2}{20}$ MHz) 0.10 μs, and integer multiples of 0.05 μs. A difference in time delay of 0.05 μs is a change in velocity of 78.5 cm/sec at a PRF of 20 KHz (pulse period of 50 μs).

$$V = \frac{\text{Ultrasound speed}}{2} \times \frac{\text{Echo digitizing period}}{\text{Pulse period}} \qquad (17)$$

$$= \frac{157,000 \text{ cm/sec}}{2} \times \frac{0.05 \text{ μs}}{50 \text{ μs}} = 78.5 \text{ cm/sec}$$

A velocity resolution of 78.5 cm/sec is much too large. With time-domain analysis, a much faster rate must be used to digitize the echo, but faster digitizing systems are very

expensive. The problem can be solved as follows. If E1 and E2 are digitized with a period of 0.05 μs (20 KHz rate), the difference (E2 − E1) will represent that digitizing rate. If E3 and E4 are digitized with a period of 0.04 μs (25 KHz rate), the difference (E4 − E3) will represent that rate. When the comparison between the two results is made over a window that is 1 μs long, a nearest neighbor comparison can be made each time the E4 − E2 echo signal is moved 0.006 μs (Fig. 13-14), which improves the velocity resolution by a factor of 8 to nearly 8 cm/sec. This velocity resolution is quite acceptable.

DOPPLER VERSUS TIME DOMAIN

Time-domain analysis is resistant to aliasing. In the example in the figures, E2 is actually delayed 0.25 μs compared with E1. Thus the result obtained with Doppler frequency analysis was aliased. The period of the 5 MHz pulse of ultrasound used is 0.2 μs so the actual phase shift was 0.25 ÷ 0.2 = 1.25. With the Doppler demodulation, this was found to be a phase angle shift of 146.4 − 96.6 = 49.8° or a phase shift of 49.8 ÷ 360 = 0.138. Because aliasing can occur, the Doppler result is consistent with a phase shift of −1.862, 0.862, 0.138, 1.138, or 2.138. If the Doppler examiner notices aliasing on the screen, baseline shift is selected to choose the proper value of 1.138. The two results, time domain and Doppler, are not exactly the same (1.25 versus 1.138) because the computational methods are different. It is not possible to say which is more accurate.

COLOR VELOCITY MEASUREMENTS WITH MEAN THRESHOLD FFT

Spectral analysis (including FFT analysis) differs from autocorrelation Doppler frequency analysis in the basic principle that leads to the method. Both direct Doppler and time-domain methods assume that there is a single, constant blood velocity present in the Doppler sample volume during the time of measurement. If that assumption is true, the Doppler or time-domain shift can be measured and displayed and there is no spectral broadening on a spectral waveform. If, however, the velocity of the blood is changing or if two or more velocities are present in the Doppler sample volume simultaneously, multiple frequencies are present in the signal and in the Doppler spectrum, the results delivered by the autocorrelation Doppler and time-domain methods are not defined, and the result that they produce is uncertain. In contrast, spectral analysis assumes that there are many Doppler frequencies associated with many velocities in the Doppler signal simultaneously. The spectrum obtained by the FFT method or by other methods shows all the frequencies present and the strength of each. Spectral analysis (which gives the strengths of multiple frequencies) cannot be used directly for determining the color (corresponding to a single frequency) of the pixel on the screen representing the Doppler sample volume.

COLOR DOPPLER FROM FTT ANALYSIS

In one color Doppler instrument, a single Doppler frequency for color display is extracted from a computed FTT spectrum. The method is circuitous. The FTT sample period is short, just 16 pulse-echo cycles rather than the 128 cycles usually used for FTT spectral waveforms but more than the 8 cycles used in autocorrelation methods or 4 cycles used in time-domain methods. The resulting spectrum consists of the Doppler frequency ranges rather than the 128 usually shown in a spectral waveform. The frequency range with the strongest signal intensity (The MODE frequency) is selected along with the adjacent higher and lower ranges. A MEAN frequency is computed from the intensities of the three adjacent ranges centered on the mode. The color used for display corresponds to the mean-adjacent-mode FTT Doppler frequency.

In the previous discussion of autocorrelation Doppler blood velocity measurement, pulses of ultrasound were transmitted into tissue, and echoes from a selected depth were phase demodulated to provide the phase and amplitude of the echo. The resulting $(E \times I)i$ and $(E \times Q)q$ values were plotted to determine the phase angle of each echo from that sample volume. In FFT spectral frequency analysis, the same process occurs. The values are plotted as $E \times I$ versus time and $E \times Q$ versus time (see Fig. 13-8). The data from Fig. 13-10 versus time are plotted on Fig. 13-15.

An FFT frequency spectrum analysis determines the strength of each possible frequency in the signal. In quadrature Doppler signals, the sine and cosine of each integer

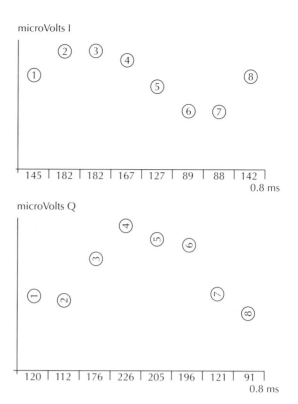

Fig. 13-15. Orienting the phase measurements for FFT analysis. The set of echoes used in Fig. 13-10 showing the combination of a stationary echo with a Doppler signal is shown with the time coordinate. The I values are shown on the upper graph vs. time; the Q values are shown on the lower graph. Both time graphs show the Doppler frequency of 1 cycle/0.8 ms.

number of cycles in the measurement period are possible from 0 cycles to half of the number of samples (pulse-echo cycles) in both the positive and negative directions (Fig. 13-16). The time over which the measurements are made (0.8 ms) determines the interval between the frequencies that are tested; a frequency of 1250 Hz (c/sec) or 1.25 KHz has a period of 0.8 ms. The relationship between angular frequency, called w, which is used to compute the sine and cosine, and the frequency in Hz is:

$$1 \text{ Hz} = 1 \text{ c/s} = 2 \times \pi \text{ radians/sec} \qquad (18)$$

or:

$$f = 2 \times \pi \times w$$

where π is 3.14159.

At the upper and lower Nyquist frequencies, where half the number of measurements equals the frequency (4wt), the positive pair of test frequencies—sin(4wt) and cos(4wt)—and the negative pair of test frequencies—sin(−4wt) and cos(−4wt)—have samples with the same magnitudes but the opposite sign; all of the cosine values are 0, so the sign is not important. The final result obtained with the positive pair will be the same as the result obtained with the negative pair because only the magnitude of the result is considered.

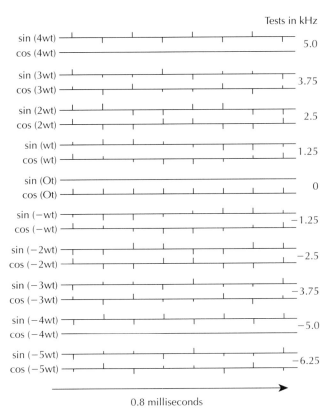

Fig. 13-16. FFT test frequencies. In FFT analysis, eight directional frequency tests, including three in the forward direction, three in the reverse direction, one test at 0, and one at the Nyquist limit, are possible. Here, the Nyquist limit test is shown twice: one at 4wt and one at −4wt; compare the two and notice that one is the negative of the other. Notice also that the cos portion of the test is 0. Compare that with the 0 frequency test (0t) in which the sin portion of the test is 0. The test at −5wt is redundant; it is a negative duplication of the 3wt test.

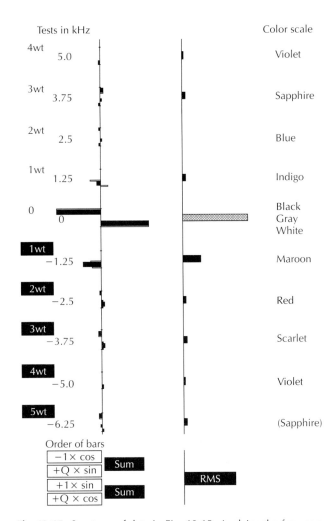

Fig. 13-17. Spectrum of data in Fig. 13-15. Applying the frequency tests in Fig. 13-16 to the data in Fig. 13-15 produces the results on the left bar graph. For each frequency test, four open bars are created. Each bar represents the sum of the eight products. Four bars are needed by the frequency test: IData × SinTest, IData × CosTest, QData × SinTest, QData × CosTest. Two of the four bars can be easily seen on the 1wt test and the −1wt test. The open bars for each frequency test are paired and added to create two solid bars, which are combined to provide the final result on the right bar graph. This is the directional Doppler frequency spectrum. Notice that when the 1wt open bars are added, because the signs are different, the sum is near 0. In contrast, the pair of open bars at −1wt have the same sign and add to form a larger sum. This step determines that the 1wt frequency in this signal represents flow in the negative direction. In this signal, a large stationary frequency was present, shown as the *hatched bar* in the spectrum at 0 frequency. This is ignored or deleted by the wall filter. The most prominent Doppler frequency here is −1wt, representing a Doppler frequency shift of −1.25 KHz. The pixel (rectangle) on the two-dimensional color flow ultrasound image will be maroon, representing slow arterial flow.

The values sin(3wt) and cos(3wt) representing 3.75 KHz are also the negative of the values representing sin(−5wt) and cos(−5wt) representing −6.25 KHz. Thus the results will be the same for the 3.75 KHz analysis as for the −6.25 KHz analysis. This duplication of results is aliasing. Only eight-independent sets of frequency tests are possible when eight samples are available, and the set on the display is selected by the examiner using the "baseline shift" function on the front panel of the instrument.

The FFT analysis can be done on a spread sheet program for demonstration purposes. In actual use, a new spread sheet would be required, 100 times/sec or more. The computation requires the same kinds of comparisons that were done before, multiplying corresponding values of the reference and the test signal and adding the results. In this case, each reference signal is represented by 8 values, and the digitized signal has 8 values. There are a total of 16 reference signals, represented as the sine and cosine of 8 frequencies (4wt, 3wt, 2wt, 1wt, 0, −1wt, −2wt, −3wt). A single frequency test of 3wt consists of comparing

sin(3wt) and cos(3wt) with the I and Q quadrature signals from Fig. 13-15. Four results are obtained. Two appropriate pairs are added, and the square root of the sum of the squares of the two results reveals the final intensity of the frequency. This is a tedious computation and it is identical to the one used to create the spectral waveform.

It is no accident that the number of frequencies in the spectrum is equal to the number of quadrature echo samples, which in turn is equal to the number of pulse-echo cycles used to determine the frequency. The underlying principle was discovered by Harry Nyquist at Bell Telephone Laboratories. It is also no accident that the spacing between the frequency bins in an FFT is equal to the inverse of the period of the measurement.

The resulting 8 frequencies (Fig. 13-17) are examined to reject the stationary echoes at 0 frequency; a spectrum of frequencies remains. Because the color flow image can only assign one color to the pixel on the image that represents the sample volume under study, a single characteristic frequency must be selected as the strongest frequency peak present or the average of the three frequency peaks adjacent to the strongest.

CHARACTERISTICS OF DOPPLER SIGNALS

In addition to the phase shift between echoes, which represents the single major component of the blood velocity approaching the transducer in the Doppler sample volume, the echoes may contain noise, multiple major velocities because of the size of the sample volume, multiple minor velocities as a result of turbulence superimposed on the major velocity, audible tissue vibrations (bruits), and changes with time in the single major component of the blood velocity. All color flow methods assume that these other components are not present. The appearance of these in color flow images probably varies from instrument to instrument.

Bruits have been characterized by Jean Primozich with one instrument as having a checkerboard appearance on a color Doppler display, with the red and blue colors correctly representing the audible bruit frequency and the checkerboard alternation between red and blue indicating the alternating choice between selecting forward and reverse colors. On a spectral waveform, the bruit appears as bidirectional harmonics.

A pair of spectral waveforms of the same signal, one taken with ensemble lengths of 128 samples and the other with ensemble lengths of 16 samples, gives the impression of similar spectral broadening (Fig. 13-18). This implies that the spectral broadening is caused by short-term factors. Another pair of waveforms, one taken directly and the other from a synthesized pair of quadrature signals created from an autocorrelation processor with an ensemble length of 16 (Fig. 13-19), shows that the waveform has much less spectral broadening after the autocorrelation processing. It also demonstrates that the peak frequencies of the spectral waveform are never represented in the color Doppler image.

A plot of the spectral broadening of the autocorrelation processed signals with different ensemble lengths versus the ensemble length (Fig. 13-20) shows that the spectral broadening decreases as the ensemble length increases. If the broadening is due to random fluctuations, the broadening will decrease as the square root of the ensemble length; if

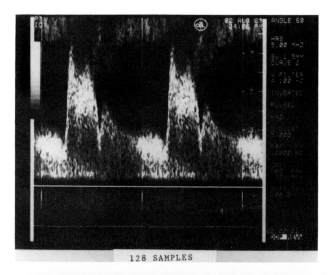

128 SAMPLES

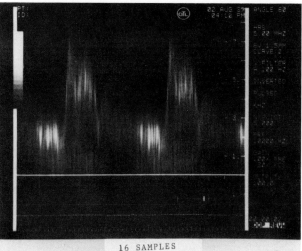

16 SAMPLES

Fig. 13-18. Effect of the number of samples on spectra. A typical spectral waveform is formed from a series of 100 spectra per second using 128 Doppler pulse-echo cycles (PRF is 12.8 KHz) for each spectrum. Reducing the number of pulse-echo cycles to 16 and holding the PRF constant will create each spectrum from a much shorter time (1.25 ms), causing the width of each frequency test to increase from 100 Hz to 800 Hz. With 128 samples, the number of frequency bins on the vertical scale is 128: 16 below the 0 line and 112 above; with 16 samples, the number of frequency bins on the vertical scale is 16: 2 below the 0 line and 14 above. The 16-sample image is filtered to hide the sharp edges of the bins. In this case, the spectral waveforms appear similar. (Courtesy Dave Rust, Advanced Technologies Laboratories, Bothel, Wash.)

the broadening is caused by changes in velocity with time, the broadening will decrease directly as the ensemble length. The line representing the square root (0.5 power) and the line representing the direct relationship (1 power) are both shown. The data points seem to fall on the square root line for times below approximately 1 ms or 20 pulse repetition cycles. At longer times, the data may fall on the direct line. This suggests that detectable velocity fluctuations have a frequency less than 1000 Hz but more than 100 Hz.

The Doppler data contain a distribution of velocities (fre-

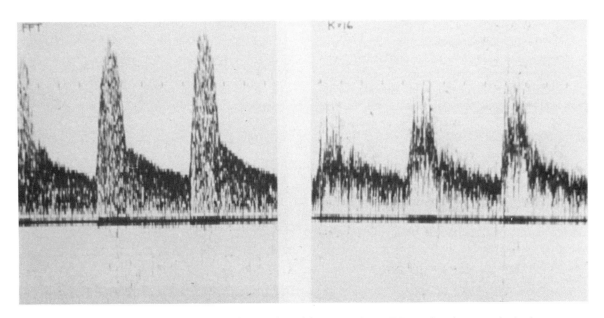

Fig. 13-19. A conventional FFT Doppler waveform *(left)* compared to an FFT waveform from a synthesized Doppler signal *(right).* Here, 16 Doppler pulse-echo cycles were used to determine the characteristic Doppler frequency as a color flow system does. The results were used to synthesize a Doppler signal that was sampled 16 times and processed as the waveform on the left to create a conventional FFT Doppler waveform on the right. The characteristic derived Doppler frequency *(right)* is never as high as the highest raw Doppler frequency *(left)*, nor as low as the lowest raw Doppler frequency. The derived Doppler does represent the middle well. (Courtesy Dave Phillips, University of Washington, Seattle, and Jeff Powers, Advanced Technologies Laboratories, Bothel, Wash.)

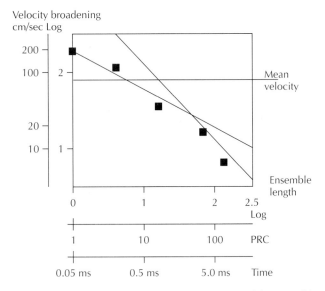

Fig. 13-20. The right panel of Fig. 13-19 was repeated for ensemble lengths of 1, 4, 16, 64, and 128 pulse-echo cycles. The spectral broadening was measured on each by measuring the maximum spread of the spectral waveform at the leading edge of peak systole. If spectral broadening is caused by statistical noise, the spectral width should decrease by the square root of the ensemble length and the slope will be -0.5. If spectral broadening is caused by changes in blood velocity during the sample time, the spectral width should decrease by the ensemble length and the slope will be -1.0. A line with slope -0.5 nearly matches the data for measurement times less than 1 ms, and a line with slope -1.0 nearly matches the data for measurement times greater than 1 ms. Thus with blood velocity near 75 cm/sec, the velocity stays nearly constant for periods of only 1 ms. (PRC, Pulse repetition cycles.)

quencies) under the maximum velocity (Fig. 13-21). This distribution can be determined with conventional FFT analysis by using 128 samples (pulse-echo cycles) for each spectrum. Time-domain, autocorrelation and pulse pair covariance, and average FFT methods attempt to determine a characteristic velocity from a small sample of the data set. Statistics suggest that if a measurement of the blood velocity is made by taking four samples from the distribution of blood velocities in the center panel, the result lies on the widest distribution of the lower panel. Repeated attempts to determine the velocity from four samples, as done with the time-domain method, result in different answers. The distribution of those answers is defined by the wider curve in the lower panel. A similar set of measurements made with 16 samples, as the average FFT method does, results in the narrower distribution in the lower panel, which is half as wide. The results in Fig. 12-20 are consistent with this statistical approach for sample periods that last less than 1 ms. Thus the number of pulse-echo cycles used by the color flow methods is too few to provide consistent answers.

The manufacturers seem to agree. Most color Doppler instruments do not display the results of the velocity component measurement on the screen. If they did, the images would look grainy rather than smooth. After the results are obtained, most systems average the color results of adjacent pixels to smooth the image and create a more attractive result. This might be unfortunate because the unsmoothed image probably contains important clues about the underlying Doppler signal strength and variability of velocity.

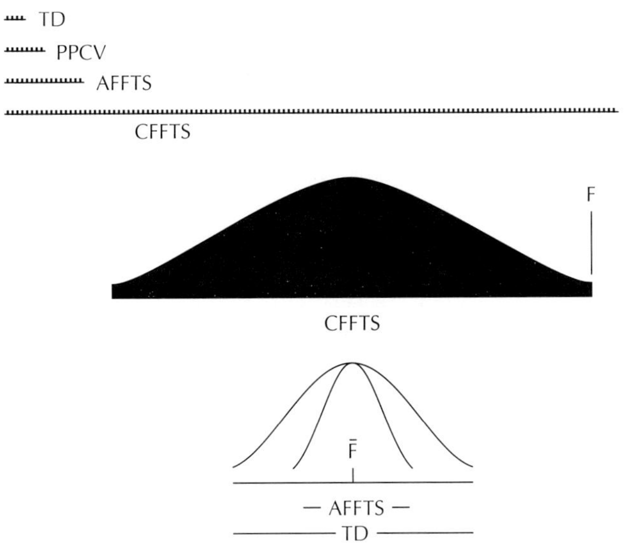

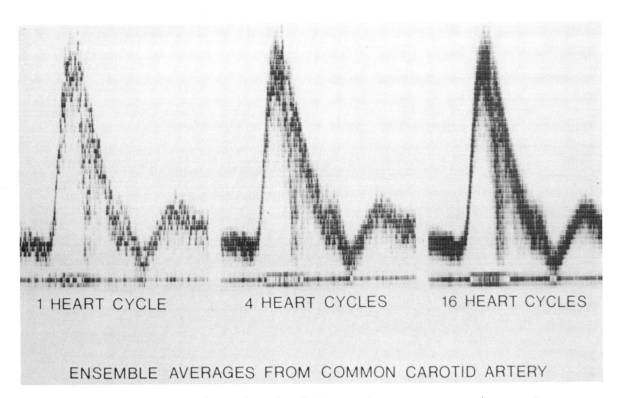

----- TD

------ PPCV

-------- AFFTS

---------- CFFTS

CFFTS

F

F̄

— AFFTS —

————— TD —————

Fig. 13-21. The solid Gaussian curve represents all frequencies present in the blood flow signal by conventional FFT waveform analysis. *F* is the frequency usually reported in a vascular Doppler examination. All three color flow methods will find a frequency near F (with the bar on top) when given the velocity data represented by the solid Gaussian curve. Using only 4 samples in time-domain analysis, the value could be anywhere under the Gaussian curve *TD;* with 16 samples, the range of likely values is narrower *(AFFTS).*

1 HEART CYCLE   4 HEART CYCLES   16 HEART CYCLES

ENSEMBLE AVERAGES FROM COMMON CAROTID ARTERY

Fig. 13-22. A conventional spectral waveform *(left)* has a noisy appearance compared a composite waveform *(right)* from averaged Doppler data. The waveforms were superimposed by aligning the ECG. (Courtesy David Phillips and F. [Buster] Greene, University of Washington, Seattle.)

Examining the spectral waveform also supports the concept that a great deal of statistical variability exists in these measurements (Fig. 13-22). A single spectral waveform, with each spectrum formed from 128 pulse-echo cycles, has a speckled appearance, which is characteristic of variability in the data. By superimposing 16 waveforms aligned by the electrocardiogram, two facts are known: (1) Statistically, the variability should be reduced. (2) Velocity excursions in the left spectral waveform might be statistical noise. However, aligning the waveforms from 16 cardiac cycles shows that these excursions are present in every cardiac cycle and are coherent (aligned) with the ECG R wave.

CONCLUSION

Although there are differences in the ways that different instruments determine the speed of blood toward (or away from) the ultrasound transducer, for the assignment of colors on color-flow images, no method is, in principle, better than another. All methods are subject to the $V \cos\theta$ term in the Doppler equation. All methods use multiple pulse-echo cycles to determine the velocity component of the blood. No method reports a value that is similar to the peak Doppler frequency usually measured from the spectral waveform; all methods report values that are much smaller than the spectral waveform value.

One critical issue in the display of color flow data is the question of how to assign priority to apparently superimposed Doppler and image data. Stationary echo strength, speed, and moving echo strength are available from all methods for use in this decision.

Although the number of color flow lines per second is usually highest with the time-domain method, next highest with the autocorrelation methods, and lowest with the FFT methods, statistical accuracy runs in the opposite order. Although the time-domain method is resistant to aliasing, variance data are not readily available from the method.

It is unfortunate that color flow displays show velocity but discard data about the strength of the Doppler signal. Jean Primozich has recently discovered the frequent appearance of dual color flow stripes associated with atherosclerotic plaques. One color stripe is in the lumen, and the other seems to pass through the plaque, creating the impression of dissection. In the B-mode image alone, the color stripe in the lumen appears in the anechoic lumen, and the other color stripe seems to be in an anechoic region beneath the plaque surface. With the spectral waveform being used to test for Doppler signal strength, the strength of the Doppler signal causing the color stripe "under the plaque" is 30 to 40 dB lower than the strength of the color stripe from the lumen, even though the other color stripes are separated by only 1 or 2 mm. The evidence suggests that a second lumen is not present, even though a color stripe appears. If the color flow signal appeared on top of a strong stationary echo, the write priority function would have suppressed the color. Such impressions from color flow images, if not confirmed by careful examination with the spectral waveform or by independent tests, can easily lead to unfortunate clinical decisions. The clinical use of a color flow examination highly depends on the skill and knowledge of the examiner.

Color displays for ultrasound are still evolving. Soon, ultrasound-generated color displays of other intraluminal hydrodynamic factors will be available, as will ultrasound-derived color displays of tissue perfusion factors. This should be another exciting decade of ultrasound instrument development.

REFERENCES

1. Eyer MK et al: Color digital echo/Doppler image presentation, *Ultrasound Med Biol* 7(1):21-31, 1981.
2. Franklin DL et al: A pulsed ultrasonic flowmeter, *Institute of Radio Engineers: Transactions in Medical Electronics* 6:204-206, 1959.
3. Hokanson DE et al: Ultrasonic arteriography: a new approach to arterial visualization, *Biomed Engineer* 6:420, 1971.
4. Koenko Z et al: Studies on ultrasonic blood-rheograph, *Brain Nerve* 72:921-935, 1960.
5. Reneman RS: Cardiovascular applications of multi-gate pulsed Doppler systems, *Ultrasound Med Biol* 12(5):357-370, 1986.
6. Satamura S: Ultrasonic Doppler method for the inspection of cardiac function, *J Acoust Soc Am* 29:1181-1185, 1957.
7. Strandness DE Jr et al: Transcutaneous directional flow detection: a preliminary report, *Am Heart J* 78(1):65-74, 1969.
8. Thomas GI et al: Noninvasive carotid bifurcation mapping: its relation to carotid surgery, *Am J Surg* 128(2):168-174, 1974.
9. White DN: *Color-coded Doppler carotid imaging.* In Bernstein EF, ed: *Noninvasive diagnostic techniques in vascular disease,* ed 3, St Louis, 1985, Mosby.

CHAPTER 14

Is color coded Doppler a waste of money?

DAVID S. SUMNER

Because of technologic advances in the late 1980s, duplex imaging and real-time color Doppler flow mapping have been combined to produce instruments that gained rapid acceptance by noninvasive vascular laboratories throughout the world. As the number and variety of these sophisticated and expensive devices proliferate, it is logical to question whether they offer significant advantages compared to conventional duplex scanning. Is the added cost justified, or have examiners been captivated and deluded by a pretty picture?

To be cost effective, color Doppler duplex scanning should excel in one or more of the following areas: (1) It should be more accurate than conventional duplex imaging, reducing the number of false-positive and false-negative errors. (2) Testing should be more rapid, enabling an increased number of examinations to be done in the limited time available in most vascular laboratories. (3) It should be versatile and widely applicable to many areas of noninvasive testing. (4) Lastly, it should be easy to use.

Color flow scanning is certainly versatile. It can be used to advantage in practically all areas of noninvasive testing, and new applications appear almost every day.[8,16] However, does color duplex improve accuracy, decrease examination time, and make testing easier? These are more difficult questions to answer, since conventional duplex scanning is highly accurate in experienced hands and is usually not excessively time consuming; the necessary skills can be acquired by most technologists. Moreover, there are few studies comparing the two modalities.

Color flow imaging offers some distinct advantages. Vessels are immediately recognized, arteries are clearly distinguished from veins, and flow is displayed over a large region and simultaneously in multiple vessels. Absence of flow, velocity changes, flow direction, and flow disturbances are evident on the color image without spectral analysis of the Doppler signal. Plaques and intraluminal clots may also be identified by encroachment on the flow map. As a result, color facilitates longitudinal scanning of vessels and the identification of vessels in cross-sectional views. It allows precise placement of the pulsed Doppler sample volume for spectral analysis, reducing the need to interrogate multiple areas. It aids in the recognition of branches, coils, kinks, aneurysms, and other anatomic variations that often prove frustrating to technologists using conventional duplex imaging. Finally, it facilitates the detection of small vessels (especially in the calf) and highly stenotic vessels in which flow velocities are low.

CEREBROVASCULAR EXAMINATIONS

The carotid bifurcation, which has been so well studied with other ultrasonic methods, offered a fertile ground for obtaining experience with color duplex imaging. The ability to actually "see" flow reversal during systole in the normal carotid bulb—a previously well-described but intangible phenomenon—was among the more intriguing early observations and suggested that the instrument had the potential of providing new dimensions to the information available with conventional scanning techniques.[36,69]

In the middle-to-severe end of the stenosis scale, color has proved useful as a rapid method for identifying the presence of flow disturbances, which can then be interrogated to obtain velocity spectra that are interpreted by using criteria identical to those used with conventional duplex imaging.[44] Visual detection of flow disturbances reduces the likelihood that a significant stenosis will be overlooked, especially when the lesion is remote from the bifurcation. One laboratory reported that the degree of stenosis measured from the color flow image itself coincided well ($\kappa = 0.81$) with that predicted by conventional duplex spectral analysis performed on the same group of patients.[20] Another report indicates that use of the green tag* to define threshold velocities from the color image is at least as accurate, and perhaps more so, as spectral analysis for diagnosing internal carotid lesions in the 60% to 99% diameter-reduction categories.[66] Color definitely expedites the examination process; the time required for a typical study is estimated to be reduced by 40%.[20,44] Even if these were the only advantages, a strong argument for the use of color could be made. The benefits of color, however, become more evident when there are distortions of the normal anatomy and at the extremes of the disease spectrum.

---

*Siemens Quantum Inc, Issaquah, Wash.

125

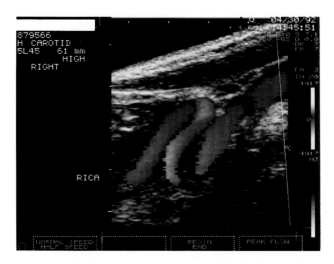

Fig. 14-1. Color duplex image of a coiled internal carotid artery. Note that hue changes from red to blue as the artery curls back on itself. In this segment the velocity vectors are oriented toward rather than away from the probe. (The head is to the left in this and all subsequent figures.)

Coils and kinks

Coiling or kinking of the internal carotid artery is common, especially in elderly hypertensive patients, and the spatial orientation of the internal and external carotid arteries is quite variable. For examiners using conventional duplex scanning, these anatomic variations can present a challenging problem, not only to ensure a thorough examination for the presence of plaque but also to identify the vessel. Although color does not obviate these problems, it definitely makes the scanning process easier and lessens the chance that a plaque will be overlooked (Fig. 14-1).[20]

Low-grade stenoses

At the lower end of the disease spectrum (diameter reductions less than 50%), where velocity criteria fail to discriminate accurately between degrees of stenosis, the technologist using conventional duplex scanning is forced to rely on rather "soft" interpretations of spectral broadening or on the appearance of the B-mode image. By outlining the dimensions of the residual lumen, color assists in the recognition of hypoechogenic plaques or thrombi that might otherwise escape detection.[11,58] In some patients with occlusions or very severe stenoses of the opposite internal carotid artery, systolic flow velocities may approach or exceed the threshold for greater than 50% diameter stenosis, despite the absence of significant disease on the ipsilateral side.[57] In these cases, absence of encroachment on the color flow map and the absence of color changes signifying localized flow disturbances suggest that velocities are spuriously high and that the artery is not significantly stenotic, thus lessening the likelihood of overclassification. The presence of reversed flow during systole in the carotid bulb on

Table 14-1. Cumulative data comparing conventional duplex scanning with arteriography for detecting total internal carotid artery occlusion (8 reports, 2314 arteries)

Duplex	Arteriography	
	Nonocclusion	**Total occlusion**
Nonocclusion	2076	23
Total occlusion	16	199

From Mattos MA et al: Identifying total carotid occlusion with color flow duplex scanning, *Eur J Vasc Surg* 6:204, 1992.
Sensitivity = 90%; specificity = 99%; positive predictive value = 93%; negative predictive value = 99%.

the side opposite the flow divider (indicated by flashes of blue) is diagnostic of a normal internal carotid artery, and its absence is highly suggestive of some plaque accumulation.[36,44,69]

Severe stenosis versus total occlusion

Noninvasive studies have been criticized for their occasional failure to differentiate between total occlusion and severe stenosis of the internal carotid artery.[1,12] This distinction is important for deciding which patients require arteriography. Errors of even a few percent in classifying disease at the upper end of the scale could have serious consequences. A survey of eight studies* documenting the results of conventional duplex scanning of 2314 internal carotid arteries revealed a cumulative positive predictive value of 93%, but the results of individual reports varied from 80% to 100% (Table 14-1). In other words, approximately 7% of internal carotid arteries thought to be occluded by conventional duplex scanning were actually patent, although most were severely stenotic. Negative predictive values tended to be better (average 99%, range 94% to 99%), but a small number of internal carotid arteries thought to be patent were really occluded. In other words, about 10% of the occluded arteries were misclassified as being patent. False-positive errors are usually caused by failure to detect flow in a severely stenotic but patent internal carotid artery in which flow velocities may be low, and false-negative errors are usually the result of mistaking a patent external carotid or one of its branches for the internal carotid.

Although the external carotid artery usually has a characteristic (high-resistance) frequency spectrum with low diastolic flow or even early diastolic flow reversal, in patients with total occlusion of the ipsilateral internal carotid artery, the external carotid spectrum may resemble that of the internal carotid artery. In these cases, color helps identify the external carotid artery by visualizing its branches.[20,35] It may also delineate a residual carotid stump, in which the absence

*References 5, 10, 18, 23, 32, 48, 59, 62.

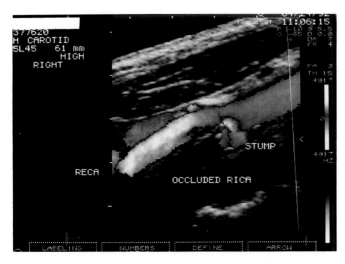

Fig. 14-2. Color duplex scan of a totally occluded internal carotid artery. The occluded portion of the internal carotid contains no color pixels but is outlined on the B-mode image. Reversed flow *(blue)* is seen in the residual stump. A small segment of the superior thyroid artery *(blue)* is also visible as it originates from the external carotid artery.

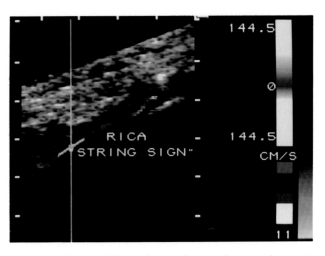

Fig. 14-3. Red pixels define the lumen of a patent but severely stenotic internal carotid artery. (From Mattos et al: Identifying total carotid occlusion with color flow duplex scanning, *Eur J Vasc Surg* 6:204, 1992.)

of color (a black image) indicates flow stagnation, and a blue color indicates flow reversal (Fig. 14-2).[47] The complete absence of color pixels in an internal carotid artery visualized on the B-mode image is the only acceptable criterion for total occlusion.

Flashes of color along the course of a nearly occluded internal carotid artery confirm its patency.[11,20,35,44] (Slow Flow* measurement capability is very helpful in these cases.) Without the aid of color, even an experienced examiner may fail to detect flow in arteries with long, very severe stenoses, those with a "string sign" on arteriography (Figs. 14-3 and 14-4).

Color also facilitates the identification of patent internal and external carotid arteries when the common carotid artery is occluded.[58] In these patients, flow in the external carotid artery is reversed (blue color), indicating that this artery is supplying collateral input to the internal carotid artery, in which flow continues in a normal antegrade direction (red color).

Vertebral arteries

Vertebral arteries, which are located deep in the neck and are surrounded by bone, may be difficult to identify and examine with conventional duplex scanning. Routine scanning of these arteries is now easily performed with the aid of color.[64] Color also immediately reveals the direction of flow. A blue image in diastole or throughout the cardiac cycle is diagnostic of an ipsilateral subclavian steal. In addition, color helps locate the junction of the vertebral and subclavian arteries.

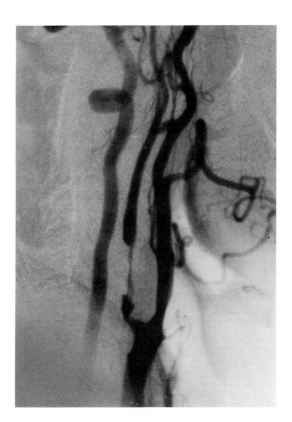

Fig. 14-4. Arteriogram of the same vessel pictured in Fig. 14-3, showing a carotid "string sign." (From Mattos et al: Identifying total carotid occlusion with color flow duplex scanning, *Eur J Vasc Surg* 6:204, 1992.)

---

*Siemens Quantum Inc, Issaquah, Wash.

Accuracy compared with conventional duplex imaging

Because the criteria used to assess the severity of carotid disease with color imaging are essentially the same as those developed for conventional duplex scanning, the results obtained with the two studies should be similar, assuming they are performed with the same degree of expertise.[46] There is evidence, however, that the advantages conferred by color may translate into a modest improvement in overall accuracy.[11,31,35,58]

Over a 2-year period ending in January 1991, 6334 carotid arteries were examined with color flow scanning in one laboratory, and 513 arteriograms were available for comparison (Tables 14-2 and 14-3).[35] A total of 43 occlusions were identified by both techniques. There were no false-positive or false-negative studies—resulting in sensitivity, specificity, and positive and negative predictive values of 100%. During the following 18 months, there was only one confirmed misdiagnosis (a patent artery was called occluded); there were no false-negative studies. This record is better than this laboratory had achieved in the past with conventional duplex scanning (sensitivity 87%, specificity 99% for total occlusion)[59] and compares favorably with historical controls (see Table 14-1).

Table 14-3 also shows that the positive and negative predictive values obtained with color flow imaging exceeded 90% for all other internal carotid arterial disease categories.

Scan results and arteriography agreed perfectly in 88% of the vessels studied. Again, this is better than the 79% concordance reported with conventional duplex scanning.[59]

In an earlier study (October 1988 through December 1989), the results of carotid examinations in two laboratories, one using color flow imaging and the other using conventional duplex scanning, were compared.[31] Although each patient was examined with only one method, the patient groups were similar, both laboratories were under the same supervision, scanning techniques were identical, technologists were equally experienced, and the scans were read by the same surgeons. Arteriograms of 206 internal carotid arteries in the conventional duplex group and of 307 internal carotid arteries in the color flow group were available for comparison. Both forms of scanning proved to be quite accurate, with sensitivities and specificities for all categories of disease closely approaching or exceeding 90%, but the κ value of color (0.82 $\pm$ 0.03) was considerably better than that of conventional scanning (0.73 $\pm$ 0.04). Arteriographic and ultrasonic classification of disease agreed perfectly in 87% of the color flow studies and in 80% of the conventional duplex examinations. Although the incidence of underclassification was similar in the two groups (conventional duplex—3.4%, color—4.6%), conventional duplex scans overclassified almost twice as many studies (17%) as color did (9%). Few carotid lesions in either group were misclassified by more than one category. By chi square analysis, the results of color flow scanning were significantly better ($p = 0.018$) than those of conventional duplex scanning.

PERIPHERAL ARTERIAL EXAMINATIONS

Although the use of conventional duplex scanning to evaluate lower extremity arteries was first described in 1985, the method was adopted by few vascular laboratories, despite its demonstrated accuracy.[24] Unlike studies of the carotid bifurcation, where disease is confined to a short and well-defined anatomic region just below the skin surface, a complete lower extremity arterial survey requires the examination of long segments of multiple arteries, portions of which are deeply located in the abdomen, pelvis, and thigh. Even when performed by skilled technologists, complete examinations proved to be prohibitively tedious and time consuming, requiring 1 to 2 hours or more.[24,26,29]

Table 14-2. Comparison of color flow duplex scanning and angiography in 513 internal carotid arteries

Color flow (% stenosis)	Arteriography (% stenosis)				
	0%-15%	16%-49%	50%-79%	80%-99%	100%
0%-15%	210	9	—	—	—
16%-49%	21	61	3	—	—
50%-79%	2	14	80	7	—
80%-99%	—	—	6	57	—
100%	—	—	—	—	43

From Mattos MA et al: Identifying total carotid occlusion with color flow duplex scanning, *Eur J Vasc Surg* 6:204, 1992.
κ = 0.833 $\pm$ 0.019; overclassified = 8.4%; underclassified = 3.7%; perfect agreement = 87.9%.

Table 14-3. Accuracy of color flow duplex examination for discriminating among categories of internal carotid artery stenosis

% Stenosis	Sensitivity	Specificity	Predictive value		Accuracy
			Positive	Negative	
≤14 vs ≥15	97%	90%	92%	96%	94%
≤49 vs ≥50	98%	95%	92%	99%	96%
≤79 vs ≥80	93%	99%	94%	98%	97%
≤99 vs 100	100%	100%	100%	100%	100%

From Mattos MA et al: Identifying total carotid occlusion with color flow duplex scanning, *Eur J Vasc Surg* 6:204, 1992.

With the introduction of color duplex scanning, there has been renewed interest in the technique. Because the color flow map helps locate and identify arteries, allows relatively long vascular segments to be visualized simultaneously, detects collaterals, reveals the absence of flow in occluded vessels, delineates areas of narrowing, and calls attention to the presence of flow disturbances, the examination is expedited and greatly simplified.[2] A single leg may be scanned from the groin to the ankle in as little as 15 to 30 minutes,[2,6,7] although complete bilateral studies usually require 45 to 90 minutes.[38,39,53] Moreover, with color, the tibial and peroneal vessels can be surveyed throughout their length in most limbs.[4,21,38,39] Scanning these infrapopliteal arteries is not feasible with conventional duplex instruments, a major drawback considering the frequency of distal arterial disease.

Most researchers maintain that the color image alone is not sufficient evidence to evaluate disease severity and that spectral analysis of all sites of flow disturbance should be obtained.[2,7,38] The velocity criteria used to predict the degree of stenosis are basically those developed for conventional duplex scanning.[24] However, at least one laboratory[39] reports excellent results based almost exclusively on flow map criteria, and others rely heavily on the color image to diagnose total occlusions.[7,38,53] Reversed flow in early diastole, an important hallmark of normal triphasic arterial flow, is easily visualized on the color image as a flash of blue sandwiched between the red color of systole and late diastole. In most of the normal arterial segments studied by Hatsukami et al,[21] there was a 94% agreement between color Doppler detection of triphasic flow and the identification of reversed flow with spectral analysis. This suggests that a negative color study alone, without hard copy spectral data, may be sufficient to rule out disease.

The accuracy data reported with color flow imaging for distinguishing occluded from nonoccluded vessels or for detecting greater than 50% stenoses of the iliac, femoral, and popliteal arteries are as good as, and perhaps somewhat better than, those obtained with conventional duplex scanning.* Sensitivities range from about 85% to over 90% and specificities from 97% to 100%. Predictive values, both positive and negative, have usually been in the 90% to 99% range. Of particular interest are the results reported by Moneta and associates[4,38] concerning the accuracy of color flow scanning for determining uninterrupted patency of the infrapopliteal arteries. In the anterior tibial and posterior tibial arteries, the sensitivity for making this determination was 90% and the specificity 92%. The accuracy in the peroneal arteries was less satisfactory but still encouraging. Similar findings have been reported by Moorehead and Arrowsmith.[39] There are no comparable data available regarding the accuracy of conventional duplex scanning in this area.

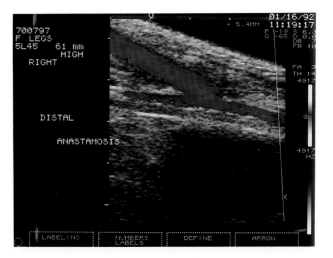

Fig. 14-5. Distal anastomosis of a saphenous vein graft to a tibial artery. Retrograde flow in the recipient artery proximal to the anastomosis is shown in *blue*. (From Sumner DS, Mattos MA, Hodgson KJ: *Surveillance program for vascular reconstructive procedures.* In Yao JST, Pearce WH: *Vascular surgery: long-term results,* Norwalk, Conn, 1993, Appleton & Lange.)

Postoperative surveillance

Color is especially valuable in postoperative follow-up studies of infrainguinal bypass grafts.* Again, the time required for a complete survey of the graft, the proximal and distal anastomoses, and the adjacent inflow and outflow arteries is reduced to about 20 minutes, or less than half that needed to perform a similar study with conventional duplex scanning.[56,63] The graft and its anastomoses are more easily located with color than with conventional duplex instruments, and longitudinal scanning is greatly simplified (Fig. 14-5).[9,30,56] Spectral analysis of Doppler signals is required only from those sites where flow disturbances appear on the color image.[45] It is no longer necessary to sample flow randomly from multiple sites or to depend on the B-mode image (which is insensitive to graft narrowing) to identify suspicious areas. Arteriovenous fistulas are also easily detected by a distortion of the flow pattern and a change in color, coupled with the demonstration of increased flow velocity above the fistula compared with that in the vessel below.[30]

Color clearly defines the interface between the flow stream and the graft wall, making it possible to estimate lumen diameter from the flow map itself.[9] In fact, Buth and associates[3] found measurement of graft diameter based on the color image to be the most sensitive indicator of low-grade stenoses.

The ratio obtained by dividing the peak systolic velocity at the site of a stenosis by that measured in a "normal" graft segment a few centimeters upstream or downstream from

---

*References 6, 7, 14, 24, 26, 29, 38, 39, 53.

*References 3, 9, 30, 34, 45, 56, 63.

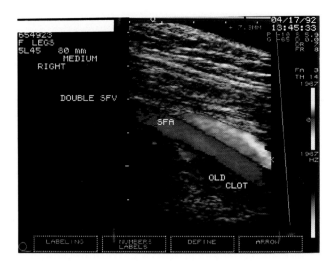

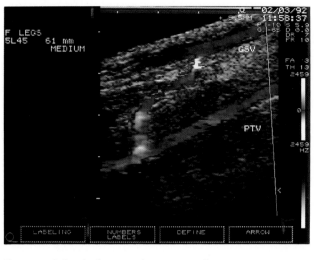

Fig. 14-6. Color duplex image of a duplicated superficial femoral vein, one channel of which is almost totally thrombosed. The other channel remains patent (*blue*), paralleling the superficial femoral artery (*SFA, red*).

Fig. 14-7. Color duplex scan showing a perforating vein connecting the posterior tibial vein (*PTV*) to the greater saphenous vein (*GSV*).

the stenosis has proved to be the most reliable method for estimating the degree of narrowing.[3,45,56] Color ensures that the normal graft segments interrogated for calculating the velocity ratio are indeed normal and that the sample volume is accurately placed in the stenotic region at the site where velocities are maximum. A velocity ratio of approximately 2:1 or more predicts greater than 50% diameter stenoses with sensitivities ranging from 83% to 95% and with specificities ranging from 92% to 100%.[3,45,56,63] Positive and negative predictive values are reported to be equally as good. In the author's experience, nonrevised saphenous vein grafts with stenoses identified by velocity ratios greater than 2:1 have a cumulative 2-year survival of only 33%. In contrast, grafts with normal color flow scans have a cumulative 4-year survival of 83%.[34]

VENOUS EXAMINATIONS

Of all vascular problems subject to noninvasive testing, none lends itself better to color flow scanning than venous disease.[17,61] Color has many advantages over duplex imaging in the diagnosis of deep venous thrombosis, both in symptomatic and in high-risk asymptomatic patients.[33,49] It facilitates identification of veins, especially small veins in the calf, which are often difficult to locate (see Figs. 97-3 and 97-10).[43,65] It displays parallel channels, lessening the need to obtain frequent cross-sectional images (Fig. 14-6). It reduces the need to evaluate venous compressibility, almost eliminates the need to assess audible Doppler signals, detects partial occlusion by visually displaying encroachment on the flow image (see Figs. 97-8 and 97-9), and simplifies longitudinal scanning. These features not only decrease the time required for a venous survey but also increase the test's accuracy (see Chapter 97).[17,60] In addition, color is as accurate as conventional duplex scanning for diagnosing

symptomatic deep venous thrombosis in femoral-popliteal veins and appears to be somewhat more accurate in the infrapopliteal area.[17,33,42,49,52] Color is probably more accurate than conventional duplex scanning for detecting asymptomatic deep venous thrombosis in above-knee veins of high-risk postoperative patients and definitely appears to be more accurate for identifying clots developing in the calf veins.[33]

Chronic venous insufficiency

Color flow imaging is singularly well adapted to the study of chronic venous insufficiency.[15,40,41] Because the direction of blood flow is evident on the color image, it is no longer necessary to evaluate audible Doppler signals or to record flow patterns to detect venous incompetence. This reduces the time required to study an individual vein from about 15 minutes to less than 5 minutes.[40] Moreover, the ability to identify specifically which veins are incompetent eliminates the need to use cumbersome and unreliable tourniquet tests to distinguish between superficial and deep venous incompetence. Although the maneuvers used to demonstrate reflux (calf muscle contraction or calf compression) are the same as those used with conventional duplex scanning, the ability to detect the direction of flow simplifies the examination process. Quantitation of reflux flow still requires the Doppler signal be recorded, but again this maneuver is facilitated by color. Since virtually all major deep and superficial veins of the thigh and calf (including perforators) can be studied, color promises to yield information not previously available (Fig. 14-7).[51] This information should be useful for deciding who needs operative treatment and in designing therapeutic approaches; it should also enhance clinicians' understanding of the pathophysiology of chronic venous disease.

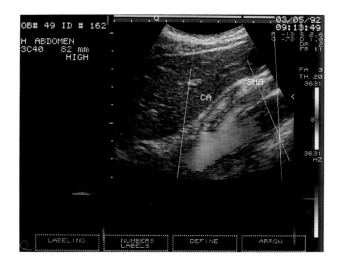

Fig. 14-8. Color flow map showing the celiac axis *(CA)* and the superior mesenteric artery *(SMA)* originating from the subdiaphragmatic aorta.

OTHER AREAS

Color flow imaging is generally acknowledged as being the best method for diagnosing peripheral arterial aneurysms and false aneurysms, which are readily distinguished from hematomas, seromas, and enlarged lymph nodes by the appearance of visible flow in the lumen.[28,54,55,68] The extent of thrombosis is clearly indicated by the distance between the B-mode image of the aneurysm wall and the lumen outlined in color. Examination of mesenteric arteries,[16,37] organ transplants,[25] the hepatic and portal circulation,[8,16,19] arteriovenous fistulas,[50,55] and vascular access sites[67] is facilitated by color, which not only makes identification of vessels easier but also reveals the direction of flow and highlights sites of possible flow disturbance (Fig. 14-8). Color makes it possible to examine the penile and testicular circulation, where the vessels are too small to be studied with conventional duplex imaging.[13,16,22]

CONCLUSION

Current reports indicate that color flow imaging is as accurate as conventional duplex scanning for identifying lesions of the carotid, venous, and arterial circulations. There is evidence suggesting that it may be more accurate, at least in some areas. Color duplex instruments have all the attributes and capabilities of conventional duplex systems plus the added feature of a real-time color flow map, which also provides supplementary diagnostic information. Color makes it possible to study vascular beds that were prohibitively difficult to examine with conventional duplex imaging, thus expanding the horizons of noninvasive investigation. Moreover, color decreases scan time, reduces frustration, and benefits less-experienced technologists by identifying vessels, sites of stenosis, and anatomic variations, advantages that should translate into improved ac-

curacy. Because of these advantages, color flow imaging is rapidly becoming the noninvasive diagnostic method of choice.[16] Color converts peripheral (vascular) scanning from a frustrating ordeal to a stimulating challenge.[2] Color, however, is no panacea; it suffers from the same artifacts that beset conventional duplex scanning plus some unique to the added technology.[16,27] To use color wisely, the examiner must be aware of these sources of error. However, color coded Doppler imaging is cost effective based on the evidence cited here.

REFERENCES

1. Bornstein NM, Beloev ZG, Norris JW: The limitations of diagnosis of carotid occlusion by Doppler ultrasound, *Ann Surg* 207:315, 1988.
2. Burnham CB: Color Doppler duplex scanning for arterial occlusive disease, *J Vasc Technol* 15:129, 1991.
3. Buth J, Disselhoff B, Sommeling C: Color-flow duplex criteria for grading stenosis in infrainguinal vein grafts, *J Vasc Surg* 14:716, 1991.
4. Caster JD et al: Accuracy of tibial artery duplex mapping (TADM), *J Vasc Technol* 16:63, 1992.
5. Cato RF et al: Carotid collateral circulation decreases the diagnostic accuracy of duplex scanning, *Bruit* 10:68, 1986.
6. Collier P et al: Improved patient selection for angioplasty utilizing color Doppler imaging, *Am J Surg* 160:171, 1990.
7. Cossman DV et al: Comparison of contrast arteriography to arterial mapping with color-flow duplex imaging in the lower extremities, *J Vasc Surg* 10:522, 1989.
8. Council on Scientific Affairs, American Medical Association: Doppler sonographic imaging of the vascular system: report of the ultrasonography task force, *JAMA* 265:2382, 1991.
9. Disselhoff B, Buth J, Jakimowicz J: Early detection of stenosis of femoro-distal grafts. A surveillance study using colour-duplex scanning. *Eur J Vasc Surg* 3:43, 1989.
10. Eikelboom BC et al: Digital video subtraction angiography and duplex scanning in assessment of carotid artery disease: comparison with conventional angiography, *Surgery* 94:821, 1983.
11. Erickson SJ et al: Stenosis of the internal carotid artery: assessment using color Doppler imaging compared with angiography, *AJR* 152:1299, 1989.
12. Farmilo RW et al: Role of duplex scanning in the selection of patients for carotid endarterectomy, *Br J Surg* 77:388, 1990.
13. Fitzgerald SW et al: Color Doppler sonography in the evaluation of erectile dysfunction: pattern of temporal response to papaverine, *AJR* 157:331, 1991.
14. Fletcher JP et al: Noninvasive imaging of the superficial femoral artery using ultrasound duplex scanning, *J Cardiovasc Surg* 31:364, 1990.
15. Foldes MS et al: Standing versus supine positioning in venous reflux evaluation, *J Vasc Technol* 15:321, 1991.
16. Foley WD, Erickson SJ: Color Doppler flow imaging, *AJR* 156:3, 1991.
17. Foley WD et al: Color Doppler ultrasound imaging of lower-extremity venous disease, *AJR* 152:371, 1989.
18. Glover JL et al: Duplex ultrasonography, digital subtraction angiography, and conventional angiography in assessing carotid atherosclerosis, *Arch Surg* 119:664, 1984.
19. Grant EG et al: Color Doppler imaging of portosystemic shunts, *AJR* 154:393, 1990.
20. Hallam MJ, Reid JM, Cooperberg PL: Color-flow Doppler and conventional duplex scanning of the carotid bifurcation: prospective, double-blind, correlative study, *AJR* 152:1101, 1989.
21. Hatsukami TS et al: Color Doppler characteristics in normal lower extremity arteries, *Ultrasound Med Biol* 18:167, 1992.
22. Hattery RR et al: Vasculogenic impotence: duplex and color Doppler imaging, *Radiol Clin North Am* 29:629, 1991.
23. Jacobs NM et al: Duplex carotid sonography: criteria for stenosis, accuracy, and pitfalls, *Radiology* 154:385, 1985.
24. Jager KA et al: Noninvasive mapping of lower limb arterial lesions, *Ultrasound Med Biol* 11:515, 1985.
25. Johnson CP et al: Evaluation of renal transplant dysfunction using color Doppler sonography, *Surg Gynecol Obstet* 173:279, 1991.

26. Kohler TR et al: Duplex scanning for diagnosis of aortoiliac and femoropopliteal disease: a prospective study, *Circulation* 76:1074, 1987.

27. Kremkau FW: Principles of color flow imaging, *J Vasc Technol* 15:104, 1991.

28. Lacy JH et al: Pseudoaneurysm: diagnosis with color Doppler ultrasound, *J Cardiovasc Surg* 31:727, 1990.

29. Legemate DA et al: Spectral analysis criteria in duplex scanning of aortoiliac and femoropopliteal arterial disease, *Ultrasound Med Biol* 17:769, 1991.

30. Londrey GL et al: Initial experience with color-flow duplex scanning of infrainguinal bypass grafts, *J Vasc Surg* 12:284, 1990.

31. Londrey GL et al: Does color-flow imaging improve the accuracy of duplex carotid evaluation? *J Vasc Surg* 13:659, 1991.

32. Martin KD et al: Is continued use of ocular pneumoplethysmography necessary in the diagnosis of cerebrovascular disease? *J Vasc Surg* 11:235, 1990.

33. Mattos MA et al: Color flow duplex scanning for the surveillance and diagnosis of acute deep venous thrombosis, *J Vasc Surg* 15:366, 1992.

34. Mattos MA et al: Does correction of stenoses identified with color duplex scanning improve infrainguinal graft patency, *J Vasc Surg* 17:54, 1993.

35. Mattos MA et al: Identifying total carotid occlusion with color flow duplex scanning, *Eur J Vasc Surg* 6:204, 1992.

36. Middleton WD, Foley WD, Lawson TL: Flow reversal in the normal carotid bifurcation: color Doppler flow imaging analysis, *Radiology* 167:207, 1988.

37. Moneta GL et al: Duplex ultrasound criteria for diagnosis of splanchnic artery stenosis or occlusion, *J Vasc Surg* 14:511, 1991.

38. Moneta GL et al: Accuracy of lower extremity arterial duplex mapping, *J Vasc Surg* 15:275, 1992.

39. Moorehead DT II, Arrowsmith D: Replacing arteriography with angiodynography in the evaluation of lower extremity peripheral vascular disease, *J Vasc Technol* 15:289, 1991.

40. Nicolaides AN, Sumner DS: *Investigation of patients with deep vein thrombosis and chronic venous insufficiency,* London, 1991, Med-Orion, pp 39-43.

41. Nicolaides AN, Christopoulos D, Vasdekis S: Progress in the investigation of chronic venous insufficiency, *Ann Vasc Surg* 3:278, 1989.

42. Persson AV et al: Use of the triplex scanner in diagnosis of deep venous thrombosis, *Arch Surg* 124:593, 1989.

43. Polak JF, Cutler SS, O'Leary DH: Deep veins of the calf: assessment with color Doppler flow imaging, *Radiology* 171:481, 1989.

44. Polak JF et al: Internal carotid artery stenosis: accuracy and reproducibility of color-Doppler-assisted duplex imaging, *Radiology* 173:793, 1989.

45. Polak JF et al: Early detection of saphenous vein arterial bypass graft stenosis by color-assisted duplex sonography: a prospective study, *AJR* 154:857, 1990.

46. Primozich JF: Color flow in the carotid evaluation, *J Vasc Technol* 15:112, 1991.

47. Quill DS, Colgan MP, Sumner DS: Carotid stump syndrome: a colour-coded Doppler flow study, *Eur J Vasc Surg* 3:79, 1989.

48. Roederer GO et al: Ultrasonic duplex scanning of extracranial carotid arteries: improved accuracy using new features from the common carotid artery, *J Cardiovasc Ultrasonography* 1:373, 1982.

49. Rose SC et al: Symptomatic lower extremity deep venous thrombosis: accuracy, limitations, and role of color duplex flow imaging in diagnosis, *Radiology* 175:639, 1990.

50. Roubidaux MA et al: Color flow and image directed Doppler ultrasound evaluation of iatrogenic arteriovenous fistulas of the groin, *JCU* 18:463, 1990.

51. Sarin S, Scurr JH, Coleridge Smith PD: Medial calf perforators in venous disease: the significance of outward flow, *J Vasc Surg* 16:40, 1992.

52. Schindler JM et al: Colour coded duplex sonography in suspected deep vein thrombosis of the leg, *Br Med J* 301:1369, 1990.

53. Schroedter WB, Holer SW: The diagnosis of lower extremity artery occlusion by color flow Doppler, *J Vasc Technol* 15:245, 1991.

54. Schwartz RA, Kerns DB, Mitchell DG: Color Doppler ultrasound imaging in iatrogenic arterial injuries, *Am J Surg* 162:4, 1991.

55. Sheikh KH et al: Utility of Doppler color flow imaging for identification of femoral arterial complications of cardiac catheterization, *Am Heart J* 117:623, 1989.

56. Sladen JG et al: Color flow duplex screening of infrainguinal grafts combining low- and high-velocity criteria, *Am J Surg* 158:107, 1989.

57. Spadone DP et al: Contralateral internal carotid artery stenosis or occlusion: pitfall of correct ipsilateral classification—a study performed with color-flow imaging, *J Vasc Surg* 11:642, 1990.

58. Steinke W, Kloetzsch C, Hennerici M: Carotid artery disease assessed by color Doppler flow imaging: correlation with standard Doppler sonography and angiography, *AJR* 154:1061, 1990.

59. Sumner DS, Spadone DE, Colgan MP: *Duplex scanning and spectral analysis of carotid artery occlusive disease.* In Ernst CB, Stanley JC: *Current therapy in vascular surgery,* ed 2, Philadelphia, 1991, BC Decker, pp 9-14.

60. Sumner DS et al: *Study of deep venous thrombosis in high-risk patients using color flow Doppler.* In Bergan JJ, Yao JST, eds: *Venous disorders,* Philadelphia, 1991, WB Saunders, pp 63-76.

61. Sumner DS et al: *Clinical application of color Doppler in venous problems.* In Yao JST, Pearce WH, eds: *Technologies in vascular surgery,* Philadelphia, 1992, WB Saunders, pp 185-200.

62. Taylor LM Jr, Loboa L, Porter JM: The clinical course of carotid bifurcation stenosis as determined by duplex scanning, *J Vasc Surg* 8:255, 1988.

63. Taylor PR et al: Colour flow imaging in the detection of femoro-distal graft and native artery stenosis: improved criteria, *Eur J Vasc Surg* 6:232, 1992.

64. Trattnig S et al: Color-coded Doppler imaging of normal vertebral arteries, *Stroke* 21:1222, 1990.

65. van Bemmelen PS, Bedford G, Strandness DE: Visualization of calf veins by color flow imaging, *Ultrasound Med Biol* 16:15, 1990.

66. Villemarette PA, Kornick AL, Hower JF Jr: Visual velocity measurement: is it a reliable method? *J Vasc Technol* 15:315, 1992.

67. Villemarette PA et al: Use of color flow Doppler to evaluate vascular access graft function, *J Vasc Technol* 13:164, 1989.

68. Villemarette PA et al: Color flow Doppler evaluation of the pulsatile mass, *J Vasc Technol* 14:18, 1990.

69. Zierler RE et al: Noninvasive assessment of normal carotid bifurcation hemodynamics with color-flow ultrasound imaging, *Ultrasound Med Biol* 13:471, 1987.

CHAPTER 15

Evaluating a pulsed Doppler duplex scanner

KIRK W. BEACH

Selecting the proper diagnostic instruments is essential for achieving an accurate and safe diagnosis. The skill of the examiner/operator is of first importance, the assurance that the instrument performs up to the design standard is of second importance, the features of the instrument are of third importance, and the brand of the instrument used is of least importance. This chapter discusses some features of vascular examinations and their relationships to instruments.

EXAMINATION TYPES

Modern ultrasonic Doppler diagnostic examinations involve all body parts, from the crown of the head to the tip of the toes. The purposes of Doppler systems are the following:

1. To locate arteries and veins
2. To detect the endpoint peripheral blood pressure measurements
3. To detect normal and abnormal arterial and venous waveforms
4. To detect local elevations in velocity associated with stenoses.
5. To detect flow disturbances in the poststenotic regions
6. To detect moving emboli
7. To measure volumetric flow rates
8. To measure the kinetic energy of blood for the computation of Bernoulli pressure changes

The development of the examination methods for arteries and veins and the training for vascular examiners has occurred in approximately this order. The last four examinations in the list are new; the other examination methods, although well established, still hold surprising secrets. Table 15-1 lists the instrument requirements for each examination type.

Table 15-1 shows that the requirements for Doppler operation are not as stringent as is often supposed. Only the last two examinations require precise quantitative measurements of velocity magnitude. Although both are common in echocardiography and are used occasionally in peripheral

vascular examinations,[5,10,11] neither is accepted practice in peripheral vascular testing. When these measurements are done in echocardiography for cardiac output and aortic valve pressure drop, the Doppler examination angle is always 0, an angle that is not possible in most peripheral vascular examinations. Because accurate measurement of velocity magnitude is not used in most vascular studies, the Doppler equation, velocity measurement versus frequency measurement, and numeric accuracy of the velocity measurement are not discussed further in this chapter.

Vascular location

Verifying the presence and determining the location of a patent blood vessel requires that a signal be detected when the Doppler points at the vessel. The three coordinates of location are longitudinal, lateral, and depth. The longitudinal coordinate has little use; the artery originates at a location proximal to the region of measurement and continues on beyond the region. The longitudinal coordinate is useful only in describing the location of bifurcations and stenoses.

The lateral location of the vessel is the most useful measurement. Every Doppler system from the first developed by Koneko and Satamura[9,16] is capable of performing this task, at least for superficial vessels. With continuous wave (CW) Doppler or a pulsed Doppler, a map of the course of the artery or vein can be created, either by drawing it on the skin or by creating a tracing on a screen.* Doppler systems for mapping the course of arteries and bifurcations have been used for over 20 years, since the method with a CW Doppler was introduced by Thomas[22] and a method using a pulsed Doppler was introduced by Hokanson.[8]

Determining the depth location of the vessel is not possible with CW Doppler but is easily done with pulsed Doppler. Tracing the depth course of a vessel was first suggested by Hokanson[8] and is now the basis of the real-time color flow imaging.[3]

Common examinations for the location of vessels include ensuring the presence of variable arteries, such as the radial and ulnar arteries; tracing the veins of the leg before har-

This work was supported by National Institutes of Health Specialized Center for Organized Research #1P50HL42270. The illustrations were prepared by Mary Pat Fitzgerald, David J. Phillips, and Jean F. Primozich.

*References 4, 8, 14, 18, 21, 22, 25.

133

Table 15-1. Doppler features required for different examination types

	Required features			
			Velocity	
Examination	Flow detection	Bidirectional detection	Quality	Quantity
Vascular location	Yes	No	No	
Vascular shape	Yes	No	No	
Pressure endpoint	Yes	No	No	
Waveform evaluation		Yes	Yes	
Elevated velocities		Yes	Yes	No
Flow disturbance		No	Yes	No
Emboli detection		No	Yes	No
Flow rates		Yes		Yes
Bernoulli pressure drop		No		Yes

vesting them for surgery; and locating arteries and veins for cannulation.

Vascular shape

Four features of vascular shape are important to diagnosis: the general vessel diameter, the diameter of stenotic regions, the presence of tortuosity, and the presence and location of bifurcations. The detection of vessel shape requires good transverse and depth resolution.

The tracing of leg veins for use in bypass surgery requires evaluating vessel size and depth as well as location. Although veins can be located and traces made by using a CW Doppler with low resolution, evaluation of the diameter requires greater lateral or depth resolution than can usually be provided by a CW Doppler. Most examiners use ultrasound B-mode imaging for the measurement of vessel diameter, although a high-resolution pulsed Doppler method can be used.

Identification of an arterial stenosis on the basis of the locations of the Doppler signals alone (without regard to Doppler frequency) requires a resolution much smaller than the vessel diameter. A high-resolution surface map of an artery contains information about the vessel width as well as the vessel course. The detection of a narrow vessel width indicates the presence of a stenosis. This method was suggested by Hokanson[8] but did not find wide acceptance until the introduction of two-dimensional, color flow imaging.

Features of the vessel course, such as tortuosity and bifurcation, can be detected with a Doppler instrument having moderate resolution, as long as the separation of the vessel segments is greater than the instrument resolution. Three-dimensional examination methods facilitate complete understanding of such structures; therefore pulsed Doppler instruments that provide depth as well as lateral information are helpful.[3]

Modern examinations of vascular shape are usually performed with a real-time, two-dimensional color flow imaging system. The display of all Doppler data in a plane permits the examiner to appreciate spatial relationships that would otherwise be difficult to visualize. Caution must be used in the interpretation of such images, since distortions caused by the time of acquisition, reflection of the ultrasound beam, and refraction of the ultrasound beam can cause significant image anomalies. Because these effects occur in all instruments, their presence is not a basis for choosing among instruments.

Pressure endpoint

The most common traditional use of ultrasonic Doppler devices in vascular examinations is to detect the endpoint during a blood pressure measurement. The systolic pressure can be measured by placing a Doppler device on an artery distal to an occlusive blood pressure cuff and noting the cuff pressure when the return of arterial flow is detected during cuff deflation. In contrast to the use of a stethoscope to auscultate Korotkoff's sounds for endpoint detection of the systolic and diastolic pressures, the Doppler method only permits the identification of the systolic pressure. Although Korotkoff's sounds can be heard during pressure measurements in some patients in arteries as far distal as the ankle, the use of Korotkoff's sounds for blood pressure measurement is most common in the brachial arteries.

One advantage of Doppler detection of the systolic blood pressure endpoint is that the signal can be amplified for examiners with impaired hearing and for those working in noisy environments. This has been particularly helpful in medical evacuation helicopters and ambulances. Because of this advantage, variability in blood pressure measurement among examiners is reduced. In addition, the Doppler signal can be obtained in most peripheral arteries, including arteries of the ankle and wrist, the digital arteries of the hand and foot, and the penile arteries. Pressure measurements in the fingers, ankles, toes, and penis are commonly used for the detection of regional ischemia.

Flow detection

Improving the signal. The success of all Doppler examinations depends on the ability of the Doppler system to

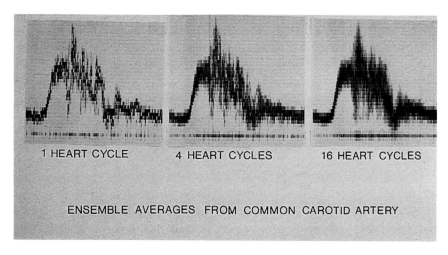

Fig. 15-1. The underlying hemodynamic data in the Doppler signal are similar to the waveform on the right averaged over several cardiac cycles. Three hemodynamic oscillations spanning the last two thirds of systole can be seen. These oscillations are coherent with the ECG R wave; if they were not, they would not appear on the average waveform. The Doppler waveform from a single cardiac cycle contains statistical noise.

detect blood flow, and Doppler systems vary in their ability to detect flow in particular arteries. The differences depend on the wavelength of the ultrasound (or the frequency of the ultrasound), the depth of the artery, the focal characteristics of the transducer, the diameter of the artery, and the method of signal processing.

For detection of flow in a sample volume by using ultrasound, a series of ultrasonic echoes (from a series of ultrasonic transmit pulses) must be obtained from the sample volume. This series of echoes contains three kinds of data: stationary information, motion information, and noise.

The stationary data are exactly the same in each echo and contain the information about the solid structures in the ultrasound beam pattern that are not moving. The stationary echoes are always strong: the range of strengths in the echo spans a dynamic range of 100 dB, or factors of 1 to 10,000,000,000. The dynamic range can be reduced to 60 dB, or factors of 1 to 1,000,000, by using a time-gain control to provide extra amplification for the echoes coming from deep in the tissue, which are weak because they have been attenuated.

Motion information is superimposed on the stationary echoes. One type of this information details blood flow. The flow information is contained in echoes from clusters of red blood cells in moving blood. The phase of the echoes is reflected from moving blood, which is coming from the depth of the sample volume, and changes in a progressive way with each successive pulse-echo cycle. The strength of the flow information is approximately 50 dB below the stationary information generating velocities about 0.003% as strong as those from the stationary echo. The relative strength of the flow signal and the stationary tissue signal can be estimated from the fact that in a B-mode image of a blood vessel, the artery lumen appears to be black while the artery walls appear white if the dynamic range of the

image is set at 45 dB and the gain controls are properly set. If the dynamic range of the B-mode image is set at 60 dB and the gains are properly set, the artery appears to have gray in it.

Noise comprises random changes in the echo data with each pulse-echo cycle. These changes do not represent blood flow and therefore do not change in a progressive way. The noise may arise from spontaneous conversion of heat into ultrasound in the tissue or from mechanical or electrical noise in the environment. The spontaneous conversion of heat into ultrasound between the frequencies of 1 MHz and 10 MHz at body temperature delivers an ultrasound intensity of about 10^{-8} mW/cm^2 to the skin,[7] a value nearly equal to echoes returning to the skin from red blood cells if the ultrasound transmit power is 1 to 10 mW/cm^2. The noise should be weaker than the flow information.

At allowable ultrasonic transmit power levels, the thermal noise emitted by tissues and other noise sources are prominent in Doppler signals because of the poor reflecting ability of red blood cells and the attenuation of overlying tissues. Examination of a spectral waveform of a single cardiac cycle (Fig. 15-1) shows the noise. If 4 or 16 consecutive heart cycles are aligned with the ECG R wave and averaged, the noise is averaged to create a much smoother waveform, which in this case, reveals hemodynamic oscillations during the last half of systole that are coherent with the ECG R wave.

For enhancing the chance of detecting the flow information, the strength of the echo containing the flow data must be increased compared to the noise. The strength of the echo from blood depends on the amount of ultrasound power transmitted into tissue, the fraction of the transmitted power that reaches the Doppler sample volume, the fraction that is reflected by blood in the sample volume back toward the ultrasound transducer, and the fraction that is able to pass through the tissue and return to the receiving ultrasound transducer. Therefore the chance of detecting flow can be increased by turning up the transmit power, thus increasing the echo strength without increasing the noise.

The fraction of ultrasound that penetrates the tissue can be increased by using a lower frequency, longer wavelength ultrasound. Frequency and wavelength are related by the speed of ultrasound in tissue:

$$C(cm/sec) = F(c/s \text{ or } Hz) \times L(cm/c) \qquad (1)$$

where C is ultrasound wave speed, F is ultrasound frequency, and L is ultrasound wavelength. Because the speed of sound in tissue is close to 150,000 cm/sec for all tissues except bone, each frequency is associated with a unique wavelength. For some purposes, it is better to think in terms of wavelength rather than frequency. The wavelength in centimeters is an indication of the size of the smallest structure that can be seen in tissue. In Fig. 15-2, the reciprocal relationship between wavelength and frequency is indicated in the horizontal scales.

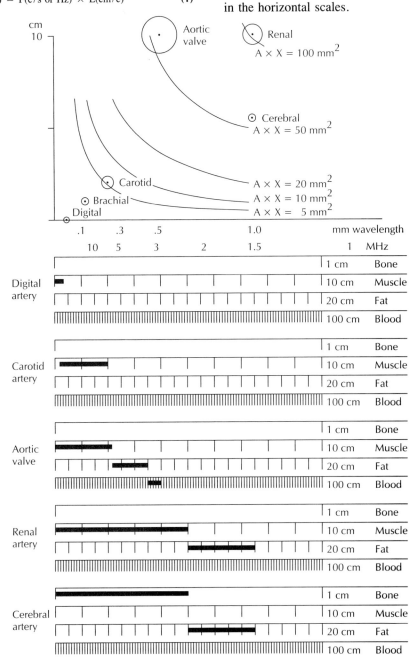

Fig. 15-2. The attenuating effects of tissues penetrated in succession are additive. The frequency dependence of attenuation and of the reflectivity of blood can be combined to determine the ultrasound frequency that return the strongest Doppler signal. Upper graph: The horizontal axis indicates the Doppler frequency and wavelength that return the strongest echo from a blood vessel, and the vertical axis shows the depth to the vessel. The size of the circle is the diameter of the blood vessel under examination, indicated by A. X is the transducer diameter. Contour lines labeled A × X are based on the ultrasound wavelength (horizontal axis) and the depth in tissue (vertical axis) assuming that the transducer is focused at the depth of interest.

Although the fraction of ultrasound that penetrates to the depth of the sample volume in tissue is increased if a longer wavelength is used, this does not necessarily increase the strength of the echo from blood. Unfortunately, the echogenicity of blood increases as the fourth power of the frequency. Thus doubling the ultrasound frequency increases the reflection strength by a factor of 16. Therefore the strongest echo from blood does not come from low-frequency, long-wavelength ultrasound that scatters poorly from red blood cells, nor from high-frequency, short-wavelength ultrasound that penetrates poorly through tissue. It comes from an intermediate frequency that balances the effect of attenuation from overlying tissue with the scattering of ultrasound by red blood cells. The ultrasound frequency that corresponds to the strongest ultrasound echo from blood at a particular depth can be found, if the attenuation factor a in the overlying tissue is known. The best ultrasound frequency F is computed by the following, which uses the derivative of the echo strength versus frequency and sets the derivative to 0:

$$F \text{ (MHz)} = \frac{20}{\ln(10)} \times \frac{1}{a \text{ (dB/MHz/cm)}} \times \frac{1}{D \text{ (cm)}} \qquad (2)$$

or

$$1/F = \ln(10)/20 \times a \times D$$

or

$$L = C/F = C \times \ln(10)/20 \times a \times D$$

where a is the attenuation coefficient with units of dB/cm/MHz and D is the thickness of the overlying tissue with attenuation a. The effects of the attenuation of different tissues and their thicknesses are cumulative. (The relationship is shown in Fig. 15-2.) The attenuation of ultrasound in solid tissue is greater than in blood, the attenuation in fat is 5 times that in blood, the attenuation in muscle is 10 times that in blood, and the attenuation in bone is 100 times that in blood. Therefore passing through 1 cm of bone or 10 cm of muscle attenuates ultrasound as much as passing through 100 cm of blood.

During examination of the aortic valve, ultrasound passes from the skin at the suprasternal notch to the aortic valve and back, moving through 2 cm of muscle, 2 cm of fat, and 5 cm of blood to reach the sample volume where the desired scattering occurs. After scattering, a portion of the ultrasound must return to the transducer passing through the same tissues. The attenuation effects of the tissues combine to determine the ultrasound frequency that will give the strongest Doppler signal from blood. This path is traced on the aortic valve scale; the path ends under 3 MHz or 0.5 mm wavelength, which is the wavelength that results in the strongest Doppler signal from blood when the sample volume is at the aortic valve. Because of the low attenuation effect of blood, 5 cm of blood has much less effect on the result than 2 cm of fat.

A similar path for the middle cerebral artery passes through 0.5 cm of bone, causing a great effect, and 5 cm of fat (brain), causing a moderate effect, to reach the middle cerebral artery. Fig. 15-2 shows that the ultrasound frequency providing the strongest echo from moving blood in the middle cerebral artery is 1.5 MHz. Similar analyses for other arteries are shown in Table 15-2.

To further enhance the chance of detecting flow information, the examiner should decrease the sample volume size until it does not include any tissue except moving blood. This decreases the stationary portion of the echo, since overlap between the sample volume and strong reflectors, which are stationary, is minimized. The size of the sample volume can be decreased in two ways: by decreasing the duration of the transmit pulse and that of the receiver gate in a pulsed Doppler and by focusing the ultrasound beams to a smaller beam pattern at the depth of the sample volume.

Most duplex scanners have a control called the *sample volume size*. This control usually affects only the sample volume length. During examinations with the ultrasound beam oblique to the artery, increasing the sample volume length causes the sample volume to extend into the regions that are shallow to the vessel and deep to the vessel. However, in some examinations the ultrasound beam is parallel to the artery axis. These include (1) examination of the aortic valve from the suprasternal notch, (2) examination of the mitral valve from the esophagus, (3) examination of the middle cerebral artery and the anterior communicating artery from the temporal view, and (4) examination of some ab-

Table 15-2. Characterisitics of vascular examinations

Vessel	Vessel diameter (A) (mm)	Diameter depth	Bone (mm)	Soft tissue (mm)	Blood (mm)	Frequency (MHz)	Wavelength (mm)	Best transducer diameter (X) (mm)	A × X = D × L (mm²)
			Depth through (D)			**Best Doppler**			
Digital	1	0.25	0	4	0	20	(0.075)	0.3	0.3
Brachial	3	0.3	0	10	0	10	(0.15)	0.5	1.5
Carotid	6	0.3	0	20	0	5	(0.3)	1.0	6.0
Femoral	6	0.3	0	20	0	5	(0.3)	1.0	6.0
Aortic valve	20	0.2	0	50	50	3	(0.5)	2.5	50.0
Renal	10	0.1	0	100	0	1.5	(1.0)	10.0	100.0
Cerebral	3	0.05	5	50	5	1.5	(1.0)	20.0	60.0

dominal arteries, such as the renal arteries from some views. In these cases, increasing the length of the Doppler sample volume will increase the volume of blood that is in the sample volume and increase the strength of the accepted echo. Increasing the length of the Doppler sample volume in transcranial Doppler examination of the middle cerebral artery is common; a typical sample volume length is greater than 10 mm.

To match the lateral dimension of the ultrasound beam with the lateral dimension of the vessel, the examiner must adjust the focus of the ultrasound beam. Unfortunately, this front panel control is not available on any Doppler instrument. Avoiding a sample volume width that is smaller than the vessel diameter increases the signal strength by increasing the number of red cells in the sample volume; avoiding a sample volume width that is greater than the vessel diameter minimizes the strength of the stationary echoes. Locating the transducer focal zone at the depth of the vessel and adjusting the sample volume size to fit the vessel are the most convenient steps. The focal zone for transmitting the ultrasound and the focal zone for receiving the echo can each be adjusted with a circular annular array transducer. With a linear or phased array scan head, the focal zones for transmitting and receiving in the lateral direction of the image can be adjusted; the focal zone in the thickness direction is fixed. Again, controls to adjust the transmit focus and the receive focus are not available.

The focal zone is the region beneath the transducer where the area of the ultrasound beam pattern is the smallest. The minimum diameter of the focal region is always larger than the wavelength of sound. The depth of the focal region can be adjusted by changing the curvature of the concave face of the transducer or, in segmented (annular array, linear array, and phased array) transducers, by electronic methods. The diameter of the focal zone is determined by three factors: (1) the location of the focal zone in depth, (2) the wavelength of ultrasound, and (3) the diameter of the ultrasound transducer. The diameter of the focal zone increases as the depth location of the focal zone (the distance from the ultrasound transducer) is increased by a change in curvature or electronic focusing of the transducer. Focal zone diameter increases as the diameter of the ultrasound transducer decreases, and it also increases as the wavelength of ultrasound increases. For a particular ultrasound wavelength and a particular depth in tissue, the diameter of the focal zone is inversely proportional to the diameter of the ultrasound transducer.

For a particular ultrasound wavelength and focal zone depth, a value equal to the diameter of the artery times the diameter of the ultrasound transducer can be computed. This value is plotted on Fig. 15-2 as curved lines marked $A \times X =$. The arterial diameter is the variable A; X refers to the transducer diameter.

The best diameter for the Doppler ultrasound transducer can be selected from Fig. 15-2, with the assumption that the ultrasound system is focused at the depth of the artery.

Both the aortic valve and the renal artery are at the same depth of 10 cm on the vertical axis. However, since the ultrasound going to the aortic valve passes through 5 cm of blood on the way to and from the sample volume and since ultrasound is not attenuated much in blood, a shorter wavelength of ultrasound can be used for the aortic valve examination compared with the renal artery examination. In addition, the size of the renal artery is much smaller than the aortic valve, requiring the width of the ultrasound beam at the sample volume depth to be small. Therefore a large-diameter transducer is required for the renal artery examination to make the ultrasound beam width small enough to match the diameter of the renal artery. An even larger diameter transducer is required because the best wavelength for getting a strong signal from the renal artery is a long wavelength and because for the same depth of focus, the transducer diameter increases with wavelength.

Table 15-2 and Fig. 15-2 contain the same data. Some relationships can be seen in Table 15-2. For all examinations except the renal and cerebral arteries, the ratio of the artery diameter to the distance from the skin is approximately 0.25. The cerebral and renal vessels are small for their depth and therefore require large-diameter transducers to control the Doppler sample volume size. Both are also beneath strong attenuators, requiring longer wavelengths for strong echoes and large-diameter transducers because the wavelength is long.

This theoretical analysis, based on principles of ultrasound physics, matches Doppler ultrasound examination practice for the majority of arteries. In Doppler evaluation of renal arteries, higher ultrasound frequencies and smaller diameter ultrasound transducers are commonly used. For difficult examinations of the deep abdominal arteries, the use of a transcranial Doppler may result in stronger Doppler signals.

Extracting and displaying the signal. Despite efforts to increase the Doppler signals by strengthening the echoes reflected by red blood cells, efforts to suppress noise, and efforts to reduce stationary echoes by limiting the size of the sample volume, stationary signals still persist in the echoes. Special methods are required to detect the Doppler signal in the presence of the stationary echo and the noise.

The pulse repetition frequency (PRF) of a standard ultrasonic pulsed Doppler used in vascular examinations ranges from 20 KHz to 3 KHz. The PRF is determined by the maximum depth in the tissue being studied.

Maximum depth (cm)	Period between pulses (ms)	PRF (KHz)
3	0.04	25
5	0.067	15
15	0.20	5

Any system will sample the echoes once for every pulse-echo cycle. The fast Fourier transform (FFT) frequency analyzer is often used in Doppler examinations to create a spectral waveform. In a typical system, the PRF is 12.8

KHz, or 12,800 pulse-echo cycles per second. The data for creating a single spectrum are gathered in 0.01 second. In that time, 128 echo samples are gathered. The spectrum consists of the intensities of 128 different frequency measurements, each 100 Hz wide spanning the frequencies from −6400 Hz to +6400 Hz, a range of 12,800 Hz. Each 100 Hz-wide frequency range that appears in the spectrum is called a *frequency bin*. The frequency resolution, 100 Hz (c/s), is equal to the inverse of the time used to gather the data (0.01 sec); in addition, the frequency range (12,800 Hz) is equal to the sample rate (or the PRF). The stationary echoes in the Doppler signal have 0 frequency. They will appear in the spectrum in the frequency bin that includes 0 frequency. That bin is 100 Hz wide and spans the distance from −50 Hz to +50 Hz. Fig. 15-3 shows a frequency spectrum from a Doppler operating at a PRF of 12.8 KHz. Thus in a standard spectrum taken over 10 ms with bins 100 Hz wide, the 0 frequency bin spans a range from −50 Hz to +50 Hz. If a bruit is present with a frequency less than 50 Hz or if a solid structure is moving at a speed of 0.3 cm/sec or less so that the Doppler frequency generated is below 50 Hz, the information will appear in the 0 frequency bin and be discarded. The numbers above are typical of FFT spectral waveform analysis.

In another FTT spectrum analyzer, a spectrum is created from a much shorter series of samples. For each spectrum, 16 pulse-echo cycles are gathered in 1.25 ms; thus each frequency bin is 800 Hz wide (1 ÷ 1.25 ms). In most spectrum analyzers, the stationary echoes in the 0 frequency bin are discarded before display of the spectrum.

One of the color Doppler imaging manufacturers uses an FFT method for detecting velocities. Each frequency analysis is done by using just 16 pulse-echo cycles to minimize the time needed to detect velocities at one place in the image. Other authors use the term *packet size* or *ensemble length* for this concept. If the PRF is 12.8 KHz, 16 samples can be gathered in just 1.25 ms. The range of the spectrum that results is from −6.4 KHz to +6.4 KHz (see Fig. 15-3).

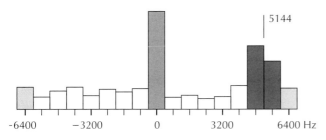

Fig. 15-3. An FFT spectrum formed from 16 pulse-echo cycles has 16 frequency bins. Seventeen are shown, but the +6400 Hz bin and the −6400 Hz bin are the same. By design, the 0 frequency bin is centered at 0, spanning frequencies from −400 Hz to +400 Hz. The 0 frequency bin contains the stationary echoes and is discarded. The Doppler frequency used to assign the color is determined by finding a group of intense frequency bins (+4800 Hz and +5600 Hz) and finding the average frequency for the group.

Because only 16 samples are gathered, only 16 frequency bins can be created; each frequency bin is now 800 Hz wide. The 0 frequency bin, centered on 0, spans the region from −400 Hz to +400 Hz. If a 7.5-MHz Doppler is used, any velocity less than 4 cm/sec directed toward the transducer or less than 8 cm/sec directed at 60° to the transducer would appear in the 0 frequency bin along with the stationary echoes and be discarded. Because some vascular flows are slower than 4 cm/sec, the manufacturer introduced "slow flow" on their instrument; they reduced the effective PRF to make the width of the 0 frequency bin smaller, which also caused the width of the total spectrum to be smaller, resulting in an increased chance of aliasing. Aliasing is not a problem if slow flow is used only in situations where velocities in the range of 4 cm/sec are expected. If slow flow reduces the PRF by a factor of 4, the velocity range at 0° changes from a range spanning between 8 cm/sec and 128 cm/sec at 60° and normal PRF to a range spanning between 2 cm/sec and 32 cm/sec at 60° at slow flow PRF.

Other color flow imaging systems use either autocorrelation methods, time-domain methods, or maximum entropy methods. All share a common feature: the Doppler frequency is determined by using the data from between 4 and 8 pulse-echo cycles. However, the data are limited. Data available for velocity analysis contain a number of components including the following:
Stationary echoes
    Fixed tissues
    Wall motion
Velocity signals
    Principal velocity
    Secondary velocities
    Turbulence
Vibrations (murmurs or bruits)
Noise
A velocity signal analysis system must be prepared to deal with any combination of these signals. Although counts vary, perhaps seven kinds of data are present. Only one pulse-echo cycle is needed to get amplitude out of the echo for the B-mode image. The difference between two pulse-echo cycles must be determined to get phase change for velocity information. If a stationary echo may be present along with the velocity information, three pulse-echo cycles are required; if wall motion is also present, four or five pulse-echo cycles are required. In short, the designers of modern frequency analysis systems have underestimated the complexity of these echo signals.

All color flow imagers show a characteristic "velocity" that is incorrectly called the *mean* value or the *average* value; it is actually a chance value somewhere between the maximum and minimum velocities. Some color Doppler systems also show "variance," usually denoted in green. The variance can only be computed if seven or more pulse-echo cycles are available; thus the time-domain system, which uses only four pulse-echo cycles, cannot determine the variance. No system expects to see bruits or murmurs;

therefore these signals appear on the image as confusing checkerboard patterns. With experience, examiners recognize the pattern. The character of a bruit is much more obvious on a spectral waveform than in a color flow pattern (Fig. 15-4). In fact, any data type that is unexpected may appear as color patterns on the screen, and it is left to the examiner to learn to recognize them. Looking at the signal with a spectral waveform is always helpful.

A bruit and the vibrating plate test phantom[24] function in the same way to produce signals that appear on Doppler displays. Wang, Bone, and Hossack[24] suggest that the number of harmonics that appears is determined by two factors: (1) the dynamic range of the spectrum analyzer and (2) the amplitude of the vibration. They state that if the amplitude of the vibration is much less than half a wavelength of ultrasound, only the lowest harmonic—the frequency of vibration—will appear. As the vibration amplitude in-

creases, the number of harmonics in the image increases. In Fig. 15-4, the bruit has the same frequency in each of the two cardiac cycles but seems to have a greater amplitude, as indicated by the appearance of more harmonics, in the second cardiac cycle.

Which kind of frequency analysis system is best for diagnosis? All appear to be equally effective. If an examiner learns to interpret images made with one kind of color flow imager, can that knowledge be directly applied to the interpretation of images made with another kind? Currently, the answer is "no."

Velocity waveform evaluation

Evaluation of the velocity waveform has been used for the diagnosis of arterial and venous obstruction since the first introduction of Doppler examination methods.[9,16] The audible detection of the phasicity of the signal demonstrates that the waveform is phasic with respiration in normal veins and biphasic or triphasic with the pulse in normal arteries supplying resting peripheral tissues.

Waveform tracings of the Doppler frequencies on the vertical axis versus time on the horizontal axis, either nondirectional or directional, make teaching easier and make the documentation of changes in a patient over time more convenient. The principal diagnostic features of an arterial waveform are a sharp systolic upslope and a dicrotic wave marking the end of systole. In addition, the dicrotic wave becomes a flow reversal at the onset of diastole in normal resting peripheral arteries. To detect the flow reversal either audibly or on a waveform, the examiner must use a bidirectional Doppler system.

Waveforms from arteries in which the flow reversal and dicrotic wave are absent and a gradual systolic upslope is present suggest that the artery has a proximal stenosis. Secondary automatic analysis of arterial waveforms has been attempted by several investigators, including the Laplace transform analysis, but the methods have not been widely accepted. The detection of the presence of reverse flow at the onset of diastole seems to be sufficient for effective diagnosis.

The trend in color flow imaging has been to discard waveform types of displays. Many examiners use a single color flow image from an unknown time in the cardiac cycle as the sole documentation of an arterial examination. In some studies a cine-loop of a cardiac cycle can be used to document periods of forward flow in the artery and periods of reverse flow, which are documented by the change in color from red to blue. An intermediate approach to documenting the time course of arterial flow between the velocity waveform and the two-dimensional color flow image is to use color M-mode to show the time behavior of the arterial signal (Fig. 15-5).

Bidirectional detection

The ability to determine the direction of the blood flow, either traveling toward the ultrasound transducer or away

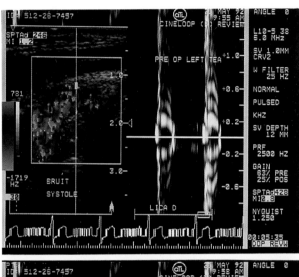

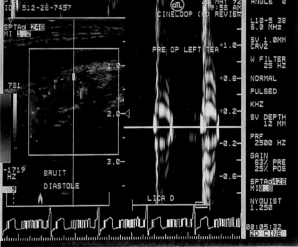

Fig. 15-4. A bruit appears on a spectral waveform as a harmonic pattern that is symmetrical above and below the 0 frequency line. The lowest harmonic (200 Hz) is the frequency that would be heard with a stethoscope. The bruit appears as a color checkerboard pattern. The number of harmonics is proportional to the amplitude of the vibration in tissue.

from it, was pioneered by Strandness and McLeod.[20] Several display techniques were created from this method. Two methods exhibit directionality on an audio Doppler signal. Meters have been used for visual observation of the direction of flow, but the common method is the familiar directional waveform with flow toward the transducer shown above a 0 axis and flow away from the transducer shown below the axis. The directional assignment on the display can be reversed. With the introduction of color flow imaging, one direction is shown in red, the other in blue.

On a directional spectral waveform display, the simultaneous presence of forward and reverse flow can be shown. Unfortunately, with single-frequency display methods like color flow imaging, when the two signals are mixed, only one color, suggesting one frequency, is shown (Fig. 15-6).

Audible Doppler frequencies can exhibit directionality by using either of two methods. The common method is to send the Doppler frequencies representing flow toward the ultrasound transducer to the right earphone or speaker and

to send the Doppler frequencies representing flow away from the ultrasound transducer to the left earphone or speaker. If flow in both directions is simultaneously present, Doppler frequencies are heard in both ears. If the examiner wishes to select flow in one direction only (e.g., to hear the arterial signal without the venous), one speaker is turned off. The other method of exhibiting directionality through the audible Doppler sound also requires separate earphones. In this method, both earphones receive all Doppler frequencies. Advancing flow arrives at the right ear before it arrives at the left ear, and receding flow arrives at the left ear first— a method that mimics the way the direction of a sound source is determined in everyday life. The difference in arrival time may be as small as 0.001 second, a fraction of one cycle of the sound.

Detection of elevated velocities

The arterial examinations based on elevated velocities at a stenosis use numeric Doppler frequency (or velocity) values compared to criteria to classify arteries as normal or abnormal. In the evaluation of the arteries of the leg, if the velocity at the stenosis is double the velocity proximal to the stenosis, the stenosis is classified as more than 50% diameter reduction. In the carotid arteries, a stenosis is identified if the velocity is greater than 125 cm/sec determined from an angle-adjusted measurement with a Doppler examination of 60°. Because these examinations are criteria based rather than theory based, they require that the measurements be consistent. However, the measurements need not be accurate. Even though the hemodynamics may be complex[12,19,26] and the frequency analyzer may provide a measurement that is in error, the correct diagnosis can be

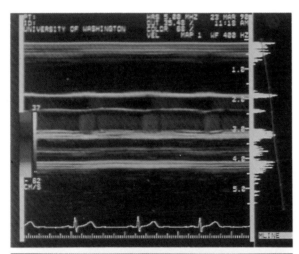

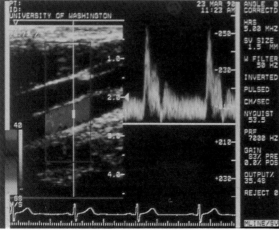

Fig. 15-5. Determining the relationship between the color on a color flow image and the frequency shown on a spectral waveform can help the examiner relate the two examinations. This can be done most easily by use of the color M-mode. ECG tracings should *always be included in vascular images.*

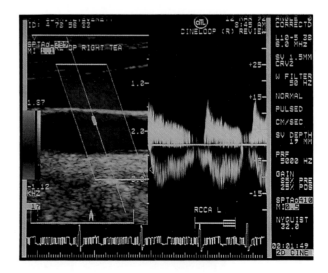

Fig. 15-6. Jugular vein from 0.8 cm to 1.6 cm, common carotid artery from 1.7 cm to 2.4 cm. Arterial walls are reflective. In this case, some of the ultrasound is reflecting from the vein/artery wall, causing reflected echoes from the venous lumen to appear superimposed at the depth of the interior of the arterial lumen. If the spectral waveform were not included in the examination, the examiner would conclude that reverse flow is present on the superficial side of the artery.

achieved as long as the criteria for diagnosis were established in the same way as the examination.

In vascular diagnosis, establishing criteria based on a series of cases with angiograms to confirm the diagnosis may take several years. By that time, the instrumentation may have evolved. This has happened several times in the last decade. If the criteria established with the old instrument are to be used for examinations performed with the new instrument, testing must be done to ensure that the two instruments perform in the same way. If the old instrument provides values that are in error and the error is consistent, no incorrect diagnoses result from using the old method. However, if a new instrument that provides correct results is introduced and used with the old criteria for diagnosis, diagnoses may be incorrect.

It is always difficult to prove that an instrument provides correct results, but it is easy to show that the instrument provides consistent results. In addition to performing Doppler examinations with the same Doppler examination angle and the same dynamic range on the spectrum analyzer, the examiner should use an instrument with the same diameter of the ultrasound transducer. A change in the transducer size will cause a change in the sample volume size, a change in the range of angles viewing the sample volume, a change in the spectral broadening, and therefore a change in the measured peak frequency.[1]

The dynamic range of the spectrum analyzer is often overlooked. It is a measure of the range of different Doppler signal intensities that can be shown on the spectral wave-form. A dynamic range setting may be 20 dB (upper row in Fig. 15-7) or 42 dB (lower row in Fig. 15-7). In signals with little spectral broadening (left column in Fig. 15-7), the dynamic range setting has little effect on the result compared with signals with great spectral broadening (right column in Fig. 15-7). In cardiac examinations, a dynamic range of 40 dB is common; in vascular examinations, 20 dB is common. The dynamic range of a spectrum analyzer is not always described by the manufacturer. Sometimes the dynamic range is adjustable with a reject control.

Detection of flow disturbance

In 1883, Reynolds[15] explored the difference between the flow in a tube described by Poiseuille (laminar) and flow in a tube described by Darcy (turbulent). The essential difference is that turbulent flow is responsible for high pressure drops along the artery; laminar flow is not. Turbulent flow mixes the fluid like a plume of smoke from a stack; laminar flow preserves a streak of dye, even if the streak must take a tortuous path. Turbulent flow leads to spectral broadening on a spectral waveform; laminar flow results in minimal spectral broadening. Complex laminar helical flows are normal in the arterial and venous system; poststenotic, randomly changing flow with rotating eddies causing high shear rates that convert flow energy into heat by the action of viscous friction are not normal.

Turbulence is easily recognized as spectral broadening on a spectral waveform of Doppler data from a single sample volume. The color of that sample volume on a color flow

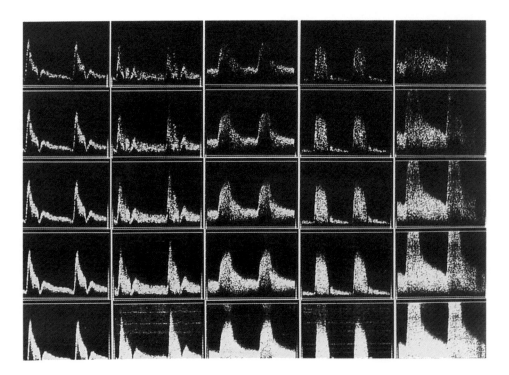

Fig. 15-7. Five spectral waveforms representing different amounts of spectral broadening are shown, with narrow spectral width on the *left* and broad spectral width on the *right*. The dynamic range of each row is different; from upper row to lower row, the ranges are: 18 dB, 24 dB, 30 dB, 36 dB, and 42 dB.

image is uncertain. If a color scale for velocity is aligned with the corresponding scale of the spectral waveform, the color displayed is the color associated with the most intense spot on the waveform. If there is no spectral broadening in the waveform, a single color is most likely. If there is great spectral broadening, many possible colors may occur. The separation of the color pattern that indicates turbulence from the pattern that indicates bruit may be impossible. When turbulence is present in a region, a mixture of colors will be displayed on the screen. Many color flow imaging systems include a method to smooth or average the colors between pixels. This tends to suppress the variation that is characteristic of turbulence.

Detection of emboli

Emboli moving through arteries can be observed on a spectral waveform by a characteristic line that spans all frequencies and is present for a short time. The sound of these emboli in the audible Doppler signal is also characteristic—it is short and contains many frequencies. Color flow systems are not designed to display this kind of information. Emboli can only be seen with Doppler ultrasound frequencies below 3 MHz when the echogenicity of blood is poor compared with the echogenicity of the emobli.

Qualitative assessment of velocity

The qualitative assessment of Doppler frequency or velocity can be performed from either the audible signal or an electronic frequency analysis. Electronic frequency analysis can determine a single Doppler frequency or the intensities of all Doppler frequencies present. Methods that determine a single Doppler frequency for each sample volume include the traditional zero-crossing waveform analyzers and the modern color flow imaging systems. The method that determines the intensity of all Doppler frequencies is spectral analysis. Accurate diagnosis can be done with any of these methods.

The first Doppler analyses used audio interpretation and spectral analysis.[9] Both permitted the observation of all Doppler frequencies. When Doppler systems were "improved" by the addition of the zero-crossing spectral waveform tracing, only a single Doppler frequency was displayed. Doppler systems were further "improved" to provide spectral waveforms that show all Doppler frequencies. Today, the further "improvement" of color flow imaging shows only a single Doppler frequency.

Measurement of volumetric flow rates

Volumetric flow rate through the aortic valve is measured routinely in echocardiography to determine cardiac output. The method consists of taking the time integral under the velocity waveform and multiplying it by the cross-sectional area of the aorta. Accurate measurement of cardiac output has not been achieved in vascular studies, and an analysis of the source of errors has not led to a resolution of the problems.[5]

To test a method for measuring volumetric flow rate, the examiner selects any bifurcation and measures the flow rate entering the bifurcation and the flow rates leaving via each branch. If the sum of the flow rates leaving each branch does not equal the flow rate entering the bifurcation, the method is not working. If the values are not equal moment by moment, the results are suspect. If any of the instruments must be calibrated, the method has no sound theoretical basis.

Bernoulli pressure drop

In the absence of turbulent flow, the mechanical energy of a fluid can be exchanged between gravitational energy related to elevation, potential energy related to pressure, and kinetic energy related to velocity. Definitions of these terms, as used by different authors, may vary. In a standing patient, the average transmural arterial pressure at the ankle is greater than the average transmural arterial pressure at the heart because of the difference in elevation. This is due to a free exchange between gravitational energy in the form of elevation and potential energy in the form of transmural pressure. In a similar way, as blood speeds up, the transmural arterial pressure decreases. As blood slows down, the transmural arterial pressure increases. This is due to a free exchange between kinetic energy in the form of velocity and potential energy in the form of pressure.

This principle is used to determine the pressure drop across a stenotic aortic valve. Only kinetic energy can be converted to heat by turbulence. Therefore if the examiner measures the kinetic energy, the maximum energy loss (to heat) that is possible is known; the maximum energy loss can be written as the maximum possible pressure drop. Distal to a stenotic aortic valve, cardiologists assume that all kinetic energy is converted to heat; therefore a measure of the kinetic energy in the jet of the aortic valve is a measure of the pressure drop across the valve. By measuring the velocity across the valve, the examiner can measure the kinetic energy and thus determine the pressure drop. The expected pressure drop is:

$$dp \ (mm \ Hg) = 4v^2(m/sec)^2 \qquad (3)$$

where dP is the pressure drop and v is the velocity. The values are striking:

Velocity	Equivalent pressure
100 cm/sec	4 mm Hg
200 cm/sec	16 mm Hg
300 cm/sec	36 mm Hg
400 cm/sec	64 mm Hg
500 cm/sec	100 mm Hg
600 cm/sec	144 mm Hg

The Bernoulli relationship shows the following: (1) for a given arterial blood pressure (as measured with a cuff), there is a maximum possible arterial velocity; (2) the maximum pressure drop across a stenosis (whether a stenotic aortic valve or any arterial stenosis) can be determined by the velocity through the stenosis; and (3) in a stenosis where the velocity is high, the Bernoulli pressure depression "sucks" on the wall of the stenosis with the calculated pressure reduction. The plaque in the stenosis may be pulled apart.[10]

The Bernoulli relationship works well in echocardiographic measurements but appears to be less reliable in vascular measurements. The difference may be that the echocardiographer uses a Doppler examination angle of 0. The vascular examiner uses angles near 60°. Only a few trials of the method in peripheral vascular diagnosis have been published.

Quantitative assessment of velocity

Although logic and the Doppler equation suggest that accurate quantitative velocity measurements should be possible in arteries, evidence suggests that only reproducible measurements are possible.

CHOOSING AMONG DIFFERENT TYPES OF INFORMATION

Although the advent of color flow imaging appeared to have carried vascular ultrasound examination to the summit of success, the frequency analysis methods of today have left the zero-crossing waveform of the 1970s in the past. The nature of both hemodynamics and ultrasound requires that a complete examination of arteries or veins use a combination of the conventional spectral waveform display: the color M-mode display and the two-dimensional color B-mode display. Each method gives a different kind of information. It is impossible to acquire or display all the kinds of hemodynamic information that are important. Table 15-3 shows some of the kinds of information available from different displays.

Of the six kinds of information available, each display is capable of showing only three or four. When the ability to acquire the data with ultrasound is compared with the ability to display the data, the most restricted portion of the information path is from the ultrasound instrument to the examiner. Ultrasonically, the single-gate pulsed Doppler that produces the spectral waveform display and the multigate ultrasonic velocimeter that produces the one-dimensional color M-mode display are identical. Thus only the lateral information is missing in those ultrasound data. However, there is no known way to show the available data from

a single ultrasound beam to the examiner, nor the data from two or three dimensions.

Some researchers argue that the display of multiple velocities and Doppler echo strength are of no diagnostic value. However, those features of the display are the key to identifying contamination of arterial flow with venous flow (or the converse) and reflective contamination in the image (Figs. 15-6 and 15-8).

If done properly, the electronic method of producing the display has little bearing on the usefulness of the display. A spectral waveform display can be created by using parallel

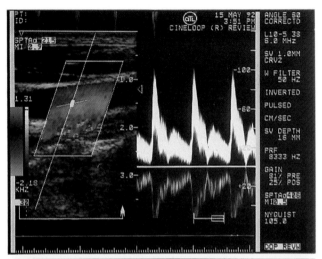

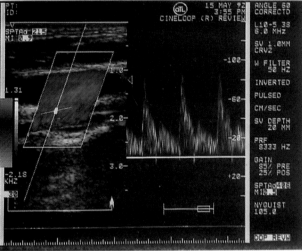

Fig. 15-8. A common carotid artery is located between the depths of 1 cm and 1.5 cm. The Doppler color extends into the tissue below because of reflection of the ultrasound at the lower arterial wall back into the arterial lumen, giving a reflected image at the greater depth. A spectral waveform shows that the Doppler signal from within the artery is strong *(upper panel)*, and that the reflected signal appearing to come from below the artery is weak *(lower panel)*. The color image gives no indication that the deeper signals are weaker. The strength of the reflected signal is about 30 dB lower than the direct arterial signal, based on the assumption that the dynamic range of the spectral waveform is 42 dB. The color outside the vessel can be suppressed by setting the right priority to reject all color signals where the B-mode image brightness is great.

Table 15-3. Hemodynamic information in ultrasound displays

Information	Spectral waveform	1-D color M-mode	2-D color B-mode
Selected velocity component	Yes	Yes	Yes
Velocity versus time	Yes	Yes	No
Velocity versus depth	No	Yes	Yes
Velocity versus lateral location	No	No	Yes
Multiple velocities	Yes	No	No
Doppler echo strength	Yes	Suppressed	Suppressed

filters, FTT, or time compression. FTT can test for 64 frequencies, 128 frequencies, or 256 frequencies. The time resolution can be 5 ms, giving a frequency resolution of 200 Hz per frequency test, or the time resolution can be 20 ms, giving a frequency resolution of 50 Hz. As long as the display is properly designed to show a frequency range equal to the Doppler PRF (the full Nyquist range), all displays are equally useful.

A color display can be created from 16 pulse-echo cycles by the FFT method (Quantum), 4 pulse-echo cycles by the time-domain method (Philips), or 8 pulse-echo cycles by the autocorrelation/pulse-pair-covariance methods (all other manufacturers). The maximum entropy method (MEM) also creates a color display and is currently being developed by at least one manufacturer. Since no quantitative information is required for the examinations, differences between the methods are of no practical importance.

In the design and setup of a color Doppler flow system, a number of choices must be made about the display method. If the image is to be recorded on a standard United States video tape recorder at 30 frames per second (25 frames per second in Europe), each image must be acquired in 33 ms. If an image with a 6-cm depth in tissue is acquired for display, each pulse-echo cycle takes 0.08 ms. A standard B-mode image uses one pulse-echo cycle for each image line, so a B-mode image could contain 416 lines. Since the lateral resolution of a standard video screen exceeds 250 lines, there are plenty of ultrasound scan lines to fill the width of the image.

If a color flow image is created, each color display line takes 4 to 16 pulse-echo cycles to create. The number of pulse-echo cycles required for each color line is the ensemble or packet length. If an ensemble length of 8 is used, only 52 color image lines can be obtained (Table 15-4). The lateral color resolution of the data gathered by the color system is only a fraction of the capability of the display screen. Because the display can show more data than the ultrasound can acquire, the instrument designer and the examiner must choose among the following:
1. Poor lateral color Doppler resolution
2. Narrow color Doppler image

Table 15-4. The lateral resolution of a two-dimensional image with a depth of 6 cm*

Image type	Ensemble length	Time per line	Lines per image
TISSUE			
B-mode	1	0.08 ms	416
VELOCITY			
Time-domain	4	0.32 ms	104
Autocorrelation	8	0.64 ms	52
FFT-mean-mode	16	1.28 ms	26

*30 frame/sec = 33 ms/frame; 6 cm deep = 80 μs/pulse-echo-cycle.

3. Slow frame (Doppler sweep) rate
4. Shallow maximum image depth
The product of these four factors is constant. If the maximum image depth is doubled, one of the other factors must be reduced in half. Because the limitation is in the ability to acquire data, no absolute solution exists.

One way to deal with the limited information is to interpolate between measurements, assuming that the values move smoothly from one to the other. This method is used by manufacturers to smooth the display. Another solution is to show the color information over a portion of the image. This is the method selected by most manufacturers.

INSTRUMENT TESTING

The rate at which ultrasonic Doppler instruments for vascular diagnosis have developed has far outpaced the rate at which effective testing methods have been developed. Some testing methods have been applied to Doppler instruments, but these have had a much greater impact as educational tools for the examiners using the instruments than as tools for the detection of flaws in the design and operation of instruments.

Phillips developed a simple test for ultrasound instruments. With a dishpan of fresh aerated water, a color flow scan head is clamped facing downward, with the face of the scan head just under the water surface. A folded bath towel in the bottom of the dish pan absorbs the ultrasound reaching that depth and thereby prevents secondary reflections from appearing in the image. Tiny air bubbles in the water are expected to rise to the surface. When the B-mode image is turned on and the gains are increased to visualize the bubbles, the air bubbles, which should be rising to the top because of their buoyancy, begin to descend, driven by the force (or pressure) of the ultrasound. The rate of the descent of the microbubbles can be increased or decreased by adjusting the transmit power. Turning on the single-gate pulsed Doppler or the color flow image also changes the speed of the bubbles. A sense of the ultrasonic transmit power can be acquired during the experiment. (The face of the scan head should be wiped from time to time to remove air bubbles. Because the water does not attenuate ultrasound, the time-gain control can be set flat.)

The examiner can stretch a sewing thread between the ends of a bow (as in a bow and arrow), submerge the thread, wipe it to remove air bubbles (a little soap or detergent might help), and move it into the field of view in front of the scan head. By aligning the thread transverse to the image plane, observing the spot on the image that represents the string in cross section, and moving the string to different locations (side to side in the image or shallow and deep in the image), the examiner can see the effects of focusing. The fact that the spot always seems wider than it is high indicates that the depth resolution is better than the lateral resolution.

If the thread is aligned parallel to the image plane and the transducer array, it should form a horizontal line on the

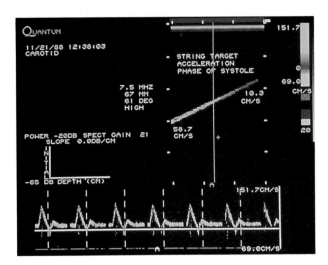

Fig. 15-9. For forming this color image, the ultrasound scan lines begin at the right (at the "key" white box in the upper right corner) and progress toward the left, reaching the left after 55 msec (at a frame rate of 18 frames per second). During that time the silk string accelerates from 10.7 cm/sec to 67.6 cm/sec. The image suggests that the silk string is accelerating.

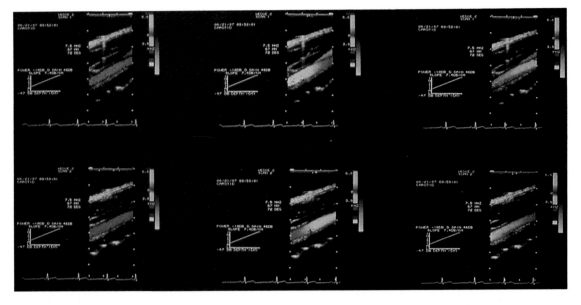

Fig. 15-10. Common carotid artery with the head on the left in all images. *Upper Row:* Three images in sequence (see ECG) spanning the time of systole taken with the first scan line on the right. *Lower Row:* Three images in sequence spanning the time of systole taken with the first scan line on the left. In the lower sequence, a systolic bolus seems to enter the image from the heart on the right (second image) and leave toward the brain on the left (third image). In the upper sequence, a systolic bolus seems to enter the image from the brain on the left (second image) and leave toward the heart on the right (third image). The impression that the length of the high-velocity blood is only a few centimeters during systole is not consistent with the fact that the onset of systole reaches the toes and brain before the end of systole occurs at the heart.

image. If the thread is aligned transverse to the image, tilted in the vertical direction to be at 45° to the image plane, an impression of the thickness of the image plane can be observed; the thicker the plane, the larger the spot appears in the vertical dimension.[6,17] The thickness of the image plane varies with depth and ranges from 2 mm to 10 mm on most instruments. The thickness of the image plane also indicates the thickness dimension of the Doppler sample volume at that depth.[2] Thus the thickness of the Doppler sample volume may be greater than the vessel diameter, contributing to the stationary echo.

Testing of the Doppler requires some kind of moving target. Vibrating targets,[24] moving strings,[1,11,23] and moving fluids have all been used. Moving fluids are a particular problem because the direction and speed are never known variables. Therefore most Doppler testing should be done with moving strings and vibrating plates. Although the frequency/velocity accuracy of the instruments can be determined by test phantoms, the importance of these to vascular testing is limited because the diagnoses do not depend on correct values, only consistent values.[1] The ability of the Doppler system to detect slow velocities compared with fast velocities can be tested with either a vibrating target or a moving string. Vibrating test targets have a limited role in the testing of color flow instruments because they have Doppler frequency shifts in both directions and the color instrument becomes confused, assigning red or blue colors at random.

A pulsatile string phantom can be useful for testing the timing effects in Doppler instruments.[13] Using this phantom with an ECG output, Phillips[13] was able to show that the timing of the ECG on the image associated with a spectral waveform was out of register. In tests of color flow imaging systems using the same string target, all the data on a color flow image are not acquired at the same time. The sweep rate is so slow (usually 50 cm/sec) that at the onset of systole, there is a considerable difference in velocity measured on the left edge of the image compared to the right (Fig. 15-9). Because the speed of pulse propagation from the heart to the foot averages approximately 1000 cm/sec, which is much faster than the blood velocity or the speed of the scan lines progressing across the image, the resultant image is quite misleading, giving the impression that a bolus of blood is present and moving from frame to frame (Fig. 15-10). If the scan head is positioned with the first scan line nearest the distal end of the artery under study, the image gives the impression that a bolus moves from the heart toward the periphery; if the scan head is flipped so that the first scan line is nearest the proximal end of the artery, the bolus appears to move toward the heart.

Testing the sensitivity of a Doppler for the detection of deep blood vessels or an extremely small residual lumen is currently not possible. The combined effects of the Doppler sample volume size and shape, the strength of the stationary echoes, the attenuating effects of the overlying tissues, the sensitivity of the Doppler, and the confounding effects of other tissue motions have not been differentiated. The best source of information about the ability of a Doppler system to function in these difficult situations is to draw on experience, carefully verifying data with confirmatory tests such as angiography.

ECG TRACINGS

Because of the importance of the pulse cycle in analyzing difficult pathology, all ultrasonic vascular examinations should include an ECG tracing to study timing.

CONCLUSION

Ultrasonic imaging systems provide a great deal of information about anatomy, but the images are far from clear. Interpretation of them depends on prior knowledge of anatomy and pathology.

Ultrasonic Doppler systems provide a great deal of information about blood flow, but data are ambiguous. Interpreting them requires a great deal of knowledge of cardiovascular anatomy, cardiovascular hemodynamics, and cardiovascular pathology. It is important to remember that the cardiovascular system includes the peripheral arteries and veins as well as the heart and lungs. Using all of this knowledge, examiners must search with physical examination methods and imaging and Doppler methods to find a set of data that matches their understanding of the anatomy, physiology, and pathology of the patient. Although each Doppler method provides additional information required for diagnosis, there is no substitute for knowledge and curiosity.

REFERENCES

1. Daigle RJ, Stavros AT, Lee RL: Overestimation of velocity and frequency values by multielement linear array Dopplers, *J Vasc Tech* 14(5):206-213, 1990
2. Deane CR et al: Accuracy of colour Doppler ultrasound velocity measurements in small vessels, *J Biomed Engineering* 13:249-254, 1991.
3. Eyer MK et al: Color digital echo/Doppler image presentation, *Ultrasound Med Biol* 7(1):21-31, 1981.
4. Franklin DL et al: A pulsed ultrasonic flowmeter, *Institute of Radio Engineers: Transactions in Medical Electronics* 6:204-206, 1959.
5. Gill RW: Measurement of blood flow by ultrasound: accuracy and sources of error, *Ultrasound Med Biol* 11(4):625-641, 1985.
6. Goldstein A: Slice thickness measurements, *J Ultrasound Med* 7:487-498, 1988.
7. Gulyaev UV, Director of the Institute of Radioengineering and Electronics Automation, lecture, Seattle, 1992, University of Washington.
8. Hokanson DE et al: Ultrasonic arteriography: a new approach to arterial visualization, *Biomed Engineering* 6:420, 1971.
9. Koenko Z et al: Studies on ultrasonic blood-rheograph, *Brain Nerve* 72:921-935, 1960.
10. Kohler TR, Strandness DE Jr: *Use of the Bernoulli principle in the peripheral circulation.* In Nicolaides S, ed: *Cardiovascular applications of Doppler ultrasonography,* London, 1987, Churchill-Livingston.
11. Kohler TR et al: Assessment of pressure gradient by Doppler ultrasound: experimental and clinical observations, *J Vasc Surg* 6(5):460-469, 1987.
12. Ku DN et al: Hemodynamics of the normal human carotid bifurcation: in vitro and in vivo studies, *Ultrasound Med Biol* 11:13-26, 1985.
13. Phillips DJ et al: Testing ultrasonic pulsed Doppler instruments with a physiologic string phantom, *J Ultrasound Med* 9(8):429-436, 1990.

14. Reneman RS et al: Cardiovascular applications of multi-gate pulsed Doppler systems, *Ultrasound Med Biol* 12(5):357-370, 1986.
15. Reynolds O: An experimental investigation of the circumstances which determine the motion of water shall be direct or sinuous, and the law of resistance in parallel channels. Part III, *Philosophical Transactions of the Royal Society of London* 174:935-982, 1884.*
16. Satamura S: Ultrasonic Doppler method for the inspection of cardiac function, *J Acoust Soc Am* 29:1181-1185, 1957.
17. Skolnick M: Estimation of ultrasound beam width in the elevation (section thickness) plane, *Radiology* 180(1):286-288, 1991.

---

*In 1883, Reynolds explored the difference between the results of Poiseuille and Darcy for fluid flow in a tube. Poiseuille's studies of blood flow in arteries, veins, and capillaries and his law that the pressure gradient along a tube is inversely proportional to the fourth power of the luminal diameter and directly proportional to the velocity through the tube (published in 1838) are well known. The studies of Darcy, which state that the pressure gradient in a tube is proportional to the square of the velocity (published in 1858), are not well known.

Darcy H: *Recherches experimentales relatives au mouvement de l'eau dans les tuyaux,* Paris, 1858, Me'm. Sevans Etrang.

18. Spencer MP: *Continuous-wave Doppler imaging of the carotid bifurcation.* In Bernstein EF, ed: *Noninvasive diagnostic techniques in vascular disease,* ed 3, St Louis, 1985, Mosby.
19. Stonebridge PA, Brophy CM: Spiral laminar flow in arteries? *Lancet* 338:1360-1361, 1991.
20. Strandness DE Jr et al: Transcutaneous directional flow detection: a preliminary report, *AHJ* 78(1):65-74, 1969.
21. Sumner DS, Moore DJ, Miles RD: *Doppler ultrasonic arteriography and flow velocity analysis in carotid artery disease.* In Bernstein EF, ed: *Noninvasive diagnostic techniques in vascular disease,* ed 3, St Louis, 1985, Mosby.
22. Thomas GI et al: Noninvasive carotid bifurcation mapping: its relation to carotid surgery, *Am J Surgery* 128(2):168-174, 1974.
23. Walker AR, Phillips DJ, Powers JE: Evaluating Doppler devices using a moving string test target, *J Clin Ultrasound* 10:25-30, 1982.
24. Wang KY, Bone SN, Hossack JM: A tool for evaluating Doppler sensitivity, *J Vasc Tech* 16(2):87-94, 1992.
25. White DN: *Color-coded Doppler carotid imaging.* In Bernstein EF, ed: *Noninvasive diagnostic techniques in vascular disease,* ed 3, St Louis, 1985, Mosby.
26. Yearwood TL, Chanderin KB: Physiological pulsatile flow experiments in a model of the human aortic arch, *J Biomechanics* 15(9):683-704, 1984.

CHAPTER 16

Processing continuous wave Doppler signals and analysis of peripheral arterial waveforms: problems and solutions

K. WAYNE JOHNSTON

In the assessment of patients with peripheral arterial occlusive disease, continuous wave (CW) Doppler velocity meters are most commonly used with a blood pressure cuff to measure limb systolic blood pressures. In addition, many vascular laboratories use them to record blood flow velocity waveforms.

This chapter describes the principles and problems of Doppler-signal processing and waveform analysis of peripheral arterial signals and outlines how these limitations can be overcome.

Representative Doppler signals must be transduced from the artery, the Doppler equipment must process the signals accurately and display a waveform that is free of artifacts, and the waveforms must be quantified accurately to obtain valid and useful clinical data. The problems in Doppler-signal processing and waveform analysis may be the result of errors introduced by (1) the Doppler equipment, (2) the vascular laboratory technologist, or (3) the patient's pathophysiologic state. In the following sections, these errors are outlined and solutions to the problems are described.

ERRORS INTRODUCED BY THE DOPPLER EQUIPMENT

The waveform recorded noninvasively from a peripheral artery with Doppler ultrasound has little or no value unless the examiner can be certain that it is proportional to the true blood flow velocity waveform in the artery. Probably the most common cause of an artifactual waveform is the use of a Doppler system that does not accurately transduce, process, display, or quantify the Doppler waveform. Errors may result from the use of an inappropriate Doppler probe, Doppler demodulation technique, Doppler signal analyzer, display system, or quantitative method for assessment of waveforms.

The Doppler probe

Clinicians have noted that superficial arteries, such as the dorsalis pedis and posterior tibial, are optimally studied by a 9 or 10 MHz Doppler probe, whereas a lower frequency

is preferable for deep vessels including the femoral and popliteal. As shown in Fig. 16-1, for a vessel of d cm depth, the optimum probe frequency (f_{opt}) in MHz is given by the following relationship[45]:

$$f_{opt} = 9/d \qquad (1)$$

If an inappropriate probe frequency is used, the signal-to-noise ratio may be poor, and as a result, it may be impossible to obtain a useful Doppler signal. Moreover, the waveform may appear to be abnormally dampened in the normal subject.

Doppler demodulation techniques

In humans, the normal peripheral arterial blood flow velocity waveform contains forward and reverse flow information. The early work with CW Doppler systems used nondirectional Doppler techniques, and thus it was necessary to determine subjectively which portions of the recorded trace correspond to forward flow and which to reverse flow.[24,54,55] This technique is associated with considerable

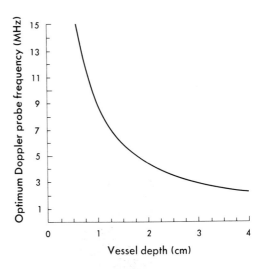

Fig. 16-1. Relationship between optimum Doppler probe frequency and vessel depth.

The secretarial assistance of Ms. P. Purdy is acknowledged.

potential error and ambiguity, and quantitative assessment of Doppler signals requires that the Doppler demodulating technique clearly separate the forward and reverse flow signals, even if they coexist.

The methods available for obtaining the Doppler frequency spectrum with directional information have been reviewed by Coghlan and Taylor[12] and Johnston et al.[24,29] Most commercially available systems make use of one of the new phase quadrature demodulation schemes[39,40,44] or other improved techniques.[37] These schemes are all limited in their ability to achieve perfect separation between the forward and reverse flow channels, and as a result, some cross talk may be present (i.e., some of the reverse flow signal may appear in the forward channel and vice versa). Because the cross talk arises from a cancellation effect, long-term drift of the circuit and aging of the components and productive tolerances can result in inadequate performance. Awareness of the potential inaccuracies that may result from cross talk has led the manufacturers of Doppler velocity meters to specify cross-talk rejections of more than 40 dB. Such high rejection values are now possible through improved designs and stringent quality control.

Doppler signal analyzer (real-time frequency analyzer)

After undistorted Doppler signals are obtained, the instrument must process and display them in a clinically useful way. The errors and limitations associated with the use of a zero-crossing detector, first moment processor, or frequency follower have been documented.[34] In particular, these techniques are associated with certain inherent errors and are not satisfactory for producing a waveform that is suitable for quantitative analysis.[27] For example, in a clinical vascular laboratory study, a zero-crossing detector system accurately recorded the velocity wave in only 15% of the femoral, 31% of the popliteal, 67% of the dorsalis pedis, and 62% of the posterior tibial artery recordings.[27] Furthermore, any recorded mean velocity waveform will be correct only if the entire vessel is uniformly insonated with ultrasound and there is no attenuation of the ultrasound beam across the vessel.

Full spectral analysis is the method of choice for processing the Doppler signals from peripheral arteries because it retains all the Doppler information and allows the examiner to determine if the waveform contains an artifact. The artifacts that can be detected may be the result of significant background noise, high-amplitude, low-frequency signals arising from arterial wall or probe movement, or signals recorded simultaneously from two arteries or an artery and vein. In early studies, frequency analysis was accomplished by an off-line method.[13] The Kay sonograph was a reliable method for processing Doppler signals, but unfortunately, only 2.5 seconds of the Doppler trace could be recorded. It was extremely time consuming, and directional Doppler information could not be displayed easily.

Real-time frequency analysis is preferable and is usually performed by fast Fourier transform (FFT) analysis. If the Doppler signals are processed by a frequency analyzer, the operator can be certain that there are no artifacts and can use different methods to display the Doppler information.

Display of Doppler waveform

After directional Doppler signals are obtained and processed by a real-time frequency analyzer, the resulting spectral information must be displayed and analyzed. Methods for displaying and recording the data include the following:

1. Doppler spectral waveform: In general, in peripheral arterial studies with CW Doppler, the gray-scale information within the waveform has little meaning and can be difficult to quantify (Fig. 16-2). Although spectral broadening is present in the region immediately downstream from a stenosis, unless the entire length of the peripheral arterial tree is examined in detail, detection of a stenosis by recording the extent of spectral broad-

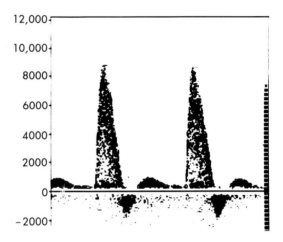

Fig. 16-2. Normal femoral artery waveform displayed by spectral analysis.

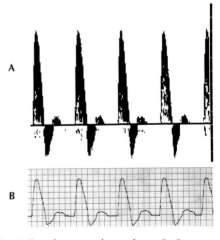

Fig. 16-3. *A,* Doppler spectral waveform. *B,* Corresponding instantaneous maximum velocity waveform.

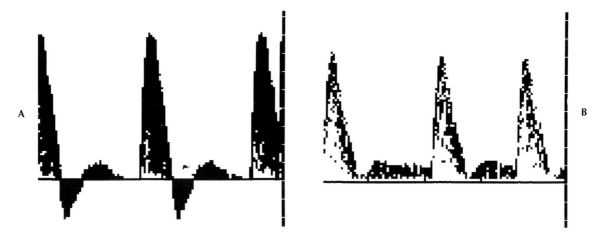

Fig. 16-4. *A,* Normal spectral waveform from bilevel display. *B,* Abnormal waveform.

ening is not generally of great practical value, in contrast to the examination of the carotid artery or peripheral arterial grafts. Consequently, only the shape of the spectral waveform is used to assess the severity of arterial disease.

2. Instantaneous maximum velocity waveform: Fig. 16-3 illustrates the correspondence between the Doppler spectral waveform and the instantaneous maximum velocity waveform derived from the outline of the spectral waveform. The instantaneous maximum velocity waveform represents the velocity of the fastest-moving red cells. This waveform is the envelope of the Doppler frequency waveform. It can be used for quantitative analysis because it is the easiest to obtain clinically and can be determined electronically from the spectral display by using a variety of algorithms.[43]

Assessment of waveforms

Waveforms can be evaluated subjectively or by quantitative analysis. Subjective evaluation of CW Doppler velocity recordings from peripheral arteries is widely used in vascular laboratories for the diagnosis and localization of occlusive peripheral arterial disease. The normal Doppler blood flow velocity waveform is triphasic, consisting of forward flow, reverse flow, and a second forward flow component (Fig. 16-4). In contrast, the waveform is dampened distal to an arterial stenosis or occlusion; that is, the amplitude of the velocity wave is decreased, the peak is delayed, and the reverse flow component is attenuated or absent.* Fig. 16-5 illustrates the progressive dampening of the waveform shape that occurs beyond stenoses. In the usual vascular laboratory study, waveforms are recorded from the femoral, popliteal, dorsalis pedis, and posterior tibial arteries (Fig. 16-6), and vascular disease is detected and regionally localized by subjective analysis. Subjective analysis may be of value in many situations, but unfortunately,

---

*References 13, 16, 19, 24, 29, 30, 58.

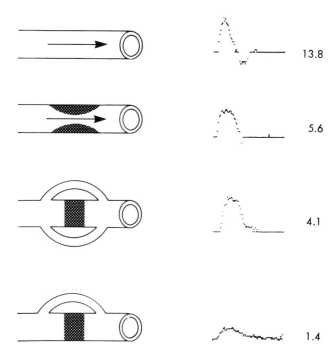

Fig. 16-5. Doppler blood flow velocity waveform is dampened by proximal arterial stenosis. *Numbers* refer to pulsatility index.

it requires experience and the results cannot be used to compare patients or to provide objective, quantitative follow-up.

Quantitative analysis of Doppler waveforms is the ideal goal. Distal to an arterial stenosis, the waveform is dampened and reduced peak amplitude, delayed peak, broadened systolic wave, and reduction or elimination of the reverse flow component are characteristic findings. Any quantitative index that incorporates one or more of these changes may be useful. As described previously, quantification is possible only if directional Doppler signals are obtained by a reliable

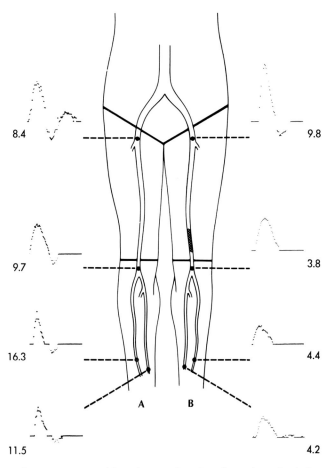

8.4

9.8

9.7

3.8

16.3

4.4

A   B

11.5

4.2

Fig. 16-6. **A,** Normal Doppler recordings from femoral, popliteal, dorsalis pedis, and posterior tibial arteries. **B,** Doppler recordings from patient with superficial femoral artery occlusion.

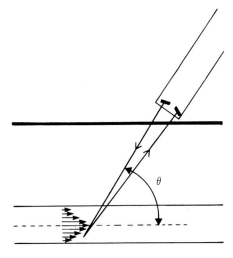

θ

Fig. 16-7. Doppler output can be converted to velocity if the angle between the ultrasound probe and axis of blood flow is known.

acteristic frequency, amplitude (frequency or velocity), and phase angle. In the same way that the amplitude of blood flow velocity waveform depends on the probe-to-vessel angle, the amplitudes of each of the Fourier harmonics and of the mean value of the wave also depend on this angle. However, because the same constant of proportionality applies to all amplitudes, the ratio from the amplitudes of each harmonic (A_n) to the mean amplitude of the wave (A_0) is independent of the probe-to-vessel angle. Fourier pulsatile index is defined by the following:

$$PI_f = \sum_{n=1}^{\infty} \frac{A_n^2}{A_0^2} \qquad (2)$$

Because both the numerator and the denominator depend on the velocity squared, the unknown constant of proportionality, which relates the maximum instantaneous frequency waveform to the maximum instantaneous velocity waveform, disappears in the calculation. Theoretically, this index is independent of the probe-to-vessel angle.[36]

Because energy is proportional to velocity squared, the Fourier pulsatility index is related to the maximum oscillatory energy of the wave divided by the energy of the mean forward flow. Distal to an arterial stenosis, the oscillatory energy of the wave is reduced, and it was therefore predicted that the Fourier pulsatility index would be reduced and would be useful for detecting occlusive arterial disease. The diagnostic value of the Fourier pulsatility index has been confirmed in clinical studies.[18,24]

Peak-to-peak pulsatility index. Because the calculation of the Fourier pulsatility index is cumbersome and time consuming, it is impractical for routine clinical use. Gosling and King[17] have suggested an alternative definition of the pulsatility index with roughly the same diagnostic sensitivity. Fig. 16-8 defines the peak-to-peak pulsatility index as:

$$PI_{p/p} = \frac{\text{Peak-to-peak velocity}}{\text{Mean velocity}} \qquad (3)$$

method and the Doppler signals are processed and displayed accurately.

The most direct way to quantify the Doppler waveform is to calibrate the waveform as velocity. However, the Doppler output can be converted to velocity only when the angle between the ultrasound probe and the axis of blood flow is known (Fig. 16-7). Even with a duplex Doppler ultrasound system, there may be significant errors in measuring this angle; certainly with a CW Doppler system, the error is too large to measure velocity accurately. Nonetheless, quantitative data can still be obtained. For any measurement from the Doppler waveform to be of value, the measurement must be independent of the probe-to-vessel angle and be clinically useful.

Fourier pulsatility index. Fourier analysis can be used to quantify the Doppler waveform.[17,18,57] Any periodic wave, including the Doppler blood flow velocity waveform, can be expressed as a series of sine waves (harmonics) that oscillate about a mean velocity. The frequencies of these sine waves are integral multiples of the fundamental frequency (i.e., the heart rate). Each sine wave has a char-

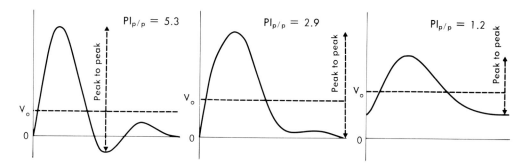

Fig. 16-8. Calculation of peak-to-peak pulsatility index.

The peak-to-peak pulsatility index is also independent of the probe-to-vessel angle, since the unknown constant of proportionality is present in both the numerator and the denominator and disappears in the calculation. The peak-to-peak pulsatility index and the Fourier pulsatility index are directly related.[30]

The pulsatility index will usually increase if the examiner progresses distally from the aorta to the pedal arteries. A second index—the dampening factor (DF)—is needed to quantify these changes and permit regional localization of occlusive arterial disease.[18]

$$DF = \frac{\text{Proximal pulsatility index}}{\text{Distal pulsatility index}} \qquad \textbf{(4)}$$

Because most clinical measurement indices decrease with increasing severity of disease, the inverse dampening factor (DF^{-1}) may be used to conform to this convention.

Clinical studies have shown that the pulsatility index is of diagnostic value.* In a typical study (see Fig. 16-6), recordings are made from the femoral, popliteal, dorsalis pedis, and posterior tibial arteries. Femoral pulsatility index and femoral, popliteal, and tibial inverse dampening factors are calculated.

Recordings were made from 224 limbs and compared to arteriographic grades to obtain the data presented in Figs. 16-9, 16-10, and 16-11. In arteriographic studies, other investigators have confirmed that the measurement of peak-to-peak pulsatility index could detect and regionally localize significant peripheral arterial occlusive disease.[1,19,20]

Because of the uncertainties of arteriographic grading, 175 aortofemoral segments were studied, and the accuracy of peak-to-peak pulsatility index was determined by comparing the systolic pressure difference between the aorta and common femoral artery as measured at the time of arteriography.[27] In Fig. 16-12, *A*, the receiver-operating characteristic (ROC) curve is shown for all pulsatility index measurements.[41,42] An aortofemoral systolic pressure difference equal to or more than 10 mm Hg was considered a positive test. The highest pulsatility index recorded from the femoral artery at the level of the inguinal ligament or 2

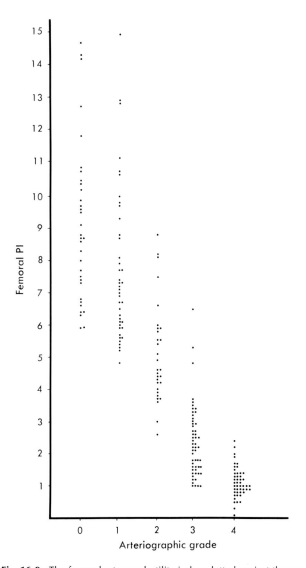

Fig. 16-9. The femoral artery pulsatility index plotted against the corresponding aortoiliac arteriographic grade. Grade 0, normal; Grade 1, intimal disease; Grade 2, less than 50% stenosis; Grade 3, greater than 50% stenosis; Grade 4, complete arterial occlusion. (Courtesy PSG Publishing Co. Inc., Littleton, Massachusetts.)

*References 11, 17-19, 23, 25, 28, 30, 31, 34, 35, 57.

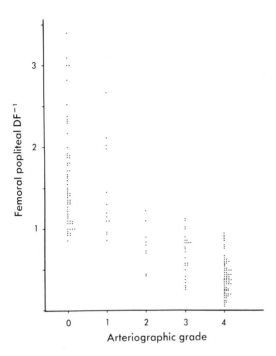

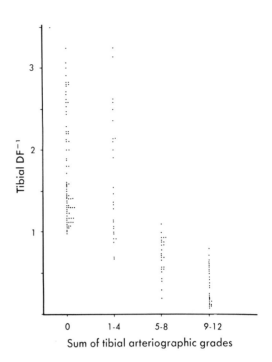

Fig. 16-10. Inverse femoral popliteal DF plotted against femoral artery arteriographic grades. (Courtesy PSG Publishing Co. Inc., Littleton, Massachusetts.)

Fig. 16-11. Inverse tibial DF plotted against sum of tibial artery arteriographic grades. (Courtesy PSG Publishing Co. Inc., Littleton, Massachusetts.)

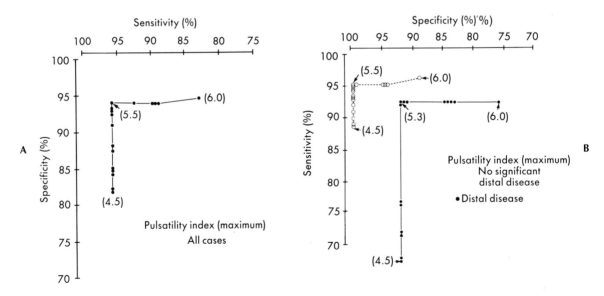

Fig. 16-12. ROC curves. An aortofemoral systolic pressure difference greater than or equal to 10 mm Hg was considered a positive test. Sensitivities and specificities are plotted for different values of pulsatility index in increments of 0.1. **A,** All cases. **B,** The effect of distal arterial occlusive disease. (From Johnston KW, Kassam M, Cobbold RSC: *Ultrasound Med Biol* 9:271, 1983.)

to 3 cm distally was used. In the ROC curve, the sensitivities and specificities are plotted in increments of 0.1 for threshold values of pulsatility index between 4.5 and 6.0. The maximum overall accuracy is approximately 95%.

The effect of distal peripheral arterial occlusive disease on the accuracy of femoral pulsatility index measurements is shown in the ROC curve plotted in Fig. 16-12, *B*. The diagnostic accuracy of the pulsatility index in patients without significant distal occlusive disease is slightly higher than for those patients with significant distal disease (i.e., patients with more than 50% stenosis or occlusion of the femoral popliteal segment or occlusion of two or three tibial arteries).

Although some research[2-4,11] has indicated that the pulsatility index is of value in diagnosing hemodynamically significant aortoiliac disease even if the patient has distal occlusive disease, other investigators[6-9,56] have suggested that the pulsatility index is strongly influenced by the severity of distal disease and that the femoral pulsatility index is less accurate when distal disease is present. Accurate reproducible measurements can be obtained only if attention is given to the technical details previously described. These factors probably explain the reason pulsatility index measurements have been less accurate in some studies.

Other indices. Although a number of indices, including transit time,[14,17,22] rise time, and rise time ratio,[22] have been suggested for quantifying Doppler ultrasound recordings, in a recent study,[32] the accuracies of the peak-to-peak pulsatility index, height-width index, path length index, and a transfer function index in the diagnosis of peripheral arterial occlusive disease were compared.

Height-width index. Height-width index (HWI) is based on the observations that waveforms recorded distal to an arterial stenosis have smaller peak forward and smaller peak reverse flow frequencies relative to the mean value and that the duration of the systolic peak is longer than that of a normal waveform. This dimensionless index is given by the following formula:

$$HWI = \frac{\text{Peak-to-peak frequency}/\text{Mean frequency}}{\text{Duration of systolic peak}/\text{Duration of cardiac cycle}} \quad (5)$$

where the systolic peak duration is measured between the half-amplitude points.

Path length index (PLI). Increased dampening on the instantaneous frequency waveform increases the total path traced out over one cardiac cycle. Consequently, the path length, normalized by mean amplitude (to remove the angle dependence) and normalized by the cardiac period (to reduce the dependence on heart rate), should be reasonably well correlated with the disease grade. The PLI is defined by:

$$PLI = \sum_{i=0}^{n-1} [(f_{i+1} - F_i)^2/\bar{f}^2 - (t_{i+1} - t_i)^2/T]^{1/2} \quad (6)$$

where the time axis has been divided into n segments, the maximum instantaneous frequency at the time t_i is f_i, f is the mean frequency, and T_0 is the total waveform duration.

Transfer function index. Researchers[10,48,49,52] have suggested that arterial occlusive disease can be diagnosed by determining the poles of the transfer function that relate the flow velocity waveform measured at two locations. Subsequently, Skidmore and Woodcock[50,51,53] proposed that the velocity waveform could fit in the frequency domain to the third-order Laplace transform. The parameters can also be obtained by fitting the waveform in the time domain to the inverse Laplace transform. Skidmore et al[52] calculated δ from the femoral Doppler recordings and investigated the sensitivity to aortoiliac disease. They concluded that δ is a sensitive index for determining the presence of aortoiliac stenosis. In addition, they also investigated the pulsatility index but found that, unlike δ, it did not seem to differentiate between stenoses of less than 50% and more than 50%.

Recordings of the Doppler spectral waveforms from the common femoral artery of 234 limbs were digitized to obtain the maximum velocity waveforms to determine the optimal index.[32] The data were analyzed on a computer, and the various indices were computed and compared with the arteriographic grades. The calculations of peak-to-peak pulsatility index, HWI, and PLI were straightforward, but the transfer function parameters were more complicated. Although the method described by Skidmore[48] was used accurately, there were significant problems with the frequency domain-fitting technique.[32] Specifically, a significant number of waveforms did not yield complex poles, there were significant discrepancies in the reconstructed waveform of certain recordings, and there were discrepancies in many of the natural frequencies as well. Because of these problems, a curve-fitting procedure in the time domain was done and δ was specifically calculated.

The accuracy of each index for detecting aortoiliac disease was determined with calculation of the ROC curves.[21] Two definitions of a positive test were used. In the first, an iliac arteriographic lesion of less than 50% or more than 50% or a complete occlusion was used; this resulted in the ROC curves in Fig. 16-13. For the second, iliac disease was defined to be present if the stenosis was either more than 50% or a complete occlusion. For this definition, the curves in Fig. 16-14 resulted. In both sets of curves, the sensitivities and specificities are plotted for different cut-off values of each index.

Coexisting femoral popliteal occlusive disease reduced the accuracy of all indices when the definition of iliac disease is a stenosis of less than 50%, more than 50%, or a complete occlusion. On the other hand, for the other definition (that is, more than 50% stenosis or a complete occlusion), the effect of femoral popliteal disease on the accuracy is less marked, particularly for peak-to-peak pulsatility index and HWI.

Although arteriography may not be the ideal standard for evaluating noninvasive Doppler data, its shortcomings are not particularly important, since all four indices in this study were calculated from the same waveforms. All the indices had very similar diagnostic accuracies. In contrast to the

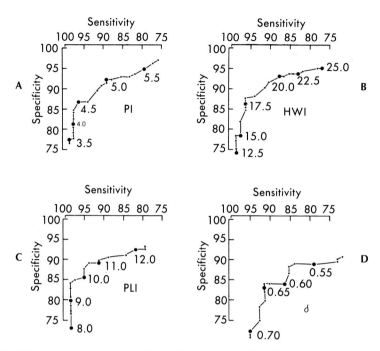

Fig. 16-13. ROC curves for **A,** PI; **B,** HWI; **C,** PLI; and **D,** δ. Iliac disease was defined as present if arteriogram showed less than 50% stenosis, greater than 50% stenosis, or complete occlusion. (From Johnston KW, Kassam M, Cobbold RSC: *Ultrasound Med Biol* 9:271, 1983.)

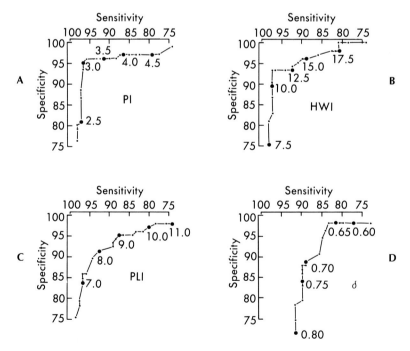

Fig. 16-14. ROC curves for **A,** PI; **B,** HWI; **C,** PLI; and **D,** δ. Iliac disease was defined as present if arteriogram showed greater than 50% stenosis or complete occlusion. (From Johnston KW, Kassam M, Cobbold RSC: *Ultrasound Med Biol* 9:271, 1983.)

previous report by Skidmore et al,[53] the index δ did not prove to be superior to pulsatility index. In view of the approximately equivalent diagnostic accuracy of the four indices studied, pulsatility index has the advantages of simplicity and ease of real-time calculation.

ERRORS INTRODUCED BY THE TECHNOLOGIST

As with most diagnostic techniques, the operator must acquire experience and appreciate the technical and physiologic limitations of Doppler signal processing and quantitative waveform analysis before representative blood flow velocity recordings can be obtained and reproducible results achieved. For example, errors in recording the femoral artery waveform may be made: (1) if only part of the artery is insonated with the CW Doppler ultrasound probe or recordings are inadvertently made from a side branch, (2) if two arteries or an artery and a vein are recorded simultaneously, or (3) if the technologist fails to realize that the Doppler signal may be attenuated if the vessel is covered with scar tissue, a hematoma, or excessive fat or it has an atherosclerotic plaque on the anterior wall. The technologist must alter the probe position and/or frequency to obtain a representative waveform recording.

If Doppler recordings are to be of quantitative diagnostic value, the technologist must be adequately trained and operate in an up-to-date technical facility. The use of frequency analysis with a real-time spectral display allows the technologist to position the probe optimally, avoid artifacts, and record representative waveforms.

PATHOPHYSIOLOGIC ERRORS
Attenuation of the Doppler signal

Ultrasound is attenuated as it passes through tissue; hence, when the distance between the probe and the vessel is increased by obesity, a hematoma from an arteriogram or operation, or scar tissue, the Doppler blood flow signals are significantly attenuated. As a result, the Doppler signals may not be distinguishable from background noise, or the waveform may appear abnormal. This problem can usually be overcome if the technologist uses the optimum Doppler probe frequency and position. Similarly, an atherosclerotic plaque on the anterior wall of the femoral artery may attenuate the ultrasound signal and give the false impression that the waveform is dampened. However, with a real-time spectral display, the operator can position the probe and obtain a representative waveform in most cases.

Variations of respiration, heart rate, and peripheral resistance

Because peripheral blood flow fluctuates with respiration, the peripheral arterial blood flow velocity waveform and thus the pulsatility index also change with respiration. However, the effect of normal respiration on pulsatility index is insignificant in most patients.

Pulsatility index is calculated by dividing the peak-to-peak height of the wave by the mean height. The mean height is the net area under the wave (forward minus reverse)

divided by the pulse length. In other words the pulsatility index varies linearly with the heart rate. This has been confirmed in a study of patients with cardiac arrhythmias,[33] but it is not a common limitation.

As with the determination of many other physiologic parameters, quantitative analysis of the Doppler waveform assumes that the patient is in a basal state. If vasodilatation occurs, limb blood flow and therefore mean velocity increase and the pulsatility index fall, even though the wave may remain very oscillatory. This problem may be minimized by examining subjects at rest, in a quiet room, and at a temperature of $21° C \pm 1° C$. No exercise should be permitted for at least 15 minutes before the examination, and subjects should be asked to refrain from smoking for 1 hour before an examination.

Minor arterial stenoses

Minor and usually asymptomatic and hemodynamically insignificant arterial stenoses are not consistently detected by calculation of the pulsatility index from Doppler velocity waveforms. However, some stenoses will only become hemodynamically significant with exercise and will not be detected in the resting state.

Major stenoses and occlusions

Major arterial stenoses and arterial occlusions cannot always be distinguished by waveform analysis. Although Gosling and King[17] suggest that the addition of transit time measurement to those of pulsatility index and inverse DF may improve this differentiation, this measurement may not be of additional value. Moreover, distinguishing severe stenosis from complete occlusion in the peripheral arteries is rarely of clinical significance and hemodynamically, a complete occlusion with good collateralization may be similar to major stenosis.

Multisegmental severe disease

With the pulsatility index and inverse DF, occlusive peripheral arterial disease can usually be detected and localized, even if more than one arterial segment is involved. However, if severe occlusive disease is present in a proximal segment and the waveforms are very dampened, meaningful quantitative measurements from the more distal segments may be impossible to attain.

Tibial artery assessment

Collateral flow between the three tibial arteries is usually quite satisfactory, so atherosclerotic occlusion of one tibial vessel cannot be detected. Nonetheless, significant occlusive tibial artery disease (disease in two or three vessels) can usually be detected by the calculation of the tibial inverse DF (see Fig. 16-11).

Recommendations for quantification with the pulsatile index

CW Doppler systems can be used to quantify the severity of peripheral arterial occlusive disease, which can lead to more precise diagnoses. However, the quantitative analysis of Doppler waveforms can be achieved only if certain recommendations are followed.

Accurate recordings can be obtained only if a Doppler probe with the proper field pattern, operating close to the optimum frequency, is used. The importance of the frequency of the Doppler probe has often been overlooked. Some investigators[7,56] have used 8 to 10 MHz probes to record Doppler signals from the femoral artery. However, obtaining a Doppler signal much above the noise level may be difficult with an 8 MHz probe, especially if the common femoral artery is deep, is surrounded by hematoma or scar tissue, or has a significant atherosclerotic plaque on the anterior wall. Although femoral recordings can be made with this high frequency, 4 to 5 MHz probes generally are preferable because they reduce the attenuation and result in a better signal-to-noise ratio.

In addition, the transmitter-receiver must have an adequate power output, good signal-to-noise ratio, and clear separation between forward and reverse flow channels to obtain an accurate reading. A high-pass filter is often used to reject wall thump artifacts. For peripheral arterial studies, this filter cut off should not exceed 100 Hz (when using 8 MHz probe) so that important reverse flow information is not lost. The presence or absence of reverse flow is a very sensitive indicator of the disease state and is reflected in the pulsatility index value. In many commercial instruments that allow both carotid and peripheral arterial studies, the wall thump filter may be set at 400 Hz to reject the wall thump artifacts experienced in the carotid artery.

A real-time frequency analyzer should be used to process the Doppler signals and obtain representative waveforms free of electronic and physiologic artifacts. Through the use of a real-time frequency analyzer, the technologist obtains both visual and audio feedback and thus can position the Doppler probe to achieve better "quality control" of the waveforms selected for analysis. Consequently, waveforms that contain artifacts caused by a poor signal-to-noise ratio, coexisting arterial or venous flow, or atypical flow patterns like those that may occur directly over a stenosis or at an arterial bifurcation can be excluded.

The maximum velocity waveform should be analyzed instead of the mean velocity waveform for several reasons.[26,27] First, the operator does not need to ensure that the vessel is completely and uniformly insonated. Instead, the operator simply searches for the largest spectral waveform while keeping the probe-to-vessel angle constant. Second, noise or coexisting arterial or venous signals may seriously affect the mean velocity waveform,* but the maximum waveform is less susceptible to these artifacts. Last, complete insonation of the vessel is required to obtain the true mean waveform but not the maximum waveform. The maximum velocity waveform can be derived directly from the envelope of the spectral waveform.[26]

---

*References 5, 15, 17, 28, 38, 46, 47.

The zero flow baseline reference must be stable at all times. Slight changes in the baseline may cause significant errors in the calculated values of pulsatility index from certain waveforms. Baseline variation resulting from electronic drift should be detected and compensated before quantification. Once the envelope of the maximum spectral waveform is obtained, prefiltering should be performed before quantification. A digital or an analogue low-pass filter with a cut off at approximately 30 Hz should be used to smooth out any spikes that may arise as a result of background noise or physiologic artifacts. Although this situation does not occur often, it will cause significant errors in the calculation of pulsatility index.

Calculation of pulsatility index can be performed in real time. The algorithm for identifying the waves without the use of an electrocardiogram trigger and for calculation of pulsatility index has been described previously.[26]

Another way to ensure accuracy is to have the technologist who performs waveform analysis be well trained, acquire experience in Doppler technique, and recognize the problems associated with waveform analysis. The use of a real-time frequency analyzer and visual display of the bidirectional Doppler information permits optimal interaction between the operator and the Doppler system and allows the technologist to obtain representative and reproducible blood flow velocity recordings.

Test conditions should be ideal. Limb blood flow and consequently Doppler blood flow velocity waveforms are affected significantly by the factors that change peripheral arterial resistance. Patients should be examined in a room with a temperature between 20° C and 22° C and after a minimum of 15 minutes rest to minimize the physiologic variations in pulsatility index.

CONCLUSION

Doppler recordings from peripheral arteries can be quantified if attention is paid to the details of Doppler signal processing methods, if the technologist is well trained and experienced, and if certain physiologic and pathologic limitations are recognized.

REFERENCES

1. Altstaedt F, Storz LW, Ruckert U: *Erste erfahrungen mit einer semiquantitativen analyse von Doppler-fluss-kurven in der gefasschirurgie.* In Kriessman A and Bollinger A, eds: *Ultrashall-Doppler-Diagnostik in der Angiologie,* Stuttgart, Germany, 1979, Thieme.
2. Archie JP: Nondimensional normalized femoral Doppler waveform indices to predict the hemodynamic significance of iliac artery stenosis, *Surg Forum* 30:191, 1979.
3. Archie JP, Feldtman RW: Intraoperative assessment of the hemodynamic significance of iliac and profunda femoris artery stenosis, *Surgery* 90:876, 1981.
4. Archie JP, Feldtman RW: Determination of the hemodynamic significance of iliac artery stenosis by noninvasive Doppler ultrasonography, *Surgery* 91:419, 1982.
5. Arts MG, Roevros JM: On the instantaneous measurement of bloodflow by ultrasonic means, *Med Biol Eng* 10:23, 1972.
6. Bagi P et al: Doppler waveform analysis in evaluation of occlusive arterial disease in the lower limb: comparison with distal blood pressure measurement and arteriography, *Eur J Vasc Surg* 4:305-311, 1990.

7. Baird RN et al: Upstream stenosis—its diagnosis by Doppler signals from the femoral artery, *Arch Surg* 115:1316, 1980.
8. Baker AR et al: Some failings of pulsatility index and damping factor, *Ultrasound Med Biol* 12:875-881, 1986.
9. Barrie WE, Evans DH, Bell PRF: The relationship between ultrasonic pulsatility index and proximal arterial stenosis, *Br J Surg* 66:366, 1979.
10. Brown JM et al: Transfer-function modelling of arteries, *Med Biol Eng Comput* 16:161, 1978.
11. Capper WL et al: Noninvasive assessment of lower limb ischemia by blood velocity waveform analysis, *S Afr Med J* 71:695-698, 1987.
12. Coghlan BA, Taylor MG: Directional Doppler techniques for detection of blood velocities, *Ultrasound Med Biol* 2:181, 1976.
13. Fitzgerald DE, Carr J: Doppler ultrasound diagnosis and classification as an alternative to arteriography, *Angiology* 26:183, 1975.
14. Fitzgerald DE, Gosling RG, Woodcock JP: Grading dynamic capability of arterial collateral circulation, *Lancet* 1:66, 1971.
15. Flax SW, Webster JG, Updike SJ: Pitfalls using Doppler ultrasound to transduce blood flow, *IEEE Trans Biomed Eng* 20:306, 1973.
16. Fronek A, Coel M, Bernstein EF: Quantitative ultrasonographic studies of lower extremity flow velocities in health and in disease, *Circulation* 53:953, 1976.
17. Gosling RG, King DH: *Continuous wave ultrasound as an alternative and complement to x-rays in vascular examinations.* In Reneman RS, ed: *Cardiovascular applications of ultrasound,* Amsterdam, 1974, North Holland.
18. Gosling RG et al: The quantitative analysis of occlusive peripheral arterial disease by a nonintrusive technique, *Angiology* 22:52, 1971.
19. Harris PL: *The role of ultrasound in the assessment of peripheral arterial disease,* doctoral dissertation, Manchester, England, 1975, University of Manchester.
20. Harris PL: The relationship between Doppler ultrasound assessment and angiography in occlusive arterial disease of the lower limbs, *Surg Gynecol Obstet* 138:911, 1974.
21. Haynes BL: How to read clinical journals. II. To learn about a diagnostic test, *Can Med Assoc J* 124:703, 1981.
22. Humphries KN et al: Quantitative assessment of the common femoral to popliteal arterial segment using continuous wave Doppler ultrasound, *Ultrasound Med Biol* 6:99, 1980.
23. Johnston KW: Role of Doppler ultrasonography in determining the hemodynamic significance of aortoiliac disease, *Can J Surg* 21:319, 1978.
24. Johnston KW, Taraschuk I: Validation of the role of pulsatility index in quantitation of the severity of peripheral arterial occlusive disease, *Am J Surg* 131:295, 1976.
25. Johnston KW, Demorais D, Colapinto RF: Difficulty in assessing the severity of aortoiliac disease by clinical and arteriographic methods, *Angiology* 32:609, 1982.
26. Johnston KW, Kassam M, Cobbold RSC: On-line identification and quantification of Doppler ultrasound waveforms, *Med Biol Eng Comput* 20:336, 1982.
27. Johnston KW, Kassam M, Cobbold RSC: Relationship between Doppler pulsatility index and direct femoral pressure measurements in the diagnosis of aortoiliac occlusive disease, *Ultrasound Med Biol* 9:271, 1983.
28. Johnston KW, Maruzzo BC, Cobbold RSC: Errors and artifacts of Doppler flowmeters and their solution, *Arch Surg* 112:1335, 1977.
29. Johnston KW, Maruzzo BC, Cobbold RSC: Inaccuracies of a zero-crossing detector for recording Doppler signals, *Surg Forum* 28:201, 1977.
30. Johnston KW, Maruzzo BC, Cobbold RSC: Doppler methods for quantitative measurement and localization of peripheral arterial disease by analysis of the blood flow velocity waveform, *Ultrasound Med Biol* 4:209, 1978.
31. Johnston KW, Maruzzo BC, Taraschuk IC: *Fourier and peak-to-peak pulsatility indices—quantitation of arterial occlusive disease.* In Taylor DEM, Whamond D, eds: *Noninvasive clinical measurement,* Tunbridge Wells, England, 1977, Pittman.
32. Johnston KW et al: Comparative study of four methods for quantifying Doppler ultrasound waveforms from the femoral artery, *Ultrasound Med Biol* 10:1, 1984.
33. Johnston KW et al: *Quantitative analysis of Doppler blood flow velocity recordings using pulsatility index.* In Nicolaides AN, Yao JST, eds: *Investigation of vascular disorders,* Edinburgh, 1980, Churchill Livingstone.
34. Johnston KW et al: *Methods for obtaining, processing and quantifying Doppler blood flow velocity waveforms.* In Nicolaides AN, Yao JST, eds: *Investigation of vascular disorders,* Edinburgh, 1981, Churchill Livingstone (in press).
35. Jorgensen JJ, Stranden E, Gjolberg T: The femoral arterial flow velocity pattern in patients with aortoiliac atherosclerosis: studies with a pulsed Doppler ultrasound flowmeter, *Acta Chir Scand* 152:257-261, 1986.
36. Kaneko J et al: Analysis of ultrasonic blood rheogram by the sound spectrograph, *Jpn Circ J* 34:1035, 1970.
37. Kassam M, Johnston KW, Cobbold RSC: *A critical assessment of heterodyne demodulation techniques for directional Doppler ultrasound.* Paper presented at the XII International Conference on Medical and Biological Engineering, part II, session 28, Jerusalem, 1979.
38. Lunt MJ: Accuracy and limitations of the ultrasonic Doppler blood velocimeter and zero-crossing detector, *Ultrasound Med Biol* 2:1, 1975.
39. Mackay RS: Noninvasive cardiac output measurement, *Microvasc Res* 4:438, 1972.
40. Maruzzo BC, Johnston KW, Cobbold RSC: *Real-time spectral analysis of directional Doppler flow signals.* Digest of XI International Conference on Medical and Biological Engineering, Ottawa, 1976.
41. McNeil BJ, Keller E, Adelstein SJ: Primer on certain elements of medical decision making, *N Engl J Med* 293:211, 1975.
42. Metz CE: Basic principles of ROC analysis, *Semin Nucl Med* 8:283, 1978.
43. Mo LY, Yun LC, Cobbold RS: Comparison of four digital maximum frequency estimators for Doppler ultrasound, *Ultrasound Med Biol* 14:355-363, 1988.
44. Nippa JH et al: Phase rotation for separating forward and reverse blood velocity signals, *IEEE Trans Sonics Ultrasonics* SU-22:340, 1975.
45. Reid JM, Baker DW: *Physics and electronics of the ultrasonic Doppler method.* In Bock J, Ossoinig K, eds: *Ultrasonographia medica,* vol 1, Vienna, 1971, Verlag Wein Medizinisch Akademie.
46. Reneman RS, Spencer MP: *Difficulties in processing of an analogue Doppler flow signal; with special reference to zero-crossing meters and quantification.* In Reneman RS, ed: *Cardiovascular applications of ultrasound,* Amsterdam, 1974, North Holland.
47. Roberts C: Ultrasound in the assessment of vascular function, *Med Prog Technol* 4:3, 1976.
48. Skidmore R: *The use of the transcutaneous ultrasonic flowmeter in the dynamic analysis of blood flow,* doctoral dissertation, Bristol, England, 1979, University of Bristol.
49. Skidmore R, Woodcock JP: Physiological significance of arterial models derived using transcutaneous ultrasonic flowmeters, *J Physiol (Lond)* 277:29, 1978.
50. Skidmore R, Woodcock JP: Physiologic interpretation of Doppler-shift waveforms. I. Theoretical considerations, *Ultrasound Med Biol* 6:7, 1980.
51. Skidmore R, Woodcock JP: Physiologic interpretation of Doppler-shift waveforms. II. Validation of the Laplace transform method for characterization of the common femoral blood-velocity/time waveform, *Ultrasound Med Biol* 6:219, 1980.
52. Skidmore R et al: Transfer function analysis of common femoral artery Doppler waveforms, *Br J Surg* 66:883, 1979.
53. Skidmore R et al: Physiological interpretation of Doppler-shift waveforms. III. Clinical results, *Ultrasound Med Biol* 6:227, 1980.
54. Stevens A, Roberts VC: *On-line signal processing of CW Doppler shifted ultrasound.* Digest of XI International Conference on Medical and Biological Engineering, Ottawa, Canada, 1976.
55. Strandness DE Jr: *Peripheral arterial disease, a physiologic approach,* Boston, 1967, Little, Brown.
56. Ward AS, Martin TP: Some aspects of ultrasound in the diagnosis and assessment of aortoiliac disease, *Am J Surg* 140:260, 1980.
57. Woodcock JP, Gosling RG, Fitzgerald DE: A new noninvasive technique for assessment of superficial femoral artery obstruction, *Br J Surg* 59:226, 1972.
58. Yao ST: Haemodynamic studies in peripheral arterial disease, *Br J Surg* 57:761, 1970.

CHAPTER 17

Blood flow disturbances and spectral analysis

DON P. GIDDENS and RICHARD I. KITNEY

The ideal noninvasive method for detecting and quantifying atherosclerosis should be able to describe the level of disease over its entire spectrum, including configuration, function, composition, and complication. Although no present single test can accomplish these goals, duplex scanning—the combination of high-resolution B-mode imaging with pulsed Doppler ultrasound—has significantly improved disease identification. It provides anatomic information and functional data on blood flow and its behavior near plaques. It is now possible, for example, to grade stenoses in rather broad categories based on peak Doppler frequency and spectral broadening.[15] On the other hand, a major weakness is the difficulty in distinguishing flow patterns induced by minimal disease from those inherent in normal vessels; this differentiation is not significantly enhanced by current imaging capability.

Despite present limitations, however, advances in disease description should be possible through a greater knowledge of arterial fluid dynamics, particularly as related to branching and poststenotic flows, and of signal analysis methods capable of extracting relevant information from Doppler-derived measurements. This chapter discusses recent advances in the understanding of arterial flow disturbances and provides examples of modern signal analysis techniques, which appear to offer promise for improvements in data processing of velocity measurements. Data obtained from laboratory and animal models are used to exhibit fundamental phenomena. This chapter also discusses problems associated with transferring this knowledge to noninvasive measurements with Doppler ultrasound and speculates on future work, which may improve clinical diagnoses.

FLUID MECHANICS

Most fluid dynamics knowledge is based on flow velocity, whereas noninvasive Doppler ultrasound measurements result in data whose frequency content is related to but not necessarily the same as flow velocity. Therefore the interpretation of Doppler-derived data requires a knowledge of the relationship between Doppler frequency and fluid velocity and of the complex flow fields that can occur in branching and stenotic vessels. In this section, the nature of poststenotic flow disturbances is examined using a simple configuration—that of an axisymmetric constriction in an

unbranched tube or vessel. The data examined are velocity results obtained with either a laser Doppler velocity meter in vitro or a hot-film anemometer in vivo. Relationships with Doppler ultrasound are also discussed.

Earlier work showed that rather mild stenoses in the descending canine thoracic aorta produced notable velocity disturbances.[14] An example of this is shown in Fig. 17-1, which displays the velocity measured at the centerline of a dog aorta by a hot-film anemometer probe located 2 cm distal to a 40% stenosis (by area reduction).[13] Disturbances in the velocity waveform are clearly seen during the deceleration phase of systole, although whether these fluctuations are turbulent is difficult to determine by visual inspection. As the degree of stenosis increases, the intensity and duration of the disturbances also increase,[14,17] until flow becomes extremely turbulent throughout the cycle.

Because of the ability to control flow conditions carefully, in vitro model studies are useful for examining the nature and evolution of poststenotic flow disturbances. An ideal instrument for such studies is the laser Doppler velocimeter (LDV), which is noninvasive and possesses far superior resolution and accuracy than Doppler ultrasound instruments. The major drawback of the LDV is its requirement of a good optical path between the instrument and sample volume. Khalifa and Giddens[18] performed a series of LDV measurements in Plexiglas tubes containing varying degrees of constriction using pulsatile flow that was representative of conditions in the dog aorta. Fig. 17-2 presents examples of velocity waveforms measured at the center line of the tube for several axial locations distal to a 50% (by area) stenosis. By carefully examining data such as these and using time series signal analysis methods, researchers found that three distinct types of flow disturbances exist:

1. A coherent structure associated with the startup process of each cycle (termed a *starting structure*)
2. Oscillations of discrete frequency originating in the shear layer formed in the diverging section of the stenosis (termed a *shear layer oscillation*)
3. Turbulent structures characterized by some degree of random velocity behavior

These disturbances are listed in the order of their occurrence as the degree of stenosis increases. For example, depending on the Reynolds number, frequency parameter, and contour,

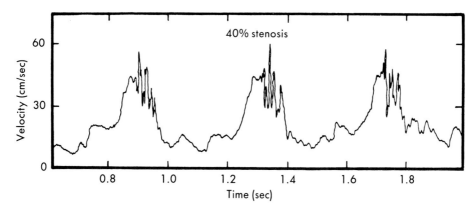

Fig. 17-1. Velocity waveforms measured distal to 40% stenosis (by area reduction) in dog aorta. Data were obtained by hot-film anemometry. (From Giddens DP, Kitney RI: Autoregressive spectral estimation of poststenotic blood flow disturbances, *J Biomech Eng* 105:401, 1983. Courtesy American Society of Mechanical Engineers.)

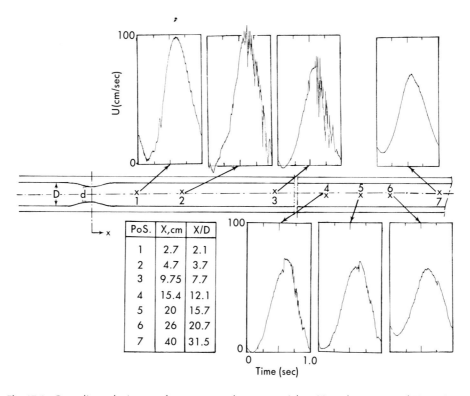

Fig. 17-2. Centerline velocity waveforms measured at seven axial positions downstream of 50% axisymmetric stenosis. Measurements were performed with laser Doppler anemometer. *U,* Measured fluid velocity; *D,* diameter of unoccluded portion of vessel; *X,* distance downstream from constriction; *PoS,* position of measurement site. (From Khalifa AMA, Giddens DP: *J Biomech* 14:279, 1981.)

a mild stenosis may result in only a starting structure with no evidence of shear layer oscillation or turbulence. Furthermore, studies by Lieber et al[24] indicate that the turbulence seen distal to mild and moderate stenoses contains ordered structures that are only pseudorandom; that is, structures that are essentially reproducible from beat-to-beat but somewhat random in their phase and amplitude.

The studies that model the dog aorta are typically at mean Reynolds numbers of about 1000, whereas the corresponding mean in the human common carotid artery is approximately 400. Therefore production of truly turbulent poststenotic flow is more difficult than in the dog aorta experiments and requires a greater degree of stenosis to produce the same effect. An extensive series of steady and pulsatile flow experiments for more moderate Reynolds number values has been completed by Ahmed[1] (see also Ahmed and Giddens[2,3]).

The discussion of flow disturbances is incomplete without consideration of a more realistic geometry. In view of the interest and importance of the carotid arteries with regard to atherosclerosis, a model bifurcation was developed based on extensive and quantitative studies of angiograms[4] and steady[4,5] and pulsatile[21,22] flow were examined through this model using flow visualization techniques and LDV instrumentation. These studies were directed toward defining normal hemodynamic behavior in the bifurcation and relating hemodynamic factors with localization of atherosclerotic lesions in humans. An important finding was that plaques localize in regions of low mean shear in the carotid bulb and not in regions of high flow velocity or shear.[27] Furthermore, when physiologic flow waveforms at appropriate Reynolds numbers were used, no turbulence was observed for the normal bifurcation.[5,21] There were, however, very strong secondary or helical flow patterns in the bifurcation, which cannot be considered flow disturbances in the true

sense because they occur for normal hemodynamic conditions. Fig. 17-3 shows the location and nature of unsteady flow phenomena that exist in carotid bifurcation under pulsatile conditions.[21] Using the LDV to measure velocity at various locations allows a quantitative assessment of velocity as a function of position and time. Fig. 17-4 presents an example, shown in a three-dimensional perspective, of the axial velocity component measured midway of the carotid bulb and in the plane of the bifurcation.[21] The two parts of the figure are two different projections of the same data, and the region of reverse flow over a large part of the bulb during systole is shown. Reverse velocity behavior has been documented in human subjects using duplex scanning instrumentation, and the similarity between model and human measurements is striking.[23] Studies are under way to examine the effects of lesions in the models, and these data will be related to similar work in humans using Doppler ultrasound.

In summary, it is now possible to make the following statements regarding the fluid dynamics of flow disturbances:

1. There are at least three distinct types of poststenotic flow disturbances that occur as the degree of stenosis

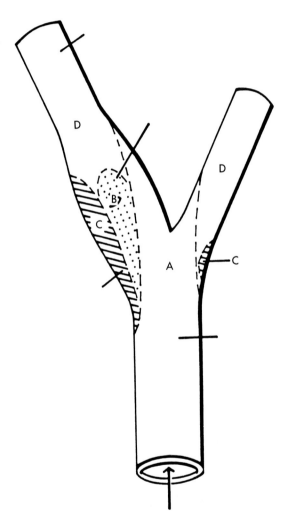

Fig. 17-3. Schematic presentation of general flow conditions at four regions in carotid bifurcation. Region *A* is one of basically axial flow. Region *B* contains evolving secondary helical structures that change direction through pulsatile cycle. Transient separation with oscillatory velocity directions characterizes region *C*, whereas region *D* has steep near-wall velocity gradients and blunt, entrance-type velocity profiles. (From Ku DN: Hemodynamics and atherogenesis at the human carotid bifurcation, doctoral dissertation, Atlanta, 1983, Georgia Institute of Technology.)

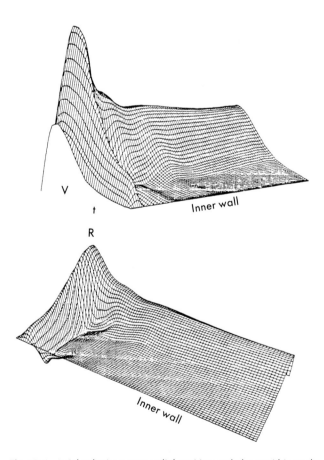

Fig. 17-4. Axial velocity versus radial position and phase within cycle as measured midway of the carotid sinus in plane of bifurcation with laser Doppler anemometer. (From Ku DN: Hemodynamics and atherogenesis at the human carotid bifurcation, doctoral dissertation, Atlanta, 1983, Georgia Institute of Technology.)

increases: starting structures, shear layer oscillations, and turbulence.

2. Because disturbances evolve during each cycle, they are nonstationary, and care must be exercised when using standard methods of time series analysis.

3. Although the normal human carotid bifurcation does not exhibit turbulence, complex secondary laminar flow patterns that may give the appearance of flow disturbances are created transiently with each beat.

4. Lowering the threshold of recognition of localized arterial disease using flow disturbance analysis is best achieved by understanding the role of coherent disturbance features, not by measurement of turbulence.

SIGNAL ANALYSIS

Because flow characteristics of interest contain recurring features on a beat-to-beat basis, most analyses of velocity data assume an underlying waveform exists that can be determined by appropriate ensemble averaging over a number of beats.[14,19] Hence a single beat in the ensemble is assumed to be of the form:

$$u(t) = U(t) + u'(t) \tag{1}$$

where U(t) is the underlying ensemble average and u'(t) is a random velocity component. The ensemble average of N beats is determined by:

$$U(t) = \frac{1}{N} \sum_{n=0}^{N-1} u(t + nP) \tag{2}$$

where P is the period of the waveform and t = 0 is the time that is referenced to the ECG signal. It should be noted that $0 \leq t \leq P$. Any waveform features that are repeatable and in phase from cycle to cycle will appear in U(t). The accuracy of this form of velocity decomposition is affected by several aspects of physiologic variability, including respiration, heart rate changes, and stroke consistency. It is possible to reduce physiologic variability somewhat by the technique of phase-shift averaging as described by Kitney and Giddens,[20] a method in which cross-correlation between U(t) and u(t) is used to minimize phase errors.

Using equations 1 and 2 along with the phase-shift averaging to construct the ensemble average, a series of 25 waveforms of the 40% occlusion data was used to form U(t) as shown in Fig. 17-5. After averaging, several disturbance structures remain in the waveform. These flow characteristics are not random in nature and in themselves would not be classified as turbulent—although they may be orderly structures that are precursors of or imbedded phasically within turbulence. Fig. 17-6 gives the square root of the corresponding ensemble average of $u'^2(t)$, that is, $\langle u'^2(t) \rangle^{1/2}$, where $\langle \rangle$ indicates ensemble average. The disturbance level is fairly low during the acceleration and peak velocity phases of systole and increases abruptly at the same time that U(t) shows obvious disturbance activity. This type of behavior in U(t) and u'(t) is seen consistently in both animal and in vitro poststenotic flow studies and emphasizes the fact that

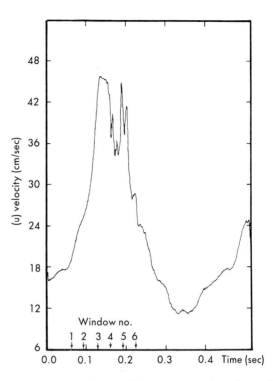

Fig. 17-5. Phase-shifted ensemble average waveform for 25 beats taken from 40% stenosis data illustrated in Fig. 17-1. Ensemble-averaged velocity is denoted by *u,* and windows are used for subsequent spectral analysis. (From Giddens DP, Kitney RI: Autoregressive spectral estimation of poststenotic blood flow disturbances, *J Biomech Eng* 105:401, 1983. Courtesy American Society of Mechanical Engineers.)

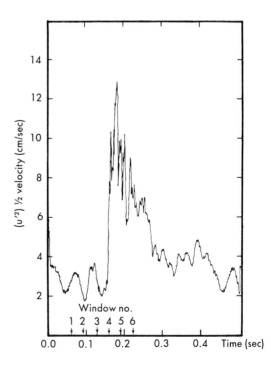

Fig. 17-6. Square root of ensemble average of u'² for 40% stenosis data of Fig. 17-1 taken over 25 beats. (From Giddens DP, Kitney RI: Autoregressive spectral estimation of poststenotic blood flow disturbances, *J Biomech Eng* 105:401, 1983. Courtesy American Society of Mechanical Engineers.)

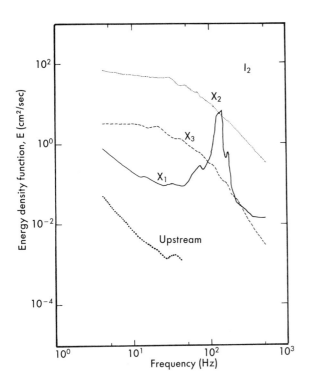

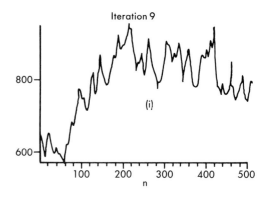

Fig. 17-8. Phase-shifted ensemble average of 100 very turbulent velocity waveforms measured distal to 88% stenosis in dog aorta with hot-film anemometer. Final ensemble average shows disturbances occurring at a discrete frequency in each cycle that survives the averaging process. Value of *n* is related to time in seconds such that time = n/2560. (From Kitney RI, Giddens DP: Analysis of blood velocity waveforms by phase shift averaging and autoregressive spectral estimation, *J Biomech Eng* 105:398, 1983. Courtesy American Society of Mechanical Engineers.)

Fig. 17-7. Energy spectra of disturbance velocity u' measured at several axial positions distal to 75% (by area) axisymmetric stenosis under pulsatile flow conditions. Spectra are calculated over 0.25-second period taken near peak systolic velocity in each cycle. Velocity was measured at tube axis using laser Doppler anemometer. (From Khalifa AMA, Giddens DP: *J Biomech* 14:279, 1981.)

flow disturbances related to localized plaques are clearly nonstationary phenomena.

Although the methods of equations 1 and 2, as shown in Figs. 17-5 and 17-6, provide a form of signal decomposition, further analysis is required to characterize the nature of the flow disturbances. One such technique is spectral analysis, in which the frequency content of a signal is determined with the objective of ultimately relating that content to physical phenomena. (The present discussion of spectral analysis deals with analyzing the *velocity* signal, not a Doppler frequency signal.)

First, spectrum estimates require data to be gathered over an interval of time that must be at least as long as the period of the lowest frequency present. Actually, for good accuracy the traditional methods of Fourier analysis require approximately five cycles of the lowest frequency present. Consequently, for flow disturbances in pulsatile flows, data must be gathered over a sufficiently long time interval within the cycle to obtain good spectrum estimates, yet the characteristics of the disturbance are changing during this interval. If the latter changes are not large during the observation time, the signal can be treated as quasi stationary—and this is the approach usually taken.

An example of the information afforded by spectral analysis of the velocity component u'(t) is given in Fig. 17-7.[18] This figure presents spectra of the energy in u'(t) as mea-

sured distal to a 75% stenosis with an LDV at several axial positions along the center line. The interval over which the spectra are calculated is a 0.25-second period taken near the peak systolic velocity in each cycle. It can be seen that at position X_1, which is two tube diameters distal to the stenosis, there is a sharp peak in the spectrum. This corresponds to an oscillation of discrete frequency arising in the poststenotic shear layer as discussed earlier. On the other hand, spectra further downstream at X_2 and X_3 show characteristically broadband turbulent shapes. The frequency content of the underlying waveform U(t) may also be of value.

Because of the transient behavior of flow disturbances during each cycle, the problem may be looked on as one of analyzing data records of short duration. For such cases, Fourier methods may lack accuracy, and linear estimation techniques[6] developed for such applications may prove valuable. Researchers have examined the potential of a class of these techniques—autoregressive methods—when applied to both underlying [U(t)][20] and random [u'(t)][13] velocities. The theory behind these methods can be found in the literature.[6,16,20,26]

An example of applying fast Fourier transform (FFT) and autoregressive (AR) methods of spectrum estimation is shown in Figs. 17-8 and 17-9. Fig. 17-8 presents an ensemble average U(t) waveform determined from hot-film anemometer measurements of velocity taken distal to an 88% (by area) stenosis in the dog aorta.[13] Flow was so turbulent that it was difficult to detect any of the individual beats in the raw data. However, by phase-shift averaging 100 beats, a well-defined U(t) waveform emerged that apparently contains distinct frequency components. Fig. 17-9 gives the spectral estimations obtained by FFT and AR methods. The fundamental peak at about 5 Hz arises from the data window used (that is, 0.20 sec). Both FFT and AR

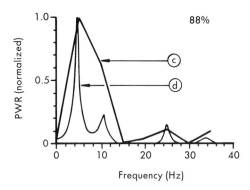

Fig. 17-9. Spectral content of curve in Fig. 17-8 as estimated by FTT and autoregressive methods. (From Kitney RI, Giddens DP: Analysis of blood velocity waveforms by phase shift averaging and autoregressive spectral estimation, *J Biomech Eng* 105:398, 1983. Courtesy American Society of Mechanical Engineers.)

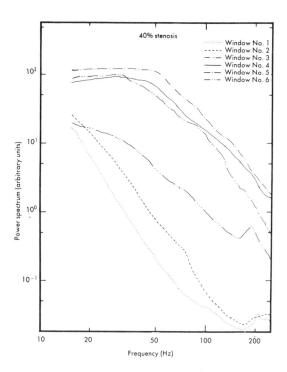

Fig. 17-10. Power spectra for disturbance velocity u' as calculated by autoregressive spectral estimation for six data windows during the cycle. Results are for 40% stenosis and give evolving spectral content of u'. (Refer to Fig. 17-6 for location of 0.064-second windows.) (From Giddens DP, Kitney RI: Autoregressive spectral estimation of post-stenotic blood flow disturbances, *J Biomech Eng* 105:401, 1983. Courtesy American Society of Mechanical Engineers.)

methods give higher frequency peaks at about 25 and 35 Hz; however, the peak at 10 Hz is not resolved by the FFT approach. Additionally, the FFT resolution is basically 5 Hz and will give no peaks other than in multiples of this value. On the other hand, the AR method provides a continuous estimate of the spectrum, resulting in better resolution.

The 40% occlusion data shown in Figs. 17-5 and 17-6 illustrate the application of the AR method to u'(t) data and the evolution of spectra during a cycle. Six "windows" are identified along the time axis. The numbers shown correspond to the locations of the centers of six windows of 0.064-second duration; each successive window is shifted by 0.032 second, resulting in a 50% overlap. The AR method was applied to the u'(t) data during each of these data windows, and the results are shown in Fig. 17-10.[13] Windows 1 and 2 give very little high-frequency activity, indicating that flow is essentially laminar and cyclically repeatable during these times, in agreement with the curve of Fig. 17-6. Window 3 begins to show an increase in high-frequency disturbances, but this is still a relatively low level. On the other hand, windows 4 to 6 display a greater amplitude of disturbance and much greater high-frequency activity than the first three windows. These later three spectra are characteristically turbulent and correspond to the high levels of disturbance seen in Figs. 17-5 and 17-6.

In summary, the following statements regarding analysis of blood velocity signals can be made:

1. Certain aspects of data interpretation are facilitated by decomposition of the velocity into an underlying waveform, U(t), determined by ensemble averaging and a random velocity component, u'(t).

2. It is impossible to obtain accurate underlying waveforms by low pass filtering (as has been suggested by others).[19]

3. Phase-shift averaging to obtain U(t) reduces physiologic variability.

4. Because data records are relatively short as a result of the evolving nature of flow disturbances, AR spectral estimation techniques offer an improvement over FFT estimates in many cases.

NONINVASIVE MEASUREMENTS

Presently, the primary means of obtaining blood velocity information is with Doppler ultrasound, most notably with pulsed Doppler ultrasound, which is guided by real-time imaging—that is, duplex scanning. However, a dilemma exists. The vast majority of fluid dynamics knowledge is based on the velocity field, whereas the output of Doppler ultrasound instruments is an amplitude- and frequency-modulated signal whose frequency content is derived from scattering by moving particles. Although the relationship between Doppler frequency and flow velocity seems straightforward, this is not the case. Unfortunately, Doppler systems suffer from Doppler ambiguity, which results from factors such as mean velocity gradient (spatial resolution), rapid variations in velocity (temporal resolution), transit time and geometric broadening, instrument bandwidth, and noise. George and Lumley[11] provide an excellent discussion of Doppler ambiguity and focus attention on laser Doppler systems, whereas Garbini et al[9,10] discuss similar considerations for ultrasonic Doppler devices. Because of the much longer wavelength of ultrasound systems, Doppler ambiguity is a central problem; perhaps as a consequence of this, most commercial Doppler ultrasound devices have tended to display Doppler spectra. Extensive clinical experience with such systems has led to diagnostic improvements, and descriptions of flow disturbances have been given in terms of "filling in the window" and "spectral broadening." However, these descriptions have not yet been properly connected to physical phenomema occurring in arterial flow, so it is perhaps more appropriate to call the output of these devices *spectral displays* rather than spectral analyses.

It is therefore important to recognize that (1) extraction of velocity information from Doppler signals arising from disturbed flows or from complex (but normal) flow patterns is not simple and that (2) spectral broadening results from many sources that are strictly instrument related, such as sample volume size, transmission frequency and bandwidth, and the resolution and accuracy of the spectrum estimator.

Although spectral broadening descriptions may be useful as an interim stage, converting to velocity information may hold more promise for diagnosis of mild to moderate lesions. This opinion is based on the fact that the vast body of fluid dynamics knowledge deals with the velocity field, not with descriptions of Doppler spectra. Thus converting the Doppler signal to fluid velocity data allows the examiner to use the full power of fluid dynamics on the interpretation of

blood flow disturbances induced by arterial disease. One approach that appears promising is to use phase lock loop (PLL) frequency tracking of the Doppler signal, in which the output of a variable frequency oscillator is caused to lock in phase with the Doppler signal and follow its frequency through a feedback system. In a series of in vitro experiments, measurements of flow disturbances were performed in pulsatile flow distal to stenoses of 50% and 75% area reduction.[12] Pulsed Doppler ultrasound (PDU) with PLL tracking was compared with data obtained from the LDV, an instrument whose ambiguity is substantially less than that for ultrasound because of its much shorter wavelength.[11] Figs. 17-11 and 17-12 give results obtained downstream of a 50% stenosis. For both U(t) and u'(t), the PDU-PLL system gave good agreement with the LDV. However, when the stenosis increased to 75% area reduction, the PDU-PLL system suffered from excessive loss in tracking, resulting in disturbance velocity measurements that were approximately 50% too large. In view of the ambiguity problems discussed earlier, this result is not surprising.

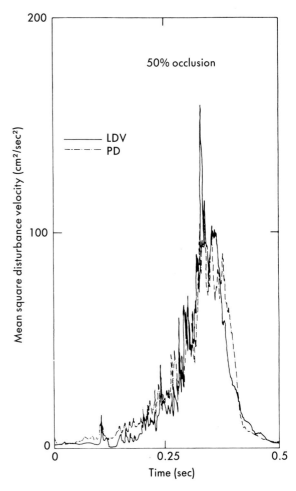

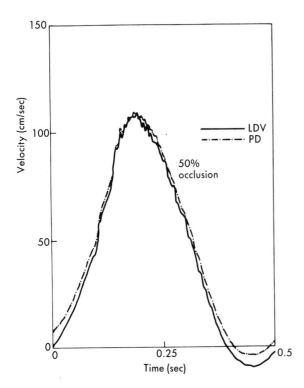

Fig. 17-11. Ensemble average axial velocity waveforms measured by pulsed Doppler *(PD)* ultrasound and laser Doppler velocity *(LDV)* meters distal to a 50% stenosis in pulsatile flow. Ultrasound data were processed by frequency tracker. (From Giddens DP, Khalifa AMA: *Ultrasound Med Biol* 8:427, 1982.)

Fig. 17-12. Ensemble averages of axial mean square disturbance velocity measured by pulsed Doppler *(PD)* ultrasound and laser Doppler velocity *(LDV)* meters distal to a 50% contoured stenosis in pulsatile flow. Ultrasound data were processed by frequency tracker. (From Giddens DP, Khalifa AMA: *Ultrasound Med Biol* 8:427, 1982.)

The PLL method may be applied to human subjects, although in such cases there is no independent method of evaluating its accuracy. Casty and Giddens[7] studied several subjects using a multichannel pulsed-Doppler system in which one of the channels was located at the center line and used to measure disturbances. Fig. 17-13 shows the results obtained from the left common carotid artery of a 65-year-old patient with failure of the aortic valve and a systolic bruit transmitted to the carotids. The presence of coherent flow disturbances during the peak phase of systole and an increase in disturbance level during the peak and deceleration phases can be seen clearly in the figures.

Another approach of converting Doppler data to velocity is that of rapid calculation of the mean value of the frequency from frequency spectra. This procedure assumes that the mean frequency may be determined from:

$$f_m(t) = \frac{\int fP(f)df}{\int P(f)df} \tag{3}$$

where $P(f)$ is the Doppler power spectrum and is assumed to represent a probability distribution function for Doppler frequency. Because equation 3 is the first moment of $P(f)$ and because the process was implemented digitally, this procedure is a digital first moment (DFM) method.[8] If appropriate windows are used, equation 3 gives excellent results when used with simulated Doppler signals.[8,25] How-

ever, again because of Doppler ambiguity, the accuracy is degraded when the method is applied to real Doppler signals. The net effects are that rapid variations in velocity cannot be followed and the output of the estimator is somewhat noisy. However, the approach may be useful when applied for detecting coherent, low-frequency velocity disturbances and has not yet been fully explored.

Finally, the following statements can be made:
1. Spectral analysis of the Doppler signal, as presently practiced, is no more than a spectral display of the audio signal whose relationship to hemodynamic phenomena is poorly understood.
2. For low to moderate levels of velocity fluctuation, frequency tracking by PLL provides reasonably accurate conversion of the Doppler signal to fluid velocity.
3. Improved methods of spectral estimation that will account for ambiguity phenomena are needed.

FUTURE DIRECTIONS

The hemodynamic behavior of normal and mildly diseased vessels is just beginning to be understood properly. Additional work is necessary in this area, particularly with regard to the three-dimensional geometries of relevant vessels. Model studies have been shown to be very important in elucidating flow behavior under controlled conditions with accurate instrumentation. These results can then be used to aid in the interpretation of data obtained under clinical conditions with noninvasive methods. Also, research should be focused on better modeling of the Doppler signal at its fundamental level and on accurate conversion to fluid velocity information so that a broader knowledge of fluid dynamics can be used on clinical measurements.

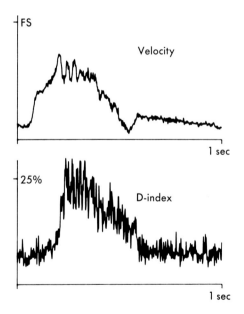

Fig. 17-13. Ensemble average waveform and disturbance velocity obtained via pulsed Doppler ultrasound from a patient with failure of the aortic valve and transmitted systolic bruit. Doppler data were processed with a frequency. *D-index* is disturbance index defined by the relation:

$$D(t) = \frac{\sqrt{<u'(t)^2>}}{\overline{U}}$$

where $\overline{U}$ is mean velocity averaged over the heart cycle and $<u'(t)^2>$ is ensemble average of the square of the disturbance velocity. (From Casty M, Giddens DP: *Ultrasound Med Biol* 10[2]:161, 1984.)

REFERENCES

1. Ahmed SA: *An experimental investigation of steady and pulsatile flow through a constricted tube,* doctoral dissertation, Atlanta, 1981, Georgia Institute of Technology.
2. Ahmed SA, Giddens DP: Velocity measurements in steady flow through axisymmetric stenoses at moderate Reynolds numbers, *J Biomech* 16:505, 1983.
3. Ahmed SA, Giddens DP: Flow disturbance measurements through a constricted tube at moderate Reynolds numbers, *J Biomech* 16:955, 1983.
4. Bharadvaj BK, Mabon RF, Giddens DP: Steady flow in a model of the carotid bifurcation. I. Flow visualization, *J Biomech* 15:349, 1982.
5. Bharadvaj BK, Mabon RF, Giddens DP: Steady flow in a model of the carotid bifurcation. II. Laser-Doppler anemometer measurements, *J Biomech* 15:363, 1982.
6. Box GE, Jenkins GH: *Time series analysis: forecasting and control,* San Francisco, 1976, Holden-Day.
7. Casty M, Giddens DP: 25 + 1 channel pulsed ultrasound Doppler velocity meter for quantitative flow measurements and turbulence analysis, *Ultrasound Med Biol* 10(2):161, 1984.
8. Craig JI, Saxena V, Giddens DP: A minicomputer-based scheme for turbulence measurements with pulsed Doppler ultrasound, *IEEE Proceedings of the third annual symposium on Computer Applications in Medical Care,* p 638, Washington, DC, 1979.
9. Garbini JL, Forster FK, Jorgensen JE: Measurement of fluid turbulence based on pulsed ultrasound techniques. I. Analysis, *J Fluid Mech* 118:445, 1982.

10. Garbini JL, Forster FK, Jorgensen JE: Measurement of fluid turbulence based on pulsed ultrasound techniques. II. Experimental investigation, *J Fluid Mech* 118:471, 1982.

11. George WF, Lumley JL: The laser-Doppler velocimeter and its application to the measurement of turbulence, *J Fluid Mech* 60:321, 1973.

12. Giddens DP, Khalifa AMA: Turbulence measurements with pulsed Doppler ultrasound employing a frequency tracking method, *Ultrasound Med Biol* 8:427, 1982.

13. Giddens DP, Kitney RI: Autoregressive spectral estimation of poststenotic blood flow disturbances, *J Biomech Eng* 105:401, 1983.

14. Giddens DP, Mabon RF, Cassanova RA: Measurements of disordered flows distal to subtotal vascular stenoses in the thoracic aortas of dogs, *Circ Res* 39:112, 1976.

15. Greene FM Jr et al: Computer-based pattern recognition of carotid arterial disease using pulsed Doppler ultrasound, *Ultrasound Med Biol* 8:161, 1982.

16. Kay SM: The effects of noise on the autoregressive spectral estimator, *IEEE Trans Acoustics Speech Signal Processing* 5:478, 1979.

17. Khalifa AMA, Giddens DP: Analysis of disorder in pulsatile flows with application to poststenotic blood velocity measurement in dogs, *J Biomech* 11:129, 1978.

18. Khalifa AMA, Giddens DP: Characterization and evolution of poststenotic flow disturbances, *J Biomech* 14:279, 1981.

19. Kitney RI, Giddens DP: Extraction and characterisation of underlying velocity waveforms in poststenotic flow, *IEE Proceedings* 129(A):651, 1982.

20. Kitney RI, Giddens DP: Analysis of blood velocity waveforms by phase shift averaging and autoregressive spectral estimation, *J Biomech Eng* 105:398, 1983.

21. Ku DN: *Hemodynamics and atherogenesis at the human carotid bifurcation,* doctoral dissertation, Atlanta, 1983, Georgia Institute of Technology.

22. Ku DN, Giddens DP: Pulsatile flow in a model carotid bifurcation, *Arteriosclerosis* 3:31, 1983.

23. Ku DN et al: Hemodynamics of the normal human bifurcation: in vitro and in vivo studies, *Ultrasound Med Biol* 11:13-26, 1985.

24. Lieber BB et al: On the discrimination between band-limited coherent and random apparent stresses in transitional pulsatile flow, *J Biomech Eng* 3:42-46, 1989.

25. Saxena V: *Turbulence measurements using pulsed Doppler ultrasound,* doctoral dissertation, Atlanta, 1978, Georgia Institute of Technology.

26. Ulrych TF, Bishop TN: Maximum entropy spectral analysis and autoregressive decomposition, *Rev Geophysics Space Physics* 13:198, 1975.

27. Zarins CK et al: Carotid bifurcation atherosclerosis quantitative correlation of plaque localization with flow velocity profiles and wall shear stress. *Circ Res* 53:502, 1983.

CHAPTER 18

Pressure measurement in the extremity

JAMES S. T. YAO

Ever since Hales[14] successfully measured mean blood pressure from the carotid artery in an unanesthetized horse in 1733, investigators have sought better and more convenient ways of measuring the same phenomenon. More than a century later, von Basch first developed an arterial occluding device to measure blood pressure in humans.[30] The use of the air-inflated arm-occluding cuff, introduced by Riva-Rocci[25] and further modified by von Recklinghausen,[31] revolutionized the method of recording blood pressure. By means of palpation of the radial pulse distal to the cuff or by the oscillometric technique, systolic blood pressure may be measured indirectly. In 1905 Korotkoff[19] proposed his auscultatory method and successfully established the basic sphygmomanometric technique for measuring brachial systolic and diastolic blood pressure.

At present the measurement of blood pressure may be classified into direct and indirect methods. The former requires placement of a needle or catheter in an artery; the latter is generally determined by placing a cuff around the part of the limb to be measured. This is done by inflating the cuff to a pressure sufficient to stop blood flow and then slowly deflating the cuff with some method to detect the pressure at which distal blood flow is resumed. Because of the noninvasive nature of the indirect technique, measurement of brachial blood pressure is now routine medical practice.

Measurement of upper extremity pressure with a conventional stethoscope seldom presents problems, except under shock conditions or in a noisy environment. The use of the stethoscope to measure lower limb pressure, however, is often difficult. Even in normal subjects, the inability to detect Korotkoff sounds in pedal arteries or even in popliteal arteries has made measurement of lower limb pressures by the conventional stethoscope a difficult procedure.[16] In the presence of arterial occlusion, the decrease of systolic pressure further limits the use of the conventional technique. Because of this limitation, various techniques are now available to aid in recording blood pressure of a lower limb noninvasively.

Supported in part by the Northwestern University Vascular Research Fund.

CURRENT INSTRUMENTATION FOR PULSE REGISTRATION

Many time-honored techniques such as the flush method, oscillometry, and volume (air or water) plethysmography are too cumbersome for clinical use. Therefore these techniques are not discussed here. Only those methods that are currently in use are reviewed.

Mercury-in-silicone-elastomer strain-gauge plethysmography

The silicone elastomer gauge filled with mercury is used to detect the change of circumference of a digit or a part of the limb to be measured. When the gauge is placed around the terminal digit (toe) of the foot, the volume changes that occur with each heartbeat produce a change in the circumference of the gauge. The pulse of a digit in a lower extremity[23,28] can be detected by balancing the gauge on a Wheatstone bridge together with an amplifier. Measurement of the systolic pressure is performed by placing a cuff proximal to the gauge. After rapid inflation of the cuff to about 20 mm Hg above the systolic pressure, the pulse signals disappear. During deflation of the cuff, the systolic pressure is recorded at the time that the pulse reappears. In the low-flow state or in vasoconstriction, pulse registration from the toe may not be apparent. Under this circumstance, a direct current (DC) mode may be used. The sudden increase in volume during deflation of the inflated cuff causes a shift of the baseline. This shift may be used as the end point for systolic pressure.

Isotope clearance

Xenon 133 injected into tissue may be used to calculate muscle flow by recording the washout curve of the isotope.[8] With the use of a cuff proximal to the site of the depot of ^{133}Xe, systolic pressure is recorded at the level during slow inflation when the washout stops. Such a pressure level represents perfusion pressure in the muscle. Similarly, Lassen and Holstein[20] have found that the flow cessation pressure measured by inflating a blood pressure cuff placed over a radioactive depot injected into the skin was nearly equal to the diastolic pressure in normal subjects. This pressure level represents skin pressure, or it may merely represent systolic pressure in small arteries, as suggested by Carter.[6]

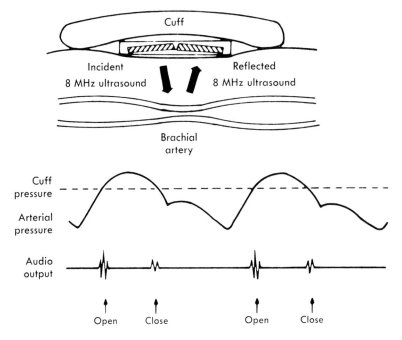

Fig. 18-1. Using ultrasound to measure vessel wall movement during deflation of the pneumatic cuff. (From Stegall HF, Kardon HB, Kemmerer WT: *J Appl Physiol* 25:793, 1968.)

Transcutaneous ultrasound techniques

Wall-motion technique. Wall-motion technique is based on the use of a specially constructed transducer to detect changes in Doppler-shifted ultrasound generated by arterial wall motion.[24] When cuff pressure is above systolic arterial pressure, the artery remains closed throughout the cardiac cycle and no signal is heard. As cuff pressure falls below systolic pressure, a short thump is heard, which splits into distinct "opening" and "closing" phases (Fig. 18-1). As cuff pressure falls further, separation between the opening and closing signals widens until a closing signal begins to encroach on the subsequent opening signal. When these two merge, cuff pressure is equivalent to diastolic pressure. Because the technique measures wall motion, it is also termed *Doppler ultrasound kinetoarteriography.*

Flow velocity detector. Arterial flow signals are now readily detected by various types of Doppler instruments with the Doppler-shift flow detection principle. These Doppler instruments range from pocket-size portable devices to the directional flow detector equipped with analogue output. When the flow probe is used like a stethoscope, the Doppler flow velocity detector greatly facilitates measurement of systolic pressure of lower limbs.

A sphygmomanometer cuff is applied just above the ankle, and a flow probe is placed over the posterior tibial artery or the dorsal artery of the foot. Flow signals cease as the cuff is inflated to 20 mm Hg or more above the brachial systolic pressure. During deflation of the cuff, a return of flow signals indicates the level of the systolic pressure at the ankle (Fig. 18-2). The flow velocity detector, however, is useful in the detection of systolic pressure only.

Photosensor technique

Measurement of skin blood pressure with photoelectric plethysmography has been reported.[24] A probe into which a lamp and a photoelectric resistance are built is placed under a cuff in direct contact with the skin, and the reflected light is recorded on a potentiometer writer. When the cuff is inflated to above systolic level, blanching of the skin occurs and pulsation disappears. During slow deflation of the cuff, a DC-register curve shift or baseline shift indicates the return of blood inflow and hence the level of skin systolic pressure. An infrared photoplethysmograph has also been introduced. This technique is particularly useful for toe pressure measurements. A DC mode is also available if pulse registration of the first toe is not feasible. Again, a shift in baseline of the DC-register curve indicates the end point of systolic pressure.

EQUIPMENT

Proper blood pressure cuffs, manometers, and control valves are prerequisites for accurate blood pressure recording.

Cuff size for recording blood pressure

Regardless of the type of instrument used, the cuff size applied to the limb is of paramount importance in achieving accurate readings. An inflatable bladder is surrounded by an unyielding cover called the *cuff.* The width of the bladder is critical. If it is too narrow (undercuffing), the blood pressure reading will be erroneously high, and if it is too wide (overcuffing), the reading may be too low. Miscuffing distorts the blood pressure reading in the arm by an average of 8.5 mm Hg.[21]

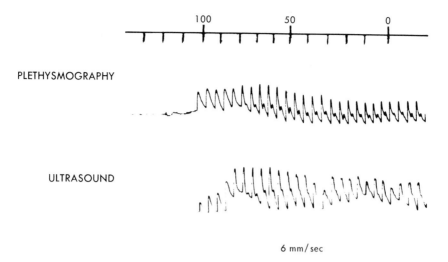

100   50   0

PLETHYSMOGRAPHY

ULTRASOUND

6 mm/sec

Fig. 18-2. Comparison of systolic pressure (in millimeters of mercury) measured by strain-gauge plethysmography and Doppler ultrasound. A systolic pressure of 100 mm Hg was recorded by both methods.

Table 18-1. Recommended bladder dimensions for blood pressure cuff

Arm circumference at midpoint* (cm)	Cuff name	Bladder width (cm)	Bladder length (cm)
5-7.5	Newborn	3	5
7.5-13	Infant	5	8
13-20	Child	8	13
17-26	Small adult	11	17
24-32	Adult	13	24
32-42	Large adult	17	32
42-50†	Thigh	20	42

From Kirkendall WM et al: Recommendations for human blood pressure determination by sphygmomanometers. Subcommittee of the AHA Postgraduate Education Committee, *Circulation* 62:1146A, 1980.

*Midpoint of arm is defined as half the distance from the acromion to the olecranon.

†In persons with very large limbs, the indirect blood pressure should be measured in the leg or forearm.

For accurate indirect measurement of blood pressure, the American Heart Association (AHA) now recommends that the cuff size be based on limb circumference.[18] It is recommended that the width of the inflatable bladder be 40% of the circumference of the midpoint of the limb or 20% wider than the diameter. The circumference of the limb, not the age of the patient, is the factor that determines cuff size. The length of the bladder should be twice its width (bladder length equal to 80% of the arm circumference). Table 18-1 outlines the recommendations for blood pressure cuff bladder dimensions made by the AHA in 1980.[18] Since the recording of ankle pressure closely parallels the recording of brachial pressure, the bladder dimension and ankle circumference must be taken into consideration for accurate measurement. For measurement of ankle blood pressure the conventional arm cuff is sufficient, although some investigators prefer a wider cuff.[29] Gundersen[13] recommends that the ankle cuff be 7 to 8 cm, the calf cuff 11 to 14 cm, and the thigh cuff 16 to 23 cm wide. Standard adult arm cuffs used in clinical medicine contain an air-inflatable rubber bladder that is 23 cm long and 12 to 12.5 cm wide, which should be sufficient for use at the ankle level. Measurements with cuffs of this size yield values that agree with intraarterial measurements.[4,23,26]

The size of the thigh cuff is important. It should be 18 to 20 cm wide. Because of the shape of the thigh, Hokanson[17] has devised a contoured thigh cuff. The bladder in this cuff is 22 cm wide and 71 cm long and is shaped to conform to the taper of the thigh. Although no study has been done to prove the superiority of the contour cuff as compared with the ordinary thigh cuff, the idea of contour cuffs is a good one and merits further application. A 19 cm cuff is useful for recording pressure of the lower thigh. Barnes[2] suggests a narrow cuff (11 cm) for upper thigh pressure measurement. In obese patients a wider cuff may be more appropriate because of the large size of the thigh.

Digital cuffs for recording finger or toe pressures may be constructed of a bladder made of Penrose drain on a backing of nylon Velcro strip[13] (Fig. 18-3). Digital cuff width varies from finger to toe, and the proper size for a finger is 2 to 2.5 cm and for a toe, 2.5 to 3 cm. According to Gundersen,[13] a 2.4 cm wide cuff was found to be the most suitable for finger pressure recording on a medium-sized man. Table 18-2 summarizes the different sizes of cuffs that should be used for recording lower limb pressure.

Obviously, for extremely obese patients or patients with odd-shaped ankles, the size of the cuff should be adjusted accordingly to avoid unusually high readings. Steinfeld et al[27] proposed that for the conically shaped obese leg, a bladder of trapezoidal design should be used so that when applied to the limb, it would conform more closely to its natural contours. The same group of investigators[1] have

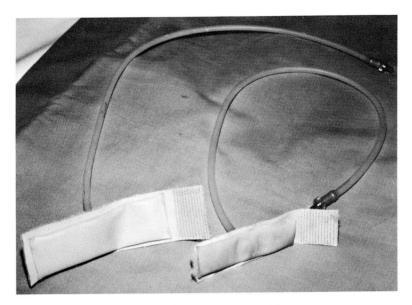

Fig. 18-3. Digital cuffs for measuring toe and finger pressures.

Table 18-2. Recommended cuff size for lower limb pressure measurement

Cuff location	Cuff size
Adult upper thigh	11 cm
Adult lower thigh	19 cm
Adult thigh (contour-type cuff)	22 cm
Adult ankle	12 cm
Adult finger	2 to 2.5 cm
Adult toe	2.5 to 3 cm

constructed a new cuff with a bladder that completely encircles the limb, thus avoiding the narrow cuff effect. In general, a large cuff should probably be used in obese patients. Error in blood pressure measurement that results from incorrect cuff size in such patients has been reported.[22]

Control valves and tubings

Defects in the control valve or air leaks may cause false or inaccurate readings. Such defects have been claimed to be a major source of error in blood pressure recording.[7] The following maneuvers should be used to test for air leaks and the function of the control valve and connecting tubes:

1. The pump should have a competent nonreturn valve and no leaks.
2. The control valve should allow the free passage of air without excessive muscular effort when the filter is clean. When closed, it should hold the mercury at a constant level. When released, it should allow a controlled fall of the mercury column.

   To test the valve, the operator rolls the cuff in its own "tail," pumps to 200 mm Hg, and waits 10 seconds, during which time the level should not fall more than 2 mm Hg. If a leak is detected, the circuit is clamped in sections to find the site; most such leaks can be traced to control valves. The operator slowly releases the valve on four occasions. During at least two of these attempts, it should be possible to control the rate of fall readily to not more than 1 mm/sec and to change to and from a faster rate at will. Ideally, this should be possible at every attempt, but a more demanding test would result in condemning nearly all sphygmomanometers, including many newer ones with the present design of control valves.

3. The connections should fit without an air leak and should come apart easily.
4. The tube should be airtight and of appropriate length.
5. The mercury tube should not be cracked. There should be a patent air vent at the top of the column.
6. The cuff should fit comfortably around the arm and stay in place when inflated. The rubber bag should be long enough to encircle the arm.

Manometers

Two types of pressure-registering systems are in general use: the mercury gravity manometer and the aneroid. Both provide accurate and reproducible results when working properly. The aneroid manometer is probably more versatile for bedside or laboratory use. If an aneroid manometer is used, efforts should be made to calibrate the instrument yearly. Such calibration can be made by interposing a Y connector in the tube from the cuff to a mercury manometer and attaching the sphygmomanometer to be tested to the free end of the connector.

MEASURING TECHNIQUES

Brachial pressure is recorded with a Doppler probe or a conventional stethoscope before lower limb pressure mea-

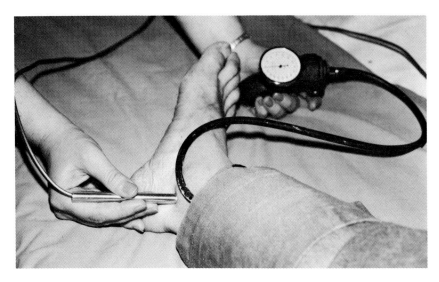

Fig. 18-4. Method of recording ankle systolic pressure.

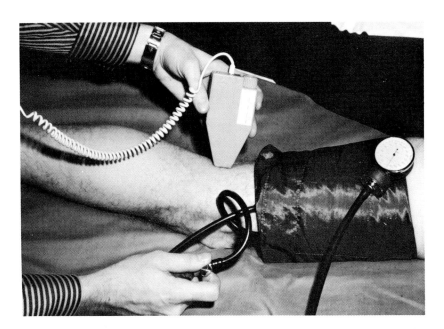

Fig. 18-5. Method of recording thigh pressure.

surement. All measurements are made with the patient in the supine position after a 10- to 15-minute period of rest.

Ankle systolic pressure

The arm pressure cuff is applied snugly above the malleolus (Fig. 18-4). The cuff is then inflated above the brachial systolic pressure (about 20 to 30 mm Hg). The end point of systolic pressure is determined by the reappearance of the pulse (an audible sound by Doppler method or pulse waveform by plethysmography). Two or three measurements should be made on each limb.

Upper thigh pressure

A narrow cuff (11 cm) is placed just below the inguinal ligament, and the Doppler probe is placed over the popliteal artery for end-point determination.

Lower thigh pressure

The thigh cuff is applied just above the knee. If the Doppler ultrasound method is used, the sound probe is placed over the popliteal artery to detect sound signals (Fig. 18-5). Placing the sensor close to the pressure cuff is critical to obtain accurate thigh pressure measurement, especially in patients with multiple-level occlusions.[11] For the plethysmographic method, the pulse registration is normally done on the big toe. The end point of the systolic pressure is determined by the same maneuver used to obtain the ankle pressure.

Toe pressure

A strain gauge or photosensor is placed on the big toe to record pulse or volume changes with the cuff placed at the base of the toe.

Postexercise measurements

Ankle pressure can be measured after exercise in a similar manner. Standard treadmill walking is used. Immediately after termination of the treadmill exercise, the patient resumes the supine position, and ankle pressure is recorded at 1-minute intervals until the pressure reaches the preexercise level.

Postischemic measurement (reactive hyperemia)

The pressure cuff applied to the thigh may be used to induce distal ischemia and to simulate the reactive hyperemia induced by exercise. The cuff is inflated to a level of 50 mm Hg above the systolic pressure for a period of 3 to 5 minutes and then abruptly deflated. Reactive hyperemia will occur immediately. Ankle systolic pressure is then recorded at 1-minute intervals until it returns to the resting pressure level.

Comparative study with intraarterial technique

Noninvasive measurement of ankle pressure with Doppler ultrasound has been compared with the intraarterial technique in normal subjects.[3] Continuous monitoring of pressure in the posterior tibial or dorsalis pedis artery showed there was good correlation ($\sqrt{} = 0.87$) between the systolic pressure values measured by the two techniques. The use of upper thigh pressure has been compared with intraarterial pressure measurements in the femoral artery.[9,10] From this analysis it was found that the upper thigh pressure does not differentiate between aortoiliac and superficial femoral artery disease.

CONCLUSION

Blood pressure is one of the measurements that is fundamental to understand the hemodynamics of occlusive arterial disease. Proper equipment, especially the size of the cuff, the dimension of the bladder, and proper measuring technique are important to achieve accurate readings. The choice of instrumentation depends on the resources of the institution. At present the Doppler ultrasound technique is probably the least expensive and the most versatile. Unlike pulse registration techniques such as plethysmography, which requires cumbersome equipment, the pocket or portable Doppler instruments allow systolic pressure recording at the bedside, in the office, in the operating room, or in the intensive care area. The technique is simple and requires little training. It can be performed readily by a nurse or competent technician. For toe pressure measurement, however, the photoplethysmograph appears to be more useful because of difficulty in recording the toe pulse.[5]

As with all measuring techniques, indirect pressure recording has its limitations. In the lower limb an important limitation is the inability of the pressure cuff to compress a heavily calcified artery. Such a condition is commonly seen in patients with diabetes mellitus or those with chronic renal failure and calcified arteries.[12,15] Because of such arterial calcification, a falsely high ankle systolic pressure may be recorded in some patients with diabetes mellitus or with chronic renal failure. In addition, when two parallel vessels of comparable size are compressed by the cuff, the measurement will reflect the pressure in the artery with the highest pressure and may not detect a significant stenotic or occlusive lesion in the other vessel.

Of pressures recorded at different levels of the lower limb, the ankle systolic pressure is probably the most reliable in detection of abnormalities. Both upper and lower thigh pressures are subject to more variation and are less sensitive in detection of arterial occlusion or stenosis.[3,9,10] Difficulties with thigh pressure measurement are caused by inability of the cuff to compress the artery completely, obesity, and inherent problems with the size and dimension of the bladder of the pressure cuff.

REFERENCES

1. Alexander M, Cohen ML, Steinfeld L: Criteria in the choice of an occluding cuff for indirect measurement of blood pressure, *Med Biol Eng Comput* 15:2, 1977.
2. Barnes RW, Wilson MR: *Doppler ultrasound evaluation of peripheral arterial disease*. A programmed audiovisual instruction, Iowa City, 1976, University of Iowa.
3. Bernstein EF et al: Thigh pressure artifacts with noninvasive techniques in an experimental model, *Surgery* 89:391, 1981.
4. Bollinger A, Barras JP, Mahler F: Measurement of foot artery blood pressure by micromanometry in normal subjects and in patients with arterial occlusive disease, *Circulation* 53:506, 1976.
5. Bone GE, Pomajzl MJ: Toe blood pressure by photoplethysmography: an index of healing in forefoot amputation, *Surgery* 89:569, 1981.
6. Carter SA: Peripheral blood flow, blood pressure and metabolism in occlusive arterial disease: application to control of surgical and medical therapy, *Scand J Clin Lab Invest* 31(suppl 128):147, 1973.
7. Conceicao S, Ward MK, Kerr DNS: Defects in sphygmomanometers: an important source of error in blood pressure recordings, *Br Med J* 1:886, 1976.
8. Dahn I, Lassen NA, Westling H: Blood flow in human muscles during external pressure or venous stasis, *Clin Sci* 32:467, 1967.
9. Flanigan DP et al: Correlation of Doppler-derived high thigh pressure and intra-arterial pressure in the assessment of aorto-iliac occlusive disease, *Br J Surg* 68:423, 1981.
10. Flanigan DP et al: Utility of wide and narrow blood pressure cuffs in the hemodynamic assessment of aortoiliac occlusive disease, *Surgery* 92:16, 1982.
11. Franzeck UK, Bernstein EF, Fronek A: The effect of sensing site on the limb segmental blood pressure determination, *Arch Surg* 116:912, 1981.
12. Gipstein RM, et al: Calciphylaxis in man. A syndrome of tissue necrosis and vascular calcification in 11 patients with chronic renal failure, *Arch Intern Med* 136:1273, 1976.
13. Gundersen J: Segmental measurements of systolic blood pressure in the extremities including the thumb and the great toe, *Acta Chir Scand* (suppl) 426:1, 1972.

14. Hales S: *Statistical essays: containing haemastaticks,* vol 2, London, 1733, W. Innys & R. Manby.

15. Hobbs JT et al: A limitation of the Doppler ultrasound method of measuring ankle systolic pressure, *Vasa* 3:160, 1974.

16. Hocken AG: Measurement of blood pressure in the leg, *Lancet* 1:466, 1967.

17. Hokanson G: Personal communication, 1976.

18. Kirkendall WM et al: Recommendations for human blood pressure determination by sphygmomanometers. Subcommittee of the AHA Postgraduate Education Committee, *Circulation* 62(5):1146A, 1980 (abstract).

19. Korotkoff NS: On the subject of methods of measuring blood pressure, *Bull Imperial Military Med Acad* 11:365, 1905.

20. Lassen NA, Holstein P: Use of radioisotopes in assessment of distal blood flow and distal blood pressure in arterial insufficiency, *Surg Clin North Am* 54:39, 1974.

21. Manning DM, Kuchirka C, Kaminski J: Miscuffing: inappropriate blood pressure cuff application, *Circulation* 68:763, 1983.

22. Maxwell MH et al: Error in blood-pressure measurement due to incorrect cuff size in obese patients, *Lancet* 2:33, 1982.

23. Nielsen PE, Bell G, Lassen NA: The measurement of digital systolic blood pressure by strain-gauge technique, *Scand J Clin Lab Invest* 29:371, 1972.

24. Nielsen PE, Poulsen NL, Gyntelberg F: Arterial blood pressure in the skin measured by a photoelectric probe and external counter pressure, *Vasa* 2:65, 1973.

25. Riva-Rocci S: Un nuovo sfigmomanometro, *Gaz Med Torino* 47:981, 1896.

26. Stegall HF, Kardon MB, Kemmerer WT: Indirect measurement of arterial blood pressure by Doppler ultrasonic sphygmomanometry, *J Appl Physiol* 25:793, 1968.

27. Steinfeld L, Alexander H, Cohen ML: Updating sphygmomanometry, *Am J Cardiol* 33:107, 1974 (editorial).

28. Strandness DE Jr, Bell W: Peripheral vascular disease. Diagnosis and objective evaluation using a mercury strain-gauge, *Ann Surg* 161(suppl 4):3, 1965.

29. Thulesius O, Gjores JE: Use of Doppler-shift detection for determining peripheral arterial blood pressure, *Angiology* 22:594, 1971.

30. von Basch S: Ueber die Messung des Blutdrucks am Menschen, *Z Klin Med* 2:79, 1881.

31. von Recklinghausen H: Ueber Blutdruckmessung beim Menschen, *Arch Exp Pathol Pharmakol* 46:78, 1901.

CHAPTER 19

Physiologic principles of ocular pneumoplethysmography

BERT C. EIKELBOOM

Soon after the introduction of the ophthalmoscope, Donders[2] (among others) studied the pulsation of the vessels at the optic disk during compression of the ocular globe with the finger. In principle the possibility of measuring blood pressure in the eye originated. It was not recognized until the beginning of this century that ophthalmic artery pressure reflects distal internal carotid artery pressure and can be used in the diagnosis of carotid stenosis.

In 1917, clinical ophthalmodynamometry originated from the springdynamometer developed by Baillart[1] in which external pressure is put on the eye during simultaneous fundoscopy. The ophthalmic artery pressure was calculated from the pressure needed to stop the pulsations in the fundus arteries. Galin[4] modified this technique by application of a suction cup to the sclera to increase ocular pressure and obliterate ocular pulsations. Gee[5-7] combined Galin's technique with ocular plethysmography and obtained a graphic reproduction of the pulsations of both eyes simultaneously at different degrees of vacuum, thus making it possible to calculate both ophthalmic artery pressures more objectively. His technique, known as *OPG-Gee,* has been used since 1973. Ever since, OPG-Gee has remained a valuable technique in the evaluation of carotid disease, even though many more sophisticated techniques have been developed in recent years. This is a result of the sound physiologic principle of pressure measurement that has proved to be valuable in assessing arterial and venous disease.

DEVELOPMENT OF INSTRUMENTATION

Gee distinguishes four phases in the development of OPG-Gee. From 1967 to 1971 two experimental machines were tested that proved to be of no clinical use. In the second phase (1971 to 1973), tests were performed with a monocular unit that produced a variable vacuum that increased in a stepwise fashion steps until pulsations disappeared. However, a few seconds after that level was reached, pulsations reappeared. This was explained by the fact that an elevated eye pressure brings along a faster outflow of ocular fluid via the Schlemm system, which results in a decrease of ocular pressure and the reappearance of ocular pulsations. Gee also recognized that since the systemic blood pressure

fluctuates, both ophthalmic artery pressures should be measured simultaneously for an accurate comparison of the left side and right side and for an accurate determination of the ophthalmic-systemic pressure ratio.

The instrument was redesigned to produce binocular registration and rapid accumulation of vacuum up to 300 mm Hg, followed by automatic gradual release over 30 seconds. This machine became commercially available in 1973 and was produced until 1978. The maximum ophthalmic artery pressure that could be measured was 110 mm Hg, and it was soon recognized that this caused a problem in patients with hypertension. This led to the development of the OPG-500, which could create a vacuum of 500 mm Hg and would allow determination of systolic ophthalmic arterial pressures up to 143 mm Hg. The original three-channel recorder was replaced by a four-channel recorder, which made simultaneous electrocardiogram (ECG) registration possible.

VALIDATION STUDIES

The correlation between the amount of vacuum applied to the eye, the resulting intraocular pressure, and the ophthalmic artery pressure was partially determined in animal and human experimental work by Gee[5-7] and was partially copied from Galin[4] (Fig. 19-1). Galin tonometrically determined the relationship between intraocular pressure and vacuum applied to the eye cup in increments of 25 mm Hg. Gee performed multiple animal experiments in which simultaneous intraoperative direct stump pressure measurements were made with OPG recordings. The level of the eye cup vacuum at which a pulse wave was first detected was noted and related to the internal carotid artery back pressure with the common and external carotid arteries clamped.

Three independent researchers proved that the ophthalmic artery pressure as measured with OPG truly reflects the distal internal carotid artery pressure. Johnston[9] investigated artificial carotid stenosis in dogs and demonstrated a good correlation between OPG pressures and direct intraarterial pressures. Eikelboom[3] compared stump pressures measured in 13 carotid endarterectomies with simultaneously determined OPG pressures. The mean difference was only 4.6%. Finally, Ricotta[10] measured arterial pressure proximal and

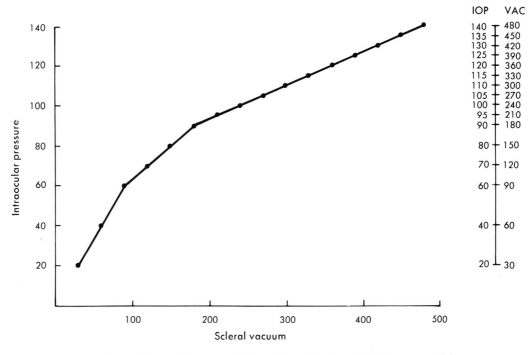

Fig. 19-1. Correlation of intraocular pressure induced by application of scleral vacuum. (All figures are in millimeters of mercury.) (From Gee W et al: *Arch Surg* 115:183, 1980. Copyright 1975, 1978, 1980, American Medical Association.)

distal to a carotid stenosis in 49 patients who had a carotid endarterectomy. He defined a drop of 5 mm Hg or more as hemodynamically significant. OPG pressures were accurate in 96% of the cases.

Ophthalmic artery pressure and carotid artery stenosis

OPG is based on pressure measurements and will detect only those obstructions that cause a reduction in arterial pressure. There is general agreement that pressure and flow are almost equally affected by a stenosis, but there is disagreement about the percentage of diameter reduction that results in a hemodynamically significant pressure reduction. Various definitions of diameter reduction between 50% and 75% have been used. In experimental situations, there is a fixed percentage of stenosis that serves as a threshold between pressure-reducing and non–pressure-reducing lesions. This is also valid lesions when pressure gradients across a stenosis are measured intraoperatively. However, it is not valid when ophthalmic artery pressures are compared with stenoses on angiograms, primarily because accurate classification of an angiogram is hard to obtain. Ophthalmic artery pressures measured with OPG might be a better standard for hemodynamic significance of a carotid stenosis than the angiographically determined percentage of stenosis. There is no fixed angiographic threshold, but there is a border zone in which a stenosis can be pressure reducing or not (Fig. 19-2). In early experience with the OPG-300, this zone was between 60% and 70% of diameter reduction.

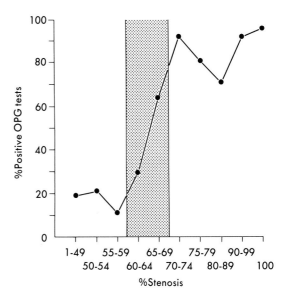

Fig. 19-2. Percentage of positive OPG tests for different degrees of carotid obstructions. Highest percentage of left and right carotid stenosis is taken.

The length of a stenosis does not influence its hemodynamic significance. The effect of two separate stenoses in the same vessel is only determined by the most severe stenosis when there is no collateral bed between the two. It does not matter which stenosis is proximal and which is distal, although this may be important in the presence of

Table 19-1. Right-left differences in intrinsic eye pressure and ophthalmic artery pressure (OAP) in patients without significant lesions on angiography[3]

1 − r intrinsic eye pressure difference	No. of patients	1 − r equal	OAPs unequal
1	3	2	1 (3 mm Hg)
2	3	2	1 (4 mm Hg)
3	6	4	2 (3 mm Hg)
4	4	4	–
10	1	1	–
TOTAL	17	13	4

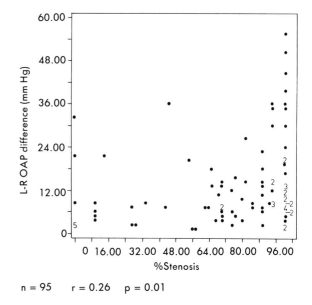

n = 95   r = 0.26   p = 0.01

Fig. 19-3. Correlation between difference in left and right ophthalmic artery pressures and severity of carotid stenosis.

combined carotid bifurcation and siphon disease. The branching of the ophthalmic artery generally originates from the distal point of the siphon, so the OPG can be used to determine the hemodynamic significance of most siphon lesions. Siphon lesions distal to the branching of the ophthalmic artery may cause an increase in ophthalmic artery pressure, but these lesions are rarely encountered. Lesions of the ophthalmic artery itself, which will cause a reduction in ophthalmic artery pressure, are rarely seen.

Central retinal artery occlusion is associated with normal ophthalmic artery pressures when determined with the OPG, whereas the pressures measured with ophthalmodynamometry are abnormal. A rare case of a reduced ophthalmic artery pressure has been described with a carotid-cavernous sinus fistula.[8] Such a fistula is characterized by an increased ocular blood flow.

Like internal carotid stenosis, lesions in the common carotid and innominate arteries may cause a reduction in ophthalmic artery pressure, although these large vessels may have larger critical diameters. However, the hemodynamic significance of a carotid lesion depends not only on the degree of stenosis but also on cardiac output, peripheral resistance, flow velocity, blood viscosity, and pulse rate.

Theoretically, intrinsic eye pressure might influence the ophthalmic artery pressure as measured with the OPG. The OPG measurements of 88 patients in whom the intrinsic eye pressure was known were studied; tonometry had been performed by an ophthalmologist. The absolute value of the intrinsic eye pressure did not influence the ophthalmic artery pressure. Even differences in intrinsic pressure between both eyes of up to 10 mm Hg did not cause unequal ophthalmic artery pressures (Table 19-1). Another factor that might influence the ophthalmic artery pressure is the position of the body, but there are no data available on OPG performed in a position other than supine. However, postural tests have been done with ophthalmodynamometry and may have some diagnostic value.[3]

A question often asked is whether the size of reduction in ophthalmic artery pressure has any value in predicting the severity of a pressure-reducing obstruction. The ability to differentiate between a severe stenosis and an occlusion is important. A group of 95 patients who had undergone

angiography was selected. They had unequal left and right pressures and did not have more than 50% stenosis on the side of the higher pressure, which excluded pressure-reducing lesions on that side. Fig. 19-3 shows the correlation between the pressure difference and the degree of carotid stenosis. Although a statistically significant correlation was found (r = 0.26), the correlation in a given patient is very low, and differentiation between stenosis and occlusion cannot be made.

Ophthalmic artery pressure and collateral circulation

The risk of cerebral damage from occlusion of the carotid artery is extremely variable and depends primarily on the availability of a collateral circulation. This does not apply only to the progression of a carotid stenosis into occlusion but also to carotid ligation, which may be necessary in embolization from surgically inaccessible carotid lesions, distal cervical aneurysms, tumor surgery, and carotid trauma. Occlusion may cause no symptoms whatsoever or may result in transitory symptoms, frank stroke, or death. These differences in clinical outcome are caused by differences in the anatomy of the many potential collateral channels, including the circle of Willis. Collateral circulation can be established at several different levels of the extracranial and intracranial blood supply. The number of potential collateral pathways increases as the location of the obstruction becomes more proximal. This is the main reason that occlusions of proximal branches of the aorta arch vessels are usually asymptomatic. Distal obstructions have fewer collateral pathways and tend to be more symptomatic. This is mainly determined by the patency of the circle of Willis, which is abnormal in about 50% of cases. Anterior and posterior communicating arteries may be stringlike or even

Table 19-2. COAP with various intracranial circulatory situations[3]

Condition	Total no.	COAP ≤60 mm Hg No.	COAP ≤60 mm Hg %	COAP >60 mm Hg No.	COAP >60 mm Hg %
Anterior communicating artery present	153	73	48	80	52
Posterior communicating artery present	45	18	40	27	60
Embryonic circle of Willis	20	14	70	6	30
Absent first part of anterior cerebral artery	18	16	89	2	11

completely absent. Several autopsy studies have shown a higher incidence of cerebral softening in patients with an abnormal circle of Willis compared with those with a normal circle.

The adequacy of collateral circulation can be assessed by means of OPG with common carotid compression,[3,6] which provides a preoperative prediction of the internal carotid artery back pressure or stump pressure. This test may be useful in assessing the risk of a carotid stenosis when there is doubt about whether to operate, for example, in a patient with an asymptomatic stenosis and a prior myocardial infarction. In patients scheduled for carotid endarterectomy, OPG with carotid compression helps predict the need for a shunt. Whenever carotid ligation is considered, preoperative knowledge about the collateral potential is essential to determine the safety of the operation.

The residual ophthalmic artery pressure on the side of carotid compression is called the *collateral ophthalmic artery pressure (COAP)* and varies greatly among patients. There may also be a considerable difference in the COAPs of both sides in an individual patient. Compression of the carotid bifurcation, if performed inappropriately over the bifurcation area, may stimulate the baroreceptors and may therefore decrease the systemic blood pressure. Experience with 5000 patients showed no such effect when carotid compression was performed low in the neck. Simultaneous automatic brachial artery pressure monitoring shows that the systemic blood pressure tends to be higher during compression than before. In 6.3% of the cases it was necessary to discontinue compression because of ischemic neurologic symptoms. Carotid occlusion should be avoided in these patients. If 60 mm Hg is taken as a threshold between good and poor collateral potential, half of the COAPs can be classified as poor and half as good.

Since the progression of carotid stenosis might coincide with an increase in COAP, whether a correlation existed between the COAP and the severity of carotid obstruction on the same side was investigated in 241 patients who underwent angiography. This was not the case ($r = 0.03$, $p = 0.623$). Since the collateral supply of a carotid territory comes mainly from the contralateral carotid artery, a correlation between the COAP and the severity of contralateral carotid disease was also investigated. Fig. 19-4 shows the results for the same 241 patients. A statistically significant

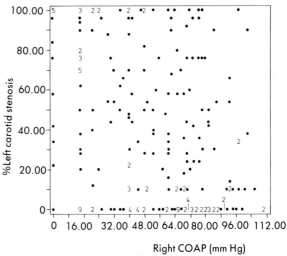

$n = 241$ $r = 0.30$ $p = <0.01$

Fig. 19-4. Correlation between right COAP and left carotid obstruction.

negative correlation was found ($r = -0.30$, $p = <0.01$), which implies that significant carotid disease diminishes the collateral circulation to the contralateral side. However, a statistically significant correlation does not imply that a prediction can be made in an individual patient, as is clearly shown by the scattergram. Whether some of the intracranial arterial distribution patterns, as shown by selective carotid and semiselective vertebral injections, correlated with differences in COAPs was also investigated. Even if the anterior or posterior communicating arteries are seen angiographically, there is no guarantee of a good collateral circulation as measured with OPG (Table 19-2).

An embryonic type of circle of Willis is accompanied by a poor collateral circulation in 70% of cases. Absence of the first part of an anterior cerebral artery may be seen by filling of the middle cerebral artery on that side only and of two anterior cerebral arteries on the other side. The COAP on the side with the two anterior cerebral arteries (the dominant side) was poor in 16 of the 18 cases (89%).

Whether differences in COAPs existed for different groups of patients according to their symptoms was also investigated. There were no differences between a control group of patients without bruits or symptoms and patients with asymptomatic bruits or nonhemispheric symptoms of transient ischemic attack. However, 84 patients who had strokes had statistically significant poorer COAPs than 134 patients who had transient ischemic attacks (t = 2.64, $p < 0.05$). This difference is especially striking, since the stroke group consisted of patients who survived strokes and whose condition was good enough to undergo angiography. Therefore the patients who had strokes with the poorest COAPs may not be included in the study. This retrospective study supports the hypothesis that a poor COAP may be a risk factor for stroke and that OPG may noninvasively identify stroke-prone patients.

REFERENCES

1. Baillart JP: La pression artérielle dans les branches de l'artère centrale de la rétine, nouvelle technique pour la déterminer, *Ann Ocul* 154:648, 1917.
2. Donders FC: Ueber die sichtbaren Erscheinungen der Blutbewegung im Auge, *Graefes Arch Opht* 1:75, 1855.
3. Eikelboom BC: *Evaluation of carotid artery disease and potential collateral circulation by ocular pneumoplethysmography,* thesis, Leiden, The Netherlands, 1981, University of Leiden.
4. Galin MA et al: Methods of suction ophthalmodynamometry, *Ann Ophthalmol* 1:439, 1970.
5. Gee W, Mehigan JT, Wylie EJ: Measurement of collateral cerebral hemispheric blood pressure by ocular pneumoplethysmography, *Am J Surg* 110:1516, 1975.
6. Gee W et al: Ocular pneumoplethysmography in carotid artery disease, *Med Instrum* 8:244, 1974.
7. Gee W et al: Simultaneous bilateral determination of the systolic pressure of the ophthalmic arteries by ocular pneumoplethysmography, *Invest Ophthalmol Vis Sci* 16:86, 1977.
8. Gee W et al: Ocular pneumoplethysmography in carotid-cavernous sinus fistulas, *J Neurosurg* 59:40, 1983.
9. Johnston CG, Bernstein EF: Quantitation of internal carotid artery stenosis by ocular plethysmography, *Surg Forum* 26:290, 1975.
10. Ricotta JJ: *Definition of extracranial carotid disease: comparison of oculo pneumoplethysmography continuous wave Doppler angiography and measurement at operation.* In Greenhalgh RM, Clifford RF, eds: *Progress in stroke research 2,* London, 1983, Pitman.

CHAPTER 20

Volume plethysmography in vascular disease: an overview

DAVID S. SUMNER

Plethysmography was first used in 1622 by Glisson[22] and in 1737 by Swammerdam[61] to study contractions of isolated muscle, but it was not until the latter half of the nineteenth century that it was applied to blood flow measurements. The first recorded attempt to determine limb blood flow with venous occlusion techniques was by François-Franck in 1876.[21] However, credit for the basic concept is usually given to Brodie and Russell,[10] who studied renal blood flow by enclosing the kidney in a chamber and then recording the increase in volume produced by clamping the renal vein. Hewlett and van Zwaluwenburg[27] applied the same principle to the measurement of blood flow in human limbs 4 years later, thus ushering in the era of venous occlusion plethysmography. Since that time, methodology has improved, new instruments have been invented, and old instruments have been perfected.[35]

BASIC PRINCIPLES

Because transient changes in the volume of most parts of the body (except the lungs) are related to their content of blood, plethysmography serves to measure changes in the volume of blood in the part being examined. However, all varieties of plethysmographs do just this—measure changes in volume. Much confusion has arisen from the idea that some plethysmographs do more or less than others. The basic differences between instruments are in the methods by which they record increases or decreases in volume, the ease with which they are used, and their stability and sensitivity.

Pulse plethysmography refers to the transient changes in volume related to the beat-by-beat activity of the left ventricle, the part that expands when arterial inflow exceeds venous outflow and contracts when the opposite occurs. More gradual changes in volume of the part are a result of dilatation or contraction of the encompassed arteries and veins, as well as expansion of the interstitial fluid space. Pulsatile information is superimposed on these gradual and sometimes periodic fluctuations in volume.

Mean blood flow can be measured by recording the rate of increase in volume that occurs when venous outflow from a part is suddenly but temporarily interrupted (venous occlusion plethysmography). Plethysmography can be used to determine blood flow only in this way. There is no way of deriving flow information from pulsatile waveforms, despite occasional claims to the contrary. The venous occlusion method has also been adapted to measure the rate of venous outflow under standardized conditions of elevated venous pressure. Here again the rate of blood flow under resting conditions is not measured, but relative venous resistance can be estimated.

INSTRUMENTATION

Although many instruments have been devised for recording plethysmographic information, they all fall into one of several categories. Some measure volume change directly by fluid displacement (water filled). Others depend on the compression of air in a closed system to produce comparable changes in pressure (air filled). Still others measure changes in the circumference of the limb (strain gauge), changes in electrical resistance (impedance), or changes in the light reflected from blood cells (photoelectric).

Water-filled plethysmographs

The earliest plethysmographs were water filled. In essence they consist of a water-filled watertight container in which the body part is immersed.[2,24,71] Any change in volume of the enclosed part displaces an equivalent quantity of water, and this displacement can be measured by a variety of means. Thus this technique provides the most direct measurement of volume change.

Many types of instruments have been constructed. Two basic varieties are shown in Figs. 20-1 and 20-2. The part to be studied is enclosed in a rigid container filled with water. Leakage is prevented by either sealing the part with cement to a rubber diaphragm at the point where it enters or leaves the container (Fig. 20-2) or by enclosing the part in a thin latex rubber sleeve or glove (Fig. 20-1). Because of hydrostatic pressure exerted by the surrounding fluid, the rubber sleeve or glove is kept in close contact with the skin. Bulging of the rubber diaphragm or sleeve at the entrance and exit points of the rigid container is avoided by means of a metal iris diaphragm.

When the enclosed part expands, water is displaced into a glass chimney, where it compresses a column of air that activates a spirometer. This in turn writes a record on a kymograph. Various types of spirometers have been used,

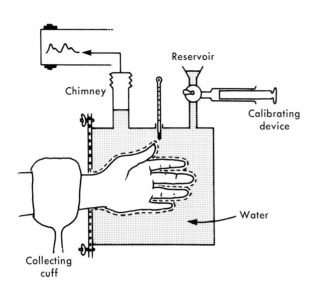

Fig. 20-1. Water-filled plethysmograph. Hand is enclosed in a loose-fitting surgical rubber glove *(dashed line)*.

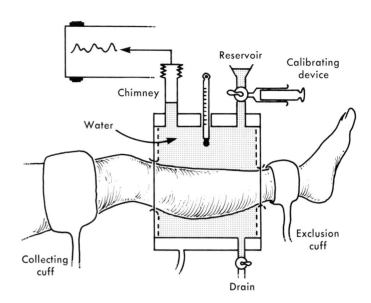

Fig. 20-2. Water-filled plethysmograph for forearm or calf. Leakage is prevented by sealing rubber diaphragms *(dashed lines)* to skin at entrance and exit. Rubber sleeve can also be used. Pneumatic exclusion cuff is used around the ankle to prevent blood flow to foot from interfering with recordings. During flow measurement, this cuff is inflated to supersystolic pressure.

including the Brodie bellows, but better results are obtained by miniature Krogh spirometers, which are counterbalanced to avoid the effect of gravity.[2] Because of the cushion of air within the bellows and chimney, the frequency response of this assembly is necessarily reduced. Optical methods for recording the fluid level in the chimney are quite accurate but have the disadvantages of requiring photosensitive paper and of not being available for immediate inspection.[38] Variations in the height of the fluid in the chimney may also be recorded by measuring the change in resistance between conductors that dip into the fluid.[13] Another method that can be used is to record changes in inductance of a coil, the core of which is floated on the fluid. Pressure changes in the enclosed air above the fluid-filled chimney may be used to activate a pressure transducer. The simplest method is to measure hydrostatic pressure changes in the fluid column by means of a sensitive pressure transducer.[36]

Calibration is achieved by adding or subtracting a known quantity of fluid to the container through a side arm (Figs. 20-1 and 20-2). By measuring the amount of liquid required to fill the container and by knowing the volume of the container, the researcher can ascertain the volume of the enclosed part.

Because blood flow rates vary widely with variations in temperature, the fluid within the container must be maintained at a constant temperature. This can be accomplished with servocontrolled heating elements immersed in the fluid or by circulating warm air or water through a jacket surrounding the container. An electric stirrer (not shown in Figs. 20-1 and 20-2) is used to ensure a constant temperature throughout the container.

Potential disadvantages of the water-filled plethysmograph include the hydrostatic pressure of the fluid, which

varies with the distance from the air-fluid interface in the chimney to the part immersed below. Ordinarily this pressure is a few centimeters of water and, consequently, does not seem to affect the recordings appreciably.[2] The necessity of enclosing the part in a rubber sleeve or of immersing the part directly in water alters the ability to sweat and may affect circulation to some degree. Air bubbles in the system or bulging of the membranes at either end of the container will cushion transient volume changes, thereby lowering the frequency response of the system and decreasing the evident volume change. Moreover, water-filled instruments are somewhat cumbersome and cannot be used conveniently to measure flow rates after exercise.

In general, however, this method of plethysmography is quite accurate and has the advantage of being the most direct technique available for evaluating changes in limb volume.

Air-filled plethysmographs

Air-filled plethysmographs measure volume changes indirectly. One class of instruments closely resembles the water-filled devices in that the part being studied is enclosed in a rigid, airtight container.[9] An increase or decrease in the volume of the part will produce a similar change in the pressure of the captive air, and this pressure change can be recorded with a suitable transducer. Unlike the water-filled instruments, those filled with air can be constructed of lighter-weight material (such as plastic) and do not require elaborate temperature-regulating features.

An even more convenient adaptation of the air-filled plethysmograph uses a pneumatic cuff that encircles a seg-

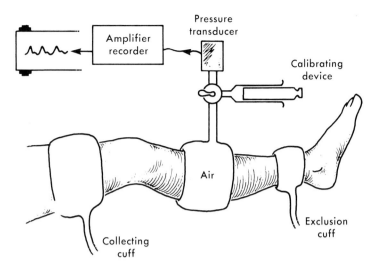

Fig. 20-3. Segmental air plethysmograph. Air-filled cuff is filled to a predetermined pressure to maintain good contact with the limb. Changes in limb volume produce corresponding changes in air pressure within the cuff.

ment of the part being examined (Fig. 20-3).[14,17,70] The cuff is kept in close approximation to the underlying skin by inflating it with air to some relatively low pressure (e.g., 40 to 65 mm Hg). Consequently, volume changes in the enclosed limbs either increase or decrease the pressure of the air entrapped within the cuff. These pressure changes are easily converted to an analogue recording by means of an attached pressure transducer. The operator can calibrate the system by injecting a known quantity of air into the cuff and noting the resulting increase in pressure. Because of the ease with which these devices can be used, they have gained widespread popularity in recent years, particularly for use in diagnostic laboratories. (For a more detailed description see Chapters 23, 59, and 112.)

In general, the frequency response of air-filled plethysmographs is not high, approximately 8 Hz.[18] However, Raines[50] states that his pulse volume recorder functions to 20 Hz without loss of amplitude. On the basis of harmonic analysis of the frequencies in pulsatile blood flow, a frequency response of 6 to 8 harmonics, or 6 to 8 times the heart rate, should produce an adequate rendition of the pulse contour.[19] Therefore these instruments are capable of providing a satisfactory, if not perfect, tracing of the pulse contour.

When the venous occlusion technique is used with air-filled plethysmographs, errors in blood flow measurement occur because of the high coefficient of expansion of air with temperature changes.[40,65] Because there is little time for the escape of heat from the instrument, expansion of the enclosed part raises the temperature of the entrapped air as it is compressed. This produces an inordinately high pressure change for each volume change and yields flow recordings that are too high.

Instruments that allow a free flow of air into or out of the plethysmograph (measuring air flow rather than pressure change) may help to avoid some of these problems.[16] A pneumotachygraph attached to the chimney is used to detect air flow. The resulting signal, which resembles an arterial flow pulse, must be integrated to provide a volume pulse recording (Fig. 20-4). According to the inventors, the system has a frequency response of 25 Hz and can record frequencies up to 35 Hz with less than a 20% loss.

Mercury strain gauge

Measurement of limb volume change by means of a mercury-filled rubber tube was first described by Whitney in 1953.[69] More recent models consist of a fine-bore silicone elastomer tube completely filled with mercury or an indium-gallium alloy that makes contact with copper electrodes at either end. The tube is wrapped around the part being studied with just enough stretch to ensure good contact. As the part expands or contracts, the length of the gauge is changed by a corresponding amount. Since the resistance of the gauge varies with its length, variations in the voltage drop across the gauge will reflect changes in limb circumference (see Fig. 22-1). Calibration is accomplished electrically or by stretching the gauge a known amount. (These methods are discussed in more detail in Chapter 22.)

Mercury-in-silicone-elastomer gauges are very sensitive and have a high frequency response. The entire system (gauge, amplifier, and recorder) is capable of reproducing the magnitude of periodic stretch without loss up to 100 Hz.[48] The system is free of resonance effects up to 30 Hz, and no significant phase shift between gauge output and stretch is apparent. Thus this instrument is particularly well adapted for accurate rendition of pulsatile phenomena. However, its extreme sensitivity makes it a bit more difficult to use in clinical practice than the air-filled devices.

A potential drawback of the mercury strain gauge is its temperature sensitivity. A change in resistance of about 1%

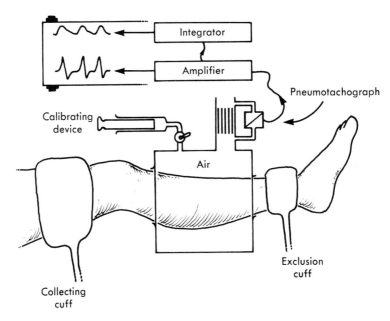

Fig. 20-4. Air-filled plethysmograph that uses pneumotachograph to measure rate of air flow produced by changing the volume of the enclosed segment. Since a flow recording is obtained, the resulting curve must be integrated to obtain the volume recording.

follows a temperature change of 10° C.[32,47] Obviously, this could introduce a measurement error if the gauge is calibrated at a temperature that differs from the temperature when the recordings are made. Since correction factors are easily applied, errors related to temperature can be avoided when a high degree of precision is required.

Impedance plethysmographs

Impedance plethysmographs indirectly detect changes in the volume of blood within a limb segment by measuring variations in electric impedance. Impedance (Z) expresses the hindrance to the passage of alternating current (I) through a conductor under the influence of a potential difference (E):

$$Z = E/I \tag{1}$$

Impedance is a vector quantity with resistive, capacitive, and inductive elements. However, in plethysmography the major portion of the impedance is resistive.

In a biologic organism, electricity is transported by the movement of ions in intracellular and extracellular fluids. Since the concentration of ions in these fluids remains relatively constant, the resistive impedance of any segment of the body is inversely proportional to its total fluid content.

In any cylindric conductor, resistance (R) is inversely proportional to its cross-sectional area (πr^2) and directly proportional to its length (L):

$$R = \rho \frac{L}{\pi r^2} \tag{2}$$

In this equation, ρ is the specific resistance of the medium between the electrodes in ohm-cm. Since volume (V) is the product of the cross-sectional area of the conductor and its length ($\pi r^2 L$), equation 2 becomes:

$$V = \rho \frac{L^2}{R} \tag{3}$$

When the volume changes from V_1 to V_2, equation 3 becomes:

$$V_1 - V_2 \quad \rho L^2 (1/R_1 - 1/R_2) \tag{4}$$
$$= \rho L^2 \left(\frac{R_2 - R_1}{R_1 R_2} \right)$$

For small changes in volume, the resistances, R_1 and R_2, are almost equal, permitting equation 4 to be simplified:

$$V_1 - V_2 \cong \rho \frac{L^2}{R} \left(\frac{R_2 - R_1}{R} \right) \tag{5}$$

Equation 12 can be substituted for $\rho L^2/R$ in equation 5 to give:

$$V_1 - V_2 \cong V \left(\frac{R_2 - R_1}{R} \right) \tag{6}$$
$$\frac{\Delta V}{V} \cong -\frac{\Delta R}{R}$$

Thus by measuring changes in resistive impedance, periodic variations in blood volume within a segment can be calculated—at least theoretically.[6,45]

Modern impedance plethysmographs use a high-frequency oscillator (22 to 250 kHz) with low currents. Although lower frequencies result in problems of contact re-

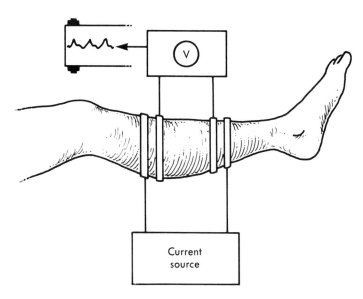

Fig. 20-5. Impedance plethysmograph. The outer two electrodes deliver a high-frequency current to the limb. Voltage drop across the limb is measured between two inner electrodes.

sistance and nonuniformity of current distribution, higher frequencies lead to subject-ground artifacts, difficulties in obtaining a high-isolation impedance, and radiofrequency interference.

Basically, two forms of instruments have been devised: the two-electrode and the four-electrode types. Because of many problems with the two-electrode system, the four-electrode design is used in most modern instruments (Fig. 20-5).[72] The outer two electrodes send current through the part, and the inner two record the decrease in voltage.

Although the impedance plethysmograph has proved to be a valuable clinical instrument, there continues to be some controversy concerning what is actually measured. Researchers have gone so far as to suggest that the entire signal is related to electrode artifact rather than volume change.[28] Others discount this theory but acknowledge the complexity of the signal source.[5,39,67] Added to the complexity is the fact that the electrical resistance of blood is affected by the orientation of red blood cells. Static blood with its random distribution of red cells has a higher resistance in the longitudinal direction than moving blood in which the red cells are oriented in the direction of flow.[66] As a result, pulse recordings with the impedance device have a more rapid upslope and a slower downslope than those made with the mercury strain gauge.[5] Similarly, the outflow curve in venous occlusion plethysmography tends to be slightly delayed.[4] These distortions are minor and do not adversely affect the clinical use of impedance plethysmography.[64]

Since the specific resistance of blood (ρ_b) is about half that of the surrounding tissues (ρ_t), one might predict that the relative change in resistance as a result of the accu-mulation of blood during venous occlusion plethysmography would exceed the relative volume change[5,55,73]:

$$\frac{\Delta V}{V} \cong -\frac{\rho_b \Delta R}{\rho_t R}$$

$$= -K\frac{\Delta R}{R} \tag{7}$$

Although some investigators have confirmed this relationship, reporting values for K that range from 0.6 to 0.8,[3,73] others have noted that the impedance method seriously underestimates flow during venous occlusion plethysmography, reporting K values of 1.6 to 3.1.* In most studies, however, simultaneous flows measured with the impedance and mechanical methods (water, air, strain gauge) have been significantly correlated (r = 0.70 to 0.93).[3,43,46,53] This suggests that an experimentally determined conversion factor (K) could be used to provide results that more nearly coincide with volume flow measurements obtained by other means. Although these disparities might prove troublesome to those trying to measure precise volume changes, they are not important when the impedance method is used to diagnose acute venous thrombosis, since this test plots venous outflow versus capacitance and cancels any errors that result from a variable K.[34,68] Indeed, because of its simplicity and reliability, impedance plethysmography has become one of the most popular methods for diagnosing deep vein thrombosis. (The theory of impedance plethysmography is more fully detailed in Chapter 21.)

Photoelectric plethysmographs

Strictly speaking, photoelectric plethysmographs are not true plethysmographs, since they do not measure volume change and are difficult to calibrate.[37] They consist of an infrared light–emitting diode and a photosensor. Blood, which is more opaque to red and near-infrared light than the surrounding tissue, attenuates light in proportion to its content in the tissue. In one type of photoplethysmograph, the part being examined is sandwiched between the light source and the sensor. Since this type of plethysmograph depends on transmitted light, its applicability is restricted to thin, relatively transparent organs, such as the earlobe. A more versatile type uses reflected light.[26,62] The light source and photosensor are mounted adjacent to one another on the same face of a small probe, which can be applied quite easily to virtually any area of the body by double-stick transparent tape (Fig. 20-6).

Pulse contours obtained when the output of the photoplethysmograph is amplified through an AC circuit are practically identical to those recorded by other methods. Thus these instruments provide a rapid, simple method for evaluating digital and supraorbital pulses.[8,42,59] DC coupling permits slower changes in the blood content of the skin to be

_____
*References 41, 43, 45, 46, 53, 63.

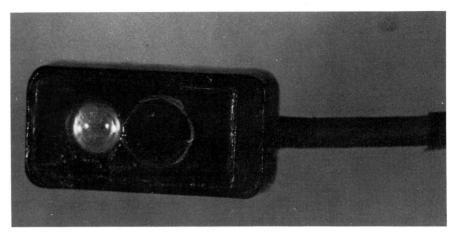

Fig. 20-6. Photoplethysmographic probe showing light-emitting diode and photoelectric sensor. (From Sumner DS: *Plethysmography in arterial and venous diagnosis.* In Zwiebel WJ, ed: *Introduction to vascular ultrasonography,* New York, 1982, Grune & Stratton.)

observed. This method of coupling is useful for measuring blood pressure in the limbs, fingers, toes, and penis.[42,52,56] Because the blood content in the skin parallels that in the calf and is correlated with venous pressure, the DC-coupled photoplethysmograph has become a popular instrument for studying limbs with venous valvular incompetence.[1]

VENOUS OCCLUSION PLETHYSMOGRAPHY

Venous occlusion plethysmography can be used to measure the total blood flow to a terminal organ (e.g., a hand, foot, finger, or toe) by means of a volume displacement apparatus as in Fig. 20-1. In this illustration the entire hand is enclosed in a watertight container so that any change in its volume can be recorded. A pneumatic cuff is applied to the arm just proximal to the container. When this cuff—often called the *collecting cuff*—is rapidly inflated well above venous pressure (usually 50 to 60 mm Hg), blood is temporarily trapped in the hand, which causes its volume to rise. The initial rate at which the volume of the hand increases is proportional to the blood flow.

The pertinent events in this process are shown in Fig. 20-7. In these diagrams the arterial inflow and the venous outflow channels are each represented by a single vessel around which is placed a collecting cuff. Blood pressures within the artery (100 mm Hg) and vein (5 mm Hg) are indicated by attached manometers. (These are added for illustrative purposes and are not necessary for measuring blood flow.) The capacitance vessels within the hand are represented by a bellows.

At rest, with the collecting cuff deflated, the baseline of the recording is relatively stable except for the periodic fluctuations caused by the arterial pulse (Fig. 20-7, *A*). When the collecting cuff is suddenly inflated to a level that exceeds venous pressure (50 mm Hg), the underlying vein is completely collapsed, thereby preventing the escape of blood from the capacitance vessels (Fig. 20-7, *B*). Because of the shape of the arterial compliance curve, a reduction

in transmural pressure (the pressure inside the vessel minus that on the outside) from 100 to 50 mm Hg will cause relatively little narrowing of the arterial lumen. This small reduction in arterial diameter is far below the critical stenosis limit; consequently, there is little or no initial change in arterial inflow or in arterial pressure. As a result of the unimpeded arterial inflow and a totally blocked venous outflow, the bellows, which represents the capacitance vessels, begins to expand. Most of the trapped blood accumulates in the venules and veins. Since the compliance of veins is great at low transmural pressures, a relatively great increase in venous volume is possible without much increase in venous pressure. Thus the initial slope of the line that depicts the volume increase of the enclosed part is almost straight, reflecting fairly accurately the arterial inflow before venous occlusion. Later, as venous pressure begins to rise, the arteriovenous pressure gradient across the vascular bed will fall, and the arterial inflow will gradually decrease.

As the veins become more distended, a stiffer portion of the venous compliance curve is reached. Less expansion of the venous wall is possible without a great increase in transmural pressure. Consequently, venous pressure rises to equal (or slightly exceed) the pressures exerted by the collecting cuff. At this point, blood again escapes from the veins, and a new equilibrium is attained, with arterial inflow and venous outflow again becoming identical (Fig. 20-7, *C*). Because of the reduction in the pressure gradient across the vascular bed (from 95 mm Hg before occlusion to 50 mm Hg at the new equilibrium point), the total flow rate is reduced.[23] The volume of the part, as depicted by the recording, becomes relatively stable at a new but higher level (Fig. 20-7, *C*).

Actually, the volume tracing will continue to rise at a very slow rate as a result of the escape of fluid through the capillary wall into the interstitial space. This is a manifestation of the elevated pressure within the capillaries, which must exceed 50 mm Hg in the present example. The elevated

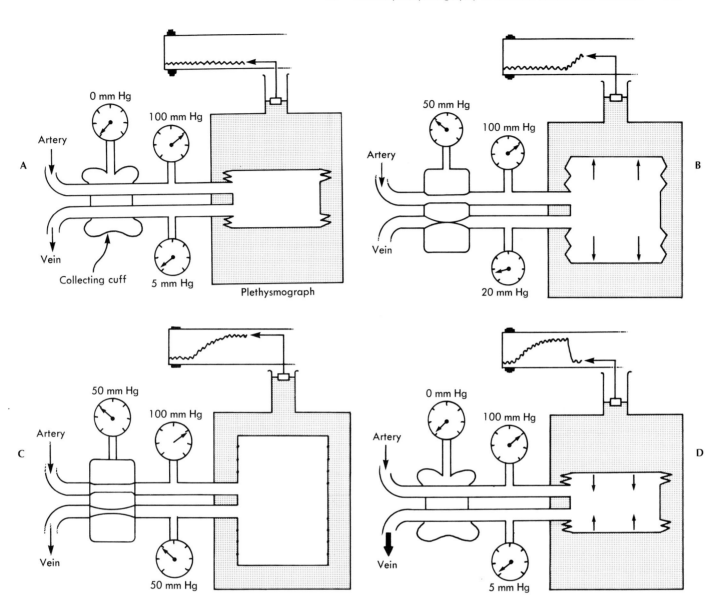

Fig. 20-7. Sequence of events responsible for the shape of the curve obtained with venous occlusion plethysmography. See text for details. *A,* Baseline recording. *B,* Early stage of venous occlusion. *C,* Late stage of venous occlusion. *D,* Cuff deflation.

capillary blood pressure upsets the Starling equilibrium; thus fluid will continue to flow into the interstitial space until a new equilibrium is established. Because of the great compliance of the interstitial space, this ordinarily requires many hours.

When the collecting cuff is suddenly deflated, there is a sudden surge of blood out through the veins (Fig. 20-7, *D*). The volume tracing falls rapidly, reaching baseline or near baseline levels.

Segmental plethysmography

When the entire organ cannot be placed in the plethysmograph or when the operator wishes to record blood flow to only a segment of a limb, it is necessary to apply a second cuff distal to the plethysmograph (Fig. 20-2). This cuff is inflated to a pressure well in excess of the arterial pressure to exclude flow from those parts of the extremity that are not enclosed in the plethysmograph.

For example, if blood flow to the forearm is being measured and no exclusion cuff has been applied to the wrist, the total arterial inflow destined for both the hand and forearm will be distributed to all the veins distal to the occlusion cuff. Since the rate of blood flow to the hand ordinarily exceeds that to the forearm, failure to apply the distal exclusion cuff will result in a spuriously high recording of forearm blood flow. The same holds true for the lower extremity: an ankle cuff must be applied when calf blood flow is being measured.

When segmental air plethysmographs (Fig. 20-3) or mercury-in-silicone-elastomer strain gauges (see Fig. 22-1) are used on the forearm or calf, it is also important to apply an exclusion cuff to the wrist or ankle. Although these devices sense flow in only that segment of the limb with which they are in direct contact, it is assumed that flow through the entire part is fairly uniform. For this reason, it is necessary only to exclude the hand or foot, which have higher flows than the forearm or calf.

Occlusion cuffs, exclusion cuffs, and inflators

The collecting cuff must be inflated rapidly to a preset pressure. This may be accomplished by connecting the cuff to an air reservoir with a wide-bore tube. The capacity of the reservoir must be large in relation to that of the cuff so that sudden inflation of the cuff will not lower the pressure in the system appreciably. Simple, inexpensive arrangements that work quite well are easily constructed from odds and ends.

Instruments specifically designed to inflate cuffs* contain a pressure regulator and two electrically operated solenoid valves. They are connected to an external air pressure source capable of delivering 20 to 100 psi. With these instruments, even large cuffs are accurately inflated or deflated to the desired pressure in about a second.

For venous occlusion and arterial flow exclusion, a variety of commercially available cuffs are suitable. Cuffs with a long bladder (40.5 cm)† can be used so that the entire circumference of the limb will be directly subjected to the air pressure. The width of the cuff can be 10 or 12.7 cm, depending on the diameter of the limb. A large contoured cuff (22 cm × 71 cm)† shaped to conform to the taper of the thigh is particularly useful for venous occlusion during studies of calf blood flow. Digit cuffs of varying lengths constructed of Penrose drains or plastic bladders backed with Velcro pile are used for venous occlusion when finger blood flow is being measured.

Venous occlusion pressures should ordinarily be about 50 to 60 mm Hg. The diastolic blood pressure in the arteries underlying the cuff should never be exceeded. When flow studies are conducted on a limb with obstructive arterial disease, it may be necessary to use a lower pressure. Ideally, the operator should experiment with several occlusion pressures to see which gives the steepest slope. In practical terms, a wide range of pressures will usually yield identical slopes.

The pressure in the exclusion cuff should always be well above the systolic pressure at the site to which the cuff is applied. Usually a pressure of 200 mm Hg will suffice. The exclusion cuff should be inflated about 30 seconds before any recordings are made.

---

*Manufactured by Hokanson, Inc, Issaquah, Wash.
†Manufactured by Hokanson, Inc, Issaquah, Wash.

Calculation of blood flow

Although absolute blood flow in terms of volume of blood per unit of time can be measured with water-filled or air-filled plethysmographs, blood flow is usually expressed in terms of volume of flow per unit volume of tissue enclosed in the plethysmograph per unit of time. Depending on the method used, flow may be expressed as cc/100 cc/min, ml/100 ml/min, or percent volume change per minute. Flow may also be reported in ml/ml/min, ml/5 ml/min, or ml/L/min. Obviously, if the total volume of the enclosed part is known, any of these measurements can be converted into ml/min.

Basically, the same methods are used to calculate blood flow whether the entire part or only a portion of it is enclosed in the plethysmograph. For determining the initial rate of filling of the part after the occlusion cuff is inflated, a line is drawn on the recording paper to connect the initial systolic peaks or diastolic valleys (Fig. 20-8). The slope of this line in terms of the arbitrary divisions (div) with which the paper is ruled is determined by measuring the number of divisions the line rises in 1 minute. Usually it is more convenient to measure the rise over a few seconds (t), divide by the number of seconds, and multiply by 60:

$$\text{Div/min} = \frac{\text{Div rise in t sec}}{\text{t sec}} \times 60 \text{ sec/min} \qquad (8)$$

Next, the calibration signal is used to convert the arbitrary divisions with which the slope is measured into volume flow per minute. This is done by dividing the calibration volume by the number of corresponding divisions and then multiplying by the division rise per minute from equation 8:

$$\frac{\text{Calibration vol}}{\text{Calibration div}} \times \frac{\text{Div}}{\text{Minutes}} = \text{Vol flow/min} \qquad (9)$$

The flow rate per 100 ml of enclosed part can be calculated by dividing the volume flow per minute by the volume of the enclosed part in milliliters and then multiplying by 100:

$$\frac{\text{Vol flow/min}}{\text{Vol of part}} \times 100 = \text{Vol flow/100 ml/min} \qquad (10)$$

The volume of the enclosed part can be measured directly by water displacement, or it can be estimated from its dimensions. (Calculation of blood flow with the mercury-in-silicone-elastomer strain gauge is discussed in Chapter 22.)

Distortion of the tracing

Ideally, the initial slope of the plethysmographic tracing after venous occlusion should describe a straight line intersecting the baseline at a definite, sharp angle (Fig. 20-9, *A*). Unfortunately, several artifacts that are commonly seen may prove perplexing.[24] Chief among these is the so-called cuff artifact, which is usually manifested by a sharp upward jump in the tracing preceding the initial slope (Fig. 20-9, *B*). This is usually caused by the displacement of tissue into the plethysmograph by the inflation of the cuff. If the jump

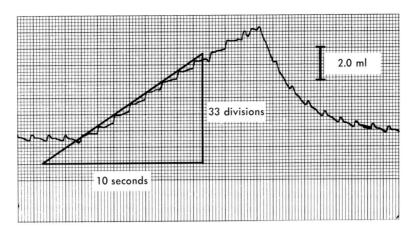

Fig. 20-8. Venous occlusion plethysmographic tracing from human calf at room temperature. Volume of calf enclosed in plethysmograph was 1200 ml. Calibration signal was 10 divisions for 2.0 ml volume increment. Blood flow is calculated as follows:

$$\frac{33 \text{ div}}{10 \text{ sec}} \times 60 \text{ sec/min} = 198 \text{ div/min}$$

$$\frac{2.0 \text{ ml}}{10 \text{ div}} \times 198 \text{ div/min} = 39.6 \text{ ml/min}$$

$$\frac{39.6 \text{ ml/min}}{1200 \text{ ml}} \times 100 = 3.3 \text{ ml/100 ml/min}$$

Fig. 20-9. Various distortions of plethysmographic pulse tracing. Arrow indicates point at which occlusion cuff was inflated. *F,* Volume of inflow; *T,* time over which it was measured; baseline, time-trace in seconds; *C,* calibration in two steps of 5 or 10 ml each; *α,* angle between traverse of recording point and baseline. See text for further explanation. (From Greenfield ADM, Whitney RJ, Mowbray JF: *Br Med Bull* 19:101, 1963.)

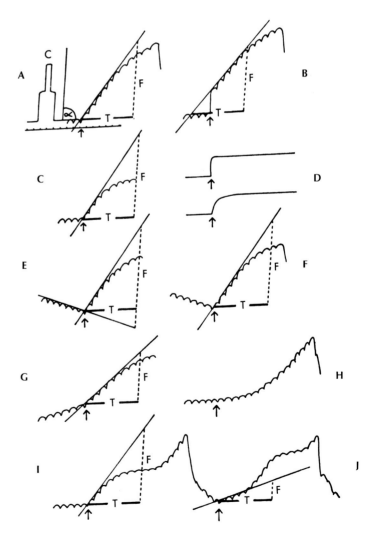

is quite abrupt so that the artifact can be clearly discriminated (Fig. 20-9, *D, top line*), the slope can be constructed in the usual fashion between the initial systolic peaks or diastolic valleys, ignoring the initial jump. If the jump is gradual, it will be difficult to tell artifact from limb expansion (Fig. 20-9, *D, bottom line*). In these cases it is best to discard the tracing and readjust the cuff and strain gauge. For determining the shape of the cuff artifact, a pressure cuff placed proximal to the venous occlusion cuff can be inflated to supersystolic pressure, after which the venous occlusion cuff is inflated. In the absence of arterial inflow, the only change in the level of the tracing will be caused by the cuff artifact (Fig. 20-9, *D*). Sometimes a negative cuff artifact is generated. This may be related to movement of the limb out of the plethysmograph. In these cases there is usually no problem in deciding where to draw the initial slope.

When the rate of arterial inflow is very high or when the venous capacity is limited, there may be no steady upward rise; rather, the pulses describe a curve with a continuously decreasing slope (Fig. 20-9, *C*). Sometimes flow is so great that the part fills within one or two beats. Such curves are rather frequently obtained in digital plethysmography. Because it may not be possible to draw an accurate tangent, flow measurements cannot be made with confidence.

Sometimes the baseline tracing rises or falls between collections. At times this may be caused by a leak in the plethysmograph or movement of the strain gauge (Fig. 20-9, *E*). An alternating baseline may be a result of fluctuation in relative arterial inflow and venous outflow. Such fluctuations can be ignored and the curve constructed as if the baseline were level (Fig. 20-9, *F* and *G*).

When, after venous occlusion, the tracing rises with an ever-increasing slope, the curve is uninterpretable and must be discarded (Fig. 20-9, *H*). Sometimes this artifact can be avoided by decreasing the gap between the plethysmograph and the occlusion cuff.

At times the curve will show differing slopes over the filling period, at first rising rapidly, then more slowly, and finally rapidly again. If this curve is duplicated simultaneously in the opposite limb, it is probably related to periodic fluctuations in blood flow. In such cases the initial slope is still valid for the flow at the instant of venous occlusion (Fig. 20-9, *I* and *J*).

Accuracy

Venous occlusion plethysmography is perhaps the most accurate noninvasive method for measuring blood flow to the limbs. Several researchers[12,20] have observed little difference in flows measured plethysmographically and those measured directly. In a series of experiments on primate limbs, Raman et al[51] found plethysmographically measured flow to be about 92% of the undisturbed flow measured electromagnetically.

Applications

Venous occlusion plethysmography finds its major application in physiologic studies of normal and diseased circulation. Although it is used in some clinical laboratories as a diagnostic tool, there are far simpler techniques that will yield equally valuable information. The validity, however, of some of these simpler techniques had to be substantiated by comparison with venous occlusion plethysmography.[60]

Occlusive arterial disease. Resting blood flow measurements are of no value in distinguishing between normal limbs and those with occlusion of major inflow arteries. Because of the capacity of the peripheral vascular bed to dilate as compensation for the increased resistance imposed by the inflow arteries, resting blood flow usually remains within normal limits (Table 20-1).[29,54,57,60] Flow begins to decrease only when there are multiple levels of obstruction and/or involvement of collateral arteries. Thus a decreased flow at normal temperatures would be found in ischemic, pregangrenous extremities. Since blood flow to the tissues (skin in particular) is quite variable and is in response to changes in temperature and sympathetic tone, peripheral

Table 20-1. Resting calf blood flow (ml/100 ml/min)

Normal	3.6 ± 1.3
Iliac occlusion	3.7 ± 2.0
Superficial femoral occlusion	3.9 ± 3.1
Combined iliac and superficial femoral occlusion	4.0 ± 1.9

Data from Hillestad[29] and Sumner and Strandness.[60]

Table 20-2. Peak reactive hyperemia flow

	Average flow (ml/100 ml/min)	Time to peak (sec)
Normal	20 to 40	5
Arterial oclusion	3 to 22	10 to 100

Data from Strandness and Sumner.[58]

vasoconstriction in all these cases must be ruled out. However, when the circulation is stressed by any mechanism that produces peripheral vasodilatation, the plethysmographic flow pattern in patients with occlusive arterial disease is quite different from that in normal individuals.

Reactive hyperemia and exercise are the two methods most commonly used to achieve maximal or near maximal peripheral vasodilatation. Reactive hyperemia is produced by arresting the circulation for 3 to 5 minutes with a pneumatic cuff inflated well above systolic pressure. This cuff is placed on the limb proximal to the venous occlusion cuff and the plethysmograph. (Fig. 22-10 shows a typical response in a normal limb. The response in an abnormal limb is obviously quite different in a number of ways [see Fig. 22-11].) First, the peak hyperemic flow is reduced in the limb with occlusive arterial disease. The time required to reach peak flow is also delayed (Table 20-2). Second, the hyperemic response is prolonged. Ordinarily more than three fourths of the excess hyperemia flow is confined to the first minute after release of the tourniquet, but in limbs with occlusive disease, less than half occurs within the first minute.[29] In spite of the prolonged hyperemic flow, the flow debt is underpaid in abnormal limbs. (Flow debt is the product of the resting blood flow and the period of ischemia.)

The normal flow response to exercise is shown in Fig. 22-12. Immediately after exercise, peak flows are attained that are often in excess of 20 to 40 ml/100 ml/min. These flows rapidly decline, usually approaching preexercise values in a few minutes. Fig. 22-13 shows the postexercise flow response in a limb with occlusive arterial disease. In these limbs, the peak flow is reduced (average of 9 to 20 ml/100 ml/min), the time required to attain peak flow is delayed (average of 3 to 7 minutes), and the hyperemic response may be prolonged well beyond 20 minutes.[30,58,60]

Clearly, these plethysmographic measurements can be used effectively to evaluate the circulation in patients with occlusive arterial disease. However, it is much easier to measure pressures, which vary in much the same way.[60] Accordingly, venous occlusion plethysmography may have little place in the diagnosis of occlusive arterial disease, although it is of great value to the clinical physiologist.[58] Venous occlusion plethysmography is helpful in evaluating the effects of vasodilators, sympathectomy, and operative procedures on calf, forearm, or finger blood flow.[42]

Vasospastic disease. Hillestad[31] and others[58] have used venous occlusion plethysmography to distinguish normal, vasospastic, and obliterative arterial disease of the hands and fingers. At normal local temperatures (32° C), hand blood flow is reduced in patients with peripheral vasospasm, but it is normal in patients with other problems that might be confused with this diagnosis. However, when the local temperature is increased to 40° C, there is a great increase in flow in the vasospastic hand, equaling the flow in the normal hand under the same conditions. In obliterative arterial disease, flow may remain stable or even drop if there is impending gangrene. A severe drop in flow may occur in the presence of arteritis. Similar studies may also be carried out on the fingers in such patients. Here again, pressure measurements are often easier to perform and may yield equally valuable information.[58]

PLETHYSMOGRAPHY IN VENOUS DISEASE

Plethysmographic techniques have been applied successfully to the diagnosis of acute deep vein thrombosis. Systems especially designed for this purpose are commercially available and are in widespread use. Although most systems use either impedance measuring devices[34,68] or air-filled cuffs,[11] much of the earlier research was done with water-filled plethysmographs or mercury strain gauges—methods that continue to be used.[7,15,25] Mercury strain gauges, photoplethysmographs, and air plethysmographs are now frequently used to confirm the presence of chronic venous insufficiency and to evaluate its severity.

PULSE PLETHYSMOGRAPHY

Sensitive plethysmographs can be used to record the periodic expansion of an organ, limb, or digit that occurs in response to the arrival of the arterial pulse wave. Because the contour and volume of these pulses have diagnostic significance, particularly in the eye and in limbs with obstructive arterial or vasospastic disease, a number of instruments capable of accurately recording the volume pulse are available commercially. Most popular are the air-cuff and mercury strain-gauge plethysmographs and the photoplethysmograph.

The moment-to-moment magnitude of volume expansion is determined by the rate at which blood flows into the part and the rate at which it simultaneously flows out. During the first part of the cycle, blood enters the part by way of the arteries more rapidly than it leaves by the veins; consequently, there is a rapid swelling of the part, producing the steep ascending limb of the pulse tracing. After peak volume is reached, blood flows out of the part more rapidly than it enters, allowing it to return to its diastolic diameter. Characteristically, the resulting descending limb of the tracing is much more prolonged than the ascending limb. Although most outflow occurs through venous channels, there is often some retrograde flow in the arteries early in diastole as a result of the arrival of a reflected wave from the periphery.

Although these periodic volume fluctuations are largely a result of passive dilatation or contraction of the vascular channels, it is not completely clear which vessels are involved. Because of the great compliance and large volume of the veins, much of the volume change may take place in these vessels.[49] This is especially true in vasodilated states. When the part is vasoconstricted, however, most of the volume expansion may be due to changes in arterial diameter.[33,44] There is also evidence that volume pulsations in the forearm and calf are largely the result of arterial expansion.[16,44]

Illustrated in Fig. 20-10 are normal volume pulses obtained from a finger, calf, and toe. After a steep systolic

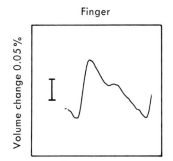
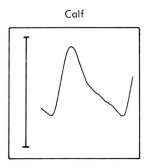
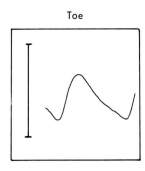

Fig. 20-10. Plethysmographic pulse tracings obtained from a normal finger, calf, and toe. Vertical bars indicate 0.05% volume change. (From Strandness DE Jr, Sumner DS: *Hemodynamics for surgeons,* New York, 1975, Grune & Stratton.)

upstroke, there is a slower downstroke that is curved toward the baseline. There is often a prominent dicrotic wave on the downslope. A strong resemblance to the arterial pressure pulse is evident. In limbs with proximal arterial obstruction, the volume of the pulse may be reduced, the systolic upslope is less rapid, the peak may be rounded, and the downslope is bowed away from the baseline.[58,59]

In any individual, when measurements are made serially, the volume of the plethysmographic pulse correlates well with blood flow.[74] On the other hand, the relative rate of blood flow from one individual to the next (or even from the same individual when measurements are not continuous) cannot be determined by comparing the volume of the plethysmographic pulse. Too many factors are involved. Disparities in pulse volume are more likely to be a result of proximal obstruction changing the shape of the wave rather than major differences in blood flow. Nevertheless, this does not obviate the value of measuring the height of the pulse excursion as a diagnostic tool.[17]

REFERENCES

1. Abramowitz HB et al: The use of photoplethysmography in the assessment of venous insufficiency: a comparison to venous pressure measurements, *Surgery* 86:434, 1979.
2. Abramson DI: *Circulation in the extremities,* New York, 1967, Academic Press, Inc.
3. Anderson FA Jr et al: Evaluation of electrical impedance plethysmography for venous volume measurements, *Proceedings of the Twenty-Ninth Annual Conference on Engineering in Medicine and Biology,* vol 18, Chevy Chase, Md, 1976, The Alliance for Engineering in Medicine and Biology.
4. Anderson FA Jr et al: Comparison of electrical impedance and mechanical plethysmographic techniques in the human calf, *Proceedings of the Twelfth Annual Meeting of the Association for the Advancement of Medical Instrumentation,* Arlington, Va, 1977.
5. Anderson FA Jr et al: Impedance plethysmography: the origin of electrical impedance changes measured in the human calf, *Med Biol Eng Comput* 18:234, 1980.
6. Barendsen GJ: *Plethysmography.* In Verstraete M, ed: *Methods in angiology,* The Hague, 1980, Martinus Nijhoff.
7. Barnes RW et al: Noninvasive quantitation of maximum venous outflow in acute thrombophlebitis, *Surgery* 72:971, 1972.
8. Barnes RW et al: Supraorbital photoplethysmography, simple accurate screening for carotid occlusive disease, *J Surg Res* 22:319, 1977.
9. Black JE: Blood flow requirements of the human calf after walking and running, *Clin Sci* 18:89, 1959.
10. Brodie TG, Russell AE: On the determination of the rate of blood flow through an organ, *J Physiol (Lond)* 32:47P, 1905.
11. Comerota AJ et al: Phleborheography: results of a ten-year experience, *Surgery* 91:573, 1982.
12. Conrad MC, Green HD: Evaluation of venous occlusion plethysmography, *J Appl Physiol* 16:289, 1961.
13. Cooper KE, Kerslake DM: An electrical recorder for use with plethysmography, *J Physiol (Lond)* 114:11, 1951.
14. Dahn I: On the calibration and accuracy of segmental calf plethysmography with a description of a new expansion chamber and a new sleeve, *Scand J Clin Lab Invest* 16:347, 1964.
15. Dahn I, Eiriksson E: Plethysmographic diagnosis of deep venous thrombosis of the leg, *Acta Chir Scand* (suppl 398):33, 1968.
16. Dahn I, Jonson B, Nilsén R: A plethysmographic method for determination of flow and volume pulsations in a limb, *J Appl Physiol* 28:333, 1970.
17. Darling RC et al: Quantitative segmental pulse volume recorder: a clinical tool, *Surgery* 72:873, 1973.
18. Dohn K: Three plethysmographs usable during functional states recording volume changes in ml per 100 ml of extremity, *Rep Steno Mem Hosp* 6:147, 1956.
19. Ferguson DJ, Wells HS: Harmonic analysis of frequencies in pulsatile blood flow, *IRE Trans Med Electronics* 6:291, 1959.
20. Formel PF, Doyle JT: Rationale of venous occlusion plethysmography, *Circ Res* 5:354, 1957.
21. François-Franck CE: Du volume des organes dans ses rapports avec la circulation du sang, *Physiol Exp (Paris)* 2:1, 1876.
22. Glisson F: *Tractatus de ventriculo intestinis* (1622). In Hyman C, Winsor T: History of plethysmography, *J Cardiovasc Surg* 2:506, 1961.
23. Greenfield ADM, Patterson GC: The effect of small degrees of venous distention on the apparent rate of blood inflow to the forearm, *J Physiol (Lond)* 125:525, 1954.
24. Greenfield ADM, Whitney RJ, Mowbray JF: Methods for the investigation of peripheral blood flow, *Br Med Bull* 19:101, 1963.
25. Hallböök T, Göthlin J: Strain-gauge plethysmography and phlebography in diagnosis of deep venous thrombosis, *Acta Chir Scand* 137:37, 1971.
26. Hertzman AB: The blood supply of various skin areas as estimated by photoelectric plethysmography, *Am J Physiol* 124:328, 1938.
27. Hewlett AW, van Zwaluwenburg JG: The rate of blood flow in the arm, *Heart* 1:87, 1909.
28. Hill RV, Jansen JC, Fling JL: Electrical impedance plethysmography: a critical analysis, *J Appl Physiol* 22:161, 1967.
29. Hillestad LK: The peripheral blood flow in intermittent claudication. V. Plethysmographic studies. The significance of the calf blood flow at rest and in response to timed arrest on the circulation, *Acta Med Scand* 174:23, 1963.
30. Hillestad LK: The peripheral blood flow in intermittent claudication. VI. Plethysmographic studies. The blood flow response to exercise with arrested and free circulation, *Acta Med Scand* 174:671, 1963.
31. Hillestad LK: Research on peripheral hemodynamics in various disease states, *Acta Med Scand* 188:191, 1970.

32. Honda N: Temperature compensation for mercury strain-gauge used in plethysmography, *J Appl Physiol* 17:572, 1962.
33. Horeman HW, Noordergraaf A: Numerical evaluation of volume pulsation in man. III. Application to the finger plethysmogram, *Phys Med Biol* 3:345, 1959.
34. Hull R et al: Impedance plethysmography: the relationship between venous filling and sensitivity and specificity for proximal vein thrombosis, *Circulation* 58:898, 1978.
35. Hyman C, Winsor T: History of plethysmography, *J Cardiovasc Surg* 2:506, 1961.
36. Hyman C, Winsor T: An electric volume transducer for plethysmographic recording, *J Appl Physiol* 21:1403, 1966.
37. Ingle FW: Calibration of the photoplethysmograph (PPG), *Proceedings of the Thirty-Fourth Annual Conference on Engineering in Medicine and Biology,* 1981.
38. Kerslake DM: The effect of the application of an arterial occlusion cuff to the wrist on the blood flow in the human forearm, *J Physiol (Lond)* 108:451, 1949.
39. Kinnen E, Hill RV, Jansen JC: A defense of electrical impedance plethysmography, *Med Res Engl* 8:6, 1969.
40. Landowne M, Katz LN: A critique of the plethysmographic method of measuring blood flow in the extremities of man, *Am Heart J* 23:644, 1942.
41. Liebman FM: Electrical impedance pulse tracings from pulsatile blood flow in rigid tubes and volume-restricted vascular beds: theoretical explanations, *Ann NY Acad Sci* 170:437, 1970.
42. Manke DA et al: Hemodynamic studies of digital and extremity replants and revascularization, *Surgery* 88:445, 1980.
43. Mohapatra SN, Arenson HM: The measurement of peripheral blood flow by the electrical impedance technique, *J Med Eng Technol* 3:132, 1979.
44. Noordergraaf A, Horeman HW: Numerical evaluation of volume pulsations in man. II. Calculated volume pulsations of forearm and calf, *Phys Med Biol* 3:59, 1958.
45. Nyboer J: *Electrical impedance plethysmography,* ed 2, Springfield, Ill, 1970, Charles C Thomas, Publisher.
46. O'Donnell JA, Hobson RW II: Comparison of electrical impedance and mechanical plethysmography, *J Surg Res* 25:459, 1978.
47. Parrish D: Appendix to Strandness DE Jr, Bell JW: Peripheral vascular disease: diagnosis and objective evaluation using a mercury strain-gauge, *Ann Surg* 161(suppl):3, 1965.
48. Parrish D, Strandness DE Jr, Bell JW: Dynamic response characteristics of a mercury-in-Silastic strain-gauge, *J Appl Physiol* 10:363, 1964.
49. Parrish D et al: Evidence for the venous origin of plethysmographic information, *J Lab Clin Med* 62:943, 1963.
50. Raines JK: *Diagnosis and analysis of arteriosclerosis in the lower limbs from the arterial pressure pulse,* doctoral dissertation, Massachusetts Institute of Technology, Cambridge, Mass, 1972.
51. Raman ER, Vanhuyse VJ, Jageneau AH: Comparison of plethysmographic and electromagnetic flow measurements, *Phys Med Biol* 18:704, 1973.
52. Ramsey DE, Manke DA, Sumner DS: Toe blood pressure, a valuable adjunct to ankle pressure measurement for assessing peripheral arterial disease, *J Cardiovasc Surg* 24:43, 1983.
53. Schraibman IG et al: Comparison of impedance and strain-gauge plethysmography in the measurement of blood flow in the lower limb, *Br J Surg* 62:909, 1975.
54. Shepherd JT: *Physiology of the circulation in human limbs in health and disease,* Philadelphia, 1963, WB Saunders Co.
55. Shimazu H et al: Evaluation of the parallel conductor theory for measuring human limb blood flow by electrical plethysmography, *IEEE Trans Biomed Eng* 29:1, 1982.
56. Støckel M et al: Standardized photoelectric technique as routine method for selection of amputation level, *Acta Orthop Scand* 53:875, 1982.
57. Strandell T, Wahren J: Circulation in the calf at rest, after arterial occlusion and after exercise in normal subjects and in patients with intermittent claudication, *Acta Med Scand* 173:99, 1963.
58. Strandness DE Jr, Sumner DS: *Hemodynamics for surgeons,* New York, 1975, Grune & Stratton, Inc.
59. Sumner DS: *Rational use of noninvasive tests in designing a therapeutic approach to severe arterial disease of the legs.* In Puel P, Boccalon H, Enjalbert A, ed: *Hemodynamics of the limbs,* ed 2, Toulouse, France, 1981, G.E.P.E.S.C.
60. Sumner DS, Strandness DE Jr: The relationship between calf blood flow and ankle blood pressure in patients with intermittent claudication, *Surgery* 65:763, 1969.
61. Swammerdam J: *Biblia naturae,* vol 3. In Woodcock, JP: *Theory and practice of blood flow measurement,* London, 1975, Butterworth & Co. Publishers, Ltd.
62. Uretzky G, Palti Y: A method for comparing transmitted and reflected light photoelectric plethysmography, *J Appl Physiol* 31:132, 1971.
63. Van den Berg JW, Alberts AJ: Limitations of electric impedance plethysmography, *Circ Res* 11:333, 1954.
64. Van De Water JM, Mount BE: *Impedance plethysmography in the lower extremity.* In Swan KG, ed: *Venous surgery in the lower extremities,* St Louis, 1975, Warren H Green, Inc.
65. Vanhuyse VJ, Raman ER: Interpretation of pressure changes in plethysmography, *Phys Med Biol* 16:111, 1971.
66. Visser KR et al: Observation on blood flow related electrical impedance changes in rigid tubes, *Pflügers Arch* 366:289, 1976.
67. Weltman G, Freedy A, Ukkestad D: A field-theory model of blood-pulse measurement by impedance plethysmography, *Ann Biomed Eng* 1:69, 1972.
68. Wheeler HB et al: Bedside screening for venous thrombosis using occlusive impedance plethysmography, *Angiology* 26:199, 1975.
69. Whitney RJ: The measurement of volume changes in human limbs, *J Physiol (Lond)* 121:1, 1953.
70. Winsor T: The segmental plethysmograph: a description of the instrument, *Angiology* 8:87, 1957.
71. Woodcock JP: *Theory and practice of blood flow measurement,* London, 1975, Butterworth & Co, Publishers, Ltd.
72. Young DG Jr et al: Evaluation of quantitative impedance plethysmography for continuous blood flow measurement. I. Electrode systems, *Am J Phys Med* 46:1261, 1967.
73. Young DG Jr et al: Evaluation of quantitative impedance plethysmography for continuous blood flow measurement. III. Blood flow determination in vivo, *Am J Phys Med* 46:1450, 1967.
74. Zweifler AJ, Cushing G, Conway J: The relationship between pulse volume and blood flow in the fingers, *Angiology* 18:591, 1967.

CHAPTER 21

Impedance plethysmography: theoretic, experimental, and clinical considerations

H. BROWNELL WHEELER, BILL C. PENNEY, and FREDERICK A. ANDERSON, Jr.

This chapter describes the theoretic, experimental, and clinical considerations involved in electric impedance plethysmography (IPG), particularly as used for the extremities. The principles are applicable to use of this technique in other regions of the body as well. Selected clinical applications of IPG are discussed briefly.

BACKGROUND

The first impedance plethysmographic measurements in biologic specimens are generally credited to Cremer in 1907.[19] Noninvasive measurements in humans with the use of skin electrodes were first reported in 1937 by Mann.[62] However, the method received its greatest clinical impetus from several publications by Nyboer, beginning in 1940.[74,76] Nyboer reported several experiments to support his theory that changes in electric impedance were a result of changes in blood volume, electrically in parallel with other tissues in the field. Using this model, he converted impedance measurements to blood volume measurements and even to blood flow measurements. Other researchers[63] subsequently used Nyboer's technique of "impedance plethysmography," as he called the method.

In IPG, skin electrodes are applied to the body region being studied. A weak, high-frequency AC current is passed through the electrodes. The current strength is so weak that it is imperceptible to the subject, and the frequency is so high that it is incapable of stimulating the heart.

Although other electrode configurations have been used, the tetrapolar configuration shown in Fig. 21-1 has become more or less standard.[85] Current is passed between two outer electrodes, and voltage changes across the field are measured through two separate inner electrodes. This electrode configuration eliminates the variable of skin resistance.

An accurate and precise theoretic basis for IPG has been described by Geselowitz[31] and others.[56,57,70] Their formulations were derived from basic electromagnetic field theory. These formulations allow prediction of the impedance change caused by a conductivity change in any known location within a four-electrode impedance field, provided that the lead vectors from current and voltage electrodes are known.

Sensitivity to conductivity changes is proportional to the scalar product* between two voltage-gradient fields. One voltage-gradient field is produced by the current passing between the current electrodes. The other voltage-gradient field is that which would be created if current were passed between the voltage electrodes (Fig. 21-2). With this theory, the sampling field can be predicted for various electrode configurations in any region of the body. These theoretic predictions can then be subjected to laboratory verifications.

THEORETIC AND EXPERIMENTAL STUDIES

Two questions must be answered to understand the nature of the impedance signal: (1) What physiologic changes contribute to segmental conductance changes? (2) What is the sampling field of the instrumentation used?

At rest, impedance changes are primarily caused by respiratory or cardiac activity. Inspiration and expiration change the volume of air in the chest and produce corresponding changes in the electric impedance. Each heartbeat produces changes in blood pressure, blood volume, and blood flow throughout the body. Synchronous changes can be observed in the conductance of almost any body segment. The question arises as to whether the conductance changes are solely a result of changes in blood volume, as proposed by Nyboer, or may also be influenced by changes in pressure, flow, or some other variable of circulatory physiology. Each of these variables has been evaluated with respect to IPG.

Some of the studies mentioned briefly herein were supported in part by grants from the National Science Foundation (GY 11514 and EPP-75-08986), the National Institutes of Health (HL-19038), the St. Vincent Hospital Research Foundation, and the Max C. Fleischmann Foundation.

*The scalar product between two electric fields is defined as the product of the magnitudes of the two fields multiplied by the cosine of the angle between them.

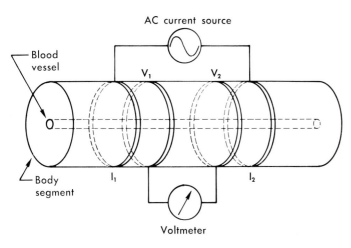

Fig. 21-1. Four-electrode IPG. Weak, high-frequency current passes between I_1 and I_2. Voltage changes are recorded between V_1 and V_2, reflecting blood volume changes in the body segment under study.

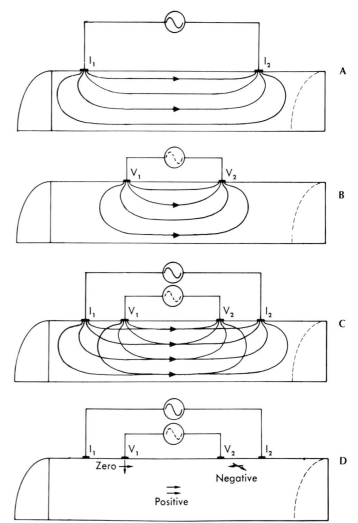

Fig. 21-2. The sampling efficiency of the four-electrode IPG can be predicted from knowledge of two electric fields. **A,** Field produced by current passing between current electrodes. **B,** Field that would be produced by current flow between voltage electrodes. Superimposing these fields, **C,** shows angles of intersection between them. Depending on these angles, **D,** shows that sensitivity will be positive, negative, or null.

Volume changes

The effect of volume changes on the impedance signal has been studied by making simultaneous IPG and volume plethysmographic measurements. Since blood velocity changes also affect the impedance signal, the relationship between blood volume and impedance changes is best studied during slow changes in venous volume.[4] This relationship has been quantified by means of air,[3] water,[114] and strain-gauge plethysmography.[98]

The responses of impedance, air, and mercury strain-gauge plethysmographs to calf volume changes produced by venous occlusion are compared in Fig. 21-3. It is common practice to display a negative impedance change as an upward deflection, which corresponds to an increase in limb volume. During venous filling the curves are essentially identical (mean correlation coefficient of 0.995). The ratio of percent volume change/percent impedance change has been found to equal the ratio of the resistivity of blood/resistivity of tissue.[98] Under most conditions this ratio falls in a narrow range (about 0.75 to 1.0).[1,98] However, a low hematocrit level or excessive tissue fluid will change this ratio.[30,44,104] For example, if the hematocrit level drops to 20% and the tissue resistivity is 165 ohm-cm, this ratio will drop to 0.55 (Fig. 21-4). Conversely, for a hematocrit level of 40% and edematous tissue with a resistivity of 110 ohm-cm, the ratio will be about 1.3. Thus blood volume changes indicated by IPG may be falsely low in markedly edematous limbs and falsely high in severely anemic patients.

Flow changes

The electrical resistance of a tube of blood is known to decrease as the blood starts flowing.[100] This phenomenon is explained by the shape and orientation of the red blood cells.[32,34,47] At the frequencies typically used in IPG (10 to 100 kHz), the red blood cells are essentially nonconducting.

Electric current encounters a higher resistance when it "sees" the full front view of a red blood cell than when it "sees" the smaller side view. Shear forces in flowing blood cause the red blood cells to turn so that their long axis is parallel to the flow. An electric current parallel to the flow will then see only the side view of the red cells. Thus blood flow reduces the electric resistivity in the direction of the flow. This phenomenon has a noticeable effect on the impedance signal whenever stationary blood begins to flow.

Previously stationary blood begins to flow rapidly when venous occlusion is released. This produces a transient difference between the impedance signal and the volume change signal measured with a mechanical plethysmograph[4] (Fig. 21-5). Similarly, rapid changes in arterial blood ve-

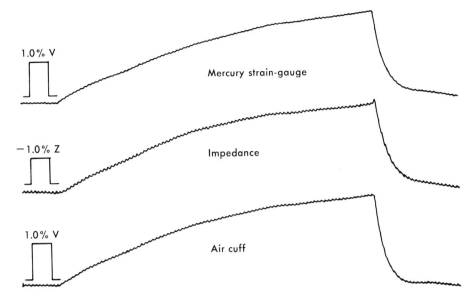

Mercury strain-gauge

1.0% V

−1.0% Z

Impedance

1.0% V

Air cuff

Fig. 21-3. Venous occlusion plethysmography recorded simultaneously by three different plethysmographic techniques.

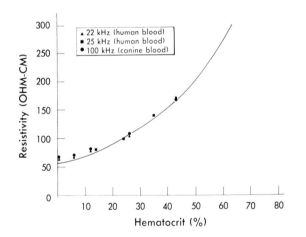

Fig. 21-4. Relationship between hematocrit and resistivity of human blood measured at two different frequencies. Data points for canine blood are similar.[30] Note that resistivity rises with hematocrit.

locity occur with each heartbeat. Differences between the pulsatile impedance and mechanical plethysmographic recordings are again noted (Fig. 21-6).[4] These differences appear when rapid changes in blood flow occur.

An in vitro model was constructed to quantify the effect of blood flow changes on the arterial impedance signal. Blood was pumped in a pulsatile fashion through a bovine carotid artery and a rigid plastic tube, which was assembled in series with a variable peripheral resistance.[83] Changes in pressure and flow in the system were measured with a pressure transducer and an electromagnetic flowmeter. Impedance changes were measured both on the artery, which was expansile, and on the rigid plastic tube, which was nonexpansile. Volume changes in the artery were recorded with

a mercury-in-silicone-elastomer strain-gauge plethysmograph. Volume changes in the rigid tube were assumed to be negligible.

When blood was pumped through the circuit, pulse contours were seen in the impedance and mercury strain-gauge measurements from the artery. A small but definite impedance pulse was also recorded from the rigid plastic tube. This was present despite the fact that a volume change could not occur in the rigid tubing. This signal was only 10% to 15% of the impedance pulse obtained from the artery, but nevertheless, it constituted a discrete signal unrelated to volume change (Fig. 21-7).

When the experiment was repeated with saline solution, pulsations were once again recorded from the artery with both IPG and strain-gauge plethysmography. However, no longer was there a detectable impedance pulse from the rigid tube. The effect previously observed with blood did *not* occur with an electrolyte solution that was free of red blood cells.

IPG is the only plethysmographic method affected by changes in blood velocity. The chief effects encountered in clinical use are (1) a modest augmentation of the arterial pulse waveform and (2) a transient "blip" at the moment the venous occlusion is released. This blood velocity effect can be a slight liability when accurate measurement of blood volume is required. It can be an asset in other situations (e.g., when measuring volume-restricted vascular beds, such as inside the teeth[63] and skull,[59] or when sampling calcified arteries). This effect also provides a larger arterial pulse signal for analysis.

Pressure changes

The relationship between pressure and impedance changes is indirect. Intravascular pressure changes cause

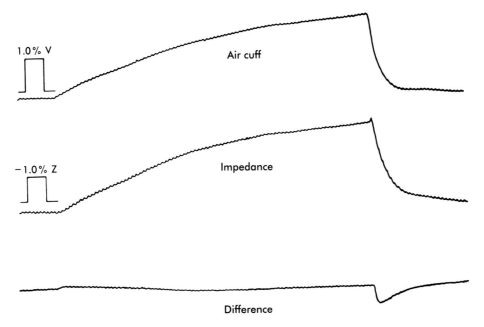

Fig. 21-5. Venous occlusion plethysmography recorded simultaneously by air cuff and impedance techniques. Difference analysis shows a slight delay in the venous outflow portion of impedance tracing.

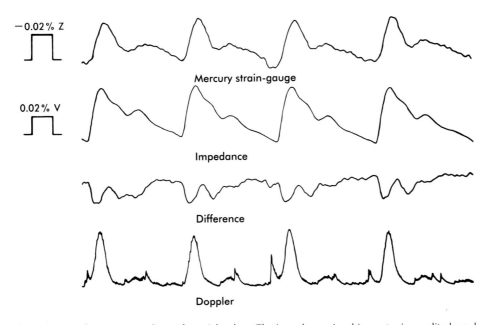

Fig. 21-6. Simultaneous recordings of arterial pulses. The impedance signal is greater in amplitude and breadth than the mercury strain-gauge tracing. Signal differences coincide with flow changes shown by the Doppler flowmeter (see text).

volume changes according to each vessel's compliance curve, and these volume changes are sensed by IPG.

Pressure changes between the skin and the electrodes can upset the polarization bilayer and change the electrode contact impedance. Although this can affect the impedance measured with the four-electrode technique, the errors pro-duced can be kept small (less than 5% of the signal of interest[79]) through proper instrument and electrode design.[32]

Sampling efficiency

Recognizing that conductance changes measured by IPG are primarily caused by blood volume changes (modified by a variable small component resulting from any rapid change in blood flow within the electric field), the next question that arises in interpreting the results of IPG is the extent of the sampling field. For example, in studying the leg the researcher needs to know whether volume changes deep within the leg are measured as efficiently as are those near the surface. The researcher also needs to know whether volume changes close to the electrodes are measured more

or less efficiently than those in the center of the sampling field. Similar questions are applicable to any indirect form of plethysmography. Since IPG has a firm theoretic basis subject to experimental verification, such questions can be answered.

Circumferential electrodes. Quantitative predictions concerning the efficiency of the electric sampling field in the lower leg have been made with theoretic formulations.[80] A uniform cylinder encircled by four narrow electrodes was used as the model for these calculations. An analytic solution for the electric field that would be produced by current flowing through either pair of electrodes was obtained with conventional mathematical methods. This solution was in a form that allowed numerical evaluation of the two voltage-gradient fields. The sensitivity to a conductivity change at any longitudinal or radial position within the electric field was then predicted by evaluating the scalar product between these two voltage-gradient fields.

The following experiment was conducted to test the predictive ability of this theoretic model for various longitudinal and radial positions within the electric field: Liverwurst and bologna were chosen for laboratory studies because they approximate uniform cylinders and their conductivity is similar to that of the leg. Circumferential electrodes were placed on these sausages, which were then encased in plaster to prevent any volume change. Small holes (0.9 cm in diameter) were drilled at specified radial positions. A conductivity change could be produced in a known location within the electric field by filling these holes with normal saline solution. Filling these holes at a constant rate produced a standard conductivity change at a constantly varying position (Fig. 21-8).

The first derivative of the impedance signal during filling provided the sensitivity as a function of time. This was converted to a function of position with the dimensions of the sausage, the placement of the electrodes, and the filling time. This procedure was followed in nine experiments, with holes in four radial positions. The results were then com-

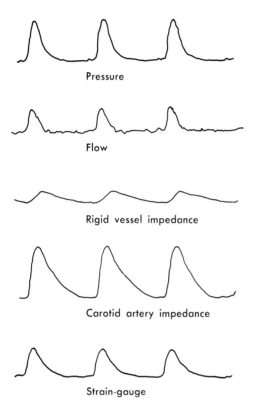

Fig. 21-7. Simultaneous tracings in the laboratory model of circulatory system designed to separate effects of volume, pressure, and flow on impedance tracing (see text).

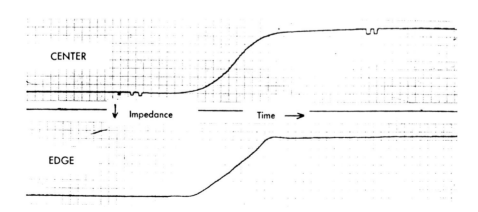

Fig. 21-8. Impedance recordings made while holes in sausages were filled at a constant rate (see text). Sampling efficiency at the center of the field is similar to but less sharp than at the edge.

pared with the theoretic predictions for sampling efficiency as a function of longitudinal position. Typical comparisons are given in Figs. 21-9 and 21-10. Experimental results conformed closely to theoretic predictions (average root-mean-square [RMS] error was 8%).

To determine whether superficial vessels are sampled more efficiently than deep vessels, that is, to determine radial sampling efficiency, researchers conducted an analogous experiment. Two pairs of electrodes were placed on each of three sausages, with separations proportional to 10 cm (the voltage field) and 18 cm (the current field) on a 37-cm circumference calf—typical electrode placement for impedance phlebography. The sausages were encased in plaster, and holes were bored at four radial positions in each. Filling each of these holes individually with saline solution and measuring the resultant impedance change allowed an experimental definition of the sensitivity-to-conductivity changes in longitudinal vessels as a function of their radial position. For this particular electrode geometry, the deep

vessels are apparently sampled with at least 80% of the efficiency obtained in more superficial vessels. Other experiments showed that if the current electrodes are moved closer to the voltage electrodes, the sampling efficiency for deep vessels is lower. As the current electrodes are moved farther away, the sampling efficiency for deep vessels increases until it approaches 100% (Fig. 21-11).

A researcher might question whether a uniform cylinder model can yield much insight about what is being measured in the human calf, which is a nonuniform mixture of bone, fat, muscle, and other tissues. To answer this question, normal saline solution has been injected into the calves of cadavers while impedance recordings were being made. Circumferential current and voltage electrodes separated by one half and one third of the maximum calf circumference, respectively, were used to make these recordings. Saline solution injections (2 ml) were made at two depths, just below the skin and deep in the muscle mass, and at seven to nine longitudinal positions. The impedance changes noted

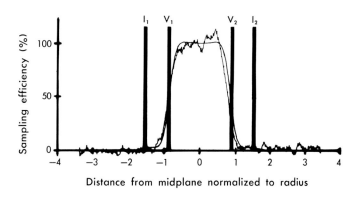

Fig. 21-9. Laboratory studies illustrating the longitudinal sampling efficiency for superficial conductivity changes. The *solid line* represents the theoretic prediction.

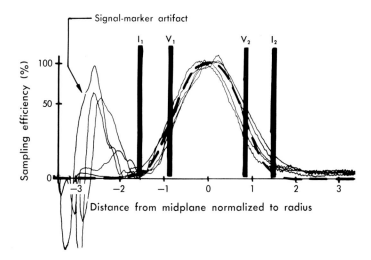

Fig. 21-10. Laboratory studies illustrating the longitudinal sampling efficiency for deep conductivity changes. The *heavy dashed line* represents the theoretic prediction.

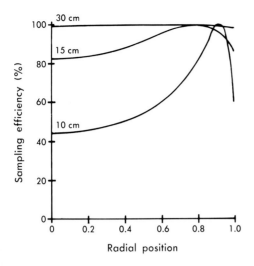

Fig. 21-11. Sampling efficiency as a function of radial position. (0 = center, 1.0 = edge; with V_1 and V_2 separated by 8 cm and I_1 and I_2 separated by 10, 15, and 30 cm.)

in each of the 20 legs were fitted to the theoretic predictions with a least-squares criterion.[5] The theoretic predictions and the experimental results display the same characteristics (Fig. 21-12).

From these and other studies, IPG measurements of the calf have been shown to represent a well-defined region that extends only slightly beyond the voltage electrodes. For the electrode configuration typically used in impedance phlebography, this region extends only about 2 cm outside the voltage electrodes (about 0.3 times the radius of the leg) (Fig. 21-13). For this same electrode configuration the sampling efficiency for deep vessels is nearly the same as that for superficial vessels. Thus in its ability to reflect deep volume changes as sensitively as superficial changes and in its ability to sample a distinctly defined region, IPG possesses the attributes of an ideal plethysmographic technique. Similar mathematical models and laboratory testing have been applied to IPG in other regions of the body.

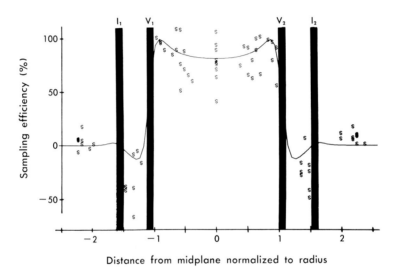

Fig. 21-12. Sampling efficiency for superficial saline injections in the lower leg of cadavers. The *solid line* represents theoretic prediction.

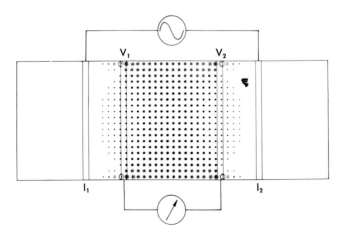

Fig. 21-13. Computer plot of sampling efficiency in four-electrode configuration simulating that used in IPG for diagnosis of deep vein thrombosis.

Spot electrodes

For some clinical applications, circumferential electrodes are less suitable than spot electrodes, such as those routinely used for electrocardiography. The field sampled by any given array of spot electrodes can be predicted from the considerations previously described. Electrode arrays can be designed for specific uses, such as sampling superficial blood vessels.

The sampling fields associated with spot electrodes on the surface of a uniform block[2,79,84,97] or cylinder[112] have been studied. Electrode size and spacing affect how quickly the sampling sensitivity attenuates with depth and position lateral to the electrodes. Two regions of negative sensitivity, each roughly hemispheric and located between a current electrode and the voltage electrode with the same polarity, have a profound influence on the size (and polarity) of the signal from a superficial vessel. By tilting the axis of the electrode array relative to the direction of the vessel, the examiner can avoid having the vessel pass through these regions of negative sensitivity. With such precautions, superficial vessels can be reliably sampled.

Imaging with IPG

Since the electric conductivity of many tissues differs, there is the theoretic possibility of forming tomographic images with IPG. This is appealing, since there would be no hazard from ionizing radiation and the image contrast could be higher than with some other imaging methods. Applications could include detecting pulmonary edema[40] and breast cancer[46] or planning and monitoring hyperthermia treatment.[69]

Initial studies have had limited success.[9,108] These studies indicate that a method must be developed to confine the electric current to a narrow path.[87] It has also been noted that the calculations involved are more difficult than in computerized tomography (CT), since they require iterative solutions.[86] Despite these problems, interest continues in this area.[72,105,115]

CLINICAL USES
Cardiac evaluation*

Thoracic IPG measurements for cardiac output determination were popularized in 1966 by Kubicek et al.[53] Since then many studies have evaluated its use. Some studies have shown good correlations,[24,29,88] whereas others show variability between subjects[7,15,39,94] and dependence on the peripheral resistance and contractile state of the heart.† Several studies conclude that it is best used for tracking relative changes in stroke volume in the same individual.[11,25,50,67]

Measurements of the cardiac synchronous change in thoracic IPG have been studied for several diagnostic purposes.[41,54,89,102] They have been used to quantify aortic or mitral valve regurgitation.[93] A number of researchers have evaluated impedance recordings made during exercise,* particularly for the determination of systolic time intervals.[33,96]

Changes in the baseline component of the thoracic IPG have been used to detect changes in thoracic fluid volume as a result of changes in pulmonary wedge pressure,[37] fluid overload,[10] and cardiac insufficiency precipitated by exercise.[8] They have also been used to give an early indication of water intoxication during transurethral resection of the prostate.[16]

Pulmonary monitoring

Thoracic IPG measurements have also been used to monitor regional lung perfusion,[17,111] fluid volume,† and ventilation.[35,38,42,52] However, the rationale used to guide electrode placement has rarely been discussed. Recently, theoretic models that allow calculation of the electric fields produced in the thorax have been developed.[51,115] These models, combined with the theoretic considerations outlined earlier, could aid the design of electrode arrays to sample selected regions of the lungs.

Neonatal monitoring

Thoracic IPG measurements taken on neonates have been used to detect apnea,[73,78,109] to detect and guide treatment of patent ductus arteriosus,[18] and to obtain indices of cardiovascular status.[27] Cephalic IPG measurements have been used to detect hydrocephalus[90] and intraventricular hemorrhage.[99] Again, there is a need for further theoretic study to guide electrode placement and interpretation of results.[61,71]

Cerebrovascular evaluation

In adults, cerebral IPG measurements have been used to detect cerebral atherosclerosis,[36,45] to obtain an index of cerebral blood flow,[43] and to detect certain psychologic disorders that may be associated with altered cerebral circulation.[22] Such measurements have not been used widely, perhaps because there are problems in interpretation of the signal.[60,64] Individual differences in the high-resistivity skull and low-resistivity scalp cause uncertainty in the proportion of the signal of intracranial origin. Although the contribution of the scalp can be made fairly small through proper electrode placement,[110] the contribution of the skull's circulation remains unknown. At present, these factors make cephalic IPG measurements unsuitable for selectively detecting occlusive disease of the arteries that feed the brain.

Peripheral arterial evaluation

IPG has been used as a convenient method of obtaining waveforms from peripheral arteries.‡ These waveforms

---

*A detailed description of the many proposed clinical applications of IPG is beyond the scope of this publication. The interested reader is referred to more comprehensive publications.[60,63,74]
†References 26, 58, 91, 95, 113.

*References 21, 28, 66, 68, 103.
†References 40, 48, 49, 65, 101.
‡References 14, 20, 55, 75, 82, 106.

have been used to detect reduced arterial compliance that results from atherosclerosis[6,44] and to study the effectivness of drug therapy.[12,13] Combined with venous occlusion during reactive hyperemia, IPG measurements have been used to estimate the severity of proximal arterial obstructions.[77]

Similar measurements can also be made with air, water, or strain-gauge plethysmographs,[23] but these mechanical plethysmographs typically have to encircle the body segment that contains the vessels to be sampled. IPG and photoplethysmography can make focal observations without encircling the region. This localized sampling ability may be of particular use in the groin, neck, and trunk.

Detection of venous thrombosis

The most widespread use of IPG has been for the detection of deep vein thrombosis. (This technique is described in more detail in Chapter 98.)

CONCLUSION

Although IPG has been actively studied since the 1930s, a firm theoretic and experimental basis has been developed only recently. It is now possible to predict the sampling efficiency for various electrode arrays in any portion of the body. This has already been accomplished with respect to the lower leg. Methods have been developed to design electrode arrays to sample a specific body region while minimizing the signal from adjacent areas.

In the past, IPG has been used primarily because of its convenience and sensitivity. The ability to make plethysmographic observations merely by applying electrodes to the skin is appealing to both the patient and the physician. The method is safe and simple. The signal is clean and free of artifacts. It can be calibrated easily, and accurate quantitation of conductance change can be ensured.

However, other types of plethysmography have also been simplified and improved. The future of IPG may relate not so much to the desirable characteristics already described, some of which are now shared by other methods of plethysmography, but rather to certain features unique to the impedance technique. These features include the ability to sample a wide variety of anatomic regions, including deep-seated organs and tissues, and to reflect changes in the blood flow as well as in blood volume. These features are not shared by conventional volume displacement plethysmographs.

The potential clinical usefulness for a noninvasive technique that can sample visceral hemodynamics has yet to be determined. Enough promising experiments have been reported to generate interest in using IPG to study the brain, heart, lungs, and kidneys, but these applications have not yet been used widely in clinical practice. It seems likely that further research, based on the established theoretic principles outlined herein, will expand the clinical usefulness of IPG considerably in years to come.

ACKNOWLEDGMENT

The authors are particularly indebted to Professor Robert Peura for his contributions to this study. We are also grateful to the biomedical engineering students from Worcester Polytechnic Institute who have participated in studying the experimental and theoretic bases of impedance plethysmography. Their interest and enthusiasm have been constantly stimulating, and their work in the laboratory has been of great technical assistance. We are particularly grateful to Craig Sherman, Steven Pareka, John Mortarelli, and John Arcuri for their participation in some of the laboratory experiments and to Dr. Nilima Patwardhan for her invaluable assistance with the cadaver studies.

REFERENCES

1. Anderson FA Jr: Impedance plethysmography in the diagnosis of arterial and venous disease, *Ann Biomed Eng* 12:79, 1984.
2. Anderson FA Jr, Penney BC, Wheeler HB: Regional impedance plethysmography: an experimental method for study of specific blood vessels. *Proceedings of the Fourteenth Annual Meeting of the Association for the Advancement of Medical Instrumentation,* Arlington, Va, 1979.
3. Anderson FA et al: Evaluation of electrical impedance plethysmography for venous volume measurements. *Proceedings of the Twenty-ninth Annual Conference on Engineering in Medicine and Biology,* vol 18, Chevy Chase, Md, 1976, The Alliance for Engineering in Medicine and Biology.
4. Anderson FA et al: Comparison of electrical impedance and mechanical plethysmographic techniques in the human calf. *Proceedings of the Twelfth Annual Meeting of the Association for the Advancement of Medical Instrumentation,* Arlington, Va, 1977.
5. Anderson FA Jr et al: Impedance plethysmography: the origin of electrical impedance changes measured in the human calf, *Med Biol Eng Comput* 18:234, 1980.
6. Arenson JS, Cobbold RSC, Johnston KW: Dual-channel self-balancing impedance plethysmograph for vascular studies, *Med Biol Eng Comput* 19:157, 1981.
7. Bache RJ, Harley A, Greenfield JC Jr: Evaluation of thoracic impedance plethysmography as an indicator of stroke volume in man, *Am J Med Sci* 258:100, 1969.
8. Balasubramanian V, Hoon RS: Changes in transthoracic electrical impedance during submaximal treadmill exercise in patients with ischemic heart disease—a preliminary report, *Am Heart J* 91(1):43, 1976.
9. Bates RHT, McKinnon GC, Seagar AD: A limitation on systems for imaging electrical conductivity distributions, *IEEE Trans Biomed Eng* 27:418, 1980.
10. Berman IR et al: Transthoracic electrical impedance as a guide to intravascular overload, *Arch Surg* 102:61, 1971.
11. Boer P et al: Measurement of cardiac output by impedance cardiography under various conditions, *Am J Physiol* 237:491, 1979.
12. Brevetti G et al: Protective effects of propranolol on the exercise-induced reduction of blood flow in arteriopathic patients, *Angiology* 30:696, 1979.
13. Brevetti G et al: Propranolol-induced reverse vascular steal in arteriopathic patients, *Angiology* 33:78, 1982.
14. Brown BH et al: Impedance plethysmography: can it measure changes in limb blood flow? *Med Biol Eng* 13:674, 1975.
15. Casthély P, Ramanathan S, Chalon J: Considerations on impedance cardiography, *Can Anaesth Soc J* 27:481, 1980.
16. Casthély P et al: Decreases in electric thoracic impedance during transurethral resection of the prostate: an index of early water intoxication, *J Urol* 125:347, 1981.
17. Cathignol D et al: Interface for pulmonary exploration real-time treatment of curves obtained by transthoracic impedance, *Med Biol Eng Comput* 16:459, 1978.
18. Cotton RB et al: Impedance cardiographic assessment of symptomatic patent ductus arteriosus, *J Pediatr* 96:711, 1980.

19. Cremer H: Ueber die Registrierung mechanischer Vorgänge auf electrischem Wege, speziell mit Hilfe des Saitengalvonometers und Saitenelektrometers, *Münch Med Wochenschr* 54:1629, 1907.

20. Derblom H, Johnson L, Nylander G: Electrical impedance plethysmography as a method of evaluating the peripheral circulation. I. Analysis of method, *Acta Chir Scand* 136:579, 1970.

21. Denniston C et al: Measurement of cardiac output by electrical impedance at rest and during exercise, *J Appl Physiol* 40:91, 1976.

22. Dixon LM, Lovett Doust JW: The diagnostic potential of rheoencephalography in psychiatry, *Psychiatr Clin* 11:219, 1978.

23. Doko S et al: Noninvasive evaluation of arterial occlusive disease, *Jpn Circ J* 47:778, 1983.

24. Edmunds AT, Godfrey S, Tooley M: Cardiac output measured by transthoracic impedance cardiography at rest, during exercise and at various lung volumes, *Clin Sci* 63:107, 1982.

25. Ehlert RE, Schmidt HD: An experimental evaluation of impedance cardiographic and electromagnetic measurements of stroke volumes, *J Med Eng Technol* 6:193, 1982.

26. Enghoff E, Lövheim O: A comparison between the transthoracic electrical impedance method and the direct Fick and the dye dilution methods for cardiac output measurements in man, *Scand J Clin Lab Invest* 39:585, 1979.

27. Freyschuss U, Noack G, Zetterström R: Serial measurements of thoracic impedance and cardiac output in healthy neonates after normal delivery and Caesarean section, *Acta Paediatr Scand* 68:357, 1979.

28. Fujinami T et al: Impedance cardiography for the assessment of cardiac function during exercise, *Jpn Circ J* 43:215, 1979.

29. Gabriel S et al: Measurement of cardiac output by impedance cardiography in patients with myocardial infarction: comparative evaluation of impedence and dye dilution methods: *Scand J Clin Lab Invest* 36:29, 1976.

30. Geddes LA, DaCosta CP: The specific resistance of canine blood at body temperature, *IEEE Trans Biomed Eng* 20:51, 1973.

31. Geselowitz DB: An application of electrocardiographic lead theory to impedance plethysmography, *IEEE Trans Biomed Eng* 18:38, 1971.

32. Gessert WL et al: Bioimpedance instrumentation, *Ann NY Acad Sci* 170:520, 1970.

33. Gollan F, Kizakevich PN, McDermott J: Continuous electrode monitoring of systolic time intervals during exercise, *Br Heart J* 40:1390, 1978.

34. Gollan F, Namon R: Electrical impedance of pulsatile blood flow in rigid tubes and in isolated organs, *Ann NY Acad Sci* 170:568, 1970.

35. Grenvik A et al: Impedance pneumography—comparison between chest impedance changes and respiratory volumes in 11 healthy volunteers, *Chest* 62:439, 1973.

36. Hadjiev D: Impedance methods for investigation of cerebral circulation, *Prog Brain Res* 35:25, 1972.

37. Haffty BG, Singh JB, Peural RA: A clinical evaluation of thoracic electrical impedance, *J Clin Eng* 2:107, 1977.

38. Hamilton LH, Rieke RJ: Ventilation monitor based on transthoracic impedance changes, *Med Res Eng* 11:20, 1972.

39. Harley A, Greenfield JC: Determination of cardiac output in man by means of impedance plethysmography, *Aerospace Med* 39:248, 1968.

40. Henderson RP, Webster JG: An impedance camera for spatially specific measurements of the thorax, *IEEE Trans Biomed Eng* 25:250, 1978.

41. Hill DW, Lowe HJ: The use of the electrical impedance technique for monitoring of cardiac output and limb blood flow during anesthesia, *Med Biol Eng* 11:534, 1973.

42. Itoh A et al: Non-invasive ventilatory volume monitor, *Med Biol Eng Comput* 20:613, 1982.

43. Jacquy J et al: Cerebral blood flow and quantitative rheoencephalography, *Electroencephalogr Clin Neurophysiol* 37:507, 1974.

44. Jaffrin MY, Vanhoutte C: Quantitative interpretation of arterial impedance plethysmographic signals, *Med Biol Eng Comput* 17:2, 1979.

45. Jenkner FL: Rheoencephalographic differentiation of vascular headaches of varying causes, *Ann NY Acad Sci* 170:661, 1970.

46. Jossinet J, Fourcade C, Schmitt M: A study for breast imaging with a circular array of impedance electrodes. *Proceedings of the Fifth International Conference on Electrical Bio-impedance,* Tokyo, 1981.

47. Kanai H, Sakamoto K, Miki M: Impedance of blood; the effects of red cell orientation, *Dig Int Conf Med Biol Eng,* vol 11, Ottawa, Ontario, Canada, 1976, National Research Council.

48. Keller G, Blumberg A: Monitoring of pulmonary fluid volume and stroke volume by impedance cardiography in patients on hemodialysis, *Chest* 72(1):56, 1977.

49. Khan MR et al: Quantitative electrical-impedance plethysmography for pulmonary oedema, *Med Biol Eng Comput* 15:627, 1977.

50. Khatib MT et al: The thoracic-impedance and thermal dilution methods of measuring cardiac output—a comparison in the dog, *Br J Anaesth* 47:1026, 1975.

51. Kim Y, Tompkins WJ, Webster JG: *A three-dimensional modifiable body model for biomedical applications.* In Cohen BA, *Frontiers of engineering in health care,* New York, 1981, IEEE Publishing.

52. Kira S et al: Transthoracic electrical impedance variations associated with respiration, *J Appl Physiol* 30:820, 1971.

53. Kubicek WG et al: Development and evaluation of an impedance cardiac output system, *Aerospace Med* 37:1208, 1966.

54. Kwoczyński J, Palko T: A trial of non-invasive diagnosis of muscular subaortic stenosis by the impedance method, *Mater Med Pol* 11:242, 1979.

55. Lee BY et al: Noninvasive hemodynamic evaluation in selection of amputation level, *Surg Gynecol Obstet* 149:241, 1979.

56. Lehr J: A vector derivation useful in impedance plethysmographic field calculations, *IEEE Trans Biomed Eng* 19:156, 1972.

57. Lehr JL: *Physiological impedance measurements—a theoretical and experimental treatment of guarded electrode and other techniques,* doctoral dissertation, Pittsburgh, 1972, Carnegie-Mellon University.

58. Lewis GK, Peura RA, Singh JB: The quantitative effect of the heart on transthoracic impedance measurement. *Proceedings of the 27th Conference on Engineering in Medicine and Biology,* vol 16, Chevy Chase, Md, 1974, The Alliance for Engineering in Medicine and Biology.

59. Lifshitz K: Rheoencephalography. I. Review of the technique, *J Nerv Ment Dis* 138:388, 1963.

60. Lifshitz K: Rheoencephalography. II. Survey of clinical applications, *J Nerv Ment Dis* 137:285, 1963.

61. Lifshitz K: Electrical impedance cephalography, electrode guarding, and analog studies, *Ann NY Acad Sci* 170:532, 1970.

62. Mann H: Study of peripheral circulation by means of an alternating current bridge, *Proc Soc Exp Biol Med* 36:670, 1937.

63. Markovich SE, ed: *International conference on bioelectrical impedance,* New York, 1970, The New York Academy of Sciences.

64. Masucci EI, Seipel JH, Kurtzke JF: Clinical evaluation of "quantitative" rheoencephalography, *Neurology (Minneap)* 20:642, 1970.

65. Meijer JH, et al: Differential impedance plethysmography for measuring thoracic impedances, *Med Biol Eng Comput* 20:187, 1982.

66. Miles DS, et al: Estimation of cardiac output by electrical impedance during arm exercise in women, *J Appl Physiol* 51:1488, 1981.

67. Miller JC, Horvath SM: Impedance cardiography, *Psychophysiology* 15(1):80, 1978.

68. Miyamoto Y, et al: Continuous determination of cardiac output during exercise by the use of impedance plethysmography, *Med Biol Eng Comput* 19:638, 1981.

69. Mochizuki A, Takada H, Saito M: Impedance computed tomography and the design of hyperthermia. *Proceedings of the Fifth International Conference on Electrical Bio-impedance,* Tokyo, 1981.

70. Mortarelli JR: A generalization of the Geselowitz relationship useful in impedance plethysmographic field calculations, *IEEE Trans Biomed Eng* 27:665, 1980.

71. Murray PW: Field calculations in the head of a newborn infant and their application to the interpretation of transcephalic impedance measurements, *Med Biol Eng Comput* 19:538, 1981.

72. Nakayama K, Yagi W, Yagi S: Fundamental study on electric impedance CT algorithm utilizing sensitivity theorem on impedance plethysmography. *Proceedings of the Fifth International Conference on Electrical Bio-impedance,* Tokyo, 1981.

73. North JB, Jennett S: Impedance pneumography for the detection of abnormal breathing patterns associated with brain damage, *Lancet* 2:213, 1972.

74. Nyboer J: *Electrical impedance plethysmography,* ed 2, Springfield, Ill, 1970, Charles C Thomas.

75. Nyboer J, Kreider MM, Hannapel L: Electrical impedance plethysmography, a physical and physiologic approach to the peripheral vascular study, *Circulation* 2:811, 1950.

76. Nyboer J et al: Radiocardiograms: electrical impedance changes of the heart in relation to electrocardiograms and heart sounds, *J Clin Invest* 19:963, 1940.

77. O'Donnell JA et al: Impedance plethysmography—noninvasive diagnosis of deep venous thrombosis and arterial insufficiency, *Am Surg* 49:26, 1983.

78. Pallett JE, Scopes JW: Recording respirations in newborn babies by measuring impedance of the chest, *Med Electron Biol Engin* 3:161, 1965.

79. Penney BC: *Development of a two channel impedance plethysmography, signal analysis techniques, and electrode arrays: with application to carotid stenosis detection,* doctoral dissertation. Worcester, Mass, 1979, Worcester Polytechnic Institute.

80. Penney BC et al: The impedance plethysmographic sampling field in the human calf, *IEEE Trans Biomed Eng* 26(4):193, 1979.

81. Penney BC: Theory and cardiac applications of electrical impedance measurements, *CRC Crit Rev Biomed Eng* 13(3):227-281, 1991.

82. Persson AV: Clinical application of electrical impedance for the study of arterial insufficiency, *Med Instrum* 13:95, 1979.

83. Peura RA et al: Influence of erythrocyte velocity on impedance plethysmographic measurements, *Med Biol Eng Comput* 16:147, 1978.

84. Peura RA et al: Regional impedance plethysmography: experimental and computer model studies for measuring single blood vessels. *Proceedings of the Fifth International Conference on Electrical Bio-impedance,* Tokyo, 1981.

85. Plonsey R, Collin R: Electrode guarding in electrical impedance measurements of physiological systems—a critique, *Med Biol Eng Comput* 15:519, 1977.

86. Price LR: Electrical impedance computed tomography (ICT): a new imaging technique, *IEEE Trans Nucl Sci* 26:2736, 1979.

87. Price LR: Imaging of the electrical conductivity and permittivity inside a patient: a new computed tomography (CT) technique, *J Soc Photo* 206:115, 1979.

88. Quail AW, Traugott FM: Effects of changing haematocrit, ventricular rate and myocardial inotropy on the accuracy of impedance cardiography, *Clin Exp Pharmacol Physiol* 8:335, 1981.

89. Rasmussen JP, Sorensen B, Kann T: Evaluation of impedance cardiography as a noninvasive means of measuring systolic time intervals and cardiac output, *Acta Anaesthesiol Scand* 19:210, 1975.

90. Reigel DH et al: Transcephalic impedance measurements during infancy, *Dev Med Child Neurol* 19:295, 1977.

91. Rubal BJ, Baker LE, Poder TC: Correlation between maximum dZ/dt and parameters of left ventricular performance, *Med Biol Eng Comput* 18:541, 1980.

92. Schieken RM et al: Effect of aortic valvular regurgitation upon the impedance cardiogram, *Br Heart J* 40:958, 1978.

93. Schieken RM et al: Effect of mitral valvular regurgitation on transthoracic impedance cardiogram, *Br Heart J* 45:166, 1981.

94. Secher NJ, Thomsen A, Arnsbo P: Measurement of rapid changes in cardiac stroke volume. An evaluation of the impedance cardiography method, *Acta Anaesthesiol Scand* 21(5):353, 1977.

95. Secher NJ et al: Measurements of cardiac stroke volume in various body positions in pregnancy and during caesarian section: a comparison between thermodilution and impedance cardiography, *Scand J Clin Lab Invest* 39:569, 1979.

96. Sheps DS et al: Continuous noninvasive monitoring of left ventricular function during exercise by thoracic impedance cardiography—automated derivation of systolic time intervals, *Am Heart J* 103:519, 1982.

97. Sherman CW et al: Impedance plethysmography: the measuring field associated with an array of small electrodes. *Proceedings of the 13th Annual Meeting of the Association for the Advancement of Medical Instrumentation,* Arlington, Va, 1979.

98. Shimazu H et al: Evaluation of the parallel conductor theory for measuring human limb blood flow by electrical admittance plethysmography, *IEEE Trans Biomed Eng* 29:1, 1982.

99. Siddiqi SF et al: Detection of neonatal intraventricular hemorrhage using transcephalic impedance, *Dev Med Child Neurol* 22:440, 1980.

100. Sigman E, Kolin A, Katz LN: Effects of motion on electrical conductivity of blood, *Am J Physiol* 118:708, 1937.

101. Smith RM, Gray BA: Canine thoracic electrical impedance with changes in pulmonary gas and blood volumes, *J Appl Physiol* 53:1608, 1982.

102. Sramek BB: Noninvasive technique for measurement of cardiac output by means of electrical impedance. *Proceedings of the Fifth International Conference on Electrical Bio-impedance,* Tokyo, 1981.

103. Takada K et al: Reliability and usefulness of impedance cardiography to measure cardiac response during exercise. *Proceedings of the Fifth International Conference on Electrical Bio-impedance,* Tokyo, 1981.

104. Trautman ED, Newbower RS: A practical analysis of the electrical conductivity of blood, *IEEE Trans Biomed Eng* 30:141, 1983.

105. Uchikawa Y, Fujimaki M, Kotani M: Analysis of the distribution of electric potentials on the body surface using electric impedance method. *Proceedings of the Fifth International Conference on Electrical Bio-impedance,* Tokyo, 1981.

106. Van de Water JM, Laska ED, Ciniero WV: Patient and operation selectivity—the peripheral vascular laboratory, *Ann Surg* 189:143, 1979.

107. Van de Water JM et al: Monitoring the chest with impedance, *Chest* 64:597, 1973.

108. Vannier MW: Imaging instruments by CT based on electrical impedance, *J Nucl Med* 22:95, 1981.

109. Walker CHM: Impedance respiratory monitoring in the newborn infant, *Biomed Eng* 3:454, 1968.

110. Weindling AM, Murdoch N, Rolfe P: Effect of electrode size on the contributions of intracranial and extracranial blood flow to the cerebral electrical impedance plethysmogram, *Med Biol Eng Comput* 20:545, 1982.

111. Weng TR et al: Measurement of regional lung function by tetrapolar electrical impedance plethysmography, *Chest* 76:64, 1979.

112. Yamada N, Sakamoto K, Kanai H: On the sensitivity of impedance plethysmography. *Proceedings of the Fifth International Conference on Electrical Bio-impedance,* Tokyo, 1981.

113. Yamakoshi K, Togawa T, Ito H: Evaluation of the theory of cardiac-output computation from transthoracic impedance plethsymogram, *Med Biol Eng Comput* 15(5):479, 1977.

114. Yamakoshi KI et al: Admittance plethysmography for accurate measurement of human limb blood flow, *Am J Physiol* 235(6):H821, 1978.

115. Yamashita Y, Takahashi T: Method and feasibility of estimating impedance distribution in the human torso. *Proceedings of the Fifth International Conference on Electrical Bio-impedance,* Tokyo, 1981.

CHAPTER 22

Mercury strain-gauge plethysmography

DAVID S. SUMNER

Although plethysmography was among the earliest methods devised for measuring blood flow, it remains one of the most useful and accurate. Much of the basic knowledge of vascular physiology and pathophysiology has been derived from plethysmographic studies. Several types of plethysmograph are currently in use, including the air, water (volumetry), impedance, photoelectric, and mercury strain-gauge varieties. Each has its advantages, but none is more generally useful than the mercury strain gauge.

In 1953, Whitney[52] first reported the use of the mercury strain gauge to measure volume changes in human limbs. Almost a decade elapsed before the method was applied in the clinical laboratory for the evaluation of peripheral vascular disease. The early reports of Holling et al[17] and Strandness et al[44] established the potential value of the technique. Largely as a result of subsequent work by Strandness and colleagues,[11,36,40,42] the method was adopted by many vascular laboratories throughout the world.

Not only is the mercury strain gauge inexpensive, relatively simple to use, and portable, it is also one of the most versatile and accurate instruments in the vascular armamentarium. Arterial blood flow can be evaluated by the venous occlusion method, pulse volumes and contours can be recorded, and segmental blood pressures can be measured even in severely ischemic extremities. The same parameters of venous disease that lend themselves to evaluation with impedance or air plethysmographs are also easily studied with the mercury strain gauge.

BASIC PRINCIPLES

Plethysmographs measure volume change, a function reflected in the derivation of the term, *plethysmograph,* from the Greek *plethysmos* (to increase) and *graphein* (to write). With the exception of the lungs, transient fluctuations in the volume of all organs of the body are totally attributable to variations in their blood content. Thus the mercury strain gauge, like all plethysmographs used in the vascular laboratory, detects and measures changes in the volume of blood in the part being examined.

Strain gauges are constructed of fine-bore silicone rubber tubes completely filled with a liquid metal conductor (mercury or an indium-gallium alloy). A tube is wrapped around the part being studied with just enough tension to ensure good contact. As the part expands or contracts, the length of the tube is altered by a corresponding amount. Because the resistance of the gauge is determined by its length, variations in the voltage drop across the gauge reflect changes in the circumference of the part to which it is applied. These variations in resistance can be accurately recorded with a variety of bridge circuits (Fig. 22-1).

A straightforward mathematical relationship makes it possible to calculate volume changes from observed changes in circumference. If one assumes that the part is a cylinder with a circular cross section and that the length of the subtended segment remains constant, the volume of the segment is:

$$V = \pi r^2 L_s \tag{1}$$

where V is volume, r is the radius of the segment, and L_s is its length. Since L_s does not change, it may be considered a unit length, and equation 1 becomes:

$$V = \pi r^2 \tag{2}$$

With venous occlusion or with each pulse, the radius of the part increases by Δr, so the new volume becomes:

$$V + \Delta V = \pi(r + \Delta r)^2 = \pi(r^2 + 2r\Delta r + \Delta r^2) \tag{3}$$

The increase in volume (ΔV) can be obtained by subtracting equation 2, the original volume (V), from equation 3, the augmented volume ($V + \Delta V$):

$$\Delta V = 2\pi r\Delta r + \pi r^2 \tag{4}$$

Dividing equation 4 by equation 2 gives the ratio of the volume change (ΔV) to the original volume (V) of the segment:

$$\frac{\Delta V}{V} = 2\frac{\Delta r}{r} + \frac{\Delta r^2}{r^2} \tag{5}$$

The circumference (C) of the part equals $2\pi r$, hence:

$$r = \frac{C}{2\pi} \tag{6}$$

and

$$\Delta r = \frac{\Delta C}{2\pi} \tag{7}$$

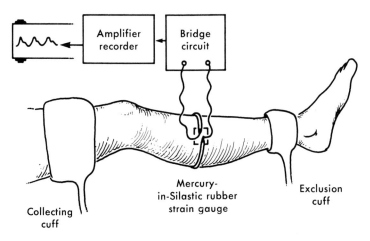

Fig. 22-1. Mercury-in-silicone-elastomer rubber strain gauge.

If equations 6 and 7 are substituted in equation 5, the following relationship between the relative change in volume and the relative change in circumference is obtained:

$$\frac{\Delta V}{V} = 2\frac{\Delta C}{C} + \left(\frac{\Delta C}{C}\right)^2 \qquad (8)$$

Because the volume changes that occur with pulsatile flow or in response to venous occlusion are minute in comparison with the original volume of the part, $(\Delta C/C)^2$ becomes vanishingly small and can usually be neglected. Therefore for all practical purposes, the relative change in the volume of the part is equivalent to twice the relative change in circumference[52]:

$$\frac{\Delta V}{V} \approx 2\frac{\Delta C}{C} \qquad (9)$$

Relative changes in the electrical resistance of the gauge $(\Delta R/R)$ are related to relative changes in gauge length $(\Delta L_g/L_g)$ by:

$$\frac{\Delta R}{R} = 2\frac{\Delta L_g}{L_g} \qquad (10)$$

Because of this, the relative change in gauge resistance equals the relative change in limb volume (see equation 9):

$$\frac{\Delta R}{R} = \frac{\Delta V}{V} \qquad (11)$$

provided that the length of the gauge (L_g) equals the circumference of the limb (C).[16,23,34,38]

This is a very important relationship because it allows for direct electric calibration of the system in terms of volume change of the part around which the gauge is stretched.

There are, however, some potential pitfalls that should be considered. The cross-section of the limbs may not be truly circular. Whitney[52] dealt with this problem and concluded that the relationship in equation 9 still holds for other geometric configurations, provided that the shape remains unaltered on expansion or contraction. When the shape is altered with volume change so that the dimensions of only one of the two orthogonal axes change, errors can be introduced. For example, if the cross-section were elliptic with the short axis being 0.8 the length of the long axis and if expansion occurred only in the long axis, equation 9 would become[52]:

$$\Delta V/V = 1.44 \, \Delta C/C$$

On the other hand, if only the short axis changed, the formula would be:

$$\Delta V/V = 3.27 \, \Delta C/C$$

Although diameter changes that are strictly limited to one axis rarely if ever occur, various parts of the limb may expand unevenly. Knox et al[23] have shown that the skin overlying the muscular compartments of the calf expands more than the skin over the tibia. When the gauge completely encircles the limb without overlap, the unequal expansion does not affect the accuracy of the results. If the gauge were too short and its ends were attached to the skin overlying the muscle, the resistance change ($\Delta R/R$) would be larger than the actual volume change of the subtended calf segment ($\Delta V/V$). If the gauge were attached only to the skin over the tibia, the calculated volume change would be too low.

Although gauges that are too short are seldom used, gauges that are too long are sometimes employed. One commercially available system uses gauges of sufficient length to fit limbs of all sizes. When these gauges are applied to the limb, there is invariably some overlap. If the overlap is placed over a muscular portion of the leg, calculated volume changes will be too large; if the overlap is over the pretibial region, calculated volume changes will be too low. According to Knox,[23] results obtained with the overlap in the two positions are appreciably different, usually varying by more than 30%. In tests used to detect deep vein throm-

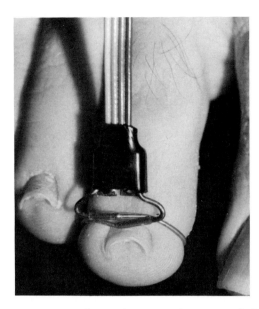

Fig. 22-2. Mercury-in-silicone-elastomer strain gauge applied to second toe. (From Sumner DS: *Digital plethysmography.* In Rutherford RB, ed: *Vascular surgery*, ed 2, Philadelphia, 1984, WB Saunders.)

bosis, in which the rate of calf volume decrease can be normalized against the increase in calf volume produced by a congesting cuff, the errors tend to cancel each other, and absolute accuracy is not required. In most other circumstances, it is desirable to select gauges that completely encircle the limb without overlap (see Chapter 97).[7]

INSTRUMENTATION

Strain gauges are constructed of fine-bore silicone rubber tubing (0.020 × 0.037 inch, 0.15 × 0.040 inch, or 0.012 × 0.025 inch) completely filled with mercury or an indium-gallium alloy. Electric contact is achieved by means of copper electrodes that are inserted a short distance into each end of the tubing. Because calves, forearms, and digits come in all sizes, gauges of differing lengths should be available. Ideally, the gauges are applied to the limb or digit with a minimal degree of stretch—about 10 g. This usually means that limb gauges must be 1 to 3 cm shorter than the circumference of the limb, and digit gauges must be 0.5 cm shorter than the circumference of the finger or toe to which they will be applied.

Digit gauges are usually constructed to form a complete circle to facilitate application to the finger or toe (Fig. 22-2). Limb gauges can be applied as a single strand, in which case the lead wires are not joined, or as a double strand, in which case the lead wires are joined and the mercury-filled silicone rubber tube is looped around the limb and hooked over the terminal (Figs. 22-3 and 22-4). Gauges loosely backed with Velcro are designed to fit multiple limb sizes. Although this arrangement permits easy application, it necessitates a certain amount of overlap, which can be a disadvantage if accurate flow readings are required.

Several matching circuits for plethysmographs are commercially available.* These instruments can be DC-coupled to a recorder to follow both slow and pulsatile volume changes or AC-coupled for pulsatile recordings only. The Hokanson and Imex plethysmographs have the advantage of permitting electric calibration. These circuits make use of the relationship of gauge resistance to limb volume given in equation 11.

Resistance changes are most accurately measured when the gauge is constructed with four lead wires, as described by Sigdell,[38] Hokanson et al,[16] and Michaux[28] (Fig. 22-4). Two lead wires are attached to each end of the mercury-filled silicone rubber tube. Current is fed to the gauge through one set of lead wires, and the voltage drop is sensed by the other set of wires, which is connected directly to the bridge circuit (Fig. 22-5, *A*). Since there is virtually no current through the wires connected to the bridge circuit, the resistance of the lead wires does not affect electric calibration. If electric calibration were attempted with two-wire gauges with the bridge circuit terminals at the ends of the lead wires (Fig. 22-5, *B*), considerable error would be introduced.

To illustrate this problem, one can assume that the resistance of each lead wire is 0.2 ohm and that of an unstretched digital gauge is 0.2 ohm. With the two-wire arrangement the resistances of the lead wires are in series with that of the gauge, giving a baseline value of 0.6 ohm (0.2 + 0.2 + 0.2). If the volume of the limb increased by 1%, the increase in resistance of the gauge would be (equation 11):

$$\Delta R = 0.2(0.01) = 0.002 \text{ ohm}$$

Consequently, the relative increase in resistance of the entire system of gauge and lead wires ($\Delta R/R$) would be:

$$0.002/0.6 = 0.003$$

or only 0.3%. Therefore electric calibration would imply an increase in volume of only 0.3% rather than the 1% increase that actually occurred—an unacceptable error. However, when the bridge circuit leads are at the end of the mercury-filled tube, the relative increase in resistance would be:

$$0.002/0.2 = 0.01$$

or 1%, an accurate value. Obviously, if measurements were made on the calf with a longer gauge having, for example, a resistance of 6 ohms, there would be much less error with the two-wire system. In this case the electric calibration would indicate a 0.9% volume increase.

Electric calibration is performed while the gauge is in situ. This avoids errors resulting from changes in temperature or stretch of the gauge that may accompany mechanical calibration performed after the gauge has been removed

---

*Parks Electronics Laboratory, Beaverton, Ore; D. Eugene Hokanson, Issaquah, Wash; Imex, Golden, Colo.

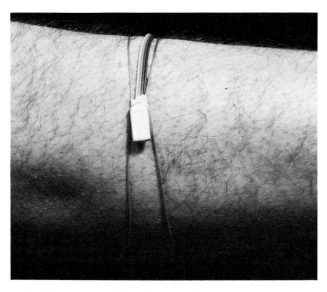

Fig. 22-3. Four-lead limb gauge applied to the calf of the leg. A mercury-filled silicone rubber tube encircles the leg and is held in place by being hooked over the "terminal."

from the limb. Regardless of the baseline stretch on the gauge, once the bridge has been balanced, a panel switch can be used to increase the output of the bridge by the same amount as a 1% increase in gauge resistance.[16] This signal is recorded for comparison with the plethysmographic data. Fig. 22-6 illustrates the 1% calibration signals obtained with the two-wire and four-wire systems and a comparison of them with a standard mechanical stretch.

Mechanical calibration may be carried out in situ by means of a calibrated screw arrangement to which the gauge is attached.[12,52] With devices of this sort, the gauge is stretched a known length, and the calibration is signal recorded. Mechanical calibration in situ has the advantages of avoiding temperature changes (which would affect the resistance of the gauge) and eliminating errors as a result of the deformability of soft tissues.[12] However, the apparatus is bulky and may not conform precisely to the curvature of the limb to which it is applied.

For most studies, it is more convenient to remove the gauge from the limb and attach it to a mechanical stretcher

Fig. 22-4. Underside of "terminal" of a four-lead gauge before it has been coated with silicone-elastomer. (From Hokanson DE, Sumner DS, Strandness ED Jr: *IEEE Trans Biomed Eng* 22[1]:25, 1975.)

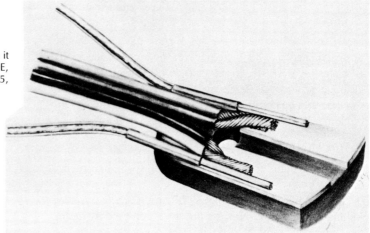

Fig. 22-5. Two ways of connecting the bridge circuit to the mercury strain gauge. *A,* Two lead wires are connected to each end of the gauge. One of the wires at each end of the gauge is connected directly to the bridge circuit. This four-lead arrangement effectively places the strain gauge at the corners of the measurement bridge. *B,* When only two leads are used, lead-wire resistances are incorporated in the bridge circuit, making electric calibration impossible.

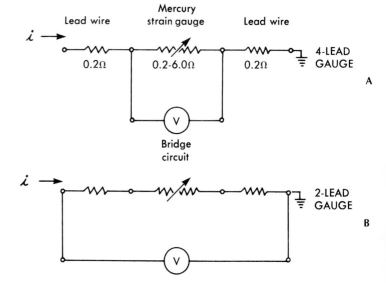

2-LEAD   4-LEAD

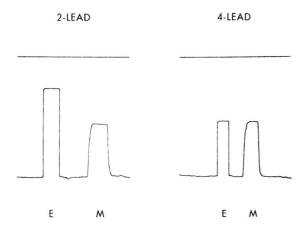

E   M   E   M

Fig. 22-6. Comparison of electric calibration with mechanical calibration using a two-lead and four-lead system. *E,* 1% electric calibration signal; *M,* signal produced by 0.5% mechanical stretch of the gauge (0.5% mechanical stretch is equivalent to 1.0% volume increase). Note that the electric calibration signal with the two-lead system is far too large, leading to significant underestimation of volume change. (From Hokanson DE, Sumner DS, Strandness DE Jr: *IEEE Trans Biomed Eng* 22[1]:25, 1975.)

bar (Fig. 22-7). The gauge is stretched manually by means of a slide arrangement on the bar until the pen of the recorder returns to baseline levels, indicating that the length of the gauge is the same as it was when it was in place on the limb. By means of a micrometer, the operator can then produce an additional known stretch of the gauge. The resulting signal is recorded for calibration purposes.

Because a 10° C change in gauge temperature causes a 1% change in resistance,[9,34] removal of the gauge from a limb where the temperature is 30° C to the surrounding air where the temperature is 20° C will introduce a significant error when absolute limb dimensions are being measured. Methods for temperature compensation have been devised to avoid these errors.[19] However, such methods are not necessary when blood flow or pulse volume is being studied, since the errors introduced by temperature change are negligible under these circumstances.[19]

MEASUREMENT OF BLOOD FLOW

By using the technique of venous occlusion plethysmography, the examiner can measure blood flow in almost any portion of a limb with the mercury strain gauge. The method is particularly applicable to flow studies on cylindric parts such as the calf, forearm, fingers, and toes.

The principle underlying venous occlusion plethysmography is simple. A volume sensor, which may be an air, water, impedance, or strain-gauge plethysmograph, is applied to the segment of the limb in which blood flow is to be measured (Fig. 22-1). A pneumatic cuff is wrapped around the limb just proximal to the volume-sensing device. When this cuff—often called the *collecting cuff*—is rapidly inflated to a pressure well in excess of that in the underlying veins, venous outflow is prevented and blood is temporarily

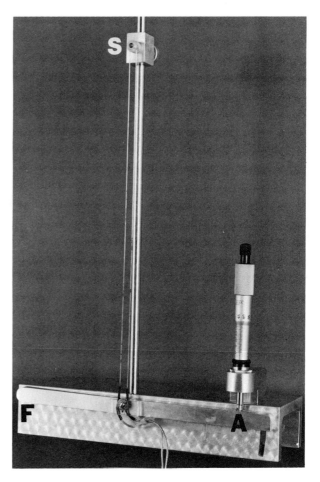

Fig. 22-7. Calibrating device ("stretcher bar") for mercury strain gauges. The ends of the gauge are secured at a point midway between the fulcrum *(F)* and the anvil *(A)*. The gauge is looped around the spindle *(S)*, which is free to slide up and down the vertical steel shaft. By manually adjusting the spindle, the operator can return the gauge to the same length that it had on the limb. The micrometer is then turned to produce the known stretch on the gauge. Because of the position of the gauge halfway between the anvil and fulcrum, the micrometer reading will be exactly twice the stretch on the gauge.

trapped in the distal part of the limb. Because the pressure applied by the cuff is significantly less than arterial blood pressure, arterial inflow continues unimpeded, which causes the volume of the limb distal to the cuff to rise. Therefore the initial rate at which the volume of the limb segment increases is proportional to the rate of arterial inflow (Phase 1, Fig. 22-8). Flow rates are usually expressed in terms of percent volume change per minute or in milliliters per 100 ml of limb volume per minute.

As the volume of blood trapped in the limb increases, venous pressure rises, the arterial-venous pressure gradient falls, the arterial inflow slows down, and the rate of limb expansion decreases (Phase 2, Fig. 22-8). After a variable length of time (depending on the rate of arterial inflow and the venous compliance), the venous pressure rises to the level of the cuff pressure, the veins underlying the cuff reopen, blood again flows out of the leg at a rate equal to

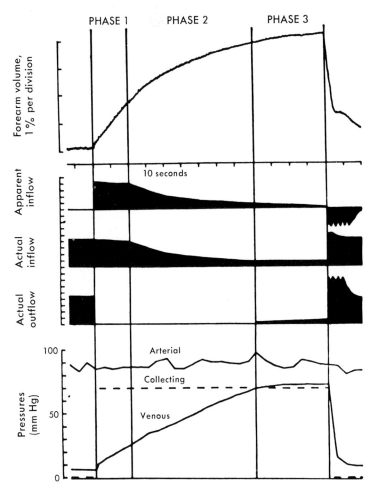

Fig. 22-8. Graph illustrating the effect of venous occlusion on forearm volume, arterial inflow, and venous outflow. Simultaneous changes in the arterial and venous pressure are also shown. The actual inflow is equivalent to the actual outflow plus the apparent inflow. The duration of occlusion was 130 seconds. (From Greenfield ADM, Patterson GC: *J Physiol [Lond]* 125:525, 1954.)

the rate of arterial inflow, and the volume of the limb becomes relatively stable (Phase 3, Fig. 22-8). When the cuff is suddenly deflated, blood rushes out of the limb, propelled by the increased pressure differential between the veins distal and proximal to the cuff; the volume of the limb rapidly returns to baseline levels. (The relevance of these volume changes to the diagnosis of venous disease is discussed in Chapter 97. In this chapter discussion is limited to the first phase of the venous occlusion tracing—that concerned with the measurement of mean arterial flow.)

Calf blood flow

All measurements should be conducted in a draft-free room at a comfortable temperature (22° C to 25° C). With the patient relaxed in a supine position, the calf is elevated slightly above heart level and maintained in that position with a pillow under the heel. Another pillow must be placed under the thigh to prevent extension of the knee and to ensure that the calf is not resting on the examining table. A large

(preferably contoured) venous occlusion cuff (22 × 71 cm)* is wrapped around the thigh just above the knee. Another pneumatic cuff (10 or 12.7 × 40.5 cm)* is wrapped around the ankle (Fig. 22-9). (This cuff is referred to as the *exclusion cuff* and is necessary to restrict the measurement to calf blood flow.) A mercury-in-silicone-elastomer strain gauge is positioned so that it encircles the calf at its widest part (Figs. 22-3 and 22-9). To conform precisely to all changes in calf circumference, the gauge should be applied with a slight amount of tension (about 10 g). Excess tension must be avoided because this will interfere with calf expansion. Ordinarily, the gauge should be 1 to 3 cm shorter than the circumference of the calf.

After the plethysmograph has been balanced so that a relatively stable baseline is evident on the recorder paper, the ankle cuff is inflated well above the systolic blood pressure. At this point, it is usually necessary to readjust the

---

*D. Eugene Hokanson, Issaquah, Wash.

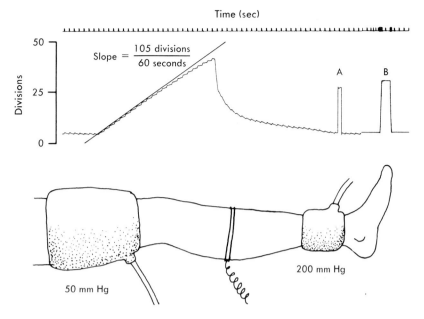

Fig. 22-9. Calf blood flow measurement with the mercury strain gauge. Electric calibration *(A)* corresponds to a 1% increase in calf volume and equals 22 divisions on the recording paper. Mechanical calibration *(B)* with a 0.2 cm stretch of the gauge produces a deflection of 26 divisions on the recording paper. The calf circumference was 34.6 cm. (From Strandness DE Jr, Sumner DS: *Hemodynamics for surgeons,* New York, 1975, Grune & Stratton.)

baseline. About 30 seconds should elapse before any recordings are made. With the recording paper running, the thigh cuff is rapidly inflated above venous pressure but below arterial diastolic pressure. Immediately, the tracing will rise above the baseline, producing a curve similar to that depicted in Fig. 22-9. When a slope of sufficient length is obtained, the thigh cuff is deflated and the tracing allowed to return to baseline before another flow recording is made. After the series of measurements is completed, the ankle cuff is deflated. A rest period of several minutes may be required before another series of measurements is made to allow the hyperemia of the part to subside.

With the tracing at baseline level, the gauge may be calibrated in situ. As described previously, a mechanical stretching device[52] may be used; if a four-lead (Hokanson) gauge and plethysmograph are being used, electric calibration is done.[16] Otherwise, the gauge is removed and attached to a "stretcher bar" (Fig. 22-7) for calibration.[34]

For most studies a venous occlusion pressure of about 50 to 60 mm Hg is appropriate. Occasionally it may be necessary to use a lower pressure when the patient has obstructive arterial disease so that the arterial diastolic pressure is not exceeded. By trying several different occlusion pressures, the researcher can select the pressure that gives the steepest slope. Usually a wide range of pressures will yield similar slopes. The venous occlusion cuff must be filled rapidly within a second or two to the predetermined level. This can be accomplished with an air reservoir or with an electrically controlled cuff inflator containing a pressure regulator and two solenoid valves.*

Frequently, the tracing will rise or fall a short distance almost instantly after the cuff is inflated. This so-called cuff artifact is usually a result of a shift of the calf skin or muscle mass produced by the cuff. If the cuff artifact is sharply defined, it will not interfere with flow measurement. Of course, the slope of the curve must not be drawn to include the artifact. Cuff artifacts can often be eliminated by readjusting the pillows or the occlusion cuff or by elevating the calf slightly.

Applications

Currently, venous occlusion plethysmography is used almost exclusively as a research tool for studying arterial physiology. Although it was initially used in diagnostic studies, far simpler methods are now available. Nonetheless, the validity of these less complicated techniques had to be substantiated by comparison with venous occlusion plethysmography.[48]

Because of the capacity of the peripheral arterioles to dilate to compensate for the increased resistance imposed by a proximal arterial obstruction, resting blood flow in limbs with arterial disease does not differ appreciably from that in normal extremities. Therefore unless the limb is severely ischemic, the level of blood flow measured at rest

---

*D. Eugene Hokanson, Issaquah, Wash.

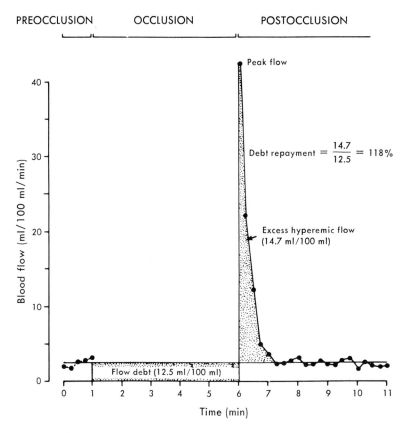

Fig. 22-10. Reactive hyperemia response in a normal human forearm after 5 minutes of ischemia. (From Strandness DE Jr, Sumner DS: *Hemodynamics for surgeons,* New York, 1975, Grune & Stratton.)

is of limited diagnostic value. However, when the circulation is stressed by any mechanism that produces vasodilatation, the plethysmographic flow pattern in patients with occlusive arterial disease is quite different from that in normal individuals.

Reactive hyperemia. For studying blood flow under conditions of maximal peripheral vasodilatation, hyperemia may be produced by reinstituting blood flow after a period of ischemia. This is an important method for evaluating the functional capacity of the circulation in patients with obstructive arterial disease.[14]

In addition to the apparatus previously discussed, a second pneumatic cuff (arterial occlusion cuff) must be placed around the thigh proximal to or over the venous occlusion cuff. After control flow measurements have been made, the arterial occlusion cuff is inflated well above arterial systolic pressure and left inflated for 5 minutes. (The proper pressure can be determined with the aid of a Doppler flowmeter.) The cuff around the ankle is inflated above systolic pressure 30 seconds before the arterial occlusion cuff is deflated. Then 10 seconds before the arterial occlusion cuff is deflated, the venous occlusion cuff is inflated to an appropriate level (usually 50 to 60 mm Hg). At time "zero" the arterial occlusion cuff is suddenly deflated, whereupon the tracing on the recording paper will rise with a very steep slope.

This tracing represents the initial flow recording at time "zero." Usually it is possible to obtain another flow recording at about 5 seconds and every 15 seconds thereafter until resting flow levels are reached.

Fig. 22-10 shows a typical reactive hyperemia response in a normal limb. Peak flow occurs within 5 seconds and reaches levels of 20 to 40 ml/100 ml/min. The response in an abnormal limb is obviously quite different (Fig. 22-11). Not only is the peak hyperemic flow reduced (range, 3 to 22 ml/100 ml/min), but the time required to reach peak flow is delayed to 10 to 100 seconds and the period of hyperemia is greatly prolonged.[14]

Exercise hyperemia. Another and perhaps more physiologic way of inducing peripheral vasodilatation is through exercise. Flexing the ankle against a foot pedal provides a method of exercising the calf with the patient in a supine position.[15] An even more physiologic way is to have the patient walk on a treadmill for a specified length of time or until the patient is forced to stop because of claudication.[48,49]

When studies are performed with the patient supine, all cuffs and gauges can be left in place so that measurements can be made immediately on cessation of exercise. However, when treadmill studies are performed, the gauge and cuffs will have to be disconnected during the exercise period and then rapidly reconnected after the patient returns to a supine

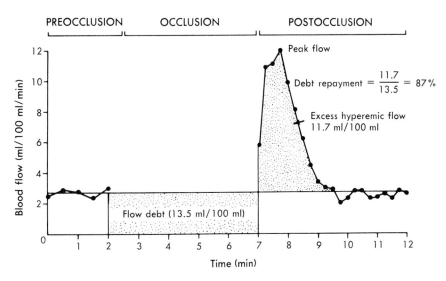

Fig. 22-11. Reactive hyperemia response in the calf of a limb with superficial artery occlusion. Note low peak flow, delay of peak flow, prolonged hyperemic response, and underpayment of flow debt. (From Strandness DE Jr, Sumner DS: *Hemodynamics for surgeons*, New York, 1975, Grune & Stratton.)

position. Since exercise hyperemia is more prolonged than reactive hyperemia, the elapsed time is not too critical.

The normal flow response to exercise is illustrated in Fig. 22-12. Immediately after exercise, peak flows in excess of 20 to 40 ml/100 ml/min are often attained. The flow rapidly declines and usually approaches preexercise levels in a few minutes. In contrast, the peak flow response in limbs with occlusive arterial disease is reduced (average, 9 to 20 ml/100 ml/min), the time required to reach peak flow is delayed (average, 3 to 7 minutes), and the hyperemic response may continue for more than 20 minutes (Fig. 22-13).[15,45,48]

Forearm blood flow

Forearm blood flow measurements are made exactly as described for calf blood flow. The venous occlusion cuff, however, need only be 10 or 12 cm wide. It is placed around the upper arm. The arterial exclusion cuff is placed around the wrist. Forearm blood flow measurements (made with the mercury strain gauge) have proved useful in assessing the peripheral vascular effects of drugs.[2,39]

Digit blood flow

Measurements of finger blood flow with the mercury strain gauge have proved useful in physiologic studies, especially in patients with vasospastic disease.[6,25,32,33] The procedure for measuring finger or toe blood flow is similar to that used for measuring calf flow. A pneumatic cuff for venous occlusion is wrapped around the proximal phalanx. Depending on the size of the digit, this cuff may be 1.5 or 2.5 cm wide (Fig. 22-14). Such cuffs are constructed of Penrose drains or a plastic bladder backed with Velcro. No distal cuff is used. The strain gauge is placed around the distal phalanx at the base of the nail. Measurements are

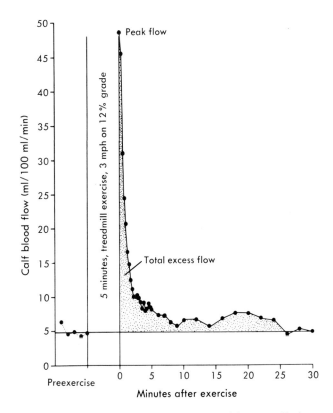

Fig. 22-12. Postexercise hyperemia in a normal human calf after 5 minutes of treadmill exercise (3 mph, 12% grade). (From Strandness DE Jr, Sumner DS: *Hemodynamics for surgeons*, New York, 1975, Grune & Stratton.)

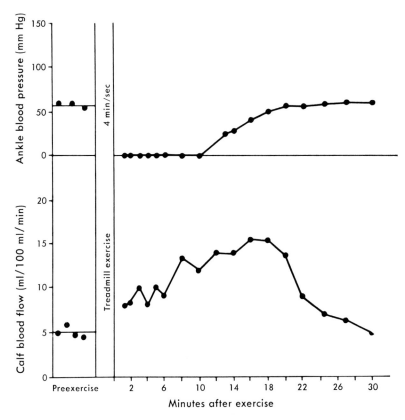

Fig. 22-13. Preexercise and postexercise calf blood flow and ankle pressure in a patient with stenosis of the iliac artery and occlusion of the superficial femoral artery. (From Sumner DS, Strandness DE Jr: *Surgery* 65:763, 1969.)

made with the hand or foot positioned comfortably, with the digits slightly above heart level.

Finger blood flow is often much higher than calf or forearm flow; consequently, the curve may rise from baseline to peak levels in one or two pulse beats, which makes accurate flow measurements difficult to obtain.[25] A cuff artifact is frequently present, and this may be difficult to eliminate. If the cuff artifact is "sharp," it is easily recognized and will present no problem. If the artifact is "rounded," it may be difficult to subtract from the actual flow tracing. In these cases the magnitude and slope of the cuff artifact can be determined by first inflating a cuff around the upper arm or leg to above systolic pressure and then inflating the venous occlusion cuff around the base of the digit. With this maneuver the rise in the baseline that occurs with no arterial inflow will become evident, and appropriate corrections can be made.

Calculation of blood flow

Blood flow is calculated from the venous occlusion tracing by connecting the initial systolic peaks or diastolic valleys of the pulsations with a straight line. This represents the slope of the flow curve (Fig. 22-9). The first step is to determine how many arbitrary divisions (div) of the recorder

paper the slope rises in 1 minute. In the example shown in Fig. 22-9 the slope is 105 div/min.

When electric calibration is used, the number of divisions corresponding to a 1% resistance change is determined. Because the calibration may have to be performed at a different recorder attenuation than that used for the flow tracing, the appropriate adjustment must be made. Since a 1% resistance change is equivalent to a 1% volume change (equation 11), flow is simply calculated as:

$$\text{Flow (ml/100 ml/min)} = \frac{\text{Slope (div/min)}}{\text{Calibration (div/1\% vol change)}} \quad (12)$$

In the example shown in Fig. 22-9, the electric calibration (A) is 22 div, and the flow is:

$$\frac{105 \text{ div/min}}{22 \text{ div/1\% vol change}} = 4.8 \text{ ml/100 ml/min}$$

The problem is slightly more complicated when mechanical calibration is used. First, one determines how many divisions on the paper correspond to a given stretch of the gauge. The stretch per division is obtained by dividing the stretch by the number of divisions. When this is multiplied by the slope, the amount of gauge stretch per minute is obtained:

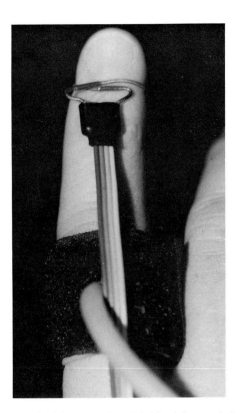

Fig. 22-14. Method for measuring digit blood flow and digit blood pressure with the mercury strain gauge and pneumatic cuff applied to the proximal phalanx. (From Sumner DS: *Noninvasive measurement of segmental arterial pressure.* In Rutherford RB, ed: *Vascular surgery,* ed 2, Philadelphia, 1984, WB Saunders.)

$$\frac{\text{Gauge stretch (cm)}}{\text{Div/gauge stretch}} \times \text{Slope (div/min)} = \qquad \textbf{(13)}$$

$$\text{Gauge stretch (cm)/min}$$

In Fig. 22-9, 26 divisions correspond to a 0.2 cm stretch of the gauge. Accordingly, the gauge stretch per minute is:

$$\frac{0.2 \text{ cm}}{26 \text{ div}} \times 105 \text{ div/min} = 0.81 \text{ cm/min}$$

Assuming that the gauge stretch per minute is equal to the circumference increase per minute, the ratio of circumference increase to the original circumference ($\Delta C/C$) can be calculated. Since the ratio of volume change to the original volume ($\Delta V/V$) is equal to twice $\Delta C/C$ (equation 9), blood flow can be calculated as follows:

$$\text{Flow (ml/100 ml/min)} = 2 \times \frac{\Delta C \text{ (cm/min)}}{C \text{ (cm)}} \times 100 \qquad \textbf{(14)}$$

It is necessary to multiply by 100 to express the flow in terms of 100 ml of tissue; otherwise, flow would be expressed as ml/1.0 ml/min.

In Fig. 22-9 the circumference of the calf is 34.6 cm. Therefore the flow is:

$$2 \times \frac{0.81 \text{ cm/min}}{34.6 \text{ cm}} \times 100 = 4.7 \text{ ml/100 ml/min}$$

The small disparity between the flows calculated from electric and mechanical calibration is a result of the inability to read the calibration signals to a fraction of a division.

Accuracy

Flow measurements made with the mercury strain gauge are subject to the same inaccuracies that occur with other instruments for venous occlusion plethysmography. In addition, the mercury strain gauge does not enclose as large a volume of tissue as does the air or water plethysmograph. Consequently, the operator has to assume that the events that take place under the strain gauge are duplicated in adjacent portions of the limb.

Despite these objections, flows measured with the mercury strain gauge are remarkably similar to those obtained with the water-filled device.[17,52] However, several studies have indicated that the mercury strain gauge tends to slightly underestimate blood flow. For example, Clarke and Hellon[3] found that the mercury strain gauge tended to underestimate flow by about 9%. Also, Lind and Schmid,[24] who made comparisons during rest and exercise, observed that the mercury strain gauge consistently gave measured flows that were about 1 ml/100 ml/min less than those measured with the water-filled plethysmograph. Eickhoff et al[10] found that the mercury strain gauge slightly underestimated calf blood flow at rest when compared with the Dohn air-filled plethysmograph; however, during hyperemia the flows measured by the two techniques were virtually identical.

MEASUREMENT OF SEGMENTAL ARTERIAL BLOOD PRESSURE

Strandness and co-workers[41,45] developed a method for measuring segmental arterial blood pressure that uses the digital mercury strain gauge as a flow sensor. Basically, it is a modification of the technique first proposed by Winsor in 1950.[53]

A pneumatic cuff is wrapped around the limb segment being studied, and a mercury strain gauge is placed around the forearm, calf, finger, or toe distal to the cuff. (A digital gauge is sufficient for most purposes; the gauge need only be placed in other locations when digital perfusion is absent.) As mentioned previously, the mercury strain gauge acts merely as a flow sensor.

Measurements are made by inflating the pneumatic cuff above systolic pressure. At this point any pulsations present in the digital plethysmographic record will disappear (Fig. 22-15). As the pressure in the cuff is gradually released, there will be a slow decline in digit volume. When the systolic pressure in the arteries underlying the cuff is reached, the digit volume will begin to increase, often rapidly. At the same time, digit pulses, if previously present, will reappear (Fig. 22-15). The point at which the digit volume increases or at which digit pulses return is the systolic pressure.

The mercury strain gauge is often applicable when other methods for sensing flow return cannot be used. For ex-

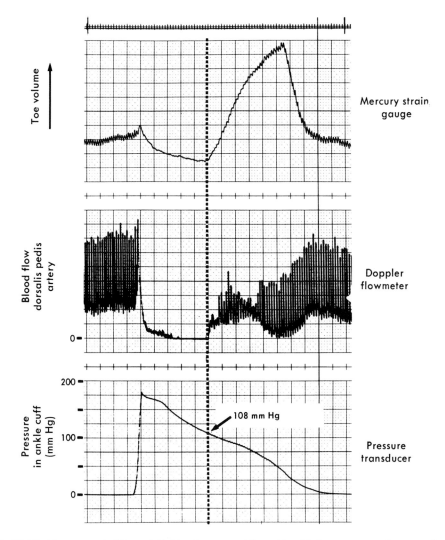

Fig. 22-15. Measurement of the systolic blood pressure at the ankle with the mercury strain gauge placed around the second toe. The Doppler flow signal is included for comparison. (From Sumner DS: *Noninvasive measurement of segmental arterial pressure*. In Rutherford RB, ed: *Vascular surgery*, ed 2, Philadelphia, 1984, WB Saunders.)

ample, the Doppler technique for measuring blood pressure may fail when there are no remaining major arterial channels that carry blood at sufficient velocity to produce a signal. Thus even in highly ischemic extremities a blood pressure can usually be obtained with the mercury strain gauge if the technologist is careful and persistent.

In the usual investigation of arterial disease of the lower extremities, the strain gauge is applied to the second toe, and pneumatic cuffs are placed around the ankle, below the knee, just above the knee, and at the upper thigh. Pressures may be recorded from all levels, beginning at the ankle. Of these pressures, the ankle pressure is the most accurate and the most significant in determining the presence or absence of obstructive arterial disease. In almost all normal limbs the ankle pressure equals or exceeds the arm pressure. On the average, the ankle systolic pressure is about 110% of the arm systolic pressure.[54] (Further discussion of the significance of leg pressures is found in other chapters.)

MEASUREMENT OF DIGITAL ARTERIAL BLOOD PRESSURE

Digital blood pressure can be measured by the same technique.[13,29] A pneumatic cuff is placed around the proximal phalanx and a mercury strain gauge around the distal phalanx (Fig. 22-14). Although finger pressures are easy to obtain, toe pressure measurements are more difficult because toes are often too short to accommodate both the cuff and the gauge comfortably. The photoplethysmograph is often more useful under these circumstances.[37]

The prognostic significance of toe blood pressures has been investigated by Holstein et al,[18] who reported that only 7 of 24 limbs (29%) with skin lesions healed when the big toe pressure was 20 mm Hg or below; 4 of 8 (50%) healed

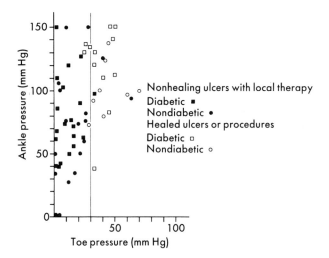

Fig. 22-16. Comparison of ankle and toe pressures in 58 limbs with healed or nonhealing ischemic ulcers or toe amputations. (From Sumner DS: *Noninvasive measurement of segmental arterial pressure.* In Rutherford RB, ed: *Vascular surgery,* ed 2, Philadelphia, 1984, WB Saunders.)

when the pressure was 30 mm Hg or greater. Similarly, Ramsey et al[37] found that 95% of distal foot lesions failed to heal when the toe pressure was less than 30 mm Hg, but 86% of such lesions healed when the toe pressure exceeded 30 mm Hg (Fig. 22-16). Thus 30 mm Hg appears to be the pressure above which healing can be anticipated. Since there is no appreciable difference between toe pressures in patients with diabetes and those without, this test may prove to be more useful than the ankle pressure, which in patients with diabetes is often distortedly high because of the presence of arterial calcification.

In patients with symptoms of cold sensitivity or ischemia of the fingers, it is important to differentiate between fixed arterial obstruction (caused by atherosclerosis, trauma, emboli, Buerger's disease, arteritis, and so on) and that resulting from vasospasm (Raynaud's disease). Digital pressures are often quite helpful in these cases.

Finger pressures in patients with arterial obstruction of the digital, palmar, or forearm arteries are consistently reduced, whereas finger pressures in patients with vasospastic conditions are normal when they are examined in a warm room (25° C). Experience has indicated that the finger pressure index (finger pressure divided by the ipsilateral brachial pressure) averages 0.97 ± 0.09 in normal individuals, 0.96 ± 0.11 in patients with vasospastic conditions, and 0.56 ± 0.27 in patients in whom obstruction is present.[47]

Nielsen and Lassen[30] have introduced an interesting test that uses the mercury strain gauge to measure pressure in fingers that have been locally cooled. This test appears to discriminate between patients with vasospastic disease, whose finger pressures drop rapidly at temperatures below 20° C to 25° C, and normal individuals, whose finger pressures drop only minimally at 10° C. It also provides an

objective method for evaluating the severity of the vasospastic process and for measuring the response to therapy.[31]

Digital arterial pressures are also useful in assessing the hemodynamics of arteriovenous fistulas.[45] When a steal is present, the digital arterial pressure is reduced with the fistula open but increases toward normal levels when the fistula is compressed.

DIGITAL PULSE PLETHYSMOGRAPHY

Digital plethysmography is among the more sensitive methods available for studying peripheral vascular disease.[1,41,46] Although almost any form of plethysmograph can be modified to record digit pulses, the mercury-in-silicone-elastomer strain gauge and the photoplethysmograph are the most useful. Because of its simplicity and high frequency response, the strain gauge remains a favorite of many clinical researchers and physiologists.

Procedure

Studies should be conducted in a warm room (22° C to 25° C) with the patient relaxed, preferably in a supine position. A strain gauge that fits snugly but not too tightly around the digit should be selected (Fig. 22-2). Because of the extreme sensitivity of the digital blood flow to variations in temperature, the hands and feet should be warm. At times it may be necessary to immerse the hands and feet in warm water for a short period before making the tracings. An electric blanket is also helpful.

The plethysmograph may be AC coupled when the examiner is concerned only with the general morphology of the pulse; however, if total changes in digit volume are being studied, it is necessary to use DC coupling.

Pulse contour

As shown in Fig. 22-17, *C,* the normal digit pulse is characterized by a sharp systolic upstroke that rises rapidly to a peak and then drops off more slowly toward the baseline. The downslope is curved toward the baseline and usually contains a more or less prominent dicrotic wave about midway between the peak and the baseline. This dicrotic wave is caused by the reflection of the arterial pulse from the periphery.

The pulse recorded distal to an arterial obstruction differs in several ways from the normal pulse (Fig. 22-17, *B*). Not only is the general shape more rounded, but the upswing is more gradual and the downslope is bowed away from the baseline. No dicrotic wave is present. In limbs with severe arterial disease (such as from ischemic rest pain or multilevel obstruction), the digital pulse may be severely reduced or entirely absent.[40]

A pulse that encompasses some of the features of both the normal and obstructive forms has been identified (Fig. 22-17, *A*).[4,40,50] This so-called peaked pulse is often found in patients with cold sensitivity, particularly in those with collagen vascular problems or some other form of anatomic digital artery disease, but may also be observed in normal

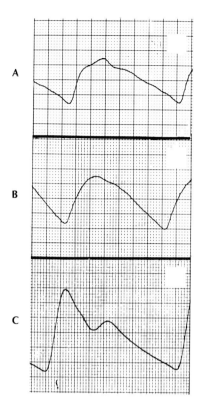

Fig. 22-17. Typical digit pulse contours. *A,* Peaked pulse. *B,* Obstructive pulse. *C,* Normal pulse. (From Sumner DS, Strandness DE Jr: *Ann Surg* 175:294, 1972.)

fingers under conditions of relative vasoconstriction.[21,33,50] The peaked pulse has a somewhat lower upswing than does the normal pulse. Near the peak there is an anacrotic notch. On the downslope the dicrotic wave is less prominent than it is in normal pulses and tends to be located closer to the peak.

By using these simple criteria, the clinician can usually diagnose significant arterial obstruction in the vessels located proximal to the site of gauge application. This includes the digital, pedal, and hand arteries, as well as those major, more proximally located arteries that are typically involved in obstructive processes. For example, the finding of an abnormal toe pulse in a patient with a normal ankle systolic pressure would tend to localize the disease to the pedal or digital arteries. Such observations can be of value in assessing the prospects for healing in a patient with ischemic lesions of the toes. If a good pulse is obtained, the prognosis may be favorable, but if pulses are flat or absent, the prospects for healing without reconstructive surgery would be remote.

The finding of a peaked or obstructive pulse in a patient with cold sensitivity is also an indication that the patient does not have primary Raynaud's disease but rather some form of obstructive arterial disease that produces a secondary Raynaud's phenomenon. Often this will turn out to be one of the collagen diseases. On the other hand, finding a

normal pulse in such a patient makes the diagnosis of primary Raynaud's disease more likely.

Analysis of the digit pulse contour

Although a number of complex methods have been devised for describing digit pulse contours, they add little to simple pattern recognition for differentiating between normal and abnormal forms. Various investigators have measured the slope of the ascending and descending limbs of the curve, the pulse width at one half its maximum excursion, the ratio of the amplitude of the dicrotic notch to peak amplitude, and the relative amplitudes at various points along the curve.[22,26,55] Although these parameters may be helpful in comparing pulses statistically, some believe that they are purely arbitrary measurements with little or no physiologic meaning.

Because the mercury strain gauge has a high frequency response (flat out to 100 Hz),[35] more rigorous analytic techniques are possible. As shown in Fig. 22-18, the pulse wave may be broken down into its harmonic components by Fourier analysis.[4,40,45] Each harmonic can be characterized in terms of its amplitude and phase angle. With progressive proximal obstructive disease, the relative amplitudes of all harmonics beyond the first tend to become more attenuated, thereby producing the rounded contour typical of the obstructive pulse. In addition, the first harmonic develops an increased phase lag, which accounts for the delayed peak. Data such as these can be handled mathematically and can be compared with data from similar studies on pressure and flow waves.[27]

When the plethysmographic pulse is electrically or mathematically differentiated, a tracing that resembles an arterial flow pulse is obtained (Fig. 22-19). Although this has led some investigators to suggest that blood flow could be measured on the basis of the pulse contour alone, the lack of a method of determining a zero flow level on the differential tracing makes such determinations unreliable.[8,51] Because the amplitude and shape of the differential tracing may change little even though flow varies widely, investigators cannot assume that the flat portion of the tracing corresponds to zero flow.

Pulse volume

Although the digit pulse may be markedly reduced or even absent in limbs with advanced arterial disease, pulse volume is only a crude indicator of the extent of arterial obstruction in less severe cases (Fig. 22-20).[5,40,55] Even in normal individuals, arterial pulse volume is extremely variable, responding to changes in local temperature and sympathetic nervous activity (Fig. 22-21).

In any given digit of the same individual, the volume of the digit pulse varies directly with the blood flow, provided that all studies are performed during the same examination period without moving the gauge.[56] Thus the pulse volume provides a convenient method for observing variation in digit blood flow during the reactive hyperemia test or in

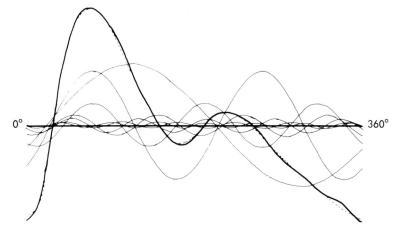

0°   360°

Fig. 22-18. Fourier analysis of normal digit volume pulse. *Heavy solid lines* indicate plethysmographically obtained pulse-wave; *light lines* are cosine waves corresponding to the first seven harmonics; *dotted lines* depict the pulse contour as reconstructed from the first seven harmonics. (From Strandness DE Jr, Sumner DS: *Hemodynamics for surgeons,* New York, 1975, Grune & Stratton.)

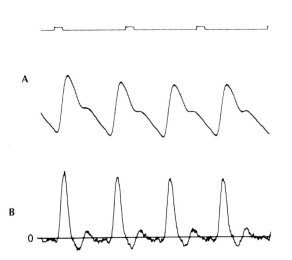

Fig. 22-19. Simultaneous recording of the digit volume pulse *(A)* and its electrical differential *(B).* Note the strong resemblance of the differentiated pulse to the arterial flow pulse. (From Strandness DE Jr, Sumner DS: *Hemodynamics for surgeons,* New York, 1975, Grune & Stratton.)

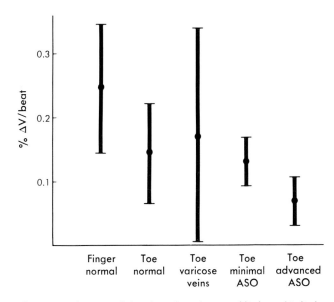

Fig. 22-20. The mean digit pulse volume in normal limbs and in limbs with arterial and venous disease. Vertical bars indicate ±1 standard deviation. (From Strandness DE Jr: *Peripheral arterial disease: a physiologic approach,* Boston, 1969, Little, Brown & Co.)

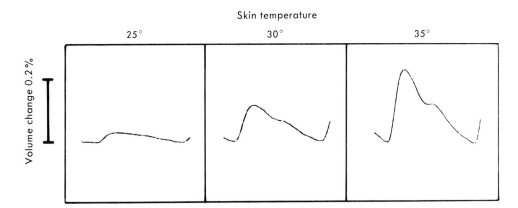

Fig. 22-21. The relationship between the digit pulse volume and skin temperature in a normal individual. Note that the contour of the pulse shows little change except during intense vasoconstriction. (From Strandness DE Jr, Sumner DS: *Hemodynamics for surgeons,* New York, 1975, Grune & Stratton.)

response to sympathetic nervous activity. However, relative estimates of blood flow from person to person or even from day to day in the same individual cannot be obtained by comparing digit pulse volumes.

Assessing sympathetic activity

Because digit blood flow is quite sensitive to sympathetic nerve impulses, the volume of the pulse may be used to follow changes in sympathetic activity. In addition, vasoconstriction of veins and arteries in response to increased sympathetic outflow will reduce the total volume of the digit.

As shown in Fig. 22-22, fingertip volume varies with respiration in the presence of normal sympathetic tone. Other deflections, known as *alpha waves,* also occur several times each minute. These waves are considerably larger than the respiratory waves. Beta and gamma waves have also been described.[1,20] Sympathectomy inhibits these responses.

When a normal individual takes a deep breath, digital volume increases momentarily and then falls precipitously to a much lower level as the total quantity of blood in the finger or toe decreases.[1,41,45] At the same time, the pulse volume decreases to a low level, gradually rising to its original amplitude over a period varying from seconds to minutes (Fig. 22-23). In the presence of a surgical sympathectomy or peripheral neuropathy that is due to diabetes, the inspiratory reflex will be absent.[43,45]

Other ways of testing the integrity of the sympathetic nervous supply to the digits include placing ice cubes on the forehead or chest and creating a painful stimulus such as a needle stick. When sympathetic innervation is intact, these stimuli will cause vasoconstriction. However, such

maneuvers have not proved to be as reliable as the "deep breath" test. Reflex vasodilatation may also be used to test for sympathetic activity. Normally, when one hand is placed in water at 40° C, the digital volume pulse on the opposite side will increase as a result of reflex inhibition of the sympathetic tone. Thus the absence of dilatation indicates absence or reduction of sympathetic innervation.

Reactive hyperemia

Creation of hyperemia after a period of ischemia is an excellent method for assessing the functional severity of peripheral arterial disease. Because acute changes in pulse volume reflect acute changes in digit blood flow with a fair degree of accuracy, digit plethysmography provides a convenient method for qualitatively assessing the reactive hyperemia response.

Reactive hyperemia is produced by inflating a pneumatic cuff placed around the ankle or upper arm to a pressure greater than systolic pressure. After the cuff has been inflated for 3 to 5 minutes, the pressure is suddenly released, and digit volume pulses are followed for the next several minutes. The volume of the largest pulse obtained during the period of reactive hyperemia is compared with the prehyperemic pulse volume.

In normal extremities the volume of the hyperemic pulse will be several times that of the control pulse (Fig. 22-24). This merely reflects the ability of the peripheral arterioles to dilate in response to a period of ischemia. However, in the presence of significant obstructive arterial disease, there may be little or no increase in pulse volume during the postischemic period (Fig. 22-24). This is explained by the

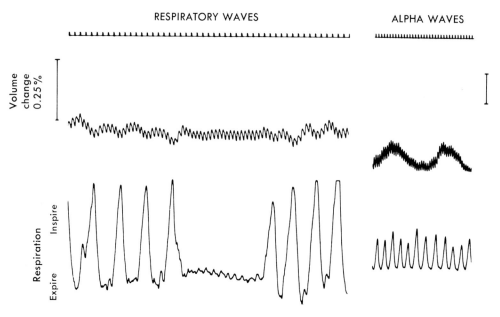

Fig. 22-22. Plethysmographic tracing from a normal fingertip. Respiratory waves and alpha waves are present. (From Strandness DE Jr, Sumner DS: *Hemodynamics for surgeons,* New York, 1975, Grune & Stratton.)

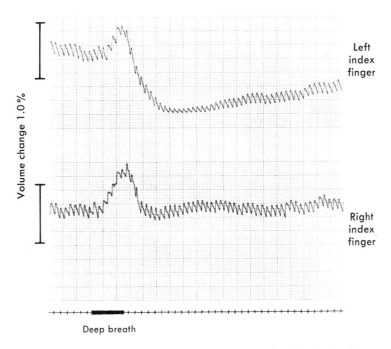

Fig. 22-23. The response of digit volume and digit pulse volume to a deep breath. Simultaneous tracings were made from index fingers of both hands in a patient who had undergone a right cervicothoracic sympathectomy several weeks before. The brief rise in volume that accompanies a deep breath is a result of temporary compression of the venous outflow. (From Strandness DE Jr, Sumner DS: *Hemodynamics for surgeons,* New York, 1975, Grune & Stratton.)

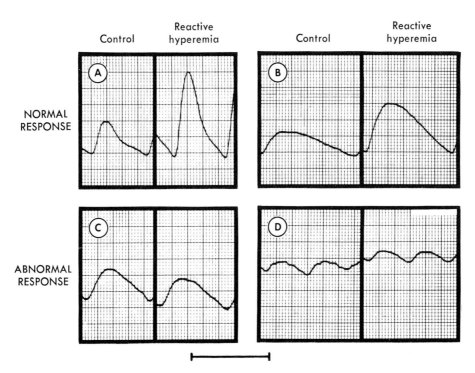

Fig. 22-24. The response of the digit volume pulse in the second toe to a 5-minute period of ischemia (reactive hyperemia test). In a normal response, the volume of the digit pulse more than doubles (upper panels). In an abnormal response, there is little change in the pulse volume. **A,** Normal circulation (pressure: arm 130, ankle 140). **B,** Superficial femoral occlusion (pressure: arm 100, ankle 80). **C,** Patient with diabetes for 20 years (pressure: arm 135, ankle 135). **D,** Multilevel disease, iliac and superficial femoral (pressure: arm 118, ankle 46). **B, C,** and **D** are recorded at twice the sensitivity used in **A.** (From Sumner DS: *Digital plethysmography.* In Rutherford RB, ed: *Vascular surgery,* ed 2, Philadelphia, 1984, WB Saunders.)

fact that the peripheral arterioles have already dilated to a considerable degree to compensate for the increased resistance imposed by the proximal arterial obstruction. Stated in another way, the magnitude of the pulse volume increase is inversely proportional to the degree of preexisting peripheral vasodilatation. When the peripheral arterioles are already dilated because of a peripheral neuropathy, there will also be little hyperemic response.

On the basis of previous experience, a surgical sympathectomy is most likely to produce a good result when the pulse at least doubles in volume in response to hyperemia. This merely indicates that the arterioles continue to have the capacity to dilate; it says nothing about the status of the sympathetic innervation. If there is little increase in pulse volume, there is less likelihood that sympathectomy will produce much increase in blood flow.

It must be emphasized that the presence or absence of reactive hyperemia has no direct relationship to the integrity of the sympathetic nervous system. Vessels in fully sympathectomized extremities retain the ability to dilate in response to a period of ischemia. Some other methods, such as the "deep breath" test or reflex vasodilatation, must be used when the examiner is concerned about sympathetic activity.

REFERENCES

1. Burch GE: *Digital plethysmography,* New York, 1954, Grune & Stratton.
2. Carabine UA et al: The effect of intravenous clonidine on the forearm circulation, *Anaesthesia* 46:1013, 1991.
3. Clarke RSJ, Hellon RF: Venous collection in forearm and hand measured by strain gauge and volume plethysmograph, *Clin Sci* 16:103, 1957.
4. Conrad MC: *Functional anatomy of the circulation to the lower extremities,* Chicago, 1971, Year Book Medical.
5. Conrad MC, Green HD: Hemodynamics of large and small vessels in peripheral vascular disease, *Circulation* 29:847, 1964.
6. Cooke et al: Sex differences in control of cutaneous blood flow, *Circulation* 82:1607, 1990.
7. Cramer M et al: Standardization of venous flow measurements by strain gauge plethysmography in normal subjects, *Bruit* 7:33, 1983.
8. Dahn I, Jonson B, Nilsén R: A plethysmographic method for determination of flow and volume pulsations in a limb, *J Appl Physiol* 28:333, 1970.
9. Eagan CJ: *The physics of the mercury strain gauge and of its use in digital plethysmography,* Technical report 60-17, Fairbanks, Alaska, 1961, Arctic Aeromedical Laboratory.
10. Eickhoff JH, Kjaer L, Siggard-Andersen J: A comparison of the strain-gauge and the Dohn air-filled plethysmograph for blood flow measurements in the human calf, *Acta Chir Scand* 502:15, 1980.
11. Gibbons GE, Strandness DE Jr, Bell JW: Improvements in design of the mercury strain gauge plethysmograph, *Surg Gynecol Obstet* 116:679, 1963.
12. Greenfield ADM, Whitney RJ, Mowbray JF: Methods for the investigation of peripheral blood flow, *Br Med Bull* 19:101, 1963.
13. Gundersen J: Segmental measurements of systolic blood pressure in the extremities including the thumb and the great toe, *Acta Chir Scand* 426(suppl):1, 1972.
14. Hillestad LK: The peripheral blood flow in intermittent claudication. V. Plethysmographic studies. The significance of the calf blood flow at rest and in response to timed arrest of the circulation, *Acta Med Scand* 174:23, 1963.
15. Hillestad LK: The peripheral blood flow in intermittent claudication. VI. Plethysmographic studies. The blood flow response to exercise with arrested and free circulation, *Acta Med Scand* 174:671, 1963.
16. Hokanson DE, Sumner DS, Strandness DE Jr: An electrically calibrated plethysmograph for direct measurement of limb blood flow, *IEEE Trans Biomed Eng* 22(1):25, 1975.
17. Holling HE, Boland HC, Russ E: Investigation of arterial obstruction using a mercury-in-rubber strain gauge, *Am Heart J* 62:194, 1961.
18. Holstein P et al: *Distal blood pressure in severe arterial insufficiency. Strain-gauge, radioisotopes, and other methods.* In Bergan JJ, Yao JST, eds: *Gangrene and severe ischemia of the lower extremities,* New York, 1978, Grune & Stratton.
19. Honda N: *Temperature compensation for the mercury strain-gauge used in digital plethysmography,* Technical report 61-28, Fairbanks, Alaska, 1961, Arctic Aeromedical Laboratory.
20. Honda N: The periodicity in volume fluctuations and blood flow in the human finger, *Angiology* 21:442, 1970.
21. Huff SE: Observations on peripheral circulation in various dermatoses, *Arch Dermatol* 71:575, 1955.
22. Koike S et al: The morphology of the digital volume pulse wave in health and hypertension recorded plethysmographically, *Jpn J Hyg* 23:60, 1968.

23. Knox R et al: Pitfall of venous occlusion plethysmography, *Angiology* 33:268, 1982.

24. Lind AR, Schmid PG: Comparison of volume and strain-gauge plethysmography during static effort, *J Appl Physiol* 32:552, 1972.

25. Manke DA et al: Hemodynamic studies of digital and extremity replants and revascularizations, *Surgery* 88:445, 1980.

26. Mathiesen FR et al: Follow-up study of patients with occlusive arterial disease. Pulse curve morphology and xenon-133 clearance, *Acta Chir Scand* 136:591, 1970.

27. McDonald DA: *Blood flow in arteries,* ed 2, Baltimore, 1974, Williams & Wilkins.

28. Michaux B et al: Calibration-free mercury strain-gauge plethysmograph, *Med Biol Eng Comput* 17:539, 1979.

29. Nielsen PE, Bell G, Lassen NA: The measurement of digital systolic blood pressure by strain-gauge technique, *Scand J Clin Lab Invest* 29:343, 1972.

30. Nielsen SL, Lassen NA: Measurement of digital blood pressure after local cooling, *J Appl Physiol* 43:907, 1977.

31. Nobin BA et al: Reserpine treatment of Raynaud's disease, *Ann Surg* 187:12, 1978.

32. Ohgi S et al: The effect of cold on circulation in normal and cold sensitive fingers, *Bruit* 9:9, 1985.

33. Ohgi S et al: Physiology of the peaked finger pulse in normal and cold-sensitive subjects, *J Vasc Surg* 3:516, 1986.

34. Parrish D: Appendix to Strandness DE Jr, Bell JW: Peripheral vascular disease: diagnosis and objective evaluation using a mercury strain gauge, *Ann Surg* 161(suppl):32, 1965.

35. Parrish D, Strandness DE Jr, Bell JW: Dynamic response characteristics of a mercury-in-Silastic strain gauge, *J Appl Physiol* 10:363, 1964.

36. Radke HM et al: Monitor of digit volume changes in angioplastic surgery: use of strain gauge plethysmography, *Ann Surg* 154:818, 1961.

37. Ramsey DE, Manke DA, Sumner DS: Toe blood pressure, a valuable adjunct to ankle pressure measurement for assessing peripheral arterial disease, *J Cardiovasc Surg* 24:43, 1983.

38. Sigdell JE: A critical review of the theory of the mercury strain-gauge plethysmograph, *Med Biol Eng* 7:365, 1969.

39. Stott DJ et al: The effects of the 5 HT2 antagonist ritanserine on blood pressure and serotonin-induced platelet aggregation in patients with untreated essential hypertension, *Eur J Clin Pharmacol* 35:123, 1988.

40. Strandness DE Jr: *Peripheral arterial disease: a physiologic approach,* Boston, 1969, Little, Brown and Co.

41. Strandness DE Jr, Bell JW: Peripheral vascular disease: diagnosis and objective evaluation using a mercury strain gauge, *Ann Surg* 161(suppl):1, 1965.

42. Strandness DE Jr, Gibbons GE, Bell JW: Mercury strain gauge plethysmography. Evaluation of patients with acquired arteriovenous fistula, *Arch Surg* 85:215, 1962.

43. Strandness DE Jr, Priest RE, Gibbons GE: Combined clinical and pathological study of diabetic and non-diabetic peripheral arterial disease, *Diabetes* 13:366, 1964.

44. Strandness DE Jr, Radke HM, Bell JW: Use of a new simplified plethysmograph in the clinical evaluation of patients with arteriosclerosis obliterans, *Surg Gynecol Obstet* 112:751, 1961.

45. Strandness DE Jr, Sumner DS: *Hemodynamics for surgeons,* New York, 1975, Grune & Stratton.

46. Sumner DS: Digital plethysmography. In Rutherford RB, editor: *Vascular surgery, ed. 2,* Philadelphia, 1984, WB Saunders.

47. Sumner DS, Lambeth A, Russell JB: Diagnosis of upper extremity obstructive and vasospastic syndromes by Doppler ultrasound, plethysmography, and temperature profiles. In Puel P, Baccalon H, Enjalbert A, eds: *Hemodynamics of the limbs,* Toulouse, France, 1979, G.E.P.E.S.C.

48. Sumner DS, Strandness DE Jr: The relationship between calf blood flow and ankle blood pressure in patients with intermittent claudication, *Surgery* 65:763, 1969.

49. Sumner DS, Strandness DE Jr: The effect of exercise on resistance to blood flow in limbs with an occluded superficial femoral artery, *Vasc Surg* 4:229, 1970.

50. Sumner DS, Strandness DE Jr: An abnormal finger pulse associated with cold sensitivity, *Ann Surg* 175:294, 1972.

51. Van De Water JM, Mount BE: *Impedance plethysmography in the lower extremity.* In Swan KG, ed: *Venous surgery in the lower extremities,* St Louis, 1975, Warren H Green.

52. Whitney RJ: The measurement of volume changes in human limbs, *J Physiol (Lond)* 121:1, 1953.

53. Winsor T: Influence of arterial disease on the systolic blood pressure gradients of the extremity, *Am J Med Sci* 220:117, 1950.

54. Yao JST: Hemodynamic studies in peripheral arterial disease, *Br J Surg* 57:761, 1970.

55. Zetterquist S et al: The validity of some conventional methods for the diagnosis of obliterative arterial disease in the lower limb as evaluated by arteriography, *Scand J Clin Lab Invest* 28:409, 1971.

56. Zweifler AJ, Cushing G, Conway J: The relationship between pulse volume and blood flow in the fingers, *Angiology* 18:591, 1967.

CHAPTER 23

Air plethysmography in arterial and venous disease

Plethysmography is derived from two Greek words: *plethysmos* (to increase) and *graphien* (to write). It indicates an instrument that records an increase in volume.

A number of methods have been used to measure volume changes: water, air, electrical impedance, mercury in rubber strain gauge, and photoelectric plethysmography. Air plethysmography has recently been developed for quantitative clinical use by calibrating the instrument to measure volume changes of the whole leg in absolute units (ml). It has found a place in both arterial inflow measurements and the assessment of chronic venous insufficiency.

THE PULSE VOLUME RECORDER
Jeffrey K. Raines

Segmental (limb and digit) plethysmographic recordings have proved to be important in the clinical evaluation of the peripheral arterial system. The segmental recordings are similar to the arterial pressure-pulse contour and reveal the degree of occlusive disease, an estimate of collateral circulation, anatomic localization of obstructive lesions, and indirectly, the level of perfusion. These measurements should not be confused with absolute blood flow, which segmental plethysmography does not measure. Plethysmographic data combined with clinical findings, segmental limb pressures, and treadmill exercise testing provide useful hemodynamic information necessary for the treatment of patients with peripheral disease.

The pulse volume recorder (PVR)* was developed through the combined efforts of the Massachusetts Institute of Technology and the Massachusetts General Hospital. It is a quantitative segmental plethysmograph designed for high sensitivity and clinical application.[9,14,15] It provides pulse volume recordings and systolic pressure measurements of the extremities, is adaptable to arterial measurements taken before and after exercise, and is capable of producing permanent records for reference. It may also be used to diagnose deep vein thrombosis in major veins of the lower and upper extremities and is now available with an attachment to measure ophthalmic systolic artery pressure. Chap-

ter 59 describes the practical clinical use of this instrument and gives examples of PVR recordings; the remainder of this section is devoted to describing the mechanics of the PVR.[13]

OPERATING PROCEDURE

With the PVR, appropriate blood pressure cuffs are placed on the extremity or digit and a measured quantity of air (75 ± 10 ml) is injected until a preset pressure (65 mm Hg) is reached. This procedure ensures that at a given pressure, the cuff volume surrounding the limb is constant from reading to reading. If this cuff setting (volume and pressure) is not met, the cuff must be reapplied at a slightly different tension. The PVR electronic package measures and records instantaneous pressure changes in the segmental monitoring cuff. Cuff pressure change reflects alteration in cuff volume, which in turn reflects momentary changes in limb volume. Cuffs are available in different sizes for all anatomic locations, including the digits. They have a neoprene bladder surrounded by a nonelastic nylon Velcro band that allows easy application.

The PVR method is simpler than making volume calibrations with application of the cuff, as has been done with other instruments.[18] Similarly, it obviates mathematical corrections for volume and pressure changes and provides PVR recordings that can be visually compared with those previously obtained. PVR recordings are taken at a chart speed of 25 mm/sec.

The major components of the PVR are illustrated in Fig. 23-1. The electronic circuit includes a pressure-sensitive silicone NPN plantar transistor with its emitter-base junction mechanically coupled to a diaphragm.[12] A differential pressure applied to the diaphragm produces a large reversible change in the gain of the transistor, which has a uniform frequency response up to 150 kHz. Additional electronic components of the PVR include (1) a sample-and-hold circuit that operates in closed-loop fashion to maintain a proper operating point for the pressure sensor, (2) logic circuits that set solenoid valve configuration according to the mode selected by the operator, and (3) a dual-limit comparator that detects and corrects for excessive differential pressures applied to the sensor.

---

*Life Sciences, Inc. Greenwich, Conn.

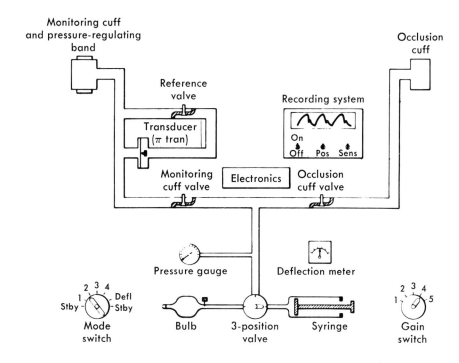

Fig. 23-1. System diagram of a PVR.

CALIBRATION

The PVR is calibrated so that a 1 mm Hg pressure change in the cuff provides a 20 mm chart deflection. If desired, maximum chart deflection may be translated (by means of cuff dynamics formulas) into volume change per cardiac cycle.

FREQUENCY RESPONSE

The frequency response of the complete device (cuff and electronic package) was tested by strapping a water-filled bladder around a rigid plastic cylinder, which in turn was encircled by an air-filled PVR monitoring cuff. A small piston-in-cylinder pump was then connected to the bladder to produce a sinusoidal pressure change in the monitoring cuff. The amplitude of these oscillations remained constant up to a pump frequency of 20 Hz, which is sufficient to evaluate the higher-frequency components of the human arterial pressure-pulse contour accurately.[10]

LINEARITY

The linearity of the system was tested by measuring cuff pressure changes as a function of cuff volume changes. This was studied over a range of mean cuff pressures varying from 20 to 200 mm Hg and with injected cuff volumes varying from 20 to 125 ml. Within the range studied, cuff pressure change was indeed a linear function of cuff volume change. This study also points out the importance of taking clinical readings at consistent cuff pressures and volumes.

CUFF DYNAMICS

It was important to understand how the pressure of the air in the cuff related to the arterial pressure and limb volume changes to aid in the development of the PVR operating procedure and the interpretation of its recordings. A number of experiments and analyses were performed.[13]

For example, a constant mass of air in the cuff is at an absolute pressure p_c in a volume V_c. Furthermore, if it is assumed that the gas undergoes an isentropic process, the following equation may be written:

$$p_c V_c^{\gamma} = \text{Constant} \qquad (1)$$

where γ is the ratio of specific heats (for air, γ is 1.4).

The pressure-measuring components of the PVR were connected to a rigid cylinder (50 ml volume) to test the validity of the isentropic assumption. Also included in the pneumatic circuit was a small piston-in-cylinder pump with a 1-ml stroke volume. The pump was used to oscillate the total volume of the system at various frequencies while measuring the pressure changes. It was found that at frequencies from 0.25 to 20 Hz (highest frequency tested), the pressure amplitude remained constant. The pressure amplitude increased approximately 34% gradually from zero frequency (isothermal) to 0.25 Hz. This experiment suggests that in the range of primary frequencies encountered in clinical use (0.5 to 1.5 Hz) the air in the cuff undergoes an isentropic process, changing from isothermal to isentropic between zero and 0.25 Hz. It can be shown that the identification of the process is not critical to the analysis, since its effect is combined with the elastic expansion of the cuff. Since the volume excursions in the cuff are a small fraction (2% maximum) of its mean volume, equation 1 can be differentiated to give:

$$\delta p_c = \frac{-\gamma \bar{p}_c}{\bar{V}_c} \delta V_c \qquad (2)$$

where p_c and V_c have been replaced by their time-mean values $\bar{p}_c$ and $\bar{V}_c$, respectively. The time-mean volume $\bar{V}_c$ is also a function of cuff pressure and the injected air mass. If the initial volume of air injected at atmospheric pressure (P_{ATM}) is V_1, the volume of air in the cuff is defined by equation 3:

$$\bar{V}_c = \frac{P_{ATM}}{\bar{p}_c} (V_1 + V_1 + V_2) - V_2 \tag{3}$$

Here V_1 is the tube volume from an internal shutoff valve in the PVR to the monitoring cuff; V_2 represents the tube volume from the shutoff valve to the syringe. V_1 and V_2 are 21 and 22 ml, respectively. The compression of the injected air is assumed to be isothermal, since it subsists for a long period of time, much longer than 4 seconds (0.25 Hz). Combining equations 2 and 3 results in:

$$\delta p_c = \frac{-\gamma \delta V_c \bar{p}_c}{(P_{ATM}/\bar{p}_c [V_1 + V_1 + V_2] - V_2)} \tag{4}$$

Another experiment was performed to investigate the validity of equation 4. The monitoring cuff was connected to the PVR electronics with a 1-ml syringe also in the pneumatic circuit. The syringe was used to change the total air volume in increments of 0.25 ml from 0.25 to 1 ml at different cuff pressures and initial injected volumes. Cuff gauge pressures at 20, 40, 60, 80, and 100 mm Hg were used with injected volumes of 25, 50, 75, and 100 ml. The results of this experiment indicated that the bladder constrained by the nylon Velcro band is not inextensible but instead expands with pressure over the monitoring cycle. The edges and corners of the bladder that are not constrained by the cuff may move and make additional volume available. The actual volume change of the air in the bladder δV_x resulting from the expansion of the cuff is defined by:

$$\delta V_x = \delta V - \delta V_c \tag{5}$$

where δV is the volume change applied to the cuff.

The ratio of $\delta V_x / \delta V$ varies with mean cuff pressures and injected volumes.[13] The extrapolations of the measurements to $p_c \rightarrow 0$ lead to $\delta V_x = \delta V$, and even at high cuff pressures the expansion is still present but to a lesser degree as the bladder becomes stiffer. The fact that wrapping an inextensible band around the cuff does not change the results suggests that end effects, not the stretching of the bladder, are the dominant factors. This observation suggests that the sensitivity of the PVR may be considerably improved by designing a cuff that absorbs all the limb volume change.

Clinical practice has indicated that improved sensitivity is not necessary; slightly modified blood pressure cuffs are adequate. Including the results of the preceding experiment, equation 4 is rewritten as:

$$\delta p_c = \frac{-\gamma \delta V \left(1 - \dfrac{\delta V_x}{\delta V}\right)}{\left[\dfrac{(P_{ATM}/\bar{p}_c [V_1 + V_1 + V_2] - V_2)}{\bar{p}_c}\right]} \tag{6}$$

Equation 6 defines the relationship of limb volume change (δV) and cuff pressure change (δp_c).

It is of interest to continue the analysis and define the relationship of cuff pressure to arterial pressure. The volume changes of the limb caused by the passage of the pressure pulse are proportional to the changes in the arterial volume δV_a encompassed by the cuff. This has been shown to be true, even in the edematous limb. Therefore:

$$\delta V = \delta V_a = C_a \delta p_a \tag{7}$$

where $C_a = \delta V_a / \delta p_a$ is the compliance of the arterial section surrounded by the cuff and p_a denotes the arterial pressure. Combining equations 6 and 7:

$$\delta p_c = \frac{\gamma C_a \delta p_a \left(1 - \dfrac{\delta V_x}{\delta V}\right)}{\left[\dfrac{(P_{ATM}/\bar{p}_c [V_1 + V_1 + V_2] - V_2)}{\bar{p}_c}\right]} \tag{8}$$

Since $\delta V_x / \delta V$ is approximately independent of δV, it follows from equation 8 that if C_a remains constant, the variations in the cuff pressure are proportional to the variations in arterial pressure and the output of the pressure-sensitive transistor will yield a good representation of the arterial pressure-pulse contour. The critical experiment to test the accuracy of this analysis is the comparison with direct intraarterial measurements. This comparison has been made with excellent correlation and is provided in Chapter 59.

DIAGNOSTIC INDICES

A number of important diagnostic parameters are contained in the pulse volume recordings.

The amplitude of the pulse volume recording with a constant pneumatic and electronic gain is a function of local pulse pressure, segmental arterial compliance, and the number of arterial vessels in the segment under investigation. These are all affected by the development of arteriosclerotic disease. Reduced pulse pressure and obliterated arterial channels are major hemodynamic parameters that affect functional perfusion.

Because the pulse volume contour is linked to the pressure-pulse contour (equation 8), the shape of the pulse volume contour contains useful hemodynamic information. Contour alterations are largely the result of changes in terminal reflection coefficients, which are a function of peripheral resistance. Peripheral resistance changes to compensate for fixed arterial resistance caused by obstructive lesions. This phenomenon has been previously described.[13,15]

CONCLUSION

This section has described the engineering development and mechanics of the PVR; its clinical application to arterial peripheral vascular disease is outlined in Chapter 59.

THE PHLEBORHEOGRAPH
John J. Cranley

Basically, four types of plethysmographs have been developed—those using water or air and, more recently, instruments using the photoelectric cell[11] or the mercury-in-rubber strain gauge.[17] The advantage of the water plethysmograph is its great accuracy in transmitting both volume and pressure changes. The disadvantages are (1) the cumbersome nature of the devices, making them impractical for routine clinical use; (2) the hydrostatic effect of water, which may inhibit swelling of the part; and (3) the reflected waves that may sometimes be seen. The advantages of air plethysmography are that it is much more convenient to use and is generally simpler in construction. However, the air plethysmograph is subject to Boyle's law, which relates pressure, volume, and temperature of a gas in a closed system, making the system sensitive to changes in temperature. The photoelectric cell cannot be calibrated volumetrically. This is also true of the mercury-in-rubber strain gauge, but this instrument is capable of measuring changes in limb circumference, which can be mathematically related to volume change in the encircled part.

The air plethysmograph is presented in this section. In the absolute sense, there cannot be a volume change in a closed system without a pressure change and vice versa. Nevertheless, the terms *pressure gauge* and *volume gauge* are useful to describe transducing devices that approach the theoretical ideal for measurement of pressure or volume changes. Thus an ideal pressure transducer would have a rigid diaphragm that is displaced to the smallest possible degree, reflecting pressure changes without corresponding volume changes. On the other hand, the true volume transducer must have a diaphragm that moves with the smallest possible pressure. Fig. 23-2 is a clinical example demonstrating these differences. The tracings are of a normal subject on whose finger an oncometer was placed. The digital pulse was recorded by two different transducers, using air followed by water transmission. In Fig. 23-2, *A*, the digital pulse is shown as recorded by the Statham P 23 AA transducer, an excellent pressure transducer. After the tracing was completed, the gauge was filled with water without moving the cup on the fingertip. There is a tremendous increase in amplification at maximum, 15 times that of air transmission (Fig. 23-2, *B*).

In Fig. 23-2, *C*, the water has been drained and the tubing from this cup attached to the Grass PT 5 volume transducer. In Fig. 23-2, *D*, this gauge has been filled with water. There is minimal difference between the tracing of the finger in air and in water with the volume transducer. This transducer

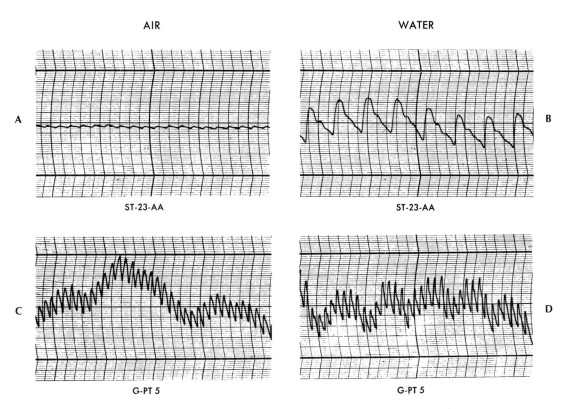

AIR   WATER

A   ST-23-AA   B   ST-23-AA

C   G-PT 5   D   G-PT 5

Fig. 23-2. **A,** Digital pulse of a normal subject recorded by Statham P 23 AA transducer using air transmission. **B,** Digital pulse recorded by Statham P 23 transducer using water transmission. Note the fifteen-fold increase in amplification compared with that in **A. D,** Digital pulse recorded by Grass PT 5 transducer using water transmission. Note the minimal increase in amplification compared with that in **C.**

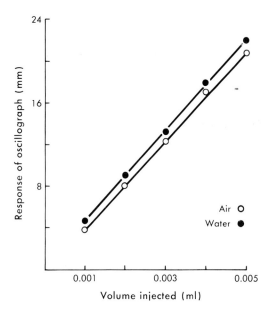

Fig. 23-3. Response of Grass PT 5 volume transducer to injection of minute amounts of air and water. Note the minimal variations. This gauge is an accurate volumetric transducer.

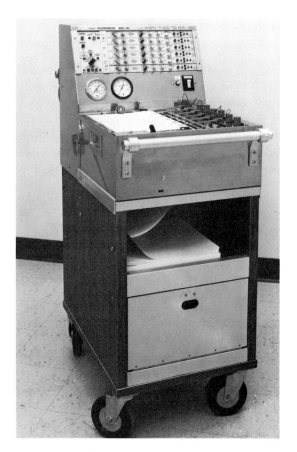

Fig. 23-4. Phleborheograph.

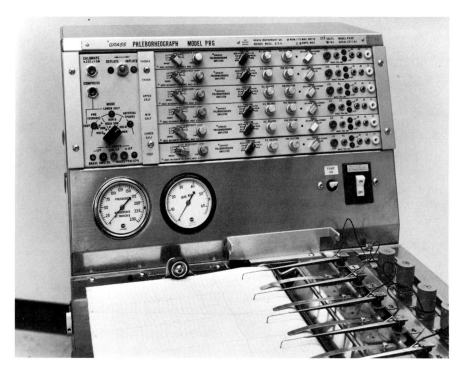

Fig. 23-5. Console of a phleborheograph.

comes close to the ideal volumetric transducer, which would give the same recording in air or water. Fig. 23-3 indicates the response of this gauge to injection of minute amounts of air and water. For all practical purposes, the response to air is similar to the response to water, and thus this volumetric transducer is accurate. With such a transducer, air plethysmography becomes practical, accurate, and convenient to use.

One study of the use of the air plethysmograph in the noninvasive diagnosis of deep vein thrombosis (DVT) was begun using the research polygraph and the Grass PT 5 volumetric transducer in conjunction with segmental pressure cuffs. This instrumentation was considered to be too sophisticated for widespread clinical use. Consequently, the manufacturer was asked to design an instrument that would be practical, convenient to use, and easy to master. The instrument progressed through several model changes before the design was considered acceptable for marketing. This final model is called the *phleborheograph* (Figs. 23-4 to 23-6). The results obtained with the polygraph and the phleborheograph are identical, suggesting that the phleborheograph is qualitatively equal to the research polygraph for

these purposes, although it is greatly simplified for use by technicians.

During the developmental period, two, four, and finally six channels were used. When two or four channels were used, the necessity of manually changing the cuffs repeatedly and recalibrating after each change unduly prolonged the test and made it more complex. The use of six channels makes it possible to apply all the cuffs at once, calibrate all of them simultaneously, and run the test without interruption. It is desirable to have all the changes in the limb recorded simultaneously, with respiratory movements measured directly from the thorax. This permits easy detection of breath-holding, exaggerated breathing, Cheyne-Stokes respiration, or sudden changes in respiratory movement in the nervous patient. Even though most patients report that the application of pressure is painless, occasionally a patient will take a quick breath each time pressure is applied. If this were not apparent in the respiratory tracing, the examiner may be misled by the significance of the sudden rise in baseline on application of pressure.

Lower extremity technique

The first channel records directly from the thorax. The cuff for the second channel is placed on the thigh just above the knee. Three cuffs are placed in close proximity to each other on the proximal lower leg. The sixth cuff is placed on the foot. The first four channels record only the volume changes. The fifth and sixth channels are alternately used to record volume change or to apply pressure to the limb. Thus when the sixth cuff is being used to apply pressure to the foot, the fifth cuff as well as all those above it are recording volumetric changes. Similarly, when the fifth cuff is being used to apply pressure to the calf, the sixth cuff records volumetric changes in the foot. The cuffs used are all currently available blood pressure cuffs. The strap of the chest cuff has been lengthened to permit its use around the epigastrium. The cuff encircling the upper thigh has also been lengthened. A cuff approximately twice as wide as the others for the foot is currently used by some physicians.

After the cuffs have been applied, an automatic inflation sequence that fills the cuffs until 10 mm Hg pressure is obtained is activated to ensure an adequate coupling between the cuff and the limb. A monitor lamp and a pressure gauge on the instrument panel indicate the inflation process. An additional lamp turns on when proper recording pressure has been reached. A paper speed of 2.5 mm/sec is usually selected for the phleborheogram. For pulse tracings a 25 mm/sec paper speed is used.

Calibration is volumetric. When the calibrating button is depressed, 0.2 ml of air is removed from each recording cuff. Amplification is adjusted so that the 0.2 ml of air results in a 2 cm downward deflection of the recording pen. By calibrating before each recording, the examiner can compare the magnitude of the respiratory waves, the emptying of the foot, or the amplitude of the digital pulses accurately when the test is recorded at different periods of time and on different subjects.

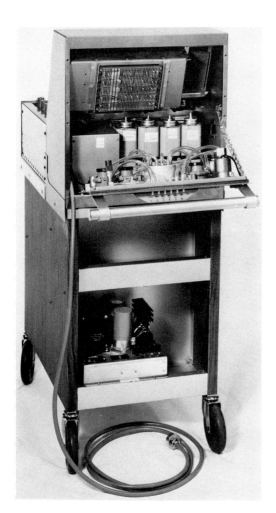

Fig. 23-6. Rear view of a phleborheograph.

Foot compression. There are two recording modes. With the selector switch on *Run A,* the sixth cuff is used for application of pressure to the foot, and all the other cuffs record volume changes. During the first period of the tracing the technician merely observes the respiratory waves and then presses the *Compress* button. This delivers three short bursts of air to the sixth cuff. Currently, 100 mm Hg is applied for approximately 0.5 seconds at intervals of 0.5 seconds. This pressure is monitored by a pressure gauge on the instrument panel and is measured at the source in the instrument. Approximately half this pressure is lost in the airway, and only 50 mm Hg pressure is delivered to the foot. This is not uncomfortable for the patient. In the normal subject, the baseline values of the tracings of the limb remain level despite the application of pressure to the foot. In the patient with DVT, compression of the foot cuff will cause congestion of blood in the limb and a rise in the baseline of the tracing.

The baseline elevation has been redefined by Comerota et al.[2] The *absolute baseline* is defined as a plot of points connecting the minimum volume of each respiratory wave, and the *dynamic baseline* represents the normal volume of the extremity that is expected at any point during the respiratory wave. (See Chapter 96 for further discussion on the diagnosis of DVT of the extremities.)

Calf compression. At the completion of *Run A,* the cuffs are deflated and the mode switch moved to *Run B.* The cuffs are reinflated, and the calibration is repeated. At the time when the *Compress* button is pressed, pressure is applied to the lower calf. In this case, 50 mm Hg is used as the source pressure, and approximately 30 mm Hg is delivered to the calf of the patient. Compression of the calf causes a rise in the baseline of the proximal tracings if there is obstruction of venous outflow. In addition, in the normal subject, compression of the calf produces some degree of emptying of the foot, which is lessened or absent in the presence of DVT.

Ankle compression. While still in the *Run B* mode, the midcalf cuff (no. 5) is moved to ankle level and is used to deliver compressions. Cuffs 1 through 4 and 6 are used for recording as they are during calf compression *(Run B₁).* Compressions are identical to those used in *Run B₁* with regard to timing, duration, and pressure.

Once again, emptying of the foot is observed as in *Run B₁.* Unlike *Run B₁,* however, the midcalf recording does not usually fall. The baseline of this recording cuff and the others remains level. If there is obstruction to venous outflow, a rise in baseline occurs. In addition, foot emptying may be reduced or absent.

Upper extremity technique

Certain modifications are necessary to record volume changes in the upper extremity. Recording cuffs are placed around the thorax, upper arm, and upper and middle forearm, along with a compression cuff on the wrist. The mode selector is turned to *Run B* and the wrist cuff is rapidly inflated to 50 mm Hg, producing compressions that pump the blood proximally. The proximal arm cuffs record any changes in volume that occur at rest or with these volume challenges. In the upper extremity, respiratory waves can persist despite complete venous occlusion, probably because of rich venous collaterals around the shoulder. Therefore a diagnosis of upper extremity deep venous occlusion is usually based on the presence or absence of baseline rise alone.[16] (Results are reported in Chapter 99.)

A six-position *Function* switch on each phleborheograph amplifier adjusts the frequency response of the system to enhance the recording as desired. The *Resp* position enables the technician to effectively filter out the pulse waves and record only the respiratory waves.

The *PRG* position provides frequency response so that pulses and respiratory waves are recorded. In the *Pulse* position the respiratory waves are filtered, and amplification is automatically increased fivefold to detail the pulse contour.

The *ECG* position provides a high-frequency response suitable for reproducing the electrocardiogram, should that be desired. A special ECG amplifier can be obtained to facilitate the ECG recording. Two DC positions are provided to facilitate Doppler studies.

An input receptacle that permits the use of special photoelectric transducers for recording pulsations in the fingertip, the ear, or the supraorbital area is included. This receptacle also accepts a unidirectional or bidirectional Doppler velocity detector.

There has been a recent modification of the phleborheo-

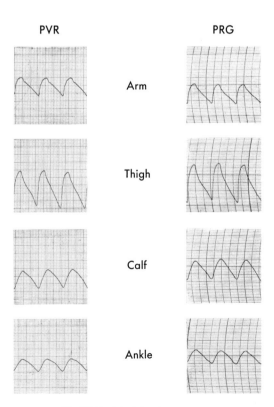

Fig. 23-7. Arterial pulse waves.

graph to make it more convenient to measure arterial pulsation. Because it measures volume changes accurately, the original phleborheograph was not convenient for measurement of arterial pulsations. The reason for this is that there are two volumetric changes occurring in the normal limb at all times. One is the amplitude of the arterial pulsation, which is what the examiner wishes to measure, and the other is the change in volume of the limb as a result of respiration, which causes the baseline to be unstable. This instability can be controlled by application of sufficient pressure to the proximal thigh to eliminate the respiratory waves.

The phleborheograph has been altered to do this. The recording cuff pressure is automatically set to 50 mm Hg, and the amplifiers are set to display the arterial pulses. This combination effectively filters out the respiratory waves. The arterial pulse waves recorded are comparable to those obtained by other pulse volume records (Fig. 23-7). This change enables the investigator to record from up to six sites simultaneously. The built-in volume calibrator used in the venous mode is also used in the arterial mode.

Other attachments make it possible to record segmental pressures on the phleborheograph by superimposing the arterial pulse, sensed by the Doppler ultrasound flow detector, on the cuff pressure waveform.

Finally, it is possible to assess the pulsatility of the arterial waves in the rectum and sigmoid for determination of the patency of the inferior mesenteric and hypogastric arteries with a rectal probe (Fig. 23-8, *B*).

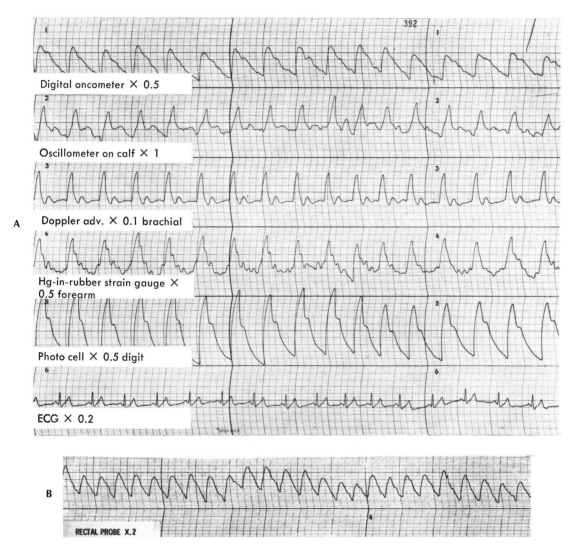

Fig. 23-8. A, Extended uses of phleborheograph. In line 1, it is being used as a digital plethysmograph with a finger oncometer. With this mechanism, the examiner can measure the amplitude of the digital pulses and relate them to the size of the enclosed finger by the water-displacement method. This may also be used to measure blood flow by the venous occlusion method. In line 2, the phleborheograph is being used in *pulse* position to record the oscillations of the calf. In line 3, it is connected to the bidirectional Doppler velocity detector with blood flowing toward the probe. In line 4, the phleborheograph is being used with a mercury-in-rubber strain gauge recording the oscillations of a limb. In line 5, it is being used with a photocell placed on the fingertip. In line 6, it is being used with an ECG module. **B,** Rectal probe in use to assess the patency of the inferior mesenteric and hypogastric arteries.

Fig. 23-8, *A* is a tracing of some of the extended uses of the phleborheograph. In the first line it is being used as a digital plethysmograph with a finger oncometer. With this mechanism the examiner can measure the amplitude of the digital pulses and relate them to the size of the enclosed finger by the water displacement method. This may also be used to measure blood flow by the venous occlusion method. The second tracing is that of the phleborheograph being used in the *Pulse* position. This setting permits the clinician to analyze pulse waves visually and measure the amplitude of the pulse wave volumetrically. The third line is a Doppler tracing with the blood flowing toward the probe in the foot, and the fourth line is a mercury-in-rubber strain-gauge tracing. The fifth line is the tracing of a digital pulse recording with a photoelectric transducer. On the sixth line an ECG module is in use. Fig. 23-8, *B* shows the rectal probe in use to assess inferior mesenteric and hypogastric arteries.

If desired, the equipment can be used to detect venous occlusion by the maximum venous outflow method (Fig. 23-9). One or more channels may be used for recording the maximum venous outflow.

The maximum calibrated sensitivity of the phleborheograph in the *PRG* mode is 0.25 ml for full-scale pen deflection, or 50 mm. In the *Pulse* mode, sensitivity is increased to 0.05 ml full scale. With the sensitivity controls at maximum the overall system sensitivity can be increased to approximately 0.15 ml full scale in *PRG* mode and 0.03 ml full scale in the *Pulse* mode. Circuitry is also provided to facilitate connection to tape recorders and computers.

During the past 12 years, more than 27,000 lower extremities have been studied at Good Samaritan Hospital,[2-8] using first the research polygraph, then the earlier models, and finally the phleborheograph. It has been possible to obtain phlebograms on 748 extremities also studied with the phleborheograph. These results (reported in Chapter 96) have been closely duplicated by others using the same technique.

The phleborheograph is an instrument specifically designed for the noninvasive diagnosis of DVT of the lower extremity. A modified technique is used for upper extremity diagnosis. It employs state-of-the-art electronics to achieve high sensitivity, is calibrated volumetrically after the cuffs have been applied to the patient, and delivers a uniform stimulus to all extremities, simultaneously recording with six channels. It is highly versatile and may be used as an amplifier and direct-writing recorder for digital plethysmography or as a recording oscillometer. It may be used with the Doppler velocity detector, the mercury-in-rubber

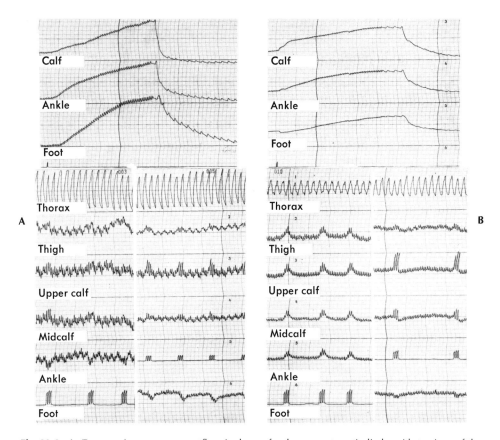

Fig. 23-9. A, *Top,* maximum venous outflow is shown for the asymptomatic limb, with tracings of the calf, ankle, and foot. *Bottom,* phleborheogram of the same asymptomatic limb. **B,** *Top,* maximum venous outflow of a patient with DVT involving the femoroiliac area. *Bottom,* phleborheogram of the same limb.

strain gauge, a photoelectric transducer, an ECG module, or a rectal probe. It is portable and of rugged construction, can be moved freely about the hospital, and is modular to permit easy servicing.

ACKNOWLEDGMENT

Throughout the developmental period of phleborheographic technique and instrumentation, consultation has been sought with F.A. Simeone, M.D., and A.M. Grass, Sc.D., on a continuing and active basis.

In addition, the following former and present Kachelmacher Research Fellows in Venous Diseases at Good Samaritan Hospital, Cincinnati, have all actively participated in and made significant contributions to the development of the phleborheograph: A.Y. Gay, Logan, Ohio; W.J. Sull, Sedalia, Missouri; A.J. Canos, Cincinnati; K. Mahalingam, Cincinnati; E.B. Ferris, Honolulu; S.L. House, Quincy, Illinois; A.J. Comerota, Temple University, Philadelphia; S.E. Cook, Bangor, Maine; L.J. Hyland, Dayton, Ohio; P.J. Sipple, Manitowoc, Wisconsin; E.D. Sullivan, New Haven, Connecticut; L.D. Flanagan and W.S. Karkow, Kachelmacher Memorial Laboratory for Venous Diseases, Good Samaritan Hospital, Cincinnati.

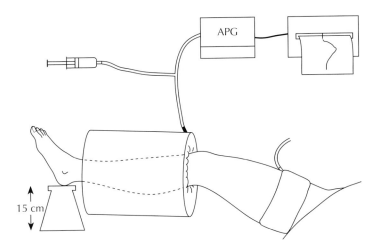

Fig. 23-10. Representation of the APG showing the venous occlusive cuff in the upper thigh position for the measurement of outflow fraction in venous disease.

QUANTITATIVE AIR PLETHYSMOGRAPHY
Nikos Labropoulos, Nicos Voltens, Miguel Leon, and Andrew N. Nicolaides

The plethysmographic methods described so far are segmental and quantitative. Quantitative air plethysmography (APG) has three advantages: it can involve the whole leg, it can express volume changes in absolute units, and it avoids tissue shifts inherent to segmental plethysmography, resulting in a higher reproducibility.

APPLICATIONS
Venous disease

The APG consists of a 35 cm long polyurethane air chamber (5 L capacity) that surrounds the whole leg and is connected to a pressure transducer, amplifier, and recorder (Fig. 23-10). The patient lies in the supine position with the knee of the leg being examined slightly flexed and elevated with the heel placed on a support 15 cm above the horizontal; the air chamber is inflated to 6 mm Hg.

Calibration is performed by depressing the plunger of the syringe (Fig. 23-10), compressing the air in the air plethysmograph (air chamber and tubing), reducing the volume of the air by 100 ml, and observing the corresponding pressure change. When the pressure in the air chamber returns to 6 mm Hg and calibration is complete, the plunger is pulled back to its original position.

The pressure of 6 mm Hg has been selected because it is the lowest pressure that ensures good contact between the air chamber and the limb, with minimum compression of the veins. Tissue movements during changes in posture and exercise are unlikely to interfere with the measurements

because the air chamber includes almost all the tissues from the knee to the ankle. The air plethysmograph is calibrated in milliliters so that consecutive measurements in the same limb are not influenced by changes in tissue volume because of increasing or decreasing edema.

Elevation of the leg results in emptying of the venous system, and when the patient stands, the refilling rate can be measured in milliliters per second and the total venous volume can be measured in milliliters. When the patient performs a tiptoe movement, the ejected volume and ejection fraction can be determined. Also, performance of 10 tiptoe movements allows the residual volume and residual volume fraction to be determined. With the patient in the horizontal resting position, the outflow in milliliter per second and outflow fraction can be measured for different thigh cuff occlusive pressures. (The technical and practical details with normal and abnormal values are discussed in Chapters 99 and 112.)

Arterial disease

Leg blood flow is measured with venous occlusion. The patient lies in the supine position with the knee of the leg being examined slightly flexed and the heel on a support, 15 cm in height as in the technique for APG in venous disease. The air chamber is inflated to 6 mm Hg. This pressure has been selected because it is the lowest pressure that ensures good contact between the air chamber and the limb, with minimum compression of the veins. Calibration is performed by depressing the plunger of the syringe (Fig. 23-11), increasing the volume of the air in the air chamber and tubing by 100 ml, and observing the corresponding pressure change. After the calibration, the plunger is pulled back to its original position when the pressure in the air chamber returns to 6 mm Hg. An 11 cm wide pneumatic tourniquet, with a bladder 40 cm long is placed just proximal to the knee and is connected to a manometer (Fig. 23-11).

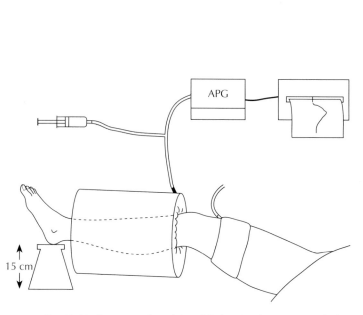

Fig. 23-11. Representation of the APG showing the venous occlusive cuff just proximal to the knee for the measurement of arterial inflow.

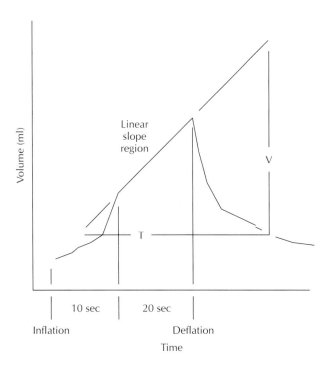

Fig. 23-12. Method of calculating the arterial inflow from the plethysmographic recording (arterial inflow = V/T).

About 10 minutes after the air chamber is inflated, when a stable leg/air chamber/room temperature gradient has been achieved and resting arterial inflow in the leg is ensured, the tourniquet is inflated *rapidly* to 50 mm Hg. An increase in leg volume is recorded for 20 seconds, and the tourniquet is then deflated. The increase in volume represents the arterial inflow to the limb. The rate of the latter can be calculated from the slope of the volume recording in milliliters per minute (Fig. 23-12). Reproducibility studies have demonstrated a coefficient of variation in the range of 3.2% to 7.6%.[1] (Chapter 60 describes the practical clinical use of APG in arterial disease.)

REFERENCES

1. Christopoulos D et al: Venous hypertensive microangiopathy in relation to clinical severity and effect of elastic compression, *J Dermatol Surg Oncol* 17:809-813, 1991.
2. Comerota AJ et al: Phleborheography—results of a ten-year experience, *Surgery* 91:573, 1982.
3. Cranley JJ: Phleborheology, *RI Med J* 58(3):111, 1975.
4. Cranley JJ: *Vascular surgery 2: peripheral venous diseases*, New York, 1975, Harper and Row.
5. Cranley JJ: *Phleborheography.* In Kempczinski RF, Yao JST, eds: *Practical noninvasive vascular diagnosis,* Chicago, 1982, Mosby.
6. Cranley JJ, Canos AJ, Mahalingam K: *Noninvasive diagnosis and prophylaxis of deep venous thrombosis of the lower extremities.* In Madden JL, Hume M, eds: *Venous thrombosis: prevention and treatment,* New York, 1976, Appleton-Century-Crofts.
7. Cranley JJ et al: A plethysmographic technique for the diagnosis of deep venous thrombosis of the lower extremities, *Surg Gynecol Obstet* 136:385, 1973.
8. Cranley JJ et al: Phleborheographic technique for diagnosing deep venous thrombosis of the lower extremities, *Surg Gynecol Obstet* 141:331, 1975.
9. Darling RC et al: Quantitative segmental pulse volume recorder: a clinical tool, *Surgery* 72:873, 1972.
10. Geddes LA: *The direct and indirect measurements of blood pressure,* Chicago, 1970, Mosby.
11. Herzman AB: Photoelectric plethysmography of fingers and toes in man, *Proc Soc Exp Biol Med* 37:529, 1937.
12. Pitran specifications, 1969, Hudson, Mass, Stow Laboratories.
13. Raines JK: *Diagnosis and analysis of arteriosclerosis in the lower limbs from the arterial pressure pulse,* doctoral dissertation, Cambridge, Mass, 1972, Massachusetts Institute of Technology.
14. Raines JK, Jaffrin MY, Rao S: A noninvasive pressure-pulse recorder: development and rationale, *Med Instrum* 7:245, 1973.
15. Raines JK, Jaffrin MY, Shapiro AH: A computer simulation of arterial dynamics in the human leg, *J Biomech* 7:77, 1974.
16. Sullivan ED, Reece CI, Cranley JJ: Phleborheography of the upper extremity, *Arch Surg* 118:1134, 1983.
17. Whitney RJ: Measurement of volume changes in human limbs, *J Physiol (Lond)* 121:1, 1953.
18. Winsor T et al: Peripheral pulse contours in arterial occlusive disease, *Vasc Dis* 5:61, 1968.

CHAPTER 24

Vascular imaging

CHRISTOPHER R.B. MERRITT

Although duplex Doppler and, more recently, Doppler color imaging (DCI) have made it possible to determine the presence or absence of flow, flow direction, flow velocity, and the character of the flow in peripheral, abdominal, and pelvic arteries and veins, Doppler represents only a part of the contribution of ultrasound in vascular diagnosis. Features of the vessels themselves and of abnormalities, including thrombus and plaque, are often as important as, and in some cases even more important than, flow characteristics. Ultrasound imaging thus plays a key role in vascular evaluation and the identification of abnormalities. In this chapter, key principles of vascular imaging are reviewed.

As with Doppler, quality imaging necessitates the understanding of basic principles and their application. Special skills in performance and interpretation of the imaging examination are required, and pitfalls await the careless or poorly trained user. Effective use of ultrasound in vascular diagnosis requires mastery of techniques to produce high-quality images. This in turn requires an understanding of the nature of ultrasound information and the methods and instruments used in its production. Artifacts and the limitations of ultrasound must be considered, along with the advantages and disadvantages of alternative approaches, and the user must have knowledge of sectional anatomy and the sonographic patterns of normal and abnormal findings necessary to establish a diagnosis. Finally, mastery of technology must be matched by clinical skills so that the sonographic findings are related to the clinical problem under evaluation.

BASIC PRINCIPLES OF ULTRASOUND IMAGING

Accurate interpretation of ultrasound images requires an understanding of the interaction of ultrasound with structures within the body as well as knowledge of the way anatomy and pathology are displayed with ultrasound. Currently, all forms of clinical diagnostic ultrasound are based on backscattered information (echoes) from interfaces within the body. Simply defined, *ultrasound* is a high-frequency mechanical vibration that passes through tissue as a pressure wave. Clinical ultrasound uses frequencies in the range of 1 to 10 MHz (1,000,000 to 10,000,000 million cycles per second), although some new intraluminal trans-

ducers are capable of operating at frequencies as high as 50 to 60 MHz. In general, frequencies used for ultrasound imaging are somewhat higher than those used for Doppler. The pressure waves produced by an ultrasound transducer travel at a velocity determined by the nature of the propagating medium. In soft tissues, the average velocity of sound propagation is approximately 1540 m/sec, although certain tissues have propagation velocities significantly less than (e.g., aerated lung and fat) or greater than (e.g., bone) those of soft tissues.

Although some ultrasound applications use a continuous ultrasound wave (e.g., continuous wave Doppler), imaging requires pulsed ultrasound. With pulsed ultrasound, the transducer introduces a series of brief bursts of acoustical energy into the body; each pulse typically consists of about three cycles. The product of the wavelength and the number of cycles in the pulse determines the pulse length, and this in turn defines the maximum resolution along the beam axis (axial resolution) (Fig. 24-1). Axial resolution is important for imaging because it determines the smallest structure that may be imaged with a given instrument and transducer. For example, a transducer operating at 5.0 MHz produces sound with a wavelength of 0.308 mm. If each pulse consists of three cycles of sound, the pulse length is slightly less than 1.0 mm, and this becomes the maximum resolution along

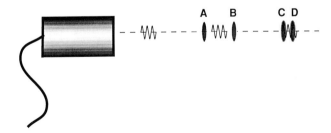

Fig. 24-1. Axial resolution. The pulse length (the wavelength times the number of cycles in the pulse) determines the maximum resolution of objects lying along the beam axis. Targets *A* and *B* are separated by a distance greater than the pulse length and will be resolved in the image as two separate structures. Targets *C* and *D* are separated by a distance less than the pulse length and will appear in the image as a single object.

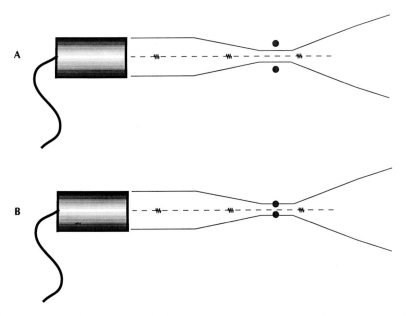

Fig. 24-2. Lateral resolution. The width of the ultrasound beam determines the maximum resolution of objects side by side in the plane perpendicular to the axis of the beam. With most transducers, focusing is used to maximize lateral resolution at a selected depth from the transducer. **A,** The width of the beam in the focal zone is less than the distance between the targets, permitting both objects to be imaged as separate structures. **B,** The distance between the targets is less than the width of the beam, and only a single object will be displayed in the image.

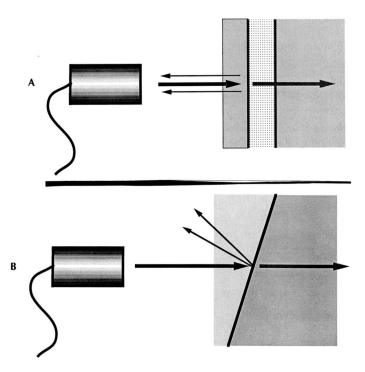

Fig. 24-3. Specular reflector. If the reflector lies near 90° to the path of the ultrasound beam **(A),** most of the reflected sound will return to the transducer. With smaller angles of incidence **(B),** the sound is reflected but little of the reflected sound returns to the transducer.

the beam axis. Image resolution is determined by not only the axial dimension of the ultrasound pulse but also the width and thickness of the ultrasound beam (lateral and elevation resolution) (Fig. 24-2). These beam characteristics are determined by the construction of the transducer and the focusing of the beam. Lateral and elevation resolution are typically less than the axial dimension of the beam. When maximal resolution is needed (as in the characterization of plaque), a high-frequency transducer with excellent focal characteristics at the depth of the plaque is required.

Reflection of sound occurs at boundaries of tissues or propagating media that have different acoustical properties. The most important properties affecting the amount of sound reflected or transmitted at a tissue boundary are the propagation velocities of sound in the adjacent media and the physical densities of the media. These parameters determine the acoustical impedance of the tissues. The greater the difference in the adjacent acoustical impedances, the greater the reflecting property of the boundary. The amount of sound reflected back to the transducer is a function of several additional properties of the reflector. If the target is smooth and large compared to the wavelength of the ultrasound used, it will behave like a mirror; such interfaces are called *specular reflectors*. A specular interface reflects sound back to the transducer only if the reflector lies near 90° to the path of the ultrasound beam. In vascular imaging, most vessel walls act as specular reflectors and are optimally imaged when insonated at angles near 90° (Fig. 24-3, *A*). With smaller angles of incidence, the sound is reflected, but

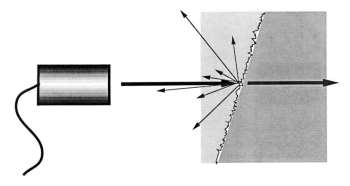

Fig. 24-4. Diffuse reflector. If the reflecting surface is irregular, there is scattering of the incident sound in many directions. Even with low incident angles, some of the sound returns to the transducer.

little of the reflected sound returns to the transducer (Fig. 24-3, *B*). Because most vessel walls behave as specular reflectors, conflicting conditions exist for optimal vessel imaging and Doppler evaluation. Imaging requires an angle of insonation near 90°, whereas Doppler requires a small angle between the sound beam and the vessel. Not all targets important in imaging are specular reflectors. Tissues, thrombus, and plaque present much smaller interfaces. When the size of the target is near the wavelength of the sound used or when the reflecting surface is irregular, there will be diffuse scattering of the incident sound. A portion of this is backscattered to the transducer and processed to provide an image (Fig. 24-4).

IMAGE DISPLAY MODES

Over the years, methods for presentation of information contained in the backscattered ultrasound signal have evolved from a simple A-mode display to high-resolution gray-scale imaging. A brief review of the features of each of these methods is appropriate to explain how current ultrasound imaging is accomplished. The backscattered ultrasound information may be processed and displayed in several ways. Thus the diagnostic image may range from a simple oscilloscope display showing the distance of a reflecting structure from the transducer (A-mode display) to a high-resolution, two-dimensional image of organs and tissue (two-dimensional B-mode), which may be shown with motion (two-dimensional real-time imaging or two-dimensional echo).

A-mode ultrasound

A-mode display is primarily of historical interest. With A-mode instrumentation, the backscattered echo is displayed as a vertical deflection on the face of an oscilloscope. The horizontal sweep of the oscilloscope indicates the time interval from the transmission of the ultrasound pulse until the return of the echo. The velocity of sound in living tissue is relatively constant, with an average value of 1540 m/sec. Therefore half the time from the initial pulse until the echo returns is the time for the sound to travel from the transducer

to the reflecting interface. The distance from the transducer to the reflecting surface can be estimated with reasonable accuracy by multiplying this time by the average velocity of sound in tissue (1540 m/sec). In this form of display the strength or amplitude of the reflected sound is indicated by the height of the vertical deflection displayed on the oscilloscope. With A-mode ultrasound, only the position and strength of a reflecting structure are recorded.

Original applications of A-mode ultrasound were for echoencephalography and as an adjunct to B-scanning in measurement and in differentiating cystic from solid masses. The A-mode display provides a dynamic presentation of the position of the reflecting interfaces in real-time and may be used as an aid in selecting sampling sites for M-mode ultrasound. The major limitation of A-mode ultrasound is that the image is essentially one dimensional and provides limited anatomic information. Interpretation of an A-mode signal therefore requires precise knowledge of the location of the tissue or object being interrogated to obtain reliable results.

M-mode ultrasound

M-mode ultrasound is used to display changes in position of reflecting structures with respect to time. M-mode displays echo amplitude and shows the position of moving reflectors. In contrast to A-mode display, in which vertical deflection of an oscilloscope tracing is used to show echo amplitude, M-mode uses the brightness of the display to indicate the relative intensity of the reflected signal. The time base of the display can be adjusted to allow for varying degrees of temporal resolution as dictated by clinical application. M-mode ultrasound was the first means of providing dynamic visualization of anatomy. A major shortcoming of M-mode display is the limiting of the field of view to the profile of the ultrasound beam. Only a small area can be interrogated at one time, and the examiner must assemble the information gathered into a composite view of the structures of interest. M-mode ultrasound is interpreted by assessing motion patterns of specific structures and determining anatomic relationships from characteristic patterns of motion. The sites for M-mode examination are limited to areas where useful anatomic landmarks can be identified. Because it portrays only the position, amplitude, and dynamics of interfaces along the essentially one-dimensional beam path, M-mode is incapable of showing shape or anatomy. M-mode is generally limited to identification of motion along the axis of the beam only and cannot evaluate motion in other directions. This limits evaluation of structures with complex three-dimensional motion. Today, the major application of M-mode display is in the evaluation of rapid motion, including valves, cardiac chamber, and vessel wall motion.

B-mode, two-dimensional, and real-time ultrasound

B-mode display uses variations in display intensity or brightness to indicate backscattered signals of differing strength. When an ultrasound image is displayed on a black background, signals of greatest intensity appear as white, absent signals are shown as black, and signals of intermediate intensity appear as shades of gray. If the ultrasound beam is moved with respect to the object being examined and the position of the reflected signal is stored, a two-dimensional image results, with the brightest portions of the display indicating structures reflecting more of the transmitted sound energy back to the transducer. Currently, most ultrasound imaging applications use this two-dimensional form of B-mode display. Since B-mode display relates the strength of a backscattered signal to a brightness level on the display device (usually a video display monitor), the operator should understand how the amplitude information in the ultrasound signal is translated into a brightness scale in the image display. Each ultrasound manufacturer offers several options for the way the dynamic range of the target is compressed for display as well as the way the transfer function assigns a given signal amplitude to a shade of gray. Although these technical details vary among machines, the way they are used (or abused) by the operator of the scanner may have a profound impact on the clinical value of the final image.

Real-time two-dimensional B-mode ultrasound is now the major method for ultrasound imaging throughout the body and is the most common form of B-mode display. Real-time ultrasound permits assessment of both anatomy and motion. A rapid series of individual two-dimensional B-mode images is generated to produce the impression of motion. When images are acquired and displayed at rates of several times per second (typically 15 to 60), the effect is dynamic; because the image reflects the state and motion of the organ at the time it is examined, the information is regarded as being shown in real-time. In cardiac applications the term *two-dimensional echocardiography* or *two-dimensional echo* is used to describe real-time B-mode imaging; in most other applications, the term *real-time ultrasound* is used.

IMAGING TRANSDUCERS

Transducers currently in use for real-time imaging may be classified by the method used for steering the ultrasound beam and the technology used for focusing the ultrasound beam. Beam steering necessary for real-time imaging may be accomplished mechanically or electronically. Electronic beam steering is used in linear array and phased array transducers and permits a variety of image display formats. Mechanically steered transducers may use single element transducers with a fixed focus or annular arrays of elements with electronically controlled focusing. (A detailed description of beam steering is beyond the scope of this chapter but is found in the works of Kremkau[1] and Powis.[3])

For real-time imaging, transducers using mechanical or electronic beam steering generate display in a rectangular or pie-shaped format. The rectangular image display has the advantage of a larger field of view near the surface but requires a larger surface area for transducer contact. For peripheral vascular examinations, linear array transducers with a rectangular image format are often used. These arrays permit a relatively long segment of the vessel to be imaged. Since most peripheral vessels run parallel to the skin surface, such transducers provide an angle of near 90° between the ultrasound beam and the vessel wall and thus are well suited for imaging the vessel wall. Sector scanners with either mechanical or electronic steering require only a small surface area for contact and are well suited for examination in which access is limited by bone or gas, as in scanning in the upper abdomen. A limitation of the sector display is the restricted display of superficial structures where the wedge-shaped format narrows.

The ability to identify subtle features with ultrasound is a function of spatial and contrast resolution. As has been noted, spatial resolution is limited by axial and lateral resolution, with axial resolution determined by wavelength and pulse length. Lateral resolution depends on the beam width at the depth of interest and is determined by the focal characteristics of the transducer. Most electronically steered transducers currently in use provide electronic focusing adjustable for depth. A more subtle determinant of image quality is the beam width in the elevation or slice thickness plane. Poor resolution in the elevation plane is a problem with many phased array transducers and is probably one factor contributing to the variable success reported in the imaging characterization of carotid plaque.[2] Currently, only annular array transducers are capable of providing dynamic focusing in this dimension of the ultrasound beam.

Unlike A-mode and M-mode, two-dimensional ultrasound allows identification of the shape and anatomy of structures as well as resolution of motion in two planes rather than one. The interpretation of two-dimensional real-time ultrasound requires an understanding of the anatomy and sonographic characteristics of the structures being examined, as well as their normal patterns of motion. To this must be added a solid knowledge of examination techniques, artifacts, and instrumentation. Although two-dimensional frame rates are limited to 30 to 60 images per second, temporal resolution is seldom a major problem with current instruments. In terms of spatial resolution, two-dimensional instruments, like all other ultrasound devices, have limits of axial and lateral resolution imposed by the pulse length and the two-dimensional profile of the ultrasound beam.

IMAGING ARTIFACTS

Perhaps more than in any other imaging method, artifacts assume great clinical importance in ultrasound. Many imaging artifacts are induced by errors in scanning technique (such as failure to image at an acceptable angle) or instrument set up (excessive gain producing artificial echoes within a vessel causing it to be regarded as occluded or insufficient gain causing a thrombosed vessel to appear patent) and are thus preventable. The importance of artifacts in influencing interpretation is twofold: they may suggest the presence of structures that are not present, causing misdiagnosis, or they may obscure important findings. In addition, artifacts may alter the size, shape, or brightness of structures. Although artifacts generally are an impediment to accurate interpretation of an image, some may aid in diagnosis. Because an understanding of artifacts is so important in the correct interpretation of ultrasound examinations and because many artifacts can be prevented by careful imaging techniques, a review of the most important artifacts is appropriate. In general, artifacts that alter ultrasound interpretation may be classified as follows:

1. Artifacts that suggest the presence of structures not actually present
2. Artifacts that remove real echoes from the display or obscure information
3. Artifacts that distort the size, shape, or brightness of a structure (displacement of echoes on the display from their proper location)

The first type of artifacts results in the display of nonstructural echoes that may interfere with diagnosis and includes reverberation, refraction, side lobes, and speckle. Recognition of these artifacts is essential for accurate interpretation of the ultrasound study. Reverberation artifacts arise when the ultrasound signal reflects repeatedly between highly reflective interfaces that are usually but not always near the transducer. This type of problem is common in the abdomen where strong interfaces exist in gas pockets within the bowel. By generating a series of equally spaced false echoes deep to the real reflectors, reverberation causes the image to contain signals that are not related to structures present at the location where the signal is displayed. Reverberations may cause diagnostic problems by hiding important image features and obscuring significant findings. A second effect of reverberation is the introduction of echoes into areas where they would not normally occur. The echoes resulting from the reverberations may give the false impression of solid structures in areas where only fluid is present. Certain types of reverberation, such as the so-called comet tail artifact (a dense tapering trail of echoes just distal to a strongly reflecting structure), may be helpful by allowing the identification of a specific type of reflector, such as a surgical clip. Reverberation artifacts should be readily recognized by experienced examiners and can often be reduced or eliminated by changing the scanning angle or transducer placement to avoid the parallel interfaces that contribute to the artifact.

Refraction causes bending of the sound beam so that targets not along the axis of the transducer are insonated. Their reflections are then detected and displayed in the image. This may cause structures that actually lie outside the volume the investigator assumes is being examined to appear in the image. Similarly, side lobes may produce confusing echoes that arise from sound beams lying outside the main ultrasound beam. Even though the structures insonated by side lobes lie outside the main beam, echoes produced by the interaction of these structures with the side lobes may be displayed in the image as artifactual specular or diffuse reflectors. Echoes associated with side lobe artifacts are of clinical importance because they may create the impression of particulate debris in fluid-filled structures such as large vessels, aneurysms, and pseudoaneurysms. Side lobes may also result in errors of measurement by reducing lateral resolution. Side lobe artifacts are seen with all types of ultrasound equipment and have been noted to be a particular problem with phased array real-time devices. As with most other artifacts, repositioning the transducer and its focal zone or use of a different transducer usually allows differentiation of artifactual from true echoes. The apparent tissue textures seen near the transducer are the result of another important artifact suggesting the presence of structures that are not present. Called *speckle,* this artifact is not directly related to tissue texture but is a result of interference effects from the distribution of scatterers in the tissue. Speckle is formed by a phase-sensitive process in which the interference of echoes arriving at the transducer at the same time produces an image pattern that resembles tissue. This may be a quite subtle and deceptive artifact, making the superficial texture of organs such as the liver appear normal when an abnormality is actually present. By repositioning the transducer to position superficial areas in the focal zone, the examiner can reduce the effects of this artifact.

The second type of artifact is one that removes real echoes from the display or obscures information. If an interface is present but not displayed in the image, important pathology may be missed. Shadowing results when there is a marked reduction in the intensity of ultrasound deep to a strong reflector or attenuator. Fortunately, this artifact is easily recognized. Shadowing results in partial or complete loss of information in the areas of shadow that occur where incoming ultrasound is highly attenuated by superficial structures. Calcified plaque is a common source of shadowing and may obscure segments of vessel lumen and plaque from view as well as interfere with Doppler measurements. Improper time gain compensation is another potential cause of loss of information from the ultrasound image. As a result of inadequate amplification, the use of a low-gain setting or excessive time (depth) gain compensation may result in failure to display echoes of clinical importance. Because many low-level echoes are near the noise levels of the equipment, considerable skill and experience are needed to adjust instrument settings to display the maximum information with the minimum noise. Critical angle effects arise when the ultrasound beam is directed onto specular reflectors at a shallow angle. Although many body structures act as diffuse scatterers and reflect sound in all directions, planar surfaces behave more like mirrors. Interfaces of this type may not be detected if the angle of incidence of the transmitted ultrasound beam is less than a certain value (the critical angle). In this case, the sound will be reflected but in a direction that prevents detection (Fig. 24-3). By adjusting the scanning angle so that the interface lies nearly perpendicular to the direction of the sound beam, examiners can more readily detect specular interfaces.

Inadequate penetration and poor resolution may also result in the loss of significant information. In ultrasound imaging, one of the fundamental compromises the operator must consider involves the relationship of depth of penetration to axial resolution. A general rule of ultrasound imaging is to select the highest transducer frequency (and thus ensure the best axial resolution) consistent with the depth of penetration needed. Careless selection of transducer frequency, as well as lack of attention to the focal characteristics of the beam, may result in loss of clinically important information because of failure to display deep low-amplitude reflectors and small targets.

In the third type, ultrasound artifacts alter the size, shape, and position of structures. These distortions affect accurate description of lesions and may impair accurate localization during biopsy or aspiration procedures. Multipath artifacts arise when the path of the returning echo is not the one expected, resulting in display of the echo at an improper location in the image. Acoustical enhancement is the result of relatively less attenuation of sound by a structure compared with normal attenuation in adjacent areas. A typical example of enhancement is the increased intensity seen deep to a cyst. This is due to the low attenuation of sound energy by the homogeneous cyst fluid compared to the surrounding solid tissues. The strong signal distal to a cyst should not be mistaken for a tissue abnormality and is useful in confirming the nature of a mass with low attenuation such as a cyst. Spatial resolution limits the ability of ultrasound to differentiate small structures. As has been noted, lateral and axial resolution are determined by the pulse length transmitted and beam profile. Improper selection of scanning frequency and transducer focus may result in two adjacent structures being visualized as a single object. Propagation speed errors occur when the actual velocity of sound in a tissue or medium differs significantly from the value assumed in the ultrasound instrument (1540 m/sec). A typical example is provided by fat, which has a slower rate of sound propagation than other tissues. The slower propagation velocity results in a longer transit time for the ultrasound signal, which is interpreted by the instrument as indicating a more distant target and results in measurement errors and an error of placement of the target in the image.

CONCLUSION

In vascular diagnosis, imaging plays an important role and complements Doppler investigations. Imaging is critical in the identification of aneurysms and dissection and plays an increasing role in the identification and characterization of atheromatous plaque. Imaging is also essential for selecting vessels for Doppler examination and to allow Doppler angle correction. Quality vascular ultrasonography thus requires a user skilled in imaging and Doppler principles and diagnostic techniques.

REFERENCES

1. Kremkau F: *Diagnostic ultrasound: principles, instruments and exercises,* Philadelphia, 1989, WB Saunders.
2. Merritt CRB, Bluth E: Commentary: the future of carotid ultrasonography, *AJR* 158:37-39, 1992.
3. Powis RL, Powis WJ: *A thinker's guide to ultrasonic imaging,* Baltimore, 1984, Urban & Schwartzenberg.

CHAPTER 25

Real-time Doppler color imaging

CHRISTOPHER R.B. MERRITT

Over the past 20 years, the development of diagnostic sonography has progressed in a series of steps, each marked by a breakthrough in instrumentation. As ultrasound technology has evolved, its clinical usefulness and range of diagnostic applications have also advanced. Doppler color imaging (DCI) represents one of the more significant recent developments in ultrasound technology. Although DCI is new, it clearly has already made valuable clinical contributions, aiding in the rapid and noninvasive determination of vessel patency, blood flow, and organ perfusion.

The quantification of blood flow in vivo has been a goal of diagnostic imaging since the turn of the century, and although Doppler ultrasound has been used clinically for more than 25 years, its role has been expanded greatly by the ability of DCI to display flow and tissue images simultaneously. On the basis of the number of published scientific articles dealing with diagnostic ultrasound, the use of both duplex Doppler and DCI has grown significantly over the past decade. DCI now accounts for almost half the scientific papers dealing with Doppler ultrasound. Although DCI initially was used for cardiac[3,5,13-17] and peripheral vascular applications,[1] the introduction of a variety of transducers, including medium- and low-frequency probes as well as transrectal and transvaginal transducers, has greatly increased its range of applications. DCI extends the applications of Doppler ultrasound well beyond the identification of stenosis, thrombosis, and occlusion of the major arteries and veins. With its convenience and graphic display, DCI now plays an important role in the diagnostic evaluation of abdominal and pelvic organs, the pregnant uterus, the breast, thyroid, prostate, and brain.[8]

In conventional B-mode imaging, only the amplitude information in the returning signal is used to generate the final display. Rapidly moving, low-amplitude targets, such as red cells moving in vessels, are usually not imaged. With conventional Doppler instrumentation, the Doppler frequency information obtained from moving red cells is displayed as an audible signal or in graphic form as a time-varying plot of the frequency spectrum of the returning signal. With DCI, Doppler frequency shifts from moving blood are displayed as a feature of the image itself. In most instruments used for DCI, the echo amplitude, phase, and

frequency are processed in real-time to generate the image. Stationary or slowly moving targets provide the basis for the B-mode image. Signal phase provides information about the presence and direction of motion, and changes in echo signal frequency relate the velocity of the target. Backscattered signals from red blood cells are displayed in color as a function of their motion toward or away from the transducer. Color saturation is used to indicate the relative velocity of the moving red cells, with less color saturation generally indicating higher Doppler frequency shifts. In addition to the color display of flow data, DCI instruments also provide range-gated, pulsed Doppler with spectral analysis. This is an important complement to the display of the less precise frequency information shown in the color image and is necessary for most quantitative studies.

APPLICATIONS OF DOPPLER COLOR IMAGING
Primary vascular evaluation

As with duplex Doppler, it is possible to determine the presence or absence of flow, flow direction, flow velocity, and character of the flow with DCI. The result has been a full range of clinical applications for DCI (box). As instrumentation evolves and new methods, including use of contrast agents, are established, this list of applications of DCI will undoubtedly expand. Currently, the uses of DCI can be divided into those in which the identification of primary vascular abnormalities is the objective and those in which DCI aids in the evaluation of organ or tissue perfusion. Primary vascular evaluation is important in examination of the carotid bifurcation, the aorta, the inferior vena cava, and the iliac, femoral, popliteal, and other peripheral arteries and veins. In these vessels, DCI is used to detect vascular occlusion, measure arterial stenosis, and identify and characterize flow disturbance and vascular abnormalities, including aneurysm, pseudoaneurysm, dissection, and arteriovenous fistulas.[2] (Most of these applications are discussed in detail in other chapters.) In the abdomen and pelvis, DCI has a role similar to that in the peripheral vascular system—that of identifying vascular occlusion, stenosis, and related flow disturbances. DCI also plays a major role in confirming arterial and venous patency following vascular reconstruction and organ transplantation.

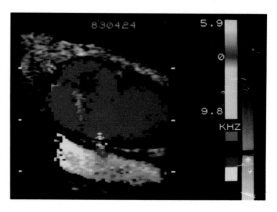

Fig. 25-1. Femoral pseudoaneurysm. Global Doppler sampling with DCI is the ideal method for identifying the presence of blood flow within pseudoaneurysms. Here the vessel from which the aneurysm arises, its communication with the pseudoaneurysm, and turbulent blood flow within the pseudoaneurysm are shown. Pulsating masses in the extremity can be evaluated rapidly and accurately, permitting differentiation of hematoma and other masses from aneurysm or pseudoaneurysm without angiography.

Carotid and peripheral arteries. Until recently, the standard method for noninvasive ultrasound imaging of the extracranial carotid and peripheral vessels has been duplex Doppler sonography. Modern instruments equipped with 7.5- to 10.0-MHz transducers allow high-resolution, real-time imaging of the vessel walls and permit identification and characterization of atheromatous plaque. Coupled with pulsed Doppler, these systems may generate quantitative data that allow highly accurate estimates of stenosis when used properly. Limitations of duplex sonography for carotid evaluation include sampling problems, competing design factors for imaging and Doppler ultrasound, aliasing, the complexity of interpretation of the Doppler data, and the considerable technical skill and time required to obtain accurate results. In addition, differentiating high-grade stenosis from total occlusion may be difficult with duplex ultrasound.[6] Shadowing due to plaque calcification and difficulty in maintaining orientation with tortuous vessels, which prevents accurate measurement of the Doppler angle and velocity calculation, are also problems in duplex carotid sonography. With DCI, the benefits of conventional duplex sonography are retained and additional capabilities are provided. (These are discussed in detail in Chapter 34.)

Other applications. Depending on the size of the patient and the amount of superimposed gas, the aorta, inferior vena cava, and iliac arteries and veins can be studied for occlusion, narrowing, dissection, or aneurysm. Flow within the femoral and popliteal arteries and veins easily is documented, and DCI has assumed an important role in the primary evaluation of patients suspected of deep venous

thrombosis.[9] The evaluation of vascular dissection, aneurysms, and pseudoaneurysms is performed quickly and accurately, and DCI can be used in lieu of angiography in selected patients (Fig. 25-1). Excellent access and visualization of dialysis fistulas for thrombosis, stenosis, and pseudoaneurysm have resulted in clinical acceptance of DCI as the initial diagnostic examination when these complications are expected.

Evaluation of abdominal and pelvic organ perfusion

The uses of duplex Doppler ultrasound in the abdomen and pelvis include identification of vessels, determination of the direction of blood flow, evaluation of narrowing or occlusion, and characterization of flow to organs and tumors. These applications are especially valuable in highly vascular organs such as the kidney, liver, spleen, placenta, and brain. Evaluation of perfusion is similarly important in transplants of the kidney, liver, and pancreas. Although most of the reported work using pulsed Doppler ultrasound has emphasized the detection of stenosis and flow disturbances in large vessels, Doppler information may also be valuable in inference of abnormalities in the peripheral vascular bed of an organ or tissue (Fig. 25-2). Changes in the spectral waveform or, in the case of color flow imaging, in the appearance of flow in diastole, provide insight into the resistance of the vascular bed supplied by the vessel and indicate alterations due to a variety of pathologic conditions. In abdominal and pelvic applications, information obtained from both large and small vessels may be of clinical value. For example, changes in large vessels identifiable by sonographic methods include flow reversal in the portal vein; the presence of portosystemic collaterals; the occlusion of portal, splenic, or renal veins; and mesenteric or renal arterial stenosis. Changes in small vessels that reflect the

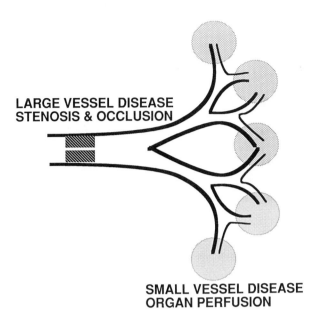

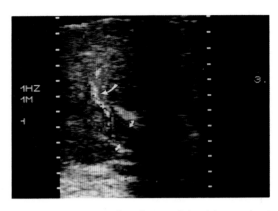

Fig. 25-3. DCI shows partial occlusion of the right portal vein. Although the main portal vein is filled with thrombus (small arrows), a small amount of flow in the residual lumen of the right portal vein is shown (large arrow).

Fig. 25-2. DCI is useful in not only the inference of the degree of stenosis of large vessels but also the identification of changes in organ perfusion due to small vessel disease. In large vessels, the contrast between the vessel wall and the lumen permits direct assessment of the degree of narrowing. Likewise, alterations in dynamic patterns of flow within smaller vessels may indicate changes in peripheral vascular resistance, often as a result of parenchymal disease.

impedance of the vascular bed may also be important in the early identification of rejection of transplanted organs and may aid in differentiation of benign from malignant masses.

Changes in tissue function are often associated with changes in blood flow, and duplex and color flow Doppler ultrasound, with their abilities to display such changes, are leading closer to the long-sought goal of noninvasive tissue characterization. Unlike early cardiac and peripheral vascular Doppler devices, current duplex Doppler systems permit scanning of abdominal and pelvic organs, allowing access to flow information at the level of small arterioles. Taylor and Burns[18] showed that semiquantitative analysis of the Doppler-shift frequency with time can be used to infer both proximal stenosis and changes in distal vascular impedance. Using pulsed Doppler sonography, numerous investigators have shown that pathologic changes in various organs and tissues, including the kidney, breast, and liver, are reflected in changes in arterial flow patterns. Although DCI has not been successful in imaging parenchymal flow in all organs, there is considerable potential for the actual imaging of organ perfusion patterns in the liver, kidney, spleen, placenta, and brain; however, some of these indications will probably require the use of ultrasound contrast agents to improve detectability of low-amplitude signals from small blood vessels.

Hepatic arteries and veins. DCI successfully visualizes normal and abnormal hepatic vessels and may aid in the characterization of hepatic masses. DCI permits prompt identification of the major hepatic veins and confirmation of their patency. This technique also frequently permits identification of flow in small or compressed hepatic veins that are not visible with gray-scale imaging alone. In the evaluation of suspected Budd-Chiari syndrome, DCI is superior to other imaging methods in terms of ease of examination and overall sensitivity. The ability of DCI to clearly differentiate vascular from nonvascular structures allows quick and accurate identification of an enlarged hepatic artery, which may be confused with the bile duct. In view of the relatively common occurrence of anatomic variation in the relationships of the vessels in the portal triad, this capability is sometimes useful.

Portal vein. Noninvasive diagnosis of thrombosis of the portal vein by means of conventional ultrasound, dynamic computed tomography, and duplex Doppler ultrasound has been reported.[7,11] Although these techniques are quite accurate, it is difficult to distinguish complete and partial occlusion. DCI permits rapid evaluation of the portal vein and is extremely effective in revealing flow in the residual lumen if a lumen is present (Fig. 25-3). Detection of the presence of collaterals (cavernous transformation), which frequently form after occlusion of the portal vein, is another application for which DCI is especially well-suited. Typical findings of cavernous transformation include numerous tubular structures exhibiting low-velocity venous flow patterns in the region of the porta hepatis. DCI also aids in the diagnosis of changes in flow in the hepatic artery that accompany this pathologic condition.

In patients with portal hypertension, DCI allows rapid determination of the direction of portal blood flow. This information is important in planning surgical treatment because the presence of hepatofugal flow indicates the need for a portocaval or mesocaval rather than a splenorenal shunt. DCI is valuable after surgery in confirming the patency of portosystemic shunts, and portosystemic collateral vessels in patients with portal hypertension are detected readily and are often found to be far more extensive than gray-scale imaging alone would suggest.

Hepatic transplantation. Doppler ultrasound is critically important in preoperative and postoperative assessment of hepatic transplant recipients. Before transplantation, the anatomy and patency of the inferior vena cava and the hepatic and portal vein must be confirmed. DCI is quite useful in this application, with a shorter examination time than that required by duplex methods. After transplantation regular Doppler evaluation of the major hepatic vessels using both spectral duplex and color flow Doppler may be performed. Early identification of thrombosis of the hepatic artery with Doppler methods may allow treatment via thrombectomy rather than retransplantation.

Splenic and mesenteric vessels. The major difficulty in Doppler assessment of the splenic and mesenteric vessels is limited visualization as a result of superimposed intestinal gas. If the patient is thin and gas is minimal, the ability of DCI to show the splenic mesenteric arteries and veins is excellent, permitting the potential diagnosis and characterization of stenosis, occlusion, or aneurysm.

Renal artery and vein. With varying degrees of success, duplex Doppler sonography aids in the diagnosis of stenosis and occlusion of the renal arteries. Because accurate evaluation demands that the entire course of each renal artery be examined, the study may be compromised in many patients because of superimposed bowel gas, bone, or fat. With DCI, normal renal arteries and veins are regularly imaged. Criteria for diagnosis of stenosis include not only the spectral changes described with duplex Doppler sonography but also direct visualization of vessel narrowing and the stenotic jet. Demonstration of a distended renal vein without evidence of flow using DCI has correlated well with results using angiography and magnetic resonance imaging in indicating renal vein thrombosis. With DCI, intrarenal vessels, including segmental, interlobar, and arcuate vessels, are visible in many patients, aiding in Doppler waveform analysis and the evaluation of renal parenchymal disease.

Renal transplants. Transplant dysfunction may result from vessel stenosis, occlusion, or parenchymal changes associated with rejection, tubular necrosis, or toxic reactions to drugs. The ability of DCI to show not only primary abnormalities in major vessels but also dynamics of flow that reflect changes in smaller vessels encourages routine postoperative use of ultrasound in the evaluation of renal transplants. Because of the superficial location of the transplanted kidney, excellent detail of intrarenal and extrarenal vessels is obtained with DCI (Fig. 25-4). The real-time display also permits a visual analogue of the pulsatility index. In the normal transplant, flow in the segmental, interlobar, and arcuate vessels continues throughout the cardiac cycle, and these vessels are seen clearly in systole and diastole. With transplant dysfunction, increased peripheral vascular resistance results in a dramatic reduction or complete cessation of diastolic flow (Fig. 25-5). In addition to providing a rapid and graphic image of flow to the transplanted kidney, pulsed spectral Doppler imaging of small intrarenal vessels

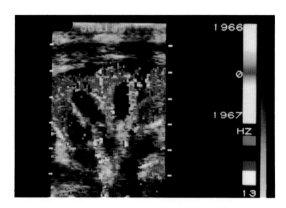

Fig. 25-4. Doppler color flow image in longitudinal view shows flow in segmental, interlobar, and arcuate arteries and intrarenal veins of a normal transplanted kidney. Because of the low impedance of the renal vascular bed, flow in these vessels normally continues through diastole.

permits accurate, angle-corrected sampling of flow in these vessels. Although studies have not clearly shown the superiority of DCI in the assessment of renal transplants, color flow imaging may provide more complete assessment, be comparable in accuracy with conventional duplex methods, and save considerable time.

Obstetric applications. Applications of DCI in obstetrics are only beginning to be explored. Imaging of uterine, placental, umbilical cord, and fetal vessels is possible throughout pregnancy (Fig. 25-6). The addition of color flow imaging to conventional Doppler methods may enhance understanding of a wide range of maternal and fetal problems.

Other uses. DCI has been used to evaluate blood flow to the thyroid, testicle, breast, and brain. High Doppler sensitivity permits imaging of normal vessels supplying the thyroid and testicle without difficulty. Abnormal flow patterns in the thyroid have been seen with Graves' disease in which a dramatic increase in vascularity of the entire gland is noted. Many thyroid masses are characterized by localized areas of increased vascularity. In the testicle, abnormal flow patterns have been seen with varicocele, torsion, and malignant tumors. The ease of examination and sensitivity of DCI in the detection of flow in small arteries and veins make this an excellent method for confirmation of varicocele (Fig. 25-7) and testicular torsion. In neonates, cerebral perfusion is seen clearly by using access provided by the open fontanel. Similar useful information related to brain flow can be obtained with intraoperative DCI. This application is particularly helpful in the intraoperative monitoring of resection of cerebral arteriovenous malformations (Fig. 25-8). Another intraoperative application that appears promising is the inspection of vessels after endarterectomy.

Evaluation of tumor neovascularity. Flow characteristics may add specificity in the ultrasound examination of masses, with display of abnormal vascular patterns associated with tumors. In this application, the information added to the

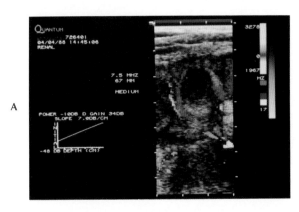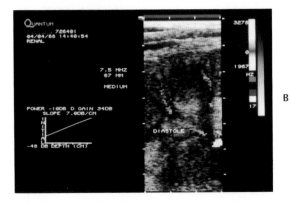

Fig. 25-5. In rejection, resistance in peripheral vessels is increased, resulting in reduced systolic flow within the segmental and interlobar arteries *(A)* and cessation of arterial flow in diastole *(B)*. Although these changes are not specific for rejection, these findings are of clinical value in the assessment of transplant dysfunction. With DCI, it is usually possible to rapidly differentiate flow disturbance caused from stenosis or occlusion of a renal artery or vein from small vessel changes, as illustrated here.

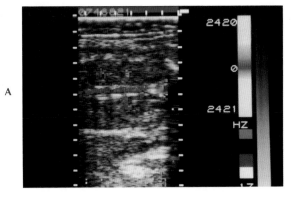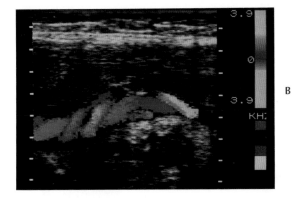

Fig. 25-6. Doppler color flow images obtained in the second trimester of pregnancy show fetal aorta and both renal arteries *(A)* and umbilical arteries and vein *(B)*.

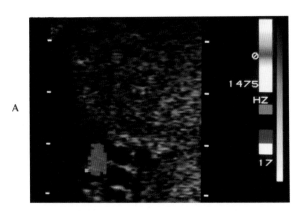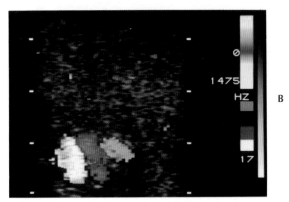

Fig. 25-7. Doppler color flow images show typical findings of testicular varicocele. *A,* A number of tubular structures are seen adjacent to the left testicle. *B,* With Valsalva maneuver, the presence of flow is confirmed, indicating the presence of a varicocele.

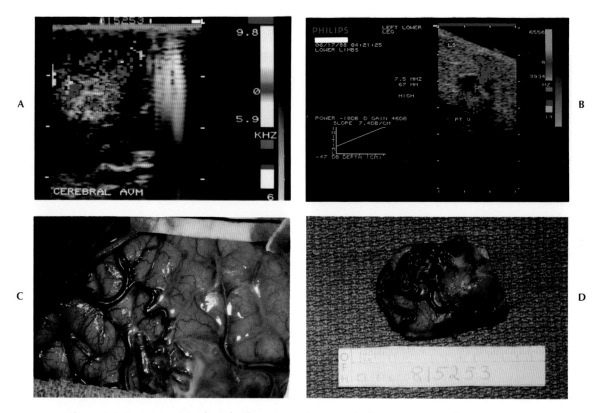

Fig. 25-8. Intraoperative Doppler color flow images show a cerebral arteriovenous malformation before *(A)* and after *(B)* operative interruption of the vascular supply to the mass. Imaging was useful in providing the neurosurgeon with immediate confirmation of the control of the major blood supply to this vascular mass. Gross pathologic findings before *(C)* and after *(D)* resection are shown.

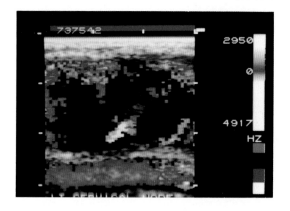

Fig. 25-9. Doppler color flow image shows tumor vascularity in an enlarged cervical lymph node. The node exhibits a marked increase in blood flow compared with that seen in a normal node. Biopsy revealed metastatic papillary thyroid carcinoma.

gray-scale tissue display by DCI may provide a long-awaited step toward sonographic characterization of tissue. Vascular changes associated with malignant tumors can be demonstrated by Doppler ultrasound. Several reports[4,12] have described characteristic signal patterns from malignant tumors when both continuous-wave and pulsed Doppler ultrasound were used. The patterns generally involve the periphery of the tumor and include a characteristic Doppler spectrum with relatively high peak systolic velocities and a preponderance

of high-power, low-frequency elements. DCI has been used to evaluate patients with tumors of the liver, kidney, breast, thyroid, and soft tisues to determine the potential for detecting tumor vascularity.[10] In the liver, many metastatic lesions show abnormal vascular patterns (Fig. 25-9). The changes include an increase in the number of vessels in the region of the tumor, the presence of vessels with irregular course or caliber, and in some cases, evidence of high-velocity flow, probably associated with arteriovenous shunting. Increased vascularity has also been seen at the periphery of tumors of the breast, testicle, thyroid, parathyroid, and soft tissues. If further study confirms that these vascular changes are relatively specific for malignant tumors, DCI and associated developments in Doppler ultrasound may have a future role in the characterization of malignant tumors.

DISCUSSION

The ultimate role of DCI in the applications described is difficult to assess fully because the technology is continuing to evolve rapidly. There are significant differences between conventional duplex Doppler ultrasound and DCI. Although duplex instrumentation has been the most widely accepted method for vascular applications, its disadvantages have slowed the acceptance of this method. DCI addresses, at least in part, several limitations of pulsed Doppler ultrasound.

Sampling

With conventional pulsed Doppler ultrasound, flow data are obtained from a small area only, and precise positioning of the Doppler sample volume is required to obtain accurate measurements. When flow disturbances are isolated to relatively small areas, the abnormality may be missed because of failure to position the sample in the small region where the stenotic jet or turbulence is present, and localized areas of severely disturbed flow can be missed or underestimated. DCI provides global Doppler sampling, eliminating the need to place the sample volume in a specific location for analysis because the Doppler flow parameters for each pixel in the entire image are displayed in real-time.

Technical skill requirements

Complex Doppler data and the need for accurate sampling and measurement of the Doppler angle make the duplex examination one of the most technically demanding ultrasound procedures performed in most departments. When Doppler ultrasound is used, the accurate estimation of velocity requires correct measurement of the angle of the sound beam from the axis of flow. The special training and skills needed to be proficient in this technique undoubtedly have slowed its acceptance. DCI greatly simplifies the measurement of the Doppler angle even in small vessels that cannot be seen clearly with conventional imaging devices and allows accurate, angle-corrected measurement of velocity in these small vessels.

Examination time

Methodical and time-consuming searching and sampling must be performed to ensure that a conventional, range-gated Doppler study has achieved reasonable sensitivity and specificity in detection of flow disturbances. As a result, duplex studies are often lengthy examinations, especially when complex vascular anatomy or advanced disease creates difficult scanning situations. With DCI, the simultaneous

real-time display of Doppler and tissue information and global Doppler sampling permit rapid evaluation, particularly when the vessel is normal, allowing a confident diagnosis to be established quickly. Because flow information is contained in the image and sampling is not necessary, less training is required for collection of basic flow data than with conventional Doppler instrumentation. When precise measurement via spectral Doppler ultrasound is necessary, the color flow display allows rapid and accurate placement of the range gate in the optimal location for measurement.

Information content

Because the Doppler signal itself has no anatomic significance, the examiner must interpret the Doppler signal and then determine its relevance in the context of the image. Components of the Doppler data that must be evaluated include the Doppler shift frequency and amplitude, the spatial distribution of frequency across the vessel, and the temporal variation of the signal. The complexity of the Doppler data undoubtedly has influenced the rate of acceptance of Doppler sonography by specialists who are accustomed to anatomically referenced images. With DCI, flow information is provided with a real-time anatomic reference and is displayed in an intuitive and highly graphic form. This markedly increases the examiner's access to the flow information being sought.

CONCLUSION

The disadvantages and limitations of DCI are few, provided the method is used in conjunction with image-analysis Doppler spectral analysis. Examiners must realize that this technology is in its infancy; the future will undoubtedly bring a number of improvements. For example, in the abdomen, gas produces a severe artifact because of the phase and frequency changes induced by the markedly reduced velocity of sound in air. Scanning of areas containing much gas is more difficult than with conventional ultrasound. The complex technology required to produce a real-time instrument with an effective combination of flow and tissue imaging is understandably expensive, but the cost may be justified by the unique capabilities of the instrumentation. Despite these limitations, DCI is already providing simple, rapid, and accurate evaluation of vessels for stenosis, occlusion, and flow disturbance, and the potential for obtaining valuable information related to organ perfusion and tumor neovascularity appears real. As with the introduction of gray-scale and real-time sonography, an exciting new dimension of sonography is possible with the advent of DCI.

REFERENCES

1. Ackroyd N et al: Colour-coded carotid Doppler imaging: an angiographic comparison of 324 bifurcations, *Aust NZ J Surg* 54:509-517, 1984.
2. Bluth EI et al: Doppler color flow imaging of carotid artery dissection, *J Ultrasound Med* 8:149-153, 1988.

3. Bommer WJ, Miller L: Real-time two-dimensional color-flow Doppler: enhanced Doppler flow imaging in the diagnosis of cardiovascular disease, *Am J Cardiol* 49:944, 1982 (abstract).

4. Burns PN et al: Ultrasonic Doppler studies of the breast, *Ultrasound Med Biol* 8:127-143, 1982.

5. Dagli SV et al: Evaluation of aortic dissection by Doppler color mapping, *Am J Cardiol* 56:497-498, 1985.

6. Dreisbach JN: Duplex ultrasound evaluation of carotid disease, *Clin Diagn Ultrasound* 13:69, 1984.

7. Merritt CRB: Ultrasonographic demonstration of portal vein thrombosis, *Radiology* 133:425-427, 1979.

8. Merritt CRB: Doppler color flow imaging, *J Clin Ultrasound* 15:591-597, 1987.

9. Merritt CRB, ed: *Doppler color imaging,* New York, 1992, Churchill Livingstone.

10. Merritt CRB, Bluth EI, Sullivan MA: *Assessment of human tumor vascularity with Doppler color flow mapping.* Paper presented at the 72nd Scientific Assembly of the Radiological Society of North America, Chicago, Dec 1, 1986.

11. Miller VE, Berland LL: Pulsed Doppler duplex sonography and CT of portal vein thrombosis, *AJR* 145:73-76, 1985.

12. Minasian H, Bamber JC: A preliminary assessment of an ultrasonic Doppler method for the study of blood flow in human breast cancer, *Ultrasound Med Biol* 8:357-364, 1982.

13. Miyatake K et al: Clinical applications of a new type of real-time two-dimensional Doppler color flow imaging system, *Am J Cardiol* 54:857-868, 1984.

14. Namekawa K et al: Imaging of blood flow using autocorrelation, *Ultrasound Med and Biol* 8:138, 1982.

15. Oritz E et al: Localisation of ventricular septal defects by simultaneous display of superimposed colour Doppler and cross sectional echocardiographic images, *Br Heart J* 54:53-60, 1985.

16. Suzuki Y et al: Detection of intracardiac shunt flow in atrial septal defect using a real-time two-dimensional color-coded Doppler color flow imaging system and comparison with contrast two-dimensional echocardiography, *Am J Cardiol* 56:347-350, 1985.

17. Switzer DF, Nanda NC: Doppler color flow mapping, *Ultrasound Med Biol* 11:403-416, 1985.

18. Taylor KJW, Burns PN: Duplex Doppler scanning in the pelvis and abdomen, *Ultrasound Med Biol* 11:643-658, 1985.

CHAPTER 26

Principles of deep Doppler ultrasonography

PETER N. BURNS

The relatively recent availability of duplex and color Doppler instruments that combine high-quality ultrasound imaging with range-gated pulsed Doppler at ultrasonic frequencies suitable for abdominal scanning has brought several exciting new areas of clinical diagnosis into view. These include the assessment of blood flow in the heart and great vessels, in the vessels and organs of the upper abdomen and pelvis, in the fetus and uteroplacental circulation during pregnancy, and in pathologically transformed circulations, such as that accompanying malignant tumors. In many circumstances, the addition of information related to blood flow has the potential to complement the role of conventional abdominal ultrasound imaging.[44,45] Therefore the abdominal Doppler sonographer must be capable of interpreting the Doppler spectrum under a relatively wide range of circumstances, and it is perhaps because of this varied nature of the application of the Doppler technique in the abdomen that there are so few firm guidelines available for its use. Although many aspects of the technique are still under development and the discussion over the precise areas in which its clinical contribution may be most significant is ongoing, a critical appreciation of the basic principles and limitations of the Doppler method applied to deep structures is an essential prerequisite for its clinical application.

INSTRUMENTATION

The basic instrument for the deep Doppler examination is the duplex scanner.[8] As in peripheral vascular work, the ultrasound image serves as a guide for the location of the Doppler sample volume. In contrast to peripheral vascular applications, however, Doppler signals in the abdomen are frequently elicited from blood vessels that are not visualized on the ultrasound image either because they are smaller than the imaging system is capable of resolving or because acoustic conditions are too poor to allow depiction of the vessel lumen itself. The ultrasound image then must demonstrate the appropriate anatomic area for the positioning of the Doppler sample volume. High-quality, real-time ultrasound imaging is therefore essential. Today, this is usually achieved with the use of several dynamically focused arrays, each of which is currently available with pulsed Doppler capability. The annular array (mechanically steered) sector scanner and the phased array (electronically steered) sector scanner are currently the two most popular instrument configurations for abdominal duplex scanning (Fig. 26-1). The linear array tends to be more popular in the Far East, where the body habitus of the patient population allows better acoustic access to the vascular structures of the upper abdomen. The curvilinear array is the newest transducer configuration for duplex scanning of the upper abdomen, combining the smaller footprint with some of the advantages of the sector scanner with the extended near field visualization afforded by the linear array. The popularity of such systems for abdominal imaging leads to one of the major compromises in the choice for instrumentation for deep Doppler: the optimal conditions for imaging and Doppler rarely coincide. One aspect of this is in the choice of transducer frequency. The mechanism by which red blood cells produce the very weak echoes the Doppler receiver detects is the Rayleigh-Tyndall process. The intensity of a Rayleigh-Tyndall scattered wave increases with the fourth power of frequency. Thus doubling the ultrasonic frequency results in an echo from blood that is 16 times stronger. This is partly responsible for a dramatic difference in performance among Doppler instruments detecting blood flow that use different ultrasonic frequencies. Attenuation in soft tissue also rises with frequency, tending to offset the advantage of the increased efficiency of scattering at higher frequencies. The optimum ultrasonic frequency with which to perform a Doppler examination is an inevitable compromise based on the strength of the echo from blood and the depth of the structure of interest. This tends to force the optimum Doppler frequency in the abdomen to below the level at which the best images are obtained. In general, the optimum frequency for a Doppler examination is below the level that is likely to be chosen for imaging the same structure. For example, the imaging examination of a pediatric abdomen may use an array whose center frequency is 5 MHz, whereas the best Doppler frequency for detecting flow in the pediatric kidney is likely to be 3 MHz. Although many modern arrays are capable of operating at a range of frequencies (and must to produce a good image), Doppler blood flow detection requires exceptionally high sensitivity, and this places an additional burden on the design of duplex receivers and the

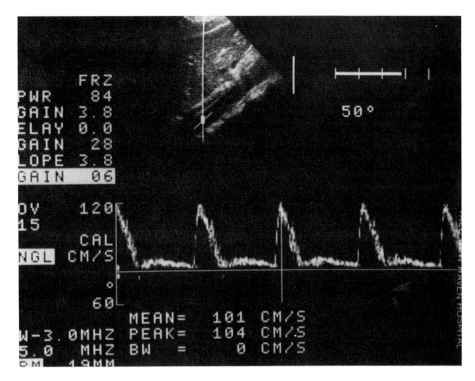

Fig. 26-1. An abdominal duplex scan. The real-time image is frozen while the sample volume is situated in the vessel of interest. The image is made with a 5-MHz annular array, and the Doppler signal is obtained from a 3-MHz plan disk transducer situated within the same probe. Notice that the sample volume is slightly smaller than the vessel diameter, therefore avoiding the effects of clutter.

transducer assemblies, especially when they operate at greater depths and use arrays. Frequently, the best pulsed Doppler performance is achieved by using single-element transducers, which usually do not produce very satisfactory images. The user must therefore be prepared to change transducers occasionally between the imaging and Doppler portion of a duplex examination.

Most duplex instruments that use mechanically moved beams permit selection of the Doppler site only after the real-time image has been frozen and stored on the screen. Electronically steered systems such as the phased sector, linear, or curvilinear arrays, however, use beams that are sufficiently agile to allow image scan lines to be acquired in rapid alteration with the Doppler data. The result is the simultaneous presentation of the Doppler spectrum and the real-time image. This time sharing (sometimes called *true duplex scanning*) is the result of some compromise; either the frame rate of the real-time image or the pulse repetition frequency of the Doppler system is reduced or some interpolation of the Doppler data is implemented during spectral analysis. The operator is usually aware that a price is being paid in performance for the provision of simultaneous Doppler and imaging.

Color Doppler instruments have recently become available for abdominal scanning.[8] They offer the potential advantage of visualization of Doppler shifts within the entire field of view of the real-time image and therefore appear to be helpful in the location or exclusion of Doppler signals, especially in sites where they may not normally be expected, such as fistulas, aneurysms, and pseudoaneurysms.[28] The color Doppler devices are inherently less sensitive to the weaker echoes scattered from low volumes of blood, so small quantities of flowing blood may be detected on duplex scanning but not with color. In addition, the difficulty of rejecting Doppler shifts from moving solid tissue within an image usually forces a higher minimum detectable Doppler shift frequency in a color system. As a result, slow flow— of which there is much in the abdomen—is detected less easily with a color system than with a duplex scanner. For these reasons, it seems prudent to use color primarily as a real-time tool with which to survey the image for flow, and the duplex (or spectral) Doppler should be used to obtain the final Doppler signal for clinical interpretation.

TECHNIQUE

Doppler examination of deep vessels is one of the more technically demanding ultrasound procedures. Like all Doppler examinations, satisfactory results rely to a great extent on the operator's coordination of hand, eye, and ear as well as experience. The nature of Doppler examination in the abdomen involves some considerations that may be new to the peripheral vascular sonographer. If duplex scanning is being used to estimate flow velocity, the beam-vessel angle must be measured. Doppler access to abdominal vessels is then confined to those scan planes containing the vessel axis, a restriction that can cause problems. For example, scanning in a midline sagittal plane to interrogate the celiac trunk or superior mesenteric artery may be inhibited by bowel gas. To help overcome this, patients can be scheduled for their examinations in the morning after an overnight fast.

Many of the problems associated with abdominal Doppler examinations have their origin in the relatively poor signal-to-noise ratio of the Doppler signals. The backscattered echo from moving blood is weak, especially if a low frequency is used; attenuation of intervening tissue and the small size of many vessels place their blood flow signals at the limit of detectability possible with current technology. Although the signal may be improved by increasing the power of the transmitted pulse into tissue, the quantity of acoustic power that is prudent to send to the body is limited. In fact, pulsed Doppler systems already emit higher spatial peak, temporal average (SPTA) powers than most other ultrasound diagnostic devices, and the current FDA guideline levels for abdominal scanning (94 mW/cm^2) are somewhat lower than the levels most duplex scanners are capable of delivering. The operator can improve the signal by attempting to optimize the acoustic conditions. This can be accomplished by positioning the transducer as near as possible to the structure of interest, minimizing the quantity of gas- or beam-distorting structures in the beam's path, and reducing clutter as much as possible.

Clutter is the intrusion of high-amplitude, low Doppler shift elements in the signal that have their origin in moving solid tissue within the sample volume.[10] Typically, such tissue will be the wall of the vessel or surrounding structures experiencing transmitted cardiac or respiratory motion. Because the echoes and hence the Doppler signal from these structures are many times stronger than that from moving blood, the Doppler detector can be overwhelmed by their presence in the signal. A low-frequency thump heard at the beginning of systole, followed by distortion of the Doppler spectrum, is a sign of clutter of cardiac origin. The sample volume should be reduced in size so as to include only blood to alleviate this artifact. For respiratory clutter, it may be helpful to ask the patient to arrest inspiration for a moment while the signal is recorded. Because the frequency of the Doppler shifts produced by these motions is quite low, clutter can be eliminated by use of the high-pass filter. However, caution should be exercised when small vessels are being interrogated or when diastolic flow velocities are being demonstrated or excluded, since these may be obliterated by too high a filter setting.

With shorter ultrasound path lengths to deep organs and vessels, there is less attenuation, but higher frequencies can be used. This has the simultaneous effect of increasing the backscattered cross section of blood, giving a stronger echo, and increasing the Doppler shift frequencies, therefore low-

ering the threshold velocity for the detection of slow flow. The advent of Doppler endosonography has made the largest contribution to the effort to gain closer access to the abdominal and pelvic structures. Although transesophageal, transrectal, transvaginal, endovascular, and endoluminal Doppler are in their infancy, color and duplex systems are already becoming available, and it is reasonable to expect that the improved acoustic access they afford to deep structures will continue to be exploited for Doppler studies.

INTERPRETING THE DOPPLER SPECTRUM
Qualitative methods

Spectral content. A survey of normal Doppler signals obtained from the major vessels of the upper abdomen and pelvis (Figs. 26-2 to 26-5) reveals a variety of waveform and spectral patterns. Many of these features have their origin in the hemodynamic conditions pertaining to that vessel. In interpreting this flow signature of a specific vessel's signal, examiners should appreciate the major factors that influence the signal's form. Thus although the waveform shape (i.e., the variation of the maximum Doppler shift frequency over the cardiac cycle) can yield information about the vascular impedance distal to the point of measurement, the content of the spectrum reflects aspects of the local flow characteristics (e.g.,whether the flow is laminar or disturbed and whether the velocity profile is flat, blunted, or parabolic). Fig. 26-6 shows signals from vessels with different velocity profiles, insonated in a manner to minimize the effects of transit time broadening. If the Doppler sample volume has a uniform sensitivity and embraces the entire vessel lumen evenly, the relative power of different frequencies reflects the relative volumes of blood moving at the corresponding velocities. In the aorta (Fig. 26-6, *A*), there is a plug flow velocity profile, that is, one in which the entire cross section of blood is moving at one velocity. There is one Doppler shift corresponding to the velocity of these laminae, and the signal shows the window, which is characteristic of the normal carotid arteries in early systole. In a smaller vessel such as in the celiac trunk (Fig. 26-6, *B*), a blunted parabolic flow profile develops in diastole as the greater proportion of blood contained in laminae adjacent to the boundary layer experience viscous loss, and the power spectrum shows a broader band of Doppler shift frequencies during diastole. In vessels less than a few millimeters in diameter, the parabolic flow profile predicted by theory leads to a flat distribution of power, with frequency up to the Doppler shift corresponding to the center stream velocity. The uniform gray of the spectral form of the ovarian artery (Fig. 26-6, *C*) is one example.

Deviations from these appearances occur with stenosis, as they do in the large peripheral vessels. However, because the normal, laminar flow signal from vessels such as the renal artery contains a range of velocities, spectral broadening alone cannot be taken as a sign of stenosis in smaller, deep-lying vessels. In fact, the flow velocity profile is only one influence on the form of the Doppler spectrum; another

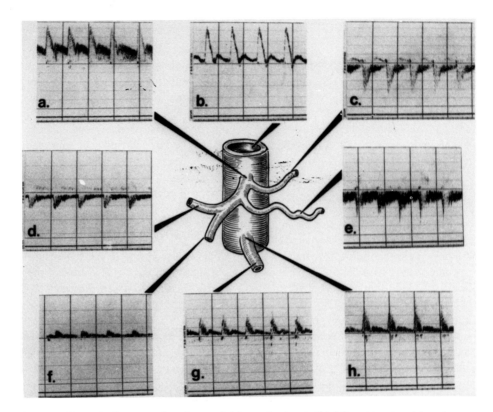

Fig. 26-2. Time-velocity spectra in celiac trunk *(a)*, proximal aorta *(b)*, left gastric artery *(c)*, and proper hepatic artery *(d)*; flow was away from the probe and hence appears below the zero line. Splenic artery *(e)*, gastroduodenal artery *(f)*, distal superior mesenteric artery (SMA) *(g)*, and proximal SMA *(h)* are shown. (From Taylor KJW et al: *Radiology* 154:487, 1985.)

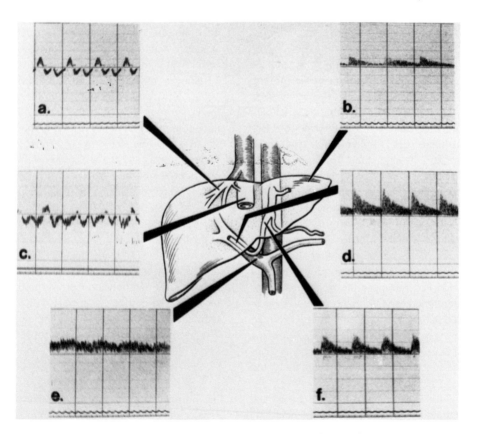

Fig. 26-3. Time-velocity spectra in right hepatic vein *(a)*, parenchymal signal *(b)*, inferior vena cava *(c)*, proper hepatic artery *(d)*, portal vein *(e)*, and hepatic artery *(f)*. (From Taylor KJW et al: *Radiology* 154:487, 1985.)

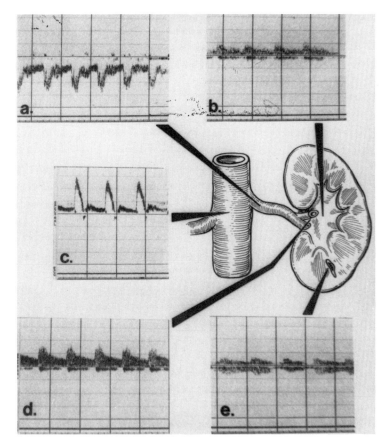

Fig. 26-4. Time-velocity spectra in proximal renal artery *(a)*; flow is away from the probe and therefore appears below the zero line. The interlobar artery *(b)*, aorta *(c)*, renal sinus *(d)*, and arcuate artery *(e)* are also shown.

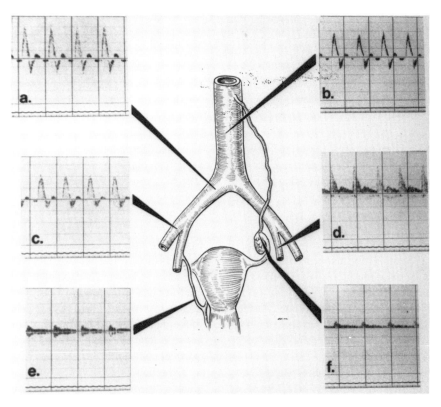

Fig. 26-5. Time-velocity spectra in the common iliac artery *(a)*, low aorta *(b)*, external iliac artery *(c)*, internal iliac artery *(d)*, uterine artery *(e)*, and ovarian artery *(f)*. (From Taylor KJW et al: *Radiology* 154:487, 1985.)

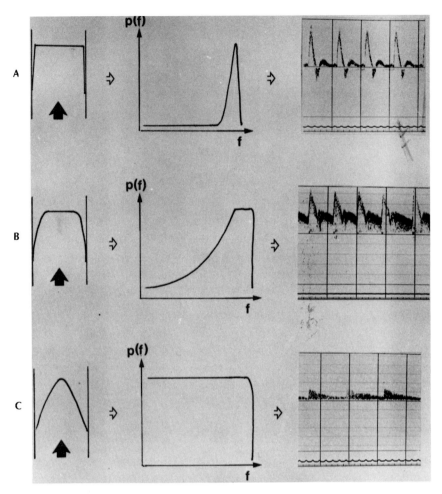

Fig. 26-6. Idealized examples of the relationship between different velocity profiles in a vessel with laminar flow *(left column),* the Doppler spectrum *(middle column)* and the resulting spectral display *(right column).* **A,** Plug flow (the aorta). **B,** Blunted parabolic flow in diastole (the celiac trunk). **C,** Parabolic flow (the ovarian artery). (From Burns PN: *Interpretation of Doppler signals.* In Taylor KJW, Burns PN, Wells PNT, eds: *Clinical applications of Doppler ultrasound,* New York, 1988, Raven Press.)

is the form of the acoustic beam itself. The sample volume is often smaller than the vessel, in which case the spectrum changes according to the velocity of those flow laminae that lie within the beam. This in turn depends on the velocity profile.[9] This explains the disquieting ability of the operator to increase or decrease the spectral width of the Doppler display from a vessel with a blunted flow profile by manipulation of the beam position. Furthermore, the beam is not uniform across its lateral dimensions. Thus, unless the vessel is small compared to the beam width, each of the flow elements probably does not contribute equally to the Doppler signal. The diagnosis of stenosis in the abdomen therefore relies on the detection of abnormally high velocities rather than of spectral broadening.

Presence of flow. Determining whether flow is present is one of the simplest but perhaps most useful applications of Doppler. The determination may be used to exclude occlusion by thrombosis or to locate the point of occlusion of a limb vessel during a pressure measurement. It can also be used to differentiate vessels from nonvascular structures that have a similar appearance on the image. An example is the differentiation of suspected biliary tract dilatation from an enlarged hepatic artery or from portal venous radicals. The recognition of splenic or hepatic arterial aneurysms and their differentiation from cysts is another application.

Confirming the absence of flow is, by its nature, a little more difficult. The lack of Doppler signal must be a consequence of lack of flow rather than the acoustical or receiver performance parameters of the system. Examiners should check that normal flow signals can be detected with the same machine settings from comparable structures at comparable depths before concluding that flow is absent at a particular location.

Direction of flow. The direction of flow is usually of diagnostic value when an occlusion has produced collateral channels whose flow direction is unusual. This is particularly useful in the evaluation of patients with suspected portal venous hypertension. The directional resolution of the

Doppler system is best when the beam-vessel angle is relatively small and the signal lies in the middle of the dynamic range of the receiver. If a mirror image of the signal is seen in the reverse-flow sideband of the display, care should be taken with the adjustment of angle and receiver gain so that a trace showing an unambiguous direction is obtained.

Identification of characteristic flow. Normal flow in various parts of the arterial circulation shows distinct characteristics according to their precise location. Characteristics of waveform shape and spectral distribution are often consequences of hemodynamic factors unique to each vessel. They allow the identification of the origin of a flow signal from the spectral display (and the aural quality of the sound) alone and are particularly useful in circumstances where the image may be ambivalent. An example is the liver, in which the Doppler signatures of the hepatic arterial, portal venous, and hepatic venous structures are quite distinct from each other and that of the biliary tree.

The addition of color

The refinement of duplex scanning to produce color-encoded flow images is one of the more exciting and one of the least well-assessed current applications of Doppler ultrasound. Although examiners may wish to view these Doppler images as depictions of vascular structures in much the same way as the findings of an angiogram are, the images are maps of one estimated Doppler parameter related to flow velocity. The information contained in these images is therefore a combination of anatomic and flow data, whose clinical interpretation requires some skill. Presently, clinical applications outside the heart in which color Doppler has been used include examination of the carotid bifurcation, lower limb arteries and veins, and abdominal vessels (especially in the kidney and the portal venous system and its collaterals); identification of aneurysms and anomalous arterial venous communications; and information about the vessels of the neonatal brain and the flow associated with solid masses.

Color Doppler imaging is clearly well suited to the investigation of the geography of flowing blood in the ultrasound image. Thus in following a vein in the leg or a portal collateral in the abdomen or in demonstrating the carotid bifurcation, the natural role of color is to create a "road map" that can be used to guide the location of the Doppler sample volume, thus increasing the speed and ease of a duplex examination. In attempting to identify and localize vascular lesions such as a stenosis, the color user relies on the effect of the lesion on the pattern of Doppler shifts. These patterns are distinct from although related to those in interpreting Doppler spectra. At present, however, criteria based on the Doppler spectrum continue to form the basis for the diagnosis of vascular disease with Doppler analysis.

Interpretation of color images is complicated by the significant role played by the machine itself in determining the content of the image. Performance of the same examination using a number of color Doppler instruments demonstrates the influence that choice of instrument design exerts on the color Doppler image. The physical method by which the machine produces the images results in some inevitable limitations on the extent of the hemodynamic information that can be extracted. Understanding color images, then, inevitably involves consideration of the way the machine processes the Doppler signals to create the color overlay. For example, the ultrasound beam must remain in one position long enough to receive echoes from the same structures during several sequential pulses so that an estimate of Doppler shift frequency can be made from the phase change in the echoes. One consequence of this limitation is that the time taken to complete one imaging frame is lengthened, thus reducing the overall frame rate; at low frame rates, different parts of the same image will be produced at different points in the cardiac cycle. Another consequence is that accurate estimation of the range of Doppler shifts occurring at a given time is not possible, rendering it difficult to gauge such signs as spectral broadening from the image. Because large changes in the direction as well as the speed of flow can occur during brief intervals of time, color imaging of arterial flow is prone to often somewhat baffling artifacts that become more severe during the imaging of progressively deeper vascular structures. These artifacts are sometimes compounded by software designed to achieve cosmetic processing of the color image, for example, to suppress artifacts from solid, moving structures.

Color flow imaging is a useful aid in the location of focal abnormalities of flow, especially when the abnormalities involve an increase in velocity. Examples include hemodynamically significant stenoses and arteriovenous fistulas.[40] Less obvious but of increasing interest clinically are the arteriovenous shunts associated with the development of solid malignant tumors. Single-gate duplex scanning indicates that very high local velocities (in excess of 1 m/sec) may be attained in such shunts, and their detection with Doppler flow imaging should enhance the ultrasound diagnosis of solid lesions. The sensitivity of color flow imaging instruments to low Doppler signal intensities (associated, for example, with the lower number of scatterers in small vessels) and low Doppler shifts (from the slower moving blood in small vessels) is a major limiting factor in the current use of these instruments in the examination of abdomen and peripheral circulation. At present, color flow imaging sensitivity, especially of flow in deep structures, is achieved at the expense of frame rate, spatial resolution, and aliasing and is generally inferior to that of the current generation of duplex scanners. Technologic developments, however, are likely to narrow this gap.

Semiquantitative methods

Disturbed flow. The characteristics that distinguish disturbed and turbulent flow from laminar flow are reflected in the content of their respective Doppler signals. In a vessel with a flat velocity profile, the spectral display shows a narrow range of Doppler shift frequencies, especially in systole. This is the origin of the window below the spectral trace in systole—a Doppler sign of laminar flow with a blunt profile. Slower-moving laminae are found toward the edge of the vessel, so the size of the window (and the contrast between laminar and disturbed flow signals) can be increased by using a small sample volume situated toward the center of the vessel. Flow disturbance produces velocity vectors with varying direction. Therefore the components of velocity along the direction of the Doppler beam change with time. The combination of many such components results in a wide range of Doppler shifts, seen as a broadening of the spectral display and a reduction in the size of the window. As the velocity increases, vortices form and the Doppler sample volume encounters rotating flow elements. Velocities and hence Doppler shifts are noticeably higher. The vortices contain simultaneous forward and reverse flow in a range of velocities. Vortex formation is time dependent in arteries; they are apparent on a Doppler trace when the critical point is attained in the upstroke of systole. Suddenly, laminar flow gives way to rotating flow, and the Doppler spectrum shows simultaneous forward and reverse velocities with a broad range of Doppler shifts. Laminar flow reappears in diastole as the Reynolds number is reduced.

As flow velocities increase, vortices are shed and travel downstream. As they move through a Doppler sample volume, they are responsible for fluctuation of Doppler shift frequency with time. These rotational components can also have their origin in geometry; a quite normal but tortuous splenic artery will often show a broad spectrum with dramatic fluctuations of maximum Doppler shift frequency. At high Reynold's numbers, turbulence ensues and may be sustained throughout the cardiac cycle. The time-velocity waveform produced by a tight stenosis is much less pulsatile than its normal counterpart. Simultaneous, disorganized forward and reverse Doppler shifts are seen, and velocities remain high throughout the cardiac cycle.

Vascular impedance and pulsatility. Analysis of pulsatile flow in the rapidly bifurcating and highly compliant vascular tree is a complex problem that only in recent years has been the subject of a coherent theory. One consequence of the structure of the arterial system readily observable to the Doppler sonographer, however, is the tendency of the waves of pressure that emanate from the heart to cause reflections from the various vascular beds into which they travel. The modification of the velocity wave by these reflections is the origin of the distinctive character of Doppler waveforms from each of the major arteries. Thus persistent diastolic flow in the internal carotid artery reflects the low resistance of the cerebrovascular bed, whereas the low or reversed diastolic flow seen in the external carotid and femoral arteries is a consequence of the higher-resistance muscular beds that they supply.

Characterization of the time-velocity waveform shape in arteries can yield information of considerable clinical interest. If the entire vessel lies within the sample volume and the flow is laminar, the contour of the maximum Doppler

shift frequency corresponds to the variation in velocity over the cardiac cycle of the fastest moving laminae of blood (usually the center stream). This waveform shape depends on the condition of the proximal circulation and that of the distal receiving bed.[19] With a given pressure waveform at the entrance of an arterial segment, however, the time-velocity waveform shape varies with the impedance of the receiving circulation,[31] a finding that is apparent from the many different waveforms in the adjacent branches of the aorta in spite of their common origin (Fig. 26-2). There are numerous examples of change in waveform as a result of physiologic activity. Best recognized is the change from high-impedance circulation of the lower limbs in the resting state to low-impedance circulation after exercise or during reactive hyperemia. Similarly, there is increased diastolic flow in the superior mesenteric artery after a meal,[1,34] in the ovarian arteries during the second half of the menstrual cycle,[44] and in the uterine arteries during pregnancy.[14,48] In each of these situations, the lowered impedance is associated with increased arterial flow as a result of functional activity.

With a given pressure waveform at the entrance of an arterial segment, the relative diastolic flow velocity changes with the impedance of the receiving circulation. Thus time-velocity waveforms with high flow in diastole (or high diastolic run off) accompany a low downstream impedance, whereas waveforms with little or reverse flow during diastole are seen when the impedance downstream is high. This effect is a direct consequence of pressure-wave propagation in a compliant vessel and is independent of volume flow rate. Because the Doppler shift frequency is proportional to flow velocity, with the constant of proportionality determined by the beam-vessel angle, the ratio of two Doppler shift frequencies is independent of angle. Such ratios may be used to define an index of pulsatility to the waveform, which is independent of probe to vessel angle and can be used as an indicator of distal impedance. The higher the distal impedance, the more pulsatile the waveform.

Several indices have been proposed that reflect the pulsatility of the maximum frequency waveform while remaining independent of probe to vessel angle (Fig. 26-7). The original pulsatility index (PI_F) was calculated from the sum of the Fourier coefficients A_i^2 normalized with respect to the DC value A_0[10]:

$$PI_F = \frac{1}{A_0^2} \sum_{i=1}^{\infty} A_i^2 \qquad (1)$$

Pulsatility index (simplified):

$$PI = \frac{A - B}{Mean} \qquad (2)$$

Pourcelot (resistance) index:

$$RI = \frac{A - B}{A} \qquad (3)$$

A:B (S:D) ratio:

$$S:D = \frac{A}{B} \qquad (4)$$

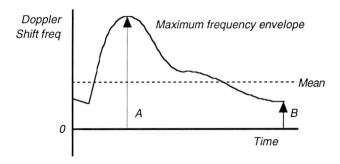

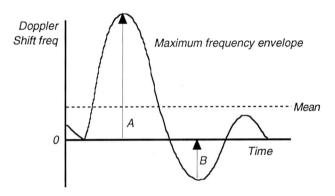

Fig. 26-7. The time-varying waveform of the maximum Doppler shift frequency in a high *(top)* and low *(bottom)* resistance circulation.

Each of these indices is a ratio of Doppler shift frequencies and therefore independent of the Doppler angle. The last three of these indices are most commonly used. A slower heart rate results in a higher pulsatility index (PI), resistance index (RI), and S:D because B and the mean of the maximum Doppler shift frequency are reduced. Although each of these indices is independent of probe to vessel angle, the PI is less susceptible to variation due to heart rate and the setting of the high-pass filter characteristic of the flowmeter, has the greatest number of degrees of freedom, and might be considered the most robust of the indices. This is, however, the only quantity of the three that requires the digitizing of the entire time-velocity waveform, making it the least convenient to measure. If the instrument used does not offer this analysis capability, a microcomputer can be used to digitize a hard cope of the trace offline. Some of the more arbitrarily conceived of these ratios behave in a particularly extravagant fashion as B becomes small. In vessels in which end-diastolic flow is zero, for example, both A:B and its variance are infinite.

As long as the circulation proximal to the point of measurement is constant, indices of pulsatility change with distal arterial impedance. Matters are complicated, however, when the proximal circulation does change. One common cause of this is the presence of a stenosis proximal to, for example, the common iliac artery. A severe stenosis has a filtering effect on pulsatile flow, rendering waveforms less pulsatile, or more dampened. Thus, peripheral vasodilatation (which reduces distal impedance) and proximal stenosis (which dampens the waveform) both have the effect of reducing pulsatility in the iliac artery signal. This may be the one reason that pulsatility analysis is of equivocal diagnostic use in the identification of iliac stenosis.

Quantitative methods

Most of the well-established applications of Doppler ultrasound are qualitative; indeed, the attraction of the color Doppler modality to many radiologists is that it comprises an essentially qualitative depiction of flow-related information. However, Doppler data bear a direct quantitative relationship to blood flow velocity. In principle, data can be used to estimate important hemodynamic variables such as pressure, impedance, and volumetric flow rate. In practice, the circumstances in which such measurements are possible are confined by physical and technical limitations. Three physiologic quantities associated with blood flow in large vessels have been found amenable to estimation with Doppler ultrasound and are local pressure difference, velocity and acceleration of flow, and volume flow rate.

Pressure difference. If blood moving along a vessel at a given flow rate encounters a region in which there is a narrowing, it will speed up. The increase in kinetic energy that a given volume of blood then experiences is equal to the loss of flow potential energy, seen as a pressure drop across the narrowing. For a given pressure drop, the increase in velocity is the same whether the volume of blood is large or small. Thus a measurement of velocity change may be used to infer the magnitude of the pressure drop. In practice, the flow of blood through a stenotic orifice is complicated by the cohesive forces that act between adjacent laminae of moving blood and that tend to resist the acceleration of a single stream within the whole lumen vessel. This effect of viscous friction or drag depends on the size of the orifice as well as the viscosity (and flow velocity) of the blood. Thus viscosity may affect the accuracy of pressure estimations made solely on the basis of flow velocity when the flow is through a relatively small orifice. In addition, if the flow rate is not constant but changing rapidly with time (e.g., in an artery during systole), the force associated with this acceleration will contribute to the drop in energy across the narrowing. These effects may be summarized by the Bernoulli equation:

$$\Delta P = \tfrac{1}{2}\rho v^2 + R_L(V) + \rho \int_s \frac{dv}{dt} ds \qquad (5)$$

where:

ΔP = The potential energy loss or pressure drop

$\tfrac{1}{2}\rho v_2$ = The kinetic energy gain due to acceleration

$R_L(v)$ = The viscous loss due to friction

$\rho \int_s \frac{dv}{dt} ds$ = The inertial gain due to a changing flow rate

In the special case where there is a steady flow and negligible viscous drag, the last two terms are 0. Using values for the density of blood, examiners can estimate the kinetic energy term from a measurement of the jet velocity:

$$\Delta P = 4(v_1^2 - v_2^2) \qquad (6)$$

where ΔP is measured in mm Hg. This relationship is frequently used in cardiac diagnosis, where the relevant characteristics of inviscid flow through a large orifice are found in several conditions (e.g., aortic stenosis), thus allowing pressure gradients to be estimated noninvasively.

Velocity and acceleration. For a given Doppler shift frequency and blood flow in a large vessel, it is a simple matter to solve the Doppler equation for velocity by using an estimate of a beam-flow angle obtained from the real-time image. Most duplex scanners provide a cursor for the direct measurement of this angle. Fig. 26-8 shows, however, that this error in the estimate of velocity resulting from the uncertainty of angle measurement greatly depends on the magnitude of the angle itself. For angles less than approximately 30°, the error is reduced to practical insignificance. For larger angles the cosine term in the Doppler equation causes a small uncertainty in the measurements of the angle to result in a large error in velocity estimation; the technique should probably not be used for angles greater than approximately 55°. For example, in a vessel lying parallel to the maternal abdomen, a satisfactory angle of insonation requires an offset Doppler system, such as a linear array with a Doppler transducer mounted on the end or attached to an articulated arm. The sector scanners with the Doppler beam originating from the apex of the field of view are the most difficult to use in this case. Linear array scanners, which use phased array technology to direct an oblique beam within the rectangular image field of view, have allowed

transducer arrays that are not specifically modified for Doppler to be used instead of the offset configuration. The need to measure the angle of insonation confines this method to vessels with axes lying in the same plane for a few centimeters of their course.

Estimating the spatial mean velocity is more problematic.[10,11,21] The sample volume must embrace the entire vessel lumen, and the mean Doppler shift frequency must be calculated. For vessels of sufficient size to be associated with velocities of interest, the lateral extent of the beam is unlikely to allow such insonation of the entire vessel. Gill[21] has shown that this limitation can be at least partially compensated by the use of a long sample at a low angle of insonation. The mean Doppler shift will then be a convolution of the spatial sensitivity of the sample volume and the velocity profile of the vessel, a quantity that will clearly change for different beams and different points in a converging or diverging field. The high-pass characteristic of the receiver further modifies the estimate of the mean frequency, from which a mean velocity may be calculated.

Flow acceleration may therefore be measured from the gradient of the velocity-time trace; facilities for this procedure are frequently incorporated into the scanner's analysis of software. Clearly, the precision of an acceleration measurement during the upstroke of systole in the aorta, for example, will be enhanced by choosing a fast sweep rate of the Doppler spectral display and a spectrum analyzer with a large, real-time bandwidth.

Volume flow measurement. Noninvasive measurement of volume flow rates in circulations such as the fetoplacental bed and the adult splanchnic system has been the goal of many researchers since the early invasive measurements were performed. All Doppler methods in current clinical use are based on measurements of the spatial mean velocity and the cross-sectional area of the vessel. The product of these two quantities is integrated over time to obtain the volume flow rate:

$$Q = \frac{1}{T} \int_0^T \int_A V. A \, dt \qquad (7)$$

Three of the most commonly used variations are the following:

1. Velocity profile method: In this method the velocity profile is measured at successive intervals throughout the cardiac cycle and integrated to give a volume flow rate. A pulsed Doppler system with a sample volume much smaller than the vessel lumen cross section is required. The sample volume is moved slowly across the vessel lumen and the velocity is calculated by using a beam-vessel angle derived from the two-dimensional image. With the circular symmetry of the profile being assumed, each velocity is multiplied by the corresponding semiannular area and the resulting flow components are summed. Multigate or infinitegate systems, which are capable of interrogating an

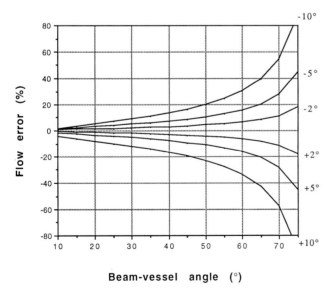

Fig. 26-8. How an error in the measurement of the angle between the beam and the flow direction causes an error in the estimate of flow velocity. Note the heavy dependence on the resulting error on the Doppler angle itself. In practice, this confines velocity measurements to Doppler angles of about 60° or less.

entire vessel at one time, can acquire the necessary data in a single heart beat and are therefore less susceptible to problems of beat-to-beat variation. For transcutaneous applications, this method seems to remain only suitable for large and accessible vessels such as the adult aorta and common carotid arteries.

2. The even insonation method: The principle of the even insonation method is shown in Fig. 26-9. The entire volume of blood whose flow rate is to be assessed is exposed to a uniform ultrasonic beam. The mean Doppler shift corresponding to the mean velocity in the sample volume is then calculated. This velocity is multiplied by the cross-sectional area of the vessels or orifice to give an instantaneous flow value. This product is then integrated into the cardiac cycle, yielding the time average rate. For arterial flow the cross-sectional area changes with time, so the product of the instantaneous mean velocity and the cross-sectional area is ideally formed at the same time. In practice, the goal of simultaneous diameter and flow velocity measurement is not attainable. The optimal ultrasonic approach for the former is perpendicular to the vessel or orifice, whereas for the latter an acute angle of approach to the direction of flow is best. Because it is difficult for two noninterfering beams to be used at the same time, operators usually measure the mean velocity and mean area separately and take their product after rather than before temporal integration. The error introduced depends on the rate of change of both the cross-sectional area and the flow velocity over the cardiac cycle. For example, a 5-mm fetal aorta may vary 20% in diameter (i.e., 40% in cross-sectional area) between systole and diastole.

A common method for the estimation of the cross-sectional area of the vessel orifice is to measure its diameter and assume circular symmetry. Because of the square dependence of area on diameter, the percentage of error in diameter measurement causes an error of approximately double that figure in the flow estimate. For example, a 1-mm uncertainty in the measurement of an 8-mm vessel produces a 25% variation in the flow circulation. For minimizing such errors, careful measurement using a consistent technique, perferably with an M-mode beam intersecting the precise location of the Doppler sampler volume, should be made. Further errors result if the vessel (e.g., a vein) is not circular in cross section. Real-time imaging could be used in this case, but ensuring that the image plane is perpendicular to the flow axis is difficult. These considerations alone limit the usefulness of such measurements in small vessels without recourse to specially designed equipment.

Because the even insonation method requires a value for the mean velocity, the difficulties described

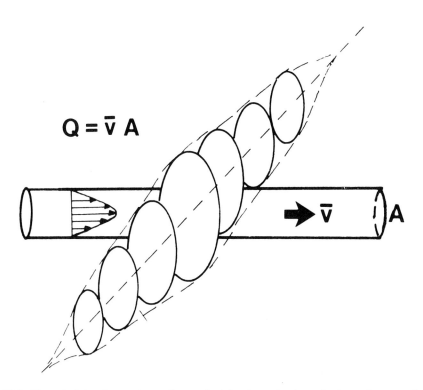

$$Q = \bar{v} A$$

Fig. 26-9. The principle of even insonation method for the estimation of volume flow rate Q. The instantaneous mean velocity v is calculated from the mean Doppler shift frequency and multiplied by the cross-sectional area A of the vessel. (From Burns PN: *Interpretation of Doppler signals.* In Taylor KJW, Burns PN, Wells PNT, eds: *Clinical applications of Doppler ultrasound,* New York, 1988, Raven Press.)

previously in obtaining a mean Doppler frequency that reflects the actual mean flow velocity in the vessel also apply. Even with a uniform beam and perfect processing of the signal to yield its mean frequency, it still will not correspond to the mean velocity. Spectral components whose presence is due to the transit time–broadening phenomenon described earlier distort the mean frequency, and the frequency dependence of attenuation due to tissue itself tends to lower the estimate of the mean velocity provided by pulsed systems. These errors are affected by factors that are hard to control, such as the ultrasonic path and system frequency and bandwidth. Electrical noise in the receiver also affects the mean frequency estimate; because the Doppler bandwidth changes over the cardiac cycle, the signal-to-noise ratio is unlikely to be constant. Finally, the assumption of the uniform scattering of ultrasound by blood is valid but not in the presence of turbulence. The results of studies on blood scattering suggest that the even insonation method should not be used in circumstances in which laminar flow may have given way to turbulence. Gill[20,21] describes a system based on the UI Octoson, which overcomes many of the disadvantages of conventional duplex systems for the estimation of volume flow, and it seems likely that use of a highly specialized instrument such as this will remain the method of choice for volume flow measurement in the adult and fetal abdomen. A linear array with an offset Doppler transducer, such as that described by Eik-Nes, Bruback, and Ulstein,[18] is a reasonable compromise for fetal measurements but suffers the usual disadvantages of linear arrays when used in the upper abdomen. For the abdomen, a modified version of a handheld, real-time duplex system can be envisaged for the quantitative measurement of splanchnic blood flow. Systems based on several methods are currently being developed (Fig. 26-10).

3. Assumed velocity profile method: Because of difficulties in achieving insonation of an entire vessel or computing the mean Doppler shift frequency, some examiners have made measurements at one point in the vessel and assumed a given velocity profile to exist over the vessel lumen. The maximum frequency is then multiplied by a numerical factor that presumably gives the mean Doppler shift frequency. Some produce this factor from empirical studies using an animal model; for these studies the factor is really a calibration constant for the particular experiment, and the physical conditions of the experiment may not correspond to those of the clinical study. Other examiners dispense with the calculation of the mean frequency and estimate its position from the subjective appearance of the spectral display. This is, however, a rather precarious procedure. The gray scale in a display bears a nonlinear relationship (usually square

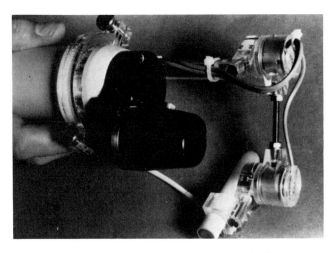

Fig. 26-10. An example of an experimental device for the measurement of volumetric flow rate. The offset transducer is an annular array, capable of producing the broad uniform beams required for the even insonation method. The imaging device is an annular array sector scanner operating at 5 MHz.

root or logarithmic) to the spectral power and can therefore mislead the operator. In some cases the assumption may be made that plug flow (i.e., a perfectly flat velocity profile) exists. This simplifies matters considerably; the spatial mean flow velocity is equal to the maximum velocity near the center of the vessel, an easy quantity to measure. The assumptions of this method probably verge on acceptability for the case of the aortic root in the normal adult. Good correlation has been reported with invasive cardiac output estimates based on dye dilution, suggesting that in the absence of cardiac disease, this may be an acceptable method for the estimation of cardiac output.

4. Attenuation-compensated method: One novel and appealing Doppler method for the measurement of volume flow rate eliminates the need to measure either the beam Doppler angle or the cross-sectional area of the vessel yet makes no severe assumptions about the velocity profile. In the attenuation-compensated flowmeter, two ultrasonic beams are used, the first with a uniform sample volume large enough to embrace the entire vessel and the second with a narrower beam along the same path.[10] The power of the backscattered Doppler signal is proportional to the number of red blood cells in the sample volume. This power is difficult to measure directly because of the attenuating effect of an unknown quantity of intervening tissue. The second, smaller sample volume (situated entirely within the vessel) provides a signal with which to compare the first, subject to the same ultrasonic path and therefore the same attenuation. The difference between the two signal power levels is accounted for entirely by the volume of blood in the large sample volume, which can thus be deduced without recourse

to the direct measurement of the vessel diameter. Furthermore, the dependence of this estimate on the beam-vessel angle is eliminated when it is multiplied by the mean Doppler shift frequency, which has an exactly reciprocal dependence on angle. Thus, in principle, volume flow may be measured without knowledge of either the vessel area or the angle of insonation. The method was proposed and results of in vitro trials were reported in 1979, but further application has awaited practical realization of the required beam geometries. These are beginning to become available, and clinical results (from flow measurements in large vessels such as the adult ascending aorta) are beginning to confirm the validity of the method.

CLINICAL APPLICATIONS

Some of the more simple applications of Doppler in the abdomen are also the most useful clinically. The clinical documentation of the presence and direction of blood flow in the otherwise relatively inaccessible renal, hepatic, splenic, and superior mesenteric circulations, for example, may allow the exclusion of vascular compromise, including thrombosis and stenosis.[2,15,30,39,42] The identification of flow characteristic to a certain circulation may aid in the identification of a structure as a vascular lesion or a transformation of a known vascular structure.[23,49] In addition, study of the Doppler signature itself can yield information related to tissue or to organ blood flow. To the extent that these signatures have characteristics unique to a specific vessel, these characteristics may be at least partly determined by the hemodynamic conditions downstream from the point of measurement.[45] Changes in the perfusion pattern of an organ system would therefore be reflected in changes in the Doppler signals seen in the large supply vessels, whether these changes are pathologic or physiologic. This hypothesis underlies the application of Doppler to the abdominal vessels; the current range of clinical applications of Doppler in the abdomen testifies to its validity.

Aorta

Flow in the aorta is marked by a clear window below systole, indicative of flow at a single velocity across the entire vessel (Figs. 26-1 and 26-2, *B*). Although some slight broadening of the spectrum is often visible in diastole when the impetus of systole is absent and some deceleration of the blood near the vessel wall is evident, plug flow is typically seen throughout the length of the aorta. Pathologic widening or narrowing of the aorta induces changes in the spectrum. Stenosis causes raised velocities, spectral broadening, and turbulence. If sufficiently abrupt, a dilatation such as that associated with an aneurysm results in flow separation and rotational motion. The appearance of such flow on color Doppler is quite striking, with the forward and reverse flow showing as a half moon of red and blue. Because of its ability to show the extent of flow, color is a suitable method with which to demonstrate the true lumen of a dissected aneurysm or to map thrombus that may not be apparent on the image.

Flow in diastole drops to zero at the approximate point in the cardiac cycle at which the aortic valve closes. Blood begins to flow again as the compliant walls of the great vessels, which expanded during systole, collapse, driving blood at the lower diastolic pressure into the peripheral circulation. Below the renal arteries, however (Fig. 26-5), a small reverse component can be seen during diastole, which becomes more marked as the bifurcation is approached. This reverse flow has its origin in the reflection of the systolic pulse of blood as it travels down the aortic tree and encounters the high impedance of the lower limb periphery. The reflections occur at the many discontinuities in vascular impedance found at the bifurcations of the arterioles, whose muscular tone varies with vasomotor activity.[9] Thus a vasoconstricted (i.e., normal) lower limb periphery causes diastolic flow reversal in the iliac arteries. Vasodilatation induced by the results of reactive hyperemia abolishes the reverse flow in these large vessels, supporting the notion that diastolic flow changes in large vessels reflect resistive variation in the microcirculation.

Celiac vessels

Flow in the celiac trunk shows spectral broadening during diastole typical of a smaller vessel (Fig. 26-2). There is persistent flow in diastole that is not changed after a meal. The hepatic and left gastric arteries are somewhat less pulsatile than the celiac artery and show a more even distribution of power with frequency (i.e., a more even grayscale) throughout the cardiac cycle. The gastroduodenal artery (Fig. 26-2, *F*) shows quite low Doppler shifts and is not always detectable. The fluctuations of the spectrum with time and the uneven distribution of power in the splenic artery signal indicate flow disturbance in this vessel, which may be related to its tortuosity.

Aneurysms can occur in the branches of the celiac trunk, most commonly in the splenic artery. Patients with chronic pancreatitis are particularly prone to these arterial aneurysms. Such aneurysms may undergo catastrophic rupture, underlining the importance of accurate diagnosis. Doppler analysis may be used to make the important differentiation between these aneurysms and cystic lesions such as pancreatic pseudocysts.[44]

Superior mesenteric artery

Flow signals in the superior mesenteric artery (SMA) can be obtained in most individuals (Fig. 26-2, *A*). When the SMA is obscured by gas in the intestine, changes in posture or ingestion of water may be helpful. The signal often shows flow disturbance near its highly curved origin with the aorta. The waveform shape in this vessel varies markedly with feeding; in the fasting state, there is typically a high-impedance pattern, with little flow in diastole and sometimes even reverse diastolic flow. This gives way in the postprandial subject to constant diastolic flow. The PI of a fasting SMA signal is about 3.5, dropping to 1.5 2 hours after a meal.[34] More quantitative studies of volumetric flow rate in the SMA have suggested that patients with the dumping syndrome after gastric surgery may experience an abnormal redistribution of splanchnic blood flow after a meal.[1] A few cases of using duplex Doppler of SMA and celiac trunk stenosis in the successful diagnosis of mesenteric angina have been reported.

The liver

Signals from the intrahepatic portions of the hepatic artery can be elicited easily by using an intercostal approach and a coronal plane. They show a waveform pattern typical of parabolic flow in a low-impedance vessel (Fig. 26-3, *D*). The portal vein displays a characteristic continuous flow pattern (Fig. 26-3, *E*), unique because of the exceptional isolation of this circulation from the proximal pump; it is buffered from the great vessels by the splanchnic bed on one side and the liver parenchyma on the other. Nonetheless, transmitted cardiac variation in the portal vein Doppler shift is discernible in most individuals. In contrast, the hepatic veins and their major branches show a distinctive triphasic signal that reflects the influence of right atrial pressure on hepatic outflow. A phase of reverse flow coinciding with regurgitation of inferior vena cava (IVC) flow in atrial systole is normal. The triphasic flow pattern is complicated in the IVC itself (Fig. 26-3, *C*) by the influence of variations in thoracic and abdominal pressure. However, the pattern of IVC flow remains similar toward the iliac veins, allowing exclusion of occlusion by thrombosis or tumor invasion or compression on the basis of continuity of an identifiable pressure pattern.

Portal hypertension. Many of the primary features of portal hypertension, including those that pose the greatest threat to the patient, are hemodynamic in nature. Doppler can be used to identify hepatofugal flow and to trace spontaneous portosystemic shunts[32] as well as the influence of portal venous congestion on the ratio of flow velocity to portal and splenic vein diameter.[29] Collateral pathways, including those that are variceal, need to be followed systematically, and protocols have been proposed to achieve this.[30,33]

Surgically established portosystemic shunts may be evaluated for patency[25] and even volumetric[21] flow rate using Doppler ultrasound. Even if the shunt itself cannot be visualized, the demonstration of hepatofugal flow within intrahepatic portal veins may be a reliable indicator of shunt patency. Transplantation of the liver[26,42,50] and pancreas[27] constitutes another area of surgical intervention in which the simple exclusion of occlusion of the major vessels by thrombosis is helpful in the monitoring of the postoperative progress. Duplex scanning is repeatable, portable, and noninvasive and therefore ideal for use in the intensive care unit.

Duplex evaluation has also proven useful in confirmation of portal vein thrombosis and associated venous collaterals, so-called cavernous transformation of the portal vein.[49] In these patients, the multiple tubular channels in the porta show a waveform characteristic of portal venous flow. Color Doppler may be helpful in the rapid identification of these structures as vascular. Finally, thrombosis of the hepatic venous system—Budd-Chiari syndrome—may be both diagnosed and excluded by using duplex or color systems, although perhaps because of the relative rarity as well as the complexity of the syndrome, no consensus as to the reliability of Doppler in this diagnosis has yet been reached.

The kidneys

Although the right renal artery can usually be examined in the supine position, the decubitus or prone translumbar approach is best for the left renal artery. All renal arteries (Fig. 26-4) show a typical low-impedance pattern, with significant diastolic flow and a broad spectrum of velocities during both systole and diastole. Signals may be obtained from the segmental, interlobar, and arcuate branches of the renal artery, even though this last class of vessels is too small to be visualized with ultrasound imaging. Doppler examination of the kidneys has been used in the diagnosis of renal artery stenosis, microvascular disease of the kidneys, fistulas, and tumors and in the assessment of renal transplant function.[37]

The prevalence of renovascular disease among patients with hypertension is estimated to be between 1% and 10%. In spite of the use of excretory urography and renal scintigraphy, definitive diagnosis and grading by measurement of a pressure gradient is generally only established by arteriography. There remains a need for a simple and noninvasive diagnostic procedure with acceptable sensitivity for the detection of renal artery stenosis (RAS). Duplex scanning of the renal vessels may be used to detect partial vascular obstruction. However, some of the signs of poststenotic flow seen routinely in superficial arteries are too unreliable to be useful in a deep vessel the size of the renal artery. Although spectral broadening and the simultaneous forward and reverse velocity of vortex flow are occasionally seen to accompany milder degrees of stenosis (Fig. 26-11), technical factors that tend to cause the normal spectrum to be broad (e.g., sample volume size and depth, a blunted flow velocity profile, vessel movement) confound the diagnostic use of these features. Thus an abnormally high velocity of blood flow in a renal artery is the main usable sign of stenosis. This high flow velocity and the turbulence that may follow it can be a local phenomenon. It is therefore necessary to ensure that the entire length of both renal arteries is scanned to exclude RAS with confidence. For these reasons, the ultrasound examination requires some practice and is still occasionally unsuccessful. Technical success rates of between 76% and 94% have been reported, although some persistence may be needed from the sonographer, with scanning times of up to 1 hour.[3,16,24] Relevant technical factors include recent oral intake, intestinal gas, scarring from previous abdominal surgery, obesity, abdominal aortic an-

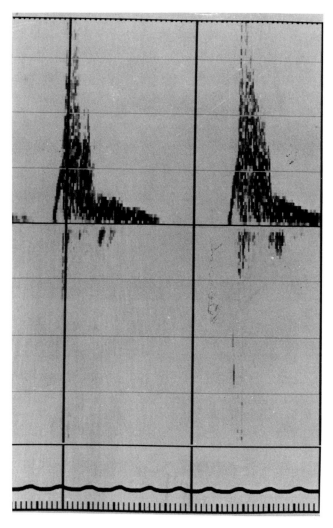

Fig. 26-11. Spectrum showing disturbed flow in renal artery stenosis. Plug flow is seen in early systole as a clear window in the time velocity spectrum. As the velocity increases, there is a sudden onset of vortex shedding (apparent as a broad spectrum), irregular spectral outline, and simultaneous forward and reversed flow. (From Burns PN: *Interpretation of Doppler signals*. In Taylor KJW, Burns PN, Wells PNT, eds: *Clinical applications of Doppler ultrasound*, New York, 1988, Raven Press.)

eurysms, ascites, and vessel calcification. Although RAS Doppler spectra may tend to have irregular waveforms with spectral broadening and a rounded or indistinct systolic peak with a slow rise time, the most reliable sign of stenosis is a localized increase in peak systolic frequency followed by a sudden decrease distally.[16,22,40] Unfortunately, it is rarely possible to estimate velocities because the Doppler angle is frequently unknown. In one study,[27] frequencies above 4 kHz when using a 3-MHz transducer yielded a sensitivity of 83% and specificity of 97% to RAS. More recently, the so-called renal-aortic ratio (RAR) has been proposed as a practical means of using the ratio of peak renal artery velocity to aortic velocity to distinguish stenotic (greater than 60% diameter reduction) from nonstenotic renal arteries. The highest peak systolic Doppler shift obtainable from each

renal artery is compared to that of the aorta at the same level. In general, the renal artery shift is no more than 1.5 times that of the aorta at peak systole; an RAR of 3.5 or more is taken to indicate a 60% or greater stenosis. In a 1986 study,[24] 90% of the duplex examinations were technically adequate, and arteriographic correlation was available for 43 renal arteries. According to these criteria, the method yields a sensitivity of 91% and a specificity of 95% to these hemodynamically significant lesions.

The transplanted kidney is superficial and an ideal organ for ultrasound scanning. The major complications of renal transplantation include RAS (12%), renal artery occlusion (12%) (generally occurring secondary to severe vascular rejection), renal vein stenosis (less common than arterial stenosis), arteriovenous fistula, and acute or chronic rejection. Assessment of many of these complications can be made with the combination of real-time imaging and pulsed Doppler.[37] Doppler signals can be readily obtained from the main renal artey and vein and the vessels to which they have been anastomosed, as well as the segmental, interlobar, and arcuate intrarenal branches. The normal arterial signals from a transplanted kidney are similar to those from a native kidney, showing a persistence of flow throughout diastole, which is indicative of a low distal impedance. Signals obtained from the renal artery near the site of anastomosis may, however, show some signs of flow disturbance. Unusual signals may also be seen within the kidney in cases of arteriovenous fistula created as a consequence of biopsy.[5,47] The confidence with which it is possible to obtain normal signals also allows the inference of total vascular occlusion when they are absent. In a series of eight such diagnoses confirmed at nephrectomy, there were no false positives or negatives.[47]

Quantitative Doppler estimates of renal flow rate have been attempted in the transplanted kidney, but the difficulty of estimating lumen area from the ultrasound views of the main renal artery generally achieved are likely to remain severe obstacles to accurate measurement. Instead, interpretation of the time-velocity spectrum itself must be relied on as the basis of assessment for vascular compromise. Severe RAS of the transplanted kidney, like that of the normal renal artery, produces isolated high Doppler shift frequencies with signs of distal turbulence that may extend into the renal sinus[37,47] (Fig. 26-12). Because of the confounding effect of flow disturbance due to surgical anastomosis or kinking of the artery, the technique is probably not suitable for assessing milder lesions. The Doppler examination is especially suited for documenting and monitoring the effect of renal artery angioplasty.[47]

Doppler changes in the renal artery accompanying acute allograft rejection were first reported as early as 1969; present techniques concentrate on analysis of the time-velocity waveform (the form of the outline of the Doppler spectrum) to detect changes in distal impedance. These changes are thought to be associated with proliferative endovasculitis or acute sclerosing vasculopathy in the renovascular bed,

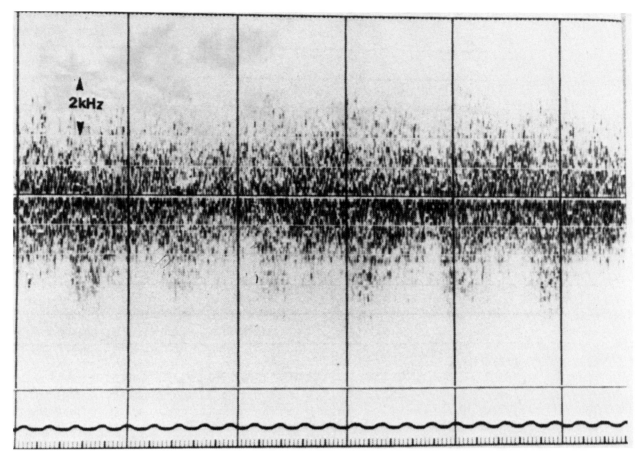

Fig. 26-12. Severe stenosis in a transplanted renal artery. Note the high velocities, the chaotic forward and reverse flow typical of turbulence, and the abolition of clear pulsatility in the waveform. This stenosis was detected by Doppler and treated by percutaneous angioplasty. (From Burns PN: *Interpretation of Doppler signals*. In Taylor KJW, Burns PN, Wells PNT, eds: *Clinical applications of Doppler ultrasound*, New York, 1988, Raven Press.)

which may accompany rejection.[4,39,43] The result is an attenuation of relative diastolic velocity and an increase in arterial pulsatility in the Doppler signal (Fig. 26-13). Pure interstitial rejection, on the other hand, leaves these vessels relatively unchanged; here the reported changes in the Doppler signal must be the result of a less direct consequence of renal dysfunction. The use of an index such as the PI allows quantitative assessment of the technique.[5,36,38] In a series of 55 patients studied within 24 hours of biopsy,[38] the normal PI for all vessels lies within the range of 1.1 to 1.26. A PI greater than 1.5 yielded a 75% sensitivity to acute rejection of all forms and a 79% sensitivity to acute vascular rejection at a specificity of 90%. The effect of important clinical complications such as acute tubular necrosis and cyclosporine toxicity on the Doppler pulsatility is not entirely clear, but experimental studies suggest that Doppler is probably not sufficiently specific to allow differentiation among all relevant entities.[4,6,38,43] Further work is required in this area. The segmental artery is perhaps the most convenient and

reproducible site from which to obtain signals for the investigation of pulsatility, and receiver-operator characteristic analysis suggests that it may also be the most accurate.[38]

Doppler tissue characterization

Traditionally, the use of Doppler has been confined to the detection of local flow characteristics such as turbulence associated with local disease such as atherosclerotic lesions. Newer applications of Doppler in the abdomen demonstrate that some information can be gained about organs in the distal circulation by looking at one point on a major vessel such as the renal artery. As this information is related to blood flow, it becomes functional, or physiologic. It is therefore natural to ask whether Doppler could be used to look at organs themselves for assessment of some characteristic related to the function of tissue. Such Doppler tissue characterization offers the possibility of assessing not only normal, physiologic changes, which may be reflected in tissue blood flow (such as in the ovary over the menstrual cycle),

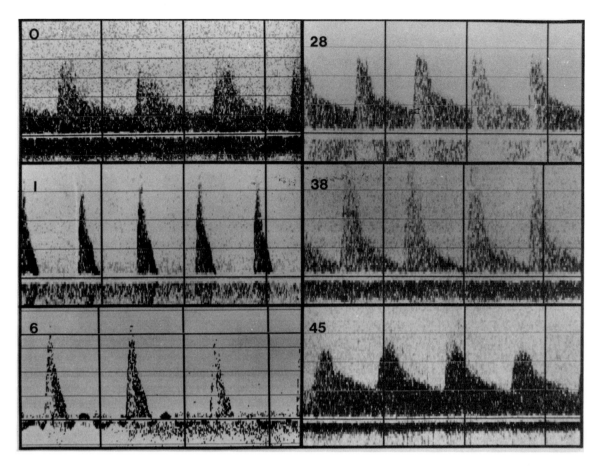

Fig. 26-13. Illustrative case of Doppler signals from the segmental artery of a transplanted kidney during an episode of acute rejection. On the day of surgery (day 0), the signal is normal. On day 1, diastolic flow has disappeared, and by day 6, reverse diastolic flow is visible. After treatment (day 2), a normal flow pattern is seen.

but also pathologic changes in tissue function that may be of diagnostic value, such as in malignant neovascularization of a developing cancer.[13]

Every malignant tumor begins life as a single aberrant cell. This cell can multiply to form a colony whose size is limited by the diffusion of oxygen and nutrients to a millimeter or so in diameter. An in situ tumor of this type in the breast or cervix can remain dormant for many years. Only when a humoral substance known as *tumor angiogenesis factor* is produced by the tumor do new blood vessels begin to proliferate from the host into the mass. This new blood supply provides the means for malignant growth as well as a path for metastatic spread to distant parts of the body. The importance of this process of tumor vascularization has led to the investigation of whether Doppler ultrasound may be able to detect the blood flow associated with a tumor. The vessels are very small, so a high-frequency system and a superficial organ is best. For example, in the breast, Doppler signals from small developing cancers have been demonstrated and their peculiar characteristics de-

scribed quantitatively.[13] These characteristics have their origin in documented features of the tumor circulation such as arteriovenous shunts and the geometry of vascular morphology.[10] They may be of help not only in the diagnosis of cancer (such neovascularization rarely happens in benign tumors) but also in studying the biology of a developing tumor; clinicians could try to see, for example, whether the tumor is responding to therapy or judge if it is aggressive or slow growing.

Explanation of these features allows Doppler ultrasound to become an adjunct to the ultrasonic investigation of abdominal lesions. Particularly sensitive duplex pulsed Doppler scanners are needed for the interrogation of deep sites for these rather weak signals. Preliminary results from assessment of tumors of the liver,[46] thyroid, skin, pancreas, and kidney[17,35] have been reported with generally optimistic conclusions. Work still needs to be done, however, to define more precisely the appropriate diagnostic criteria for specific tumor sites and to establish those areas in which the clinical contribution of the technique is likely to be greatest.

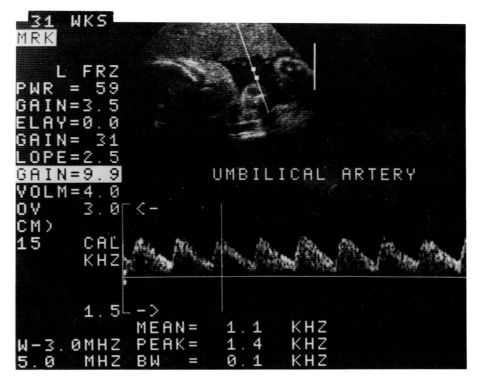

Fig. 26-14. Typical signals from the umbilical cord artery of a fetus at 31 weeks. Note the persistent flow throughout diastole that characterizes placental arterial blood flow in the normal pregnancy during the last trimester.

Obstetric Doppler

Ultrasound imaging has established its preeminence in antenatal diagnosis through its ability to depict anatomic change and hence follow fetal growth. In contrast, Doppler ultrasound, by virtue of its ability to detect blood flow, offers the potential to study functional and hence physiologic change. One important question is whether Doppler may help distinguish the fetus that is small for gestational age but otherwise healthy from the small for gestational age fetus that is suffering from deprivation of oxygen and nutrition in utero and hence is at risk for obstetric and neonatal complications.

In physiologic terms, the most useful blood flow parameter to measure may well be the volumetric flow rate through the fetal umbilical circulation.[7] Ultrasound can accomplish this measurement in the umbilical vein but only at the risk of substantial errors if careful attention is not paid to physical technique. In general, specialized instrumentation is necessary for the accurate measurement of blood flow rate with Doppler ultrasound. Results do show, however, significant differences in flow rate between fetuses with intrauterine growth retardation and normal fetuses. Furthermore, the severity of subsequent morbidity has been shown to relate to the magnitude of the flow deficit through the placenta. The measurement also seems to anticipate the detection of fetal compromise by conventional means, although by no great margin.

One method of detecting related flow changes, which may be more practical in a clinical setting, is the analysis of the shape of the time-velocity waveform itself (Fig. 26-14). Pulsatility indices from the umbilical cord and maternal uterine arteries have yielded promising clinical results to date. Some recent results suggest that Doppler examinations may be sensitive to the subgroup of small for gestational age fetuses who are suffering privation in utero and are thus at particular risk.[48]

Finally, Doppler signals can be detected from the arterial uterine and uteroplacental circulations. The normal evolution of the placenta in pregnancy includes a dramatic lowering in resistance to uterine flow, which occurs during the second trimester. This process appears to be modified in such cases as toxemia of pregnancy; this clue may hold promise in the future for an early screening examination with Doppler ultrasound of patients who have pregnancy-induced hypertension.[14,48]

NEW METHODS

Generally speaking, the sensitivity of color flow imaging instruments to *low* Doppler signal intensities associated with the lower number of scatterers in small vessels and *slow* Doppler shifts from the slower moving blood in small vessels is a major limiting factor in their current use in the abdomen and peripheral circulation. In addition, the spatial resolution of color instruments limits the definition of ve-

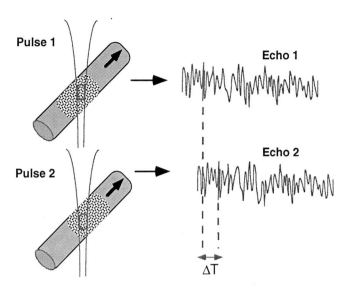

Fig. 26-15. The principle of the time-domain speckle-tracking method for the production of color images. Random fluctuations present in the echo form a small volume of blood create a speckle pattern that moves at the same velocity as the blood itself. The cross-correlation technique compares consecutive echoes, looking for displacement of the pattern along the axis of the beam. Velocity is calculated by dividing the distance moved by the period between pulses. Note that the method yields an estimate of the component of velocity in the direction of the ultrasound beam, just as Doppler methods do. The time-domain method overcomes an evident compromise in color Doppler methods, whereby spatial resolution and accuracy of velocity estimation are conflicting requirements. Time-domain methods use short pulses similar to those used for imaging and hence are able to achieve high spatial resolution.

locity detail within a large vessel and the ability to localize low flow structures. At present, color flow imaging sensitivity, especially of flow in deep structures, can only be achieved at the expense of spatial resolution and frame rate and is generally inferior to that of current duplex scanners. Likewise, color spatial resolution is inferior to that of the gray-scale image. Technologic developments, however, are likely to narrow these gaps. One of the more promising of these is the use of the time-domain, speckle-tracking methods for the production of color images (Fig. 26-15). These methods do not rely directly on the Doppler shift for the detection of motion; instead they track the movement of structure in the ultrasound image. The principle is quite simple: the echo from blood is the combined result of many small echoes from the individual scatterers, which are the red blood cells themselves. These account for a grainy, specklelike structure within the blood that would be visible on the image if the echo from blood were stronger, much as speckle within the parenchyma of the liver is seen. With flow, this pattern moves at the same speed as the blood. By comparing the pattern of the ultrasound (usually at the radiofrequency level of the receiver) at a particular location in the beam at one time to that obtained a moment later at the same location, the examiner can measure the distance the speckle has moved and infer the blood velocity. This

method, like Doppler, yields only the component of velocity along the ultrasound beam. Just as for a Doppler image, the beam-flow angle must be known to measure true velocity. This method seems to be particularly suited to the production of high-resolution color images; the cross-correlation method works best with the short pulses that give high axial resolution. Under these conditions the technique is also immune from aliasing, the artifact so familiar to pulsed Doppler users. It is possible, however, that the current price for these advantages may be a lower sensitivity to low flow states. Exciting possibilities for the future of the correlation method include two-dimensional Doppler images (albeit with much reduced lateral velocity resolution) and quantitative (perhaps volumetric flow) color imaging.

In the future, it is likely that a combination of these techniques will be applied toward the production of high-resolution images of low or slow flow. An important role in the detection of low volumes of blood will be played by ultrasound contrast agents, an intravenous injection of a small quantity of which is capable of increasing the echo from deep arterial vessels by a factor of 50 or more. This is one method to raise the received echo intensity of ultrasound scattered from small quantities of blood deep in the body to levels detectable at the skin surface. When this is attained, color flow imaging can be applied to the issue of blood velocity and blood flow imaging itself at the parenchymal level. Quantitative and deep color Doppler is in its infancy at present, with many technical problems still needing to be overcome before specific clinical applications are achievable. However, these and other developments in Doppler technology are likely to ensure that the current proliferation of clinical problems to which ultrasonographers have addressed Doppler methods will be sustained in the foreseeable future.

CONCLUSION

Deep Doppler analysis presents a stimulating challenge to the vascular sonographer. Although the technique is demanding on both the operator and the equipment and there are relatively few firm guidelines available for the interpretation of studies, the rewards for successful application of the technique are high. Future developments in instrumentation are certain to encourage the development of Doppler examination of smaller and deeper vessels. For example, fundamental limitations such as the low signal strength from the blood echo itself might be overcome with the refinement of ultrasound contrast agents that can be injected into the peripheral vascular system and that remain stable for a sufficient length of time to recirculate for the duration of an ultrasound examination. Color Doppler is likely to become a more suitable modality for the detection of the low flow velocities found in organ parenchyma. Finally, quantitative flow-measuring methods await development to allow the Doppler method to be extended into the area of true physiologic measurement of abdominal blood flow.

REFERENCES

1. Aldoori MI et al: Increased flow in the superior mesenteric artery in dumping syndrome, *Br J Surg* 72:389-390, 1985.
2. Alpern MB et al: Porta hepatis: duplex Doppler US with angiographic correlation, *Radiology* 162:53-56, 1987.
3. Avasthi PS, Voyles WF, Greene ER: Noninvasive diagnosis of renal artery stenosis by echo-Doppler velocimetry, *Kidney Int* 25:824-829, 1984.
4. Berland LL, Lawson TL, Adams MB: Evaluation of canine renal transplants with pulsed Doppler duplex sonography, *J Surg Res* 39:433-438, 1985.
5. Berland LL et al: Evaluation of renal transplants with pulsed Doppler duplex sonography, *J Ultrasound Med* 1:215-222, 1982.
6. Buckley AR et al: The distinction between acute renal transplant rejection and cyclosporine nephrotoxicity: value of duplex sonography, *AJR* 149:521-525, 1987.
7. Burns PN: *Doppler flow estimations in the fetal and maternal circulations: principles, techniques and some limitations.* In Maulik D, McNellis D, eds: *Doppler ultrasound measurement and maternal-fetal hemodynamics,* Ithaca, New York, 1987, Perinatalogy Press.
8. Burns PN: Physical principles of Doppler ultrasound and spectral analysis, *J Clin Ultrasound* 15:567-590, 1987.
9. Burns PN: *Hemodynamics.* In Taylor KJW, Burns PN, Wells PNT: *Clinical applications of Doppler ultrasound,* New York, 1988, Raven Press.
10. Burns PN: *Interpretation of Doppler signals.* In Taylor KJW, Burns PN, Wells PNT: *Clinical applications of Doppler ultrasound,* New York, 1988, Raven Press.
11. Burns PN, Jaffe CC: Quantitative Doppler flow measurements: techniques, accuracy and limitations, *Radiol Clin North Am* 23(4):641-657, 1985.
12. Burns PN, Taylor KJW, Blei AT: Doppler flowmetry and portal hypertension, *Gastroenterology* 92:824-826, 1987.
13. Burns PN et al: Ultrasonic Doppler studies of the breast, *Ultrasound Med Biol* 8(2):127-143, 1982.
14. Campbell S et al: New Doppler technique for assessing uteroplacental blood flow, *Lancet*:657-677, 1983.
15. Dalen K et al: Imaging of vascular complications after hepatic transplantation, *AJR* 150:1285-1290, 1988.
16. Dubbins PA: Renal artery stenosis: duplex Doppler evaluation, *Br J Radiol* 59:225-229, 1986.
17. Dubbins PA, Wells PNT: Renal carcinoma: duplex Doppler evaluation, *Br J Radiol* 59:231-236, 1986.
18. Eik-Nes SH, Bruback AO, Ulstein MK: Measurement of human fetal blood flow, *Br Med J* 280:283-284, 1980.
19. Evans DH: Some aspects of the relationship between instantaneous volumetric blood flow and continuous wave Doppler ultrasound recordings. I. The effect of ultrasonic beam width on the output of maximum, mean and rms frequency processors, *Ultrasound Med Biol* 8:605-609, 1982.
20. Gill RW: Pulsed Doppler with B-mode imaging for quantitative blood flow measurement, *Ultrasound Med Biol* 5:223-235, 1979.
21. Gill RW: Measurement of blood flow by ultrasound: accuracy and sources of error, *Ultrasound Med Biol* 11:625-641, 1985.
22. Greene ER, Avasthi PS, Hodges JW: Noninvasive Doppler assessment of renal artery stenosis and hemodynamics, *J Clin Ultrasound* 15:653-659, 1987.
23. Helvie MA et al: The distinction between femoral artery pseudoaneurysms and other causes of groin masses: value of duplex Doppler sonography, *AJR* 150:1177-1180, 1988.
24. Kohler TR et al: Noninvasive diagnosis of renal artery stenosis by ultrasonic duplex scanning, *J Vasc Surg* 4:450-456, 1986.
25. Lafortune M et al: Hemodynamic changes in portal circulation after portosystemic shunts: use of duplex sonography in 43 patients, *AJR* 149:701-706, 1987.
26. Letourneau JG et al: Abdominal sonography after hepatic transplantation: results in 36 patients, *AJR* 149:299-303, 1987.
27. Letourneau JG et al: Ultrasound and computed tomography in the evaluation of pancreatic transplantation, *Radiol Clin North Am* 25(2):345-355, 1987.
28. Mitchell DG et al: Femoral artery pseudoaneurysm: diagnosis with conventional duplex and color Doppler US, *Radiology* 165:687-690, 1987.
29. Moriyasu F et al: "Congestion index" of the portal vein, *AJR* 146:735-739, 1986.
30. Nelson RC et al: Comparison of pulsed Doppler sonography and angiography in patients with portal hypertension, *AJR* 149:77-81, 1987.
31. Norris CS et al: Noninvasive evaluation of renal artery stenosis and renovascular resistance, *J Vasc Surg* 1:192-201, 1984.
32. Ohnishi K et al: Direction of splenic venous flow assessed by pulsed Doppler flowmetry in patients with a large splenorenal shunt: relation to spontaneous hepatic encephalopathy, *Gastroenterology* 89:180-185, 1985.
33. Patriquin H et al: Duplex Doppler examination in portal hypertension: technique and anatomy, *AJR* 149:71-76, 1987.
34. Qamar MI et al: Transcutaneous Doppler ultrasound measurement of superior mesenteric artery blood flow in man, *Gut* 27:100-105, 1984.
35. Ramos I et al: Detection of tumor vascular signals in renal masses by Doppler ultrasound, *Radiology* 168:633-637, 1988.
36. Rifkin MD et al: Evaluation of renal transplant rejection by duplex Doppler examination: value of the resistive index, *Am J Roentgenol* 148:759-767, 1987.
37. Rigsby CM, Burns PN: *Renal duplex sonography.* In Taylor KJW, Burns PN, Wells PNT, eds: *Clinical applications of Doppler ultrasound,* New York, 1988, Raven Press.
38. Rigsby CM, Burns PN, Weltin G: Quantitation of Doppler signals in renal allografts: comparison of normal and rejecting transplants with pathologic correlation, *Radiology* 162:39-42, 1987.
39. Rigsby CM et al: Renal allografts in acute rejection: evaluation using duplex sonography, *Radiology* 158:375-378, 1986.
40. Rittgers SE, Norris CS, Barnes RW: Detection of renal artery stenosis: experimental and clinical analysis of velocity waveforms, *Ultrasound Med Biol* 11:3, 523-531, 1985.
41. Sato S et al: Splenic artery and superior mesenteric artery blood flow: nonsurgical Doppler US measurement in healthy subjects and patients with chronic liver disease, *Radiology* 164:347-352, 1987.
42. Segel MC et al: Hepatic artery thrombosis after liver transplantation: radiologic evaluation, *AJR* 146:137-141, 1986.
43. Steinberg HV et al: Renal allograft rejection: evaluation by Doppler US and MR imaging, *Radiology* 162:337-342, 1987.
44. Taylor KJW, Burns PN: Duplex Doppler scanning in the pelvis and abdomen, *Ultrasound Med Biol* 11:4, 643-658, 1985.
45. Taylor KJW et al: Blood flow in deep abdominal and pelvic vessels: ultrasonic pulsed-Doppler analysis, *Radiology* 154:487-493, 1985.
46. Taylor KJW et al: Focal liver masses: differential diagnosis with pulsed Doppler US, *Radiology* 164:643-647, 1987.
47. Taylor KJW et al: Vascular complications in renal allografts: detection with duplex Doppler US, *Radiology* 162:31-38, 1987.
48. Trudinger BJ, Giles WB, Cook CM: Uteroplacental blood flow velocity time waveforms in normal and complicated pregnancy, *Br J Obstet Gynaecol* 92:39-45, 1985.
49. Weltin G et al: Duplex Doppler: identification of cavernous transformation of the portal vein, *AJR* 144:999-1001, 1985.
50. Wozney P et al: Vascular complications after liver transplantation: a 5-year experience, *AJR* 147:657-663, 1986.

CHAPTER 27

Noninvasive evaluation of the cutaneous circulation

ARNOST FRONEK

Despite the skin's accessibility, there is no ideal method that permits a quantitative evaluation of skin perfusion. The only exception is the determination of digital (or toe) blood flow, which can be measured by venous occlusive plethysmography (see Chapter 97). Since skin blood flow is the most essential component of digital blood flow, the two can be equated. The need to determine skin perfusion at other sites, however, poses serious difficulties, especially if a quantitative evaluation is desired.

There are several indications for the determination of skin perfusion: (1) to determine optimal amputation level, (2) to evaluate vasospastic conditions, (3) to evaluate vasoactive or rheologic drugs that may have an effect on skin circulation, and (4) to predict the effectiveness of sympathectomy. Methods that can be considered in this category include the following:

1. Skin thermometry
2. Thermal conductance
3. Thermal clearance
4. Transcutaneous partial tension of oxygen (Po_2)
5. Laser Doppler flux
6. Skin arterial blood pressure
7. Epicutaneous ^{133}Xe clearance
8. Venous occlusion plethysmography
9. Photoplethysmography

Venous occlusion plethysmography and photoplethysmography are not discussed in this chapter because they are covered elsewhere in this text. In this chapter, only general aspects of skin temperature measurements are discussed. (A detailed evaluation is also discussed in Chapter 102.)

SKIN THERMOMETRY

Skin temperature is one of the best-known indices of skin perfusion. However, its value is limited when it is compared with superior techniques. These limitations are based on physical as well as physiologic considerations.

Skin temperature is determined by many factors, which include room temperature, humidity, circulation of the air, state of metabolic and nervous activity, vasomotor and audiomotor activity, previous exposure to nicotine, and type of food ingested. It is difficult to keep all these factors constant, especially during routine diagnostic examination

conditions. On the other hand, temperature differences among various sites of the body are more meaningful because the results are somewhat normalized. However, this does not prevent misinterpretations, since some vascular regions are under different vasomotor control than others, such as toes or fingers and thigh or arm. In addition, absolute temperature measurements are much less useful than relative temperature measurements (topographic gradients) and dynamic skin temperature tests (temporal gradients).

An example of the limited diagnostic value of absolute temperature measurements is the finding of a highly non-linear correlation between blood flow and skin temperature.[29] Relatively small increases in blood flow, starting with low skin temperature, result in significant increases in skin temperature, whereas a similar increase in blood flow corresponds to a minute temperature increase once the 28° C threshold is reached.

Skin thermometry can be subdivided into contact thermometry, with a thermocouple, thermistor, or liquid crystals; and noncontact thermometry (infrared thermography), with imaging and nonimaging techniques.

Contact thermometry

Thermocouples. Widely used in the past, thermocouples are being used slightly more today after having been displaced by the more sensitive thermistors. If two different metals are joined, such as copper and constantan, a temperature-dependent potential develops.[19,37] For instance, the combination of copper and constantan has a thermoelectric sensitivity of 40 μV for each degree Celsius. This relatively small voltage compelled earlier investigators to use high-sensitivity galvanometers, which were impractical in daily laboratory routine. Low-sensitivity but more rugged recording devices required high-gain direct current (DC) amplification, which was not a simple task before the advent of operational amplifiers.

Thermistors. The electric resistance of some metals, especially alloys, exhibits considerable temperature dependence. Alloys with a high temperature coefficient of resistivity are selected as the base material for thermistors. In contrast to most metals such as platinum, which have a positive thermal coefficient, thermistors are composed of different metallic oxides, which have a negative thermal coefficient—with increasing temperature, the resistance decreases.

Thermocouples versus thermistors. Thermocouples usually require DC amplification when used with simple and rugged recording or monitoring devices. The availability of low-drift, high-gain, semiconductor amplifier systems has triggered a renewed interest in these instruments. Their advantages are linearity and sturdiness of the probe.

The thermistors usually need very little if any amplification because of their high thermal coefficient. Although the temperature-resistance relationship is exponential, this is usually not a serious problem. First, the range of biologic application is almost linear; second, if an extended range is needed for greater laboratory versatility, linearization can be achieved electronically.

No distinct advantages can be seen between thermocouples and thermistors for skin temperature measurement, and a choice may be made strictly on a technical basis.

Liquid crystals. Liquid crystals represent an inexpensive but far less sensitive alternative to infrared thermography. These substances behave mechanically like liquids but display the optical properties of crystals.[31] By mixing cholesteric substances in different proportions, specific temperature-color relationships can be produced.[93] The cholesteric liquid can be applied to the skin as a spray or as a reusable tape.[71] This method has the potential for inexpensive skin temperature scanning; the changing color combinations, as a function of changing temperature, can be photographed. The liquid crystal method has not yet found wide application in vascular diagnosis, although some early reports confirm ease of application and reliability.[35,36,71]

Infrared thermography

The skin constantly emits a certain amount of infrared energy, and interestingly, its optical properties vary significantly with the wavelength.[38,107,112] To visible light, human skin is partially reflective and partially transparent. This also applies somewhat to the near infrared spectrum. However, in the far infrared region (around 10 μm) the skin behaves almost as a perfect absorber, and it is a perfect emitter of infrared energy. Thermographic instruments usually consist of an optical system, infrared detector, processing system, and display.[80] The radiation emitted by the skin is picked up by a temperature scanning and detecting system that is synchronized with the display; this results in a picture of the scanned temperatures. The usual thermal sensitivity is around 0.1° C, with a frame time of about 2 seconds (time required to take one picture).

Some instruments include color coding as a function of temperature, whereas others use different grades of black and white. A display of the isotherm, the line connecting the same temperature points, is a useful improvement.

Diagnostic value. Despite the sophisticated electronics and the elegant application of complex physical principles, the same limitations described for the contact skin temperature methods apply to infrared thermography, with some exceptions. Thermography offers a quick overview of the temperature points in the examined area more rapidly than temperature mapping, especially when the isotherm display is used. Although skin temperatures can be determined quickly, the cost effectiveness of the test remains questionable because of the limited value of skin temperature in the diagnosis of vascular disease.

THERMAL CONDUCTANCE
Principle

It can be shown mathematically that if a heat source is surrounded by an infinite mass of material, under steady-state conditions, heat production is equal to heat loss[12]:

$$J^2 \times R = 4 \times \pi \times r \times k \times \Delta t \tag{1}$$

where:

J = Electric current of the heating system
R = Electric resistance of the heating system
r = Radius of the sphere
k = Thermal conductivity of the surrounding material
Δt = Temperature elevation of the sphere

From this it follows that thermal conductance (k) is derived as follows:

$$k = \frac{J^2 R}{4\pi r \Delta t} \tag{2}$$

Thermal conductance depends on the thermal conductivity of the underlying tissue and on the flow rate of blood. Provided that the first factor can be subtracted, k is proportional to blood flow rate.

Early studies

Practically all flow determination methods with thermal conductivity are based on Gibbs' description[39] of a "blood-flow recorder" with a heated thermocouple. This instrument was originally designed to measure blood flow in vessels and served as a basis for future modifications of this approach.[10,11,45,50,51]

The application of Gibbs' principle to noninvasively measure skin blood flow was first suggested by Burton[10] but was developed and analyzed by Hensel et al[49,50-51] and Golenhofen et al.[41,42] Theoretical analysis combined with model experiments are described by Vendrik and Vos.[106] Harding et al[47] pursued the idea of maintaining a constant temperature difference by means of a servocontrol system, which compensates for the loss of heat caused by changes in blood flow rate. The changes in power are then related to flow fluctuations. This system is currently used in some commercially available transcutaneous Po_2 meters, which use the heating coil to obtain information about relative flow changes. A detailed technical description of this principle is given by McCaffrey and McCook.[74]

Renewed interest in this type of noninvasive skin blood flow measurement was initiated by Holti et al in attempting to evaluate patients with Raynaud's disease, as well as new

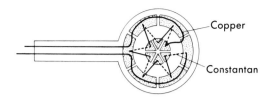

Copper

Constantan

Fig. 27-1. Thermal conductance probe with copper and constantan junctions. (From Holti G, Mitchell KW: *Clin Exp Dermatol* 3:189, 1978.)

vasoactive drugs.[40,54-56] The design is essentially based on a report by Van de Staak et al,[105] in which the temperature difference between a heated copper disk at the center of the probe and an unheated, concentric copper anulus at its periphery is measured. Both temperature-sensing elements are in direct contact with the skin (Fig. 27-1). When a temperature equilibrium is established, a temperature difference of about 2° C is maintained. Changes in blood flow produce temperature changes in the tenths of 1° C. When blood flow decreases, less heat is removed from the center plate, which leads to an increased temperature difference, and vice versa. A similar system was described by Challoner[13] and was also tested with a model flow system. Brown et al,[9] using a system described by Holti and Mitchell,[56] subjected the method to theoretical analysis and concluded that constant thermal flux caused by thermal conductivity was equal to 38 mW, whereas that caused by blood flow was only about 7 mW. This explains the requirements for high electronic stability of the system and for consideration of special precautions, such as not placing the probe in the vicinity of large vessels to accurately measure the small changes in temperature that result from changes in cutaneous blood flow.

THERMAL CLEARANCE

All the previously described methods that measure thermal conductance are expressed in cal $\times$ cm^{-1} $\times$ sec^{-1} $\times$ °C^{-1}. Because of complex factors that influence the final reading, besides the desired flow-related thermal conductance, the measurements cannot be expressed in absolute values. Betz and Apfel[5] attempted to quantify these measurements and to express the results in absolute values by introducing the concept of "thermal clearance," similar to the clearance technique in which radioisotope tracers are used.[5,76-78] In principle a certain amount of heat is injected into the tissue for a short time (slug heating), and the temperature "disappearance" curve is recorded. A normalization with thermal clearance under zero flow rate conditions is required. Under these conditions the temperature field (U_{slug}) of the perfused and unperfused tissue is related as follows:

$$\frac{U_{slug\ \phi}}{U_{slug\ o}} = e^{-\frac{\phi \times t}{\lambda}} \qquad (3)$$

where ϕ is blood flow and λ is the partition coefficient for heat; indices ϕ and o correspond to perfused and unperfused

tissue, respectively. A similar approach was described by Baptista[2] and included skin flow applications. Unfortunately, his technique yields only a "peripheral blood circulatory index," and no absolute skin blood flow values are available.

All heat conductance techniques have one disadvantage in common: they do not offer absolute flow rate values. On the other hand, if relative flow change information is sufficient for a given project, thermal conductance is a suitable flow-related index that can be monitored with relatively inexpensive instrumentation.

However, thermal clearance may supply quantitative flow information. It does not require expensive equipment but has not yet been developed for clinical application. Some doubts exist about whether the resolution will be good enough for such a relatively low-perfusion vascular bed as the skin. Further experimental information is needed.

TRANSCUTANEOUS Po$_2$ DETERMINATION
Principle

A modified Clark-type platinum oxygen electrode is used to monitor Po$_2$ from the surface of the skin during heat-induced local vasodilatation.

Physiologic and physicochemical notes

The first impetus for transcutaneous Po$_2$ (tcPo$_2$) monitoring can be traced back to a report in which an electrolytic solution at 45° C was equilibrated with the arterial Po$_2$ after a finger was immersed for a sufficient time.[4] Although Evans and Naylor[27] found that the Po$_2$ on the surface of the skin was close to zero, this value could be increased up to 30 mm Hg by vasodilatation. The finding that drug-induced vasodilatation increases transcutaneously monitored Po$_2$[59] led to the development of a combined electrode probe that incorporated a heater system.[62,65] This represented the single most decisive improvement toward further acceptance of the method. A similar system in which a heated cathode is used was described by Eberhard et al.[23] Standardized vasodilatation is important because beyond 43° C skin temperature, the ratio of tcPo$_2$ to arterial Po$_2$ remains constant and is close to 1.[60]

The electrode design is based on the original Clark oxygen electrode,[17] which uses three 15 μm platinum cathodes surrounded by a common silver ring anode (Fig. 27-2). The temperature of the heating coil adjacent to the anode is controlled by a servosystem sensed by a thermistor constantly monitoring the actual skin temperature. Theoretically, this closed-loop heater control system should be capable of monitoring relative skin perfusion changes (see previous discussion on thermal conductance), but available systems do not reflect these changes adequately,[26,115] despite initially encouraging reports.[62,64,95] The probe designed primarily for tcPo$_2$ monitoring obviously does not fulfill the requirements for measuring exact heat consumption, as documented by a number of authors.[7,9,49,104] The electrolytic solution that covers the electrodes is retained by a thin Teflon

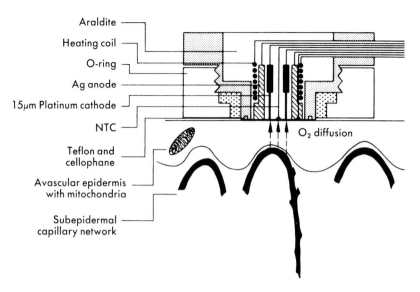

Fig. 27-2. Transcutaneous Po_2 electrode with heating coil. (From Huch A, Huch R: *Technical, physiological and clinical aspects of transcutaneous Po_2 measurements.* In Taylor DEM, Whamond J, eds: *Noninvasive clinical measurements,* Baltimore, 1977, University Park Press. By permission of Pitman Publishing, Ltd.)

membrane. The 95% response time of this system is about 10 seconds, whereas another system[23] requires about 50 seconds because of a thicker membrane, which, on the other hand, reduces the oxygen consumption of the electrodes.

With the use of the polarographic principle, it can be shown that the resulting current (J) is determined by the following equation[89]:

$$J = \frac{n \times F \times A \times P_m}{V_T \times a} Po_2 \qquad (4)$$

where:

n = Equivalents/mole
F = Faraday's constant
A = Cathode area
a = Membrane thickness
P_m = Membrane permeability
V_T = Correction for temperature

Clinical application

In view of the thin skin of newborn babies, they are obvious candidates for $tcPo_2$ monitoring and comparisons with direct Po_2 determinations.[57,59,63,66] A review of the application of $tcPo_2$ measurements in obstetrics and neonatology was published by Huch et al[61] in 1979 with encouraging results, although some limitations must be recognized. First, the specific effects of some anesthetics must be considered.[43,44,94] These effects can be reduced significantly with proper design of the electrode, reducing membrane permeability and changing polarization voltage to −600 mV.[22] Unfortunately, results are less reliable in cases of increased sympathetic tone and with decreased body temperature.[30]

Determination of $tcPo_2$ was successfully applied in plastic surgery to evaluate skin oxygen supply.[68]

Tønnesen[103] reported very low $tcPo_2$ values (close to zero) in patients with severe arterial occlusive disease. The severity of ischemic disease and changes in leg position were well correlated with ^{99m}Tc clearance. A more systematic study, in which $tcPo_2$ values were correlated with limb position in normal control subjects, concluded that the $tcPo_2$ values varied with changes of arteriovenous pressure differences (mainly changes in hydrostatic pressure) but suddenly dropped to zero at a certain perfusion level.[113] This phenomenon, also described by Tønnesen,[103] can be explained in several ways, but one of the most plausible explanations may be that this may occur at a moment of a zero, or negative, balance between oxygen supply and oxygen consumption by the tissue and the electrodes.

Matsen et al[73] presented $tcPo_2$ values from 13 normal subjects and nine patients with peripheral arterial disease. The $tcPo_2$ values were lower in the patient group at the below-knee (BK) and foot levels. The authors concluded that all patients with a $tcPo_2$ below 20 mm Hg required some surgical procedure (e.g., vascular reconstruction, amputation), reflecting the extreme severity of the disease.

Franzeck et al[34] compared the $tcPo_2$ in a normal control group (24 subjects) to that of 69 patients with various degrees of arterial occlusive disease. The mean BK values in the control group were 56.8 ± 9.9 mm Hg (standard deviation), whereas the average value in the patient group was significantly lower, 31.7 ± 18.1 mm Hg (Fig. 27-3). In view of the relatively wide scatter, however, an attempt was made to investigate the effect of postocclusive reactive hyperemia (PORH) on the $tcPo_2$ response. Fig. 27-4 illustrates the typical time course of the PORH response in a normal control subject. The $tcPo_2$ value drops to zero within 3 minutes, and reperfusion is very rapid. The halftime of the response, the time it takes until 50% of the initial $tcPo_2$ is reached, was 60.4 ± 15.2 seconds. The average halftime in the patient group was 130.6 ± 69.2 seconds. A representative tracing is shown in Fig. 27-5 in which one can see not only that the slope of the reperfusion part of the curve is shallower but also that there is a considerable delay between cuff pressure release and the inflection point of the reperfusion curve. This delay seems to indicate severely compromised skin perfusion, since either it takes so long for the oxygen molecules to reach the surface of the skin or the amount of oxygen supplied is so small that it does not adequately cover the low oxygen requirements of the tissue and the electrode. It is possible that both factors are responsible.

In summary, although the $tcPo_2$ level is related to skin blood flow, this relationship is complex and cannot be used directly to measure skin blood flow, at least at present. On the other hand, it is a very sensitive indicator of oxygen availability in the skin.

It therefore seemed appropriate for Franzeck et al[32-34] to investigate the usefulness of the $tcPo_2$ determination as a predictor of amputation stump healing. Patients were divided into three categories (A, successful amputation; B, prolonged healing; and C, failure). As seen in Fig. 27-6, the mean $tcPo_2$ value in 26 patients in group A was 36.5 ± 17.5 mm Hg, whereas in six patients with a failed amputation (group C), values were between 0 and 3 mm Hg. Additional experience with this method revealed some false-positive and false-negative results and led the investigators to increase the sensitivity and specificity of the test

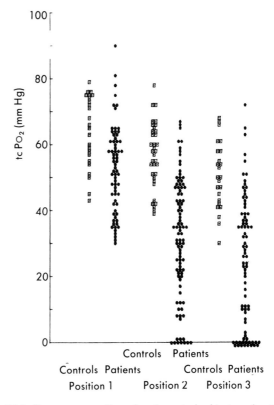

Fig. 27-3. Transcutaneous Po_2 values in control subjects and patients with peripheral arterial occlusive disease. Position 1, chest; position 2, below knee; position 3, dorsum of foot. (From Franzeck UK et al: *Surgery* 91:156, 1982.)

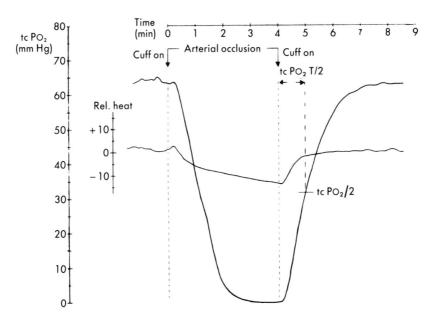

Fig. 27-4. Postocclusive reactive hyperemia response in control subject. (From Franzeck UK et al: *Surgery* 91:156, 1982.)

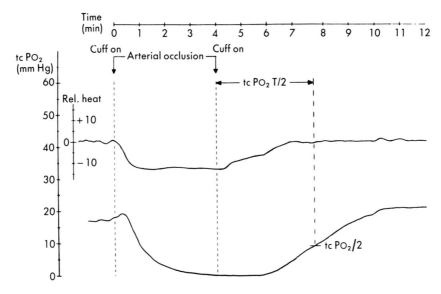

Fig. 27-5. Postocclusive reactive hyperemia response in patient with arterial occlusive disease. (From Franzeck UK et al: *Surgery* 91:156, 1982.)

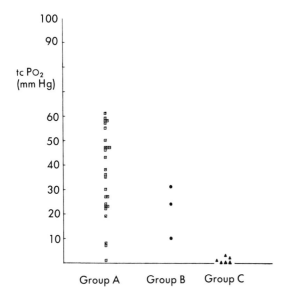

Fig. 27-6. Transcutaneous Po_2 values in patients with excellent amputation stump healing (group A), delayed healing (group B), and failure of healing (group C). (From Franzeck UK et al: *Surgery* 91:156, 1982.)

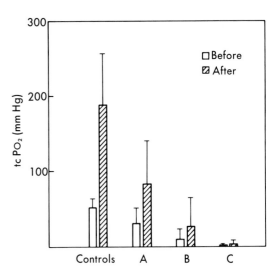

Fig. 27-7. Response to 100% O_2 breathing in control subjects and groups A, B, and C from Fig. 27-6. (From Franzeck UK et al: *Surgery* 91:156, 1982.)

by adding the $tcPo_2$ response to 100% oxygen inhalation for 10 minutes to the initial resting $tcPo_2$ determination. Fig. 27-7 illustrates the increase in $tcPo_2$ values in normal control subjects and in different groups of patients. Although there is a striking difference in all categories, there was a false-positive result and a false-negative result in groups A and C, respectively.

White et al[109] analyzed the predictive value of $tcPo_2$ in the success of spontaneous wound healing and amputation stump healing in 25 patients. They concluded that $tcPo_2$ values below 40 mm Hg predicted a poor chance of ulcer or stump healing. A postoperative improvement of $tcPo_2$ level correlated well with the long-term effectiveness of vascular bypass procedures.

Hauser and Shoemaker[48] reported an interesting decrease in their regional perfusion index (RPI) ($tcPo_2$ of the extremity divided by $tcPo_2$ of the chest) after standardized exercise in patients with intermittent claudication. No significant reduction was observed in asymptomatic patients, despite objective evidence of arterial occlusive disease. In a related study, using an implanted silicone elastomer tubing that is permeable to oxygen, Jussila and Niinikoski[67] observed a decrease in PO_2 in the perfused fluid after mild exercise (tiptoeing), whereas no drop was evident after successful arterial reconstruction. With more general applications in mind, Chang et al[15] used this invasive, implanted silicone elastomer tubing technique to evaluate the optimal conditions for postoperative wound healing. Conclusions from both invasive studies are relevant to the future application of $tcPO_2$ monitoring.

Evaluation

To place the potential value of $tcPO_2$ monitoring in proper perspective, it is necessary to consider all factors that may influence the recorded $tcPO_2$ level. These include factors related to (1) morphology, especially of the skin; (2) physiology; and (3) methodology.

Morphologic factors include the diffusing capacity of the skin, thickness of various skin layers, and histologic structure of the cutaneous vasculature. The last factor may be age dependent, which may explain why decreased $tcPO_2$ values have been observed in the chest region of older patients.[34,43]

Physiologic factors include cardiac output; degree of sympathetic stimulation, which may be a main source of discrepancies between arterial and transcutaneous PO_2; state of arteriovenous shunts; and oxygen consumption of the epidermis.

Methodologic factors include the effect of increased local temperature on skin blood flow and on the hemoglobin-binding curve, oxygen consumption by the electrode, and the effect of membrane quality and thickness.

Finally, the observed $tcPO_2$ value is the end result of all these factors, although the most decisive one influencing the final balance is local oxygen availability, which is ultimately a function of blood flow. Therefore $tcPO_2$ will probably become a useful technique to evaluate both oxygen availability and skin viability.

LASER DOPPLER FLUX MEASUREMENT
Relationship of skin histology to cutaneous blood flow determination

Some basic histologic principles that relate to the skin must be considered to evaluate the possibilities and limitations of laser Doppler perfusion (LDP) monitoring. Despite the great variability of the skin structure, which results from topographic differences (finger, forearm, foot), there is a general pattern. The epidermis is completely devoid of vascularization; it is usually a 40 to 50 μm keratin layer, which may reach a thickness of up to 400 μm in the fingertips.[110] The microvascular structure starts with the feeding arterioles, which end up in a hairpinlike system of capillaries that rise from the papillae of the corium to return to the subpapillary venous plexus. In contrast to the vertical takeoff of the capillaries, the larger vessels in the lower dermis run parallel to the skin surface.[46,90,96] In some sites, especially those involved in thermoregulation, arteriovenous anastomoses ($\sim$40 μm in diameter) are present and effectively shunt the capillary system if the anastomoses are dilated.

Physical principles

In contrast to the insonation of an exactly defined vessel cross section with Doppler ultrasound, the detection of the Doppler shift signal from the cutaneous microcirculation is far more complex. First, because of the microscopic dimensions of the capillaries, relatively low-frequency ultrasonic energy cannot be used. Second, the energy beam that impinges on the microcirculatory system does not face a uniform, geometrically well-defined vasculature but rather a network of vessels crisscrossing the measurement sample site.

The selection of a very narrow monochromatic light source (laser) helped limit the difficulties posed by the complexities of skin microvasculature. However, even the application of a single, narrow-frequency light source did not solve other inherent difficulties. The incident light source reaches the capillaries and red blood cells (RBCs) at a variety of different angles because of the random orientation of the capillary loops. In addition, significant scattering occurs before the beam reaches the capillary. All this is repeated by the reflected beam on its path back to the pickup system. The incident light usually penetrates to a depth of 1.5 mm, but the actual depth of penetration is a function of technical parameters, such as power density of the source and aperture, and of anatomic variables, such as skin pigmentation, thickness of the epidermis, and topographic differences. However, the recorded Doppler-shifted signal corresponds to an average velocity obtained under an average angle. To complicate the matter, the resulting signal, at least in the available systems, also depends on the number of RBCs in the sample volume because of the type of signal processing currently used. The resulting signal is therefore a product of the number of RBCs moving in the sample volume and the mean velocity of the moving RBCs. Because it is neither velocity nor flow, the term *blood cell flux* has been suggested[83,84,98]:

$$\text{Flux} = \text{Red cell volume fraction} \times \text{Velocity} \qquad (5)$$

Historical notes

In 1964, Cummins et al[20] suggested that by applying a highly coherent monochromatic light source (laser) previously developed by Schawlow and Townes,[92] even the movement of macromolecules could be detected if a proper heterodyning technique (mixing of two close frequencies and using their difference) was used. Yeh and Cummins[114] documented that with this approach, even very low flow velocities could be detected ($\sim$0.07 mm/sec). Riva et al[86] applied this principle to the determination of retinal blood flow in the rabbit. In model experiments with glass capillaries, they found a remarkable difference in the recorded frequency spectrum: a flat plateau with a sharp falloff point when polystyrene spheres were used, whereas the falloff frequency was less exactly defined when RBCs were used as reflecting particles, probably because of additional light scattering caused by the different RBC geometry. In subsequent studies, Tanaka et al[100,101] reported additional improvement in the signal-to-noise ratio when autocorrelation with retinal vessel application was used. Laser Doppler velocimetry was then directly applied in experimental microcirculatory research by Einav et al[24,25] and Mishina et al[75] by bringing the laser beam to the examined microvessels through a special microscope system. Le-Cong and Zweifach[70] applied the advantages of the coherent, monochromatic light source to measure not only velocities but also microvascular dimensions. Their system, however, used the interference measurement rather than the Doppler shift signal.

Noninvasive application to monitor blood flow was first demonstrated by Stern,[97] who used a spectrum analyzer to process the Doppler-shifted signals from the fingertip. In a subsequent comprehensive theoretical and experimental analysis, Stern et al[98] obtained a good correlation with ^{133}Xe washout studies in normal subjects who were subjected to ultraviolet-induced local hyperemia. In all these studies, root-mean-square (RMS) bandwidth of the Doppler signal was found to correlate with actual flow measurements:

$$F = \int_0^\infty \omega^2 P(\omega)d\omega \tag{6}$$

where F indicates the Doppler "flow parameters" and $P(\omega)$ denotes the power spectrum of the Doppler signal.

The advantage of this type of signal processing is its relative simplicity, although the amount of reflected energy also influences the resulting signal. Replacement of the photomultiplier type by a photodiode facilitated the more widespread use of the system because of its portability.[108] A similar system was later described by Nilsson et al,[81-84] who improved the signal-to-noise ratio by using a differential optical system, which feeds a split fiberoptic output into two identical photodiode systems (Fig. 27-8). This helps reduce the signals that originate from stationary reflection sites, whereas the Doppler-shifted signals are amplified because their uniqueness precludes cancellation of the signal in the differential amplifier. Signal processing is performed in a similar way by using the RMS detection and subtracting the noise-generated signals[83]:

$$\text{RMS (blood flow)} = \sqrt{\text{RMS}^2_{\text{(total)}} - \text{RMS}^2_{\text{noise}}} \tag{7}$$

A more comprehensive theoretical analysis of optimal signal processing was published by Bonner et al[6,7] and Nilsson et al.[83]

The advantage of autocorrelation was recently emphasized by Cochrane et al[18] in an experimental and theoretical study. Investigators using the laser Doppler system in retinal artery velocimetry reported acceptable results with simpler signal processing with a logarithmic correlation of the power output versus frequency output.[8,86,88]

Clinical application

Although the resulting signal is a product of velocity and RBC volume, which makes it difficult to calibrate or even to compare with existing techniques, the ease, convenience, and noninvasiveness of this method have already resulted in many studies in which this technique is used as a prime tool to evaluate various aspects of skin perfusion.

Powers and Frayer[85] reported an application in plastic

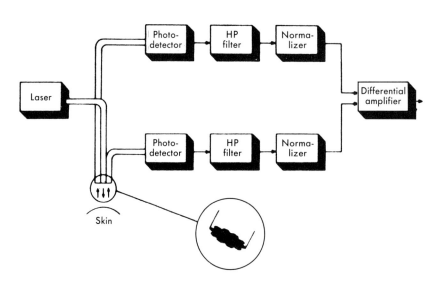

Fig. 27-8. Compensated laser Doppler fluxmeter. (From Nilsson GE, Tenland T, Oberg PA: Evaluation of a laser Doppler flowmeter for measurement of tissue blood flow, *IEEE Trans Biomed Eng* 27:597, 1980.)

surgery, although there is no systematic study that correlates output with flap viability. Holloway[52] found a significant increase in blood flow induced by needle trauma, whereas the increase caused by histamine was lower than that induced by needle trauma. These changes were significantly smaller if vasodilatation (local heating) preceded the intervention. Salerud et al[91] systematically investigated the spontaneous rhythmic microcirculatory variations previously described in both animals[14] and clinical studies.[28] Although the coefficient of variation was low in model experiments, the spatial differences in the forearm and temporal variations from day to day were significant.[102] A preliminary study by Low et al[72] indicated the usefulness of using laser Doppler flux metering in combination with standardized tests (e.g., inspiratory gasp, Valsalva's maneuver, cold stimulus) to separate disorders of the autonomic nervous system.

Evaluation

The advantages of laser Doppler flux metering include its noninvasive application, continuous readout, and ease of operation. The main disadvantage is the absence of calibration and the inability to express results in units generally used in fluid mechanics, such as velocity and flow rate. Although the flux, RBC volume fraction multiplied by velocity, is of interest if overall questions of perfusion are investigated, an output related only to velocity or flow would be preferable. This question may be solved with appropriate signal processing.

SKIN ARTERIAL PRESSURE

In contrast to the generally accepted and highly informative arterial segmental pressure, which reflects the pressure in large arteries of the extremities, the application of skin blood pressure is still in its infancy, despite the clinical importance of skin perfusion pressure in determining skin viability, as in amputation level assessment and objective evaluation of patients with Raynaud's syndrome.

In 1967, Dahn et al[21] used the effect of counterpressure on radioisotope clearance from the skin. The pressure at which the clearance stopped was considered the skin perfusion pressure. This method is invasive, since it requires the injection of a radioactive substance such as ^{133}Xe; in addition, it is time consuming and cumbersome. Lassen and Holstein[69] established the clinical value of the counterpressure technique—monitoring the effect of the increasing cuff pressure on some index of skin circulation underneath the cuff—and concluded that a skin perfusion pressure of 20 mm Hg or less predicts very poor healing for an amputation stump.

Chawatzas and Jamieson[16] described a very simple but subjective technique to estimate skin perfusion pressure: observation of the blanching and reddening of the skin through a transparent sphygmomanometric cuff. Nielsen et al[79] described an objective and simple technique to determine "systolic skin pressure" (SSP). A flat photoelectric probe is placed beneath a standard inflation cuff in direct contact with the skin, and it records the reflected light from the skin. The skin becomes pale at suprasystolic pressures; during release of the cuff pressure, reddening of the skin results in a change in the recorded signal. The authors used the DC mode of operation so that a change in baseline might be considered the moment of blood return to the cutaneous vascular system, the SSP. In a group of normal control subjects the SSP thus obtained was close to the diastolic pressure measured in the arm by auscultation: diastolic arm pressure, 78.2 mm Hg; SSP, 85.8 mm Hg. In a group of patients with hypertension, however, the difference between SSP and diastolic arm pressure was more pronounced: diastolic arm pressure, 106.3 mm Hg; SSP, 129.9 mm Hg. Holstein et al[53] compared SSP in 13 normal subjects with intraarterial blood pressure obtained from the posterior tibial artery with an ultralow-compliance transducer.[3] Again the SSP was only slightly higher, 84.3 mm Hg, when compared with the direct diastolic pressure of 72 mm Hg. This method will probably become an important examination technique in establishing the optimal level for dysvascular amputation.

CONCLUSION

Despite the number of methods available and the accessibility of the skin, there is no single technique that completely fulfills the basic requirements for evaluating skin perfusion, that is, to determine accurately the state of skin perfusion both quantitatively and noninvasively. Of the methods described, the last three appear to have the potential to be more widely used under clinical conditions. Each reflects a different aspect of skin perfusion: transcutaneous PO_2 determination reflects oxygen availability on the surface of the skin, laser Doppler velocity metering output is a function of RBC velocity, and skin systolic pressure relates to the diastolic blood pressure in the large arteries. Further clinical experience will help in identifying which of these techniques is most helpful in evaluating the hemodynamics of the cutaneous circulation.

REFERENCES

1. Aschoff J, Wever R: Die Anisotropie der Haut für den Wärmetransport, *Pflügers Arch* 269:130, 1959.
2. Baptista AM: A simple thermal method for the study of the peripheral blood circulation and applications, *Microvasc Res* 2:123, 1970.
3. Barras JP: Direct measurement of blood pressure by transcutaneous micropuncture of peripheral arteries—use of a new developed isovolumetric manometer, *Scand J Clin Lab Invest* 128(suppl):153, 1973.
4. Baumberger JP, Goodfriend RB: Determination of arterial oxygen tension in man by equilibrium through intact skin, *Fed Proc* 10:10, 1951.
5. Betz E, Apfel H: *Wärmeleitmessung und Wärmeclearance mit Thermoelementen und Thermistoren.* In Hild R, Spann G, eds: *Therapiekontrolle in der Angiologie*, Baden-Baden, West Germany, 1979, G. Witzstrock Publishers.
6. Bonner R, Nossal R: Model for laser Doppler measurements of blood flow in tissue, *Appl Optics* 20:2097, 1981.
7. Bonner RF et al: *Laser-Doppler continuous real-time monitor of pulsatile and mean blood flow in tissue microcirculation.* In: Chen SH, Chu B, Nossal R, eds: *Scattering techniques applied to supramolecular and nonequilibrium systems*, NATO ASI series B, 73:685, New York, 1981, Plenum Press.

8. Brein KR, Riva CE: Laser Doppler velocimetry measurement of pulsatile blood flow in capillary tubes, *Microvasc Res* 24:114, 1982.

9. Brown BH et al: A critique of the use of a thermal clearance probe for the measurement of skin blood flow, *Clin Phys Physiol Meas* 1:237, 1980.

10. Burton AC: The direct measurement of thermal conductance of the skin as an index of peripheral blood flow, *Am J Physiol* 129:326, 1940.

11. Burton AC, Edholm OG: *Man in a cold environment,* London, 1955, S. Arnold.

12. Carslaw HS: *The mathematical theory of the conduction of heat in solids,* London, 1921, Macmillan Publishers.

13. Challoner AVJ: Accurate measurement of skin blood flow by a thermal conductance method, *Med Biol Eng* 13:196, 1975.

14. Chambers R, Zweifach BW: The topography and function of the mesenteric circulation, *Am J Anat* 75:173, 1944.

15. Chang N et al: Direct measurement of wound and tissue O_2 tension in post operative patients, *Ann Surg* 197:470, 1983.

16. Chawatzas D, Jamieson C: A simple method for approximate measurement of skin blood pressure, *Lancet* 1:711, 1974.

17. Clark LC Jr: Monitor and control of blood and tissue oxygen tensions, *Trans Am Soc Artif Intern Organs* 2:41, 1956.

18. Cochrane T, Earnshaw JC, Love AHG: Laser Doppler measurement of blood velocity in microvessels, *Med Biol Eng Comput* 19:589, 1981.

19. Cromwell FJ, Weibell FY, Pfeiffer EA: *Biomedical instrumentation and measurements,* ed 2, Englewood Cliffs, NJ, 1980, Prentice-Hall, Inc.

20. Cummins HZ, Knable N, Yeh Y: Observation of diffusion broadening of Rayleigh scattered light, *Phys Rev Lett* 12:150, 1964.

21. Dahn I, Lassen NA, Westling H: Blood flow in human muscles during external pressure or venous stasis, *Clin Sci* 32:467, 1967.

22. Eberhard P, Mindt N: Interference of anesthetic gases at skin surface sensors for oxygen and carbon dioxide, *Crit Care Med* 9:717, 1981.

23. Eberhard P, Hammacher K, Mindt W: Methode zur kutanen Messung des Sauerstoffpartialdruckes, *Biomed Tech* 18:212, 1973.

24. Einav S et al: Measurements of velocity profiles of red blood cells in the microcirculation by laser Doppler anemometry (LDA), *Biorheology* 12:207, 1975.

25. Einav S et al: Measurement of blood flow in vivo by laser Doppler anemometry through a microscope, *Biorheology* 12:203, 1975.

26. Enkema L Jr et al: Laser Doppler velocimetry vs. heater power as indicators of skin perfusion during transcutaneous O_2 monitoring, *Clin Chem* 27:391, 1981.

27. Evans NTS, Naylor PFD: The systemic oxygen supply to the surface of human skin, *Respir Physiol* 3:21, 1967.

28. Fagrell B, Fronek A, Intaglietta M: A microscope-television system for studying flow velocity in human skin capillaries, *Am J Physiol* 233:H318, 1977.

29. Felder D et al: Relationship in the toe of skin surface temperature to mean blood flow measured with a plethysmograph, *Clin Sci* 13:251, 1954.

30. Fenner A et al: Transcutaneous determination of arterial oxygen tension, *Pediatrics* 55:224, 1975.

31. Ferguson JL: Liquid crystals, *Sci Am* 211:77, 1964.

32. Franzeck UK et al: Transcutaneous pO_2 measurements in health and peripheral arterial occlusive disease, *Bibl Anat* 20:688, 1981.

33. Franzeck UK et al: *Transkutane pO_2—Messungen bei der peripheren arteriellen Verschlusskrankheit, Mikrocirculation und Arterielle Verschlusskrankheiten,* München, 1981, Karger.

34. Franzeck UK et al: Transcutaneous pO_2 measurements in health and peripheral arterial occlusive disease, *Surgery* 91:156-63, 1982.

35. Gautherie M: Application des cristaux liquides cholestériques á la thermographie cutanée, *J Physique* 30(suppl):11-2, 1969.

36. Gautherie M, Quenneville Y, Gros CH: Thermographie cholestérique, *Pathol Biol* 22:553, 1974.

37. Geddes LA, Baker LE: *Principles of applied biomedical instrumentation,* ed 2, New York, John Wiley & Sons, Inc.

38. Gershon-Cohen J, Haberman-Brueschke JD, Brueschke EE: Medical thermography, *Radiol Clin* 3:403, 1965.

39. Gibbs FA: A thermoelectric bloodflow recorder in the form of a needle, *Proc Soc Exp Biol NY* 31:141, 1933.

40. Gillon R, Holti G, Mitchell KM: Measurement of nutrient skin blood-flow using the thermal clearance rate and cinerecordings of stereoscopic capillary microscopy, *Biorheology* 13:262, 1976.

41. Golenhofen K: Blood flow of muscle and skin studied by the local heat clearance technique, *Scand J Clin Lab Invest* 19(suppl 99):79, 1967.

42. Golenhofen K, Hensel H, Hildebrandt G: *Durchblutungsmessung mit Wärmeleitelementen,* Stuttgart, 1963, G. Thieme.

43. Gøthgen I, Jacobsen E: Transcutaneous oxygen tension measurement. I. Age variation and reproducibility, *Acta Anaesthesiol Scand* 67(suppl):66, 1978.

44. Gøthgen I, Jacobsen E: Transcutaneous oxygen tension measurement. II. The influence of halothane and hypotension, *Acta Anaesthesiol Scand* 67(suppl):71, 1978.

45. Grayson J: Internal calorimetry in the determinations of thermal conductivity and bloodflow, *J Physiol* 118:54, 1952.

46. Greenfield ADM: *The circulation through the skin.* In II. Circulation, Hamilton WF, ed: *Handbook of physiology* 1963, Washington, DC, American Physiology Society.

47. Harding DC, Rushmer RF, Baker DW: Thermal transcutaneous flowmeter, *Med Biol Eng* 5:623, 1967.

48. Hauser CJ, Shoemaker WC: Use of a transcutaneous pO_2 regional perfusion index to quantify tissue perfusion in peripheral vascular disease, *Ann Surg* 197:337, 1983.

49. Hensel H: Messkopf fur Durchblutungsregistrierung an Oberflächen. *Pflügers Arch* 268:604, 1959.

50. Hensel H, Bender F: Fortlaufende Bestimmung der Hautdurchblutung am Menschen mit einem elektrischen Wärmeleitmesser, *Pflügers Arch* 263:603, 1956.

51. Hensel H, Ruef J, Golenhofen K: Fortlaufende Registrierung der Muskeldurchblutung am Menschen mit der Calorimetersonde, *Pflügers Arch* 259:267, 1954.

52. Holloway GA: Cutaneous blood flow responses to injection trauma measured by laser Doppler velocimetry, *J Invest Dermatol* 74:1, 1980.

53. Holstein P, Nielsen PE, Barras JP: Blood flow cessation at external pressure in the skin of normal human limbs (photoelectric recordings compared to isotope washout and to local intra-arterial blood pressure), *Microvasc Res* 17:71, 1979.

54. Holti G: The copper-tellurite-copper thermocouple adapted as skin thermometer, *Clin Sci* 14:137, 1955.

55. Holti G: The assessment of the nutrient skin bloodflow with special reference to measurement of the thermal clearance rate, *Biorheology* 11:208, 1974.

56. Holti G, Mitchell KW: Estimation of the nutrient skin bloodflow using a segmental thermal clearance probe, *Clin Exp Dermatol* 3:189, 1978.

57. Huch R, Huch A: Transcutane Überwachung des arteriellen pO_2 in der Anesthesie. Einsatzfähikeit der Methode am Beispiel von Kurznarkosen, *Anaesthesist* 23:181, 1974.

58. Huch A, Huch R, Lübbers DW: Quantitative polarographische Sauerstoffdruckmessung auf der Kopfhaut des Neugeborenen, *Arch Gynakol* 207:443, 1969.

59. Huch R, Huch A, Lübbers DW: Transcutaneous measurement of blood PO_2 (tcPO_2)—method and application in perinatal medicine, *J Perinat Med* 1:183, 1973.

60. Huch A, Huch R, Lucey YF: Continuous transcutaneous blood gas monitoring, *First Int Symp Birth Defects Orig Art Series* 15:1, 1979.

61. Huch R, Huch A, Rolfe P: Transcutaneous measurement of pO_2 using electrochemical analysis. In Rolfe P, editor: *Non-invasive physiological measurements,* vol 1, London, 1979, Academic Press.

62. Huch R, Lübbers DW, Huch A: Quantitative continuous measurement of partial oxygen pressure on the skin of adults and new-born babies, *Pflügers Arch* 337:185, 1972.

63. Huch R, Lübbers DW, Huch A: Reliability of transcutaneous monitoring of arterial PO_2 in new-born infants, *Arch Dis Child* 49:213, 1974.
64. Huch A, Lübbers DW, Huch R: Der periphere Perfusionsdruck: eine neue, nicht-invasive Messgrösse zur Kreislanfüberwachung von Patienten, *Anaesthesist* 24:39, 1975.
65. Huch A et al: *Eine schnelle, beheizte Pt-Oberflächenelektrode zur kontinuierlichen Überwachung des PO_2 beim Menschen,* Stuttgart, 1972, Vortrag Medizin-Technik.
66. Huch A et al: Continuous transcutaneous oxygen tension measured with a heated electrode, *Scand J Clin Lab Invest* 31:269, 1973.
67. Jussila EJ, Niinikoski J: Effect of vascular reconstructions on tissue gas tensions in calf muscles of patients with occlusive arterial disease, *Ann Chir Gynaecol* 70:56, 1981.
68. Knote G, Bohmert H: Determination of the viability of skin regions in danger of necrosis by means of transcutaneous polarographic measurement of oxygen pressure, *Fortschr Med* 95:640, 1977.
69. Lassen NA, Holstein P: Use of radioisotopes in assessment of distal blood flow and distal blood pressure in arterial insufficiency, *Surg Clin North Am* 54:39, 1974.
70. Le-Cong P, Zweifach BW: In vivo and in vitro velocity measurements in microvasculature with a laser, *Microvasc Res* 17:131, 1979.
71. Lee BY, Trainor FS, Madden JL: Liquid crystal tape: its use in the evaluation of vascular diseases, *Arch Phys Med Rehab* 54:96, 1973.
72. Low PA et al: Evaluation of skin vasomotor reflexes by using laser Doppler velocimetry, *Mayo Clin Proc* 58:592, 1983.
73. Matsen FA III et al: Transcutaneous oxygen tension measurement in peripheral vascular disease, *Surg Gynecol Obstet* 150:525, 1980.
74. McCaffrey TV, McCook RD: A thermal method for determination of tissue blood flow, *J Appl Physiol* 39:170, 1975.
75. Mishina H, Koyama T, Asakura T: Velocity measurements of blood flow in the capillary and vein using a laser Doppler microscope, *Appl Optics* 14:2326, 1975.
76. Müller-Schauenburg W: Über einen Ansatz fur Trennung von Wärmeleitung und Wärmeabtransport durch des Blut—ein neues Verfahren zur quantitativen Messung der Lokalen Gewebsdurchblutung, thesis, University of Tübingen, 1972.
77. Müller-Schauenburg W, Betz E: *Gas and heat clearance comparison and use of heat-transport for quantitative local blood flow measurements.* In Brock M et al, eds: *Cerebral blood flow,* New York, 1969, Springer-Verlag.
78. Müller-Schauenburg W et al: Quantitative measurement of local blood flow with heat clearance, *Basic Res Cardiol* 70:547, 1975.
79. Nielsen PE, Poulsen HL, Gyntelberg F: Arterial blood pressure in the skin measured by a photoelectric probe and external counterpressure, *Vasa* 2:65, 1973.
80. Nilsson K: Evaluation of infra-red thermography in experimental biology and medicine, *Adv Microcirc* 3:67, 1970.
81. Nilsson GE, Tenland T, Oberg PA: *Continuous measurement of capillary blood flow by light beating spectroscopy,* Proceedings of the Conference on Transducers and Measurements, Madrid, Oct. 10-14, 1978.
82. Nilsson GE, Tenland T, Oberg PA: *Laser Doppler flowmetry—a noninvasive method for microvascular studies,* Thirteenth Annual International Conference on Bioengineering, Jerusalem, Aug. 19-24, 1979.
83. Nilsson GE, Tenland T, Oberg PA: A new instrument for continuous measurement of tissue blood flow by light beating spectroscopy, *IEEE Trans Biomed Eng* 27:12, 1980.
84. Nilsson GE, Tenland T, Oberg PA: Evaluation of a laser Doppler flowmeter for measurement of tissue blood flow, *IEEE Trans Biomed Eng* 27:597, 1980.
85. Powers EW III, Frayer WW: Laser Doppler measurement of blood flow in the microcirculation, *Plast Reconstr Surg* 61:250, 1978.
86. Riva CE, Grunwald JE, Sinclair SH: Laser Doppler measurement of relative blood velocity in the human optic nerve head, *Invest Ophthalmol Vis Sci* 22:241, 1982.
87. Riva C, Ross B, Benedek GB: Laser Doppler measurements of blood flow in capillary tubes and retinal arteries, *Invest Ophthalmol Vis Sci* 11:936, 1972.
88. Riva CE et al: Bi-directional LDV system for absolute measurement of blood speed in retinal vessels, *Appl Optics* 18:2301, 1979.
89. Rolfe P: Arterial oxygen measurement in the newborn with intravascular transducers, *IEE Med Electr Monogr* 18-22, London, 1976, Peter Perigrinus.
90. Ryan JJ: *Structure and shape of blood vessels of the skin.* In Jarrett A, ed: *The physiology and pathophysiology of the skin,* vol 2, London, 1973, Academic Press.
91. Salerud EG et al: Rhythmical variations in human skin blood flow, *Int J Microcirc Clin Exp* 2:91, 1983.
92. Schawlow AL, Townes CH: Infrared and optic lasers, *Physiol Rev* 112:1940, 1958.
93. Selawry AS, Selawry HS, Holland JF: Use of liquid cholesteric crystals for thermographic measurement of skin temperature in man, *Mol Cryst* 1:495, 1966.
94. Severinghaus JW et al: Oxygen electrode errors due to polarographic reduction of halothane, *J Appl Physiol* 31:640, 1971.
95. Severinghaus JW et al: Workshop on methodological aspects of transcutaneous blood gas analysis, *Acta Anaesthesiol Scand* 68:1, 1978.
96. Sparks HV: *Skin and muscle.* In Johnson PC, ed: *Peripheral circulation,* New York, 1978, John Wiley & Sons.
97. Stern MD: In vivo evaluation of microcirculation by coherent light scattering, *Nature* 524:56, 1975.
98. Stern MD et al: Continuous measurement of tissue blood flow by laser Doppler spectroscopy, *Am J Physiol* 232:H441, 1977.
99. Strandness ED Jr, Summer DS: *Hemodynamics for surgeons,* New York, 1975, Grune & Stratton.
100. Tanaka T, Benedek GB: Measurement of the velocity of blood flow (in vivo) using a fiber optic catheter and optical mixing spectroscopy, *Appl Optics* 14:180, 1975.
101. Tanaka T, Riva C, Ben-Sira I: Blood velocity measurements in human retinal vessels, *Science* 186:830, 1974.
102. Tenland T et al: Spatial and temporal variations in human skin blood flow, *Int J Microcirc Clin Exp* 2:81, 1983.
103. Tønnesen KH: Transcutaneous oxygen tension in imminent foot gangrene, *Acta Anaesthesiol Scand* 68:107, 1978.
104. Tremper K, Huxtable RF: Dermal heat transport analysis for transcutaneous O_2 measurement, *Acta Anaesthesiol Scand* 68:48, 1978.
105. Van de Staak WJBM, Brakkee AJM, De Rijke-Herweijer HE: Measurements of the thermal conductivity of the skin as an indication of skin bloodflow, *J Invest Dermatol* 51:149, 1968.
106. Vendrik AJH, Vos JJ: A method for the measurement of the thermal conductivity of human skin, *J Appl Physiol* 11:211, 1957.
107. Wallace JD, Cade CM: *Clinical thermography,* Cleveland, 1975, CRC Press.
108. Watkins DW, Holloway GA Jr: An instrument to measure cutaneous blood flow using the Doppler shift of laser light, *IEEE Trans Biomed Eng* 25:28, 1978.
109. White RA et al: Noninvasive evaluation of peripheral vascular disease using transcutaneous oxygen tension, *Am J Surg* 144:68, 1982.
110. Whitton JT, Everall JD: The thickness of the epidermis, *Br J Dermatol* 89:467, 1973.
111. Winsor T: Vascular aspects of thermography, *J Cardiovasc Surg* 12:379, 1971.
112. Winsor T, Bendezer J: Thermography and the peripheral circulation, *Ann NY Acad Sci* 121:135, 1964.
113. Wyss CR et al: Dependence of transcutaneous oxygen tension on local arteriovenous pressure gradient in normal subjects, *Clin Sci* 60:499, 1981.
114. Yeh Y, Cummins HZ: Localized fluid flow measurements with an He-Ne laser spectrometer, *Appl Physiol Lett* 4:176, 1964.
115. Zick GL, Holloway GA Jr, Piraino DW: *Simultaneous measurement of tcPO$_2$ and capillary blood flow,* Proceedings of the International Conference of Vital Parameter Determination during Extracorporeal Circulation, Nijmegan, The Netherlands, 1980.

CHAPTER 28

Laser Doppler flowmetry: principles of technology and clinical applications

ANDREW N. NICOLAIDES and GIANNI BELCARO

Noninvasive optical methods to evaluate skin flow have been used for many years. The most popular is photoplethysmography, which records variations in the blood volume of the skin. With the exception of time measurements (e.g., refilling time, pulse rate), only qualitative data may be obtained. Quantitative data are difficult to obtain and standardize, and attempts at calibration have been unsuccessful. Fluctuations in venous volume caused by postural changes or motion artifacts alter the signal and make the interpretation of skin flow variations difficult. As a result, photoplethysmography has been used mainly to evaluate a specific aspect of vascular disease, such as the pulsatility of skin flow in Raynaud's disease or the refilling time after venous emptying after an exercise test. Light beam photoplethysmography penetrates the skin for variable depths (2 to 6 mm), and the reflected signal may include a variety of skin circulatory elements without separation. The photoplethysmography probes are not easily applied to the evaluation of organs such as the intestine or the parenchymatous organs (e.g., liver, spleen, muscle).

Laser Doppler flowmetry (LDF), a more sophisticated method, has been developed in the last 15 years from a research tool to a clinical diagnostic technique that may be used to assess tissue viability and perfusion.[1-4] The fundamental principle of LDF as applied to the measurements of tissue perfusion have been described in detail in several publications.[4-8,15] Measurement of blood flow velocity in single, large vessels and the measurement of skin perfusion can be obtained with LDF. However, the technology required for these two applications is completely different. In this chapter only the measurement of microvascular perfusion is discussed.

THEORY OF LASER DOPPLER FLOWMETRY

A detailed technical description of the method is beyond the scope of this chapter. However, some simple concepts are needed to understand the method, its applications, and possible limitations. Most commercially available laser Doppler instruments use helium-neon gas or gallium aluminum arsenide elements to produce a weak laser beam with low tissue penetration. This type of laser light does not damage the tissues under evaluation or produce an increase in tissue temperature. Most tissues (e.g., skin) are relatively opaque because they contain particles that refract (scatter) light in random directions. At the microvascular level, blood constitutes only a small fraction of tissue volume, so most light scattering is due to small particles and stationary tissue elements. Only moving objects in the sample volume (i.e., blood cells) will cause a Doppler shift in the light frequency. The scattering angles and red cell velocities are variable and can be determined only in a statistical sense.[23] Therefore the LDF signal is a stochastic representation of the number of cells in the sample volume multiplied by their velocities.

Advantages. The technology of LDF using coherent laser light overcomes some problems observed with other optical and nonoptical methods used to evaluate skin perfusion. The helium-neon laser, which emits a red light and is used in many LDF instruments, detects very small changes in the wavelength of the laser light as a result of red blood cell movements (Doppler effect), well below the resolution of the optical spectroscope.[1,3]

The frequency distribution of the signal is defined by computerized spectral analysis of the output, resulting in a power spectrum with a separation between the noise and the true signal due to blood cell motion. Some components of the LDF signal are caused by external biologic or instrumental elements (e.g., vibration) and some to internal factors (mainly electronic noise). The LDF photodetector signal contains all the Doppler-shifted frequencies arising from the laser interaction with moving particles in the tissue as well as static components. Elaborate electronic processing and filtering are used to transform the LDF signal into a physiologically reproducible parameter such that the LDF output varies linearly with the bloodflow within the sample volume.

The total power in the backscattered signal depends on the number of moving particles producing a laser Doppler frequency shift. Therefore a laser Doppler flowmeter must be capable of measuring the mean frequency shift in the signal. Some laser Doppler flowmeters digitize the signal and analyze it with a fast Fourier transform from which the mean frequency shift can be measured. Other systems use analogue signal-processing circuitry.

Electronic components are needed to normalize the signal and to compensate for noise. In most instruments the noise level remains relatively stable and can theoretically be extracted from the LDF output by subtracting a constant offset. Different technical solutions have been applied in low-noise lasers or laser diodes.[4,5,13,14] (More specific technical information and details on the structure of laser Doppler flowmeters can be found in other reports.[2,3,5,6])

TERMINOLOGY

The output from the LDF is referred to as *flux* instead of flow, which requires some explanation. The difference in the terminology is explained by Almond.[1] If blood is replaced with saline that does not contain particles, Doppler shift is produced. A method that measures volume flow of the fluid, such as venous occlusion plethysmography, would measure approximately the same value of flow as if blood were present. With saline, a laser Doppler flowmeter would give a zero output because there are no scattering particles to produce a Doppler shift. However, in most physiologic and clinical situations even with a variable relationship between the cellular and fluid elements, LDF flux and volume flow have a good correlation. In other words, flux is the product of the number of cells times the mean velocity and is proportional to flow.

CALIBRATION

Many studies have demonstrated a good correlation between LDF measurements and other methods of blood flow measurements.[1,13,23] Some studies have shown a poor correlation between LDF and isotopic methods (e.g., xenon clearance[7]) in the presence of arteriovenous shunts[8] or when measurements are made in bone.[10]

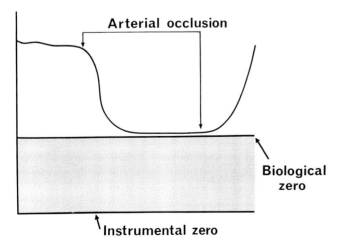

Fig. 28-1. The instrumental and biologic zero.

The major problem at this stage is that there is no gold standard, particularly in the skin, against which LDF can be compared. Because each type of LDF instrument gives its own values, it is difficult to compare results that are obtained with instruments from different manufacturers. Relative changes (i.e., before and after treatment, after thermal or postural changes, or after arterial occlusion to cause reactive hyperemia) are clinically more useful than absolute flux measurements. A universal calibration does not appear possible at the moment because several factors, including light penetration, diffusion, and reflection, make the calibration relevant only to the tissue being examined. Despite these limitations, LDF has many positive aspects that have progressively enlarged its application from purely experimental and clinical physiology to clinical practice (see Chapter 63).

The instrumental baseline and the biologic zero

The flux zero baseline is obtained by positioning the probe against a white surface. An instrumental zero is different from the biologic zero, which may be due to Brownian motion and can be obtained from the skin by complete occlusion of the arterial supply (Fig. 28-1).[9-21]

When blood flow in the skin is completely abolished, the LDF signal decreases to 20% to 50% of the normal tissue flux measurement. The relative ratio between the normal resting flux state and the occlusion state values is variable from region to region and also from organ to organ. In a fingertip the ratio is 5% to 7%, and in closely related areas the biologic zeroes are very similar.[21]

The origin of the signal responsible for the biologic zero is not clearly understood. Studies on excised tissue have shown an elevated baseline from the instrumental zero even several hours after excision. However, the elevated biologic zero disappeared after a few days. Freezing tissues abolishes the biologic zero baseline by lowering the values to a level similar to the instrumental baseline.[21] In situations of inflammation of human skin, the biologic zero is increased to approximately 50% to 70%.[9] The clinical implications of these findings are still not clear, and further studies are required. However, in the practical clinical evaluation of limbs, particularly in low perfusion states, each measurement should be associated with an estimation of the instrument zero baseline as well as the biologic zero.

PROBLEMS OF LDF IN CLINICAL PRACTICE

LDF is noninvasive and does not interfere with the microcirculation when measuring local blood flow.[23] LDF is also particularly useful because it produces a continuous output that can be used for prolonged monitoring of tissue viability, such as after plastic surgery or to record skin flow perfusion during sleep or in the newborn. These techniques are impossible to obtain with any other noninvasive technique. LDF monitoring is also relatively stable, reproducible, and easy to learn and apply, although variations in resting values have been emphasized by several authors.

The technology of clinically usable LDF instruments is continuously improving. Multiple-channel systems capable of measuring distant tissue areas at the same time are now produced by different manufacturers. LDF imagers[21] and multiwavelength systems[1] are currently being developed and may be used for more accurate and interesting physiologic clinical applications.

LDF has been extensively used for clinical physiologic evaluations and in clinical practice in humans. The technique is easy and noninvasive and has become popular, but at times the interpretation of clinical results has been uncritical.[9]

As stated previously, LDF measures minute particle motion. In living tissue, such particles include mainly blood cells that constitute the major component of the LDF output. In situations of altered microcirculation or alteration of the blood hematocrit (e.g., in inflammation or leukemia), the number of particles can change, producing a different output. Thus the LDF signal can be considered a stochastic representation of the motion of all particles in the sample volume.[16,18,23] This measurement cannot be correctly defined as flow, however; in certain tissues and under certain conditions, it may be proportional and closely related to flow[9] as measured with isotopic methods. Another reason true volume flow cannot be measured is because the precise sampling volume is not easy to determine.[9,13]

For the reasons discussed, the LDF output signal recorded has been defined as flux, but possibly the most correct expression in clinical application should be *relative perfusion units*.[9] Additional terms used to express output signal such as volt or mV, arbitrary units, and other terms need to be unified. This is difficult at the moment because there is no dialogue concerning a common standard among manufacturers. The term *flow* may be used to express a concept that is more familiar to most physicians when referring to flow in certain contexts and considering the limitations.

Depth of measurements and volume in the skin

The sensitivity of the reflected LDF measurements decreases exponentially with the distance from the probe.[23] The estimated theoretical average depth of sampling in the skin is 0.14 mm, but in artificial models, it has been estimated to be 1.5 mm.[9] However, these values have little importance in clinical applications. There is also evidence that in intestinal models the measuring depth can be greater than 6 mm and that the signal output can be increased from 85% to 100% by placing a mirror on the opposite intestinal wall.[2] These observations suggest that the measuring depth is not a fixed value for the skin but probably a continuous variable as in other tissues.

As reported by Fagrell,[9] the microcirculation, particularly skin microcirculation, can be considered to consist of a small, superficial, thin layer characterized by the presence

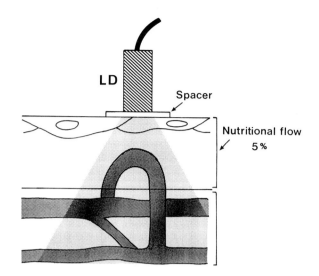

Fig. 28-2. The nutritional flow consists of approximately 5% of the total skin blood flow. A polycarbonate spacer may be theoretically useful to increase the nutritional flux component within the laser Doppler total output.

of nutritional capillaries and a deep, thicker layer with thermoregulatory vessels. The nutritional capillaries are the most superficial (0.1 to 0.5 mm from the skin surface), and in normal conditions, only a very small amount of the total skin blood flow (5% to 10%) passes through them (Fig. 28-2). In the subpapillary, mostly thermoregulatory bed (0.05 to 2.0 mm in depth), the most common vessels are venules (95%), with a small portion being arterioles. In this bed at least 95% of skin blood flow can be responsible for the LDF output, whereas in the nutritional bed, only a small percentage of flow (5% to 10%) contributes to the global output. LDF measurements in the skin measuring 1 to 2 mm of skin depth therefore record a signal in which the thermoregulatory flow component is predominant and the nutritional flow is a small component. New microprobes may reduce the measuring depth and provide a means of selective evaluation of the most relevant superficial nutritional capillaries, but clinically relevant data are not yet available.

Using polycarbonate (Delrin) spacers between the probe and the skin surface may allow examiners to record the more superficial flux (increasing the proportion of the nutritional flux component). The spacers have the same optical density as the skin and may be useful to separate the most superficial skin flux from the total skin flux, which is obtained by placing the probe directly on the skin. A different biological zero is also obtained with the spacers. It appears that the new biological zero obtained with the spacers is significantly different (higher) in patients with diabetes than that obtained in normal subjects.

VASOMOTION

Because LDF measures flux continuously, flux motion can also be easily evaluated. During LDF monitoring in normal conditions the skin vessels in the microcirculation fill up with blood rhythmically as a consequence of pressure and flow changes due to cardiac action respiration and vaso-motion. The LDF output is therefore variable.

Flux motion patterns are markedly changed in patients with peripheral vascular disease, who frequently display a high-frequency flux motion component. The prevalence of high-frequency motion waves is significantly increased in low perfusion states and is proportionally more evident with increasingly severe ischemia.

The presence of high-frequency flux motion waves at the forefoot has been evaluated by Hoffman et al[11] before and after percutaneous transluminal angioplasty. In successfully treated patients a significant decrease in high-frequency flux waves was observed after angioplasty. The persistence of such waves after angioplasty was associated with severe persisting chronic ischemia. Different patterns of vasomotor waves were also detected by Hoffman[11] in different conditions of perfusion. Flux motion in normal individuals was characterized by low-frequency and pulsatile flux waves. Occasionally, an additional high-frequency wave component appeared in the recording. Flux motion patterns in ischemia showed almost no pulsatile flux waves, whereas high-frequency waves were frequently observed in severe ischemia. In the most severe cases of ischemia, no flux motion was observed. In contrast, patients with intermittent claudication showed variable patterns (excluding the last pattern with no vasomotion).

With frequency analysis, it appears possible to qualitatively differentiate degrees of ischemia. Although there is little doubt that the alteration of vasomotion in low- or high-perfusion states is clinically relevant to indicate microcirculatory disturbances, no definite clinically practical application has been found based on the analysis of vasomotion.

CONCLUSION

The use of LDF is increasing in the fields of physiology and pharmacology and in the practical daily clinical evaluation of vascular disease. The monitoring of the effects of treatment on the microcirculation appears to be one of the most promising fields for the application of LDF. Further technical development of LDF combined with extensive clinical research application may make this method one of the most interesting noninvasive fields of investigation in vascular disease.

REFERENCES

1. Almond NE: *Laser Doppler flowmetry: instrumentation theory and practice.* In Belcaro G et al, eds: Med-Orion (in press).
2. Almond NE, Jones DP, Cooke ED: Noninvasive measurement of the human peripheral circulation: relationship between laser Doppler flowmeter and photoplethysmograph signals from the finger, *Angiology* 39:819, 1988.
3. Almond NE et al: *A laser Doppler blood flowmeter used to detect thermal entrainment in normal persons and patients with Raynaud's phenomenon.* In Spence VA, Sheldon CD, eds: *Practial aspects of skin blood flow measurement,* London, 1985, Biological Engineering Society.
4. Boggett D, Blond J, Rolfe P: Laser Doppler measurement of blood flow in skin tissue, *J Biomed Eng* 7:225, 1985.
5. Bonner RF, Nossal R: Model for laser Doppler measurements of blood flow in tissue, *Applied Optics* 20:2097, 1981.
6. Bonner RF et al: Laser Doppler continuous realtime monitor of pulsatile and mean blood flow in tissue microcirculation. In Chen S, Chu B, Nossal R, eds: *Nato Advanced Study Institute, Series B, Physics, Scattering techniques applied to supramolecular and non-equilibrium systems,* New York, 1981, Plenum Press.
7. Borgos JA: TSI's LDV blood flowmeter. In Shepherd A, Oberg P, eds: Laser Doppler blood flowmetry, Boston, 1990, Kluver Academic.
8. Engelhart M, Kristensen JK: Evaluation of cutaneous blood flow responses by [133]Xenon washout and a laser Doppler flowmeter, *J Invest Dermatol* 80:12, 1983.
9. Fagrell B: *Problems using laser Doppler on the skin in clinical practice.* In Belcaro G et al, eds: Med-Orion (in press).
10. Hellem S et al: Measurement of microvascular blood flow in cancellous bone using laser Doppler flowmetry and ^{133}Xe clearance, *Int J Oral Surg* 12:165, 1983.
11. Hoffman U et al: *Skin blood flux in peripheral arterial occlusive disease.* In Belcaro G et al, eds: *Laser-Doppler flowmetry: experimental and clinical applications,* Med-Orion (in press).
12. Holloway GA, Watkins DW: Laser Doppler measurement of cutaneous blood flow, *J Invest Dermatol* 69:306, 1977.
13. Johnson JM et al: Laser Doppler measurement of skin blood flow: comparison with plethysmography, *J Appl Physiol Respirat Environ Exercise Physiol* 56:798, 1984.
14. Nilsson GE, Tenlan T, Oberg PA: Evaluation of a laser Doppler flowmeter for measurement of tissue blood flow, *IEEE Trans Biomed Eng* 27:597, 1980.
15. Obeid AN et al: Depth discrimination in laser Doppler skin blood flow measurement using different lasers, *Med Biol Eng Comput* 26:415, 1988.
16. Obeid AN et al: A critical review of laser Doppler flowmetry, *J Med Eng Technol* 14:178, 1990.
17. Riva C, Ross B, Benedek GB: Laser Doppler measurement of blood flow in capillary tubes and retinal arteries, *Investigative Ophthalmology* 11:936, 1972.
18. Stern MD: In vivo evaluation of microcirculation by coherent light scattering, *Nature* 254:56, 1975.
19. Stern MD et al: Continuous assessment of tissue blood flow by laser Doppler spectroscopy, *Am J Physiol* 232:H441, 1977.
20. Tonneson KH, Pederson LJ: *Laser Doppler flowmetry: problems with calibration.* In Belcaro G et al, eds: Med-Orion (in press).
21. Wardell K, Jakobbson A, Nilsson GE: *A laser Doppler imager for microcirculatory studies.* A meeting of the 1st European Laser Doppler Users, Oxford, England, March 1991.
22. Weis GH, Nossal R, Bonne RF: Statistics of penetration depth of photons re-emitted from irradiation tissue, *J Mod Optics* 36:349-359, 1989.
23. Winsor T et al: Clinical application of laser Doppler flowmetry for measurement of cutaneous circulation in health and disease, *Angiology* 10:727, 1987.

PART THREE

AREAS OF APPLICATION: DETECTION, QUANTITATION, AND PREDICTION

Introduction

D. EUGENE STRANDNESS, Jr., and BERT C. EIKELBOOM

Since publication of the third edition in 1985, many changes have occurred that have a direct impact on the use of noninvasive testing for this area of the circulation. First, the indirect tests have generally been replaced by duplex scanning because the results with this method are so superior. The technology, particularly as related to duplex scanning, has evolved to the point where many consider the results to be as accurate as arteriography for many applications other than screening, including assessment of the extracranial vessels. For example, increasing numbers of studies have shown that duplex scanning can be used as the sole study before carotid endarterectomy. This represents a major departure from the conventional approach, which is still the most commonly practiced. It is also apparent that if surgeons take this approach, they must be confident of the accuracy of the scanning procedure.

The other major development has been the reporting of the results of the randomized trials that examined the role of carotid endarterectomy for the treatment of both patients with symptomatic and those with asymptomatic cerebrovascular disease. It is now clear that the operation is much more effective in the prevention of stroke in patients with symptoms when compared with conventional medical therapy. These results have finally placed the operation on very solid ground as an effective method of stroke prevention.

Now that the results with the surgical treatment of high-grade stenoses (greater than 70% diameter reduction) are well established, the role for screening by the use of duplex scanning becomes even more important. Since nearly all patients will be studied by this modality first, it is essential that the results permit proper segregation of those patients who will be best treated by means of surgery. For example,

if a patient with symptoms of stenosis is misclassified into a stenosis category of less than 70% diameter reduction when there is a higher grade lesion present, it is likely that the patient would be treated by nonoperative means and be placed at considerable risk for a stroke. Further, there is no proof at this time that plaque morphology other than the degree of stenosis should be used as the basis for clinical decisions.

For asymptomatic patients, it has been the practice in this country to offer surgery for the high-grade lesions (greater than 80% diameter reduction). The Veterans Administration Trial of asymptomatic patients has shown that for patients with a more than 50% diameter reduction and a positive oculoplethysmograph, surgery is better than medical therapy for the prevention of transient ischemic events and strokes. The National Institutes of Health trial of patients who have no symptoms has not yet reported their results. Until this trial is completed, the guidelines previously mentioned should still be followed.

In conclusion, it appears that the place of noninvasive testing and in particular duplex scanning has assumed a central role in the evaluation of carotid bifurcation disease. This includes the postoperative patient, although carotid restenosis has been shown to be a relatively benign process. It is not yet possible to be so definitive about the role of duplex scanning in the evaluation of vertebrobasilar insufficiency. It is very difficult to relate symptoms in this subset of patients to the findings from any of the noninvasive testing procedures. It is likely that a combination of duplex scanning and transcranial Doppler may provide more definitive answers, but we must await the results of further studies.

CHAPTER 29

The clinical spectrum of ischemic cerebrovascular disease

EUGENE F. BERNSTEIN

Stroke is the third leading cause of death in the United States after heart disease and cancer. It is the second leading cause of death in patients over the age of 70. However, stroke is more greatly feared than most other serious diseases because only about 25% of patients who have a stroke die and three times as many patients survive with varying and often greatly disabling degrees of neurologic deficit. Both physically and emotionally, a major stroke that results in permanent hemiplegia and aphasia drains the most important qualities of life. Frequently, the patient is committed to a nursing home or has a bedridden existence with little hope of significant improvement or recovery. In the last three decades a great deal of new information has been obtained concerning the pathogenesis of this disease. Emphasis has shifted from the recognition and treatment of the advanced state of major neurologic involvement to those conditions that precede a major stroke episode and to those diagnostic and management tools that may be used to significantly reduce the likelihood of a major stroke.

Pathogenesis

Ischemic cerebrovascular disease is usually the end result of progressive atherosclerosis in the arterial system leading to the brain. Thus all factors known to be significant in the pathogenesis of atherosclerosis are pertinent to this problem, including heredity, high cholesterol and triglyceride levels, obesity, diabetes, smoking, and states of high anxiety and stress. The development of an intimal plaque that contains atheromatous material is usually the first recognizable pathologic evidence of this disease and is now a frequent finding in young adults in Western society. Progression of the intimal atheromatous lesion then occurs, followed by necrosis of some central contents of the atheroma. This is presumably because inadequate nutrition results in an increasing diffusion barrier that prevents oxygen and glucose from reaching the depths of the lesion. In addition, subintimal hemorrhage contributes to the development of thicker lesions in the necrotic interior of the atheroma. Such necrotic deeper portions of the plaque may then break through the intimal lining, which results in the release of plaque contents to the arterial bloodstream. This atheroembolic material is then deposited at a distant site, which if in the central nervous system, may provoke neurologic signs or result in physical findings that are indicators or warnings of the future potential of a major stroke. The cavitary lesion in the plaque that results from the release of atheroembolic plaque material is referred to as an ulcer and may then be the site of swirling blood, leading to the deposition of platelet fragments and thrombi. Subsequent embolic episodes may therefore contain not only atheromatous material but also varying amounts of platelet clumps and fibrin clots. It is this triad of embolic contents—atheroma, platelets, and fibrin—that justifies the current medical approach to the treatment of this condition.

In addition to the embolic mechanism that is believed to be the most common cause of a stroke and the warning sign of a future stroke, the atheromatous lesion may progress to obstruct most or all of the lumen of the artery. Larger plaques are more likely to become ulcerated, cavernomatous, and associated with subintimal hemorrhage and may eventually lead to thrombosis. Thus an ischemic stroke may result either from inadequate blood flow to the brain or from a large embolus. Early detection of stroke potential has centered around the identification of evolving atherosclerotic lesions in vessels that feed the brain and around the detection of symptoms caused by such lesions, although such symptoms may appear insignificant or may be entirely transient.

Although atherosclerosis is generally considered to be a diffuse systemic arterial disease, there is a clear predisposition to more severe localized disease at certain selected sites, including the coronary arteries, the branches of the aortic arch, the bifurcations of the carotid arteries, the infrarenal abdominal aorta, and the superficial femoral arteries. Of these, the bifurcation of the carotid arteries is an area in which atherosclerotic disease tends to be particularly severe and segmentally localized. Recent research has confirmed the concept that ischemic cerebrovascular stroke is most frequently a result of atherosclerosis in the neck or the arch of the aorta. The precise location and segmental nature of this process is the basis for the surgical approach to the treatment of these conditions, since effective surgical procedures can be performed on well-localized, discrete lesions.

Temporal classification

The clinical stages of ischemic cerebrovascular disease are summarized in the box below, ranging from the patient who is free of symptoms with only a minimally detectable shallow plaque or shallow ulceration in an artery leading to the brain to the patient with a full, complete, and permanent stroke. Asymptomatic disease may be defined as an identifiable pathologic state associated with the increased likelihood of a future stroke. Such patients are identified by the presence of a cervical bruit or by noninvasive vascular or angiographic procedures that document the existence of carotid bifurcation stenosis or ulceration.

A transient ischemic attack (TIA) is an episode of focal, visual, motor, or sensory loss that persists for less than 24 hours. Most of these episodes are much shorter, usually lasting for 5 to 30 minutes. They are painless, involve no loss of consciousness, are generally associated with a rapid onset and resolution, and may be a result of one of a variety of factors (see the box below). If the neurologic symptoms persist for more than 24 hours but eventually resolve completely, the event is referred to as a reversible ischemic neurologic deficit (RIND). If the deficit persists permanently, the patient has had a stroke. During the time interval that neurologic symptoms are changing, the condition is described as a progressing stroke or stroke in evolution. Once the patient's neurologic condition has become stable with a persisting neurologic deficit, the condition is referred to as a completed stroke.

Because the temporal classification that is in general clinical use fails to include data regarding the history of prior events in the ipsilateral or contralateral hemispheres, does not include information regarding the location and magnitude of cerebral arterial disease, and does not coincide with existing European classifications of stroke, a new classification system has been proposed (Table 29-1).

The CHAT classification of vascular disease was designed to separate various current *(C)* and historical *(H)* presentations of disease and their separate angiographic *(A)* and target *(T)* organ manifestations from each other to identify specific factors or groups of factors that would be important in determining appropriate management approaches or prognosis. When initially described, the system provided information about the improved outlook of patients with amaurosis fugax compared with those with cortical TIA, both of which had previously been grouped within the overall classification of TIA.[15,68] In addition, patients who are free of symptoms with prior contralateral symptoms were shown to have a different outlook than those with a completely negative contralateral history of cerebrovascular disease.

The CHAT classification system was adopted by the Subcommittee on Reporting Standards for Cerebrovascular Disease of the SVS/ISCVS in 1988.[6] More recently, a CHAT analysis has documented that each clinical presentation of cerebrovascular disease leading to carotid endarterectomy was associated with a differing risk factor complex regarding the probability of late postoperative stroke.[16] Thus CHAT appears to be a clinically useful classification of stroke-prone patients.

Differential diagnosis of acute cerebral deficit

Although the vast majority of acute cerebrovascular problems are of vascular etiology, a number of systemic, neurologic, and cardiogenic diseases may also produce such symptoms (see box below). Since the specific identification of a large number of these entities can lead to a satisfactory management and therapy plan, the physician should under-

---

CEREBROVASCULAR DISEASE—TEMPORAL CLASSIFICATION

Asymptomatic—bruit, stenosis, ulceration
Transient ischemic attack (TIA)
Reversible ischemic neurologic deficit (RIND)
Progressing stroke
Completed stroke

CAUSES OF ACUTE CEREBRAL DEFICIT

All patients
⌐——————→ Nonvascular (e.g., tumor)—5%
Vascular causes—95%
⌐——————→ Hemorrhagic—14%
Ischemic—81%
⌐——————→ Cardiogenic—12%
│ Other—4%
↓
Cerebrovascular
disease—65%

From Easton JD et al: *Curr Probl Cardiol* 8:1, 1983.

DIFFERENTIAL DIAGNOSIS OF ACUTE CEREBRAL DEFICIT

Cerebrovascular atherosclerosis
Cardiogenic embolism—valvular, ventricular cavity, tumor, and paradoxic
Arteriopathy—inflammatory (systemic collagen diseases, Takayasu's disease, or infections) or noninflammatory (fibromuscular hyperplasia, spontaneous and traumatic dissection, cerebral angiopathies, or neoplasm)
Vasospasm—migraine or hypertensive encephalopathy
Subarachnoid hemorrhage
Coagulopathies and hyperviscosity syndromes
Trauma
Systemic hypotension
Metabolic disturbances
Drug reactions

Table 29-1. The CHAT classification of stroke

C Current status (<1 yr)		H History (>1 yr)	A Artery		T Target	
Symptoms	Vascular territory	Symptoms vascular territory	Site	Pathology	Site	Pathology
0 — Asymptomatic	a — Carotid ocular (amaurosis fugax)	Same categories as current status	0 — No lesion	a — Arteriosclerosis	0 — No lesion	h — Hemorrhage
1 — Brief stroke TIA (<24 hr)	b — Carotid cortical	Current clinical	1 — Appropriate lesion	c — Cardiogenic embolus	1 — Appropriate lesion	i — Infarct
2 — Temporary stroke with full recovery (24 hr to 3 wk)	c — Vertebrobasilar	1-5 a-c	2 — Lesion only in another vascular pathway	d — Dissection	2 — Lesion only in another vascular territory	j — Lacunar
3 — Permanent stroke, minor (>3 wk)	d — Other focal		3 — Combined, appropriate lesion and lesion in another vascular pathway	e — Aneurysm	3 — Combined, appropriate lesion and lesion in another vascular territory	m — AVM
4 — Permanent stroke, major (>3 wk)	c — Diffuse	Subscript s is used to indicate prior operation		f — Fibromuscular		n — Neoplasm
5 — Nonspecific dysfunction				r — Arteritis		q — Other
6 — Improving stroke				t — Trauma		r — Retinal embolism
7 — Fluctuating stroke						
8 — Deteriorating stroke						

From Baker ID et al: *J Vasc Surg* 8:721, 1988.
AVM, Arteriovenous malformation; significant, 50% stenosis or disease thought to be the source of symptoms.

Table 29-2. Frequency of symptoms in TIA

Symptoms	Patients (%)
CAROTID ARTERY DISTRIBUTION	
Paresis (monoparesis, hemiparesis)	61
Paresthesia (monoparesis, hemiparesis)	57
Monocular visual	32
Paresthesia (facial)	30
Paresis (facial)	22
VERTEBROBASILAR DISTRIBUTION	
Binocular visual	57
Vertigo	50
Paresthesia	40
Diplopia	38
Ataxia	33
Paresis	33

Table 29-3. Arterial classification of symptomatic cerebrovascular disease

Artery	Symptoms
Ophthalmic	Amaurosis fugax
Middle cerebral	
Anterior cortical branch	Contralateral sensory and motor loss of face, arm, and hand
	Nonfluent aphasia (dominant hemisphere)
Posterior cortical branch	Homonymous hemianopsia
	Fluent aphasia (dominant hemisphere)
Proximal middle cerebral or lenticulostriate branch	Internal capsule
	Unilateral motor and sensory findings of face, arm, and leg
Vertebrobasilar	Diplopia
	Bilateral facial sensory loss
	Bilateral extremity weakness
	Vertigo
	Ataxia

take a methodical and complete workup of any patient with an abrupt cerebral deficit.

THE TIA

Symptoms associated with transient ischemic episodes may generally be classified by the arterial circulation involved. In the anterior circulation from the carotid system, the most frequently observed symptoms include amaurosis fugax (transient monocular blindness) and numbness, weakness, or paralysis of an arm or leg or both (Table 29-2). In addition, lesions in this portion of the brain may be accompanied by dysphasia or aphasia, headache, dizziness, blackouts, buzzing noises, mental deterioration, memory loss, coma, and convulsions. In contrast, patients whose pathologic condition resides in the vertebrobasilar or posterior portion of the brain frequently complain of bilateral visual disturbances, dysarthria, dysphasia, drop attacks, and bilateral sensory deficits. In addition, they may experience vertigo, headaches, bilateral visual disturbances, loss of consciousness, monoparesis, shifting paralysis, or cerebellar ataxia. The relative frequency of these complaints as assessed by the Canadian Cooperative Study Group[23] is in Table 29-1. A further localization of the symptom complexes associated with carotid artery distribution and the middle cerebral artery is summarized in Table 29-3, although occlusions of other vessels with variable collateral circulatory compensation may yield similar symptom complexes. The symptom complex associated with the lenticulostriate branches of the internal capsule is important. This complex results in lacunar infarction, which is generally manifested by unilateral motor and sensory findings in the face, arm, and leg and explains the absence of large-vessel atherosclerotic disease on an angiogram.

Natural history of a TIA

The natural history of patients who have experienced a TIA has been intensively studied in the last 2 decades. Outcome for such patients is based primarily on the symp-

Table 29-4. Prognosis following TIA without treatment

Author and year	Patients (no.)	Average follow-up (mo)	Stroke (%)
Fisher,[48] 1958	23	?	34
Baker,[10] 1962	20	20	25
Siekert,[113] 1963	160	60	32
Acheson,[2] 1964	151	48	62
Marshall,[83] 1965	158	60	43
Pierce,[91] 1965	20	11	10
Baker,[10] 1966	30	41	23
Baker,[8] 1968	79	41	22
Friedman,[51] 1969	23	27	35
Goldner,[54] 1971	111	?	38
Ziegler,[140] 1973	135	36	16
Whisnant,[183] 1973	198	60	32
Toole,[126] 1975	56	66	19
Olsson,[96] 1976	124	21	15
Canadian Cooperative,[23] 1978	139	26	14
Loeb,[80] 1978	94	78	12
Sorenson,[114] 1983	102	25	11
Bousser,[18] 1983	204	36	18

tom complex and on the full spectrum of causes in the box at the bottom. The box lists the differential diagnoses of acute cerebral deficits. Approximately one third of the patients with a TIA will have sustained a complete stroke episode within 5 years (Table 29-4). The likelihood of stroke is greatest within the first month after a TIA, during which approximately 5% of the patients will sustain a stroke. The incidence of stroke then decreases gradually, with an overall likelihood of 12% within 1 year and 20% within 2 years. The ominous nature of these data dictates the need for an urgent and complete workup of the patient who has experienced a TIA.

The box identifies the even more severe implications of the presence of retinal cholesterol crystals (Hollenhorst's plaques).[101] Although these patients are technically free of symptoms and since many have not experienced transient monocular blindness, they are clearly at high risk for stroke and should undergo a similar workup.

Approximately 25% of patients who sustain a permanent stroke and do not die are then faced with the likelihood of further stroke episodes, which may result in the progressive loss and deterioration of their residual neurologic function. Table 29-5 summarizes the available data on the incidence of ischemic strokes after a single stroke episode, from which it appears that the likelihood of recurrent stroke varies from 6% to 11% per year. Thus the continuing risk for further neurologic erosion argues for identifying a course of management that will minimize future strokes. The practical problem, however, is that many of these patients have already lost so much neurologic function that they are no longer independently capable of managing their lives. Under these circumstances the additional risks required to attempt to preclude further strokes often do not appear justifiable. Nevertheless, those patients who have recovered from a stroke with a small permanent deficit that has left them relatively capable of functioning independently are at as great a risk of further stroke as if they had experienced a TIA and should be considered in the same workup category as patients who have sustained a TIA or RIND.

Workup of the patient with symptoms

The evaluation of patients with a single TIA, RIND, or small stroke should include a complete history, physical examination, and basic workup for systemic, cardiac, and neurologic disease. This workup should include a complete blood count, urinalysis, prothrombin time, partial thromboplastin time, chest x-ray examination, cerebrospinal fluid examination, antinuclear antibody (ANA) level, erythrocyte sedimentation rate, and computerized tomographic (CT) scan (Fig. 29-1). Patients who present with amaurosis fugax should be seen by an ophthalmologist and should have an erythrocyte sedimentation rate test to rule out great cell arteritis. All patients with evidence of cardiac disease that may be a potential embolic source should also have cardiac consultation and appropriate cardiac evaluation. Patients with evidence of systemic disease, including an increased erythrocyte sedimentation rate, anemia, or thrombocytosis, should undergo further studies including ANA, cerebrospinal fluid examinations, and protein electrophoresis levels. A CT scan should be performed in all patients with symptomatic cerebrovascular disease because it may provide information regarding the presence of a mass lesion such as a tumor. The CT scan may also permit identification of an ischemic infarction (a hypodense area) or a hemorrhagic lesion (a hyperdense area). It may also demonstrate a mass effect secondary to edema surrounding an embolic lesion and may permit the diagnosis of a lacunar stroke.

In the absence of evidence of cardiogenic emboli or systemic disease, a presumptive diagnosis of cerebrovascular disease should be made.[36] Cerebrovascular disease is responsible for the transient episode in approximately 65% of patients with such symptoms. A decision must then be made regarding the suitability of the patient as a candidate for carotid surgery, with the further workup directed toward that goal. Patients who are considered to be at inordinately high risk for cerebrovascular surgery should be treated with antiplatelet or anticoagulant therapy. Good-risk patients should continue on the management algorithm path in Fig. 29-1. Several satisfactory options exist for their further workup. In the first, the patient is sent to the vascular laboratory to obtain evidence of a carotid artery lesion producing significant hemodynamic stenosis. In the presence of such data, angiography will confirm the presence of ca-

---

PROGNOSIS AFTER DETECTION OF RETINAL CHOLESTEROL EMBOLI

208 patients, mean age 64 years of age, 86% male, 97% followed for 6 +2 years, 70 followed for 10+ years
75% (157) had TIA or stroke
45% (94) had stroke
28% (58) had stroke ipsilateral to the retinal embolus

From Pfaffenbach DD, Hollenhorst RW: *Am J Ophthamol* 75:66, 1973.

Table 29-5. Likelihood of recurrent stroke

Author	Patients (no.)	Mean follow-up (mo)	Ischemic strokes (%/year)	Lethal strokes (%/year)
Baker[7]	62	13	6	3
Baker[8]	60	11	11	9
Hill (phase I)[65]	71	10	7	0
Hill (phase II)[65]	65	31	11	1
McDowell[86]	99	34	8	2
Enger[39]	49	23	11	3

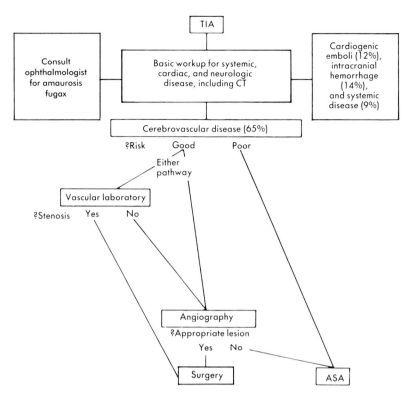

Fig. 29-1. Scheme for workup of patient with TIA. *CT,* Computed tomography; *ASA,* acetyl salicylic acid.

rotid stenosis. In straightforward cases with a well-defined carotid lesion, formal contrast angiography may be necessary. Patients with anatomically appropriate lesions are candidates for surgical therapy.

Role of angiography. Carotid angiography is the appropriate, definitive diagnostic procedure for all patients with a symptomatic acute cerebrovascular event with complete or nearly complete recovery. In addition, selected patients with chronic cerebral ischemia (based on multivessel occlusive disease) or with asymptomatic carotid stenosis (defined by a vascular laboratory study) are also candidates for angiography.

Formal cerebrovascular angiography is generally performed through a femoral puncture with a catheter placed in the arch of the aorta, after which injections are performed and x-ray films are obtained in two planes. Selective injections into both carotid arteries are also routine. In addition, the subclavian arteries are selectively injected when the patient has vertebral artery symptoms. All studies should also include intracranial views to identify the possibility of tandem lesions in the upper portion of the internal carotid artery and other intracranial lesions that may be the cause of the patient's symptoms. With modern techniques the risks of cerebral angiography for the evaluation of cerebrovascular symptoms are quite low and carry an expected stroke rate of approximately 1% and a low anticipated mortality rate of 1% (Table 29-6).

The clinical correlation of significant symptoms with the

Table 29-6. Complications of cerebral angiography

Author	Year	Patients (no.)	Stroke (%)	Mortality (%)
Swanson[117]	1977	464	1.1	?
Mani[82]	1978	1702	0.1	0
Faught[43]	1979	147	5.4	0
Link[79]	1979	162	0	0
Allen[3]	1981	154	2.0	0
Harrison[58]	1982	188	1.1	?

angiographic demonstration of appropriate carotid bifurcation stenosis or occlusion is very high.[13,37,44,55,59] Symptoms such as amaurosis fugax or the presence of retinal emboli have a likelihood of a significant carotid artery lesion in over 90% of the patients. On the other hand, when all patients with carotid system TIAs undergo angiography, fully 25% of the angiograms appear normal (Table 29-7). In these patients the workup for other causes, including systemic collagen disease, neurologic conditions, and cardiogenic emboli, should be intensified. A total of 20% of these patients have a minimal irregularity on angiography, and these lesions are consistent with an embologenic pathogenesis. Such patients should be candidates for carotid endarterectomy. Approximately 10% of patients with TIA will have occlusion of the appropriate internal carotid system as determined by angiography. Under these circumstances a

Table 29-7. Angiographic correlations in carotid TIA

	Angiographic classification			
Author and year	Normal (%)	Minimal disease (%)	Stenosis ≥ 25% (%)	Occlusion (%)
Ramirex-Lassepas, 1973[106]	17	←———— 69 ————→		14
Lemak, 1976[77]	43	←———— 49 ———→		8
Harrison, 1976[58]	45	10	40	5
Pessin, 1977[100]	←——— 42 ———→		46	12
Eisenberg, 1977[38]	9	0	73	15
Marti-Vilalta, 1979[84]	27			
Link, 1979[79]	8	←———— 89———→		3
Ueda, 1979[129]	11	14	59	16
Van Oudenarrden, 1980[131]	24	32	←———— 44 ————→	
Thiele, 1980[121]	13	40	←———— 47 ————→	
Barnett, 1980[13]	22	27	35	13
Russo, 1981[110]	55	19	15	11
Muuronen, 1981[93]	49	10	37	4
ESTIMATED MEAN	27%	19%	44%	10%

Adapted from Easton JD et al: *Curr Probl Cardiol* 8:1, 1983.

Table 29-8. Distribution of extracranial arterial occlusive diseases in 4748 patients with stroke symptoms

	Stenosis (%)	Occlusion (%)
Innominate	4.2	0.6
Common carotid (left)	4.8	4.4
Subclavian (left)	12.4	2.5
Carotid bifurcation (right)	33.8	8.5
Carotid bifurcation (left)	34.1	8.5
Vertebral (right)	18.4	4.0
Vertebral (left)	22.3	5.7

careful search must be made for the possibility of embologenic lesions from the contralateral carotid bifurcation or symptoms associated with chronic cerebral ischemia that might benefit from an extracranial-to-intracranial bypass. Although such patients do constitute a higher risk group for surgery, in good hands the surgical approach still offers the best outlook in the prevention of recurrent stroke.

The most important and largest source of data concerning the diagnostic rewards of complete cerebrovascular angiography in patients with stroke symptoms was presented by Fields et al[45] in a joint study that included four-vessel angiography in 4748 patients with stroke symptoms. In 19.4% of the patients, no lesions were identified. However, in 74.5%, significant and appropriate lesions in a surgically accessible area were identified, although multiple lesions were present in two thirds of the patients (Table 29-8). Carotid bifurcation stenosis was the most common localized lesion associated with stroke symptoms, followed by stenosis of vertebral origin and left subclavian stenosis. On the other hand, occlusion of any of these vessels was relatively uncommon.

Therapeutic alternatives. The major alternatives available to patients who have had a transient ischemic episode or a mild stroke with good recovery include anticoagulation therapy, antiplatelet aggregation therapy, and surgery. Anticoagulation therapy is suggested as appropriate for patients who have had a TIA because it inhibits the development and propagation of thrombi in association with plaques and ulcers.[37,85,88,119] A summary of the major trials of anticoagulation therapy in the treatment of TIA is presented in Table 29-9. Data indicate that anticoagulation therapy was beneficial in most but not all of the studies. However, the incidence of cerebral hemorrhage associated with anticoagulation therapy increases with time and is estimated to be at least 2% per year. Therefore the general consensus has been that anticoagulation is appropriate only in patients who require a short period of therapy, perhaps up to 6 months, during which the likelihood of stroke after a TIA episode is greatest.[37,53] In general, anticoagulation therapy is limited to those patients who are not surgical candidates or those who refuse surgery. Data regarding use of anticoagulation therapy in patients with progressing stroke also suggest benefits (Table 29-10) and justify advocating the use of these drugs during the immediate period of stroke in evolution.[24] On the other hand, anticoagulation therapy for completed stroke clearly has an adverse effect on outcome, since the risks of serious hemorrhage exceed the benefits of minimizing recurrent stroke (Table 29-11).

Platelet antiaggregation agents have also been used in the treatment of patients with TIA and have been evaluated in a number of prospective randomized trials. The United States and Canadian multicentered studies, which are summarized in Table 29-12, are considered the most valid. In the U.S. study, when the incidence of TIA, stroke, or death was used as an end point, there was a significant benefit for the patient group treated with aspirin.[45] However, when stroke alone was evaluated, the benefits were not significant. In the Canadian study the results were similar.[23] When TIA, stroke, and death were evaluated, the results indicated some benefit for the aspirin treatment group at a borderline significance. However, when stroke alone was evaluated, there was no difference between the control group and the treated group. This was also true when stroke alone was evaluated in men. The major benefits of aspirin therefore appear to be in inhibiting the likelihood of further TIA and in decreasing the incidence of death from cardiac disease. Additional studies involving the use of sulfinpyrazone or dipyridamole alone or together with aspirin did not appear to significantly improve the end results for TIA, stroke, or death.

Surgery is the third alternative for the treatment of cerebrovascular occlusive disease. The goals of carotid surgery are to prevent future strokes and prolong life. It also may relieve symptoms, particularly in those patients who are subject to continuing TIAs. Currently accepted indications for surgery include TIAs (plus reversible ischemic neurologic deficits) and prior stroke with significant recovery and a current minimal neurologic deficit.[15,116,123,132] Other indications include symptomatic subclavian steal, chronic

Table 29-9. Anticoagulation for TIA

Author and year	Ischemic stroke (%)	
	Treatment	Control
Randomized studies		
Baker, 1961[7]	5	0
Baker, 1962[10]	6	25
Pierce, 1965[91]	6	10
Baker, 1966[9]	7	23
MEAN	5	17
Nonrandomized studies		
Fisher, 1958[49]	3	35
Siekert, 1963[113]	7	32
Friedman, 1969[51]	0	35
Toole, 1975[126]	29	13
Olsson, 1965[96]	0	6
Gallhofer, 1979[52]	8	21
Link, 1979[79]	0	—
Terent, 1980[119]	8	31
Olsson, 1980[96]	2	—
Buren, 1971[20]	3	—
MEAN	6	28

Table 29-10. Anticoagulation for progressing stroke

Type of study	Patients (no.)	Ischemic stroke (%)	
		Treatment	Control
Randomized	304	23	46
Nonrandomized	269	21	57

From Easton JD et al: *Curr Probl Cardiol* 8:1, 1983.

Table 29-11. Anticoagulation for completed stroke

Author and year	Ischemic stroke (%)		Serious hemorrhage (%)	
	Treatment	Control	Treatment	Control
Baker, 1961[7]	5	6	13	4
Baker, 1962[10]	17	25	24	0
Hill, Phase I, 1962[65]	13	6	1	0
Phase II, 1962	33	29	18	0
McDowell, 1965[86]	21	21	12	2
Enger, 1965[39]	10	20	6	0

Table 29-12. Aspirin for TIA

Source	Patients (no.)	End point events	Events (%)		
			Treatment	Control	p value
U.S. Multicenter Study, 1977[45]	178	TIA, stroke, death	17	38	0.01
		Stroke, death	7	16	NS
		Stroke	5	11	NS
Canadian Cooperative Study, 1978[23]	585	TIA, stroke, death	57	66	0.05
		Stroke, death	18	22	0.05
		Stroke	15	14	NS
		Stroke, death (males)	17	24	0.01
		Stroke (males)	14	16	NS

NS, Not significant.

cerebral ischemia from multivessel occlusive disease, and select asymptomatic carotid stenosis.[59,99,105] Recent data concerning the risk of carotid endarterectomy for patients with TIAs indicate that the procedure should be performed when the mortality rate is approximately 1% and stroke risk is 5% or less (Table 29-13). In addition, data regarding the late results of carotid endarterectomy for patients with TIAs indicate a reduction of the expected natural history stroke rate of 5% to 7% per year to less than 2% per year (Table 29-14).[11] Such results assume morbidity and mortality data in the currently reported ranges.

Each of the three multicenter, prospective, randomized trials reported in 1991 confirmed a highly statistically valid advantage for surgery over medical treatment alone in those patients with symptoms who also had appropriate carotid stenoses of 70% or more (50% in the Veterans Administration study). In the North American Symptomatic Carotid Endarterectomy trial, there was a 5:1 benefit in favor of surgery ($p < 0.001$), and the benefit increased with increasing degrees of stenosis from 70% to 99% (Table 29-15). In the European Carotid Surgery trial, a similar benefit of surgery was observed for stenoses of 70% to 99%. No benefit was observed with lesions of 0% to 20%, and those with 30% to 60% stenoses are still being recruited and

Table 29-13. Risk of carotid endarterectomy for TIA

Author and year	Operations (no.)	Mortality (%)	Stroke (%)
Schechter and Acinapura,* 1979[112]	200	1.0	1.0
Duke, 1979[33]	70	1.4	5.7
Bouchier-Hayes, 1979[16]	34	—	5.9
Haynes and Dempsey,* 1979[61]	276	1.1	4.0
Pinkerton and Gholkar,* 1979[103]	100	0	4.0
White, 1981[135]	104	1.0	1.9
Whisnant, 1982[134]	151	1.0	3.0
Asiddao, 1982[5]	94	0	4.3
Modi, 1983[89]	249	0.4	1.6
Bernstein, 1983[14]	152	0	2.6
NASCET, 1991[94]	328	0.6	2.1
ECST, 1991[42]	455	0.9	2.9
VA Symptomatic, 1991[130]	91		
AVERAGE		1.2	4.8

*Minority of patients had small strokes, most had TIAs.

Table 29-14. Late results of carotid endarterectomy for TIA

Author and year	Patients (no.)	Average follow-up (mo)	Late stroke* (%)	Late death* (%)
Young, 1969[139]	95	12 to 60	3.2	10.5
Fields, 1970[45]	150	42	4.0	15.3
Thompson, 1970[122]	289	6 to 156	5.4	27.3
Wylie, 1970[138]	129	48	5.7	14.6
DeWeese, 1973[30]	102	60	10.6	34.3
Chung, 1974[25]	58	48	—	20.1
Nunn, 1975[94]	168	39	7.7	31.0
Toole, 1975[125]	77	46	6.9	18.2
McNamara, 1977[87]	52	10	0.0	7.7
Fields, 1977[47]	60	24	13.3	—
Cornell, 1978[27]	65	32	3.1	—
Pinkerton, 1979[103]	85	25	0.0	?
Bouchier-Hayes, 1979[16]	57	12 to 72	3.5	7.0
Ericsson, 1980[41]	143	22	7.0	?
Whisnant, 1982[134]	150	72	—	—
Harrison, 1982[57]	58	50	17.2	?
Bernstein, 1983[14]	152	45	6.0	19.0

*The aggregate estimates were as follows: stroke, 1.8% per year; death, 5% per year.

followed up with uncertain results. The third study, the VA Symptomatic trial, was similar. Thus there are firm, current, statistically sound data in favor of surgery as the best treatment for the patient with symptomatic high-grade stenosis.

Whether carotid endarterectomy is appropriate in patients who are free of symptoms is clearly more controversial.* Since such patients are at less risk than patients who have sustained a TIA (Table 29-16), the tolerance for perioper-

*References 19, 21, 26, 28, 56, 60, 92, 109, 118.

ative morbidity and mortality must be less, and the responsibility of the surgical team therefore greater. Data addressing the risk of carotid endarterectomy in asymptomatic patients are presented in Table 29-17 and indicate that the acceptable mortality rate should be 1% or less and the acceptable operative stroke rate 2% or less. Long-term results of such procedures in asymptomatic patients appear to justify their continued use by selected teams. The available data (Table 29-18) suggest the stroke rate after prophylactic carotid surgery is approximately 1% per year, significantly less than would be expected with other forms of treatment. However, it seems clear that survival after carotid endarterectomy for any of these indications is significantly less than that for the general population, primarily as a result of myocardial disease.[63,107,128]

Three additional multicenter clinical trials are currently under way to ascertain the value of carotid endarterectomy in the patient who is free of symptoms. In each of these, a minimal stenosis of 50% is required for entry (60% in ACAS). Two of these trials have closed their acquisitions, and the third (ACAS) is still recruiting cases. In all, the mandatory follow-up will preclude a definitive conclusion before 1994. Until then, decisions regarding asymptomatic stenosis will have to be made on the basis of local surgeon

Table 29-15. Symptomatic carotid artery trials

	NASCET	ECST	VA
Patients (total)	1212	2518	189
(70%-99%)	659	778	189 (>50%)
No. of centers	50	80	16
Total stroke			
Medical	22%	28%	19%
Surgical	13%	6%	8%
p value	0.001	0.001	0.01

NASCET, North American Symptomatic Carotid Endarterectomy trial, *ECST,* European Carotid Surgery trial; *VA,* Veterans Administration cooperative trial on symptomatic carotid stenosis.

Table 29-16. Prognosis of symptomatic carotid artery disease

Author and year	Patients (no.)	Mean follow-up (yr)	TIA (%)	Stroke (%/yr)
BRUIT				
Kagan, 1976[72]	124	4	?	1
Kartchner, 1977[74]	1130	2	1.5	1.5
Thompson, 1978[125]	138	4	6.5	4.5
Heyman, 1980[64]	72	6	?	2.3
Dorazio, 1980[32]	97	7	1.6	2.7
Wolf, 1981[137]	171	4	1	3
Busuttil, 1981[22]	58	2.5	8.2	2.1
STENOSIS				
Kartchner, 1977[74]	143	2	2.5	6.0
Moll, 1979[90]	29	2	0	0
Barnes, 1981[12]	19	1	8	2.5 (1.9%)
Busuttil, 1981[22]	45	2.5	11.6	3.0
Humphries, 1976[67]	168	2.6	15	2
Johnson, 1978[71]	22	2	9	0
Levin, 1980[78]	147	0 to 20	12	1 (0%)
Podore, 1980[104]	28	5	14	7
Durwood, 1982[34]	67	4	13	3
ULCERATION				
Type A (small single ulceration)				
Kroener, 1980[75]	63	3		1
Dixon, 1982[31]	72	4		0.9
Type B (larger ulcers)				
Kroener, 1980[75]	24	3		0
Dixon, 1982[31]	54	4		4.5
Type C (compound ulcers)				
Dixon, 1982[31]	27	4		7.5

Table 29-17. Risk of carotid endarterectomy in asymptomatic patients

Author and year	Operations (no.)	Operative mortality rate (%)	Perioperative stroke rate (%)
Young, 1969[139]	33	3	0
Javid, 1971[20]	56	4	2
DeWeese, 1973[30]	50	0	4
Kanaly, 1977[73]	21	0	0
Easton, 1977[35]	11	0	18
Thompson, 1978[123]	167	0	1
Hertzer, 1978	95	1.1	4.2
Moore, 1979[91]	78	0	3
Whitney, 1980	279	1.1	2.2
Crowell, 1981[28]	30	0	0
White, 1981[135]	44	0	0
Assidao, 1982[5]	13	0	15
Burke, 1982[21]	70	3	1
Modi, 1983[89]	74	3	3
Bernstein, 1983[14]	87	0	3
Towne, 1990	211	1.9	2.4
Anderson, 1991	120	0	0
Fleischlag, 1992[50]	141	0	2

Table 29-18. Late results of carotid endarterectomy for asymptomatic disease

Author and year	Operations (no.)	Mean follow-up (yr)	Stroke (%)	Death (%)
Javid, 1971[70]	49	3	4	31
Lefrak, 1974[76]	34	5	3	44
Kanaly, 1977[73]	9	2	0	36
Thompson, 1978[123]	132	4.5	5	33
Moore, 1979[91]	72	6	1	42
Jausseran, 1979[69]	47	2.5	4	4
Thevenet, 1979[120]	92	4.5	4	18
Burke, 1982[21]	57	3.5	2	26
Bernstein, 1983[14]	87	3.8	3	25
Fleischlag, 1992[50]	141	4.7	0	32

and institutional experience and on the guidelines detailed previously.

In summary, the three alternative therapeutic modalities for threatened stroke include anticoagulation therapy, aspirin, and carotid artery surgery.[37,108] Each appears to have its own specific role and indication. Good-risk patients who have a TIA with appropriate carotid artery lesions should undergo angiography and surgery. Poor-risk patients or those who refuse surgery should be considered candidates for anticoagulation therapy, particularly in the period of time during an acute progressing stroke or in the first few months after a TIA. Antiplatelet aggregation therapy remains the mainstay for other patients who are not candidates for surgery, although data justifying its widespread use for the suppression of strokes are not statistically significant or convincing.

CONCLUSION

Ischemic stroke is a major life-threatening and disabling event. Recent information implicates atherosclerotic disease of the aortic arch and carotid arteries as a major source of atheroembolic and flow-inhibiting factors that are the most important pathogenic mechanisms for stroke. An appropriate workup must include efforts to detect systemic, hematologic, neurologic, and cardiogenic causes of such episodes, particularly when the patient has significant residual independent neurologic capability. Identification of a specific clinical entity should permit the design of treatment plan to minimize future neurologic destructive episodes. For the patient with atherosclerotic carotid bifurcation disease a management plan that includes complete cerebrovascular angiography and that selects appropriate patients for surgery seems to provide the greatest potential for minimizing future risk of stroke.

REFERENCES

1. ACAS (Asymptomatic Carotid Artery Stenosis Study): A prospective multicenter review of morbidity/mortality in carotid endarterectomy (abstract), *Stroke* 17:146, 1986.
2. Acheson J, Hutchinson EC: Observations of the natural history of transient cerebral ischemia, *Lancet* 2:871, 1964.

3. Allen GS, Preziosi TJ: Carotid endarterectomy: a prospective study of its efficacy and safety, *Medicine* 60:298, 1981.
4. Anderson RJ et al: Carotid endarterectomy for asymptomatic carotid stenosis: a ten year experience with 120 procedures in a fellowship training program, *Ann Vasc Surg* 5(2):111-5, 1991.
5. Asiddao CB et al: Factors associated with perioperative complications during carotid endarterectomy, *Anesth Analg* 61:631, 1982.
6. Baker JD et al: Suggested standards for reports dealing with cerebrovascular disease, *J Vasc Surg* 8:721-9, 1988.
7. Baker RN: An evaluation of anticoagulant therapy in the treatment of cerebrovascular disease: report of the Veterans Administration cooperative study of atherosclerosis, *Neurology* 11:132, 1961.
8. Baker RN, Ramseyer JC, Schwartz W: Prognosis in patients with transient cerebral attacks, *Neurology* 18:1157, 1968.
9. Baker RN, Schwartz W, Rose AS: Transient ischemic attacks—a report of a study of anticoagulant treatment, *Neurology* 16:841, 1966.
10. Baker RN et al: Anticoagulant therapy in cerebral infarction, *Neurology* 12:823, 1962.
11. Bardin JA et al: Is carotid endarterectomy beneficial in prevention of recurrent stroke? *Arch Surg* 117:1401, 1982.
12. Barnes RW et al: Natural history of symptomatic carotid disease in patients undergoing cardiovascular surgery, *Surgery* 90:1075, 1981.
13. Barnett HJM: The pathophysiology of transient cerebral ischemic attacks, *Med Clin North Am* 63:649, 1979.
14. Bernstein EF et al: Life expectancy and late stroke following carotid endarterectomy, *Ann Surg* 198:80, 1982.
15. Bernstein EF, Browse NL: The CHAT classification of stroke, *Ann Surg* 209:242-8, 1989.
16. Bernstein EF et al: CHAT analysis of the influence of specific risk factors on late results after carotid endarterectomy, *J Vasc Surg* 16:575-587, 1992.
17. Bouchier-Hayes D, DeCosta A, MacGowan WAL: The morbidity of carotid endarterectomy, *Br J Surg* 66:433, 1979.
18. Bousser MG et al: "AICLA" controlled trial of aspirin and dipyridamole in the secondary prevention of athero-thrombotic cerebral ischemia, *Stroke* 14:5, 1983.
19. Brewster DC et al: Rational management of the asymptomatic carotid bruit, *Arch Surg* 113:927, 1978.
20. Buren A, Ygge J: Treatment program and comparison between anticoagulants and platelet aggregation inhibitors after transient ischemic attack, *Stroke* 12:578, 1981.
21. Burke PA et al: Prophylactic carotid endarterectomy for asymptomatic bruit: a look at cardiac risk, *Arch Surg* 117:1222, 1982.
22. Busuttil RW et al: Carotid artery stenosis—hemodynamic significance and clinical course, *JAMA* 245:1438, 1981.
23. Canadian Cooperative Study Group: A randomized trial of aspirin and sulfinpyrazone in threatened stroke, *N Engl J Med* 299:53, 1978.
24. Carter AB: Anticoagulant treatment in progressing stroke, *Br Med J* 2:70, 1961.
25. Chung WB: Long-term results of carotid artery surgery for cerebrovascular insufficiency, *Am J Surg* 128:262, 1974.
26. Cooperman M, Martin EW, Evans WE: Significance of asymptomatic carotid bruits, *Arch Surg* 113:1339, 1978.
27. Cornell WP: Carotid endarterectomy: results in 100 patients, *Ann Thorac Surg* 25:121, 1978.
28. Crowell RM, Ojemann RG: Carotid endarterectomy. In Hoff JT, editor: *Practice of surgery,* Hagerstown, Md, 1981, Harper & Row.
29. Crowell RM et al: Carotid endarterectomy in high risk patients with cardiopulmonary disease (abstract), *Stroke* 12:123, 1981.
30. DeWeese JA et al: Results of carotid endarterectomy for transient ischemic attacks five years later, *Ann Surg* 178:258, 1973.
31. Dixon S et al: Natural history of nonstenotic asymptomatic ulcerative lesions of the carotid artery, *Arch Surg* 117:1493, 1982.
32. Dorazio RA, Ezzet F, Nesbit NJ: Long-term follow-up of asymptomatic carotid bruits, *Am J Surg* 140:212, 1980.
33. Duke LJ et al: Carotid arterial reconstruction: ten-year experience, *Am Surg* 45:281, 1979.
34. Durwood QJ, Ferguson GG, Barr HWK: The natural history of asymptomatic carotid bifurcation plaques, *Stroke* 13:459, 1982.
35. Easton JD, Sherman DG: Stroke and mortality rate in carotid endarterectomy: 228 consecutive operations, *Stroke* 8:565, 1977.
36. Easton JD, Sherman DG: Management of cerebral embolism of cardiac origin, *Stroke* 11:433, 1980.
37. Easton JD et al: Diagnosis and management of ischemic stroke. I. Threatened stroke and its management, *Curr Probl Cardiol* 8:1, 1983.
38. Eisenberg RL et al: Relationship of transient ischemic attacks and angiographically demonstrable lesions of carotid artery, *Stroke* 8:483, 1977.
39. Enger E, Boyesen S: Long-term anticoagulant therapy in patients with cerebral infarction: a controlled clinical study, *Acta Scand* 178(suppl 438):1, 1965.
40. Ennix CL et al: Improved results of carotid endarterectomy in patients with symptomatic coronary disease: an analysis of 1,546 consecutive carotid operations, *Stroke* 10:122, 1979.
41. Ericsson BF, Takolander RJ: Operative treatment of carotid artery stenosis, *Lakartidningen* 77:893, 1980.
42. European Carotid Surgery Trialists' Collaborative Group. MRC European Carotid Surgery Trial: Interim results for symptomatic patients with severe (70-99%) or with mild (0-29%) carotid stenosis, *Lancet* 337:1235-1243, 1991.
43. Faught E, Trader SD, Hanna GR: Cerebral complications of angiography for transient ischemia and stroke: prediction of risk, *Neurology* 29:4, 1979.
44. Fazekas JF, Alman RW, Sullivan JF: Management of patients with vertebral-basilar insufficiency, *Arch Neurol* 8:215, 1963.
45. Fields WS et al: Joint study of extracranial artery occlusion. V. Progress report of prognosis following surgery or non-surgical treatment for transient ischemic attacks and cervical artery lesions, *JAMA* 211:1993, 1970.
46. Fields WS et al: Controlled trial of aspirin in cerebral ischemia. II. Surgical results, *Stroke* 9:308, 1978.
47. Fields WS et al: Controlled trial of aspirin in cerebral ischemia, *Stroke* 8:301, 1977.
48. Fisher CM: Use of anticoagulants in cerebral thrombosis, *Neurology* 8:311, 1958.
49. Fisher CM: Anticoagulant therapy in cerebral thrombosis and cerebral embolism: a national cooperative study, interim report, *Neurology* 11:119, 1961.
50. Freischlag JA, Hanna D, Moore WS: Improved prognosis for asymptomatic carotid stenosis with prophylactic carotid endarterectomy, *Stroke* 23:479-82, 1992.
51. Friedman GD et al: Transient ischemic attacks in a community, *JAMA* 210:1428, 1969.
52. Gallhofer B, Ladurner G, Lechner H: Prognosis of prophylactic anticoagulant treatment in ischemic stroke, *Eur Neurol* 18:145, 1979.
53. Genton E et al: Report of the Joint Committee for Stroke Facilities. XIV. Cerebral ischemia: the role of thrombosis and antithrombotic therapy, *Stroke* 8:150, 1977.
54. Goldner JC, Whisnant JP, Taylor WF: Long-term prognosis of transient cerebral ischemic attacks, *Stroke* 2:160, 1971.
55. Goldstone J, Moore WS: A new look at emergency carotid artery operations for the treatment of cerebrovascular insufficiency, *Stroke* 9:599, 1978.
56. Grotta J, Fields WS, Kwee K: Prognosis in patients with asymptomatic carotid bruits due to nonstenotic lesions (abstract), *Ann Neurol* 12:85, 1982.
57. Harrison MJG, Marshall J: Angiographic appearance of carotid bifurcation in patients with completed stroke transient ischemic attacks, and cerebral tumor, *Br Med J* 1:205, 1976.
58. Harrison MJB, Marshall J: Prognostic significance of severity of carotid atheroma in early manifestations of cerebrovascular disease, *Stroke* 13:567, 1982.
59. Hart RG et al: Diagnosis and management of ischemic stroke. II. Selected controversies, *Curr Probl Cardiol* 8:1, 1983.
60. Harward TRS et al: Natural history of asymptomatic ulcerative placques of the carotid bifurcation, *Am J Surg* 146:209, 1983.
61. Haynes CD, Dempsey RL: Carotid endarterectomy: review of 276 cases in a community hospital, *Ann Surg* 189:758, 1979.
62. Hertzer NR et al: Internal carotid back pressures, intraoperative shunting, ulcerated atheromata, and the incidence of stroke during carotid endarterectomy, *Surgery* 83:306-312, 1978.
63. Hertzer NR, Lees CD: Fatal myocardial infarction following carotid endarterectomy, *Ann Surg* 194:212, 1981.

64. Heyman A et al: Risk of stroke in asymptomatic persons with cervical arterial bruits: a population study in Evans County, Georgia, *N Engl J Med* 302:838, 1980.

65. Hill AB, Marshall J, Shaw DA: Cerebrovascular disease: trial of long-term anticoagulant therapy, *Br Med J* 2:1003, 1962.

66. Hobson RW et al: Role of carotid endarterectomy in asymptomatic carotid stenosis: a Veterans Administration Cooperative Study, *Stroke* 17:534-539, 1986.

67. Humphries AW et al: Unoperated asymptomatic significant carotid artery stenosis: a review of 182 instances, *Surgery* 80:695, 1976.

68. Hye RJ, Dilley RB, Browse NL, Bernstein EF: Evaluation of a new classification of cerebrovascular disease (CHAT), *Am J Surg* 154:104-110, 1987.

69. Jausseran JM et al: *Justification des indications chirurgicales dans les arteriopathies cerebrales extracraniennes asymptomatiques.* In Courbier R, ed: *Arteriopathies cerebrales extracraniennes asymptomatiques,* Lyons, France, 1979, Documentation Medicale Oberval.

70. Javid H et al: Carotid endarterectomy for asymptomatic patients, *Arch Surg* 102:389, 1971.

71. Johnson N et al: Carotid endarterectomy: a follow up study of the contralateral nonoperated carotid artery, *Ann Surg* 188:748, 1978.

72. Kagan A et al: *Epidemiologic studies on coronary artery disease and stroke in Japanese men living in Japan, Hawaii, and California.* In Scheinberg P, ed: *Cerebrovascular disease,* New York, 1976, Raven Press.

73. Kanaly PJ et al: The asymptomatic bruit, *Am J Surg* 134:821, 1977.

74. Kartchner M, McRae LP: Non-invasive evaluation and management of the "asymptomatic carotid bruit," *Surgery* 82:840, 1977.

75. Kroener JM et al: Prognosis of asymptomatic ulcerating carotid lesions, *Arch Surg* 115:1387, 1980.

76. Lefrak EA, Guinn GA: Prophylactic carotid artery surgery in patients requiring a second operation, *South Med J* 67:185, 1974.

77. Lemak NA, Field WS: The reliability of clinical predictors of extracranial artery disease, *Stroke* 4:377, 1976.

78. Levin SM, Sondheimer FK, Levin JM: The contralateral diseased but asymptomatic carotid artery: to operate or not? *Am J Surg* 140:203, 1980.

79. Link H et al: Prognosis in patients with infarction and TIA in carotid territory during and after anticoagulant therapy, *Stroke* 10:529, 1979.

80. Loeb C, Priano A, Albano C: Clinical features and long-term follow-up of patients with reversible ischemic attacks (RIA), *Acta Neurol Scand* 57:471, 1978.

81. Manelfe C et al: Investigation of extracranial cerebral arteries by intravenous angiography: report of 1,000 cases, *Am J Neuroradiol* 3:287, 1982.

82. Mani RL, Eisenberg RL: Complications of catheter cerebral arteriography: analysis of 5,000 procedures. II. Relation of complication rates to clinical and arteriographic diagnoses, *AJR* 131:867, 1978.

83. Marshall J: *Treatment of completed stroke.* In Millikan CH, Siekert RG, Whisnant JP, eds: *Cerebral vascular diseases: Fourth Princeton Conference,* New York, 1965, Grune & Stratton.

84. Marti-Vilalta JL et al: Transient ischemic attacks: retrospective study of 150 cases of ischemic infarct in the territory of the middle cerebral artery, *Stroke* 10:259, 1979.

85. McDevitt E et al: Use of anticoagulants in treatment of cerebral vascular disease, *JAMA* 166:592, 1958.

86. McDowell F, McDevitt E: *Treatment of the completed stroke with long-term cerebral vascular diseases.* In Millikan CH, Siekert RG, Whisnant JP, eds: *Cerebral vascular diseases: Fourth Princeton Conference,* New York, 1964, Grune & Stratton.

87. McNamara JO et al: The value of carotid endarterectomy in treating transient cerebral ischemia of the posterior circulation, *Neurology* 27:682, 1977.

88. Millikan CH: *Anticoagulant therapy in cerebrovascular disease.* In Millikan CH, Siekert RH, Whisnant JP, eds: *Cerebral vascular diseases,* New York, 1961, Grune & Stratton.

89. Modi JR, Finch WT, Sumner DS: Update of carotid endarterectomy in two community hospitals: Springfield revisited (abstract), *Stroke* 14:128, 1983.

90. Moll FL, Eikelboom BC, Vermeulen FEE: *The value of OPG-Gee in a prospective follow-up study of patients with asymptomatic carotid bruits.* In Courbier R, ed: *Arteriopathies cerebrales extracraniennes asymptomatiques,* Lyons, France, 1979, Documentation Medicale Oberval.

91. Moore WS et al: Asymptomatic carotid stenosis: immediate and long-term results after prophylactic endarterectomy, *Am J Surg* 138:228, 1979.

92. Moore WS et al: Natural history of non-stenotic, asymptomatic ulcerative lesions of the carotid artery, *Arch Surg* 113:1352, 1978.

93. Muuronen A, Kaste M: Outcome of 314 patients with transient ischemic attacks, *Stroke* 13:24, 1982.

94. NASCET Collaborators: Beneficial effect of carotid endarterectomy in symptomatic patients with high-grade carotid stenosis, *N Engl J Med* 325:445-53, 1991.

95. Nunn DB: Carotid endarterectomy: analysis of 234 operative cases, *Ann Surg* 182:733, 1975.

96. Olsson JE, Mulle R, Berneli S: Long-term anticoagulant therapy for TIAs and minor stroke with minimum residuum, *Stroke* 7:444, 1976.

97. Olsson JE et al: Anticoagulant vs. antiplatelet therapy as prophylactic against cerebral infarction in transient ischemic attacks, *Stroke* 11:4, 1980.

98. Ortega G et al: Postendarterectomy carotid occlusion, *Surgery* 90:1093, 1981.

99. Patterson RH: Risk of carotid surgery with occlusion of the contralateral carotid artery, *Arch Neurol* 30:188, 1974.

100. Pessin MS et al: Clinical and angiographic features of carotid transient ischemic attacks, *N Engl J Med* 296:358, 1977.

101. Pfaffenbach DD, Hollenhorst RW: Morbidity and survivorship of patients with embolic cholesterol crystals in the ocular fundus, *Am J Ophthalmol* 75:66, 1973.

102. Pierce JMS, Gubbay SS, Walton JM: Long-term anticoagulant therapy in transient cerebral attacks, *Lancet* 1:6, 1965.

103. Pinkerton JA, Gholkar V: Carotid endarterectomy: 100 consecutive operations, *Mo Med* 76:585, 1979.
104. Podore PC et al: Asymptomatic contralateral carotid artery stenosis: a five-year follow-up study following carotid endarterectomy, *Surgery* 88:748, 1980.
105. Prioleau WH, Aiken AF, Hairston P: Carotid endarterectomy: neurologic complications as related to surgical techniques, *Ann Surg* 185:678, 1977.
106. Ramirez-Lassepas M, Sandok BA, Burton RC: Clinical indicators of extracranial carotid artery disease in patients with transient symptoms, *Stroke* 4:537, 1973.
107. Riles TS, Lopelman I, Imparato AM: Myocardial infarction following carotid endarterectomy: a review of 683 operations, *Surgery* 85:249, 1979.
108. Roden S et al: Transient cerebral ischemic attacks—management and prognosis, *Postgrad Med J* 57:275, 1981.
109. Ropper AH, Wechsler R, Wilson LS: Carotid bruit and the risk of stroke in elective surgery, *N Engl J Med* 307:1388, 1982.
110. Russo LS: Carotid system transient ischemic attacks: clinical, racial and angiographic correlations, *Stroke* 12:470, 1981.
111. Sandok BA et al: Guidelines for the management of transient ischemic attacks, *Mayo Clin Proc* 53:665, 1978.
112. Schechter DC, Acinapura AJ: Panoperative safeguards for carotid endarterectomy, *NY State J Med* 79:54, 1979.
113. Siekert RG, Whisnant JP, Millikan CH: Surgical and anticoagulant therapy of occlusive cerebral vascular disease, *Ann Intern Med* 48:637, 1963.
114. Sorenson PS et al: Acetylsalicylic acid in the prevention of stroke in patients with reversible cerebral ischemic attacks: a Danish cooperative study, *Stroke* 14:15, 1983.
115. Stanford JR, Lubow M, Vasko JS: Prevention of stroke by carotid endarterectomy, *Surgery* 83:259, 1978.
116. Sundt TM, Sandok BA, Whisnant JP: Carotid endarterectomy: complications and preoperative assessment of risk, *Mayo Clin Proc* 50:301, 1975.
117. Swanson PD et al: A cooperative study of hospital frequency and character of transient ischemic attacks. II. Performance of angiography among six centers, *JAMA* 237:2002, 1977.
118. Taylor GW et al: *Doppler detection of carotid disease in patients with peripheral vascular disease.* In Courbier R, ed: *Arteriopathies cerebrales extracraniennes asymptomatiques,* Lyons, France, 1979, Documentation Medicale Oberval.
119. Terent A, Andersson B: The outcome of patients with transient ischemic attacks and stroke treated with anticoagulants, *Acta Med Scand* 208:359, 1980.
120. Thevenet A: *Resultats a longue terme de l'endarterectomie carotidienne pour stenose asymptomatique.* In Courbier R, ed: *Arteriopathies cerebrales extracraniennes asymptomatiques,* Lyons, France, 1979, Documentation Medicale Oberval.
121. Thiele BL et al: Correlation of arteriographic findings and symptoms in cerebrovascular disease, *Neurology* 30:1041, 1980.
122. Thompson JE, Austin DJ, Patman RD: Carotid endarterectomy for cerebrovascular insufficiency: long-term results in 592 patients followed up to 13 years, *Ann Surg* 172:663, 1970.
123. Thompson JE, Patman RD, Talkington CM: Asymptomatic carotid bruit: long-term outcome of patients having endarterectomy compared with unoperated controls, *Ann Surg* 188:308, 1978.
124. Thompson JE, Talkington CM: Carotid endarterectomy, *Ann Surg* 184:1, 1976.
125. Toole JF et al: Transient ischemic attacks due to atherosclerosis: a prospective study of 160 patients, *Arch Neurol* 32:5, 1975.
126. Toole JF et al: Transient ischemic attacks: a prospective study of 225 patients, *Neurology* 28:746, 1978.
127. Towne JB, Weiss DG, Hobson RW: First phase report of Veterans Administration asymptomatic carotid stenosis study—operative morbidity and mortality, *J Vasc Surg* 11:252-9, 1990.
128. Turnipseed WD, Berkoff HA, Belzer FO: Postoperative stroke in cardiac and peripheral vascular disease, *Ann Surg* 192:365, 1980.
129. Ueda K, Toole JF, McHenry LC: Carotid and vertebrobasilar transient ischemic attacks: clinical and angiographic correlation, *Neurology* 29:1094, 1979.
130. VA Symptomatic Carotid Stenosis Group: Carotid endarterectomy and prevention of cerebral ischemia in symptomatic carotid stenosis, *JAMA* 266:3289-3294, 1991.
131. van Oudenaarden WF, Tans JTJ, Hoogland PH: Angiographical findings and risk factors in cerebral ischemia, *Eur Neurol* 19:376, 1980.
132. Whisnant JP, Matsumoto N, Elveback LR: Transient cerebral ischemic attacks in a community, *Mayo Clin Proc* 48:194, 1973.
133. Whisnant JP, Matsumoto N, Elveback LR: The effect of anticoagulant therapy on the prognosis of patients with transient cerebral ischemic attacks in a community, *Mayo Clin Proc* 48:844, 1973.
134. Whisnant JP, Sandok BA, Sundt TM: Endarterectomy for transient cerebral ischemia: long-term survival and stroke probability (abstract), *Stroke* 13:113, 1982.
135. White JS et al: Morbidity and mortality of carotid endarterectomy: rates of occurrence in asymptomatic and symptomatic patients, *Arch Surg* 116:409, 1981.
136. Whitney DG, Kahn EM, Estes JW, Jones CE: Carotid artery surgery without a temporary indwelling shunt, *Arch Surg* 115:1393-1399, 1980.
137. Wolf PA et al: Asymptomatic carotid bruit and risk of stroke: the Framingham Study, *JAMA* 245:1441, 1981.
138. Wylie EJ, Ehrenfeld WK: *Extracranial occlusive cerebrovascular disease: diagnosis and treatment,* Philadelphia, 1970, WB Saunders.
139. Young JR et al: Carotid endarterectomy without a shunt, *Arch Surg* 99:293, 1969.
140. Ziegler DK, Hassanein R: Prognosis in patients with transient ischemic attacks, *Stroke* 4:666, 1973.

CHAPTER 30

Distribution of intracranial and extracranial arterial lesions in patients with symptomatic cerebrovascular disease

BRIAN L. THIELE and D. EUGENE STRANDNESS, Jr.

In any evaluation of the accuracy of noninvasive methods used to identify extracranial vascular disease, arteriography remains the standard against which these techniques are compared. The current study was conducted to determine the frequency, distribution, and types of lesions in a group of patients with symptomatic cerebral ischemia. These arteriograms were reviewed not only to determine the frequency of hemodynamically significant lesions at the carotid bifurcation but also to perform a more detailed examination of the location of identifiable atherosclerotic disease in the intracranial and extracranial vessels, with particular reference to the presence of potential embolic sources. Although the distribution of atherosclerotic disease in patients with cerebral ischemia was addressed by a national cooperative study,[3] a correlation between arteriographic findings and symptoms was not possible, and no data were presented regarding the morphology of the arteriographic lesions.

Lesion morphology has become increasingly important with the recognition that embolization from the carotid bifurcation may be responsible for symptoms of cerebral and retinal ischemia in a higher proportion of patients than was previously envisaged.[6] Not only have potentially embolic lesions received greater attention in patients with symptomatic cerebrovascular disease, but Moore et al[8] have presented evidence to suggest that the presence of ulcerated lesions is a significant factor in predicting which asymptomatic lesions will subsequently become symptomatic.

The widespread use of the indirect, noninvasive methods designed to detect hemodynamically significant lesions has focused attention on the role of such lesions in producing transient or permanent neurologic deficits. Since the relative roles of potentially embolic and hemodynamically significant lesions in the pathogenesis of cerebral ischemia can only be determined by prospective studies, this evaluation represents an attempt to assess the relative importance of these two processes in producing symptoms.

The frequency of tandem lesions or abnormalities of the intracerebral collateral circulation in the various patient groups was also examined. Although the role of the collateral circulation and tandem disease is well recognized in

limb ischemia, the importance of these abnormalities in the pathogenesis of cerebral ischemia remains to be documented. Evidence for the importance of isolated siphon lesions in producing symptoms of transient cerebral ischemia is accumulating from the published reports of the relief of such symptoms in patients who have undergone extracranial-intracranial bypass. In addition, observations of the frequency of deficiencies of the circle of Willis made from autopsy examinations have also served as a basis for speculation on the importance of this anomaly in contributing to cerebral ischemia.

METHODS OF STUDY

All patients with symptoms that suggested cerebral ischemia underwent arteriographic study of the extracranial and intracranial vasculature via the percutaneous Seldinger technique. Initially, views were obtained of the arch and origins of the extracranial arteries; then selective catheterization of the carotid arteries was performed, and biplane views of the cervical carotid and intracranial vessels were obtained. Injection was also performed at the arch level with lateral head films to visualize the anterior and posterior intracranial circulation. The radiographs were independently examined by two radiologists, who reported stenoses in one of five grades. Grade I represented a normal carotid bifurcation, grade II represented stenoses with less than 10% diameter reduction, grade III represented stenoses of 10% to 49% diameter reduction, grade IV represented stenoses of 50% to 99% reduction, and grade V represented complete occlusion. The radiologists were also asked to comment on the presence or absence of irregularity, ulceration, and specifically smoothness of plaques. This evaluation was performed for all areas of both the extracranial and intracranial vessels. The presence of the anterior and posterior communicating arteries was also determined from the anteroposterior and lateral head studies. On the basis of these reports, lesions were classified as occlusions, hemodynamically significant lesions (greater than 50% diameter reduction), or potentially embolic lesions (irregular or ulcerated).

Only patients who had well-documented classic symp-

toms of transient or permanent cerebral ischemia were included in the study. According to this classification, four groups of patients were available for study: the first group had amaurosis fugax alone; the second group had hemispheric symptoms, with or without amaurosis fugax; the third group had vertebrobasilar symptoms; and the final group had fixed neurologic deficits. This last group consisted of patients whose neurologic deficits had initially exceeded 24 hours but subsequently resolved partially or completely before their studies. The time span between onset of symptoms and arteriography varied from 4 weeks to 1 year.

DISTRIBUTION OF SYMPTOMS

Included in the study were 109 patients with well-documented symptoms who underwent arteriography. The distribution of symptoms is shown in Table 30-1. A total of 9 patients initially had amaurosis fugax alone, and 19 patients had a combination of amaurosis fugax and hemispheric symptoms. By combining these two groups, 28 arteriograms of patients with amaurosis fugax were available for study. In addition, 47 patients had symptoms of transient hemispheric ischemia alone, and with the 19 patients in the preceding group, provided a total of 66 arteriograms for evaluation of the transient hemispheric symptoms. Also studied were 29 patients who had experienced fixed neurologic deficits and 5 patients with vertebrobasilar symptoms.

RESULTS
Amaurosis fugax

The arteriographic findings in the group of patients with amaurosis fugax are summarized in Table 30-2. In all cases the findings were those in the carotid bifurcation appropriate to the patient's symptoms. Of the 28 patients studied, only 2 (7% of the group) had no lesion demonstrated at the bifurcation. A total of 10 patients (36% of the group) had lesions that were considered potentially embolic but not associated with flow-reducing stenoses. Of the remaining 16 patients, 5 (18%) had smooth, hemodynamically significant lesions and 11 (39%) had a combination of hemodynamically significant and potentially embolic lesions. By combining the second and fourth groups, the number of potentially embolic lesions in this group of patients totaled 21 (75%), and by combining the third and fourth groups, 16 patients (57%) had hemodynamically significant stenoses. In view of the small number of negative arteriograms, it could be concluded that amaurosis fugax is a highly specific symptom for carotid bifurcation disease and that potentially embolic lesions are more common than hemodynamically significant lesions.

Hemispheric symptoms

The results obtained from the group of patients with hemispheric symptoms are listed in Table 30-3. There were 47 patients in the group, and in 6 (13%), no lesion was demonstrated at the bifurcation. A total of 19 patients (40%)

Table 30-1. Distribution of symptoms in 109 patients with symptomatic cerebrovascular disease

Symptoms	Patients (no.)
Amaurosis fugax only	9
Amaurosis fugax and hemispheric symptoms	19
Hemispheric symptoms only	47
Fixed neurologic deficits	29
Vertebrobasilar symptoms	5

Table 30-2. Distribution of angiographic lesions in 28 patients with amaurosis fugax

Type of lesion	Patients (no.)	Percentage
No lesion	2	7
Potentially embolic only	10	36
Hemodynamically significant*	16	57
Potentially embolic†	21	75

*Includes 5 smooth (18%) and 11 ulcerated or irregular (39%) hemodynamically significant lesions (50% or greater diameter reduction).
†Includes all ulcerated or irregular lesions regardless of degree of stenosis.

Table 30-3. Distribution of angiographic lesions in 47 patients with hemispheric symptoms

Type of lesion	Patients (no.)	Percentage
No lesion	6	13
Potentially embolic only	19	40
Hemodynamically significant*	22	47
Potentially embolic†	37	79

*Includes 4 smooth (9%) and 18 ulcerated or irregular (38%) hemodynamically significant lesions.
†Includes all ulcerated or irregular lesions regardless of degree of stenosis.

had potentially embolic lesions not associated with flow-reducing lesions, 4 patients (9%) had smooth stenoses that were considered hemodynamically significant, and the remaining 18 patients (38%) had stenoses of greater than 50% diameter reduction associated with irregularity or ulceration. In a form of analysis similar to that used for the preceding group, by combining the second and fourth groups, the number of patients with potentially embolic lesions totaled 37 (79% of the group), and by combining the third and fourth groups, the number of patients with hemodynamically significant lesions totaled 22 (47%). Thus hemispheric symptoms were not as specific for carotid bifurcation disease as amaurosis fugax was, but potentially embolic lesions occurred more frequently than hemodynamically significant ones.

Hemispheric symptoms and amaurosis fugax

The types and distribution of lesions in the group with hemispheric symptoms and amaurosis fugax are summarized in Table 30-4. Of the 66 patients with this symptom complex, 6 (9%) had no lesion visualized at the bifurcation, 27 (41%) had potentially embolic lesions only, 5 (8%) had smooth, hemodynamically significant lesions only, and 28 (42%) had a combination of hemodynamically significant and potentially embolic lesions. Further breakdown of this group revealed that 56 (85%) had potentially embolic lesions, and 33 (50%) had hemodynamically significant lesions of the appropriate carotid bifurcation.

Fixed neurologic deficits

Patients with fixed neurologic defects were characterized by diffuse atherosclerotic changes in both the intracranial and extracranial vessels (Table 30-5). A total of 8 patients (28%) had hemodynamically significant lesions only, and in 7 of these patients, complete occlusion of the appropriate internal carotid artery was present. In addition, 13 patients (45%) had ulcerated lesions associated with a stenosis of greater than 50% diameter reduction, and 5 patients (17%) had ulcerated or irregular lesions associated with minimal degrees of stenosis. The incidence of hemodynamically significant lesions was 72%, whereas that of potentially embolic lesions was 62%. A surprising finding was the relative infrequency of complete occlusions of the internal carotid artery (7 of 29 patients, or 24%). Compared with those patients who experienced transient ischemic symptoms, patients in the fixed neurologic deficit group had a higher proportion of hemodynamically significant lesions.

Vertebrobasilar symptoms

There were only 5 patients with vertebrobasilar symptoms, so no significant conclusions could be drawn from an analysis of the location and distribution of lesions. In addition, because of the nonlocalizing nature of their symptoms, it would be impossible to attach significance to a lesion in either carotid artery. Therefore these have been excluded from this analysis.

RELATIONSHIP BETWEEN ULCERATION AND STENOSIS

The results from the preceding study were then evaluated to determine whether ulcerated lesions were more commonly associated with hemodynamically significant lesions. Tables 30-6 and 30-7 detail the relative frequency of ulceration and its relationship to hemodynamically significant lesions. Of the 104 patients who underwent arteriograms, 56 (54%) were considered to have hemodynamically significant lesions on the appropriate side. Ulcerated lesions predominated in this group and were three times as common as smooth lesions (41% versus 13%). Table 30-7 details the frequency of ulcerated lesions in all the arteriograms with the degrees of stenosis divided into two groups, hemodynamically significant or insignificant. Potentially embolic lesions occurred in 74% of the patient population, but surprisingly, irregularity or ulceration occurred with almost equal frequency whether the degree of stenosis was considered hemodynamically significant or not (41% versus 33%). Thus although ulceration frequently accompanied hemodynamically significant lesions, it occurred with almost equal frequency regardless of the degree of stenosis.

Table 30-4. Distribution of angiographic lesions in 66 patients with both hemispheric symptoms and amaurosis fugax

Type of lesion	Patients (no.)	Percentage
No lesion	6	9
Potentially embolic only	27	41
Hemodynamically significant*	33	50
Potentially embolic†	55	84

*Includes 5 smooth (8%) and 28 ulcerated or irregular (42%) hemodynamically significant lesions.
†Includes all ulcerated or irregular lesions regardless of degree of stenosis.

Table 30-5. Distribution of angiographic lesions in 29 patients with fixed neurologic deficits

Type of lesion	Patients (no.)	Percentage
No lesion	0	
Potentially embolic only	5	17
Hemodynamically significant*	21	72
Potentially embolic†	18	62

*Includes 7 occlusions and 1 smooth and 13 ulcerated (45%) hemodynamically significant lesions.
†Includes all ulcerated or irregular lesions regardless of degree of stenosis.

Table 30-6. Relationship between ulceration and hemodynamically significant lesions

Type of lesion	Degree of stenosis	Percentage
Smooth lesions	>50% diameter reduction	13
Irregular lesions	>50% diameter reduction	41
ALL LESIONS	>50% diameter reduction	54

Table 30-7. Relationship between ulceration and degree of stenosis

Type of lesion	Degree of stenosis	Percentage
Irregular lesions	>50% stenosis	41
Irregular lesions	<50% stenosis	33
TOTAL POTENTIALLY EMBOLIC LESIONS		74

Finally, the frequency of smooth lesions as identified arteriographically was determined in the total patient population; these results are shown in Table 30-8. Only 18% of the patients had smooth lesions, and in this group, hemodynamically significant lesions were twice as common as nonhemodynamically significant lesions (13% versus 5%). The remaining 8% of the total patient sample had no lesions identified by arteriography.

INTRACEREBRAL VASCULAR ANOMALY OR DISEASE

In addition to the type and location of lesions in the extracranial vessels, the frequency of intracerebral atherosclerotic lesions and anomalies of the collateral circulation was also assessed. The prevalence of intracerebral disease or anomaly was determined in each of the patient groups, namely, patients with transient ischemia, patients with fixed neurologic deficits, and patients with vertebrobasilar symptoms (Table 30-9). In the 66 patients with hemispheric and/or ocular transient ischemia, 29% had intracerebral abnormalities, as evidenced by siphon disease or the absence of one or more communicating arteries. In contrast, in the 29 patients with fixed neurologic deficits, the same abnormality was found in 90% of the patient group. All 5 patients with vertebrobasilar symptoms had either anomalies of the intracerebral collateral circulation or evidence of siphon disease.

CONTRALATERAL DISEASE

A similar analysis of the location and type of lesions in the contralateral carotid bifurcation was performed to determine the frequency of hemodynamically significant lesions that could adversely affect the results of the indirect, noninvasive tests. The frequency of hemodynamically significant lesions in the ipsilateral external carotid artery was also determined because of the potential of these lesions to interfere with testing. Hemodynamically significant lesions were present in the contralateral internal carotid artery in 29% of the 104 patients studied (Table 30-10). Of these hemodynamically significant lesions in the internal carotid artery, 41% (12 patients) were complete internal carotid occlusions. A further 17% had hemodynamically significant lesions of the contralateral external carotid artery. Potentially embolic lesions occurred in 30% (31 patients). Approximately 15% (15) of the patients also had hemodynamically significant lesions of the ipsilateral external carotid artery. In 40 patients (39%) a hemodynamically significant lesion existed in one or more of the extracranial vessels that would function as collaterals for a lesion in the internal carotid artery.

DISCUSSION

Although the foregoing study was initiated as part of the assessment of the accuracy of noninvasive methods of detecting extracranial vascular disease, it also serves as a means of studying the detailed distribution and morphology of atherosclerosis in these vessels. These data can be used not only for this purpose but also to examine some additional questions. The first area addressed by these studies is the

appropriateness and potential accuracy of the indirect, noninvasive tests currently used in evaluation of extracranial vascular disease. In patients with well-documented symptoms the frequency of hemodynamically significant lesions was of interest, since many indirect methods are designed to detect only such stenoses. In half of the patients with transient hemispheric symptoms with or without ocular ischemia, hemodynamically significant lesions were found on the side appropriate for the symptoms. Thus if researchers disregarded all the factors that may influence the pressure and flow direction in the retina and periorbital vessels and also assumed that the noninvasive methods used were 100% accurate, only half of the patients with symptom-producing lesions could be identified. The hemodynamics of the ocular and periorbital vascular system are also influenced by flow-reducing lesions in the contralateral carotid system and the ipsilateral external carotid artery. In the patient population with localizing cerebral ischemia, one third (39%) had potential flow-reducing lesions in these sites. Since it is not possible to accurately predict the hemodynamic disturbances that occur as the result of lesions visualized arteriographically, these findings remind physicians of the diffuse dis-

Table 30-8. Distribution of smooth lesions in patients with symptomatic cerebrovascular disease

Type of lesion	Degree of stenosis	Percentage
Smooth lesions	>50% diameter reduction	13
Smooth lesions	<50% diameter reduction	5
TOTAL SMOOTH LESIONS		18

Table 30-9. Incidence of intracerebral disease or anomaly in patients with symptomatic cerebrovascular disease

Type of symptom	Percentage
Transient ischemia	29
Fixed neurologic deficits	90
Vertebrobasilar symptoms	100

Table 30-10. Incidence of contralateral disease of the carotid bifurcation in 104 patients with symptomatic cerebrovascular disease

Type of lesion	Percentage
Potentially embolic	30
Hemodynamically significant (internal carotid disease)*	29
Hemodynamically significant (external carotid disease)	17

*Occlusions of 12 patients were complete.

tribution of atherosclerosis in patients with cerebral ischemia and also question the validity of those tests in which distant changes are used to identify the location of proximal lesions. Thus although the indirect tests may indicate that there is an abnormality in the orbital circulation, the inference that it is a result of ipsilateral carotid disease will be valid if this is the only pathologic condition involved. An analogy to this situation can readily be drawn from the noninvasive assessment of lower limb ischemia in which reductions in ankle pressure are an extremely reliable guide to the presence of hemodynamic disturbance[2] but are inaccurate in predicting the location of the responsible lesion. On the basis of these findings, the lack of sensitivity and specificity of these indirect methods was not surprising.

The next question raised by these studies relates to the pathogenesis of cerebral ischemia and its relation to abnormalities in the intracranial circulation. The demonstration by Moore et al[8] of the importance of the overtly ulcerated lesion as a major predisposing factor for the development of cerebral ischemia is confirmed by these studies. Meaningful statistical analysis cannot be applied to these figures because of the number of variables involved, although some of the results do warrant an attempt at interpretation. If the frequency of potentially embolic lesions between the asymptomatic and symptomatic sides is compared (30% versus 75%), the difference strongly suggests that ulceration or irregularity is associated with the presence of symptoms. When a comparison of the frequency of smooth lesions and potentially embolic lesions on the symptomatic side was made, embolic lesions were four times as common as smooth lesions (74% versus 18%); this further reinforces the view that the pathogenesis of cerebral ischemia is strongly related to the presence of potentially embolic lesions of the carotid bifurcation. Attempts at statistical analysis of these results are hampered by the frequency of overlap of hemodynamically significant and ulcerated lesions and the influence that unknown variables may have. Nevertheless, this study suggests that the ulcerated lesion is of major significance in symptomatic cerebral ischemia.

The current treatment of asymptomatic carotid lesions may also be influenced by these arteriographic findings, since high-grade stenoses are generally thought to predispose to occlusion of the internal carotid artery and the production of fixed neurologic deficits. Of the 29 patients with fixed neurologic deficits in this study, only 7 had internal carotid occlusions. Although these patients did have a higher frequency of hemodynamically significant lesions than the group with transient ischemic symptoms, the major differ-

ence in the two groups was the presence of siphon disease or an abnormality of the collateral vessels in the circle of Willis. It is recognized that traumatic internal carotid occlusion can occur without the production of neurologic deficits, particularly in patients with adequate collateral circulation. Conversely, the development of neurologic deficits in such patients is thought to be related to a congenital absence of communicating vessels in the circle of Willis. It therefore seems reasonable to suggest that disease or abnormality of the intracerebral circulation plays a major role in determining which patients will have transient ischemic attacks and which patients will have fixed neurologic deficits with atherosclerosis. Thus a factor that should be evaluated in future studies of the natural history of cerebrovascular disease is the role of disease or anomalies of the intracerebral vessels. This is particularly important in view of one current approach to patients with asymptomatic lesions, in which the decision for surgical treatment is influenced almost solely by the angiographic demonstration of a high-grade stenosis.

Finally, the demonstration that only 24% of those patients with fixed neurologic deficits had complete occlusions of the appropriate internal carotid artery highlights the need for identification of the patients who still have patent internal carotid arteries that may subsequently be responsible for the development of recurrent symptoms. The observation that 76% of the patients with fixed neurologic deficits still have patent internal carotid arteries on the appropriate side may partly explain the mechanism of recurrent strokes.

SUMMARY

This detailed arteriographic study suggests that in patients with symptoms of cerebral ischemia, isolated disease of a single cervical carotid artery is unusual and that as in other areas of the body, the atherosclerotic process is usually diffuse by the time symptoms occur. This diffuse location of lesions limits the use of indirect test methods as a means of accurately identifying bifurcation disease. This study also provides presumptive evidence to support the view that the majority of symptoms of transient cerebral ischemia occur as a result of embolization from the carotid bifurcation.

In patients with fixed neurologic deficits, the demonstration of a high frequency of siphon lesions or abnormalities of the vessels in the circle of Willis suggests that the status of the intracranial collateral circulation may be a significant factor in the pathogenesis of fixed neurologic deficits associated with carotid bifurcation atherosclerosis.

ACKNOWLEDGMENT

We acknowledge the assistance of the following individuals: Dr. P.M. Chikos, Assistant Professor, Dr. J.D. Harley, Associate Professor, and Dr. J.H. Hirsch, Assistant Professor, of the Department of Radiology, University of Washington School of Medicine; and Dr. J.V. Young, Research Fellow, Department of Surgery, University of Washington School of Medicine. We also acknowledge the help of the Departments of Surgery and Radiology, Veterans Administration Medical Center and University Hospital, Seattle, Washington.

REFERENCES

1. Blackshear WM et al: A prospective evaluation of oculoplethysmography and carotid phonoangiography, *Surg Gynecol Obstet* 48:201, 1979.
2. Carter SA: Response of ankle systolic pressure to leg exercise in mild or questionable arterial disease, *N Engl J Med* 287:578, 1972.
3. Hass WK et al: A joint study of extracranial arterial occlusion. II. Arteriography, techniques, sites, and complications, *JAMA* 203:961, 1968.
4. Horenstein S et al: Arteriographic correlates of transient ischemic attacks, *Trans Am Neurol Assoc* 97:132, 1972.
5. Janeway R, Toole JF: Vascular anatomic status of patients with transient ischemic attacks, *Trans Am Neurol Assoc* 97:137, 1972.
6. Kollarits CR, Lobow M, Hissong SL: Retinal strokes. I. Incidence of carotid atheroma, *JAMA* 222:1273, 1972.
7. Millikan CH: The pathogenesis of transient cerebral ischemia, *Circulation* 32:438, 1965.
8. Moore WS et al: Natural history of nonstenotic asymptomatic ulcerative lesions of the carotid artery, *Arch Surg* 113:1357, 1978.
9. Pessin MS et al: Clinical and angiographic features of carotid transient ischemic attacks, *N Engl J Med* 296(7):358, 1977.

CHAPTER 31

Basic and practical aspects of cerebrovascular testing

R. EUGENE ZIERLER

The objective evaluation of the blood supply to the brain in a living patient was first reported in 1927 when Moniz described a technique for performing cerebral arteriography.[30] Despite this development, the carotid arterial system received relatively little clinical attention until 1968, when the Joint Study of Extracranial Arterial Occlusion reported that the most common site of stenosis in the cerebral circulation was the carotid bifurcation, particularly the origin of the internal carotid artery.[18] At the time of the joint study, cerebral arteriography was the only diagnostic method that could be used to classify the severity of carotid artery disease. However, due to its invasive nature, arteriography is not suitable for screening patients who are free of symptoms or for performing serial follow-up studies to determine the natural history of disease of the carotid bifurcation. In addition, arteriography is a strictly anatomic investigation that gives no information on the physiologic consequences of observed lesions.

Over the past two decades, problems associated with arteriography have prompted the development of a variety of noninvasive methods for the evaluation of cerebrovascular disease. Because the tests are noninvasive, they can be used to show both the extent of disease at an initial time and the subsequent changes that occur. The ideal noninvasive test could be used to distinguish normal from diseased arteries, classify the spectrum of disease, detect progression of disease, show the structural features of atherosclerotic plaque, and assess the potential of the collateral circulation to maintain cerebral blood flow. Although no single noninvasive test has all these capabilities, many of these goals can be achieved with currently available methods.[51]

INDIRECT TESTS

Noninvasive tests for extracranial carotid artery disease can be direct or indirect (box). Indirect tests rely on pressure or flow changes in the distal branches of the internal and external carotid arteries to indicate the presence of lesions at the carotid bifurcation.[2] Because pressure and flow are not significantly reduced in the carotid system until the diameter of the lumen is narrowed by 50% or more, indirect tests can detect only severely stenotic or occlusive lesions. Furthermore, the test results are either positive (a lesion is

present) or negative (no lesion is present). Therefore these tests cannot be used to distinguish normal from minimally diseased arteries or high-grade stenosis from occlusion, and thus grading of disease is not possible.

Periorbital Doppler examination

The first indirect test used in the clinical setting was periorbital Doppler examination.[45] Because the ophthalmic artery is the first intracranial branch of the internal carotid, occlusive disease at the level of the arch and bulb can be evaluated by detecting changes in blood flow patterns about the eye. The periorbital Doppler examination uses a directional, continuous wave Doppler system to detect flow in the branches of the ophthalmic artery that supply the ipsilateral forehead. Blood flow in the periorbital arteries is normally from the inside to the outside of the orbit. In the presence of a hemodynamically significant carotid lesion, the periorbital branches of the external carotid become an important source of collateral flow to the ipsilateral hemisphere of the brain. When this occurs, flow is reversed in the periorbital arteries, and the source of collateral flow to the hemisphere can be detected using a series of compression maneuvers.[4] The principal advantage of the periorbital

---

NONINVASIVE TESTS FOR EXTRACRANIAL CAROTID ARTERY DISEASE

Indirect tests

Periorbital Doppler examination
Oculoplethysmography
  Fluid filled
  Air filled (OPG-Gee)

Direct tests

Ultrasonic arteriography
B-mode imaging
Duplex scanning
  B-mode imaging
  Pulsed Doppler flow detection
  Spectral waveform analysis
  Color flow imaging

Doppler test is that it requires inexpensive equipment and is relatively simple to perform. Although abnormal results are a good indicator of a hemodynamically significant carotid lesion, in cases of stenoses of the common or external carotid artery and efficient collateral pathways, the results are often false-negative.[26] Thus this test is most reliable when the results are abnormal.

Oculoplethysmography

When a plaque that reduces distal pressure is present in the carotid system, flow through the collateral pathways should delay arrival of the ocular pulse and reduce ocular perfusion pressure. Kartchner et al[22] introduced an indirect test that is based on detecting the difference in pulse arrival times between the two eyes. Ocular pulsations were sensed through saline-filled tubes connected to plastic cups applied to the corneas. External carotid pulsations were detected by photoplethysmograph transducers clipped on each ear. Pulse waveforms from the eyes and ears could then be compared electronically, and any delay or distortion could be noted. Because of the extremely variable and inconsistent results reported with this type of oculoplethysmography, this method is now considered to be unsuitable for diagnostic purposes.[7,23]

The air-filled oculoplethysmographic system developed by Gee has been the most widely used.[16] This instrument measures ophthalmic artery pressure through suction cups, which are placed on the sclera. The ocular pulsations normally seen are temporarily obliterated by applying a negative pressure of 300 to 500 mm Hg to the cups. The pressure in the system is gradually decreased until the ocular pulsations reappear. Criteria for interpretation are based on the difference between the pressures in the two eyes and the relationship between pressures in the ophthalmic and brachial arteries.[11] Experience with ocular pneumoplethysmography has shown its accuracy in detecting carotid lesions that reduce the diameter of the carotid artery more than 65%. In addition, the rate of false-negative results is generally lower than that seen with the periorbital Doppler examination.[15]

DIRECT TESTS

With direct tests, carotid disease can be detected by examining the site of involvement. The goal is to detect and classify lesions of the extracranial arteries.[46] Direct tests include carotid phonoangiography, quantitative phonoangiography, and continuous wave Doppler scanning.[2] However, the techniques that use pulsed wave Doppler ultrasound and B-mode imaging have emerged as the most accurate and reliable for classification of carotid bifurcation disease.

Ultrasonic arteriography

The first pulsed wave Doppler imaging system was described in 1971.[32] This method, called *ultrasonic arteriography,* used a directional 5-MHz pulsed wave Doppler transducer mounted on a position-sensing arm. The transducer had six range gates that could be placed at various depths in tissue from which flow could be detected. When flow was detected, a spot corresponding to its location was stored on the oscilloscope screen. In this way, a two-dimensional flow image of the carotid bifurcation could be created by moving the Doppler transducer slowly over the neck.

Although it was hoped that ultrasonic arteriography would provide diagnostic information comparable to that obtained by contrast arteriography, the quality of the flow images was limited. The best use of such studies was for detection of the branches of the carotid bifurcation, which facilitated placement of the sample volume to acquire useful velocity signals. When the combination of flow imaging and spectral waveform analysis was used to classify the severity of stenosis of the internal carotid artery, the results agreed with those of contrast arteriography in about 85% of cases.[3] The main limitations of ultrasonic arteriography are that it provides no direct information on arterial wall anatomy and does not allow the examiner careful control of the incident angle of the pulsed Doppler beam.

B-mode imaging

The usefulness of visualizing the arterial wall with B-mode ultrasound has led to attempts to use imaging alone to classify the spectrum of carotid artery disease. It appears that B-mode imaging is accurate for assessing lesions of minimal to moderate severity but most accurate for high-grade stenoses or occlusions.[9] B-mode imaging has also been used to evaluate the surface and histologic features of carotid bifurcation lesions, with varying degrees of success.[20,36,38] Because the acoustic properties of noncalcified plaque, thrombus, and flowing blood are similar, it may be difficult to determine the size of the arterial lumen by using a B-mode image. In addition, calcified atherosclerotic plaques produce acoustic shadows that prevent complete visualization of the arterial wall. These limitations are largely overcome by combining B-mode imaging with flow-detection techniques, such as spectral waveform analysis and color flow imaging.

Duplex scanning

Duplex scanning enhanced the diagnostic capabilities of noninvasive testing by making it possible to obtain anatomic and physiologic information directly from sites of vascular disease (Fig. 31-1). This approach is based on the concept that arterial lesions produce disturbances in blood flow patterns that can be characterized by analyzing Doppler flow signals. In conventional duplex scanning, the B-mode image is used to place a pulsed wave Doppler sample volume within the artery of interest, and the local flow pattern is assessed by analyzing the spectral waveform. Although the B-mode image may be useful for detecting anatomic variants and thickening or calcification of the arterial wall, classification of the severity of arterial disease is based on the interpretation of pulsed wave Doppler spectral waveforms.

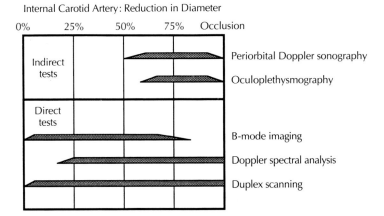

Internal Carotid Artery: Reduction in Diameter

Fig. 31-1. Range of internal carotid artery stenosis detected by the various indirect and direct noninvasive tests for extracranial carotid artery disease.

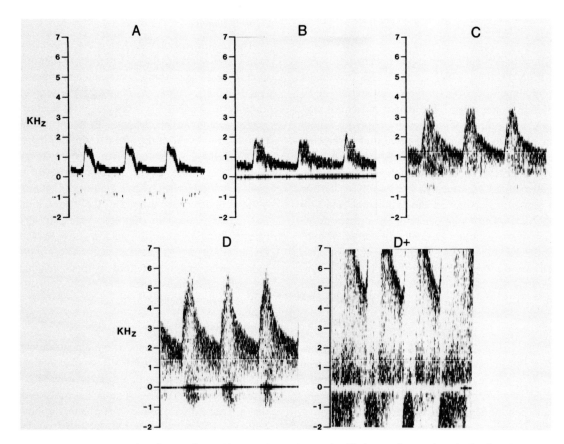

Fig. 31-2. Examples of internal carotid spectral waveforms classified according to the criteria given in Table 31-1. *A,* Normal; *B,* 1% to 15% diameter reduction; *C,* 16% to 49% diameter reduction; *D,* 50% to 79% diameter reduction; *D+,* 80% to 99% diameter reduction. (From Zierler RE, Strandness DE Jr: *Noninvasive dynamic and real-time assessment of extracranial cerebrovasculature.* In Wood JH, ed: *Cerebral blood flow: physiologic and clinical aspects,* New York, 1987, McGraw-Hill.).

Table 31-1. Criteria for classification of internal carotid artery disease by duplex scanning with spectral waveform analysis of pulsed Doppler signals

Arteriographic lesion		
Grade	Reduction in diameter (%)	Spectral criteria*
A	0	Peak systolic frequency <4 KHz, no spectral broadening
B	1-15	Peak systolic frequency <4 KHz, spectral broadening in deceleration phase of systole only
C	16-49	Peak systolic frequency <4 KHz, spectral broadening throughout systole
D	50-79	Peak systolic frequency ≥4 KHz, end-diastolic frequency <4.5 KHz
D+	80-99	End-diastolic frequency ≥4.5 KHz
E	100 (occlusion)	No internal carotid flow signal, flow to zero in common carotid artery

*Criteria are based on a pulsed Doppler with a 5-MHz transmitting frequency, a sample volume that is small relative to the internal carotid artery, and a 60% beam-to-vessel angle of insonation. Approximate angle-adjusted velocity equivalents are 4 KHz = 125 cm/sec and 4.5 KHz = 140 cm/sec.

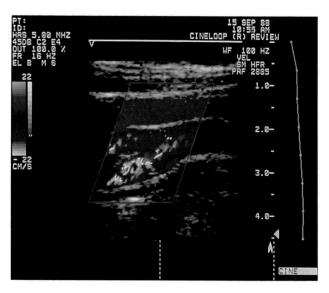

Fig. 31-3. Color flow image of a carotid bifurcation shows flow in the common, internal, and external carotid arteries. Arterial flow is represented primarily by shades of *red* and *yellow*. Flow in the adjacent internal jugular vein appears as *blue*.

The features of the spectral waveform used to classify arterial lesions include spectral broadening and peak systolic frequency. Spectral waveform criteria or velocity patterns for classification of the degree of stenosis of the internal carotid artery have been developed and validated by a series of comparisons with independently interpreted contrast arteriograms.[14,25,40] (An example of currently used criteria is given in Table 31-1 and illustrated in Figure 31-2.) These criteria distinguish between normal and diseased internal carotid arteries with a specificity of 84% and a sensitivity of 99%. The accuracy for detecting 50% to 99% reduction in diameter or occlusion is 93%.

Color flow imaging is an alternative method of displaying the Doppler information obtained during duplex scanning. The color flow image enables visualization of moving blood in the plane of the B-mode image (Fig. 31-3). As discussed in Chapter 34, color flow images can be extremely helpful for detecting vessels, particularly when the vessels are small, deeply located, or anatomically complex.[53] Changes in the color flow image may suggest the presence of turbulence associated with high-grade arterial lesions. However, because the color assignments typically represent mean rather than peak blood flow velocities, it is difficult to classify disease severity on the basis of color flow images alone. Therefore even when color flow imaging is used, spectral waveforms are still necessary for accurate classification.

Some degree of variability is unavoidable in any physiologic evaluation, such as duplex scanning or arteriography. In duplex scanning of the carotid artery, the greatest variability has been noted for the categories of normal, minimal, and moderate stenosis (designated as *A*, *B*, and *C* lesions

in Table 31-1). Agreement is much better for classification of lesions that reduce the diameter by at least 50%.[24] Interpretation of carotid arteriograms is subject to the same variability when the arteries are normal or disease is minimal.[8] In general, agreement between the results of duplex scanning and arteriography is equivalent to the agreement between two radiologists interpreting the same arteriograms.

CLINICAL APPLICATIONS

The primary role of noninvasive testing has been the selection of patients for arteriography and carotid endarterectomy. Considerations for patients who are free of symptoms differ from those for patients who have typical signs and symptoms of cerebral ischemia. Although the treatment of asymptomatic carotid disease remains controversial, detection of severe stenoses of the internal carotid artery has been emphasized. Ultrasound has been used to assess plaque composition and ulceration; however, the results have been variable, and the interpretation of B-mode images is highly subjective.[36-38,44]

Duplex scanning provides a safe and cost-effective alternative to arteriography for screening and follow-up examinations of patients with cerebrovascular lesions. One of the most common reasons for requesting a carotid duplex scan is for evaluation of a bruit in the neck. In 100 patients with 165 asymptomatic bruits, duplex scanning showed a normal internal carotid artery in 12 cases (7%), less than 50% reduction in diameter in 83 cases (50%), a 50% or greater reduction in 61 cases (37%), and occlusion in 9 cases (6%).[13] Thus although the majority of neck bruits are associated with some degree of carotid disease, relatively few are related to severe stenosis of the internal carotid arteries.

The chief concern in patients with asymptomatic carotid disease is the natural history of the lesions. Therapeutic decisions for these patients must take into account not only the severity of carotid disease but also the expected clinical outcome if no specific intervention is used. In a serial follow-up study of 167 patients with asymptomatic neck bruits, duplex scanning showed progression of disease in 60% of the internal carotid arteries.[42] The mean annual rate of progression to a greater than 50% reduction in diameter was 8%, and the mean annual rate for development of ipsilateral neurologic symptoms (transient ischemic attack or stroke) was 4%. A strong correlation was found between an 80% to 99% reduction in diameter of the internal carotid artery as shown by duplex scanning and the occurrence of neurologic symptoms or occlusion of the internal carotid artery. Patients with lesions of this severity had a 46% prevalence of one or more of these events, whereas those with less severe lesions had only a 1.5% prevalence. The mean interval between detection of an 80% to 99% reduction in diameter and an event was 4.9 months. This study[41] showed that the degree of stenosis as shown by duplex scanning could be used to predict clinical outcome in patients who were free of symptoms. In a separate study, further attempts were made to define risk in patients with high-grade carotid lesions.[29] This study indicated that stenoses with end-diastolic frequencies greater than 6.5 kHz were more likely to be associated with neurologic symptoms than those with lower end-diastolic frequencies; end-diastolic frequencies greater than 6.0 kHz correlated with an increased risk of occlusion of the internal carotid artery.

Inasmuch as the finding of an asymptomatic 80% to 99% reduction in diameter of the internal carotid artery appears to identify a group of patients who are at high risk for neurologic symptoms or occlusion of the internal carotid artery, the clinically important issue is whether this risk can be reduced by surgical or pharmacologic intervention. Although this question will ultimately be answered by randomized clinical trials, follow-up data are available on 129 patients with severe stenoses (80% to 99% reduction in diameter) of the internal carotid artery, of which 56 were treated by carotid endarterectomy and 73 were followed up without surgery.[28] No significant differences were found between the two groups for characteristics such as age, diabetes mellitus, hypertension, ischemic heart disease, and aspirin use. During 24 months of follow-up, neurologic symptoms and occlusion of the internal carotid artery were significantly more frequent in the patients who did not have surgery (48%) than in the patients who had endarterectomy (9%). Although the patients in this study were not assigned randomly to treatment groups, the results strongly suggest that endarterectomy improves the natural history of asymptomatic high-grade stenosis of the internal carotid artery, provided that the perioperative complication rate is extremely low. These studies suggest that in patients without

symptoms with less than 80% reduction in diameter of the internal carotid artery, it is safe to wait 6 months between follow-up examinations. If neurologic symptoms or progression to an 80% to 99% reduction in diameter occurs, carotid endarterectomy should be considered.

The purpose of screening patients with lateralizing neurologic symptoms is to detect lesions in the appropriate extracranial carotid system that could reduce hemispheric blood flow or be the source of cerebral emboli. Although it is generally accepted that moderate stenoses of the cartoid artery can be responsible for the signs and symptoms of cerebral ischemia, most patients with symptoms have severe stenoses. In the recently reported North American Symptomatic Carotid Endarterectomy Trial (NASCET), surgery was highly beneficial for patients with recent hemispheric transient ischemic attacks or mild strokes and 70% to 99% reduction in diameter of the ipsilateral internal carotid artery.[35] Because of the striking difference in favor of surgical treatment, it was recommended that patients with symptomatic 70% to 99% reductions in diameter be considered for endarterectomy. Virtually the same conclusions were reached by the European Carotid Surgery Trialists' Collaborative Group.[12]

On the basis of the results of these clinical trials, patients with symptoms of severe stenoses of the carotid artery should be treated by endarterectomy unless their medical condition makes the risk of surgery prohibitive. The management of patients with symptoms of moderate stenoses remains unsettled. If duplex scanning shows that the carotid artery is normal, other causes should be sought for the cerebral ischemia.[34,50]

A question frequently raised concerns the management of patient without symptoms who requires cardiac or other major surgery and in whom noninvasive studies show high-grade stenosis of the carotid artery. The studies that reviewed this issue did not show a consistent relationship between perioperative neurologic events and the degree of stenosis of the internal cartoid artery.[5,21,48] Therefore in this setting, prophylactic carotid endarterectomy cannot be recommended. However, high-grade stenoses are associated with an increased risk of neurologic symptoms and carotid occlusion. For these patients, carotid endarterectomy should be performed after coronary bypass grafting procedures have been done.

Follow-up with duplex scanning of patients after carotid endarterectomy has provided information on the prevalence and clinical significance of recurrent stenosis of the carotid artery. Although symptomatic recurrent stenosis occurs in only about 5% of patients, the overall anatomic prevalence is in the range of 9% to 21%.[6,19,33,52] In addition to showing that asymptomatic recurrent stenosis is relatively common after carotid endarterectomy, serial duplex scanning has also shown that the lesions developing during the first 2 years after surgery may regress. The recurrent lesions that persist generally remain stable, and progression to occlusion of the internal carotid artery is rare. Since the prevalence of neurologic signs and symptoms does not appear to be significantly different in those patients with recurrent stenosis from those patients without such stenosis, a conservative approach is justified.[19]

With continued improvements in the accuracy and reliability of carotid duplex scanning, there has been increasing interest in using the clinical evaluation and duplex findings alone as the basis for decisions about performing carotid endarterectomy. This approach avoids the expense and risk of arteriography.* Carotid bifurcation lesions suitable for endarterectomy include high-grade stenoses (80% to 99% reduction in diameter) in patients without symptoms and moderate to severe stenoses (more than 70% reduction) in patients with hemispheric neurologic symptoms. Although duplex scanning is useful for assessment of the carotid bifurcation, it does not provide direct information on lesions that involve the proximal aortic arch branches or the intracranial circulation. However, clinical experience has shown that lesions proximal or distal to the carotid bifurcation contributing to cerebral ischemia are rare and do not appear to adversely affect the outcome of carotid endarterectomy.[1,27,41,43] In addition, most stenoses of the proximal brachiocephalic vessels are associated with common carotid flow abnormalities or unequal blood pressures in the arms. Although the indications for carotid surgery without arteriography remain controversial, the results of arteriography rarely influence clinical decisions when a technically adequate duplex scan shows an ipsilateral 50% to 99% reduction in diameter in a patient with hemispheric neurologic symptoms or an 80% to 99% reduction in a patient who is free of symptoms.[10] Arteriography is most likely to be of value for when the duplex scan is technically inadequate, for atypical lesions that appear to extend beyond the carotid bifurcation, and for reductions in the diameter of the internal carotid artery that are less than 50% and in patients with neurologic symptoms.

---

*References 10, 17, 31, 39, 47, 49.

REFERENCES

1. Akers DL, Bell WH, Kerstein MD: Does intracranial dye study contribute to evaluation of carotid artery disease? *Am J Surg* 156:87, 1988.
2. Bandyk DF, Thiele BL: Noninvasive assessment of carotid artery disease, *West J Med* 139:486, 1983.
3. Barnes RW et al: Noninvasive ultrasonic angiography: prospective validation by contrast arteriography, *Surgery* 80:328, 1976.
4. Barnes RW et al: The Doppler cerebrovascular examination: improved results with refinements in technique, *Stroke* 8:468, 1977.
5. Barnes RW et al: The natural history of asymptomatic carotid disease in patients undergoing cardiovascular surgery, *Surgery* 90:1075, 1981.
6. Bernstein EF, Torem S, Dilley RB: Does carotid restenosis predict an increased risk of late symptoms, stroke, or death? *Ann Surg* 212:629, 1990.
7. Blackshear WM et al: A prospective evaluation of oculoplethysmography and carotid phonoangiography, *Surg Gynecol Obstet* 148:201, 1979.
8. Chikos PM et al: Observer variability in evaluating extracranial carotid artery stenosis, *Stroke* 14:885, 1983.
9. Comerota AJ et al: Real-time B-mode carotid imaging: a three-year multicenter experience, *J Vasc Surg* 1:84, 1984.
10. Dawson DL, Zierler RE, Kohler TR: Role of arteriography in the preoperative evaluation of carotid artery disease, *Am J Surg* 161:619, 1991.
11. Eikelboom B et al: Criteria for interpretation of oculopneumoplethysmography (Gee), *Arch Surg* 118:1169, 1983.
12. European Carotid Surgery Trialists' Collaborative Group: MRC European carotid surgery trial: Interim results for symptomatic patients with severe (70-99%) or with mild (0-29%) carotid stenosis, *Lancet* 337:1235, 1991.
13. Fell G et al: Importance of noninvasive ultrasonic Doppler testing in the evaluation of patients with asymptomatic carotid bruits, *Am Heart J* 102:221, 1981.
14. Fell G et al: Ultrasonic duplex scanning for disease of the carotid artery, *Circulation* 64:1191, 1981.
15. Gee W: Carotid physiology with ocular pneumoplethysmography, *Stroke* 13:666, 1982.
16. Gee W, Mehigan JT, Wylie EJ: Measurement of collateral hemispheric blood pressure by ocular pneumoplethysmography, *Am J Surg* 130:121, 1975.
17. Geuder JW et al: Is duplex scanning sufficient evaluation before carotid endarterectomy? *J Vasc Surg* 9:193, 1989.
18. Hass WK et al: Joint study of extracranial arterial occlusion II: arteriography, techniques, sites, and complications, *JAMA* 203:159, 1968.
19. Healy DA et al: Long-term follow-up and clinical outcome of carotid restenosis, *J Vasc Surg* 10:662, 1989.
20. Hennerici MG et al: Detection of early atherosclerotic lesions by duplex scanning of the carotid artery, *JCU* 12:455, 1984.
21. Ivey TD et al: Management of patients with carotid bruit undergoing cardiopulmonary bypass, *J Thorac Cardiovasc Surg* 87:183, 1984.
22. Kartchner MM, Mcrae LP, Morrison FD: Noninvasive detection and evaluation of carotid occlusive disease, *Arch Surg* 106:528, 1973.
23. Kartchner MM et al: Oculoplethysmography: an adjunct to arteriography in the diagnosis of extracranial carotid occlusive disease, *Am J Surg* 132:728, 1976.
24. Kohler T et al: Sources of variability in carotid duplex examination: a prospective study, *Ultrasound Med Biol* 4:571, 1985.
25. Langlois YE et al: Evaluating carotid artery disease: the concordance between pulsed Doppler/spectrum analysis and angiography, *Ultrasound Med Biol* 9:51, 1983.
26. Lye CR, Sumner DS, Strandness DE Jr: The accuracy of the supraorbital Doppler examination in the diagnosis of hemodynamically significant carotid disease, *Surgery* 79:42, 1976.
27. Mackey WC, O'Donnell TF, Callow AD: Carotid endarterectomy in patients with intracranial vascular disease: short-term risk and long-term outcome, *J Vasc Surg* 10:432, 1989.
28. Moneta GL et al: Operative versus nonoperative management of asymptomatic high-grade internal carotid artery stenosis: improved results with endarterectomy, *Stroke* 18:1005, 1987.
29. Moneta GL et al: Asymptomatic high-grade internal carotid artery stenosis: is stratification according to risk factors or duplex spectral analysis possible? *J Vasc Surg* 10:475, 1989.
30. Moniz E: L'encephalographie arteriel, son importance dans la localisation des tumeurs cerebrales, *Rev Neurol* 2:72, 1927.
31. Moore WS et al: Can clinical evaluation and noninvasive testing substitute for arteriography in the evaluation of carotid artery disease? *Ann Surg* 208:91, 1988.
32. Mozersky DJ et al: Ultrasonic arteriography, *Arch Surg* 103:663, 1971.
33. Nicholls SC et al: Carotid endarterectomy: relationship of outcome to early restenosis, *J Vasc Surg* 2:375, 1985.
34. Nicholls SC et al: Diagnostic significance of flow separation in the carotid bulb, *Stroke* 20:175, 1989.
35. North American Symptomatic Carotid Endarterectomy Trial (NASCET) Investigators: Clinical alert: Benefit of carotid endarterectomy for patients with high-grade stenosis of the internal carotid artery. National Institute of Neurological Disorders and Strike, Stroke and Trauma Division, *Stroke* 22:816, 1991.
36. O'Donnell TF et al: Correlation of B-mode ultrasound imaging and arteriography with pathologic findings at carotid endarterectomy, *Arch Surg* 120:443, 1985.
37. O'Leary et al: Carotid bifurcation disease: prediction of ulceration with B-mode US, *Radiology* 162:523, 1987.
38. Reilly LM et al: Carotid plaque histology using real-time ultrasonography: clinical and therapeutic implications, *Am J Surg* 146:188, 1983.
39. Ricotta JJ et al: Is routine angiography necessary prior to carotid endarterectomy? *J Vasc Surg* 1:96, 1984.

40. Roederer GO et al: Ultrasonic duplex scanning of extracranial carotid arteries: improved accuracy using new features from the common carotid artery, *J Cardiovasc Ultrasonogr* 1:373, 1982.

41. Roederer GO et al: Is siphon disease important in predicting outcome of carotid endarterectomy? *Arch Surg* 118:1177, 1983.

42. Roederer GO et al: The natural history of carotid arterial disease in asymptomatic patients with cervical bruits, *Stroke* 15:605, 1984.

43. Schuler JJ et al: The effect of carotid siphon stenosis on stroke rate, death, and relief of symptoms following elective carotid endarterectomy, *Surgery* 92:1058, 1982.

44. Seeger JM, Klingman N: The relationship between carotid plaque composition and neurologic symptoms, *J Surg Res* 43:78, 1987.

45. Strandness DE Jr: *Historical aspects*. In *Duplex scanning in vascular disorders,* New York, 1990, Raven Press, pp 1-24.

46. Thiele BL et al: Correlation of arteriographic findings and symptoms in cerebrovascular disease, *Neurology* 30:1041, 1980.

47. Thomas GI et al: Carotid endarterectomy after Doppler ultrasonic evaluation without angiography, *Am J Surg* 151:616, 1986.

48. Turnipseed WD et al: Postoperative stroke in cardiac and peripheral vascular disease, *Ann Surg* 192:365, 1980.

49. Wagner WH et al: The diminishing role of diagnostic arteriography in carotid artery disease: duplex scanning as definitive preoperative study, *Ann Vasc Surg* 5:105, 1991.

50. Zierler RE, Kohler TR, Strandness DE Jr.: Duplex scanning of normal or minimally diseased carotid arteries: correlation with arteriography and clinical outcome, *J Vasc Surg* 12:447, 1990.

51. Zierler RE, Strandness DE Jr: *Noninvasive dynamic and real-time assessment of extracranial cerebrovasculature.* In Wood JH, editor: *Cerebral blood flow: physiologic and clinical aspects,* New York, 1987, McGraw-Hill.

52. Zierler RE et al: Carotid artery stenosis following endarterectomy, *Arch Surg* 117:1408, 1982.

53. Zierler RE et al: Noninvasive assessment of normal carotid bifurcation hemodynamics with color-flow ultrasound imaging, *Ultrasound Med Biol* 13:471, 1987.

CHAPTER 32

Duplex scanning of aortic arch branches and vertebral arteries

ROB G.A. ACKERSTAFF

Ultrasonic duplex scanning with spectral analysis of a pulsed Doppler signal is a reliable technique for the detection of atherosclerosis of the cervical carotid arteries.[4] With this noninvasive technique, it is possible to identify normal vessels and those with disease involvement in the internal carotid artery.[6,11,12,22,45] For the external carotid artery, the duplex method differentiates reasonably well between non-hemodynamically and hemodynamically significant stenosis.[2,14] However, only brief attention has been paid to the investigation of the innominate-subclavian-vertebral arterial system. This is surprising because the vertebral arteries are often as large as or sometimes larger than the internal carotid arteries where they penetrate the dura and because they supply the vital centers of the brainstem. This omission may be because the innominate and subclavian arteries are more deeply located and because a large part of the vertebral artery is inaccessible to ultrasound if it is obscured by bone in its cervical segment. Moreover, the presence of numerous other vessels, especially in the lower neck, makes it difficult to be certain that the Doppler signal detected does arise from the vertebral artery. The difficulties of vertebral arteriography and the sometimes dramatic complications after this radiologic procedure also contribute to the limited knowledge of the clinical significance of atherosclerosis of the vertebrobasilar arterial system.[17] More importantly, physicians have failed to comprehend the frequency of atherosclerosis of the innominate-subclavian-vertebral arterial system and its relationship to cerebral ischemia. Nevertheless, transient ischemic attacks are not rare. In his textbook on cerebrovascular disorders, Toole[36] stated that 10% to 30% of transient ischemic attacks involve the vertebrobasilar territory. Although there is lack of consensus among clinicians about the treatment of patients with atherosclerosis of the innominate-subclavian-vertebral arterial system, it is well known that severe obstructive disease of the extracranial part of the vertebral arteries can lead to a neurologic deficit of the posterior circulation.[16,28,30] Some studies even indicate that involvement of the vertebral arteries is significant in increasing stroke risk in patients with atherosclerosis of the carotid system.[23,34] In patients with focal neurologic deficit of the anterior circulation, the nidus of thromboembolism may be located in the innominate artery.[27] Finally, interest in revascularizing highly stenosed vertebral arteries requires the detection, grading, and postoperative follow-up of the lesions of this part of the cerebral vasculature with a reliable noninvasive technique.[13,29,35,38]

Continuous wave (CW) Doppler sonography is currently used to investigate the innominate, subclavian, and vertebral arteries in many laboratories. However, only a few authors have carried out validation studies by comparing their results with contrast arteriography.[26,33] Correct identification of the vertebral arteries is not always possible with CW Doppler, so the role of this method in predicting stenoses at the site of the origin of the vertebral artery is of little value.[41,44] It was not always possible to ensure that the signals originated from the vertebral artery, and there were times when the investigators must have mistakenly recorded signals from other arteries. Many of these problems can be circumvented by using a duplex system, which allows visualization of arterial walls and detection of flow velocities at specific sites within the imaged vessels.

For the innominate-subclavian-vertebral arterial system, B-mode imaging provides an anatomic road map from which the exact location and course of the vessels can be identified. In many cases the B-mode image provides information about atheromatous deposits within and along diseased arteries. Direction of blood flow in the vertebral arteries has been described, and quantitative vertebral artery flow measurements in patients with vertebrobasilar ischemia have been performed.[8,9,10,37,43] However, in most studies the investigation of the vertebral arteries is restricted to the cervical segment, and the examination of the ostium and the prevertebral segment is performed only in a few studies with a relatively small number of cases.[4,19,20,39] Because of interest in atherosclerosis of the extracranial contribution to the posterior cerebral circulation in patients with symptoms and those who were free of symptoms, the arch branches and the prevertebral segment of the vertebral artery were routinely investigated with duplex scanning. The results of duplex scanning were compared with those of intraarterial contrast angiography in 584 arteries.[1,2,5,25] In patients with a possible history of vertebrobasilar ischemia, the cervical segment of the vertebral artery up to the level of the atlas was also investigated. More recently, after the introduction

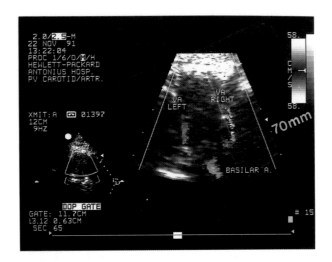

Fig. 32-1. A B-mode image of the intradural segments of the vertebral arteries and the caudal part of the basilar artery. The image is made by a suboccipital approach with a 2.5-MHz transducer. Between the *VA* (vertebral artery), the foramen magnum is visualized. In this case, the vertebrobasilar conjunction is located at a depth of 75 mm.

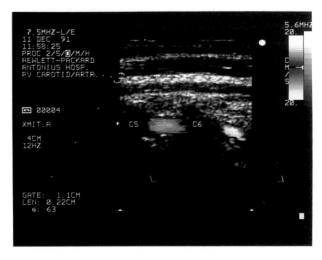

Fig. 32-2. The vertebral artery and vein imaged between the transverse processes of the sixth and fifth cervical vertebrae.

of transcranial duplex scanning with color flow imaging, the intradural segments of the vertebral artery and the basilar artery were also investigated (Fig. 32-1).

METHODS

During the first part of the study, mechanical real-time ultrasonic scanners (ATL Mark V and MK 600*) with multifrequency transducers (7.5 MHz, 5 MHz short focus, and 5 MHz medium focus) were used. The spectral resolution of the single-gate pulsed Doppler system was evaluated by Hoeks and coworkers[24] and published in an earlier report.[1] More recently an HP Sonos 1000 system† with linear array and phased array transducers with color flow imaging was used. In addition to audible interpretation, real-time spectral analysis of the Doppler signals was used to evaluate the degree of stenosis. The hard copy output displayed the Doppler-shifted frequencies, the direction of flow, and the amplitude of the back-scattered signal in shades of gray.

During the examination the patient lies in the supine position with the head on a small pillow. The preferred position for the investigator is at the patient's head. During the first part of the study,[1] the innominate and subclavian arteries are examined through the supraclavicular fossa. These vessels are followed in a distal direction until the vertebral artery is found. With this approach, it is important to note the close proximity of the vertebral artery to a number of other arteries of similar size, which makes correct identification of the vertebral artery difficult. In most cases, however, it is possible to identify the ostium and the course

of the vertebral artery. Because images and Doppler recordings can be mistakenly produced by other arteries, the procedure has been modified. The approach to the vertebral artery was changed to direct visualization of the artery itself. With practice, it is fairly easy to obtain an image of the cervical segment of the vertebral artery between the transverse processes of the cervical vertebrae (Fig. 32-2). The acoustic shadows of the transverse processes are easily identified by placing the probe on the lateral side of the neck a few centimeters above its base between the trachea and the sternocleidomastoid muscle. The transverse processes appear as echogenic masses with acoustic shadowing, and the vertebral artery is seen between them as an anechoic structure bounded by echogenic walls. Once the vertebral artery is located, the Doppler cursor line is placed across the vessel and the sample volume is widened to encompass the entire diameter of the vessel. The diameter of the arterial lumen is measured, and attention should be paid to the shape of the velocity pattern and, particularly, to the diastolic component. Unlike the internal carotid arteries, the vertebral arteries are often unequal in size. The vertebral vein lies in close proximity to the artery. However, it is easy to differentiate the venous signals from the arterial signals by their characteristic features.

By scanning along the longitudinal axis of the neck, the examiner can obtain an image of the vertebral artery before it enters its bony canal just caudal to the sixth cervical vertebra. With careful positioning of the probe, it is possible to follow the course of the vertebral artery to its origin from the subclavian artery. The vertebral artery often has a typical flat curve just distal to its origin, and the subclavian artery is usually then visualized in an oblique or transverse plane (Fig. 32-3).

A decision about the state of the prevertebral arterial segment and the origin of the vertebral artery is made only

---

*Advanced Technology Laboratories, Bethel, Wash.
†Hewlett Packard, Palo Alto, Calif.

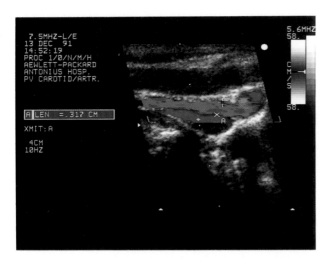

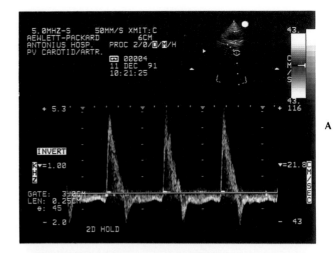

A

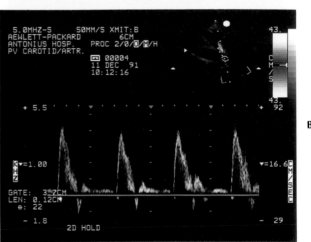

B

Fig. 32-3. The most proximal segment of a vertebral artery with its origin from the subclavian artery. The subclavian artery is shown on the right side in a transverse plane. The diameter of the vertebral artery is 32 mm.

Fig. 32-4. The sonograms of the Doppler signals of *A,* subclavian and *B,* innominate arteries.

when this portion of the vessel can be followed along its entire length. In most cases it is possible to locate the origin of the vertebral artery. It is usually possible to position the angle of the Doppler beam to about 60° with the long axis of the artery and to obtain a reliable Doppler measurement. However, in some cases, it may not be possible to obtain an optimum angle of insonation with the artery. In these cases, it may be difficult to obtain a reliable velocity waveform.

The operator always attempts to measure the angle of the Doppler beam relative to the long axis of the vessel. The sample volume must be placed near the center stream in large vessels such as the innominate or subclavian artery, to avoid detection of velocities and eddies close to the vessel wall. Under normal conditions with a laminar flow during systole, the red blood cells are moved forward with approximately the same velocity. The Fourier transform of the Doppler signal recorded from center stream shows a narrow band of frequencies with a clean window below the systolic peak (Fig. 32-4). With regard to the much smaller arteries, such as the vertebral arteries, the entire vessel is insonated, including reflections from the slowly moving red blood cells near the vessel wall. This results in an increase of the spectral width, with obliteration of the systolic window (Fig. 32-5). The velocity patterns of vertebral arteries are typical of those feeding a low-resistance circulation. The velocity pattern evaluation includes the peak systolic frequencies, the degree of spectral broadening, and the direction of flow (forward, zero, or reverse flow). The finding of reverse flow in the vertebral artery is a sign of significant stenosis in the innominate or subclavian artery proximal to the origin of the vertebral artery. In vertebral arteries, flow reversal is sometimes cardiac-cycle dependent.[42]

According to the characteristic spectral changes of the

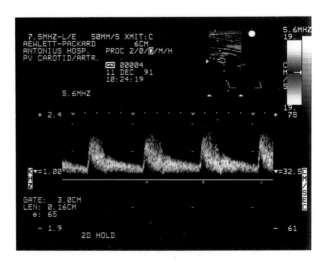

Fig. 32-5. The sonogram of the Doppler signals of a normal vertebral artery. Since the sample volume is large relative to the vessel diameter, there is usually spectral broadening during systole.

Doppler signal recorded in the vertebral artery, three categories can be defined:

1. *Normal:* Antegrade flow, peak frequencies less than 4 kHz, and moderate spectral broadening during systole without striking turbulence (Fig. 32-5)
2. *Abnormal:* Antegrade flow, peak frequencies more than 4 kHz, increased spectral broadening, and striking turbulence during systole (Fig. 32-6)
3. *Total occlusion:* Usual acquisition of an image of the vertebral artery, no detection of flow

The 4-kHz peak frequency is only applicable with the use of a transducer with a nominal frequency of 5 MHz and an angle of insonation of 60°. It is important to emphasize that in these studies, a normal signal suggested the finding of a normal vessel or one with a stenosis of less than 50%. An abnormal Doppler signal suggested a vessel with a stenosis of 50% to 99%. For the innominate and subclavian arteries the criteria are somewhat different. The flow patterns from these arteries show a steep systolic wave and, after the onset of diastole, a brief period of flow reversal.

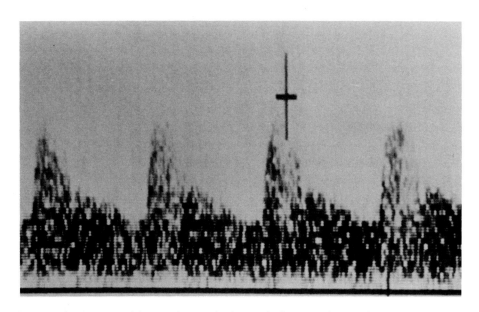

Fig. 32-6. The sonogram of the Doppler signals of a vertebral artery with a significant stenosis at the site of the ostium. Note the increased peak frequencies (cross 5.3 kHz) and spectral broadening.

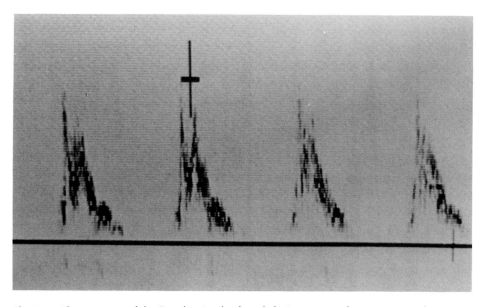

Fig. 32-7. The sonogram of the Doppler signals of a subclavian artery, a few centimeters downstream to a significant stenosis. Note the irregular outline and loss of high frequencies (cross 3.1 kHz).

During late diastole, there is no significant forward flow present in the subclavian artery (Fig. 32-4, *A*). The innominate artery, however, often shows a forward flow component during diastole (Fig. 32-4, *B*). Under normal conditions the peak systolic frequencies obtained from the arch arteries are often greater than 4 kHz. If the sample volume is placed near the center stream, the recorded Doppler signals are clean. With increasing stenosis, turbulence will develop, which will produce a harsh Doppler signal. If the obstructive lesion is in or near the origin of the innominate or subclavian artery, it is not always possible to place the sample volume near the stenotic area. A few centimeters downstream to a significant stenosis, the outline of the velocity pattern is irregular and the spectrum often reveals loss or dropout of some higher frequencies (Fig. 32-7). In the event of a total occlusion of the innominate or subclavian artery, a low-frequency monophasic signal will be detected. The finding of asymmetry of the velocity pattern between sides is extremely important in determining the status of the origin of the great vessel.

Patients normally underwent four-vessel arteriography. The arteriographic studies were either conventional or intraarterial digital subtraction procedures. In many patients, selective studies of the innominate-subclavian-vertebral arterial system, as well as biplane carotid angiography, were performed. The narrowest diameter within the stenosis was measured and compared with the normal diameter of the artery either distal or proximal to the filling defect. This was converted into an estimate of the extent of the diameter reduction. The results of the duplex study were classified as normal or abnormal. The results of the classification procedures were not only expressed as the proportion of correct classification (overall accuracy) but also as diagnostic sensitivity and specificity; the positive and negative predictive values were also calculated (Table 32-1).

RESULTS
Innominate artery

Direct visualization of the origin of the innominate artery from the aorta was possible only in slender patients with the use of a 5-MHz transducer. However, investigation of the more distal part of this artery was usually no problem. In 10% of the patients the innominate artery was located too deeply to make it possible to complete the study. Only a few patients (0.25%)[18] have an abnormal origin of the

right subclavian artery directly from the aorta distal to the origin of the left subclavian artery. It is possible to obtain velocity signals 2 to 4 cm distal to the origin of the innominate artery. Since the more significant atherosclerotic lesions are located in the most proximal part of the innominate artery, close to its origin, it is necessary to detect flow disturbances distal to the stenosis as an indication of disease. With lesser degree of stenosis (less than 50%), the transition to a normal flow pattern takes place quickly. In the case of a stenosis with a diameter reduction of 50% to 60% at the site of the origin of innominate artery, the velocity patterns will return to normal approximately 3 cm downstream[31] of the origin of the artery. Therefore atherosclerotic lesions of the innominate artery with a diameter reduction of less than 50% will not give rise to disturbed velocity signals in the distal part of this artery and cannot be detected with ultrasonic duplex scanning.

Subclavian arteries

Investigation of the subclavian arteries is possible in nearly all patients. In patients with a significant stenosis in the innominate artery, it may be difficult to distinguish the flow disturbances induced by this lesion from the disturbances induced by a lesion at the site of the origin of the right subclavian artery. Duplex scanning of the right subclavian artery is the most difficult part of the investigation. The most proximal part of the right subclavian artery makes a posterolateral curve from which it is difficult to obtain satisfactory Doppler signals due to the difficulty of obtaining a suitable angle of insonation. This may occur in about 15% of patients. In most of these cases, however, the proximal part of the right subclavian artery can be imaged fully, and an atherosclerotic lesion at the site of the origin can usually be seen.

In a few patients, it was possible to image the origin of the left subclavian artery, and in almost all patients the Doppler signals were recorded roughly 1 to 4 cm downstream to the origin of this artery. In spite of this, the accuracy was better for the left subclavian artery than for the right. Atherosclerotic lesions of the left subclavian artery are more diffuse than those in the right subclavian artery. In many patients the lesions extend to the origin of the left vertebral artery. This is probably the reason for the relatively low number of false-negative results in the investigation of the left subclavian artery.

Table 32-1. Sensitivity, specificity, positive and negative predictive values, and overall accuracy for identifying a stenosis of 50% or more

Artery	Sensitivity (%)	Specificity (%)	PPV (%)	NPV (%)	Overall accuracy
Innominate	98	99	75	100	99
Right subclavian	76	99	75	96	95
Left subclavian	91	98	78	99	97
Vertebral	80	97	87	94	93

PPV, Positive predictive value; *NPV*, negative predictive value.

Extracranial vertebral artery

After the introduction of modern transducers with relatively high spatial resolution, imaging of the cervical segment of the vertebral artery has been possible in almost all patients. An occlusion of the vertebral artery could be correctly identified, and confusion with a hypoplastic or intracranially occluded vertebral artery was not a problem. Only in obese patients or young children is it difficult to identify the artery. The assessment of coiling and kinking of the vertebral artery by osteoarthritic spurs, as well as the evaluation of atherosclerotic lesions in the cervical segment, can now be assessed accurately.

The investigation of the prevertebral segment of the vertebral artery is more difficult. It is important, however, because the majority of atherosclerotic lesions involving this artery are located at its origin. This part of duplex scanning of the innominate-subclavian-vertebral arterial system needs extra attention. Although the skill of the sonographers has increased and the introduction of a transducer with a transmitting frequency of 7.5 MHz improved the spatial resolution of the image significantly, the failure rate of the investigation of the origin of the vertebral artery only decreased from 23% during the first years to 20% during the last years of one study.[25] In some cases this was due to the tortuosity of the artery, which could be misleading. Although the vertebral artery is easily located just proximal to the transverse process of the sixth cervical vertebra, it may be impossible to follow the artery proximally to its origin. In most of these cases the origin was too deeply located, which prevented acquisition of a good image. This also made it more difficult to obtain good Doppler signals. In other cases there were variations in the location of the origin of the artery. It is more common on the left side. In patients in whom the investigation of the ostium of the vertebral artery was possible, duplex scanning had a high sensitivity (80%), specificity (97%), and overall accuracy (93%) for the detection of an obstructive lesion with a diameter-reducing stenosis of 50% or more. Most false-positive test results occurred in patients with severe multivessel disease in whom the vertebral artery served as a major collateral for the cerebral circulation. In these cases it was difficult to distinguish disturbances of the sonographic pattern secondary to high flow from those induced by a significant stenosis.[5] When a vertebral artery showed a low flow state, as in cases of marked hypoplasia or a vertebral artery with an intracranial occlusion, a decision concerning the state of its ostium was also impossible. In these cases the velocities were too low, and a stenosis was easily underestimated. Significant lesions (greater than 50% diameter reduction) in the remaining part of the prevertebral segment of the vertebral artery were rare (0.7%). In most of these cases, however, the results of duplex scanning were in accordance with those of arteriography.

Intracranial vertebral and basilar arteries

Direct investigation of the intradural segment of the vertebral artery and the basilar artery is generally performed with standard transcranial Doppler sonography.[15,33,40] The probe is placed suboccipitally in the region of the foramen magnum, and the patient's head is flexed slightly forward. Most authors describe this procedure as simple and easily learned. For the detection of intracranially located stenotic lesions of the vertebral and basilar arteries, sonographic criteria such as a local increase of blood flow velocities and spectrum distribution at the baseline have been used by several investigators. In general, for the assessment of significant stenosis in the intracranial segments of the vertebrobasilar arterial system, standard transcranial Doppler sonography is valid only when this technique is used in combination with selective arteriography. However, as a result of frequent anatomic variations of the posterior circulation, it is often difficult to ascertain the vessel from which the Doppler signals are obtained. Transcranial duplex scanning with color flow imaging (Fig. 32-1) will probably prove to be more practical and reliable in the near future.

CONCLUSION

The vertebral artery is the most difficult part of the extracranial posterior cerebral circulation to examine accurately with noninvasive techniques. It is recognized that with nonimaging systems, correct identification of the vertebral artery is not always possible and that the role of this method in predicting stenoses is of little value. The main challenge is to document that segment of the vertebral artery most commonly involved. Recent studies have shown that with adequate skill and patience of the operators, the innominate and subclavian arteries and the cervical and prevertebral segments of the vertebral artery can be displayed with real-time, pulsed-echo methods. Instruments that produce pie-shaped sector scans would appear to be advantageous for imaging the arch branches and vertebral artery origin, since these instruments have a small scan head, which is amenable to imaging poorly accessible structures. Ultrasonographic duplex scanning appears to be the most successful and accurate technique by which to diagnose noninvasively atherosclerotic lesions of the vertebral arteries. With this technique, it is easy to visualize the cervical segment of the vertebral artery, and the direction of flow can be determined without the use of special tests. A reliable investigation of the prevertebral segment and the ostium of the vertebral artery is possible in more than 80% of cases. Some studies[7,20,21] claim more rapid identification and a higher success rate if color flow imaging is used. For the detection of a stenosis of greater than 50% in the arch branches and at the site of the origin of the vertebral artery, duplex scanning has high sensitivity, specificity, and overall accuracy. Nevertheless, this technique has several disadvantages. The most important is that satisfactory displays of the origin of the vertebral artery cannot be achieved in all patients. In addition, it is obvious that in those arteries in which the examination is successfully completed, only a limited spectrum of disease involvement can be identified. Finally, the intradural segment of the vertebral artery and the basilar artery at present are investigated with nonimaging Doppler techniques. Accuracy of the ultrasonographic examination of this segment of the posterior circulation may be improved by the introduction of simultaneous B-mode and color flow imaging.

REFERENCES

1. Ackerstaff RGA: *Ultrasonic duplex scanning in atherosclerotic disease of the vertebrobasilar arterial system: a non-invasive technique compared with contrast arteriography,* thesis, Utrecht, 1985, Elinkwijk BV.
2. Ackerstaff RGA, Eikelboom BC, Moll FL: Investigation of the vertebral artery in cerebral atherosclerosis, *Eur J Vasc Surg* 5:229-235, 1991.
3. Ackerstaff RGA et al: The accuracy of ultrasonic duplex scanning in carotid artery disease, *Clin Neurol Neurosurg* 84:211-220, 1982.
4. Ackerstaff RGA et al: Ultrasonic duplex scanning in atherosclerotic disease of the innominate, subclavian, and vertebral arteries: a comparative study with angiography, *Ultrasound Med Biol* 10:409-418, 1984.
5. Ackerstaff RGA et al: Ultrasonic duplex scanning of the prevertebral segment of the vertebral artery in patients with cerebral atherosclerosis, *Eur J Vasc Surg* 2:387-393, 1988.
6. Archie JP: A simple, non-dimensional, normalized common carotid Doppler velocity wave-form index that identifies patients with carotid stenosis, *Stroke* 12:322-324, 1981.
7. Bartels E, Fuchs HH, Flügel KA: Color Doppler imaging of vertebral arteries: a comparative study with duplex ultrasonography. In Oka M et al, eds: *Recent advantages in neurosonology,* Amsterdam, 1992, Elsevier Science Publishers.
8. Bendick PHJ, Glover JL: Vertebrobasilar insufficiency: evaluation by quantitative duplex flow measurements, *J Vasc Surg* 5:594-600, 1987.
9. Bendick PHJ, Glover JL: Hemodynamic evaluation of vertebral arteries by duplex ultrasound, *Surg Clin North Am* 70:235-244, 1990.
10. Bendick PHJ, Jackson VP: Evaluation of the vertebral arteries with duplex sonography, *J Vasc Surg* 3:523-530, 1986.
11. Blackshear WM et al: Carotid artery velocity patterns in normal and stenotic vessels, *Stroke* 11:67-71, 1980.
12. Bodily KC et al: Spectral analysis of Doppler velocity patterns in normals and patients with carotid artery stenosis, *Clin Physiol* 1:365-374, 1981.
13. Brachereau A, Magnan PE: Results of vertebral artery reconstruction, *J Cardiovasc Surg* 31:320-326, 1990.
14. Breslau PJ: Ultrasonic duplex scanning in the evaluation of carotid artery disease, thesis, Voerendaal, Heerlen, 1982, *Schrijen-Lipperts BV.*
15. Budingen HJ, Stuadacher TH: Die Identifizierung der Arteria Basilaris mit der transkraniellen Doppler-Sonographie, *Ultraschall Med* 8:95-101, 1987.
16. Caplan LR: *Vertebrobasilar occlusive disease.* In Barnett AS et al, editors: *Stroke,* New York, 1986, Churchill Livingstone.
17. Cornelius P et al: Clinical utilization of quantitative vertebral flow measurements, *J Vasc Technol* 15:235-240, 1991.
18. Daseler EH, Anson BJ: Surgical anatomy of the subclavian artery and its branches, *Surg Gynecol Obstet* 108:149-174, 1959.
19. Davis PC et al: A prospective comparison of duplex sonography versus angiography of the vertebral arteries, *Am J Neuroradiol* 7:1059-1064, 1986.
20. De Bray JM: Le duplex des axes verébro-sous-claviers, *J Echographie Méd Ultrasons* 12:141-151, 1991.
21. Frattnig S et al: Color-coded Doppler imaging of normal vertebral arteries, *Stroke* 21:1222-1225, 1990.
22. Hames TK et al: The validation of duplex scanning and continuous wave Doppler imaging: a comparison with conventional angiography, *Ultrasound Med Biol* 11:827-834, 1985.
23. Hennerici M, Rautenberg W, Mohr S: Stroke risk from symptomless extracranial arterial disease, *Lancet* 1180-1183, 2, 1982.
24. Hoeks APG et al: Methods to evaluate the sample volume of pulsed Doppler systems, *Ultrasound Med Biol* 10:261-264, 1984.
25. Jak JG et al: A six year evaluation of duplex scanning of the vertebral artery. A non-invasive technique compared with contrast angiography, *J Vasc Technol* 13:26-30, 1989.
26. Karnik R et al: Validity of continuous-wave Doppler sonography of the vertebrobasilar system, *Angiology* 38:556-561, 1987.
27. Lord RSA, Berry NA: Atherosclerotic ulceration of the brachocephalic artery, *Aust N Z J Surg* 44:370-374, 1974.
28. Naritomi H, Sakai F, Meyer JS: Pathogenesis of transient ischemic attacks within the vertebrobasilar arterial system, *Arch Neurol* 36:121-128, 1979.
29. Perry MO: Symposium: surgery of the vertebral artery, *J Vasc Surg* 2:620-642, 1985.
30. Pessin MS, Caplan LR: *Heterogeneity of vertebrobasilar occlusive disease.* In Kunze K et al eds: *Clinical problems of brainstem disorders,* Stuttgart, 1986, Thieme Verlag.
31. Reneman RS, Spencer MP: Local Doppler audio spectra in normal and stenosed carotid arteries in man, *Ultrasound Med Biol* 5:1-11, 1979.
32. Ringelstein EB: *Neue Anwendungsmóglichkeiten der Dopplersonographie am hinteren Hirnkreislauf bei degenerativer Gefässkrankheit, angiotherapeutischen Eingriffen und epidemiologischen Untersuchungen,* Aachen, 1981, Habilitationsschrift.
33. Schneider PA et al: Noninvasive evaluation of vertebrobasilar insufficiency, *J Ultrasound Med* 10:373-379, 1991.
34. Sindermann F: Krankheitsbild und Kollateralkreislauf bei einseitigem und doppelseitigem Carotisverschluss, *J Neurol Sci* 5:9-25, 1967.
35. Thevenet A, Ruotolo C: Surgical repair of vertebral artery stenosis, *J Cardiovasc Surg* 25:101-110, 1984.
36. Toole JF: *Cerebrovascular disorders,* New York, 1984, Raven Press.
37. Touboul PJ et al: Duplex scanning of normal vertebral arteries, *Stroke* 17:921-923, 1986.
38. van Schill PEJ et al: Long-term clinical and duplex follow-up after proximal vertebral artery reconstruction, *Angiology* 43:961-968, 1992.
39. Visona A et al: The echo-Doppler (duplex) system for the detection of vertebral artery occlusive disease: comparison with angiography, *J Ultrasound Med* 5:247-250, 1986.
40. Vole D et al: Transcranial Dopplersonography of the vertebro-basilar system, *Acta Neurochir (Wien)* 90:136-138, 1988.
41. von Reutern GM, Budeingen HF, Freund HJ: Dopplersonograpfische Diagnostik von Stenosen und Verschlussen der VErtebraliarterien und Sublcavian-Steal-Syndromes, *Arch Psychiatrie Nervenkrankheiten* 222:209-222, 1976.
42. von Reutern GM, Pourcelot L: Cardiac cycle-dependent alternating flow in vertebral arteries with subclavian artery stenosis, *Stroke* 9:229-236, 1978.
43. Walker DW, Acker JD, Cole CA: Subclavian steal syndrome detected with duplex pulsed Doppler sonography, *Am J Neuroradiol* 3:615-618, 1982.
44. White DM, Ketelaars CEJ, Cledgett PR: Noninvasive techniques for recording of vertebral artery flow and their limitations, *Ultrasound Med Biol* 6:315-327, 1980.
45. Zwiebel WJ: Spectrum analysis in carotid sonography, *Ultrasound Med Biol* 13:625-636, 1987.

CHAPTER 33

Accuracy and potential pitfalls of continuous wave carotid Doppler frequency analysis

K. WAYNE JOHNSTON

Frequency analysis of continuous wave (CW) Doppler signals is a widely used method for diagnosing extracranial carotid artery disease because it can reliably detect moderate and severe stenoses.[3-5,19] Although duplex Doppler systems and color flow imaging systems with pulsed wave Doppler signals are now the most common direct methods for carotid evaluation, the CW Doppler technique still has a role, particularly in smaller laboratories, because of its simplicity, relatively low cost, and good clinical accuracy.*

The purposes of this chapter are to review the changes in the Doppler spectral waveform produced by a stenosis, to describe the CW carotid Doppler technique and the clinical results, and to identify ways to avoid problems that limit the accuracy of this method.

CHANGES IN THE DOPPLER SPECTRAL WAVEFORM PRODUCED BY A STENOSIS

Spectral recordings provide diagnostic information by displaying the velocity changes that occur in the region of a stenosis. At the site of a stenosis the peak frequency is increased,[5,8,12,19] and beyond the stenosis, the spectrum of Doppler frequencies is broadened because of the presence of disturbed or turbulent flow.[1,5,8,17] In Fig. 33-1 frequency analysis recordings from an in vivo model illustrate the two abnormalities that are of value in detecting carotid artery stenoses. First, the Doppler frequency increases at the site of the stenosis, and second, the Doppler spectrum is broadened beyond the stenosis where the flow is disturbed.

Peak frequency increase

The relationship between the peak Doppler frequency and the severity of the stenosis has been studied both in vitro and clinically. As illustrated in Fig. 33-2, from the results obtained with a pulsatile flow in vitro model[8] with a nominal flow rate of 225 ml/min and a 4-MHz probe kept at a constant angle of 60°, it can be seen that the peak frequency is directly related to the percentage area of stenosis. The comparable clinical results are shown in Fig. 33-

3, in which the peak Doppler frequency is plotted against the percentage of internal carotid diameter stenosis measured from arteriograms in 397 cases.

The reason for the increased Doppler frequency at the site of a stenosis is well understood.[5,8] In a nonbranched artery, the volumetric flow is the same at all points along the artery, and since the cross-sectional area is reduced at the stenosis, the mean velocity increases. Clinical recordings such as those illustrated in Fig. 33-4 clearly show that the maximum peak frequency is detected directly over the stenosis.

Spectral broadening and spectral broadening index

In a normal carotid Doppler recording, there is a clear window beneath the systolic peak; at this point, the flow velocity profile is nearly flat. Beyond a stenosis where the flow is disturbed, the clear window is obliterated (i.e., the spectrum is broadened) because the directions of the flow vectors change with respect to the angle of insonation.

Although spectral broadening can be graded subjectively, the limitations of the method of assessment are well known. Kassam et al[11] reviewed the problems of quantifying the Doppler spectrum and identified the relative stability of the maximum and mean Doppler frequencies in contrast to the variability of the mode and minimum frequencies. For these reasons, it has been postulated that it would be more accurate to quantify spectral broadening by the measurement of an index that is based on the difference between the maximum and mean frequencies, divided by the maximum frequency. This index has the theoretic advantage with the handheld CW Doppler technique because the probe-to-vessel angle is unknown. Thus the spectral broadening index (SBI) was defined as follows:

$$\text{SBI} = \frac{\text{Fmax} - \text{Fmean}}{\text{Fmax} \times 100} \qquad (1)$$
$$= \frac{100 - \text{Fmean}}{\text{Fmax} \times 100}$$

where Fmax is the maximum frequency and Fmean is the mean frequency recorded at peak systole.

---

*References 1, 5, 7, 8, 14, 17, 19.

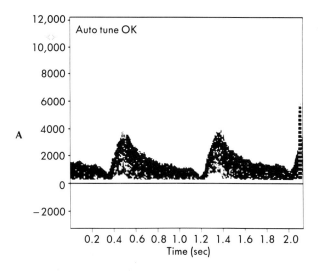

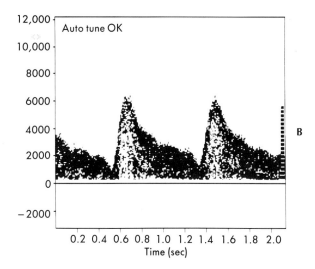

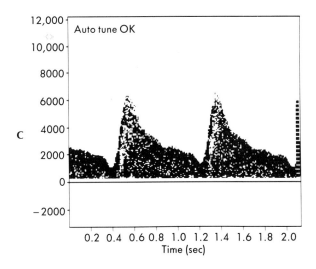

Fig. 33-1. Frequency analysis recordings from in vitro model. **A,** Normal. **B,** Peak frequency is increased at site of stenosis. **C,** Spectral broadening is present beyond stenosis. (Note that spectral waveforms produced in this model have been found to be nearly identical to those seen in human carotid artery.)

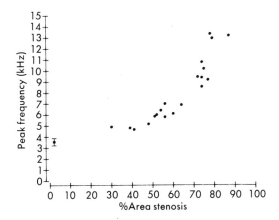

Fig. 33-2. In vitro results showing relationship between percentage of stenosis and peak Doppler frequency.

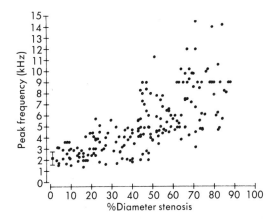

Fig. 33-3. Clinical results showing relationship between peak Doppler frequency and percentage of internal carotid diameter stenosis (i.e., minimum residual lumen diameter divided by diameter of distal internal carotid). Normal peak frequency ± standard deviation is shown (2.2 ± 0.6 kHz, N = 149).

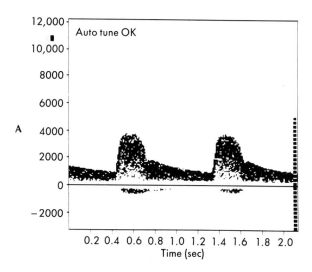

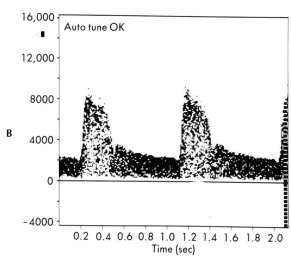

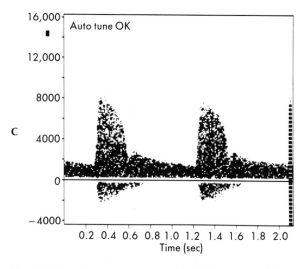

Fig. 33-4. Recordings from patient with 60% stenosis of diameter of internal carotid artery. *A,* Normal. *B,* Directly over stenosis. *C,* 1 cm beyond stenosis.

The initial validation of the SBI was performed in a rigid tube pulsatile flow model that produced waveforms virtually identical to those observed in the human carotid artery.[8] A close linear relationship between the severity of arterial stenosis and the SBI was observed. It was shown that the SBI was potentially affected by other factors, including the flow rate, the recording site in relationship to the site of the stenosis, the shape of the stenosis, and the timing in the cardiac cycle when the recording is made. Nevertheless, in these in vitro studies the major determinant factor of the SBI was the severity of the stenosis.

CAROTID DOPPLER TECHNIQUE

CW Doppler frequency analysis studies of the carotid artery are performed with a 5-MHz CW Doppler velocity meter and a real-time frequency analyzer (SP-25).* The technologist holds the Doppler probe and maintains a probe-to-skin angle that is as constant as possible, usually between 45° and 60°. Representative recordings are made at 0.5 to 1.0 cm increments along the common carotid and internal carotid axis. At each site the probe is positioned to obtain waveforms that are free of artifacts and show the least amount of spectral broadening under the peak. Two measurements are made: the peak frequency and the spectral broadening index.

CLINICAL RESULTS

A prospective multicenter study has determined the accuracy of the CW Doppler technique for the evaluation of carotid stenosis.[10] In this study the Doppler examinations were performed by technologists who were not aware of the results of the angiograms. The results of the angiograms were interpreted by physicians who were blinded to the results of the Doppler study. The severity of the carotid stenosis was measured as the ratio of the minimum residual lumen diameter at the stenosis in either of the two views to the distal internal carotid artery diameter in the same view.[2]

A total of 337 Doppler examinations of the carotid artery were performed in 170 patients by nine different technologists in the three participating centers. A total of 7 patients had unilateral angiograms or underwent study of only one side by Doppler frequency analysis for technical reasons. Thus 333 sides were available for analysis.

There was not significant difference in accuracy among the three participating centers or the nine technologists. Normal values from 15 cases are as follows: peak frequency from low internal carotid of 2.3 ± 0.8 Hz (for a 5-MHz probe) and SBI of 38 ± 9.6. Note that the maximum peak frequency is invariably recorded from a different site than the SBI.

Accuracy of peak frequency

The maximum peak frequency measured from any of the three internal carotid artery recordings on each side was

---

*Medasonics, Inc, Mountainview, Calif.

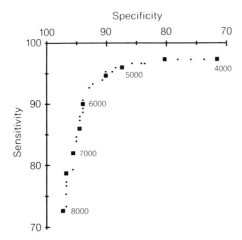

Fig. 33-5. Receiver operating characteristics curve for maximum peak frequency recorded from the internal carotid artery. Angiographic evidence of stenosis greater than 45% was considered a positive test. A 5-MHz probe had been used. (From Johnston KW et al: *J Vasc Surg* 4:493, 1986.)

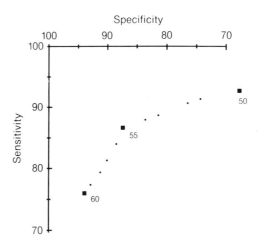

Fig. 33-6. Receiver operating characteristic curve for the maximum spectral broadening index recorded from the internal carotid artery. (From Johnston KW et al: *J Vasc Surg* 4:493, 1986.)

used to determine the accuracy of peak frequency. As illustrated in the receiver operating characteristic (ROC) curve[9,15,16] in Fig. 33-5, as the peak frequency threshold level is increased, the sensitivity decreases but the specificity increases. With a 5-MHz transmitting frequency, the maximal accuracy was 92.2% and was obtained with a peak frequency cutoff threshold value of 5500 Hz. For a peak frequency value of 5500 Hz, the sensitivity was 94.7%, specificity was 92%, positive predictive value was 88.8%, negative predictive value was 95.4%, and the kappa statistic was 0.84.

Accuracy of SBI

The maximum value of the SBI recorded from the internal carotid artery had an overall accuracy of 87.1% when the diagnostic cutoff threshold value was 55%. The ROC curve is shown in Fig. 33-6. For a cutoff value of 55% the sensitivity was 86.7%, specificity was 87.4%, positive predictive value was 85.0%, negative predictive value was 88.9%, and the kappa statistic was 0.74.

Relationship between peak frequency and SBI

When both the peak frequency and the SBI were abnormal (i.e., peak frequency greater than 5500 Hz and SBI greater than 55%), carotid stenosis greater than 45% was present in 117 of 122 cases. When both SBI and peak frequency were normal, a carotid stenosis greater than 45% was present in 5 of 149 cases. When the SBI was more than 55% but peak frequency was less than 5500 Hz, a significant carotid stenosis was present in 3 of 17 cases. When peak frequency was greater than 5500 Hz but the SBI was less than 55%, a significant stenosis was present in 18 of 25 cases.

As described by Sackett,[18] the standard measurements of accuracy from ROC curves have two specific shortcomings.

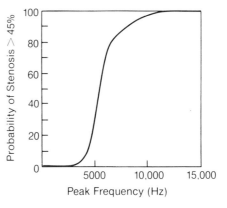

Fig. 33-7. For each value of peak frequency, the probability that the individual patient has stenosis greater than 45% is plotted. A 5-MHz probe had been used. (From Johnston KW et al: *J Vasc Surg* 4:493, 1986.)

They are difficult to apply to the results obtained in the study of an individual patient and they do not take into account the degree of abnormality of the measured test results. The use of a single cutoff value estimates the risk of disease for only two groups of patients, those with measurements above the cutoff value and those with measurements below it. Within each group, this approach will overestimate the risk for some patients and underestimate it for others. These limitations can be overcome by calculating the likelihood ratio. The *likelihood ratio* is defined as the ratio of the relative frequency with which a particular test result is seen in patients who have carotid stenosis greater than 45% to the relative frequency with which it is seen in patients who have carotid stenosis less than 45%. Fig. 33-7 shows the percentage probability that an individual patient has a stenosis greater than 45% for each value of peak frequency. Fig. 33-8 shows the percentage chance that a patient has stenosis greater than 45% for each value of SBI. Peak frequency measurements and SBI can be combined to more precisely define the chances that an individual patient has a significant carotid artery stenosis (Fig. 33-9).

In summary, the results of this prospective multicenter study confirm the initial observations of Brown et al[3-5] and those of Spencer and Reid,[19] showing that frequency analysis of CW Doppler recordings can accurately diagnose moderate and severe stenoses or occlusions but not minor stenoses.

AVOIDING POTENTIAL PITFALLS OF THE CAROTID DOPPLER TECHNIQUE

When the CW Doppler method is used for the diagnosis of carotid arterial occlusive disease, accurate and reproducible results can be obtained if several technical details are observed.

Technologist

The technologist must be experienced and well trained so that representative waveforms free of artifacts can be recorded. For example, the common, internal, and external carotid arteries are usually distinguished by the morphologic differences in the shape of their waves, and failure to correctly identify the arteries can lead to serious errors in diagnosis. Also, as in vitro and clinical studies have demonstrated, measurements of peak frequency will be variable unless the technologist holds the Doppler probe at a relatively constant angle and carefully locates the site of the maximum velocity change,[13] which is found directly over the stenosis. Thus the accuracy of the CW carotid Doppler technique strongly depends on the skill of the technician.

Doppler probe

A 5-MHz probe with uniform beam characteristics and an adequate depth of penetration should be used. With an 8- to 10-MHz probe, it has been noted that the Doppler signal may be weak and that there may be a large amount of background noise. This is the result of signal attenuation in patients who have a deep vessel, scar tissue in the neck, or a significant plaque present on the anterior wall of the

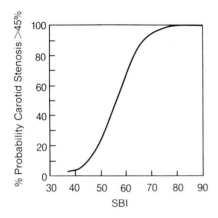

Fig. 33-8. For each value of spectral broadening index (SBI), the probability that the individual patient has stenosis greater than 45% is plotted. (From Johnston KW et al: *J Vasc Surg* 4:493, 1986.)

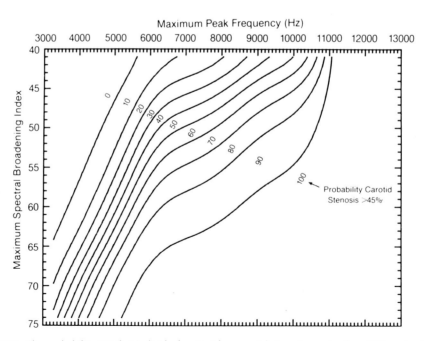

Fig. 33-9. The probability (%) that individual patient has carotid stenosis greater than 45% on basis of measurements of peak frequency and spectral broadening index. Contour lines are in 10% increments. A 5-MHz probe had been used. (From Johnston KW et al: *J Vasc Surg* 4:493, 1986.)

vessel. Ideally, the ultrasound beam produced by the Doppler probe should uniformly insonate the vessel cross section. The beam pattern of commercially available probes has been mapped, and it has been shown that some have very wide beam patterns that do not uniformly insonate the vessel.[6] In some clinical vascular laboratory studies, it has been noted that the clear window under the systolic peak of a normal recording could not be identified if certain probes were used. In contrast, other probes allowed accurate evaluation of the severity of spectral broadening. Thus if the probe beam pattern is not ideal and distorts the spectral waveform, the subtle changes produced by minor flow disturbances may be masked.

Doppler velocity meter

The Doppler velocity meter should be of high quality and have excellent separation between the forward and reverse flow channels. With the CW Doppler technique, there is a risk that coexisting venous flow may be recorded along with the arterial signal. With an inferior Doppler velocity meter, the forward and reverse flow signal will appear along with the arterial signal, and as a consequence, accurate evaluation of the spectral waveform is impossible.

Frequency analyzer

A real-time frequency analyzer should be used to give the technologist the benefit of both audio and visual feedback to determine whether the probe is positioned optimally to obtain representative recordings. One of the fundamental problems of frequency analysis is the variability of instantaneous spectrums which may be a result of the inherent random nature of the Doppler signal itself or of the sampling and processing errors introduced by the frequency analyzer. By averaging consecutive spectra, examiners can reduce this variability. In the future, with improved methods of spectral estimation, the accuracy of individual spectral recordings may be improved.

Recording sites and quantification

Five or six recordings are made at 0.5 to 1.0 cm increments along the common carotid/internal carotid axis. The external and internal carotid arteries must be clearly differentiated by making separate external carotid artery recordings.

The maximum peak frequency and the maximum SBI recorded from the internal carotid artery are used for quantification. Note that the maximum peak frequency and the maximum SBI are seldom recorded at the same site. In vitro the SBI is not affected significantly by changes in the flow rate or by the presence of a bulb.

Incomplete vessel insonation

Incomplete insonation of the artery by the ultrasound beam will result in distortion of the spectrum and consequently an error in the measured SBI. Fortunately, this problem can be minimized by moving the probe laterally across the vessel and by searching for the site where the Doppler effect is maximal (i.e., the site at which the audio signal is loudest and the signal-to-noise ratio is best).

ACKNOWLEDGMENTS

The author acknowledges the financial grant support of the Canadian Heart and Stroke Foundation and the secretarial assistance of Ms. Pam Purdy.

REFERENCES

1. Barnes RW et al: Noninvasive ultrasonic carotid angiography: prospective validation by contrast arteriography, *Surgery* 80:328, 1976.
2. Brown PM, Johnston KW: The difficulty of quantifying the severity of carotid stenosis, *Surgery* 92:468, 1982.
3. Brown PM, Johnston KW, Douville Y: Detection of occlusive disease of the carotid artery with continuous-wave Doppler spectral analysis, *Surg Gynecol Obstet* 155:183, 1982.
4. Brown PM, Johnston KW, Kassam M: Real-time Doppler spectral analysis for the measurement of carotid stenosis. In Diethrich EB, ed: *Non-invasive cardiovascular diagnosis*, ed 3, Littletown, Mass, 1982, PSG Publishing.
5. Brown PM et al: A critical study of ultrasound Doppler spectral analysis for detecting carotid disease, *Ultrasound Med Biol* 8:515, 1982.
6. Douville Y et al: Critical evaluation of continuous wave Doppler probes for carotid studies, *J Clin Ultrasound* 11:83, 1983.
7. Douville Y et al: An in vitro model and its application for the study of carotid Doppler spectral broadening, *Ultrasound Med Biol* 9:347, 1983.
8. Douville Y et al: An in vitro study of carotid Doppler spectral broadening, *Ultrasound Med Biol* 9:347, 1983.
9. Haynes BL: How to read clinical journals. II. To learn about a diagnostic test, *Can Med Assoc J* 124:703, 1981.
10. Johnston KW et al: Quantitative analysis of continuous-wave Doppler spectral broadening for the diagnosis of carotid disease: results of a multicenter study, *J Vasc Surg* 4:493, 1986.
11. Kassam M et al: Quantification of carotid arterial disease by Doppler ultrasound, *IEEE Ultrasonics Symposium* 675, 1982.
12. Keagy BA et al: Evaluation of the peak frequency ratio (PFR) measurement in the detection of internal carotid artery stenosis, *J Clin Ultrasound* 10:109, 1982.
13. Lally M, Johnston KW, Cobbold RSC: Limitations in the accuracy of peak frequency measurements in the diagnosis of carotid disease, *J Clin Ultrasound* 12:403, 1984.
14. Maruzzo BC, Johnston KW, Cobbold RSC: Real-time spectral analysis of directional Doppler flow signals, *Digest of XI International Conference on Medical and Biological Engineering*, Ottawa, 168, 1976.
15. McNeil BJ, Keller E, Adelstein SJ: Primer on certain elements of medical decision making, *N Engl J Med* 293:211, 1975.
16. Metz CE: Basic principles of ROC analysis, *Semin Nucl Med* 8:283, 1978.
17. Rittgers SE, Thornhill BM, Barnes RW: Quantitative analysis of carotid artery Doppler spectral waveforms—diagnostic value of parameters, *Ultrasound Med Biol* 9:255, 1983.
18. Sackett DL: Interpretation of diagnostic data. 5. How to do it with simple maths, *Can Med Assoc J* 129:947, 1983.
19. Spencer MP, Reid JM: Quantitation of carotid stenosis with continuous wave (CW) Doppler ultrasound, *Stroke* 10:326, 1979.

CHAPTER 34

Real-time color flow Doppler carotid imaging

R. EUGENE ZIERLER

Ultrasonic duplex scanning, first described in 1974, has become the standard noninvasive method for examining the extracranial carotid artery.[1,13] This technique evaluates arterial anatomy with B-mode imaging and hemodynamic patterns by spectral analysis of pulsed Doppler flow signals. The small sample volume of the pulsed Doppler system allows characterization of flow patterns at specific sites in the arterial lumen. In the standard approach to duplex scanning, a single pulsed Doppler sample volume is used, and flow patterns within the imaged vessels are evaluated by manually positioning the sample volume at the points of interest.

One of the principal limitations of the standard approach is that only a small region of the arterial lumen can be evaluated at any one time. The single pulsed Doppler sample volume must be moved serially to various sites within the B-mode image to obtain complete information on flow patterns. This process can be tedious, and flow disturbances that are confined to a small section of the vessel may be overlooked. In addition, the complex three-dimensional features of flow in the bifurcation of the common carotid artery are difficult to appreciate with the single sample volume technique.

This chapter describes initial clinical experience with real-time color flow duplex imaging of the extracranial carotid artery. Color flow instruments display a real-time color image of blood flow superimposed on a two-dimensional, B-mode tissue image. With a color scale to indicate the magnitude and direction of blood flow, the flow patterns in normal and diseased carotid arteries can be visualized with remarkable temporal and spatial detail.

SPECTRAL ANALYSIS AND COLOR FLOW IMAGING

In the standard approach to carotid duplex scanning, the B-mode image is used to locate the arteries and facilitate placement of the pulsed Doppler sample volume. The severity of disease is then determined by spectral analysis of the pulsed Doppler signals. Spectral waveforms are represented with Doppler shift frequency or velocity on the vertical axis, time is represented on the horizontal axis, and amplitude is indicated by a gray scale. The amplitude of the signal is proportional to the number of blood cells passing through the sample volume. Experience has shown that arterial lesions are associated with flow patterns that can be characterized by spectral analysis. Normal center stream arterial flow is laminar, so the corresponding spectral waveforms show a narrow band of frequencies. Arterial lesions disturb this normal pattern and result in spectral waveforms with a wider range of frequencies and amplitudes. This increased width of the frequency band is called spectral broadening. Severe stenoses produce high-velocity jets that appear in spectral waveforms as increased peak systolic frequencies. As discussed in Chapter 31, a set of criteria has been developed for classification of internal carotid artery stenoses with contrast arteriography as the standard test.[3,6,10,11] This approach can distinguish between normal and diseased internal carotid arteries with a sensitivity of 99% and a specificity of 84%. The overall accuracy for identifying 50% to 99% diameter stenosis and occlusion is 93%.[10]

Real-time color flow imaging is an alternative to spectral analysis for displaying the pulsed Doppler information obtained by duplex scanning. Although spectral analysis evaluates the entire frequency and amplitude content of the signal at a selected site, color flow imaging provides a single estimate of the Doppler shift or flow velocity for each site within the B-mode image. Thus spectral waveforms actually give considerably more information on flow at each individual site than color flow imaging. The main advantage of the color flow display is that it presents flow information on the entire image, even though the amount of data for each site is reduced.

Because of these differences, it is often difficult to compare the Doppler information obtained by spectral analysis to that based on color flow imaging. Spectral waveforms contain a range of frequencies and amplitudes, which allow determination of flow direction and parameters such as mean, mode, peak, and bandwidth. In contrast, color assignments for the color flow image are based on flow direction and a single mean or average frequency estimate. Consequently, the peak Doppler frequency shifts or velocities seen with spectral analysis are generally higher than the frequencies or velocities indicated by color flow imaging.

Color flow imaging is based on pulsed Doppler ultrasound and is therefore subject to the same physical limitations as pulsed Doppler imaging with spectral analysis. For example, since the Doppler frequency shift depends on the beam-to-vessel angle, color assignments will be accurate only if this angle is properly set and remains constant along the length of a vessel. Unfortunately, blood vessels are seldom straight, so color differences may represent either true velocity changes or variations in the frequency shift

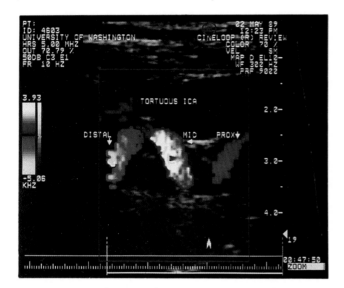

Fig. 34-1. Color flow image of a tortuous internal carotid artery *(ICA)*. Changes in color from shades of red to shades of blue result from different angles between the flow stream and the ultrasound scan lines; no color appears when the angle approaches 90°.

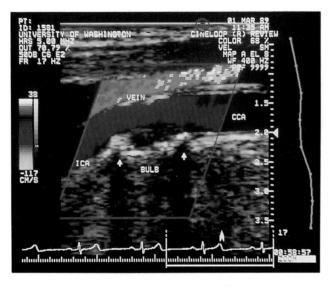

Fig. 34-2. Color flow image of a common carotid artery *(CCA)*, internal carotid artery *(ICA)*, and internal jugular vein *(VEIN)*. Flow in the arterial direction is represented by shades of red and in the venous direction by shades of blue. An atherosclerotic plaque, indicated by thickening of the vessel wall and shadowing due to calcification, is present along the posterior wall of the carotid bulb *(BULB)*. The carotid lumen appears widely patent.

that result from changes in the Doppler angle. This potential source of error should always be considered when color flow images are interpreted (Fig. 34-1). Another problem that can occur in both spectral analysis and color flow imaging is the pulsed Doppler artifact called *aliasing*. Aliasing in spectral analysis produces an abrupt loss of the waveform above the Nyquist limit, with the missing portion appearing below the baseline as flow in the reverse direction. This appears to indicate that the blood underwent a sudden and discontinuous change in speed and direction. When aliasing is present in a color flow image, high-velocity jets are assigned colors that indicate flow in the direction opposite to arterial flow. (More detailed discussions of color flow imaging are presented in Chapters 12 and 13.)

Shades of two distinct colors, typically red and blue, are used to indicate direction of flow relative to the ultrasound scan lines. The display is generally set up by the examiner to show flow in the arterial direction as red and flow in the venous direction as blue (Fig. 34-2). Variations in the Doppler frequency shift or flow velocity are then indicated by changes in color, with lighter shades representing higher flow velocities. The specific features of the color flow image vary considerably among the commercially available ultrasound instruments. However, a single sample volume pulsed Doppler analyzer and a spectrum analyzer are also included as part of the color flow instrument to allow detailed evaluation of flow patterns at selected arterial sites.

EXAMINATION TECHNIQUE

The basic examination technique with a color flow instrument is similar to that for standard duplex scanning. First, the common carotid artery is imaged low in the neck and followed distally to its bifurcation. The internal and external carotid arteries can usually be identified according to their typical location, with the internal carotid posterolaterally and the external carotid anteromedially. The bulb may be seen as a dilatation of the arterial lumen at the origin of the internal carotid artery (Fig. 34-3). Flow patterns are most easily visualized when the arteries are scanned in longitudinal section. Occasionally, transverse scans are useful for showing unusual anatomic relationships among the various carotid branches. Particular care is taken to completely visualize the flow pattern in the carotid bulb or proximal internal carotid artery. Abnormal flow disturbances such as high-velocity jets and poststenotic turbulence are also noted.

NORMAL CAROTID FLOW PATTERNS

The color flow duplex scanner has been used to evaluate flow patterns in normal carotid bifurcations.[12] Peak systolic flow velocity in the common carotid artery is higher in the center stream than near the vessel wall, as indicated by the predominance of lighter color shades in the middle of the lumen. The lower flow velocities present during diastole are associated with darker shades in the center stream. A small, transient region of reverse flow is often observed in the common carotid artery adjacent to the vessel wall. This

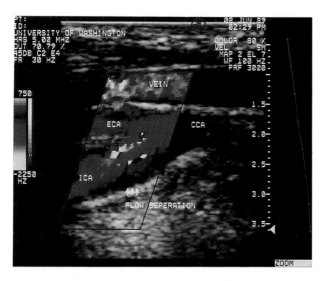

Fig. 34-3. Color flow image of a normal carotid bifurcation showing the common carotid artery *(CCA)*, external carotid artery *(ECA)*, internal carotid artery *(ICA)*, and internal jugular vein *(VEIN)*. An area of flow separation is present along the posterior wall of the carotid bulb.

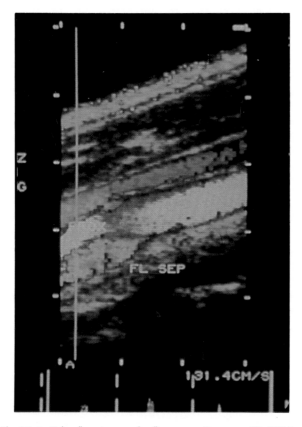

Fig. 34-4. Color flow image of a flow separation zone *(FL SEP)* in a normal internal carotid artery. Flow separation occurs along the outer wall of the carotid bulb, appearing as an oval blue area at peak systole. Continuous forward flow is present adjacent to the separation zone along the flow divider in the proximal internal carotid artery *(PROX)*. The pulsed Doppler sample volume is in the area of forward flow. The external carotid artery is not in the image plane.

reverse flow component is a consequence of the flow deceleration that occurs across the carotid lumen in late systole or early diastole, which slows the higher velocities in the center stream and briefly reverses the lower velocities near the arterial wall.

The carotid bulb occupies a variable portion of the distal common and proximal internal carotid arteries. A zone of boundary-layer separation or flow separation is normally present near the origin of the internal carotid artery (Fig. 34-3).[2] This zone is located along the posterior or outer wall of the bulb on the side opposite the flow divider. Since flow direction in the separation zone is primarily in the reverse direction, the zone usually appears as an oval-shaped blue area. Fig. 34-4 shows the typical appearance of the separation zone. The size of the separation zone fluctuates during the cardiac cycle and is largest around peak systole. During diastole, the separation zone often appears as a dark area, which represents very low flow velocities. These separation zones are limited to the bulb and are not present in the distal internal carotid artery. Continuous forward flow is present in the bulb along the flow divider. A smaller zone of flow separation is occasionally found near the origin of the external carotid artery. The features of separation zones in normal carotid bifurcations have been delineated by model studies and clinical pulsed Doppler examinations.[4,5,7,9]

ABNORMAL CAROTID FLOW PATTERNS

Initial clinical experience with color flow instruments has concentrated on the qualitative evaluation of flow patterns associated with carotid artery disease.[14] Color flow imaging provides a means for visualizing not only the center stream flow pattern but also the interface between the arterial wall and flowing blood. Although carotid arteries with minimal disease generally have normal center stream flow patterns, disturbed flow can sometimes be observed adjacent to the vessel wall. As shown in Fig. 34-2, accumulation of atherosclerotic plaque results in a gradual filling in of the carotid bulb. As this occurs, the normal diverging and converging geometry of the carotid bulb is lost, and the separation zone disappears. Thus mild to moderate lesions of the carotid bifurcation are characterized by absence of the normal separation zone in the bulb and disturbances in the color flow image near the vessel wall.

Stenoses that narrow the carotid artery diameter by 50% or more are associated with distinct changes in the center stream flow pattern. The color flow image of a severe internal carotid stenosis is shown in Fig. 34-5. Although flow in the prestenotic segment appears relatively normal, a high-velocity stenotic jet is seen as a narrowing in the flow stream with aliasing of the color flow image. The mosaic color pattern in the poststenotic segment is typical of the turbulent flow immediately distal to a severe stenosis and is analogous to the broadening of poststenotic spectral waveforms.

Color flow imaging has also been useful for identifying unusual anatomic features of the carotid bifurcation such as tortuosity or kinking (Fig. 34-1). These features can be

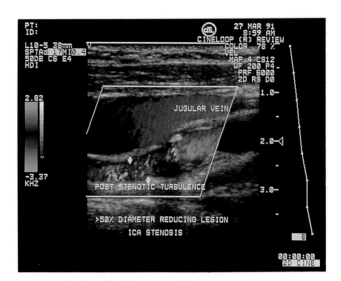

Fig. 34-5. Severe internal carotid artery *(ICA)* stenosis. The color flow image shows normal flow in the prestenotic segment, a high-velocity jet with aliasing, and poststenotic turbulence.

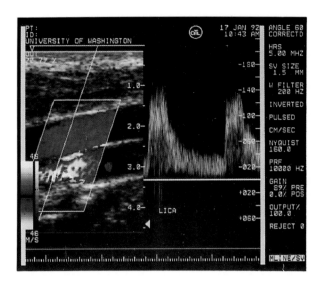

Fig. 34-7. Color flow image and spectral waveform taken from a left internal carotid artery *(LICA)* with a 50% to 79% diameter stenosis. Although the color flow image suggests an abnormal flow pattern, classification of stenosis severity is based on the features of the spectral waveform.

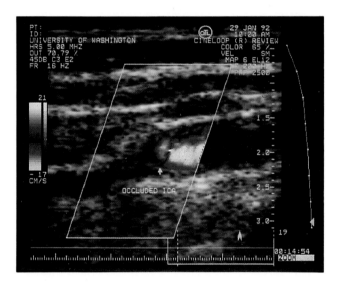

Fig. 34-6. Occluded internal carotid artery *(ICA)*. Occlusion is indicated by failure to visualize flow on the color image distal to the bifurcation. The small blue area represents transient reversal of flow at the site of occlusion.

difficult to recognize with standard duplex scanning techniques. Internal carotid occlusion is indicated by failure to identify flow in that vessel, common carotid flow velocity decreasing to zero in late diastole, and presence of flow in the external carotid artery. In addition, the site of occlusion in the proximal internal carotid can often be visualized (Fig. 34-6). Audible bruits are occasionally seen in color flow images as speckled areas of red and blue that extend beyond the arterial wall into the adjacent tissue.

CLINICAL APPLICATIONS

Color flow imaging systems offer several potential advantages over the standard approach to duplex scanning. With

areas of flow within a B-mode image displayed, the branches of the carotid bifurcation can be easily identified. This facilitates recognition of localized flow disturbances and areas of flow separation.[12] Although it is possible to characterize these flow patterns with standard duplex scanning techniques, it is usually not practical because of the longer examination time required. Thus it is expected that color flow imaging will shorten the examination time and reduce the need for evaluating flow patterns at multiple sites with a single pulsed Doppler sample volume.

As previously discussed, the color flow instrument also functions as a standard duplex scanner, and the criteria for interpretation of spectral waveforms must still be used to classify the extent of carotid disease (Fig. 34-7). However, the color flow image may enhance the accuracy of spectral analysis by allowing optimal positioning of the pulsed Doppler sample volume at sites of disease. Although there are currently no definitive criteria for interpretation of color flow images alone, certain waveform features such as spectral broadening appear to be associated with distinct color patterns.

To determine whether color flow imaging actually improves the accuracy of carotid duplex scanning, a study was conducted in two vascular laboratories: one laboratory had a color flow imaging instrument and the other laboratory had only a standard duplex scanner.[8] A total of 307 internal carotid arteries were evaluated by color flow imaging and arteriography, and 206 internal carotid arteries were evaluated by standard duplex scanning and arteriography. Perfect agreement between the noninvasive test result and the arteriogram occurred in 87% of the color flow examinations and 80% of the standard duplex scans. In addition, significantly fewer arteries were overclassified by one disease category when color flow imaging was used. Although this comparative study supported the overall accuracy of both duplex techniques, there was a strong trend toward improved diagnostic results with color flow imaging. This difference was attributed to more precise placement of the pulsed Doppler sample volume when the color flow image was used as a guide.

Duplex scanning is now generally regarded as the preferred method for noninvasive evaluation of the carotid bifurcation. Clinical applications include screening of patients for carotid artery disease, monitoring patients with previously documented lesions, and follow-up of patients after carotid endarterectomy. Although the diagnostic role of color flow imaging has not been clearly established, the advantages of this technology are extremely appealing. Those who prefer images over spectral information will be impressed by the visual effect of the color flow display. However, since the overall accuracy of the standard duplex approach is already quite favorable, the additional value of color flow imaging in routine noninvasive carotid testing may be relatively small. Color flow imaging is most likely to be helpful in selected patients who have atypical arterial anatomy or suspected internal carotid occlusion.

REFERENCES

1. Barber FE et al: Ultrasonic duplex echo-Doppler scanner, *IEEE Trans Biomed Eng* 21:109, 1974.
2. Bharadvaj BK, Mabon RF, Giddens DP: Steady flow in a model of the human carotid bifurcation. Part I. Flow visualization, *J Biomechanics* 15:349, 1982.
3. Fell G et al: Ultrasonic duplex scanning for disease of the carotid artery, *Circulation* 64:1191, 1981.
4. Ku DN, Giddens DP: Pulsatile flow in a model carotid bifurcation, *Arteriosclerosis* 3:31, 1983.
5. Ku DN et al: Hemodynamics of the normal human carotid bifurcation: in vitro and in vivo studies, *Ultrasound Med Biol* 11:13, 1985.
6. Langlois YE et al: Evaluating carotid artery disease—the concordance between pulsed Doppler/spectrum analysis and angiography, *Ultrasound Med Biol* 9:51, 1983.
7. LoGerfo FW, Nowak MD, Quist WC: Structural details of boundary layer separation in a model human carotid bifurcation under steady and pulsatile flow conditions, *J Vasc Surg* 2:263, 1985.
8. Londrey GL et al: Does color-flow imaging improve the accuracy of duplex carotid evaluation? *J Vasc Surg* 13:659, 1991.
9. Phillips DJ et al: Flow velocity patterns in the carotid bifurcations of young, presumed normal subjects, *Ultrasound Med Biol* 9:39, 1983.
10. Roederer GO et al: Ultrasonic duplex scanning of extracranial carotid arteries—improved accuracy using new features from the common carotid artery, *J Cardiovasc Ultrasonography* 1:373, 1982.
11. Roederer GO et al: A simple spectral parameter for accurate classification of severe carotid disease, *Bruit* 8:174, 1984.
12. Spadone DP et al: Contralateral internal carotid artery stenosis or occlusion: pitfall of correct ipsilateral classification—a study performed with color-flow imaging, *J Vasc Surg* 11:642, 1990.
13. Strandness DE Jr: Ultrasound in the study of atherosclerosis, *Ultrasound Med Biol* 12:453, 1986.
14. Zierler RE et al: Color-flow ultrasound imaging of the normal and diseased carotid bifurcation, *Dynamic Cardiovasc Imaging* 1:34, 1987.
15. Zierler RE et al: Noninvasive assessment of normal carotid bifurcation hemodynamics with color-flow ultrasound imaging, *Ultrasound Med Biol* 13:471, 1987.

CHAPTER 35

Importance of carotid plaque morphology

LINDA M. REILLY

The controversy surrounding carotid endarterectomy centers around the risk associated with the procedure compared with the risk associated with the atheromatous lesion. If it were possible to consistently identify the patient with occlusive disease of the carotid bifurcation in whom a neurologic event would occur if the patient were left untreated, the risk-benefit ratio of carotid endarterectomy would be altered dramatically. Unfortunately, the features associated with carotid atheroma that reliably predict neurologic risk have not been defined because the mechanisms of cerebral ischemia production by carotid atheroma are incompletely understood. Initial efforts to identify the clinically significant carotid lesion emphasized flow reduction as the cause of neurologic symptoms, and thus the degree of stenosis resulting from a lesion was thought to be the basis for the risk of neurologic events.[11] However, a highly variable correlation between lesion size and the presence of symptoms,[32,39] as well as the increasing evidence of the embolic causes of most strokes,[20] began to focus attention on the role of plaque structure itself in the production of cerebral ischemia.

Although Fisher[12] observed that hemorrhage within carotid plaques was common as early as 1954, plaque ulceration—with its embolic potential—was first emphasized as most predictive of neurologic risk.* In 1974, Houser et al[16] again reported the frequent finding of hemorrhage in carotid plaques and concluded that it represented a partial dissection originating at the site of an ulceration. In 1979, Imparato et al[17] reported the results of a clinicopathologic study of carotid atheroma that implicated intraplaque hemorrhage as the only gross morphologic characteristic occurring significantly more frequently in symptomatic lesions than in asymptomatic ones. Their careful analysis of specimens showed that these intramural hemorrhages were often completely encompassed by an unbroken fibrointimal cap. They concluded that ulceration more likely resulted from thinning and breakdown of the overlying intima that was due to the contained hemorrhage rather than from the mechanism proposed by Houser et al and postulated that the hemorrhage

itself originated from ruptured vasa vasorum. Shortly thereafter, Lusby et al[27] published their microscopic analysis of plaque and confirmed the relationship of plaque hemorrhage to both neurologic symptoms and the appearance of intimal ulceration. Thus plaque hemorrhage seemed to offer an important refinement in the ability to identify the clinically significant carotid lesion and also offered a plausible mechanism for the pathogenesis of the ulcerated plaque, which had already been associated with the appearance of symptoms.

The two reports by Imparato et al[17] and Lusby et al[27] were based on pathologic studies, one on gross morphology and the other on both gross and microscopic analysis. Plaque morphology must be identified preoperatively to be used to assess clinical risk and to determine the necessity for surgery. Imparato et al[17] concluded that a rational therapeutic regimen for carotid occlusive disease would not be possible until patients could be classified according to the pathologic changes in plaque, diagnosed noninvasively.

NONINVASIVE DETECTION OF INTRAPLAQUE HEMORRHAGE

In 1979, Edwards et al[8] described the characteristic angiographic appearance of subintimal hematoma of the carotid artery as a sharply marginated, rounded, often eccentric filling defect with smooth contours and abrupt limitations. They found this radiographic image in 7 of 12 specimens (58.3%) with plaque hemorrhage. Their study was flawed by the fact that 41.6% of the specimens with hemorrhage did not conform to this picture, by the small number of specimens, and by the failure to provide any comparative description of the angiographic appearance of specimens without hemorrhage. Furthermore, angiography is a luminal imaging technique and obviously provides only inferential data on plaque structure or content. Subsequent studies comparing conventional angiography with duplex scanning in the evaluation of carotid plaque morphology have confirmed the inferiority of angiography in this area.[1,37] Nonetheless, the study by Edwards was the first attempt to diagnose plaque hemorrhage preoperatively.

In contrast to angiography, ultrasound imaging was rec-

---

*References 4, 10, 21, 28, 38, 43.

333

ognized to be a noninvasive technique with the unique potential to assess both luminal features and arterial wall structure. Although it was already well established as a method of detecting flow abnormalities and determining the severity of stenosis, the first report of the ultrasonographic characterization of carotid plaque composition did not appear until 1983. In that study, Reilly et al[34] reported the results of both gross and microscopic analysis of the plaque content of 50 endarterectomy specimens compared with a blinded interpretation of the preoperative sonograms. They identified two distinct ultrasound echo patterns produced by carotid atheroma: heterogeneous and homogeneous. The homogeneous pattern was characterized by a uniform appearance of high- or medium-level echoes with or without acoustic shadowing. The heterogeneous pattern was a mixture of high-, medium-, and low-level echoes (mostly low- and medium-level) and often showed an area contained within the plaque with the same echogenicity as blood.

Among the 36 heterogeneous lesions in this study, 30 (83.3%) contained intraplaque hemorrhage. The 6 false-positive studies resulted from plaque content that consisted of large amounts of lipid, cholesterol, loose stroma, proteinaceous deposits, or a combination of these. Of the 14 homogeneous lesions, 11 (78.6%) were smooth fibrous plaques with no detectable intraplaque hemorrhage. The 3 false-negative studies resulted from very small foci (less than 2 mm) of old, organized hemorrhage. All specimens with histologically proven surface ulceration demonstrated the heterogeneous ultrasound pattern preoperatively, and no lesion with a heterogeneous echo pattern was a smooth fibrous plaque. There was a statistically significant correlation between the heterogeneous ultrasound pattern and the presence of hemorrhage ($p = 0.00008$, Fisher's exact test, one-tailed), as well as with the presence of ulceration ($p = 0.011$, Fisher's exact test, one-tailed), when compared with the homogeneous ultrasound pattern. Overall, duplex scanning detected intraplaque hemorrhage with an accuracy of 82% (41 of 50), a sensitivity of 91% (30 of 33), and a specificity of 65% (11 of 17).

Subsequently, seven additional studies* were conducted to investigate the ability of ultrasound imaging to diagnose plaque hemorrhage noninvasively (Table 35-1). Five of these studies were prospective, and in all seven the histologic analysis of the plaque specimens was performed by a reviewer who had no knowledge of the interpretation of the ultrasound images. The same two ultrasound echo patterns produced by the carotid atheroma were described in five of these studies, although O'Donnell et al[29] used the term *nonhomogeneous* instead of heterogeneous. Gray-Weale et al[15] subdivided the ultrasound images into four different categories from most echolucent (type 1) to most echogenic (type 4), but for purposes of statistical analysis, they recombined them into only two groups. In the seventh study, Widder et al[42] separated their analysis into two categories, plaque density (echogenic versus echolucent) and plaque structure (hetereogeneous versus homogeneous). In four of these studies, no statistical analysis was performed,[1,15,29,42] but sufficient data are included in the articles to allow statistical assessment.

A statistically significant correlation between the duplex ultrasound heterogeneous echo pattern and intraplaque hemorrhage is confirmed by the data in six of the seven studies (Table 35-1). In general, the sensitivity achieved in these studies greatly exceeded the specificity. This uniformly high false-positive rate results from a similar heterogeneous ultrasonographic appearance for plaques with a substantial content of lipid, cholesterol, proteinaceous debris, loose stroma, or extensive calcification. Two recent histopathologic studies,[9,25] representing essentially the same data from a group of investigators published in two different journals, documented that the most common component of the plaques they analyzed was an eosinophilic-staining amorphous material that contained various amounts of cholesterol. These authors suggest that this material has been incorrectly classified as old or degenerating hemorrhage in other studies. It is clear that the heterogeneous ultrasound

*References 1, 6, 15, 29, 33, 40, 42.

Table 35-1. Correlation of ultrasound plaque appearance and presence of intraplaque hemorrhage

Author	N	Sensitivity (%)	Specificity (%)	Accuracy (%)	p Value*
Reilly et al[34]	50	90.9	64.7	82.0	0.00008
Ratliff et al[33]	42	72.2	41.7	54.8	NSS
O'Donnell et al[29]	79	93.1	84.0	87.3	0.0001†
Bluth et al[6]	53	94.4	88.6	90.6	<0.005
Weinberger et al[40]	54	97.1	50.0	79.6	<0.01
Aldoori et al[1]	27	90.5	83.3	88.9	0.0014†
Gray-Weale et al[15]	244	89.2	60.3	79.9	0.0001†
Widder et al[42]	165	80.5	56.5	62.4	0.0001†
	119	96.0	45.2	52.1	0.0013†
TOTAL‡	549	89.9	67.8	80.7	

NSS, Not statistically significant.
*All statistical analysis by chi-square contingency analysis with Yates' continuity correction, except for Weinberger et al: Fisher's exact test, one-tailed.
†Analysis of data provided in authors' manuscript.
‡Excluding results of Widder et al.

echo pattern is *not* specific for plaque hemorrhage but that it does have a substantial correlation with it.

Two studies reported notably poor specificity, sensitivity, and accuracy. The study by Widder et al[42] suffers from a high incidence of poor-quality ultrasound images, which appears to be related to suboptimal equipment used at the start of the study. In addition, the separation of plaque density and plaque structure into two distinct categories would predictably worsen the results, since these two features are essentially combined into the definition of heterogeneous and homogeneous in the other published series. Widder et al[42] acknowledge this by claiming that combining parameters may improve results. The combination of echolucency and heterogeneous structure increased the positive predictive value for the detection of intraplaque hemorrhage to at least 62%.[44] This was an improvement from 43% and 26%, respectively, for the two features assessed independently. In spite of the fact that the authors concluded that ultrasound scanning could not reliably detect intraplaque hemorrhage, mainly because it could not be distinguished from atheromatous debris in the plaque, statistical analysis of their raw data demonstrates a significant correlation between echolucency and intraplaque hemorrhage ($p = 0.0001$, chi-square analysis), and between heterogeneous structure and intraplaque hemorrhage ($p = 0.0013$, chi-square analysis).

Only the study by Ratliff et al[33] showed no significant correlation between intraplaque hemorrhage and the appearance of the preoperative ultrasound scan. They concluded that "the only component of atheromatous lesions of the internal carotid that can be characterized from the B-scan is calcification" and theorized that since "calcium deposits within intimal plaque are responsible for marked attenuation of transmitted ultrasound . . . the dark area in heterogeneous lesions might be interpreted as intraplaque hemorrhage by some observers." This study differs from the other six studies in one significant aspect. The authors divided the specimens into those with a *low content* and those with a *high content* of plaque hemorrhage, whereas the other studies characterized specimens as those with *any* plaque hemorrhage and those with *none*. This variation in the analysis of specimens makes it difficult to determine the significance of the negative results in Ratliff's series.[33]

Overall, pooling the results of all of the studies (except for the study by Widder et al[42]) yields an accuracy of 80.7% (443 of 549), a sensitivity of 89.9% (287 of 319), and a specificity of 67.8% (156 of 230) when sonographic imaging is used to determine carotid plaque histology and, specifically, to identify intraplaque hemorrhage preoperatively. (The data from the study by Widder et al[42] cannot be included without double-counting the specimens because of the different methodology for categorization of the ultrasound images.) These data support the conclusion that ultrasound imaging is an acceptably reliable method for the noninvasive determination of plaque content.

The rapid application of ultrasound imaging to the di-agnosis of intraplaque hemorrhage resulted from its preexisting widespread use in the routine assessment of extracranial cerebrovascular disease. Its safety (noninvasiveness, lack of radiation exposure) and low cost make it the ideal choice for the sequential study of these lesions. Despite these obvious advantages, which give ultrasound imaging favored status for characterization of the structure of carotid plaque, it is not the only technique that has been studied. Culebras et al[7] reported the use of computed tomography to detect plaque hemorrhage. In this study, discrete, lucent defects seen within the carotid plaque correlated with the histologic demonstration of plaque hemorrhage in 13 of 15 lesions with such lucent defects. Unfortunately, only 4 specimens without lucent defects as determined by computed tomographic scan were available for histologic analysis, but 3 of these had no evidence of intraplaque hemorrhage. No statistical analysis was performed on these preliminary data, and no further studies or follow-up data have published.

Perhaps more intriguing is the potential use of magnetic resonance imaging to assess the content of atherosclerotic plaques. Presently, this technique, modified to produce an image analogous to an angiogram (magnetic resonance angiography), is being used with increasing frequency to assess carotid stenosis, but no attempts to perform plaque content analysis have been undertaken. Nonetheless, the concept of keying the scan to the presence of a specific ion or element might allow precise and consistent detection of intraplaque hemorrhage. An obvious concern with magnetic resonance technology is the cost.

CLINICAL SIGNIFICANCE OF CAROTID INTRAPLAQUE HEMORRHAGE

The ability to detect intraplaque hemorrhage noninvasively is only important if intraplaque hemorrhage is clinically significant, that is, if it has some correlation with the development of neurologic symptoms. Since the first report of Imparato et al[17] 13 years ago, many studies have investigated the relationship between plaque hemorrhage and neurologic signs and symptoms of cerebral ischemia. Unfortunately, these studies are more notable for their differences than for their similarities. Thus the question, What is the clinical significance of carotid intraplaque hemorrhage? remains difficult to answer.

Studies of the association of plaque hemorrhage and neurologic symptoms have generally focused on one of three possible correlations: (1) the presence of any hemorrhage in the plaque, (2) the presence of acute or recent hemorrhage (less than 6 weeks old) in the plaque, or (3) hemorrhage accounting for more than half of the plaque content (Table 35-2). The original article by Imparato et al[17] actually focused on this last possible correlation. Ironically, the data in that study, when subjected to statistical analysis, show no significant correlation between what the investigators termed significant plaque hemorrhage and neurologic signs and symptoms. The authors themselves pointed out that the random method of selecting specimens (the study group of

69 was a subgroup of 850 available specimens) invalidates any meaningful statistical analysis, and therefore they did not include those results in the article. In only two subsequent reports (Table 35-2) was the size of intraplaque hemorrhage with respect to the development of symptoms studied, and opposite conclusions were reached.[14,26] Bassiouny et al[5] also investigated plaque hemorrhage size and found no correlation with symptoms, but all plaque hemorrhages in their series were quite small, averaging only 1% to 2.5% of the plaque area. Feeley et al[9] also encountered small-volume plaque hemorrhages in their specimens, averaging 1% to 2%, with a maximum hemorrhage content of 13%. The reason for the very small hemorrhages in these two studies, in comparison with the large hemorrhages usually seen in the majority of studies, is not clear.

The series of Lusby et al[27] first introduced the concept that the age of the plaque hemorrhage might be the factor that determined neurologic risk (Table 35-2). In their prospective, consecutive, blinded study, acute or recent plaque hemorrhage (less than 6 weeks old) occurred significantly more often among symptomatic lesions than among asymptomatic ones ($p < 0.005$, chi-square analysis). Similar results were later reported by Fryer et al.[14] Ammar et al[3] also showed a significant correlation between the presence of acute or recent hemorrhage and the onset of symptoms, although they did not include these data or statistical analysis in their original report. In contrast, four studies could find no correlation between age of plaque hemorrhage and symptoms.[5,9,26,34] The carefully conducted retrospective analysis by Lennihan's group[26] used a different definition of acute and recent hemorrhage (less than 4 weeks old) and also required a match between the time of onset of symptoms and the age of the plaque hemorrhage, which is a reasonable stipulation. The three studies with a positive correlation made no similar attempt to match age of hemorrhage with the time that symptoms appeared. Feeley et al[9] and Bassiouny et al[5] are the only investigators to consistently observe very small foci of hemorrhage in their specimens, and this difference may have had some impact on their negative results. Additionally, both of these studies involved a rel-

Table 35-2. Clinicohistopathologic studies of carotid atheroma

Reference	N	Frequency of plaque hemorrhage		Correlation of plaque hemorrhage and neurologic symptoms (*p* value)*
		N	%	
PRESENCE OF ANY INTRAPLAQUE HEMORRHAGE				
Imparato et al[18]	376	115	30.6	<0.02
Persson[30]	160	131	81.8	0.0001†
Fisher and Ojemann[13]	141	47	33.3	0.007†
Fryer, Myers, and Appleberg[14]	91	78	85.7	0.0009†
Lusby et al[27]	79	77	97.5	NSS†
Reilly et al[34]	50	33	66.0	NSS
Ricotta et al[35]	84	34	40.5	NSS
Ammar et al[2]	95	83	87.3	NSS
Lennihan et al[26]	198	96	48.5	NSS
Bassiouny et al[5]	45	33	73.3	NSS
PRESENCE OF INTRAPLAQUE HEMORRHAGE >50% OF THE PLAQUE				
Fryer, Myers, and Appleberg[14]	91	43	47.3	0.0026†
Imparato, Riles, and Gorstein[17]	69	45	65.2	NSS†
Lennihan et al[26]	198	21	10.6	NSS
PRESENCE OF ACUTE OR RECENT INTRAPLAQUE HEMORRHAGE				
Lusby et al[27]	79	56	70.9	<0.005
Ammar et al[2]	95	44	46.3	0.0437†
Fryer, Myers, and Appleberg[14]	91	67	73.6	0.0027†
Reilly et al[34]	50	20	40.0	NSS
Lennihan et al[26]	198	46	23.2	NSS†
Bassiouny et al[5]	45	Not stated	Not stated	NSS
Feeley et al[9]	52	28	53.8	NSS†
PRESENCE OF MULTIPLE INTRAPLAQUE HEMORRHAGES				
Ammar et al[3]	95	47	49.5	<0.05

NSS, Not statistically significant.
*All statistical analysis by chi-square contingency analysis with Yates' continuity correction, except for Fryer, Myers, and Appleberg[14]; any plaque hemorrhage: Fisher's exact test, one-tailed.
†Analysis of data provided in the authors' manuscript.

atively small sample size. This was also true of a later study by Lusby's group[27] and may have caused the failure of that study to confirm the positive correlation that was originally reported.

The most popular area of investigation has been the possible correlation between the presence of any plaque hemorrhage and the onset of neurologic symptoms (Table 35-2). In their second large clinicopathologic series, Imparato's group[18] found a significant relationship between these two features, independent of the size of the hemorrhage. Because this study was based only on gross morphology, it included no data on the age of the subintimal hemorrhages. Subsequently, work by Persson et al[30,31] and Fryer, Myers, and Appleberg[14] confirmed the correlation between *any* plaque hemorrhage and the risk of neurologic symptoms. In a fourth report, Fisher and Ojemann[13] stated that they found no correlation between plaque hemorrhage and symptoms (the statistical method was not specified) and concluded that "hemorrhage into plaque posed little or no threat in the present series." However, review of their data shows that 28 of 57 symptomatic plaques contained hemorrhage (49.1%), whereas only 6 of 33 asymptomatic lesions (18.2%) did. With chi-square analysis, this is significant at a *p* value of 0.007. In contrast to the results of these four studies, six other reports, which investigated a possible association between any plaque hemorrhage and the patient's clinical status, failed to show any statistically significant correlation.*

One final area of study has been the significance of multiple intraplaque hemorrhages in the production of signs and symptoms. In many studies,[2,14,26,27,34] investigators have observed that a single plaque often contains hemorrhages of various ages, which indicates repeated episodes of plaque hemorrhage. To date, only Ammar et al[3] have studied the importance of this feature, and they found that it was correlated with the clinical status of the patient (Table 35-2). No confirmatory studies have yet appeared.

In summary, conflicting results have been reported for almost every feature of plaque hemorrhage that has been postulated to have clinical significance. A number of methodologic factors that vary from study to study (Table 35-3) undoubtedly contribute significantly to the inconsistency of the reported results. Among these, the most obvious are the study design, the definition of "symptomatic," the prevalence of severe stenosis in the study population, and the symptom-surgery interval.

Less than half of the recent studies were prospective. Two studies were clearly retrospective, which is particularly important for the otherwise well-designed study of Lennihan et al,[26] in which no significant correlation was found between any feature of plaque hemorrhage (e.g., presence, size, age) and clinical status. Of particular concern in a retrospective study is the accurate symptomatic classification of the patient, the lack of opportunity for special specimen processing with histologic stains designed to discretely determine the presence and features of plaque hemorrhage, and the lack of any in situ or gross morphologic assessment of the specimen. Although some authors[9,13,25] argue that gross plaque assessment to determine the presence of hemorrhage can be

---

*References 2, 5, 26, 27, 34, 35.

Table 35-3. Studies investigating correlation of intraplaque hemorrhage and neurologic symptoms: comparison of methodologies

| Reference | Study design | | Plaque assay method | | | Definition of symptomatic | Prevalence of critical stenosis (%) | Symptom-surgery interval (mean) |
	Prospective	Consecutive	Gross/microscopic	Blinded	Special stains			
Imparato, Riles, and Gorstein[17]	No	No	Both	Unknown	No	Focal	70	Unknown
Lusby et al[27]	Yes	Yes	Both	Yes	Yes	Focal + NLS	>23	All sxs: 3 weeks
Imparato et al[18]	Yes	Yes (10.5%)*	Gross	No	No	Focal	55	Unknown
Reilly et al[34]	Yes	Yes	Both	Yes	Yes	Focal + NLS	30	TIA: 4 weeks CVA: 16 weeks
Ricotta et al[35]	Unknown	Yes (16%)*	Both	Unknown	No	Focal	Unknown	Unknown
Persson[30]	Unknown	Yes	Both†	Unknown	No	Focal	Unknown	Unknown
Ammar et al[2]	Yes	Yes	Both	Yes	Yes	Focal	Unknown	All sxs: 4 weeks
Fisher and Ojemann[13]	Unknown	Unknown	Microscopic	Unknown	Yes	Focal	63‡	TIA: <4 weeks CVA: unknown
Lennihan et al[26]	No	Yes	Microscopic	Yes	No	Focal	72	Unknown§
Fryer, Myers, and Appleberg[14]	Unknown	Yes (17.3%)*	Both	Unknown	Yes	Unknown	Unknown	Unknown
Bassiouny et al[5]	Unknown	Unknown	Both	Yes	Yes	Focal	73	All sxs: 4 weeks
Feeley et al[9]	Unknown	Unknown	Both	Yes	Yes	Unknown	"High"	All sxs: 16 weeks

Unknown, Cannot be determined from the data in the manuscript; *TIA,* transient ischemic attack; *CVA,* cerebrovascular attack; *NLS,* nonlocalizing symptoms; *sls,* symptoms.
*Percentage of specimens excluded because of inadequate data or operative fragmentation.
†Both for 35.6% of specimens; gross only for the remainder.
‡Data reported as size of residual lumen (in mm); 63% represents those specimens with a residual lumen ≤1 mm.
§Data reported as number of patients per time interval; mean (overall or by symptom type) not available.

misleading, others[18] believe that it is the optimal method, particularly when used to identify regions of the specimen that require microscopic review.[29] It seems reasonable to conclude that both approaches should be used and that neither should stand alone unless the entire specimen is routinely examined histologically with serial sections obtained at close intervals, as in the study by Fisher and Ojemann.[13] Furthermore, the determination of plaque hemorrhage should be performed by a reviewer who has no knowledge of the patient's clinical status. When gross specimen review only is undertaken and performed in the operating room by the treating surgeon (as was the case in the second and larger study by Imparato's group[18,36]), it seems unlikely that this requirement can be met. If there is any consistent feature that distinguishes the studies that investigate the relationship of any plaque hemorrhage to neurologic signs and symptoms, it is the issue of the plaque assessment by someone who has no knowledge of the patient's clinical status. Almost all of the studies that *failed* to show a correlation used blinded assessment (one was unknown), whereas in almost all of the studies in which a significant correlation was observed, whether the review was blinded could not be determined, and in one case it clearly was not.

It is clear that the definition of *symptomatic* has not been consistent among studies and that the inconsistency has centered on the classification of patients with nonfocal or nonlocalizing symptoms. For the most part, the studies usually included only patients with focal symptoms and regarded all others as being free of symptoms (8 of 12 studies) (Table 35-3). This approach is supported by data from studies in which it was possible to compare all symptoms, focal symptoms, and nonfocal symptoms, in relationship to plaque hemorrhage.[18,35] Imparato et al[18] found that plaque from patients with focal symptoms had a significantly greater prevalence of hemorrhage than plaque from patients with nonfocal symptoms. Thus plaques from patients who were free of symptoms and those from patients with nonlocalizing symptoms are similar in the frequency of plaque hemorrhage. Therefore studies that combine focal and nonfocal symptoms in the same group[34] may mask a significant correlation between focal symptoms and plaque hemorrhage.

Several groups[5,18,24,26,36] have clearly shown a significant correlation between high-grade stenosis and intraplaque hemorrhage. The more severe the stenosis, the more likely it is that hemorrhage will be found in the atheroma. Therefore if the prevalence of severe stenosis is high in all segments of the study group,[5,9,17,26] a significant correlation between plaque hemorrhage and neurologic symptoms may be masked. The majority of patients without symptoms only undergo endarterectomy if they have a severe stenosis. Consequently, the prevalence of plaque hemorrhage in the subgroup of patients without symptoms who are selected for surgery may be much greater than it is among *all* patients without symptoms. Bassiouny et al[30] found a statistically greater incidence ($p < 0.05$, chi-square analysis) of intraplaque hemorrhage (12 of 14, 86%) in asymptomatic lesions

removed at carotid endarterectomy (mean cross-sectional area reduction of 89% ± 2%), when compared with asymptomatic lesions removed at autopsy (7 of 17, 41%) from age-matched subjects who had no history of cerebrovascular symptoms (mean cross-sectional area reduction of 34% ± 4%). Therefore comparison of the prevalence of plaque hemorrhage among patients with symptoms who were selected for operation with that of patients without symptoms who were selected for operation will not yield the same results as a comparison of all patients with symptoms with all patients without symptoms.

Finally, the observation of hemorrhage of various ages in some specimens suggests that hemorrhage into a plaque can be followed by healing and possibly resolution of that hemorrhage.* Therefore a long interval between onset of symptoms and surgery may result in an underestimation of the frequency of plaque hemorrhage in symptomatic lesions. Unfortunately, many of the clinicopathologic studies failed to provide any data regarding this symptom-surgery interval (Table 35-3).

Nonoperative studies

A significant disadvantage of the aforementioned studies is that they are all operative studies. By definition, patients selected for operation are not the same as patients who are treated nonoperatively. Thus observations derived only from the subgroup of patients who had surgery may not be applicable to the group of patients with cerebrovascular disease as a whole. Only three nonoperative series that investigated the clinical significance of plaque hemorrhage have been published[19,22-24] (Table 35-4). Because the absence of any specimens in these three studies prevented histologic confirmation of the presence of intraplaque hemorrhage, the clinical status of the patients was correlated instead with the sonographic appearance of the plaque (heterogeneous or homogeneous, Leahy et al[23,24]; calcific, dense, or soft, Johnson et al[19]; type 1-echolucent to type 4-echogenic, Langsfeld et al[22]). In two of the series,[19,23,24] the study group consisted of patients who were referred to a vascular laboratory for evaluation of suspected cerebrovascular disease. Langsfeld et al[22] had two patient groups, one referred to the laboratory for suspected cerebrovascular disease and one composed of patients who had undergone carotid endarterectomy and whose contralateral, asymptomatic carotid artery was being studied. In the series by Leahy et al[24] the patients were studied with duplex scanning once, and the sonographic appearance of the plaque was correlated with their symptomatic status at that time. In the other two studies, all patients were free of symptoms at the time of the initial scan. Johnson et al[19] followed up their patients clinically over 3 years, and the ultrasonographic appearance of the plaque was correlated with the development of symptoms during the follow-up period. Langsfeld et al[22] repeated the duplex scans at specified intervals (3, 6, and 12 months

---

*References 3, 14, 15, 26, 27, 34.

Table 35-4. Correlation of ultrasound plaque appearance and neurologic symptoms

Reference	N	p value*
Johnson et al[19]	297	0.0003†
Leahy et al[23,24]	108	<0.05
Langsfeld, Gray-Weale, and Lusby[22]	289	<0.001
Reilly et al[34]	50	NSS
Bluth et al[6]	53	NSS

NSS, Not statistically significant.
*Chi-square contingency analysis with Bonferroni correction (Johnson et al); with Yates' continuity correction (Leahy et al); statistical method not stated (Langsfeld et al).
†Analysis of data provided in authors' manuscript.

after enrollment and every year thereafter). None of the studies specified whether the clinical assessment and ultrasound scan interpretation were performed in a blinded manner.

Johnson et al[19] found that soft plaque (equivalent to heterogeneous plaque) had the highest associated prevalence of subsequent neurologic events (51 of 89, 57.3%). Calcific plaque had the lowest prevalence (4 of 90, 4.4%), and dense plaque (equivalent to homogeneous plaque) was intermediate in the frequency of neurologic symptoms (31 of 118, 26.3%). No statistical analysis was provided; however, chi-square analysis with the Bonferroni correction for multiple pair-wise comparisons shows that in this series, any ultrasound plaque type is significantly different from each of the other two in the frequency of neurologic symptoms (p = 0.0003). Unfortunately, the observed rate of neurologic events for the entire group of patients was so high in this study (86 of 297, 29.0%) that it suggested an inadvertent selection bias for the study group as a whole. This may have resulted from the large proportion of high-grade lesions (greater than 75% stenosis) in this series (121 of 297, 40.7%). The neurologic event rate for this category of stenosis was 58.7% (71 of 121), whereas it was only 8.5% (15 of 176) for less severe stenoses. An additional shortcoming is the failure of the authors to specify whether all of the observed neurologic events were ipsilateral to the lesions that were being followed up. Leahy et al[23,24] did find a statistically significant correlation between the heterogeneous plaque and the presence of ipsilateral (focal) hemispheric symptoms (p < 0.05, chi-square analysis). In the study by Langsfeld et al,[22] the group of patients that initially underwent carotid endarterectomy had a significantly greater frequency of type 1 or type 2 plaques (heterogeneous or echolucent) on the symptomatic side than on the non-operated, asymptomatic side (p < 0.001, statistical method not specified). In this study, 80% of the neurologic events were focal hemispheric symptoms, whereas 20% were non-localizing symptoms. The authors further found that patients with asymptomatic lesions had a significantly greater risk of subsequently experiencing symptoms if their plaque was

a type 1 or 2 at the time of the initial ultrasound study (p < 0.02, statistical method not specified). However, they were not able to document any correlation between increasing echolucency of the plaque during follow-up and the subsequent onset of symptoms.

Since only one of the groups[42] had previously established the accuracy of their laboratory in correlating the ultrasound image with plaque hemorrhage and since the overall false-positive rate for detecting plaque hemorrhage with duplex scanning is 32.2%, the results of these three studies raise the intriguing possibility that it is the heterogeneous plaque, independent of the presence of intraplaque hemorrhage, that is the clinically significant factor. In fact, data in the study by Feeley et al[9] show a significant correlation between plaques containing amorphous material mixed with cholesterol and neurologic symptoms (p = 0.017, Fisher's exact test, one-tailed). Additionally, Widder et al[42] found that both plaque hemorrhage and what they termed atheromatous debris in the plaque independently exhibited a close correlation to ipsilateral neurologic symptoms. Therefore the heterogeneous-appearing plaque may represent an unstable atheroma that is undergoing structural changes. It may have an increased potential for plaque breakdown with or without overlying thrombus formation, and subsequent microembolization or macroembolization of plaque contents or thrombus, producing neurologic symptoms, may occur more frequently.

There have been two other studies[6,34] that included sufficient data to allow analysis of the ultrasound appearance of the plaque in comparison to the patient's clinical status (Table 35-4). Neither of these studies showed any significant correlation. In both studies, ultrasound interpretation was performed by reviewers who had no knowledge of the clinical status of the patient. Both negative studies had considerably smaller patient cohorts than any of the positive studies.

Thus the controversy continues. Despite considerable interest and investigation, identification of those features of carotid atheroma that correlate with clinical risk has not been achieved. The most recent prospective trials of the efficacy of carotid endarterectomy have once again focused attention on diameter reduction as the most clinically relevant feature of carotid bifurcation lesions and have included no data regarding plaque composition. Nonetheless, carotid lesions can be distinguished easily by ultrasonography, and plaque hemorrhage can be detected reliably by noninvasive methods. Therefore the resolution of this debate is feasible and requires only a large enough, appropriately designed, and well-conducted study.

REFERENCES

1. Aldoori MI et al: Duplex scanning and plaque histology in cerebral ischemia, *Eur J Vasc Surg* 1:159, 1987.
2. Ammar AD et al: Intraplaque hemorrhage: its significance in cerebrovascular disease, *Am J Surg* 148:840, 1984.
3. Ammar AD et al: The influence of repeated carotid plaque hemorrhages on the production of cerebrovascular symptoms, *J Vasc Surg* 3:857, 1986.

4. Bartynski WS, Darbouze P, Nemir P: Significance of ulcerated plaque in transient cerebral ischemia, *Am J Surg* 141:353, 1981.

5. Bassiouny HS et al: Critical carotid stenoses: morphologic and chemical similarity between symptomatic and asymptomatic plaques, *J Vasc Surg* 9:202, 1989.

6. Bluth EI et al: Sonographic characterization of carotid plaque: detection of hemorrhage, *AJR* 146:1061, 1986.

7. Culebras A et al: Computed tomographic evaluation of cervical carotid complications, *Stroke* 16:425, 1985.

8. Edward JH et al: Atherosclerotic subintimal hematoma of the carotid artery, *Radiology* 133:123, 1979.

9. Feeley TM et al: Histologic characteristics of carotid artery plaque, *J Vasc Surg* 13:719, 1991.

10. Fields WS: Selection of patients wth ischemic cerebrovascular disease for arterial surgery, *World J Surg* 3:147, 1979.

11. Fisher M: Occlusion of the internal carotid artery, *Arch Neurol Psychiatry* 65:346, 1951.

12. Fisher M: Occlusion of the carotid arteries, *Arch Neurol Psychiatry* 72:187, 1954.

13. Fisher CM, Ojemann RG: A clinico-pathologic study of carotid endarterectomy plaques, *Rev Neurol* 142:573, 1986.

14. Fryer JA, Myers PC, Appleberg M: Carotid intraplaque hemorrhage: the significance of neovascularity, *J Vasc Surg* 6:341, 1987.

15. Gray-Weale AC et al: Carotid artery atheroma: comparison of preoperative B-mode ultrasound appearance with carotid endarterectomy specimen pathology, *J Cardiovasc Surg* 29:676, 1988.

16. Houser OW et al: Atheromatous disease of the carotid artery: correlation of angiographic, clinical, and surgical findings, *J Neurosurg* 41:321, 1974.

17. Imparato AM, Riles TS, Gorstein F: The carotid bifurcation plaque: pathologic findings associated with cerebral ischemia, *Stroke* 10:238, 1979.

18. Imparato AM et al: The importance of hemorrhage in the relationship between gross morphologic characteristics and cerebral symptoms in 376 carotid artery plaques, *Ann Surg* 197:195, 1983.

19. Johnson JM et al: Natural history of asymptomatic carotid plaque, *Arch Surg* 120:1010, 1985.

20. Kannel WB et al: Vascular disease of the brain—epidemiologic aspects: the Framingham study, *Am J Pub Health* 55:1355, 1970.

21. Kroener JM et al: Prognosis of asymptomatic ulcerating carotid lesions, *Arch Surg* 115:1387, 1980.

22. Langsfeld M, Gray-Weale AC, Lusby RJ: The role of plaque morphology and diameter reduction in the development of new symptoms in asymptomatic carotid arteries, *J Vasc Surg* 9:548, 1989.

23. Leahy AL et al: Duplex scanning for noninvasive assessment of both carotid luminal diameter and atheromatous plaque morphology, *Ann Vasc Surg* 1:465, 1986.

24. Leahy AL et al: Duplex ultrasonography and selection of patients for carotid endarterectomy: plaque morphology or luminal narrowing? *J Vasc Surg* 8:558, 1988.

25. Leen EJ et al: "Haemorrhagic" carotid plaque does not contain haemorrhage, *Eur J Vasc Surg* 4:123, 1990.

26. Lennihan L et al: Lack of association between carotid plaque hematoma and ischemic cerebral symptoms, *Stroke* 18:879, 1987.

27. Lusby RJ et al: Carotid plaque hemorrhage: its role in production of cerebral ischemia, *Arch Surg* 117:1479, 1982.

28. Moore WS, Hall AD: Importance of emboli from carotid bifurcation in pathogenesis of cerebral ischemic attacks, *Arch Surg* 101:708, 1970.

29. O'Donnell TF Jr et al: Correlation of B-mode ultrasound imaging and arteriography with pathologic findings at carotid endarterectomy, *Arch Surg* 120:443, 1985.

30. Persson AV: Intraplaque hemorrhage, *Surg Clin North Am* 66:415, 1986.

31. Persson AV, Robichaux WT, Silverman M: The natural history of carotid plaque development, *Arch Surg* 118:1048, 1983.

32. Pessin MS et al: Clinical and angiographic features of carotid transient ischemic attacks, *N Engl J Med* 296:358, 1977.

33. Ratliff DA et al: Characterization of carotid artery disease: comparison of duplex scanning with histology, *Ultrasound Med Biol* 11:835, 1985.

34. Reilly LM et al: Carotid plaque histology using real-time ultrasonography: clinical and therapeutic implications, *Arch Surg* 146:188, 1983.

35. Ricotta JJ et al: Angiographic and pathologic correlates in carotid artery disease, *Surgery* 99:284, 1986.

36. Riles TS et al: The significance of intramural hemorrhage in the carotid bifurcation plaque, *Stroke* 13:124, 1982.

37. Rubin JR, Bondi JA, Rhodes RS: Duplex scanning versus conventional arterography for the evaluation of carotid artery plaque morphology, *Surgery* 102:749, 1987.

38. Thiele BL, Strandness DE Jr: Distribution of intracranial and extracranial arterial lesions in patients with symptomatic cerebrovascular disease. In Bernstein EF, editor: *Noninvasive diagnostic techniques in vascular disease*, St Louis, 1982, Mosby.

39. Thiele BL et al: Correlation of arteriographic findings and symptoms in cerebrovascular disease, *Neurology* 30:1041, 1980.

40. Weinberger J et al: Atherosclerotic plaque at the carotid artery bifurcation: correlation of ultrasonographic imaging with morphology, *J Ultrasound Med* 6:363, 1987.

41. Widder B: Impact of ultrasound methods on decision making for carotid and EC/IC bypass surgery. In Aichner F, Gerstenbrand F, Grcevic N, editiors: *The present state in clinical neuroimaging*, New York, 1989, Gustav Fischer.

42. Widder B et al: Morphological characterization of carotid artery stenoses by ultrasound duplex scanning, *Ultrasound Med Biol* 16:349, 1990.

43. Wood EH, Correll JW: Atheromatous ulceration in major neck vessels as a cause of cerebral embolism, *Acta Radiol* 9:520, 1969.

CHAPTER 36

Principles and applications of transcranial Doppler sonography

SHIRLEY M. OTIS and E. BERND RINGELSTEIN

After the original report by Miyazaki and Kato[42] in 1965 on the use of Doppler ultrasonography for the assessment of extracranial cerebral vessels and the rapid development of this technique, it was only a matter of time before Doppler ultrasound would be applied to the intracranial vessels. Nevertheless, it was not until 1982 that Aaslid, Markwalder, and Nornes[6] developed a transcranial Doppler device with

---

CLINICAL APPLICATIONS OF TCD

- Diagnosis of intracranial occlusive disease (individual and epidemiologic aspects)
- Auxiliary test for extracranial occlusive disease in inconclusive extracranial tests
- Evaluation of hemodynamic effects of extracranial occlusive disease on intracranial blood flow (e.g., internal carotid artery occlusion, subclavian steal)
- Detection and identification of feeders of arteriovenous malformations
- Preoperative compression tests for evaluation of collateralizing capacities of circle of Willis
- Detection of right-to-left shunts in the heart (e.g., patent foramen ovale) and paradoxical embolism
- Intermittent monitoring and follow-up of
    Vasospasm in subarachnoid hemorrhage and migraine
    Spontaneous or therapeutically induced recanalization of occluded vessels
    Establishment of collateral pathways after occluding interventions
    Occlusive disease during anticoagulative or fibrinolytic therapy
- Continuous monitoring during
    Neuroradiologic interventions (e.g., balloon occlusion, embolization)
    Short-term pharmacologic trials of vasoactive drugs and anesthetics
    Carotid endarterectomy (shunt)
    Cardiac surgery (ischemic encephalopathy? embolism?)
    Increasing intracranial pressure
    Evolution of brain death
- Functional tests
    Stimulation of cerebral vasomotors with CO_2 or other vasoactive drugs (e.g., acetacolamide)
    External stimulation of visual cortex
- Neuropsychologic tasks for hemispheric dominance (with simultaneous bilateral and TCD recording)

---

a pulse sound emission of 2 MHz that could penetrate successfully the skull and accurately measure both blood flow direction and velocities in the basal cerebral vessels and in the circle of Willis. During the last several years, this technique has turned out to be an amazingly useful tool in the whole field of neurosonology. It has become possible to record intracranial hemodynamic changes directly and with an excellent tissue resolution, thus establishing this technique as an important noninvasive method for assessing cerebral hemodynamics and cerebral blood flow.

A principal problem in the application of transcranial Doppler (TCD) ultrasonography has been the unclear relationship between cerebral blood flow and the flow velocities within the basal cerebral arteries. However, these limitations can be overcome, and relative changes in blood flow velocity nicely reflect the relative changes in regional cerebral blood flow.[31,52] Besides its noninvasiveness and low cost, the decisive advantage of TCD as a method for the evaluation of cerebral blood flow is the optimal time resolution of the measurements.[2,9] Relative changes in cerebral blood flow can now be measured objectively and immediately and for as long and as often as desired. This makes TCD an attractive tool for monitoring, particularly during neurosurgical, cardiac, and cerebrovascularization operations, both for knowledge of the immediate status of cerebral blood flow and for reducing the occurrence of postoperative cerebral complications.[21,38,40,49] The abrupt or short- and long-lasting effects of any external mechanical manipulation or functional stimulation of the intracranial circulation can be assessed in real-time as can the pathophysiology of cerebral circulation in acute stroke.[54,62] The box lists the already established applications of TCD sonography in clinical and experimental settings.

EXAMINATION TECHNIQUES
General prerequisites

Before a TCD examination is performed, two prerequisites should be fulfilled: (1) the status of the extracranial arteries must be completely known, and (2) the patient must be lying supine and comfortably to preserve a stable position of the probe and to avoid major fluctuations in the carbon dioxide pressure. The examiner must also deal with two main anatomic considerations: The number and extent of so-called acoustic windows or foramina within the skull that can be penetrated with the ultrasound beam are sometimes limited and/or not easily identified, and the arteries of the base of the skull are extremely variable in respect to size, development, site, and course.*

The problem of acoustic properties of the skull has been well studied, and transmission of the ultrasound beam through the cranium depends on the structure of the skull itself.[67] The skull consists of three layers of bone, each of which influences the beam in a different manner. The middle layer (diploë) has the most important effect on the attenuation and scattering of the sound, whereas the outer and inner tables, made of so-called ivory bone, are more important for refraction. Because of the essential absence of bony spicules in the temporal region, this is an attractive area for ultrasound evaluation. Grolimund[20] has performed a number of in vitro experiments to determine the effect of the skull bone on Doppler ultrasound. His experiments have shown that a wide range of energy loss occurs in different skull samples and that the power loss depends on the thickness of the skull. In no case was the power measured behind the skull greater than 35% of the transmitted power. He further showed that the skull has the effect of an acoustic lens and that the refraction of the beam depended more on variation of bone thickness than on the angle of insonation. His data suggested that it would be advantageous to use ultrasound lenses with longer focal lengths to improve the sensitivity, particularly at depths of 5 and 10 cm.

Transcranial Doppler devices

Commercial systems that use a 2-MHz Doppler ultrasound device of pulsed, range-gated design and with good directional resolution are available. For transcranial application the primary consideration is a good signal-to-noise resolution. This is one reason the available instruments developed for transcranial application have larger and less-defined sample volume than most other pulsed Doppler instruments. The former have a decreased bandwidth in an attempt to improve the signal-to-noise ratio. Additional requirements are transmitting power between 10 and 100 mW/cm² sec, adjustable Doppler gate depth, pulse repetition frequency up to 20 kHz, focusing of the ultrasonic beam at distances of 40 and 60 mm, and on-line, time-averaged velocity and peak systolic velocity produced by spectroanalysis of backscattered Dopper signals.[1] Instruments include the first commercially available transcranial Doppler, TCD-64,† and the recently developed Transpect Transcranial Doppler.‡ Both systems include a special 2-MHz transducer for continuous monitoring that can be attached to the head by a specially developed headband or helmet. Also available is the TransScan,† a three-dimensional transcranial

imaging system with velocity color-coding and mapping capabilities.[1] Recently, B-mode imaging with duplex systems has become available to visualize both the intracranial arteries and the surrounding brain tissue.[8,63]

Acoustic windows

Four different approaches[53] have been described to insonate the intracranial arteries: transtemporal, transorbital, suboccipital, and submandibular (Fig. 36-1).[1]

Transtemporal approach. In the transtemporal approach, the probe is placed on the temporal plane, cephalad to the zygomatic arch and immediately anteriorly and slightly superior to the tragus of the ear conch (Figs. 36-2 and 36-3, *1*). This site is usually the most promising. A more posterior window immediately over and slightly dorsal to the first one may be more appropriate in a minority of cases; this is the optimal site for insonation of the P2 segment of the posterior cerebral arteries (Fig. 36-3, *2*). In some patients, more frontally located temporal windows may be present (Fig. 36-3, *3*). With these preauricular, transtemporal approaches, the beam can be angulated anteriorly or posteriorly relative to a frontal plane running through the corresponding probe positions on either side of the head. The anterior orientation of the beam allows insonation of the M1 and M2 segments of the middle cerebral arteries, the C1 segment of carotid siphon, and the A1 segment of the anterior cerebral artery, including the anterior communicating artery (Fig. 36-4, *A*). The posteriorly angulated beam insonates the P1 and P2 segments of the posterior cerebral artery, the top of the basilar artery, and the posterior communicating arteries (Fig. 36-4, *B*).

Transorbital approach. The ophthalmic artery can be insonated at depths of 45 to 50 mm whereas the C3 segment

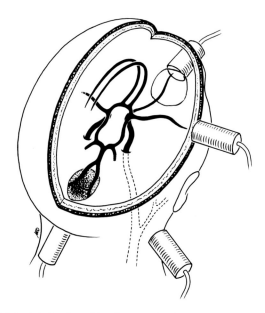

Fig. 36-1. Relationship of the ultrasound probes at the available acoustic windows and their relationship to the basal cerebral arteries.

*References 6, 7, 48, 49, 53, 62.
†EME, Ueberlingen, West Germany.
‡Medasonics, Mountainview, Calif.

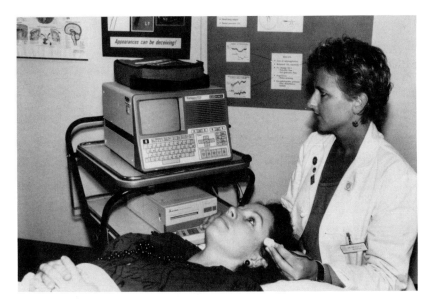

Fig. 36-2. Transtemporal approach for insonation of the middle cerebral artery (M1 and M2 segment), anterior cerebral artery (A1 segment), distal carotid siphon, posterior cerebral artery (P1 and P2 segments), top of the basilar artery, and the posterior communicating artery if it is acting as a collateral channel.

(anterior knee of the carotid siphon) is normally met at insonation depths of 60 to 65 mm (Figs. 36-5 and 36-6, *A*). At slightly greater insonation depths of 70 to 75 mm, the C2 segment shows flow away from the probe (downward deflection), and the C4 segment shows flow toward the probe (upward deflection), provided that the angulation of the beam is nearly sagittal via the supraorbital fissure or via the infraorbital fissure, with a slightly oblique approach (Fig. 36-6, *B*). During a strongly oblique approach with the probe placed at the superior outer quadrant of the eyelids and the beam angulated medially, the ultrasound beam penetrates the optic canal and is aimed at the contralateral arteries (i.e., anterior cerebral artery, supraclinoidal carotid siphon, proximal middle cerebral artery). Typical insonation depths are listed in Table 36-1.

Suboccipital approach. The suboccipital approach is essential for screening the vertebral basilar access in its whole length (Fig. 36-7, *A*). The probe is placed exactly between the squama ossis occipitalis and the palpable spinous process of the first cervical vertebra with the beam aimed at the bridge of the nose and an insonation depth of 65 mm. The patient may be seated with the head flexed or lying with the head turned laterally (Fig. 36-8). The distal vertebral arteries are tracked in both directions with small insonation depths (35 to 50 mm), and by angulating the beam strongly to one side, the examiner can screen the extradural part of the vertebral arteries on the posterior arch of the atlas (flow toward the probe). The top of the basilar artery is normally reached at depths of 95 to 125 mm with flow directed away from the probe (Fig. 36-7, *B*).

Submandibular approach. The submandibular approach completes the examination in the sense that the retroman-

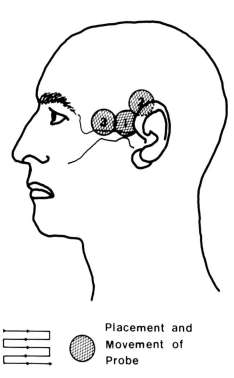

Placement and Movement of Probe

Fig. 36-3. Available temporal acoustic windows and placement of the probe: *1*, preauricular position; *2*, posterior window; and *3*, anterior window. The probe should be placed first in the preaural region to identify the middle cerebral artery. Subtle meandering movements of the probe should be performed in each position. If position 1 is not successful, position 2 should be tried before position 3.

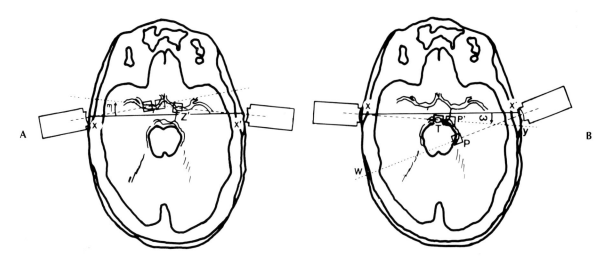

Fig. 36-4. Position of the probe in the temporal region to insonate the anterior and posterior part of the circle of Willis. **A,** Line XX' indicates a frontal plane that runs through the regular placement of the probe on either side and, simultaneously, perpendicular to the sagittal midline of the skull. Z' indicates the site of the intracranial bifurcation of the internal carotid artery. The X'Z distance was 63 ± 5 mm. μ indicates the angle with which the probe is more anteriorly aimed at the middle and anterior cerebral arterial segments. This angle was 6° ± 1.1°. **B,** Omega indicates the angle with which the beam is directed more posteriorly to insonate the top of the basilar artery *(T)* and the P1 segments *(P')* on both sides. This angle was 4.6 ± 1.2°. The bifurcation of the basilar artery could be insonated at depths of 78 ± 5 mm, corresponding to the distance X'T or X'T, respectively. Y indicates the fictional point where the pathway of the beam then transits the contralateral skull (i.e., approximately 2-3 cm behind the external acoustic meatus). The P2 segments *(P)* also can be insonated if the beam is directed even more posteriorly and slightly caudally (line X,P). W lies approximately 5 cm behind the contralateral external acoustic meatus.

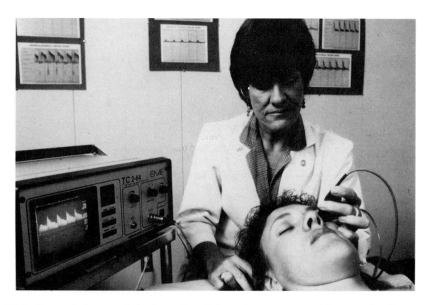

Fig. 36-5. Transorbital approach for insonation of the various segments of the carotid siphon (C1-C4), the ophthalmic artery, and via the optic canal, the contralateral anterior cerebral artery.

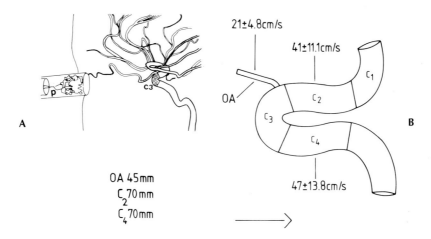

Fig. 36-6. Insonation of the ophthalmic artery (OA) and carotid siphon via the transorbital approach. ***A,*** Probe location and relationship to the ophthalmic artery and carotid siphon. Representative insonation depths are also given. ***B,*** Normal flow velocity values within various segments of the carotid siphon and ophthalmic artery.

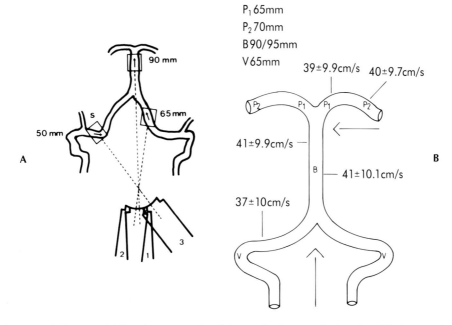

Fig. 36-7. A, Transcranial Doppler sonography of the vertebral system via the suboccipital approach. ***B,*** Representative insonation depths and normal flow velocity values within the distal vertebral arteries and the basilar trunk. The P1 and P2 velocities are measured transtemporally.

dibular and more distal, extradural parts of the internal carotid artery (C5-C6 segment) can be evaluated (Fig. 36-9, *A*). This particular examination is helpful as a complementary test to extracranial studies and helps avoid overlooking chronic occlusions of the internal carotid artery in cases with abundant collateralization via the external carotid artery. The beam is directed slightly medially and posterior to the longitudinal axis of the body where the internal carotid artery regularly can be tracked up to 80 to 85 mm, where it bends medioanteriorly to form the siphon (Fig. 36-9, *B*).

Diagnostic measurements

The primary diagnostic measurements for identifying cerebral arteries are (1) the insonation depth, (2) the direction of blood flow at that depth, (3) the flow velocities (mean time of flow velocity and systolic or diastolic peak flow velocities), (4) site of the probe's position (temporal, orbital, suboccipital, and submandibular), (5) direction of the ultrasonic beam (posterior, anterior, caudad, or cephalad), (6) the "traceability" of vessels, and (7) response to carotid compression.[1,49]

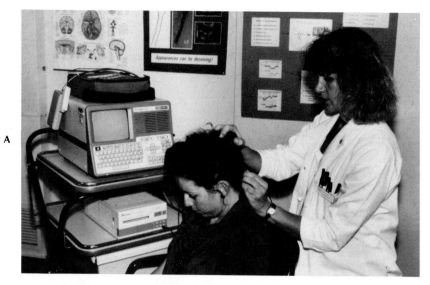

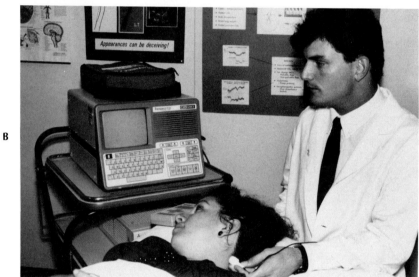

Fig. 36-8. The suboccipital approach for insonation of the distal vertebral arteries and the basilar trunk. **A,** Patient in the sitting position with head forward flexed. **B,** Alternative method of examination with the patient supine and head turned comfortably to one side.

Initial examination. Generally, it is most convenient to start with the middle cerebral artery on either side at an insonation depth of 50 to 55 mm and then to track the basal arterial network step by step in various directions. Proof of traceability of the middle cerebral artery is decisive for its unequivocal identification. This is also true for the other basal arterial vasculature. Traceability refers to the fact that the middle cerebral artery (and usually other arteries) can be tracked in incremental steps from more shallow depths (e.g., 35 mm) to deeper sites (e.g., 55 mm) without changes in the character of the flow profile and direction. When the middle cerebral artery is tracked medially (65 to 70 mm), an abrupt change in the direction of flow indicates insonation of the A1 segment of the anterior cerebral artery. Flow

toward the probe at this step is usually registered from the carotid siphon (Fig. 36-10).

When the beam is angulated more posteriorly during a transtemporal approach, the P1 segment of the posterior cerebral artery can be picked up most readily at an isonation depth of 65 to 70 mm and can then be tracked over the top of the basilar artery (75 mm) to the contralateral posterior cerebral artery (P1, 80 to 85 mm). The criteria of traceability include display of a bilateral blood flow at the top of the basilar artery and the change of flow direction within the contralateral posterior cerebral artery. These are important features for identification of the posterior cerebral arteries without resorting to the use of compression tests. Generally, depending on the clinical situation being evaluated, exam-

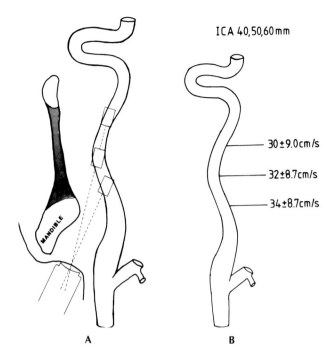

ICA 40,50,60 mm

— 30±9.0 cm/s

— 32±8.7 cm/s

— 34±8.7 cm/s

A   B

Fig. 36-9. *A,* Transcranial Doppler sonography of the petrous portion of the internal carotid artery (ICA) via the submandibular approach. The ICA can be tracted from depths of 25 to 80 mm corresponding to the C4- and C5-segments of the ICA. *B,* Representative insonation depths and normal flow values within the distal intracranial ICA.

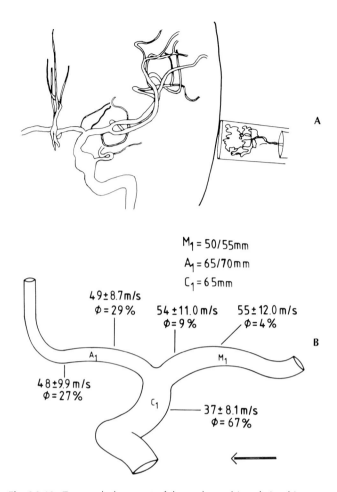

A

$M_1 = 50/55$ mm

$A_1 = 65/70$ mm

$C_1 = 65$ mm

49±8.7 m/s
$\phi = 29\%$

54±11.0 m/s
$\phi = 9\%$

55±12.0 m/s
$\phi = 4\%$

B

A_1 M_1

48±9.9 m/s
$\phi = 27\%$

C_1

37±8.1 m/s
$\phi = 67\%$

Fig. 36-10. Temporal placement of the probe and its relationship to the middle cerebral artery (MCA). *A,* The beam axis is in line with the M2, M1, and A1 segments of the cerebral vasculature. *B,* Representative insonation depths and normal flow values within the MCA, the anterior cerebral artery, and the distal part of the internal carotid artery.

inations via the orbital, suboccipital, or submandibular pathways follow.

Flow velocity measurements. The mean flow velocities and standard deviations of various vessel segments at representative insonation depths are shown in Table 36-1 for different age groups. Normal flow velocity values in adults show good correlation between different investigators (Table 36-2), revealing good interobserver agreement.* The highest velocities are almost always found in the middle or anterior cerebral arteries. The posterior cerebral arteries and the basilar arteries have lower Doppler shifts than the middle cerebral artery in normal subjects. This variation, however, does not reflect differences in cerebral blood flow but differences in the ratios of territorial blood flow and diameter of the feeding artery.[18]

Flow velocities in the basal cerebral arteries show a consistent decrease with increasing age (Table 36-1).[21,26,50] These findings correlate well with age-related changes seen in studies of cerebral blood flow.[29,30] This underlines the validity and sensitivity of the ultrasound method as an intraindividually close semiquantitative estimate of cerebral blood flow on the basis of velocity data.

Vessel identification. Identification of vessels is primarily based on the window of foramina used, the angulation of

*References 5, 7, 17, 22, 53, 55.

the beam, the depth of insonation, the direction of blood flow relative to the probe, and the traceability of the vessel segments. However, in pathologic conditions and in many individuals, particularly the elderly, compression tests may be required for the unequivocal identification of certain arterial segments.[6,37,47,53] Compression tests during TCD examinations can be performed on the common carotid arteries, low in the neck (with two fingers) (Fig. 36-11, *A*), or on the vertebral arteries at the mastoidal slope (Figs. 36-11 and 36-12). Little risk of creating embolism from plaques in the carotid arteries exists if compression is performed only after knowledge of B-mode imaging of the carotid arteries and by an experienced investigator.[59,64] Generally, compression maneuvers strictly for arterial identification are not necessary; however, these compression maneuvers are extremely valuable in the assessment of collateral pathways. Figs. 36-13 and 36-14 show the ways flow is affected in intracranial arteries during compression maneuvers. Re-

Table 36-1. Normal values of mean blood velocity (cm/sec) for cranial arteries*

Age (yr)	MCA (M1)	ACA (A1)	PCA (P1)	BA	VA
10-29	70 ± 16.4	61 ± 14.7	55 ± 9.0	46 ± 11	45 ± 9.8
30-49	57 ± 11.2	48 ± 7.1	42 ± 8.9	38 ± 8.6	35 ± 8.2
50-59	51 ± 9.7	46 ± 9.4	39 ± 9.9	32 ± 7.0	37 ± 10
60-70	41 ± 7.0	38 ± 5.6	36 ± 7.9	32 ± 6.7	35 ± 7.0
Insonated depth (mm)	50-55	60-65	60-65	90-95	60-65

MCA (M1), middle cerebral artery (M1 segment); *ACA (A1),* anterior cerebral artery (A1 segment); *PCA (P1),* posterior cerebral artery (P1 segment); *BA,* basilar artery; *VA,* vertebral artery.
*Velocities are given as means plus or minus the standard deviation.

Table 36-2. Normal values of mean blood velocity (cm/sec) for the middle, anterior, posterior and basilar arteries

Author	Middle	Anterior	Posterior	Basilar
Aaslid, Huber, Nornes[5]	62 ± 12	51 ± 12	44 ± 11	48 mean
DeWitt, Wechsler[16]	62 ± 12	52 ± 12	42 ± 10	42 ± 10
Harders[22]	65 ± 17	50 ± 13	40 ± 9	39 ± 9
Hennerici et al[27]	58 ± 12	53 ± 10	37 ± 10	36 ± 12
Ringelstein et al[53]	55 ± 12	49 ± 9	40 ± 10	41 ± 10
Russo et al[55]	65 ± 13	48 ± 20	35 ± 18	45 ± 10

Values are given as means plus or minus the standard deviation.

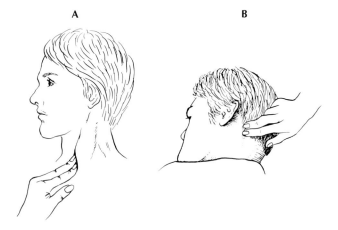

Fig. 36-11. Compression tests.
A, Compression of the common carotid artery low in the neck.
B, Compression of the vertebral artery at the mastoid slope.

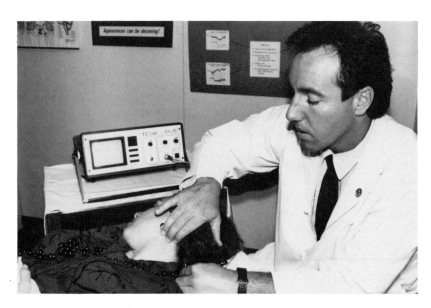

Fig. 36-12. Supine patient with head turned and neck flexed allowing access to the intracranial vertebral by way of the foramen magnum, and compression of the vertebral artery at the mastoid.

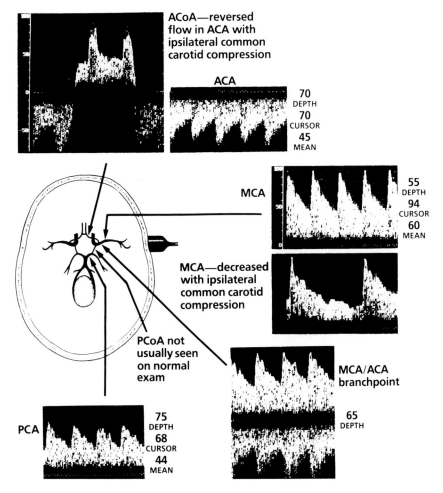

Fig. 36-13. Transcranial Doppler sonography of the basilar intracranial arteries from the transtemporal approach, their normal location, and their response to compression of the common carotid artery.

sponses include (1) no reaction at all, (2) increase of flow velocity, (3) decrease of flow velocity, (4) reversal of flow, (5) alternating flow direction (to and fro), and (6) cessation of flow (Table 36-3).

Functional tests

Because of its excellent time resolution of flow velocity measurements, TCD is ideal for functional tests with rapid changes of cerebral perfusion. Such tests are aimed primarily at the evaluation of the reserve mechanism of the cerebral vasculature by using various stimuli such as hypocapnia or hypercapnia, increased or reduced systemic arterial pressure, and hypoxia. The response of cerebral circulation to carbon dioxide has been demonstrated by many (Fig. 36-15).* During changing concentrations of carbon dioxide, the relationship between cerebral blood flow and volume flow within a large basal artery is a linear one provided that the carbon dioxide does not affect the diam-

eters of the large proximal arterial segments themselves. It has been shown that the effect of carbon dioxide is restricted mainly to the peripheral arterial vascular bed, in particular the small cortical vessels.[28] Thus intraindividual changes in flow velocity during TCD directly reflect changes in volume flow.[44,52] Velocities measured from the middle cerebral artery with different concentrations of carbon dioxide showed a biasymptotic S-shaped curve (Fig. 36-16).

Intactness of vasomotor reserve implies that a drop in perfusion pressure can be counterbalanced by vasodilatation of cortical arteriole to maintain a sufficient blood supply. This reserve may become exhausted if the resistant vessels of the brain are already maximally dilated.[11,41,52] In this state, they are refractory to any further vasodilatory stimuli, and hypercapnia cannot increase blood flow. This condition would be critical because ischemic brain injury would occur if perfusion pressure were reduced further for whatever reason. Carbon dioxide reactivities permit the study of the reaction of cerebral arteries in different pathologic situations and measurement of cerebral vascular reserve. These tests

---

*References 9, 11, 24, 31, 34, 41, 44, 52, 68.

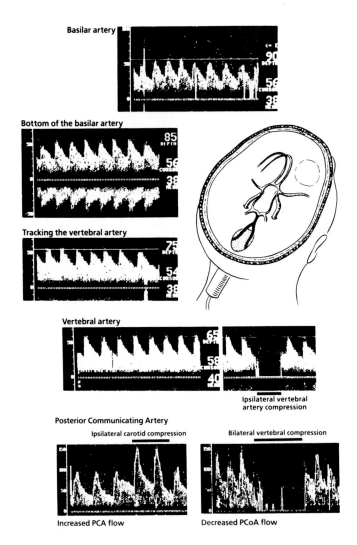

Fig. 36-14. Transcranial Doppler examination of the vertebrobasilar circulation, normal vessel location, and the effects of compressive maneuvers.

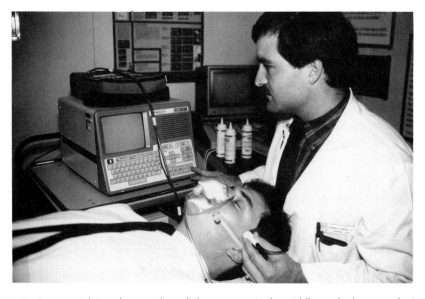

Fig. 36-15. Transcranial Doppler recording of changes seen in the middle cerebral artery velocity flow related to CO_2 administration.

Table 36-3. Effects of compression tests of the common carotid arteries on various vessel segments and their diagnostic meanings*

Insonated vessel segment	Findings at rest	Effect of ipsilateral CCA compression test	Effect of contralateral CCA compression test	Functional meaning of compression test
MCA M1/M2	Normal flow velocity, flow toward probe	↓ or ↓↓ or [STOP]	Ø or [↓↓]	Confirmation of vessel identity
ACA (A1)	Normal flow velocity, flow away from probe	[↓↓↓] or [STOP] or ∩ or ∩ with D or [↑↑ with D and flow toward probe]	[Ø] or ↑ or ↑↑ with or without D	Confirmation of vessel identity, presence or absence of potential anterior collateral pathway
ACoA	No signal available	↑↑ with D and flow toward probe	↑↑ with D and flow away from the probe	Confirmation of existence of ACoA
	Indistinguishable from contralateral ACA	Ø or ↑ or ↑↑	[↓↓↓] or [STOP] or ∩ or ∩ with D	See ACA
	Indistinguishable from ipsilateral ACA	See ACA	Ø or ↑ or ↑↑	See ACA
PCA (P1)	Normal flow signal, flow toward probe	Ø or ↑ or ↑↑	Ø or ↑	Confirmation of vessel identity, presence or absence of potential posterior collateral pathway
PCA (P2)	Normal flow signal, flow away from probe	Ø or ↓, or ↓↓ or [STOP] if ICA supplied	Ø or [↓↓]	Confirmation of vessel identity and type of PCA supply, differentiation of basilar and/or ICA blood supply
PCoA (transtemporal or transorbital)	No signal available. Indistinguishable from PCA or MCA branches without compression maneuvers. Alternating flow	In nonembryonal type: with D or ↑↑ with D. With flow toward probe in vicinity of PCA. With flow toward probe during transorbital insonation. In embryonal type: ↓ or ↓↓ or ∨ or ∩	No reactions observed thus far	Confirmation of existence of PCoA, differentiation of posterior and anterior collateral pathway; differentiation of basilar or ICA blood supply
DVA	Normal flow signal away from probe	Ø or ↑	Ø or ↑	Confirmation of existence of vessel
BA	Normal flow signal away from probe	Ø or ↑ or [↑↑↑]	Ø or ↑ or [↑↑↑]	Confirmation of existence of posterior collateral pathway, conclusive differentiation from carotid vascular tree within large insonation depths
ICA, C2-4 segments of siphon, transorbital approach	Normal flow toward probe, away from probe, or bidirectional	STOP or ↓↓ and/or [↑↑ with D]†	0 or ↑	Exclusion of silent ICA occlusion, analysis of potential collateral pathways
ICA-C1, transtemporal approach	Low-frequency flow toward probe. Indistinguishable from MCA (M1)	STOP or ↓↓	Ø or ↑	Analysis of potential collateral pathways
				Analysis of potential collateral pathways, differentiation from MCA often possible

CCA, Common carotid artery; *MCA*, middle cerebral artery; ↓, slight decrease of flow velocity; ↓↓, strong decrease of flow velocity; [], very rare event; Ø, no effect; *ACA*, anterior cerebral artery; *D*, ∩, ∩, reversal of flow toward or away from transducer; local distortion of blood flow due to relative stenosis; ↑, slight increase of flow velocity; ↑↑, strong increase of flow velocity; *ICA*, internal carotid artery; ∨, alternating flow; *DVA*, distal vertebral artery; *BA*, basilar artery. *P1*, precommunicating part of PCA; *P2*, postcommunicating part of PCA; *ACoA*, anterior communicating artery; *PCA*, posterior cerebral artery; *PCoA*, precommunicating part of PCA.

*This list reflects our present experience, but may not be complete. It refers to findings in normal subjects.

†Due to jet of PCoA collateral channel, overlap of ↓↓ and ↑↑ signals is possible.

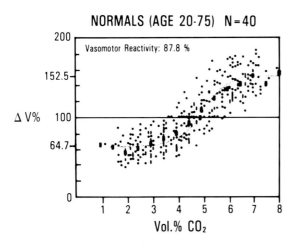

NORMALS (AGE 20-75) N = 40

Fig. 36-16. Vasomotor reactivity in 40 normal subjects (ages 20-75 years). Changes in blood flow velocity during CO_2-induced hypercapnia (upper curve) and hypocapnia (lower curve). Average change was 87.8% (52.5% and 35.3% for hypercapnia and hypocapnia, respectively).

are useful in evaluating the hemodynamic impact of extracranial occlusive carotid disease and other conditions of reduced cerebral perfusion, such as seen in migraine, hypoxia, high altitude, blunt head trauma, and acute stroke. In general, any kind of alteration of brain vasculature or brain injury in which vasodilatation may play a pathogenic role can be quantified.

The pulsatility index has been found to be a sensitive index of diastolic runoff (i.e., with increased peripheral vasodilatation, diastolic runoff would be expected to increase and the index decrease). The pulsatility index of the middle cerebral artery has been studied by Lindegaard et al[37] in carotid stenosis. They found that it was more sensitive than flow velocity because it presumably reflected a combination of reduced partial pressure (decreased flow in the middle cerebral artery) and lowered cerebrovascular resistance. With these various ratios, TCD can indirectly measure cerebral perfusion pressure in flow accurately.

CLINICAL APPLICATIONS
Intracranial vascular disease

Doppler ultrasound has been widely accepted as an accurate, noninvasive method for diagnosis of carotid extracranial disease. TCD is an extension of the use of these techniques to the intracranial arteries. The detection of intracranial stenosis by using TCD was first reported in 1983 by Spencer and Whisler,[62] who used basically similar criteria for stenosis as those for carotid bifurcation disease. Since then, a number of authors have reported similar findings.[26,32,36,43,51]

The most obvious clinical advantage of TCD is the rapid screening of the acute stroke patient for intracranial high-grade stenosis or complete occlusion. Normal TCD findings in these patients have a considerable clinical impact.

The typical features of a circumscribed stenosis of a large

basal cerebral artery are acceleration of flow (increased flow velocity), disturbed flow (spectral broadening and enhanced systolic low frequency echo components), and covibration phenomena (vibration of vessel wall and surrounding soft tissue).[36,51] As in extracranial disease, mild stenosis increases peak velocity with little change in the rest of the Doppler pattern, whereas moderate or severe stenosis leads to greater increase in peak velocity with spectral broadening, increased diastolic velocity, and turbulent flow. A post-stenotic drop in peak velocity is usually seen as well (Fig. 36-17).

Occlusion of the middle cerebral artery can be assessed by the lack of the artery's signal in spite of the presence of echoes from the posterior and/or anterior cerebral arteries or the distal carotid siphon. Dislocation of the middle cerebral artery because of intracerebral hematoma or tumor must be excluded by computed tomography because this may mimic absence of the flow signal of the artery at the site where it is regularly expected to occur. The absence of signals from the middle cerebral artery in its expected location while good signals are obtained from the anterior and posterior cerebral arteries also indicates an intact temporal window but occlusion of the middle cerebral artery. Information is now available about the sensitivity and specificity of TCD in the detection of intracranial lesions.[36] A major problem has been the strong variations in sensitivity and specificity of TCD from one vessel segment to another. This means that the measurements of validity must be calculated separately for the carotid siphon; the various segments in the middle, anterior, and posterior cerebral arteries; and particularly, the vertebral and basilar arteries. Recently, investigators have reported success in detecting stenosis in the middle cerebral artery carotid siphon and the vertebrobasilar arterial system.[26,32,36,43,51] Particularly in the vertebrobasilar arterial system, accuracy remains a problem because (1) the course and site of the arteries are unpredictable, (2) often the junction of the vertebral arteries cannot be reliably identified, (3) absence of the vertebral artery flow signal on one side may not represent disease, and (4) an occlusion of one vertebral artery will not necessarily produce intracranial flow abnormalities. In addition, segmental occlusion of the basilar artery and top of the basilar occlusions may not necessarily lead to upstream flow abnormalities, and with the deeper insonation depths (90 mm), the signal-to-noise ratio becomes poor.

Noninvasive demonstration of intracranial arterial occlusion is a valuable clinical tool. However, a variety of typical errors can occur: (1) misinterpretation of hyperdynamic collateral channels as stenosis, (2) displacement of arteries because of a space-occupying lesion, (3) misinterpretation of physiologic variables in the circle of Willis, (4) misdiagnosis of vasospasm as stenosis, and (5) misinterpretation of reactive hyperemia as stenosis. With increasing experience, many of these problems have been alleviated. For instance, the sonographic differentiation of vasospasm and stenosis can be made because vasospasm is usually more

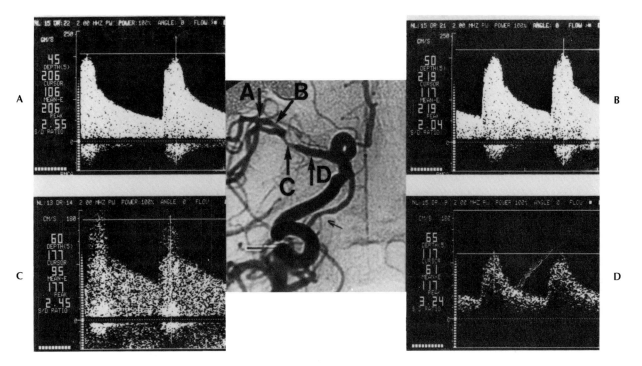

Fig. 36-17. Angiographic display of middle cerebral artery stenosis and associated changes in the transcranial Doppler velocity spectra. *A* and *B* demonstrate poststenotic turbulence seen distal to the area of stenosis. *C* demonstrates the velocity spectral changes of increased peak systolic and diastolic frequencies, spectral broadening, and turbulent flow with vessel wall vibration (bRUIT). *D* shows normal MCA spectra proximal to the area of stenosis.

generalized than atherosclerosis, often occurs bilaterally and in several arterial distributions, and changes progressively over time.[5,49] In these cases, it has been helpful to follow the patients with daily reexaminations. In addition, serial examinations of patients with acute infarcts with occlusion of the middle cerebral artery may show recanalization.[14,15,54]

In embolic middle cerebral artery occlusions, recanalization has been shown to occur in two thirds of the patients within 72 hours.[54] Intermittent close-meshed TCD monitoring of these patients helps to define the therapeutic time window for beneficial fibrinolytic treatment.

Other conditions exist that are difficult to distinguish from intracranial stenosis. Increased velocity and turbulence are seen in intracranial arteries that are providing collateral flow.[26] Increased velocity also occurs in intracranial arteries supplying arteriovenous malformation.[26,27,37,57,60] In these cases the increases in velocity are generally seen throughout the course of the involved arteries, which distinguishes them from localized areas of increased velocity due to stenosis.

Effects of extracranial occlusive disease

Identification of collateral flow in patients with extracranial carotid disease is now possible by TCD. The various pathways and number of functional collaterals are variable and until recently were assessed only by angiography. The patency of the circle of Willis can be tested by recording the changes in blood velocity and flow direction in the basal cerebral arteries in response to compression of the common carotid artery. Significant changes occur in the intracranial circulation because of extracranial flow-limiting disease. Velocity in the middle cerebral artery decreases ipsilateral to severe carotid stenosis or occlusion, and the pulsatility index generally decreases because of the vasodilatation in the distal arterial circulation ipsilateral to the stenosis.[26,37,65] Increased velocities and turbulence in the collateral arteries are accentuated during compression of the common carotid artery. A functional anterior communicating artery can be shown by reversal in flow direction in the proximal anterior cerebral artery contralateral to a significant stenosis. Increased velocity in the anterior cerebral artery contralateral to the stenosis in the internal carotid artery with reversal of the direction of flow in the ipsilateral anterior cerebral artery suggests collateral circulation from the contralateral internal carotid artery via the anterior communicating artery. Similar findings are shown in the posterior cerebral artery, revealing functional collateral flow from the posterior circulation via the posterior communicating artery. These findings have also been recorded in the basilar artery in patients with severe bilateral carotid disease, with collateral flow being supplied by both hemispheres from the posterior circulation. Correlation with angiography basically is good; however, angiography may not functionally show reversal of flow, depending on the pressure of injection of contrast material.[37] Many researchers believe that TCD may provide a much more accurate indication of functional collateral flow.

Evaluation of hemodynamic disturbances within the carotid artery/middle cerebral artery pathway is of particular interest in patients with subtotal stenosis or occlusions of the internal carotid artery both unilaterally and bilaterally. Although the main mechanism of stroke is thromboembolism rather than low flow, a small subgroup of patients do experience transient ischemic attacks, permanent stroke, or progressive ischemic eye disease because of critically reduced blood flow.[12,13,50,52] This subgroup of patients may benefit from recanalization vascular surgery, including external-internal carotid bypass surgery. The identification of these individuals is based on the detection of an exhausted cerebral vascular reserve. The carbon dioxide responsiveness of the cerebral arteries is a reliable indicator of the collateral reserve capacity in those patients who have severe carotid arterial disease.[9,19,44,48,68] TCD evaluation of the flow velocity within the middle cerebral artery can easily be used to measure the carbon dioxide reactivity of the cerebral vasomotor reserve in the periphery.[52,68] The vasomotor reserve is reduced dramatically in those patients who have unilateral or bilateral occlusion of the internal carotid artery. A reduction to less than 34% is strongly associated with hemodynamically induced ischemic brain or eye symptoms (low-flow infarction), positional transient ischemic attacks, and chronic ischemic eye disease.

Subclavian steal mechanism is the classic paradigm to study hemodynamic disturbance in the vertebrobasilar system in man. Rapid flow changes due to any kind of restriction of blood flow in the vertebral artery can be measured directly within the basilar artery. Under resting conditions, blood flow within the basilar artery is rarely critically impaired, even if the steal is continuous. However, if the contralateral feeding vertebral artery is also diseased, blood flow in the basilar artery may become reduced. During hyperemia testing of the stealing arm, velocity and direction of flow within the basilar trunk may become less or more affected (Figs. 36-18 and 36-19). Essentially, subclavian steal is a benign condition, and even in patients with symptoms, most vertebrobasilar symptoms are caused by cerebral microangiopathies rather than flow disturbance.[49] Blood flow in the basilar artery is extremely resistant to any critical changes due to subclavian steal mechanism. In rare cases, however, TCD has convincingly identified individuals for beneficial recanalizations.

Monitoring of cerebral vasospasm

Spasm of cerebral arteries is a complication seen with subarachnoid hemorrhage and is a significant cause of morbidity and mortality. The first application of TCD was to detect and monitor vasospasm due to subarachnoid hemorrhage.[4,6] Angiography is generally performed to localize the existence of aneurysm before surgery and is helpful in assessing the existence of vasospasm, but it cannot be performed repeatedly to provide continuous monitoring of the development of vasospasm. TCD allows noninvasive detection of vasospasm and continuous monitoring. A close correlation has been observed between increased flow velocities within the spastic basal arteries (middle, posterior, and anterior cerebral arteries) and severity of the subarachnoid hemorrhage.[21-23,58] This correlation was true with respect to the size and extent of the blood clot, the clinical state of the patients, and the angiographically documented severity of the spasm (if Doppler shift was greater than 3

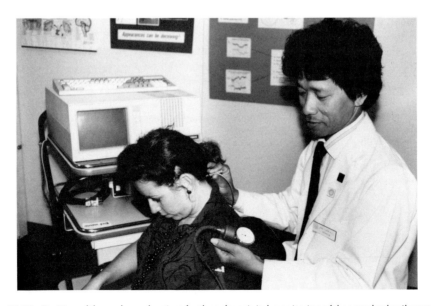

Fig. 36-18. Position of the probe and patient for the suboccipital monitoring of the vertebrobasilar arteries during hyperemic testing for subclavian steal syndrome.

kHz or 120 cm/sec); the side with the more severe flow changes during TCD corresponded to the main location of the blood clot and presumed site of the aneurysm. A steep increase in flow velocity within the first few days (greater than 20 cm/sec per day) after the hemorrhage was associated with poor prognosis. Usually, a velocity exceeding 200 cm/sec in the middle cerebral artery in patients with vasospasm had associated critical reduction in cerebral blood flow (Table 36-4). Also of clinical interest was the time course of development of vasospasm. Generally, vasospasm associated with subarachnoid hemorrhage occurred between 4 and 14 days after the hemorrhage; however, an increased velocity on TCD often preceded the onset of symptoms by hours to days. This ability to detect vasospasm before symptoms appear allows clinical determination of possible pro-

phylactic treatment. TCD is becoming an important technique in the diagnosis, monitoring, and treatment of vasospasm, and the transcranial information is being used to determine the timing of operation and to evaluate the effect of new medical treatments.[25] Recently, it even became possible to combine TCD with color-coded B-mode imaging of the brain.[8]

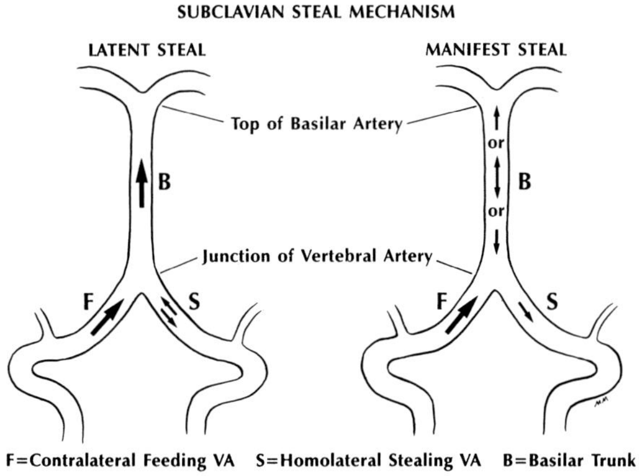

Intraoperative monitoring

The unique advantage of TCD over other techniques of measurement of regional cerebral blood flow is the complete noninvasiveness of TCD and its potential to detect rapid alterations of blood supply in an on-line fashion. Although TCD records only the mean flow velocity of the blood column within the basal arteries, this variable closely reflects the true volume flow when measured both simultaneously and individually.[49] In the past, any alteration of the cerebral circulation could not be detected except by means of repeat angiography or measurements of blood flow that had to be performed off line. This kind of examination cannot be regarded as monitoring in a strict sense, since data must be stored for later interpretation. This lack of suitable methods for monitoring regional cerebral blood flow led to the measurement of electrophysiologic variables that provided information about abnormal metabolism occurring only as a result of reduced cerebral perfusion. In contrast, TCD monitoring delivers immediate information about cerebral perfusion, thus anticipating potential hazards or allowing rapid modification of therapy. TCD monitoring has been used during endarterectomy, open heart surgery with cardiopulmonary bypass, and intensive care therapy. Continuous monitoring in these situations can be accomplished by several types of permanent temporal probes mounted on the patient's head and fixed with bands or helmetlike constructions (Fig. 36-20). So far, however, most of them have resulted in considerable artifact signals, and handheld positioning of the probe has remained the method of choice. In most studies the M1 segment of the middle cerebral artery is insonated at a depth of 50 or 55 mm (Fig. 36-21). TCD monitoring can be performed by either repeated examinations at short intervals or continuously over a longer period. Most experience with TCD monitoring has been accumulated during carotid endarterectomy.[17,46,48,50] Blood flow ve-

SUBCLAVIAN STEAL MECHANISM

LATENT STEAL   MANIFEST STEAL

Top of Basilar Artery

Junction of Vertebral Artery

F=Contralateral Feeding VA   S=Homolateral Stealing VA   B=Basilar Trunk

Fig. 36-19. Schematic drawing of the flow conditions in the various vertebrobasilar vessel segments in patients with subclavian steal mechanism. With latent steal, flow in the feeding vertebral artery *(F)* is increased during brachial hyperemia and is normal in the basilar trunk *(B)*. By contrast, the blood column shows an alternating flow direction in the stealing vertebral artery *(S)*. During manifest steal, blood flow in *S* is continuously reversed. This leads to an unaffected, alternating, or reversed blood flow within the basilar trunk. During transcranial Doppler sonography, each of the three vessel segments can be differentiated clearly by means of the segment's characteristic flow changes during brachial hyperemia. (From Ringelstein EB: *A practical guide to transcranial Doppler sonography.* In Weinberger J, ed: *Noninvasive assessment of the cerebral circulation in cerebrovascular disease,* New York, 1988, Alan R. Liss.)

Table 36-4. Clinical meaning of increased flow velocites in middle cerebral artery after subarachnoid hemorrhage

Flow velocity in middle cerebral artery	Mean time-averaged peak velocity (cm/sec)	Clinical consequences
Normal or unspecifically increased	≤80	Should be observed further
Subcritically accelerated	>80-120	Moderate vasospasm, preventive therapy indicated
Critically accelerated	>120-140	Severe vasospasm, consequent treatment necessary
Highly critical flow acceleration	>140	Severe vasospasm, consequent treatment necessary Delayed ischemic deficit highly probable

Modified from Harders A: *Neurosurgical applications of transcranial Doppler sonography,* New York, 1986, Springer-Verlag.

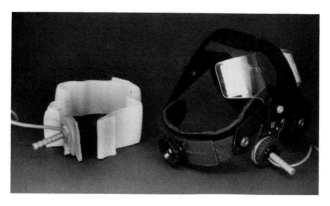

Fig. 36-20. Two representative types of permanent temporal headbands to fix the TCD probe over the temporal area during continuous monitoring. Note both are equipped with "joy sticks" to allow readjustment during the operative procedures.

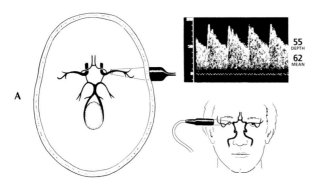

A

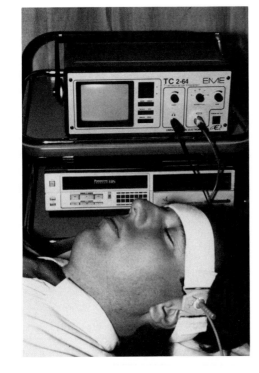

B

Fig. 36-21. *A,* Transcranial Doppler insonation of the MCA through the transtemporal window recording the M1 segment of the MCA at an insonation depth of 55 mm. *B,* Transcranial Doppler monitoring probe and head device adjusted to the temporal window with the angle of insonation adjusted by a joy stick, which can be removed and the probe locked in position.

locity in the middle cerebral artery during carotid clamping has a linear correlation with measurement of stump pressure (Fig. 36-22). It has been shown that during intraoperative clamping of the carotid artery, flow in the middle cerebral artery is far less affected than was expected, raising the possibility that shunts may be inserted too often. When stump pressure was used as a reference, a velocity greater than 10 cm/sec during clamping reportedly correlated with adequate collateral circulation.[46] A reduction in velocity of 65% or less from preclamp values was found to be consistent with adequate collateral flow.[48] Preliminary experience with combined somatosensory-evoked potential monitoring and TCD velocity monitoring of the middle cerebral artery during carotid endarterectomy has shown that complete absence of any measurable flow in the middle cerebral artery is necessary to alter the somatosensory evoked cortical response.* From a pathophysiologic point of view, these findings suggest that most postoperative neurologic deficits in these patients are the result of acute thrombosis and/or operative-related embolism rather than hypoperfusion. The effect of removal of plaques and stenosis in the carotid bifurcation on velocity in the middle cerebral artery can also be measured. It has been shown that the average velocity was only slightly increased postoperatively when compared with preoperative values, again indicating that removal of the stenosis is only rarely of hemodynamic significance. The effects of preoperative manual compression of the common carotid artery on blood flow in the middle cerebral artery are also predictive of the intraoperative events during cross-clamping of the exposed carotid bifurcation. A close relationship between preoperative and intraoperative velocity in the middle cerebral artery and flow reduction is evident.

TCD monitoring during open heart surgery with cardiopulmonary bypass has revealed a number of disturbances that occur in cerebral blood flow as a result of the extracorporeal bypass (a pumping technique that severely alters

---

*Ringelstein EB et al: Unpublished data.

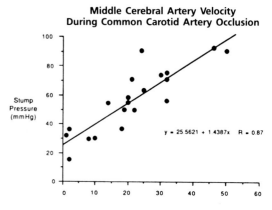

Fig. 36-22. Blood flow velocity in the middle cerebral artery during carotid clamping shows a linear correlation with measurement of stump pressure.

physiologic blood flow).[38-40, 55] During artificial maintenance of the arterial circulation, hypoxic brain damage and perioperative strokes may occur. However, transcranial measurements have thrown considerable doubt on the theory that postoperative encephalopathy is caused by critical hypoperfusion. On the contrary, accidental cerebral hyperperfusion may play a more decisive role, as well as loss of cerebral autoregulation and/or microemboli (Fig. 36-23). These monitoring studies have provided information on cerebral autoregulation and carbon dioxide reactivity during cardiopulmonary bypass. Preoperatively, TCD may identify patients at high risk for ischemic encephalopathy with the help of the carbon dioxide inhalation test for assessing the autoregulatory capacity of the brain arterials. Studies have shown that there is impaired autoregulation but sustained carbon dioxide reactivity and that the increase in cerebral blood flow during bypass is proportional to the amount of hemodilution.[38,39]

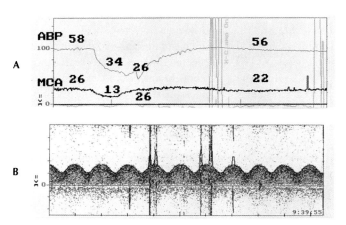

Fig. 36-23. Transcranial Doppler monitoring during open heart surgery. *A,* Loss of autoregulation demonstrated by the corresponding drop in MCA velocity with decrease in mean arterial blood pressure *(ABP). B,* Typical artifactual-appearing emboli recorded during pusatile bypass flow.

TCD monitoring during intensive care therapy is a wide and as yet still unexplored field. Monitoring may be informative and possibly beneficial for the patient's outcome in subarachnoid hemorrhage with vasospasm, as mentioned earlier, and in high- and low-pressure hydrocephalus, increased intracranial pressure, low-flow states associated with extracranial occlusive disease, myocardial failure or valvular disease, and impending brain death. TCD monitoring may provide further information on the pathophysiology of various abnormal conditions as well as being helpful for therapeutic intervention. Hyperperfusion and hypoperfusion phenomena after blunt injury of the head is another exciting field for TCD monitoring, particularly with respect to the prognostic impact of these findings.[48] Carbon dioxide reactivity may be an indicator of prognosis in that strict control of cerebral blood flow may lead to reduction in cerebral injury. Recently, Aaslid and Lindegaard[3] have described a new measurement extracted from the ultrasound profiles that is highly indicative of cerebral perfusion pressure and thus of the momentary intracranial pressure. If this approach becomes accepted, it will be of utmost interest for the large group of intensive care patients who have elevations in intracranial pressure, from whatever cause, and will perhaps indicate more effective therapeutic regimens in these life-threatening conditions.

Brain death

The accurate diagnosis of brain death has become more important in light of transplantation of kidneys or other organs and with respect to ethical limitations of intensive care measurements. In patients with brain death, a characteristic and diagnostic flow pattern has been recorded by TCD for the basal intracranial arteries[3,35,48,66] (Fig. 36-24). Determination of brain death is based on three variables: the clinical criteria, electroencephalographic criteria, and angiographic evidence of intracranial circulatory arrest.[10] This arrest, resulting in a negative cerebral perfusion pressure, results in a characteristic reflux phenomenon during late systole after antegrade injection of the blood into the

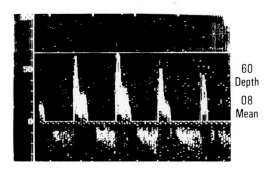

Left Middle Cerebral Artery

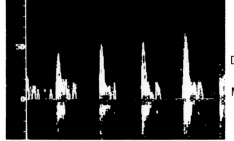

Left Extracranial Common Carotid Artery

Fig. 36-24. Changes in the left middle cerebral and extracranial common carotid arteries seen on transcranial Doppler sonography in brain death. The characteristic reflux phenomenon seen during late systole is shown.

vascular tree. This to-and-fro movement is easily noted in the TCD flow velocity waveform. Depending on the cardiac output, flow profiles may vary from sharp and pulsatile to dampened with sluggish acceleration and deceleration of the blood column. TCD monitoring may replace other more invasive methods used to show circulatory arrest.

Arteriovenous malformations and fistulas

Although arteriovenous malformation is a developmental abnormality, the arteries and veins involved in supplying the blood to the malformation are essentially normal and are the usual vessels that supply that region of the brain. The arteries that exclusively or partially feed arteriovenous malformations can be identified unequivocally with TCD by means of their significant flow abnormalities, namely increased flow velocity, reduced pulsatility, and reduced responsiveness to carbon dioxide.[21,25,60] This high velocity and low pulsatility index seen in the feeding arteries and their response to carbon dioxide allow location and evaluation of the hemodynamic state of the malformations. Flow velocities as high as 280 cm/sec can be measured in these feeders, and under carbon dioxide stimulation, pure angioma feeders show either no changes in flow velocity or only a slight increase of diastolic flow velocities during hypercapnia. These vessels are totally unresponsive to hypocapnia. Severe reduction of pulsatility is indicated by a diastolic-systolic ratio greater than 74% or a low resistant index less than 0.27.[25] Obviously, a striking hemispheric difference of flow velocities is also noted in side-to-side comparisons. Arteries that contribute only a little to the malformation may not be identified by changes in velocity and pulsatility index but will show decreased responsiveness to carbon dioxide. A linear relationship between mean flow velocity and the diameter of the feeder vessel and volume of the angioma is noted, as well as a negative linear relationship to the length of the feeder. Draining veins associated with the angioma can be identified by their pulsatile flow near the vicinity of the angioma but complete lack of flow changes during Valsalva maneuvers.[25]

TCD reexamination after radiation[57] or surgery for angioma may be particularly helpful to detect feeders of residual arteriovenous malformation and identify the severe changes in flow due to bleeding. Flow velocities in former feeders drop dramatically below the velocities of normal vessels and gradually adopt again the flow characteristics of normal brain-supplying arteries.[23]

Clinically, TCD is helpful in making the primary diagnosis of arteriovenous malformation and deciding if angiography is needed. Other types of intracranial-arteriovenous shunts of small size can also be detected, such as carotid siphon cavernous sinus fistulas and dural fistulas, which are detected by their high flow velocities and severely disturbed flow at the site. In addition, TCD may be helpful in the follow-up of patients undergoing other types of treatment, such as local radiation or embolization.[5,49]

CONCLUSION

The tremendous potential of TCD is becoming more apparent as more and more investigators from different backgrounds are reporting on its uses in different clinical settings. Because of its noninvasive characteristics and excellent time resolution, detailed and repeated investigations of intracranial cerebral blood flow can be monitored. The usefulness of TCD in early detection of vasospasm and its possible use in altering and planning therapies has been clearly documented.[5,23,54,58] Intraoperative monitoring in carotid endarterectomy and cardiopulmonary bypass may improve and minimize surgical mortality and possibly provide further information on the efficacy of these procedures.[17,38,51,56] In patients with cerebral vascular disease, TCD monitoring of the intracranial and cerebral collateral circulation and cerebral vascular reserve promises to result in improved treatments and therapies.[32,36,43,52,53] Measurements of regional cerebral blood flow and combined information on intracranial and extracranial circulation are becoming available and should lead to better understanding and treatment in various conditions, as well as allow repeated studies of the natural progression of disease. Intensive care monitoring in brain injury, brain death, and increased intracranial pressure should enhance understanding and treatment of these critical situations.[3,37,54] TCD may become an important research tool for the evaluation of cerebral blood flow in experimental animals and humans in outer space or at high altitudes because of its excellent time resolution and extreme sensitivity to flow changes.[45]

Recent advances now enable clinicians to penetrate the available ultrasound windows and skull foramina with B-mode imaging (Fig. 36-25). This represents a major break-

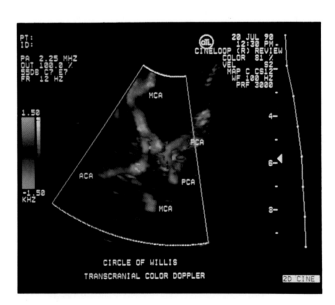

Fig. 36-25. Intracranial B-mode imaging of the circle of Willis demonstrating views of the anterior and posterior cerebral arteries. (Courtesy ATL, Bothell, Washington.)

through in intracranial arterial diagnosis and allows combination of the anatomic imaging information and Doppler physiologic flow information. This duplex color system promises to have the same dramatic effect on intracranial vessel identification and diagnosis as it has in the extracranial carotid examination.

REFERENCES

1. Aaslid R, ed: *Transcranial Doppler ultrasound,* New York, 1986, Springer-Verlag.
2. Aaslid R: Visually evoked dynamic blood flow response of the human cerebral circulation, *Stroke* 18:771, 1987.
3. Aaslid R, Lindegaard KF: *Cerebral hemodynamics.* In Aaslid A, ed: *Transcranial Doppler sonography,* New York, 1986, Springer-Verlag.
4. Aaslid R, Nornes H: Musical murmurs in human cerebral arteries after subarachnoid hemorrhage, *J Neurosurg* 60:32, 1984.
5. Aaslid R, Huber P, Nornes H: Evaluation of cerebrovascular spasm with transcranial Doppler ultrasound, *J Neurosurg* 60:37, 1984.
6. Aaslid R, Markwalder TM, Nornes H: Non-invasive transcranial Doppler ultrasound recording of flow velocity in basal cerebral arteries, *J Neurosurg* 57:769, 1982.
7. Arnolds DJ, Von Reutern GM: Transcranial Doppler sonography: examination technique and normal reference values, *Ultrasound Med Biol* 12:115, 1986.
8. Becker G et al: Diagnosis and monitoring of subarachnoid hemorrhage by transcranial color-coded real-time sonography, *Neurosurgery* 28:814-820, 1991.
9. Bishop CFR et al: The effect of internal carotid artery occlusion on middle cerebral artery blood flow at rest and response to hypercapnia, *Lancet* 1:710, 1986.
10. Black PM: Brain death, *N Engl J Med* 299:338-344, 1978.
11. Bullock R et al: Cerebral blood flow and CO_2 responsiveness as an indicator of collateral reserve capacity in patients with carotid arterial disease, *Br J Surg* 72:348, 1985.
12. Caplan LR, Sergay S: Positional cerebral ischemia, *J Neurol Neurosurg Psychiatry* 39:385, 1976.
13. Carter JE: Chronic ocular ischemia and carotid vascular disease, *Stroke* 16:721, 1985.
14. Del Zoppo GJ, Otis SM: *Thrombolytic therapy in acute stroke.* In Comerota AR, ed: *Thrombolytic therapy,* Orlando, Fla, 1988, Grune & Stratton.
15. Del Zoppo GJ, Zeumer H, Harker LA: Thrombolytic therapy in stroke: possibilities and hazards, *Stroke* 17:595, 1986.
16. De Witt LD, Wechsler H: Transcranial Doppler, *Stroke* 19:915-921, 1988.
17. Edelmann M, Ringelstein EB, Richert F: Transcranial Doppler sonography for monitoring of the middle cerebral artery blood flow velocity during carotid endarterectomy, *Rev Bras Angiol Clin Vasc* 16:96, 1986.
18. Frackowiak RSJ et al: Quantitative measurements of cerebral blood flow and oxygen metabolism in man using 15-oxygen and positron emission tomography: theory, procedure and normal values, *J Comput Assist Tomogr* 4:727, 1980.
19. Gibbs JN et al: Evaluation of cerebral perfusion reserve in patients with carotid artery occlusion, *Lancet* 1:310, 1984.
20. Grolimund P: *Transmission of ultrasound through the temporal bone.* In Aaslid R, ed: *Transcranial Doppler sonography,* New York, 1986, Springer-Verlag.
21. Harders A: *Monitoring of hemodynamic changes related to vasospasm in the circle of Willis after aneurysm surgery.* In Aaslid R, ed: *Transcranial Doppler sonography,* New York, 1986, Springer-Verlag.
22. Harders A: *Neurosurgical applications of transcranial Doppler sonography,* New York, 1986, Springer-Verlag.
23. Harders A, Gilsbach JM: Time course of blood velocity changes related to vasospasm in the circle of Willis measured by transcranial Doppler ultrasound, *J Neurosurg* 66:718, 1987.
24. Harper AM, Glass HI: Effect of alterations in the arterial carbon dioxide tension on the blood flow through the cerebral cortex at normal and low arterial blood pressures, *J Neurol Neurosurg Psychiatry* 28:449, 1966.
25. Hassler W: Hemodynamic aspects of cerebral angiomas, *Acta Neurochir* 37(suppl):38, 1986.
26. Hennerici M, Rautenberg W, Schwartz A: Transcranial ultrasound for the assessment of intracranial arterial flow velocity, part 2, *Surg Neurol* 27:523, 1987.
27. Hennerici M et al: Transcranial Doppler ultrasound for the assessment of intracranial arterial flow velocity. Part 1. Examination technique and normal values, *Surg Neurol* 27:439, 1987.
28. Huber P, Hauda J: Effect of contrast material, hypercapnia, hyperventilation, hypertonic glucose and papaverine on the diameter of the cerebral arteries: angiographic determination in man, *Invest Radiol* 2:17, 1987.
29. Kennedy C, Sokoloff L: An adaptation of the nitrous oxide method to the study of the cerebral circulation in children: normal values for cerebral blood flow and cerebral metabolic rate in childhood, *J Clin Invest* 36:1130, 1957.
30. Kety SS: Human cerebral blood flow and oxygen consumption as related to aging, *J Chronic Dis* 3:478, 1956.
31. Kety SS, Schmidt CF: The effects of altered tensions of carbon dioxide and oxygen on cerebral blood flow and oxygen consumption of normal young men, *J Clin Invest* 27:484, 1948.
32. Kirkham FJ, Levin SD, Neville BGR: Bedside diagnosis of stenosis of the middle cerebral artery, *Lancet* 1:797, 1986.
33. Kirkham FJ et al: Transcranial measurement of blood velocities in the basal cerebral arteries using pulsed Doppler ultrasound: velocity as an index of flow, *Ultrasound Med Biol* 12:15-21, 1986.
34. Klingelhöfer J, Sander D: CO_2-reactivity test as an indicator of autoregulatory capacity and prognosis in severe cerebral disease, *Stroke* (in press).
35. Lewis RR et al: Investigation of brain death with Doppler-shift ultrasound, *JR Soc Med* 76:308, 1983.
36. Ley Pozo J, Ringelstein EB: Noninvasive detection of occlusive disease of the carotid siphon and middle cerebral artery, *Ann Neurol* 28:640-647, 1990.
37. Lindegaard R et al: Assessment of intracranial hemodynamics in carotid artery disease by transcranial Doppler ultrasound, *J Neurosurg* 63:890, 1985.
38. Lundar T et al: Cerebral perfusion during nonpulsatile cardiopulmonary bypass, *Ann Thorac Surg* 40:144, 1985.
39. Lundar T et al: Dissociation between cerebral autoregulation and carbon dioxide reactivity during nonpulsatile cardiopulmonary bypass, *Ann Thorac Surg* 40:582, 1985.
40. Lundar T et al: Cerebral carbon dioxide reactivity during nonpulsatile cardiopulmonary bypass, *Ann Thorac Surg* 41:525, 1986.
41. Markwalder TM et al: Dependency of blood flow velocity in the mddle cerebral artery on end-tidal carbon dioxide partial pressure: a transcranial ultrasound Doppler study, *J Cereb Blood Flow Metab* 4:368, 1984.
42. Mull M, Aulich A, Hennerici M: Transcranial Doppler ultrasonography versus arteriography for assessment of the vertebrobasilar circulation, *J Clin Ultrasound* 18:539-549, 1990.
43. Niederkorn R, Neumayer K: Transcranial Doppler sonography: a new approach in the noninvasive diagnosis of intracranial brain artery disease, *Eur Neurol* 26:65, 1987.
44. Norrving B, Nilsson B, Risberg J: rCBF in patients with carotid occlusion: resting and hypercapnic flow related to collateral pattern, *Stroke* 13:155, 1982.
45. Otis SM et al: Relationship of cerebral blood flow regulation to acute mountain sickness, *J Ultrasound Med* 8:143-148, 1989.
46. Padayachee TS et al: Monitoring middle cerebral artery blood velocities during carotid endarterectomy, *Br J Surg* 73:98, 1986.
47. Padayachee TS et al: Transcranial measurement of blood velocities in the basal cerebral arteries using pulsed Doppler ultrasound: a method of assessing the circle of Willis, *Ultrasound Med Biol* 12:5, 1986.
48. Ringelstein EB: *Transcranial Doppler monitoring.* In Aaslid R, ed: *Transcranial Doppler sonography,* New York, 1986, Springer-Verlag.
49. Ringelstein EB: *A practical guide to transcranial Doppler sonography.* In Weinberger J, ed: *Noninvasive assessment of the cerebral circulation in cerebrovascular disease,* Frontiers of Clinical Neuroscience Series, New York, 1988, Alan R Liss.
50. Ringelstein EB, Zeumer H, Angelou D: The pathogenesis of strokes from internal carotid artery occlusion: diagnostic and therapeutical implications, *Stroke* 14:867, 1983.

51. Ringelstein EB et al: Transkranielle Dopplersonographie der hirnversorgenden. Arterien: atraumatische Diagnostik von Stenosen und Verschlussen des Karotissiphin und der A. cerebri media, *Nervenarzt* 56:296, 1985.
52. Ringelstein EB et al: Noninvasive assessment of CO_2 induced cerebral vasomotor reactivity in normals and patients with internal carotid arterial occlusion, *Stroke* 19:963-969, 1988.
53. Ringelstein EB et al: Transcranial Doppler sonography. Part I. Anatomical landmarks and normal velocity values, *Ultrasound Med Biol* 16:745-761, 1990.
54. Ringelstein EB et al: Type and extent of hemispheric brain infarctions and clinical outcome in early and delayed middle cerebral artery recanalization, *Neurology* (in press).
55. Russo G et al: Transcranial Doppler ultrasound: examination technique and normal reference values, *J Neurosurg Sci* 30:97, 1986.
56. Schneider PA et al: Transcranial Doppler (TCD) in the management of extracranial cerebrovascular disease: implications in diagnosis and monitoring, *J Vasc Surg* 7:223, 1988.
57. Schwartz A, Hennerici M: Noninvasive transcranial Doppler ultrasound in intracranial angiomas, *Neurology* 36:626, 1986.
58. Seiler RW et al: Relation of cerebral vasospasm evaluated by transcranial Doppler ultrasound to clinical grade and CT-visualized subarachnoid hemorrhage, *J Neurosurg* 64:594, 1986.
59. Silverstein A, Doniger D, Bender MB: Manual compression of the carotid vessels, carotid sinus hypersensitivity and carotid artery occlusions, *Ann Intern Med* 52:172, 1960.
60. Sommer C, Müllges W, Ringelstein EB: Noninvasive assessment of intracranial fistulas and other small arteriovenous malformations, *Neurosurgery* (in press).
61. Spencer MP: *Transcranial Doppler ultrasound imaging using duplex ultrasonic imaging.* Paper presented at 1st International Conference on Transcranial Doppler Sonography, Consiglio Nazionale della Richerche, Rome, 1986.
62. Spencer MP, Whisler D: Transorbital Doppler diagnosis of intracranial arterial stenosis, *Stroke* 17:916, 1986.
63. von Reutern GM, et al: Transcranial Doppler ultrasonography during cardiopulmonary bypass in patients with severe carotid stenosis or occlusion, *Stroke* 19:674-680, 1988.
64. Webster JE, Gurdjian FJ: Observations upon response to digital carotid artery compression, *Neurology* 7:757, 1957.
65. Wechsler LR et al: The effects of endarterectomy on the intracranial circulation studied by transcranial Doppler, *Neurology* 37:317, 1987.
66. Werner C et al: Transcranial Doppler sonography as a supplement in the detection of cerebral circulatory arrest, *J Neurosurg Anesthesiol* 2:159-165, 1990.
67. White DN, Curry GR, Stevenson RJ: The acoustic characteristics of the skull, *Ultrasound Med Biol* 4:225, 1978.
68. Widder B et al: Transcranial Doppler CO_2-test for the detection of hemodynamically critical carotid artery stenoses and occlusions, *Eur Arch Psychiatry Neurol Sci* 236:162, 1986.

CHAPTER 37

Intraoperative monitoring with transcranial Doppler sonography

ROB G.A. ACKERSTAFF and TORBEN V. SCHROEDER

During both carotid endarterectomy and heart surgery with cardiopulmonary bypass, cerebral blood flow (CBF) is variable and unsuspected ischemia to the brain may result. For determination of when this occurs, several techniques of monitoring cerebral function during these surgical interventions have been developed. These include measurements of CBF, electroencephalography (EEG), and more recently transcranial Doppler (TCD) ultrasonography. CBF monitoring should permit an accurate assumption concerning the adequacy of brain oxygenation. However, it is an indirect monitor and lacks the specificity of the EEG in identifying cerebral ischemia. For this reason and because the techniques for measuring CBF are relatively complex, the routine monitoring of CBF during surgery is not common practice. It is only performed in a few institutions and is largely limited to patients undergoing carotid endarterectomy.* On the other hand, there is a good correlation between the cortical blood flow and the frequency content of the EEG. In general, slow wave activity appearing in the EEG will parallel a decrease in regional CBF (rCBF).[10,50] Suppression of electrical activity in the EEG during surgery indicates severe hypoxia,[9] the early phase of air embolism,[9,32] or borderline low CBF and likely hypotension.[10,50] Thus during the critical periods of both carotid surgery and cardiopulmonary bypass (CPB), continued surveillance of the brain by an EEG appears to be a reliable method of determining the adequacy of CBF.[31,55] This method is not infallible because similar EEG changes can also result from variation in the level of anesthesia and from hypothermia. Use of the standard 16-channel EEG is admittedly clumsy and expensive. It generates large amounts of paperwork and requires an experienced neurophysiologist to continuously observe and interpret the changes that might occur. Therefore most institutions find it impractical to monitor all patients undergoing carotid endarterectomy or heart surgery with EEG.

The introduction of TCD in 1982[1] offered a new, noninvasive, continuous technique for monitoring the cerebral circulation during surgery. Although TCD is not a measure of CBF, changes in flow are reflected by changes in flow velocity. Autoregulation of CBF and carbon dioxide reactivity is assumed to act on vessels distal to the mainstem of the basal cerebral arteries. The diameter of the proximal middle cerebral artery (MCA) is assumed to remain constant.[13,19,54] Changes of the blood flow velocity in the MCA would therefore be a relatively good indicator of changes of MCA volume flow during variations in cerebral perfusion pressure as well as in the partial pressure of arterial carbon dioxide.[6,58] Comparative studies of MCA flow velocity measured with TCD and internal carotid artery flow recorded electromagnetically in humans have demonstrated a close correlation between these two variables.[28] Finally, several studies have demonstrated that TCD is sensitive to the detection of cerebral microemboli that occur during carotid and heart surgery.[37,53]

The best method for assessing brain function during surgery under general anesthesia is the EEG. Measurement of CBF is an available technique that has proved useful as an investigational tool but is unlikely to become popular as a clinical tool. TCD seems to be a reliable, noninvasive technique. It is a relatively new technique, however, and its clinical value must be shown in properly designed studies in which the TCD data can be compared with the EEG and rCBF measurements.

INTRAOPERATIVE MONITORING DURING CAROTID SURGERY

The EEG expert system

In an effort to reduce at least some of the drawbacks of continuous EEG monitoring during surgery, St. Antonius Hospital in the Netherlands developed an expert system to process the EEG in patients undergoing carotid endarterectomy and open heart surgery. The automatic EEG monitoring system has been described in detail in earlier reports.[40-42] Briefly, the system provides continuous acquisition and recording of the EEG of both hemispheres and data concerning the blood pressure, temperature, carotid cross-clamping, and anesthesia during surgery. The EEG is recorded with frontoparietal and temporooccipital derivations of both sides and is immediately transmitted to video in the operating theater and the neurophysiology department. Clinically relevant features are extracted from the EEG data, and abnormal activity results in the generation of an automatic warning and alarm signal. Trends in the patient data

---

*References 3, 5, 15, 20, 34, 36, 57.

are presented graphically, and instantaneously measured data are numerically displayed. A continuous recording of blood pressure registration makes it possible to relate to their data the extracted EEG data. This assists in adjusting the blood pressure to maintain adequate CBF. The neurophysiologist can compare these data with the on-line EEG, which is helpful in identifying EEG artifacts. During carotid endarterectomy the asymmetry between the hemispheres is continuously calculated by comparing the number of zero-crossings of the EEG on both sides. This is numerically displayed. Asymmetry between the hemispheres of greater than 15% is considered severe enough to justify the use of a shunt.

Since 1971, about 1200 carotid endarterectomies have been performed with the EEG expert system. The reliability of the system with respect to the detection of intraoperative stroke has been evaluated.[27] Transient EEG asymmetry that reversed after placement of a shunt occurred in 32 of 230 endarterectomies (13.9%). This was not associated with intraoperative stroke. Persistent EEG asymmetry on the side undergoing surgery developed in eight cases, and four of these patients had a major stroke. The detection rate of intraoperative major stroke with the system was 80% sensitivity and 99% specificity, and the diagnostic gain was 47.8%. In contrast, minor strokes were not detected by the EEG expert system. In most of these cases the infarcts were small and deeply located. Using the morphologic analysis of the brain infarct on computed tomography (CT) scan to establish the pathogenesis of stroke in carotid surgery, Krul et al[26] revealed that 43% of intraoperative infarcts were probably hemodynamic in etiology. This proportion is significantly higher than observed in the natural history of spontaneous stroke.[43] The remaining 57% was probably of thromboembolic origin and occurred during manipulation of the carotid arteries by the surgeon.

Measurement of regional cerebral blood flow

For more than two decades, researchers at the Rigshospitalet in Copenhagen have been working with intraoperative xenon[133] rCBF determinations in the study of the cerebral hemodynamics in patients with carotid artery disease.[8,48] On the basis of these data and the experience from the Mayo Clinic (see Chapter 41), a critical level of rCBF of 20 ml/100 g/min has been established. Below this level, EEG abnormalities appear with increasing frequency. The rCBF measurements were performed with the intraarterial xenon[133] technique. Four scintillation detectors were positioned over the ipsilateral MCA territory. A bolus of 1 mCi xenon[133] in saline was injected into the common carotid artery with the external carotid artery clamped. After three heart beats, the internal carotid artery was also clamped. Clearance was followed for 2 minutes, and rCBF was calculated from a monoexponential fit of the first minutes' decay curve. Flow was presented as an average of the four values.

TCD monitoring

For the TCD studies a pulsed Doppler system with a relatively large sample volume (axial width 10 to 20 mm, lateral width 5 mm) is used. The sample volume is gated at a depth of 45 to 55 mm from the temporal bone to insonate the main stem of the MCA. The TCD transducer is fixed in place with a head strap. Ipsilateral common carotid compression can be carried out to ensure that the artery being insonated is the MCA. Video recordings of the Doppler spectra and audio signals of Doppler ultrasound are recorded from the time the patient is intubated until the end of anesthesia. It is very important to make the Doppler audio signal available to the personnel in the operating room throughout the entire procedure. Most studies have addressed the MCA mean velocity, determined as the maximum velocity (Doppler spectrum envelope) averaged over the cardiac cycle. Changes in blood flow velocity before and during carotid cross-clamping as well as after release of the clamps (Fig. 37-1) are compared with changes in the EEG and rCBF.

RESULTS
Hemodynamic aspects

To monitor cerebral function during carotid endarterectomy more reliably, many institutions have introduced continuous TCD registration of the blood flow velocities of the ipsilateral MCA,[16,17,34,38,44] some as an addition to neuro-

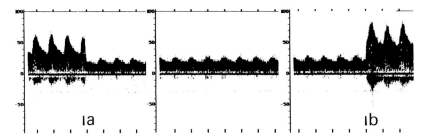

Fig. 37-1. The mean velocity during carotid endarterectomy decreased immediately from 44 to 22 cm/sec when the internal carotid artery was cross-clamped (↑ a), remained constant during clamping, and increased to 60 cm/sec after declamping (↑ b).

physiologic monitoring.[20,57] TCD recordings provide direct information about the cerebral circulation and are sensitive to the detection of cerebral microemboli.[53]

In the study from Copenhagen, 44 patients were simultaneously monitored with EEG, rCBF, and TCD during carotid endarterectomy.[23] During cross-clamping of the carotid artery, only a modest correlation was found between the rCBF values and MCA velocities (r = 0.51, Fig. 37-2). All 13 patients who had a rCBF of less than 20 ml/100 g/min were identified by a MCA velocity of less than 30 cm/sec. However, another 12 patients also had MCA velocities of less than 30 cm/sec with an rCBF greater than 20 ml/100 g/min. With respect to the detection of a rCBF of less than 20 ml/100 g/min at cross-clamping, a MCA velocity of 30 cm/sec had a sensitivity of 100%, a specificity of 61%, and an overall accuracy of 73%. Of the 13 patients who had a rCBF of less than 20 ml/100 g/min, 3 also demonstrated EEG abnormalities on cross-clamping. In these patients, the rCBF values were 10, 11, and 15 ml/100 g/min, respectively, and the corresponding MCA velocities were 10, 18, and 26 cm/sec, respectively (Fig. 37-2). Only 2 other patients had a rCBF of less than 15 ml/100 g/min.

Previous experience relating TCD to rCBF and EEG during carotid surgery has been limited. Halsey et al[16,17] reported a significant correlation between MCA velocity and rCBF, but this was obtained entirely due to measurements at rCBF of less than 20 ml/100 g/min. In agreement with the Copenhagen experience, they found rCBF measurements to be more specific for EEG abnormalities than were absolute MCA velocities.

The relatively poor correlation between the absolute values of MCA velocity and rCBF at cross-clamping is probably caused by biologic and methodologic variability. This can be partially eliminated by considering the relative decrease of the MCA velocity. In this study, the MCA velocity during carotid clamping (Vc) is expressed as a fraction of the MCA velocity shortly before clamping (Vp). By using a Vc/Vp ratio of less than 0.6, 89% of the patients having a rCBF above or below 20 ml/100 g/min during clamping were correctly identified (Fig. 37-3). Similarly, with a cutoff ratio of 0.4, 43 of 44 patients (98%) were correctly categorized according to the appearance of EEG abnormalities.

When both the EEG expert system and TCD monitoring are used in 139 carotid endarterectomies, the percentage of decrease of the MCA blood flow velocity at cross-clamping was compared with the calculated asymmetry of the EEG. In this study, the only criterion used to select patients in need of a shunt was an EEG asymmetry of more than 15% (severe asymmetry). ROC analysis of the TCD data (Fig. 37-4) revealed that a 60% decrease (Vc/Vp=0.4) of the MCA mean velocity resulted in a sensitivity of 94% and a specificity of 93%. With a cut-off value of 0.4 for the Vc/Vp ratio, there was only one false-negative study, and in 6.5% of the cases the necessity of a shunt was overestimated. Other studies relating the relative changes of MCA

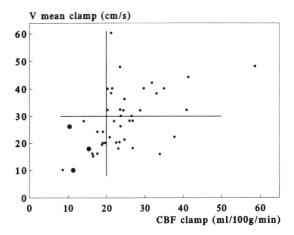

Fig. 37-2. The MCA mean velocity and rCBF during cross-clamping of the internal carotid artery in 44 patients. The 3 patients who developed EEG abnormalities are denoted with a large dot. (From Jorgensen LG, Schroeder TV: Transcranial Doppler for detection of cerebral ischaemia during carotid endarterectomy, *Eur J Vasc Surg* 6:142-147, 1992.)

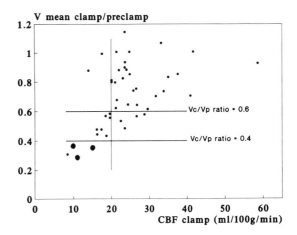

Fig. 37-3. The MCA mean velocity during cross-clamping of the internal carotid artery is expressed as a fraction of the preclamp velocity (Vc/Vp ratio) and rCBF during cross-clamping in 44 patients. The 3 patients who developed EEG abnormalities are denoted with a large dot. (From Jorgensen LG, Schroeder TV: Transcranial Doppler for detection of cerebral ischaemia during carotid endarterectomy, *Eur J Vasc Surg* 6:142-147, 1992.)

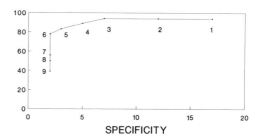

Fig. 37-4. The ROC curve of MCA mean velocity for various values of Vc/Vp ratio as threshold criteria for the selective use of a shunt. *1,* Vc/Vp = 0.50; *2,* Vc/Vp = 0.45; *3,* Vc/Vp = 0.40; *4,* Vc/Vp = 0.35; *5,* Vc/Vp = 0.30; *6,* Vc/Vp = 0.25; *7,* Vc/Vp = 0.20; *8,* Vc/Vp = 0.15; *9,* Vc/Vp = 0.10.

velocities with EEG[39] or somatosensory evoked potentials[57] have revealed similar results.

Stump pressure measurement is the most frequently used method for assessing the need for a temporary indwelling shunt. Correspondingly, a relatively large number of studies have related the MCA velocity during cross-clamping to stump pressure.[2,3,23,34,47] Although a significant correlation has been reported in all studies, the ability to predict stump pressure based on the MCA velocity has varied in individual cases. Moreover, the interpretation of these data is hampered by the same uncertainty of the accuracy of stump pressure measurements.

Another hemodynamic aspect of TCD monitoring during carotid surgery relates to the use of a shunt. In up to 15% of the cases, shunt malfunction may occur due to thrombosis, kinking, or intimal dissection.[2,3,34,38] Continuous monitoring of MCA velocities may instantaneously detect malfunction of the shunt, which allows for correction before irreversible ischemic damage has occurred.

Thromboembolic aspects

The introduction of continuous TCD monitoring of the basal cerebral arteries during other interventions has renewed interest in the detection of cerebral microemboli during carotid surgery.[21,53] Earlier reports[38] have demonstrated that TCD monitoring of the MCAs will detect air embolism with Doppler ultrasound in the intracranial arteries during cardiopulmonary bypass. In the course of monitoring of carotid endarterectomies,[52,53] it became apparent that signals identical to the qualities of gas bubble emboli were occurring during arterial dissection but before arteriotomy. It was clear these signals were not from air emboli, since the arteries had not been opened. It was concluded that the signals were caused by emboli that were called *formed element emboli*. These particulate emboli were also detected in patients with implanted prosthetic valves and atrial fibrillation.[4,56]

With the use of modern spectral analyzers, much has been learned about the audio features of such emboli. They cause short transients in the spectral waveform, usually less than 0.1 seconds in duration and ranging 3 to 60 dB above the background of the Doppler blood velocity spectrum. They appear at random throughout the cardiac cycle, and their duration in the spectrum is inversely proportional to their velocity. Although they are essentially unidirectional, they can cause bidirectional artifacts if they overload the preamplifier (Fig. 37-5). The most important characteristic is most likely that they sound like harmonic chirps, whistles, or clicks, depending on their velocity, which makes emboli characteristic to the listener.

In a study of 130 carotid endarterectomies performed with simultaneous EEG and TCD monitoring,[21] embolization was detected in 75 episodes in 55 patients. Embolization signals varied from a single embolus during insertion of a needle for stump pressure measurement to massive embolization for 5 minutes after release of the clamps. This was the only patient in whom embolization resulted in an intra-

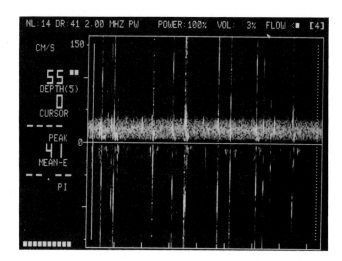

Fig. 37-5. The sonogram of the left MCA Doppler signal during non-pulsatile CPB. Many artifacts of the Doppler signal (monodirectional as well as bidirectional) are demonstrated. This patient had thousands of cerebral microemboli during CPB and died 11 days postoperatively from an intracerebral hematoma in the left MCA territory.

operative stroke of thromboembolic origin. None of the remaining patients with evidence of embolization on TCD showed signs of cerebral ischemia, either clinically or on the postoperative CT scan of the brain. In only 2 cases with massive embolization did the EEG show transient, diffuse slow-wave activity with the maximum change in the ipsilateral hemisphere. Otherwise, the time of cerebral embolization was not detected by the EEG expert system. The risk of dislodging atheromatous debris or introducing air by insertion of the shunt was found to be low. In only 19% of the cases in which an indwelling shunt was used were cerebral emboli detected by the TCD. In 8 cases, emboli were detected in the MCA on release of the clamps of the external carotid artery before the internal carotid artery was unclamped. In these cases the emboli probably entered the basal cerebral arteries via the periorbital collateral circulation.

INTRAOPERATIVE MONITORING DURING CARDIAC SURGERY

Although the risk of central nervous system complications during cardiac surgery has decreased since the 1960s, permanent brain damage is still among the most feared complications after cardiac surgery. This decrease is partly an effect of improved monitoring and surgical techniques, along with the introduction of membrane oxygenators and in-line filtration that decrease the release of microaggregates into the circulation. Today, open heart operations are associated with a 2% to 5% risk of stroke and 12% risk of diffuse encephalopathy.[11] Cardiopulmonary bypass still poses a significant risk for cerebral damage, with its incidence depending on the criteria used. In studies using psychometric tests,[35,49,51] subtle changes in personality have been described in 20% to 65% of the patients after coronary bypass graft surgery. Although several investigations indicated that many patients recover 2 to 12 months postoperatively, even transient disturbances of brain function should be considered as potentially harmful.

In some patients, specific causes such as a left ventricular mural thrombus, dysrhythmias, a brittle aorta, massive air embolization, or significant hemodynamic instability can be identified. However, in most cases the cause of the brain damage has not been identified. Knowledge concerning the cerebral circulation during cardiopulmonary bypass is scarce. Several invasive and noninvasive techniques have been applied to evaluate cerebral function during heart surgery, including rCBF measurements by xenon injection,[14,18] EEG,[7,25,46] and TCD.[24,29,59] The EEG may be useful for detecting the time of onset of focal or global brain ischemia intraoperatively and may provide clues to the mechanism of injury. In a study that used the expert EEG system,[7] diffuse major EEG abnormalities were generally related to hemodynamic instability and resulted in a diffuse encephalopathy. Focal EEG abnormalities were more often related to massive embolization and often resulted in stroke. However, not all focal abnormalities could be explained by the intraoperative EEG findings, and fast rewarming was usually associated with diffuse EEG abnormalities that are of no clinical relevance. Moreover, some patients with normal intraoperative EEG findings were found to have a stroke in the recovery room.[46] More recently, the simultaneous use of EEG and TCD monitoring during cerebrovascular surgery has revealed that tens to hundreds of cerebral microemboli detected by the TCD may not result in EEG abnormalities.[21,22] The impact of cerebral microemboli on brain function and morphology is still not well understood. The intraoperative use of TCD in combination with a microcomputer produces a simple and sensitive tool to quantitate cerebral microemboli.[12,45]

There is also considerable discussion about the effect of cardiopulmonary bypass on cerebral autoregulation. Some studies have described a loss of cerebral autoregulation with hyperperfusion of the brain during CPB.[18,29,30] In other series, cerebral autoregulation was maintained during hypothermia, and CBF was dependent on temperature and intraarterial carbon dioxide tension.[33,58] These differences are probably related to the pH management during hypothermia (alpha-stat versus pH-stat). If the blood gases are measured at 37° C and corrected to the estimated brain temperature, a relative hypercapnia is induced with hypothermia, and CBF becomes pressure dependent. With the alpha-stat policy, a coupling between cerebral metabolism and blood flow is maintained. Although the two policies of acid-base management introduce significant biologic differences, the superiority of either management in terms of cerebral protection remains to be proved.

CONCLUSION

Because of its high temporal resolution and noninvasive character, TCD monitoring during carotid endarterectomy

and cardiac surgery has many attractive features. It reveals additional information about the cerebral circulation, particularly during surgical manipulations of the carotid bifurcation. If made audible in the operating room, it provides instantaneous information to the surgeon. During carotid surgery, it may immediately detect shunt malfunction due to kinking or thrombosis and allow for correction before irreversible ischemic damage has occurred.[2,3,38] If used in combination with EEG monitoring and/or rCBF measurements, more reliable criteria for the selective use of a shunt can be defined. Concerning cerebral embolization surgeons have been guided by the emboli signals and have tried to avoid further embolization. After the introduction of TCD monitoring to the EEG expert system, the intraoperative stroke rate during carotid endarterectomy decreased.[21]

TCD monitoring during cardiac surgery is still in a more experimental phase. The clinical relevance of continuous monitoring of the blood flow velocities in the basal cerebral arteries, the quantification and discrimination of cerebral microemboli, and the impact of embolization on brain function and morphology still have to be evaluated in properly designed studies.

The use of TCD monitoring during surgery has limitations. The major obstacle to routine intraoperative use arises from problems of obtaining interpretable signals from the basal cerebral arteries, either because the temporal window may not be identified or because of other technical difficulties. These problems occur in 10% to 20% of the patients studied. The results vary with the patients' age, sex, and race; the equipment used; and the experience of the sonographer.[2,3,5,15] Sometimes the insonated artery is not the MCA but the carotid syphon or a significant cerebral collateral. There may be problems with the automatic calculation of mean velocity because of a poor signal-to-noise ratio, especially at low velocities. Finally, surgeons' manipulations may move the transducer, and the frequent use of electrocautery may preclude a reliable measurement.

REFERENCES

1. Aaslid R, Markwalder TM, Nornes H: Noninvasive transcranial Doppler ultrasound recording of flow velocity in basal cerebral arteries, *J Neurosurg* 57:769-774, 1982.
2. Bass A et al: Intraoperative transcranial Doppler: limitations of the method, *J Vasc Surg* 10:549-553, 1989.
3. Benichou H et al: Pre- and intraoperative transcranial Doppler: prediction and surveillance of tolerance to carotid clamping, *Ann Vasc Surg* 5:21-25, 1991.
4. Berger M et al: Detection of subclinical microemboli in patients with prosthetic aortic valves, *J Cardiovasc Tech* 9:282-283, 1990.
5. Bernstein EF: Role of transcranial Doppler in carotid surgery, *Surg Clin North Am* 70:225-234, 1990.
6. Bishop CCR et al: Transcranial Doppler measurements of middle cerebral artery blood flow velocity: a validation study, *Stroke* 17:913-915, 1986.
7. Boezeman EHJF, Simons AJR, Leusink JA: *Automatic EEG monitoring in cardiac surgery.* In Willer AE, Rodewald G, eds: *Impact of cardiac surgery on the quality of life: neurological and psychological aspects,* New York, 1989, Plenum Press.
8. Boysen G: Cerebral hemodynamics in carotid surgery, *Acta Neurol Scand* 49(suppl):1-84, 1973.
9. Cloche R et al: Morphology and evolution of the EEG in acute cerebral anoxia (42 cases), *Electroenceph Clin Neurophys* 25:89, 1968.

10. Freeman J, Ingvar DH: Influence of tissue hypoxia upon the EEG-cerebral blood flow relationship, *Electroenceph Clin Neurophys* 23:395, 1967.

11. Furlan AJ, Breuer AC: Central nervous system complications of open heart surgery, *Stroke* 15:912-915, 1984.

12. Gibby GL, Ghani GA: Computer-assisted Doppler monitoring to enhance detection of air emboli, *J Clin Monitor* 4:64-73, 1988.

13. Giller CA et al: Diameter changes in cerebral arteries during craniotomy, *J Cardiovasc Tech* 9:301, 1990.

14. Goviers AV et al: Factors and their influence on regional cerebral blood flow during nonpulsatile cardiopulmonary bypass, *Ann Thorac Surg* 38:592-600, 1984.

15. Halsey JH: Effect of emitted power on waveform intensity in transcranial Doppler, *Stroke* 21:573-578, 1990.

16. Halsey JH, McDowell HA, Gelman S: Transcranial Doppler and rCBF compared in carotid endarterectomy, *Stroke* 17:1206-1208, 1986.

17. Halsey JH et al: Blood velocity in the middle cerebral artery and regional cerebral blood flow during carotid endarterectomy, *Stroke* 20:53-58, 1989.

18. Henriksen L, Hjelms E, Lindeburgh T: Brain hyperperfusion during cardiac operations: cerebral blood flow measured by intra-arterial injection of xenon 133: evidence suggestive of intraoperative microembolism, *J Thorac Cardiovasc Surg* 86:202-208, 1983.

19. Huber P, Handa J: Effect of contrast material, hypercapnia, hyperventilation, hypertonic glucose and papaverine in the diameter of cerebral arteries: angiographic determination in man, *Invest Radiol* 2:17-32, 1967.

20. Jansen C, Ackerstaff RGA, Eikelboom BC: *The use of transcranial Doppler in carotid artery disease.* In Yao JS, Pearce WH, eds: *Technologies in vascular surgery,* Philadelphia, 1991, WB Saunders.

21. Jansen C et al: Carotid endarterectomy with simultaneous EEG and transcranial Doppler monitoring, *Stroke* (submitted for publication).

22. Jansen C et al: *Simultaneous EEG and TCD monitoring during carotid endarterectomy.* In Oka M et al, eds: *Recent advances in neurosonology,* Amsterdam, 1992, Elseviers.

23. Jørgensen LG, Schroeder TV: Transcranial Doppler for detection of cerebral ischaemia during carotid endarterectomy, *Eur J Vasc Surg* 6:142-147, 1992.

24. Kaps M et al: Pulsatile flow pattern in cerebral arteries during cardiopulmonary bypass: an evaluation based on transcranial Doppler ultrasound, *J Cardiovasc Surg* 30:16-19, 1989.

25. Kritikou PE, Branthwaite MA: Significance of changes in cerebral electrical activity at onset of cardiopulmonary bypass, *Thorax* 32:534-538, 1977.

26. Krul JMJ et al: Site and pathogenesis of infarcts associated with carotid endarterectomy, *Stroke* 20:324-328, 1989.

27. Krul JMJ et al: Stroke-related EEG changes during carotid surgery, *Eur J Vasc Surg* 3:423-428, 1989.

28. Lundar T et al: Cerebral perfusion during nonpulsatile bypass, *Ann Thorac Surg* 40:144-150, 1985.

29. Lundar T et al: Dissociation between cerebral autoregulation and carbon dioxide reactivity during nonpulsatile cardiopulmonary bypass, *Ann Thorac Surg* 40:582-587, 1985.

30. Lundar T et al: Some observations on cerebral perfusion during cardiopulmonary bypass, *Ann Thorac Surg* 39:318-323, 1985.

31. Messick JM et al: Correlation of regional cerebral blood flow (rCBF) with EEG changes during isoflurane anaesthesia for carotid endarterectomy: critical rCBF, *Anesthesiology* 66:344-349, 1987.

32. Meyer JS et al: Monitoring cerebral blood flow, metabolism and EEG, *Electroenceph Clin Neurophys* 22:497-508, 1967.

33. Murkin JM et al: Cerebral autoregulation and flow metabolism coupling during cardiopulmonary bypass: the influence of pCO_2, *Anesthesia Algesia* 66:825-832, 1987.

34. Naylor AR et al: Transcranial Doppler monitoring during carotid endarterectomy, *Br J Surg* 78:1264-1268, 1991.

35. Newman S: The incidence and nature of neuropsychological morbidity following cardiac surgery, *Perfusion* 4:93-100, 1989.

36. Padayachee TS et al: Monitoring middle cerebral artery blood flow velocity during carotid endarterectomy, *Br J Surg* 73:98-100, 1986.

37. Padayachee TS et al: The detection of microemboli in the middle cerebral artery during cardiopulmonary bypass: a transcranial Doppler ultrasound investigation using membrane and bubble oxygenerators, *Ann Thorac Surg* 44:298-302, 1987.

38. Padayachee TS et al: Monitoring cerebral perfusion during carotid endarterectomy, *J Cardiovasc Surg* 31:112-114, 1990.

39. Powers AD, Smith RR, Graeber MC: Transcranial Doppler monitoring of cerebral blood flow velocities during surgical occlusion of the carotid artery, *Neurosurgery* 25:383-389, 1989.

40. Pronk RAF: *EEG processing in cardiac surgery,* thesis, Krips Repro, Meppel, The Netherlands, 1982.

41. Pronk RAF, Simons AJR: *Automatic recognition of abnormal EEG activity during open heart and carotid surgery,* Amsterdam, 1982, Elsevier, Biomedical Press.

42. Pronk RAF, Simons AJR: Processing of the electroencephalogram in cardiac surgery, *Comp Program Biomed* 18:181-190, 1984.

43. Ringelstein EB, Zeumer H, Schneider R: Der Beitrag der zerebralen Computertomographie zur Differentialtypologie und Differentialtherapie des ischaemischen Grosshirninfarktes, *Fortschr Neurol Psychiat* 53:315-336, 1985.

44. Ringelstein EB et al: Transkraniell-sonographisches Monitoring des Blutflusses der A. cerebri media während rekanalisierender Operationen an der extrakraniellen A. carotis interna, *Nervenarzt* 56:423-430, 1985.

45. Russell D et al: *The intensity of the Doppler signal caused by arterial emboli depends on emboli size.* In Oka M et al, eds: *Recent advances in neurosonology,* Amsterdam, 1992, Elseviers Science Publishers (in press).

46. Salerno TA et al: Monitoring of electroencephalogram during open-heart surgery: a prospective analysis of 118 cases, *J Thorac Cardiovasc Surg* 76:97-100, 1978.

47. Schneider PA et al: Transcranial Doppler in the management of extracranial cerebrovascular disease: implications in diagnosis and monitoring, *J Vasc Surg* 7:223-231, 1988.

48. Schroeder T: Hemodynamic significance of internal carotid artery disease, *Acta Neurol Scand* 77:353-372, 1988.

49. Shaw PJ, Bates D, Cartlidge NEF: Early intellectual dysfunction following open-heart surgery, *Q J Med* 255:59-68, 1986.

50. Slug T, Ingvar DH: Regional cerebral blood flow and EEG frequency content, *Electroenceph Clin Neurophys* 23:395, 1967.

51. Sotaniemi KA, Joulasmaa A, Hokkanen ET: Neuropsychologic outcome after open-heart surgery, *Arch Neurol* 38:2-8, 1981.

52. Spencer MP: *Doppler detection of cerebral arterial emboli.* In Newell D, Aaslid R, eds: *Transcranial Doppler,* 1991, Raven Press (in press).

53. Spencer MP et al: Detection of middle cerebral artery emboli during carotid endarterectomy using transcranial Doppler ultrasonography, *Stroke* 21:415-423, 1990.

54. Strandgaard S, Paulson OB: Cerebral autoregulation, *Stroke* 15:413-416, 1984.

55. Sundt TM et al: Correlation of cerebral blood flow and electroencephalic changes during carotid endarterectomy, *Mayo Clin Proceed* 56:533-543, 1981.

56. Tegeler ChH et al: Microembolic detection in stroke associated with atrial fibrillation, *J Cardiovasc Tech* 9:283-284, 1990.

57. Thiel A et al: Transcranial Doppler sonography and somatosensory evoked potential monitoring in carotid surgery, *Eur J Vasc Surg* 4:597-602, 1990.

58. van der Linden J et al: Transcranial Doppler-estimated versus thermodilution-estimated cerebral blood flow during cardiac operations: influence of temperature and arterial carbon dioxide tension, *J Cardiovasc Surg* 102:95-102, 1991.

59. von Reutern GM et al: Transcranial bypass in patients with severe carotid stenosis or occlusion, *Stroke* 19:674-680, 1988.

CHAPTER 38

Three-dimensional transcranial Doppler scanning

FERNAND RIES

Angiography remains the ultimate method of morphologically imaging intracranial vessels. However, the risks inherent in this invasive investigation and the tendency to limit surgery in cerebrovascular disease[13] have led to restricted indications for its application and thus to a marked decrease in the number of angiograms performed. The development of a 2-MHz ultrasound probe with a pulsed and focused ultrasound beam[9] able to overcome the bone barrier of the skull was the first and essential step to a noninvasive assessment of the basal intracranial arteries, which has now led to the possibility of using color duplex scanning in transcranial ultrasound imaging.

Indications and limitations of conventional transcranial Doppler (TCD) sonography have been described in Chapter 36. When the variability and complexity of the circle of Willis and of the main stems of intracranial vessels are considered,[26,41] the handheld device poses two specific problems: vessel identification and documentation. Thus statements about pathologic findings as well as description of collateral pathways may be unreliable. When the handheld probe is used, identification of vessels is influenced by the following factors: insonation window, position of the probe, the chosen depth of insonation, the direction of flow, and typical frequency patterns (including optional compression tests). Thus no morphologic information about the highly variable vessel course is provided. Also, follow-up investigations may be comparing different points of insonation, particularly if hemodynamic changes in the circle of Willis have occurred in the intervening time. Moreover, there is no facility for documenting the actual insonation window or the insonation angle. Finally, the Doppler signals are generally not available for further processing, such as recalculation of pulsatility indices or reconstruction of the insonated vessel tree.

Since the first report about TCD via handheld probes, attempts have been made to obtain morphologic information about the insonated vessel segment in addition to the hemodynamic assessment. A first device, which provided a two-dimensional mapping in either a single coronal or a single horizontal plane,[1,2] finally led to the development of the so-called three-dimensional "trans-scan" TCD system.[*4,35] This system offers a simultaneous representation of the insonated vessel in three projection levels; it is, in fact, a "multiprojection sample volume position documentation."[3] The newest mapping software allows the display of insonated vessels in a three-dimensional view and the rotation of represented vessel segments in any direction. Results in clinical applications are considered in this chapter in terms of indications, reliability, problems, and limitations of the method.

METHOD AND EXAMINATION TECHNIQUE
Principles and technical devices

The three-dimensional TCD system uses a pulsed, range-gated 2-MHz ultrasonic transducer similar to the one in handheld systems. Technical specifications are described in the box. A concave polystyrene lens at the face of the probe focuses the ultrasound beam. The sample volume can be moved in steps of 1.5 mm; the optimum focusing depth is about 55 to 60 mm, and the maximum insonating depth depending on the pulse repetition frequency (PRF) is 150 mm. The axial length of the sample volume varies from 2 to 15 mm, increasing proportionally to the burst width. The lateral extension of the sample volume of about 4 to 6 mm in diameter is largely influenced by ultrasound scattering through the skull, increasing with a higher ultrasound emission energy. The actual emission energy is expressed as a percentage of the spatial-peak, time-averaged energy (SPTA; in the United States, the SPTA approved by the Food and Drug Administration is 240 mW/cm²). It can be increased up to 190% for insonating in increased depths inside the cranium, since at least 60% and in the worst case 100% of this energy is reflected or absorbed by the skull and scalp.[15] On the other hand, the emission energy should be reduced to the lowest degree in case of insonation through the transorbital window or open fontanels or after craniotomy.

In the trans-scan device, two identical 2-MHz ultrasound probes are fixed in a system of rods and socket joints on

---

*Eden Medical Electronics EME, Überlingen, Germany and Kent, Washington.

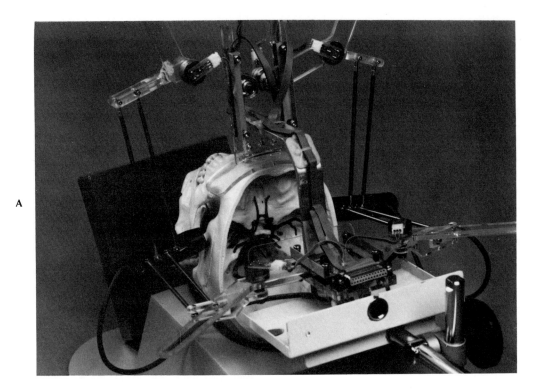

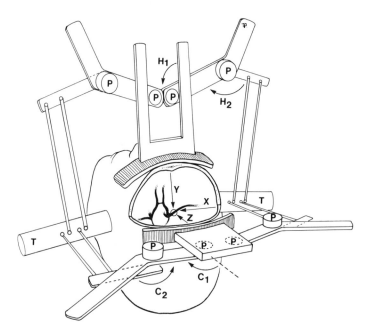

Fig. 38-1. *A,* Coordinate system in three-dimensional scanning. Headpiece holding the ultrasound transducers is shown in use on a model with a display of the circle of Willis. *B,* Principle of the three-dimensional coordinate system. *x, y, z,* Coordinate axes; *x,* insonation depth; *C1, C2, H1, H2,* angles for computer read out of axes y and z; *P,* potentiometer; *T,* 2-MHz transducer. Circle corresponds to position of the sample volume. (For explanation, see text.)

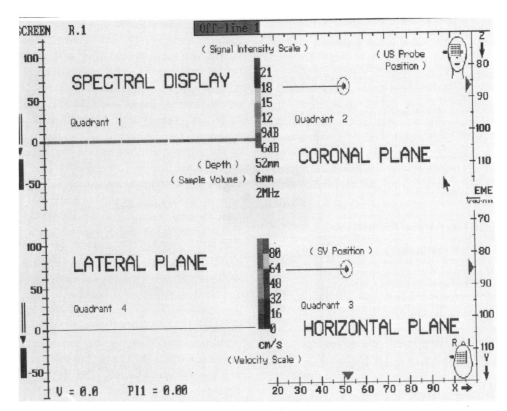

Fig. 38-2. Computer screen with four quadrants for display of color-coded spectral analysis (top left and upper scale), and three projection levels with coronal (top right), horizontal (bottom right), and lateral (bottom left) planes. Lower color-coding scale for mean flow velocity and flow direction; red/yellow, toward the probe; blue/green, away from the probe. *SV,* Sample volume position (circle) with insonation depth (triangular cursor on axis) and direction (line).

both sides of a headpiece, which is placed over the skull of the supine patient (Fig. 38-1, *A*). Reference points are the glabella and the bregma. Every change of the probe position in the five possible degrees of freedom is measured by potentiometers and transmitted to a computer. The point of intracranial insonation is instantly represented in a coordinate system of three projection levels: x = temporal insonation depth, y = glabella to sample volume, and z = bregma to sample volume (Fig. 38-1, *B*). When insonation is through a temporal window, these projections simultaneously represent the coronal (or anteroposterior) x-z plane, the horizontal x-y plane, and the lateral (or sagittal) y-z plane, as represented in different quadrants of the computer display (Fig. 38-2). The transnuchal approach allows the representation of vertebrobasilar vessel segments in the lateral and horizontal plane when using a different software (Fig. 38-3).

Joining the insonation points in minimal steps of 1.5 mm leads to a rough representation of the vessel segments on the actually insonated side. A true three-dimensional representation of the circle of Willis has to be pictured mentally by the investigator, combining the information from each view.

Spectral waveforms displaying blood flow velocities as

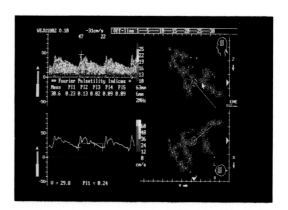

Fig. 38-3. Occipital scan in a young woman shows the vertebral arteries *(Vert),* the basilar artery *(Basil),* with the anterior inferior cerebellar artery *(AICA)* to the origin of posterior cerebral arteries. Top right, lateral view; bottom right, horizontal view; bottom left, enveloping pulse curve (lateral view omitted).

well as flow direction are color-coded for each distinct insonation point. The amplitudes of the reflected frequency power spectra are color coded in reference to a dB scale, which uses 3-dB steps. The color-coded dB scale on the trans-scan system offers, for the first time in Doppler technique, the possibility to quantify the signal amplitude in dB, as was done in assessing the signal enhancement after the application of ultrasound contrast media.[38] The data registered during the investigation are stored; they may be recalled later as a complete display or as single pulse curves for further assessment. Colored print-outs are available on an inkjet printer.

Examination technique and normal findings

Compared with a conventional handheld TCD examination, the only change in insonation technique is that the 2-MHz probe is fixed in the system of rods while moved by hand. Insonation depths and flow velocity values correspond to those found in conventional TCD examination.[11,21,43] However, insonating with a generally smaller sample volume, obtaining additional information, and handling the coordinate system may cause difficulties, at least for beginners of this technique. In this case a preexamination with the handheld probe, available either on the conventional TCD or on the trans-scan system, may help in determining the adequate ultrasonic window and in identifying the main vessels. When considering still lacking numbers on the sensitivity and specificity of three-dimensional TCD compared with the conventional handheld device, the mapping technique[23] was shown to provide a better visual comprehension of the complex three-dimensional circle of Willis and thus improves the investigator's understanding of the spatial relationship of different vessel segments; the examination time may be shortened and the identification of insonated vessel segments is improved.

In conventional TCD, normal findings must be supported by typical insonation parameters as well as empirically established hemodynamic characteristics. Identification of vessels depends on the skill of the investigator. In the presence of atypical features, such as anatomic variations and collateralization, vessel identification is more difficult and may require compression tests,[43] which may be omitted by using transcranial mapping.[30] The main difference in TCD scanning compared to handheld investigation is in the simultaneous visual orientation on the insonated vessel segment by the spatial representation on the computer screen.

The most frequent technical limitation concerns the unsuccessful temporal approach because of a thick skull. The rate of success in insonating the basal cerebral arteries depends mainly on the experience of the investigator and the amount of time devoted to the investigation. In a group of 326 patients with cerebrovascular disease preexamined by conventional TCD, sufficient signals were not found in at least one hemispheric side in about 5% of the patients, which corresponds to the results obtained by the handheld device.[6,16,21] Failure to yield fair signals from the orbital and

transnuchal approach most probably will be caused by anatomic variations, subtotal stenosis, or occlusion.

The first step in examining with the three-dimensional device is the correct positioning of the patient, since a slight shift of the head in either direction may lead to a major displacement of the sample volume in reference to the circle of Willis. Thus reproducibility of the insonating conditions is critical. The position of the sample volume and the angle of the ultrasound beam are displayed on the screen (Fig. 38-2). After the appropriate ultrasonic window is determined, the Doppler investigation normally begins with the representation of the middle cerebral artery (MCA). In general, the representation of the M1-segment of the MCA at about 45 to 60 mm depth does not cause problems. A first advantage of using three-dimensional TCD is apparent in the identification of the carotid bifurcation, with flow directions both toward and away from the probe. The carotid siphon shows below the bifurcation in the coronal projection, whereas it may be displayed either just before or behind the internal carotid artery (ICA) bifurcation in the horizontal projection, depending on the placement of the head. The insonation of the A1-segment of the anterior cerebral artery at a depth of about 60 to 75 mm with a flow direction away from the probe may be continued to the anterior communicating artery and even to the contralateral anterior cerebral artery. Although significant signal attenuation will occur, the contralateral MCA can be insonated in about 15% of cases, giving mostly weak signals with flow direction away from the probe (Fig. 38-4).

The three-dimensional scanning system demonstrates one of its greatest advantages in discriminating the anterior part of the circle of Willis from the posterior part, which is also insonated from the rear part of the temporal window, but by using a more posterior insonating direction. In insonating

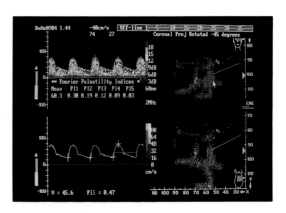

Fig. 38-4. Display of the circle of Willis in a 64-year-old man with bilateral occlusion of the internal carotid artery. Insonation is from the left temporal window. Sample volume (circle) on left posterior communicating artery. Coronal projection is rotated downward, thus displaying the posterior collateral circulation. Note weak signals (reduced size and brightness of dots) in insonation of both middle cerebral arteries from the left side.

the junction of the posterior cerebral artery and the posterior communicating artery at a depth of about 65 to 70 mm, the mapping displays flow directions toward the probe in the proximal part (P1-segment) of the posterior cerebral artery, and away from the probe in the distal part (P2-segment). The posterior communicating artery is generally insonated in normal patients slightly posterior to the distal internal carotid artery with weak signals and inconstant flow directions. Compression of the homolateral common carotid artery leads to an increasing flow in the homolateral posterior communicating artery toward the probe. The latter artery can be displayed clearly in case of carotid lesions requiring a posterior collateral circulation (Fig. 38-4).

Special software permits the scanning of the vertebro-basilar system in a lateral and horizontal plane. This part often shows tortuosities and important anatomic variations, which may create difficulties when the course of the basilar segment is assessed by using conventional TCD.[12] The basilar artery can be followed from about 70 to 75 mm, including the display of cerebellar branches of the basilar artery. The bifurcation into both posterior cerebral arteries is seen at a depth of about 100 to 115 mm (Figs. 38-3 and 38-4).

After the Doppler data have been recorded, postprocessing may lead to a better representation or expanded information. Calculation of pulsatility indices may complete the hemodynamic assessment.

CLINICAL APPLICATIONS AND PATHOLOGIC FINDINGS

Indications for three-dimensional TCD examinations largely meet those for conventional TCD.[16,20,32,52] Furthermore, the classification of transcranial Doppler signals in three-dimensional TCD depends on the same measurements (i.e., flow direction; absolute systolic, mean, and diastolic flow velocities; fast Fourier frequency analysis of the flow pattern). Thus the problem of detecting low-grade stenosis, such as atherosclerotic plaques, remains unchanged. However, the trans-scan system offers the possibility of assigning abnormal signals to defined, even smaller vessel segments. The representation of turbulent flow and flow acceleration is improved by the display in a color-coded amplitude-to-frequency range, leading to better documentation and discrimination of these pathologic signals. Moreover, an optimized signal-to-noise ratio leads to a better spatial resolution and to less scattering of the ultrasound beam. With conventional TCD, a direct quantitative assessment of the absolute flow volume is not possible.[24] The brightness and the size of the color dots correspond to the amplitude of the reflected ultrasound signal; thus they may be considered an indirect index of peripheral flow.

Stenotic and occlusive intracranial vascular lesions

TCD is a logical supplement to extracranial continuous wave Doppler sonography and duplex scanning because both normal and pathologic extracranial findings require further intracranial assessment. The importance of a noninvasive technique suitable for use in follow-up studies has increased with restricted indications for surgery in occlusive cerebrovascular disease, such as carotid endarterectomy or extracranial-intracranial artery bypass.[17] For example, the TCD demonstration of an intracranial MCA stenosis (Fig. 38-5) or occlusion[28,29] does not necessarily lead to an invasive angiographic investigation because the latter may have no surgical consequence. A possible recanalization, especially in thrombosis of the MCA, can be assessed noninvasively. If vascular surgery is done, intraoperative monitoring[31,42,45] and preoperative and postoperative follow-up studies[17] will show eventual hemodynamic changes, as demonstrated by the three-dimensional technique for extracranial-intracranial bypass[14] (Fig. 38-6) or internal carotid dissection (Fig. 38-7).

The criteria for evaluation of the severity of intracranial vascular lesions are the same as those for evaluation of extracranial lesions.[36] However, collateralization in the circle of Willis may lead to abnormally increased flow velocities and turbulences, especially in the communicating arteries. The resulting functional stenosis is often difficult to differentiate from a real stenotic lesion. In this case, compression tests should be useful.[43]

The nearby microcirculation may have a more pronounced effect on pulsatility characteristics as in extracranial assessment. This may lead to an indirect evaluation of lesions located distally from the insonated vessel segments, such as microangiopathy. First results with a newly developed effective pulsatility range (EPR), defined as a mean blood flow velocity minus the amplitude between peak systolic and end diastolic flow velocities, allow a highly significant discrimination between patients with multiinfarct dementia and patients with Alzheimer-type dementia.[39]

Hemodynamic effect of extracranial vascular lesions

The hemodynamic effect of vascular lesions in the extracranial segment of the carotid system has to be assessed intracranially because a purely morphologic approach is insufficient. A significant correlation can be shown between the grade of extracranial carotid stenosis and changes in pulsatility as measured for various pulsatility indices (PI) in the homolateral middle cerebral artery (Fig. 38-8)[37,48] (with the use of the Gosling PI [defined as peak systolic minus end-diastolic flow velocities, divided by mean flow velocity], the mean-accentuated SAM-index [sum of amplitude plus mean], and the harmonics 1 and 2 according to a fast Fourier transform analysis). Thus hemodynamic changes are reflected by a mathematical description of the pulse curve. It was shown by three-dimensional TCD that collateralization, mostly occurring in high-grade stenosis and in more than one collateral system, does not restore pulsatilities found in normal reference values.[37] Assessment of CO_2-induced cerebral vasomotor response[46] or after hyperventilation can be completed by including pulsatility evaluation.[43] The pulsatility transmission index (PTI) used by Lindegaard et al[27] is based on the comparison of the

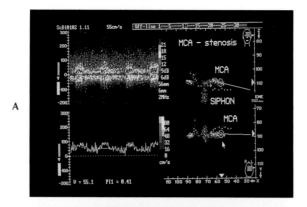

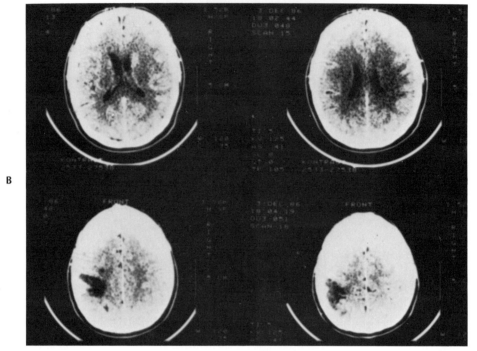

Fig. 38-5. A 42-year-old man with left hemispheric transient ischemic attack. *A,* Left temporal insonation of a high-grade stenosis of left middle cerebral artery. Increase in velocity in the upper (top right) and posterior (bottom right) branch corresponds to the stenotic vessel segment in presence of an early MCA bifurcation. Frequency spectral analysis (top left) shows turbulent flow and velocity up to 200 cm/sec. *B,* Computed tomography scan of the same patient shows hypodensity in area supplied by posterior MCA branch in left hemisphere.

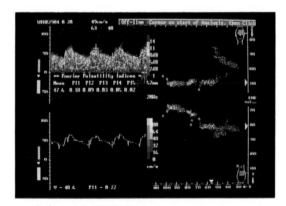

Fig. 38-6. Left temporal insonation in a 44-year-old woman after extracranial-intracranial artery bypass surgery in presence of extracranial occlusion of left internal carotid artery; no representation of left carotid siphon. Cross-filling of left anterior cerebral artery. Sample volume *(circle)* on left middle cerebral artery shows orthograde filling (yellow/red). Example for insufficient hemodynamic indication for bypass surgery.

lesion side with the nonlesion side; there is a limitation in the frequent cases of bilateral vascular lesions.

Arteriovenous malformations

The spatial resolution of the three-dimensional TCD system limits the morphologic representation of arteriovenous malformations to angiomas, giant aneurysms, and carotid-cavernous sinus fistulas. High-flow angiomas are diagnosed easily on the basis of typical Doppler signals (reduced pulsatility, high systolic and end-diastolic velocities, musical murmurs) in conventional TCD.[49] The trans-scan system provides a rough morphologic representation, including feeder arteries. Thus noninvasive preoperative and postoperative evaluations can be made to assess the effect of embolization or proton-beam irradiation.[50] "Musical murmurs," probably due to high-frequent vibrations of the vessel

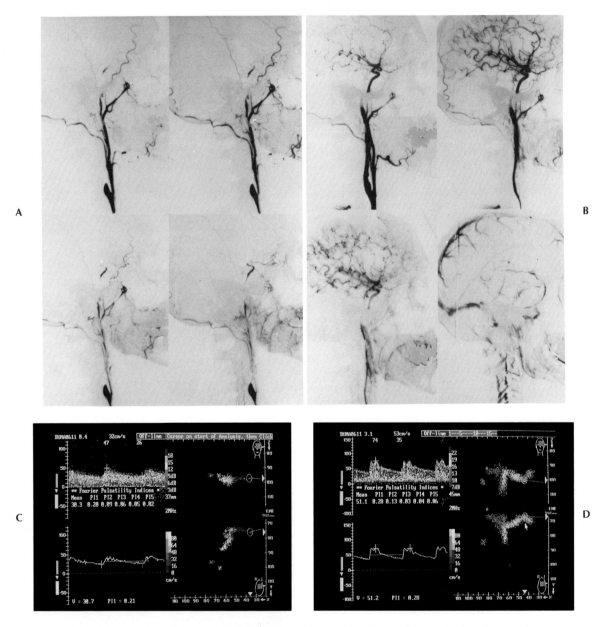

Fig. 38-7. Traumatic dissection of left internal carotid artery in a 45-year-old man. Decision for vascular surgery (combined endarterectomy and transluminal angioplasty) was made after dramatic neurologic deterioration corresponding to increasing grade of stenosis (Doppler follow-up and angiographic control). Contrast angiograms (lateral view) show *A,* high-grade stenosis of left middle cerebral artery (MCA), cross-filling of A1 segment of left anterior cerebral artery (ACA) before surgery, and *B,* patent left internal carotid artery with remaining wall irregularities after surgery. Corresponding TCD displays with *C,* reduced pulsatility of left MCA (top left), no display of left carotid siphon and left ACA, increased velocities and dot brightness in collateralizing left posterior communicating artery (PCoA). *D,* Display after surgery with normalized pulsatility and absolute flow velocities, insonation of left carotid siphon and orthograde left ACA, but no more display of left PCoA (bottom right).

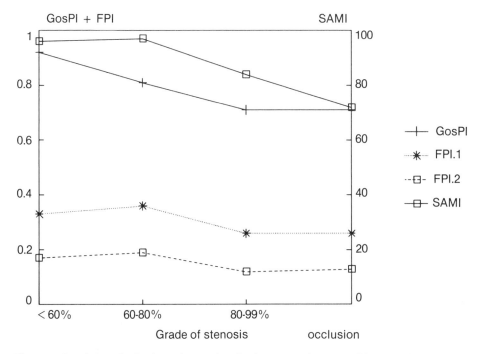

Fig. 38-8. Correlation of pulsatility indices and grade of extracranial stenosis of the internal carotid artery. Numbers are dimensionless. *GosPI,* Gosling pulsatility index; *FPI.1 and FPI.2,* first and second harmonics in fast Fourier transform; *SAMI,* sum of amplitude plus mean velocity index.

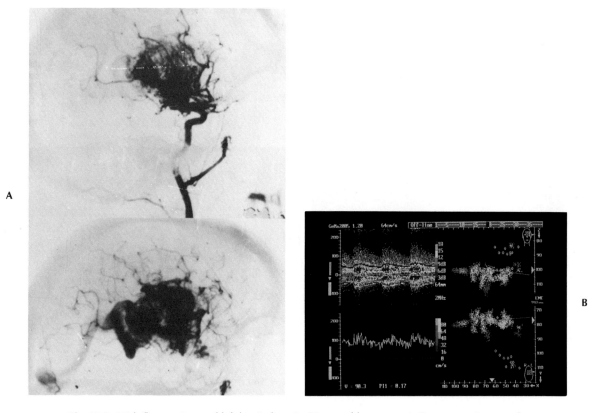

Fig. 38-9. High-flow angioma of left hemisphere in 35-year-old woman. *A,* Contrast angiogram after detection by TCD sonography with a handheld probe. *B,* Three-dimensional display 1 year after proton-beam irradiation. Right temporal insonation: abnormally high velocities in remaining angioma and display of musical murmurs as symmetrical bands of low frequency (top left).

wall,[6] show as symmetrical small bands of low frequencies (Fig. 38-9).

Aneurysms as the source of bleeding in subarachnoid hemorrhage generally remain undetected by TCD, but further improvement of spatial resolution (e.g., by using ultrasound contrast media) may lead to imaging of midsize aneurysms by three-dimensional TCD. The severity and extent of spasms[7,8,18,51] can be assessed in a more detailed way, thus enabling a better therapeutic management. Although

morphologic representation of small aneurysms is generally not possible with three-dimensional TCD, giant aneurysms are shown with their approximate size, depending on the amount of aneurysmal thrombosis. In the case of a giant ophthalmic aneurysm, the effect of a balloon embolization and the iatrogenic occlusion of the homolateral internal carotid artery, leading to an extensive collateral circulation, has been documented (Fig. 38-10). Follow-up is indicated in case of carotid-cavernous sinus fistulas, considering the

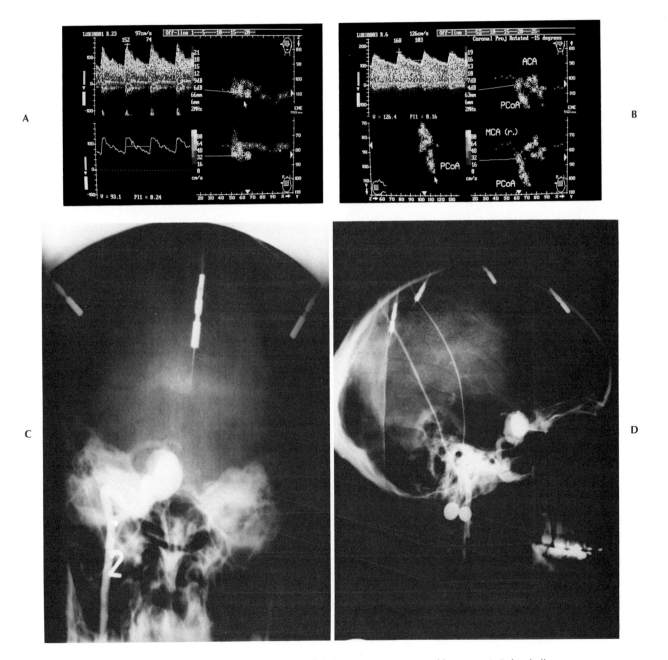

Fig. 38-10. Giant aneurysm at origin of right ophthalmic artery in 28-year-old woman. ***A,*** Before balloon embolization (cluster of dots, top and bottom right), high pulsatility and turbulent flow (top left) are seen in area of aneurysm. ***B,*** Thrombosis of right internal carotid artery after balloon embolization leads to collateralization over both right anterior cerebral artery (pulse curve in top left) and right posterior communicating artery. ***C,*** Contrast angiograms show balloons in giant aneurysm in anteroposterior projection and ***D,*** in lateral projection.

possible spontaneous occlusion of such fistulas. In case of balloon embolization or surgery on the internal carotid artery, hemodynamic changes and sufficient collateral supply can be evaluated.

Vertebrobasilar circulation

Occipital three-dimensional scanning permits a morphologic assessment of the vertebrobasilar circulation.[22] The possibility of detecting a basilar thrombosis at an early stage without the topologic uncertainty of conventional TCD may lead to a better therapeutic management, including early thrombolysis. In case of a subclavian steal phenomenon,[12,25] hemodynamic abnormalities such as a possible flow reversal[34,44] in the basilar artery can be documented regularly. Further applications for a trans-scan TCD examination of the posterior circulation may include functional tests, such as registration of hemodynamic changes following visually evoked potentials.[5]

Intracranial pressure monitoring

Intracranial pressure monitoring by TCD[7] reflects hemodynamic deterioration preceding intracranial circulatory arrest as in brain death[19,47] as well as temporary pressure increase.[18] Typical intracranial Doppler signs include abnormal high pulsatilities with reduced systolic velocities and absent or reversed diastolic flow. The respiratory cycle may be superimposed on systolic peaks.[33] Legal implications in this diagnostic field require documentation and quantification of hemodynamic parameters in terms of pulse curve characteristics, such as offered by three-dimensional TCD. Pitfalls, such as mass lesions responsible for displacing major intracranial vessels, can be taken into account in three-dimensional representation.

PROBLEMS, LIMITATIONS, AND PERSPECTIVES
Technical problems and pitfalls

As previously mentioned, technical problems may arise because of inadequate positioning of the patient's head. The fixation of the ultrasonic probe in the system of rods may be difficult for beginners. As the sample volume is potentially smaller than in conventional TCD and is moved in steps of 1.5 mm, the problem of finding and following a definite vessel segment may arise. The same feature may cause confusion in case of a parallel representation of two smaller branches, for example of the MCA. This often leads to a confusing multitude of color dots on the screen. Therefore saving only optimal signals from fewer vessel segments facilitates the morphologic identification of the basal cerebral arteries. Changing the dot size afterward may improve the plotting.

The posterior circulatory pathways are often hidden behind the carotid system; rotating the coronal projection up or down leads to a view from above or below the circle of Willis. The color-coded velocity scale must be chosen according to the maximum mean flow velocities, thus revealing spots of acceleration typical for stenosis or spasm.

Pitfalls mainly occur in misinterpretations of the insonated vessel segments, especially in the presence of anatomic variations or collateral flow acceleration. The posterior communicating artery may be regarded as a supraclinoidal stenosis of the carotid siphon, or the supplying anterior cerebral artery, in case of a cross-filling, may be considered as an A1-segment stenosis. A mass lesion, for instance, one caused by an intrahemispheric hemorrhage or by edema, can displace the MCA, thus leading to an incorrect diagnosis of occlusion or intracranial circulatory arrest. The same holds true in case of total ultrasound absorption and reflection by a thick skull. Methodologic errors include failure to detect low-grade stenoses and lesions in distal vessel branches because these are out of range of TCD insonation.

Ultrasound signal and pulse-curve characteristics

The optimal representation of the pulse curve is a compromise between the lowest possible gain presenting no artifacts and the optimal (i.e., the lowest possible) emission energy according to the insonating conditions. A high-gain factor is equal to an insufficient signal-to-noise ratio and vice versa. The intensity of the Doppler signal greatly depends on the grade of reflection and absorption of the ultrasound energy by the skin and the skull. In a thick skull, the resulting pulse curve may be inadequate for a detailed evaluation, since a higher gain and a high emission energy are necessary. This leads to an increased ultrasound scattering and thus to a bigger sample volume and a change in focus. According to the Nyquist theorem, the aliasing phenomenon (registration of the maximum Doppler shift) will occur at one-half the pulse repetition frequency (PRF) or 6.17 kHz (see box below). The PRF determines the maximum Doppler shift (shown as the maximum velocity scale) that can be measured. Exceeding frequencies would be displayed in the reversed display. By increasing the insonation depth, or in the case of abnormal high velocities, a technically insufficient pulse curve with overlying artifacts may result. Thus high velocities can only be measured in a shallow depth with a high PRF. The three-dimensional trans-

---

TECHNICAL SPECIFICATIONS OF THE THREE-DIMENSIONAL TRANS-SCAN TCD SYSTEM

- 2-MHz pulsed ultrasound emission frequency (1 kHz of Doppler shift represents 39 cm/sec blood flow velocity)
- Pulse repetition frequency range of 1.54 kHz to 12.34 kHz
- Burst width range from 2 to 20 ms
- Spatial-peak, time-averaged energy of 240 mW/cm²
- Emission energy adjustment from 2% to 190%
- Depth setting in steps of 1.5 mm up to 150 mm
- Maximal blood flow velocity scale from −250 to +350 cm/sec
- Sample volume size of 2 to 15 mm axial length
- Fast Fourier transform Doppler display with 64 points, time resolution of 6 ms, and display of 200 spectral lines

scan system uses a simulation device that permits the display of blood flow velocities within the frequency range of $+PRF$ to $-PRF/2$.

According to the equation for the measurement of Doppler frequency shift and assuming an habitual angle of insonation between 0° and 30° (to be estimated on the screen), the error in converting the Doppler frequency shift into blood flow velocity is not greater than 13%.[3]

Signal enhancement

The main problem in TCD sonography is the result of the extremely high ultrasound reflection. Higher emission energies are prohibited because of possible biologic effects, such as heat production and cavitation. Therefore further improvements of the method require a better signal-to-noise ratio within the range of the actual emission energy. One possible solution is to enhance the signal by using air microbubbles as a powerful reflecting agent.[38] First experiences with this contrast agent in clinical studies give perspectives of even smaller sample volumes as well as perfect pulse curves on low-gain scales[40] (Fig. 38-11). Doppler signals that currently are too weak to be considered may be detected and represented by three-dimensional TCD (e.g., in hyperostosis and subtotal intracranial stenosis or severe spasm). Improvements on the electronic level are required to adapt technical devices, including signal processing and Doppler transducers, to such a signal enhancement (e.g., by offering different focusing depths and several sizes of sample volume). A truly three-dimensional representation of the circle of Willis is conceivable.

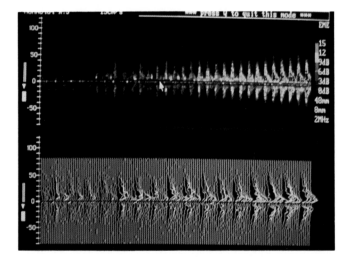

Fig. 38-11. Signal enhancement of an insufficient native TCD signal in a 68-year-old woman. After the intravenous injection of 10 ml of a galactose-air microbubble suspension (300 mg microparticles/ml suspension), the left middle cerebral artery shows with a continuous increase of the amplitude of the Doppler signal (upper display), reaching 15 dB with reference to the color-coded dB scale (right margin of display). Lower part shows the amplitude to frequency spectrum for the signals marked by the blue line in the upper display.

CONCLUSION

In comparison with conventional TCD by means of a handheld TCD probe, the three-dimensional trans-scan system allows the assignment of hemodynamic parameters to define vessel segments in a rough morphologic representation. Stenotic vascular lesions and arteriovenous malformations can be evaluated in terms of their hemodynamic and morphologic characteristics. Preoperative and postoperative examinations can be used for assessment and follow-up studies in various neurosurgical and neuroradiologic indications. Functional tests are more reliable because vessels can be identified reliably. Even in the case of a TCD examination with a handheld probe, such as in intraoperative or intensive care monitoring, the facilities of the trans-scan system may have an advantage for a sophisticated hemodynamic assessment.

The three-dimensional trans-scan system is the first noninvasive method for the diagnosis of intracranial vascular disease that considers and even quantifies hemodynamic and morphologic parameters. Thus it is an extension of existing cerebrovascular diagnostic methods; it can anticipate, expand, and sometimes replace information provided by angiography, especially when no surgical therapy is intended. Further developments, such as the application of a signal-enhancing agent or progress in electronic processing, may lead to an unexpected qualitative improvement of the Doppler signal and thus of spatial resolution.

REFERENCES

1. Aaslid R: *Transcutaneous evaluation of intracranial arterial flow.* Proceedings of the Application of Doppler Ultrasound in Medicine, International Congress, Düsseldorf, Germany, May 1984.
2. Aaslid R: Transcranial Doppler flow mapping. Proceedings of the Ultrasound Diagnosis of Cerebrovascular Disease Symposium, Seattle, May 1985.
3. Aaslid R, ed: *Transcranial Doppler sonography,* New York, 1986, Springer-Verlag.
4. Aaslid R: *Five years of TCD: a look back. Two years of TCD scanning: a look forward.* International workshop on three-dimensional transcranial Doppler scanning, Bonn, Germany, Nov 1987.
5. Aaslid R: Visually evoked dynamic blood flow responses of the human cerebral circulation, *Stroke* 18:771-775, 1987.
6. Aaslid R, Nornes H: Musical murmurs in human cerebral arteries after subarachnoid hemorrhage, *J Neurosurg* 60:32-36, 1984.
7. Aaslid R, Huber P, Nornes H: Evaluation of cerebrovascular spasm with transcranial Doppler ultrasound, *J Neurosurg* 60:37-41, 1984.
8. Aaslid R, Huber P, Nornes H: A transcranial Doppler method in the evaluation of cerebrovascular spasm, *Neuroradiology* 28:11-16, 1986.
9. Aaslid R, Markwalder TM, Nornes H: Noninvasive transcranial Doppler ultrasound recording of flow velocity in basal cerebral arteries, *J Neurosurg* 57:769-774, 1982.
10. Aaslid R et al: *Estimation of cerebral perfusion pressure from arterial blood pressure and transcranial Doppler recordings.* In Miller J et al, eds: *Intracranial pressure VI,* Heidelberg, Germany, 1986, Springer-Verlag.
11. Arnolds B, von Reutern GM: Transcranial Doppler sonography: examination technique and normal reference values, *Ultrasound Med Biol* 12:115-123, 1986.
12. Buedingen HJ, Staudacher T: Die Identifizierung der Arteria basilaris mit der transkraniellen Doppler-Sonographie, *Ultraschall* 8:205-212, 1987.
13. EC/IC Bypass Study Group: Failure of extracranial-intracranial arterial bypass to reduce the risk of ischemic stroke, *N Engl J Med* 313:1191-1200, 1985.

14. Fritz WL, Klein HJ: Three-dimensional Doppler sonographic monitoring of patients with extraintracranial arterial bypass, *J Vasc Tech* 14:77-81, 1990.

15. Grolimund P: *Transmission of ultrasound through the temporal bone.* In Aaslid R, ed: *Transcranial Doppler sonography,* New York, 1986, Springer-Verlag.

16. Grolimund P, Seiler RW, Mattle H: Moeglichkeiten und Grenzen der transkraniellen Doppler-Sonographie, *Ultraschall* 8:87-95, 1987.

17. Harders A, Gilsbach JM: Transcranial Doppler sonography and its application in extracranial-intracranial bypass surgery, *Neuro Res* 7:129-141, 1985.

18. Harders A, Gilsbach JM: Time course of blood flow velocity changes related to vasospasm in the circle of Willis measured with the noninvasive transcranial Doppler method, *J Neurosurg* 66:718-728, 1987.

19. Hassler W, Steinmetz H, Gawlowski J: Transcranial Doppler ultrasonography in raised intracranial pressure and in circulatory arrest, *J Neurosurg* 68:745-751, 1988.

20. Hennerici M, Rautenberg W, Schwartz A: Transcranial Doppler ultrasound for the assessment of intracranial arterial flow velocity. Part 2. Evaluation of intracranial disease, *Surg Neurol* 27:523-532, 1987.

21. Hennerici M et al: Transcranial Doppler ultrasound for the assessment of intracranial arterial flow velocity. Part 1. Examination technique and normal values, *Surg Neurol* 27:439-448, 1987.

22. Hennerici M et al: *Doppler examination of the intracranial vertebrobasilar system,* abstract, 4th Toronto Stroke Workshop, Toronto, Canada, Sept 1988.

23. Katz ML, Smalley KJ, Comerota AJ: Transcranial Doppler: prospective evaluation of handheld vs mapping technique, *J Vasc Tech* 14:69-71, 1990.

24. Kirkham FJ et al: Transcranial measurement of blood velocities in the basal cerebral arteries using pulsed Doppler ultrasound: velocity as an index of flow, *Ultrasound Med Biol* 12:15-21, 1986.

25. Klingelhöfer J et al: Transcranial Doppler ultrasonography of carotid-basilar collateral circulation in subclavian steal, *Stroke* 19:1036-1042, 1988.

26. Krayenbühl H, Yasargil MG: *Die zerebrale Angiographie für Klinik und Praxis,* Stuttgart, Germany, 1979, Thieme Verlag.

27. Lindegaard KF et al: Assessment of intracranial hemodynamics in carotid artery disease by transcranial Doppler ultrasound, *J Neurosurg* 63:890-898, 1985.

28. Lindegaard KF et al: Doppler diagnosis of intracranial artery occlusive disorders, *J Neurol Neurosurg Psychiat* 49:510-518, 1986.

29. Mattle H et al: Transcranial Doppler sonographic findings in middle cerebral artery disease, *Arch Neurol* 45:289-295, 1988.

30. Niederkorn K et al: Three-dimensional transcranial Doppler blood flow mapping in patients with cerebrovascular disorders, *Stroke* 19:1335-1344, 1988.

31. Padayachee TS et al: Monitoring middle cerebral artery blood flow velocity during carotid endarterectomy, *Br J Surg* 40:144-150, 1985.

32. Ries F: Transkranielle Doppler-Sonographie. Eine neue nicht-invasive Methode in der Diagnostik cerebrovaskulärer Erkrankungen, *Aktuelle Neurologie* 13:207-215, 1986.

33. Ries F, Moskopp D: Value of the transcranial Doppler technique (TCD) for the determination of brain death, *Neurosurg Rev* 12:302-306, 1989.

34. Ries F, Solymosi L, Klar J: Noninvasive assessment of a carotid-subclavian steal syndrome treated by PTA, *J Neurorad* 33:221, 1991.

35. Ries F, Solymosi L, Moskopp D: 3-D transcranial Doppler scanning: a non-invasive adjunction or substitution of cerebral angiography? *J Cardiovasc Ultrason* 7:121-122, 1988.

36. Ries F et al: Evaluation of the hemodynamic effect of extra- and intracranial cerebrovascular lesions by 3-D transcranial Doppler scanning, *J Cardiovasc Ultrason* 7:78, 1988.

37. Ries F et al: Is pulsatility a reliable index of intracranial hemodynamic changes in CVD? *J Cardiovasc Technol* 8:159-160, 1989.

38. Ries F et al: Air microbubbles as a signal enhancing agent in transcranial Doppler sonography: a pilot study, *J Neuroimaging* 1:173-178, 1991.

39. Ries F et al: Differentiation of multi-infarct and Alzheimer dementia by intracranial hemodynamic parameters, *Stroke* 24:228-235, 1993.

40. Ries F et al: A transpulmonary contrast medium enhances the transcranial Doppler signal in humans, *J Neurol* 239:56, 1992.

41. Riggs HE, Rupp R: Variations in form of circle of Willis, *Arch Neurol* 8:8-14, 1963.

42. Ringelstein EB: *Transcranial Doppler monitoring.* In Aaslid R, ed: *Transcranial Doppler sonography,* New York, 1986, Springer-Verlag.

43. Ringelstein EB: *Transcranial Doppler sonography.* In Poeck K, Ringelstein EB, Hacke W, eds: *New trends in diagnosis and management of stroke,* Berlin, 1987, Springer-Verlag.

44. Ringelstein EB, Zeumer H: Delayed reversal of vertebral artery blood flow following percutaneous transluminal angioplasty for subclavian steal syndrome, *Neuroradiology* 26:189-198, 1984.

45. Ringelstein EB et al: Transkraniell-sonographisches Monitoring des Blutflusses der A. cerebri media während rekanalisierender Operationen an der extrakraniellen A. carotis interna, *Nervenarzt* 56:423-430, 1985.

46. Ringelstein EB et al: Noninvasive assessment of CO_2-induced cerebral vasomotor response in normal individuals and patients with internal carotid artery occlusions, *Stroke* 19:963-969, 1988.

47. Ropper AH et al: Transcranial Doppler in brain death, *Neurology* 37:1733-1735, 1987.

48. Schneider PA et al: Effect of internal carotid artery occlusion on intracranial hemodynamics: transcranial Doppler evaluation and clinical correlation, *Stroke* 19:589-598, 1988.

49. Schwartz A, Hennerici M: Non-invasive transcranial Doppler sonography in intracranial angioma, *Neurology* 36:626-635, 1986.

50. Seiler RW: *TCD scanning in the management of arteriovenous malformations.* International Workshop on 3-D Transcranial Doppler Scanning, Bonn, Germany, Nov 1987.

51. Seiler RW et al: Relation of cerebral vasospasm evaluated by transcranial Doppler ultrasound to clinical grade and CT-visualized subarachnoid hemorrhage, *J Neurosurg* 64:594-600, 1986.

52. Wechsler LR, Ropper AH, Kistler JP: Transcranial Doppler in cerebrovascular disease, *Stroke* 17:905-912, 1986.

CHAPTER 39

Prediction of stroke with transcranial Doppler scanning

CEES JANSEN, BERT C. EIKELBOOM, and ROB G.A. ACKERSTAFF

The principle that signals emitted from an ultrasound source and reflected by moving erythrocytes undergo a frequency shift in direct proportion to the velocity of the moving red cells has been used to study the bloodstream in arteries for the past 25 years. Examination techniques with continuous wave and pulsed wave Doppler systems of 4-MHz frequency or more have made an accurate study of blood flow velocities in extracranial arteries possible. At this frequency range, however, recording flow velocities of intracranial arteries is impossible because of attenuation by the skull. In 1982, Aaslid and colleagues[2] solved this problem with the use of lower (2 MHz or less) frequencies, which enabled them to record blood flow velocities from intracranial vessels through thin areas of the skull. (The principles and applications of transcranial Doppler [TCD] sonography are reviewed in Chapter 36.)

Although the advantages of TCD ultrasonography, such as its noninvasive nature, its small and relatively inexpensive bedside equipment, and its sensitivity to detect flow velocities and thromboembolism in real-time, are convincing, the clinical value of TCD is subject of much debate.[5,16,43] This common problem occurs in other new diagnostic tools as well when skilled technicians develop them before doctors validate a suitable clinical application for them. A new tool like TCD has to prove its value by experimental work and by comparison with other techniques to be financially worthwhile.

Recently, the established use of TCD has been limited to the following: (1) the detection of severe intracranial stenosis; (2) assessment of collateral circulation in patients with known regions of severe stenosis or occlusion; (3) evaluation and follow-up of patients with vasoconstriction, particularly after subarachnoid hemorrhage; (4) detection of arteriovenous malformations (AVMs), their major supply arteries, and flow patterns; and (5) intracranial velocity changes in brain death.* Although the application of TCD is not yet established in migraine patients; or in monitoring during carotid endarterectomy, coronary bypass, or other surgical procedures; in the evaluation of intracranial aneu-

rysms; in assessing autoregulation; and in vasculopathies like Moya-Moya disease, the technique is under study and seems promising in most cases.[3,26,47,48,62] In this chapter, the application of TCD as a predictor of stroke, in both symptomatic and asymptomatic individuals, is discussed.

NATURAL HISTORY OF STROKE

With the possible exception of the noninvasive or invasive imaging of carotid artery stenosis in patients without symptoms, there seems to be no technical test to predict stroke in individuals. Symptoms such as amaurosis fugax or transient ischemic attacks (TIAs) in the carotid or vertebrobasilar distribution do predict impending ischemia in those patients who are at risk, but unfortunately, just a few (20%) of those who will develop a brain infarct experience these early signs of stroke.[15] Recent investigations have shown that from a clinicopathologic point, there is no clear difference between patients with TIAs or small cerebral infarcts.[14,42,64] Another subgroup of patients with cerebral infarcts on computed tomography (CT) without clinical symptoms makes the situation more complicated than it seemed a few years ago.[33] With new diagnostic and noninvasive techniques such as duplex scanning of the carotid arteries and recently established treatment strategies such as carotid endarterectomy in selected cases and pharmacologic treatment (e.g., aspirin, ticlopedin, warfarin) in others, the prediction of stroke has gained major importance.

After a correct diagnosis of amaurosis fugax, TIA, or minor stroke, which has to be made by a neurologist[32] and exclusion of vasculitis, intrinsic blood coagulation disorders, and intracranial mass lesions such as subdural hematomas, tumors, and AVMs, the search for carotid artery disease, intracranial artery disease, and cardiac embolism should begin immediately. TCD has a place in the screening of these conditions.

After the diagnosis of an asymptomatic carotid stenosis as a result of routine cardiologic or neurologic examinations, the picture is probably more complicated: the risk of stroke in unselected patients with asymptomatic stenosis is low, but there may be a subgroup of individuals without symptoms with a greater risk of stroke; treatment is therefore indicated after appropriate diagnosis.

---

*References 16, 25, 27, 30, 34-38, 55-57, 60.

ASSESSMENT OF STROKE RISK IN EXTRACRANIAL CAROTID ARTERY DISEASE

Recently, the collaborators of the North American Symptomatic Carotid Endarterectomy Trial[45] and the European Carotid Surgery Trial[22] published their results on the effects of carotid endarterectomy in patients at risk for ischemic stroke who had experienced signs and symptoms suggesting impending ischemia (e.g., amaurosis fugax, TIA, or minor stroke in the carotid territory) as a result of atherosclerosis of the ipsilateral carotid artery. Both studies showed a beneficial effect from the surgery in patients with a linear internal diameter reduction of the affected artery of more than 70%. Carotid endarterectomy should be recommended to these patients provided a skilled vascular surgeon, who has a record of low intraoperative and postoperative stroke rate, is available to perform the surgery. Surgery is the usual management for patients with symptoms, but there is the question of whether patients without symptoms with significant carotid artery disease should also be recommended for surgery.[18,51] Because many of these patients are not actually asymptomatic but have "silent" infarcts on CT or have suffered TIAs during sleep, there may be a considerable stroke rate. Initially, Bogousslavsky and Regli[9] found an association between cerebral infarcts with transient signs and occlusion of the internal carotid artery. However, in a subsequent study of 57 patients with TIA, including 16 with a cerebral infarct on CT scan, no specific underlying cause was found.[10] Others found an association between carotid stenosis or carotid plaque ulceration and cerebral infarction.[23,41,66] In general, patients with asymptomatic carotid stenosis have a remarkably low risk of stroke.[7,19,54] During the last 10 years, however, evidence from widespread application of noninvasive testing has shown that a subgroup of patients exists with hemodynamically significant lesions who have an annual stroke risk of 4% to 12%.[11,28,40] In these studies, many of the neurologic events were unheralded strokes. Nevertheless, it is still not known if these stroke rates justify the risk of carotid endarterectomy. If criteria can be found to define a subgroup of patients with progressive carotid artery disease who will develop a stroke, the controversy over carotid endarterectomy in patients without symptoms can be resolved by prospective studies.

In patients with an endangered cerebral circulation caused by progressive asymptomatic stenosis, there are two important risk factors that can be assessed by simple noninvasive diagnostic tools, such as the electroencephalogram, oculopneumoplethysmography, and TCD[20,21,39]: first, a lack of sufficient collateral circulation via the circle of Willis and second, an exhausted potential of cerebral precapillary vessels to dilate and compensate for a reduced cerebral blood flow.[8,53,59,65]

Both factors are related to carotid artery stenosis.[31] Evaluation of the transorbital collateral circulation between the external and internal carotid arteries can also be accomplished with TCD. Via the transorbital approach, the ophthalmic artery is an easily accessible vessel that reflects hemodynamic alterations due to cerebrovascular disease. A direct relationship exists between the ophthalmic systolic pressure, as measured with oculopneumoplethysmography, and the ophthalmic artery blood flow velocity measured by TCD.[58] Great variability in collateral potential can be demonstrated in individual patients by TCD registration of blood flow velocities in different arterial segments during temporary compression of the common carotid artery.[46,52] Before this procedure is carried out, duplex scanning should be used to detect severe atherosclerotic plaques in the common carotid artery wall, thereby preventing severe thromboembolism resulting from this diagnostic maneuver. A pulse detector is attached to the ipsilateral ear lobe to control the adequacy of compression. This TCD technique promises to help identify collateral channels.[44,56] The principles of testing the collaterals in the circle of Willis by common carotid artery compression are shown in Fig. 39-1. The effects of ipsilateral and contralateral common carotid artery compression are demonstrated for the three different cerebral arteries (middle cerebral artery [MCA], anterior cerebral artery [ACA], and posterior cerebral artery [PCA]) on the right side and four different types of circles. Type 1 circle of Willis is the complete circle with an anterior communicating artery (ACoA) and on both sides a posterior communicating artery (PCoA). Type 2 or the anterior type lacks an ipsilateral PCoA; Type 3 or the posterior type lacks the ACoA; Type 4 is the incomplete circle without ACoA or ipsilateral PCoA. Fig. 39-1 also shows the hemodynamic changes that occur when the ipsilateral extracranial carotid artery becomes occluded. Keunen[31] found a direct relationship between the severity of the extracranial carotid artery stenosis, a reversed direction of the periorbital blood flow, and an incomplete circle of Willis. There are indications that patients with an incomplete circle of Willis and progressive carotid artery disease have a greater risk of stroke. In 34 patients with carotid artery occlusion, there were 8 complete, 21 partial, and 5 incomplete circles.[31] As is shown in Fig. 39-2, stroke occurred in 1 (12%), 14 (67%), and 5 (100%) patients, respectively.

The vasomotor reactivity (VMR) is defined as the potential of the precapillary vessels to dilate in response to a decrease of cerebral blood flow as an essential part of cerebral autoregulation. The VMR can be measured by TCD when the patient breathes carbogen, a mixture of oxygen (95%) and CO_2 (5%) through an anesthesiologic mask. CO_2 causes a rapid dilatation of precapillary arterioles and thus an increase in blood flow velocity as measured by TCD. The VMR is calculated as the relative change in mean blood flow velocity in the MCA at normocapnic conditions and after 2 minutes of carbogen inhalation per absolute change in end tidal CO_2 as measured in the expired air. With the use of intravenous acetazolamide, the VMR can also be assessed.[59] The VMR of patients with an occlusion of the internal carotid artery shows a significant decrease.[8,53,65] More important is the observation that the VMR is particularly decreased in patients with a linear carotid artery di-

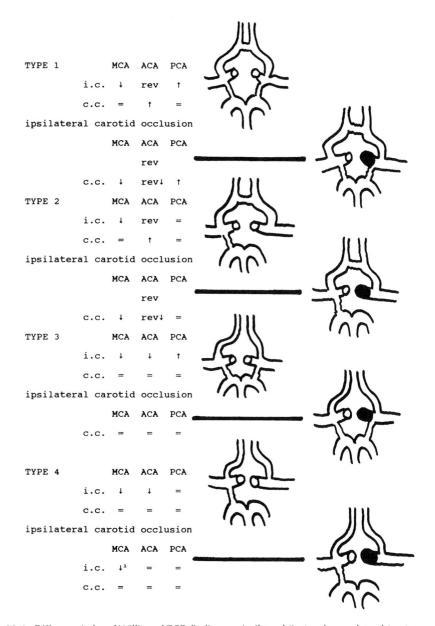

Fig. 39-1. Different circles of Willis and TCD findings on ipsilateral *(i.c.)* and contralateral *(c.c.)* common carotid artery compression. *MCA,* Middle cerebral artery; *ACA,* anterior cerebral artery; *PCA,* posterior cerebral artery; =, no change; ↓, decrease; ↑, increase; *rev,* reversed flow direction. Superscript one denotes that collateral circulation via the external carotid artery is present.

ameter reduction of 80% or more who have inadequate cerebral collateral circulation.[13,31] This decreased VMR in occlusive vascular disease can be associated with a local increased oxygen extraction ratio,[29] which is in accordance with positron emission tomography (PET) scan studies in patients with internal carotid artery occlusion and compensatory maximal vasodilatation of the precapillary vessels.[49] Other researchers also found a relationship between the VMR and the clinical status of patients with occlusive cerebrovascular disease.[53,65] They noted an increased frequency of TIAs or strokes in patients with decreased VMR, which could be reproduced by Keunen.[31]

In conclusion, it appears that a correlation exists between the extent of extracranial atherosclerosis, the integrity of the circle of Willis, the VMR, and the neurologic condition of the patient. This suggests that TCD is a useful tool in the detection of patients without symptoms who are at risk and that the risk of the natural course outweighs the risk of carotid endarterectomy. Prospective studies are necessary to validate these suggestions.[17]

The effectiveness of medical treatment in patients without symptoms with cervical bruits is also unknown. A promising study is under way, but unfortunately, the patients in the study are not tested for collateral potential or vasoreactive capacity.[6]

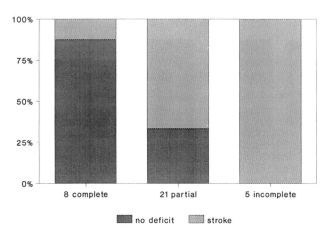

Fig. 39-2. Relationship between the collateral circulation via the circle of Willis and ipsilateral stroke in 34 patients with an occlusion of the internal carotid artery. Complete circles (type 1): $n = 8$, 12% stroke; partial circles (types 2 and 3): $n = 21$, 67% stroke; incomplete circles (type 4): $n = 5$, 100% stroke.

ASSESSMENT OF INTRACRANIAL STENOSIS AND OCCLUSION

Although the risk of stroke is relatively high if significant intracranial lesions are present,[12] the incidence of such lesions is relatively low, and therefore arteriography is frequently negative. When the risks of selective intraarterial angiography are considered, the new possibilities offered by TCD to investigate the basal cerebral circulation are an attractive alternative. TCD offers the potential of detection of significant (more than 65%) stenosis of the carotid siphon and the main stem of the MCA. For the assessment of stenosis in these segments of the intracranial arterial tree, sonographic criteria, such as local increase of blood flow velocities, a spectrum distribution with increased low-frequency components, and the occurrence of musical murmurs, have been used by several authors. Because blood flow velocities vary with age, sex, carbon dioxide tension, cerebral vascular resistance, intracranial pressure, and blood pressure,[4,24,63] it is not prudent to use rigid average velocity values for the diagnosis of vascular obstructive disease. Comparison of velocities between the left and right sides of the arterial system in one patient and comparison with the other arterial segments can offer a clue about a correct diagnosis. Validation of the results with angiographic data is described in only one study. In a group of 133 consecutive patients, Ley-Pezo and Ringelstein[34] reported remarkably good agreement between the findings of TCD and selective cerebral arteriography.

The diagnostic accuracy for the detection of stenosis or occlusion was presented in terms of sensitivity, specificity, positive and negative predictive values (arteriography being the gold standard), and a chance-corrected measure of agreement (kappa). For both the carotid siphon and the main stem

of the MCA, these parameters exceeded 90% and kappa was close to $+1$. In other studies, however, differentiation from vasospasm or high blood flow velocities in collateral pathways, such as the anterior or posterior communicating arteries, remains difficult.[1,25] One of the most important reasons sonographers must be aware of the extent of atherosclerosis of the extracranial arteries is so that they understand the phenomenon of cross-filling by collaterals via the circle of Willis. Presently, TCD seems to be a valid method for screening lesions in the carotid siphon and main stem of the MCA, but more studies must be undertaken to assess its value in comparison with arteriography.

ASSESSMENT OF STROKE RISK FROM CARDIAC THROMBOEMBOLISM

In patients with stroke or those under the age of 45 with transient neurologic symptoms, cardiac thromboembolism ranks high as a direct cause. A wide variety of cardiac diseases, such as valvular disorders, prosthetic valves, atrial fibrillation, cardiomyopathy, akinetic segments, ventricular hypertrophy, and septal defects, are directly associated with stroke. Recently, the unique properties of pulsed Doppler equipment to detect emboli in the basal cerebral arteries in a variety of conditions were described by Spencer and others.[47,50,61] Theoretically, these observations open new perspectives for the detection of cardiac emboli in patients with TIAs and in patients with known cardiac disease who are free of symptoms. Frequency, number, and other physical properties of emboli can be used to assess the risk of stroke in these patients. New and challenging studies on this subject must be undertaken soon.

CONCLUSION

There is increasing evidence that the detection of both hemodynamic changes and thromboembolic phenomena by TCD offers new possibilities to predict stroke in individual patients. The assessment of blood flow velocities in the basal cerebral arteries and changes within during compression of the common carotid artery provides information about the collaterals in the circle of Willis. This can be used as a predictor of stroke in patients with significant extracranial carotid artery disease, especially when these data are used in combination with the assessment of the VMR by TCD. Furthermore, TCD can be used for the diagnosis of stenosis or occlusion of the carotid siphon or the main stem of the MCA. Finally, the sensitivity of TCD to detect emboli will lead to new studies on the pathogenesis of thromboembolic cerebrovascular disease.

REFERENCES

1. Aaslid R, Huber P, Nornes H: A transcranial Doppler method in the evaluation of cerebrovascular spasm, *Neuroradiology* 26:11-16, 1986.
2. Aaslid R, Markwalder TM, Nornes H: Noninvasive transcranial Doppler ultrasound recording of flow velocity in basal cerebral arteries, *J Neurosurg* 57:769-774, 1982.
3. Ackerstaff RGA et al: Cerebral function monitoring during carotid endarterectomy by simultaneous electroencephalography and transcranial Doppler sonography, *J Cardiovasc Technol* 9:310-311, 1990.

4. Ackerstaff RGA et al: Influence of biological factors in changes in mean cerebral blood flow velocity in normal aging: a transcranial Doppler study, *Neurol Res* 12:187-192, 1990.

5. American Academy of Neurology, Therapeutics and Technology Assessment Subcommittee: Assessment: transcranial Doppler, *Neurology* 40:680-681, 1990.

6. Asymptomatic Cervical Bruit Study Group: Natural history and effectiveness of aspirin in asymptomatic patients with cervical bruits, *Arch Neurol* 48:683-686, 1991.

7. Barnes RW et al: Late outcome of untreated asymptomatic carotid disease following cardiovascular operations, *J Vasc Surg* 2:843-849, 1985.

8. Bishop CC et al: The effect of internal carotid artery occlusion on middle cerebral artery blood flow, at rest and in response to hypercapnia, *Lancet* 1:710-712, 1986.

9. Bogousslavsky J, Regli F: Cerebral infarction with transient signs (CITS): do TIAs correspond to small deep infarcts in internal carotid artery occlusion? *Stroke* 15:536-539, 1984.

10. Bogousslavsky J, Regli F: Cerebral infarct in apparent transient ischemic attack, *Neurology* 35:1501-1503, 1985.

11. Bogousslavsky J, Despland PA, Regli F: Asymptomatic tight stenosis of the internal carotid artery: long-term prognosis, *Neurology* 36:861-863, 1986.

12. Bogousslavski J et al: Atherosclerotic disease of the middle cerebral artery, *Stroke* 17:1112-1120, 1986.

13. Brown MM et al: Reactivity of the cerebral circulation in patients with carotid occlusion, *J Neurol Neurosurg Psychiat* 49:899-904, 1986.

14. Caplan LR: Are terms such as completed stroke or RIND of continued usefulness? *Stroke* 14:431-433, 1983.

15. Caplan LR, Stein RW: *Stroke: a clinical approach,* London, 1986, Butterworth.

16. Caplan LR et al: Transcranial Doppler ultrasound: present status, *Neurology* 40:696-700, 1990.

17. CASANOVA Study Group: Carotid surgery versus medical therapy in asymptomatic carotid stenosis, *Stroke* 22:1229-1235, 1991.

18. Chambers BR, Norris JW: The case against surgery for asymptomatic carotid stenosis, *Stroke* 15(6):964-967, 1984.

19. Chambers BR, Norris JW: Outcome in patients with asymptomatic neck bruits, *N Engl J Med* 315:860-865, 1986.

20. Eikelboom BC, Vermeulen FEE: *The value of ocular pneumoplethysmography versus angiography in the determination of the potential collateral hemispheric circulation.* In Diethrich G, ed: *Noninvasive cardiovascular diagnosis,* ed 2, Littleton, Mass, 1981, PSG Publishing.

21. Eikelboom BC et al: Recognizing stroke prone patients with a poor collateral circulation, *Eur J Vasc Surg* 1:381-384, 1987.

22. European Carotid Surgery Trialists' Collaborative Group: MRC European carotid surgery trial: interim results for symptomatic patients with severe (70-99%) or with mild (0-29%) stenosis, *Lancet* 337:1235-1243, 1991.

23. Grigg MF et al: The significance of cerebral infarction and atrophy in patients with amaurosis fugax and transient ischemic attack in relation to internal carotid artery stenosis, *J Vasc Surg* 2:215-222, 1980.

24. Grolimund P, Seiler RW: Age dependency of the flow velocity in the basal cerebral arteries—a transcranial Doppler ultrasound study, *Ultrasound Biol* 14:191-198, 1988.

25. Grolimund P, Seiler RW, Aaslid R: Evaluation of cerebrovascular disease by combined extracranial and transcranial Doppler sonography: experience in 1039 patients, *Stroke* 18:1018-1024, 1987.

26. Halsey J et al: Blood velocity in the middle cerebral artery and regional cerebral blood flow during carotid endarterectomy, *Stroke* 20:53-58, 1989.

27. Hennerici M, Rautenberg W, Schwartz A: Transcranial Doppler ultrasound for the assessment of intracranial arterial flow velocity. Part 2. Evaluation of intracranial arterial disease, *Surg Neurol* 27:523-532, 1987.

28. Hennerici M et al: Natural history of asymptomatic extracranial arterial disease: results of a long-term prospective study, *Brain* 110:777-791, 1987.

29. Herold S et al: Assessment of cerebral haemodynamic reserve: correlation between PET parameters and CO_2 reactivity measured by the intravenous 133 Xenon injection technique, *J Neurol Neurosurg Psychiat* 51:1045-1050, 1988.

30. Jansen C, Ackerstaff RGA, Eikelboom BC: *The use of transcranial Doppler in carotid artery disease.* In Yao JST, Pearce WH, eds: *Technologies in vascular surgery,* Philadelphia, 1991, WB Saunders.

31. Keunen RWM: *Transcranial Doppler sonography of the cerebral circulation in occlusive cerebrovascular disease,* thesis, Nijmegen, The Netherlands, 1990, Benda BV.

32. Koudstaal PJ et al: Diagnosis of transient ischemic attacks: improvement of interobserver agreement by a check list in ordinary language, *Stroke* 17:723-728, 1986.

33. Koudstaal PJ et al: Transient ischemic attacks with and without a relevant infarct on computed tomographic scans cannot be distinguished clinically, *Arch Neurol* 48:916-920, 1991.

34. Ley-Pozo J, Ringelstein EB: Noninvasive detection of occlusive disease of the carotid siphon and middle cerebral artery, *Ann Neurol* 28:640-647, 1990.

35. Lindegaard KF et al: Assessment of intracranial hemodynamics in carotid artery disease by transcranial Doppler ultrasound, *J Neurosurg* 63:890-898, 1985.

36. Lindegaard KF et al: Doppler diagnosis of intracranial artery occlusive disorders, *J Neurol Neurosurg Psychiat* 49:510-518, 1986.

37. Lindegaard KF et al: Evaluation of cerebral AVMs using transcranial Doppler ultrasound, *J Neurosurg* 65:335-344, 1986.

38. Mattle H et al: Transcranial Doppler ultrasonographic findings in middle cerebral artery disease, *Arch Neurol* 45:289-295, 1988.

39. Moll FL et al: Dynamics of collateral circulation in progressive asymptomatic carotid disease, *J Vasc Surg* 3:470-474, 1986.

40. Moneta GL et al: Operative versus nonoperative management of asymptomatic high-grade internal carotid artery stenosis: improved results with endarterectomy, *Stroke* 18:1005-1010, 1987.

41. Murros KE et al: Cerebral infarction in patients with transient ischemic attacks, *J Neurol* 236:182-184, 1989.

42. Nicolaides A, Zukowski A: *The place of computerized tomographic brain scanning in the classification of ischaemic cerebral disease.* In Courbier R, ed: *Basis for a classification of cerebral arterial diseases,* Amsterdam, 1985, Excerpta Medica.

43. Norris JW: Does transcranial Doppler have any clinical value? *Neurology* 40:329-331, 1990.

44. Norris JW, Krajewski A, Bornstein NM: The clinical role of the cerebral collateral circulation in carotid occlusion, *J Vasc Surg* 12:113-118, 1990.

45. North American Symptomatic Carotid Endarterectomy Trial Collaborators: Beneficial effect of carotid endarterectomy in symptomatic patients with high-grade stenosis, *N Engl J Med* 325:445-453, 1991.

46. Padayachee TS et al: Transcranial measurement of blood velocities in the basal cerebral arteries using pulsed Doppler ultrasound: a method of assessing the circle of Willis, *Ultrasound Med Biol* 12:5-14, 1986.

47. Padayachee TS et al: The detection of microemboli in the middle cerebral artery during cardiopulmonary bypass: a transcranial Doppler ultrasound investigation using membrane and bubble oxygenators, *Ann Thorac Surg* 44:298-302, 1987.

48. Padayachee TS et al: Transcranial Doppler assessment of cerebral collateral during carotid endarterectomy, *Br J Surg* 74:260-262, 1987.

49. Powers WJ, Raichle ME: Positron emission tomography and its application to the study of cerebrovascular disease in man, *Stroke* 16:361-376, 1985.

50. Pugsley W: The use of Doppler ultrasound in the assessment of microemboli during cardiac surgery, *Perfusion* 4:115-122, 1989.

51. Quinones-Baldrich WJ, Moore WS: Asymptomatic carotid stenosis: rationale for management, *Arch Neurol* 42:378-382, 1985.

52. Ringelstein EB: *A practical guide to transcranial Doppler sonography.* In Weinberger J, ed: *Noninvasive imaging of cerebrovascular disease,* New York, 1989, Alan R Liss.

53. Ringelstein EB et al: Noninvasive assessment of CO_2-induced cerebral vasomotor response in normal individuals and patients with internal carotid artery occlusions, *Stroke* 19:963-969, 1988.

54. Roederer GO et al: The natural history of carotid arterial disease in asymptomatic patients with cervical bruits, *Stroke* 15:605-613, 1984.

55. Ropper A, Kehne S, Wechsler L: Transcranial Doppler in brain death, *Neurology* 37:1733-1735, 1987.

56. Schneider PA et al: Effect of internal carotid artery occlusion on intracranial hemodynamics: transcranial Doppler evaluation and clinical correlation, *Stroke* 19:589-593, 1988.

57. Schneider PA et al: Transcranial Doppler in the management of extracranial cerebrovascular disease: implications in diagnosis and monitoring, *J Vasc Surg* 7:223-231, 1988.

58. Schneider PA et al: Noninvasive assessment of cerebral collateral blood supply through the ophthalmic artery, *Stroke* 22:31-36, 1991.

59. Schroeder T: Cerebrovascular reactivity to acetazolamide in carotid artery disease: enhancement of side-to-side asymmetry indicates critically reduced perfusion pressure, *Neurol Res* 8:231-236, 1986.

60. Sloan MA et al: Sensitivity and specificity of transcranial Doppler ultrasonography in the diagnosis of vasospasm following subarachnoid hemorrhage, *Neurology* 39:1514-1518, 1989.

61. Spencer MP et al: Detection of middle cerebral artery emboli during carotid endarterectomy using transcranial Doppler ultrasonography, *Stroke* 21:415-423, 1990.

62. von Reutern G et al: Transcranial Doppler ultrasonography during cardiopulmonary bypass in patients with severe carotid stenosis or occlusion, *Stroke* 19:674-680, 1988.

63. Vriens EM et al: Transcranial pulsed Doppler measurements of blood velocity in the middle cerebral artery: reference values at rest and during hyperventilation in healthy volunteers in relation to age and sex, *Ultrasound Med Biol* 15:1-18, 1989.

64. Waxman S, Toole JF: Temporal profile resembling TIA in the setting of cerebral infarction, *Stroke* 14:433-437, 1983.

65. Widder B et al: Transcranial Doppler CO_2 test for the detection of haemodynamically critical carotid artery stenoses and occlusions, *Eur Arch Psychiatr Neurol Sci* 236:162-168, 1986.

66. Zukowski AJ et al: The correlation between carotid plaque ulceration and cerebral infarction seen on CT scan, *J Vasc Surg* 1:782-786, 1984.

CHAPTER 40

Do we really need transcranial Doppler in the vascular laboratory?

JOHN W. NORRIS

It is almost 10 years since insonation of the cerebral circulation became feasible[1] and about 5 years since commercially available transcranial Doppler (TCD) machines came into general use. TCD has found a secure and clinically valuable place in several areas of neurosurgical practice. The measurement of blood flow velocities (BFVs) of the middle cerebral (MCA) and anterior cerebral arteries has permitted close monitoring of the cerebral vasospasm that may occur after subarachnoid hemorrhage.[9] The increase in BFV in the affected cerebral arteries is sensitive enough to reflect the course of arterial vasospasm. Abnormal velocities will persist for days after arteriographic findings have returned to normal. Similarly, it can be used to monitor the graded extracranial occlusion of the carotid artery by clamp in those cases in which craniotomy is neither desirable nor feasible.[5]

In the diagnosis of brain death, TCD may prove as sensitive as any other method but is noninvasive, and inexpensive, quick, and easy to perform.[21] It is also valuable for detecting the raised intracranial pressure that may occur in cerebral trauma[13] and may be used to diagnose arteriovenous malformations and monitor the effectiveness of ablation.[10]

It is more difficult to define the role of TCD in vascular surgery, however. A major disadvantage affecting the usefulness of any surgical diagnostic procedure is a significant degree of technical failure, particularly if alternative procedures are available. Because TCD is very operator dependent, this may explain the wide range of failure to insonate one or both temporal "windows," the major portals for ultrasonic scanning of the cerebral circulation. The documented failure rate varies between 6% and 35%,[4,12] and failure to observe the course of individual vessels may yield false-positive diagnoses of occlusion.[12,17]

As found for neurosurgical procedures, the major value of TCD in vascular surgery is to monitor cerebral perfusion, especially when angiography has already demonstrated the nature of the underlying disease. For example, in patients with unilateral carotid occlusion or high-grade stenosis and in those with contralateral carotid stenosis, it is helpful to determine how dependent the cerebral hemispheres are on

the remaining patent extracranial vessels. This can be readily determined by monitoring the BFVs of the MCA over each cerebral hemisphere while the patent carotid artery is compressed (Fig. 40-1).[19] This does not exclude the possibility of thromboembolism from a patent but narrowed carotid artery, nor does it exclude the possibility that over time, the dependency of the cerebral hemisphere on collaterals may change because of disease arising at new sites. However, it does give information concerning the hemodynamic state existing at the moment of the TCD evaluation.

MONITORING CAROTID SURGERY

Neurovascular monitoring using TCD during carotid endarterectomy is undergoing critical appraisal. Although electroencephalography (EEG) is probably the most common and easy method available, there is good evidence that the EEG changes observed during carotid clamping have little relevance to prognosis, including any immediate complications when the patient awakes from surgery. For instance, in a recent study of 458 consecutive carotid endarterectomies, 7 of 10 patients with immediate strokes and all 5 with immediate minor deficits had no change in their EEGs from the time of the baseline reading to the end of the surgical procedure.[14] Similar disappointing results were

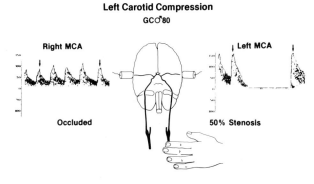

Left Carotid Compression
GC♂80

Right MCA

Occluded

Left MCA

50% Stenosis

Fig. 40-1. In an 80-year-old man (*GC*) with unilateral carotid occlusion, compression of the patent carotid artery produced complete obliteration of ipsilateral MCA flow but had no effect on contralateral flow in the occluded side (i.e., the patent hemisphere was completely dependent on the patent carotid artery). (From Norris JW, Krajewski A, Bornstein NM: *J Vasc Surg* 12:113-118, 1990.)

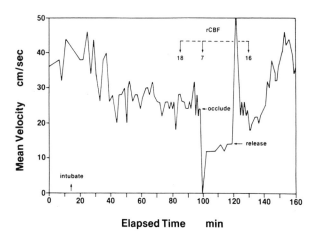

Fig. 40-2. Continuous record of mean blood flow velocity in middle cerebral artery with contralateral internal carotid artery occlusion. The electroencephalogram was suppressed ipsilaterally during clamping (occlude). This case suffered no clinical disability. *rCBF,* Regional cerebral blood flow in ml/100 g/min. (From Halsey JH et al: *Stroke* 20:53-58, 1989.)

found in a recent study of sensory evoked potentials (SEPs), in which 4 patients awoke with strokes yet had shown no change in their SEPs during the procedure.[11]

A recent study of TCD monitoring during carotid surgery yielded generally disappointing results.[2] Temporal windows could not be adequately insonated in 13% of the patients, and in another 27%, technical difficulties precluded obtaining meaningful results. Consequently, only 60% of the patients had results that could be evaluated. (In fact, one problem in assessing the published results of surgical procedures is that the authors commonly do not always include consecutive patients, inadvertently omitting their technical failures and so biasing their results in favor of the procedure.) In those patients in whom complete TCD evaluations were obtained during surgery, no information was obtained that would have changed the management protocol. In the one patient sustaining a postoperative stroke, there was no change in TCD values that might have alerted the surgeon to the developing problem during the procedure.

There are two reasons for these paradoxical findings concerning the worth of TCD during carotid artery surgery. First, clamping of the extracranial carotid artery during carotid endarterectomy for periods of usually 20 to 30 minutes appears to have little effect on cerebral tissue, whatever evidence the neurovascular monitor (e.g., EEG) may show of severely disturbed cerebral function or disastrous decrease in cerebral blood flow (CBF) (Fig. 40-2).[8] Surgeons who operate without shunts have the same perioperative incidence of cerebral ischemia as those using shunts and monitors.[2] Second, most strokes that occur after carotid surgery are embolic and do not stem from cerebral damage due to hypoperfusion sustained during surgery.[15]

HYPERPERFUSION SYNDROME

One of the most perplexing but fortunately rare complications of carotid endarterectomy is the postoperative hyper-

perfusion syndrome. The frequency of this complication is estimated to occur in less than 1% of the procedures, although minor manifestations may be much more common. In this syndrome, the patient experiences severe headache, sometimes seizures, uncontrollable hypertension, and occasionally, cerebral hemorrhage, usually 1 to 2 weeks after an otherwise uneventful carotid procedure. In one series, this occurred in 8 (0.4%) of 1930 procedures.[24] In such patients, the carotid artery operated on has always shown a severe degree of carotid stenosis (greater than 75%), and this is presumably associated with a chronically ischemic cerebral hemisphere. When the offending stenosis is removed, there is "hyperperfusion" leading to cerebral edema and hemorrhage. In one patient who underwent autopsy, the affected hemisphere showed extensive pathologic changes similar to those seen in patients with acute hypertensive encephalopathy.[3] The blood vessels were normal in the contralateral cerebral hemisphere.

Using TCD, Powers and Smith[22] documented BFV increases in the MCA of 100% to 400% after endarterectomy, which then returned to normal over the next few days. A small asymptomatic hemorrhage in the ipsilateral thalamus was seen on the magnetic resonance imaging scan in one case. In one unreported case, high BFVs in the MCA persisted for more than 2 weeks after surgery, fortunately without incident apart from severe vascular headache.

MONITORING CEREBRAL EMBOLI

Air bubbles are much more powerful deflectors of ultrasound waves than are red blood cells, and making use of this principle, Gillis, Peterson, and Karagianes[16] used Doppler detection of gas emboli in the pulmonary artery to monitor decompression sickness. This method was later applied to the detection of presumed gas emboli in the brain circulation during cardiopulmonary bypass operations[20] and carotid endarterectomy.[25] Air bubble emboli were detected by TCD in 35 (38%) of 91 patients on release of the common carotid clamp during carotid surgery (Fig. 40-3).[25] Formed-element emboli both appeared during and after the carotid surgical procedure but, of greater interest, formed spontaneously *before* the procedure. Hence this technique might be used to assess activity of the carotid plaque.

The significance of these emboli is uncertain. Although originally deemed innocuous,[20] subsequent data have indicated that continuing, spontaneous embolism occurring after surgery may be an index of more serious and even devastating cerebral embolism.[25] Similarly, Doppler has proved to be a sensitive method for detecting experimentally introduced clots, platelets, atheromatous fragments, fat, and air emboli in the rabbit aorta.[23]

This technique is also used to detect right-to-left cardiac shunting through a patent foramen ovale as a cause of stroke or transient ischemic attack (TIA). Contrast echocardiography has shown that as much as 50% of young patients have such shunting of blood at the atrial level, and this may serve as a source of paradoxical cerebral embolism.[27] When

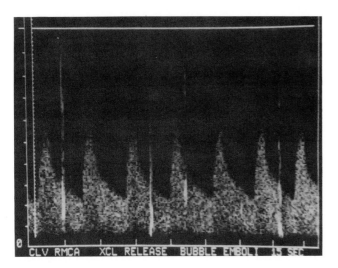

Fig. 40-3. Transcranial Doppler spectrogram showing typical bubble emboli (vertical bright linear transients) after the carotid clamp was removed during endocarterectomy. (From Spencer MP et al: *Stroke* 21:415-423, 1990.)

a TCD monitor is used simultaneously with two-dimensional echocardiography, air bubbles introduced through a vein can be detected passing through the heart and into the brain.[26]

EVALUATION OF PATIENTS WITH TRANSIENT ISCHEMIC ATTACKS AND STROKE

The use of TCD in patients suffering from acute cardiovascular events has so far proved disappointing and is of limited use in the evaluation of patients with intracranial vascular stenoses and occlusions. One problem is that the BFVs in the circle of Willis branches relate poorly to CBF. BFVs may be increased in the presence of vasospasm even though CBF is low, or it may be decreased when the contracting arterial lumen reaches a critical degree of narrowing.[17]

In an attempt to relate BFV of the MCA to both acute metabolic depression and the luxury perfusion that occurs in acute cerebral infarction, the clinical status, BFV of the MCA, and single photon emission computerized tomographic (SPECT) images of cerebral perfusion in 299 patients were compared.[18] In the first 160 consecutive patients, the cerebral circulation was not adequately insonated in 21 (13%) patients. In the remaining 139 patients, 94 (68%) were normal, 17 (12%) showed increased BFVs, and 28 (20%) showed reduced BFVs in the MCA. However, the SPECT findings in these patients showed no relationship to the BFV in the MCA, in that a high CBF on SPECT may be associated with high, low, or normal BFVs in the MCA. Patients with a high or low BFV in the MCA had significantly more severe strokes than did those with a normal BFV in the MCA.

One can conclude from these findings that BFV in the

MCA reflects only the status of intracranial (or extracranial) carotid stenoses or occlusions and not metabolic activities or changes in CBF. However, because there is little or no indication to perform cerebral angiography in cases of completed stroke, there is no gold standard for comparison in most cases.

Kushner et al[15] compared TCD findings to those seen on intraarterial digital angiograms obtained in 42 patients in the acute stage of cerebral hemisphere infarctions. They found a high correlation between absent or suppressed MCA flow shown by TCD and MCA occlusion revealed by angiography. The abnormal TCD values tended to be associated with more extensive cerebral infarcts. Halsey[7] evaluated BFV in the MCA in 15 patients within 12 hours of acute ischemic strokes and found that those with low BFVs (less than 30 cm/sec) did more poorly.

There are several studies that attempted to relate angiographic and TCD findings in the context of cerebrovascular disease. In a comparison similar to the one just described, TCD and angiographic findings were compared in 48 patients with carotid ischemic cerebral lesions within 4 hours of the ictus.[28] Again, MCA occlusions were commonly detected, as was diverted flow in other pathways through the circle of Willis.

The mapping of lesions in the vertebrobasilar system is not as easy as that in the carotid arteries. In a study of 58 patients, Mull et al[16] concluded that the TCD results were valid only when used in combination with cerebral angiography findings.

CONCLUSION

TCD is still in its infancy, in terms of both technological development and experience with the spectrum of its uses. Although its ability to detect intracranial stenoses and occlusions may assist in identifying the origins of cerebral ischemia, its value in monitoring various forms of cardiac and neurovascular surgery has not been fully defined.

New forms of real-time color-coded TCD represent a major avenue for progress[4] and may come to be a preferred form of intracranial vascular imaging, even over magnetic resonance imaging.

REFERENCES

1. Aaslid R, Markwalder TM, Nornes H: Noninvasive transcranial Doppler ultrasound recording of flow velocity in basal cerebral arteries, *J Neurosurg* 57:769-774, 1982.
2. Bass A et al: Intraoperative transcranial Doppler: limitations of the method, *J Vasc Surg* 10:549-553, 1989.
3. Bernstein M, Fleming JFR, Deck JHN: Cerebral hyperperfusion after carotid endarterectomy: a cause of cerebral hemorrhage, *Neurosurgery* 15:50-56, 1984.
4. Bogdahn U et al: Transcranial color-coded real-time sonography in adults, *Stroke* 21:1680-1688, 1990.
5. Giller CA et al: Transcranial Doppler ultrasound as a guide to graded therapeutic occlusion of the carotid artery, *Neurosurg* 26:307-311, 1990.
6. Gillis MF, Peterson PL, Karagianes MT: In vivo detection of circulating gas emboli associated with decompression sickness using the Doppler flowmeter, *Nature* 217:965-966, 1968.
7. Halsey JH: Prognosis of acute hemiplegia estimated by transcranial Doppler ultrasonography, *Stroke* 19:648-649, 1988.

8. Halsey JH et al: Blood velocity in the middle cerebral artery and regional cerebral blood flow during carotid endarterectomy, *Stroke* 20:53-58, 1989.

9. Harders AG: *Monitoring hemodynamic changes related to vasospasm in the circle of Willis after aneurysm surgery.* In Aaslid R, ed: *Transcranial Doppler sonography,* Vienna, 1986, Springer-Verlag.

10. Harders AG: *Neurosurgical applications of transcranial Doppler sonography,* Vienna, 1986, Springer-Verlag.

11. Horsch S, De Vleeschauwer P, Ktenidis K: Intraoperative assessment of cerebral ischemia during carotid surgery, *Stroke* 22:548, 1991.

12. Kaps M et al: Transcranial Doppler ultrasound findings in middle cerebral artery occlusion, *Stroke* 21:532-537, 1990.

13. Krajewski A et al: Doppler monitoring in cerebral trauma, *Can J Neurol Sci* 15:241, 1988.

14. Kresowik TF et al: Limitations of electroencephalographic monitoring in the detection of cerebral ischemia accompanying carotid endarterectomy, *Stroke* 22:1103, 1991.

15. Kushner MJ et al: Transcranial Doppler in acute hemispheric brain infarction, *Neurology* 41:109-113, 1991.

16. Mull M, Aulich A, Hennerici M: Transcranial Doppler ultrasonography versus arteriography for assessment of the vertebrobasilar circulation, *J Clin Ultrasound* 18:539-549, 1990.

17. Norris JW: Does transcranial Doppler have any clinical value? *Neurology* 40:329-331, 1990.

18. Norris JW, Zhu CZ: *Transcranial Doppler: a new test for cerebral embolism?* In Yao JST, Pearce WH, eds: *Technologies in vascular surgery,* New York, 1991, WB Saunders.

19. Norris JW, Krajewski A, Bornstein NM: The clinical role of the cerebral collateral circulation in carotid occlusion, *J Vasc Surg* 12:113-118, 1990.

20. Padayachee TS et al: The detection of microemboli in the middle cerebral artery during cardiopulmonary bypass: a transcranial Doppler ultrasound investigation using membrane and bubble oxygenators, *Ann Thorac Surg* 44:298-302, 1987.

21. Petty GW et al: The role of transcranial Doppler in confirming brain death: sensitivity, specificity, and suggestions for performance and interpretation, *Neurology* 40:300-303, 1989.

22. Powers AD, Smith RR: Hyperperfusion syndrome after carotid endarterectomy: a transcranial Doppler evaluation, *Neurosurgery* 26:56-60, 1990.

23. Russel D et al: Detection of arterial emboli using Doppler ultrasound in rabbits, *Stroke* 22:253-258, 1991.

24. Solomon RA et al: Incidence and etiology of intracerebral hemorrhage following carotid endarterectomy, *J Neurosurg* 64:29-34, 1986.

25. Spencer MP et al: Detection of middle cerebral artery emboli during carotid endarterectomy using transcranial Doppler ultrasonography, *Stroke* 21:415-423, 1990.

26. Teague SM, Sharma MK: Detection of paradoxical cerebral echo contrast embolization by transcranial Doppler ultrasound, *Stroke* 22:740-745, 1991.

27. Webster MWI et al: Patent foramen ovale in young stroke patients, *Lancet* 2:11-12, 1988.

28. Zanette EM et al: Comparison of cerebral angiography and transcranial Doppler sonography in acute stroke, *Stroke* 20:899-903, 1989.

CHAPTER 41

Cerebral blood flow measurements during carotid endarterectomy

THORALF M. SUNDT, JR.

In collaboration with Nicolee C. Fode, RN, MS, Robert E. Anderson, BS, Joseph M. Messick, Jr., MD, and Frank W. Sharbrough, MD*

From January 1972 through December 1990, 2887 carotid endarterectomies were performed in patients with carotid ulcerative-stenosis disease on the neurovascular surgical service at the Mayo Clinic. These patients were routinely monitored with intraoperative cerebral blood flow (CBF) measurements and continuous electroencephalograms (EEGs). The EEG was found to be a sensitive monitor of neurologic function. No patients awoke after the operative procedure with a new neurologic deficit that was not predicted by EEG. The critical CBF (flow required to maintain normal EEG findings) varied somewhat with the anesthetic agent but approximated 30% of normal CBF of 50 ml/100 g/min. Shunts were usually placed if flow fell below 18 to 20 ml/100 g/min during occlusion for endarterectomy in patients who were anesthetized with enflurane or halothane and below 15 ml/100 g/min for patients who were anesthetized with combined isoflurane-fentanyl anesthesia.

Patients were categorized into four groups before surgery according to medical, neurologic, and angiographically determined risk factors. Baseline and occlusion CBF values were significantly lower in the highest risk group in comparison with similar measurements in the lowest risk group. Occlusion flow rate less than 10 ml/100 g/min was recorded in 8% of patients with grade 1 risk, 15% with grade 2, 19% with grade 3, and 28% with grade 4. Shunts were used in approximately 40% of the patients. This varied slightly according to the anesthetic agent used: halothane in 42%, enflurane in 46%, and isoflurane in 36%. Occlusion flow rate below the critical level was found in 24.9% of all patients (0 to 4 ml/100 g/min in 3%, 5 to 9 ml/100 g/min in 7%, and 10 to 14 ml/100 g/min in 14%). In an additional 15% of patients with borderline flow rates (15 to 20 ml/100 g/min) shunts were often used, some of these because of a preexisting EEG abnormality related to a preoperative infarct. Shunts were required in 54% of patients who were neurologically unstable before surgery but in only 29% of patients who were neurologically stable before the operation. Saphenous vein patch grafts were used in more than 90% of the operative procedures. This chapter describes the use of intraoperative CBF measurements in carotid artery surgery.

Intraoperative monitoring techniques were adopted almost 20 years ago after the results of endarterectomy without monitoring were analyzed and found to be unacceptable. At that time the overall morbidity-mortality rate was less than 5% but was associated with a group of patients at lower risk than those who are currently undergoing surgery at this institution. Although the arterial procedure itself seldom took longer than 15 to 20 minutes, a number of patients awoke after surgery with either a major or minor neurologic deficit; some were transient, and others were permanent. Although ever cognizant of the risk of intraoperative embolization, the surgeons did not believe that these deficits were attributable to that cause. Furthermore, a postoperative internal carotid artery occlusion rate approaching 3% was documented in more than 100 patients operated on without patch grafting (the identification of the occlusion in two patients by a reduction in the postoperative retinal artery pressure measurement led to prompt reconstruction of the endarterectomy with patch grafting before the development of a neurologic deficit). A reappraisal led to the decision to perform a more meticulous endarterectomy and to patch graft routinely. Coupled with this approach was the need to provide cerebral protection by indwelling shunts, either routinely or selectively, during the period of carotid occlusion, since the period of occlusion for patch grafting would obviously be longer.

This chapter relates the results of the intraoperative correlation of continuous EEGs with intermittent CBF measurements. Results and complications of the operative procedure have been previously reported in detail.[41,48] Attention is focused on intraoperative complications and those complications that follow surgery specifically related to the phenomenon of cerebral hyperperfusion.

---

*Mayo Clinic and Medical School, Rochester, Minn.

METHODS

This report includes all patients who were operated on for carotid stenosis by one neurovascular surgical service between January 1, 1972, and January 1, 1991. Surgery was performed by one of five staff surgeons or by a chief resident with one of those staff surgeons acting as first assistant. Approximately 58% of the operations were performed on one surgeon's service. During the entire period of the report, patients were classified into one of four categories on the basis of preoperative risk factors.

Preoperative risk factors

Early in the study, certain preoperative risk factors were correlated with specific types of complications.[35,44] The following represent the major but by no means the only considerations in determining the patient's surgical risk:

1. Medical risk factors: Presence of symptomatic coronary artery disease (angina pectoris) or myocardial infarction within 6 months of the date of surgery, severe hypertension (blood pressure greater than 180/110 mm Hg), chronic obstructive pulmonary disease, physiologic age more than 70 years, and severe obesity

2. Neurologic risk factors: Progressive neurologic deficit, presence of a deficit for less than 24 hours before surgery, frequent daily transient ischemic attacks, or symptoms of generalized (as opposed to focal) cerebral ischemia

3. Angiographically determined risks: Coexisting stenosis of the internal carotid artery in the siphon area, extensive involvement of the vessel to be operated on with the plaque extending more than 3 cm distally in the internal carotid artery or 5 cm proximally in the common carotid artery, bifurcation of the carotid artery at the level of the second cervical vertebra in conjunction with a short or thick neck, occlusion of the opposite internal carotid artery, evidence of a soft thrombus extending from the ulcerative lesion or small vessel occlusions from multiple emboli, and a slowed intracranial circulation time as determined by angiography

The degree of stenosis per se was not considered a risk factor.

Classification of patients

On the basis of the foregoing general risk factors, it is possible to create a system for grading a patient's potential risk for surgery.[44] Although a given patient does not always fit neatly into a particular group, this system does provide a framework for comparative purposes. The patients were categorized as follows:

Grade 1: Neurologically stable (no neurologic risk factors) with no major medical or angiographically determined risks, with unilateral or bilateral ulcerative-stenotic disease

Grade 2: Neurologically stable with no major medical risks but with significant angiographically determined risks

Grade 3: Neurologically stable with major medical risks with or without significant angiographically determined risks

Grade 4: Major neurologic risks with or without associated major medical or angiographically determined risks, with angiograms frequently showing both a slowed flow and multiple small vessel occlusions

Preoperative evaluation

All patients underwent detailed medical and neurologic examinations before surgery. Before 1988, most patients had preoperative retinal artery pressure (RAP) measurements along with, in some instances, digital subtraction angiograms (DSAs). Over the past 3 years, however, these studies have been replaced with oculoplethysmography and duplex scanning. These two studies are used as screening procedures. They are not considered to be substitutes for formal angiography. Only in rare instances have patients been accepted for surgery without undergoing formal angiography, and in those isolated cases, DSAs have been available.

Intraoperative monitoring

Anesthesia. The anesthetic technique used has been reported previously. The depth of anesthesia was carefully controlled to get a sensitive EEG tracing, and the arterial carbon dioxide tension ($Paco_2$) was held constant to create comparable conditions for the comparison of CBF measurements. There was considerable variation of CBF with the anesthetic agent. The mean ($\pm$SD) baseline $Paco_2$ values were 40 $\pm$ 5 torr with halothane, 40 $\pm$ 5 torr with enflurane, and 39 $\pm$ 3 torr with isoflurane-fentanyl. The mean ($\pm$SD) baseline mean arterial pressure (MAP) determinations were 135 $\pm$ 21 torr with halothane, 126 $\pm$ 19 torr with enflurane, and 125 $\pm$ 35 torr with isoflurane-fentanyl.

Cerebral blood flow measurements. Regional CBF (rCBF) measurements were determined from clearance curves obtained from the extracranial detection of intraarterially injected xenon 133. The technique has been described in detail previously.[46] All instruments for recording counts were located in an adjacent monitoring room (Fig. 41-1). No cumbersome equipment was present in the operating suite. The indicator was injected through a no. 27 needle into the common carotid artery with the external carotid artery temporarily occluded. Each injectate contained 200 to 300 µCi ^{133}Xe diluted to 0.2 to 0.3 ml total volume with physiologic saline solution. Customarily, three measurements were obtained: one before occlusion, one during occlusion, and one after restoration of flow. If a shunt was used, a fourth measurement and sometimes a fifth were obtained with the shunt in place.

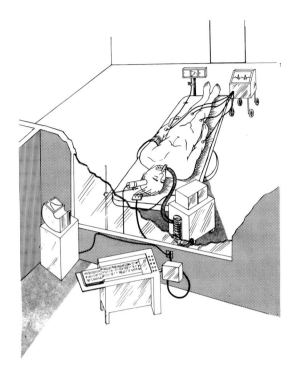

Fig. 41-1. Equipment arranged for simultaneous cerebral blood flow measurements and electroencephalograms during an operative procedure. All cumbersome equipment and paraphernalia are housed in an adjacent monitoring room so as not to encroach on the working space of the surgical or anesthesia teams.

Operative technique

A saphenous vein patch graft was used routinely except in patients with particularly large vessels. A shunt was always placed when both the EEG and the CBF indicated cerebral ischemia during the period of occlusion and frequently placed if the CBF was marginal, even if the EEG pattern remained unchanged. This latter indication for shunting was particularly important in patients with a preoperative cerebral infarction and abnormal EEG findings, since changes on the EEG are more difficult to identify and since these individuals appear to have a lower tolerance for ischemia. A shunt was never placed until the normal lumen of the vessel was visualized beyond the limits of the plaque. If a temporal artery pulse was not present after flow had been restored, the origin of the external carotid artery was temporarily occluded, and the shelf of elevated plaque or intima, which was invariably present at the distal limit of the resection, was excised through a separate short arteriotomy in that vessel. Routinely, 4000 to 5000 units of heparin was given before occlusion of the vessels, and this heparin was not reversed.

Postoperative monitoring

All patients underwent detailed neurologic examination when they awakened from anesthesia. They remained in the intensive care unit for 24 hours, during which time post-operative RAPs and oculoplethysmography measurements were obtained.

In the past, most patients remained in the hospital for 6 or 7 days while they underwent postoperative EEGs. This is no longer the current practice. Patients are usually discharged from the hospital on the third or fourth postoperative day, which makes it difficult to obtain postoperative EEGs. Currently, patients undergo routine postoperative duplex ultrasound study on approximately the third day after surgery.

RESULTS
Cerebral blood flow versus anesthetic agent and patient category

Table 41-1 summarizes intraoperative CBF measurements in 2731 patients with primary carotid stenosis and correlates these measurements with the anesthetic agent used during the operation and the patient's preoperative risk category. Data from 156 patients are not included because an anesthetic agent other than halothane, enflurane, or isoflurane-fentanyl was used, or because the endarterectomy was performed as the result of an acute occlusion or recurrent disease.

The discrepancy between the number of patients with postocclusion flow and those with baseline flow relates to technical problems in delivering the indicator to the brain in patients with a very high-grade stenosis (99.9%) or a physiologic occlusion.

There is a statistically significant difference among the baseline flow measurements in comparable grades of risk in patients who were operated on under these three anesthetic agents. There is also a significant difference between the baseline and occlusion flows in the patients of grade 4 risk compared with those of better risk (grades 1 and 2) who were operated on under the same anesthetic agent.

Correlation of EEG and CBF measurements

The severity of EEG changes observed with varying degrees of ischemia is illustrated in Fig. 41-2. Table 41-2 summarizes changes that are seen in the EEG with carotid occlusion according to the anesthetic agent used. It should be noted that in patients with a low CBF, shunting was often performed before the development of an EEG change. In such cases the plaque was usually removed from the distal internal carotid artery before the shunt was placed so that the period of occlusion before placement of a shunt approximated 2 to 4 minutes.

Cerebral blood flow and stump pressure

Stump pressures were measured in 100 consecutive patients to correlate these measurements with the occlusion CBF. These data are summarized in Fig. 41-3.

Embolic complications

Embolic complications during the operation are easily identified by a very dramatic change in the EEG. There

Table 41-1. Cerebral blood flow according to anesthetic used and patient grade of risk

Time of measurement	Grade 1		Grade 2		Grade 3		Grade 4	
	N	CBF ± SD	N	CBF ± SD	N	CBF ± SD	N	CBF ± SD
Halothane (480 cases)								
Baseline	157	62 ± 26	91	58 ± 28	143	51 ± 21	82	48 ± 21
Occlusion	157	35 ± 18	89	30 ± 18	145	26 ± 16	78	24 ± 13
Shunt	43	44 ± 15	44	52 ± 17	66	43 ± 17	48	42 ± 12
Postocclusion	158	69 ± 27	92	69 ± 26	145	61 ± 23	85	60 ± 22
Enflurane (883 cases)								
Baseline	313	50 ± 18	197	44 ± 18	204	42 ± 18	145	37 ± 21
Occlusion	311	28 ± 13	195	23 ± 13	200	21 ± 11	143	18 ± 11
Shunt	105	39 ± 15	102	35 ± 11	109	36 ± 13	91	35 ± 14
Postocclusion	317	51 ± 18	200	50 ± 19	211	48 ± 19	155	51 ± 22
Isoflurane (1368 cases)								
Baseline	359	34 ± 15	325	32 ± 18	413	30 ± 13	213	25 ± 13
Occlusion	354	22 ± 11	316	18 ± 12	398	18 ± 9	205	15 ± 10
Shunt	88	27 ± 10	128	30 ± 10	145	27 ± 10	130	26 ± 10
Postocclusion	363	39 ± 16	332	40 ± 16	436	35 ± 15	237	41 ± 34

N, Number of cases; *CBF*, cerebral blood flow; *SD*, standard deviation.

Table 41-2. Cerebral blood flow during carotid occlusion

Flow (mg/100 g/min)	Percent of cases anesthetized with a specific agent *not having* EEG change			Percent of cases anesthetized with a specific agent *having* EEG change		
	Halothane	Enflurane	Isoflurane	Halothane	Enflurane	Isoflurane
0-4	0	0.2	1.6	2.5	3	4.5
5-9	0.2	0.2	6	4.5	9	6
10-14	2	6	14	9	8.8	5
15-19	5	11	17	9	5.5	2
20-24	10	14.5	16.9	0	0	0.5
25-29	12	12	11	0	0	0
30+	46	30	16	0	0	0
TOTAL	75	74	82	25	26	18

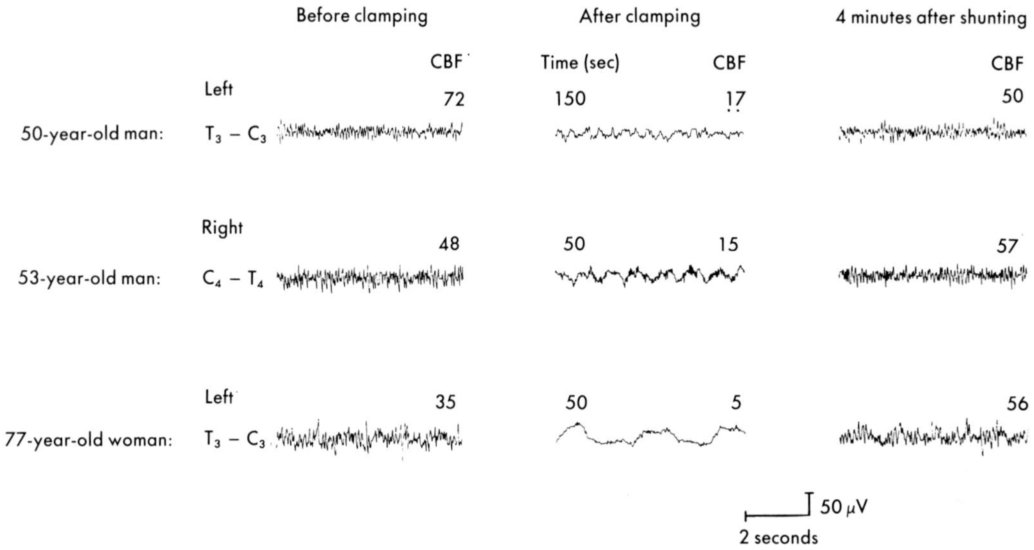

Fig. 41-2. Correlation between electroencephalograms and cerebral blood flow measurements during carotid endarterectomy. The severity of the EEG change parallels the reduction in cerebral blood flow.

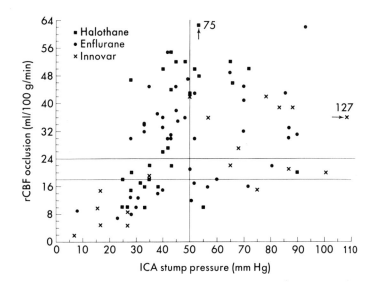

Fig. 41-3. Scattergram of occlusion regional cerebral blood flows *(rCBF)* plotted against the internal carotid artery *(ICA)* stump pressures. The vertical line represents the stump pressure of 50 torr (considered critical level). Two horizontal lines represent the critical flow level (rCBF ≤ 18 ml/100 g/min) and margin zone (rCBF 18 to 24 ml/100 g/min). Regression lines for each anesthetic agent were calculated. For enflurane, $rCBF_{occl}$ = 0.51 (stump pressure) ± 9.94, r = 0.43. For enflurane, $rCBF_{occl}$ = 0.26 (stump pressure) ± 16.51, r = 0.39. For isoflurane (fentanyl), $rCBF_{occl}$ = 0.27 (stump pressure ± 0.93, r = 0.68.)

were 22 embolic complications during the surgery, for an incidence of less than 1%. One half of these led to only a transient EEG change, but one half were associated with a major or minor neurologic deficit.

There were eight cases of emboli through a functioning shunt during the operation in this series. Four of these were major events relating to proximal atherosclerosis and, in retrospect, might possibly have been avoided with more experience. The other four embolic complications were minor: two patients regained normal EEG findings before awakening from anesthesia and had normal neurologic function in the recovery room; two patients retained minor deficits.

There were 14 embolic complications not related to shunts. Of these, 12 occurred during the exposure of the vessel (2 with induction of anesthesia), and 2 developed as the patient was awakening from anesthesia. A total of 6 of these led to a transient EEG change, and 8 led to a neurologic complication.

DISCUSSION
Monitoring and shunting during surgery

Between January 1972 and January 1991, 2887 endarterectomies for carotid stenosis were performed with the intraoperative monitoring techniques described. The correlation of CBF measurements with EEGs in these cases has been excellent, as indicated in Table 41-2, which summarizes data from 2731 patients (grades 1 to 4) operated on under halothane, enflurane, or isoflurane-fentanyl. Occlusion flow rate was between 0 and 4 ml/100 g/min in 124 patients, between 5 and 9 ml/100 g/min in 268, and between 10 and 14 ml/100 g/min in 444. With the xenon washout technique, flow less than 5 ml/100 g/min is difficult to quantitate and can be equated with zero flow. Thus 4 or 5 patients would definitely have sustained a cerebral

infarction without shunting because of inadequate collateral flow. Another 9% to 10% of these patients, those with flow rates between 5 and 9 ml/100 g/min, probably would have sustained an infarction with any prolonged period of occlusion. Patients with flow between 10 and 14 ml/100 g/min, who represent 16% of the group, may not have withstood the period of ischemia. Shunts were also used in a large number of patients with flows between 15 and 20 ml/100 g/min for fear that the EEG would fail to reveal regions of focal ischemia in the deep white matter or basal ganglia with these borderline flow rates or because of a preoperative region of infarction or ischemia. Occasionally, patients with flow rates greater than 20 ml/100 g/min also received shunts if they had a preexisting EEG abnormality related to preoperative infarct, since it has been demonstrated that these patients are particularly vulnerable to marginal flow.* Shunts are usually not inserted until the plaque has been removed from the distal internal carotid artery except in cases in which flow is less than 5 ml/100 g/min or in which there has been a dramatic and catastrophic change in EEG patterns. (Usually these are simultaneous events—one does not occur without the other.)

In a total of 1099 of the 2731 endarterectomies performed under these three anesthetic agents, cerebral protection was provided by indwelling shunts during the operations. However, there was a statistically significant difference in the frequency of shunt usage according to both the grade of risk and the anesthetic agent used. Thus shunts were placed in 42% and 46% of patients who were operated on under halothane and enflurane, respectively, compared with only 36% of patients who were operated on under isoflurane (often supplemented with fentanyl).

There was also a statistically significant difference in

---

*References 9, 17, 18, 24, 35, 51.

blood flow among patients categorized according to the anesthetic agent used. The highest flow rates were seen with halothane and the lowest with isoflurane (supplemented in many cases with fentanyl). An analysis of the data in Table 41-1 shows significant differences in baseline and postocclusion CBF in patients who were operated on under the three agents studied (p less than 0.001). Halothane was associated with higher flow rates than enflurane, which in turn was associated with higher flow rates than isoflurane. Halothane occlusion and shunt flow rates were also significantly higher when compared with enflurane and isoflurane, but there were less striking differences between the latest two agents. The use of fentanyl with isoflurane skews these comparisons.

In comparing CBF according to the grade of patient risk, there were statistically significant differences in the baseline and occlusion flow rates in grade 4 compared with grade 1; values in patients with grade 4 flow rates were lower (p less than 0.001). There were no differences in the postocclusion flow values.

Shunts were required in only 28% of patients who were grade 1 candidates for surgery but were required in 56% of those who were grade 4 candidates for surgery. Furthermore, both the baseline and occlusion flow rates were lower in the patients at higher risk. This leads to the conclusion that the microembolic and hemodynamic theories for transient ischemic attacks and infarctions are not mutually exclusive. Areas of brain functioning on a marginal flow of 40% to 50% of normal are particularly vulnerable to the effects of emboli.

Conversely, Whisnant et al[53] performed a detailed multivariant analysis of a group of patients with transient ischemic attacks who were operated on between 1970 and 1974 and found that no patients with high occlusion flow rates had an intraoperative or postoperative stroke. Furthermore, this group had no stroke in 4.5 years of follow-up evaluation, which indicated that the prognosis is good in individuals with high collateral flow.

Critical flow and ischemic tolerance

The critical flow rate required to maintain a normal EEG pattern may be higher than that required to maintain basic cell metabolism, so even with a state of physiologic paralysis, cell death is prevented and recovery is possible after a certain period of latency. Some biologic variation in the critical flow required to maintain cell viability has been found. Data from studies by Sundt et al[45,47] and the studies of Boysen et al[5] show that the critical flow for the former ranges between 15 and 20 ml/100 g/min, and laboratory studies suggest that the critical flow for the latter in primates is between 10 and 15 ml/100 g/min.[2] It follows that the ischemic tolerance of neural tissue is proportional to both the duration and severity of flow reduction. The precise length of time that these reduced flows can be tolerated before cellular injury occurs is unknown.[1,2]

Intraoperative cerebral blood flow measurements with intraarterially injected xenon are a great deal more reliable than blood flow measurements with the inhalation xenon technique in which the true severity of ischemic lesions is not identified. With the intraarterial injection technique a representative amount of indicator arrives in the area predestined for ischemia before occlusion of the vessel, and thus measurements are based on the clearance of indicator from the true region of ischemia.[15] With the systemic administration of xenon, intravenously or by inhalation, artifact in these measurements develops related to "look-through," in which the blood flow probe measures from normally perfused tissue deep to the area of ischemia, since the obstructions to the arterial inflow prevent the indicator from arriving in the ischemic zone.[15]

CBF measurements in the laboratory animal are difficult because of the small size of the brain and the even smaller areas of brain subjected to ischemia. Furthermore, the common laboratory animals—the dog, cat, and rat—have excellent collateral circulations over the cortex, so areas of ischemia often lie remote from the area of measurement. The primate unfortunately remains the only animal in which CBF measurements comparable to those in human beings can be acquired. In these animals it is very difficult to perform accurate measurements of CBF throughout a period of prolonged ischemia and salvage the particular animal for a long-term preparation to determine the ultimate areas of infarction. Thus it is necessary to extrapolate from one study to another and measure blood flow,[15] energy metabolites,[42] and zones of infarction in different preparations[52] and then cross-correlate the results.

The squirrel monkey makes an excellent model for focal incomplete cerebral ischemia, and some early studies on this subject suggested that the animals could tolerate a 60% to 70% reduction in CBF for approximately 1 hour. This did not exclude microinfarctions, since nonuniform characteristics of flow in areas of incomplete ischemia were readily apparent in the microcirculation.[52] During this time of incomplete ischemia, there was a steady decrease in adenosine triphosphate levels and a rise in lactate levels.[43] However, these animals were operated on under barbiturate anesthesia, and at that time the protective effects of this agent were not understood. Thus this tolerable period of 1 hour might be a good bit shorter in the awake animal; studies by other investigators suggest that this is indeed the case.[11,22]

During the period of these investigations (1965 to 1972) the investigators believed that seldom if ever would CBF fall below a critical level of cell viability during carotid endarterectomy. Collateral flow from one source or another would be able to sustain a flow of at least 10 to 15 ml/100 g/min, particularly if the patient were protected with an elevated blood pressure. With greater experience the investigators found that this was not the case. In some patients, hemispheric blood flow falls to essentially zero with carotid occlusion, approximating quite closely the situation of cardiac arrest or animal decapitation in which both clinical experience and laboratory data[28] suggest that within 4 to 9 minutes of zero flow, irreparable brain damage begins to occur.

The laboratory confirmation of the clinical impressions had to await the studies of Symon et al[1,2,6,7,50] in the Rhesus monkey. This group established that blood flow less than 15 ml/100 g/min results in paralysis of neuronal activity and that flow less than 10 ml/100 g/min results in ionic shifts that may be irreversible if allowed to persist. The true level of tolerance for ischemia in patients with flow between 5 and 10 or 10 and 15 ml/100 g/min is unknown, but recent studies stress the variability and focality of histologic changes in these levels.[7,22] There is some recent evidence that incomplete ischemia, which is associated with a greater degree of acidosis than is complete ischemia because of continued glycolysis, has complications uniquely related to its acidosis.[37]

Skillful general anesthesia

Possibly the most sensitive monitor of neurologic function is the awake patient, and some very experienced surgeons still use this method of monitoring.[20] Other surgeons prefer general anesthesia because it is safe in the hands of competent anesthesiologists, protects the patient's airway, facilitates high exposure of distal internal carotid artery lesions, and improves the comfort of both the patient and the surgeon. However, to date, barbiturates are the only anesthetic agents that have unequivocally been proved to protect the brain and improve tissue tolerance to ischemia.[19,25,26,29,30] Experience suggests that the critical flow is lower with isoflurane. Data from Michenfelder's laboratory[27,31] support this theory.

Short occlusion time

Some surgeons believe that rapid performance of endarterectomy is fraught with hazard. The plaque must be removed meticulously from the vessel, with no lip of intima distally to serve as a source of dissection and no stump of the external carotid artery to serve as a source of emboli. According to the experience of some surgeons the best reconstruction of the vessel is achieved with a saphenous vein patch graft, which extends the period of occlusion approximately 15 minutes. The only series of patients operated on without patch angioplasty routinely undergoing postoperative angiograms (by an experienced and respected group) is reported to demonstrate a 20% occlusion rate of the external carotid artery and a 4% occlusion rate of the internal carotid artery.[12]

Hyperperfusion syndromes

The most common complication after endarterectomy is related to the group of high-risk patients, in which there has been a very marked increase in CBF during the operative procedure.[47] This usually occurs several days after surgery in patients with a low baseline CBF measurement before endarterectomy and a greater than or equal to 200% increase in flow after endarterectomy. This paralysis of autoregula-

tion leads to an ipsilateral hemispheric hyperperfusion and associated vascular headaches. Fortunately, in most patients this seems to be limited to unilateral headache. However, in some patients it has been associated with paroxysmal lateralizing epileptiform discharges, cerebral hemorrhage, and migraine variants. Most of these patients, except those with headaches alone, have undergone angiography at the time of the complication, and in none of them has major intracranial vessel occlusion been identified. Hemorrhage into an area of previous infarction is a well-known complication of endarterectomy.[8,56] However, these hyperperfusion syndromes have occurred in patients without a major area of infarction. These complications have not been frequently reported,[55] which leads to the concern that they might be uniquely related to the policy of not reversing the heparin given at surgery, a policy based on the protective effects of heparin on the thrombogenic surface of a freshly endarterectomized vessel.[13] Alternatively, without CBF monitoring, these complications might not be recognized as unique by other groups and attributed to a different mechanism.

Comments

Experience can be defined as a compilation of complications. Experience of most of the outstanding pioneers in this field led them to conclude that routine shunting[10,21,51] or some form of monitoring (awake patient or internal carotid artery back pressure)[17,32] with selective shunting was advisable. It was the experience of these individuals that a number of complications occurred that could not be attributed to embolic events. Those who are now second-generation surgeons and who shared the disappointments of their first-generation mentors vividly recall certain types of complications so frequent that they were not anecdotal. One of these, in patients operated on under local anesthesia, was the onset of an acute and profound hemiplegia with carotid occlusion that was irreversible with restoration of flow 20 to 30 minutes thereafter.

There is no room for a cavalier attitude toward carotid endarterectomy. It can be a relatively easy operation or an extremely difficult procedure. In either case, it remains a dangerous operation with intraoperative risks of embolization or infarction from inadequate flow during the period of occlusion and postoperative risks of occlusion or embolization[14,32,33,51] from vessels inadequately reconstructed or from complications of cerebral hyperperfusion after the restoration of a normal perfusion pressure to a vascular bed with paralyzed autoregulation.[47]

Effects of endarterectomy

It is important to note that measurements were of CBF, not flow through the artery, and were performed under static, controlled conditions. Even in cases in which there was not a major change in CBF,[5] when electromagnetic arterial flow probes along with simultaneous CBF measurements were used, an increase in arterial flow and the contribution to total CBF from the vessel operated on was found if a high-grade stenosis was present.

The cerebral hemispheric arterial circulation can be divided into two general types of arteries: (1) the conducting vessels, consisting of the internal carotid artery and its major trunks, which divide into a network of interlacing and anastomosing smaller branches of the brain's surface, and (2) the penetrating or nutrient arterioles, which arise on the surface of the brain from the conducting vessels and enter the brain parenchyma.[38] In normal human beings there is only a 10% to 15% drop in perfusion pressure between the origin of the internal carotid artery and the penetrating vessels.[3] The conducting vessels can be regarded as a pressure equalization reservoir that is modulated by the sympathetic nervous system.[16,49] True cerebral autoregulation probably resides in the penetrating arterioles, which apparently are modulated by an intrinsic nervous system that originates in the brainstem.[4,23,36,39] Those arterioles must be supplied with an adequate perfusion pressure to function normally. The normalization of RAPs after endarterectomy indicates that the restoration of a normal perfusion pressure permits the parenchymal arterioles to return to a more normal tone from one of maximal dilatation, and thus the brain's autoregulatory ability is restored.

The microembolic[40,54] and hemodynamic theories[34] for transient ischemic attacks and infarcts are not mutually exclusive. Areas of brain that function on a marginal flow of 40% to 50% of normal are particularly vulnerable to the effects of emboli. Furthermore, plaque deposits that cause a severe degree of stenosis, which therefore represent a significant hemodynamic lesion, are more likely to develop deep ulcer craters than those of lesser severity.

Thus endarterectomy in a patient with a high-grade stenosis and ulceration (1) removes a source of emboli, (2) restores a normal distal perfusion pressure and the capability for normal autoregulation, (3) increases flow through the artery and, depending on collateral flow, increases CBF, and (4) prevents progression of the stenosis to occlusion.

REFERENCES

1. Astrup J, Siesjo BK, Symon L: Thresholds in cerebral ischemia: the ischemic penumbra, *Stroke* 12:723, 1981.
2. Astrup J et al: Cortical evoked potential and extracellular K$^+$ and H$^+$ at critical levels of brain ischemia, *Stroke* 8:51, 1977.
3. Bakay L, Sweet WH: Cervical and intracranial intra-arterial pressures with and without vascular occlusion, *Surg Gynecol Obstet* 95:67, 1952.
4. Bates D et al: The effect of lesions in the locus coeruleus on the physiological responses of the cerebral blood vessels in cats, *Brain Res* 136:431, 1977.
5. Boysen G: Cerebral hemodynamics in carotid surgery, *Acta Neurol Scand* (suppl) 52:1, 1973.
6. Branston NM, Hope DT, Symon L: Barbiturates in focal ischemia of primate cortex: effects of blood flow distribution, evoked potential and extracellular potassium, *Stroke* 10:647, 1979.
7. Branston NM, Strong AJ, Symon L: Extracellular potassium activity, evoked potential and tissue blood flow: relationship during progressive ischaemia in baboon cerebral cortex, *J Neurol Sci* 32:305, 1977.
8. Bruetman ME et al: Cerebral hemorrhage in carotid artery surgery, *Arch Neurol* 9:458, 1963.
9. Callow AD, O'Donnell TF: *Electroencephalogram monitoring in cerebrovascular surgery.* In Bergan JJ, Yao JS, eds: *Cerebral vascular insufficiency,* New York, 1983, Grune & Stratton, 327-341.
10. Crawford ES et al: Surgical treatment of occlusive cerebrovascular disease, *Surg Clin North Am* 46:873, 1966.
11. Crowell RM et al: Temporary occlusion of the middle cerebral artery in the monkey: clinical and pathological observations, *Stroke* 1:439, 1970.
12. Diaz FG et al: Early angiographic changes after carotid endarterectomy, *Neurosurgery* 10:151, 1982.
13. Dirrenberger RA, Sundt TM Jr: Carotid endarterectomy: temporal profile of the healing process and effects of anticoagulation therapy, *J Neurosurg* 48:201, 1978.
14. Giannotta SL, Dicks RE, Kindt GW: Carotid endarterectomy: technical improvements, *Neurosurgery* 7:309, 1980.
15. Hanson EJ Jr, Anderson RE, Sundt TM Jr: Comparison of ^{85}krypton and ^{133}xenon cerebral blood flow meaurements before, during, and following focal incomplete ischemia in the squirrel monkey, *Circ Res* 36:18, 1975.
16. Harper AM et al: The influence of sympathetic nervous activity on cerebral blood flow, *Arch Neurol* 27:1, 1972.
17. Hays RJ, Levinson SA, Wylie EJ: Intraoperative measurement of carotid back pressure as a guide to operative management of carotid endarterectomy, *Surgery* 72:593, 1972.
18. Hertzer NR et al: Internal carotid back pressure, intraoperative shunting, ulcerated atheromata, and the incidence of stroke during carotid endarterectomy, *Surgery* 83:306, 1978.

19. Hoff JT et al: Barbiturate protection from cerebral infarction in primates, *Stroke* 6:28, 1975.
20. Imparato AM et al: Cerebral protection in carotid surgery, *Arch Surg* 117:1073, 1982.
21. Javid H et al: Seventeen-year experience with routine shunting in carotid artery surgery, *World J Surg* 3:167, 1979.
22. Jones TH et al: Thresholds of focal cerebral ischemia in awake monkeys, *J Neurosurg* 54:773, 1981.
23. Langfitt TW, Kassell NF: Cerebral vasodilatation produced by brainstem stimulation: neurogenic control vs. autoregulation, *Am J Physiol* 215:90, 1968.
24. Matsumoto GH et al: EEG surveillance as a means of extending operability in high risk carotid endarterectomy, *Stroke* 7:554, 1976.
25. Michenfelder JD: The interdependency of cerebral functional and metabolic effects following massive doses of thiopental in the dog, *Anesthesiology* 41:231, 1974.
26. Michenfelder JD: Cerebral protection by barbiturate anesthesia: use after middle cerebral artery occlusion in Java monkeys, *Arch Neurol* 33:345, 1976.
27. Michenfelder JD: Personal communication, 1982.
28. Michenfelder JD, Theye RA: The effects of anesthesia and hypothermia on canine cerebral ATP and lactate during anoxia produced by decapitation, *Anesthesiology* 33:430, 1970.
29. Michenfelder JD, Theye RA: Effects of fentanyl, droperidol, and innovar on canine cerebral metabolism and blood flow, *Br J Anaesth* 43:603, 1971.
30. Michenfelder JD, Theye RA: Cerebral protection by thiopental during hypoxia, *Anesthesiology* 39:510, 1973.
31. Michenfelder JD et al: Isoflurane when compared to enflurane and halothane decreased the frequency of cerebral ischemia during carotid endarterectomy, *Anesthesiology* 67:336-340, 1987.
32. Murphey F, Maccubbin DA: Carotid endarterectomy: a long-term follow-up study, *J Neurosurg* 23:156, 1965.
33. Perdue GD: Management of post-endarterectomy neurologic defects, *Arch Surg* 117:1079, 1982.
34. Pessin MS et al: Mechanisms of acute carotid stroke, *Ann Neurol* 6:145, 1979.
35. Phillips MR et al: Carotid endarterectomy in the presence of contralateral carotid occlusion: the role of EEG and intraluminal shunting, *Arch Surg* 114:1232, 1979.
36. Raichle ME et al: Central noradrenergic regulation of cerebral blood flow and vascular permeability, *Proc Natl Acad Sci USA* 72:3726, 1975.
37. Rehncrona S, Rosen I, Siesjö BK: Brain lactic acidosis and ischemic cell damage: biochemistry and neurophysiology, *J Cereb Blood Flow Metab* 1:297, 1981.
38. Saunders RL, Bell MA: X-ray microscopy and histochemistry of the human cerebral blood vessels, *J Neurosurg* 35:128, 1971.
39. Sahlit NM et al: Carbon dioxide and cerebral circulatory control. III. The effects of brainstem lesions, *Arch Neurol* 17:342, 1967.
40. Siekert RG, Whisnant JP, Millikan CH: Surgical and anticoagulant therapy of occlusive cerebral vascular disease, *Ann Intern Med* 48:637, 1963.
41. Sundt TM Jr: *Occlusive cerebrovascular disease: diagnosis and surgical management*, Philadelphia, 1987, WB Saunders.
42. Sundt TM Jr, Grant WC, Garcia JH: Restoration of middle cerebral artery flow in experimental infarction, *J Neurosurg* 31:311, 1969.
43. Sundt TM Jr, Michenfelder JD: Focal transient cerebral ischemia in the squirrel monkey: effect on brain adenosine triphosphate and lactate levels with electrocorticographic and pathologic correlation, *Circ Res* 30:703, 1972.
44. Sundt TM Jr, Sandok BA, Whisnant JP: Carotid endarterectomy: complications and preoperative assessment of risk, *Mayo Clin Proc* 50:301, 1975.
45. Sundt TM Jr et al: Cerebral blood flow measurements and electroencephalograms during carotid endarterectomy, *J Neurosurg* 41:310, 1974.
46. Sundt TM Jr et al: Monitoring techniques for carotid endarterectomy, *Clin Neurosurg* 22:199, 1975.
47. Sundt TM Jr et al: Correlation of cerebral blood flow and electroencephalographic changes during carotid endarterectomy, *Mayo Clin Proc* 56:533, 1981.
48. Sundt TM Jr et al: Prospective study of the effectiveness and durability of carotid endarterectomy, *Mayo Clin Proc* 65:625-635, 1990.
49. Symon L: A comparative study of middle cerebral pressure in dogs and macaques, *J Physiol (Lond)* 19:449, 1967.
50. Symon L: The relationship between CBF, evoked potentials and the clinical features in cerebral ischaemia. Proceedings of the Twenty-third Scandinavian Neurological Congress, *Acta Neurol Scand* (suppl 78) 62:175, 1980.
51. Thompson JE: Complications of carotid endarterectomy and their prevention, *World J Surg* 3:155, 1979.
52. Waltz AG, Sundt TM Jr: The microvasculature and microcirculation of the cerebral cortex after arterial occlusion, *Brain* 90:681, 1967.
53. Whisnant JP, Sandok BA, Sundt TM Jr: Carotid endarterectomy for unilateral carotid system transient cerebral ischemia, *Mayo Clin Proc* 58:171, 1983.
54. Whisnant JP et al: Effect of anticoagulants on experimental cerebral infarction, *Circulation* 20:56, 1959.
55. Wilkinson JT, Adams HP Jr, Wright CB: Convulsions after carotid endarterectomy, *JAMA* 244:1827, 1980.
56. Wylie EJ, Heim MF, Adams JR: Intracranial hemorrhage following surgical revascularization for treatment of acute stroke, *J Neurosurg* 21:212, 1964.

CHAPTER 42

Other noninvasive techniques in cerebrovascular disease

ROBERT W. BARNES

Currently, the three noninvasive techniques most frequently used for screening cerebrovascular disease are duplex scanning, with or without Doppler color flow; ocular pneumoplethysmography (OPG-Gee); and transcranial Doppler. In addition, several other noninvasive techniques have been used to detect extracranial carotid artery disease. Indirect techniques include supraorbital photoplethysmography (PPG), carotid compression tonography, ophthalmodynamometry (ODM), pneumatic tonometry or oculocerebrovasculometry (OCVM), ophthalmomanometry Doppler (OMD), and facial thermography. Direct techniques include radionuclide arteriography or carotid scanning and computerized tomography (CT). Although many if not most of these techniques are now only of historical interest, they are included here for purposes of reference and completeness.

INDIRECT TECHNIQUES
Supraorbital photoplethysmography

Technique. The photoelectric plethysmography was originally described by Hertzman,[17] and the use of the photoplethysmograph (PPG) to detect extracranial carotid occlusive disease was independently reported by Howell,[19] Fuster et al,[12] and Heck and Price.[15] The original photoelectric transducers contained an incandescent light source, which was beamed into the superficial layers of the skin. The light reflected from the skin was then received by a photoelectric cell. The principle underlying this method was that the amount of backscattered light varied with the amount of blood in the superficial circulation of the skin. A voltage output of the photoelectric cell permitted recording of pulsatile fluctuations in the microcirculation of the skin. However, the incandescent light absorption by blood was somewhat influenced by the saturation of hemoglobin, and the light source also potentially heated the superficial layers of the skin. Refinements in transducer design led to the development of an infrared light-emitting diode and adjacent phototransistor,* which was not affected by hemoglobin saturation and did not cause heating of the skin. It was first used in a prospective study of patients undergoing contrast arteriography for suspected cerebrovascular disease.[2,3]

In this method, two PPG transducers are placed above

the medial aspect of each eyebrow and affixed using clear, two-sided plastic tape. The transducers are connected to a two-channel recorder to permit continuous recording of the supraorbital pulse amplitude. The supraorbital region of the forehead is normally supplied by the frontal and supraorbital arteries, which are terminal branches of the ophthalmic artery. While recording bilateral supraorbital pulsations, the technologist first sequentially compresses the branches of each external carotid artery (superficial temporal, infraorbital, and facial arteries) and then each common carotid artery. Carotid compression is applied low in the neck to avoid stimulating baroreceptors and prevent dislodging emboli from a diseased carotid bifurcation. Using this technique, several thousand common carotid compressions have been carried out without a single instance of stroke or cardiac arrest.

Normally, the supraorbital pulse amplitude is not significantly diminished by compression of the external carotid artery branches. Occasionally, the pulse amplitude is slightly reduced, but this should be no more than 33% below the resting pulse amplitude. Greater attenuation of the supraorbital pulsation suggests a significant stenosis (greater than 50% diameter reduction) or occlusion of the extracranial internal carotid artery. Normally, the supraorbital pulse amplitude is diminished only with compression of the ipsilateral common carotid artery. In the presence of extensive carotid occlusive disease, failure of ipsilateral common carotid compression to attenuate the supraorbital pulse implies the existence of intracranial collateral circulation. Collateral circulation from the contralateral carotid artery via the circle of Willis may be documented if contralateral carotid compression results in diminution of supraorbital pulsation. If sequential compression of each common carotid artery fails to alter supraorbital pulsation, this indicates intracranial collateral circulation achieved via the vertebrobasilar system.

Results. The accuracy of supraorbital PPG was established in a prospective screening of 78 consecutive patients undergoing contrast arteriography for suspected cerebrovascular disease.[3] PPG results were abnormal for all 20 occluded internal carotid arteries and all 16 vessels with substantial (greater than 50%) stenosis. Only 10 of 44 vessels with less than 50% stenosis showed abnormal PPG

---

*Medasonics, Mountain View, Calif.

findings. False-positive results were obtained for 8 (11%) of 76 arteries that were normal according to contrast arteriography. When compared with the results of periorbital Doppler ultrasound in this same group of patients,[2] supraorbital PPG proved to be more sensitive (100% versus 94%) but less specific (89% versus 96%). When the two techniques were used in combination and the results agreed, they were 100% sensitive in detecting significant carotid stenosis or occlusion and 97% specific in identifying arteries that were normal on angiograms; however, the techniques rarely detected nonobstructive carotid stenosis (less than 50%).

Supraorbital PPG provides simple, rapid, and objective hard-copy data about the simultaneous status of both internal carotid systems. It is not influenced by the presence of bilateral carotid disease of balanced severity and does not require ocular anesthesia. The greatest limitation to the method is the frequent false-positive result. Supraorbital PPG has been used for continual monitoring of ophthalmic artery flow dynamics during carotid endarterectomy.[13] The ratio of supraorbital pulse amplitude before and during carotid clamping correlates well with the carotid back (stump) pressure ($r = 0.87$; $p < 0.001$). The supraorbital PPG assesses the adequacy of blood flow through the carotid shunt as well as the integrity of the carotid endarterectomy site after closure of the arteriotomy.

Carotid compression tonography

Technique. Carotid compression tonography records volume adjustments within the eye in association with carotid compression. The technique was originally described by Barrios and Solis.[4] In this method, an electronic recording tonometer (Mueller*) registers ocular pulse and pressure on a standard recorder. Once the tracing is stabilized, sequential compression of the ipsilateral and contralateral carotid artery is performed. The same test is repeated for the opposite eye. Three variables are used to interpret the tests: (1) comparison of the pulse amplitudes between each eye, (2) determination of the slope of recovery of ocular pressure on release of carotid compression, and (3) assessment of the intraocular pressure responses to compression of the contralateral carotid artery. Normally, ipsilateral carotid compression elicits a rapid fall in intraocular pressure, which recovers rapidly on release of the compression. In addition, intraocular pressure is normally not affected by compression of the contralateral carotid artery. In the presence of a hemodynamically significant obstruction of the extracranial internal carotid artery, the ocular phase amplitude may be diminished, the recovery time for the return of intraocular pressure to the baseline is delayed, and the intraocular pressure may be diminished on compression of the contralateral carotid artery.

Results. Cohen et al[8] reported the results of carotid compression tonography in 122 patients who also underwent

carotid arteriography because of suspected cerebrovascular disease. The sensitivity of the test in detecting hemodynamically significant stenosis or occlusion of the internal carotid artery was 92% in a group of 82 patients with greater than 50% stenosis or occlusion of the artery shown on arteriograms. Carotid compression tonography was normal in 75% of 40 patients with insignificant or no demonstrable abnormality on the carotid arteriogram.

Hertzer et al,[16] from the same center as Cohen's group, reported on a follow-up study that examined the correlation of carotid compression tonography with cerebral arteriography in 300 patients. The sensitivity of the test was 88% (160/182) and the specificity was 69% (81/118) for detecting or excluding carotid stenosis that exceeded 50%. It showed a positive predictive value of 81% (160/197) and a negative predictive value of 78% (81/103). This test seems to have many of the same attributes as supraorbital PPG in that it is fairly sensitive but somewhat nonspecific. The technique is objective and relatively inexpensive, but like other indirect noninvasive techniques, it is insensitive to nonobstructive carotid occlusive disease of less than 50% diameter reduction.

Ophthalmodynamometry

Technique. As originally described by Baillart,[1] ODM involves measuring the gram force applied to the eye necessary to obliterate arterial pulsations in the branches of the retinal artery (systolic pressure) or to create maximal pulsation in these vessels (diastolic pressure). The vessels are observed through an ophthalmoscope, and the gram force applied by the foot plate of the ophthalmodynamometer is read from the scale on the instrument.

Results. ODM has been widely used by ophthalmologists, but the results have been less accurate than those yielded by newer noninvasive screening techniques. In a study of 45 patients conducted by Kobayashi et al,[23] a significant difference in retinal artery pressure between the two eyes was seen in only 74% of patients with at least one severely stenotic carotid artery. Even in patients with minimal disease of the opposite vessel, only 80% manifested a significant difference in retinal artery pressure. On the other hand, significant differences in retinal artery pressure were found in only 55% of the patients studied who had severe bilateral carotid occlusive disease. Sanborn et al[31] carried out a prospective study comparing the results of ODM with carotid arteriography in 94 arteries of 47 patients. The sensitivity for detecting greater than 50% carotid stenosis was 48%, and the specificity for excluding such disease was 93%. In a modified technique of suction ODM in which a scleral vacuum cup was used, the sensitivity was 88% and the specificity was 61%. Samples et al[30] correlated the results of ODM with the cerebral angiography findings in 100 patients. They found the sensitivity for detecting greater than 90% carotid stenosis was 71% and the specificity was 90%. The positive and negative predictive values were 83% and 81%, respectively. From these data, ODM would appear to

---

*V. Mueller & Co, Chicago, Ill.

be a less accurate screening technique than other periorbital or direct carotid methods.

Pneumatic tonometry

Technique. Pneumatic tonometry,[25] or OCVM, combines a pneumatic applanation tonometer with a vacuum system for increasing intraocular pressure, which allows more direct measurement of ophthalmic artery pressure than can be achieved by OPG-Gee. The pressure at which ocular pulsations cease during progressive increases in intraocular pressure induced by incremental increases in the vacuum applied to the sclera is graphically and digitally recorded as the intraocular pressure. The device also permits comparison of the amplitude of each ocular phase.

Results. Langham et al[25] determined that ophthalmic artery systolic pressures in normal control subjects averaged 89.0 ± 2.1 mm Hg, which was $66\% \pm 1\%$ of the brachial artery systolic pressure (a value similar to that measured by OPG-Gee). In 20 patients with stenosis of the internal carotid artery that was 95% or greater as documented by arteriography, the mean ophthalmic artery pressure was 49.9 ± 4.1 mm Hg, and this represented $33\% \pm 3\%$ of the brachial systolic pressure. In a subsequent prospective study that consisted of 60 patients undergoing arteriography, Langham and Preziosi[24] reported that the sensitivity, specificity, and accuracy of ophthalmic/brachial arterial pressure ratios in identifying or excluding carotid stenosis that was 50% or greater were 89%, 80%, and 86%, respectively. Russell et al[29] found that OCVM was 100% sensitive but only 36% specific in detecting or excluding stenosis of the internal carotid artery of 50% or greater in a small series of 19 arteries visualized arteriographically.

Ophthalmometry Doppler

Technique. OMD estimates the blood pressure in the supraorbital or frontal arteries.[32] A chamber with an aperture is hermetically applied to the orbital borders. A contained Doppler probe is then positioned over one of the periorbital arteries, and the pressure within the chamber is increased until the Doppler signal disappears at the systolic pressure of the periorbital artery.

Results. Strauss et al[32] compared the results of OMD with cerebral angiography findings in 102 patients with occlusion (n = 50) or greater than 60% stenosis (n = 52) of the internal carotid artery. The mean (± 1 SD) Doppler ophthalmic pressure was 69 ± 15 mm Hg ipsilateral to an occlusion and 86 ± 18 mm Hg ipsilateral to greater than 60% stenosis. Using an ophthalmic/brachial pressure index of 0.60 as the lower limit of normal, the sensitivity of OMD was 98% for carotid occlusion and 71% for carotid stenosis that exceeded 60%.

Thermography

Technique. Because the supraorbital region of the forehead is normally supplied by blood from the internal carotid arteries via ophthalmic artery branches, this area of the face normally has a slightly higher temperature than other areas. Asymmetric coolness of one supraorbital area may therefore indicate significant obstruction of the ipsilateral internal carotid artery. Although direct temperature measurement with thermistor thermometry is possible,[28] most investigations of supraorbital temperature have involved the use of infrared thermography.[33] In this test, the patient is permitted to accommodate to a constant-temperature room. The thermograph analyzes the infrared energy emission from the skin of the face. Polaroid photographic recordings of the oscilloscope image represent heat energy as proportional shades of gray. Thermograms may be obtained with the subject at rest or while undergoing provocative maneuvers such as forehead cooling or compression of the superficial temporal arteries. Normally the thermal patterns on the forehead are symmetric. Abnormal thermograms are defined as those with temperature asymmetry in the supraorbital region of $0.7°$ C or greater.

Results. Capistrant and Gumnit[7] reported on the accuracy of conventional facial thermography and also described the results obtained with provocative tests of facial cooling and temporal artery compression in patients undergoing contrast arteriography. Using routine thermography, the sensitivity of the test was only 57% in the 30 patients with significant carotid occlusive disease. Test results were abnormal in only 5 of 14 patients with carotid stenosis and 12 of 16 with internal carotid occlusion. The specificity was 92%, with 5 false-positive results in 65 patients without significant carotid disease. When thermography was performed with the superficial temporary artery compressed, the sensitivity increased to 83% in the 30 patients with significant carotid occlusive disease. The specificity was 92% for the 59 patients without significant carotid disease. When forehead cooling was used as a provocative test, sensitivity was 81% and specificity, 84%. These results suggest that the findings of facial thermography do correlate with the presence of carotid occlusive disease, especially when provocative tests are performed, but the technique does not have the accuracy of some of the other indirect screening techniques and is not economically feasible for the mass screening of healthy individuals.

DIRECT TECHNIQUES
Radionuclide arteriography

Technique. Radionuclide angiography furnishes rapid-sequence, dynamic-flow images of injected isotope before static brain imaging is done. The radionuclide sodium pertechnetate ^{99m}Tc is injected rapidly by the intravenous route, and serial Polaroid photographs are then obtained with a gamma camera positioned over the head and neck of the patient. Sequential dynamic flow images can reveal the course of the isotope as it travels up the carotid and vertebral arteries and subsequently through the cerebral circulation. Although it is not possible to achieve good resolution of the vascular defects with this technique, it can reveal delay in cerebrovascular flow and maldistribution of flow.

Results. Radionuclide angiography is a useful adjunct to static brain imaging; however, the limited resolution and relatively low sensitivity make this technique less accurate than other noninvasive screening techniques. Its reported sensitivity to hemodynamically significant extracranial carotid disease averages 60%, and its specificity is approximately 90%.[10,20] In the presence of internal carotid occlusion, its sensitivity is only about 75%, and in the presence of carotid stenosis, the sensitivity drops to about 50%. The technique is expensive and should only be considered as an adjunct to brain scanning in a patient with symptoms of carotid disease.

Radionuclide carotid scanning

Technique. In contrast to dynamic flow scanning, a static carotid artery scan can detect the localized accumulation of isotope-labeled particles, such as fibrinogen or platelets, at areas of thrombosis or ulceration of the cervical carotid artery. A variety of preparations have been used, including ^{99m}Tc sulfur colloid–albumin aggregates,[27] ^{123}I or ^{131}I fibrinogen,[21,26] and ^{99m}Tc or ^{111}In autologous platelets.[9,14] After injection of the radionuclide-labeled particles, the cervical area over the carotid arteries is scanned with a scintillation detector. Areas of increased radioactivity suggest localization of the labeled particles at sites of vascular injury, atherosclerotic ulceration, or carotid thrombosis.

Results. To date, most studies of static radionuclide carotid scanning have involved experimental animals in whom carotid trauma or ulceration was induced. The findings of a few clinical studies have suggested potential application of these techniques.[14,26] However, future prospective clinical trials that include validation with contrast arteriography or carotid endarterectomy are necessary before the true value of these techniques in humans is established.

Computed tomography

Technique. CT evaluation involves scanning a portion of the body with a narrow beam of x rays from different multiple angles at equally spaced intervals. The attenuation of the x-ray beam is measured by photon detectors, and the absorption values of tissues are calculated by computer. X-ray absorption coefficients, or densities, are then calculated for blocks of tissue and displayed as a matrix of numerous white, gray, or black pixels on a cathode ray tube.[18] The major impact of CT scanning in the assessment of cerebrovascular disease is its ability to detect intraparenchymal hemorrhage and intracranial lesions that may cause symptoms that mimic stroke.[6] The technique has been used for the direct assessment of cervical carotid arteries to identify carotid calcifications in patients suffering transient ischemic attacks.[11]

Results. The indirect application of CT scanning suggests that results are normal in most patients with transient ischemic attacks and that scans will show abnormal findings within at least 48 hours in patients who have suffered stroke.[22] In a small series, all 17 patients with transient ischemic attacks and angiographically abnormal arteries showed carotid calcification on CT scans of the neck.[11] Of 3 patients with normal arteries, the cervical tomograms were normal; however, further clinical investigations, including the use of contrast-enhanced CT scans, must be carried out before the clinical value of this technique is established.

CONCLUSION

The noninvasive techniques reviewed in this chapter can no longer be considered state-of-the-art methods in the evaluation of patients for extracranial cerebrovascular disease. Although these modalities are much less expensive and simpler to use than those used currently, they are limited by their insensitivity to carotid disease of less than 50% to 75% diameter reduction and they do not distinguish operable carotid stenoses from inoperable occlusions. Despite these limitations, these methods have made creative and physiologic contributions in the history of noninvasive diagnostic methodology for screening cerebrovascular disease. Some of the current sophisticated techniques may similarly assume a place of obscurity as continued advances in this field are made.[5]

REFERENCES

1. Baillart P: La pression arterielle dans les branches de l'artere centrale de al retine: nouvelle technique pour la determiner, *Ann Ocul (Paris)* 154:648, 1917.
2. Barnes RW et al: Doppler ultrasound and supraorbital photoplethysmography for noninvasive screening of carotid occlusive disease, *Am J Surg* 134:183, 1977.
3. Barnes RW et al: Supraorbital photoplethysmography: simple accurate screening for carotid occlusive disease, *J Surg Res* 22:319, 1977.
4. Barrios RR, Solis C: Carotid-compression tonographic test: its application in the study of carotid-artery occlusions, *Am J Ophthalmol* 62:116, 1966.
5. Bone GE, Barnes RW: Limitations of the Doppler cerebrovascular examination in hemispheric cerebral ischemia, *Surgery* 3:11, 1977.
6. Campbell JK: Use of computerized tomography and radionuclide scan in stroke, *Stroke* 4:57, 1973.
7. Capistrant JD, Gumnit RJ: Detecting carotid occlusive disease by thermography, *Stroke* 4:57, 1973.
8. Cohen DN et al: Carotid compression tonography, *Stroke* 6:257, 1975.
9. Davis HH et al: Scintigraphic detection of atherosclerotic lesions and venous thrombi in men by indium-111-labeled autologous platelets, *Lancet* 1:1185, 1978.
10. Foo D, Henrickson L: Radionuclide cerebral blood flow and carotid angiogram: correlation in internal carotid artery disease, *Stroke* 8:39, 1977.
11. Frisen L et al: Detection of extracranial carotid stenosis by computed tomography, *Lancet* 1:1319, 1979.
12. Fuster B et al: Extracranial internal and external carotid territories as mapped by photoelectric photoplethysmography, *Acta Neurol Lat Am* 15:1, 1969.
13. Garrett WV, Slaymaker EE, Barnes RW: Noninvasive perioperative monitoring of carotid endarterectomy, *J Surg Res* 26:255, 1979.
14. Grossman ZD et al: Platelets labeled with oxine complexes of Tc99m and In-111. II. localization of experimentally induced vascular lesions, *J Nucl Med* 19:488, 1978.
15. Heck AF, Price TR: Opacity pulse propagation measurements in humans: atraumatic screening for carotid artery occlusion, *Stroke* 1:411, 1970.
16. Hertzer NR, Santoscoy TG, Langston RH: Accuracy of carotid compression tonography in the diagnosis of carotid artery stenosis: correlation with arteriography in 300 patients, *Clev Clin Q* 47:79, 1980.
17. Hertzman AB: Blood supply of various skin areas as estimated by the photoelectric plethysmography, *Am J Physiol* 124:328, 1938.

18. Hounsfield GN: Computerized transverse axial scanning (tomography). I. Description of system, *Br J Radiol* 46:1016, 1973.

19. Howell WL: Photosensor monitoring of supraorbital blood flow, *Med Ann DC* 36:730, 1967.

20. Jhingran SG, Johnson PC: Radionuclide angiography in the diagnosis of cerebrovascular disease, *Neurology* 14:265, 1973.

21. Kaufman HH et al: Radioiodinated fibrinogen for clot detection in a canine model of cervical carotid thrombosis, *J Nucl Med* 19:370, 1978.

22. Kinkel WR, Jacobs L: Computerized axial transverse tomography in cerebrovascular disease, *Neurology* 26:924, 1976.

23. Kobayashi S, Hollenhorst RW, Sundt TM: Retinal arterial pressure before and after surgery for carotid artery stenosis, *Stroke* 2:569, 1971.

24. Langham ME, Preziosi TJ: Non-invasive diagnosis of mild to severe stenosis of the internal carotid artery, *Stroke* 15:614, 1984.

25. Langham ME, To'mey KF, Preziosi TJ: Carotid occlusive disease: effect of complete occlusion of internal carotid artery on intraocular pulse/pressure relation and an ophthalmic arterial pressure, *Stroke* 12:759, 1981.

26. Mettinger KL et al: Detection of atherosclerotic plaques in carotid arteries by the use of ^{123}I-fibrinogen, *Lancet* 1:242, 1978.

27. Pollack EW et al: Arterial scan versus radiographic angiography in detection of shallow arterial ulcers, *Am Surg* 43:242, 1977.

28. Price TR, Heck AF: Correlation of thermometry and angiography in carotid arterial disease, *Arch Neurol* 26:450, 1972.

29. Russell JB et al: Oculocerebrovasculometry: a new procedure for the measurement of the ophthalmic artery pressure, *Bruit* 4:34, 1980.

30. Samples JR, Trautmann JC, Sundt TM Jr: Interpretation of results of compression ophthalmodynamometry, *Stroke* 13:655, 1982.

31. Sanborn GE et al: Clinical-angiographic correlation of ophthalmodynamometry in patients with suspected carotid artery disease: a prospective study, *Stroke* 12:770, 1981.

32. Strauss AL et al: Doppler ophthalmic blood pressure measurement in the hemodynamic evaluation of occlusive carotid artery disease, *Stroke* 20:1012, 1989.

33. Wood EH: Thermography in the diagnosis of cerebrovascular disease, *Radiology* 83:540, 1964.

CHAPTER 43

Oculoplethysmography and ocular pneumoplethysmography

BERT C. EIKELBOOM

Indirect tests were once the most widely used techniques in noninvasive cerebrovascular testing. They were easy to apply and quite accurate for detecting hemodynamically significant carotid artery disease. Indirect tests focus on the vessels in or around the eye. There are two plethysmographic techniques: oculoplethysmography as developed by Kartchner (OPG-K) and ocular pneumoplethysmography as developed by Gee (OPG-G). The first publications date from the early 1970s.[4] Both techniques have flourished from the late 1970s through the 1980s but have been replaced almost completely by duplex scanning. OPG-G survived the longest because it measures arterial pressure in a noninvasive way and it still has certain capabilities that make it a valuable technique. OPG-K has virtually disappeared from use, but a short description is supplied for historical interest.

OCULOPLETHYSMOGRAPHY

OPG-K is based on the principle that arterial obstruction leads to a delay in the pulse-arrival time. Plethysmographic tracings are obtained from both eyes and both earlobes. In this method, fluid-filled suction cups are applied to both eyes and photoelectric cells are mounted on the earlobes with earclips. Internal carotid artery stenosis imparts a phase shift between the pulses arriving at both eyes, and the earlobe pulses can detect external and bilateral carotid disease.

OPG-K was quite good at detecting unilateral stenosis or occlusion but not so effective with bilateral disease. Moreover, it could not distinguish between stenosis and total occlusion of the internal carotid artery. The same was true for OPG-G. Therefore the technique was used in combination with carotid phonoangiography (CPA), which could provide a graphic representation of carotid bruits. Bruits appear in the presence of 40% to 50% carotid stenosis, and their amplitude increases until an 80% stenosis is reached, at which time they start to diminish. Progressive stenosis causes the bruit to extend from systole into diastole. When the results of OPG-K and CPA were compared, OPG was found to be more sensitive and CPA, more specific. Most authors combined the two techniques but results differed widely. These differences were due in part to the degree of stenosis used as the threshold for deciding a positive or negative test. This ranged from 40% to 60%, which is slightly lower than the threshold that was usually adopted for OPG-G.

A review of the literature of both OPG techniques reveals a sensitivity of 70% and a specificity of 88% for OPG-K.[4] This clearly was not good enough to justify its continued use, especially when compared with duplex scanning.

OCULAR PNEUMOPLETHYSMOGRAPHY

The development and physiologic principles of OPG-G are described in Chapter 19, but the following are practical details on its technique, interpretation, and applications.

Technique

Before OPG is performed, the patient's medical history is taken, with particular regard to the reason for referral and the presence of hypertension, allergies, or any ophthalmologic contraindications to the test, including a history of retinal detachment, unstable glaucoma, recent eye surgery, lens implants, and conjunctivitis. If there is any doubt, the patient's ophthalmologist should be consulted.

The patient is informed that the procedure causes little discomfort, although a dimming or loss of vision may be experienced for several seconds. The patient should be instructed to focus on a fixed point and to avoid blinking while the test is under way. The patient is next placed in a supine position, and two drops of a topical anesthetic are applied to each eye, with any excess wiped off with a tissue to avoid aspiration of fluid into the tubing of the eyecups. Blood pressure is measured in each arm by an ordinary sphygmomanometer, and the side with the highest pressure is taken as the reference reading. An automatic blood pressure monitor may be used for simultaneously measuring the systemic blood pressure and ophthalmic artery pressure. A simultaneous electrocardiogram (ECG) recording can also be obtained by the OPG instrument, but this is rarely helpful in routine OPG testing.

The eyecups are then placed on the sclera, lateral to the cornea. Slight pressure is maintained manually to keep the eyecups in the proper position until the vacuum is applied by activating the foot switch. A choice must be made between vacuums of 300 and 500 mm Hg. The former is used in normotensive patients and the latter in hypertensive patients. After the chosen vacuum is reached, the record switch is pushed and the vacuum is automatically released in about 30 seconds. Then the technician or physician must determine whether the tracings for both the left and right eyes show the appropriate onset of pulsations. The first ocular pulsations are used for measuring the ophthalmic artery pressure (OAP) from the calibrated ruler overlay. In extremely hypertensive patients, even a 500 mm Hg vacuum may not be sufficient to obliterate ocular pulsations, and thus no real OAPs can be determined. Blinking may produce artifacts that can make it difficult to determine the appearance of the first two arterial pulsations. To solve this problem in most patients, the examiners should repeat the test with the patient's eyes closed.

Occasionally several small pulsations may appear before the amplitude of pulsations increases. In this event, the first pulse that is followed by a pulse of greater amplitude should be used for calculating the OAP. Another artifact can arise

as the result of incorrect placement of the eyecup. This may produce an initial pulse with a large amplitude that is not preceded by the usual gradual progression in amplitude (Fig. 43-1). The test should be repeated after the eyecup is properly positioned.

OPG may also be performed with the common carotid artery compressed to obtain information about the collateral circulation. In more than 10,000 patients this technique is found to be a safe maneuver if performed low in the neck to prevent dislodging atheromatous debris from the carotid bifurcation and stimulating the baroreceptors. The OAPs are measured in the same way as previously described; the pressure on the side of compression is called the *collateral ophthalmic artery pressure* (COAP). Some experience is necessary to perform carotid compression reliably. A photoplethysmograph placed on the compression side of the earlobe is helpful for checking whether complete occlusion is achieved and maintained. Compression should be released

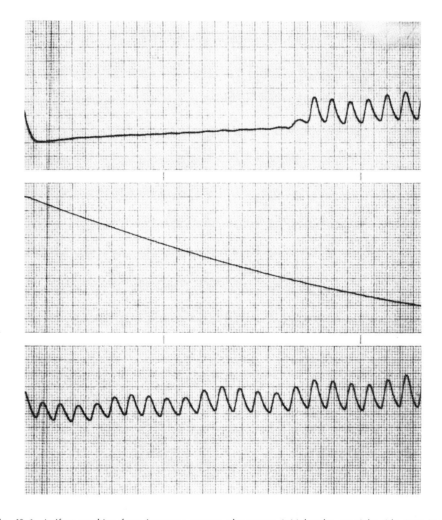

Fig. 43-1. Artifact resulting from incorrect eyecup placement. Initial pulse on right side *(top)* is not preceded by the usual gradual progression in amplitude. (From Gee W: *Ocular pneumoplethysmography* [*OPE-Gee*]. In Kempczinski RF et al, eds: *Practical noninvasive vascular diagnosis*, Chicago, 1982, Mosby.)

gradually to avoid the sudden return of blood flow. The OPG instrument can record ocular pulsations at high paper speed, which makes it possible to determine the pulse arrival time. Overall, the value of this procedure is limited. Following the test, there may be some scleral erythema where the eyecup was placed, but this is not serious. Patients are told that this does not require treatment and will disappear spontaneously. Patients are also told that their eyes may remain anesthetic for up to 2 hours after the test and that they should not rub their eyes.

Interpretation of findings

The OPG recording yields three pieces of information: the OAP between the two sides, the ophthalmic/systemic pressure (OP/SP) ratio, and the pulse amplitude. There has been a lack of unanimity in the literature concerning the criteria that should be used to classify the test as normal or abnormal. Different criteria have been published by several laboratories, creating confusion among the users of the instrument. The choice of criteria is important, as this greatly influences the accuracy of the test. These different criteria were applied to the OPG results obtained from 200 patients with angiographically evaluated carotid arteries, and McDonald's criteria were found to be the most suitable for clinical use.[5] In his system, the OPG result is considered abnormal if there is a left-to-right OAP difference of 5 mm Hg or more or if the OP/SP ratio is less than 0.66. These criteria yield the best balance between sensitivity and specificity, as shown by the receiver operating characteristic (ROC) curve for the different criteria (Fig. 43-2). Better sensitivities can only be reached at the cost of lower specificities, which is not acceptable, since the test is of greatest value for patients with asymptomatic bruits and vague or nonhemispheric symptoms. Gee's criteria also yield good results but are more cumbersome. He considers a left-to-right difference of 5 mm Hg or more or an OAP of less than 39 plus an SP of 0.43 as abnormal.

The pulse amplitude should only be used as a determining factor for those hypertensive patients in whom even a vacuum of 500 mm Hg does not obliterate the ocular pulsations, and thus no OAP can be measured. A difference in amplitude of 2 mm or more between the first pulsation of the left and that of the right eye indicates a hemodynamically significant carotid lesion on the side of the lower amplitude. Although the amplitude is lower for carotid arteries with hemodynamically significant lesions than for those without such lesions, application of this criterion when actual OAPs can be determined will reduce the test's specificity.[6]

Results

The results obtained with OPG in detecting hemodynamically significant carotid lesions depend on not only the criteria used for interpreting the test but also on the criteria used to interpret the arteriogram. Reading arteriograms is more subjective than reading OPG curves, as confirmed by the reportedly high intraobserver and interobserver variability. Accurate measurement of the degree of stenosis is difficult, and in addition, many authors do not state whether the vessel diameter within the stenosis is compared with the estimated diameter of the bulbs or with the distal internal carotid artery. Confusion also exists about transverse diameter stenosis versus cross-sectional stenosis. For example, how should a stenosis of 60% seen in the lateral projection with none visible in the anteroposterior projection be classified? Other kinds of questions also arise. How should weblike stenoses be classified? Are the hemodynamic consequences of a 60% lesion in the common carotid artery the same as those of a 60% lesion in the siphon, which is a much smaller vessel? Did the angiogram completely visualize the whole pathway from the aortic arch to the ophthalmic artery? Obviously, innominate artery lesions as well as siphon lesions may cause a reduction in OAP. Nevertheless, this is only rarely considered in the literature on OPG results.

Degrees of stenosis varying from 50% to 75% have been used as the threshold between normal and abnormal, but the results of OPG are then influenced by the stenosis threshold chosen. The sensitivity will be higher when the threshold is high, but specificity will be low. This relationship is shown graphically in the ROC curve in Fig. 43-2. Comparing the results obtained by different researchers is also hampered by the fact that some researchers present data in terms of patients and others in terms of arteries. Nonetheless, a survey of the existing literature on OPG has been conducted, and the findings indicate that sensitivities range from 70% to 92% and specificities from 80% to 100%, with a mean sensitivity of 86% and a mean specificity of 92%.[4] An overall accuracy of approximately 90% can be expected if a fixed angiographic threshold is used as the standard.

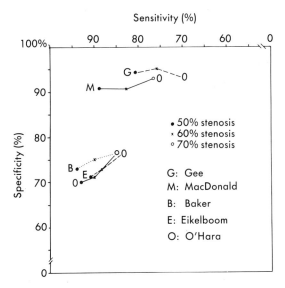

Fig. 43-2. Sensitivity and specificity by using different criteria for interpretation of OPG and different angiographic thresholds for hemodynamically significant stenosis. (From Eikelboom BC et al: *Arch Surg* 118:1169, 1983.)

Some believe, however, that this fixed threshold does not exist and that OPG may sometimes more accurately define the significance of a lesion than angiography.

Unfortunately, in the event of an abnormal OPG, no distinction can be made between hemodynamically significant stenosis and occlusion. However, an interesting observation has been made in patients with carotid occlusion on one side and significant stenosis on the other side. As expected, the OAP was generally lower on the side of the occlusion, but this is not always the case. Several cases of lower OAP on the side of the stenosis have been documented. This also suggests that OPG reflects the functional significance of a lesion better than angiography.

Areas of application

The primary application of OPG is for the detection of hemodynamically significant carotid lesions. Symptoms of cerebrovascular insufficiency or asymptomatic bruits can be indications for testing. It is well known, however, that carotid stenosis may exist in the absence of a bruit. OPG has been used as a screening device for the detection of hemodynamically significant carotid disease in 500 consecutive patients with symptoms of peripheral obstructive arterial disease. There were carotid bruits in 130 patients (26%). The OPG was abnormal in 86 patients (14%), and half of the patients had no bruit. In summary, the OPG results were abnormal in 43 of 370 (12%) of the patients with peripheral arterial disease who had no bruits.

The findings from another OPG screening study have been published for 500 patients scheduled for cardiac operations.[1] Bruits were present in 32 patients (6%), and a total of 18 patients (3%) had abnormal OPG measurements. Similar to the peripheral arterial disease group, half of these patients had a bruit and half did not. Therefore 9 of 468 cardiac patients (2%) without bruits had abnormal OPG findings. This leads to the conclusion that normal OPG findings occur more frequently in patients with peripheral arterial disease. Despite these drawbacks, OPG can be used to document the natural history of carotid disease. A prospective follow-up study has been conducted in 400 patients with asymptomatic carotid bruits. At the first examination, a pressure-reducing lesion was identified by OPG in 47 patients (11.8%), 9 of whom proved to have carotid occlusion. During a mean follow-up of 3 years, the test became abnormal in 44 patients (11%).

Several investigators have shown that patients with an abnormal OPG are at a much higher risk of stroke compared to those with a normal OPG. Busuttil et al[2] observed 215 patients with a history of stroke, transient ischemic attacks, or asymptomatic bruits. They found the incidence of stroke and death was 16.2% in patients with hemodynamically significant stenosis, but it was only 2.2% in patients with nonhemodynamically significant OPG-negative lesions. A further step in recognizing stroke-prone patients can be made by performing OPG during carotid compression. Those patients who show clinical signs of cerebral ischemia during compression and those who have COAPs less than 60 mm Hg are at high risk when a stenosis progresses to occlusion. Aggressive surgical therapy may be indicated in these patients, especially since the risk of inadequate collateral circulation remains during progression of asymptomatic carotid stenosis.[10]

OPG and an electroencephalogram (EEG) recorded during carotid compression can predict preoperatively which patients will need a shunt during carotid endarterectomy.[7] In one study, these tests were performed in 208 patients.[7] Insertion of a shunt was based on intraoperative test clamping with EEG control and was necessary in 29 patients (14%). The sensitivity of preoperative OPG and EEG was 93% and the specificity, 73%. Preoperative prediction of the stump pressure is also of great value when carotid ligation or resection is planned to identify those patients who are susceptible to cerebral ischemia.[3]

After carotid endarterectomy has been performed, OPG is used to document early patency. OPG should be carried out in the recovery room if the patient exhibits an immediate postoperative neurologic deficit and can differentiate between early thrombosis and intracranial hemorrhage. If the OPG is abnormal on the operated side, thrombosis has probably occurred and the patient is immediately taken back to the operating room without losing time to perform angiography. However, special criteria for the interpretation of the OPG findings during this period may have to be applied.[11] The reasons for this phenomenon have not yet been established. After a patient has undergone carotid endarterectomy, OPG is performed once a year to detect possible restenosis. A 5% incidence of restenosis and occlusions was found after a mean follow-up of 2.5 years.[7]

The outcome of an extracranial-intracranial bypass operation for carotid occlusion can also be evaluated by OPG. OAPs are determined both with and without compression of the bypass. The difference between these pressures then represents the contribution of the bypass to the intracranial perfusion pressure, which averaged 12.8 mm Hg in 13 patients who underwent this operation for unilateral internal carotid occlusion.

OPG can also be used to determine the ocular blood flow. It is calculated as the product of pulse rate, calibrated ocular pulse amplitude, and a constant of 0.0016.[9] The ocular blood flow reflects the stroke volume of the heart, and its measurement by OPG can be used for the hemodynamic assessment of cardiac pacing[8] in that it is a simple method for documenting the effect of ventricular versus atrioventricular sequential pacing. A final application of OPG is for the assessment of comatose patients with head injuries. Ocular blood flow reflects cerebral blood flow, and this can reveal alterations in brain compliance as a result of cerebral edema. A bilateral reduction in ocular blood flow of less than 0.53 mm/min may be incompatible with cerebral survival.[9] Serial OPG studies may be useful for the simple documentation of changes in brain compliance and may influence therapeutic decisions.

Is there still a role for OPG?

Because duplex scanning now appears to be the best screening test now available, OPG is superfluous in the routine evaluation of carotid artery disease. Duplex scanning is better for determining the absence or presence of disease and quantifies the degree of stenosis. Occasionally, OPG may still have a role in patient care, however. There is a trend to perform carotid endarterectomy without obtaining a preoperative angiogram, and a sensible application of OPG is therefore to confirm the ultrasound diagnosis of a major stenosis. When no pressure drop is found, duplex scanning may have overestimated the disease and it may then be wise to perform an angiogram.

The main application of OPG at this time is probably for the purpose for which it was developed: to investigate a patient's collateral reserve. However, there is not enough evidence to validate the concept that it can identify patients at increased risk for stroke. Nevertheless, OPG remains a good tool for research in this important area, as shown by recently published comparisons with transcranial Doppler[12] and cerebral blood flow mapping.[13] OPG still provides valuable pathophysiologic information in a very simple way.

REFERENCES

1. Balderman SC et al: Noninvasive screening for asymptomatic carotid artery disease prior to cardiac operation, *J Thorac Cardiovasc Surg* 85:427, 1983.
2. Busuttil RW et al: Carotid artery stenosis: hemodynamic significance and clinical course, *JAMA* 245:1438, 1981.
3. Ehrenfeld WK, Stoney RJ, Wylie EJ: Relation of carotid stump pressure to safety of carotid artery ligation, *Surgery* 93:299, 1983.
4. Eikelboom BC: Ocular pneumoplethysmography (OPG-Gee) and oculoplethysmography (OPG-Kartchner): review and perspectives, *Int Angiol* 4:15, 1985.
5. Eikelboom BC et al: Criteria for interpretation of ocular pneumoplethysmography (Gee), *Arch Surg* 118:1169, 1983.
6. Eikelboom BC et al: Pulse amplitude as a diagnostic criterion in OPG-Gee, *Bruit* 7:50, 1983.
7. Eikelboom BC et al: Recognizing stroke prone patients with a poor collateral circulation, *Eur J Vasc Surg* 1:381, 1987.
8. Gee W: Ocular pneumoplethysmography in cardiac pacing, *PACE* 6:1268, 1983.
9. Gee W et al: Ocular pneumoplethysmography in head-injured patients, *J Neurosurg* 59:46, 1983.
10. Moll FL et al: Dynamics of collateral circulation in progressive asymptomatic carotid disease, *J Vasc Surg* 3:470, 1986.
11. Ortega G et al: Postendarterectomy carotid occlusion, *Surgery* 90:1093, 1981.
12. Schneider PA et al: Noninvasive assessment of cerebral collateral blood supply through the ophthalmic artery, *Stroke* 22:31, 1991.
13. Steed DL, Yongas H, Webster MW: Is there still a role for OPG in the noninvasive vascular lab? *J Cardiovasc Surg* 32:62, 1991.

CHAPTER 44

Periorbital Doppler velocity evaluation of carotid obstruction

EDWIN C. BROCKENBROUGH

Obstruction to blood flow through the internal carotid artery invokes collateral blood supply from the circle of Willis and the reversal of flow in the ophthalmic artery. These collateral pathways serve to ameliorate the effects of the restricted carotid blood flow. In addition, they provide a simple means by which carotid obstruction may be diagnosed. Using a Doppler ultrasonic velocity detector, the clinician can examine flow in these vessels and determine the status of functioning collateral pathways. The technique for this examination has been developed over many years, and it has proved to be a reliable method for detecting hemodynamically significant carotid obstruction.

In 1967, the early commercial methods of the Doppler velocity detectors were introduced.[5] The concept of the supraorbital Doppler test for identifying carotid obstruction was developed in conjunction with another diagnostic technique for carotid disease, which was called *ocular plethysmography*.[6] Both tests were based on the principle of compressing collateral vessels feeding the ophthalmic artery as a means of recognizing the abnormal flow patterns associated with internal carotid obstruction. In 1968, the Doppler test became more refined when direction capability was added. As experience in the field grew, it became apparent that the frontal, supraorbital, and angular arteries were each important to an understanding of the vagaries of collateral circulation, hence adoption of the more descriptive term *periorbital Doppler examination*.

A number of other investigators have made similar observations. Maroon et al[11] independently described "ophthalmosonometry" in 1969. Müller[12] expanded on this concept in 1972 and stressed the importance of retrograde flow in the frontal artery as a diagnostic sign of internal carotid occlusion. Machleder and Barker[10] used the periorbital test in 1972 and emphasized its usefulness in recognizing unsuspected carotid obstruction. In 1975, Barnes and Wilson[2] published a very comprehensive treatment of this subject, adding many of their own observations as well as reviewing in detail the principles involved. Following is a status report on the periorbital test—the anatomy and principles on which the test is based, the technique of the examination, the information that can be derived, and the role of the test in the spectrum of noninvasive diagnostic tests of the cerebrovascular system.

ANATOMIC BASIS OF THE PERIORBITAL EXAMINATION

The blood flow through the internal carotid artery is distributed almost entirely to intracranial vessels, with the ophthalmic artery the one exception. This ophthalmic artery passes into the orbit, gives rise to a number of intraorbital branches, and then terminates in three branches that surface on the face: the nasal, frontal, and supraorbital branches (Fig. 44-1). The nasal artery becomes the angular artery, which descends along the lateral border of the nose and communicates with the facial branch of the external carotid artery. The frontal and supraorbital arteries turn upward and pass into the subcutaneous tissue of the forehead, where they communicate with branches of the superficial temporal artery. These communications serve as collateral pathways in the event of internal carotid obstruction. Other communications between the ophthalmic artery and branches of the external carotid artery occur through the ethmoid and lacrimal branches. Although these are not accessible for Doppler examination, they should be considered when assessing a patient with possible obstruction because of their contribution to the collateral blood supply. In addition to the periorbital anastomoses, the other major collateral pathway is the anterior communicating artery of the circle of Willis. It is through this pathway that crossover circulation from the opposite internal carotid artery is accomplished.

TECHNIQUE

The examination consists of detecting flow in the periorbital vessels, noting the quality and direction of the velocity signals, and determining the response of these signals to the compression of different arteries about the face and neck.

The Doppler equipment used for the examination should have directional capability, and the probe should be small enough to permit the separate examination of each of these small vessels. The examination is begun with the patient supine and the eyes gently closed. The probe is then placed at the inner canthus of the eye and the maximum flow signal is identified. The probe is then moved along this signal toward the rim of orbit; this is where the frontal artery is examined. The probe is then moved laterally to the supraorbital notch, where the supraorbital signal is identified. The angular artery may be found over the lateral aspect of the nose. It is the smallest of the three vessels and is usually

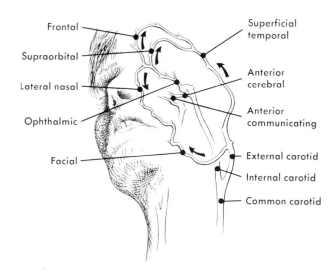

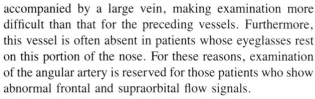

Fig. 44-1. Arteries of significance to the periorbital Doppler test. The normal flow pattern is shown by arrows.

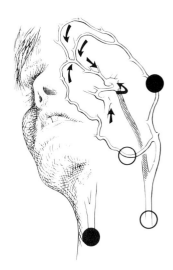

Fig. 44-2. Carotid occlusion, or high-grade stenosis—dominant periorbital collaterals. This is the flow pattern seen in over 90% of patients with this condition.

accompanied by a large vein, making examination more difficult than that for the preceding vessels. Furthermore, this vessel is often absent in patients whose eyeglasses rest on this portion of the nose. For these reasons, examination of the angular artery is reserved for those patients who show abnormal frontal and supraorbital flow signals.

If the Doppler probe is held at the proper angle, the direction of flow can usually be determined reliably. However, in some instances, a tortuous artery may alter the probe angle in relation to the vessel, and the observed direction of flow may be reversed. Compression techniques help to minimize errors of this sort.

After locating the frontal and supraorbital arteries and noting the direction and quality of the flow signals, the examiner compresses the superficial temporal artery in front of the ear, just above the zygoma. In most patients, there is a slight augmentation of the frontal and supraorbital signals, but in some normal individuals, there is no change elicited by this maneuver. If the signals are diminished or obliterated when the temporal artery is compressed, the flow may be assumed to be retrograde. The facial artery is then compressed along the lower border of the mandible and its effect on the frontal artery noted. These maneuvers are then repeated on the opposite side. Finally, common carotid compression is performed to identify crossover circulation. Compression is applied low in the neck, well away from the carotid bifurcation, and is maintained for only one or two heart beats. During compression, the probe is usually held at the inner canthus of the eye, where the maximum flow signal is located. Normally the signal at this point is obliterated or greatly diminished by ipsilateral carotid compression and is not affected by contralateral carotid compression. When the ipsilateral carotid is compressed, the residual flow signals on both sides should be about the same. Although there is undoubtedly some inherent risk of

dislodging an embolus during carotid compression, the risk of complications is low if the compression is deft and brief.

During the examination, the examiner should hold the probe steady, and this is facilitated by resting the hand holding the probe on the patient's forehead and bridge of the nose. The probe should also be held lightly, since even a modest pressure from the tip of the probe can obliterate flow in these small vessels. In this regard, the examiner must resist the tendency to press with the probe while compressing the temporal or facial vessels with the opposite hand.

PATTERNS OF COLLATERAL BLOOD FLOW

A variety of patterns of collateralization is seen around the orbit in the presence of internal carotid obstruction. Following are some examples.

Dominant periorbital collaterals

The pattern of dominant periorbital collaterals is the most common (Fig. 44-2), constituting over 90% of all abnormal examination results. It is usually associated with high-grade stenosis or total occlusion of the internal carotid artery. The examiner first notices that there is asymmetry between the two sides. The signal on the obstructed side may be either dampened and have only a single component or loud and continuous. The direction indicator on the Doppler instrument shows that the direction of flow in the periorbital vessels is reversed. Furthermore, the periorbital signals are obliterated or diminished during temporal and facial artery compressions. In some instances, a reversed signal may be converted to a normal directional signal by these compressions. Finally, there is usually evidence of some crossover flow during common carotid compression. Ipsilateral common carotid compression evokes a prominent residual signal that may be either antegrade or retrograde, depending on

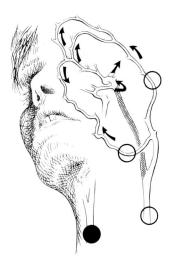

Fig. 44-3. Carotid occlusion, or high-grade stenosis—dominant crossover collaterals. This pattern is sometimes seen in long-standing carotid obstruction. The key diagnostic maneuver is contralateral carotid compression.

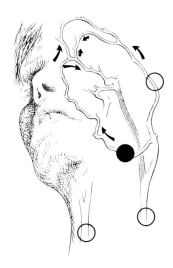

Fig. 44-4. Carotid occlusion, or high-grade stenosis—dominant facial artery collateral. The key diagnostic maneuver is facial artery compression.

whether the dominant collateral supply travels through the opposite internal carotid or the opposite external carotid artery, respectively. Compression of the contralateral carotid artery usually increases the retrograde flow in the periorbital vessels.

Dominant crossover collaterals

The pattern of dominant crossover collaterals is the next most common finding (Fig. 44-3) and is usually seen in patients with long-standing occlusion of the internal carotid artery or in patients with a common carotid artery occlusion. The examiner first notices asymmetry between the two sides and usually detects an abnormal signal on the affected side. The flow is noted to be coming from within the orbit, but with compression of the common carotid artery on the affected side, the periorbital flow signals are augmented in a normal direction. The diagnosis is confirmed with contralateral common carotid compression, which eliminates the crossover supply and usually produces a reversal of flow in the periorbital vessels.

Dominant facial artery collateral

A dominant facial artery collateral is occasionally present (Fig. 44-4). In this variant of the pattern shown in Fig. 44-2, the facial artery supplies not only retrograde flow to the angular artery but also flow to the frontal, and sometimes the supraorbital, vessel. This results in normal directional flow in these vessels, so the response to temporal artery compression may be normal. The diagnosis is made when compression of the facial artery diminishes or obliterates the frontal and supraorbital signals as well as the angular signal.

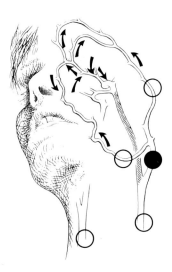

Fig. 44-5. Carotid occlusion, or high-grade stenosis—dominant intraorbital collaterals. This is a rare cause for diagnostic error. The key diagnostic maneuver is selective compression of the external carotid artery.

Dominant intraorbital collaterals

Occasionally, communications within the orbit may provide sufficient flow to produce normal directional signals in the periorbital vessels (Fig. 44-5). These anastomoses probably occur between the orbital branches of the ophthalmic (anterior and posterior ethmoid, lacrimal) and branches of the internal maxillary (sphenopalatine, middle meningeal) arteries. This variant has been observed on several occasions in patients with long-standing internal carotid artery occlusion. It is fortunate that this is a rare condition, since the results of standard compression techniques may suggest nor-

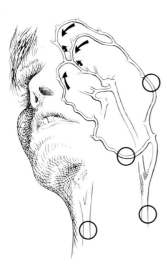

Fig. 44-6. Carotid stenosis—critically balanced flow in the periorbital vessels. Bidirectional flow may be identified.

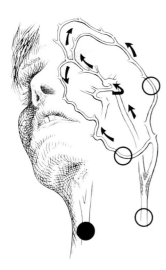

Fig. 44-7. Combined internal and external carotid stenosis—normal directional periorbital flow may be present. The key diagnostic maneuver is contralateral carotid compression.

mal blood supply. The diagnosis can be made by selectively compressing the external carotid artery, which will obliterate or diminish the periorbital signals. With a little practice, this compression can be accomplished satisfactorily while the temporal artery is assessed for completeness using the Doppler probe.

Balanced internal carotid and external carotid artery supply

Usually a sign of early hemodynamic obstruction of the internal carotid artery, the balanced internal carotid and external carotid artery supply (Fig. 44-6) occurs in patients whose stenosis does not yet cause complete periorbital reversal. In this pattern, the examiner first notices asymmetry between the two sides. The signal on the affected side goes in the normal direction during systole but reverses in late diastole. In this balanced state, small changes in collateral flow or peripheral resistance may shift the periorbital flow from one direction to the other. For example, compression of the contralateral common carotid artery may result in periorbital flow reversal. If administered sublingually, nitroglycerin will bring about a progressive reduction in the normal directional component and progressive increase in the reversed component. Occasionally, this balanced state stems from stenosis of both the external and internal carotid arteries or from stenosis of the common carotid artery at the bifurcation (Fig. 44-7). In either of these situations, however, there is usually evidence of collateralization from the opposite side that may be demonstrated during contralateral carotid compression.

DIAGNOSTIC CRITERIA

Based on the observations made during the periorbital Doppler examination, the examiner can be reasonably confident about the presence or absence of collateral blood flow. If there is collateral circulation, this implies the existence of hemodynamically significant carotid obstruction. However, total occlusion of the carotid artery cannot be distinguished from high-grade stenosis. It must also be emphasized that the periorbital examination cannot disclose some clinically significant but nonobstructive lesions. Collateralization around the orbit can usually be recognized when the diameter of the internal carotid is reduced by 65% to 70%. This corresponds to a mean pressure gradient across the lesion of 10 to 12 mm Hg or greater.[17]

The most reliable signs of collateralization are retrograde flow from the temporal and facial arteries and evidence of crossover flow from the opposite carotid artery. Doppler changes that are not diagnostic but strongly suggestive include asymmetry between the two sides, dampened velocity signals, and a change from the normal two-component signal to either a systolic or continuous signal.

Retrograde flow

Retrograde flow can be identified both by the direction indicated on the Doppler instrument and by compression of the facial and temporal arteries. Occasionally the periorbital vessels are supplied from the contralateral temporal and facial arteries, which must be compressed to confirm the source.

Crossover flow

Abnormal blood supply via the anterior communicating artery is diagnosed by compressing the contralateral common carotid artery. If there is normal directional periorbital flow, the Doppler signals are either diminished or reversed by this maneuver. Likewise, compression of the ipsilateral common carotid artery does not obliterate the periorbital signals and may even augment them.

If there is reversed periorbital flow, opposite carotid artery compression augments the reversed flow. Compression of the ipsilateral carotid artery results in normal directional periorbital flow.

Asymmetric signals

Although asymmetry between the two sides is not diagnostic, it does suggest abnormal flow and alerts the examiner to look carefully for other signs of collateralization. The asymmetry is caused by one of the following signal abnormalities:

1. Dampened flow signal: Whether the direction is normal or reversed, the periorbital flows on the side of an obstructed carotid artery are less brisk than on the opposite normal side.
2. Single-component flow signal: As an obstructing lesion begins to reduce flow in the internal carotid artery, one of the first Doppler changes is loss of the diastolic component of the periorbital signal.
3. Bidirectional flow signal: As the stenosis progresses, the flow signal becomes bidirectional, with reversed flow detectable at the end of diastole. In this balanced state, changes in peripheral resistance may shift the flow in either direction. This can be demonstrated by administering sublingual nitroglycerin to the patient. Over 1 or 2 minutes, the antegrade component diminishes and the retrograde component increases. Flow can be completely reversed by this technique, making it useful as a provocative test for lesions of borderline significance. This response is considered to result from lowering the peripheral resistance in the intracranial distribution to a greater extent than the resistance in the external carotid distribution.
4. Continuous flow signal: Occasionally, a nearly continuous signal can be heard in the periorbital vessels, resembling the sound of an arteriovenous fistula. This is often observed in the presence of an acute internal carotid occlusion and suggests that a high-pressure gradient exists between the external and internal carotid arteries.

DIAGNOSTIC ACCURACY

The purpose of the periorbital Doppler examination is to identify functioning collateral pathways around the orbit and, by inference, hemodynamically significant carotid obstruction. An accuracy of 95% or better is realistic and can be achieved by a careful and reasonably astute examiner. Using essentially the same approach, Barnes and Wilson[2] reported a 98.7% overall diagnostic accuracy in a series of 76 patients undergoing angiography. These investigators encountered two false-negative diagnoses (5%) among 38 carotid arteries with occlusion or stenosis of 75% or greater. Reports from other institutions have varied somewhat, but in general, the findings have been similar.[4,7-9,13-16]

There are a number of possible sources of error in the examination, and the examiner should be aware of these to ensure the best accuracy. It is important that the anatomy of the periorbital vessels be well understood and that at least the frontal and supraorbital vessels be identified in each patient. The flow signals should be located just beneath the rim of the orbit and the probe angled toward the direction of flow so that the direction of flow can be accurately assessed. As mentioned earlier, the probe must be held steady, particularly when the compressions are performed. It is also essential that the examiner avoid pressing too firmly with the probe and possibly obliterating the flow signal.

Anatomic variants that might lead to diagnostic errors have been illustrated. For example, occasionally a reversed flow in the supraorbital artery will be found in normal individuals, even when care is taken to identify the vessel in this supraorbital notch. The reason for this phenomenon is not certain, but this single abnormality should not lead to an interpretation of error if the remainder of the examination findings are normal. The lateral palpebral artery may sometimes be misidentified as the supraorbital artery, and because the palpebral artery arises from a branch of the temporal artery, compression may elicit a false-positive response.

When interpreting the results of the examination, the examiner should resist the temptation to render a precise anatomic diagnosis. The observed data only provide information concerning collateralization about the orbit, and the basis for this collateralization can only be inferred from these findings. Although most patients with periorbital collateralization do have carotid obstruction in the neck, obstruction at the level of the carotid siphon or the ophthalmic artery can also yield positive findings. In fact, as already pointed out, the distinction between total occlusion of the internal carotid and high-grade stenosis cannot be made from these observations alone. In addition, the diagnosis is almost never based on a single abnormal finding. There are usually two or more abnormalities, and these abnormalities must be consistent with one another. If there is an unexplained finding or if the findings are inconsistent, the examiner should persist with compressions (e.g., contralateral, facial, and temporal compressions), until the collateral pathways are delineated.

ROLE OF THE PERIORBITAL DOPPLER EXAMINATION

With the more recent advent of duplex scanning, flow velocity analysis, transcranial Doppler sonography, and other sophisticated techniques, the periorbital examination has become a less important tool in the modern vascular laboratory. Primary use of the periorbital examination may be as a component of a comprehensive noninvasive cerebrovascular evaluation.[18] The periorbital Doppler findings help to distinguish obstructing from nonobstructing lesions and also serve to increase the confidence with which the overall interpretation is made.

Because the periorbital examination is relatively simple and can be performed with portable equipment either at the patient's bedside or in the office, it remains a useful test for the clinical vascular surgeon.[1] Furthermore, using the same instrumentation, it is possible to gain considerable information from the direct assessment of the carotid bifurcation using a handheld probe.[3] The internal and external carotid signals can be easily recognized using this method and zones of increased flow velocity identified. Thus the examiner can perform a reasonably reliable screening examination that is both quick and inexpensive.

Fewer than one half of the patients with clinically significant carotid disease will manifest Doppler signs of collateralization about the orbit. For this reason, a normal periorbital examination alone should not be relied on to rule out disease in a patient with symptoms who might be a candidate for carotid surgery. On the other hand, the finding of functioning collaterals in patients without symptoms may be a useful criterion for identifying patients with critical stenosis who are at high risk for suffering a stroke.

CONCLUSION

The periorbital Doppler test is a relatively simple method for identifying functioning collateral pathways around the orbit. The presence of a flow-restricting carotid obstruction may be inferred from these findings. If the techniques are carried out as described, the correlation between the Doppler evidence for collateralization and the angiographic evidence for significant obstruction should be 95% or better. The periorbital Doppler test cannot detect nonobstructing lesions that may be of clinical significance and, for this reason, is used to best advantage as a component of a more comprehensive noninvasive cerebrovascular evaluation. In this setting, the periorbital Doppler information distinguishes between obstructing and nonobstructing lesions and helps the practitioner make a diagnosis with greater confidence. The periorbital Doppler test by itself is useful as an office or bedside screening test for carotid obstruction and can assist in identifying the patient without symptoms with high-grade stenosis who is at risk for suffering stroke.

REFERENCES

1. Baker JD: How vascular surgeons use noninvasive testing, *J Vasc Surg* 4(3):272-276, 1986.
2. Barnes RW, Wilson MR: *Doppler ultrasonic evaluation of cerebrovascular disease,* Iowa City, 1975, University of Iowa Press.
3. Barnes RW, Nix L, Rittgers SE: Audible interpretation of carotid Doppler signals: an improved technique to define carotid artery disease, *Arch Surg* 116(9):1185-1189, 1981.
4. Bone GE, Dickinson D, Pomajzl MJ: A prospective evaluation of indirect methods for detecting carotid atherosclerosis, *Surg Gynecol Obstet* 152(5):587-592, 1981.
5. Brockenbrough EC: *Screening for the prevention of stroke: use of a Doppler flowmeter.* Information and Education Resource Support Unit, Washington/Alaska Regional Medical Program, 1969.
6. Brockenbrough EC, Lawrence C, Schwenk WG: Ocular plethysmography: a new technique for the evaluation of carotid obstructive disease, *Rev Surg* 24:299, 1967.
7. Chambers BR, Merory JR, Smidt V: Doppler diagnosis in cases of acute stroke, *Med J Aust* 150(7):382-384, 1989.
8. Lewis RR, Padayachee TS, Gosling RG: Ultrasound screening for internal carotid disease. II. Sensitivity and specificity of a single site periorbital artery test, *Ultrasound Med Biol* 10(1):17-25, 1984.
9. Lynch TG et al: Comparison of continuous-wave Doppler imaging, oculopneumoplethysmography, and the cerebrovascular Doppler examination, *Circulation* I106-I111, 1982.
10. Machleder HI, Barker WF: Stroke on the wrong side: use of the Doppler ophthalmic test in cerebral vascular screening, *Arch Surg* 105:943, 1972.
11. Maroon JC, Pieroni DW, Campbell RL: Ophthalmosonometry, an ultrasonic method for assessing carotid blood flow, *J Neurosurg* 30:238, 1969.
12. Müller HR: The diagnosis of internal carotid artery occlusion by directional Doppler sonography of the ophthalmic artery, *Neurology* 22:816, 1972.
13. O'Leary DH et al: Noninvasive testing for carotid artery stenosis. II. Clinical application of accuracy assessments, *AJR* 138(1):109-111, 1982.
14. Padayachee TS, Lewis RR, Gosling RG: Ultrasound screening for internal carotid disease. I. The temporal artery occlusion test—which periorbital artery? *Ultrasound Med Biol* 10(1):13-16, 1984.
15. Schneider PA et al: Noninvasive assessment of cerebral collateral blood supply through the ophthalmic artery, *Stroke* 22(1):31-36, 1991.
16. Seneviratne BI et al: Rapid Doppler screening test for internal carotid disease, *Aust NZ J Med* 16(4):481-485, 1986.
17. Sillesen H et al: Doppler examination of the periorbital arteries adds valuable hemodynamic information in carotid artery disease, *Ultrasound Med Biol* 13(4):177-181, 1987.
18. Spencer JP et al: *Cerebrovascular evaluation using Doppler C-W ultrasound.* Proceedings of the World Federation of Ultrasound in Medicine and Biology, San Francisco, August 1976.

CHAPTER 45

Natural history of carotid stenosis

TIMOTHY C. HODGES and D. EUGENE STRANDNESS, JR.

Since its inception in the early 1950s, carotid endarterectomy has been a controversial treatment for carotid artery stenosis.[1,16,24] Part of the early debate surrounding the role of this operation arose because of a poor understanding of the natural history of carotid stenosis. Data concerning the evolution of carotid bifurcation atherosclerosis were not available because suitable study methods were lacking. It was impossible to predict which patients were at risk for an ischemic event on the basis of the findings yielded by examination of a carotid artery lesion at a single point in time, making it difficult to predict which patients would benefit from surgery. With the introduction of ultrasonic duplex scanning, new information is beginning to emerge about the progression of carotid plaques, the risk of neurologic ischemic events, and the outcome after carotid endarterectomy.

METHODS OF DETECTING CAROTID ARTERY DISEASE
Physical examination

Before the availability of sensitive noninvasive tests, physical examination was the only way to screen patients for possible carotid arterial disease. The finding of a carotid bruit has been the subject of several studies. Auscultation of the cervical region is recommended as an initial screening test for all patients who are seen because of a history of transient ischemic attacks (TIAs) or stroke, those with evidence of atherosclerosis elsewhere in the body, and those over 40 years of age. Most modern studies cite the results of bruit detection obtained with the stethoscope and describe the problems inherent in interpreting the findings. Ziegler et al[34] reported on 199 subjects with ischemic cerebrovascular disease (excluding major strokes) and a cervical carotid bruit who underwent cervical angiography. The method of bruit detection was designed to closely resemble that used in a routine physical examination. The authors cited a false-negative rate of 73% (carotid stenosis present with minimal bruit) and a false-positive rate of 10% (moderate to loud bruit present without evidence of arterial stenosis), and concluded that a carotid bruit is an unreliable indicator of carotid disease. David et al[5] challenged this finding by reporting that 75% of their patients with a TIA and a carotid bruit had demonstrable internal carotid artery

stenosis shown by arteriogram, whereas 65% of the patients without symptoms but with a bruit had internal carotid artery stenosis as well. They did point out, however, that the absence of a bruit does not exclude the presence of significant carotid stenosis. Cooperman et al[3] related their similar experience with 60 patients who had audible carotid bruits. These authors found a 35% incidence of neurologic events (TIAs or stroke) versus a 16% incidence in those without bruits. None of these studies demonstrated that either the presence or absence of a carotid bruit as an isolated finding carried a high degree of sensitivity or specificity for the existence of carotid stenosis. Given the difficulties in relating the presence of a bruit to the degree of stenosis, it is unlikely that this method can ever be used for conducting natural history studies.

Arteriography

Arteriography was the only objective means of detecting carotid artery stenosis for many years and remains the standard for comparison with other methods. In a joint cooperative study of arteriography, Hass et al[10] published their experience with 3788 four-vessel (cervical and vertebral) examinations and cited a 1.2% major and a 5.3% to 14.3% minor complication rate during the 7 years of the study. As the study progressed, the complication rate declined because of increased familiarity with the methods. Modern approaches, such as digital subtraction arteriography (DSA) and the use of nonionic contrast agents, appear to have reduced the complications associated with performing standard arteriography without sacrificing important information.[4] In a review of the diagnostic accuracy of DSA, Sumner et al[30] reported a cumulative sensitivity and specificity of 92%. Riles et al[25] performed arteriography on 990 carotid arteries to try and relate neurologic symptoms and bruits to the degree of stenosis. In 505 arteries with detectable bruits, a linear relationship between the incidence of bruit and degree of stenosis was found, although the correlation between the presence of a bruit and neurologic symptoms was poor. The potential risks and discomfort associated with arteriography limit its current use to patients being considered for surgery. The method is not suitable for screening or serial studies.

Ultrasonic duplex scanning

Because of the relative insensitivity of cervical bruits in identifying carotid artery disease, attempts have been made to develop a noninvasive diagnostic method for patients at risk for carotid stenosis. Kartchner and McRae[17] described oculoplethysmography and carotid phonoangiography and tried to use the difference between ocular and earlobe pulse timing to differentiate between internal and external carotid artery stenosis in patients with asymptomatic cervical bruits. This method failed to determine the intracranial or extracranial site of the stenosis and could not distinguish occluded arteries from those with severe flow-limiting lesions.

This pulse delay method has now been largely replaced by the ocular pneumoplethysmography technique developed by Gee,[9] in which suction cups are applied to the sclerae and a negative pressure is generated that eliminates ocular pulsations. With the reduction of pressure in the cups, the point at which pulsations reappear can be used to calculate the pressure in the ophthalmic artery. This approach has been extensively tested and found accurate for detecting high-grade carotid stenosis. Although useful for follow-up studies, this plethysmographic method also has major limitations. It cannot distinguish between stenosis and occlusion, and once a test result is positive, the test is of little further use in documenting changes in the status of a bifurcation lesion.

For conducting natural history studies, these methods have been replaced by the ultrasonic duplex scanner, which has proved to be the most useful noninvasive method for the evaluation of extracranial cerebrovascular disease. Modern commercially available devices operate by combining B-mode imaging with pulsed Doppler velocity measurements to describe flow within the vessel lumen. B-mode images are generated via piezoelectric crystals within the ultrasonic transducer, which generates a pulse echo at a known frequency. The pulse travels at a given speed, depending on the tissue media, and is reflected by tissue interfaces of varying density (i.e., the interface between flowing blood and the arterial wall) (Fig. 45-1). The time between the pulse emission and its reflection to the transducer indicates the relative depth of the interface, and the strength of the returned signal determines the acoustic reflectivity of the tissue; higher reflectivity is represented on the video screen as a higher-intensity (brighter) region (Fig. 45-2). Determination of flow within the vessel is based on the Doppler principle, which states that any moving object in the path of an emitted sonic beam will alter the frequency of the reflected beam in a predictable manner. The Doppler signal then undergoes a fast Fourier transform to yield a video display of frequency versus time (Fig. 45-3). In 1981, Fell et al[8] reported their initial results in the duplex scanning of patients with asymptomatic bruits and cited a sensitivity of 97% but a specificity of only 37%. Further refinement of this technique by Roederer et al[29] in 1984 yielded a stenosis classification system that was based on peak systolic frequency and spectral waveform characteristics, and this

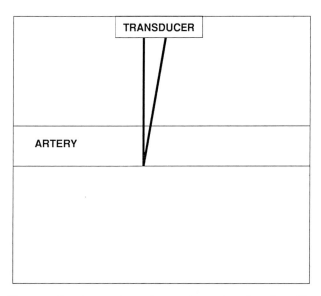

Fig. 45-1. The ultrasound transducer emits a pulse echo reflected by the artery wall. The travel time in both directions determines the depth of the reflection, and the strength of the reflection determines the intensity.

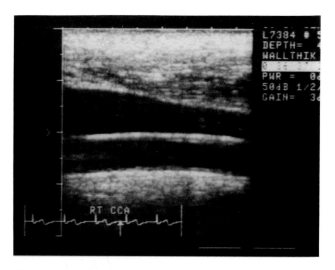

Fig. 45-2. B-mode image of a common carotid artery. The internal jugular vein is superior to the artery.

was associated with a false-positive rate of 12% and a false-negative rate of 16%. By 1987, the identification of additional variables such as end-diastolic velocity and better analysis of the Doppler waveform made it possible for Taylor and Strandness[31] to achieve a sensitivity of 99% and a specificity of 84%, as compared with conventional angiography (Fig. 45-4). An excellent description of the technique and its application can be found in a review by Langlois et al.[18]

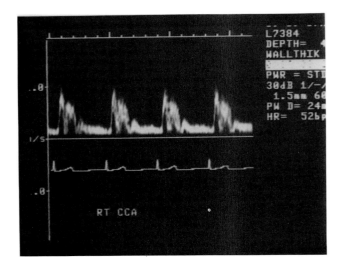

Fig. 45-3. A processed Doppler signal as frequency versus time.

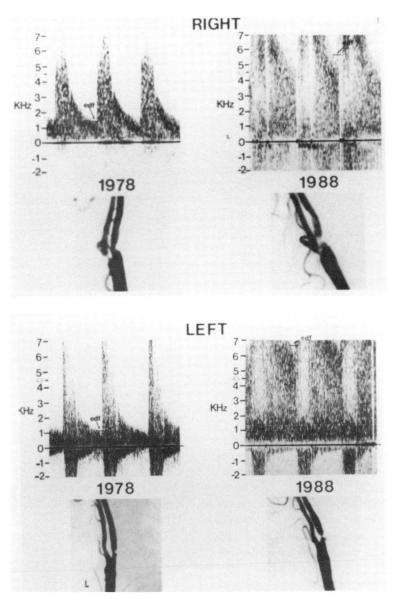

Fig. 45-4. Correlation of duplex scanning with arteriography. This patient developed a greater than 80% stenosis over 10 years. (From Strandness DE: *Duplex scanning in vascular disorders,* New York, 1990, Raven Press.)

NATURAL HISTORY STUDIES
Carotid bruit

Just as the finding of a carotid bruit once was used to diagnose carotid stenosis, it was also tested as a means for observing the natural history of the disease. In a rural community study (Evans County, Georgia), Heyman et al[13] conducted a survey of 1620 subjects 45 years of age and older and found that males with asymptomatic cervical bruits were at a significant increased risk for stroke. However, the correlation between bruit site and the hemisphere affected was poor. They suggested that although a carotid bruit is a marker for atherosclerosis, it is a poor predictor of which hemisphere will be affected when a stroke occurs. The Framingham study data reported by Wolf et al[33] in 1981 confirmed that carotid bruits can serve as markers for increased stroke risk but only as a sign of generalized atherosclerosis. Chambers and Norris[1] determined that patients with asymptomatic carotid bruits were at a greater risk for a myocardial ischemic event than a cerebral ischemic event. In one of the few long-term studies of patients with asymptomatic carotid bruits who did not undergo endarterectomy, Dorazio et al[6] found an 11% incidence of TIAs and a 19% incidence of stroke in 90 subjects who were observed over 5 to 13 years. A similar prognosis was described by Thompson et al[32] who reported a 28% incidence of TIAs and a 19% incidence of stroke over 10 years in 102 patients who did not undergo operation versus a 1.7% incidence of neurologic events in those who did.

Arteriography

Javid et al[14] conducted the only study based on repeat arteriograms obtained over 1 to 9 years from 93 subjects with carotid stenosis of less than 60% diameter reduction. They found disease progression in 51 patients, 32 of whom had shown progression in their stenosis of greater than 25% per year. Risk factors associated with disease progression include hypertension, persistent symptoms, a localized carotid bruit, and a bifurcation stenosis of greater than 25%.

Ultrasonic duplex scanning

The development of duplex scanning techniques provided the best opportunity to study the natural history of carotid atherosclerosis. In January 1980, a prospective study was begun to observe the course of a consecutive series of patients with asymptomatic midcervical bruits. Over a 30-month period, 203 patients were examined, with 162 available for follow-up. Patients were seen at 6-month intervals for the first year and at 12-month intervals thereafter. Pertinent medical history was obtained and a standard duplex examination was performed at each visit. Based on the features previously described, Roederer et al[27] classified the carotid stenosis in these patients into one of six categories: (1) normal, (2) 1% to 15% stenosis, (3) 16% to 49%, (4) 50% to 79%, (5) 80% to 99%, and (6) occlusion. Using life-table analysis, the annual rate of symptom development (e.g., carotid occlusion, TIA, stroke) was 4%. Progression

to 80% or greater diameter reduction was significantly correlated with the development of symptoms ($p = 0.00001$), but only 1.5% of the patients with less than 80% stenosis suffered complications. Moneta et al[20] examined the risk factors and the duplex characteristics that put patients with a greater than 80% diameter-reducing lesion at highest risk of suffering a neurologic event. Outcome could not be related to age, gender, aspirin use, smoking, hypertension, diabetes, or cardiac disease. However, it was noted that patients with end-diastolic frequencies at the site of stenosis that exceeded 6.5 kHz were more likely to have an adverse neurologic event.

Other natural history studies have also been undertaken at the University of Washington using long-term duplex studies as their basis. In 1986, Nicholls et al[22] examined 212 patients with internal carotid artery occlusion and found that the annual stroke rate in the territory of the occluded artery was 3%, with the presence of hypertension and diabetes increasing the risk of stroke. Before the widespread use of the duplex scanner, Durward et al[7] at the University of Western Ontario identified 73 patients with angiographically confirmed asymptomatic carotid stenosis in the artery contralateral to a prior endarterectomy. Of these, 30% went on to exhibit new cerebral ischemic symptoms, but the distribution was approximately equal between the operated side, the unoperated side, and the vertebrobasilar system. Roederer et al[28] examined the progression of disease in the carotid arteries contralateral to the endarterectomy. They found that the mean annual rate for progression to greater than 50% stenosis was 7.4% and that a strong association between the development of symptoms and progression to greater than 80% stenosis existed. Based on these findings, they recommended endarterectomy for patients without symptoms only when the lesion progressed to that level. Recently this policy was examined by Hatsukami et al,[11] who observed 200 patients for a mean period of 54 months after endarterectomy. Progression to 80% to 99% stenosis was found to occur at a rate of 1.2% per year on the unoperated side. Only 6 patients suffered stroke during the follow-up period. The authors concluded that a protocol of serial duplex examinations was appropriate and that in such patients, surgery should be undertaken only when symptoms or a stenosis of greater than 80% occur.

THERAPEUTIC RESULTS

Carotid endarterectomy is now an established therapy in the treatment of carotid stenosis. In centers with appropriate resources, Jonas and Hass[16] calculated that a perioperative stroke complication rate after surgery for TIAs should be less than 2.9% to successfully demonstrate the superiority of surgical over medical management. At the University of Washington Medical Center and the Seattle Veterans Administration Medical Center, the outcome for 115 patients with asymptomatic high-grade (80% to 99%) carotid stenosis was examined over a 4-year period.[19] A total of 56 carotid endarterectomies were performed in this group. Life-table analysis at 24 months revealed a higher rate of stroke (19% versus 4%), TIAs (28% versus 5%), and carotid occlusion (29% versus 0%) in the nonoperated group. The perioperative stroke rate was 1.8%, and there was no differen in the death rates between the operated and nonoperated groups. Roederer et al[26] determined that the degree of narrowing of the carotid siphon had no bearing on the outcome of endarterectomy. After the conclusion of a 7-year follow-up study, Healy et al[12] reported the results of 200 consecutive patients who had undergone carotid endarterectomy at the University of Washington Medical Center and the Seattle Veterans Administration Medical Center. The perioperative stroke rates were dependent on the indication for operation: 2.8% in those patients operated for stroke, 2.3% for TIAs, and 1.3% for asymptomatic high-grade stenosis. Using duplex scanning surveillance, Zierler et al[35] reported a postoperative high-grade restenosis rate of 19%, which is much higher than would be expected based on the observed recurrence of clinical symptoms. The lesion responsible for this is myointimal hyperplasia. It develops within months postoperatively and stabilizes after the first year. Recurrent stenoses after that time are usually due to atherosclerosis. Because most of the stenoses in this repoort were not associated with neurologic events, the authors concluded that myointimal hyperplastic lesions and atherosclerotic plaques differ in terms of their ability to produce ischemic cerebral events.

Recently, the results of two multicenter trials have supported the benefits of carotid endarterectomy in the treatment of carotid atherosclerotic stenosis. In February 1991, the North American Symptomatic Carotid Endarterectomy Trial (NASCET) determined that carotid endarterectomy was significantly more beneficial than medical management for patients with symptomatic high-grade (70% to 99%) carotid stenosis.[25] In the same month, the investigators participating in the European Carotid Surgery Trial (ECST) reported that surgery had shown a clear benefit over medical management in 778 patients showing symptoms with 70% to 99% carotid stenosis.[2] They found that although the perioperative stroke rate was 7.5% according to life-table analysis, operated patients faced an additional 2.8% risk of stroke over the following 3 years, but this risk was 16% in nonoperated patients ($p < 0.00001$).

CONCLUSION

The ultimate goal of carotid surgery for atherosclerosis is the prevention of stroke. Those patients with carotid stenosis have generalized atherosclerosis, and their risk of death from myocardial ischemia is higher than that for the general population. Nevertheless, the morbidity and mortality from stroke are signficant, and stroke prevention is made possible by carotid endarterectomy. The clinical history and physical examination are the first steps in evaluating the patient who is at risk for carotid stenosis. The finding of a bruit or a history consistent with TIAs or stroke should prompt further

assessment using duplex scanning. The advantage of this noninvasive screening test is that it allows clinical decisions to be made on the basis of the characterization of flow within the vessel lumen. Because of the higher risk of neurologic ischemic events described earlier, cervical angiography and carotid endarterectomy are recommended for patients without symptoms who are otherwise suitable for operation and who are found to have 80% to 99% stenosis during duplex examination. Those with less narrowing are closely monitored by duplex scans performed every 6 to 12 months. If the stenosis progresses to greater than 80%, endarterectomy is offered to the patient.

REFERENCES

1. Chambers B, Norris J: The case against surgery for asymptomatic carotid stenosis, *Stroke* 15:964, 1984.
2. Chambers B, Norris J: Outcome in patients with asymptomatic neck bruits, *N Engl J Med* 315:860, 1986.
3. Cooperman M, Martin E, Evans W: Significance of asymptomatic carotid bruits, *Arch Surg* 113:1339, 1978.
4. Crummy A: *Peripheral arteriography: some current considerations.* In Strandness DE et al, eds: *Vascular diseases: current research and clinical applications,* Orlando, Fla, 1987, Harcourt Brace Jovanovich.
5. David T et al: A correlation of neck bruits and arteriosclerotic carotid arteries, *Arch Surg* 107:729, 1973.
6. Dorazio R, Ezzet F, Nesbitt N: Long-term follow-up of asymptomatic carotid bruits, *Am J Surg* 140:212, 1980.
7. Durward QJ, Ferguson GG, Barr H: The natural history of asymptomatic carotid bifurcation plaques, *Stroke* 13:459, 1982.
8. Fell G et al: Importance of noninvasive ultrasonic-Doppler testing in the evaluation of patients with asymptomatic carotid bruits, *Am Heart J* 102:221, 1981.
9. Gee W, Mehigan JT, Wylie EJ: Measurement of collateral cerebral hemispheric blood pressure by ocular pneumoplethysmography, *Am J Surg* 130:121-125, 1975.
10. Hass W et al: Joint study of extracranial arterial occlusion. II. Arteriography, techniques, sites and complications, *JAMA* 203:961, 1968.
11. Hatsukami TS et al: Fate of the carotid artery contralateral to endarterectomy, *J Vasc Surg* 11:244, 1990.
12. Healy DA et al: Immediate and long-term results of carotid endarterectomy, *Stroke* 20:1138, 1989.
13. Heyman A et al: Risk of stroke in asymptomatic persons with cervical arterial bruits, *N Engl J Med* 302:838, 1980.
14. Javid H et al: Natural history of carotid bifurcation atheroma, *Surgery* 67(1):80, 1970.
15. Jonas S: Can carotid endarterectomy be justified? No, *Arch Neurol* 44:652, 1987.
16. Jonas S, Hass WK: An approach to the maximal acceptable stroke complication rate after surgery for transient cerebral ischemia (TIA), *Stroke* 10:104, 1979.
17. Kartchner M, McRae L: Noninvasive evaluation and management of the "asymptomatic" carotid bruit, *Surgery* 82:840, 1977.
18. Langlois YE, Roederer GO, Strandness DE: Ultrasonic evaluation of the carotid bifurcation, *Echocardiography* 4:141, 1987.
19. Moneta GL et al: Operative versus nonoperative management of asymptomatic high-grade internal carotid artery stenosis: improved results with endarterectomy, *Stroke* 18:1005, 1987.
20. Moneta GL et al: Asymptomatic high grade internal carotid artery stenosis: is stratification according to risk factors or duplex spectral analysis possible? *J Vasc Surg* 10:475, 1989.
21. MRC European Carotid Surgery Trial: Interim results for symptomatic patients with severe (70-99%) or with mild (0-29%) carotid stenosis, *Lancet* 337:1235, 1991.
22. Nicholls SC et al: Carotid artery occlusion: natural history, *J Vasc Surg* 4:479, 1986.
23. North American Symptomatic Carotid Endarterectomy Trial Collaborators: Beneficial effects of carotid endarterectomy in symptomatic patients with high-grade carotid stenosis, *N Engl J Med* 325:445, 1991.

24. Patterson R: Can carotid endarterectomy be justified? Yes, *Arch Neurol* 44:651-652, 1987.
25. Riles T et al: Symptoms, stenosis, and bruit, *Arch Surg* 116:218, 1981.
26. Roederer GO et al: Is siphon disease important in predicting outcome of carotid endarterectomy? *Arch Surg* 118:1177, 1983.
27. Roederer GO et al: Evolution of carotid arterial disease in asymptomatic patients with bruits, *Stroke* 15:605, 1984.
28. Roederer GO et al: Natural history of carotid artery disease on the side contralateral to endarterectomy, *J Vasc Surg* 1:62, 1984.
29. Roederer GO et al: A simple spectral parameter for accurate classification of severe carotid disease, *Bruit* 8:174, 1984.
30. Sumner D et al: Digital subtraction angiography: intravenous and intra-arterial techniques, *J Vasc Surg* 2(2):244, 1985.
31. Taylor D, Strandness DE: Carotid artery duplex scanning, *J Clin Ultrasound* 15:635, 1987.
32. Thompson J, Patman D, Persson AV: Management of asymptomatic carotid bruits, *Am Surg* 42:77, 1976.
33. Wolf P et al: Asymptomatic carotid bruit and risk of stroke: the Framingham study, *JAMA* 245:1442, 1981.
34. Ziegler DK et al: Correlation of bruits over the carotid artery with angiographically demonstrated lesions, *Neurology* 21:860, 1971.
35. Zierler RE et al: Carotid artery stenosis following endarterectomy, *Arch Surg* 117:1408, 1982.

CHAPTER 46

Arterial wall thickness with high-resolution B-mode imaging

DAVID L. DAWSON and D. EUGENE STRANDNESS, JR.

The noninvasive nature of ultrasound scanning makes it a useful tool for detecting arterial disease, but the usual duplex scanning methods are inadequate for some research applications. The pulsed Doppler cannot detect early changes in the artery wall because there are no distinct changes in flow that can be used to differentiate normal from minimally diseased vessels, but with improvements in imaging, it has become possible to examine the artery wall to identify early changes. This method is being used increasingly in clinical laboratories to investigate the development of atherosclerosis.

Changes in the thickness of the arterial wall are thought to represent the earliest sonographic evidence of developing atherosclerosis. Measurements of the double line representing intima-media thickness (IMT) are one way of assessing changes in wall thickness (Fig. 46-1). Although useful, this technique requires that the operator decide where to make the measurement. A system has been developed that permits computerized analysis of high-resolution B-mode images of arterial walls. The images are acquired from a plane where a vein and artery are adjacent and have an echogenic vessel wall complex located between two hypoechoic lumen regions. This echogenic region includes all layers of both the artery and the vein. If the vein is thin and does not vary in thickness because of arterial disease, the computer-generated measurement of the distance from lumen to lumen indirectly represents the total arterial thickness (Fig. 46-2). When used to assess arterial segments not affected by focal atherosclerotic disease (plaques), this measurement can then be used to evaluate generalized wall thickness changes in both normal subjects and patients with arterial disease.

USES OF B-MODE IMAGING IN ARTERIAL IMAGING
Vessel identification

The principal application of the B-mode image in conventional duplex scanning is for identifying blood vessels and examining the anatomic features of the region being examined. Specific identification of the vessel by B-mode imaging permits accurate placement of the pulsed-Doppler sample volume. This is the key advantage of duplex scanning over simpler continuous wave Doppler instruments. In clinical practice, the Doppler data (e.g., waveform characteristics, spectral width, and amplitude of the systolic and diastolic frequency shift) obtained from areas of disease have proved to be effective means of establishing the degree of stenosis. Doppler findings have been shown to correlate with the arteriographic grading of stenosis severity.[19,22,38]

Grading the severity of arterial disease on the basis of Doppler information has proved useful for several reasons: (1) the criteria for grading stenoses are quantifiable, (2) comparable interpretations can be made by different examiners, (3) interpretable Doppler spectra are often obtainable even when there is a suboptimal image, and (4) Doppler-derived information has proved reliable for clinical decision-making.[14,21]

Gross pathologic changes

In some ways, B-mode imaging and arteriography provide similar information: they can localize atherosclerotic plaques, measure residual lumen width, and identify vessel wall irregularities. The B-mode image, however, may be more sensitive for detecting minimal and moderate disease (less than 50% stenosis). Arteriography provides only a picture of the luminal surface, whereas ultrasound identifies some of the changes in the wall secondary to atherosclerosis.[32]

The displayed B-mode image lends itself to direct measurement, and all modern scanners have electronic caliper functions and software packages for making distance measurements. The dimensions of arterial lesions can be directly determined. However, for grading the severity of clinically significant stenoses, B-mode imaging lacks the accuracy of either duplex scanning with pulsed Doppler spectral waveform analysis or arteriography.* Conversely, duplex scanning is less accurate for grading minimal stenoses. Wall irregularities or lesions that are not associated with abrupt or large changes in luminal diameter may also not be associated with increased blood flow velocities. Grading the

---

This work was supported in part by grant HL 42270-03 from the National Institutes of Health, Bethesda, Md.

*References 19, 20, 22, 24, 38, 43.

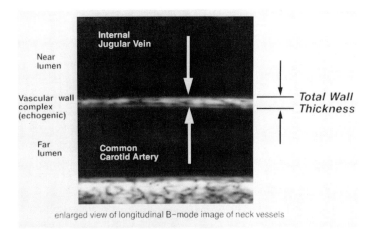

enlarged view of longitudinal B–mode image of neck vessels

Fig. 46-1. This B-mode image of the common carotid artery and adjacent internal jugular vein shows the low echo density vessel lumens and the echogenic vessel wall complex. In this normal 32-year-old subject, the intima-media double line can be seen in both the near and far arterial walls, though the far wall double line is clearer. No distinct sonographic features identify the outer boundary of the arterial adventitia. In the vascular wall complex, the outer arterial adventitia and vein have homogeneous echogenicity. In the opposite arterial wall the outer adventitia blends imperceptibly with the surrounding soft tissue echo pattern.

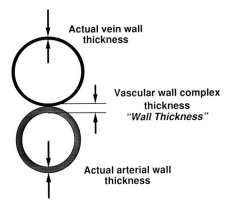

Fig. 46-2. Wall thickness measured between the venous and arterial blood-intima interfaces enables total arterial wall thickening to be assessed but assumes the vein wall is thin with respect to that of the artery, not changing in thickness with arterial disease, and relatively constant.

severity of spectral broadening caused by flow disturbance in areas of less severe disease remains subjective and difficult to quantify accurately.

Arterial wall features

Plaque ulceration. Many investigators have postulated that ulceration in carotid artery plaques is important in the pathogenesis of thromboembolic disease and that therefore the detection of arterial ulcers would be useful diagnostically. However, there is no evidence to support this assertion. In multicenter trials, the ability of both B-mode imaging and arteriography to identify ulceration in atheromatous lesions has been disappointing.[13,23,32]

Plaque composition. Efforts to stratify patients' risk of exhibiting future thromboembolic symptoms have prompted

attempts to correlate the composition of plaques with their sonographic appearance. Plaques identified by B-mode imaging can be characterized as either homogeneous or heterogeneous. Homogeneous plaques exhibit a uniform echo pattern and a smooth covering. Heterogeneous plaques have a nonuniform echo pattern and anechoic areas within the lesion, calcification that results in shadowing, and an irregular surface. Reilly et al[31] examined specimens removed at the time of carotid endarterectomy and found that 91% of the heterogeneous lesions had intraplaque hemorrhage and 100% of the ulcerated lesions displayed a heterogeneous ultrasound appearance. In 82% (41 of 50) of the specimens, ultrasound had correctly identified the existence of intraplaque hemorrhage. However, large amounts of lipid in the lesions can also mimic the appearance of intraplaque hemorrhage. Bluth et al[4] encountered similar results when they prospectively evaluated the ability of ultrasound to detect intraplaque hemorrhage in carotid lesions. The correlation of the sonographic and pathologic findings (heterogeneous appearance and intraplaque hemorrhage) with the presence of embolic symptoms was poor, however. In the patients with heterogeneous plaques, 65% had symptoms, but 52% of those with homogeneous plaques were symptomatic. Thus to date, the plaque features revealed by ultrasound have not been of great importance in clinical decision making. Stenosis severity as indicated by velocity changes remains the best predictor of those carotid lesions most likely to be the source of clinical events.[33]

Plaque thickness. The thickness of atherosclerotic plaques undoubtedly has an important bearing on the severity of disease, and it is well known that the risk of thromboembolic events in patients with carotid artery disease depends on the severity of the carotid artery stenosis. This holds true for both asymptomatic and previously symptomatic lesions.[23,33]

Plaque thickness, which is measured with high-resolution ultrasound, correlates with the arteriographic assessment of stenosis severity, but in a study by Dempsey et al,[11] the plaque thickness at the carotid bifurcation was found to be an even better predictor of transient ischemic attacks. It is theorized that thicker plaques are more likely to have intraplaque hemorrhage or necrosis, and the flow disturbance produced at the site of stenosis may then lead to further platelet accumulation and deposition of thrombus. Material from either the contents or surface of the plaque can then embolize and cause symptoms.

Some investigators have used the summation of plaque thicknesses from several arbitrarily defined locations to yield a "plaque score," from which they grade the severity of atherosclerosis in the carotid arteries.[10,16]

Arterial wall thickness. Pignoli,[28] at the University of Milan, was the first to correlate the sonographic features of the arterial wall to thickness measurements obtained in fixed specimens. He found a characteristic double line on images of normal or moderately diseased arteries and determined that the distance from the leading edge of the first line to the leading edge of the second line represented the combined thicknesses of the intima and media of the arterial wall. The bright ultrasound reflections are generated by the changes in acoustic impedance between the blood-filled lumen and the intima, followed by the transition from the outer media to the adventitia. As these interfaces act as specular reflectors when imaged *en face,* the double line of Pignoli is best seen with the scan head placed orthogonally to the vessel. This orientation also exploits the superior axial (depth) resolution of the ultrasound instruments. Because linear array transducers have a wider aperture than sector scan heads, they produce this specular reflection over a longer vessel segment and can more clearly image this double line.

The IMT measurement requires no special equipment or technique and has been used by a number of investigators.* The double line is easiest to demonstrate and measure in the common carotid artery because this vessel is straight, superficial, and parallel to the skin. However, it can also be seen in most large and medium-sized arteries in the trunk and extremities. Although the double line is often seen in both the superficial and deep arterial wall, measurements of IMT are most accurate when limited to the deep wall.[29,40,41]

The width of the intima-media double line is useful to know but represents only a partial measurement of the total arterial wall thickness. Currently there is no noninvasive technique that can measure the total thickness of all layers of an artery because there are no distinct sonographic features that identify the outer boundary of the adventitia, which blends imperceptibly with the surrounding soft tissue echo pattern.

DETECTION OF SUBCLINICAL CHANGES IN THE ARTERIAL WALL
Early changes of atherosclerosis

For the detection of the earliest atherosclerotic changes in arteries, only noninvasive studies using ultrasound techniques are of any value. Arteriography is inappropriate as a screening method for clinical research in an asymptomatic population. Other methods, such as angioscopy or intravascular ultrasound, are also associated with risk, discomfort, or costs that are too high to warrant their use for clinical screening or most research applications. Current computerized tomography and magnetic resonance imaging systems lack the resolution needed for assessing small changes in the arterial wall. The "gold standard" method for making vascular diagnosis—contrast arteriography—may be insensitive to the earliest arterial changes of atherosclerosis, since luminal size may be preserved by dilatation of the arterial diameter during the early stages of wall thickening.[15,42] The research group at the University of Washington and others have hypothesized that the determination of wall thickness changes may be the best means of detecting and quantifying the early development of atherosclerosis.

Identification of high-risk individuals

The early identification of patients with minimal atherosclerosis might allow the initiation of intervention at a stage when the disease could be reversed. Risk-factor modification could then be directed at those most likely to benefit from it. This would be more likely to succeed in such patients than it would in those patients with far-advanced complicated plaques since there is much doubt that such lesions can regress. Simple sonographic screening to detect the early changes in the arterial wall would be a useful tool for identifying those patients who would most likely benefit from early interventions such as a lipid-lowering regimen.

The association between clinically significant carotid artery disease and coronary artery disease has been known for a while. Craven et al[7] carried out B-mode ultrasound assessment of the common and internal carotid artery thickness in 510 patients who also underwent coronary angiography. The sonographic evidence of carotid artery disease, even in the absence of hemodynamically significant or symptomatic internal carotid stenosis, was found to be a strong, consistent, and independent marker for coronary artery disease (at least 50% stenosis in one or more coronary arteries) in patients over 50 years of age. They concluded that data from carotid ultrasound imaging can supplement clinical risk-factor assessment in identifying those at risk for having coronary artery disease. The small changes in the wall thickness of the carotid artery that are now measurable with high-resolution ultrasound may thus be a relatively simple way of quantifying the systemic arterial effects of a generalized atherogenic process.

Noninvasively detected lower extremity atherosclerosis, even in subjects who do not display symptoms, is associated

---

*References 1, 5, 6, 18, 27, 29, 30, 36, 40, 41.

with a four to five times higher mortality rate than for those without detectable arterial disease. The significance of peripheral artery disease was found to be independent of other cardiovascular risk factors when subjected to multivariate analysis.[9]

Natural history of atherosclerosis

The outcomes in patients with atherosclerotic diseases, including coronary artery disease, are currently being evaluated in NIH-funded, multicenter, population-based cohort studies, such as the Cardiovascular Health Study and the Atherosclerosis Risk in Community Study.[1,9]

Clinical trials

In addition to use in epidemiologic studies of atherosclerosis development in large populations, measurements of arterial wall thickening offer promise as surrogate end points for prospective studies and clinical trials. A primary end point assesses clinical benefit, whereas surrogate end points are an index of a part of the disease process.[6,41] Quantifiable surrogate end points that reflect the disease process may yield statistically meaningful results for smaller and shorter clinical trials. Using "hard" primary end points (for example, events such as myocardial infarction or death) requires large numbers of patients to be observed for many years, but changes in arterial walls may occur earlier and be quantified.

Measurement techniques sensitive to changes in arterial wall thickness of less than 1 mm can detect progression or regression of vessel abnormalities far earlier than would be recognized solely through the presence or absence of symptoms.

The direct assessment of arterial changes allows treatment regimens to be tested in selected patients who remain free of symptoms. Patients with hyperlipidemia frequently have demonstrable atherosclerosis before they develop symptoms.[34] The amount of atherosclerosis,[11] as defined by the severity of arterial wall or surface changes, can therefore be assessed before and after a therapeutic trial. The effects of lipid-lowering drugs in preventing or reversing arterial changes can be evaluated, even in younger patients who are symptom free.

In addition to detecting changes in the thickness of the common carotid artery wall resulting from atherosclerosis, there is a potential role for reliable and quantitative assessments of vessel wall thickness in other sites of the circulation. Intimal thickening in vascular grafts and recurrent stenoses after endarterectomy are serious clinical problems. A means of quantifying the pathologic changes is necessary if the results of new pharmacologic interventions are to be accurately evaluated.

TOTAL ARTERIAL WALL THICKNESS MEASUREMENT
Methods

Because no direct sonographic measurement of arterial wall thickness is possible, a strategy that involves indirectly measuring the total arterial thickness by measuring the lumen-to-lumen distance of both the artery and its adjacent vein can be used. This lumen-to-lumen measurement of the echogenic vascular wall complex ("total wall thickness") yields a sonographic approximation of the complete thickness of the arterial wall. This method exploits the clear definition of the lumen-intima and intima-lumen interfaces seen with conventional B-mode imaging techniques. It is also assumed that atherosclerosis does not affect the thickness of the venous wall. Factors that diffusely affect changes in the arterial wall structure can thus be examined.

The imaging plane must pass through both the artery and adjacent vein to measure total wall thickness (Figs. 46-3 and 46-4), and the selected scan plane must intersect the axes of both vessels to avoid tangential sectioning of the wall. Because of the method of image analysis and to take advantage of the superior depth resolution of ultrasound, the vessel wall complex is oriented horizontally in the image.

The total wall thickness measurement system has two components (Fig. 46-5). First, B-mode images are acquired and the composite video output is stored on videotape. These images are then captured and digitized, and the region of the image that contains the vascular wall complex is selected and analyzed. The software algorithms used have focused on overall vessel wall thickening; details of wall irregularity are not evaluated (Fig. 46-6).

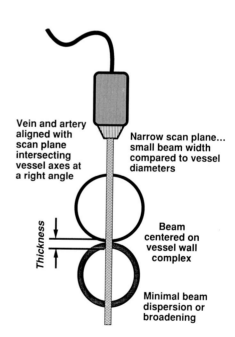

Fig. 46-3. A narrow, well-focused scan plane and proper alignment of the scan plane with the vessels are needed to measure total wall thickness. This alignment can be confirmed with rotation of the transducer to image the vessels in transverse section. Because refraction and other effects degrade lateral resolution, vessel wall features are best demonstrated with the scan plane rotated to image the vessels in longitudinal section.

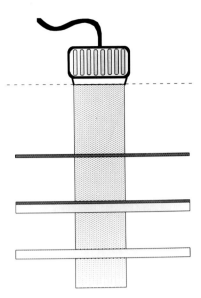

Fig. 46-4. Positioning the transducer 90° to the vessels optimizes image quality and reduces measurement variability.

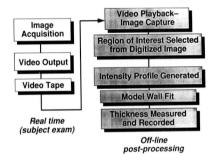

Fig. 46-5. Flow chart illustrating the components of the total wall thickness measurement system.

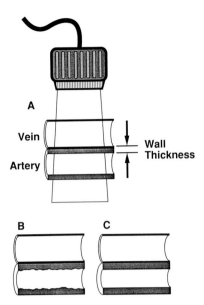

Fig. 46-6. Imaging and measurement of total wall thickness. **A,** Because image brightness (echo strength) is averaged over a selected horizontal segment of the image, uniform thickening with wall irregularity **(B)** may not be distinguished from that with smooth luminal surfaces **(C).** Identifying extremely fine details of wall irregularity depends on image quality. Excluding such considerations makes a measurement technique more robust and therefore usable in a greater number of images.

In the second component, offline analysis of the video images is performed using a custom software routine on a computer with an image-processing board. The captured images are digitized and displayed on a monitor, and the operator selects the measurement locations by positioning cursors on the screen (Figs. 46-7 and 46-8). Within the image region selected, an image profile is generated. The average pixel intensity (or echo strength) in each horizontal video line is plotted across the depth axis. This plot includes the low echo–near lumen, the vessel wall complex, and the low echo–far lumen. Using a least-squares regression algorithm, the intensity profile is fit to an idealized wall model, and the thickness is calculated from this.

One advantage of this line-by-line analysis of average echo intensity is that it does not depend directly on the resolution of the ultrasound system. (*Resolution* is the minimum distance between points that is required to identify the points as separate.) This computerized thickness measurement technique looks for transitions from low to high

and from high to low echo intensity within the selected region and identifies the transitions in echo strength as the locations of the interfaces. Because it does not require point-to-point discrimination, its accuracy can theoretically exceed the resolving power of the ultrasound instrument. Another advantage of the method is that the intensity information is averaged over each horizontal video line. Even if there is degradation of the video image quality due to tape tracking errors during tape playback, the recorded information in each line of the video field is preserved and measurements of total wall thickness do not suffer.

Total arterial wall thickness can be measured in several locations. In almost all cases, the superficial femoral (Fig. 46-9) and common carotid arteries can be successfully imaged and measured. These vessels are large, have segments that are straight, and have a parallel accompanying vein. These vessels were chosen for study after initial research showed the practicality of their measurement and because the carotid and femoral arteries are common sites where atherosclerosis develops.

Standard scanning techniques are used to acquire the images, and instrumentation and scanning methods are optimized for the region being studied. Studies have used an Acuson 128 duplex scanner with a 7.5-MHz linear array transducer for imaging, but this method of offline image processing and computer measurement is applicable with any high-resolution scanner (Fig. 46-10).

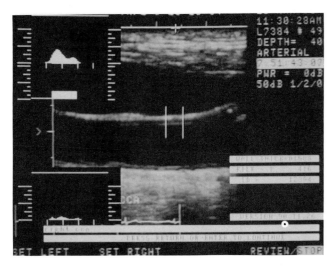

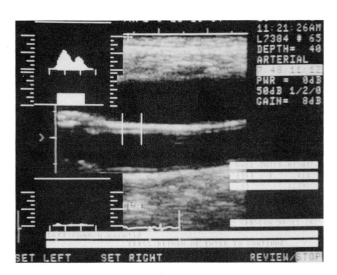

Fig. 46-7. This computer-processed image superimposes measurement information over the recorded B-mode image of the common carotid artery and internal jugular vein. The operator has selected the thickness measurement site, the region between the two parallel vertical lines that cross the vascular wall complex. The curve in the upper left is a histogram displaying pixel brightness (echo strength) averaged across each horizontal video line. The block below the brightness curve is the computer's model of the wall, from which the thickness measurement is made. The wall thickness measurement and identifying data are displayed on the monitor and recorded to a data file or other output device.

Fig. 46-8. This common carotid artery shows wall thickening. The intima-media double line appears widened in both the near and far arterial walls. The total wall thickness is significantly greater than age-matched controls. The thickening of the intima-media can also be recognized by the prominent second peak in the brightness profile shown in the upper left.

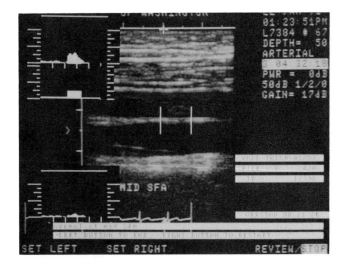

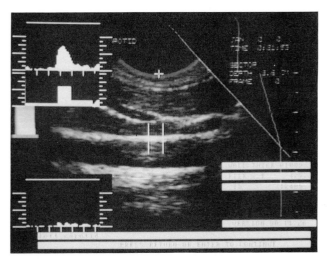

Fig. 46-9. Wall thickness measurement in a normal superficial femoral artery. The total thickness in this subject measures 0.125 mm. Scanning from the anteromedial thigh, the vein is deep to the artery (a valve cusp is visible in the vein lumen). The intima-media double line can be seen in the deep wall of the artery, and this is also reflected in the intensity profile (upper left).

Fig. 46-10. A sector scanning transducer can also be used with the total wall thickness measurement system. The measurement is made in the middle of the image as arterial wall features are best imaged with the incident ultrasound at 90° to the vessel wall. The intima-blood interface acts as a specular reflector and produces a brighter B-mode image where the scan lines intersect the vessel at a right angle.

Validation

Beach et al[3] initially described the technique of validation in 1989. These investigators demonstrated that the thickness of a variety of test materials, measured with this total wall thickness measurement technique correlated well to the caliper-measured physical thicknesses.

The repeatability of the total wall thickness measurements obtained from normal vessels that could be clearly imaged was assessed. The computer and software algorithm, as well as the variability introduced by the operator in selecting regions to be measured, was examined by repeatedly measuring thicknesses from the same recorded image. In addition, the repeatability of the technologist's selection of a scan plane and imaging location was evaluated through the repeated image acquisition at the same anatomic location.

The right and left common carotid arteries were each imaged 10 times, and 10 measurements were made from each image; the mean thickness values obtained were 1.22 and 1.24 mm, respectively. Within-image repeatability is reflected by the standard deviation for multiple measurements of a single image. The average standard deviations for the 10 series of measurements were 0.04 and 0.07, respectively, for the right and left common carotids. Scan head repositioning adds 15% to 40% more noise to the measurement data spread. The 95% confidence intervals are only 0.3 mm wide, and most measurements fall in a ±1 video pixel range. The findings from these variability studies suggest that differences in thickness of less than 0.1 mm can be detected with this technique, but serial studies require unvarying instrument setup and special techniques to ensure correct scan head repositioning. However, it is also important to keep in mind that these were normal vessels and that irregularities in the vessel wall or poor image quality will add to the variability in measurements.

Limitations of wall thickness measurements

Although IMT can be measured on images obtained with standard ultrasound techniques, the methods used have varied among different investigators. These differences in measurement strategies must be recognized when comparing different studies and consist of the following: First, thickness measurements may be made at a single location, or the measurements from several locations may be summed or averaged. Second, some investigators measure the thickness between two selected points on the double lines; others trace the double lines along a selected segment and then use a computer to calculate the average and maximum thickness. Third, although far-wall double lines are the most distinct, some investigators measure both the near and far walls. Fourth, scan plane and measurement point selection protocols may differ between centers.

When multiple locations are measured, several values are often averaged, thus detracting from the point accuracy of the test. If some of the measurement points of the protocol are not well visualized, these values may be excluded from the averages reported, thus potentially biasing the data.

Because atherosclerotic plaques are eccentric and irregular, any ultrasound technique that requires positioning the transducer and scanning from a predetermined location or scanning limited to a specific plane through the vessel is a poor tool for characterizing focal plaque. Figs. 46-11 and 46-12 illustrate this problem. The thickness of the arterial wall at a location that has changes other than concentric thickening varies depending on the scan plane used. A thicker measurement is obtained if the plane intersects the middle rather than the edge of the plaque.

A measurement of total wall thickness can accurately

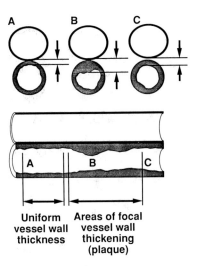

Fig. 46-11. Total wall thickness measurements can provide an assessment of generalized arterial changes even in a subject with established atherosclerosis if there are areas of the artery that have uniform vessel wall thickness (**A**). Areas with focal thickening of the artery wall (plaque formation) (**B** and **C**) are less representative and subject to measurement variability because of the eccentric and irregular nature of atherosclerotic plaque formation.

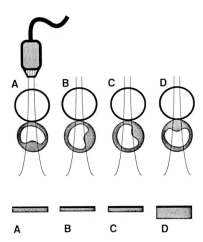

Fig. 46-12. The measurement of total arterial wall thickness is feasible only when the scan plane intersects the artery and adjacent vein at 90°. There would be little or no difference in the measured thicknesses of **A, B,** and **C** because eccentric plaque is not situated on the part of the artery's circumference where the measurement is taken. Only in **D** would the plaque's thickness contribute to the measured total wall thickness.

reflect changes in arterial morphology only when it is used to measure changes in vessels before focal plaque formation. If used in a subject who already has atherosclerotic plaques, meaningful measurements of total wall thickness can only be acquired if the anatomic locations examined are not affected by plaque development (Fig. 46-13).

Although common carotid artery total wall thickness can be measured, the total wall thickness measurement techniques do not work well at many other sites. Imaging and measurement of the superficial femoral artery in the mid-

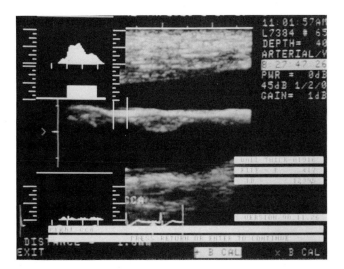

Fig. 46-13. If there is established atherosclerotic disease with the formation of focal areas of plaque (such as in this common carotid artery), wall thickness measurements may reflect local changes in the arterial wall rather than any systemic effects. The measurement site chosen here, however, is separated from the prominent near-wall plaque, and it may better reflect the generalized changes in arterial wall thickness occurring with atherosclerosis.

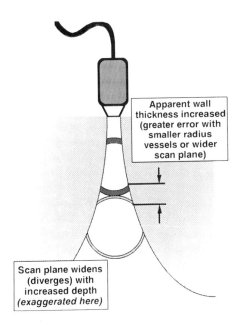

Apparent wall thickness increased (greater error with smaller radius vessels or wider scan plane)

Scan plane widens (diverges) with increased depth (exaggerated here)

Fig. 46-14. Measurement errors are potentially introduced if the scan plane intersecting the vascular wall complex is wide in relation to the vessel diameters. Using a transducer with a wide beam or scanning smaller diameter vessels (such as the posterior tibial or the brachial arteries) or deeply situated vessels may degrade wall thickness measurement accuracy.

thigh have proved quite satisfactory, but in the adductor canal region, depth and myofascial tissue planes frequently degrade image quality and compromise the accuracy of measurements. Because of vessel curvature and an inconstant relationship with the accompanying vein, brachial and popliteal arteries are frequently not measurable. Small vessels

such as the posterior tibials at the ankle level are easily imaged, but the small diameter of the vessels with respect to both their wall thickness and the imaging ultrasound beam width limits reliable measurement of the total vessel wall thickness (Fig. 46-14).

The technique of total wall thickness measurement is not designed to measure plaque thickness but only the combined arterial and venous wall thickness at one point on the circumference of the artery. Total wall thickness is measured only in locations free of focal plaque. At first this strategy may seem to contradict the usual clinical objective. Vascular diagnostic techniques assess disease where it is the most severe, since the detection, localization, and characterization of the severity of stenoses are what is needed for planning treatment. For research purposes, however, the detection of small subclinical changes becomes important, and thus the difference in approach.

COMPUTERIZED IMAGE ANALYSIS IN VASCULAR DIAGNOSIS

The value of any system that examines early arterial disease depends on its ability to objectively analyze image features and reliably quantify the severity of pathologic changes. Computerized image analysis and computer-assisted measurement of image features have been used to lessen any subjective observer variability.

Salonen et al[3] compared the intraobserver and interobserver variability of IMT measurements obtained using operator-positioned electronic calipers on images of the common carotid arteries of 10 middle-aged subjects. Among the four scanning technologists and physicians who participated in this study, they found a mean absolute difference between repetitive measurements of less than 0.1 mm. In a two-way analysis of variance, 96% of the variation in IMT measurement was attributable to interobserver variability and 4% to intraobserver variability. This suggests that the observer-dependent recognition of vessel wall features in the B-mode image can be quite consistent, but despite close communication and cooperation, individuals from even a single research group can exhibit subtle differences in their interpretation of images. This reinforces the need for developing an automated image-analysis system that uses simple and reliable algorithms for the measurement of arterial wall features.

Computer-assisted evaluation of arteriographic features

To reproducibly quantify subclinical changes in arterial disorders, investigators in the United States and Europe have used computer-aided image analysis of the arteriographic features of vessel walls.[8] Using computer-analyzed femoral arteriograms to estimate the decrease in arterial luminal volume, Olsson[26] evaluated a small group of subjects being treated for hyperlipidemia. Studies obtained at 6-month intervals demonstrated objective improvement after 1 year. Barndt et al,[2] at the University of Southern California, studied changes in early femoral artery atherosclerosis in 25 hyperlipidemic patients. Because only 1 of their patients had claudication, clinical end points were not sensitive enough to assess therapeutic responses. These investigators measured arterial wall edge roughness, detected by a computerized image-processing system, in combination with observations by a radiologist, to compare pretreatment and posttreatment femoral arteriograms. Use of the computerized "image dissector" yielded an objective and quantifiable index of minimal and moderate arterial wall irregularity. Follow-up angiographic studies obtained at an average interval of 13 months showed that lowering elevated blood pressure and serum lipid levels with diet and drug therapy brought about regression of early atherosclerotic changes. In a randomized, controlled trial, Duffield et al[12] used a computer-generated edge-irregularity index with visual interpretation of serial arteriographic studies to assess femoral artery atherosclerosis in 24 hyperlipidemic patients with intermittent claudication. Patients were observed for a mean of only 19 months, but by using arteriographic assessment as an end point, they were able to show that the therapy instituted to normalize LDL-cholesterol levels slowed the progression of disease by 60% compared to controls.

Arteriographic studies have several limitations. Besides the discomfort and morbidity risk involved, arteriography has several technical requirements that must be considered when it is used for the serial evaluation of arterial disease: (1) the films must be biplanar to assess the three-dimensional nature of atherosclerotic changes; (2) contrast concentration, doses, and injection rates must be constant from study to study; (3) patient positioning must be identical from visit to visit; and (4) all radiographic and film parameters must be the same.

Computer-assisted evaluation of sonographic features

Computer-assisted measurements of the arterial IMT—Pignoli's double-line measurement—have been developed by several groups. Image capture and computer-aided measurements have facilitated this measurement, allow IMT measurement along segments (rather than points) of the arterial wall, and permit direct recording of large amounts of measurement information into computer files, which can be retrieved later for data analysis. Offline computerized analysis of IMTs allows a single center to interpret ultrasound data gathered from several institutions. The Atherosclerosis Risk in Communities Study and the Cardiovascular Health Study, now ongoing, are using computerized routines to automate the calculation of IMT and lumen width.[1,25]

In the Cardiovascular Health Study, digitized images have luminal, media-adventitia, and adventitia-periadventitia interfaces that are manually outlined by a trained reader. By outlining these interfaces over a short segment (rather than making single point-to-point measurements), examiners can obtain calculations of thickness and lumen dimensions as well as their mean and maximum values.[25] The computer calculates the measurements, and the reader remains responsible for identifying the interfaces. The inter-reader variability in producing these measurements, however, is less than the variability introduced during repeated image acquisition, whether by one or more sonographers. A mean difference of only 0.10 ± 0.14 mm SD was obtained in repeated measurements of the maximum thickness of the far wall of the common carotid artery. This approaches the depth resolution capabilities of the 6.7-MHz ultrasound probes used in this study.

Several other research groups employ similar computer-assisted IMT measurement methods and use operator-controlled input devices (e.g., mouse, digitizing tablet) to mark the location of features of interest (such as the edges of the intima-media double lines) on digitized ultrasound images. Wendelhag et al[39,40] in Gothenberg, Sweden, measure the carotid artery IMT, luminal diameter, and plaque area. This method measures the mean and maximum thickness of a 10-mm segment of the intima-media complex in the deep wall of the artery. Repeat measurements obtained from 50 subjects yielded a coefficient of variation for mean and maximum thickness of 10.2% and 8.9%, respectively. This system was also used by Persson et al[27] to measure both carotid and femoral arteries. They found a similar reproducibility with a 10.0% coefficient of variation for IMT measurements of the common carotid artery. The superficial femoral arteries could not be as well imaged, and they found the intima-media double lines were less distinct. The coefficient of variation for the femoral artery was 16.2%. In both studies, repeated measurements of luminal diameter and plaque area displayed more variability than measurement of the IMT.

Pignoli et al[28,29] measure IMT in the deep wall, summing measurements from nonoverlapping images to get an average IMT for the entire common carotid artery. With repeated measures, they found that the average difference in duplicate thickness determinations was 4.6%.

Using similar techniques for offline image capture and computer-aided measurement, Finnish investigators have reported making point-to-point measurements of IMT that have exhibited excellent repeatability.[35] In their technique, three measurements from the far wall of both common carotid arteries where the IMT appears thickest are averaged. To test their method, they performed repeated scanning and calculations of IMT 1 week apart in 49 male subjects, and the mean difference in the IMT measured was found to be only 0.03 ± 0.09 mm SD. A single technologist performed the scans and a single observer made the measurements. Eliminating interobserver variability is an important part of optimizing measurement accuracy.

Results of multicenter studies

The need for more objective means of quantifying sonographic measurements of arterial wall features was demonstrated by a multicenter trial that examined the capabilities of high-resolution B-mode imaging for detecting and categorizing atherosclerotic lesions. Although O'Leary et al[24] evaluated five centers and found moderately good within-reader agreement on serial measurements of B-mode scans of diseased carotid arteries, between-reader agreement was poor. For example, the mean absolute difference in repeated measurements of total lesion width (plaque thickness) was 0.81 mm when performed by a single observer, but averaged 1.3 mm when two readers were involved. The repeatability of B-mode measurement was inferior to that of arteriography. This was in large part due to B-mode images being measured from static recorded images and the observer making the measurements not examining the vessel in real-time. These investigators noted that IMT measurement variability was reduced when the measurements were done in real-time by the scanning technologist or physician. Slight changes in transducer position or scanning technique can also alter images significantly. Automating measurements could decrease interobserver measurement variability, but by its nature, ultrasound scanning is still operator dependent for scan head positioning and image selection.

Future application within instrument software packages

Digital signal processing, image enhancement, digitized color and gray-scale display, and computerized data processing are the norm in modern arteriography and sonography systems. The image-processing and measurement software routines that have been used by investigators to measure wall thickness and other B-mode features could all be incorporated into future generations of ultrasound scanners. This would allow direct analysis of the raw data acquired by the imaging system. To date, however, all these specialized programs are run on desktop computer systems with capture of video images and offline processing.

FACTORS AFFECTING CAROTID ARTERY THICKNESS
Intima-media thickness

Age. The arterial wall thickening that occurs with aging is a consistent observation, and several studies have identified it as the principal factor associated with increasing wall thickness. Based on measurements of the carotid artery IMT, several studies have demonstrated an increase in thickness with age.[16-18,30,37]

Gender. Patient sex does not appear to be an independent factor associated with arterial wall thickening.[30]

Hypertension. In a study of 12 patients with untreated, newly diagnosed hypertension (diastolic blood pressure ranging from 95 to 106), the IMT of the common carotid artery was identical to that of age-matched controls, although echocardiographic findings of left ventricular thickening were noted, thus furnishing objective evidence of the cardiovascular significance of hypertension.[17] Kawamori et al[18] found blood pressure had no significant effect on carotid artery IMT in nondiabetic Japanese but, when multivariate regression analysis was applied, found a small increase in IMT in diabetic subjects with hypertension compared to nonhypertensive diabetics. Another Japanese study also found no correlation between hypertension and wall thickening.[16]

Hyperlipidemia. In a cross-sectional population-based study conducted in Eastern Finland, Salonen et al[37] examined 412 men, ages 42, 48, 54, and 60 years. Overall, 37% showed intima-media thickening (defined as an IMT greater than 1.2 mm), and this appeared to be age related. An elevated LDL-cholesterol level was associated with IMT thickening in this population, and this remained an independent predictor of carotid disease, even when age; body mass; serum LDL-, HDL_2-, and HDL-cholesterol levels; plasma fibrinogen concentration; cigarette-smoking years; and years of hypertension were accounted for in a multivariate regression model.

Wendelhag et al[39,40] compared the carotid artery IMTs obtained in 53 subjects with familial hypercholesterolemia to those obtained from 53 control subjects matched for age, gender, and body habitus. They found a significantly greater IMT in the hypercholesterolemic patients. Over a 10-mm segment of the carotid artery, the mean IMT was 0.13 mm greater, and the maximum IMT averaged 0.20 mm more in those with familial hypercholesterolemia.

Diabetes mellitus. Diabetes is associated with an increased IMT in the carotid arteries. In those with diabetes, the IMT is greater than that in age-matched controls. This arterial wall thickening seems to be greater in diabetics with poor glucose control or those requiring insulin.[18]

Smoking. The effect of cigarette smoking on IMT as a single controlled variable has not been studied, and there are no clear data to show that smokers have thicker arterial walls than nonsmokers.[16,30,40] However, an increased rate of wall thickening in smokers has been observed.[35] Cigarette smoking also seems to have an effect when combined with elevated serum lipid levels. In a study of patients with type IIa hyperlipidemia, Poli et al[30] found a significantly greater common carotid artery IMT in smokers than in nonsmokers.

Factors affecting progression of disease. Ultrasound techniques are especially useful for performing serial evaluations to monitor the natural history of arterial disease. Salonen and Salonen[35] monitored the course of 100 middle-aged Finnish men over a 2-year period and assessed the progression of common carotid arterial wall thickness. An increase in IMT was seen in 83% of the subjects and regression in 9%. The mean IMT increased by 12% over the 24 months of follow-up. They identified age, serum LDL-cholesterol levels, smoking, blood leukocyte count, and platelet aggregation as predictors of atherosclerosis progression, but blood pressure (or a history of hypertension) and serum HDL-cholesterol levels showed no association with the change in IMT at the end of 2 years.

UNIVERSITY OF WASHINGTON STUDIES: WALL THICKNESS PROJECT DATA

After performing initial pilot studies, total wall thickness measurements were used to evaluate both normal volunteers and those with established or subclinical atherosclerosis. Strict selection criteria were used to define the normal controls, who consisted of 71 volunteers without symptoms

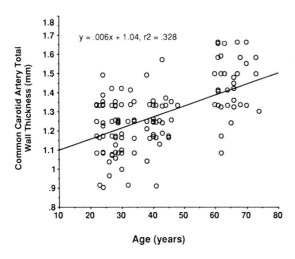

$y = .006x + 1.04, r2 = .328$

Fig. 46-15. The total wall thickness of the common carotid artery increases with age in normal individuals.

Table 46-1. Age and gender effects on total wall thickness in the common carotid artery

Age (yr)	Gender	n	Mean common carotid artery total thickness (mm)	Standard error
20-35	Male	19	1.19	0.04
NS	Female	24	1.22	0.03
60-75	Male	8	1.52	0.05
$p = 0.058$*	Female	11	1.39	0.04

NS, Not significant.
*Two-tailed test comparing males and females.

confirmed to be free of identifiable atherosclerosis according to history, ankle pressures, duplex scans of carotid and extremity arteries, and other clinical criteria. Serum lipid levels were also tested, and no one with hyperlipidemia was included in the control group.

One study goal was to evaluate lower extremity arterial disease, so 38 patients with intermittent claudication were recruited. These subjects had ankle/arm indices of less than 0.90 at rest along with other objective evidence of lower extremity occlusive disease.

A third group consisted of 19 subjects without symptoms but with focal atherosclerotic disease evident on duplex scans.

Age was found to be the most significant factor associated with carotid total wall thickening (Fig. 46-15). In the normal subjects examined, total wall thickness increased an average of 0.6% each year. Carotid thickness was significantly greater in those 60 to 75 years of age compared with normal subjects 20 to 35 years old. The younger group showed no gender-related difference in the thickness observed but among those 60 to 75 years old, the carotid arteries in men averaged 0.13 mm thicker than those in women, a difference that approached statistical significance (Table 46-1).

The total thickness measurements correlated poorly with electronic caliper–measured IMTs obtained in the same vessels. Although there was a general trend toward increased total wall thickness with intima-media thickening, intrasubject correlation between total wall thickness and IMT was poor. This may reflect the asymmetry of the thickening process, since the IMTs were measured on the far wall and the total thickness is only measurable in the near wall.

Based on these findings, carotid artery thickening, even in the absence of carotid bifurcation disease, might be a marker for generalized atherosclerotic disease. This same association is not shown for lower extremity arterial occlusive disease. When the findings for normal patients who

have claudication or have subclinical atherosclerosis are compared, the mean values for total carotid thickness were equivalent. Future studies under consideration include examining total wall thickness in the context of coronary artery disease, hyperlipidemia, hypertension, and diabetes.

CONCLUSION

Measurements of arterial wall thickness have been put to use in a number of studies, including several major clinical trials currently under way. Studies of the development and prevalence of early atherosclerosis using high-resolution B-mode ultrasound imaging of vessel wall features have shown that increasing IMT and total wall thickness are associated with recognized atherosclerosis risk factors. The assumption that arterial wall thickening, in either a population or an individual, is in fact atherosclerosis or that it correlates with the subsequent development of symptomatic arterial occlusive lesions remains to be proved.

Total thickness and IMT are different measurements that have been used to assess early arterial disease, but they may be sensitive to different factors that affect arterial wall structure. Lumen-lumen total wall thickness measurements are practical and can detect wall thickening. Computer-image analysis facilitates accurate and objective measurement of this distance.

The carotid artery thickens with age in normal individuals, and this thickening is greater in men than in women. Any definition of a "normal" value for arterial wall thickness must therefore take into consideration that thickness increases with aging, even in subjects who are free of detectable atherosclerotic disease or risk factors.

REFERENCES

1. ARIC Investigators: The Atherosclerosis Risk in Community (ARIC) study: designs and objectives, *Am J Epidemiol* 129:687-702, 1989.
2. Barndt R Jr et al: Regression and progression of early femoral atherosclerosis in treated hyperlipoproteinemic patients, *Ann Intern Med* 86:139-146, 1977.
3. Beach KW et al: An ultrasonic measurement of superficial femoral artery wall thickness, *Ultrasound Med Biol* 15:723-728, 1989.
4. Bluth EI et al: Sonographic characterization of carotid plaque: detection of hemorrhage, *AJR* 146:1061-1065, 1986.
5. Bond MG, Mercuri M, Tandg R: *Research B-mode ultrasonography: clinical trials.* In Bernstein EF, ed: *Proceedings of the Sixth San Diego Symposium on Vascular Diagnosis,* San Diego, 1992.

6. Bond MG et al: Detection and monitoring of asymptomatic atherosclerosis in clinical trials, *Am J Med* 86:33-36, 1989.
7. Craven TE et al: Evaluation of the associations between carotid artery atherosclerosis and coronary artery stenosis: a case-control study, *Circulation* 82:1230-1242, 1990.
8. Crawford D et al: Computer densitometry for angiographic assessment of arterial cholesterol content and gross pathology in human atherosclerosis, *J Lab Clin Med* 89:378-392, 1977.
9. Criqui M, Coughlen S, Fronek A: Non-invasively diagnosed peripheral arterial disease as a predictor of mortality: results from a prospective study, *Circulation* 72:768-773, 1985.
10. Crouse JR et al: Evaluation of a scoring system for extracranial carotid atherosclerosis extent with B-mode ultrasound, *Stroke* 17:270-275, 1986.
11. Dempsey RJ, Diana AL, Moore RW: Thickness of carotid artery atherosclerotic plaque and ischemic risk, *Neurosurgery* 27:343-348, 1990.
12. Duffield RGM et al: Treatment of hyperlipidaemia retards progression of symptomatic femoral atherosclerosis, *Lancet* 2:639-642, 1983.
13. Edwards J et al: Angiographically undetected ulceration of the carotid bifurcation as a cause of embolic stroke, *Radiology* 132:369-373, 1979.
14. Gelabert HA, Moore WS: Carotid endarterectomy without angiography, *Surg Clin North Am* 70:213-223, 1990.
15. Glagov S et al: Compensatory enlargement of human atherosclerotic coronary arteries, *N Engl J Med* 316:1371-1375, 1987.
16. Handa N et al: Ultrasonic evaluation of early carotid atherosclerosis, *Stroke* 21:1567-1572, 1990.
17. Jogestrand T, Lemne C, de Faire U: *Noninvasive assessment of vessel wall change in patients with hypertension.* Presented at Ultrasound in the Management of Peripheral Vascular Disease, Stockholm, Sweden, Oct 3-4, 1991.
18. Kawamori R et al: Prevalence of carotid atherosclerosis in diabetics: ultrasound high-resolution B-mode imaging of the carotid arteries, *Diabetes Care* 15(10):1290-1294, 1992.
19. Kohler TR et al: Duplex scanning for diagnosis of aortoiliac and femoropopliteal disease: a prospective study, *Circulation* 76:1074-1080, 1987.
20. Kohler TR et al: Variability in measurement of specific parameters for carotid duplex examination, *Ultrasound Med Biol* 13:637-642, 1987.
21. Kohler TR et al: Can duplex scanning replace arteriography for lower extremity arterial disease? *Ann Vasc Surg* 4:280-287, 1990.
22. Langlois Y et al: Evaluating carotid artery disease: the concordance between pulsed Doppler/spectrum analysis and angiography, *Ultrasound Med Biol* 9:51-63, 1983.
23. North American Symptomatic Carotid Endarterectomy Trial Collaborators: Beneficial effect of carotid endarterectomy in symptomatic patients with high-grade carotid stenosis, *N Engl J Med* 325:445-453, 1991.
24. O'Leary DH et al: Measurement variability of carotid atherosclerosis: real-time (B-mode) ultrasonography and angiography, *Stroke* 18:1011-1017, 1987.
25. O'Leary DH et al: Use of sonography to evaluate carotid atherosclerosis in the elderly: the cardiovascular health study, *Stroke* 22:1155-1163, 1991.
26. Olsson AG et al: Regression of computer estimated femoral atherosclerosis after pronounced serum lipid lowering in patients with asymptomatic hyperlipidaemia, *Lancet* 1:1311, 1982.
27. Persson J et al: Noninvasive quantification of atherosclerotic lesions: reproducibility of ultrasonographic measurement of arterial wall thickness and plaque size, *Arterioscler Thromb* 12:261-266, 1992.
28. Pignoli P: Ultrasound B-mode imaging for arterial wall thickness measurement, *Atheroscler Rev* 12:177-184, 1984.
29. Pignoli P et al: Intimal plus medial thickness of the arterial wall: a direct measurement with ultrasound imaging, *Circulation* 74:1399-1406, 1986.
30. Poli A et al: Ultrasonographic measurement of the common carotid artery wall thickness in hypercholesterolemic patients: a new model for the quantification and follow-up of preclinical atherosclerosis in living human subjects, *Atherosclerosis* 70:253-261, 1988.
31. Reilly LM et al: Carotid plaque histology using real-time ultrasonography: clinical and therapeutic implications, *Am J Surg* 146:188-193, 1983.
32. Ricotta JJ et al: Multicenter validation study of real-time (B-mode) ultrasound, arteriography, and pathologic examination, *J Vasc Surg* 6:512-520, 1987.
33. Roederer GO et al: The natural history of carotid arterial disease in asymptomatic patients with cervical bruits, *Stroke* 15:605-613, 1984.
34. Ruhn G, Erikson U, Olsson A: Prevalence of femoral atherosclerosis in asymptomatic men with hyperlipoproteinaemia, *J Intern Med* 225:317-323, 1989.
35. Salonen R, Salonen JT: Progression of carotid atherosclerosis and its determinants: a population-based ultrasonographic study, *Atherosclerosis* 81:33-40, 1990.
36. Salonen R, Haapanen A, Salonen JT: Measurement of intima-media thickness of common carotid arteries with high-resolution B-mode ultrasonography: inter- and intra-observer variability, *Ultrasound Med Biol* 17:225-230, 1991.
37. Salonen R et al: Prevalence of carotid atherosclerosis and serum cholesterol levels in eastern Finland, *Arteriosclerosis* 8:788-792, 1988.
38. Taylor DC, Strandness DE Jr: Carotid artery duplex scanning, *J Clin Ultrasound* 15:635-644, 1987.
39. Wendelhag I, Wiklund O, Wikstrand J: Arterial wall thickness in familial hypercholesterolemia: ultrasound measurement of intima-media thickness in the common carotid artery, *Arterioscler Thromb* 12:70-77, 1992.
40. Wendelhag I et al: Ultrasound measurement of wall thickness in the carotid artery: fundamental principles and description of a computerized analysing system, *Clin Physiol* 11:565-577, 1991.
41. Wikstrand J, Wiklund O: Frontiers in cardiovascular science: quantitative measurement of atherosclerotic manifestations in humans, *Arterioscler Thromb* 12:114-119, 1992.
42. Zarins K, Zatina M, Glagov S: *Correlation of postmortem angiography with pathologic anatomy: quantitation of atherosclerotic lesions.* In Bond M et al, eds: *Clinical diagnosis of atherosclerosis,* New York, 1983, Springer-Verlag.
43. Zwiebel WJ et al: Correlation of high-resolution, B-mode and continuous-wave Doppler sonography with arteriography in the diagnosis of carotid stenosis, *Radiology* 149:523-532, 1983.

CHAPTER 47

Arterial wall changes with atherogenesis: ultrasound measurement of asymptomatic atherosclerosis

RONG TANG, MICHELE MERCURI, and M. GENE BOND

Atherosclerosis, the leading cause of disability and mortality in the populations of most countries, is an arterial disease that produces lumen narrowing and obstruction and that may ultimately lead to myocardial, cerebral, and leg ischemia. The findings from pathologic studies have confirmed that symptoms occur only when the atherosclerotic lesions, which may have existed for years or even decades, reach an advanced stage.[81] During the intervening period, lipid accumulates in the arterial wall, and this is followed by the proliferation of extracellular connective tissue elements, such as collagen and elastin. The initiation of atherogenesis and the mechanisms that govern it are still not well understood; however, several hypotheses explaining the pathogenesis of atherosclerosis have been proposed, including the lipid* and response-to-injury hypotheses.† The process begins in the intima, where plasma lipoproteins accumulate to form a fatty streak, which may later become advanced plaques. It has been suggested that this progression could be retarded by treatment with antiatherogenic agents.[12,51] Alpha-blockers, angiotensin-converting enzyme inhibitors,[19,60] beta-blockers,[78] and calcium channel antagonists[77,84] have all exhibited such antiatherogenic activity in animal model experiments. Therefore the detection and assessment of atherosclerosis during its early and asymptomatic stages might provide a powerful tool that can be used to investigate epidemiologic issues and assess the effects of various interventional therapies.

Several methods are currently used to evaluate the extent and severity of atherosclerosis, but arteriography is the only method now available that can evaluate coronary atherosclerosis. Because of its invasive nature, however, arteriography involves some risk and should not be used to routinely evaluate asymptomatic subjects. In addition, arteriography images the arterial lumen from only a limited number of angles and cannot reveal the identity of intramural plaque components, such as necrosis and hemorrhage. It is also limited in its ability to detect early atherosclerotic le-

sions because during the early stages of plaque formation, the artery may enlarge to compensate for increasing wall thickness.* This compensatory change may be accompanied by a larger than normal lumen.[85] In monitoring lumen changes over time, therefore, such findings could be misinterpreted to represent atherosclerotic regression. Studies have also shown that arteriography frequently underrepresents the severity of lesions or fails to identify significant lumen narrowing.[38,82]

Bond et al[11] have demonstrated that the coronary arteries of cynomolgus monkeys fed an atherogenic diet dilated during the early phases of plaque formation without a resultant decrease in lumen diameter. Armstrong et al[4] obtained comparable results from a similar experiment that focused on the iliac and femoral arteries of two nonhuman primate species. During these experiments, the intima of the hindlimb arteries was observed to thicken as the atherosclerosis progressed, but lumen size was not significantly reduced. Furthermore, hemodynamic studies showed that blood flow in these atherosclerotic arteries was only slightly compromised. The same phenomenon occurs in human arteries.[31,71,85] Glagov et al[31] have shown that human coronary arteries enlarge as the plaque area increases, but the lumen area of these vessels does not decrease until the disease involves 40% of the length of the internal elastic lamina. Zarins et al[85] also found that the size of the left arterior descending coronary artery increases as the plaque area enlarges. In the most severely diseased distal portion of these arteries, the lumen area was approximately twice the size of the least-diseased vessel segment.

The optimal method to assess atherosclerosis is one that images both the arterial wall and the lumen. Ultrasound methods have been used in clinical laboratories for more than 20 years and allow for the noninvasive morphologic evaluation of atherosclerosis and the related hemodynamic changes.[20,64] B-mode ultrasound imaging enables the examiner to visualize both the arterial lumen and wall.[5] Although once considered unreliable because of its low res-

---

*References 16, 17, 26, 34, 35, 40, 41, 68.
†References 24, 25, 27, 29, 42, 61, 67, 68.

*References 4, 11, 31, 71, 80, 85.

olution,[8,22,37,56] technical advancements have now made B-mode ultrasonography superior to angiography in detecting and quantifying early to moderate atherosclerotic lesions that do not significantly narrow lumen diameter.[42] Furthermore, ultrasonography has the potential for identifying specific plaque characteristics, which are often more relevant than lumen stenosis in explaining clinical sequelae,[36,49,62,69] especially in the presence of intraplaque hemorrhage and ulceration of the surface.[9,36,45,48,62,79]

ARTERIAL WALL STRUCTURE

The walls of normal elastic and muscular arteries consist of three distinct morphologic layers that differ in their cellular and extracellular composition. The intima constitutes the inner layer and extends from a continuous monolayer of endothelial cells that line the lumen to an extracellular layer of elastic tissue—the internal elastic lamina. Endothelial cells orient their long axis in the direction of blood flow, thereby creating a pivotal interface between the blood and the vessel wall. These cells perform a variety of specific functions that maintain vessel wall integrity and function and thus ensure normal blood flow. The thickness of this layer usually ranges from 15 to 100 μm. The intima becomes enriched with cholesterol ester during atherogenesis and with aging.[43,76] In normal arteries, the thickest layer is the media, which comprises spirally arranged smooth muscle cells, elastin, collagen, and proteoglycans. Smooth muscle cells occupy 40% to 50% of the medial area in large elastic arteries and 80% to 85% of the medial area in muscular arteries such as the coronaries.[28] These cells act in conjunction with elastin to bring about vessel wall tension and function. The outer arterial layer is the adventitia, which is separated from the media by the external elastic lamina. The adventitia consists of fibroblasts and loose collagenous tissue that contains a network of capillaries and nerves supplying the arterial wall. The adventitia provides both longitudinal and circumferential support for the artery.

TYPES OF ATHEROSCLEROTIC LESIONS

It is generally agreed that there are three types of lesions that represent the spectrum of atherosclerosis: fatty streaks, fibrous plaques, and complicated plaques. The fatty streak is the earliest lesion visible to the naked eye and appears in the abdominal aorta shortly after birth, enlarging rapidly during the second decade of life. By 30 years of age, 30% to 50% of the aortic surface is covered by this fatty streak,[30,47] which is composed of multiple layers of intimal smooth muscle cells and macrophages containing lipid inclusions.[2] These lesions are flat or slightly raised and are found beneath an intact endothelium. Controversy still exists about whether fatty streaks are precursors to fibrous plaques. A lesion that is thought to be transitional between the fatty streak and fibrous plaque has been described. It is also slightly raised, but microscopically may be found to contain focal necrosis and extracellular lipid, similar to the composition of fibrous plaque.[44,46]

Fibrous plaques, which are considered the next stage in atherosclerosis development, consist of large accumulations of smooth muscle cells surrounded by collagen, proteoglycans, elastic fibers, and varying amounts of intracellular and extracellular lipids, including cholesterol monohydrate crystals, cholesterol esters, fatty acids, lysolecithin, sphingomyelin, and triglycerides.[44] The fibrous plaque may be large enough to narrow the lumen and compromise blood flow.[32]

The complicated lesion is an advanced fibrous plaque that has degenerated and contains a variable amount and combination of necrosis, minerals, hemorrhage, and cholesterol monohydrate crystals. The core of this lesion is unstable and is covered by a fibromuscular cap made up of smooth muscle cells and collagen. This cap may become very thin as the size of the necrotic core increases, and thus may rupture when exposed to shear stress or transient sudden changes in blood pressure. Rupture of these lesions results in arterial thrombosis, thromboembolism, or both, thus producing the characteristic clinical sequelae.[45,62]

B-MODE IMAGING OF THE ARTERIAL WALL

The ultrasound image of a normal artery contains three distinctly echoic interfaces on both the near and far walls. Fig. 47-1 is a longitudinal B-mode image of a carotid artery. The first interface on the wall nearest the transducer is generated by the boundary between the periadventitia and adventitia (interface 1[13]); the second, by the adventitia-media boundary (interface 2[49]); and the third, by the intima-lumen boundary (interface 3[49]). The interfaces of the far wall are the mirror image of those on the near wall: the lumen-intima boundary (interface 4[58]), the media-adventitia (interface 5[58]), and the adventitia-periadventitia (interface 6[13]). This information[13,15,50,58,63] can be used to determine arterial wall thicknesses, that is, the intima-media thickness (IMT) or total wall thickness.[13,15,49,58,63]

The measurement of arterial wall thickness using ultrasound imaging was first validated for the arterial far wall by Pignoli et al.[58] They identified a double-line pattern in the ultrasound images of all the common carotid arteries, as well as all of the relatively normal aortic specimens they studied. This *double-line pattern* is characterized by two parallel echogenic lines separated by a hypoechoic space. These studies demonstrated that interface 4 represented the boundary between the lumen and the intimal surface and interface 5 was the boundary between the media and the adventitia. The B-mode measurement of the distance between interfaces 4 and 5 was directly correlated with the thickness of the intima plus media, as determined by both gross and microscopic methods.

The near-wall measurement was validated by Mercuri et al,[49] who compared the intima plus media measurements obtained from an in vitro model of the near wall with those obtained when the same arterial specimen was scanned as a far-wall model. The near-wall measurements were slightly less than those obtained from the far wall, but there was a high correlation (r = 0.93) between the two. The reproduc-

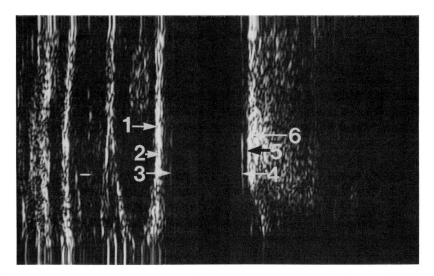

Fig. 47-1. Longitudinal B-mode ultrasound image of the carotid artery. On the near wall, interface 1 is generated by the boundary between periadventitia and adventitia, interface 2 is generated by the adventitia-media boundary, and interface 3 is generated by the intima-lumen boundary. On the far wall, interfaces 4, 5, and 6 are generated by the lumen-intima, the media-adventitia, and the adventitia-periadventitia boundary, respectively.

ibility of near-wall thickness measurements as described by correlation coefficients was 0.92 in the in vitro aortic model, 0.98 in the in vitro carotid model, and 0.87 in common carotid arteries examined in vivo.

When assessing the IMT of the far wall, examiners make measurements from the leading edge of interface 4 to the leading edge of interface 5. Conversely, for near-wall measurements, the intima-lumen interface is located at the echoic boundary of interface 3. Therefore it is sometimes difficult to determine visually the precise location of this boundary. A specific algorithim is needed that can be used to automatically identify the intima-lumen boundary using gray-scale level peak intensities.

In an in vivo animal model, Bond et al[15] compared arterial wall thicknesses and lumen diameters obtained by B-mode ultrasonography with the data acquired by arteriography and microscopic study of pathologic specimens. Almost all of the measurements obtained by B-mode ultrasound in the primate study were larger than those yielded by microscopic study. The absolute differences for lumen diameter and wall thickness were 0.30 and 0.56 mm, respectively, and the correlation coefficients were 0.42 and 0.41, respectively. Compared with the findings yielded by arteriography, B-mode lumen diameters were smaller, with a mean difference of -1.0 mm (r = 0.69). The variance between these measurements may have resulted from limitations stemming from the axial resolution of the ultrasound instrument, changes in arterial size due to tissue processing, or the pressure used to inject contrast media during arteriography. The absolute differences between two replicate examinations in measuring wall thickness and lumen diameter with

B-mode ultrasonography were 0.97 and 0.23 mm, respectively. These investigators concluded that these small differences resulted from slight changes in the cardiovascular status of the animals at the time of the two examinations and from making measurements at slightly different times during each pulse cycle.

To define the validity and reliability of B-mode ultrasonography in evaluating atherosclerosis in human beings, investigators participating in a multicenter National Heart, Lung and Blood Institute[53,63,75] project compared lesion width and lumen diameter obtained by ultrasound, arteriography, and pathologic examination.[40,53,54] The results showed that ultrasound revealed the presence of some lesion in half of the 345 arteries defined as normal by arteriography. Compared with the findings from the pathology examination, ultrasound showed the best correlation in terms of measuring lesion width (mean difference, -1.1 mm), but arteriography showed the best correlation with regard to measuring lumen diameter (mean difference, -0.1 mm). This project also analyzed the measurement variability of ultrasonography and arteriography. Using a standardized protocol, the arterial images of B-mode sonography and arteriography were read by the same or different reader multiple times. The within-reader and between-reader variabilities for B-mode ultrasonography were similar to those calculated for the contrast studies in terms of lesion width. The within-reader correlation coefficients were 0.74 and 0.72 for ultrasonography and arteriography, respectively, and the between-reader correlation coefficients were 0.56 and 0.64, respectively. Both the within- and between-reader correlation coefficients of lumen diameter measurement from arteriography were 0.85 but were 0.77 and 0.62, respectively, for B-mode ultrasonography. Results from this study suggest that arteriography is better than B-mode ultrasonography for measuring lumen diameter but that B-mode ultrasonography is superior for detecting lesion width.

EPIDEMIOLOGIC STUDIES AND INTERVENTIONAL TRIALS WITH B-MODE IMAGING

Because of the validity and reliability of B-mode ultrasonography in the noninvasive measurement of arterial wall characteristics, it has been applied in epidemiologic and clinical studies to evaluate atherosclerosis risk factors and determine the impact of medical intervention. Poli et al[59] used this method to evaluate the common carotid arteries of 36 hypercholesterolemic patients and 31 controls. The values of right and left common carotid far-wall IMTs examined at three different angles constituted the primary outcome measure. This study identified a link between increased plasma cholesterol concentrations and increased arterial IMTs and demonstrated a positive correlation with cigarette smoking, gender, and age. These findings have been confirmed by Crouse et al[23] and later by the Kuopio Ischemic Heart Disease (KIHD) Risk Factor Study.[71,73,74] In particular, the KIHD study identified the distribution of the IMTs of the common carotid artery among Eastern Finnish men aged 42, 48, 54, and 60 years according to several cardiovascular risk factors: cigarette smoking, systolic and diastolic blood pressure, serum low-density lipoprotein (LDL) and high-density lipoprotein (HDL) cholesterol levels, history of ischemic heart disease, diabetes, obesity, plasma fibrinogen concentration, platelet aggregability, and white blood cell count. They found that the degree of carotid atherosclerosis (categorized as no atherosclerosis, intima-media thickening, nonstenotic plaque, and stenosis) was associated with age, the serum LDL cholesterol concentration, and smoking[70,74] and, based on the findings gleaned from a 2-year follow-up, concluded that these factors as well as systolic blood pressure and white blood cell count were major determinants of changes in the common carotid arteries.[71-73] Male smokers showed a 14% greater IMT than did nonsmokers; men with a high serum cholesterol concentration had a 10% greater IMT than did those with lower levels; and men with systolic hypertension had a 9% greater IMT that did those with no systolic hypertension.

Epidemiologic studies

Currently there are two large ongoing multicenter epidemiologic studies under way in the United States that are using B-mode ultrasonography to detect and monitor carotid thickness. The Atherosclerosis Risk in Communities (ARIC) Study[3] is a four-center prospective cohort study designed to investigate the prevalence, distribution, and etiology of carotid atherosclerosis and its clinical sequelae in 1600 adults aged 45 to 64 years living in four states. This study is examining the variations in the disease and cardiovascular

risk factors in terms of race, gender, location, and time. Carotid artery wall thickness is evaluated with B-mode ultrasound scanning performed by trained and certified sonographers who scan both carotid arteries.[14] For the purposes of this study, the extracranial carotid artery has been divided into three segments: the distal 1.0-cm straight portion of the common carotid artery, the carotid bifurcation, and the proximal 1.0-cm of the internal carotid artery. The end points in the study are to determine near- and far-wall mean and maximum IMTs and lumen diameter derived from the measurement of the distance between interfaces 2 and 3, 4 and 5, and 3 and 4. In repeated quality control scans, the intrasonographer reliability coefficient for the wall thickness of combined right and left carotid arteries has ranged from 0.74 to 0.92, and the between-reader reliability coefficient for the mean lumen diameter, minimum lumen diameter, and wall thicknesses has ranged from 0.78 to 0.98. The intrareader reliability also fell in the same range.[66]

This study has identified 386 subjects with carotid artery wall thickening and an equal number of matched controls without arterial wall thickening to compare the association between arterial wall thickness and risk factors for carotid artery atherosclerosis.[39] The investigators have found that the mean values of total cholesterol, LDL cholesterol, total triglycerides, blood pressure, and years of cigarette smoking were significantly higher in subjects with arterial wall thickening than in the controls, whereas the mean HDL cholesterol level was significantly lower in the patients than in the controls.

The other large ongoing epidemiologic study currently under way in the United States is the Cardiovascular Health Study (CHS),[55] and its objective is to investigate risk factors for coronary heart disease and stroke. This is a four-center study consisting of 5000 men and women, aged 65 and older, from four communities. Carotid sonography is performed during a baseline examination and again 3 years later. At each examination, the largest lesions in the right and left internal carotid arteries are measured from three angles (anterooblique, lateral, and posterooblique) and from a single lateral view of the distal 1.0 cm of the common carotid artery. The carotid bifurcation is incorporated into the internal carotid segment. The end points used in this study are to determine the maximum and mean near- and far-wall IMTs and minimum lumen diameter. In addition, the appearance of the intimal surface, the plaque morphology, and the density characteristics of the lesion are recorded. The intersonographer correlation coefficients for wall thickness have ranged from 0.43 to 0.55 and, for lumen diameter, from 0.55 to 0.57. The interreader correlation coefficients for wall thicknesses have ranged from 0.74 to 0.91 and, for lumen diameter, from 0.68 to 0.85. The range of reliability coefficients for intrareader measurement of usual thickness have been 0.14 to 0.68 and, for lumen diameter, 0.53 to 0.58. The variability of internal carotid artery measurement has been greater than that of the common carotid arteries because this segment is neither straight nor parallel to the skin surface. The data derived from this study, however, do suggest that carotid sonography is a reproducible method for studying carotid atherosclerosis in cohort studies.

Interventional trials

B-mode ultrasonography is also being used in interventional trials to determine whether several different pharmacologic treatments can slow the progression of asymptomatic carotid atherosclerosis.

The Asymptomatic Carotid Artery Plaque Study (ACAPS)[65] is a collaborative, double-blind, placebo-controlled interventional trial undertaken to determine the effect of two treatments, aspirin and lovastatin, in retarding the progression of early atherosclerotic lesions in the carotid arteries. The study population consists of 919 high-risk, asymptomatic, hypercholesterolemic participants. The primary end point of this 3-year trial is to determine the mean maximum IMT for the near and far walls of each segment.

The Pravastatin, Lipids, and Atherosclerosis in the Carotid (PLAC-II) Study[23a] is also a double-blind, placebo-controlled interventional trial designed to determine the effectiveness of pravastatin, an HMG-CoA reductase inhibitor, in reducing atherosclerosis in hyperlipidemic patients with coronary artery disease who have asymptomatic stenosis of the carotid arteries. All patients in this study have severe coronary artery atherosclerosis, as defined by history and coronary arteriography.

The Carotid Atherosclerosis Italian Atherosclerosis Study (CAIUS)[18] is a 3-year multicenter, double-blind, placebo-controlled trial with the goal of determining the effect of pravastatin on the progression of carotid atherosclerosis in moderately hypercholesterolemic asymptomatic patients. This study is monitoring 300 patients who have at least one uncomplicated atherosclerotic plaque, defined as an IMT of between 1.3 and 3.5 mm in the common carotid, carotid bifurcation, or internal carotid arteries on either the right or left side.

The Multicenter Isradipine/Diuretic Atherosclerosis Study (MIDAS)[1,51] is also a randomized, double-blind, active-controlled trial that is comparing the effects of a diuretic and calcium antagonist in reducing the progression rate of early carotid atherosclerosis in hypertensive patients. This 3-year study consists of 883 hypertensive men and women aged 40 years or older with a carotid IMT determined at baseline and semiannually using B-mode ultrasound imaging.

Ultrasound protocols. Each of the ultrasound protocols used in the four interventional trials is similar. The carotid artery has been divided into three segments: the distal common carotid artery, the carotid bifurcation, and the proximal internal artery. The primary end point of the studies is to determine the mean maximum IMTs of the near and far walls of every segment. Trained and certified sonographers and readers scan and measure the largest IMT from 12

standard sites, with examinations done every 6 months during the active treatment period. Unlike the KIHD study, these epidemiologic studies and interventional trials are quantifying all thickness in the carotid bifurcation and internal carotid arteries at sites that, when diseased, may result in clinical sequelae. Quality control procedures are performed routinely in the interventional clinical trials to reduce the error of the method. The sonographers and readers are centrally trained to perform standardized ultrasound protocols to ensure that valid and reliable measurements can be obtained. After initial certification, sonographers and readers are routinely evaluated, both quantitatively and qualitatively, to confirm their proficiency and efficiency. All the instruments used in these studies are calibrated as closely as possible, and routine preventive maintenance is done to continuously maintain a high image quality. As a result, the reliability of data sets has proved excellent. Replicate baseline mean maximum IMTs from repeat scans and readings in the MIDAS[50] have proved to be highly consistent, with a mean absolute difference of 0.11 mm. The absolute intrasonographer and intersonographer differences were 0.11 and 0.12 mm, with correlation coefficients of 0.74 and 0.68, respectively. Intrareader and interreader absolute differences were 0.09 and 0.11 mm, with correlation coefficients of 0.82 and 0.71, respectively. These data demonstrate that B-mode ultrasound imaging can furnish reliable information in trials that assess the progression of peripheral atherosclerosis and the effectiveness of therapy to slow the process.

B-MODE IMAGING TO ASSESS PLAQUE MORPHOLOGY

In addition to measuring wall thickness, B-mode ultrasound may be able to characterize the plaque type or its components.* Using B-mode gray scale patterns, several investigators have suggested it has potential for identifying the existence of intraplaque hemorrhage, citing a 90% accuracy, 94% sensitivity, and 88% specificity.[9] Weinberger et al[83] have also found that 97% of hemorrhagic plaques are heterogeneous and that 77% of these heterogeneous plaques contain intraplaque hemorrhage. It is still controversial whether B-mode ultrasound can recognize plaque ulceration.[9,10,21] Bluth et al[10] could not establish any sonographic characteristics that could differentiate between plaques with and without ulceration and suggested that plaque surface characteristics could not be used as a valid method to identify ulceration. This finding was supported by Barry et al,[6] who reported that when surface irregularity was used as a criterion for identifying plaque ulceration, sensitivity was 81% and specificity was 33%. The diagnostic specificity increased to 85% and the sensitivity decreased to 17% when a clearly visible crater was considered to denote an ulcerated lesion. Comerota et al[21] have shown that the diagnostic sensitivity for correctly identifying ulceration was influenced by the degree of lumen stenosis, with a 77% sensi-

---

*References 6, 7, 9, 10, 21, 33, 36, 52, 57, 62, 69.

tivity in lumens with 50% or less stenosis and 41% sensitivity in lumens with stenosis exceeding 50%. They therefore concluded that B-mode ultrasonography could not reliably identify ulceration in high-grade lesions.

Other attempts have been made to quantitatively define tissue characteristics using ultrasound. Picano et al[57] and Barzilai et al,[7] using radiofrequency signal analysis, were able to differentiate calcified plaques from normal and fibrotic lesions. However, this method has not been extrapolated for use in in vivo studies. Mercuri et al[48] have proposed an alternative in vitro approach that uses analysis of the gray-scale level distribution to define morphologic differences. To test this method, digitized B-mode images of three classes of arterial specimens (normal, fibrotic, and complicated) were evaluated quantitatively, and their gray-scale level intensities and distribution were defined with a computerized system. The average and maximum intensities revealed significant differences among the three classes of lesions.

CONCLUSION

B-mode ultrasound has been and is currently being used in the performance of basic research, epidemiologic studies, and clinical trials. Data from these studies have shown that the method is reliable and valid for describing and measuring arterial wall thicknesses of both normal and atherosclerotic vessels on the basis of known morphology. The method is noninvasive and therefore can be used not only to select those patients who are at risk for the development of atherosclerosis but also to identify those individuals who have the disease. Furthermore, the precision of the method, both in terms of scanning and reading, can be established routinely, unlike other more costly and invasive methods. Most importantly, B-mode ultrasound can visualize the arterial wall itself, at least in superficial vessels, and may constitute a powerful tool for monitoring the progression of atherosclerosis.

ACKNOWLEDGMENT

We kindly acknowledge Jennifer FitzSimons and Tammy Nail for their assistance in preparing this manuscript.

REFERENCES

1. Applegate WB, Byington RP: MIDAS, the multicenter isradipine/diuretic atherosclerosis study: design features and baseline data, *Am J Hypertens* 4:114s-117s, 1991.
2. Aqel NM et al: Identification of macrophages and smooth muscle cells in human atherosclerosis using monoclonal antibodies, *J Pathol* 146:197-204, 1985.
3. ARIC Investigators: The atherosclerosis risk in communities (ARIC) study: design and objectives, *Am J Epidemiol* 29(4):687-702, 1989.
4. Armstrong ML et al: Structural and hemodynamic responses of peripheral arteries of macaque monkeys to atherogenic diet, *Arteriosclerosis* 5:336-346, 1985.
5. Barber FE et al: Ultrasonic duplex echo-Doppler scanner, *IEEE Trans Biomed Eng* 21:109-113, 1974.
6. Barry R, Pienaar C, Nel CJ: Accuracy of B-mode ultrasonography in detecting carotid plaque hemorrhage and ulceration, *Ann Vasc Surg* 4:446-470, 1990.
7. Barzilai B et al: Quantitative ultrasonic characterization of the nature of atherosclerotic plaques in human aorta, *Circ Res* 60:459-463, 1987.
8. Blue SK et al: Ultrasonic B-mode scanning of extracranial vascular disease, *Neurology* 22:1079-1085, 1972.
9. Bluth EI et al: Sonographic characterization of carotid plaque: detection of hemorrhage, *AJR* 146:1061-1065, 1986.
10. Bluth EI et al: The identification of ulcerative plaque with high resolution duplex carotid scanning, *J Ultrasound Med* 7:73-76, 1988.
11. Bond MG, Adams MR, Bullock BC: Complication factors in evaluating coronary artery atherosclerosis, *Artery* 9:21-29, 1981.
12. Bond MG et al: New perspective for clinical evaluation of atherosclerosis, *Drug Dev Res* 6:127-134, 1985.
13. Bond MG et al: Detection and monitoring of asymptomatic atherosclerosis in clinical trials, *Am J Med* 86(suppl):33-36, 1989.
14. Bond MG et al: High resolution B-mode ultrasound scanning methods in the atherosclerosis risk in communities study (ARIC), *J Neuroimag* 1:68-73, 1991.
15. Bond MG et al: Ultrasound imaging of atherosclerotic lesions in arteries of animals: validity and reproducibility (in preparation).
16. Brown MS, Goldstein JL: Lipoprotein metabolism in the macrophage: implication for cholesterol deposition in atherosclerosis, *Annu Rev Biochem* 52:223-261, 1983.
17. Brown MS, Goldstein JL: How LDL receptors influence cholesterol and atherosclerosis, *Sci Am* 251:58-66, 1984.
18. CAIUS Group: *Carotid atherosclerosis Italian ultrasound study (CAIUS): a protocol for non-invasive evaluation of atherosclerosis.* Presented at the 9th International Symposium on Atherosclerosis, Oct 1991, Rosemont, Ill.
19. Chobanian AV et al: Antiatherogenic effect of captopril in the Watanabe heritable hyperlipidemic rabbit, *Hypertension* 15:327-331, 1990.
20. Comerota AJ, Cranley JJ, Cook SE: Real-time B-mode carotid imaging in diagnosis of cerebrovascular disease, *Surgery* 89:718-729, 1982.
21. Comerota AJ et al: The preoperative diagnosis of the ulcerated carotid atheroma, *J Vasc Surg* 11:505-510, 1990.
22. Cooperberg PL et al: High resolution real-time ultrasound of the carotid bifurcation, *J Clin Ultrasound* 7:13-21, 1979.
23. Crouse JR et al: Risk factors for extracranial carotid artery atherosclerosis, *Stroke* 18:990-996, 1987.
23a. Crouse JR et al: Provastatin, lipids, and atherosclerosis in the carotid arteries: design features of a clinical trial with carotid atherosclerosis outcome, *Controlled Clin Trials* 13:495-506, 1992.
24. Deuell TF et al: Chemotaxis of monocytes and neutrophils to platelet-derived growth factor, *J Clin Invest* 69:1046-1049, 1982.
25. Faxon DP et al: Restenosis following transluminal angioplasty in experimental atherosclerosis, *Arteriosclerosis* 4:189-195, 1984.
26. Feldman DL, Hoff HF, Gerrity RG: Immunohistochemical localization of apoprotein B in aortas from hyperlipidemic swine: preferential accumulation in lesion-prone areas, *Arch Pathol Lab Med* 108:817-822, 1984.
27. Friedman RJ, Moor S, Singal DP: Repeated endothelial injury and induction of atherosclerosis in normal lipidemic rabbits by human serum, *Lab Invest* 32:404-415, 1975.
28. Gabella G: Structural apparatus for force transmission in smooth muscles, *Physiol Rev* 64:455-477, 1984.
29. Gajdusek C et al: An endothelial cell derived growth factor, *J Cell Biol* 85:467-472, 1980.
30. Geer JC: Fine structure of human aortic intimal thickening and fatty streak, *Lab Invest* 14(10):1764-1783, 1965.
31. Glagov S et al: Compensatory enlargement of human atherosclerotic coronary arteries, *N Engl J Med* 316:1371-1375, 1987.
32. Glagov S et al: Hemodynamics and atherosclerosis: insights and perspectives gained from studies of human arteries, *Arch Pathol Lab Med* 112:1018-1030, 1988.
33. Goes E et al: Tissue characterization of atheromatous plaques: correlation between ultrasound image and histologic findings, *J Clin Ultrasound* 18:611-617, 1990.
34. Goldstein JL, Brown MS: The LDL receptor defect in familial hypercholesterolemia: implications for pathogenesis and therapy, *Med Clin North Am* 66:335-362, 1982.
35. Goldstein JL et al: Receptor-mediated endocytosis: concepts emerging from the LDL receptor system, *Annu Rev Cell Biol* 1:1-39, 1985.
36. Gray-Weal AC et al: Carotid atheroma comparison of preoperative B-mode ultrasound appearance with carotid endarterectomy pathology, *J Cardiovasc Surg* 29:676-681, 1988.

37. Green PS et al: Real-time ultrasonic imaging system for carotid arteriography, *Ultrasound Med Biol* 3:129-142, 1977.

38. Harrison DG et al: The value of lesion cross-sectional area determined by quantitative coronary angiography in assessing the physiologic significance of proximal left anterior descending coronary arterial stenosis, *Circulation* 69:1111-1119, 1984.

39. Heiss G et al: Carotid atherosclerosis measured by B-mode ultrasound in populations: association with cardiovascular risk factors in the ARIC study, *Am J Epidemiol* 134:250-256, 1991.

40. Hoff HF: Apolipoprotein localization in human cranial arteries, coronary arteries and the aorta, *Stroke* 7:390-393, 1976.

41. Hoff HF: Localization of apolipoproteins in human carotid artery plaque, *Stroke* 6(5):531-534, 1975.

42. Jorgensen L et al: Focal aortic injury caused by cannulation: increased plasma protein accumulation and thrombosis, *Acta Pathol Microbiol Scand* 82(A):637-647, 1974.

43. Katz SS: The lipids of grossly normal human aortic intima from birth to old age, *J Biol Chem* 256:12275-12280, 1981.

44. Katz SS, Shipley GG, Small DM: Physical chemistry of the lipids of human atherosclerotic lesions: demonstration of a lesion intermediate between fatty streaks and advanced plaques, *J Clin Invest* 58:200-211, 1976.

45. Lusby RJ et al: Carotid plaque hemorrhage: its role in production of cerebral ischemia, *Arch Surg* 117:1479-1488, 1982.

46. McGill HC Jr: *Questions about the natural history of human atherosclerosis,* Prepared for the Workshop of the Evolution of Human Atherosclerotic Plaque, Sept 20-27, 1986, Rockville, Md.

47. McGill HC, Strong JP: The geographic pathology of atherosclerosis, *Annu NY Acad Sci* 149:923-927, 1968.

48. Mercuri M, Bond MG: B-mode ultrasound characterization of atherosclerosis, *J Cardiovasc Tech* (in press).

49. Mercuri M, Tang R, Bond MG: Validity and reproducibility of B-mode ultrasound imaging in measuring arterial near walls, *Circulation* 84:II-541, 1991.

50. Mercuri M et al: Consistency of B-mode ultrasound measurements of carotid atherosclerosis: the MIDAS baseline examinations. Presented at the 9th International Symposium on Atherosclerosis, Oct 1991, Rosemont, Ill.

51. MIDAS Research Group: Multicenter isradipine diuretic atherosclerosis study (MIDAS): design features, *Am J Med* 86(suppl):37-39, 1989.

52. O'Donnell TF Jr et al: Correlation of B-mode ultrasound imaging and arteriography with pathologic findings at carotid endarterectomy, *Arch Surg* 120:443-449, 1985.

53. O'Leary DH et al: Measurement variability of carotid atherosclerosis: real-time (B-mode) ultrasonography and angiography, *Stroke* 18:1011-1017, 1987.

54. O'Leary DH et al: Extracranial atherosclerosis in a general population: the Framingham heart study, *Stroke* 19:143, 1988.

55. O'Leary DH et al: The use of sonography to evaluate carotid atherosclerosis in the elderly: the cardiovascular health study, *Stroke* 22:1155-1163, 1991.

56. Olinger CP: Ultrasonic carotid echoarteriography, *Am J Roentgenol Radium Ther Nucl Med* 106:282-291, 1969.

57. Picano E et al: Time domain echo pattern evaluations from normal and atherosclerotic arterial walls: a study in vitro, *Circulation* 77:654-659, 1988.

58. Pignoli P et al: Intimal plus medial thickness of the arterial wall: a direct measurement with ultrasound imaging, *Circulation* 74:1399-1406, 1986.

59. Poli A et al: Ultrasonographic measurement of the common carotid arterial wall thickness in hypercholesterolemic patients, *Atherosclerosis* 70:253-261, 1988.

60. Powell JS et al: Inhibitors of angiotensin-converting enzyme prevent myointimal proliferation after vascular injury, *Science* 245:186-188, 1989.

61. Reidy MA: A reassessment of endothelial injury and arterial lesion formation, *Lab Invest* 53:513-520, 1985.

62. Reilly LM et al: Carotid plaque histology using real-time ultrasonography: clinical and therapeutic implications, *Am J Surg* 146:188-193, 1983.

63. Ricotta JJ et al: Multicenter validation study of real-time (B-mode) ultrasound, arteriography, and pathologic examination, *J Vasc Surg* 6:512-520, 1987.

64. Ricotta JJ et al: *Validation of real-time (B-mode) ultrasound, arteriography and pathology: sensitivity and specificity.* In Glagov S, Newman WP, Schoffer SA, eds: *Pathobiology of the human atherosclerotic plaque,* ed 1, New York, 1990, Springer-Verlag.

65. Riley WA et al: *Noninvasive measurement of carotid atherosclerosis: reproducibility.* Presented at the 63rd Scientific Session of the American Heart Association, Nov 1990, Dallas, Tex.

66. Riley WA et al: High resolution B-mode ultrasound reading methods in the atherosclerosis risk in communities (ARIC) cohort, *J Neuroimag* 1:168-172, 1991.

67. Ross R, Raines EW, Bowen-Pope DF: The biology of platelet-derived growth factor, *Cell* 46:155-169, 1986.

68. Ross R et al: A platelet-dependent serum factor that stimulates the proliferation of arterial smooth muscle cells in vitro, *Proc Natl Acad Sci USA* 71:1207-1210, 1974.

69. Rubin JR, Bondi JA, Rhodes RS: Duplex scanning versus conventional arteriography for the evaluation of carotid artery plaque morphology, *Surgery* 102:749-755, 1987.

70. Salonen JT, Salonen JT: Association of serum low density lipoprotein cholesterol, smoking and hypertension with different manifestations of atherosclerosis, *Intl J Epidemiol* 19:911-917, 1990.

71. Salonen R, Salonen JT: Progression of carotid atherosclerosis and its determinants: a population-based ultrasonography study, *Atherosclerosis* 81:33-40, 1990.

72. Salonen R, Salonen JT: Carotid atherosclerosis in relation to systolic and diastolic blood pressure: Kuopio ischemic heart disease risk factor study, *Ann Med* 23:23-27, 1991.

73. Salonen R, Salonen JT: Determinants of carotid intima-media thickness: a population-based ultrasonography study in Eastern Finnish Men, *J Intern Med* 229:225-231, 1991.

74. Salonen R et al: Prevalence of carotid atherosclerosis and serum cholesterol levels in Eastern Finland, *Arteriosclerosis* 8:788-792, 1988.

75. Schenk EA et al: Multicenter validation study of real-time ultrasonography, arteriography, and pathology: pathologic evaluation of carotid endarterectomy specimens, *Stroke* 19:289-296, 1988.

76. Smith EB, Evans PH, Downham MD: Lipid in the aortic intima: the correlation of morphological and chemical characteristics, *J Atheroscler Res* 7:171-186, 1967.

77. Sowers JR et al: Hypertension and atherosclerosis: calcium antagonists as antiatherogenic agents, *J Vasc Med Biol* 2:1-6, 1990.

78. Spence JD et al: Hemodynamic modification of aortic atherosclerosis: effects of propranolol vs hydralazine in hypertensive hyperlipidemic rabbits, *Atherosclerosis* 50:325-333, 1984.

79. Sterpetti AV, Hunter WJ, Schultz RD: Importance of ulceration of carotid plaque in determining symptoms of cerebral ischemia, *J Cardiovasc Surg* 32:154-158, 1991.

80. Stiel GM et al: Impact of compensatory enlargement of atherosclerotic coronary arteries on angiographic assessment of coronary heart disease, *Circulation* 80:1603-1609, 1989.

81. Sumner DS: *Correlation of lesion configuration with functional significance.* In Bond MG et al, eds: *Clinical diagnosis of atherosclerosis: quantitative methods of evaluation,* ed 2, New York, 1983, Springer-Verlag.

82. Thomas AC et al: Potential errors in the estimation of coronary arterial stenosis from clinical arteriography with reference to the shape of the coronary arterial lumen, *Br Heart J* 55:129-139, 1986.

83. Weinberger J et al: Atherosclerotic plaque at the carotid artery bifurcation: correlation of ultrasonographic imaging with morphology, *J Ultrasound Med* 6:363-366, 1987.

84. Weinstein DB, Heider JG: Protective action of calcium channel antagonists in atherosclerosis and experimental vascular injury, *Am J Hypertens* 2:205-212, 1989.

85. Zarins CK et al: Differential enlargement of artery segments in response to enlarging atherosclerotic plaque, *J Vasc Surg* 7:386-394, 1988.

CHAPTER 48

Carotid disease in preoperative patients: perioperative and late stroke risk

ROBERT W. BARNES

The surgical therapy of carotid artery disease has come under increased scrutiny in recent years, and the comparative efficacies of carotid endarterectomy and medical therapy for both symptomatic and asymptomatic carotid occlusive disease are being evaluated by several prospective, randomized clinical trials. In the meantime, decisions concerning the management of these patients are subject to the personal experience and bias of both surgeons and nonsurgeons. Asymptomatic carotid artery disease may exist in patients who have an incidentally detected carotid bruit, an angiographic lesion contralateral to symptomatic disease, or a carotid obstruction (preoperative patients) found before a major operation. Despite the controversy about the role of carotid endarterectomy in preventing stroke, it has been recommended that patients who have severe carotid obstruction undergo this procedure before they have coronary or peripheral vascular reconstructions.[22] The validity of this approach has never been supported by the findings of prospective, randomized trials, however. This chapter reviews the literature on various alternatives in the management of asymptomatic carotid artery disease in patients undergoing major cardiovascular operations, none of whom underwent prophylactic endarterectomy. Finally, a method of evaluating and managing the patients is presented in the form of an algorithm.

REVIEW OF LITERATURE

A total of 54 reports published from 1972 to 1991 that addressed the issue of managing asymptomatic carotid artery disease in the preoperative patient were reviewed; 42 were retrospective studies and 12 were prospective studies. As is often the case, the findings of 81% of the retrospective studies favored prophylactic carotid endarterectomy, whereas only 50% of the prospective studies supported such an approach.

Staged carotid–coronary artery procedure

Table 48-1 lists the outcomes in patients who underwent staged carotid artery endarterectomy followed by coronary artery bypass grafting. All but 4 of the 17 studies were retrospective. Of the 446 patients who had staged carotid–

coronary artery procedures, the perioperative morbidity included stroke in 2.5%, myocardial infarction in 9.0%, and death in 8.8%.

Concomitant carotid–coronary artery procedures

Table 48-2 lists the reported results in patients who underwent simultaneous endarterectomy and bypass grafting. Of the 37 studies, 6 were prospective. The resulting morbidity seen in the 2279 patients who had concomitant carotid and coronary artery procedures included stroke in 3.8%, myocardial infarction in 3.5%, and death in 4.8%. Combining the outcomes in the 2725 patients from the 29 studies (Tables 48-1 and 48-2), reporting the results of either staged or concomitant endarterectomy and bypass grafting yields an overall stroke rate of 3.6%, with myocardial infarction occurring in 4.6% and death in 5.5%.

Nonoperative management

Table 48-3 lists the outcomes in patients with carotid disease who underwent major cardiovascular operations without antecedent or concomitant carotid endarterectomy. Of the 21 studies, 9 were prospective. The surgical procedures consisted exclusively of coronary bypass grafts in 13 reports, peripheral vascular reconstructions in 4, and both coronary and vascular procedures in 4. Only the study by Ropper et al[50] included patients who underwent both general surgery as well as coronary or vascular procedures. In the total of 960 patients who did not have prophylactic endarterectomy for the treatment of carotid disease but did undergo major surgery, the perioperative stroke rate was 3.5% and the mortality rate was 7.3%.

The risk of an asymptomatic carotid bruit was the subject of five studies.[11,19,50,53,54] Of the total of 2255 patients who made up those studies, 355 (15.7%) had an asymptomatic bruit. A total of 19 patients (0.8%) who did not undergo prophylactic endarterectomy suffered perioperative stroke, and this occurred in 17 (0.9%) of the 1900 patients who did not have bruits and in only 2 (0.6%) of the 355 patients who did.

In the 13 reports of patients who had bypass grafting without prophylactic endarterectomy performed for known

Table 48-1. Perioperative risks of patients undergoing staged carotid endarterectomy and coronary artery bypass grafting

Reference	Year	Design	No. of patients	Stroke (%)	Myocardial infarction (%)	Death (%)
Bernhard et al[6]	1972	Retrospective	15	6.7	26.7	33.3
Lefrak and Guinn[33]	1974	Retrospective	34	2.9	14.7	17.6
Urschel et al[56]	1976	Retrospective	24	4.2	4.2	0
Mehigan et al[37]	1977	Retrospective	25	4.0	4.0	8.0
Morris et al[40]	1978	Retrospective	35	0	8.6	20.0
Hertzer et al[25]	1978	Retrospective	59	3.4	10.2	1.7
Ennix et al[18]	1979	Retrospective	77	5.2	14.3	18.2
Crawford et al[14]	1980	Retrospective	40	0	5.0	5.0
O'Donnell et al[43]	1983	Retrospective	13	0	7.7	0
Balderman et al[2]	1983	Prospective	8	0	0	0
Ivey et al[28]	1984	Prospective	5	0	ND	ND
Rosenthal et al[51]	1984	Retrospective	14	0	7.1	7.1
Berkoff and Turnipseed[5]	1984	Retrospective	2	0	0	0
Cosgrove et al[12]	1986	Prospective	24	0	ND	0
Newman et al[41]	1987	Retrospective	28	0	0	0
Hertzer et al[27]	1989	Prospective	24	4.2	4.2	4.2
Faggioli et al[20]	1990	Retrospective	19	0	ND	0

ND, No data.

Table 48-2. Perioperative risks of patients undergoing simultaneous prophylactic carotid endarterectomy and coronary artery bypass grafting

Reference	Year	Design	No. of patients	Stroke (%)	Myocardial infarction (%)	Death (%)
Bernhard et al[6]	1972	Retrospective	16	0	0	0
Urschel et al[56]	1976	Retrospective	8	0	0	0
Oakies et al[42]	1977	Retrospective	16	6.3	6.3	6.3
Mehigan et al[37]	1977	Retrospective	24	12.5	0	8.3
Morris et al[40]	1978	Retrospective	44	2.2	0	4.5
Dalton et al[15]	1978	Retrospective	25	0	0	4.5
Hertzer et al[25]	1978	Retrospective	115	4.3	10.4	4.3
Ennix et al[18]	1979	Retrospective	51	0	3.9	5.9
Crawford et al[14]	1980	Retrospective	48	2.1	2.1	2.1
Rice et al[47]	1980	Retrospective	54	1.9	0	0
Robertson and Fraser[48]	1981	Retrospective	26	3.8	ND	ND
Craver et al[13]	1982	Retrospective	68	1.5	1.5	0
Schwartz et al[52]	1982	Retrospective	73	1.4	0	11.0
Hertzer et al[26]	1983	Retrospective	331	4.5	6.3	5.7
Emery et al[17]	1983	Retrospective	42	0	0	4.8
O'Donnell et al[43]	1983	Retrospective	22	4.5	9.1	4.5
Balderman et al[2]	1983	Prospective	1	0	0	0
Jones et al[30]	1984	Retrospective	132	1.5	0.8	3.0
Brener et al[7]	1984	Prospective	29	3.4	ND	3.4
Ivey et al[28]	1984	Prospective	4	25.0	ND	25.0
Rosenthal et al[51]	1984	Retrospective	24	0	0	0
Berkoff and Turnipseed[5]	1984	Retrospective	16	6.3	0	6.3
Perler et al[45]	1985	Retrospective	37	0	2.7	8.1
Babu et al[1]	1985	Retrospective	62	3.2	3.2	4.8
Lord et al[34]	1986	Retrospective	78	6.4	3.8	6.4
Cosgrove et al[12]	1986	Prospective	72	5.6	ND	5.6
Brener et al[8]	1987	Prospective	28	0	ND	17.9
Newman et al[41]	1987	Retrospective	10	10.0	0	0
Lubicz et al[35]	1987	Retrospective	40	10.0	ND	5.0
Vermeulen et al[57]	1988	Retrospective	168	7.1	ND	3.0
Perler et al[45]	1988	Retrospective	63	3.2	3.2	11.1
Cambria et al[10]	1989	Retrospective	71	4.2	2.8	2.8
Hertzer et al[27]	1989	Prospective	170	5.3	ND	5.3
Jausseran et al[29]	1989	Retrospective	18	0	5.6	5.6
Duchateau et al[16]	1989	Retrospective	82	7.3	ND	7.3
Minami et al[38]	1989	Retrospective	116	1.7	1.7	1.7
Maki et al[36]	1989	Retrospective	95	2.1	ND	4.2

ND, No data.

Table 48-3. Perioperative risks of patients undergoing major cardiovascular operations without antecedent or concomitant carotid endarterectomy

Reference	Year	Design	Operation	No. of patients	Stroke (%)	Death (%)
Treiman et al[53]	1973	Retrospective	Vascular	40	0	ND
Carney et al[11]	1977	Retrospective	Vascular	35	0	ND
Evans and Cooperman[19]	1978	Retrospective	Vascular	92	0	ND
Treiman et al[54]	1979	Retrospective	Vascular	84	1.2	ND
Turnipseed et al[55]	1980	Prospective	Coronary, vascular	76	3.9	ND
Breslau et al[9]	1981	Prospective	Coronary	18	0	ND
Barnes et al[3]	1981	Prospective	Coronary, vascular	85	3.5	10.6
Kartchner and McRae[32]	1982	Retrospective	Coronary, vascular	41	17.1	4.9
Ropper et al[50]	1982	Prospective	General, coronary, vascular	104	1.0	ND
Ogren et al[44]	1983	Retrospective	Coronary	20	5.0	ND
Balderman et al[2]	1983	Prospective	Coronary	2	50.0	0
Ivey et al[28]	1984	Prospective	Coronary	16	0	ND
Rosenthal et al[51]	1984	Retrospective	Coronary	8	0	0
Berkoff and Turnipseed[5]	1984	Retrospective	Coronary	3	33.3	0
Furlan and Craciun[23]	1985	Retrospective	Coronary	29	3.4	ND
Gravlee et al[24]	1985	Retrospective	Coronary	3	0	0
Cosgrove et al[12]	1986	Prospective	Coronary	36	11.1	2.8
Brener et al[8]	1987	Prospective	Coronary	64	1.6	15.6
Newman et al[41]	1987	Retrospective	Coronary	12	0	0
Hertzer et al[27]	1989	Prospective	Coronary	104	5.3	1.9
Faggioli et al[20]	1990	Retrospective	Coronary	88	4.5	4.5

ND, No data.

carotid disease, perioperative stroke occurred in 20 (5.0%) of the total 403 patients.

In the 12 studies documenting the severity of carotid artery disease using either noninvasive techniques or angiography, the prevalence of perioperative stroke was 5.2% in the total 524 patients with carotid stenosis 50% or greater who did not undergo prophylactic endarterectomy.

Prospective perioperative and follow-up findings

In 1979, a prospective cohort study was begun to investigate the prevalence and natural history of asymptomatic carotid artery disease in patients undergoing major cardiovascular operations. One experienced nurse-technologist screened all 449 patients who were candidates for bypass grafting (324 patients) or peripheral arterial reconstruction (125 patients) at either the Medical College of Virginia or the Richmond Veterans Administration Medical Center. The study comprised 382 men and 67 women. All patients were evaluated for the presence of asymptomatic cervical bruit and underwent periorbital and direct carotid continuous wave Doppler screening to determine whether there was extracranial carotid obstruction that reduced the diameter of the artery by 50% or more. Patients with cerebrovascular symptoms or a history of carotid surgery were excluded from the study. No patient who had carotid obstruction detected underwent prophylactic endarterectomy, and all

had the coronary or peripheral vascular reconstruction that was indicated by the clinical findings.

The prevalence of asymptomatic bruits and Doppler evidence of carotid obstruction, as well as the perioperative outcomes of the 449 patients in the study, have been reported.[3] There was an asymptomatic cervical bruit in 44 patients (9.8%), and this constituted 18.4% of the patients with peripheral arterial disease and 6.4% of the patients with coronary artery disease. Doppler evidence of carotid obstruction that reduced the lumen by 50% or more was noted in 63 patients (14.0%), and this represented 18.4% of the patients with peripheral vascular disease and 12.3% of the patients with coronary artery disease. Carotid bruit, Doppler evidence of carotid obstruction, or both findings were found in 85 patients, and this constituted 28.8% of the patients with peripheral arterial disease and 15.1% of those with coronary artery disease. The correlation between cervical bruit and Doppler evidence of carotid obstruction that involved 50% or more of the artery was inconsistent; only 36.9% of the patients with a bruit actually had severe carotid obstruction, and only 27.3% of the patients with Doppler evidence of severe obstruction had a bruit.

Although no prophylactic endarterectomies were performed, perioperative neurologic deficits occurred in only 8 (1.8%) of the 449 patients. Deficits occurred in 1.6% of the patients undergoing peripheral vascular reconstruction and in 1.9% of those who had coronary bypass grafting. Transient ischemic attacks accounted for three of these deficits; strokes occurred in 5 patients, only 1 of whom had shown preoperative Doppler evidence of carotid stenosis of 50% or more. A total of 10 perioperative deaths (2.2%) occurred, and 8 were due to myocardial infarction. Death was significantly more common in patients with carotid disease (10.6%) than in those who had no bruit or Doppler evidence of carotid obstruction (0.3%; $p < 0.01$).

The late follow-up findings in 67 patients in this study with asymptomatic carotid disease who survived cardiovascular operation without neurologic deficit have also been reported.[4] Prophylactic carotid endarterectomy was not performed until patients displayed symptoms. In a follow-up study that extended to 61 months (mean, 35 months), a neurologic deficit developed in 22 patients (32.8%), and this represented 55.6% of the patients with peripheral arterial disease and 17.5% of the patients with coronary artery disease. Transient ischemic attacks occurred in 7 patients (10.4%), only 3 of whom had shown carotid artery disease preoperatively. The prevalence of late postoperative stroke was 22.2% in patients who underwent peripheral arterial reconstruction and only 2.5% in patients who had coronary bypass grafting. Doppler evidence of the late progression of carotid disease was noted in 19.6% of the patients and consisted of increasing stenosis in 13.7% and progression to carotid occlusion in 5.9%. In addition, 2 of the 3 patients with carotid occlusion suffered fatal strokes, and both had shown preoperative evidence of contralateral asymptomatic carotid occlusion. There were late postoperative deaths in 11 (16.4%) of the 67 patients, and these occurred in 25.9% of the patients who had peripheral arterial reconstruction and in only 10.0% of those who had coronary bypass grafting.

DISCUSSION

The indications for performing carotid endarterectomy are controversial, both for patients experiencing symptoms and for those with asymptomatic carotid disease.[58] Until the results of ongoing clinical trials are available, clinicians must make management decisions based on their own experience and the published experience of others. This review has attempted to compile the available data that either support or refute performing prophylactic endarterectomy in patients undergoing a major operation, usually a cardiovascular procedure. The results of this overview suggest that there is little justification for doing prophylactic endarterectomy preoperatively, a practice originally recommended by Fields.[21]

The discovery of an asymptomatic cervical bruit often prompts the decision to carry out further noninvasive screening or angiography. However, the presence of a bruit is a fallible guide to severe carotid obstruction, as shown by the study of Barnes et al[3] and the report published by Kartchner and McRae.[31] Although noninvasive studies have become an accurate means of evaluating extracranial carotid disease

minus the risk and expense of angiography, this technology has contributed to an increase in the detection of severe asymptomatic carotid disease and an inherent rise in the number of prophylactic endarterectomies performed. Fortunately, some investigators have also used noninvasive diagnostic techniques to define prospectively the natural history of asymptomatic carotid disease, including that in patients about to undergo major surgery.* Although such prospective studies account for less than one fourth of the literature published to date, the findings in one half of them fail to endorse the use of prophylactic endarterectomy in patients about to have major surgery, whereas 80% of the retrospective studies favor such a practice.

Despite the low systemic perfusion pressure during cardiopulmonary bypass, the prevalence of perioperative stroke in patients undergoing coronary bypass grafting is relatively low, usually less than 2%. Furthermore, some strokes may actually be due to complications of cardiopulmonary bypass and not to carotid disease. The role of systemic anticoagulation in reducing the risk of perioperative stroke during coronary bypass grafting and peripheral vascular reconstructions is unknown. All but one study[50] of carotid disease in the preoperative patient has involved patients undergoing cardiovascular operations. Such patients exhibit a higher prevalence of carotid disease than that seen in the general population, particularly patients who have peripheral arterial disease, as noted in the study of Barnes et al.[3]

The timing of carotid artery endarterectomy and coronary artery bypass grafting is a matter of controversy. Although the procedures generally have been staged to reduce perioperative morbidity, the observations gleaned from this overview suggest that performing endarterectomy before bypass grafting results in an increased number of both perioperative myocardial infarctions and deaths after the carotid procedure.

The review of the study suggests that the risk of perioperative stroke in patients who do not have prophylactic carotid endarterectomy before major cardiovascular surgery is not significantly greater than that in patients who do undergo this procedure. In particular, the risk of stroke in patients with asymptomatic carotid bruit who have peripheral arterial reconstruction is the same as that in patients without bruit.[11,19,50,53,54] The risk of perioperative stroke (5.0%) in patients who underwent coronary bypass grafting without endarterectomy did not differ much from the stroke rate (3.6%) in patients who did have endarterectomy before or at the same time as coronary bypass grafting. Whether the 5.2% preoperative stroke rate in patients with carotid stenosis of 50% or more who did not have endarterectomy is significantly greater than that in patients who did not undergo endarterectomy cannot be determined from these published series.

The follow-up reported by Barnes et al[4] is the only study to date that describes the late postoperative course in patients

---

*References 3, 8, 9, 20, 27, 28, 49, 55.

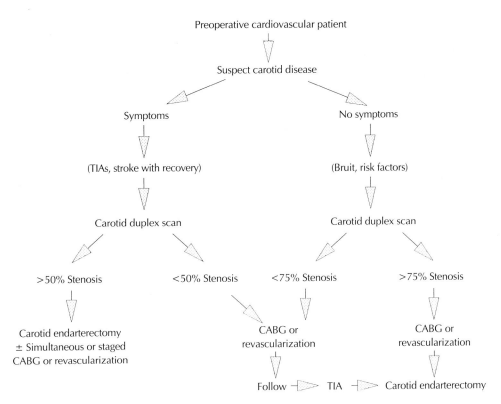

Fig. 48-1. Algorithm for evaluation and management of carotid disease in the preoperative patient. (*TIA,* Transient ischemic attack; *CABG,* coronary artery bypass graft.)

with untreated carotid artery disease who underwent major cardiovascular surgery. The findings in this study suggest that there is a significant incidence (33%) of late neurologic deficits in such patients, two thirds of which are transient ischemic attacks. Only one stroke occurred in the territory of the severe carotid disease that was documented preoperatively. Progression of carotid disease was documented by Doppler ultrasound in 20% of the patients during a mean follow-up period of 35 months. Of three patients in whom carotid occlusion developed, two suffered fatal strokes. The occlusion of the contralateral carotid artery had been documented preoperatively in both these patients. The major risk stemming from asymptomatic carotid disease in this study, however, was not a neurologic deficit but coronary artery disease. The risk of both preoperative and late postoperative deaths due to myocardial infarction was significantly higher in patients with carotid disease than in those without such disease.

Fig. 48-1 is an algorithm that shows a current approach to the evaluation and management of patients with suspected carotid artery disease before they undergo a major operation. Cerebral arteriography is performed if the patient has symptomatic carotid disease consisting of ocular or hemispheric transient ischemic attacks or stroke with recovery. If a carotid stenosis is found, either staged or concomitant carotid endarterectomy and the intended coronary artery bypass grafting are performed. The procedures may be staged for

patients scheduled to undergo peripheral arterial reconstruction.

Carotid disease may be suspected in patients with no cerebrovascular symptoms if an asymptomatic bruit or known atherosclerotic risks for stroke are found. In such a case, a noninvasive study is performed, preferably with a combined B-mode and Doppler (duplex) scanner. If severe carotid stenosis (75% or more) is detected, the patient should undergo the cardiovascular operation followed by staged endarterectomy. This approach to treatment is based on the findings reported by Moneta et al[39] that indicated a more favorable outcome in patients undergoing carotid endarterectomy than in those in whom the natural history of the severe carotid stenosis was merely monitored by Doppler scanning. If a carotid stenosis of less than 75% is found, the patient should undergo the cardiovascular operation as planned and then be carefully watched for the occurrence of late postoperative transient ischemic attacks that might warrant prophylactic endarterectomy. Patients whose noninvasive carotid studies are normal should undergo the intended cardiovascular operation.

CONCLUSION

Although carotid endarterectomy is the second most common cardiovascular operation performed in the United States, the past decade has witnessed much controversy over its efficacy. Until prospective clinical trials validate this procedure, clinicians must make their decisions based on their own experience and the published experiences of others. The role of endarterectomy in the treatment of patients about to have major cardiovascular surgery has been the subject of a large body of literature, most of which is retrospective and supports the use of endarterectomy. However, increasing numbers of prospective studies have failed to justify the practice of routine endarterectomy before or concomitant with major cardiovascular operations. Such prospective studies, which have taken advantage of the capability of noninvasive techniques, have revealed the prevalence and natural history of carotid disease in the perioperative patient. Although untreated carotid artery disease does not appear to significantly contribute to an increased risk of perioperative stroke, it does mark the patient who is at significantly increased risk of perioperative and late postoperative death, usually as the result of coronary artery disease. In addition, patients in the late postoperative period with a natural history of untreated asymptomatic carotid disease are at increased risk of suffering neurologic deficits, especially transient ischemic attacks. If carefully screened for, these deficits should prompt the decision to perform prophylactic endarterectomy before stroke develops. Thus, the recognition of asymptomatic carotid disease and then careful follow-up in patients about to have major cardiovascular surgery is recommended as a rational alternative to performing routine endarterectomy.

REFERENCES

1. Babu SC et al: Coexisting carotid stenosis in patients undergoing cardiac surgery: indications and guidelines for simultaneous operations, *Am J Surg* 150:207, 1985.
2. Balderman SC et al: Noninvasive screening for asymptomatic carotid artery disease prior to cardiac operation, *J Thorac Cardiovasc Surg* 85:427, 1983.
3. Barnes RW et al: The natural history of asymptomatic carotid disease in patients undergoing cardiovascular surgery, *Surgery* 90:1075, 1981.
4. Barnes RW et al: Late outcome of untreated asymptomatic carotid disease following cardiovascular operations, *J Vasc Surg* 2:843, 1985.
5. Berkoff HA, Turnipseed WD: Patient selection and results of simultaneous coronary and carotid artery procedures, *Ann Thorac Surg* 38:172, 1984.
6. Bernhard VM, Johnson WD, Peterson JJ: Carotid artery stenosis, association with surgery for coronary artery disease, *Arch Surg* 105:837, 1972.
7. Brener BJ et al: A four-year experience with preoperative noninvasive carotid evaluation of two thousand twenty-six patients undergoing cardiac surgery, *J Vasc Surg* 1:326, 1984.
8. Brener BJ et al: This risk of stroke in patients with asymptomatic carotid stenosis undergoing cardiac surgery: a follow-up study, *J Vasc Surg* 5:269, 1987.
9. Breslau PJ et al: Carotid arterial disease in patients undergoing coronary artery bypass operations, *J Thorac Cardiovasc Surg* 82:765, 1981.
10. Cambria RP et al: Simultaneous carotid and coronary disease: safety of the combined approach, *J Vasc Surg* 9:56, 1989.
11. Carney WI et al: Carotid bruit as a risk factor in aortoiliac reconstruction, *Surgery* 81:567, 1977.
12. Cosgrove DM, Hertzer NR, Floyd DL: Surgical management of synchronous carotid and coronary artery disease, *J Vasc Surg* 3:690, 1986.
13. Craver JM et al: Concomitant carotid and coronary artery reconstruction, *Ann Surg* 195:712, 1982.
14. Crawford ES, Palamara AE, Kasparian AS: Carotid and noncoronary operations: simultaneous, staged, and delayed, *Surgery* 87:1, 1980.
15. Dalton ML et al: Concomitant coronary artery bypass and major noncardiac surgery, *J Thorac Cardiovasc Surg* 75:621, 1978.
16. Duchateau J et al: Combined myocardial and cerebral revascularization: a ten-year experience, *J Cardiovasc Surg* 30:715, 1989.
17. Emery RW et al: Coexistent carotid and coronary artery disease: surgical management, *Arch Surg* 118:1035, 1983.
18. Ennix CL Jr et al: Improved results of carotid endarterectomy in patients with symptomatic coronary disease: an analysis of 1,546 consecutive carotid operations, *Stroke* 10:122, 1979.
19. Evans WE, Cooperman M: The significance of asymptomatic unilateral carotid bruits in peroperative patients, *Surgery* 77:521, 1978.
20. Faggioli GL, Curl GR, Ricotta JJ: The role of carotid screening before coronary artery bypass, *J Vasc Surg* 12:724, 1990.
21. Fields WS: Neurologic disorders related to alterations in blood pressure, *Cardiovasc Res Cent Bull* 2:65, 1964.
22. Fields WS: Selection of stroke patients for arterial reconstructive surgery, *Am J Surg* 125:527, 1973.
23. Furlan AJ, Craciun AR: Risk of stroke during coronary artery bypass graft: surgery in patients with internal carotid artery disease documented by angiography, *Stroke* 16:797, 1985.
24. Gravlee GP et al: Coronary revascularization in patients with bilateral internal carotid occlusions, *J Thorac Cardiovasc Surg* 90:921, 1985.
25. Hertzer NR et al: Staged and combined surgical approach to simultaneous carotid and coronary vascular disease, *Surgery* 84:803, 1978.
26. Hertzer NR et al: Combined myocardial revascularization and carotid endarterectomy: operative and late results in 331 patients, *J Thorac Cardiovasc Surg* 85:577, 1983.
27. Hertzer NR et al: Surgical staging for simultaneous coronary and carotid disease: a study including prospective randomization, *J Vasc Surg* 9:455, 1989.
28. Ivey TD et al: Management of patients with carotid bruit undergoing cardiopulmonary bypass, *J Thorac Cardiovasc Surg* 87:183, 1984.
29. Jausseran JM et al: Single staged carotid and coronary artery surgery: indications and results, *J Cardiovasc Surg* 30:407, 1989.
30. Jones EL et al: Combined carotid and coronary operations: when are they necessary? *J Thorac Cardiovasc Surg* 87:7, 1984.
31. Kartchner MM, McRae LP: Noninvasive evaluation and management of "asymptomatic" carotid bruit, *Surgery* 82:840, 1977.
32. Kartchner MM, McRae LP: Carotid occlusive disease as a risk factor in major cardiovascular surgery, *Arch Surg* 117:1086, 1982.
33. Lefrak EA, Guinn GA: Prophylactic carotid artery surgery in patients requiring a second operation, *South Med J* 2:185, 1974.
34. Lord RS et al: Rationale for simultaneous carotid endarterectomy and aortocoronary bypass, *Ann Vasc Surg* 1:201, 1986.
35. Lubicz S et al: Combined carotid and coronary surgery, *Aust NZ J Surg* 57:593, 1987.
36. Maki HS, Keuhner ME, Ray JF III: Combined carotid endarterectomy and myocardial revascularization, *Am J Surg* 158:443, 1989.
37. Mehigan JT et al: A planned approach to coexistent cerebrovascular disease in coronary artery bypass candidates, *Arch Surg* 112:1403, 1977.
38. Minami K et al: Management of concomitant occlusive disease of coronary and carotid arteries using cardiopulmonary bypass for both procedures, *J Cardiovasc Surg* 30:723, 1989.
39. Moneta GL et al: Operative versus nonoperative management of asymptomatic high-grade internal carotid artery stenosis: improved results with endarterectomy, *Stroke* 18:1005, 1987.
40. Morris GC Jr et al: Management of coexistent carotid and coronary artery occlusive atherosclerosis, *Cleve Q J* 45:125, 1978.
41. Newman DC et al: Coexistent carotid and coronary arterial disease, *J Cardiovasc Surg* 28:599, 1987.
42. Oakies JE et al: Myocardial revascularization and carotid endarterectomy: a combined approach, *Ann Thorac Surg* 23:560, 1977.
43. O'Donnell TF Jr et al: The impact of coronary artery disease on carotid endarterectomy, *Ann Surg* 198:705, 1983.
44. Ogren CO et al: The role of noninvasive cerebrovascular testing in patients undergoing coronary artery surgery, *Bruit* 7:22, 1983.
45. Perler BA, Burdick JF, Williams GM: The safety of carotid endarterectomy at the time of coronary artery bypass surgery: analysis of results in a high-risk patient population, *J Vasc Surg* 2:558, 1985.
46. Perler BA et al: Should we perform carotid endarterectomy synchronously with cardiac surgical procedures? *J Vasc Surg* 8:402, 1988.
47. Rice PL et al: Experience with simultaneous myocardial revascularization and carotid endarterectomy, *J Thorac Cardiovasc Surg* 79:922, 1980.

48. Robertson JT, Fraser JC: *Evaluation of carotid endarterectomy with and without coronary artery bypass surgery.* In Mossy J, Reinmuth OM, eds: *Cerebrovascular disease,* New York, 1981, Raven Press.

49. Roederer GO et al: The natural history of carotid arterial disease in asymptomatic patients with cervical bruits, *Stroke* 15:605, 1984.

50. Ropper AH, Wechsler LR, Wilson LS: Carotid bruit and the risk of stroke in elective surgery, *N Engl J Med* 307:1286, 1982.

51. Rosenthal D et al: Carotid and coronary arterial disease, *Am Surg* 50:233, 1984.

52. Schwartz RL et al: Simultaneous myocardial revascularization and carotid endarterectomy, *Circulation* 66(suppl):97, 1982.

53. Treiman RL et al: Carotid bruit: significance in patients undergoing an abdominal aortic operation, *Arch Surg* 106:803, 1973.

54. Treiman RL et al: Carotid bruit: a follow-up report on its significance in patients undergoing an abdominal aortic operation, *Arch Surg* 113:1138, 1979.

55. Turnipseed WD, Berkoff HA, Belzer FO: Postoperative stroke in cardiac and peripheral vascular disease, *Ann Surg* 192:365, 1980.

56. Urschel HC, Razzuk MA, Gardner MA: Management of concomitant occlusive disease of the carotid and coronary arteries, *J Thorac Cardiovasc Surg* 72:829, 1976.

57. Vermeulen FE et al: Simultaneous extensive extracranial and coronary revascularization, *Eur J Cardiothorac Surg* 2:113, 1988.

58. Winslow CM et al: The appropriateness of carotid endarterectomy, *N Engl J Med* 318:721, 1988.

CHAPTER 49

Management of symptomatic and asymptomatic carotid stenosis: results of current randomized clinical trials

ROBERT W. HOBSON II

Defining the therapeutic benefit of carotid endarterectomy in asymptomatic and symptomatic carotid occlusive disease has constituted a controversial issue in the management of patients with vascular disease. Recently published data obtained in three randomized clinical trials have demonstrated the efficacy of carotid endarterectomy in symptomatic patients with high-grade carotid stenosis.[19,37,47] However, the results of two major clinical trials in patients with asymptomatic carotid stenosis have yet to be finalized and published.[2,26]

The more important debate concerning indications for carotid endarterectomy has focused on the efficacy of operative intervention in patients with asymptomatic carotid stenosis. The rationale for using carotid endarterectomy as a primary treatment for transient ischemic attacks (TIAs) and stroke in patients with high-grade asymptomatic carotid stenosis is based on several assumptions: (1) such patients can be identified by accurate noninvasive studies[33] and the progression from less severe to significant stenosis can be documented[42]; (2) arteriographic confirmation can be obtained virtually free of the risk of death and with a low stroke risk[27,43]; (3) the annual occurrence rate of TIAs, accompanied by positive computed tomographic (CT) findings[3,39] or frank stroke, is relatively high in this subset of patients, perhaps ranging from less than 3% to as much as 5%[12,13]; and (4) carotid endarterectomy can be performed with low combined stroke morbidity and operative mortality, preferably less than 2% to 5% (Table 49-1).

CATEGORIZATION OF PATIENTS AND DETERMINATION OF ASYMPTOMATIC STENOSIS

Data supporting the first assumption that noninvasive means can be used to reliably dated and monitor the progression of asymptomatic stenosis have been reviewed amply. A major problem in the assessment of asymptomatic carotid stenosis has been agreeing on the definition of "significant" carotid stenosis. In the past, the term *carotid bruit* was used to denote transient neurologic events or stroke. Although a bruit may be indicative of a carotid stenosis varying between 20% and 30% to 95% or greater, all carotid bruits obviously do not imply the existence of hemodynamically significant

lessons. Kartchner and McRae[30] reported that only 36% of their 668 patients with cervical bruits had a hemodynamically significant carotid stenosis. This impression was confirmed by Roederer et al,[42] who reported that more then half of the arteries with an associated bruit that they evaluated did not have hemodynamically significant stenoses, as determined by duplex scanning techniques. Hennerici et al,[21] Ziegler et al,[50] and Riles et al[40] have concluded that the clinical evaluation of bruits does not provide reliable information regarding the presence of hemodynamically significant carotid stenosis. Furthermore, significant carotid occlusive disease is not always accompanied by a bruit. Jain et al[28] reported that 50% of their patients with hemodynamically significant stenoses had no associated cervical bruits, whereas Barnes et al[4] observed cervical bruit in only 27% of their patients with noninvasively obtained evidence of hemodynamically significant obstruction.

The definition of asymptomatic but clinically significant carotid stenosis is usually formulated in terms of the magnitude of stenosis present at the carotid bifurcation and the proximal internal carotid artery. Convention as well as the findings of laboratory studies documenting reductions in distal pressure and flow have generally defined hemodynamically significant stenoses as those causing a 50% or greater reduction in the luminal diameter of the artery shown by biplanar arteriography, or those constituting a 75% reduction in the artery's cross-sectional area. These definitions identify the threshold levels of hemodynamic significance. The percentage of the stenosis is determined by comparing the least transverse diameter at the stenosis with the diameter of the distal uninvolved internal carotid artery where the arterial walls become parallel. The percentage may then be expressed as the function of either the diameter or the cross-sectional area (Fig. 49-1).

Noninvasive techniques have been used to identify patients with asymptomatic carotid stenosis and have included indirect hemodynamic testings such as the cerebrovascular Doppler examination[8] as well as the oculoplethysmographic determination of ocular pulse delay[32] or ophthalmic artery pressure.[20] Although these techniques can detect hemodynamically significant stenoses, they cannot distinguish high-

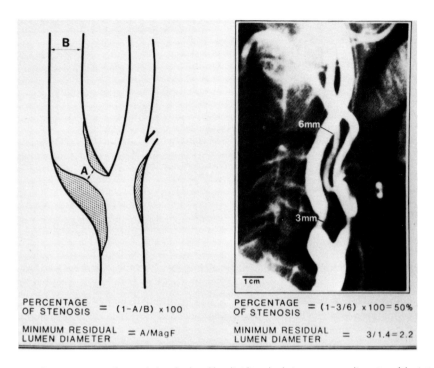

$$\text{PERCENTAGE OF STENOSIS} = (1 - A/B) \times 100$$

$$\text{MINIMUM RESIDUAL LUMEN DIAMETER} = A/\text{MagF}$$

$$\text{PERCENTAGE OF STENOSIS} = (1 - 3/6) \times 100 = 50\%$$

$$\text{MINIMUM RESIDUAL LUMEN DIAMETER} = 3/1.4 = 2.2$$

Fig. 49-1. The percentage of stenosis is calculated by dividing the least transverse diameter of the internal carotid artery at the stenosis *(A)* by the diameter of the distal, uninvolved artery *(B)*. The minimum residual lumen diameter is equivalent to the least transverse diameter *(A)* divided by the magnification factor (MagF) of the arteriogram. The example *(right)* illustrates a 50% stenosis by diameter and a minimum residual lumen diameter of 2.2. (From Lynch TG, Hobson RW: *Vascular surgery: principles and practice,* New York, 1987, McGraw-Hill.)

Table 49-1. Morbidity and mortality associated with carotid endarterectomy for asymptomatic carotid disease in different studies

Author	No. of operations	Mortality	Morbidity Transient	Morbidity Permanent
Thompson et al[45]	167	0	2 (1.2%)	2 (1.2%)
Moore et al[36]	78	0	2 (2.6%)	0
Hertzer et al[22]	95	1 (1.1%)	—	4 (4.2%)
Whitney et al[48]	279	3 (1.1%)	5 (1.8%)	6 (2.2%)
Javid et al[29]	65	1 (1.5%)	1 (1.5%)	1 (1.5%)
Anderson et al[1]	120	0	2 (1.7%)	0
Veterans Administration Clinical Trial[46]	211	4 (1.9%)	2 (0.9%)	5 (2.4%)

grade stenosis from total occlusion and cannot quantitate lesser degrees of stenosis. Consequently, direct investigation of the carotid bifurcation using spectral analysis[7,41] and ultrasound imaging of the cervical carotid artery[14,25] has become increasingly important in the analysis of these cases. O'Leary et al[38] assessed the impact of noninvasive testing on patient management and demonstrated an increase in the number of positive arteriograms and a reduction in the incidence of less significant findings that were directly related to the clinical application of duplex scanning.

These noninvasive techniques must eventually be evaluated in terms of a reference standard, such as arteriography, or perhaps through direct pathologic analysis of the resected carotid plaque. Performance of these studies is then judged on the basis of sensitivity and specificity as well as positive and negative predictive values. Each laboratory is responsible for these determinations, which must be gathered carefully and reassessed periodically. In this way, the noninvasive laboratory can make important contributions to the identification of patients with asymptomatic stenosis, who in the context of satisfactory operative risk factors may be considered candidates for arteriography and prophylactic carotid endarterectomy.

The safety of arteriography has improved with the use

of newer types of contrast media as well as the application of intraarterial digital subtraction arteriographic techniques. One study examining the complications of arteriography encountered at six university medical centers in patients seen because of TIAs reported a stroke risk of less than 1%, and this was generally associated with a transfemoral route of catheterization.[43] Recent analysis of data[27] from the VA Cooperative Study on Asymptomatic Carotid Stenosis demonstrated a stroke rate of 0.4% without mortality in patients with asymptomatic stenoses as well as with asymptomatic stenoses contralateral to a symptomatic lesion. Consequently, arteriography has proved to be safe in asymptomatic patients and causes a complication rate that permits aggressive surgical management in such patients.

TIAs, when accompanied by positive CT scans or frank stroke, occur at relatively high annual rates in patients with significant but asymptomatic carotid stenosis. Furthermore, the presumption that a clinical TIA is innocuous awaits further clinical investigation. Some authors[3,39] have reported that CT scans are positive in 30% to 40% of the cases of transient neurologic events. Consequently, the concept that a transient neurologic event is of no or only minor clinical consequences[17] may be erroneous because it also becomes an index for patients at greatest risk of suffering stroke during the first month after their initial TIA.[15]

Several authors have used noninvasive techniques to identify the risk of subsequent stroke in that subset of patients with hemodynamically significant but asymptomatic stenoses. Kartchner and McRae[31] reported a 12% stroke rate after 2 years in a group of asymptomatic patients with hemodynamically significant stenoses identified by one oculoplethysmographic technique. Cullen et al[16] used ophthalmic artery pressure to identify 77 patients with hemodynamically insignificant stenosis and 29 with hemodynamically significant stenosis. Clinical follow-up at 18 months revealed that 11% of those patients without significant stenoses had become symptomatic, whereas 24% with significant stenoses had become symptomatic. Moneta et al[34] reported on 129 patients who were separated into two groups: those undergoing carotid endarterectomy and those treated nonoperatively. Life-table analysis up to 24 months in this study demonstrated a higher rate of TIAs (28% versus 5%; $p = 0.008$), internal carotid occlusion (29% versus 0%; $p = 0.003$), and stroke (19% versus 4%, $p = 0.08$) in the group treated nonoperatively. None of the strokes was preceded by TIAs, eight of nine occurred within 9 months of the diagnosis of a high-grade lesion, and none occurred in the 10 patients who refused operation because of coexisting medical problems. In the patients who were treated surgically, there was one perioperative stroke (1.8%) and no hospital deaths.

Moore et al[35] reported similar data for their group of patients with asymptomatic stenoses of 50% or greater. In the nonoperated group, the stroke rate was 21% compared

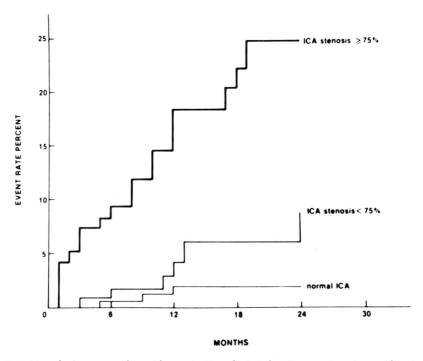

Fig. 49-2. Neurologic events and carotid stenosis. Neurologic ischemic events in patients with an internal carotid stenosis greater than 75% occur at a rate of 15% per year. In patients with stenoses of less than 75%, however, the rate is 3% per year, and in patients without evidence of disease the rate is 2% per year. (From Chamber BR, Norris JW: The case against surgery for asymptomatic carotid stenosis, *Stroke* 15:964-967, 1984.)

with 8% in the operated group ($p < 0.05$). Chambers and Norris[12,13] have reported data on 500 patients obtained in their study of asymptomatic cervical bruits. Ischemic cerebrovascular events occurred annually in 18% of the patients with area stenoses of greater than 75%; 12% of these were TIAs and 6% were strokes, about half of them ipsilateral to the stenosis. In those patients with stenoses of less than 75%, neurologic events occurred at a rate of less than 3% per year (Fig. 49-2). Their data and those from other reports have confirmed the association of high-grade stenosis with an increased risk of TIAs and stroke. Although the annual stroke rates in patients with carotid bruit alone have been low,[23,49] long-term studies examining the incidence of stroke and transient neurologic events in an asymptomatic population with high-grade stenosis have not been well documented.

In the absence of data from multicenter, prospectively randomized clinical trials on carotid endarterectomy in the asymptomatic population, the justification for performing prophylactic endarterectomy is based on the supposition that its associated complications are less than the morbidity and mortality expected in the nonoperated population. Consequently, the surgical experience of all practitioners who recommend endarterectomy in these patients must be well documented. Multiple reports in the literature have documented the relative safety of operation in these patients. Thompson et al[45] reported a less than 2% incidence of perioperative morbidity and no operative deaths in their patient population. The immediate and long-term results of carotid endarterectomy in asymptomatic patients have also been evaluated by Moore et al,[36] who reported no operative deaths or perioperative strokes in a series of 78 operations as well as a 95% stroke-free status in surviving patients. Recently a group of investigators reported similar results. No perioperative strokes or deaths were encountered among 120 consecutive patients who underwent endarterectomies for high-grade asymptomatic carotid stenosis. Table 49-1 summarizes data from several clinical series that evaluated the results of carotid endarterectomy in asymptomatic patients. These data are generally consistent with the operative stroke and mortality rates recommended by Barnett, Plum, and Walton.[6] Pending the availability of outcome data from prospective trials such as the current VA protocol[27] or the NIH-sponsored Asymptomatic Carotid Artery Stenosis Study,[2] the viewpoints expressed in recent editorials[24,44] seem appropriate. They suggest that it is the responsibility of the operating surgeons to report the local operative complication rates so that this can be taken into consideration before carotid endarterectomy is recommended in patients with asymptomatic stenosis.

PROSPECTIVE RANDOMIZED CLINICAL TRIALS

A principal response among the vascular surgery community to Barnett's description[5] of the efficacy of carotid endarterectomy as a matter of "clinical disarray" has been to perform randomized clinical trials. Although most vascular surgeons agree on the relatively precise indications for operative intervention, many of the surgical concepts have been challenged because results from clinical trials confirming the efficacy of carotid endarterectomy have been lacking and because of the misperception that the higher operative complication rates reported from some centers[9,18] reflect the experience nationwide. However, the recently published findings from randomized clinical trials in patients with symptomatic carotid occlusive disease[19,37,47] have confirmed the efficacy of operation in patients with high-grade stenosis (greater than 70%) who have had ipsilateral TIAs or stroke with minimal disability.

Perhaps the most important clinical trial (box) has been the North American Symptomatic Carotid Endarterectomy Trial (NASCET).[37] In an analysis of 659 patients with TIAs or nondisabling strokes occurring within the 120 days preceding presentation and with ipsilateral carotid stenosis of 70% to 99%, the cumulative risk of an ipsilateral stroke occurring by 24 months of follow-up was 26% for the 331 medically treated patients and 9% for the 328 surgically treated patients, yielding an absolute risk reduction of 17% ($p < 0.001$). The corresponding incidences of major or fatal ipsilateral stroke were 13.1% and 2.5% for the medically and surgically treated groups, respectively; this translates into an absolute risk reduction of 10.6% or a greater than 5:1 benefit in favor of operation ($p < 0.001$). The NASCET investigators concluded that carotid endarterectomy was highly beneficial for patients with recent hemispheric or retinal TIAs or those with nondisabling stroke in the presence of ipsilateral high-grade carotid stenosis. However, these investigators have also made a plea for the continued randomization of symptomatic patients with stenoses of between 30% and 69%, since the relative merits of medical and surgical management currently are not well defined. Furthermore, this study found that the incidence of stroke in the medically treated group increased significantly as the degree of stenosis increased for those patients with 70% to 79%, 80% to 89%, and 90% to 99% stenoses.

CLINICAL TRIALS OF THE EFFICACY OF CAROTID ENDARTERECTOMY FOR SYMPTOMATIC AND ASYMPTOMATIC CAROTID STENOSIS

Symptomatic carotid stenosis

1. North American Symptomatic Carotid Endarterectomy Trial (NASCET)[37]
2. European Carotid Surgery Trialists' (ECST)[19] Collaborative Group
3. VA Cooperative Trial on Symptomatic Carotid Stenosis[47]

Asymptomatic carotid stenosis

1. VA Cooperative Trial on Asymptomatic Carotid Stenosis[26]
2. NIH Asymptomatic Carotid Atherosclerosis Study (ACAS)[2]
3. Carotid Artery Stenosis with Asymptomatic Narrowing: Operation Versus Aspirin (CASANOVA)[11]

The results of another clinical trial on symptomatic carotid occlusive disease, the European Carotid Surgery Trial, were also published in 1991.[19] These investigators randomized patients into a uniform protocol; however, each center was allowed its own preference regarding the selection of patients considered eligible for randomization. Although some considered this a methodologic flaw, the results of the study essentially confirmed those of the NASCET. Among a cohort of 778 patients with stenoses in the 70% to 99% range, the risk of surgical stroke or death, ipsilateral ischemic stroke, or any other stroke was 12.3% for the surgical group and 21.9% for the medical group at 3 years of follow-up; this represented an absolute risk reduction of 9.6% ($p < 0.01$). The incidence of more significant disabling or fatal stroke was 6% in the surgically treated group and 11% in the medically treated group ($p < 0.05$). These investigators also studied 374 patients with stenoses of 0% to 29% and concluded that carotid endarterectomy offered no benefit in these patients. The results of carotid endarterectomy in patients with 30% to 69% stenoses remain uncertain.

Finally, a third randomized trial that studied patients with symptomatic carotid stenosis and also published in 1991 was the VA trial,[47] which consisted of 189 patients with TIAs or nondisabling stroke and ipsilateral stenosis of 50% or greater. During a mean follow-up of 11.9 months, the incidence of stroke or crescendo TIA was 7.7% in the surgical group and 19.4% in the medical group, for an absolute risk reduction of 11.7% ($p = 0.028$). The differences between groups in terms of stroke alone were not significant, but the smaller sample size and shorter period of follow-up were responsible for these results. However, these results are viewed as confirming the high clinical risk of stroke in the patient with crescendo TIAs. As found in the NASCET, an increased risk of stroke was also observed in patients with stenoses of 70% or more.

Results from these randomized clinical trials have influenced the management of patients with a history of recent TIA or nondisabling stroke. The referral of symptomatic patients for noninvasive vascular testing to establish the severity of stenosis is therefore advocated. If this confirms severe stenosis (70% or more), carotid endarterectomy is recommended for those better-risk patients, to be performed at those centers reporting a low operative risk of permanent stroke and death. Primary treatment with antiplatelet agents or in some instances coumadin, with referral for carotid endarterectomy only if break-through symptoms appear while on this treatment, is no longer an acceptable clinical option.

Concerning the indications for operation in patients with asymptomatic carotid stenosis, investigators from the Carotid Artery Stenosis with Asymptomatic Narrowing: Operation Versus Aspirin (CASANOVA) trial[11] randomized 410 patients to receive either operative or optimal medical management. After a mean follow-up of 3 years, these investigators were unable to demonstrate any significant difference in event rates between the medically and surgically treated groups of patients. However, higher-risk patients were excluded from the study and referred preferentially for carotid endarterectomy. This group included patients with stenoses of 90% or greater as well as patients who had noninvasive evidence of significant progression of their stenoses. Coupled with a qualitative flaw in the randomization protocol, the results of this trial should be regarded as inconclusive pending the publication of the findings from the VA trial[26] and the NIH-sponsored trial.[2]

Investigators from the VA trial have randomized 440 high-risk adult male patients to undergo either optimal medical management plus carotid endarterectomy or optimal medical management alone, with both groups receiving antiplatelet medication. All stenoses were confirmed arteriographically and shown to reduce the diameter of the arterial lumen by 50% or more, in conjunction with a positive OPG-Gee (oculopneumoplethysmography as described by Gee) or duplex scan. Primary end points for the study included TIA, stroke, and death. Data from this trial have been submitted for publication and indicate that carotid endarterectomy significantly reduces the incidence of neurologic events in adult male patients with arteriographically defined asymptomatic carotid stenoses. Although this trial's smaller sample size causes it to lack sufficient weight to address the question of the procedure's efficacy in preventing stroke and death, analysis of these end points awaits further investigation in a clinical trial with larger sample sizes.[5] Regardless, both trials can confirm the efficacy of carotid endarterectomy only if the operative complication rates can be kept at or below 5%[46] but preferably below a recommended 3%.[10]

These randomized clinical trials that examine the outcome of treatment for symptomatic and asymptomatic stenosis serve to underscore the validity of some of the prior retrospective analyses demonstrating the efficacy of operative intervention. Their importance, however, is derived from the multicenter and cooperative nature of the clinical methodology as well as the acknowledgment that any difference in clinical characteristics between treatment groups is unbiased. However, the results of these trials cannot anticipate every clinical scenario confronted in daily practice. Surgical judgment will continue to be required in analyzing the individual patient's risk factors as well as the likely morbidity and mortality of a particular surgical group following carotid endarterectomy. However, once these important aspects of the decision-making process are acknowledged, 1991 should be remembered as a momentous year for confirming the efficacy of operative intervention in patients with symptomatic carotid stenosis, and 1993 should provide results that further clarify the case for performing carotid endarterectomy in patients with asymptomatic carotid stenosis.

REFERENCES

1. Anderson RJ et al: Carotid endarterectomy for asymptomatic carotid stenosis: a ten-year experience with 120 procedures in a fellowship training program, *Ann Vasc Surg* 5(2):111-115, 1991.
2. ACAS (Asymptomatic Carotid Artery Stenosis Study): A prospective multicenter review of morbidity/mortality in carotid endarterectomy, *Stroke* 17:146, 1986 (abstract).
3. Awad I et al: Focal parenchymal lesions in transient ischemic attacks: correlation of computed tomography and magnetic resonance imaging, *Stroke* 17:399-403, 1985.
4. Barnes RW et al: The natural history of asymptomatic carotid disease in patients undergoing cardiovascular surgery, *Surgery* 90:1075-1083, 1981.
5. Barnett HJM: *Carotid endarterectomy: a challenge for scientific medicine*. In Norris JW, Hachinski VC, eds: *Prevention of stroke*, New York, 1991, Springer-Verlag.
6. Barnett HJM, Plum F, Walton JN: Carotid endarterectomy: an expression of concern, *Stroke* 15:941-943, 1984.
7. Blackshear WM et al: Detection of carotid occlusive disease by ultrasonic imaging and pulsed Doppler spectrum analysis, *Surgery* 86:698-706, 1979.
8. Brockenbrough EC: *Screening for the prevention of stroke: use of the Doppler flowmeter*, Washington/Alaska Regional Medical Program Brochure, 1970.
9. Brott T, Thalinger K: The practice of carotid endarterectomy in a large metropolitan area, *Stroke* 15:950-955, 1984.
10. Callow AD et al: Carotid endarterectomy: what is its current status? *Am J Med* 85:835-838, 1988.
11. The CASANOVA Study Group: Carotid surgery versus medical therapy in asymptomatic carotid stenosis, *Stroke* 22:1229-1235, 1991.
12. Chambers BR, Norris JW: The case against surgery for asymptomatic carotid stenosis, *Stroke* 15:964-967, 1984.
13. Chambers BR, Norris JW: Outcome in patients with asymptomatic neck bruits, *N Engl J Med* 315:860-865, 1986.
14. Comerota AJ et al: Real-time B-mode carotid imaging: a three year multicenter experience, *Vasc Surg* 1:84-95, 1984.
15. Committee on Health Care Issues, American Neurological Association: Does carotid endarterectomy decrease stroke and death in patients with transient ischemic attacks? *Ann Neurol* 22:72-76, 1987.
16. Cullen SJ et al: Clinical sequelae in patients with asymptomatic carotid bruits, *Circulation* 68(suppl II):83-87, 1983.
17. Dyken MD: Carotid endarterectomy studies: a glimmering of science, *Stroke* 17:355-357, 1986.
18. Easton JD, Sherman DG: Stroke and mortality rate in carotid endarterectomy: 228 consecutive operations, *Stroke* 8:565-568, 1977.
19. European Carotid Surgery Trialists' Collaborative Group, MRC European Carotid Surgery Trial: Interim results for symptomatic patients with severe (70-99%) or with mild (0-29%) carotid stenosis, *Lancet* 337:1235-1243, 1991.
20. Gee w et al: Ocular pneumoplethysmography in carotid artery disease, *Med Instrum* 8:244-248, 1974.
21. Hennerici M et al: Incidence of asymptomatic extracranial disease, *Stroke* 12:750-758, 1981.
22. Hertzer NR et al: Internal carotid back pressures, intraoperative shunting, ulcerated atheromata, and the incidence of stroke during carotid endarterectomy, *Surgery* 83:306-312, 1978.
23. Heyman W et al: Risk of stroke in asymptomatic persons with cervical arterial bruits: a population study in Evans Country, Georgia, *N Engl J Med* 302:838-841, 1980.
24. Hobson RW, Towne J: Carotid endarterectomy for asymptomatic carotid stenosis, *Stroke* 20:575-576, 1989 (editorial).
25. Hobson RW et al: Comparison of pulsed Doppler and real-time B-mode echo arteriography for noninvasive imaging of the extracranial carotid arteries, *Surgery* 87:286-293, 1980.
26. Hobson RW et al: Role of carotid endarterectomy in asymptomatic carotid stenosis: a Veterans Administration Cooperative Study, *Stroke* 17:534-539, 1986.
27. Hobson RW et al: Arteriography for asymptomatic carotid stenosis, *Stroke* 20:135, 1989.
28. Jain KM et al: Clinical screening of preoperative patients for carotid occlusive disease by oculoplethysmography, *Am Surg* 192:679-685, 1980.
29. Javid H et al: Carotid endarterectomy for asymptomatic patients, *Arch Surg* 102:389-391, 1971.
30. Kartchner MM, McRae LP: Noninvasive evaluation and management of the "asymptomatic" carotid bruit, *Surgery* 82:840-847, 1977.
31. Kartchner MM, McRae LP: *The clinical use of oculoplethysmography and carotid phonoangiography*. In Baker WH, ed: *Diagnosis and treatment of carotid artery disease*, Mt Kisco, NY, 1979, Futura.
32. Kartchner MM, McRae LP, Morrison FD: Noninvasive detection and evaluation of carotid occlusive disease, *Arch Surg* 106:528-535, 1973.
33. Lynch TG, Hobson RW: *Noninvasive cerebrovascular diagnostic techniques*. In Wilson SE, et al, ed: *Vascular surgery: principles and practice*, New York, 1987, McGraw-Hill.
34. Moneta GL et al: *Duplex ultrasound assessment of venous diameters, peak velocities, and flow patterns*. Presented at Vascular Symposium, February, 1988, San Diego, Calif.
35. Moore DJ et al: Noninvasive assessment of stroke risk in asymptomatic and nonhemispheric patients with suspected carotid disease, *Ann Surg* 202:491-504, 1985.
36. Moore WS et al: Asymptomatic carotid stenosis: immediate and long-term results after prophylactic endarterectomy, *Am J Surg* 138:228-233, 1979.
37. NASCET Collaborators: Beneficial effect of carotid endarterectomy in symptomatic patients with high grade carotid stenosis, *N Engl J Med* 325:445-453, 1991.
38. O'Leary DH et al: The influence of noninvasive tests on the selection of patients for carotid angiography, *Stroke* 16:264-267, 1985.
39. Perrone P et al: CT evaluation in patients with transient ischemic attack: correlation between clinical and angiographic findings, *Eur Neurol* 18:217-221, 1979.
40. Riles TS et al: Symptoms, stenosis and bruit, *Arch Surg* 116:218-220, 1981.
41. Rittgers SE, Thornhill BM, Barnes RW: Quantitative analysis of carotid artery Doppler spectral waveforms: diagnostic value of parameters, *Ultrasound Med Biol* 9:255-264, 1983.
42. Roederer GO et al: The natural history of carotid arterial disease in asymptomatic patients with cervical bruits, *Stroke* 15:605-613, 1984.
43. Swanson PD et al: A cooperative study of hospital frequency and character of transient ischemic attacks. II. Performance of angiography among six centers, *JAMA* 237:2202-2206, 1977.
44. Thompson JE: Don't throw out the baby with the bath water, *J Vasc Surg* 4:543-546, 1986 (editorial).
45. Thompson JE, Patman RD, Talkington CM: Asymptomatic carotid bruit: long-term outcome in patients having endarterectomy compared with unoperated controls, *Ann Surg* 188:308-316, 1978.
46. Towne JB, Weiss DG, Hobson RW: First phase report of Veterans Administration asymptomatic carotid stenosis study—operative morbidity and mortality, *J Vasc Surg* 11:252-259, 1990.
47. VA Symptomatic Carotid Stenosis Group: Carotid endarterectomy and prevention of cerebral ischemia in symptomatic carotid stenosis, *JAMA* 266:3289-3294, 1991.
48. Whitney DG et al: Carotid artery surgery without a temporary indwelling shunt, *Arch Surg* 115:1393-1399, 1980.
49. Wolf PA et al: Asymptomatic carotid bruit and the risk of stroke, *JAMA* 245:1442-1445, 1981.
50. Ziegler DK et al: Correlation of bruits over the carotid artery with angiographically demonstrated lesions, *Neurology* 21:860-865, 1971.

CHAPTER 50

Intraoperative assessment of carotid endarterectomy

DENNIS F. BANDYK

The controversy regarding carotid endarterectomy has properly focused on indications for the procedure and outcome analysis compared with the "best" medical treatment. The efficacy of carotid surgery depends on both appropriate patient selection and achievement of technical precision during the repair. Practice guidelines have been recommended for the appropriate use of carotid endarterectomy; seven prospective randomized trials are currently being conducted to define those patient groups most likely to benefit from surgical intervention.[8] The North American Symptomatic Carotid Endarterectomy Trial (NASCET) has concluded that for patients with symptoms who have 70% or greater internal carotid stenosis, carotid bifurcation endarterectomy significantly reduced stroke (5% versus 12%).[9] This observed benefit of carotid endarterectomy is highly dependent on perioperative morbidity (stroke and death rate). Operative stroke rates greater than 3% in patients who are full of symptoms with high-grade internal carotid artery (ICA) stenosis or greater than 7% in patients with symptoms would negate the early benefit of surgery when compared with the natural history of the disease with or without medical treatment. Both retrospective and prospective randomized trials of carotid endarterectomy have clearly indicated that perioperative thrombosis of the repair accounts for greater than one half of the operative strokes and deaths.[2,13,14] Recurrent carotid stenosis that is due to myointimal hyperplasia has a more benign natural history than an atherosclerotic plaque, but it is one cause of late ischemic stroke.[15] Some investigators have hypothesized that postrepair myointimal lesions may have their origin in a technically imperfect reconstruction. Follow-up studies have shown that recurrent neurologic symptoms and progression to ICA occlusion are associated with high-grade myointimal or recurrent atherosclerotic stenoses. This chapter reviews the data supporting routine intraoperative assessment of carotid endarterectomy that aims to diminish neurologic complications of carotid surgery and to prolong durability of the reconstruction.

INTRAOPERATIVE TECHNIQUES

The goal of carotid endarterectomy is to remove an obstructing lesion and reconstruct an arterial segment void of anatomic and hemodynamic abnormalities. Despite careful operative technique, experienced vascular surgeons occa-

sionally miss vascular defects (e.g., intimal flaps, luminal thrombus-platelet aggregation, stricture, adventitial bands) that occur in the course of carotid repair. Many of these abnormalities escape detection by visual inspection and palpation of the repair for a pulse deficit or bruit during their preocclusive phase. If left undetected, these lesions can result in stroke by platelet aggregation, thrombus embolization, vessel thrombosis (inadequate cerebral flow), or postrepair recurrent occlusive lesions. In 1967, Blaisdell et al[4] illustrated the fallibility of clinical assessment by routine completion arteriograms, which revealed unsuspected defects in 25% of cases. A number of investigators have subsequently confirmed this observation by using arteriography, alone or in combination with ultrasound techniques (e.g., continuous wave Doppler examination, pulsed Doppler spectral analysis, duplex ultrasonography). Regardless of the diagnostic modality, intraoperative monitoring has consistently demonstrated severe defects in the internal or common carotid artery that warranted immediate correction in 2% to 8% of all repairs (Table 50-1). The percentage of patients with residual repair abnormalities in whom a postoperative stroke would develop if the defect were left uncorrected is not known, but prudent surgical practice dictates that detection and revision of a technical problem at the primary operation are best. The sequelae of an ICA thrombosis are frequently catastrophic, which justifies all efforts to ensure technical perfection before skin closure.

Most surgeons rely on imaging or Doppler flow detection techniques to exclude technical error and confirm the presence of unobstructed blood flow. Although contrast arteriography is the accepted standard for intraoperative arterial imaging, the technique is cumbersome and invasive and is associated with a risk of subintimal injection, embolization, and allergic reaction. Portable studies can produce a marginal quality image for interpretation. For these reasons, Doppler ultrasound techniques have been applied for the initial evaluation of technical adequacy. The diagnostic accuracy of Doppler signal analysis is high (sensitivity and specificity greater than 90%), particularly if pulsed Doppler spectral analysis is performed. The examination technique is simple, and the instruments are widely available and relatively inexpensive. The Doppler probe is moved along the area of arterial reconstruction, with special attention

Table 50-1. Intraoperative evaluation of carotid endarterectomy

Author	Evaluation	No. of operations	Defects corrected (%) ICA/CCA	ECA	Ischemic infarction (%)
Zierler[16] (1984)	Angiography/PD spectral analysis	150	5	2	0
Barnes[3] (1986)	Audible CW Doppler	125	8	4	0
Dilley[6] (1986)	Angiography/B-mode imaging	158	8	9	0
Lane[7] (1987)	Duplex scanning	175	2	6	0.5
Bandyk[2] (1988)	Angiography/PD spectral analysis	250	4	3	0.4
Schwartz[12] (1988)	Duplex scanning	84	8	2	0
Cato[5] (1991)	Conventional/color duplex scanning	73	7	7	0
Bandyk[1] (1991)	Color duplex	67	4	7	0
Roon[10] (1992)	Angiography	535	2	—	0.7

ICA, Internal carotid artery; *CCA,* common carotid artery; *ECA,* external carotid artery; *CW,* continuous wave; *PD,* 20-MHz pulsed Doppler.

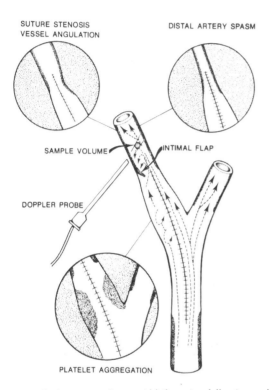

Fig. 50-1. Velocity patterns in carotid bifurcation following endarterectomy and commonly encountered vascular defects that can be detected by the presence of blood flow turbulence. Downstream from the intimal flap in the internal carotid artery, flow disturbances are identified by pulsed Doppler spectral analysis. The sample volume of pulsed Doppler is positioned in the center of the flow stream.

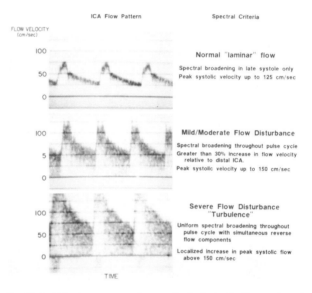

Fig. 50-2. Velocity spectra and spectral criteria for the three categories of flow disturbance in the internal carotid artery.

directed to those locations where technical errors are known to occur, such as endarterectomy end points and vascular clamp sites (Fig. 50-1). Spectral analysis of midstream flow in animal models has characterized the spectral changes that develop downstream of graded arterial stenoses, anastomotic sites, and surgically constructed technical errors (e.g., intimal flaps, luminal thrombosis). As the severity of the obstructing lesion increased, spectral broadening and blood flow velocity also increased. Although abnormalities of the

Doppler flow signal are readily apparent by audible interpretation, quantitative spectral analysis permits the development of diagnostic criteria that are important for objective intraoperative decision making. With pressure and flow-reducing lesions, spectral broadening is present throughout the pulse cycle, and peak systolic flow velocity components exceed 150 cm/sec. Visual inspection of the velocity spectra and calculation of peak systolic velocity, obtained by high-frequency (20 MHz) pulsed Doppler probe or duplex scanning, permit classification of blood flow patterns into three categories: normal laminar flow, mild to moderate flow disturbance, and severe flow disruption or turbulence (Fig. 50-2). When a significant residual flow abnormality is identified, angiography is recommended to delineate the abnormality before reexploration of the repair. The presence of a severe residual flow disturbance indicates a vascular defect and should not be ignored. Anatomic defects that require revision will be confirmed in greater than 90%

of those arteries.[4] Doppler spectral analysis is particularly useful in the detection of platelet aggregation within the endarterectomy site, since abnormalities of this type are frequently subtle or not visualized at all on arteriography (Fig. 50-3).

Recently, intraoperative duplex ultrasonography has been advocated because of its capability to provide both anatomic (high-resolution, real-time B-mode imaging) and hemodynamic (midstream pulsed Doppler spectral analysis) information.[1,5,7,12] Improvements in linear array scan head design and electronic signal processing, including color-coded velocity displays, have made duplex scanning feasible in the operating room and an ideal modality for the assessment of carotid bifurcation reconstructions. A distinct advantage of duplex scanning compared with Doppler flow analysis alone is that the structure of the anatomic defects associated with severe flow disturbance can usually be determined from the real-time B-mode imaging, and an immediate decision can be made regarding the need for operative revision. B-mode imaging alone is limited in providing only anatomic information, and the severity of the hemodynamic derangement is an important consideration in the decision to reopen a carotid artery. B-mode imaging is sensitive in detecting small intimal defects and flaps; however, most investigators have not repaired these minor lesions, and outcome of the procedure has not been adversely influenced.[11] Reluctance

to use duplex scanning during surgery has been attributed to the complexity of the examination and interpretation, cost and availability of instruments, and the erroneous assumption that arteriography is superior. In a comparison of high-resolution B-mode imaging and operative exploration with arteriography, Dilley and Bernstein[6] documented a 5.3% false-negative rate with arteriography. With the development of color Doppler transducers designed for intraoperative use, the validity of these concerns should be questioned. Since duplex scanning has become the standard by which patients both with and without symptoms are initially evaluated for the presence and severity of extracranial carotid occlusive disease, it is only natural that this instrumentation be adapted to confirm technical adequacy at operation. A comparison of intraoperative and early postoperative duplex findings indicates that the majority of abnormalities identified by duplex scanning within 3 months of carotid endarterectomy represent residual rather than recurrent stenosis.[5]

Intraoperative color duplex imaging

Color duplex instrumentation with a 7.5- to 10-MHz linear array transducer has been used for intraoperative studies. Studies were conducted with the transducer covered by a sterile disposable plastic sleeve that contained acoustic gel. The probe was positioned by the surgeon in the cervical incision directly over the exposed carotid repair. Sterile

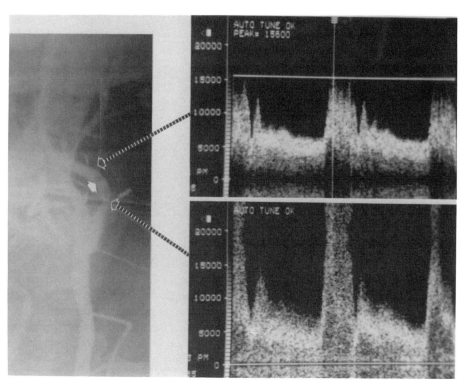

Fig. 50-3. Operative arteriogram *(left)* and velocity spectra *(right)* show severe flow disturbance (peak velocity greater than 20 KHz, 152 cm/sec) in proximal internal carotid artery caused by fibrin-platelet aggregates *(arrow)* in the endarterectomized arterial segment.

saline solution was instilled into the incision for acoustic coupling. Participation of a vascular technologist familiar with the instrumentation is important during intraoperative scanning. As the surgeon scans the arterial repair, the technologist adjusts the instrument to optimize the color-coded image, the Doppler beam angle and sample volume, and the recorded velocity spectra. Vessel walls should be imaged at 90°, but blood flow patterns should be assessed at Doppler beam angles of less than 65°. Familiarity with ultrasonographic vascular anatomy, good three-dimensional hand-eye coordination, and the ability to visualize the arterial repair in multiple planes (longitudinal, transverse, oblique) are essential elements of duplex imaging. The pitfalls and limitations of the technique are largely related to lack of familiarity with the instrumentation, transducer size, recognition of abnormal flow patterns, and correct measurement of duplex-derived blood flow velocities. Although the cost of color duplex scanners is significant ($100,000 to $150,000) and few facilities can justify dedicated operating room equipment, instruments used in the vascular diagnostic laboratory can be transported to the operating room on the basis of a scheduled appointment and predicted scanning time.

At the Medical College of Wisconsin, pulsed Doppler spectral analysis and duplex scanning (conventional and color) have been used to assess the technical adequacy of over 400 carotid repairs (Tables 50-2 and 50-3). The ultrasound examination can be directed to specific regions of the repair (e.g., endarterectomy end points, site[s] of occluding clamps) where technical problems are likely to occur. When a severe flow disturbance is detected, the structure of the vascular defect can frequently be determined and a decision regarding revision be made (Fig. 50-4). B-mode imaging alone is not recommended because it only provides anatomic information and the hemodynamic significance of imaged vascular defects is equally important. Color Doppler imaging does facilitate the intraoperative scanning of carotid repairs by permitting a global survey of the flow pattern in the imaged arterial segment. Uniformity of the color-coded flow field during systole and the absence of anatomic defects in the B-mode image are characteristic of a normal study. In 70 consecutive carotid endarterectomies, a residual defect was identified in one ICA, two common carotid arteries (CCAs), and five external carotid arteries (ECAs) (10% of repairs); all lesions were verified by exploration or arteriography. The duplex criterion for revision was identification of an anatomic lesion (e.g., lumen reduction, intimal flap) in the region of severe flow disturbance (spectral broadening, peak systolic velocity greater than 150 cm/sec). No perioperative strokes occurred, and all CCAs and ECAs were patent as determined by postoperative color duplex examinations performed at 3 months.

The benefits of intraoperative duplex imaging compared with arteriography include comparable or higher accuracy, safety, ease of repeated use after reexploration, and low cost. Color Doppler studies are sensitive to minor vascular defects and variations in anatomy that alter blood flow streamlines. Some surgeons have reported vascular defects in as many as 30% of repairs, but only one third appeared to justify reexploration. The flow patterns produced by patch angioplasty are predictable and should not be regarded as abnormal. Familiarity with ultrasonographic vascular anatomy, good hand-eye coordination skills, and the ability to visualize the arterial repair in three dimensions are essential aspects of imaging. Color Doppler imaging in combination with pulsed Doppler spectral analysis can eliminate the need

Table 50-2. Incidence of ICA/CCA restenosis relative to intraoperative study

| Intraoperative ultrasound | No. | Life-table analysis | | |
		1 mo	1 yr	4 yr
Normal	336	0.6%	3.2%	8.3%*
Flow abnormality	74	7%	13%	20%
Not done	51	10%	18%	26%

U/S, Duplex scanning or pulsed Doppler spectral analysis.
*p <0.007 compared with flow abnormality and not done.

Table 50-3. Incidence of stroke relative to type and outcome of intraoperative studies

| Intraoperative ultrasound | No. | Life-table analysis | | |
		1 mo	1 yr	4 yr
Normal	336	1.2%	1.2%	3.7%
Flow abnormality	74	2.7%	2.7%	4.9%
Not done	51	0%	2.5%	8%

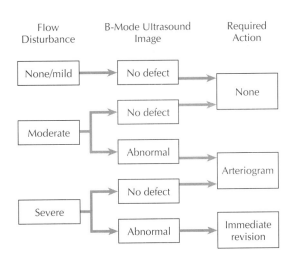

Fig. 50-4. Diagnostic algorithm for intraoperative duplex imaging of carotid artery repairs.

for arteriography, and decisions regarding technical adequacy or the need for revision can be safely based on the results of duplex scanning. In a series of 410 consecutive carotid endarterectomies, a normal intraoperative ultrasound study ($n = 336$) was associated with a perioperative stroke rate of 1% and an incidence of late ICA stenosis/occlusion of 8% at 4 years (life-table analysis, Table 50-2). In contrast, when the surgeons permitted a residual flow abnormality to remain without connection ($n = 74$) in the ICA or CCA, the perioperative stroke rate was similar (2.7%; $p > 0.05$), but the incidence of late ICA stenosis/occlusion increased to 20% at 4 years ($p < 0.01$).

Routine intraoperative imaging can assist in the construction of durable carotid repairs. The experience and technical skill of the surgeon should not preclude the use of objective intraoperative assessment after carotid endarterectomy.

REFERENCES

1. Bandyk DF, Govostis DM: Intraoperative color flow imaging of "difficult" arterial reconstructions, *Video J Color Flow Imaging* 1:13-20, 1991.
2. Bandyk DF et al: Turbulence occurring after carotid bifurcation endarterectomy: a harbinger of residual and recurrent carotid stenosis, *J Vasc Surg* 7:261-274, 1988.
3. Barnes RW et al: Recurrent versus residual carotid stenosis: incidence detected by Doppler ultrasound, *Ann Surg* 203:652-660, 1986.
4. Blaisdell FW, Lin R, Hall AD: Technical result of carotid endarterectomy—arteriographic assessment, *Am J Surg* 114:239-246, 1967.
5. Cato R et al: Duplex scanning after carotid reconstruction: a comparison of intraoperative and postoperative results, *J Vasc Tech* 15:61-65, 1991.
6. Dilley RB, Bernstein EF: A comparision of B-mode real-time imaging and arteriography in the intraoperative assessment of carotid endarterectomy, *J Vasc Surg* 4:457-463, 1986.
7. Lane RJ et al: The application of operative ultrasound immediately following carotid endarterectomy, *World J Surg* 11:593-597, 1987.
8. Moore WS et al: Carotid endarterectomy: practice guidelines, *J Vasc Surg* 15:469-479, 1992.
9. North American Symptomatic Carotid Endarterectomy Trial (NASCET) Investigators: Clinical alert: benefit of carotid endarterectomy for patients with high-grade stenosis of the internal carotid artery, *Stroke* 22:816-817, 1991.
10. Roon AJ, Hoogerwerf D: Intraoperative arteriography and carotid surgery, *J Vasc Surg* 16:239-243, 1992.
11. Sawchuck AP et al: The fate of unrepaired minor technical defects detected by intraoperative ultrasound during carotid endarterectomy, *J Vasc Surg* 9:671-676, 1989.
12. Schwartz RA et al: Intraoperative duplex scanning after carotid artery reconstruction: a valuable tool, *J Vasc Surg* 7:620-624, 1988.
13. Towne JB, Bernhard VM: Neurologic deficit following carotid endarterectomy, *Surg Gynecol Obstet* 154:849-852, 1982.
14. Towne JB, Weiss DG, Hobson RW: First phase report of cooperative Veterans Administration asymptomatic carotid stenosis—operative morbidity and mortality, *J Vasc Surg* 11:252-259, 1990.
15. Washburn WK et al: Late stroke after carotid endarterectomy: the role of recurrent stenosis, *J Vasc Surg* 15:1032-1037, 1992.
16. Zierler RE, Bandyk DF, Thiele BL: Intraoperative assessment of carotid endarterectomy, *J Vasc Surg* 1:73-83, 1984.

CHAPTER 51

Fate of unrepaired defects after carotid endarterectomy

ROBERT COURBIER, MICHEL FERDANI, and MICHEL REGGI

Although carotid endarterectomies are performed frequently, routine operative angiographic control is not commonly practiced. Residual lesions may remain and may not be detected, possibly leading to complications soon after surgery.

Monitoring techniques that have been proposed for operative completion studies include arteriography,[4,9,21] B-mode imaging,[12] and direct angioscopy.[19] Sensitivity of these methods varies in the detection of residual lesions that can either deteriorate, remain stable, or even regress. The threshold of the potential risk of a given residual lesion is difficult to determine: if no risk of complication is present, it would be unnecessary to extend the operation of carotid endarterectomy by reoperation and additional clamping and cerebral ischemia. Hertzer[17] advocated the use of simple magnifying loupes instead of ultrasonic or radiologic controls. However, a satisfactory external appearance to the naked eye does not rule out the possibility of internal stenosis. The danger that a residual lesion can deteriorate is always possible.

MATERIAL AND METHODS

This prospective study included 80 consecutive patients who underwent a total of 94 carotid endarterectomies. The appearance of residual lesions and their outcomes were studied. A total of 58 patients were followed up for more than 2 years and reexamined at 1 and 2 years. Clinical staging was done according to the Marseilles classification in stages I, II, and III. Carotid endarterectomy was performed while patients were under general anesthesia. A shunt was placed when the stump pressure in the internal carotid artery (ICA) was below 50 mm Hg and the pressure curve was nonpulsatile or whenever the contralateral ICA was occluded. Direct sutures with no patch were routine. A dilator was always used to calibrate the ICA.

Completion of arteriography was performed with a portable device. Injection of 5 ml of 60% diatrizoate was monitored on a television screen. The image of the carotid bifurcation was recorded on videotape. This technique has been described in detail elsewhere.[9] A second intraarterial angiogram was performed 12 months later by digital subtraction technique, and the results were classified according to the degree of stenosis[20] as follows:

Category 0—0% to 19% stenosis
Category I—20% to 58% stenosis
Category II—60% to 79% stenosis
Category III—80% to 90% stenosis
Category IV—thrombosis, occlusion

B-mode imaging was performed 10 days, 180 days, and 1 year after arteriography. It was focused on the main axis of the common carotid artery (CCA), the bulb, and the ICA. Findings were classified as follows:

E1—Normal appearance
E2—Smooth and homogeneous plaque
E3—Rough and homogeneous plaque
E5—Rough and heterogeneous plaque
E6—Thrombosis

No anticoagulants were administered after surgery.

RESULTS

A total of 94 endarterectomies (14 bilateral) were performed on 80 patients (52 men and 28 women). Ages of these patients ranged from 46 to 84 years (mean age, 71.4 ± 7.9 years). The preoperative clinical stages (Marseilles classification)[8] of these patients were as follows:

Grade 0—39 (40.4%)
Grade IA—52 (55.3%)
Grade II—2 (2.2%)
Grade IIIA—2 (2.2%)

Among patients with 0 classification, 19 had asymptomatic unilateral lesions, 19 had asymptomatic bilateral lesions, and all had high-grade stenosis. Bilateral lesions were asymptomatic on both sides in six cases, and in seven cases they were associated with contralateral stage I lesions.

Arteriography was performed during the procedure (Table 51-1) and at 1 year (Table 51-2). B-mode imaging was performed about 10 days after the procedure (Table 51-3) and then at 1 year (Table 51-4). The decision whether to reoperate immediately or to accept the residual lesions was made on the basis of completion operative arteriographic findings (Table 51-5). Immediate reoperation was undertaken in four cases (one endarterectomy of the external

Table 51-1. Intraoperative angiography

Grade/stenosis	CCA	ICA	ECA
0—Normal	86	88	77
IA	8	4	9
II	—	1	5
IIIA	—	1	3
TOTAL	94	94	94

Table 51-2. Arteriographic control (at 1 year)

Grade/stenosis	CCA	ICA	ECA
0—Normal	87	83	80
I	7*	5	4
II		6	2
III			4
IV—Thrombosis			4
TOTAL	94	94	94

*Shelf aspect disappears; small irregularities persist.

Table 51-3. B-mode imaging after 10 days

Aspect/grade		CCA		ICA	
Normal	E1	81		79	
or			84		83
subnormal	E2	3		4	
	E3	3		3	
Abnormal	E4	2	10	5	11
	E5	5		3	
	E6	0		0	
		94		94	

Table 51-4. B-mode imaging after 1 year

Aspect/grade		CCA		ICA	
Normal	E1	61		65	
or			73		68
subnormal	E2	12		3	
	E3	11		9	
Abnormal	E4	3	21	17	26
	E5	7		0	
	E6	0		0	
		94		94	

Table 51-5. Changes in arteriographic appearance (after 1 year)

Lesion	Intraoperative angiography	Lesion on angiography control		
		Aggravation	Stable	Improvement
CCA				
Normal	86	5*	81	0
Accepted	8	0	2	6
Corrected	0	0	0	0
ICA				
Normal	88	10	78	0
Accepted	3	0	0	3
Corrected	3	0	0	3
ECA				
Normal	77	7	70	0
Accepted	16	5	5	6
Corrected	1	1	0	0

*Shelf aspect disappeared; small irregularities persist.

carotid artery [ECA], one endarterectomy of the ICA, and two saphenous vein grafts of the ICA). All but one of the procedures that involved the ICA were uneventful.

Despite normal arteriographic findings, a completed stroke was observed in three cases. One hemiplegic patient who underwent emergency surgery (stage II) did not improve. No patients died during the operation or during the first year of follow-up. All patients were reexamined.

After arteriography at 1 year, all patients were free of symptoms. Five patients with low-grade stenosis of the ICA (grade I) did not undergo reoperation. In six cases, post-operative stenoses of the ICA (grade II) were detected, and

all were caused by intimal hyperplasia. Results of completion operative arteriography had been normal in each of these cases. In one patient an operation was contraindicated because of untreated coronary artery lesions. Four saphenous vein bypasses (Figs. 51-1 and 51-2) were performed with uneventful recovery. One patient underwent percutaneous transluminal angioplasty and died in the immediate post-operative period.

DISCUSSION

Intraoperative assessment of carotid endarterectomy is necessary to detect residual lesions that might place the patient

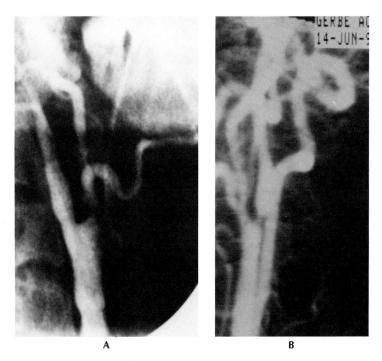

A   B

Fig. 51-1. ***A,*** Intraoperative arteriography showing slightly narrowed ECA and a normal ICA. ***B,*** After 1 year, there are normalization of the ECA, high-grade stenosis of the ICA, and a need for reoperation.

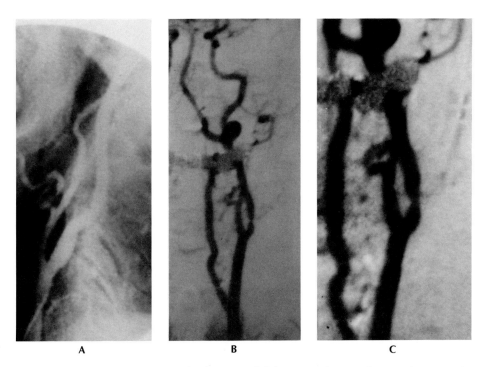

A   B   C

Fig. 51-2. ***A,*** Intraoperative arteriography showing a slightly narrowed ECA and a normal ICA. ***B,*** After 1 year, there is normalization of the ECA and asymptomatic high-grade stenosis of the ICA. ***C,*** after 18 months, there are high-grade stenosis of the ICA and the need for reoperation.

at risk. Late postoperative studies in which the status of the artery is not documented immediately after surgery are of little value.

Method of intraoperative control angiography

Routine angiographic controls during peripheral artery surgery have been performed for many years. Recently, intraoperative assessment has also been done during carotid artery surgery.[9] Arteriographic findings allow immediate correction of technical defects during the same period of anesthesia. Were such control to be performed in the first few days after surgery, it could still lead to reoperation but would expose the patient to high risks in the interval.

Portable digital subtraction angiography devices now provide excellent image quality. With this technique, the cervical and intracranial segments of the ICA can be visualized simultaneously. The physician can determine whether a postoperative stroke is caused by an embolus or a flow reduction. No allergic reactions to the contrast agent were observed whether general or regional anesthesia was employed. The risk of irradiation is negligible. Ramalanjaona[22] demonstrated that the cumulative dose of radiation was hazardous for the surgeon only after 20,000 endarterectomies a year.

Ultrasonic imaging, which avoids exposure to x-rays, provides highly detailed images and detects more technical defects than arteriography does. Dilley and Bernstein,[11] using both techniques in 158 patients, concluded that they were complementary. Because sterilization of the ultrasonic transducer is time consuming, several B-mode imaging transducers are needed if several carotid procedures are to be performed on the same day. The size of these probes often makes them difficult to use in the open wound of the neck. In addition, the only part of the operative field that can be visualized is the carotid bifurcation, since the intracranial portion of the internal carotid artery is not visualized by ultrasonography.

Angioscopy, which has been used mainly for peripheral endoscopic surgery,[19] has recently been adopted for the intraoperative assessment of carotid endarterectomy, but the risk of dislodging residual intimal fragments greatly limits the use of this technique. In a series of 76 cases, Mehigan and De Campli[19] reoperated five times, which resulted in a prolongation of clamp time from 2 to 15 minutes. They did not believe that the two strokes observed were a result of the angioscopic technique. They concluded that an intimal flap of more than 5 mm to 10 mm in length could fold over and occlude the artery. Obviously, such a lesion cannot be neglected.

Fate of residual lesions

The reported incidence of restenosis varies widely depending on the screening method used.[16-18] The choice of a control technique depends on its sensitivity and specificity. The "acceptability" of a residual lesion identified on a completion study must be on the basis of the surgeon's judgment about the functional status of the patient and the problems encountered during the procedure before and/or after clamping. Objective examination of x-ray images of accepted lesions is an important responsibility of the surgeon, who is the only one capable of evaluating the film and the risk-benefit balance of reopening the carotid bifurcation.

In this study, because only lesions that had been evolving for 1 year after endarterectomy were tabulated, it was possible to discount the role of slowly evolving atheroma and to focus on the fate of intimal hyperplasia. An "acceptable" residual lesion can deteriorate, stabilize, or regress.

Progression of the lesions may lead to stenosis but rarely to thrombosis of the ICA. The incidence of thrombosis is higher for the ECA. Habozit[15] observed no thrombosis after a 2-year follow-up of 17 cases. Evolving lesions are usually detectable within 3 to 6 months after the operation.[6] Bandyk[2] assessed 250 carotid arteries intraoperatively by pulsed Doppler spectral analysis and arteriography. Of this total, 182 arteries presented no residual lesion, stenosis, or thrombosis after 3 months. After 1 year, significant stenosis was observed in only 5% of the cases and after 2 years in only 9%. At the same follow-up times, stenosis was observed in 8%, 18%, and 21% of the remaining 68 arteries that displayed residual lesions.

The highly variable incidence of stenosis after endarterectomy is indicated by the timing of the first control study. When frequent controls were performed at close intervals in the short-term follow-up, stenosis developed and then regressed. Nicholls[20] reported nine cases of postoperative stenoses (62%) that showed a 5% to 15% diameter reduction, which then progressed to a range of 16% to 49% before returning to the 5% to 15% category. Sanders,[23] who monitored healing after endarterectomy by duplex scanning, found that 79% of cases of stenoses developing because of intimal hyperplasia in the 6 months after the procedure diminished or disappeared before the end of the first year. However, 40% of the arteries with stenoses that were greater than or equal to 40% after 3 months continued to progress after 1 year.[3,26]

Low-grade, smooth, residual lesions remain stable. In the CCA, a "healed" image with low-grade stenosis is often observed after disappearance of the proximal "shelf." Smoothness of the wall resulting from a tight suture does not create turbulence in blood flow and does not lead to further complications.

Spontaneous regression without any treatment has been noted frequently. By 1970, Schultz[25] had reported regression of stenosis in 50 patients with persistence of a stenotic "pantaloon aspect" at the origin of the endarterectomy. Although Diaz[10] claimed that this type of lesion could regress, Baker,[1] who assessed 133 patients after surgery by using Doppler spectral analysis and oculoplethysmography (OPG), observed a decrease in stenosis in only seven cases and a return to normal in two cases. Using ultrasonography, Zierler[27] studied 32 cases of restenosis of the ICA. In serial follow-up of 22 patients with restenosis, the stenosis was stable in 12 cases and had regressed in 9 cases. Nicholls[20] observed 12 cases of stenoses that decreased from the 16% to 49% category to the 1% to 15% category. The concept of spontaneous regression of carotid plaque was proposed by Hennerici[16] on the basis of the results of B-mode scanning. Habozit[15] observed complete regression in 3 of 18 stenoses (16%). Similar findings have previously been reported.[9] In the present study, regression was noted in six patients with lesions in the CCA and three patients with involvement of the ICA.

Using intraoperative B-mode imaging, Sawchuk[24] observed minor defects in 18 of 80 arteries (21 defects in all). Stenosis involved the ICA in four cases, the CCA in nine cases, and the ECA in eight cases. In seven patients the flap was located in the ICA; it measured 1 mm in length in one case, 2 mm in four cases, and 3 mm in two cases; it caused 20% stenosis in each case. Of these 19 flaps, 16 normalized at 27 months, and 2 stenoses disappeared 1 month later.

Regression can be observed in all three arteries of the carotid bifurcation. In the CCA, this can be explained in two ways. First, the proximal residual shelf may disappear (Fig. 51-3) because the blood flow pushes the flap back against the wall.[13] Second, the difference in diameter between the healthy and endarterectomized segments of the artery (Fig. 51-4) may be concealed as the fibrin deposit accumulates.

In the ECA the direction of the blood flow tends to increase the defect (Fig. 51-3). The thicker structure of this artery makes it impossible to taper the endarterectomy. For these reasons, secondary thrombosis is more frequent in the ECA even if surgical defects are corrected immediately.

In the ICA, regression and disappearance of defects are possible (Fig. 51-5). An irregularity caused by a stitch that takes an undue "bite" of the wall or a small flap can remodel and become smooth (Fig. 51-6), but a hemodynamically significant stenosis almost inevitably becomes more severe (Fig. 51-7).

As demonstrated in animals,[20] regression represents a remodeling of the smooth muscle cells that proliferate in response to the arterial injury of endarterectomy. Since the role of platelet-derived growth factor has been well documented,[7] it is reasonable to expect that use of anti-platelet-derived growth factor agents might be an effective means of preventing restenosis.

No systematic correlation has been noted between the persistence of a defect and the occurrence of symptoms. Green[14] found that 12.5% of patients with high-grade residual lesions had clinical manifestations in the first 6 months, but Callow[5] reported that only 1% to 2.5% of cases became symptomatic. It is widely recognized that these early stenoses are related to healing. Sawchuk[24] observed no difference in the stroke rate in the patients with normal or abnormal intraoperative controls.

The acceptability of residual lesions detected by intraoperative arteriography differs in the three branches of the carotid bifurcation. In the CCA, a residual shelf is acceptable unless its length is more than 5 mm, which may present a risk of thrombosis, or embolism caused by blood flow turbulence. In the ICA, an irregularity caused by a stitch at the top or a narrowing because of a defect is acceptable as long as the resulting stenosis is less than 30%. A flap or an

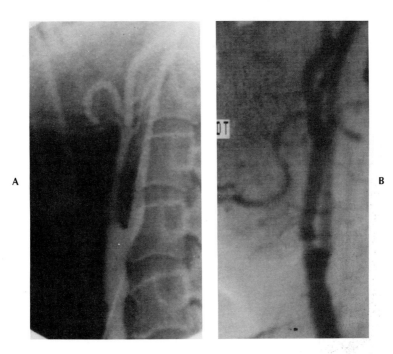

Fig. 51-3. A, Intraoperative arteriography showing slightly narrowed CCA and ECA. **B,** After 1 year, there are normalization of the CCA and stenosis of the ECA.

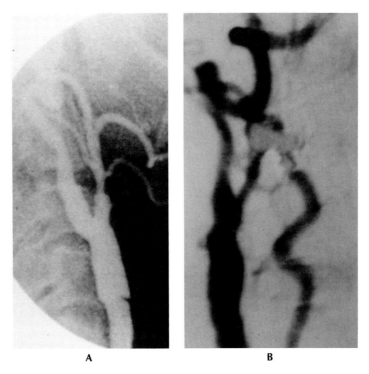

Fig. 51-4. *A,* Intraoperative arteriography showing "pantaloon aspect" on the carotid bifurcation and a flap on the CCA. *B,* After 1 year, there is normalization of the lesions.

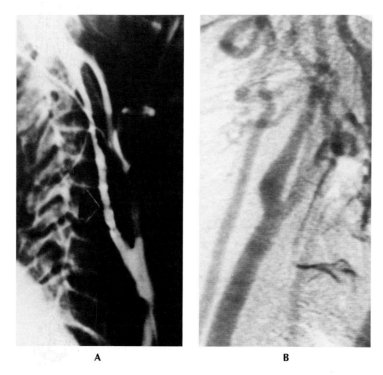

Fig. 51-5. *A,* Intraoperative arteriography showing a difficult endarterectomy due to the extent of the stenosis and arterial spasm. Also seen is the irregular appearance of the ICA extending upwards. *B,* After 1 year, there is complete normalization.

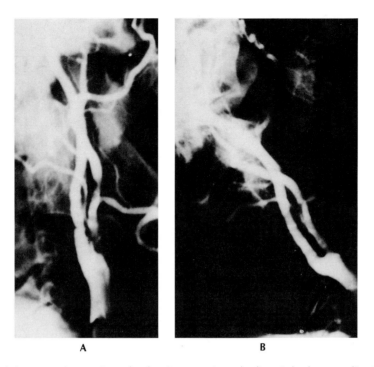

A   B

Fig. 51-6. **A,** Intraoperative arteriography showing stenosis on the first stitch of a suture line in the ICA and high-grade stenosis of the ECA. **B,** After 1 year, there are normalization of the ICA, stenosis of the ECA, and no need for reoperation.

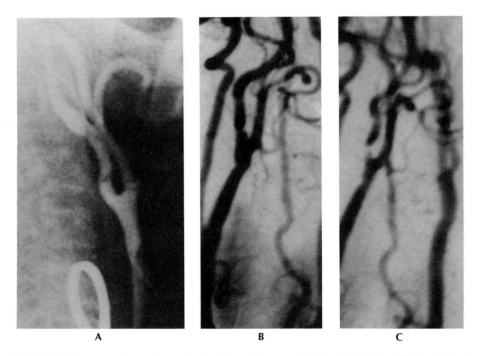

A   B   C

Fig. 51-7. **A,** Intraoperative arteriography showing an "accepted" lesion of the ICA and ECA. **B,** After 6 months, there are normalization of the ECA and asymptomatic stenosis of the ICA. **C,** After 1 year, there are high-grade stenosis of the ICA and the need for reoperation.

extensive irregularity should be corrected immediately. The most dangerous lesion in terms of immediate thrombosis is an extensive irregularity in the unobstructed zone (calcareous infiltration). Immediate saphenous vein bypass to eliminate that thrombogenic segment is indicated. In the ECA, stenosis greater than 50% should be corrected if the artery downstream is flexible and uninvolved.

In deciding whether to reoperate immediately after endarterectomy, the surgeon must consider the patient's condition and any problems encountered during the first part of the procedure. Correction is not necessary every time a lesion is detected by arteriography. Unrepaired lesions that are detected by intraoperative arteriography have a relatively favorable prognosis. On the basis of experience and a review of the literature, an aggressive approach is taken only for lesions that carry a high risk of rapid deterioration.

The most sensitive B-mode imaging techniques do not have a clear-cut advantage over angiography, since they detect more small lesions for which immediate repair is not necessary. Although this method is advocated by some surgical teams, the fate of accepted defects proves that immediate reoperation is not obligatory for all lesions. For carotid surgery, the method of control technique is not as important as the routine use of some form of intraoperative monitoring.

REFERENCES

1. Baker WH et al: Durability of carotid endarterectomy, *Surgery* 94:112-115, 1983.
2. Bandyk DF et al: Accuracy of duplex scanning in the detection of stenosis after carotid endarterectomy, *J Vasc Surg* 8:696-702, 1988.
3. Bandyk DF et al: Turbulence occurring after carotid bifurcation endarterectomy: a harbinger of residual and recurrent carotid stenosis, *J Vasc Surg* 7:261-274, 1988.
4. Blaisdell FW: Routine operative arteriography following carotid endarterectomy, *Surgery* 83:114-115, 1978.
5. Callow AD, O'Donnell TF: *Recurrent carotid stenosis—frequency, clinical implications and some suggestions concerning etiology.* In Bergan J, Yao J, eds: *Reoperative arterial surgery,* New York, 1980, Grune & Stratton.
6. Clagett GP et al: Etiologic factors for recurrent carotid artery stenosis, *Surgery* 93:313-318, 1983.
7. Clowes AW, Reidy MA, Clowes MM: Kinetics of cellular proliferation after arterial injury, *Lab Invest* 49:327-333, 1983.
8. Courbier R: Basis for an international classification of cerebral arterial diseases, *J Vasc Surg* 4:179-183, 1986.
9. Courbier R et al: Routine intraoperative carotid angiography: its impact on operative morbidity and carotid restenosis, *J Vasc Surg* 3:343-350, 1986.
10. Diaz FZ, Patel S, Boulos R: Early arteriographic changes following carotid endarterectomy, *Neurosurgery* 10:457-463, 1982.
11. Dilley RB, Bernstein EF: A comparison of B-mode real-time imaging and arteriography in the intraoperative assessment of carotid endarterectomy, *J Vasc Surg* 4:457-463, 1986.
12. Flanigan DP et al: Intraoperative ultrasonic imaging of the carotid artery during carotid endarterectomy, *Surgery* 100:893-899, 1986.
13. Gonzalez LL, Partusch L, Wirth P: Non-invasive carotid artery evaluation following endarterectomy, *J Vasc Surg* 1:403-408, 1984.
14. Green RM et al: The clinical course of residual carotid arterial disease, *J Vasc Surg* 13:112-120, 1991.
15. Habozit B: *Suivi anatomique de l'endarériectomie carotidienne.* In Kieffer E, Bousser MG, eds: *Indications et résultats de la chirurgie Carotidienne,* Paris, 1988, AERCV.
16. Hennerici M et al: Incidence of asymptomatic extracranial arterial disease, *Stroke* 12:750-758, 1981.
17. Hertzer N et al: The fate of unrepaired minor technical defects detected by intraoperative ultrasonography during carotid endarterectomy, *J Vasc Surg* 9:671-676, 1989.
18. Kieny R et al: *Les resténoses carotidiennes aprés endartériectomie.* In Kieffer E, Bousser MG, eds: *Indications et résultats de la chirurgie Carotidienne,* Paris, 1988, AERCV.
19. Mehigan JT, De Campli WM: *Angioscopic control of carotid endarterectomy.* In Moore WS, Ahn SS, eds: *Endovascular surgery,* 1989, WB Saunders.
20. Nicholls SC et al: Relationship of outcome to early restenosis, *J Vasc Surg* 2:375-381, 1985.
21. Paredero del Bosque V et al: Intraoperative assessment of carotid endarterectomy, *J Card Vasc Surg* 30:89-94, 1989.
22. Ramalanjaona GR, Pearce WH, Ritenour ER: Radiation exposure risk to the surgeon during operative angiography, *J Vasc Surg* 4:224-228, 1986.
23. Sanders M et al: Residual lesions and early stenosis after carotid endarterectomy: a serial follow-up study with duplex scanning and intravenous digital subtraction angiography, *J Vasc Surg* 5:731-737, 1987.
24. Sawchuk AP et al: The fate of unrepaired minor technical defects detected by intraoperative ultrasonography during carotid endarterectomy, *J Vasc Surg* 9:671-676, 1989.
25. Schutz H, Fleming JFR, Awerbuck B: Arteriographic assessment of carotid endarterectomy, *Ann Surg* 171:509-521, 1970.
26. Thomas M, Otis SM, Rush M: Recurrent carotid artery stenosis following endarterectomy, *Ann Surg* 200:74-79, 1984.
27. Zierler RE et al: Carotid artery stenosis following endarterectomy, *Arch Surg* 117:1408-1415, 1982.

CHAPTER 52

Recurrent carotid artery stenosis

EUGENE F. BERNSTEIN

Carotid endarterectomy was introduced in 1951 and was considered a remarkably durable procedure until the 1976 report by Stoney and String,[35] which showed that 1.6% of patients required another procedure on the same artery. About that time, noninvasive methodology for studying the carotid bifurcation became available. The initially used indirect methods were rapidly replaced by duplex scanning, which permitted a detailed and direct examination of the patient who had undergone carotid surgery. Since 1980, data obtained by use of duplex scanning have documented that carotid restenosis (more than 50% of the lumen cross section) occurs in a significant number of patients. Concerns about the potential subsequent development of cerebral symptoms or carotid occlusion have stimulated the frequent postoperative reassessment of patients after carotid endarterectomy and resulted in some reoperations.[5,8,22] Postoperative duplex screening has been advised every 3 months, and there is controversy regarding the indications for reoperation.

This chapter summarizes experience with patients in whom carotid endarterectomy was technically successful, as documented by completion angiography, and in whom restenosis was documented. In addition, the results of a controlled study to prevent carotid restenosis with preoperative and intraoperative administration of aspirin and Persantin, which have provided an additional base regarding the need for postoperative surveillance, are presented. Finally, the literature is reviewed to aid in forming clinically acceptable and appropriate guidelines for the postoperative screening of patients after carotid reconstruction.

RESIDUAL VERSUS RECURRENT CAROTID STENOSIS

An important aspect of the problem of carotid restenosis is related to the condition of the carotid bifurcation at the completion of the surgical procedure. Thus residual lesions that have not been corrected adequately by the surgeon may predispose the patient to hemodynamic or anatomic conditions initiating or enhancing the restenotic process. To avert this sequence and to document the technical quality of carotid reconstruction, some surgeons routinely perform a completion evaluation procedure before they leave the operating room so that an unsatisfactory reconstruction can

be repaired at the same sitting. Methods for carotid completion examination have included various techniques of angiography, Doppler velocity studies, and angioscopy. Barnes,[3] Sanders,[34] and Zierler[40] have emphasized the importance of intraoperative control studies, and the course of specific lesions that have been permitted to remain after identification by such methods has been carefully characterized by Courbier[11] and Sanders.[34] These authors emphasize that most reports regarding the incidence of carotid restenosis have failed to document the state of the vessels at the end of surgery and therefore may well be confusing residual with recurrent disease. Unfortunately, completion studies are still uncommon after carotid surgery, although several current techniques can be performed with a minimum of time, effort, risk, and expense and offer the surgeon and patient an opportunity to improve the results of surgery.

INCIDENCE OF CAROTID RESTENOSIS

Duplex ultrasound reports document an overall incidence of carotid restenosis (usually including undiscovered residual disease) ranging from 6.4% to 23.9%, with a mean of 12.9%, on the basis of 21 studies (Table 52-1). In the same reports, from 0 to 9.7% of these patients are identified as having symptoms (mean 3.5%), although the spectrum of symptoms, whether they are persistent or new and their severity, is infrequently detailed. In these retrospective studies, factors that have commonly been found to be associated with a higher incidence of restenosis include female gender, youth, persistent smoking, hypertension, and hyperlipidemia.

LATE STROKE AND SURVIVAL

Because the importance of the restenotic lesion is determined by the clinical course of these patients, a retrospective study was done of experience with 507 consecutive patients who underwent 566 carotid endarterectomies for whom completion angiography had indicated a satisfactory outcome of surgery.[5] In addition, postoperative duplex scans were done at 3 days (before hospital discharge); at 1, 3, 6, and 12 months; and annually thereafter. Adequate data were obtained from 484 carotid operations with a mean follow-up period of 42 months. In 49 arteries (10.1%), a lesion

Table 52-1. Incidence of carotid restenosis

Author and year	Operations (no.)	Restenosis	
		Symptomatic (%)	Total (%)
Kremen, 1980[25]	173	1.7	9.8
Turnipseed, 1980[38]	80	2.5	11.3
Cantelemo, 1981[7]	199	4.5	12.0
Zierler, 1982[40]	89	5.5	19.0
Salvian, 1983[33]	105	4.8	11.4
Thomas, 1984[37]	257	1.6	8.9
Colgan, 1984[9]	80	1.3	12.5
Pierce, 1984[32]	75	2.7	6.7
O'Donnell, 1985[29]	276	1.4	12.3
Keagy, 1985[24]	122	—	22.1
Zbornikova, 1986[39]	113	9.7	23.9
Glover, 1987[17]	155	2.1	14.8
Barnes, 1987[3]	47	0	6.4
Sanders, 1987[34]	75	—	8.0
De Groote, 1987[13]	310	3.9	13.3
Ouriel, 1987[30]	102	5.9	18.6
Sundt, 1988[36]	99	2.0	7.6
Mattos, 1988[27]	117	6.0	14.5
Bernstein, 1990[5]	484	1.3	10.1
Cook, 1990[10]	76	2.6	18.2
Atnip, 1990[2]	184	1.6	6.0

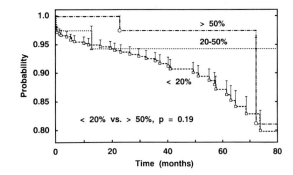

Fig. 52-1. Life-table analysis of the effect of varying degrees of carotid restenosis on the probability of remaining free of stroke after carotid endarterectomy. (From *Ann Surg* 212:629-636, 1990.)

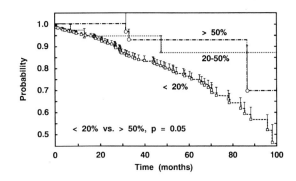

Fig. 52-2. Analysis of the effect of carotid restenosis on the probability of survival after carotid endarterectomy. (*Ann Surg* 212:629-636, 1990.)

characterized as greater than 50% stenosis was identified during at least one evaluation after carotid endarterectomy. A total of 8 of these vessels were occluded. Each of these patients had a normal postoperative duplex scan before hospital discharge. The incidence of restenosis in females (13.9%) was significantly greater than in males (8.0%) ($p = 0.003$). More modest lesions ranging from 20% to 50% were identified in 40 other arteries (8.3%). The mean time for the appearance of more than 50% restenosis was 4.6 months, and the mean time to reach the maximum level of restenosis was 12.3 months.

Kaplan-Meier life-table analyses were performed for the end points of ipsilateral stroke and survival. The probability of remaining stroke free was no greater in those patients with restenosis (Fig. 52-1), and in fact, the outlook for the patients with restenosis was somewhat better than that for those with persistently normal carotid arteries. In addition, the patients with restenosis had a better life expectancy ($p = 0.05$), as indicated in Fig. 52-2. Female gender was not associated with a higher rate of late ipsilateral stroke or early death.

When ipsilateral stroke and death were combined as end points, the difference between the restenosis group and the normal subjects became more significant ($p = 0.03$, Fig. 52-3). Finally, when transient hemispheric symptoms were combined with stroke and death as end points, the likelihood of symptom-free survival was greater in those patients with any degree of restenosis than in those who remained normal ($p = 0.08$, not significant, Fig. 52-4).

An analysis with the end point of time to stroke was performed by using the Cox proportional hazards regression model. The risk of stroke increased with age and was higher among patients with diabetes and smokers. Women were at greater risk of stroke than men, patients with bilateral operations were at less risk than those with unilateral operations, and those with restenosis were at less risk of stroke than those without restenosis ($p = 0.005$). Stepwise analysis showed that only age and smoking were statistically significant predictors of stroke ($p = 0.0002$).

Analyses for survival showed that the mortality risk increased with age, was higher for male patients than for female patients, was higher among patients with diabetes and smokers, and was higher among patients who had bilateral operations. However, the mortality risk was less among those with restenosis than those without restenosis ($p = 0.01$). A more refined stepwise analysis showed that only age and diabetes were statistically significant predictors of death ($p = 0.0008$). Thus the study indicated that carotid restenosis was not a clinical predictor of serious neurologic or lethal consequence.

Similar results have also been reported by others. Healy examined a group of 78 patients with carotid restenosis at the University of Washington, where the prevalence of restenosis at 7 years was 31%.[20] By life-table analysis, the

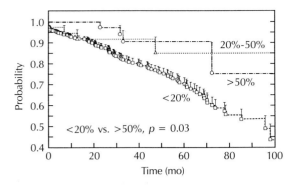

Fig. 52-3. Effect of carotid restenosis on the probability of remaining both alive and stroke free. (From *Ann Surg* 212:629-636, 1990.)

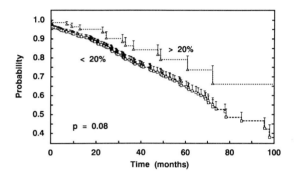

Fig. 52-4. Effect of carotid restenosis on the probability of remaining free of any subsequent cerebrovascular event (transient ischemic attack, stroke, or death). (From *Ann Surg* 212:629-636, 1990.)

Table 52-2. Effect of patch graft closure on carotid restenosis

Author and year	Cases (no.)	Mean follow-up (mo)	>50% restenosis (%)	Material
Deriu, 1984[14]	60	6-36	0	PTFE
Little, 1984[26]	50	1	0	SV
Sundt, 1986[36]	89	24	4	SV
Archie, 1986[1]	100	12	0	SV
Hans, 1987[19]	66	34	4.5	SV
Ouriel, 1987[30]	70	17	5.7	Dacon
Hertzer, 1987[21]	917	21	2.7	SV
Mattos, 1988[27]	19	15	10.5	PTFE
Eikelboom, 1988[16]	67	12	3.5	SV
Bernstein, 1990[5]	80	42	12.5	Mostly PTFE
Hans, 1991[18]	90	55	15.9	SV

PTFE, Teflon; *SV,* saphenous vein.

cumulative incidence of transient ischemic attack (TIA), stroke, and survival was not statistically different in the patients with restenosis. According to Healy's data, the incidence of late stroke in those patients with restenosis was 3% at 7 years, compared with 16% in those without restenosis. Again, at 7 years after surgery, 67% of the patients with restenosis were alive, compared with 62% of those without restenosis.

Cook[10] also studied the incidence of hemispheric transient episodes, late stroke, and survival; he found that the incidence of ipsilateral hemispheric symptoms was not significantly different (in the restenosis patients) from that in the group with mild stenosis or no stenosis ($p = 0.30$). By life-table analysis, the risk of stroke and TIA was the same in both cohorts after 5 years. Also, 5-year survival without stroke or TIAs in patients with significant restenosis did not differ significantly from that in patients without recurrent stenosis (Wilcoxon $p = 0.78$).

PRIMARY PATCH GRAFT CLOSURE

In some cases, patch closure of a carotid endarterectomy is dictated by a long incision into a small internal carotid artery or by other technical features of the endarterectomy. In addition, primary closure of the carotid incision with a patch has been advocated by some authors as a method of preventing recurrent stenosis. In the initial reports of primary patching, very few cases of restenosis were observed (Table 52-2), but as more data with longer-term follow-up have been collected, an increasing incidence of restenosis has been observed, even with primary patch closure (see Table 52-2).

In one study, patch closure was performed at the time of endarterectomy in 80 arteries. In general this procedure was used for small arteries and difficult reconstructions and especially in female patients for whom the predilection to restenosis was known. Restenosis developed in 10 of these 80 patients (12.5%) and was more common in female patients (16.1%) than in male patients (9.2%). Patch material (saphenous vein or Teflon) did not affect the incidence of restenosis. The somewhat higher rate of restenosis in this group of patients with primary patch closure may reflect their selection as the cases most prone to restenosis but does indicate that patch closure does not absolutely prevent restenosis.

The argument against routine carotid patch closure includes the fact that such procedures involve longer carotid occlusion time, a longer suture line, and the use of a patch material that may add its own complications. For example, saphenous vein patches have an incidence of late patch disruption, infection, or aneurysm formation, which has been estimated at 1%, often with a catastrophic outcome.

Hertzer[21] conducted a prospective trial of vein patch angioplasty in 801 patients who underwent 917 consecutive operations at the Cleveland Clinic. The cumulative 3-year incidence of greater than 30% restenosis was 9% in the vein patch group and 31% in the group without patch ($p = 0.007$), and various recurrent defects were documented in 4.8% of the patch group and 14% of the nonpatch group. Operative stroke was less common in the patch group (0.7%) than in the nonpatch group (3.1%), and the mortality rate during surgery was the same in both groups. Ipsilateral late stroke occurred in 2.7% of the nonpatch group and 2.0% of the patch group, and survival at 3 years was 80% in the patch group and 87% in the nonpatch group. Reoperation was required in 0.7% of the patients in the patch group and 1.5% of those in the nonpatch group.

A contemporary, prospective, randomized trial of primary carotid patching was conducted by Eikelboom in Holland.[16] Duplex scanning revealed restenosis at 1 year in 3.5% of patients in the patch group and 21% of those with primary closure ($p = 0.006$). These data were also supported by the results of earlier studies by Imparato[22] and Sundt.[36] In summary, several investigators have evaluated the advantages of routine carotid patch closure and have reported a decrease in the incidence of postoperative restenosis, but clinical data have not been adequate to define a significant decrease in the incidence of late stroke and/or early death with this approach. Probably for this reason, routine carotid patch closure has not been adopted by most surgeons at this time.

PREOPERATIVE ASPIRIN AND DIPYRIDAMOLE

On the basis of the theory that platelet activation stimulates the smooth muscle cell hyperplasia observed in carotid restenosis, a prospective, randomized study was performed in 183 patients who underwent carotid endarterectomy to test the effects of preoperative aspirin and dipyridamole in the prevention of carotid restenosis.[6] Both intention-to-treat (all patients randomized) and efficacy (all patients who actually completed the study) analyses were performed and failed to demonstrate any benefit for the aspirin/dipyridamole group. In fact, more early restenosis occurred among those patients who received aspirin and dipyridamole, and the cumulative number of such restenoses was slightly but not statistically higher throughout the follow-up period.

IMPLICATIONS FOR POSTOPERATIVE SCREENING AND REOPERATION

The data reviewed herein indicate that although carotid restenosis is fairly common, it is only rarely associated with clinically important symptoms, including TIA, stroke, and related early death. For this reason, the identification of carotid restenosis appears much less important than was thought in the past. At present, in the patient who is free of symptoms, a single postoperative baseline duplex study at 1 month after surgery, a study at 6 months, and then one study annually are recommended. New symptoms, transient or permanent, are an indication for more frequent study, as is the development of known restenosis greater than 80%.

Indications for reoperation should be conservative and limited to those patients with ipsilateral symptoms and an anatomically appropriate lesion or the development of progressively more severe stenosis that reaches a level of 90% or greater and is a threat to internal carotid occlusion. According to experience and the collected data from the literature (Table 52-3), reoperation for restenosis should be indicated in a very small percentage of patients (1% to 3%)

Table 52-3. Surgery for carotid restenosis

Author and year	Operations (no.)	Death (%)	Stroke (%)
Clagett, 1983[8]	29	0	3.4
Das, 1985[12]	65	3.1	1.5
Piepgras, 1986[31]	57	0	10.4
Barttlet, 1987[4]	116	1.7	2.6
Kazmiers, 1988[23]	14	0	0
Edwards, 1989[15]	106	0	0.9
Bernstein, 1990[5]	10	0	0
Nitzberg, 1991[28]	27	0	3.4

within the first 3 years after surgery. Subsequently, the gradual development of recurrent atherosclerotic lesions will slowly increase the expected incidence of symptomatic recurrent carotid bifurcation lesions.

Thus asymptomatic carotid restenosis is a relatively common but usually benign process. Patients with such restenosis are less likely to have late transient symptoms or stroke and are less likely to die than patients who do not have restenosis. Antiplatelet therapy and patch closure do not prevent restenosis. Postoperative screening is probably not indicated more frequently than every 6 to 12 months, and surgery should be reserved for those patients in whom recurrent symptoms or critical stenoses that appear prone to progress to occlusion develop.

REFERENCES

1. Archie JP Jr: Prevention of early restenosis and thrombosis-occlusion after carotid endarterectomy by saphenous vein patch angioplasty, *Stroke* 17:901-904, 1986.
2. Atnip RG et al: A rational approach to recurrent carotid stenosis, *J Vasc Surg* 11:511-516, 1990.
3. Barnes RW et al: Recurrent versus residual carotid stenosis: incidence detected by Doppler ultrasound, *Ann Surg* 203:652-660, 1987.
4. Bartlett FF et al: Recurrent carotid stenosis: operative strategy and late results, *J Vasc Surg* 452:456, 1990.
5. Bernstein EF, Torem S, Dilley RB: Does carotid restenosis predict an increased risk of late symptoms, stroke or death? *Ann Surg* 212:629-636, 1990.
6. Bernstein EF et al: *Preoperative aspirin and dipyridamole in the prevention of carotid artery restenosis: a controlled trial.* In Veith FJ, ed: *Current critical problems in vascular surgery,* St Louis, 1991, Quality Medical.
7. Cantelmo NL et al: Noninvasive detection of carotid stenosis following endarterectomy, *Arch Surg* 116:1005-1008, 1988.
8. Clagett GP et al: Etiologic factors for recurrent carotid artery stenosis, *Surgery* 93:313-318, 1983.
9. Colgan MP, Kingston V, Shanik G: Stenosis following carotid endarterectomy, Arch Surg 119:1033-1035, 1984.
10. Cook JM, Thompson BW, Barnes RW: Is routine duplex examination after carotid endarterectomy justified? *J Vasc Surg* 12:334-340, 1990.
11. Courbier R et al: Routine intraoperative carotid angioplasty: its impact on operative morbidity and carotid restenosis, *J Vasc Surg* 3:343-350, 1986.
12. Das MB, Hertzer NR, Ratliff NB: Recurrent carotid stenosis: a 5-year series of 65 reoperations, *Ann Surg* 202:28-35, 1988.
13. DeGroote RD et al: Carotid restenosis: long-term noninvasive follow-up after carotid endarterectomy, *Stroke* 18:1031-1036, 1987.
14. Deriu GP et al: The rationale for patch graft angioplasty after carotid endarterectomy: early and long-term follow-up, *Stroke* 15:972-979, 1984.

15. Edwards WH Jr, Mulherin JL, Martin RS III: Recurrent carotid artery stenosis: resection with autogenous vein replacement, *Ann Surg* 209:662-669, 1989.

16. Eikelboom BC et al: Benefits of carotid patching: a randomized study, *J Vasc Surg* 7:240-247, 1988.

17. Glover JL et al: Restenosis following carotid endarterectomy: evaluation by duplex ultrasonography, *Stroke* 18:1031-1036, 1987.

18. Hans SS: Late follow-up of carotid endarterectomy with venous patch angioplasty, *Am J Surg* 162:50-54, 1991.

19. Hans SS, Girishkumar H, Haus B: Venous patch grafts and carotid endarterectomy, *Arch Surg* 122:1134-1138, 1988.

20. Healy DA et al: Long-term follow-up and clinical outcome of carotid restenosis, *J Vasc Surg* 10:662-669, 1989.

21. Hertzer NR et al: A prospective study of vein patch angioplasty during carotid endarterectomy: three-year results for 801 patients and 917 operations, *Ann Surg* 206:628-635, 1987.

22. Imparato AM et al: Intimal and neointimal fibrous proliferation causing failure of arterial reconstructions, *Surgery* 72:1007-1017, 1972.

23. Kazmers A et al: Reoperative carotid surgery, *Am J Surg* 156:346-352, 1988.

24. Keagy BA et al: Incidence of recurrent or residual stenosis after carotid endarterectomy, *Am J Surg* 149:722-725, 1985.

25. Kremen JE et al: Restenosis or occlusion after carotid endarterectomy, *Arch Surg* 114:608-610, 1980.

26. Little JR, Bayerton BS, Furlan AF: Saphenous vein patch grafts in carotid endarterectomy, *J Neurosurg* 61:743-747, 1984.

27. Mattos MA et al: Is duplex follow-up cost effective in the first year after carotid endarterectomy? *Am J Surg* 156:91-95, 1988.

28. Nitzberg RS et al: Long-term follow-up of patients operated on for recurrent carotid stenosis, *J Vasc Surg* 13:121-127, 1991.

29. O'Donnell TF Jr et al: Ultrasound characteristics of recurrent carotid disease: hypothesis explaining the low incidence of symptomatic recurrence, *J Vasc Surg* 2:26-41, 1985.

30. Ouriel K, Green RM: Clinical and technical factors influencing recurrent carotid stenosis and occlusion after endarterectomy, *J Vasc Surg* 5:702-706, 1987.

31. Piepgras DG et al: Recurrent carotid stenosis, *Ann Surg* 203:205-213, 1988.

32. Pierce GE et al: Incidence of recurrent stenosis after carotid endarterectomy determined by digital subtraction angiography, *Am J Surg* 148:848-854, 1984.

33. Salvian A et al: Cause and noninvasive detection of restenosis after carotid endarterectomy, *Am J Surg* 146:29-34, 1988.

34. Sanders EACM et al: Residual lesions and early recurrent stenosis after carotid endarterectomy, *J Vasc Surg* 5:731-737, 1987.

35. Stoney RJ, String ST: Recurrent carotid stenosis, *Surgery* 8:597-605, 1977.

36. Sundt MT et al: Correlation of postoperative and two year follow-up angiography with neurological function in 99 carotid endarterectomies in 85 consecutive patients, *Ann Surg* 203:90-100, 1988.

37. Thomas M et al: Recurrent carotid artery stenosis following endarterectomy, *Ann Surg* 200:74-79, 1984.

38. Turnipseed WD, Berkoff HA, Crummy A: Postoperative occlusion after carotid endarterectomy, *Arch Surg* 115:573-574, 1980.

39. Zbornikova V et al: Restenosis and occlusion after carotid surgery assessed by duplex scanning and digital subtraction angiography, *Stroke* 17:1137-1142, 1986.

40. Zierler RE et al: Carotid artery stenosis following endarterectomy, *Arch Surg* 117:1408-1415, 1982.

Introduction

R. EUGENE ZIERLER and DENNIS F. BANDYK

Although the clinical features of peripheral arterial disease are well known, noninvasive tests have assumed an increasingly important role in defining both the anatomic extent of arterial lesions and the degree of physiologic abnormality that they produce. The earliest noninvasive diagnostic tests for arterial disease of the extremities were indirect methods that were capable of identifying changes in pressure or flow but did not provide any detailed information on the location and severity of the responsible lesions. These methods were usually based on measurements of limb blood pressure or analysis of plethysmographic tracings or continuous wave Doppler signals. The simplest and most widely used of the indirect methods is ankle pressure measurement with a pneumatic cuff and Doppler flow detector. Although indirect techniques have been quite helpful in the clinical setting, their value is limited by the inability to delineate arterial anatomy.

The limitations of the indirect methods have been largely overcome by direct evaluation of the peripheral arteries with ultrasonic duplex scanning. Since duplex scanning emerged over a decade ago as the preferred noninvasive test for extracranial carotid artery disease, advances in ultrasound technology have expanded its applications to the vessels of the abdomen and extremities. This combination of B-mode imaging and spectral analysis of pulsed Doppler signals provided the first opportunity to accurately characterize arterial disease without resorting to arteriography. The recent addition of color flow imaging has enhanced the abilities of duplex scanning, particularly in the evaluation of small vessels such as the tibial and peroneal arteries.

The clinical role of noninvasive tests can be considered in three categories: screening, definitive diagnosis, and follow-up. An ideal screening test is one that is rapid, accurate, and low in cost; is simple to perform; and does not expose the patient to any significant risk or discomfort. Screening for lower extremity arterial disease is readily accomplished in most patients by ankle pressure measurement and calculation of an ankle-arm index. This provides an assessment of the presence and overall severity of arterial occlusive disease. When definitive diagnostic information is required, duplex scanning can be used to evaluate specific arterial segments. The results of lower extremity duplex scanning

can then serve as the basis for initial clinical decisions. For example, duplex scanning can identify patients who are good candidates for percutaneous transluminal angioplasty, permitting more selective and efficient use of arteriography. In most clinical situations, arteriography serves as an adjunct to radiologic or surgical intervention; arteriography should rarely be necessary for diagnosis alone. The purpose of follow-up testing is to detect progressive or recurrent disease, either in a previously treated arterial segment or at some other site. Although this is similar to screening, it is essential that follow-up testing be able to differentiate between arterial lesions at various anatomic locations. Thus duplex scanning is the preferred method for follow-up after direct intervention.

The chapters in this section provide a broad and detailed overview of the important indirect and direct noninvasive diagnostic tests for peripheral arterial disease. Since the fundamental principles of these techniques have been discussed earlier, these chapters emphasize specific clinical applications. In addition to the indirect tests based on pressure, velocity, and volume measurements, some less common or specialized methods are also covered. These include laser Doppler techniques, air plethysmography, and measurement of transcutaneous oxygen tension. The chapters on peripheral arterial duplex scanning include discussions of screening before intervention, intraoperative assessment, and postoperative surveillance.

It seems likely that future developments in the field of noninvasive testing for peripheral arterial disease will focus on sophisticated ultrasonic imaging techniques that permit measurement of arterial wall thickness and three-dimensional reconstructions of vascular lesions. As these methods are refined, the diagnostic information they provide will more closely resemble the results of arteriography, and the issue of whether arteriography is really necessary will continue to be debated. However, duplex scanning is relatively expensive and time consuming, so it is impractical to perform this test on all patients with signs or symptoms of peripheral arterial disease. Therefore even though progress is inevitable, the simple indirect tests will continue to play a role in the noninvasive arterial evaluation.

CHAPTER 53

Clinical problems in peripheral arterial disease: is the clinical diagnosis adequate?

STEFAN A. CARTER

The diagnosis of arterial obstruction should be made by clinical assessment backed by laboratory data. In the majority of patients with occlusion or narrowing of the arterial supply to the extremities, clinical assessment is adequate to detect even milder degrees of narrowing, to estimate the relative severity of the disease, and to decide on the general approach to management. In addition, the major site of obstruction may frequently be localized. This chapter reviews methods of clinical diagnosis of peripheral arterial disease and in the concluding section relates the roles of clinical diagnosis and laboratory investigation.

HISTORY

The history should be taken first; when carefully elicited, it will often indicate to the physician the presence or absence of arterial obstruction and its severity even before the physical examination is begun. However, a negative history does not rule out the presence of arterial obstruction. Many patients with long-standing obstruction have no symptoms, particularly if they lead a sedentary existence or if their exercise tolerance is limited more by another condition such as cardiac or pulmonary disease or by other limb disease.

Symptoms of peripheral arterial disease

The symptoms of peripheral arterial disease include pain, impotence, coldness, and Raynaud's phenomena. (Raynaud's phenomena are discussed on p. 477 and in Chapter 74.)

Since the pain secondary to arterial disease has specific characteristics, the time taken by the physician to elicit these characteristics and the circumstances under which the pain occurs is well spent because it will usually allow determination of whether the symptom is caused by arterial disease.

Pain associated with exercise. Pain during exercise (walking), or intermittent claudication, occurs when blood flow to the skeletal muscle is insufficient to meet the metabolic demands of the exercising muscle; it is thought to be related to the accumulation of metabolites. The discomfort is variously described as cramps, tiredness, tightness, aching, or pain. The important characteristics are that the pain is absent during the first part of the walk, begins after a relatively constant distance has been traversed, and disappears within a few minutes after the patient stops walking. The distance the patient walks before the onset of the discomfort can vary from a fraction of one city block to half a mile or more, depending on the severity of the condition. The distance may also vary to some extent depending on the speed of walking, the type of terrain, and the presence of an incline. It is of value to try to ascertain whether the discomfort disappears rapidly when the patient stops walking and stands still. However, many individuals do not like to stop in the middle of the street and will try to reach their destination and sit down, since it appears that relief is obtained faster when the patient sits. This may be because of lower intramuscular pressure in the legs in the sitting position, which impedes arterial inflow to a lesser extent than in a standing position in which the muscles of the legs contract to some extent to maintain posture. Intermittent claudication practically never occurs solely from standing and should not be confused with pain in the feet caused by weight bearing, which may occur in various other disorders.

The usual site of claudication is in the muscles of the leg distal to the knee. This is frequently the case not only in patients with obstruction at the level of the thigh but also in those with aortoiliac disease. Other patients with aortoiliac obstruction may experience hip, thigh, or lower back claudication with or without more distal discomfort. In patients with very distal disease, for example, when only branches of the popliteal artery are involved, discomfort brought on by exercise tends to involve the foot and may have atypical features.

In some patients, spinal or other neuromuscular disorders mimic intermittent claudication. For example, compression of the cauda equina during walking may result in pain.[24,33,41,76] For this reason the term *pseudoclaudication* has been coined. The physician may obtain clues as to the presence of such conditions by inquiring whether similar pain occurs when the patient is sitting, lying, or standing or whether it is brought on by certain movements such as bending. The nature of the discomfort may also be different.

Table 53-1. Features of the history in patients with intermittent claudication caused by arterial disease and patients with pseudoclaudication

History of discomfort	Arterial disease	Pseudoclaudication
Onset	Occurs after walking a distance	Produced by walking, prolonged standing, straightening or bending, or turning the back (even in bed)
Nature	Cramp, tiredness, ache, squeezing	Tingling, weakness, clumsiness
Relation to distance walked	Constant	Variable
Relief	Within minutes after cessation of walking (while standing)	May have to sit or lie down for 15 minutes or longer

An important point is that patients with pseudoclaudication often have to sit or even lie down to obtain relief, and a considerable period of time, for example, 15 minutes or much longer, may be necessary for the discomfort to disappear. Table 53-1 summarizes the features of intermittent claudication caused by arterial disease and of pseudoclaudication produced by spinal conditions. Characteristics of pain that are not typical of vascular disease should arouse suspicion that another cause may be present.

Neurologic examination, examination of the spine, electromyography, determination of nerve conduction velocity, noninvasive tests of arterial function, angiography, and myelography may be needed to distinguish the respective roles of the spinal and arterial pathologic conditions, especially if the two coexist.[33,47] However, it is relevant that in a study of 52 patients with diagnostic problems in whom various tests of spinal and vascular status were carried out, at least 70% could have been diagnosed by critical assessment of the patients' symptoms.[33]

Pain at rest. When arterial obstruction is more severe, patients may complain of pain in the limb at rest. This occurs when blood flow is insufficient to meet even the relatively low metabolic demands of the resting tissue. The characteristic features of ischemic pain at rest are its distal distribution and relation to posture. The pain usually involves the toes and the foot. Pain proximal to the ankle may also be present if there is severe pain in the foot and toes. However, pain limited to the more proximal parts of the limb is not caused by arterial disease unless there is skin breakdown and ulceration that give rise to local pain. In the absence of ulceration, pain at rest in the upper parts of the legs, thighs, or hips is practically never caused by chronic ischemia.

Ischemic pain is increased or occurs only when patients are supine, and they are awakened frequently by the pain during the night. Relief is often obtained by putting the limb down over the side of the bed or by sitting up. These manifestations are related to postural changes in the hydrostatic pressure in the vessels of the lower limbs and to changes in central blood pressure. The important factor in the occurrence of the nocturnal pain is the decrease in the mean arterial blood pressure during sleep. The decrease is associated with about a 30% lower forefoot blood flow in limbs with ischemic pain at rest compared with the flow in the supine position when patients are awake.[39] When the patient is in the supine position, the collateral vessels are distended less and thus have smaller radii. This results in a greater resistance and lower distal blood pressure and flow. Conversely, when the patient assumes the dependent position, the increased hydrostatic pressure, which is due to the weight of the long column of blood, distends the collateral vessels and leads to lower resistance, higher distal blood pressure and blood flow, and the relief of pain.[16,29,49] The effects of changes in the distension of the collateral vessels are also demonstrated by the finding of increased flow and pressure in the feet in limbs with occlusion of the superficial femoral artery during external application of negative pressure to the thigh.[2] Another mechanism that contributes to increased flow in the feet when patients are upright is related to the vasoconstriction in the skin and muscles of the thigh in response to the assumption of the upright posture. This vasoconstriction results in lower blood flow through the collateral arteries and thus in a smaller pressure drop during the flow through them.[1] This in turn leads to a higher arterial pressure distal to the occlusion and higher blood flow in the ischemic tissues.[1] Some patients do not obtain relief from the pain by sitting up, but walking slowly around the room alleviates the pain. The relief is brought about by the activation of the venous muscle pump, which reduces venous pressure and results in the increase of 200% to 300% in the arteriovenous pressure gradient available to cause blood flow through the foot.[30]

A more severe form of pain at rest may be caused by ischemic neuropathy, which can result from damage to the nerves by ischemia. This intense pain may consist of paroxysms of sharp shooting pain superimposed on the more constant diffuse pain, and the relationship to posture may be lost.

Impotence. Male patients with proximal arterial disease may experience impotence related to absent or decreased erection. A demonstration of decreased penile systolic pressure is helpful in determining the presence of significant arterial obstruction in the blood supply of the penis and thus provides evidence that the symptom may be related to an impairment of arterial circulation.[28]

Coldness. Patients with arterial obstruction may complain of coldness of the extremities, although coldness is not a specific symptom of organic arterial obstruction. History of asymmetric coldness in one of the limbs or in some of the digits is a more likely indication of the presence of arterial disease.

Other aspects of history

The physician should also inquire about evidence of arterial disease in other vascular beds, since arteriosclerosis obliterans—the most common cause of arterial obstruction in the limbs—is a diffuse disease and frequently involves coronary vessels, the arteries supplying the brain, and other organs at times. Therefore patients should be questioned about a history of myocardial infarction, angina, and cerebrovascular disease. The presence of risk factors that increase the likelihood of development of arteriosclerotic complications should be ascertained by determining the presence or absence of hypertension, diabetes mellitus, smoking, and hyperlipidemia. The presence of arterial disease in other vascular beds is important to assess because it increases the surgical risk, which should be considered if reconstructive surgery is contemplated. The elimination or treatment of risk factors is important because it tends to improve prognosis by decreasing mortality and risk of amputation.[38]

Other less common causes of arterial obstruction should be kept in mind. For example, patients should be asked whether they experience migraine headaches because medications that may be used in the treatment of migraine, such as ergot or methysergide, may result in arterial occlusion, which is reversible if the drug is discontinued early.[12,44,61] Intermittent claudication occasionally has been reported in patients with severe anemia,[58] pheochromocytoma,[67] or amyloidosis,[25] without organic obstruction in the main arterial pathways. Moreover, buttock claudication may rarely result from isolated bilateral internal iliac arterial obstruction.[35] In such cases, examination of the peripheral arteries and ankle pressure at rest and in response to exercise will be normal. Patients may complain of pain during intercourse, and in male patients, penile pressure is expected to be reduced. However, neurogenic or orthopedic causes of the symptoms must be excluded before considering the diagnosis of intermittent claudication due to arterial obstruction limited to the internal iliac vessels.

PHYSICAL EXAMINATION
Palpation of peripheral pulses

At rest. Palpation of pulses is the mainstay of physical examination, and its importance cannot be overemphasized. To acquire this simple skill, trainees must take time to practice palpation. In feeling for a pulse, the examiner must persist and try repeatedly after slightly altering the position of the palpating fingers, the pressure applied, and the po-

sition of the examined limb. If there is doubt as to the presence or absence of the patient's pulse, counting the pulse introduces an element of objectivity to an otherwise subjective examination. The examiner should count the pulse aloud for 10 to 12 beats while an assistant who feels an easily palpable pulse such as the radial pulse reports whether the examiner is keeping in rhythm with the patient's pulse. If an assistant is not available, the patient may be asked to do Valsalva's maneuver to alter the heart rate to determine whether the change can be detected. Alternatively, the physician's own pulse rate may be altered by breath-holding or exercise. If the pulse cannot be counted in this manner, it is probably absent. Without these precautions, the examiner is liable to mistake the pulse in the examiner's own finger or at times repetitive movements of the patient's tendon for the patient's pulse. If the pulse is palpable, the examiner must decide whether it is diminished, since a diminished pulse indicates the presence of a proximal occlusive or stenotic process. The pulse distal to an arterial obstruction has diminished amplitude and increased upstroke time. To decide whether the pulse is diminished, the examiner may consider the quality of the pulse itself, but comparison with the contralateral pulse or with the corresponding pulse in the upper limb is more helpful. If the pulse is weaker than in the contralateral limb, there is strong evidence of the presence of a proximal occlusive or stenotic process. However, since the disease may be bilateral, the examiner should also compare the pulse in the lower limbs with an upper limb pulse. In normal subjects the arterial pressure wave becomes more peaked during distal propagation, its upstroke time shortens, and the amplitude increases, mainly because of the increase in the systolic pressure.[9,46] Therefore inappropriate conclusions might be drawn if proximal pulses in the lower limbs were compared with distal pulses in the upper limbs. The examiner should compare the femoral and popliteal pulses with the brachial pulse, and the pedal pulses with the radial or ulnar pulses.

In an examination of a patient's arterial system, all of the accessible arteries should be palpated. In the arterial supply to the brain, carotid pulses should be palpated carefully, preferably in the lower part of the neck, so as not to press over the area of carotid bifurcation and stimulate sensitive baroreceptors in the carotid sinus, which could result in bradycardia or asystole. Superficial temporal and facial pulses should also be felt. A decrease in these pulses may be caused by obstruction of the external carotid artery. However, asymmetry of the superficial temporal or facial arteries may be caused by an increase in the size of these vessels on the side of an internal carotid obstruction, when the flow in them tends to compensate for absent or diminished flow through the internal carotid system.

Unless the patient's abdomen is very large or there is guarding, the width of the abdominal aorta should be estimated to detect the presence of an abdominal aneurysm. The possibility of increased arterial width should also be considered when the lower abdominal quadrants, the groins, and the popliteal fossae are palpated because of the possibility of aneurysms of the iliac, femoral, and popliteal arteries. In a patient in whom both femoral pulses are absent or markedly diminished, deep palpation over the epigastrium to detect the presence of the aortic pulse may be of value, since absence of the epigastric pulsation suggests the presence of high obstruction of the abdominal aorta,[65] whereas in the more common obstruction in the region of the aortic bifurcation, the epigastric pulse is usually easily palpable.

In the lower extremities, femoral, popliteal, dorsalis pedis, and posterior tibial pulses should be felt routinely. The femoral pulse can often be followed down the thigh along the course of the superficial femoral artery. Except in very large extremities, the pulse can be followed at least approximately 10 cm distal to the groin and often all the way to the region of the adductor canal. This is done by proceeding gradually along the course of the vessel, finger-breadth by finger-breadth, using deep palpation with both hands. If the pulse stops short at the groin or high in the thigh and especially if the finding is unilateral, an occlusion of the common femoral artery that tends to render the limb more ischemic or a high obstruction of the superficial femoral artery near the division of the common femoral artery may be suspected rather than the more common site of occlusion in the adductor canal. One method is to feel all the pulses with the patient supine. In the case of the popliteal pulse the examiner places the fingers of both hands behind the patient's knee to palpate in the popliteal fossa while counterpressure is applied on the front of the knee with the thumbs and/or the thenar eminences of the hands. The pressure applied and the position of the fingers may have to be altered slightly. In some patients the pulse may be felt more readily if the knee is flexed to a slight extent while the examiner searches for the pulse. The best place to start palpation is below the level of the knee joint where there is less tissue between the skin and the bone and the vessel can be compressed against the flat posterior surface of the tibia.[32] However, in some patients who may have occlusion of the popliteal artery in the popliteal fossa, the pulse may be palpable only in the upper part of the popliteal space above the level of the joint.

The dorsalis pedis artery usually arises from the anterior tibial artery, but in some patients it may originate from the peroneal artery and take a more lateral course on the dorsum of the foot. At times the dorsalis pedis pulse cannot be felt if the ankle is excessively plantar flexed[37] or if the patient's feet are very cold. Palpation in front of the ankle between the malleoli in patients in whom posterior tibial and dorsalis pedis pulses may be absent may reveal the presence of a good quality pulse, which indicates that at least the peroneal or the anterior tibial artery is patent down to that level. Since the dorsalis pedis artery is congenitally absent in 5% to 10% of normal individuals,[4,37,51] absence of the dorsalis pedis pulse does not by itself signify arterial disease. Absence of the posterior tibial pulse is more significant because these vessels are rarely absent as a result of congenital anomaly.[4,15,51]

In the upper limbs, palpation should include the subclavian, axillary, brachial, radial, and ulnar pulses. The Allen test provides evidence as to the patency of the wrist arteries into the palms. It is important to avoid pitfalls that at times may lead to a false-positive result of the Allen test.[25] The ulnar artery more often than the radial artery may be compressed by stretching the skin over it with the examiner's fingers. Excessive dorsiflexion of the wrist when the patient makes a fist may compress the radial and ulnar vessels where they cross the wrist and may lead to a false-positive test result. In addition, if the patient's hand is opened and the fingers are extended forcibly, the skin may be stretched taut over the palm, which may lead to relative pallor because of interference with circulation through the compressed small vessels in the stretched skin.

The principle of the Allen test may also be used in assessing patency of the dorsalis pedis and posterior tibial arteries into the foot.[25] Elevation of the foot instead of clenching of the fist is used to produce pallor of the skin.

After exercise. If a patient has palpable pulses and the examiner is not sure whether they are diminished, it may be helpful to ask the patient to walk or do other exercise and then repeat the palpation. If a proximal stenosis is responsible for the findings, distal pulses will usually further decrease or disappear as a result of the exercise, and marked pallor of the foot may develop. This phenomenon is caused by pronounced vasodilatation in the vessels of the skeletal muscle, which leads to increased flow through the stenosis with resulting loss of pressure energy, fall in distal pressure, and disappearance of pulses.[18,23,43] Pallor of the foot develops because the flow is preferentially diverted from the skin to the proximal and vasodilated skeletal muscle.[23]

Maneuvers to detect arterial compression. Palpation of the radial artery, or if the radial pulse is absent or diminished, palpation of the ulnar or brachial pulse, is carried out during "shoulder girdle maneuvers" to detect compression by structures in the thoracic outlet. The maneuvers include palpation of the pulse during hyperabduction, during the costoclavicular maneuver (exaggerated military position), and during the Adson or scalene maneuver. Details of the various maneuvers are given in classic textbook descriptions.[26,80] Compression is demonstrated by marked diminution or disappearance of the pulse. However, such a finding does not prove that symptoms are caused by compression in the thoracic outlet, since these tests show positive results in a significant proportion of normal subjects who are free of symptoms.[80] If the maneuver reproduces the patient's symptoms, it suggests that they are caused by the compression, but the diagnosis must be based on an overall evaluation of the patient.

Disappearance of the pedal pulses during active plantar flexion or during forced passive dorsiflexion of the ankle may provide a clue to the presence of the popliteal artery entrapment.[17,55]

Estimation of skin temperature

Although it is difficult to estimate the absolute temperature of the skin, differences of 1° C to 2° C between sites can easily be detected by palpation. Maintained asymmetric difference in the skin temperature of the corresponding sites of the distal parts of the limbs favors the presence of arterial obstruction. In addition, lower temperature of individual digits suggests the presence of local interference with blood flow. However, since severe obstruction in the arterial tree is required before resting blood flow is significantly decreased, the absence of coldness does not rule out mild or moderate arterial disease.

Although skin temperature of the acral part of the limb (e.g., the foot) may be lower distal to the site of the obstruction, collateral circulation at the level of the occlusion tends to increase and may lead to a local increase in skin temperature. When the popliteal artery is occluded, collateral circulation develops around the knee by way of the geniculate system. This is frequently manifested by increased skin temperature of one or both sides of the knee on the involved side,[31] and at times the enlarged geniculate vessels may be palpable on the side of the knee joint. Therefore the finding of a cold foot with a warm knee strongly suggests an occlusion of the popliteal artery. Similarly, the skin of the lower thigh, usually on the medial aspect, is often warmer in limbs with occlusion of the superficial femoral artery in the adductor canal.

Auscultation

At rest. Auscultation is an important part of the physical examination of the arterial system but tends to be neglected and underestimated. Murmurs or bruits may be produced by arteriovenous fistulae, aneurysms, or vascular tumors.[22,34,82] More frequently, a bruit indicates the presence of an arterial stenotic lesion and may allow localization of a lesion or lesions and distinction between a complete occlusion and a stenosis. Auscultation should be carried out over both sides of the neck and supraclavicular fossae, and if there are symptoms or suggestion of arterial disease in the arterial supply to the upper limbs, it should also be carried out in the axillary and upper brachial regions. Auscultation should also include listening over all quadrants of the abdomen, in some cases over the back, in the groins, along the length of the medial aspect of the thighs over the course of the superficial femoral arteries, and in the popliteal fossae. If the presence of an arteriovenous malformation is suspected, auscultation over more distal parts of the extremities should be included. Auscultation of the chest is important to reveal murmurs that might be transmitted to the neck, supraclavicular fossae, or epigastrium.

It is important not to exert excessive pressure with the diaphragm of the stethoscope because the vessel may be compressed, which would result in an artifactual bruit. This tends to occur over superficial vessels such as the common femoral arteries in the groin and the popliteal vessels. It is more difficult to create an artifactual bruit over the lower abdomen or the thigh, and the examiner may apply a fair amount of pressure initially to be sure that good apposition is present so that a soft bruit will not be missed. If a bruit is heard, the pressure should be relaxed to ascertain whether it disappears.

The frequency of bruits will depend on the population studied. In over 300 patients with peripheral arteriosclerosis obliterans who were referred for assessment to the Vascular Laboratory at St. Boniface General Hospital in Winnipeg, Manitoba, abdominal bruits were found in 30%, a bruit in one or both groins in 48%, a bruit over the thigh distal to the groin in 26%, and a popliteal bruit in 11%.[10] Widmer et al[79] used auscultation together with other tests to screen about 2000 factory workers for arterial disease. They found that the presence of bruits was a useful sign in detecting arterial disease, which indicates that it may provide an easy and valuable screening method for population studies. Although bruits over some sites, especially in the neck and supraclavicular regions, over the epigastrium, and at times in the region of the groins, may be found in apparently normal, usually young, subjects and in hyperkinetic states,[34,54,57,63,78] consideration of the clinical condition, the age of the subject, details of the physical findings, and the effect of exercise will usually suggest whether the bruit is functional or is likely to be caused by pathologic conditions. Pathologic bruits as compared with functional bruits are longer and may extend into diastole, particularly after exercise.[27,34,57,64] Bruits over the flanks, the lower abdominal quadrants, and the region of the adductor canal are rarely functional.[63,78] In addition, bruits over the thigh in the region of the adductor canal (likely a result of early atherosclerotic lesions) may be found in limbs in which the ankle systolic pressure at rest is within normal limits.[10]

After exercise. Exercise of the extremity usually increases the intensity and duration of the bruit and thus is helpful in confirming the finding when the bruit is soft or difficult to hear at rest. In the presence of a mild arterial narrowing, there may be no bruit at rest when the blood flow is relatively low. Increased flow after exercise by increasing velocity through and distal to the stenosis results in increased turbulence and often in an audible bruit, thus unmasking the presence of a stenotic lesion.[7,27,60,70]

Distinction between a complete occlusion and a stenosis is of value in patients in whom emboli from aneurysms, ulcerated plaques, or areas of poststenotic dilation in the proximal part of the arterial tree may lead to localized small vessel occlusions in the distal part of the limb, which are manifested by localized ischemic areas such as cyanotic digits[40] or irregular patches of discoloration with associated symptoms.[42] Demonstration of a bruit after exercise in such a case demonstrates the presence of a patent pathway through which embolization can occur.[10] Auscultation after exercise may also be of help in localizing the lesions, for example, when there are multiple stenoses, by allowing more precise localization of the maximum intensity of the bruits. A change in hemodynamics as a result of drug administration may also change the characteristics of the bruits and be of practical value.[73,74]

Maneuvers to detect arterial compression. In examining patients for the presence of compression in the thoracic outlet, it is helpful to auscultate in the paraclavicular region. During the maneuvers referred to earlier in the section on the palpation of pulses, systolic bruits may be heard as the subclavian artery is compressed. They usually disappear together with the distal pulse as the maneuver is completed.[26] The bruit can be heard transiently as the maneuver is reversed. Such examinations may be helpful in assessing patients with suspected thoracic outlet syndrome, but the presence of bruits during the maneuvers does not prove that the symptoms are caused by outlet compression because these findings also occur in a significant number of subjects who are free of symptoms.

Other maneuvers to localize the site of bruits. Dowell and Sladen[21] drew attention to an interesting and valuable maneuver aimed at the localization of bruit-producing lesions. The "bruit-occlusion test" consists of manual compression of an artery distal to the bruit. If the bruit disappears, stenosis is likely to be present proximally in the compressed artery or in its parent vessel. Conversely, if the bruit is unchanged or increases, the site of the lesion is likely to be in an unoccluded branch of the parent vessel. A decrease in the bruit may be caused by stenosis of the parent vessel or may indicate a multiple origin. A change in the intensity of the bruit is usually most noticeable during the first few beats after compression and after release of the efferent vessel. For example, if caused by the stenosis at the takeoff of the superficial femoral artery, a bruit in the groin will disappear when the superficial femoral artery is compressed a few inches distally, may decrease in intensity if it is in the common femoral or external iliac artery, and will remain unchanged or increase if located in the profunda femoris artery. The same procedure can be applied to the elucidation of bruits in other parts of the arterial tree.

In a patient who has a bruit in the right supraclavicular fossa and lower part of the neck and a murmur in the right second interspace, marked diminution of the bruit over the supraclavicular area and disappearance from the second interspace during compression of the upper brachial artery confirm the absence of aortic stenosis and the presence of a stenotic lesion in the subclavian or innominate artery. Disappearance of an abdominal bruit in the paraumbilical region on the compression of the right femoral artery in the groin indicates that it originates in the abdominal aorta or the right common or external iliac vessels and not in a visceral aortic branch. Auscultation of the abdominal bruits can be carried out during bilateral femoral compression. A bruit that originates in the aortoiliac region may disappear or may only decrease because of flow continuing through patent internal iliac vessels. On the other hand, if the bruit does not change or becomes louder, it is likely that it originates from a side branch of the abdominal aorta such as a renal, celiac, or mesenteric artery. Accentuation of a carotid

bruit may be produced by compression of the contralateral carotid artery.[34,64]

Significance of arterial auscultation in peripheral vascular disease was demonstrated by correlation of the auscultatory findings with systolic pressure measurements in 309 patients with arterial obstruction and in 149 subjects without arterial disease.[10] Examination for bruits after limb exercise and during compression maneuvers provided additional important information. The findings of the study confirmed that auscultation over the peripheral arteries should be an integral part of the physical examination of patients for arterial disease, since it often provides valuable information about the presence and location of arterial lesions. In a number of cases, bruits that result from early arterial lesions may be found before the onset of symptoms and even in the presence of normal resting ankle pressures.[10]

Inspection

Trophic changes in the skin. Chronic severe impairment of blood flow leads to changes in the skin that can be noted by inspection. Since the flow is usually decreased to the greatest extent in the most distal part of the limb, such trophic changes are commonly found in the toes and feet. They include thinning of the skin, attenuation or disappearance of the skin ridges on the plantar aspects of the distal phalanges of the digits, thickening of the nails, dryness and scaliness, and loss of hair on the toes. Absence of hair on the more proximal parts of the limbs is of little significance, since it occurs frequently in patients without arterial disease. The presence of abnormal discoloration in the supine position may indicate local ischemia. Persistent cyanosis usually indicates severe ischemia or a preinfarction stage. Scattered, irregular cyanotic areas, at times resembling livedo reticularis, may be caused by multiple small emboli of thrombotic or atheromatous material from proximal ulcerated plaques, sites of poststenotic dilatation, or aneurysms.[40,42]

Chronic ulcers or gangrenous lesions are also most commonly found on the toes and feet but may occur more proximally as a result of injury in limbs with severe arterial obstruction. Skin cracking, which may lead to a chronic lesion, should be sought in the skin of the heels and between the toes. Ulcers secondary to venous insufficiency are commonly found in the region of the ankle, most often on the medial aspect. They are usually associated with induration of the skin caused by fibrosis of subcutaneous tissue and with brown pigmentation of the skin of the ankle or lower leg. Painful hypertensive ischemic ulcers occur in the leg, often on the lateral aspect of the ankles.[69]

Positional color changes. Observation of changes in the color of the skin with changes in the position of the limb is useful in assessing the severity of arterial obstruction. With the patient in the supine position, the examiner lifts the patient's legs with the knees straight as far above the bed as possible without causing discomfort to the patient. The soles of the feet and the toes are observed for the development of pallor. Deathly pallor develops in the presence of severe arterial obstruction, whereas lesser degrees of pallor signify milder disease. It is important to observe the elevated feet for at least a minute or longer, since the pallor may not develop for some time. After observation for pallor is completed, the patient is asked to sit up with the feet over the side of the bed hanging loosely. The feet are observed for the development of increased rubor. Relaxation of smooth muscle in the walls of the small vessels of the skin because of severe ischemia leads to the accumulation of a greater volume of blood in these small vessels when hydrostatic pressure is increased in the dependent position and thus results in a deeper color. The dependent rubor is an important sign in the assessment of patients with chronic arterial occlusion. The finding of pronounced rubor signifies the presence of at least fairly severe arterial obstruction, whereas its absence indicates that arterial obstruction, if present, is not severe.

Venous filling time. It is convenient to combine observations for positional color changes with a determination of the venous filling time. When the patient sits up and hangs the legs over the side of the bed, the dorsum of the foot is observed for the time it takes for the veins to fill. This represents a rough index of blood flow to the foot and normally varies from less than 10 seconds to 20 seconds or more. Although several textbooks indicate 10 or 15 seconds as the upper limit of normal, this is true only if there is peripheral vasodilatation and a high blood flow. When there is vasoconstriction because of coldness or nervousness, the venous filling time in normal subjects may be 20 seconds or longer. The finding of a difference of 5 or more seconds between the filling times of the two feet provides strong evidence of the presence of obstruction or of more severe obstruction on the side with the longer filling time. In the presence of venous insufficiency, however, the veins of the foot may fill from above, and the test results can be misleading.

The venous filling time is often within normal limits in the presence of significant arterial obstruction. Marked prolongation suggests the presence of at least fairly severe obstruction, but it may also occur in the presence of pronounced peripheral vasoconstriction when patients are cold or if they have a tendency to vasospasm in the absence of organic obstruction.

Other aspects of the physical examination

Since symptoms in the lower limbs may be caused by a number of conditions other than arterial disease, it may be worthwhile to examine the extremities for the presence of several other conditions. Neurologic examination with testing of the tendon jerks and sensation may demonstrate abnormalities because of neuropathy (e.g., in diabetics) or because of nerve root compression that results from disease of the spine. Tenderness may suggest the presence of phlebitis or of a muscular abnormality, although calf muscle tenderness may be present in patients with intermittent clau-

dication, especially if the arterial occlusion is relatively recent or sometimes if the patient has walked long distances despite claudication. Increased temperature of the skin overlying the joints may be caused by an active arthritic condition. Edema may point to venous or lymphatic obstruction, although hydrostatic edema may be present in patients with severe arterial disease who may sleep for protracted periods of time with their limbs in a dependent position.

PERIPHERAL ARTERIAL DISEASE OF THE UPPER EXTREMITIES

Although arterial disease in the vessels supplying the upper limbs is less common than in the lower extremities, arterial obstruction from the subclavian to the digital arteries occurs as a result of atherosclerosis,[13] Takayasu's disease,[81] embolism,[81] thoracic outlet syndromes,[19,75,81] complications of diagnostic arterial catheterization,[19] thromboangiitis obliterans,[81] trauma,[19,75,81] and various conditions that affect more distal arteries of the hand or digits.[75,81] An obstruction of the subclavian arteries by arteriosclerosis obliterans is common in older subjects, and the left subclavian artery is affected more frequently than the right.[13] Such obstruction may be asymptomatic and manifested only by an unequal brachial pressure in the two upper limbs. However, since the involvement of the subclavian arteries may be bilateral, it may result in abnormally low blood pressure in both brachial regions; in such a case brachial blood pressure measurement may result in an erroneous interpretation of the patient's central blood pressure. This consideration makes it mandatory to listen for the presence of bruits in the paraclavicular regions, which if present, may provide clues as to the presence of stenotic lesions in the subclavian vessels and abnormally low brachial blood pressures. Patients with arterial obstruction in the upper extremities may have symptoms of claudication, pain at rest, and skin ulceration or gangrene. The characteristics of the symptoms and principles of physical examination of the lower extremities discussed earlier apply to the assessment of patients with disease of the arterial supply of the upper limbs.

Raynaud's phenomena are symptoms of peripheral arterial disease that predominantly affect the acral parts of the extremities and especially the digits. They consist of episodes of white or cyanotic discoloration, usually of the fingers or toes, which may involve a part of the digit or the whole digit and at times more proximal parts of the hands and feet. Raynaud's phenomena are thought to be a result of spasm or critical closure of digital arteries and probably of smaller distal vessels. The vasospastic episodes are precipitated by exposure of the extremities or of the body to cold and, at times, by emotional upsets. Although episodes may involve the toes, they occur more frequently in the fingers. Such episodes may be secondary to a variety of primary conditions that include connective tissue disorders, trauma, arteriosclerosis or thromboangiitis obliterans, exposure to drugs and toxic substances, and use of vibratory tools. In some patients the symptoms are primary and not related to another disorder.

The diagnosis of Raynaud's phenomena is made by history of the characteristic episodic discoloration. Although a number of physiologic tests to objectively document Raynaud's phenomena have been described, varying proportions of false-negative results occur with virtually all types of tests, including assessment of responses of blood flow, skin temperature, and local systolic pressures to a cold challenge. Thus Raynaud's phenomena continue to be elusive in some patients in laboratory studies, and this parallels the clinical experience of the inability to consistently provoke the attacks in the physician's office by putting patients' limbs under cold water.

Although demonstration of a primary condition to which Raynaud's phenomena might be secondary is often made by a combination of careful clinical assessment and various laboratory studies, in some patients the vasospastic attacks may precede the development of other manifestations of the primary disorder by a number of years. Certain clues in the clinical assessment may suggest that Raynaud's phenomena are secondary to other pathologic conditions. They include unilateral vasospastic attacks or episodes that consistently involve only some digits of an extremity, evidence of organic arterial obstruction, the presence of severe ischemia or necrosis, and the recent onset of severe symptoms.

ROLE OF CLINICAL ASSESSMENT IN MANAGEMENT AND FOLLOW-UP

Decisions concerning management of the patient are based on the results of the clinical findings and, as may be indicated, laboratory assessment of the individual patient in the context of the knowledge of the natural history of the disease. Patients with arteriosclerosis obliterans in the vessels supplying the extremities are more likely to have an underlying involvement of the vessels supplying other vascular beds. Many patients eventually die of cardiac or cerebral complications of atherosclerosis.* Therefore the search for underlying disease in other vascular beds and assessment for the presence of risk factors are of primary importance. The factors that adversely influence prognosis include diabetes, smoking, hypertension, and hyperlipidemia.

Despite frequent development of further obstructive lesions in the arterial tree of the same or contralateral limb,[5,72] the prognosis for the limbs is good in nondiabetic patients with intermittent claudication, and the amputation rate is between 1% and 2% per year or 10% to 12% at 10 years.[5,56,68] The prognosis in patients with diabetes mellitus and claudication is not as good, and the rate of amputation has been estimated at two to three times that in persons without diabetes.[36,68] In the majority of patients who have intermittent claudication, the symptoms improve.[5,53,68,77] Considerable improvement often occurs gradually after the occurrence of an occlusive process or its progression. The symptomatic improvement may be paralleled by a gradual

increase in the ankle systolic pressure[8] and in maximal blood flow, which may continue for a year or longer.[6] Numerous studies also indicate that walking exercise training is frequently followed by a great improvement in walking ability,[66] and about 75% of the patients with claudication achieve remarkable walking ability despite moderately severe arterial obstruction.[11]

The relatively benign prognosis for limbs with intermittent claudication and the potential for good walking ability have to be taken into account in making decisions about the advisability of arterial reconstructive surgery, since these patients may have an increased surgical risk related to the underlying arteriosclerotic involvement of the vessels supplying the heart and brain. On the other hand, the presence of persistent pain at rest or unhealed ulceration and gangrene warrants a more aggressive surgical approach.

Patients with arterial occlusive disease to the extremities should be followed up at regular intervals by clinical assessment and when indicated by noninvasive laboratory tests. Development of pain at rest or skin breakdown is usually associated with progression of the arterial obstruction. In addition, an increase in the severity of intermittent claudication suggests progression. However, since severity of the claudication is also greatly influenced by the amount of walking that the patients perform, it is not uncommon for patients, especially those who live in cold northern climates, to experience more severe symptoms when they resume walking in the spring after being inactive during the winter without any progression of the arterial disease. Absence of the progression may be ascertained by physical examination and confirmed by noninvasive pressure measurements. On the other hand, the severity of the arterial obstruction may increase before a change in clinical manifestations occurs and may also be demonstrated by pressure measurements.[8,72]

CONCLUSION

Previous sections of this chapter reviewed clinical assessment of patients for peripheral arterial disease. When carried out carefully by experienced clinicians, the clinical diagnosis is adequate in the majority of patients. The clinician's experience, ability, and willingness to take time to carry out the clinical assessment are important. Errors in diagnosis occur when assessment is carried out by less experienced personnel.[3] Comparisons of the results of clinical diagnosis and noninvasive testing of arterial disease have been published. Significant correlations exist between physical findings and the results of the physiologic studies,[45,50] but the latter provide more quantitative data. One study reported a significant percentage of false-positive and false-negative results obtained by clinical assessment when noninvasive hemodynamic testing was used as a criterion of the arterial disease.[52] In another study in which angiographic findings were used as a criterion, clinical diagnosis by experienced vascular surgeons was as useful as the results of vascular laboratory testing.[3] It seems that it is not an important issue

---

*References 14, 20, 36, 48, 62, 68, 71, 77.

whether clinical diagnosis or laboratory studies are better because most physicians will agree that the patient should be thoroughly evaluated clinically and that laboratory studies should be carried out as needed to improve the assessment and assist in the diagnosis or management. The finding of false-negative history is to be expected because many patients with complete occlusion of the main artery to the limb may be free of symptoms if they are limited in their ability to exercise by another condition. The sensitivity of the physical examination to detect an arterial lesion will depend on the thoroughness of the procedure (e.g., whether arterial auscultation is carried out over various sites, before and after exercise, and with compression maneuvers). Auscultation after exercise and auscultation during arterial compression are worthwhile methods for detecting milder stenotic lesions and for localizing the origin of bruits. Bruits may occur at times at rest or after exercise in the presence of minor stenotic lesions and in limbs in which systolic pressures may be within normal limits.[10] Such bruits could be referred to as "clinically false-positive" information. Yet this type of examination may be useful in screening for early atherosclerotic lesions and may be applied to population studies[79] for the purpose of preventive health measures, perhaps in combination with simple noninvasive testing.[59]

There is no doubt that laboratory investigations are needed in the evaluation of patients with arterial disease and might include both noninvasive testing and angiography. Angiography is most important in providing detailed information about the anatomy of the diseased arteries when planning surgery or other endovascular interventions, but because it is associated with a small but significant incidence of complications, it should never be used just to make a diagnosis.

Noninvasive testing is useful and of great practical importance in the assessment and management of patients with peripheral arterial disease. It provides quantitative, objective documentation of arterial obstruction and of its severity, against which the progress of the disease can be gauged in individual patients and in the determination of its natural history. Laboratory measurements are especially valuable in the assessment and diagnosis of patients with pseudoclaudication or with other conditions, such as diabetic neuropathy, especially when these conditions coexist with arterial obstruction. Systolic pressure measurement in the penis is of value in the assessment of arterial obstruction that may cause impotence. Noninvasive testing is helpful in the management of patients by estimating the chances of healing of skin lesions and of elective surgical procedures in limbs with arterial obstruction and of amputation sites. The tests may assist in selecting patients for specific medical and surgical therapies. Physiologic measurements will also provide new data of value in research, which are necessary to gain a better understanding of the pathophysiology of disease and to develop improved diagnostic and therapeutic methods.

REFERENCES

1. Agerskov K: Influence of thigh blood flow upon the arterial pressure gradient over the collateral arteries in patients with occlusion of the superificial femoral artery, *Cardiovasc Res* 16:304, 1982.
2. Agerskov K et al: External negative thigh pressure: effect upon blood flow and pressure in the foot in patients with occlusive arterial disease, *Dan Med Bull* 37:451, 1990.
3. Baker WH et al: Diagnosis of peripheral occlusive disease, *Arch Surg* 113:1308, 1978.
4. Barnhorst DA, Barner HB: Prevalence of congenitally absent pedal pulses, *N Engl J Med* 278:264, 1968.
5. Bloor K: Natural history of arteriosclerosis of the lower extremities, *Ann R Coll Surg Engl* 28:36, 1961.
6. Bollinger A: Kollateraldurchblutung bei Verschlüssen der Gliedmassenarterien, *Angiologica* 3:293, 1966.
7. Bühler F, Da Silva A, Widmer LK: Die Arterienauskultation zur Früherfassung der Atherosklerose, *Schweiz Med Wochenschr* 98:1932, 1968.
8. Carter SA: Clinical measurement of systolic pressures in limbs with arterial occlusive disease, *JAMA* 207:1869, 1969.
9. Carter SA: Effect of age, cardiovascular disease, and vasomotor changes on transmission of arterial pressure waves through the lower extremities, *Angiology* 29:601, 1978.
10. Carter SA: Arterial auscultation in peripheral vascular disease, *JAMA* 261:1682, 1981.
11. Carter SA et al: Walking ability and ankle systolic pressures: observations in patients with intermittent claudication in a short-term walking exercise program, *J Vasc Surg* 10:642, 1989.
12. Conley JE, Boulanger WJ, Mendeloff GL: Aortic obstruction associated with methysergide maleate therapy for headaches, *JAMA* 198:808, 1966.
13. Crawford ES et al: Surgical treatment of occlusion of the innominate, common carotid, and subclavian arteries: a 10 year experience, *Surgery* 65:17, 1969.
14. Criqui MH, Coughlin SS, Fronek A: Noninvasively diagnosed peripheral arterial disease as a predictor of mortality: results from a prospective study, *Circulation* 72:768, 1985.
15. Criqui MH et al: The sensitivity, specificity, and predictive value of traditional clinical evaluation of peripheral arterial disease: results from noninvasive testing in a defined population, *Circulation* 71:516, 1985.
16. Dahn I et al: On the conservative treatment of severe ischemia, *Scand J Clin Lab Invest* 19(suppl 99):160, 1966.
17. Darling RC et al: Intermittent claudication in young athletes: popliteal artery entrapment syndrome, *J Trauma* 14:543, 1974.
18. DeWeese JA: Pedal pulses disappearing with exercise, *N Engl J Med* 262:1214, 1960.
19. Dick R: Arteriography in neurovascular compression at the thoracic outlet, with special reference to embolic patterns, *Am J Roentgenol Radium Ther Nucl Med* 110:141, 1970.
20. Dormandy J et al: Fate of the patient with chronic leg ischaemia, *J Cardiovasc Surg* 30:50, 1989.
21. Dowell AJ, Sladen JG: The bruit-occlusion test: a clinical method for localizing arterial stenosis, *Br J Surg* 65:201, 1978.
22. Edwards EA, Levine HD: Peripheral vascular murmurs, *Arch Intern Med* 90:284, 1952.
23. Edwards EA, Cohen NR, Kaplan MM: Effect of exercise on the peripheral pulses, *N Engl J Med* 260:738, 1959.
24. Evans JG: Neurogenic intermittent claudication, *Br Med J* 2:985, 1964.
25. Fairbairn JF II: *Clinical manifestations of peripheral vascular disease.* In Juergens JL, Spittell JA Jr, Fairbairn JF II: *Peripheral vascular diseases,* ed 5, Philadelphia, 1980, WB Saunders.
26. Fairbairn JF II, Campbell JK, Payne WS: *Neurovascular compression syndromes of the thoracic outlet.* In Juergens JL, Spittell JA Jr, Fairbairn JF II: *Peripheral vascular diseases,* ed 5, Philadelphia, 1980, WB Saunders.
27. Garrison GE, Floyd WL, Orgain ES: Exercise in the physical examination of peripheral arterial disease, *Ann Intern Med* 66:587, 1967.
28. Gaskell P: The importance of penile blood pressure in cases of impotence, *Can Med Assoc J* 105:1047, 1971.
29. Gaskell P, Becker WJ: The erect posture as an aid to the circulation in the feet in the presence of arterial obstruction, *Can Med Assoc J* 105:930, 1971.

30. Gaskell P, Parrott JC: The effect of a mechanical venous pump on the circulation of the feet in the presence of arterial obstruction, *Surg Gynecol Obstet* 146:582, 1978.

31. Gaylis H: Warm knees and cold feet; a new sign in arterial occlusion, *Lancet* 1:792, 1966.

32. Ger R: Palpation of the popliteal pulse, *Surgery* 60:615, 1966.

33. Goodreau JJ et al: Rational approach to the differentiation of vascular and neurogenic claudication, *Surgery* 84:749, 1978.

34. Harvey WP: Some newer or poorly recognized findings on clinical auscultation. (I), *Mod Conc Cardiovasc Dis* 37:85, 1968.

35. Hodgson KJ, Sumner DS: Buttock claudication from isolated bilateral internal iliac arterial stenoses, *J Vasc Surg* 7:446, 1988.

36. Hughson WG, et al: Intermittent claudication: factors determining outcome, *Br Med J* 1:1377, 1978.

37. Ison JW: Palpation of dorsalis pedis pulse, *JAMA* 206:2745, 1968.

38. Janzon L, et al: Intermittent claudication and hypertension: ankle pressure and walking distance in patients with well-treated and nontreated hypertension, *Angiology* 32:175, 1981.

39. Jelnes R: Why do patients with severe arterial insufficiency get pain during sleep? *Scand J Clin Lab Invest* 47:649, 1987.

40. Karmody AM et al: "Blue toe" syndrome, *Arch Surg* 111:1263, 1976.

41. Kavanaugh GJ et al: "Pseudoclaudication" syndrome produced by compression of the cauda equina, *JAMA* 206:2477, 1968.

42. Kazmier FJ et al: Livedo reticularis and digital infarcts: a syndrome due to cholesterol emboli arising from atheromatous abdominal aortic aneurysms, *Vasc Dis* 3:12, 1966.

43. Keitzer WF et al: Hemodynamic mechanism for pulse changes seen in occlusive vascular disease, *Surgery* 57:163, 1965.

44. Kempczinski RF, Buckley MJ, Darling RC: Vascular insufficiency secondary to ergotism, *Surgery* 79:597, 1976.

45. Krähenbuhl B, Rohr J: Artères pèrphèriques: palpation manuelle et examen par la méthode de Doppler, *Schweiz Med Wochenschr* 104:240, 1974.

46. Kroeker EJ, Wood EH: Comparison of simultaneously recorded central and peripheral arterial pressure pulses during rest, exercise and tilted position in man, *Circ Res* 3:623, 1955.

47. Lamerton AJ et al: "Claudication" of the sciatic nerve, *Br Med J* 286:1785, 1983.

48. Lassila R, Lepantalo M, Lindfors O: Peripheral arterial disease—natural outcome, *Acta Med Scand* 220:295, 1986.

49. Lezack JD, Carter SA: Systolic pressures in arterial occlusive disease with special reference to the effect of posture, *Clin Res* 17:638, 1969.

50. Lorentsen E: The plantar ischemia test (contribution to the discussion about local blood pressure measurements in patients with peripheral arterial insufficiency), *Scand J Clin Lab Invest* 31(suppl 128):149, 1973.

51. Ludbrook J, Clarke AM, McKenzie JK: Significance of absent ankle pulse, *Br Med J* 1:1724, 1962.

52. Marinelli MR et al: Noninvasive testing vs. clinical evaluation of arterial disease, *JAMA* 241:2031, 1979.

53. McAllister FF: The fate of patients with intermittent claudication managed nonoperatively, *Am J Surg* 132:593, 1976.

54. McLoughlin MJ, Colapinto RF, Hobbs BB: Abdominal bruits, *JAMA* 232:1238, 1975.

55. Miles S et al: Doppler ultrasound in the diagnosis of the popliteal artery entrapment syndrome, *Br J Surg* 64:883, 1977.

56. Naji A: Femoropopliteal vein grafts for claudication analysis of 100 consecutive cases, *Ann Surg* 188:79, 1978.

57. Pennetti V, Di Renzi L: On some phonoarteriographic aspects of peripheral arterial murmurs due to hyperactivity and to obliterating arteriopathies, *Angiologica* 7:8, 1970.

58. Pickering GW, Wayne EJ: Observations on angina pectoris and intermittent claudication in anaemia, *Clin Sci* 1:305, 1934.

59. Prineas RJ et al: Recommendations for use of noninvasive methods to detect atherosclerotic peripheral arterial disease—in population studies, *Circulation* 65:1561, 1982.

60. Provan JL, Moreau P, MacNab I: Pitfalls in the diagnosis of leg pain, *Can Med Assoc J* 121:167, 1979.

61. Rackley CE et al: Vascular complications with use of methysergide, *Arch Intern Med* 117:265, 1966.

62. Reunanen A, Takkunen H, Aromaa A: Prevalence of intermittent claudication and its effect on mortality, *Acta Med Scand* 211:249, 1982.

63. Rivin AU: Abdominal vascular sounds, *JAMA* 221:688, 1972.

64. Royle JP: Auscultation of peripheral arteries, *Med J Aust* 2:488, 1969.

65. Sako Y: Arteriosclerotic occlusion of the midabdominal aorta, *Surgery* 59:709, 1966.

66. Saltin B: *Physical training in patients with intermittent claudication.* In Cohen LS, Mock MB, Ringquist I, eds: *Physical conditioning and cardiovascular rehabilitation,* New York, 1981, John Wiley & Sons.

67. Scharf Y et al: Intermittent claudication with pheochromocytoma, *JAMA* 215:1323, 1971.

68. Schatz IJ: *The natural history of peripheral arteriosclerosis.* In Brest AN, Moyer JH, eds: *Atherosclerotic vascular disease: a Hahnemann symposium,* New York, 1967, Appleton-Century-Crofts.

69. Schnier BR, Sheps SG, Juergens JL: Hypertensive ischemic ulcer, *Am J Cardiol* 17:560, 1966.

70. Schoop W: Frühdiagnose stenosierender Arterienveränderungen, *Dtsch Med Wochenschr* 92:1723, 1967.

71. Smith GD, Shipley MJ, Rose G: Intermittent claudication, heart disease risk factors, and mortality, *Circulation* 82:1925, 1990.

72. Strandness DE Jr, Stahler C: Arteriosclerosis obliterans: manner and rate of progression, *JAMA* 196:1, 1966.

73. Strano A, Di Renzi L: Stethoacoustic findings on peripheral arteries and phonoarteriographic records in normal young subjects during the intravenous infusion of adrenalin, *Angiology* 21:678, 1970.

74. Ueda H et al: Quantitative assessment of obstruction of the aorta and its branches in "aortitis syndrome," *Jpn Heart J* 7:3, 1966.

75. Velayos ED et al: Clinical correlation analysis of 137 patients with Raynaud's phenomena, *Am J Med Sci* 262:347, 1970.

76. Verstraete M: Pseudo-intermittent claudication, *Angiologia* 7:212, 1970.

77. Verstraete M: Current therapy for intermittent claudication, *Drugs* 24:240, 1982.

78. Widmer LK, Glaus L: Zur Epidemiologie des Verschlusses von Gliedmassenarterien, *Schweiz Med Wochenschr* 100:761, 1970.

79. Widmer LK et al: Zur Häufigkeit des Gliedmassenarterienverschlusses bei 1864 berufstätigen Männern, *Schwiez Med Wochenschr* 97:102, 1967.

80. Wright IS: *Neurovascular syndromes of the shoulder girdle.* In *Vascular diseases in clinical practice,* ed 2, Chicago, 1952, Mosby.

81. Yao JST et al: A method for assessing ischemia of the hand and fingers, *Surg Gynecol Obstet* 135:373, 1972.

82. Zoneraich S, Zoneraich O: Diagnostic significance of abdominal arterial murmurs in liver and pancreatic disease, *Angiology* 22:197, 1971.

CHAPTER 54

Basic and practical aspects of peripheral arterial testing

ANDREW N. NICOLAIDES

Symptoms such as pain on walking, cold feet, and blue toes are common complaints suggestive of ischemia. The internist or vascular surgeon must first exclude the presence of osteoarthritis, sciatica, or venous insufficiency. Although this may be easy in the majority of patients, it can be difficult when ischemia is mild and especially when arthritis may coexist. Evidence of peripheral ischemia, such as nutritional changes, cold feet, and absent pulses, will confirm the suspicion of arterial disease noted in the history. Rest pain, especially at night, will make the diagnosis even easier, and an urgent admission to the hospital and arteriography will be arranged with the expectation of early revascularization. However, in some patients with claudication, such clearcut evidence of ischemia may be absent because nutritional changes do not exist and all the peripheral pulses are present when the patient is examined at rest (see Chapter 53).

Careful examination reveals four main groups of patients with the following conditions: (1) absent or weak femoral pulses suggesting that at least aortoiliac disease is present, (2) absent foot pulses but normal femoral pulses suggesting femoropopliteal disease, (3) normal foot and femoral pulses at rest that become weak or disappear during exercise with a variable number of minutes elapsing before their return, and (4) normal foot and femoral pulses at rest not altered by exercise. In the 1960s, these were the basic observations to consider before a decision could be made that arterial disease was present or that it was of such severity that reconstruction would be justified if judged to be feasible by the arteriogram. At that time, arteriography was an invariable sequel to the clinical examination. However, the noninvasive investigations recently developed supplement the history and clinical examination and in many patients allow clinical decisions without resorting to angiography.

The purpose of this chapter is to analyze the surgeon's approach to the diagnosis of arterial disease, the decision to proceed to arteriography, vascular reconstruction, and the selection of the correct procedure in light of information obtained from noninvasive investigations. The discussion is developed through a series of questions a surgeon should consider regarding a patient with symptoms suggesting arterial disease.

IS THERE ARTERIAL DISEASE?

The value of the history and clinical examination and particularly the examination of pulses in determining the presence of arterial disease has been discussed. If the pulses are absent, the clinical examination alone is enough to determine the presence of arterial disease; the noninvasive tests are not necessary to make a diagnosis, and their use is mainly to document the presence and degree of disease. In the presence of weak pulses the noninvasive tests are also unnecessary, but they can provide objective confirmation. The ankle pressure at rest will be enough for this and is useful in obese patients or in the presence of ankle edema when the pulses may not be easily palpable. However, in the presence of normal pulses and pain on walking the noninvasive tests are necessary to determine the presence or absence of disease. In such patients the ankle pressure should be measured both at rest and after exercise because it is possible to have normal pulses and a normal ankle pressure at rest, with a fall in ankle pressure after exercise as the sole indicator of disease (see Chapters 55 and 61).

It is now well established that the fall in ankle pressure after a standardized exercise test on a treadmill (see Chapter 61) and the disappearance of pulses and pulse reappearance time during reactive hyperemia (see Chapter 62) are the most sensitive measures of the presence and severity of occlusive arterial disease. A study of 400 patients referred to an outpatient clinic with pain on walking has demonstrated the relative accuracy of the pulses, pressure index at rest, and ankle pressure after exercise in relation to the presence of significant arterial disease.[5] The presence or absence of foot pulses at rest, the pressure index at rest, and the ankle pressure after exercise were recorded in the more symptomatic of the two limbs of all 400 patients. A standard procedure was followed. The patient first rested on a couch for 30 minutes. The brachial and ankle pressures were measured, and the patient walked on a treadmill at 4 km/hr for a maximum of 5 minutes or until stopped by claudication. The brachial and ankle pressures were measured 1 minute after the end of exercise and then every 2 minutes until they returned to the preexercise level. Aortography was the objective arbiter of the presence of arterial

481

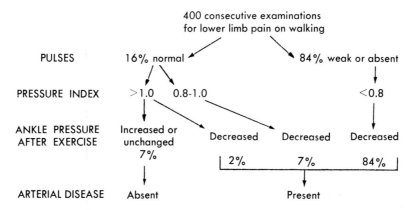

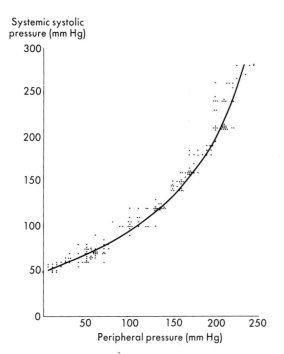

Fig. 54-1. The value of pulses, pressure index, and ankle pressure after exercise in determining the presence or absence of arterial disease.

Fig. 54-2. Relationship between systemic and peripheral systolic pressures. Regression tends to be a straight line through the origin in normotensive patients only.

disease; a lesion causing more than 40% stenosis in diameter was considered significant. It can be seen from Fig. 54-1 that the ankle pressure after exercise was the most sensitive index of the presence or absence of significant disease and that relying on the pulses alone would have resulted in the wrong diagnosis in 9% of patients. Whenever the exercise ankle pressure was increased or unchanged, the aortogram was normal and the symptoms were the result of other conditions such as osteoarthritis, sciatica, and venous insufficiency. Thus an *increase* in ankle pressure after exercise is a definite indicator of the absence of hemodynamically sig-

nificant arterial disease, and patients can be saved from any further unnecessary vascular investigations.

Although the pressure index has been used in vascular surgery for many years, it is only recently that it has been realized that the relationship between brachial systolic and ankle systolic pressures is nonlinear.[1] Belcaro et al[1] have studied 200 patients who had cardiac catheterization by measuring aortic or brachial pressure and ankle systolic pressure using Doppler ultrasound. These measurements were done during catheterization for cardiac investigation, during operations, and in the intensive care unit. None of the patients had peripheral arterial disease. A nonlinear relationship was found between the systemic pressure and the systolic ankle pressure. For systemic pressure of less than 100 mm Hg or greater than 200 mm Hg, the ankle pressure was on average 25% lower. For systemic pressure 100 mm Hg to 200 mm Hg, the ankle pressure was the same or slightly higher (Fig. 54-2). These data indicate that in normal limbs the pressure index at rest is 1.0 to 1.2 when the systolic brachial pressure is between 100 and 200 mm Hg, but in patients with hypotension or hypertension, it may be less than 1.0. This is an important observation that will prevent vascular surgeons from making erroneous diagnoses of arterial disease in the presence of hypertension or hypotension.

WHAT IS THE SEVERITY OF THE DISEASE?

From the history and clinical examination, it is possible to classify patients into three groups: patients with mild disease and mild claudication, patients with moderate disease and severe claudication, and patients with severe disease with a limb in danger. A more precise classification is very difficult without objective quantitative assessment. The information provided by the vascular laboratory is essential because it provides such a quantitative measure of the severity of the disease.

The measurement of ankle pressure became simple in the late 1960s with the development of instruments that could detect flow in small vessels distal to a pneumatic

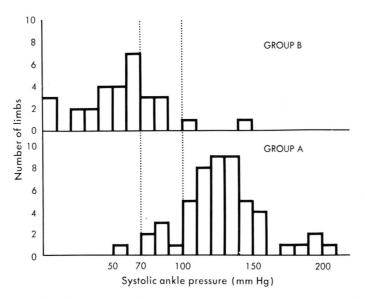

Fig. 54-3. The relationship of ankle pressure to the pressure or absence of foot pulses.

cuff[2,3,14,16] (see Chapters 18 and 55). It is now realized that the grading of pulses as normal, weak, or absent by palpation lacks precision, however sensitive and trained the examiner's fingers may be.

The relationship of systolic ankle pressure to the presence or absence of foot pulses was determined in the following study.[11] Limbs of 82 patients in the ward were randomly selected and examined by two observers. They were classified as group A if any of the foot pulses were palpable and as group B if both foot pulses (posterior tibial and dorsalis pedis) were absent. The examiners were not aware of the angiographic findings or the operation proposed for these patients. The ankle pressure was subsequently determined by a third person who did not know the previous findings. Pulses were present in 52 limbs (group A) and absent in 30 limbs (group B). The distribution of the two groups in relation to ankle pressure is shown in Fig. 54-3. Pulses were palpable in 50 (96%) of 52 limbs with an ankle pressure greater than 100 mm Hg and only in 1 (4%) of 23 limbs with ankle pressures less than 70 mm Hg. Pulses were palpable in 6 (50%) of 12 limbs with ankle pressures between 70 and 100 mm Hg. These results demonstrate that palpation is a very crude screening test with relatively little quantitative value. Thus when the ankle systolic pressure is 110 mm Hg, foot pulses may be graded as normal, though this pressure may be only 60% of the brachial systolic pressure (180 mm Hg) in a patient with claudication. At a pressure of 70 mm Hg the foot is not in immediate danger, but at a pressure of 30 mm Hg it is, yet palpation may reveal cold feet with absent pulses in both cases.

The decrease in ankle pressure after a standard period of exercise and the time taken for it to return to the preexercise level (recovery time) are good indicators of the severity of the disease, whereas the time of onset of claudication

is an accurate measure of the patient's incapacity (see Chapter 61).

WHERE IS THE DISEASE?

There are good reasons why the examiner must determine whether the disease is in the aortoiliac or femoropopliteal segment, is distal to the popliteal artery, or is in more than one segment. In the case of aortoiliac reconstruction or angioplasty, the results are good; iliac vessels or grafts remain patent for many years, and the patients remain free of symptoms. However, the results of femoropopliteal or more distal reconstruction are not as good; the primary failure rate is significant, and at least 30% to 50% of grafts become occluded in 5 years, with a resultant limb loss in a significant number of patients. Although the patency rates after angioplasty are similar, the morbidity rate is much lower, and provided the lesions are short (less than 5 to 10 cm long), angioplasty is offered as a means of relieving claudication. Grafting distal to the inguinal ligament is reserved for severe incapacitating claudication (walking distance less than 25 m) or critical limb ischemia. This is in contrast to aortoiliac reconstruction, which because of the lasting results, is offered to most patients with claudication.

Often the surgeon cannot decide by clinical observation alone whether in a patient with obvious superficial femoral occlusion and femoral pulses there is also an added element of aortoiliac disease. Simple auscultation may reveal a bruit at the common femoral artery, but its significance may not be certain.

A clue about the site and extent of disease can be obtained from the recovery time (i.e., the time taken for the decreased ankle pressure after exercise to return to the preexercise level). A recovery time of less than 5 minutes means that there is a single lesion only and that this is most probably

in the femoropopliteal segment.[16] A recovery time between 5 and 10 minutes suggests a single lesion also, but this is usually in the aortoiliac region. A recovery time that is longer than 10 minutes suggests multiple occlusions.

The recordings of Doppler velocity tracings from the common femoral artery together with velocity tracings from the ankle and the measurements made from them (see Chapters 9, 16, and 56) will supplement the pressure measurements and recovery time and help to localize the disease. The principle involved is the fact that velocity tracings distal to a stenosis or occlusion are damped. In the majority of cases, it is possible to localize disease by visual inspection of such tracings and to classify limbs into the following four groups: (1) no disease, (2) aortoiliac disease only, (3) femoropopliteal disease only, and (4) disease with combined aortoiliac and femoropopliteal lesions. In the past a number of techniques that analyze the Doppler velocities from the common femoral including the pulsatility index, Laplace transform function, and principal component analysis had been used to characterize the aortoiliac segment.[4] With the advent of duplex scanning and particularly color flow imaging, these techniques have become obsolete. At present, visual inspection of the Doppler velocity tracings is adequate to classify limbs into the four categories mentioned.[8] Duplex scanning is then used to confirm whether the aortoiliac segment is normal, to grade any stenoses in the aortoiliac or femoropopliteal segment, to determine the extent of occlusions in the superficial femoral artery if any, and to assess their suitability for angioplasty.

IS THE AORTOILIAC SEGMENT NORMAL?

After identifying the presence of occlusive arterial disease, the surgeon should determine whether the aortoiliac segment is normal (i.e., whether the disease is confined to the superficial femoral artery) because disease confined to the superficial femoral artery is a very benign condition. In one vascular laboratory, 250 patients with superficial femoral artery occlusion and an aortoiliac segment that was either normal or had less than 30% stenosis in diameter have been followed up.[7] There was a clinical improvement in 92% of patients with an increase in the mean pressure index from 0.4 to 0.6. Deterioration occurred in only 8%; 4 of these patients required operations and 3 were successful. Only 1 patient had amputation.

As previously mentioned, the femoral pulse and presence or absence of bruits may offer clues about the presence of aortoiliac disease. However, if the Doppler velocity tracings from the common femoral artery are triphasic,[9] they will confirm that the aortoiliac segment is normal. This will be sufficient to enable the surgeon to decide that the disease is distal to the inguinal ligament.

GRADING OF STENOTIC LESIONS WITH DUPLEX SCANNING

Duplex scanning with color flow imaging enables the examiner to rapidly scan an arterial segment and localize a stenosis by the change in color (usually toward white) as a result of high velocities. The change in peak systolic velocity (PSV) at the site of a suspected lesion compared with the PSV proximal and distal to the lesion in the same arterial segment is used to indicate the degree of stenosis. This is based on the principle that the total amount of flow at one point of an arterial segment is the same as at a point just proximal or distal to it. Flow is the product of velocity and cross-sectional area. Thus the velocity increases in the presence of reduced cross-sectional area. A PSV ratio (PSV at one point/PSV at another point) greater than 2.5 can detect a lesion producing greater than 50% angiographic diameter stenosis with a sensitivity of 84% and a specificity of 96%. Absence of a Doppler signal indicates occlusion. Aortoiliac occlusion can be detected with a sensitivity of 100% and a specificity of 100%; occlusion in the femoropopliteal segment can be detected with a sensitivity of 91% and a specificity of 99%.[6] The presence of a biphasic or triphasic signal indicates a diameter reduction of less than 50% (positive predictive value of 94%).

Because of the accuracy of this method, patients can be deemed suitable for angioplasty on the basis of results of the duplex scan; radiologists have agreed to accept patients for such a procedure without a preliminary angiogram. However, only patients in whom the clinical examination, the treadmill test, and Doppler waveforms suggest a stenosis at a particular site, which with adequate treatment, could relieve the patient's symptoms, are referred for duplex scanning.

THE FINAL DECISION

The final decision of whether to recommend an operation is determined by weighing of the severity of symptoms, by the incapacity experienced by the patient, and by the danger to the limb if operation is not done against the risk of reconstruction and both the long- and short-term results of reconstruction. The clinician must assess how long the reconstruction (or angioplasty) will last, particularly if operating for mild or moderate claudication. Finally, the clinician should be able to say what the short-term results will be. A patient will not be grateful after a successful arterial reconstruction if angina or pain from an osteoarthritic hip is still just as incapacitating. The clinician should assesss the severity of these conditions and decide whether these symptoms can be relieved too, since these conditions coexist with arterial disease in many patients. For example, the surgeon may decide that a patient should have a coronary reconstruction first with subsequent arterial reconstruction.

Many patients with lower limb ischemia have occult myocardial ischemia. They may have a history of one or more myocardial infarctions or of angina that disappeared when the distance to onset of claudication decreased. In one physician's practice, 50% of those with claudication have electrocardiographic evidence of myocardial ischemia during exercise, although only 3% experience angina.[15] It has been found that although their walking ability may be lim-

ited, they are able to exercise on a bicycle ergometer and raise their heart rate to a level that will give meaningful electrocardiographic results. In addition, the ability to diagnose the presence of one-, two-, or three-vessel coronary disease noninvasively by electrocardiographic chest-wall mapping during bicycle ergometry[10,13] offers the chance to select the high-risk group that is responsible for the perioperative mortality rate (3% to 5%) and the late mortality rate, which can be as high as 30% at 2 years. A 7-year follow-up study with the use of life-table analysis has demonstrated that a negative stress test or a stress test that indicates single-vessel coronary disease was associated with 83% of patients being event free compared with 53% of patients in whom the electrocardiographic chest-wall mapping stress test indicated multivessel disease (logrank test, $p < 0.05$).[12]

REFERENCES

1. Belcaro G, Nicolaides AN: The variation of pressure index in relation to systemic systolic blood pressure, *Br J Surg* 70:693, 1983.
2. Carter SA: Indirect systolic pressures and pulse waves in arterial occlusive disease of the lower extremities, *Circulation* 37:624, 1968.
3. Carter SA: Clinical measurement of systolic pressures in limbs with arterial occlusive disease, *JAMA* 207:1869, 1969.
4. Johnston KW, Tarashuk I: Validation of the role of pulsatility index in quantitation of the severity of peripheral arterial occlusive disease, *Am J Surg* 131:295, 1976.
5. Koliopoulos P: *The relationship of pressure measurements before and after exercise to the severity of arterial disease,* master's thesis, Athens, Greece, 1981, Athens University.
6. Legemate DA et al: Spectral analysis criteria in duplex scanning of aortoiliac and femoropopliteal arterial disease, *J Ultr Med Biol* (in press).
7. Levien L et al: *The natural history of superficial femoral artery occlusion,* abstract presented to the Vascular Society of Great Britain and Ireland, Oxford, England, Dec 18, 1979.
8. Myers KA, Williams MA, Nicolaides AN: *The use of Doppler ultrasound to assess disease in arteries to the lower limb.* In Salmasi AM, Nicolaides AN: *Cardiovascular applications of Doppler ultrasound,* London, 1989, Churchill Livingstone.
9. Nicolaides AN et al: The value of Doppler blood velocity tracings in the detection of aortoiliac disease in patients with intermittent claudication, *Surgery* 80:774, 1976.
10. Nicolaides AN et al: *Coronary and carotid arterial disease in patients with peripheral arterial disease.* In Bell PRF, Jamieson CW, Ruckley CV, eds: *Surgical management of vascular disease,* London, 1992, WB Saunders.
11. Poller M, Nicolaides AN: Unpublished data, 1977.
12. Sonecha TN: *The noninvasive detection and prevalence of occult "high risk" atherosclerotic disease,* thesis, London University, 1992.
13. Sonecha TN et al: Noninvasive detection of coronary artery disease in patients presenting with claudication, *Int Angiol* 2:79, 1990.
14. Strandness DE Jr, Bell JW: An evaluation of the hemodynamic response of the claudicating extremity to exercise, *Surg Gynecol Obstet* 119:1237, 1964.
15. Vecht RJ et al: Resting and treadmill electrocardiographic findings in patients with intermittent claudication, *Int Angiol* 1:119, 1982.
16. Yao JST, Hobbs JT, Irvine WT: Ankle systolic pressure measurements in arterial disease affecting the lower extremities, *Br J Surg* 56:675, 1969.

CHAPTER 55

Role of pressure measurements

STEFAN A. CARTER

In collaboration with Eugene R. Hamel*

Blood flow to an organ is determined by the difference in pressure between the large arteries and veins and by the resistance to flow of a given vascular bed. Under normal conditions the resistance to flow depends primarily on the degree of vasoconstriction in the microcirculation. Large and distributing arteries offer relatively little resistance to flow, and the mean pressure does not fall much between the aorta and small arteries of the limbs such as the radial or the dorsal artery of the foot.[129] Although the mean pressure falls slightly, the amplitude of the pressure wave and the systolic pressure actually increase as the wave travels distally because of the presence of increasing stiffness of the walls of the arteries toward the periphery and the presence of the reflected waves.[129,226]

Encroachment on the lumen of an artery by an atherosclerotic plaque or a stenosis may result in diminished pressure and flow distal to the lesion, but since arteries offer relatively little resistance to flow compared with the microcirculation, the encroachment on the lumen has to be relatively extensive before changes in hemodynamics become manifest. Studies in humans and experimental animals indicate that about 90% of the cross-sectional area of the aorta has to be encroached on before there is a change in the distal pressure and flow, whereas in smaller arteries such as the iliac, femoral, carotid, and renal arteries, the "critical stenosis" varies from 70% to 90%.[151,203] Experiments with graded stenoses in animals indicate that although the diastolic pressure does not fall until the stenosis is severe, decrease in systolic pressure is a sensitive index of the fall in mean pressure and of the altered shape and amplitude of the pressure wave distal to the stenosis.[240] Studies in humans indicate that systolic pressure measured at rest is a far more sensitive index of the occlusive or stenotic process than a measurement of blood flow.[74,139]

The presence of occlusive arterial disease in the extremities may be demonstrated in the majority of patients by a careful history and physical examination as outlined elsewhere. Precise information about the site and severity of the lesions may be obtained by angiography or duplex scanning. However, clinical assessment is subjective and provides only qualitative information. Angiography is invasive and may result in complications, and it and duplex scanning do not give information about the overall degree of functional impairment.[61,125,127] Measurement of systolic pressure, which can be performed by noninvasive methods easily and repeatedly, provides a quantitative, objective, and sensitive index of the occlusive process and complements the information obtained by clinical assessment and, where appropriate, by angiography or duplex scanning.

This chapter reviews information that can be obtained from measurements of systolic pressures, examines their limitations, and surveys the application of the measurements to the diagnosis, follow-up, and management of patients with disease of the arterial supply to the extremities.

PRINCIPLES AND LIMITATIONS OF NONINVASIVE MEASUREMENTS
Principles

Technical details of the measurements of blood pressure are discussed elsewhere in this volume. The method of noninvasive measurement uses pneumatic cuffs, which are applied around the extremity. Pressures may be measured anywhere the cuffs can be applied around the limb. Cuffs have to be of proper size because otherwise, inaccurate high or low readings may be obtained.[80,83] The cuffs are inflated to a pressure sufficient to stop blood flow into the distal part of the limb. During slow deflation of the cuff, some method is used to detect the pressure in the cuff at which the flow into the distal part of the limb resumes. That pressure represents the systolic pressure at the level of the cuff. Various methods have been used to detect the resumption of blood flow. They include volume,[74] air,[205] photocell,[191,236] and strain-gauge plethysmography,[215] the appearance of oxyhemoglobin in the light reflected from the skin[76]; "visual flush" technique[29]; ultrasonic flow detectors[30,210]; capacitance pulse pickups[29]; and isotope clearance.[135] When care-

Supported by grants-in-aid from the Manitoba Heart, Manitoba Medical Service, and St. Boniface General Hospital Research Foundations.
*Vascular Laboratory, St. Boniface General Hospital, Winnipeg, Manitoba, Canada.

fully performed, all these techniques appear to give accurate estimations of the systolic pressures as judged by the results of intraarterial measurements,[20,89,165,210] they agree with one another,[29,30,80,135,247] and the reproducibility of the measurements is comparable to that of the routine measurements of brachial blood pressure by auscultation.[29,38,91,161,182] However, it cannot be overemphasized that to obtain valid measurements, meticulous attention to detail is necessary. During measurements the patient and the extremities should be comfortably warm. Pressures are measured routinely with the patient in the supine position. Any deviation from this position, which could result in a difference between the level of the heart and the limb segment in which the pressure is measured, would require correction for the differences in the hydrostatic level.[156] Careful attention must be given to the maintenance of the instruments that detect the resumption of blood flow and to the mercury manometers or other pressure transducers. Proper deflation rates of the cuff pressures during measurements, appropriate width and length of the cuffs, and the use of a sufficient number of replicate measurements are necessary to obtain acceptable reproducibility.

It was previously reported that single replicate determinations of systolic pressures could differ from the mean of three or more measurements by up to 11 mm Hg for the auscultatory brachial pressure and up to 14 mm Hg for the ankle and thigh pressures.[29] Expressed as ratios of the lower limb to brachial systolic pressure, these differences corresponded to 0.09 and 0.13 for the ankle and thigh pressure measurements, respectively. Measurements in the lower limbs repeated on another day within 1 month varied by an average of 0.06, with maximal deviations up to 0.16 when expressed as fractions of the brachial systolic pressures. These data were obtained with the use of capacitance pulse pickups to measure pressures in the lower limbs. However, similar results were obtained for ankle and digital pressures in other laboratories with various techniques.* Therefore when individual patients are followed up or the effects of treatment are evaluated, small differences in the peripheral pressures should not be considered significant.

Limitations

Noninvasive measurements of pressures are influenced by a number of factors and have limitations. These factors and limitations must be kept in mind or the results may be interpreted incorrectly and lead to improper evaluation of the arterial status of the patient. Lack of awareness of such limitations may be partly responsible for conflicting reports on some of the practical applications of the pressure measurements.

Effect of the interruption of blood flow by the measuring cuff. Inflation of the cuff around the limb interrupts blood flow into the part of the limb under and distal to the cuff and therefore tends to decrease blood flow in the vessels proximal to the cuff. This decrease in flow leads to a smaller fall in pressure along the vessels proximal to the cuff and tends to increase the measured pressure, an effect especially important in the presence of proximal stenotic lesions. Such effects are more pronounced when measurements are carried out at the more proximal sites in the extremities and the flows to a relatively large tissue mass are interrupted.

Effect of the girth of the limb. When the girth of the limb is large in relation to the width of the cuff, the pressure in the cuff may not be transmitted completely to the vessels in the central part of the limb and the measured pressures may be greatly exaggerated. Such exaggerated pressures are commonly encountered in the measurements at the level of the thighs (see p. 492).

Effect of the rigidity of the arterial walls. In a certain percentage of cases, rigidity of the arterial walls, usually caused by Mönckeberg's sclerosis, may interfere with pressure measurements. Calcification may lead to "incompressibility" of the arterial walls in the legs so that it may be impossible to stop the flow even with cuff pressures of 300 mm Hg or more.[29,215] In some instances the flow will be stopped, but the required pressure is greater than the blood pressure because additional force is needed to deform the stiff arterial walls, and falsely high pressure values may be obtained.[32,228] Theoretical considerations indicate that increased elastic stiffness modulus, increased wall thickness to radius ratio, and viscoelasticity contribute to this phenomenon.[64,196] Falsely high brachial pressure measurements as a result of arterial rigidity have also been reported.[208,225] The frequency with which arterial rigidity interferes with valid measurements of the systolic pressures when blood pressure cuffs are used has not been established. Earlier reports suggested that the frequency may be 1% or less,[29,101] whereas more recent publications report an incidence of about 3%, 10%, or higher.[63,136,150,232,236] An evaluation of the incidence of falsely high pressures is complicated by differences in the criteria for what is considered to be normal pressure in various laboratories, by exaggerated values in limbs with large girth, and in some cases by difficulties in determining the presence of functionally significant arterial lesions from angiograms. Medial calcification occurs most frequently in patients with diabetes,[60,150] but has also been reported in those undergoing long-term corticosteroid therapy, in patients undergoing renal dialaysis,[109] and in those who have undergone renal transplantation.[93] Neuropathy and surgical sympathectomy promote medial calcification in diabetic and nondiabetic patients.[60,86] It was impossible to assess from x-ray films whether arterial calcification will interfere with the measurement of the systolic pressure.[32] Bone and Pomajzl[23] found no correlation between the extent to which the noninvasive method overestimated the pressure obtained by intraarterial measurements and the extent of roentgenographic density of arterial calcification.

Certain clues may suggest that falsely high pressures are measured. Such clues may be noted by the technicians who perform the measurements and taken into account when

---

*References 7, 32, 67, 119, 133, 161, 170, 236.

reporting and interpreting the data. These clues include the following:

1. An unusually high ankle/brachial artery pressure ratio (i.e., one exceeding 1.3 or 1.35) may be reported.
2. When ultrasonic flow detectors are used, a much higher pressure may be required to stop the flow during inflation of the cuffs (closing pressure) than the pressure at which the flow resumes during deflation (opening pressure). In 80 patients with arterial occlusive disease, it was found that the closing ankle pressure was significantly higher than the opening pressure ($p < 0.001$) at times by 50 mm Hg or more. There was no significant difference in the case of brachial pressure measurements. Similar findings were reported by Thulesius and Länne.[229] Theoretical considerations indicate that in addition to wall rigidity, viscoelasticity may also contribute to this phenomenon.[64]
3. The progression of the segmental systolic pressures measured along the extremities may be abnormal. Noninvasive measurements show pressures that are higher in the more proximal parts of the limbs because of larger limb girth. The presence of an arterial obstruction will further contribute to the finding of lower pressures at the more distal sites. When this progression is altered and a considerably higher pressure is found distally, there is a fair likelihood that falsely high pressures are present.[71]
4. The arterial flow sounds that are heard when an ultrasonic flow detector is used to measure systolic pressure may not appear to correspond to the pressure values. Ordinarily in limbs with normal or near-normal hemodynamics, triphasic or biphasic flow sounds are heard, whereas in the presence of a significant obstruction, single sounds are present and their volume varies inversely with the severity of the obstruction.[228]
5. When pressure measurements are repeated over a period of time in patients who are in a stable condition, the results vary little.[29,108] Finding a large increase during follow-up without apparent reason should alert the physician or technician that development of increased arterial rigidity may be resulting in a falsely high pressure.

When it is suspected that ankle pressure may be overestimated because of the rigidity of the arterial walls or when it cannot be measured at all, certain measures can be used in the assessment of the patient. Recording pressures at several levels proximal to the ankle may be helpful,[71] although finding a falsely high pressure at one level increases the chances that measurements at other levels may also be incorrect. Elevation reactive hyperemia test may be helpful in estimating distal perfusion pressure when ankle pressure measurement is not reliable.[85] Falsely high pressures are known to occur at the level of the forefoot[204] and proximally. On the other hand, calcification of the arteries of the toes

is less extensive and less frequent and in the experience of several investigators,[23,223,236] does not appear to interfere with the measurements. Therefore measurement of the pressure in the toes is of special value and should be used routinely for evaluation of limbs with severe ischemia, in patients with diabetes, and in the assessment of the results of surgery and other endovascular interventions.

Externally recorded pressure pulse waves* or the flow waves obtained with the Doppler ultrasonic method[70,71,73,87,117] may also be of practical value in assessing the circulation of patients in whom arterial rigidity may interfere with the pressure measurements. The use of waveform analysis for that purpose is based on reports that in the majority of patients with peripheral arterial disease, the measurements of pressures and arterial wave recordings appear to give comparable results and to correlate well.[29,116,150]

Obstruction in parallel vessels. When two or more parallel vessels of comparable size are under the cuff, the measurement will usually reflect the pressure in the artery with the highest pressure and will not detect stenotic or occlusive lesions in the other vessels.[29] Therefore the measurements will not detect isolated obstruction in the internal iliac, profunda femoris, tibial, peroneal, ulnar, or individual digital arteries nor interruption of one of the palmar or plantar arches.

Effects of changes in the vasomotor tone. Changes in the vasomotor state affect arterial pressures. When blood flow is increased during peripheral vasodilatation induced by body heating, exercise, or reactive hyperemia, more pressure energy is used in causing flow through stenotic lesions, collaterals, and small distal vessels, and therefore distal blood pressure is reduced. Conversely, when the flow is lower at rest or when the patient is cool, the pressure tends to be higher. These considerations explain why pressures measured at rest may be within normal limits in limbs with mild stenotic lesions and why ankle and particularly digital pressures may be altered significantly by changes in the vasomotor tone. In addition, a high tone of the smooth muscle in the wall of the smaller distal arteries of the limbs may result in an artifactual reduction of the measured systolic pressure. These phenomena are discussed further in the sections that deal with these measurements.

FINDINGS IN ARTERIAL DISEASE OF THE LOWER EXTREMITIES

Systolic pressure in the lower limb has to be compared with an index of the pressure proximal to the site of the occlusive or stenotic process to demonstrate the presence of arterial disease in the lower extremities. For that purpose, brachial systolic pressure measured by the ausculatory technique is usually used, and the leg pressure is expressed as a percentage of the brachial systolic pressure[29,30] or as the ratio of the lower limb to the brachial pressure, a so-called systolic pressure index.[228,247] Since arterial disease may occur

---

*References 29, 136, 150, 177, 190, 223.

in the vessels supplying the upper limbs, it is important that pressures be measured in both arms. Brachial pressure in the arm with the higher pressure value should be used for the calculation of the lower limb systolic pressure index. In addition, examination for the presence of supraclavicular bruits should be carried out to identify patients who may have bilateral arterial disease in the upper limbs. Failure to identify such patients may lead to erroneous conclusions if the pressure in the lower limb is compared with an abnormally low brachial blood pressure.

Ankle pressures

Although segmental measurements of blood pressure at various levels in the limbs proximal to the ankles may provide additional information of practical value and measurements of pressures in the toes are superior for the evaluation and practical applications in certain groups of patients, systolic pressure measured at the level of the ankles has been used most frequently for a routine assessment of the occlusive process in the lower extremities. Measurements with cuffs of the standard 12 cm width give values that agree well with intraarterial measurements.[20,165,210] Ankle pressures reflect the overall occlusive process in the main proximal arteries, which may be amenable to arterial reconstruction, except for disease of individual vessels distal to the division of the popliteal artery. In the absence of disease in more proximal arteries, ankle pressure may be normal when one or two of the popliteal branches are occluded.[29] For example, a normal pressure may be measured in the presence of the occlusion of the anterior and posterior tibial arteries when there is a large peroneal vessel free of disease.[29] However, when ankle pressures are measured with ultrasonic flow detectors, a clue may be obtained about disease in the individual tibial branches. A difference of more than 15 mm Hg between pressures measured by detecting flow over the dorsal artery of the foot and the posterior tibial artery suggests a lesion in the vessel that gives the lower pressure, although a smaller difference does not rule it out.[30] These considerations should also be kept in mind when interpreting pressure measurements at the level of the calf.

Blood flow measured at rest is often within normal limits in limbs with an arterial occlusive process.[74,139] In contrast to flow measurements, resting systolic pressures have been reported by Naumann,[159] Winsor,[243] and Gaskell[74] to be diminished, and this finding has since been confirmed by numerous reports. Strandness and co-workers* in a series of publications successfully applied pressure measurements to the assessment and follow-up of patients with peripheral vascular disease. Because of systolic amplification, ankle pressure is almost always greater than brachial pressure in the absence of a significant narrowing. Although some reports give ankle pressures of 90% of the brachial pressure or less as the lower limit of normal,[228] it is likely that the presence of mild stenotic lesions in patients who are free

of symptoms or the use of too wide a cuff[228] is responsible for the low readings, and therefore a more correct lower limit of normal is 97% of the brachial pressure.[29,30,247] Experience with a large number of cases suggests that the lower limit of normal for the ankle pressures, measured with the use of blood pressure cuffs, may increase with age. This is supported by the finding that the difference between the thigh or calf pressure and the brachial pressure is greater in older patients.[15] In subjects of the age usually associated with arteriosclerosis obliterans, ankle pressures that are equal to or even a few millimeters of mercury greater than brachial pressures may be associated with a mild arterial disease.[31,34] The apparent increase in the pressure in the legs as compared with that in the arm in older patients may be related to the greater increase in stiffness of the walls of the leg arteries with aging.[238] This could result in some overestimation of the pressure in the lower limbs.[15] Intraarterial measurements actually indicate that systolic amplification in the aortoiliac axis[179] and in the arteries of the lower limbs[33] does not increase with age.

Correlation with angiography. Carter[29,30] and Yao et al[247] correlated measurements of ankle systolic pressures with angiographic documentation of the disease in large series of cases. Fig. 55-1 shows that ankle pressures are always abnormal in limbs with complete arterial occlusion. In most cases they do not exceed 80% of the brachial pressure, but in some limbs with well-developed collateral pathways, pressures may range from 80% to 90%. In limbs with a single complete occlusion, the pressure is usually 50% or more of the brachial pressure, whereas in those with two or more occlusions in series, it is usually less than 50%. The presence of some overlap is not surprising because of differences in length, diameter, and number of collateral pathways. For example, it is often observed that soon after an acute arterial occlusion, the ankle pressure may be quite low, often less than 50% of the brachial pressure. However, over a period of time as the collateral circulation and symptoms improve, the pressure increases to values greater than 50%.

In limbs with arterial stenosis, pressures range from about 50% of the brachial levels to values within normal limits. This is also not surprising, since the degree of narrowing varies and considerable encroachment on the lumen has to be present before there are appreciable effects on distal flow and pressure.[161,203] In the majority of patients with stenotic lesions and normal ankle pressures shown in Fig. 55-1, there were no symptoms.[30]

Effect of changes in blood flow. It is known that the decrease in pressure across an arterial narrowing or across collateral pathways, which bypass an arterial occlusion, depends on the rate of blood flow. This has been well documented by studies on the "critical arterial stenosis" in experimental animals and humans.[151,197,203] The pressure drop increases with increased blood flow, which may be produced by vasodilatation in the peripheral resistance vessels in the limb distal to the site of the arterial obstruction. An increase

---

*References 12, 13, 206, 207, 211, 212, 214-218, 224.

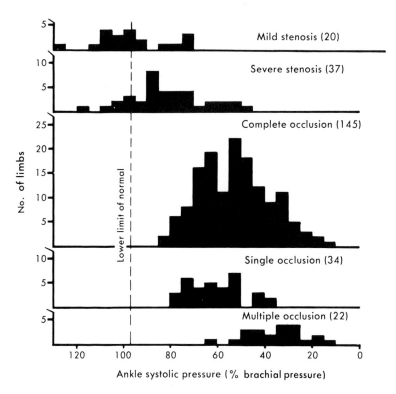

Fig. 55-1. Correlation of ankle systolic pressures measured at rest with angiographic findings. Numbers in parentheses indicate number of limbs. (From Carter SA: *JAMA* 207:1869, 1969.)

in blood flow may result in a pressure gradient in a case of a mild narrowing, when there is no pressure drop under resting or low flow conditions. Since blood flow through the skin of the extremities increases manyfold when there is need to eliminate heat as part of the function of the regulation of the body temperature, the question of whether physiologic changes in cutaneous blood flow might influence pressure measurements in limbs with arterial disease arises.[88,193] Body heating and cooling was performed using a modification of the technique of Gibbon and Lowdis in a group of patients with peripheral arterial disease to study the effect of changes in skin blood flow.[84,141] The presence of large changes in blood flow was confirmed by large changes in digital skin temperature, which averaged 9° C. Considerable changes in the ankle and toe pressures were found. The differences in the ankle index between heating and cooling exceeded 0.15 in over 30% of the limbs and in the toe index in 50% of the limbs.[39] Significant effects of temperature on distal systolic pressures have also been reported by other centers.[91,162] Since differences in body temperature may result in significant effects on distal systolic pressures, it is important not to carry out routine pressure measurements when the patients or their extremities are cold. The use of a preliminary period of warming in routine testing should improve reproducibility of the measurements.[39]

Changes in blood flow through the large muscle mass of a lower limb in response to various interventions can result in larger changes in blood flow and have profound effects on distal arterial pressure. Distal pressures have been measured after exercise and in response to reactive hyperemia. Types of exercise used include walking at a fixed rate in a corridor,[143] walking on a treadmill at various speeds and elevations,* toe stands[28] and step test,[42] and flexion-extension exercise of the ankle.[31] Cappelen and Hall[28] demonstrated a large decrease in the intraarterially recorded pressure from the dorsal artery of the foot in limbs with intermittent claudication during exercise. Strandness et al[124,209,212,224] studied changes in ankle blood pressure and calf blood flow in response to exercise in normal limbs and in limbs of patients with arterial disease at various levels. Fig. 55-2 shows that in the presence of a severe arterial stenosis, there is a profound drop in ankle pressure after exercise that takes several minutes to return to the preexercise level. The time course of the return of the pressure closely parallels the time course of the postexercise hyperemia shown by the calf blood flow. The extent of the postexercise pressure drop and the time required for it to return to the preexercise level depend on the number, severity, and level of the stenotic or occlusive lesions.[43,139,212,224,246] Thus measurements of pressure after exercise provide more physiologic information about circulation in limbs with arterial disease than do measurements taken at rest. Similar changes in pressure in limbs with arterial disease occur during re-

---

*References 124, 139, 209, 212, 214, 224, 246.

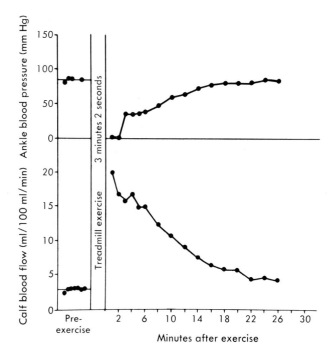

Fig. 55-2. Effect of exercise on ankle systolic pressure and calf blood flow in a limb with severe arterial stenosis. (From Sumner DS, Strandness DE Jr: *Surgery* 65:763, 1969.)

active hyperemia produced by a period of occlusion of blood flow to the limb with thigh cuffs inflated to suprasystolic pressures.[22,54,115] The degree of postexercise or reactive hyperemia also depends on the severity of the exercise or the period of ischemia. When ischemia is prolonged or the exercise is strenuous, ankle systolic pressure will decrease to some extent even in normal limbs,[148,209] and a positive brachial-to-ankle pressure difference may develop.[31,148]

Demonstration of the presence of mild arterial disease. Fig. 55-1 shows that in some patients with an arterial stenosis, ankle pressure may be within normal limits. Although the majority of such patients do not have symptoms, patients with symptoms consistent with intermittent claudication may occasionally have ankle pressures that, at rest, are greater than the brachial pressure.[31,211] Measurement of pressure after exercise is then of assistance in deciding whether the symptoms are a result of arterial disease.[214] Fig. 55-3 shows changes in the ankle pressure and the brachial-ankle pressure difference in such a patient. The ankle pressure was higher than the brachial pressure at rest but fell profoundly after supine exercise, which consisted of flexion-extension of the ankle for 2½ minutes at a rate of one per second, and took several minutes to return to preexercise level. Although ankle pressure after exercise decreased in relation to the brachial pressure in 34 of 37 limbs of normal subjects, it remained higher than the brachial pressure in 30 of these limbs.[31] The greatest brachial-ankle pressure difference after exercise in the normal group was 7 mm Hg. Statistical evaluation of the results in the normal limbs in-

dicates that after this type of exercise, the brachial-ankle difference should be less than 9 mm Hg. A difference of 9 to 16 mm Hg represents a borderline response, and more than 16 mm Hg is abnormal. Ankle pressures at rest were normal in 7 of 14 limbs with mild arterial disease and in 13 of 18 with questionable arterial disease.[31] All 14 limbs with mild arterial disease showed abnormal responses to exercise. Among the limbs with questionable disease, 11 had an abnormal response, 4 responses were borderline, and 3 were within normal limits.

A correlation exists between the brachial-ankle difference at rest and after exercise. In older patients if ankle pressure at rest is less than 110% of the brachial pressure, the response to exercise is often abnormal; if it is 115% or more at rest, then the response is usually within normal limits. Measurements after supine exercise may have some advantage as compared with testing after walking, since the first measurement can usually be obtained within 10 to 20 seconds after cessation of exercise, and a longer time may be necessary to obtain the first measurement after walking. In some patients with mild stenotic lesions the drop in ankle pressure may be quite transient and difficult to demonstrate if the first measurements are not obtained quickly. Simultaneous measurement of brachial pressure increases the usefulness of the test because, on occasion, ankle pressure may show little change after exercise, but a simultaneous increase in the brachial pressure would indicate that an abnormal brachial-ankle pressure difference had developed.

There is considerable interest in the measurements of distal systolic pressures in response to exercise and reactive hyperemia. Large numbers of patients are tested by these methods in vascular laboratories,[137] and various studies compare the results of pressure measurements after different forms and intensities of exercise and during reactive hyperemia.[6,107,145,147,241] There are advantages and disadvantages in the various methods of testing. Measurements during reactive hyperemia do not require the patient to walk, can be carried out in laboratories that do not possess treadmills, and are generally less time-consuming, but the decrease in pressure is much more transient than after exercise. Measurement after exercise may separate more completely patients with mild disease from normal subjects and is preferable for the assessment of patients with "pseudoclaudication" and normal resting ankle pressures.[107] In patients who had femoropopliteal bypass surgery, application of suprasystolic pressures over the graft for a considerable period of time may not be advisable at least in the early postoperative period.[107] There is no doubt that measurements after exercise or during reactive hyperemia are useful in making the diagnosis in patients with mild or questionable arterial disease. Disappearance of previously palpable pulses or development or increase in the intensity of arterial bruits is a clinical counterpart to the increased blood flow after exercise.[10,34] However, measurement of ankle pressure provides a more objective and quantitative method. A normal pressure response can rule out arterial disease as the cause of

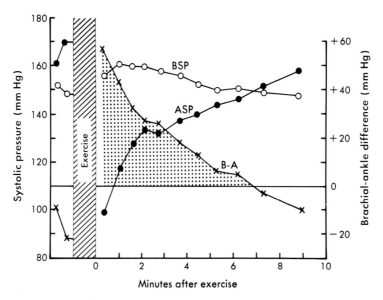

Fig. 55-3. Response of ankle and brachial systolic pressure to leg exercise in a patient with questionable arterial disease. Scale on left is for ankle systolic pressure (*ASP,* solid circles) and brachial systolic pressure (*BSP,* open circles); scale on right is for brachial minus ankle pressure difference. *B-A,* Crosses; dotted area indicates positive difference. (From *N Engl J Med* 287:578, 1972.)

symptoms and is particularly useful in the diagnosis of patients with pseudoclaudication who may develop pain in the limbs on walking as a result of spinal or neuromuscular disorders.[63,107] Measurements after stress are of value in such cases and in other selected patients and provide physiologic information about the functional state of the circulation that may be of interest for research purposes and special applications. However, in the majority of patients with clinically significant arterial obstruction, measurements of pressure at rest are sufficient to demonstrate the presence and to assess the severity of the obstruction, and the measurements after stress are not needed for clinical purposes.[181] This is also corroborated by close correlation between the brachial-ankle pressure difference at rest and after exercise.[31,41,147]

Cholesterol crystal or atherothrombotic embolization from the sites of ulcerated atherosclerotic lesions in the proximal but patent arterial tree can occlude small muscular arteries, as documented by muscle biopsies.[5,122] Although intermittent claudication primarily caused by occlusion of the small muscular arteries appears to be rare, measurement of blood flow after exercise may demonstrate an abnormality in such cases.[75]

Pressures proximal to the ankles

Winsor[243] reported in 1950 on segmental measurements at various levels in the upper and lower limbs in 10 young normal subjects and showed that the measurements were abnormal in patients with arterial disease. A large number of reports have since appeared. However, such measurements are affected by various artifacts more than by ankle pressures. Also, differences in the techniques and width of

cuffs used in the various studies can affect the results and further limit the practical usefulness of such studies.*

Thigh pressures. Relatively greater range of variation in the girth and shape of the thigh contributes to a fairly large range of values found in normal subjects and patients with arterial disease. In the majority of studies, systolic pressures at the level of the thigh were found to be higher than brachial systolic pressure. There is little doubt that thigh pressures tend to be overestimated because cuff pressure may not be transmitted completely to the vessels in the central part of this wide region of the limb. Intraarterial pressure measurements show that femoral pressure at the groin corresponds closely to the brachial systolic pressure,[183] but systolic pressure increases distally in the limb, with pressures in the dorsal artery of the foot and the posterior tibial artery being consistently greater than femoral pressure.[33,129,134] Therefore "true" pressures in the upper part of the thigh should be only slightly greater than brachial pressure, but the difference would be expected to increase in the lower part of the thigh and distally.

A review of the published results suggests that cuffs of the standard width of 12 cm or narrower, even if the bladder is long, tend to overestimate thigh pressure considerably.[51,72] Cuffs 15 to 18 cm in width with a long bladder appear to give values that correspond reasonably well with the pressures that would be expected on the basis of intraarterial findings. Since considerable taper of the circumference of the thigh in some subjects makes it difficult to apply wider cuffs, the 15 cm cuff may provide a better fit in such cases

*References 14, 29, 51, 72, 144, 205.

and therefore more consistent results, even though the values may be overestimated to some extent.[29,126] Bell et al[14] reported that thigh pressure did not differ significantly from the brachial (− 22 to + 28 mm Hg) in 30 normal subjects. They used an 18 cm wide cuff but did not state where along the thigh the cuff was applied. When a 15 cm cuff was used at the lower thigh (above the knee), it was found that the pressure averaged 116% of the brachial pressure in 24 subjects without peripheral vascular disease, with the lower limit of normal 107% of brachial pressure.[29] Although assessment of the vessels proximal to the groin is very important for practical decisions regarding surgical management, it cannot always be made reliably by noninvasive methods.

The pressure at the upper thigh is greatly influenced by the size of the limb and the width of the measuring cuffs, and normal standards have to be determined by each laboratory. It is helpful to measure the circumference of the limb at the site of the measurement and to take it into account in the interpretation of the results. In one laboratory, 12 cm wide cuffs are used at the upper thigh, and according to experience, the pressure at the upper thigh must exceed the brachial pressure by 30 mm Hg if it is to be considered normal. It appears that the main value of the measurements at the upper thigh is to exclude hemodynamically significant aortoiliac occlusive disease at rest when the pressure is clearly normal.[65] However, such pressures measured at rest do not rule out mild proximal lesions. Measurements during reactive hyperemia or after intraarterial injection of vasodilating agents are needed for that purpose.[25,42]

If the pressure at the upper thigh is lower than that of the arm or significantly lower than that of the opposite limb, significant obstruction is present at or proximal to the upper thigh. The obstruction might be proximal to the groin or in the upper part of the thigh, especially in limbs with obstruction of the proximal part of the superficial femoral artery and a poorly developed or diseased profunda artery. If the pressure at the upper thigh is equal to or only slightly higher than the arm pressure and there is little difference between the two lower limbs, the presence of an obstruction at or proximal to the upper thigh cannot be ruled out.[213] Consideration of all information including clinical findings, pressure at the upper thigh, pressure gradients distally along the limb, and angiography results may help elucidate the problem. If it is important to assess the arteries proximal to the groin more precisely to make therapeutic decisions, other methods may have to be used in individual patients. The techniques that may be useful include comparison of intraarterial pressures measured in the femoral and brachial arteries[25,42,92,237] and recording of blood flow velocity waves from over the femoral arteries.[70,116] An abnormally low thigh pressure usually indicates the presence of disease at or proximal to that level, but normal pressure may not rule out disease of the superficial femoral artery, depending on the placement of the cuffs and the site of the occlusion. When

the superficial femoral artery is occluded near its origin and the deep femoral artery enlarges to provide collateral circulation to the distal part of the limb, a cuff at the thigh that overlies the superficial femoral occlusion may give pressure values within normal limits because the measurement gives the high pressure in the enlarged deep femoral artery.[29]

Calf pressures. In 30 normal subjects, with the cuffs applied just below the knees, Bell et al[14] found pressures to average 5 mm Hg above the brachial (range − 16 to + 28 mm Hg) when an 18 cm wide cuff and digital plethysmography were used. Cutajar et al[51] used a standard 12 cm cuff and Doppler ultrasonic flow detector in another group of 30 normal subjects and found the pressure to average 117% of the brachial pressure, with a range of 100% to 140%. Similar results were reported by Fronek et al.[72]

Pressure gradients. Abnormal differences between pressures measured at the upper thigh, above the knee (low thigh), at the calf, and at the ankle may provide information about the number and site of the occlusive or stenotic lesions. Findings to date have been correlated with angiographic documentation of the disease.[15,29,72,94,215] Despite the differences in the size of the cuffs and the techniques used in different studies, most investigators agree that a gradient of less than 20 mm Hg between contiguous sites along the extremity is normal. Usually, gradients of 20 to 30 mm Hg would be considered borderline, and those greater than 30 mm Hg, abnormal.[9,215] Cuff artifacts are probably responsible for the apparently "normal" gradients without an arterial lesion. In the presence of an obstruction, these and other measurement artifacts can at times seriously affect segmental pressure measurements and the apparent pressure gradients. When there is a proximal lesion, the level at which the cuff is applied to measure pressure in the extremity distal to the lesion could affect the measurements and contribute to an apparent gradient.[134] For example, blood flow through collaterals bypassing an iliac occlusion would be lower when a thigh cuff is inflated than during inflation of an ankle cuff, since flow through a large part of the limb would be cut off during the measurement of thigh pressure. This would tend to increase the pressure measured at the thigh and increase the thigh-ankle difference. In addition, falsely low pressures may at times be measured in the presence of arterial obstruction distal to the cuffs,[16] and the measurements can be affected by the type of flow-sensing device and the site at which it is applied.[68] Below the knee, the presence of three branches of the popliteal artery in parallel and the capacity for extensive collateral interconnections in this part of the limb may result in normal gradients from the calf to the ankle in the presence of an extensive occlusive process.[211] It is desirable to measure brachial pressure by ausculation simultaneously with the lower limb pressures and to make corrections for changes in the brachial pressure.[72] When the patient's thigh is large, inflation of the cuff to a high pressure may cause considerable discomfort and result in an increase in the central and peripheral blood pressure.[14,29] Differences of more than 15 to 20 mm Hg between pressures in the two lower limbs measured at the same level are also indicative of arterial disease.[72]

Pressures distal to the ankles

Since ankle pressures may not provide information about disease in the individual branches of the popliteal artery, do not reflect arterial disease that may be present in the small vessels distal to the ankle, and can give falsely high values in the presence of medial calcification, there is considerable interest in the measurement of the more distal pressures.

Foot pressures. Winsor[243] reported on measurements with 13 cm wide cuffs applied to the ankle and the foot in 10 young normal individuals and found that the average difference between the ankle and foot pressures was 17 mm Hg, although the range of values was not given. He found that the difference was increased in some patients with peripheral arterial disease. Hirai and Shionoya[98] studied 50 limbs of patients with thromboangiitis obliterans with angiographic documentation of occlusion of the arteries distal to the popliteal bifurcation and without evidence of more proximal disease. They measured foot pressures with 6 cm wide cuffs and photoelectric plethysmography and found that the pressures averaged between 50 and 60 mm Hg lower than brachial systolic pressure, although they did not report data in subjects without arterial obstruction. In all limbs the difference exceeded 20 mm Hg with a range of more than 20 to about 100 mm Hg. The average difference between ankle and foot systolic pressures was approximately 40 mm Hg, although individual values of the differences were not given. The difference between foot and toe pressure in the same study was significantly greater in those patients who had foot claudication and averaged 40 to 50 mm Hg, although it appears that there was considerable overlap between pressures in limbs with and without foot claudication.

Gaskell[78] studied foot pressures in the limbs of 59 normal subjects 19 to 59 years of age and in 43 patients with arterial disease and angiographic visualization of limb arteries, including the vessels down to and including the foot. A spectroscopic method was used to determine systolic end point during deflation of contoured 9 cm wide cuffs wrapped around the forefoot. Foot pressures were compared with ankle systolic pressures. On the basis of this study the difference between the ankle and foot pressures in normal subjects should be less than 30 mm Hg. A larger difference is abnormal. Since pressure differences along the distal parts of the lower and upper limbs may be increased in hypertension even in the absence of arterial obstruction, abnormally high ankle-to-foot pressure differences could be present in patients with hypertension, although further data to establish this theory are needed. In patients with additional significant obstruction in the proximal arteries, low ankle pressures, and low blood flows in the feet, differences between ankle and foot pressures of less than 30 mm Hg may be associated with obstruction of the foot arteries. Foot pressures have also been reported to give falsely high values

in some cases with medial calcification.[204] Measurements of foot pressures may be of special value in the assessment of distal arterial obstruction when pressures cannot be measured in the toes because of previous amputations or the presence of skin lesions.

Toe pressures. There are many reports on the pressures measured in the toes. Measurements in patients with arterial disease were reported as early as 1934.[66] Conrad and Green[49] found that systolic pressures in the second toe were decreased in patients with severe arterial disease and that the brachial-toe pressure difference was increased. They reported that in normal subjects there was no significant difference between the brachial and toe pressures. However, they used a 1 cm wide cuff, which is too narrow and which probably gave values to high for the pressures in the digits. Pressures measured with pneumatic cuffs will be overestimated if the cuff is too narrow and may be underestimated if it is too wide.[80,83,141] There appears to be a range of cuff widths in which the measured pressure does not change much. This was shown for the toes,[141] fingers,[80] and the brachial region[83]; in the last case the findings were compared with intraarterial recordings. In the second toe, systolic pressures show little change with cuffs between 2 and 3 cm in width.[141] Since a certain length of the digit is needed to apply the sensing device distal to the cuff, the 2 cm cuff was used in some studies.[38,141,142] It was also found that a 3 cm cuff on the big toe gave values comparable to those from the 2 cm cuff on the second toe.[38]

Since cuffs are usually applied at the base of the toe, the measurements cannot detect disease in the vessels situated more distally near the tip of the digit. In addition, since digits have two main lateral arteries, occlusion of only one of these vessels would not be detected.[58] Comparison of measurements in the toes with the cuff applied at the base and 1 cm distally along the digit showed no significant differences in normal subjects, indicating that there is no steep fall in the pressure along the toe and that small differences in the exact positioning of the cuff are not important as long as the proximal edge of the cuff is not more than 1 cm from the base of the digit.[141]

Measurements are carried out with the patients in a supine position, and the toes are then higher relative to the level of the heart than the sites at which pressures are measured proximally in the lower and upper limbs. This difference in level corresponds to an average difference of 9 mm Hg in hydrostatic pressure.[141] One does not correct for the difference in level because the uncorrected values reflect the transmural pressure that exists when the patients are in bed in the supine position. The very low values recorded in some patients with severe occlusive disease emphasize the importance of treatment by having the limbs in the dependent position, which results in increase in hydrostatic pressure.[38,141] The near zero or unmeasurable toe pressures in some patients indicate that there may be little or no blood flow in their toes in the supine position.[38]

In normal subjects toe pressures are always found to be

lower than ankle pressures and usually lower than brachial systolic pressures.[141] Validity of these findings would require comparison with direct pressure measurements, which are not available. However, data on the relationship of the toe pressures to proximal pressures[38,41] are similar to those obtained in intraarterial studies in vessels of comparable size in dogs.[221] Also, a single report on measurement of intraarterial pressure in a finger artery showed that finger pressure was lower than the brachial pressure.[165] The decrease in systolic pressure between the ankle and the toe must be a result of smaller diameter of the arteries of the feet, which results in damping of the pressure wave and greater resistance, which leads to a loss of some of the pressure energy during flow through the foot.

Since the arteries of the feet offer a greater resistance to flow than do the more proximal conduit vessels, the change in pressure along the foot is affected by changes in blood flow to a greater extent than are the more proximal pressures. In normal subjects systolic pressure in the second toe decreased during body heating as compared with body cooling, and the ankle-toe and brachial-toe pressure differences showed opposite changes; that is, they increased during body heating and decreased during body cooling.[141] Other researchers reported similar changes in pressures with changes in the vasomotor tone in the digits of the lower[49,168] and upper extremities.[57,81] Measurements in patients with arterial disease are usually carried out under normal resting conditions. Normal values were determined by studying pressures in 45 subjects without peripheral vascular disease whose ages ranged from 18 to 70 years.[38] Measurements were carried out with the subjects supine at a room temperature of about 21° C, with the trunk covered by an electric blanket to prevent excessive body cooling. The lower limit of normal for the toe pressure was found to be 50 mm Hg and 64% of the brachial systolic pressure. For the ankle-toe gradient the upper limit of normal was 70 mm Hg.

In patients with hypertension but without peripheral vascular disease, the systolic pressures in the toes are higher, as are the ankle-toe pressure gradients.[38] Therefore an ankle-toe pressure gradient of more than 70 mm Hg may not signify arterial obstruction in the presence of systemic hypertension. However, toe pressures expressed as a ratio of the toe pressure to the brachial pressure are not different in patients with hypertension, and therefore this parameter, if abnormal, indicates the presence of proximal arterial disease whether or not hypertension exists.[38]

Correlation of measurements of toe pressures with angiographic findings in 102 limbs showed that the pressures were abnormal in 97% of limbs with arterial occlusion and in 74% of limbs with stenotic lesions,[38] indicating that these pressures represent a valid index of the occlusive process. Since they reflect disease in the smaller distal vessels of the limb, which is not the case with the pressures measured more proximally, they are of special value in assessing the overall extent and severity of disease whether or not there is concomitant involvement of the larger proximal arter-

ies.[38,104,142,191,223] Measurement of toe pressures also allows assessment of the occlusive process in those cases in which arterial calcification interferes with the measurement of the more proximal pressures.[104,223,236] In addition to the measurements in patients with arteriosclerosis obliterans, toe pressures have been successfully applied to the assessment of the occlusive process in thromboangiitis obliterans and Raynaud's phenomenon.[38,98] In these conditions arterial lesions are usually situated in the smaller distal vessels,[58,146,200] and ankle pressures may be normal.[38,223] As discussed in detail in the section on the prognosis for healing, it is important to carry out the measurements with the patients and their limbs comfortably warm[39] because, in the presence of vasospasm or high tone in the smooth muscle of the digital arteries, values that are artifactually too low and do not represent an organic occlusive process, may be recorded.[37,91,134,199]

Systolic pressures in the toes have also been studied by Gundersen[90,91] and numerous other investigators.* Their results are similar to those presented earlier.

Skin pressures

Nielsen et al[167] and Holstein and Lassen[102] reported on measurements of "skin" blood pressures. The method consists of detecting the pressure in the cuff at which blood flow in the skin directly under the cuff begins. A photoelectric probe or clearance of an isotope can be used for this purpose. Skin pressures are lower than the systolic pressures. Although they correlate well with the diastolic pressure in normotensive subjects,[102] they are higher in the presence of hypertension.[167] The measurements probably represent systolic pressure in small vessels of the skin. As will be discussed later, they may be of value in predicting prognosis for healing.

Table 55-1 shows guidelines for interpretation of pressures at various levels in the lower limbs. However, the values will depend on the size of the cuffs used, the girth of the limb, and the vasomotor state of the limb.

Relation to symptoms

Intermittent claudication. The absolute levels of ankle systolic pressure show wide variation in patients with claudication. It has been reported that claudication can occur in normotensive patients with ankle pressures as high as 100 mm Hg.[75] Raines et al[190] found that average ankle systolic pressures at rest in patients with "limiting claudication" was 77 mm Hg with a large range of values. Fig. 55-4 shows distribution of ankle pressures in 160 patients with claudication studied in one laboratory. There is no significant difference between patients with and without diabetes. The presence of hypertension among the group accounts for some of the high pressures and the mean of 95 mm Hg. Since ankle pressure falls markedly with exercise in the

---

*References 103, 104, 113, 135, 161, 164, 168, 182, 191, 204, 223, 232, 236.

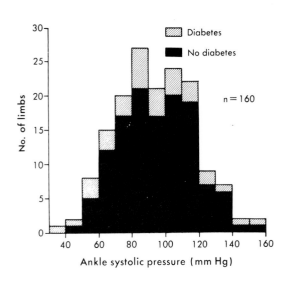

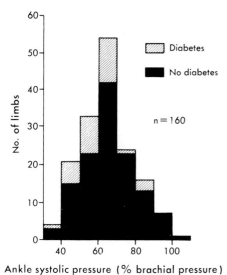

Fig. 55-4. Absolute values of the ankle systolic pressure measured at rest in limbs with intermittent claudication. *n,* Number of limbs.

Fig. 55-5. Ankle systolic pressure expressed as a percentage of the brachial systolic pressure in limbs with intermittent claudication. *n,* Number of limbs.

Table 55-1. Systolic pressure values in the lower extremities at rest

Pressure (mm Hg)	Normal	Borderline	Abnormal
Difference between right and left limbs at same level	Below 15	15-20	Above 20
Upper thigh–brachial difference	Above 30	Below 30	Below 30
Gradients along lower limbs proximal to ankle	Below 20	20-30	Above 30
Ankle (% of brachial)	Above 103*	97-103	Below 97
Ankle-foot difference†	Below 30	30	Above 30 (? less than 30)‡
Ankle-toe difference†	Below 65	65-70	Above 70 (? 60)‡
Toe	Above 50	50	Below 50
Toe (% of brachial)	Above 64	64	Below 64

*In the presence of a mild stenosis, response to exercise may be needed to demonstrate abnormality.
†May be above normal in patients with hypertension without arterial obstruction.
‡With severe proximal disease and low flows.

presence of a proximal stenosis or occlusion, absolute ankle pressures at rest do not reflect the hemodynamic situation during exercise when claudication occurs. The relationship of the ankle pressure to brachial blood pressure is a better index of the occlusive process. Yao[245] reported in 1970 that in 213 limbs with claudication, ankle systolic pressure averaged 59% of the brachial pressure with a range of 20% to 100%. Similar average ankle pressures between 57% and 65% of the brachial pressure and wide ranges were reported by Cutajar et al,[51] Lennihan and Mackereth,[137] and others,[9,227] and agree with the experience of Carter et al, which is illustrated in Fig. 55-5. As discussed earlier, in an occasional patient with claudication and a normal ankle pressure at rest, the response to exercise is necessary to demonstrate the hemodynamic abnormality. The wide range of pressure values found in patients with claudication is related in part to the variations in the site, length, and number of the occlusive or stenotic lesions and the devel-

opment of collateral circulation. However, other factors are likely to contribute as well.

Loretsen[144] and Yao et al[248] found correlation coefficients of less than 0.5 between ankle pressures and the maximal walking distance, even though the correlation with resting ankle pressure was as good as or better than with hyperemic muscle blood flow. To further investigate the relationship of the pressures to the walking ability, brachial and ankle systolic pressures were measured at rest and after a standard walk on a treadmill at 2 mph on a 7% grade in 28 patients with claudication. The maximal walking time correlated significantly with ankle systolic pressure and brachial-ankle pressure difference at rest and after exercise, as well as with the return time of the ankle systolic pressure ($p < 0.01$). Figs. 55-6 and 55-7 show brachial-ankle pressure differences at rest and after the standard walk plotted against the maximal walking distance. Eight patients with occlusive disease who were able to walk half a mile or more without

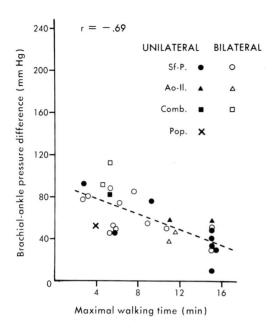

Fig. 55-6. Relationship of maximal walking time to brachial minus ankle pressure difference measured at rest in limbs with intermittent claudication. Maximal walking time was determined on a treadmill at 2 mph and on a 7% elevation. Calculated regression line and correlation coefficient *(r)* are shown. *Sf-P,* Superficial femoropopliteal; *Ao-II,* aortoiliac; *Comb,* combined aortoiliac and superficial femoropopliteal; *Pop,* popliteal.

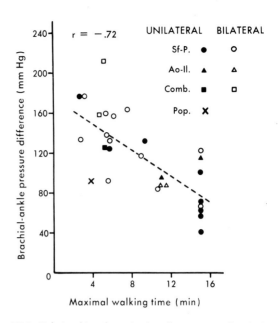

Fig. 55-7. Relationship of maximal walking time to brachial minus ankle pressure difference 3 minutes after a standard 5-minute walk on a treadmill at 2 mph and on a 7% elevation. Calculated regression line and correlation coefficient *(r)* are shown. *Sf-P,* Superficial femoropopliteal; *Ao-II,* aortoiliac; *Comb,* combined aortoiliac and superficial femoropopliteal; *Pop,* popliteal.

having to stop had resting ankle systolic pressure that ranged from 72 to 112 mm Hg or 61% to 93% of the brachial pressure. Their brachial-ankle pressure difference at rest varied from 10 to 58 mm Hg, and at 3 minutes after exercise, from 41 to 122 mm Hg. The highest correlation of -0.72 was with brachial-ankle pressure difference after exercise, but the correlation coefficients with this difference at rest (-0.69) and with ankle systolic pressure index at rest (0.66) were nearly as high. These findings indicate that severity of the occlusive process as determined by the measurements of the ankle and brachial systolic pressures at rest and after walking is an important determinant of the walking ability of patients with intermittent claudication. The large remaining variability must be caused by other factors such as differences in motivation, in the distribution of the available blood flow to the more ischemic muscle groups, or in the ability of the muscle to extract oxygen and nutrients from the available blood flow.[3,52] Some of these factors may in turn be influenced by the amount of exercise the patients perform in their daily lives.[41,198]

Because ankle pressures do not reflect arterial obstruction in the distal part of the extremity and may be falsely exaggerated by arterial rigidity, measurements of systolic pressures in the toes have been assuming a more prominent role in the assessment of patients. Like the ankle pressures, the digital pressures in patients with intermittent claudication show wide variation. Carter and Lezack[38] reported in 1971 that systolic pressure in the toes averaged 62 mm Hg and

43% of brachial systolic pressure in patients with intermittent claudication secondary to arteriosclerosis obliterans. There was no significant difference between patients with and without diabetes. However, in patients with claudication that resulted from thromboangiitis obliterans, the pressures were lower and averaged 30 mm Hg and 24% of the brachial pressure. This finding may be a result of more severe distal arterial obstruction in this group of patients. These findings have been confirmed by other researchers.[191,223,232,236] Figs. 55-8 and 55-9 show distribution of the systolic pressure in the toes in limbs with intermittent claudication studied in one laboratory.

Rest pain and skin lesions. Patients with a more advanced occlusive process manifested by pain at rest or lesions of the skin have lower pressures. Yao[245] found an average ankle systolic pressure index of 0.26 in 77 patients with pain at rest, with a range from values near 0 to 0.65, and similar findings have been reported by others.[9,51,137,223,227] Raines et al[190] found that absolute ankle systolic pressure averaged 36 mm Hg in limbs with pain at rest and 52 mm Hg in those with lesions of the skin, again with a wide range of values.

The wide range of values in patients with symptoms and signs of severe ischemia is related to the following considerations. As indicated previously, ankle pressures may not reflect disease in the branches of the popliteal artery below the knee nor in the smaller vessels distal to the ankles. Such distal disease may be present because of the basic disease

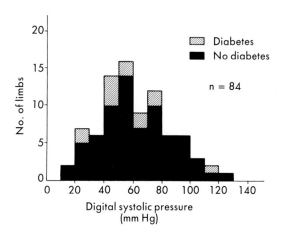

Fig. 55-8. Absolute values of the systolic pressure measured in the second toe in limbs with intermittent claudication. *n,* Number of limbs.

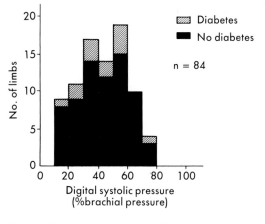

Fig. 55-9. Systolic pressure measured in the second toe expressed as a percentage of the brachial systolic pressure in limbs with intermittent claudication. *n,* Number of limbs.

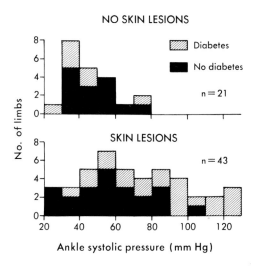

Fig. 55-10. Absolute values of the ankle systolic pressure in limbs with severe rest pain, without and with skin lesions. *n,* Number of limbs.

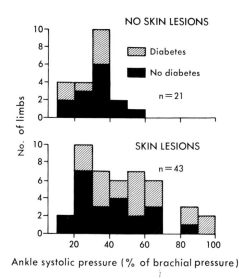

Fig. 55-11. Ankle systolic pressure expressed as a percentage of the brachial systolic pressure in limbs with severe rest pain, without and with skin lesions. *n,* Number of limbs.

process, as a result of thrombosis secondary to local trauma, infection, or stasis[48]; and in some cases, thromboembolism or atheroembolism from complicated atherosclerotic plaques located proximally in the arterial tree.[5,122] Also, ankle systolic pressures could be overestimated in some patients with arterial calcification, and this is more likely to happen in the presence of diabetes.[29,190,215] Figs. 55-10 and 55-11 show our findings of the ankle systolic pressure given in millimeters of mercury and expressed as percentage of the brachial pressure, respectively. In limbs with rest pain but without skin breakdown, pressure is usually less than 40% of the brachial pressure and less than 60 mm Hg. Patients with diabetes do not differ from those without diabetes ($p > 0.2$). In the limbs with skin lesions the range of values is greater, and some limbs have ankle pressures that are nearly normal. Although there is considerable overlap, pres-

sures are significantly higher in the limbs of patients with diabetes ($p < 0.01$ for absolute values and $p < 0.02$ for percentage of brachial pressure).

Systolic pressures measured in the toes correlate better with the presence of severe ischemia.[36] It was reported previously that in patients with rest pain, with or without ischemic skin lesions, systolic pressures in the toes averaged 33 mm Hg and 21% of the brachial systolic pressure.[38] There was no significant difference between diabetic and nondiabetic patients. Fig. 55-12 shows that in 96% of limbs with severe rest pain with or without skin lesions, the pressures were less than 30 mm Hg. The two high digital pressures in the group with skin lesions were in patients with lesions that involved a single toe and not the one in which the pressure was measured. Similar results were reported by other researchers.[90,191,223,232,236] The findings demonstrate that

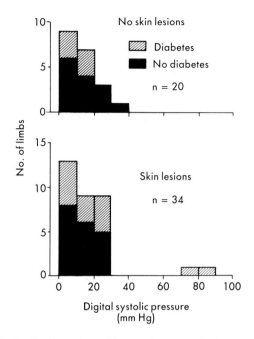

Fig. 55-12. Absolute values of the systolic pressure in the toes in limbs with severe rest pain, without and with skin lesions. *n*, Number of limbs.

systolic pressures measured in the toes correlate better than do ankle pressures with clinical evidence of severe ischemia, and they seem to provide a better index of the overall occlusive process, which may include obstruction in the more distal vessels of the extremity. The somewhat higher average pressure in limbs with skin lesions may be because of the lesions developing as a result of a precipitating cause, such as trauma in some limbs with relatively less severe disease. Higher ankle pressure found in some patients with diabetes and ischemia may be a result of the overestimation of the systolic pressure because of arterial calcification, but it can also be caused, at least in part, by the presence of more extensive distal disease in patients with diabetes.[47,219] The finding of higher ankle-toe pressure differences in some patients with diabetes and in the majority of patients with symptoms due to thromboangiitis obliterans,[38] whose disease is primarily in the small distal vessels of the extremities[201] but who are not known to have calcified arteries, also supports this contention.

APPLICATION TO THE ASSESSMENT AND MANAGEMENT OF DISEASE OF THE LOWER EXTREMITIES
Diagnosis and follow-up of patients

Previous parts of the chapter demonstrated that measurements of pressures provide a quantitative, reproducible, and sensitive method for determination of the presence and severity of the occlusive process in limbs with arterial disease. Since the measurements are noninvasive and can be performed easily and repeatedly, they lend themselves well to the follow-up of individual patients and to the documentation of the natural history of the disease.

Although in the majority of patients the diagnosis can be made on the basis of history and physical examination, several reports indicate that changes in pressures frequently occur before there are clear changes in the clinical findings.* For example, development of obstruction in the arterial tree after diagnostic catheterization has been documented by pressure measurements even in the absence of symptoms.[11,18] Measurement of pressure is of special value in those patients who may have symptoms in the extremities caused by a spinal, arthritic, or muscular disorder that may mimic arterial disease or coexist with it[63,107] and in those with mild disease.[31] Measurement of ankle pressure at rest will document the presence or absence of proximal disease in most cases, but in some patients with mild stenotic lesions the response of pressure to exercise may have to be determined. The finding of normal or nearly normal pressure will usually eliminate the need for angiography. Addition of pressure measurements in the toes is necessary when more proximal pressures are incorrect because of medial calcification. Also, since toe pressures provide information about the obstruction in the more distal vessels of the limbs than do ankle pressures, they should be used as a routine test in all limbs with severe ischemia at rest and for the assessment of the presence and severity of arterial disease in patients with diabetes, thromboangiitis obliterans, or Raynaud's phenomenon.[38]

Even when disease is obvious by clinical assessment, measurement of pressure provides a baseline against which future changes in the disease process can be monitored. Studies of reproducibility of the measurements indicate that changes in ankle and toe pressure indices are significant if they exceed about 0.15, whereas differences of 0.10 to 0.15 are of borderline significance.[6,29,91,161] If a patient with known arterial disease has a change in symptoms, measurement of pressure can be of assistance in deciding whether the change or new symptom is caused by the progression of the disease.

Natural history of disease

Progression of the occlusive process. Measurements of ankle pressures have been applied to the study of the progression of the occlusive process.[138,216] Development of disease in the second limb in patients with unilateral occlusive process is frequent.[216] Patients often show objective improvement during the first year after the onset of symptoms, and then there are no significant changes in many cases over periods of up to 4 years[138] or longer.[158] These reports provide objective evidence that supports the findings of previous clinical studies that prognosis in limbs with arteriosclerosis obliterans is generally good.[19,24,200] Patients with disease that involves the femoral and popliteal arteries showed a more variable clinical course than did those with localized superficial femoral block.[138] There was little or no deterioration in limbs with good runoff on angiography, whereas signif-

---

*References 30, 138, 158, 212, 216, 217.

icant deterioration occurred over 3 years in the group with poorest runoff. Limbs with poor runoff that eventually required amputation had significantly lower ankle pressures expressed as percentage of the brachial pressure than did those with poor runoff that did not require amputation. Serial pressure measurements often showed deterioration without an obvious clinical change, suggesting that surgical intervention in such cases might improve limb salvage.[138] A low incidence of progression of disease in patients with isolated lesions above the inguinal ligament and in those with combined proximal and distal disease was found in the majority of patients who were followed up with pressure measurements.[138,158,216]

Measurements of systolic pressure in the toes have also been applied to the study of the progression of the arterial obstruction and are essential for evaluation of severe ischemia. Paaske and Tønnesen[182] showed that prognosis for limb salvage was poor when toe systolic pressure index was less than 0.08 and improved at higher values. The study also showed the importance of the follow-up of patients with repeated measurements, since some patients with initially low pressures showed an increase in the measurements over a 2-year period and did not experience rest pain or skin breakdown. Other studies reported similar findings.[32,36] The results indicate that toe pressures provide important information that is helpful in making decisions about the management of individual patients on a more rational basis.

Population studies. Since pressure measurements provide a sensitive index of arterial obstruction and can be performed easily and repeatedly, their value in the study of the prevalence of arterial disease in population studies was recognized by the American Heart Association[187] and used by a number of researchers. The brachial-ankle pressure difference was found to correlate significantly with smoking, hypertension, and hyperlipedemia in patients with intermittent claudication.[110] The researchers suggested that such measurements could be used to quantitate the severity of the arteriosclerotic process and to evaluate the relationship to the factors that influence its progression. Ankle pressure measurements were used to estimate prevalence of peripheral arteriosclerotic disease[50,95,202] and were applied to the study of the prevalence of arteriosclerosis obliterans in patients with diabetes mellitus.[12,13,180] Toe pressures were found to correlate with the risk of amputation and with death.[4,111,169,182] These and similar studies provide important information on the prevalence of arterial disease in various patient subgroups, the relationship to smoking, prognosis, and the results of various therapeutic interventions.

It is important to realize that the sensitivity of the pressure measurements to detect an early arteriosclerotic process will depend on the criteria used. The evidence discussed earlier in this chapter indicates that mild stenotic lesions may be present in limbs with a resting ankle pressure that lies between 100% and 115% of the brachial systolic pressure. Assessment of the response of the ankle pressure to exercise would be required to demonstrate such mild stenotic lesions.

Also, as emphasized by the American Heart Association,[187] the noninvasive studies should be combined with clinical assessment. There is evidence that auscultation for bruits, especially over the superficial artery in the region of the adductor canal in the thigh at rest and after exercise, is a sensitive index of mild arterial lesions. Such bruits may be present in limbs with normal systolic pressures.[34]

Medical therapy

Measurements of pressure can be used to guide and evaluate medical therapy. Segmental pressure measurements have been reported to be helpful in the management of a patient with arterial occlusion secondary to ergotism that may regress spontaneously[123] and to assist in the treatment of severe ischemia with drug-induced systemic hypertension by monitoring distal systolic pressure.[91,131] The use of dependent position in the treatment of severe ischemia of the limbs is supported by the findings that in the presence of severe occlusion the increase in the ankle[79] and digital[140] pressures with dependency is greater than the increase in hydrostatic level, at least in part because of the distension of the collateral vessels. The effect of changes in the distension of the collateral vessels was demonstrated by the finding of increased flow and pressure in the feet in limbs with occlusion of the superficial femoral artery during external application of negative pressure to the thigh.[2] Also, vasoconstriction in the tissues of the thigh in response to the assumption of the upright posture leads to lower blood flow through collateral vessels and thus to a smaller pressure drop during flow through them. This in turn leads to a higher arterial pressure distal to the occlusion and higher blood flow through the distal ischemic tissues.[1] Combination of the upright posture with intermittent venous compression may increase blood flow in the presence of arterial obstruction by increasing the arteriovenous pressure gradient across the foot. Significant increases in skin blood flow measured with the xenon clearance method occurred when a mechanical venous pump was used in patients with arterial obstruction in the sitting position, but only when arterial obstruction was severe, as indicated by the ankle pressure of 60 mm Hg or less.[82]

Vasodilators have been shown to decrease digital blood pressure distal to occlusion and are probably not indicated, particularly in the presence of severe ischemia.[91] Walking on a raised heel did not change the response of ankle systolic pressure to exercise nor the walking time of patients with claudication.[44] On the other hand, treatment with clofibrate resulted in a significant improvement in the response of ankle pressure to exercise in a group of patients with intermittent claudication and high plasma fibrinogen level.[186] Similarly, defibrination by subcutaneous injections of ancrod for 5 weeks was followed by improvement of the symptoms and statistically significant increases in resting ankle pressure and its response to exercise, which improved by 25% or more.[56] In a study of patients with intermittent claudication, cessation of smoking was followed by significant improvement of the walking distance, resting ankle pressures, and ankle pressures after exercise, whereas patients who continued to smoke showed no significant changes.[188]

Numerous reports indicate that exercise improves walking ability of patients with intermittent claudication. The mechanism of improvement is not clear, but it is likely that several factors may contribute to the remarkable walking ability that many patients achieve in the exercise programs.[41,198] Some studies reported increases in blood flow in response to training,[3,131] whereas others did not.[250] Similarly, early clinical studies reported increases in the ankle systolic pressure at rest and in response to exercise after training,[206,207] whereas more recent studies showed only modest increases.[41,45] Remarkable walking ability may be achieved in about 75% of patients with intermittent claudication.[41] Good walking ability may be achieved in patients with obstruction either proximal or distal to the inguinal ligament, in patients with combined disease, in patients with and without ischemic heart disease and diabetes, and in patients taking β-blocking drugs. Similar degrees of improvement were also observed in patients with widely varying severity of obstruction as assessed by systolic pressure measurements. Good walking ability was achieved by patients whose ankle systolic pressures were as low as 55 mm Hg and ankle index of 0.40 and toe systolic pressures as low as 30 mm Hg.[41]

Prognosis for healing

The use of pressure measurements to determine prognosis for healing is one of its most important practical applications. Patients with severe ischemia and skin lesions in whom arterial reconstruction may be associated with a significant risk because of the associated cardiovascular disease present a common clinical problem. If the lesion were to heal without surgery, the risk to life could be avoided. In other patients arterial reconstruction may not be feasible because disease is too extensive. In such cases one often persists with conservative management in the hope that the lesion will heal. In many patients, however, the conservative approach fails and amputation is carried out, often after a long period of suffering and hospitalization. In 1973 it was demonstrated that measurements of distal systolic pressures can be helpful in making decisions in such cases.[32] If ankle pressure was less than 55 mm Hg, healing did not take place and major amputation had to be carried out in diabetic and nondiabetic patients. The chances for healing were good in nondiabetic patients when the ankle pressure was greater than 55 mm Hg, whereas in the diabetic patients the chances for healing were uncertain even with high ankle pressures. This finding is not surprising because of the frequency of severe obstruction in the small distal vessels of the limbs in the diabetic patients and higher incidence of medial calcification that may render ankle pressure unreliable. On the other hand, toe pressures correlated well with healing in the limbs of both diabetic and nondiabetic patients. Chances of healing were uncertain when the pressure was less than 30

mm Hg and good when it was higher. Slightly lower chances of healing in the diabetic patients are probably related to the impairment of the tissue reparative processes by the metabolic disorder, increased susceptibility to infection, and neuropathy. Similar results have since been obtained in numerous studies. Raines et al[190] reported that healing was unlikely when ankle pressure was less than 55 mm Hg and that higher pressures were required for healing to occur in diabetic patients. Scandinavian researchers[103,132,134,176,182] applied measurements of toe and skin blood pressures extensively to the assessment of prognosis for healing with similar results and Sumner recently reviewed the evidence.[223] Table 55-2 summarizes the relationship of the pressure measurements to the prognosis for healing of skin lesions of the toes or feet on the basis of a large combined experience in Copenhagen and in the author's laboratory. The results in the table are based on studies in which cuffs 25 to 29 mm in width were used on the hallux or 2 cm wide cuffs were used on the second toe. The results may be somewhat different if measurements are carried out by using a different cuff width.

The finding that a distal arterial pressure of about 30 mm Hg is necessary to achieve healing of skin lesions is in agreement with the findings on the relationship of the toe systolic pressures to the healing of distal amputations of the feet and toes.[23,191,204,223] Another situation in which systolic pressures may be used to estimate the chances of healing is elective surgery in the feet of patients with arterial obstruction, for the purpose of correcting bunions, hammer toes, or other pathologic conditions, for example, excising neuromas. When there is clinically evident arterial obstruction, there may be reluctance to consider surgery, and patients may be left at times with significant disability. Experience with orthopedic procedures in the feet of patients with arterial disease showed that healing occurred without difficulties in all cases.[37a] Although the degree of arterial obstruction estimated by distal systolic pressure measurements was mild in many cases, the ankle pressure was decreased in some to 60 to 70 mm Hg, and in four cases

Table 55-2. Relationship of systolic pressure to prognosis for healing of skin lesions of the toes or feet

Pressure (mm Hg)	Probability of healing (%)	
	No diabetes	Diabetes
Ankle		
Below 55	0	0
55 to 90	85	45
Above 90	100	85
Toe		
Below 20	25	29
20 to 30	73	40
30 to 55	100	85
Above 55	100	97
Skin		
Below 20	0	0

the digital systolic pressures were 40 to 60 mm Hg. This experience and the other data on the relationship of pressures to healing suggest that when systolic pressure exceeds 30 mm Hg in the toes of nondiabetic subjects and 55 mm Hg in diabetic patients, elective surgery can probably be safely done, although there is a need for the study of a larger number of cases.

It seems reasonable that a pressure of about 30 mm Hg in the small arteries is usually needed to maintain an effective arteriovenous pressure difference and to provide adequate nutritional blood flow and thus promote healing. Although adequate blood flow and oxygen delivery to the tissues are the important parameters necessary for healing, they depend on the available driving pressure and peripheral resistance in the microcirculation. There is evidence that when the ability of the small vessels to vasoconstrict is abolished by local heating or ischemia, the flow and oxygen delivery depend primarily on the available arterial pressure, which is reflected in the distal systolic pressure measurements. This concept is supported by the finding of a good correlation between transcutaneous measurements of oxygen tension in limbs with arterial obstruction and distal systolic pressures[46,62,239] and by corresponding correlations between ischemia, pressures, and other measurements of digital circulation.[113] The questions of why healing occurs in some limbs in which the measured pressures are even lower[32,103,182] and why some patients with very low pressures may have no symptoms remain.[38,103] Several considerations may be relevant. Technical factors, for example, too tight application of the measuring cuffs, might result in falsely low pressures, since the digital arteries with low pressures might be compressed or even closed more easily by a tightly applied cuff. During measurements, usually carried out with the patient in the supine position, the toes are higher than the level of the heart, which results in an average decrease in the measured pressure of 9 mm Hg.[141] Therefore it is likely that when patients lie in a different position, the digital pressure is slightly higher. Also, it has been shown that when limbs with severe arterial obstruction are in a dependent position, the increase in digital pressure is greater than expected from the difference in hydrostatic level,[1,140] which should result in an increased arteriovenous pressure gradient. The digital pressures will also vary with the changes in the hemodynamic state of the patient. If a patient's central blood pressure is relatively low during the measurements and high at other times, lower systolic pressure measured in the toes during the test would not represent higher pressures that may otherwise exist.

As discussed earlier in this chapter, distal blood pressures are known to vary with changes in blood flow and vasomotor tone. They are higher when blood flow proximal to the site of the measurement is lower and conversely decrease when there is peripheral vasodilatation and blood flow increases.[57,141] For example, in the presence of a strong vasodilating stimulus, higher blood flow proximal to the toe could result in a relatively low digital pressure, which would suggest a poorer prognosis than actually might be present. It is possible that in some limbs with lesions and arterial obstruction, pronounced vasodilatation and relatively high flows might be present as a result of inflammation, ischemia,[152,153] or neuropathy[59] in the presence of toe pressures below 30 mm Hg. If such a situation is suspected, the use of some index of distal blood flow can provide important information. Test modalities that may be used for this purpose include recording of digital pulse volume changes by using strain-gauge or photocell plethysmography[177,211] or measurements of skin temperature,[157] measurement of skin blood flow,[149] or determination of transcutaneous oxygen tension.[27,120,244]

Although peripheral vasoconstriction induced by body cooling was shown to be associated with higher digital pressure,[57,141] local cold, whether produced by local cooling or low blood flow related to intense sympathetic vasoconstriction, may result in decreases of measured digital pressure in some subjects. Such an effect was demonstrated in the fingers and toes of patients with Raynaud's syndrome and in some normal subjects.[37,40,128,170,171] The loss of measurable digital pressure or an "artifactual" decrease in such cases is thought to be due to the effect of temperature on the smooth muscle of the main digital arteries and the delayed opening of these vessels during or after the deflation of the pressure cuffs.[40] Thus decrease in temperature may exert two opposing effects on the pressure measured in the digits. Vasoconstriction in the microcirculation in response to cold decreases flow and the frictional pressure energy losses and thus increases digital pressure.[57,141] On the other hand, local cold can result in delayed opening of the digital arteries during pressure measurements and thus in underestimation of the digital pressure. The net effect of temperature in an individual subject probably depends on the relative balance between these two opposing effects and the "sensitivity" of the digital vessels to low temperature. Marked sensitivity of digital pressure to temperature can be used to demonstrate vasospasm in patients with Raynaud's syndrome and occurs in some normal subjects.[37,40,170] Similar decreases were recently demonstrated in the toe pressure at low temperature in limbs with arteriosclerotic arterial obstruction.[199] These various phenomena indicate that it is of utmost importance to measure distal pressures with the patients and their extremities comfortably warm and to avoid measurements during pronounced vasoconstriction or vasodilatation. A preliminary period of warming with an electric blanket for about 20 minutes should be used, especially when the weather is cool in moderate and severe climates.[38] Also, repetition of the pressure measurements during follow-up is important, because in some patients subsequent testing may show an increase in pressure and suggest a better prognosis.[103,182]

APPLICATION TO THE ASSESSMENT AND MANAGEMENT OF DISEASE OF THE UPPER EXTREMITIES

Disease in the arteries supplying the upper limbs is less common than in the lower extremities, but the occlusive process in the arterial tree from the subclavian to the digital vessels occurs as a result of atherosclerosis,[26,114] Takayasu's disease,[249] embolism,[249] thoracic outlet syndromes,[55,235,249] complications of diagnostic arterial catheterization,[8,55,112] thromboangiitis obliterans,[200] trauma,[55,235,249] and various conditions that affect small distal arteries of the hand or digits.[146,235,249] As in the case of the lower limbs, measurements of systolic pressures in the upper limbs provide information about the presence, site, and severity of the stenotic or occlusive process and thus aid in the diagnosis and management of patients.

Obstruction in the main arterial pathways

An occlusive or stenotic process in the subclavian or axillary artery will result in a decrease of the brachial blood pressure. There are many publications that deal with obstruction of the subclavian arteries, including those about patients with subclavian steal syndrome.[184] Results of pressure measurements in 15 limbs with subclavian stenosis or occlusion studied in one laboratory, combined with the data from five published reports,[26,114,185,189,234] show that the difference in the brachial systolic pressures between the two arms averaged 41 ± SD 14 mm Hg (range 20 to 70) in 21 cases of subclavian stenosis and 64 ± SD 25 (range 24 to 130) in 29 cases with a complete occlusion. The difference exceeded 50 mm Hg in 23 cases with occlusion and in only 3 with a stenosis. Although it has been stated that differences in pressure of more than 30 mm Hg between the two arms are indicative of the disease,[134] studies of blood pressure differences between the two arms in large series of subjects[192,220] suggest that differences greater than 15 mm Hg should arouse suspicion. At times the difference in the blood pressure between the two arms may underestimate the severity of the disease, since the disease may be bilateral and a milder lesion may exist in the limb with the higher pressure. A comparison with pressure measurement in the lower limbs may provide a more accurate assessment of the significance of the occlusive process to the upper extremities in such cases.[249] Arm exercise will result in the drop of pressure distal to a hemodynamically significant lesion, and this procedure may be of additional help in the assessment of patients.[234,249] Lamis et al[130] reported that distal segmental pressure measurements after hyperemia were helpful in the evaluation of the donor subclavian or innominate vessels before axillo-axillary bypass graft for occlusion of the contralateral subclavian artery.

Among six cases of obstruction in the axillary region we found differences in blood pressure between the two arms that ranged from 40 to 68 mm Hg in four patients, whereas in two who sustained an injury to the axillary region at a relatively young age and who had few or no symptoms, the difference was only 20 mm Hg and was not increased by exercise. This finding might be explained by the potential for the development of abundant collateral circulation in the shoulder region.[249]

With increased use of arterial catheterization for diagnostic purposes, complications that result in the obstruction of the brachial artery are becoming one of the more common causes of the occlusive process of the arteries of the upper limbs.[112] Among 10 patients with obstruction in the brachial region who were referred to one laboratory, in 8 the obstruction was secondary to a diagnostic catheterization. The mean difference between brachial pressures was only 11 ± SD 12 mm Hg (range −2 to 36), and it exceeded 20 mm Hg in only two patients. On the other hand, the difference in forearm pressure averaged 44 ± SD 15 mm Hg (range 30 to 79). The difference between brachial pressures did not reflect the severity of the occlusive process. The situation here is similar to that in the thigh, where high pressures may be measured in the presence of the obstruction of the superficial femoral artery because of the enlargement of the deep femoral artery. In the upper limb an enlarged deep brachial artery was probably responsible for relatively high pressures recorded in the arms of these patients. Determination of forearm or wrist pressures with a Doppler ultrasonic flow detector over the radial and ulnar vessels may at times give different readings over the two vessels. This was the case in one patient in this series in whom a much lower pressure recorded with the Doppler flow detector over the radial artery was caused by thrombotic occlusion of this vessel in addition to the brachial occlusion. All patients whose obstruction was secondary to arterial catheterization had symptoms consistent with intermittent claudication and associated coldness of the hand. The pressures in the fingers were also reduced. An abnormally large difference between the blood pressures in the two upper limbs that is not associated with an obstructive arterial lesion may occur in patients with supravalvular aortic stenosis. It has been suggested that asymmetric jet effects lead to the observed pressure difference.[69]

Finger pressures in the assessment of distal diseases including Raynaud's phenomenon

Systolic pressures in the fingers have been measured for at least 80 years, and earlier studies were reviewed by others.[66,80] After correction for the difference in level between fingers and toes in the supine position, pressures in the fingers were found to be, on the average, 13 mm Hg higher than in the toes.[141] Gaskell and Krisman[80] studied the effect of various cuff widths and found that cuffs 3 to 4 cm wide appeared to give consistent results. Although there are differences in the results of various studies related, at least in part, to differences in the techniques and possibly to differences in the vasomotor state of the subjects,[57,81,141,166] finger pressures are generally lower than brachial pressures except at times under the condition of pronounced peripheral vasoconstriction.[57,58,81,141] Intraarterial measurements indicate that there is also amplification of the systolic pressure along the arteries of the upper limbs,[129] although it may not be as pronounced as in the lower limbs. The report of a direct measurement from a finger artery indicates that a decrease in pressure occurs between the wrist and the finger.[165] Similar to the findings in the lower limbs, increased brachial-to-digit pressure differences may be found in patients with hypertension without an occlusive arterial process.[81]

Effect of changes in the vasomotor tone. In general, pressures in the fingers behave in a similar way to those measured in the toes. In an elegant study in 1939, Doupe et al[57] demonstrated that finger pressures decreased during peripheral vasodilatation and increased during vasoconstriction and that the difference between the brachial and finger pressures showed opposite changes. Similar results were reported by Gaskell and Krisman[81] and by Lezack and Carter.[141] However, when the fingers are cold, high tone in the digital arteries may result in delayed opening of these vessels during deflation of the blood pressure cuffs and thus in artifactually diminished values or loss of measurable finger pressure.[40] These phenomena can be used to assess patients for Raynaud's phenomena as discussed below, but they dictate that measurements to assess for the presence of organic arterial obstruction must not be carried out when the hands are cold.

Organic obstruction. Downs et al[58] carried out a careful study of pressure measurements in the fingers of normal subjects and patients with angiographically demonstrated occlusive process in the arteries of the hands and fingers with 38 mm wide cuffs applied around the proximal phalanx. Their findings were that systolic finger pressures of less than 70 mm Hg, wrist-digit gradients of more than 30 mm Hg, and brachial-finger differences of more than 35 to 40 mm Hg strongly suggest the presence of an occlusive process at or proximal to the digit. Also, differences between simultaneously measured pressures in the corresponding fingers should not exceed 15 mm Hg.

Measurements of finger pressures in normal subjects and in patients with arterial obstruction were also reported by Gundersen[90,91] and others.[96,164,166] Their results are similar, but some differences are related to the use of a narrower 24 mm wide cuff[91,167,168] as compared with the 38 mm cuffs used in the study of Downs et al.[58] Hirai[96] studied a large number of normal subjects and patients with arterial disease by using a 24 mm wide cuff to measure pressures at both the proximal and intermediate phalanges of the fingers. He did not find significant differences between the measurements at the proximal and middle phalanges despite a previous report, which indicated that the pressure at the middle phalanges is about 5 mm Hg lower than that at the base of the digit.[99] He also reported that brachial-finger differences should not exceed 20 mm Hg in normal subjects less than 50 years of age and 25 mm Hg in older subjects without arterial disease. The differences between the findings of Hirai and Downs et al[58] might be a result of the use of different cuff widths and of the different vasomotor state of the subjects, since Hirai did not specify the conditions under which the measurements were carried out, whereas Downs et al studied subjects who were kept warm by means of an electric blanket. It is necessasry for each laboratory to apply and develop appropriate normal standards according to the techniques and procedures that are used, although to assess the presence and severity of the organic arterial obstruction, the measurements in the limbs and particularly in the digits should be carried out with the patients and extremities at least comfortably warm.

Measurements of systolic pressures in the fingers to assess arterial obstruction have limitations similar to those discussed with respect to the assessment of the obstruction in the lower limbs and the more proximal disease in the upper limbs. If only one of the two digital arteries is occluded, the measured pressure will be normal.[58,96] Also, if obstruction is present in the digital arteries in the distal part of the finger, the obstruction may be detected only if the cuff is placed at the intermediate phalanx and normal values are obtained at the proximal phalanx. In cases of very distal disease even measurements at the intermediate phalanx may be normal, and the evidence of obstruction may only be obtained by assessment of distal blood flow or skin temperature.[35]

Hirai found normal finger pressure in all 184 fingers with at least one normal arterial pathway to the digit as assessed by angiography.[96] Among 203 fingers with occlusion of both digital arteries or more proximal vessels supplying the digit, abnormal pressures were recorded in 173 digits. In 30 fingers with "falsely negative" results there were no symptoms in the majority. Such normal findings are a result of the occasional development of very large collateral channels that may form connections between two occluded digital arteries,[58] the presence of other large collateral pathways within the palm, very distal obstructions in the digit, and the uncertainty of the evaluation of the angiographic findings in relatively small arteries of the hands and fingers.[96] Such false negative results are relatively infrequent, usually not associated with severe impairment of blood flow, and may be taken into account in the interpretation of the results. These considerations therefore do not detract from the value of pressure measurements in the digits in the functional assessment of the arterial obstruction to the fingers.

Prognosis for healing. Pressure measurements in the fingers may be of value in assessing prognosis for healing. A study of 23 patients showed that chances for early healing were high when finger systolic pressure exceeded 55 mm Hg, the brachial-finger pressure difference was less than 50 mm Hg, and the maximal difference among the fingers was less than 30 mm Hg.[35] Early healing was also likely when finger temperature of 10° C or more above room temperature was achieved during body heating. However, slow healing over a period of up to a year or more occurred in all digits in which the pressure exceeded 25 mm Hg.[35]

Cold sensitivity. Although digital pressures usually increase during peripheral vasoconstriction, in patients with cold sensitivity abnormally low digital pressures may be recorded when the patient or the extremities are cold, because excessive force is exerted by the smooth muscle in the digital arteries in such cases.[134] This phenomenon has been applied to the study of patients with cold sensitivity in the elegant studies of Krähenbuhl et al[128] and Nielsen and Lassen.[171]

The method uses measurement of systolic pressure in locally cooled fingers. In normal subjects the pressure in the locally cooled digits was reported to fall by an average of only 15% when the local temperature was lowered to 10° or 5° C, whereas in patients with Raynaud's phenomena it fell precipitously, often to unobtainable values, indicating closure of the digital arteries.[170,230] The frequency of the occurrence of digital artery closure with local cooling was increased by the addition of body cooling.[170] This interesting technique gave an early promise of providing a sensitive and specific test for the diagnosis of Raynaud's phenomena, and some studies reported good separation between normal subjects and patients.[100,170] However, other reports indicate that subjects without Raynaud's phenomena may at times exhibit abnormal decrease in the finger pressure with local cooling at times even to zero,[40,128,173] and in other studies more than 20% of patients with Raynaud's phenomena did not show an abnormal response.[40,230] Also, in patients with Raynaud's phenomena, abnormal responses and closure may occur during body cooling without local cooling of the fingers.[40] The method appears to provide an interesting research tool and has been used to assess these vessels in patients with arterial obstruction,[97,174] hypertension, and diabetes[231] and to evaluate the effect of various therapeutic interventions.[163,172,175] However, the diagnosis of Raynaud's phenomena can usually be made easily on the basis of clear history of typical episodic discoloration. Therefore from a practical point of view, the measurements of finger pressures in response to local cooling are probably needed only for objective documentation of the vasospastic condition in the cases of occupational disease in which there is a question of compensation.

OTHER APPLICATIONS
Assessment of procedures to eliminate arterial obstruction

Organic arterial occlusions or stenosis may be eliminated by surgery, by percutaneous transluminal dilatation, or by other endovascular interventions. Pressure measurements have been used in the assessment of the results of these procedures and attempts made to apply the measurements to help select patients for treatment. The use of pressures in relation to the surgical treatment is dealt with in detail in Chapters 60 to 66. There are reports of successful use of the measurements to assess the results of transluminal angioplasties,* but these and numerous other studies on this subject are not reviewed in detail. It is clear, however, that the measurements are useful in the assessment of patients before surgery or angioplasty, in the immediate and long-term follow-up after the procedures, and in the objective evaluation of the results.[160,169,176,194,195,233] The methods, criteria, and use of the measurements are essentially similar

to those discussed in earlier sections of this chapter. Measurements of toe pressures should be applied routinely to the assessment of the results in limbs of patients with diabetes and in limbs with severe ischemia.[38]

The role of the measurements in predicting the chances of success of specific procedures is also discussed in other chapters. Pressure measurements by themselves may not be able to predict with complete accuracy the chances of success of treatment, which may also be influenced by the nature and extent of the obstruction, the techniques and materials used, and other factors; therefore, such expectations may be unrealistic.[222]

Healing of major amputations

Healing of major amputations is discussed in detail in Chapter 64. Although pressure measurements at the ankles and at more proximal sites in the lower limbs have been used in attempts to predict healing of below-knee and above-knee amputations, the results are not as consistent as in the case of healing of lesions in the feet and toes, distal amputations, and elective surgery of the toes and feet discussed earlier in this chapter. These findings should not be surprising. Toe pressures are a good index of perfusion pressure close to the level of the lesion or surgery in the feet. On the other hand, ankle and proximal pressures may not reflect the perfusion pressure in the small skin vessels in the areas in which healing after major amputations has to occur, and those pressures may also be unreliable in the presence of medial calcification. It appears that measurements of skin perfusion pressures at the sites of amputation may represent a more appropriate index for prediction of healing of these more proximal procedures. Good results with the use of this method have been reported.[105,106] Measurements of cutaneous blood flow with the xenon clearance method[149] and of transcutaneous oxygen tension[27] have also been found useful in predicting healing of major amputations. These techniques are discussed in other chapters.

Penile pressure in the assessment of impotence

Gaskell[77] was the first to report on the use of measurements of systolic blood pressure in the penis in normal young men, patients with occlusive arterial disease in the extremities but without impotence, and patients with impotence. He found that in the absence of arterial obstruction, systolic pressure in the penis should not be less than the mean brachial blood pressure taken as the diastolic plus one third of the pulse pressure. According to this criterion, there were only two patients who had abnormally low penile pressures and claimed to be potent and only one patient with a normal pressure and impotence. Numerous studies of penile pressure measurements in the assessment of impotence have appeared since. In most studies the ratio of the penile systolic to the brachial systolic pressure has been reported and not the difference between mean brachial pressure and penile systolic pressure, which was used by Gaskell. In a study of 97 patients at the Vascular Laboratory at St. Boniface Gen-

---

*References 17, 118, 121, 178, 194, 242.

eral Hospital in Winnipeg a good correlation was found between penile/brachial systolic pressure index and the difference between the penile systolic and brachial mean pressure, with the correlation coefficient of 0.93 ($p < 0.001$). A zero difference between penile systolic and brachial mean pressures corresponded to the penile systolic pressure index of 0.72. Therefore lower pressures suggest the presence of arterial obstruction in the arterial supply of the penis, and this is in agreement with other reports.[154,155] The relationship of penile blood pressure to the occurrence of impotence is complex, since there are a number of other factors that may affect the erectile function. This subject is discussed in detail in Chapter 97.

Popliteal artery entrapment

Popliteal artery entrapment may be responsible for a history of intermittent claudication in young patients, although routine physical examination may show normal peripheral pulses before complications occur. The diagnosis should be suspected if pedal pulses disappear or diminish markedly with sustained active plantar flexion or with passive dorsiflexion at the ankle. Recording of abnormal pulse waves and of diminished ankle systolic pressure will corroborate the diagnosis.[53]

Coarctation

Comparison of the ankle and brachial systolic pressures can be used to assess patients with coarctation and to evaluate the efficacy of surgical treatment. Bollinger et al[21] found that the difference between the brachial and ankle systolic pressures at rest averaged 70 mm Hg in 12 patients. Patients with coarctation of the thoracic aorta did not have intermittent claudication, despite the significant difference in pressures between the upper and lower limbs. The peak calf blood flow after 3 minutes of ischemia was normal in patients with coarctation,[21] suggesting that extensive collateral circulation that develops early in life is able to provide adequate blood flow to the exercising muscles of the lower extremities. In four patients with coarctation, it was found that after exercise of the lower limbs, the ankle systolic pressure showed little or no change.

Peripheral arteriovenous fistula

Systolic pressure measurements have been applied to the study of the circulation in limbs distal to arteriovenous fistulas. Distal to a large fistula, ankle pressures are decreased at rest and show an abnormal fall in response to exercise that resembles the response in limbs with occlusive arterial process.[211,218] Compression of the fistula results in an increase of the ankle pressure. Noninvasive testing for assessment of arteriovenous fistula is discussed in detail in Chapter 71.

CONCLUSION

As is well known, noninvasive measurements of brachial blood pressure with pneumatic cuffs were introduced during the nineteenth century and have been an essential tool in the clinical assessment and treatment of patients. Noninvasive measurements of systolic pressure in the fingers and in the lower limbs including the toes were carried out beginning early in this century. These early reports are referred to in the 1934 paper by Formijne.[66] In 1950 Winsor[243] reported on the segmental pressure measurements in the upper and lower limbs in normal subjects and patients with arterial obstruction, and in 1956, Gaskell[74] demonstrated that ankle systolic pressures measured at rest were a better index of the arterial obstruction than measurements of blood flow at rest and as good as measurements of blood flow in response to reactive hyperemia. The advent of extensive use of arterial surgery led to increased interest in the development of noninvasive methods for assessment of patients with peripheral arterial disease. The pioneering work of Strandness, which began in the early 1960s and has continued since, provided a major stimulus for the interest and further development of noninvasive pressure measurements by other researchers. As a result, pressure measurements have become an accepted method of evaluation of patients with arterial disease in diagnostic laboratories throughout the world. Some investigators became interested in the measurements of pressures in the toes in the mid-1960s[140,141] and applied them to the assessment of arterial obstruction and estimation of the chances of healing of skin lesions.[32,38] These studies, those by Gundersen,[90,91] and those by others* led to the documentation of the value of such distal measurements in the assessment and treatment of patients. In 1971 Gaskell[77] reported on the use of penile systolic pressure in the assessment of impotence, and other similar studies followed. The increasing interest in the use of pressure measurements to assess peripheral arterial disease is illustrated by the large number of papers, symposia, and courses on this subject during the past 15 to 20 years. Extensive work of numerous researchers has allowed a better assessment of the value and specific applications of the measurements and their limitations.

The ankle systolic pressure measured at rest often provides a good index of the presence and severity of the arterial obstruction in the main arterial channels proximal to the division of the popliteal artery. Ankle pressures, however, are not reliable in some patients in whom tibial arteries are "incompressible," usually because of medial calcification. This occurs in patients with diabetes mellitus, in those undergoing renal dialysis, and probably in some elderly patients without those conditions. With these limitations in mind, ankle pressure equal to the brachial systolic pressure should be used as a practical guideline for the lower limit of normal. However, mild stenotic lesions may be present in the limbs, in which ankle pressure exceeds brachial pressure by up to about 15%, and at times there may be associated symptoms of intermittent claudication. Measurements

---

*References 103, 104, 113, 135, 161, 166, 168, 182, 191, 204, 223, 232, 236.

of pressures after exercise or during reactive hyperemia are useful in the demonstration of such mild stenotic lesions and in the differentation of the causes of symptoms in patients who may have pseudoclaudication associated with neurospinal disorders, especially when arterial disease coexists. However, measurements after stress do not usually add practical information to the resting ankle pressure measurements if these are clearly abnormal. Measurements after stress should not be a part of a routine assessment of all patients with arterial disease. Measurements of segmental pressures at different levels have not fulfilled the promise of early enthusiastic reports. The results of these more proximal measurements are affected severely by various artifacts. The most useful information they may provide is evidence for the absence of significant obstruction proximal to the groin when the pressure at the upper thigh is considerably higher than brachial systolic pressure (by at least 30 mm Hg), in the presence of a strong femoral pulse, and in the absence of bruits. When the upper thigh pressure is lower, the presence of significant proximal lesions cannot be ruled out without resorting to other methods, including invasive pressure measurements. Segmental measurements frequently do not provide reliable information about the site of the obstruction and the number of lesions along the arterial tree of the extremity. The value of the ankle pressure by itself can give a reasonably good indication as to whether there is a single lesion or multiple sites of obstruction.

Since ankle and more proximal pressures may be falsely high in limbs with medial calcification and do not provide evidence about obstruction in the more distal vessels of the limbs, measurements of systolic pressures in the toes that are not subject to these limitations have been shown clearly to be of great value. Measurements of toe pressures should be a routine test for assessment of arterial disease in patients with diabetes and in others, especially those with severe ischemia. In the absence of extensive or deep-seated infection, such as osteomyelitis, systolic pressures in the toes are an excellent index of healing of skin lesions, amputations, and elective surgical procedures in the toes and feet of patients with arterial disease. Pressures of 30 mm Hg or greater indicate excellent prognosis for healing in nondiabetic patients and good prognosis in diabetic patients, with a pressure of 55 mm Hg assuring healing in nearly 100% of cases—even in the diabetic patients. These findings fit well with physiologic concepts, since pressure of 30 mm Hg probably approaches the value of arterial pressure necessary to provide a minimum pressure gradient for an effective tissue blood flow. Together with other techniques, measurements of penile systolic pressures are of value in the assessment of impotence.

Measurements of pressures provide an objective and quantitative method for the assessment of the presence and severity of the arterial obstruction in the extremities and are of value in the follow-up of individual patients, in population studies to assess the natural history and prevalence of arterial disease, and in the evaluation of results of specific treatments. Pressure measurements are important in the long-term assessment of the results of various interventions aimed at the restoration of arterial patency. They provide important data about the functional hemodynamic status of the extremity, which is the important determinant of the prognosis and limb preservation. It is important to keep in mind that although the hemodynamic status is affected by the presence and degree of arterial obstruction and the patency at the site of the intervention, it is not equivalent to the anatomic data. Also, the hemodynamic status is determined not only by the patency of the intervention but also by the presence or progression of arterial disease, which may be situated proximally or distally in the arterial tree. The anatomic information can only be obtained by angiography or duplex scanning. Both anatomic and hemodynamic information is needed to provide a better understanding of the effects of treatments and their interaction with the basic disease process.

It appears that noninvasive pressure measurements may not be able to reliably predict the success of various therapies, although their role in conjunction with other methods remains to be fully elucidated. Such a finding should not be surprising, since pressure in the main arterial channels is not the only factor that affects the success of therapeutic procedures. This consideration also applies to the healing of major amputations, although measurements of skin pressure, which probably reflects pressure in the small arteries supplying the areas in question, appear to be a good predictor, as pressure measurements in the toes are in the case of healing in the distal parts of the extremities.

There is abundant evidence that noninvasive pressure measurements are extremely useful in the assessment, follow-up, and treatment of patients with arterial disease and provide an objective method for the evaluation of results of therapeutic procedures. Judicious use of the measurements for routine assessment of patients is not only justified but necessary. Careful attention to the techniques and the use of the appropriate normal standards is of critical importance, since the normal range of values may be different when different techniques, and particularly when cuffs of different widths, are used in the measurements. Also, care has to be exercised in evaluating benefits of therapy when the resulting changes in pressure are relatively small and may be within the range of variability of the measurements. Various limitations of specific measurements must be kept in mind when interpreting the results and applying them to the assessment and treatment of patients. It must also be emphasized that the measurements should not be used as a substitute for careful clinical assessment but only in conjunction with it.

ACKNOWLEDGMENT

I wish to thank all members of the technical, nursing, and secretarial staff of the Vascular Laboratory of St. Boniface General Hospital for their excellent help over the past 30 years, students who participated in our research, and numerous colleagues in our and other medical centers for the stimulation and motivation of my interest in the role of pressure measurements.

REFERENCES

1. Agerskov K: Influence of thigh blood flow upon the arterial pressure gradient over the collateral arteries in patients with occlusion of the superficial femoral artery, *Cardiovasc Res* 16:304, 1982.
2. Agerskov K et al: External negative thigh pressure: effect upon blood flow and pressure in the foot in patients with occlusive arterial disease, *Dan Med Bull* 37:451, 1990.
3. Alpert JS, Larsen OA, Lassen NA: Exercise and intermittent claudication, *Circulation* 39:353, 1969.
4. Andersen HJ et al: The ischaemic leg: a long-term follow-up with special reference to the predictive value of the systolic digital blood pressure. Part I. No arterial reconstruction, *Thorac Cardiovasc Surgeon* 37:348, 1989.
5. Anderson WR: Necrotizing angitis associated with embolization of cholesterol, *Am J Clin Pathol* 43:65, 1965.
6. Baker JD: Poststress Doppler ankle pressures, *Arch Surg* 113:1171, 1978.
7. Baker JD, Dix D: Variability of Doppler ankle pressures with arterial occlusive disease: an evaluation of ankle index and brachial-ankle pressure gradient, *Surgery* 89:134, 1981.
8. Baker RJ, Chunprapagh B, Nyhus LM: Severe ischemia of the hand following radial artery catheterization, *Surgery* 80:449, 1976.
9. Baker WH, Barnes RW: Revitalizing the ischemic limb, *Geriatrics* 28:56, 1973.
10. Barner HB et al: Intermittent claudication with pedal pulses, *JAMA* 204:958, 1968.
11. Barnes RW et al: Complications of percutaneous femoral arterial catheterization, *Am J Cardiol* 33:259, 1974.
12. Beach KW, Strandness DE Jr: Arteriosclerosis obliterans and associated risk factors in insulin-dependent and non-insulin-dependent diabetes, *Diabetes* 29:882, 1980.
13. Beach KW, Brunzell JD, Strandness DE Jr: Prevalence of severe arteriosclerosis obliterans in patients with diabetes mellitus, *Arteriosclerosis* 2:275, 1982.
14. Bell G et al: Indirect measurement of systolic blood pressure in the lower limb using a mercury-in-rubber strain gauge, *Cardiovascular Res* 7:282, 1973.
15. Bell G et al: Measurements of systolic pressure in the limbs of patients with arterial occlusive disease, *Surg Gynecol Obstet* 136:177, 1973.
16. Bernstein EF et al: Thigh pressure artifacts with noninvasive techniques in an experimental model, *Surgery* 89:319, 1981.
17. Blebea J et al: Laser angioplasty in peripheral vascular disease: symptomatic versus hemodynamic results, *J Vasc Surg* 13:222, 1991.
18. Bloom JD et al: Defective limb growth as a complication of catheterization of the femoral artery, *Surg Gynecol Obstet* 138:524, 1974.
19. Bloor K: Natural history of arteriosclerosis of the lower extremities, *Ann R Coll Surg Engl* 28:36, 1961.
20. Bollinger A, Barras JP, Mahler F: Measurement of foot artery blood pressure by micromanometry in normal subjects and in patients with arterial occlusive disease, *Circulation* 53:506, 1976.
21. Bollinger A, Mahler F, Gruentzig A: Peripheral hemodynamics in patients with coarctation, normotensive and hypertensive arteriosclerosis obliterans of the lower limbs, *Angiology* 22:354, 1971.
22. Bollinger A, Mahler F, Zehender O: Kombinierte Druck- und Durchflussmessungen in der Beurteilung arterieller Durchblutungsstörungen, *Dtsch Med Wochenschr* 95:1039, 1970.
23. Bone GE, Pomajzl MJ: Toe blood pressure by photoplethysmography: an index of healing in forefoot amputation, *Surgery* 89:569, 1981.
24. Boyd AM: The natural course of arteriosclerosis of the lower extremities, *Proc R Soc Med* 55:591, 1962.
25. Brener BJ, et al: Measurement of systolic femoral arterial pressure during reactive hyperemia: an estimate of aortoiliac disease, *Circulation* 50(suppl):259, 1974.
26. Bryant LR, Spencer FC: Occlusive disease of subclavian artery, *JAMA* 196:109, 1966.
27. Burgess EM et al: Segmental transcutaneous measurements of Po_2 in patients requiring below-the-knee amputation in peripheral vascular insufficiency, *J Bone Joint Surg* 64A:378, 1982.
28. Cappelen C Jr, Hall KV: The effect of obstructive arterial disease on the peripheral arterial blood pressure, *Surgery* 48:888, 1960.
29. Carter SA: Indirect systolic pressures and pulse waves in arterial occlusive disease of the lower extremities, *Circulation* 37:624, 1968.
30. Carter SA: Clinical measurement of systolic pressures in limbs with arterial occlusive disease, *JAMA* 207:1869, 1969.

31. Carter SA: Response of ankle systolic pressure to leg exercise in mild or questionable arterial disease, *N Engl J Med* 287:578, 1972.
32. Carter SA: The relationship of distal systolic pressures to healing of skin lesions in limbs with arterial occlusive disease, with special reference to diabetes mellitus, *Scand J Clin Lab Invest* 31(suppl 128):239, 1973.
33. Carter SA: Effect of age, cardiovascular disease, and vasomotor changes on transmission of arterial pressure waves through the lower extremities, *Angiology* 29:601, 1978.
34. Carter SA: Arterial auscultation in peripheral vascular disease, *JAMA* 261:1682, 1981.
35. Carter SA: Finger systolic pressures and skin temperatures in severe Raynaud's syndrome: the relationship to healing of skin lesions and the use of oral phenoxybenzamine, *Angiology* 32:298, 1981.
36. Carter SA: The definition of critical ischaemia of the lower limb and distal systolic pressures, *Br J Surg* 70:188, 1983.
37. Carter SA: The effect of cooling on toe systolic pressures in subjects with and without Raynaud's syndrome in the lower extremities, *Clin Physiol* 11:253, 1991.
37a. Carter SA: Elective foot surgery in limbs with arterial disease, *Clin Orthop* (in press).
38. Carter SA, Lezack JD: Digital systolic pressures in the lower limb in arterial disease, *Circulation* 43:905, 1971.
39. Carter SA, Tate RB: The effect of body heating and cooling on the ankle and toe systolic pressures in arterial disease, *J Vasc Surg* 16:148, 1992.
40. Carter SA, Dean E, Kroeger EA: Apparent finger systolic pressures during cooling in Raynaud's syndrome, *Circulation* 77:988, 1988.
41. Carter SA et al: Walking ability and ankle systolic pressures: observations in patients with intermittent claudication in a short-term walking exercise program, *J Vasc Surg* 10:642, 1989.
42. Castaneda-Zuniga W et al: Hemodynamic assessment of obstructive aortoiliac disease, *Am J Roentgenol* 127:559, 1976.
43. Chamberlain J, Housley E, Macpherson AIS: The relationship between ultrasound assessment and angiography in occlusive arterial disease of the lower limb, *Br J Surg* 62:64, 1975.
44. Chavatzas D, Jamieson CW: The doubtful place of the raised heel in patients with intermittent claudication of the leg, *Br J Surg* 61:299, 1974.
45. Clifford PC et al: Intermittent claudication: is a supervised exercise class worthwhile? *Br Med J* 280:1503, 1980.
46. Clyne CAC et al: Oxygen tension on the skin of ischemic legs, *Am J Surg* 143:315, 1982.
47. Conrad MC: Large and small artery occlusion in diabetics and nondiabetics with severe vascular disease, *Circulation* 36:83, 1967.
48. Conrad MC: Abnormalities of the digital vasculature as related to ulceration and gangrene, *Circulation* 38:568, 1968.
49. Conrad MC, Green HD: Hemodynamics of large and small vessels in peripheral vascular disease, *Circulation* 29:847, 1964.
50. Criqui MH et al: The prevalence of peripheral arterial disease in a defined population, *Circulation* 71:510, 1985.
51. Cutajar CL, Marston A, Newcombe JF: Value of cuff occlusion pressures in assessment of peripheral vascular disease, *Br Med J* 2:392, 1973.
52. Dahllöf AG et al: Metabolic activity of skeletal muscle in patients with peripheral arterial insufficiency, *Eur J Clin Invest* 4:9, 1974.
53. Darling RC et al: Intermittent claudication in young athletes: popliteal artery entrapment syndrome, *J Trauma* 14:543, 1974.
54. Delius W: Hämodynamische Untersuchungen über den systolischen Blutdruck und die arterielle Durchblutung distal von arteriellen Gefässverschlüssen an den unteren Extremitäten, *Z Kreislaufforsch* 58:319, 1969.
55. Dick R: Arteriography in neurovascular compression at the thoracic outlet, with special reference to embolic patterns, *Am J Roentgenol Radium Ther Nucl Med* 110:141, 1970.
56. Dormandy JA, Goyle KB, Reid HL: Treatment of severe intermittent claudication by controlled defibrination, *Lancet* 1:625, 1977.
57. Doupe J, Newman HW, Wilkins RW: The effect of peripheral vasomotor activity on systolic arterial pressure in the extremities of man, *J Physiol* 95:244, 1939.
58. Downs AR et al: Assessment of arterial obstruction in vessels supplying the fingers by measurement of local blood pressures and the skin temperature response test—correlation with angiographic evidence, *Surgery* 77:530, 1975.

59. Edmonds ME, Roberts VC, Watkins PJ: Blood flow in the diabetic neuropathic foot, *Diabetologia* 22:9, 1982.
60. Edmonds ME et al: Medial arterial calcification and diabetic neuropathy, *Br Med J* 284:928, 1982.
61. Edwards WS, Carmichael JD: Aorto-iliac reconstruction without preoperative aortogram, *Ann Surg* 165:853, 1967.
62. Eickhoff JH, Engell HC: Transcutaneous oxygen tension (tcPO₂) measurements on the foot in normal subjects and in patients with peripheral arterial disease admitted for vascular surgery, *Scand J Clin Lab Invest* 41:743, 1981.
63. Evans JG: Neurogenic intermittent claudication, *Br Med J* 2:985, 1964.
64. Fenton TR, Carter SA, Vaishnav RN: Collapse and viscoelasticity of diseased human arteries, *J Biomechanics* 17:789, 1984.
65. Flanigan DP et al: Utility of wide and narrow blood pressure cuffs in the hemodynamic assessment of aorto-iliac occlusive disease, *Surgery* 92:16, 1982.
66. Formijne P: Investigation of the patency of peripheral arteries, *Am Heart J* 10:1, 1934.
67. Fowkes FGR et al: Variability of ankle and brachial systolic pressures in the measurement of atherosclerotic peripheral arterial disease, *J Epidemiol Community Health* 42:128, 1988.
68. Franzeck UK, Bernstein EF, Fronek A: The effect of sensing site on the limb segmental blood pressure determination, *Arch Surg* 116:912, 1981.
69. French JW, Guntheroth WG: An explanation of asymmetric upper extremity blood pressures in supravalvular aortic stenosis, *Circulation* 42:31, 1970.
70. Fronek A, Coel M, Bernstein EF: Quantitative ultrasonographic studies of lower extremity flow velocities in health and disease, *Circulation* 53:957, 1976.
71. Fronek A, Coel M, Bernstein EF: The importance of combined multisegmental pressure and Doppler flow velocity studies in the diagnosis of peripheral arterial occlusive disease, *Surgery* 84:840, 1978.
72. Fronek A et al: Noninvasive physiologic tests in the diagnosis and characterization of peripheral arterial occlusive disease, *Am J Surg* 126:205, 1973.
73. Fronek A et al: Ultrasonographically monitored postocclusive reactive hyperemia in the diagnosis of peripheral arterial occlusive disease, *Circulation* 48:149, 1973.
74. Gaskell P: The rate of blood flow in the foot and calf before and after reconstruction by arterial grafting of an occluded main artery to the lower limb, *Clin Sci* 15:259, 1956.
75. Gaskell P: Laboratory tests of circulation in the limbs, *Manitoba Med Rev* 45:540, 1965.
76. Gaskell P: The measurement of blood pressure, the critical opening pressure, and the critical closing pressure of digital vessels under various circumstances, *Can J Physiol Pharmacol* 43:979, 1965.
77. Gaskell P: The importance of penile blood pressure in cases of impotence, *Can Med Assoc J* 105:1047, 1971.
78. Gaskell P: Personal communication, 1979.
79. Gaskell P, Becker WJ: The erect posture as an aid to the circulation in the feet in the presence of arterial obstruction, *Can Med Assoc J* 105:930, 1971.
80. Gaskell P, Krisman AM: An auscultatory technique for measuring the digital blood pressure, *Can J Biochem Physiol* 36:883, 1958.
81. Gaskell P, Krisman AM: The brachial to digital blood pressure gradient in normal subjects and in patients with high blood pressure, *Can J Biochem Physiol* 36:889, 1958.
82. Gaskell P, Parrott JCW: The effect of a mechanical venous pump on the circulation of the feet in the presence of arterial obstruction, *Surg Gynecol Obstet* 146:583, 1978.
83. Geddes LA, Tivey R: The importance of cuff width in measurement of blood pressure indirectly, *Cardiovasc Res Cent Bull* 14:69, 1976.
84. Gibbon JH, Landis EM: Vasodilatation in lower extremities in response to immersing forearms in warm water, *J Clin Invest* 11:1019, 1932.
85. Gilfillan RS, Leeds FH, Spotts RR: The prediction of healing in ischemic lesions of the foot. A comparison of Doppler ultrasound and elevation reactive hyperemia, *J Cardiovasc Surg* 26:15, 1985.
86. Goebel FD, Füessl HS: Mönckeberg's sclerosis after sympathetic denervation in diabetic and non-diabetic subjects, *Diabetologia* 24:347, 1983.
87. Gosling RG, King DH: Arterial assessment by Doppler-shift ultrasound, *Proc R Soc Med* 67:447, 1974.
88. Greenfield ADM, Shepherd T, Whelan RF: The proportion of the total hand blood flow passing through the digits, *J Physiol* 113:63, 1951.
89. Grüntzig A, Schlumpf M, Bollinger A: *Direkt und indirekt gemessner Druckgradient bei Stenosen der Becken- und Oberschenkelarterien.* In Kriessman A, Bollinger A, eds: *Ultraschall-Doppler-Diagnostik in der Angiologie,* Stuttgart, 1978, Georg Thieme Verlag.
90. Gundersen J: Diagnosis of arterial insufficiency with measurement of blood pressure in fingers and toes, *Angiology* 22:191, 1971.
91. Gundersen J: Segmental measurements of systolic blood pressure in the extremities including the thumb and the great toe, *Acta Chir Scand* 426(suppl):1, 1972.
92. Haimovici H, Escher DJ: Aortoiliac stenosis, *Arch Surg* 72:107, 1956.
93. Hällgren R et al: Arterial calcification and progressive peripheral gangrene after renal transplantation, *Acta Med Scand* 198:331, 1975.
94. Heintz SE et al: Value of arterial pressure measurements in the proximal and distal part of the thigh in arterial occlusive disease, *Surg Gynecol Obstet* 146:337, 1978.
95. Hiatt WR et al: Diagnostic methods for peripheral arterial disease in the San Luis Valley diabetes study, *J Clin Epidemiol* 43:597, 1990.
96. Hirai M: Arterial insufficiency of the hand evaluated by digital blood pressure and arteriographic findings, *Circulation* 58:902, 1978.
97. Hirai M: Cold sensitivity of the hand in arterial occlusive disease, *Surgery* 85:140, 1979.
98. Hirai M, Shionoya S: Intermittent claudication in the foot and Buerger's disease, *Br J Surg* 65:210, 1978.
99. Hirai M, Nielsen SL, Lassen NA: Blood pressure measurement of all five fingers by strain gauge plethysmography, *Scand J Clin Lab Invest* 36:627, 1976.
100. Hoare M et al: The effect of local cooling on digital systolic pressure in patients with Raynaud's syndrome, *Br J Surg* 69(suppl):S27, 1982.
101. Hobbs JT et al: A limitation of the Doppler ultrasound method of measuring ankle systolic pressure, *Vasa* 3:160, 1974.
102. Holstein P, Lassen NA: Radioisotope clearance technique for measurement of distal blood pressure in skin and muscles, *Scand J Clin Lab Invest* 31(suppl 128):143, 1973.
103. Holstein P, Lassen NA: Healing of ulcers on the feet correlated with distal blood pressure measurements in occlusive arterial disease, *Acta Orthop Scand* 51:995, 1980.
104. Holstein P, Sager P: Toe blood pressure in peripheral arterial disease, *Acta Orthop Scand* 44:564, 1973.
105. Holstein P, Dovey H, Lassen NA: Wound healing in above-knee amputations in relation to skin perfusion pressure, *Acta Orthop Scand* 50:59, 1979.
106. Holstein P, Sager P, Lassen NA: Wound healing in below-knee amputations in relation to skin perfusion pressure, *Acta Orthop Scand* 50:49, 1979.
107. Hummel BW et al: Reactive hyperemia vs. treadmill exercise testing in arterial disease, *Arch Surg* 113:95, 1978.
108. Hutchison KJ, Williams HT: Calf blood flow and ankle systolic blood pressure in intermittent claudication monitored over five years, *Angiology* 29:719, 1978.
109. Ibels LS et al: Arterial calcification and pathology in uremic patients undergoing dialysis, *Am J Med* 66:790, 1979.
110. Janzon L et al: The arm-ankle pressure gradient in relation to cardiovascular risk factors in intermittent claudication, *Circulation* 63:1339, 1981.
111. Jelnes R et al: Fate in intermittent claudication: outcome and risk factors, *Br Med J* 293:1137, 1986.
112. Jeresaty RM, Liss JP: Effects of brachial artery catheterization on arterial pulse and blood pressure in 203 patients, *Am Heart J* 76:481, 1968.
113. Jogestrand T, Berglund B: Estimation of digital circulation and its correlation to clinical signs of ischaemia—a comparative methodological study, *Clin Physiol* 3:307, 1983.
114. Johnson CD, Zirkle TJ, Smith LL: Occlusive disease of the vessels of the aortic arch, *Calif Med* 108:20, 1968.
115. Johnson WC: Doppler ankle pressure and reactive hyperemia in the diagnosis of arterial insufficiency, *J Surg Res* 18:177, 1975.
116. Johnston KW: Role of Doppler ultrasonography in determining the hemodynamic significance of aortoiliac disease, *Can J Surg* 21:319, 1978.

117. Johnston KW, Taraschuk I: Validation of the role of pulsatility index in quantitation of the severity of peripheral arterial occlusive disease, *Am J Surg* 131:295, 1976.

118. Johnston KW, Colapinto RF, Baird RJ: Transluminal dilation, *Arch Surg* 117:1604, 1982.

119. Johnston KW, Hosang MY, Andrews DF: Reproducibility of non-invasive vascular laboratory measurements of the peripheral circulation, *J Vasc Surg* 6:147, 1987.

120. Karanfilian RG et al: The value of laser Doppler velocimetry and transcutaneous oxygen determination in predicting healing of ischemic forefoot ulcerations and amputations in diabetic and nondiabetic patients. *J Vasc Surg* 4:511, 1986.

121. Kaufman SL et al: Hemodynamic measurements in the evaluation and follow-up of transluminal angioplasty of the iliac and femoral arteries, *Radiology* 142:329, 1982.

122. Kazmier FJ et al: Livedo reticularis and digital infarcts: a syndrome due to cholesterol emboli arising from atheromatous abdominal aortic aneurysms, *Vasc Dis* 3:12, 1966.

123. Kempczinski RF, Buckley CJ, Darling RC: Vascular insufficiency secondary to ergotism, *Surgery* 79:597, 1976.

124. King LT, Strandness DE Jr, Bell JW: The hemodynamic response of the lower extremities to exercise, *J Surg Res* 5:167, 1965.

125. Knox WG, Finby N, Moscarella AA: Limitations of arteriography in determining operability for femoropopliteal occlusive disease, *Ann Surg* 161:509, 1965.

126. Kotte JH, Iglaner A, McGuire J: Measurements of arterial blood pressure in arm and leg: comparison of sphygmomanometric and direct intra-arterial pressures with special attention to their relationship in aortic regurgitation, *Am Heart J* 28:476, 1944.

127. Kottke BA, Fairbairn JH II, Davis GD: Complications of aortography, *Circulation* 30:843, 1964.

128. Krähenbühl B, Nielsen SL, Lassen NA: Closure of digital arteries in high vascular tone states as demonstrated by measurement of systolic blood pressure in the fingers, *Scand J Clin Lab Invest* 37:71, 1977.

129. Kroeker EJ, Wood EH: Beat-to-beat alterations in relationship of simultaneously recorded central and peripheral arterial pressure pulses during Valsalva maneuver and prolonged expiration in man, *J Appl Physiol* 8:483, 1956.

130. Lamis PA, Stanton PE Jr, Hyland L: The axillo-axillary bypass graft, *Arch Surg* 111:1353, 1976.

131. Larsen OA, Lassen NA: Medical treatment of occlusive arterial disease of the legs, *Angiologia* 6:288, 1969.

132. Lassen NA, Holstein P: Use of radioisotopes in assessment of distal blood flow and distal blood pressure in arterial insufficiency, *Surg Clin North Am* 54:39, 1974.

133. Lassen NA, Krähenbühl B, Hirai M: Occlusion cuff for routine measurement of digital blood pressure and blood flow, *Am J Physiol* 232:H338, 1977.

134. Lassen NA, Tönnesen KH, Holstein P: Distal blood pressure (editorial), *Scand J Clin Lab Invest* 36:705, 1976.

135. Lassen NA et al: Distal blood pressure measurements in occlusive arterial disease, strain gauge compared to xenon-133, *Angiology* 23:211, 1972.

136. Lazarus HM et al: *Doppler ankle pressures and stiff arteries*. In Diethrich EB, ed: *Noninvasive cardiovascular diagnosis: current concepts*, Baltimore, 1978, University Park Press.

137. Lennihan R Jr, Mackereth MA: Ankle blood pressures as a practical aid in vascular practice, *Angiology* 26:211, 1975.

138. Lewis JD: Pressure measurements in the long-term follow-up of peripheral vascular disease, *Proc R Soc Med* 67:443, 1974.

139. Lewis JD et al: Simultaneous flow and pressure measurements in intermittent claudication, *Br J Surg* 59:418, 1972.

140. Lezack JD, Carter SA: Systolic pressures in arterial occlusive disease with special reference to the effect of posture, *Clin Res* 17:638, 1969.

141. Lezack JD, Carter SA: Systolic pressures in the extremities of man with special reference to the toes, *Can J Physiol Pharmacol* 48:469, 1970.

142. Lezack JD, Carter SA: The relationship of distal systolic pressures to the clincial and angiographic findings in limbs with arterial occlusive disease, *Scand J Clin Lab Invest* 31(suppl 128):97, 1973.

143. Lorentsen E: Blood pressure and flow in the calf in relation to claudication distance, *Scand J Clin Lab Invest* 31:141, 1973.

144. Lorentsen E: Calf blood pressure measurements. The applicability of a plethysmographic method and the results of measurements during reactive hyperaemia, *Scand J Clin Lab Invest* 31:69, 1973.

145. Lorentsen E: The vascular resistance in the arteries of the lower leg in normal subjects and in patients with different degrees of atherosclerotic disease, *Scand J Clin Lab Invest* 31:147, 1973.

146. Lynn RB, Steiner RE, Van Wyk FAK: Arteriographic appearance of the digital arteries of the hands in Raynaud's disease, *Lancet* 1:471, 1955.

147. Mahler F, Schlumpf M, Bollinger A: *Knöchelarteriendruck nach standardisierter Gehbelastung bei Gesunden und bei Patienten mit arterieller Verschlusskrankheit*. In Kriessman A, Bollinger A, eds: *Ultraschall-Doppler-Diagnostik in der Angiologie*, Stuttgart, 1978, Georg Thieme Verlag.

148. Mahler F et al: Postocclusion and postexercise flow velocity and ankle pressures in normals and marathon runners, *Angiology* 27:721, 1976.

149. Malone JM et al: The "Gold Standard" for amputation level selection: xenon-133 clearance, *J Surg Res* 30:449, 1981.

150. Matesanz JM, Patwardhan N, Herrmann JB: A simplified method for evaluating peripheral arterial occlusive disease in a clinical vascular laboratory, *Angiology* 29:791, 1978.

151. May AG et al: Critical arterial stenosis, *Surgery* 54:250, 1963.

152. McEwan AJ, Ledingham IM: Blood flow characteristics and tissue nutrition in apparently ischaemic feet, *Br Med J* 3:220, 1971.

153. McEwan AJ, Stalker CG, Ledingham IM: Foot skin ischaemia in atherosclerotic peripheral vascular disease, *Br Med J* 3:612, 1970.

154. Metz P: Erectile function in men with occlusive arterial disease in the legs, *Dan Med Bull* 30:185, 1983.

155. Metz P, Bengtsson J: Penile blood pressure, *Scand J Urol Nephrol* 15:161, 1981.

156. Mitchell PL, Parlin RW, Blackburn H: Effect of vertical displacement of the arm on indirect blood-pressure measurement, *N Engl J Med* 271:72, 1964.

157. Montgomery H, Naide M, Freeman NE: The significance of diagnostic tests in the study of peripheral vascular disease, *Am Heart J* 21:780, 1941.

158. Mozersky DJ, Sumner DS, Strandness DE Jr: Long-term results of reconstructive aortoiliac surgery, *Am J Surg* 123:503, 1972.

159. Naumann M: Der Blutdruck in der Arteria dorsalis pedis in der Norm und bei Kreislaufstörungen, *Z Kreislaufforsch* 31:36, 1939.

160. Nicolaides AN, Fernandes e Fernandes J, Angelides NA: *The effect of profundaplasty on ankle pressure and walking distance: an objective assessment using Doppler ultrasound and a treadmill*. In Diethrich EB, ed: *Noninvasive cardiovascular diagnosis: current concepts*, Baltimore, 1978, University Park Press.

161. Nielsen PE: Digital blood presure in patients with peripheral arterial disease, *Scand J Clin Lab Invest* 36:731, 1976.

162. Nielsen PE: Digital blood pressure in normal subjects and patients with peripheral arterial disease, *Scand J Clin Lab Invest* 36:725, 1976.

163. Nielsen PE, Nielsen SL: Digital arterial tone in hypertensive subjects treated with cardioselective and non-selective beta-adrenoreceptor blocking agents, *Dan Med Bull* 28:76, 1981.

164. Nielsen PE, Rasmussen SM: Indirect measurement of systolic blood pressure by strain gauge technique at finger, ankle and toe in diabetic patients without symptoms of occlusive arterial disease, *Diabetologia* 9:25, 1973.

165. Nielsen PE, Barras JP, Holstein P: Systolic pressure amplification in the arteries of normal subjects, *Scand J Clin Lab Invest* 33:371, 1974.

166. Nielsen PE, Bell G, Lassen NA: The measurement of digital systolic blood pressure by strain gauge technique, *Scand J Clin Lab Invest* 29:371, 1972.

167. Nielsen PE, Poulsen HL, Gyntelberg F: Skin blood pressure measured by a photoelectric probe and external counterpressure, *Scand J Clin Lab Invest* 31(suppl 128):137, 1973.

168. Nielsen PE et al: Reduction in distal blood pressure by sympathetic nerve block in patients with occlusive arterial disease, *Cardiovasc Res* 7:577, 1973.

169. Nielsen PH et al: The ischaemic leg: a long-term follow-up with special reference to the predictive value of the systolic digital blood pressure. Part II. After arterial reconstruction, *Thorac Cardiovasc Surgeon* 37:351, 1989.

170. Nielsen SL: Raynaud phenomena and finger systolic pressure during cooling, *Scand J Clin Lab Invest* 38:765, 1978.

171. Nielsen SL, Lassen NA: Measurement of digital blood pressure after local cooling, *J Appl Physiol* 43:907, 1977.

172. Nielsen SL, Olsen N, Henriksen O: Cold hypersensitivity after sympathectomy for Raynaud's disease, *Scand J Thor Cardiovasc Surg* 14:109, 1980.

173. Nielsen SL, Sørensen CJ, Olsen N: Thermostatted measurement of systolic blood pressure on cooled fingers, *Scand J Clin Lab Invest* 40:683, 1980.

174. Nielsen SL et al: Raynaud's phenomenon in arterial obstructive disease of the hand demonstrated by locally provoked cooling, *Scand J Thor Cardiovasc Surg* 12:105, 1978.

175. Nobin BA et al: Reserpine treatment of Raynaud's disease, *Ann Surg* 187:12, 1978.

176. Noer I, Tønnesen KH, Sager P: Preoperative estimation of run off in patients with multiple level arterial obstructions as a guide to partial reconstructive surgery, *Ann Surg* 188:663, 1978.

177. Oliva I, Roztocîl K: Toe pulse wave analysis in obliterating atherosclerosis, *Angiology* 34:610, 1983.

178. O'Mara CS et al: Hemodynamic assessment of transluminal angioplasty for lower extremity ischemia, *Surgery* 89:106, 1981.

179. O'Rourke MF et al: Pressure wave transmission along the human aorta, *Circ Res* 23:567, 1968.

180. Osmundson PJ: A prospective study of peripheral occlusive arterial disease in diabetes. II. Vascular laboratory assessment, *Mayo Clin Proc* 56:223, 1981.

181. Ouriel K et al: A critical evaluation of stress testing in the diagnosis of peripheral vascular disease, *Surgery* 91:686, 1982.

182. Paaske WP, Tønnesen KH: Prognostic significance of distal blood pressure measurements in patients with severe ischaemia, *Scand J Thor Cardiovasc Surg* 14:105, 1980.

183. Pascarelli EF, Bertrand CA: Comparison of blood pressures in the arms and legs, *N Engl J Med* 270:693, 1964.

184. Patel A, Toole JF: Subclavian steal syndrome—reversal of cephalic blood flow, *Medicine (Baltimore)* 44:289, 1965.

185. Piccone VA Jr, Karvounis P, LeVeen HH: The subclavian steal syndrome, *Angiology* 21:240, 1970.

186. Postlethwaite JC, Dormandy JA: Results of ankle systolic pressure measurements in patients with intermittent claudication being treated with clofibrate, *Ann Surg* 181:799, 1975.

187. Prineas RJ et al: Recommendations for use of noninvasive methods to detect atherosclerotic peripheral arterial disease—in population studies, *Circulation* 65:1561A, 1982.

188. Quick CR, Cotton LT: The measured effect of stopping smoking on intermittent claudication, *Br J Surg* 69(suppl):S24, 1982.

189. Rahman A, Rodbard S: Timing of the arterial sounds in the subclavian steal syndrome, *Arch Intern Med* 125:1027, 1970.

190. Raines JK et al: Vascular laboratory criteria for the management of peripheral vascular disease of the lower extremities, *Surgery* 79:21, 1976.

191. Ramsey DE, Manke DA, Sumner DS: Toe blood pressure a valuable adjunct to ankle pressure measurement for assessing peripheral arterial disease, *J Cardiovasc Surg* 24:43, 1983.

192. Reinle E: Über Blutdruckdifferenzen zwischen rechtem und linkem Arm, *Schweiz Med Wochenschr* 93:1616, 1963.

193. Roddie IC, Shepherd JT, Whelan RF: The contribution of constrictor and dilator nerves to the skin vasodilatation during body heating, *J Physiol* 136:489, 1957.

194. Rutherford RB: Standards for evaluating results of interventional therapy for peripheral vascular disease, *Circulation* 83(suppl I):I-6, 1991.

195. Rutherford RB et al: Suggested standards for reports dealing with lower extremity ischemia, *J Vasc Surg* 4:80, 1986.

196. Sacks AH: Indirect blood pressure measurements: a matter of interpretation, *Angiology* 30:683, 1979.

197. Sako Y: Value of flowmeter and pressure measurements during vascular surgery: clinical and experimental, *Surg Clin North Am* 47:1383, 1967.

198. Saltin B: *Physical training in patients with intermittent claudication.* In Cohen LS, Mock I, Ringquist MB, eds: *Physical conditioning and cardiovascular rehabilitation,* New York, 1981, John Wiley & Sons.

199. Sawka AM, Carter SA: The effect of temperature on digital systolic pressures in the lower limb in arterial disease, *Circulation* 85:1097, 1992.

200. Schatz IJ: *The natural history of peripheral arteriosclerosis.* In Brest AN, Moyer JH, eds: *Atherosclerotic vascular disease: a Hahnemann symposium,* New York, 1967, Appleton-Century-Crofts.

201. Schatz IJ, Fine G, Eyler WR: Thromboangiitis obliterans, *Br Heart J* 28:84, 1966.

202. Schroll M, Munck O: Estimation of peripheral arteriosclerotic disease by ankle blood pressure measurements in a population study of 60-year-old men and women, *J Chronic Dis* 34:261, 1981.

203. Schultz RD, Hokanson DF, Strandness DF Jr: Pressure-flow and stress-strain measurements of normal and diseased aortoiliac segments, *Surg Gynecol Obstet* 124:1267, 1967.

204. Schwartz JA et al: Predictive value of distal perfusion pressure in the healing of amputation of the digits and the forefoot, *Surg Gynecol Obstet* 154:865, 1982.

205. Siggaard-Andersen J et al: Blood pressure measurements of the lower limb. Arterial occlusions in the calf determined by plethysmographic blood pressure measurements in the thigh and at the ankle, *Angiology* 23:350, 1972.

206. Skinner JS, Strandness DE Jr: Exercise and intermittent claudication. I. Effect of repetition and intensity of exercise, *Circulation* 36:15, 1967.

207. Skinner JS, Strandness DE Jr: Exercise and intermittent claudication. II. Effect of physical training, *Circulation* 36:23, 1967.

208. Sprague DH, Kim DI: Pseudohypertension due to Mönckeberg's arteriosclerosis, *Anesth Analg* 57:588, 1978.

209. Stahler C, Strandness DE Jr: Ankle blood pressure response to graded treadmill exercise, *Angiology* 18:237, 1967.

210. Stegall HF, Kardon MB, Kemmerer WT: Indirect measurement of arterial blood pressure by Doppler ultrasonic sphygmomanometry, *J Appl Physiol* 25:793, 1968.

211. Strandness DE Jr: *Peripheral arterial disease. A physiologic approach,* Boston, 1969, Little, Brown.

212. Strandness DE Jr: Exercise testing in the evaluation of patients undergoing direct arterial surgery, *J Cardiovasc Surg* 11:192, 1970.

213. Strandness DE Jr: *Common pitfalls in the noninvasive evaluation of lower extremity renal insufficiency.* In Diethrich EB, ed: *Noninvasive cardiovascular diagnosis: current concepts,* Baltimore, 1978, University Park Press.

214. Strandness DE Jr, Bell JW: An evaluation of the hemodynamic response of the claudicating extremity to exercise, *Surg Gynecol Obstet* 119:1237, 1964.

215. Strandness DE Jr, Bell JW: Peripheral vascular disease: diagnosis and objective evaluation using a mercury strain gauge, *Ann Surg* 161(suppl 4):1, 1965.

216. Strandness DE Jr, Stahler C: Arteriosclerosis obliterans. Manner and rate of progression, *JAMA* 196:1, 1966.

217. Strandness DE Jr, Sumner DS: Applications of ultrasound to the study of arteriosclerosis obliterans, *Angiology* 26:187, 1975.

218. Strandness DE Jr, Gibbons GE, Bell JW: Mercury strain gauge plethysmography. Evaluation of patients with acquired arteriovenous fistula, *Arch Surg* 85:215, 1962.

219. Strandness DE Jr, Priest RE, Gibbons GE: Combined clinical and pathologic study of diabetic and nondiabetic peripheral vascular disease, *Diabetes* 13:366, 1964.

220. Sturm A Jr, Puentes F, Scheja HW: Ursachen der Blutdruckdifferenzen zwischen dem rechten und linken Arm, *Dtsch Med Wochenschr* 95:1914, 1970.

221. Sugiura T, Freis ED: Pressure pulse in small arteries, *Circ Res* 11:838, 1962.

222. Sumner DS: Presidential address: noninvasive testing of vascular disease—fact, fancy, and future, *Surgery* 93:644, 1983.

223. Sumner DS: *Noninvasive assessment of peripheral arterial occlusive disease.* In Rutherford RB, ed: *Vascular surgery,* ed 3, Philadelphia, 1989, WB Saunders.

224. Sumner DS, Strandness DE Jr: The relationship between calf blood flow and ankle blood pressure in patients with intermittent claudication, *Surgery* 65:763, 1969.

225. Taguchi JT, Suwangool P: "Pipestem" brachial arteries. A cause of pseudohypertension, *JAMA* 228:733, 1974.

226. Taylor MG: *Wave travel in arteries and the design of the cardiovascular system.* In Attinger EO, ed: *Pulsatile blood flow,* New York, 1964, McGraw-Hill.

227. Thulesius O: *Beurteilung des Schweregrades arterieller Durchblutungsstörungen mit dem Doppler-Ultraschallgerät.* In Bollinger A, Brunner U, eds: *Aktuelle Probleme in der Angiologie,* Bern, 1971, Hans Huber.

228. Thulesius O, Gjöres JE: Use of Doppler shift detection for determining peripheral arterial blood pressure, *Angiology* 22:594, 1971.

229. Thulesius O, Länne T: *The importance of arterial compliance and tone for the determination of ankle systolic pressure,* Paper presented at the Thirteenth World Congress of the International Union of Angiology, Rochester, Minn, 1983.

230. Thulesius O, Brubakk A, Berlin E: Response of digital blood pressure to cold provocation in cases with Raynaud's phenomena, *Angiology* 32:113, 1981.

231. Thulesius O, Valmin K, Todoreskov R: Response of finger systolic blood pressure to cold provocation in cases with hypertension and diabetes, *Clin Physiol* 2:513, 1982.

232. Tønnesen KH et al: Classification of peripheral occlusive arterial diseases based on symptoms, signs, and distal blood pressure measurements, *Acta Chir Scand* 146:101, 1980.

233. Tooke J: European consensus document on critical limb ischaemia, *Vasc Med Rev* 1:85, 1990.

234. Toole JF, Tulloch EF: Bilateral simultaneous sphygmomanometry. A new diagnostic test for subclavian steal syndrome, *Circulation* 33:952, 1966.

235. Velayos ED et al: Clinical correlation analysis of 137 patients with Raynaud's phenomenon, *Am J Med Sci* 262:347, 1970.

236. Vincent DG et al: Noninvasive assessment of toe systolic pressures with special reference to diabetes mellitus, *J Cardiovasc Surg* 24:22, 1983.

237. Weismann RE, Upson JF: Intra-arterial pressure studies in patients with arterial insufficiency of lower extremities, *Ann Surg* 157:501, 1963.

238. Wezler K, Standl R: Die normalen Alterskurven der Pulswellengeschwindigkeit in clastischen und muskulären Arterien des Menschen, *Z Biol* 97:265, 1936.

239. White RA et al: Noninvasive evaluation of peripheral vascular disease using transcutaneous oxygen tension, *Am J Surg* 144:68, 1982.

240. Widmer LK, Staub H: Blutdruck in stenosierten Arterien, *Z Kreislaufforsch* 51:975, 1962.

241. Wilbur BG, Olcott C IV: *A comparison of three modes of stress on Doppler ankle pressures.* In Diethrich EB, ed: *Noninvasive cardiovascular diagnosis: current concepts,* Baltimore, 1978, University Park Press.

242. Wilson SE, Wolf GL, Cross AP: Percutaneous transluminal angioplasty versus operation for peripheral arteriosclerosis, *J Vasc Surg* 9:1, 1989.

243. Winsor T: Influence of arterial disease on the systolic blood pressure gradients of the extremity, *Am J Med Sci* 220:117, 1950.

244. Wyss CR et al: Transcutaneous oxygen tension as a predictor of success after amputation, *J Bone Joint Surg* 70A:203, 1988.

245. Yao JST: Haemodynamic studies in peripheral arterial disease, *Br J Surg* 57:761, 1970.

246. Yao JST: Exercise testing using Doppler ultrasound and xenon clearance techniques, *Angiology* 26:528, 1975.

247. Yao JST, Hobbs JT, Irvine WT: Ankle systolic pressure measurements in arterial disease affecting the lower extremities, *Br J Surg* 56:676, 1969.

248. Yao JST et al: A comparative study of strain-gauge plethysmography and Doppler ultrasound in the assessment of occlusive arterial disease of the lower extremities, *Surgery* 71:4, 1972.

249. Yao JST et al: A method for assessing ischemia of the hand and fingers, *Surg Gynecol Obstet* 135:373, 1972.

250. Zetterquist S: The effect of active training on the nutritive blood flow in exercising ischemic legs, *Scand J Clin Lab Invest* 25:101, 1970.

CHAPTER 56

Quantitative velocity measurements in arterial disease of the lower extremity

ARNOST FRONEK

The application of the Doppler principle to ultrasonic examination of the arterial system represents the single most important stimulus in the development of the vascular laboratory. Early publications[14,47,48] were quickly followed by additional reports that recognized the potential of the Doppler ultrasonic velocity meter (Doppler meter) for the objective analysis of arterial occlusive disease.[46,52,53,54] In addition to a simple auscultatory analysis of the Doppler signals, the advantages of recorded output were immediately used. The limitations of the early nondirectional Doppler instruments were eliminated when McLeon[36,37] described an approach to determine the direction of blood flow. When the limitations of McLeod's original recommendation to detect flow direction were recognized, a number of alternative technical solutions were subsequently reported (see Chapter 16).

The first reports demonstrating the usefulness of Doppler examination of the arterial system interpreted the recorded signals on a qualitative basis using pattern recognition. Even today this type of interpretation is the most widely used for a number of reasons. First, the differences between normal and pathologic tracings of advanced stages of arterial occlusive disease are so clear that additional signal analysis seems unnecessary and time consuming. However, qualitative evaluation only uses a fraction of the information contained in the recorded Doppler signal, especially in less advanced or borderline cases.

The biggest obstacle to quantitating Doppler signals is that the Doppler frequency shift depends on the angle between the ultrasonic beam and the main velocity vector (see Chapter 9). As will be described, two developments, the introduction of special probes that determine the angle of the ultrasonic beam[17,21,42] and the application of the duplex principle (see Chapter 57), have opened new avenues for Doppler quantitation.

SEMIQUANTITATIVE DOPPLER SIGNAL EVALUATION

Gosling et al[18,19] and Woodcock et al[57] described a pulsatility index (PI) that is insensitive to the angle of the probe. The PI is a ratio of the peak-to-peak Doppler velocity amplitude to the mean Doppler velocity value:

$$PI = \frac{Peak\text{-}to\text{-}peak}{Mean} \qquad (1)$$

The ranges of PI values given are abdominal aorta 2 to 6, common femoral artery 5 to 10, popliteal artery 6 to 12, and posterior tibial artery 7 to 15. The PI is essentially not influenced by variations of the Doppler beam angle.[20] Originally the values used for the calculation of the PI were obtained on the basis of a Fourier analysis, with the expectation that this approach, although more complex, would be sensitive even to minute changes in hemodynamics.[58] However, the Fourier analysis added little to the accuracy of the method.[57] Since then the PI has been calculated on the basis of simple Doppler system tracings without Fourier analysis.

In addition to the PI, Gosling et al described two other indices to increase the overall sensitivity and specificity of the examination. The damping factor (DF) measures the degree of attenuation of the Doppler signal, which is expressed as a ratio of two adjacent PIs as follows:

$$DF = \frac{PI \ (proximal \ site)}{PI \ (distal \ site)} \qquad (2)$$

The normal range of DF measured from the femoral artery to the popliteal artery is 0.79 ± 0.30 and measured from the popliteal artery to the posterior tibial artery is 0.94 ± 0.35.

The transit time (T) is defined as the time it takes for the Doppler signal to travel from one measurement site to another. Since the velocity signal is a function of the driving pressure, which is practically synchronous with the arterial wall displacement, the results are inversely related to the pulse wave velocity (PWV) as the following:

$$PWV = \frac{l}{T} \qquad (3)$$

where l is the distance between two measurement sites and T is the time for the pulse to travel from the proximal to the distal sensing site. The published values of T measured from the femoral artery to the popliteal artery are 42.2 ± 4.8 ms and measured from the popliteal artery to the posterior tibial artery are 40.1 ± 4.6 ms. The T and mean blood pressure relationship confirms this assumption. A classification based on these three indices to identify the approximate topography and severity of the disease has been developed.

These results have been confirmed by a number of other researchers who found the PI as informative as the Fourier pulsatility index[27,28] and who also found a good correlation of PI with angiographic findings.[22,26,28] On the other hand, there are several reports[3,8,56] concluding that there is a poor relationship between the PI and the severity of the disease, although it is generally accepted that a low PI is a confirmation of very severe arterial occlusive disease. Demorais and Johnston[10] found a good correlation of the PI with intraoperative femoral artery pressure values. However, most researchers concluded that the diagnostic value of the transit time is limited.

Humphries et al[24] found a good correlation of Gosling's indices with angiographic findings, although their accuracy in detecting moderate stenoses was unsatisfactory. They found, however, that a rise-time ratio (distal-proximal rise time) yields results at least as accurate as the PI and is easier to obtain.

The clinical need to determine the hemodynamic significance of aortoiliac obstruction stimulated a number of researchers to search for other helpful indices. Archie and Feldman[1,2] used a minimum-maximum ratio referring to the recorded Doppler signals, whereas Nicolaides et al[39] used a slightly modified PI labeled waveform index (RI) and found little correlation with the severity of disease. Flanigan et al,[13] in a carefully designed experimental study, demonstrated that although femoral artery PI tends to decrease with increasing degrees of stenosis, it only occurs after similar changes in pressure are demonstrated. Most important, these results were seriously influenced by concomitant changes in the superficial femoral artery, which is a factor neglected in previous studies. This circumstance reduces the accuracy of the velocity-based conclusions under clinical conditions. In another study, Segard et al[49] found that the diagnosis of aortoiliac artery obstruction can be determined accurately on the basis of the Doppler velocity signal. Accuracy, however, decreased in the presence of a concomitant superficial artery obstruction.

Fitzgerald et al[11,12] developed a classification of lower extremity arterial occlusive disease using a combination of PI, DF, and T. Although their results were compared grossly with angiography, there is no information on the influence of distal obstruction on the monitored values.

The influence of superficial femoral artery obstruction on common femoral velocity data can be explained by the effect of distal resistance on the reverse velocity component of the femoral artery velocity pulse. It has been shown in a number of experimental[43,52] and clinical studies[31,34] that increased resistance leads to an increase in the reverse velocity component, whereas peripheral vasodilatation, whether pharmacologic or physiologic (post-occlusive reactive hyperemia), leads to its reduction or even complete disappearance. It is therefore understandable that a combination of proximal and distal resistance changes (e.g., iliac and superficial femoral artery stenosis) may produce challenging diagnostic problems.

QUANTITATIVE FLOW VELOCITY DETERMINATION

As previously noted, one of the prerequisites for the quantitative assessment of flow velocities in the arteries of the lower extremities is the simultaneous recording of the Doppler-shifted signals and the beam velocity angle. In the future this will be possible by using either multiple crystal probes[7,17,21,41,42] or duplex systems[7] (see Chapter 57). At the present time these systems, with the exception of the duplex scanner, are not commercially available, although the need for some degree of quantification is urgent in the daily diagnostic routine. Fronek et al[15] reported absolute flow velocity values from the femoral, posterior tibial, and dorsalis pedis arteries using a precalibrated Doppler velocity metering system[55] (Fig. 56-1). A calibration curve was first obtained with a 0.5% Sephadex suspension (substituting blood) circulating in polyethylene tubing. The probe position was adjusted to yield the maximum deflection for a given flow velocity (scanning the tubing and then changing the angle until maximum output was obtained). Under these conditions, excellent linearity was obtained up to about 60 cm/sec with most commercially available Doppler meters[50] (Fig. 56-2). Under clinical conditions, highly reproducible results have been obtained with the same approach (maximum amplitude search by scanning the artery horizontally, and after a maximum signal obtained, varying the angle of the probe again until a maximum signal was recorded). The probe was then fixed in position with a magnetic clamp. It is possible to introduce artifacts (e.g., by careless positioning, probe movement), but reproducible tracings can be obtained routinely by a skilled vascular technician (Fig. 56-3).

Table 56-1 summarizes the data obtained under these conditions in 39 normal subjects.[15] These values are close to those obtained by Risøe and Wille.[44] Nimura et al,[40] however, obtained far higher values, which would also imply unacceptably high blood flow values.[44]

In addition to peak flow, reversed, and mean velocity, a number of calculated indices proved to be useful, that is, deceleration and peak-mean velocity ratio (Table 56-2 and Fig. 56-4). These velocity measurements are especially valuable in combination with other findings or are suggestive of disease where other measurements (e.g., segmental pressure) may be falsely negative, as when vessel compliance is reduced and upper thigh pressure is erroneously normal or even elevated.[16]

QUALITATIVE EVALUATION OF DOPPLER VELOCITY SIGNALS

The Doppler-shifted signal obtained from the main arteries (femoral, popliteal, posterior tibial, and dorsalis pedis) of the lower extremity can be useful even without quantitative evaluation.[4,5,30,52] Generally accepted criteria of disease are reduction of amplitude, absence of reversed velocity component (especially in the femoral artery), rounded peak velocity, and a shallow, descending portion of the velocity tracing.

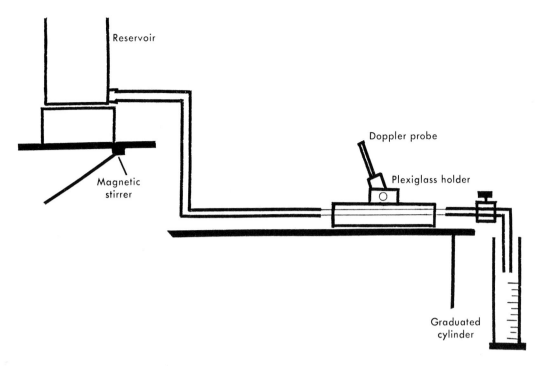

Fig. 56-1. Apparatus for in vitro calibration of Doppler flow probe (Parks 806).

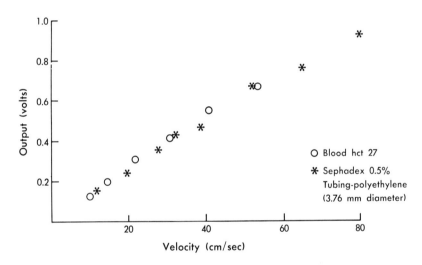

Fig. 56-2. Relationship of velocity to output voltage as determined with the Parks 806 Doppler Directional Meter. Note the excellent linearity when either blood or Sephadex is used.

Two special qualitative signs specific for two different lesions have been described. Fitzgerald et al[12] described a high-frequency signal with a specific ripple that could be recognized by Doppler auscultation or that produced a doublehump on the Doppler tracing in patients with abdominal aneurysm. Nicolaides et al[39] described a special disturbance in the femoral artery velocity tracing after exercise in cases of significant aortoiliac disease. Unfortunately, statistics on the accuracy of both of these findings are not available.

In addition to this pattern recognition, auscultatory evaluation of the Doppler signal is important, especially where recording facilities are not available. Under these circumstances, special attention must be given to any significant changes in the normal audio spectrum and particularly to signals with an unusually high pitch, coarse or rough sounds, monotonous sounds, and weak signals.[4] Much like cardiologic auscultation, this type of Doppler signal evaluation requires considerable training and experience.

Table 56-1. Normal velocity values

	Peak forward velocity (cm/sec)	Peak reverse velocity (cm/sec)	Mean velocity (cm/sec)	Acceleration (cm/sec²)	Deceleration (cm/sec²)	Peak velocity/ mean velocity	Acceleration/ deceleration
Femoral artery n = 78 extremities	40.7 ± 10.9*	6.5 ± 3.6	9.8 ± 5.3	353.0 ± 113.1	250.9 ± 60.0	4.8 ± 1.6	1.4 ± 0.2
Posterior tibial artery n = 78	16.0 ± 10.0	2.0 ± 2.3	4.0 ± 3.5	145.0 ± 73.3	129.8 ± 75.7	4.8 ± 2.5	1.2 ± 0.1
Dorsalis pedis artery n = 73	16.8 ± 5.7	1.3 ± 2.2	3.4 ± 1.6	160.5 ± 55.3	137.0 ± 54.5	6.0 ± 4.1	1.3 ± 0.5

*Mean ± standard deviation.

Table 56-2. Velocity measurement in patients with angiographic evidence of arterial disease

	Peak forward velocity (cm/sec)	Peak reverse velocity (cm/sec)	Mean velocity (cm/sec)	Acceleration (cm/sec²)	Deceleration (cm/sec²)	Peak velocity/ mean velocity	Acceleration/ deceleration
FEMORAL ARTERY							
Normal (n = 78)	40.7 ± 10.9	6.5 ± 3.6	9.8 ± 5.3	353.0 ± 113.1	250.0 ± 60.0	4.8 ± 1.6	1.4 ± 0.2
Group I (n = 14)	25.8 ± 9.4*	3.5 ± 3.5	8.9 ± 2.9	260.7 ± 176.6	122.9 ± 75.6*	3.1 ± 1.1*	2.0 ± 1.1
Group II (n = 27)	30.3 ± 15.4*	4.2 ± 4.4	8.9 ± 4.2	352.5 ± 193.8	181.0 ± 117.0*	3.6 ± 0.8*	2.2 ± 1.1
Group III (n = 70)	20.9 ± 11.2*	0.8 ± 1.9*†	7.9 ± 4.2	208.5 ± 166.2*	91.0 ± 70.7*†	2.7 ± 0.8*	2.7 ± 1.6*
POSTERIOR TIBIAL ARTERY							
Normal (n = 78)	16.0 ± 10.0	2.0 ± 2.3	4.0 ± 3.5	145.0 ± 73.7	129.8 ± 75.7	4.8 ± 2.5	1.2 ± 0.1
Group I (n = 14)	13.4 ± 11.5	2.2 ± 2.9	4.4 ± 3.3	165.7 ± 191.8	79.2 ± 62.4	3.0 ± 0.76	1.9 ± 0.9
Group II (n = 25)	13.3 ± 6.6	1.2 ± 1.5	7.4 ± 7.0*	121.7 ± 59.5	77.2 ± 82.9*	2.8 ± 1.1*	1.8 ± 0.7*
Group III (n = 66)	11.7 ± 8.2*	0.4 ± 1.1*†	5.2 ± 4.2	89.6 ± 64.7*	43.0 ± 40.2*†	2.1 ± 0.8*	2.5 ± 1.5*
DORSALIS PEDIS ARTERY							
Normal (n = 73)	16.8 ± 5.7	1.3 ± 2.2	3.4 ± 1.6	160.5 ± 55.3	137.9 ± 54.5	6.0 ± 4.1	1.3 ± 0.5
Group I (n = 13)	14.7 ± 6.4	2.0 ± 2.4	4.7 ± 2.4	168.2 ± 121.4	79.9 ± 50.8*	3.4 ± 1.5	2.0 ± 0.8
Group II (n = 27)	11.4 ± 9.2*	0.9 ± 1.9*	4.3 ± 3.2	116.9 ± 93.4*	71.8 ± 55.0*	2.6 ± 0.9*	2.0 ± 1.1
Group III (n = 60)	6.9 ± 6.5*	0.2 ± 0.5*	3.6 ± 3.4	68.9 ± 65.9*	28.9 ± 20.8*†	2.0 ± 0.7*	2.6 ± 1.4*

*Control group vs. I, II, or III. Significant at $p < 0.01$.
†Group III vs. I and II. Significant at $p < 0.01$.

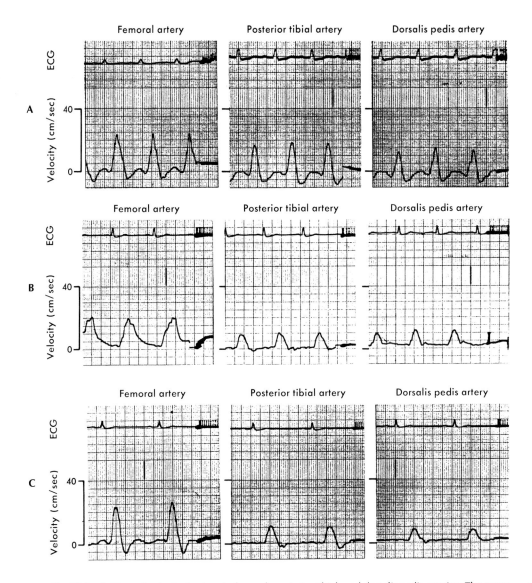

Fig. 56-3. **A,** Normal velocity tracings in femoral, posterior tibial, and dorsalis pedis arteries. The paper speed is 25 mm/sec, and at the end of each tracing, it is reduced to 1 mm/sec for recording the mean velocity. Note the sharp upslope, downslope, and prominent reverse component in all three vessels. Peak forward velocity is less in the posterior tibial and dorsalis pedis arteries when compared with the femoral artery. **B,** Velocity tracings from the femoral, posterior tibial, and dorsalis pedis arteries in a patient with aortoiliac stenosis. The paper speed is 25 mm/sec, and at the end of each tracing, it is reduced to 1 mm/sec for recording the mean velocity. Note the prolonged upslope, downslope, and absence of the reverse component in all three vessels. In the femoral artery, the tracing signal also does not return to zero baseline. The presence of changes in all three vessels is indicative of disease above the femoral artery level. **C,** Velocity tracings from the femoral, posterior tibial, and dorsalis pedis arteries in a patient with femoropopliteal stenosis. The paper speed is 25 mm/sec, and at the end of each tracing, it is reduced to 1 mm/sec for recording the mean velocity. The upslope, downslope, peak forward, and reverse velocities are normal in the femoral artery tracing but abnormal or absent in the posterior tibial and dorsalis pedis arteries. These changes are consistent with disease in the superficial femoral artery.

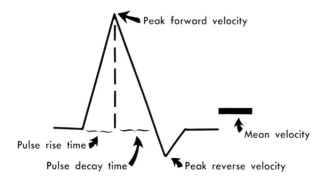

$$\text{Acceleration} = \frac{\text{Peak velocity}}{\text{Pulse rise time}}$$

$$\text{Deceleration} = \frac{\text{Peak velocity}}{\text{Pulse decay time}}$$

Fig. 56-4. Normal velocity signal. Pulse rise time, peak forward velocity, pulse delay time, peak reverse velocity, and mean velocity are measured directly from the tracing. Acceleration, deceleration, and peak velocity/mean velocity are then calculated from the measured variables.

Profunda femoris artery Doppler examination. Becker et al[6] describe a set of maneuvers to identify the course and patency of the profunda femoris artery using a 4-MHz Doppler velocity meter. These results were confirmed by Luizy et al.[30] Because this artery is important as a supply route to the distal part of the leg in cases of superficial femoral artery obstruction,[35,38] this test may help in planning both angiography and surgery.

Popliteal artery Doppler examination. Although the assessment of the popliteal artery velocity signal is considered an important part of the complete arterial evaluation, there are few reports describing normal and pathologic values of popliteal artery flow velocity. This is probably because examination of the popliteal artery is somewhat more difficult than examination of the other limb arteries, but it is not beyond the standard training capacity of a good technician. It is helpful to examine the patient lying on one side with the knees slightly bent, using the same maneuver described for all other arteries (e.g., scanning for maximum amplitude). Under those conditions the normal values summarized in Table 56-3 can be expected.

The determination of popliteal artery flow velocity has also been reported under dynamic conditions after exercise.[32] The reproducibility was good, and correlation with venous occlusion plethysmography yielded a straight line up to about 20 ml/min/100 ml (the Doppler output was expressed in frequency).

Pedal arch Doppler examination. Patency of tibial artery grafts primarily depends on patency of the pedal arch.[9,25] In view of the difficulties in adequately visualizing the pedal arch angiographically,[23,29,51] Roedersheimer et al[45] began to systematically examine the feasibility of a functional Doppler evaluation of the pedal arch. They identified three Doppler examination sites—dorsalis pedis artery, posterior tibial artery, and deep plantar artery (in the first metatarsal space). An Allen type of test was used to determine which tibial vessel was communicating with the pedal arch. While listening to or recording the pedal arch signal in the first metatarsal space, the examiner alternately compressed the inflow arteries at the malleolar level. Compression of the remaining tibial artery, which is analogous to the Allen test, resulted in the disappearance of the pedal arch signal. If more than one tibial artery communicated with the pedal arch, compression of one tibial vessel resulted in attenuation, but not in disappearance of the pedal arch signal. In addition, greater attenuation after one tibial artery is compressed suggests that it is the preferred artery to receive the bypass graft.

Aneurysm. Fitzgerald et al[12] described typical changes at the level of and below aortic and femoral aneurysms. They observed a special rippling effect that could also be identified acoustically. Unfortunately, the tracings presented in the original publications were obtained with a nondirectional Doppler velocity meter, so that evaluation is difficult. Additional information from other investigators is not currently available.

CONCLUSION

Application of the Doppler principle to flow velocity determination represents one of the most important contributions to angiology in the last three decades. It has developed from single pattern recognition to more quantitative evaluation criteria. The application of frequency analysis and the future commercial availability of double crystal probes should reduce the difficulty of probe/velocity angle determination and permit more reliable quantitation of flow velocity determination in the arterial system of the lower extremities.

Table 56-3. Popliteal artery flow velocity values

Parameter	Normal value	Standard deviation
Peak (cm/sec)	29.3	±5.9
Decay time (ms)	117.3	±18.3
Deceleration (cm/sec)	253.2	±47.0
Peak/mean	8.6	±6.3
Reversal (cm/sec)	10.2	±2.9
Mean velocity (cm/sec)	4.4	±2.3

REFERENCES

1. Archie JP, Feldman RW: Intraoperative assessment of the hemodynamic significance of iliac and profunda femoris artery stenosis, *Surgery* 90:76, 1981.
2. Archie JP, Feldman RW: Determination of the hemodynamic significance of iliac artery stenosis by noninvasive Doppler ultrasonography, *Surgery* 91:419, 1982.

3. Baird RN et al: Upstream stenosis: its diagnosis by Doppler signals from the femoral artery, *Arch Surg* 115:1316, 1980.

4. Barnes RW, Russell HE, Wilson MR: *Doppler ultrasonic evaluation of arterial disease*, audiovisual instruction, Iowa City, Iowa, 1975, University of Iowa Press.

5. Barsotti J et al: L'effet Doppler son utilisation en pathologie et chirurgie vasculaire peripherique, *Nouv Presse Med* 2677, 1972.

6. Becker F, Demercière, Perrin M: Examen de l'artère fémorale profunde par vélocimétrie ultrasonique, *Doppler Ultrason* 1:63, 1980.

7. Blackshear WM Jr et al: Detection of carotid occlusive disease by ultrasonic imaging and pulsed Doppler spectrum analysis, *Surgery* 86:698, 1979.

8. Bone GE: The relationship between aortoiliac hemodynamics and femoral pulsatility index, *J Surg Res* 32:228, 1982.

9. Dardik H, Ibrahim IM, Dardik I: Evaluation of glutaraldehyde tanned human umbilical cord vein as a vascular prosthesis for bypass to the popliteal, tibial and peroneal arteries, *Surgery* 83:577, 1979.

10. Demorais D, Johnston KW: Assessment of aortoiliac disease by noninvasive quantitative Doppler waveform analysis, *Br J Surg* 68:789, 1981.

11. Fitzgerald DE, Carr J: Doppler ultrasound diagnosis and classification as an alternative to arteriography, *Angiology* 26:183, 1975.

12. Fitzgerald DE et al: Detection of arterial aneurysms with Doppler ultrasound, *J Irish Coll Phys Surg* 5:11, 1975.

13. Flanigan DP et al: Femoral pulsatility index in the evaluation of aortoiliac occlusive disease, *J Surg Res* 31:392, 1981.

14. Franklin D, Schlegel WM, Rushmer RF: Blood flow measured by Doppler frequency shift of back-scattered ultrasound, *Science* 134:564, 1961.

15. Fronek A, Coel M, Bernstein EF: Quantitative ultrasonographic studies of lower extremity flow velocities in health and in disease, *Circulation* 53:953, 1976.

16. Fronek A, Coel M, Bernstein EF: The importance of combined multisegmental pressure and Doppler flow velocity studies in the diagnosis of peripheral arterial occlusive disease, *Surgery* 84:840, 1978.

17. Furuhata H et al: An ultrasonic Doppler method designed for the measurement of absolute blood velocity values, *Jpn J Med Elec Bioeng* 16:264, 1978.

18. Gosling RG, King DH: *Continuous wave ultrasound as an alternative and complement to x-rays in vascular examinations*. In Reneman RS, ed: *Cardiovascular applications of ultrasound*, Amsterdam, 1974, North Holland.

19. Gosling RG, King DH: *Ultrasonic angiology*. In Harcus AW, Addenson L, ed: *Arteries and veins*, Edinburgh, 1975, Churchill Livingstone.

20. Gosling RG et al: The quantitative analysis of occlusive peripheral arterial disease by a nonintrusive ultrasonic technique, *Angiology* 22:52, 1971.

21. Hansen LP, Cross G, Light LH: *Beam-angle independent Doppler velocity measurement*. In Woodcock Y, ed: *Clinical blood flow measurement*, New York, 1976, Pitman Medical.

22. Harris PL et al: The relationship between Doppler ulrasound assessment and angiography in occlusive arterial disease of the lower limbs, *Surg Gynecol Obstet* 138:911, 1974.

23. Hishida Y: Peripheral arteriography using reactive hyperemia, *Jpn Circ J* 27:349, 1963.

24. Humphries KN et al: Quantitative assessment of the common femoral to popliteal arterial segment using continuous wave Doppler ultrasound, *Ultrasound Med Biol* 6:99, 1980.

25. Imparato AM et al: The results of tibial artery reconstruction procedures, *Surg Gynecol Obstet* 138:33, 1974.

26. Johnston KW, Maruzzo BC, Cobbold RSC: Doppler methods for quantitative measurement and localization of peripheral arterial disease by analysis of the blood flow velocity waveform, *Ultrasound Med Biol* 4:209, 1978.

27. Johnston KW, Maruzzo BC, Taraschuk IC: *Fourier and peak-to-peak pulsatility indices: quantitation of arterial occlusive disease*. In Taylor DEM, Whamond J, eds: *Non-invasive clinical measurement*, Baltimore, 1977, University Park Press.

28. Johnston KW, Taraschuk I: Validation of the role of pulsatility index in quantitation of the severity of peripheral arterial occlusive disease, *Am J Surg* 131:295, 1976.

29. Kahn PC et al: Reactive hyperemia in lower extremity arteriography: an evaluation, *Radiology* 90:975, 1968.

30. Kriessmann A, Bollinger A: *Ultraschall Doppler-Diagnostik in der Angiologie*, Stuttgart, 1979, Georg Thieme.

31. Lee BY, Castillo HT, Madden JL: Quantification of the arterial pulsatile blood flow wave form in peripheral vascular disease, *Angiology* 21:595, 1970.

32. Lubbers J et al: A continuous wave Doppler velocimeter for monitoring blood flow in the popliteal artery, compared with venous occlusion plethysmograph of the calf, *Pflugers Arch* 382:241, 1979.

33. Luizy L et al: Exploration de l'artere femorale profunde par U.S. Doppler continue en 4MHz, *J Echo Méd Ultrasonore* 2:37, 1981.

34. Mahler F et al: Postocclusion and post-exercise flow velocity and ankle pressures in normals and marathon runners, *Angiology* 27:721, 1976.

35. Martin P et al: On the surgery of atherosclerosis of the produnda femoris artery, *Surgery* 71:182, 1972.

36. McLeod FD: Directional Doppler demodulation, *Proc Conf Med Biol* 27:1, 1967.

37. McLeod FD: Calibration of CW and pulsed Doppler flowmeters, *Proc Conf Engr Med Biol* 12:271, 1970.

38. Morris GC et al: Surgical importance of the profunda femoris artery, *Arch Surg* 82:52, 1961.

39. Nicolaides AN et al: The value of Doppler blood velocity tracings in the detection of aortoiliac disease in patients with intermittent claudication, *Surgery* 80:774, 1976.

40. Nimura Y et al: Studies on arterial flow pattern instantaneous velocity spectrums and their phasic changes with directional ultrasonic Doppler technique, *Br Heart J* 36:899, 1974.

41. Peronneau PP et al: Debitmetrie sanguine par ultrasons: developpement et applications experimentales, *Europ Surg Res* 1:147, 1969.

42. Peronneau PP et al: *Theoretical and practical aspects of pulsed Doppler flowmetry: real-time application to the measure of instantaneous velocity profiles in vitro and in vivo*. In Reneman RS, ed: *Cardiovascular applications of ultrasound*, Amsterdam, 1974, North Holland.

43. Pritchard WH et al: A study of flow pattern responses in peripheral arteries to the injection of vasomotor drugs, *Am J Physiol* 138:731, 1943.

44. Risøe C, Wille SØ: Blood velocity in human arteries measured by a bidirectional ultrasonic Doppler flowmeter, *Acta Physiol Scand* 103:370, 1978.

45. Roedersheimer RL, Feins R, Gree RM: Doppler evaluation of the pedal arch, *Am J Surg* 142:601, 1981.

46. Rushmer RF, Baker DW, Stegall HF: Transcutaneous Doppler flow detection as a nondestructive technique, *J Appl Physiol* 21:554, 1966.

47. Satomura S: Study of the flow patterns in peripheral arteries by ultrasonics, *J Acoust Soc Jpn* 15:151, 1959.

48. Satomura S, Kanako Z: *Ultrasonic blood rheograph*, Proceedings of the Third International Conference on Medical Electronics, London, 1960.

49. Segard M, Carey P, Fronek A: *Doppler velocity indices and topographic diagnosis of peripheral arterial occlusive disease*, Proceedings of the Symposium on Noninvasive Diagnostic Techniques in Vascular Disease, San Diego, 1982.

50. Shoor PM, Fronek A, Bernstein EF: Quantitative transcutaneous arterial velocity measurements with Doppler flowmeters, *Arch Surg* 114:911, 1979.

51. Soulen RL et al: Angiographic criteria for small-vessel bypass, *Radiology* 107:513, 1973.

52. Strandness DE, Sumner DS: *Ultrasonic techniques in angiology*, Berne, Switzerland, 1975, Hans Huber.

53. Strandness DE et al: Ultrasonic flow detection: a useful technique in the evaluation of peripheral vascular disease, *Am J Surg* 113:311, 1967.

54. Strandness DE et al: Transcutaneous directional flow detection: a preliminary report, *Am Heart J* 78:65, 1969.

55. Thangavelu M, Fronek A, Morgan R: Simple calibration of Doppler velocity metering, *Proc San Diego Biomed Symp* 16:1, 1977.

56. Ward AS, Martin TP: Some aspects of ultrasound in the diagnosis and assessment of aortoiliac disease, *Am J Surg* 140:200, 1980.

57. Woodcock JP, Gosling RG, Fitzgerald DE: A new noninvasive technique for assessment of superficial femoral arterial obstruction, *Br J Surg* 59:226, 1972.

58. Woodcock JP et al: *Physical aspects of blood-velocity measurement by Doppler-shifted ultrasound*. In Roberts C, ed: *Blood flow measurement*, London, 1972, Sector.

CHAPTER 57

Duplex scanning for the evaluation of lower limb arterial disease

TED R. KOHLER

Although the diagnosis of arterial occlusive disease of the lower extremities can usually be made on the basis of a thorough history and physical examination alone, localization and quantification of disease requires some form of additional testing. Arteriography is considered the diagnostic standard, but it is expensive, invasive, and not suitable for routine screening or follow-up examinations. It may also be misleading because atherosclerotic lesions tend to be eccentric and can be missed on uniplanar views. Although the most sensitive method for detecting significant stenoses is direct measurement of pressure gradients at the time of angiography, this is not always anatomically possible. Interpretation of the angiograms is also subject to observer variability.[22,23] For these reasons, many forms of noninvasive testing have been devised to quantify and localize occlusive disease. The simplest of these is measurement of blood pressure in the ankle by using continuous wave Doppler ultrasound. This provides a rough estimate of the severity of disease, but it does not provide anatomic information and lacks sensitivity, particularly in patients with medial calcinosis. Measurement of segmental blood pressure provides some anatomic information but is not accurate enough to use for planning therapy. Because it is easy to obtain a continuous wave Doppler waveform from the common femoral artery, efforts have been made to diagnose aortoiliac disease by analysis of this signal. Velocity cannot be calculated without measurement of the Doppler angle, so angle-independent parameters, such as the Laplace transform[21] and the pulsatility index,[9] are used. Although use of the pulsatility index has gained some popularity, this measurement is affected by the presence of distal as well as proximal occlusive disease and therefore lacks specificity.[1,2,17,25] It may also fail to detect proximal stenoses because the Doppler waveform can return to normal within several vessel diameters downstream from the lesion. Indirect noninvasive tests for arterial disease of the lower extremities suffer from the same limitations of all indirect testing: they are unable to distinguish near-total from total occlusion, they do not localize stenoses to specific arterial segments, and they cannot categorize minimal and mild stenoses accurately.

Duplex scanning overcomes many of the drawbacks of arteriography and indirect noninvasive testing. It obtains velocity information directly from sites of disease. Stenosis causes an increase in flow velocity and turbulence, which appears as broadening of the velocity waveform on duplex scanning. Because early duplex scanners used 5-MHz ultrasound, which can penetrate only a few centimeters beneath the skin, only superficial arteries such as the carotids could be studied. Therefore during the first decade after development of duplex scanning, emphasis was placed on diagnosis of carotid artery stenosis. A widely accepted classification scheme that separates carotid disease into six categories of narrowing, ranging from normal to total occlusion, was developed based on the extent of spectral broadening and increase in velocity.

Several advances in duplex technology have made study of deep abdominal structures possible. Transducers that use low-frequency (as low as 2.5 MHz) ultrasound were developed with appropriate focal lengths for deep studies. The length of the sample volume was made variable. This allows continuous acquisition of Doppler information from abdominal structures that may move with respiration and makes it easier to obtain signals from small, deep arteries, such as the renal and mesenteric vessels. The spectrum analyzers have been improved to provide higher-quality spectral waveforms. This is particularly important for abdominal studies, which rely heavily on the spectral patterns for identification of vessels difficult to image. Computer-based calculation of velocity from the frequency shift makes comparison of velocity patterns much simpler. This was not necessary for studies of the carotid artery, which used frequency shift rather than velocity, because these vessels could be studied using a standard Doppler angle and transmitting frequency. Arteries in the lower extremities are studied with transducers of different frequencies depending on the depth of the vessel and may not be studied at the same Doppler angle because of anatomic constraints. Calculation of velocity adjusts for different Doppler angles and transmitting frequencies, but it introduces two new sources of error. First, it assumes that the velocity of flow follows the axis of the visualized vessel, and this is not always correct, particularly at bends or kinks. Second, because the cosine of the Doppler angle is used in the calculation, errors in the measurement of the angle are magnified greatly as the angle approaches 90°. Therefore it is good practice to use Doppler angles no greater than 70°.

Stenoses in arteries supplying the extremities produce increases in velocity and spectral broadening, as do stenoses in the carotid system. However, several distinctive features of the carotid system made it necessary to develop independent criteria for classification of arterial disease in the extremities. First, the widening of the carotid bulb is unique and produces flow separation, which is used to identify normal arteries. Second, because the cerebral circulation has a low vascular resistance, flow in the internal carotid artery is always forward. Although forward flow throughout the cardiac cycle is present in other low-resistance vascular beds, such as the splenic, renal, and mesenteric arteries post cibum, velocity waveforms of normal arteries in the extremities have a reverse velocity component in early diastole followed by a second forward flow component (Fig. 57-1); that is, they are triphasic. In young persons, the second forward component may even be followed by a second reverse phase. The presence of reverse flow in arteries in the lower extremity is caused by the higher resistance of this vascular bed and may be abolished in normal arteries when resistance is lowered by drugs, exercise, or reactive hyperemia after temporary occlusion of inflow with a thigh cuff. As arteries narrow, the reverse diastolic velocity is gradually

lost, and the end-diastolic velocity increases. In both animal and clinical experiments, the magnitude of this diastolic velocity has been found to correlate with the degree of stenosis better than any other velocity parameter.[16] Loss of the reverse velocity component occurs when stenoses become hemodynamically significant (diameter is reduced 50% or more).[12]

Carotid artery disease is classified on the basis of specific frequency-shift cutoff points: peak systolic velocity greater than 4 kHz indicates 50% reduction in diameter, and end-diastolic frequency greater than 4.5 kHz indicates an 80% reduction in diameter. It has not been possible to associate specific levels of velocity with the degree of stenosis in other arterial systems. Velocity varies with the size of the artery and the amount of flow through it and is affected by stenosis proximal and distal to the site of interest. For these reasons, velocities are compared with those of adjacent, proximal, normal segments.

The earliest studies of femoral arteries with the duplex scanner showed the normal triphasic waveform.[3] It was noted that the reverse velocity component is less pronounced in the profunda circulation compared with the common and superficial femoral arteries, indicating decreased resistance to this vascular bed. Loss of reverse flow during reactive hyperemia produced by 3 minutes of occlusion via a thigh cuff was also noted. Attention was then focused on the

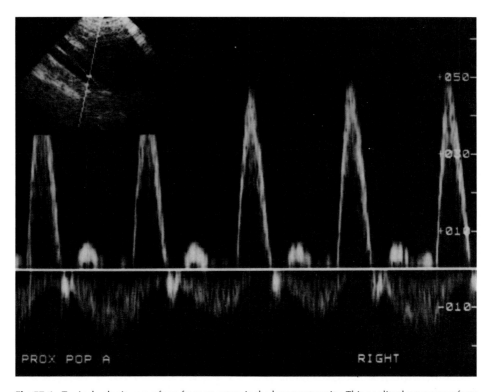

Fig. 57-1. Typical velocity waveform from an artery in the lower extremity. This popliteal artery waveform is triphasic, with a brief reverse flow component in early diastole. Superimposed is the low, reverse velocity, monophasic signal from the popliteal vein. The B-mode image is in the insert, upper left. (From Kohler TR et al: Duplex scanning for diagnosis of aortoiliac and femoropopliteal disease, *Circulation* 5:1074-1080, 1987. Used with permission of the American Heart Association, Inc.)

carotid arteries until deep Doppler examination became possible.

TECHNIQUE

Examination of abdominal arteries is complicated by bowel gas, obesity, or recent surgery. Proper preparation of the patient can reduce bowel gas. Patients are asked to avoid fatty foods on the evening before the examination. On the morning of the study, they are requested to limit oral intake to only a small amount of fluid with necessary medications. Some centers include a bowel preparation, which may be as mild as a single suppository or as vigorous as the preparation used before barium enema. With adequate preparation, approximately 90% of aortoiliac segments can be examined.

The study is begun with the patient supine and the transducer placed just below the xyphoid. A 2.5- or 3-MHz transducer is usually required, but a 5-MHz probe may occasionally be used for asthenic individuals. The aorta is visualized in sagittal section. The origin of the superior mesenteric artery can usually be seen with little difficulty. The renal arteries come off the posterolateral aspect of the aorta just below the superior mesenteric artery and then run farther posterolaterally to the kidneys. The aorta is followed distally to the iliac bifurcation, and the iliac system is followed to the groin. The internal iliac arteries are difficult to identify individually, and their examination may be facilitated by starting at the groin level and working proximally.

Vessels at the groin and below can be studied with higher-frequency transducers for better image quality. The origin of the profunda femoris and the superficial femoral artery to the knee are studied. The patient then can be turned to the supine position with the knees slightly flexed to facilitate study of the popliteal and proximal tibial arteries. It is difficult to study the proximal and middle parts of the tibial arteries, and classification of disease in these vessels is usually not possible. Patency of tibial arteries can be assessed most easily with color flow imaging.

Waveforms are recorded from standard locations: the aorta; common and external iliac arteries; common and deep femoral arteries; the proximal, middle, and distal superficial femoral artery; and the popliteal artery. In addition, any sites of increased velocity or flow disturbance are recorded. It is important to obtain velocity waveforms from the center of the vessel to avoid spectral broadening caused by the steep velocity gradient at the wall. Because abnormal waveforms can return to normal within several vessel diameters,[24] the entire length of each vessel studied must be examined to avoid missing sites of localized stenosis. Although areas of calcification and apparent plaque may be seen on the B-mode image and should be noted, it is not yet possible to estimate the severity of disease from the image alone. Although a complete examination may take several hours, studies directed to a single extremity or site may take as little as 30 minutes.

THE USE OF COLOR FLOW IMAGING

Examination of abdominal and lower extremity arteries and veins is simplified when flow can be visualized by color mapping.[27] Small vessels, such as tibial arteries and calf veins, are more easily located,[26] and unusual anatomy is more readily identified with this technique. Color imaging can be used to identify sites of occlusion, wall irregularities, increased velocities associated with stenosis, poststenotic turbulence, bruits, triphasic waveforms, and collateral vessels. The ability to visualize flow along the length of the vessel may improve placement of the sample volume for formal spectral analysis, thus increasing the overall accuracy of duplex scanning. Normal arteries can be recognized when their triphasic flow patterns are apparent on the color images. However, it is not yet possible to measure the degree of stenosis from color information alone; disease classification still requires conventional analysis of the velocity waveforms. Much of the potential information from the Doppler-shifted signal, such as the degree of spectral broadening, is lost. Color mapping provides only a single velocity parameter, which is typically a mean or average frequency estimate that is less than the peak or maximum frequency displayed on the spectral waveform. Color imaging is subject to the same physical principles of conventional spectral analysis, including aliasing, which may be seen as apparent changes in direction, and dependence on the angle of insonation, which may result in color changes caused by changes in direction of flow rather than changes in velocity. Finally, the relatively slow frame rate of image acquisition for color scanning results in spatial and temporal distortion. For example, one portion of the vessel may be imaged during systole and another during diastole, resulting in the appearance of a velocity change along the length of the vessel. This may be misinterpreted as a change caused by luminal narrowing, when in fact it is the result of signal acquisition at different times during the cardiac cycle. However, when combined with spectral analysis, color flow duplex imaging provides accurate and relatively rapid classification of lower extremity arterial occlusive disease.

Table 57-1. Arterial diameters and peak velocities measured by duplex scanning in 55 healthy subjects

Artery	Diameter ± SD (cm)	Velocity ± SD (cm/sec)
External iliac	0.79 ± 0.13	119.3 ± 21.7
Common femoral	0.82 ± 0.14	114.1 ± 24.9
Superficial femoral (proximal)	0.60 ± 0.12	90.8 ± 13.6
Superficial femoral (distal)	0.54 ± 0.11	93.6 ± 14.1
Popliteal	0.52 ± 0.11	68.8 ± 13.5

SD, Standard deviation.
Modified from Jager KA, Ricketts HJ, Strandness DE Jr: *Duplex scanning for the evaluation of lower limb arterial disease.* In Bernstein EF, ed: *Noninvasive diagnostic techniques in vascular disease,* St Louis, 1985, Mosby.

Jager et al[7] began the study of arteries in the lower extremity by establishing normal values for diameter and velocity in 55 healthy subjects (30 men, 25 women) with an age range of 20 to 80 years (Table 57-1). They found that the peak aortic velocity decreases with increasing age. Arteries tend to be smaller in women than in men, but the velocities are not significantly different. After normal waveforms and velocity parameters were established, diseased segments were studied. As in carotid arteries, stenoses in peripheral arteries could be recognized by the increase in velocity and spectral broadening (Fig. 57-2).

Comparisons were made between duplex scans and arteriograms, and a classification scheme for diagnosis of arterial disease in the lower extremity was established (Table 57-2). Typical waveforms are shown in Fig. 57-3. Normal arteries have narrow, triphasic velocity waveforms and no

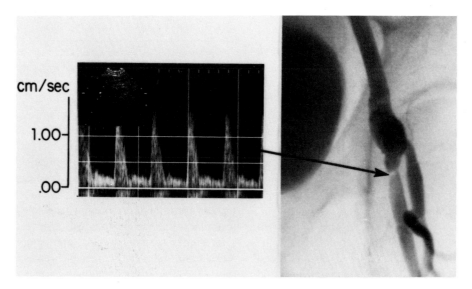

Fig. 57-2. Velocity waveform from a stenosis of a left aortofemoral anastomosis shows typical findings of a hemodynamically significant stenosis: spectral broadening, loss of reverse flow in diastole, and increased peak systolic velocity. (From Kohler TR et al: Duplex scanning for diagnosis of aortoiliac and femoropopliteal disease, *Circulation* 5:1074-1080, 1987, by permission of the American Heart Association, Inc.)

Table 57-2. Classification criteria for estimating severity of stenosis in peripheral arteries

Classification	Criteria
Normal	Triphasic waveform, no appreciable spectral broadening
1%-19% reduction in diameter	Normal waveform with slight spectral broadening and peak velocities increased less than 30% more than those in proximal adjacent segment
20%-49% reduction in diameter	Spectral broadening filling clear window under systolic peak, peak velocity less than 100% more than that of next most proximal segment
50%-99% reduction in diameter	Peak systolic velocity 100% more than that in proximal adjacent segment and reverse velocity component usually absent in stenosis; monophasic waveform and reduced systolic velocity beyond stenosis
Occlusion	No flow in imaged artery; monophasic, preocclusive "thump" heard proximal to occlusion; velocities markedly diminished and waveforms monophasic beyond stenosis

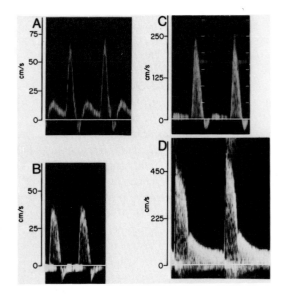

Fig. 57-3. Typical velocity waveforms for the various categories of arterial occlusion in the lower extremity. (From Kohler TR et al: Duplex scanning for diagnosis of aortoiliac and femoropopliteal disease, *Circulation* 5:1074-1080, 1987. Used with permission of the American Heart Association, Inc.)

increases in velocity. Minimal disease (0% to 19% reduction in diameter) causes mild spectral broadening only. Moderate stenosis (20% to 49% reduction in diameter) produces more spectral broadening (the clear area under the systolic peak may be completely obscured), and peak systolic velocity is increased by as much as 100% above that of the adjacent, proximal segment.

Significant stenoses of a reduction in diameter of 50% or more are generally associated with decreased pressure and flow. For this reason, proximal and distal waveforms have decreased velocities and often monophasic waveforms. The reverse velocity component is absent at the site of stenosis. Peak systolic velocity is increased by more than 100%, and spectral broadening is usually marked. Sometimes the proximal or distal abnormal waveform is obtained before the site of stenosis is identified. In this situation the abnormal waveform is probably in a segment proximal to the stenosis if the systolic upstroke is abnormally steep. Total occlusions are identified by the absence of flow in visualized arterial segments. Proximal and distal waveforms are markedly abnormal, with extremely low-velocity, monophasic waveforms. There may be only a preocclusive "thump" in the proximal segment.

After these criteria were developed, Jager et al[8] applied them prospectively in 30 patients with arterial disease in the lower extremity who were evaluated by angiography and duplex scanning. There were 338 arterial segments in 54 extremities. Arteriography was considered the reference standard, even though this technique may occasionally miss significant stenoses and is known to have considerable observer variability. To estimate the variability of arteriography, Jager et al studied the agreement between two different radiologists' interpretation of these angiograms. Agreement between duplex scanning and arteriography was exact in 76% of the segments. The best agreement was achieved for the iliac arteries. Results were not affected by the presence of multisegment disease. The kappa statistic was used to evaluate the degree of concordance between different classification techniques. It takes into account the amount of agreement expected by chance alone and can range from 1 for perfect agreement to 0 for random agreement only.[4] Kappa was 0.69 for duplex scanning and 0.63 for two different radiologists' readings of the arteriograms. For detecting hemodynamically significant stenosis (50% reduction in diameter), duplex scanning had a sensitivity of 77%, a specificity of 98%, a positive predictive value of 94%, and a negative predictive value of 92%.

After these encouraging experimental trials, duplex scanning was used routinely for evaluation of symptomatic aortoiliac and femoropopliteal occlusive disease. Initial results included 155 duplex scans performed between July 1984 and February 1987.[11] A total of 32 patients had arteriography within 3 months of the duplex scan. In this group, 393 arterial segments were studied. Table 57-3 shows the comparison between the results of duplex scanning and arteriography. For the purposes of this comparison, two segments

Table 57-3. Duplex scanning versus arteriography for classifying 393 arterial segments

		0%	1%-19%	20%-49%	50%-99%	100%
A	0%	161	16	9	6	1
N						
G	1%-19%	16	12	4	3	0
I						
O	20%-49%	20	10	14	12	0
G						
R	50%-99%	6	3	9	32	1
A						
M	100%	2	0	0	2	54

From Kohler TR et al: Duplex scanning for diagnosis of aortoiliac and femoropopliteal disease, *Circulation* 5:1074-1080, 1987. Used with permission of the American Heart Association, Inc.

that were graded as less than 50% reduction in diameter by arteriography nonetheless were categorized as greater than 50% reduction because significant pressure gradients (greater than 15 mm Hg at rest) were measured across them. It was assumed that the hemodynamically significant stenoses were missed on uniplanar views. Results were very similar to the earlier studies of Jager et al. Kappa was 0.55 for duplex scanning versus arteriography. Agreement was exact in 69% of the segments and was within one category in 87%. For the clinically important distinction between greater than or less than 50% reduction in diameter, duplex scanning had a sensitivity of 82%, a specificity of 92%, a positive predictive value of 80%, and a negative predictive value of 93%. A total of 18 segments were graded as greater than 50% reduction in diameter by arteriography and less than 50% reduction by duplex scanning. In 5 of these, velocities were reduced significantly because the segment involved was downstream from a totally occluded vessel. This points out the difficulty of diagnosing stenoses in low-flow segments beyond or near occlusions. Recognition of this difficulty should improve the sensitivity of duplex scanning.

Sensitivity and specificity for each arterial segment are given in Table 57-4. Duplex scanning was particularly accurate for diagnosis of disease in the iliac arteries (sensitivity 89%, specificity 90%). Iliac disease is the most difficult to study by any other technique. The ability of duplex scanning to diagnose disease accurately in this segment is this technique's most significant contribution. It allows the clinician to identify patients who may benefit from angioplasty and to determine before operative intervention whether inflow is adequate to the groin level. Kappa values were poor for the deep femoral artery. This segment can be difficult to study. With continued experience, the laboratory involved has become more confident in obtaining and interpreting waveforms from the profunda femoris artery. A total of 10 aortoiliac and femoropopliteal bypass grafts were studied. Duplex scanning correctly identified 7 normal grafts and 2 graft stenoses and missed 1 graft stenosis.

Table 57-4. Sensitivity and specificity for predicting >50% diameter-reducing stenoses

Artery	n	Sensitivity	Specificity
Aorta*	25	1.00	1.00
Iliac	110	0.89	0.90
Common femoral	50	0.67	0.98
Superficial femoral	123	0.84	0.93
Profunda	48	0.67	0.81
Popliteal	37	0.75	0.97
All segments	393	0.82	0.92
Bypass grafts	10	0.67	1.00

From Kohler TR et al: Duplex scanning for diagnosis of aortoiliac and femoro-popliteal disease, *Circulation* 5:1074-1080, 1987. Used with permission of the American Heart Association, Inc.

*No aortic segments had >50% stenosis in the study group.

CLINICAL APPLICATIONS: CAN DUPLEX SCANNING REPLACE ANGIOGRAPHY?

Duplex scanning fulfills an important role in clinical practice in initial diagnosis, treatment planning, and follow-up after intervention. It is unique among noninvasive tests in its ability to locate sites of stenosis accurately, distinguish between tight stenoses and occlusions, and grade the severity of stenosis into multiple levels. The data reviewed in this chapter show that duplex scanning can be used to classify arterial occlusive disease in the lower extremity with an accuracy comparable to that of two different radiologists interpreting the same arteriograms. This technique is physiologic and based on assessment of flow velocity and can therefore complement arteriography, which is an anatomic study. Occasionally, duplex scanning identifies stenoses that may be missed on arteriography. The high negative predictive value of this technique (93%) means that a normal duplex scan virtually excludes significant occlusive disease. This is important when determining whether a patient needs bypass of a proximal aortoiliac segment before a more distal revascularization.

Duplex scanning before arteriography can identify specific segments for the arteriographer to study. This often allows more rapid arteriography with less contrast medium and greater attention to diseased segments. Multiple views can be obtained when initial studies do not show a previously identified stenosis. Thus the sensitivity of arteriography is increased. The arteriographer and patient can be prepared before the examination for the possibility of angioplasty. Indications for arteriography have been altered somewhat on the basis of a laboratory's ability to identify potential candidates for angioplasty by using duplex scanning. Arteriography may be recommended for patients with moderate symptoms with discrete iliac stenoses amenable to angioplasty even if their symptoms are not severe enough to warrant surgical intervention.

Angiography is still performed routinely before revascularization for lower extremity occlusive disease, but this practice may be modified as duplex scanning improves. The

role of angiography before aneurysm or carotid surgery has already changed. Many surgeons have limited their use of preoperative angiography in patients with abdominal aortic aneurysms to those with specific indications, such as evidence of possible renal artery occlusive disease (significant hypertension or impaired renal function), presence of lower extremity arterial occlusive disease, suspected mesenteric ischemia, suspected suprarenal extension of the aneurysm, or suspected thoracic aneurysm.[5] These indications have been further reduced by the use of duplex scanning to rule out renal, iliac, or mesenteric artery occlusive disease. Similarly, many groups are limiting the use of angiography before carotid artery surgery.[15,19] In a retrospective study, preoperative carotid angiography was found to be useful in only 13% of cases, and the need for this additional study was evident from results of the duplex scan.[6]

The routine use of preoperative angiography before lower extremity revascularization has also been questioned.[13,18,20] Before the advent of reliable duplex examination of lower extremity arteries, Shearman et al[20] found that clinical examination of the femoral pulse could reliably establish adequacy of inflow in most cases, and continuous wave Doppler examination could determine patency of the tibial vessels at the ankle. They used an intraoperative angiogram to establish the exact site for distal anastomosis. Preoperative angiography was used only when it was needed to define the extent of aortoiliac disease.

The recent development of duplex scanning has made the argument against routine angiography before lower extremity revascularization even more compelling. A study was done to determine if clinical decisions based on duplex scan results would be significantly different from those based on angiograms.[11] In a retrospective study, six vascular surgeons made two different treatment plans for each of 29 patients based on simple clinical information. For each patient, one treatment plan was based on the patient's duplex scan report and the other treatment plan on the angiogram report. The cases were presented in random order, with the surgeons being blinded as to whether the anatomic information came from the duplex scan or angiogram. Disease severity in the study patients ranged from mild claudication to gangrene, with both simple and tandem stenoses. Clinical decisions based on duplex scanning and angiography were remarkably similar. Discrepancies in disease estimation by the two different techniques resulted in significantly different clinical decisions in 17% of the patients. Most of these errors would have been eliminated by providing more complete clinical information. For example, one significant error occurred when duplex scanning missed a femoropopliteal graft stenosis. Clinicians caring for the patient suspected the stenosis because of the patient's decreasing ankle pressures. Clearly, the best approach combines a detailed history, physical examination, noninvasive testing with duplex scanning, and selective angiography.

How, then, should duplex scanning be incorporated into the management of patients with lower extremity occlusive disease? The first thing the clinician must determine is whether the patient requires intervention. This is a clinical decision based on the presence of disabling claudication or threatened limb viability as evidenced by the patient's tissue loss or pain at rest. If the general medical condition warrants intervention, the clinician must determine whether flow to the level of the groin is adequate. Presence of a strong femoral pulse indicates adequate inflow. If this is in question, a normal duplex scan reliably excludes the possibility of a significant iliac stenosis (negative predictive value of 96%).[10] Duplex scanning can also identify aortoiliac lesions that may be amenable to angioplasty as well as abnormalities that indicate extensive disease. In either case, angiography is necessary before intervention. Establishment of improved inflow may be adequate to treat patients with claudication or pain at rest. Infrainguinal reconstruction is required to treat tissue loss in most cases and to treat claudication when inflow is adequate. Duplex scanning is helpful in planning these reconstructions. It can assess popliteal and tibial patency but does not give adequate detail to allow determination of the exact level of distal anastomosis for lower extremity bypass.[14] In this situation, either preoperative or intraoperative angiography is still required.

In addition to its usefulness in preoperative planning, duplex scanning is invaluable for following the results of intervention and is the first practical technique for performing long-term studies of the progression of disease. Increases in velocity may be noted before ankle blood pressures decline or symptoms recur. Duplex scanning has been helpful for follow-up of direct surgical revascularization, including femoropopliteal, aortofemoral, renal, and visceral reconstructions, as well as angioplasty.

REFERENCES

1. Baird RN et al: Upstream stenosis: its diagnosis by Doppler signals from the femoral artery, *Arch Surg* 115:1316, 1980.
2. Barrie WE, Evans DH, Bell PRF: The relationship between ultrasonic pulsatility index and proximal arterial stenosis, *Br J Surg* 66:366, 1979.
3. Blackshear WM, Phillips DJ, Strandness DE Jr: Pulsed Doppler assessment of normal human femoral artery velocity patterns, *J Surg Res* 27:73, 1979.
4. Cohen J: A coefficient of agreement for nominal scales, *Educ Psychol Measurement* 20(1):37, 1960.
5. Couch NP et al: The place of abdominal aortography in abdominal aortic aneurysm resection, *Arch Surg* 118:1029-1034, 1983.
6. Dawson DL, Zierler RE, Kohler TR: Role of arteriography in the preoperative evaluation of carotid artery disease, *Am J Surg* 161:619-624, 1991.
7. Jager KA, Ricketts HJ, Strandness DE Jr: *Duplex scanning for the evaluation of lower limb arterial disease.* In Bernstein EF, ed: *Noninvasive diagnostic techniques in vascular disease,* St Louis, 1985, Mosby.
8. Jager KA et al: Noninvasive mapping of lower limb arterial lesions, *Ultrasound Med Biol* 11:515, 1985.
9. Johnson KW, Kassam M, Cobbold RSC: Relationship between Doppler pulsatility index and direct femoral pressure measurements in the diagnosis of aortoiliac occlusive disease, *Ultrasound Med Biol* 10:1, 1984.
10. Kohler TR et al: Duplex scanning for diagnosis of aortoiliac and femoropopliteal disease, *Circulation* 76:1074, 1987.
11. Kohler TR et al: Can duplex scanning replace arteriography for lower extremity arterial disease? *Ann Vasc Surg* 4:280-287, 1990.
12. Kohler TR et al: Assessment of pressure gradient by Doppler ultrasound: experimental and clinical observations, *J Vasc Surg* 6:460-469, 1987.
13. Michel JB et al: Pathophysiological role of the vascular smooth muscle cell, *J Cardiovasc Pharmacol* 16(suppl)1:S4-S11, 1990.
14. Moneta GL et al: Accuracy of lower extremity arterial duplex mapping, *J Vasc Surg* 15:275-284, 1992.
15. Moore WS et al: Can clinical evaluation and noninvasive testing substitute for arteriography in the evaluation of carotid artery disease? *Ann Surg* 208:91-94, 1988.
16. Nicholls SC et al: Diastolic flow as predictor of arterial stenosis, *J Vasc Surg* 3:498, 1986.
17. Reddy DJ et al: Limitations of the femoral artery pulsatility index with aortoiliac artery stenosis: an experimental study, *J Vasc Surg* 4:327, 1986.
18. Ricco JB et al: The use of operative prebypass arteriography and Doppler ultrasound recordings to select patients for extended femorodistal bypass, *Ann Surg* 198:646-653, 1983.
19. Ricotta JJ et al: Is routine angiography necessary prior to carotid endarterectomy? *J Vasc Surg* 1:96-102, 1984.
20. Shearman CP et al: Noninvasive femoropopliteal assessment: is that angiogram really necessary? *Br Med J* 293:1086-1089, 1986.
21. Skidmore R, Woodcock JP: Physiological interpretation of Doppler-shift waveforms. II. Validation of the Laplace transform method for characterization of the common femoral blood-velocity/time waveform, *Ultrasound Med Biol* 6:219, 1980.
22. Slot HB, Strijbosch L, Greep JM: Interobserver variability in single plane aortography, *Surgery* 90:497, 1981.
23. Thiele BL, Strandness DE Jr: Accuracy of angiographic quantification of peripheral atherosclerosis, *Prog Cardiovasc Dis* 26:223, 1983.
24. Thiele BK et al: *Pulsed Doppler waveform patterns produced by smooth stenosis in the dog thoracic aorta.* In Taylor DEM, Stevens AL, eds: *Blood flow theory and practice,* New York, 1983, Academic Press.
25. Thiele BL et al: A systematic approach to the assessment of aortoiliac disease, *Arch Surg* 118:477, 1983.
26. van Bemmelen PS, Bedford G, Strandness DE Jr: Visualization of calf veins by color flow imaging, *Ultrasound Med Biol* 16:15-17, 1990.
27. Zierler RE: Duplex and color-flow imaging of the lower extremity arterial circulation, *Sem Ultrasound CT MR* 11:168-179, 1990.

CHAPTER 58

Color duplex imaging of peripheral arterial disease before angioplasty or surgical intervention

THOMAS M. KERR and DENNIS F. BANDYK

Historically the evaluation of patients with peripheral arterial occlusive disease consisted of a careful history and physical examination, indirect noninvasive hemodynamic testing, and arteriography. This approach, although adequate for initial decision making regarding intervention, relied on invasive testing for lesion localization and characterization. The hemodynamic significance of diseased arterial segments, in particular the aortoiliac segment, frequently cannot be reliably assessed from a single-plane angiographic image, and direct measurement of pressure gradients by catheter is not usually feasible for lesions distal to the puncture site. The validated accuracy of duplex ultrasonography for lesion localization and quantitation of abnormal blood flow hemodynamics suggests that this technique could have important applications in peripheral arterial testing before intervention. In busy vascular laboratories, it has not been practical to perform extensive arterial mapping using conventional duplex scanning, but the recent development of color Doppler technology facilitates this task. When used appropriately, duplex instrumentation can differentiate stenosis from occlusion, grade stenosis severity, and determine the extent of occlusive disease. When physicians are provided with this information, the type of intervention required (e.g., endovascular versus direct surgical repair/bypass) can be predicted accurately. Unnecessary diagnostic arteriography may be avoided, and in selected patients, surgical intervention may be implemented without preliminary angiographic evaluation.

Endovascular technology, such as percutaneous transluminal balloon angioplasty (PTA) catheters, atherectomy devices, and laser-based instrumentation, has altered the management of focal arterial lesions (e.g., stenoses, short occlusions) by providing a less invasive therapy compared with direct surgical repair. Patients formerly relegated to exercise training programs and drug therapy for intermittent claudication are now being offered this "nonoperative" intervention. Because of this modification in treatment philosophy, it is now more important than ever that accurate, noninvasive methods be used to screen for patients who might benefit from endovascular therapy. When patients with lifestyle-limiting claudication are subjected to arteri-

ography, only one-third are found to have lesions suitable for PTA. Indirect noninvasive peripheral arterial tests (e.g., Doppler-derived pressure measurements, velocity waveform analysis) are incapable of localizing specific sites of lesions or discriminating between stenosis and occlusion. Confirming the technical adequacy of PTA procedures is also difficult with indirect methods. Color Doppler imaging can assess peripheral arterial anatomy in real-time and, like conventional duplex ultrasonography, is the only noninvasive modality that affords both lesion localization and quantitation of stenosis severity.

The diagnostic accuracy of duplex scanning in peripheral arterial testing has reached levels comparable to the more established applications, such as venous[6,16,17,23] and cerebrovascular testing.[4] Published diagnostic criteria applying color duplex scanning to peripheral arteries of the lower extremity have a sensitivity and specificity exceeding 90% for the detection of stenosis exceeding 50% or occlusion.[5,18,22,26] In contrast, arteriography, which is the accepted gold standard of arterial testing, has important limitations. Even with biplanar views, arteriography can overestimate or underestimate the hemodynamic significance of eccentric lesions. The lack of standardized angiographic techniques contributes to significant variability in interpretation.[32,33] Kohler et al[19] demonstrated that agreement of peripheral arterial duplex scanning with arteriography was similar to the variance noted when two radiologists interpreted the same arteriograms. Other factors that preclude the use of arteriography as a routine screening technique include the requirement for catheterization, contrast allergy, nephrotoxicity, arterial intimal damage, atheroemboli, potential pseudoaneurysm formation at puncture sites, and most importantly, patient discomfort and cost.

Ongoing advances in duplex instrumentation have resulted in better image resolution, probe technology, and user-friendly scanners. It is now possible to record detailed anatomic and hemodynamic information with an accuracy that rivals routine arteriographic studies.[12,33,34] In some applications, the data provided by duplex scanning may surpass those from angiography in usefulness. Several reports have documented the ability of duplex scanning to demonstrate patent infrageniculate and plantar arteries not visualized by conventional arteriography in up to one third of limbs with critical ischemia.[11,29] When duplex scanning was used to screen patients for PTA, 45% of the patients were found to be suitable candidates. When a focal lesion was identified and judged amenable for PTA, essentially all patients (94%) were able to successfully undergo the procedure.[9] These preliminary observations indicate that duplex scanning should become the standard method for screening before an angiographic study, thus eliminating unnecessary invasive diagnostic studies.

The addition of color Doppler to duplex instrumentation has transformed peripheral arterial imaging from a time-consuming, tedious task to an efficient, practical examination. It is appropriate to use duplex imaging routinely when abnormal ankle-brachial systolic pressure indexes (ABIs) have been recorded in patients displaying symptoms, particularly if the severity of limb ischemia warrants intervention. Duplex-derived information can also supplement preliminary arteriographic studies that are poor in quality or when the hemodynamic significance of imaged abnormalities is equivocal. In patients with impaired renal function (serum creatinine level greater than 2 mg%), preliminary duplex imaging can identify normal arterial segments and thus permit a limited angiographic study with less contrast media. Duplex scanning has already replaced invasive contrast studies in a number of clinical applications, such as the diagnosis of acute deep venous thrombosis, identification of high-grade (reduction in diameter of 80% or more) internal carotid stenosis, and the diagnosis of peripheral artery aneurysms. It is thus axiomatic that duplex technology be appropriately applied in the preinterventional stage of symptomatic peripheral arterial occlusive disease. This approach has been instituted in highly selective situations, such as the evaluation and treatment of iatrogenic arterial lesions, diagnosis of pseudoaneurysm, and infrainguinal graft surveillance; however, the full potential of duplex scanning before intervention remains to be exploited. Color duplex scanning can be integrated into diagnostic algorithms of peripheral arterial testing to aid in defining treatment options before arteriography, resulting in a safer, cost-effective evaluation process.

LOWER LIMB ARTERIAL OCCLUSIVE DISEASE

The type and extent of vascular laboratory testing performed on patients with suspected limb ischemia should be dictated by the presenting of symptoms (e.g., intermittent claudication, pain at rest) and the physical examination (e.g., inspection, pulse palpation, auscultation). The combination of arterial systolic pressure measurements and Doppler or plethysmographic waveform analysis is valuable in confirming occlusive disease and grading the severity of ischemia (Table 58-1).[30] In general, measurements of ABI and toe systolic pressure are adequate for categorization of ischemia severity. Toe systolic pressures, which are measured with photoplethysmographic methods, are especially helpful in patients with insulin-dependent diabetes mellitus in which the presence of calcified, incompressible tibial vessels produces erroneously high ABIs. When intervention is warranted, it is useful to further stratify patients according to the level of disease (e.g., aortoiliac, femoropopliteal, multilevel) and determine whether the hemodynamic abnormality is the result of stenosis or occlusion. A number of studies have demonstrated good correlation between duplex scanning and arteriography in the detection of hemodynamically significant lesions (Table 58-2).[5,18,22,26] On the basis of this level of diagnostic accuracy, duplex scanning can be selectively integrated into the preintervention diagnostic algorithm. Patients with atypical exertional leg pain should undergo exercise testing to confirm the hemodynamic deficit (e.g., fall in ankle systolic pressure to less than 50 mm Hg) associated with true intermittent claudication to distinguish it from the pseudoclaudication syndrome. When the level of limb ischemia is severe (ABI less than 0.5, toe systolic pressure less than 40 mm Hg), stress testing is not recommended because further delineation of vascular symptoms is unlikely.[30]

Patients with mild to moderate claudication will usually have a resting ABI greater than 0.6 and a toe pressure greater than 60 mm Hg. Duplex scanning of the symptomatic limb or limbs is not required unless symptoms preclude daily activities. These patients should be treated medically (e.g., atherosclerosis risk-factor reduction, smoking and dietary counseling, cardiac evaluation) and followed at 6- to 12-month intervals by serial ABIs and toe pressure measure-

Table 58-1. Clinical categories of chronic limb ischemia

Grade	Category	Clinical description	Objective criteria
0	0	Asymptomatic	Normal treadmill/stress test, completion of treadmill testing,* AP after exercise <50 mm Hg but >25 mm Hg less than BP
	1	Mild claudication	
I	2	Moderate claudication	Between categories 1 and 3
	3	Severe claudication	Inability to complete treadmill exercise, AP after exercise <50 mm Hg
II	4	Ischemic rest pain	Resting AP<40 mm Hg, TP <30 mm Hg
	5	Minor tissue loss	Resting AP<60 mm Hg, TP <40 mm Hg
III	6	Major tissue loss	Same as category 5

AP, Ankle pressure; *BP*, brachial pressure; *TP*, toe pressure.
*Five minutes at 2 mph on 12% incline.

Table 58-2. Comparison of arteriography to color duplex imaging in detecting hemodynamically significant lesions*

Author	Iliac	CFA	DFA	SFA	POP	TB
Moneta et al[26]	89/99†	76/99	83/97	87/98	67/99	90/2
Cossman et al[5]	81/98	70/97	71/95	97/92	79/97	50/8
Langsfeld et al[22]‡	82/93	—	—	—	—	—
Kohler et al[18]‡	89/90	67/98	67/81	84/93	75/97	—

CFA, Common femoral artery; *DFA,* deep femoral artery; *SFA,* superficial femoral artery; *POP,* popliteal artery; *TB,* posterior tibial artery (according to Moneta et al[26]) trifurcation (according to Cossman et al[5]).
*Hemodynamically significant lesions are those with stenosis exceeding 50%.
†Sensitivity/specificity
‡No color duplex imaging.

ments unless symptoms worsen dramatically. However, it is appropriate to recommend duplex examination of patients with severe claudication or individuals who experience no improvement in exertional leg pain after a 3-month exercise program. The goal of further testing is to characterize the occlusive lesions and plan intervention.

Preintervention duplex imaging technique

Patients should be examined after a fast of 8 to 12 hours to minimize the presence of intestinal gas that obscures imaging of the aortoiliac segment. Scanning begins by imaging the infrarenal aorta with a 2- to 3-MHz transducer to document any aneurysmal or occlusive changes. Color Doppler imaging permits rapid location of sites of stenosis by the presence of lumen narrowing and a color-coded "flow jet." At sites of disordered flow, center stream pulsed Doppler spectral analysis (Doppler angle corrected) should be performed, with the clinician noting the velocity waveform configuration and changes in peak systolic and end-diastolic velocities in the vicinity of imaged lesions. A stenosis exceeding 70% can be diagnosed if the peak systolic velocity is greater than 160 cm/sec and there is an increase in peak systolic velocity of 100% with respect to the arterial segment proximal to the stenosis.[2] Duplex interrogation is performed distal to the aortic bifurcation with scanning of the common iliac, external iliac, common femoral, profunda femoris, superficial femoral, popliteal, and tibial arteries. A range of transducers (5 to 10 MHz) can be used to image arteries distal to the inguinal ligament, depending on artery depth and blood flow velocity. The aortoiliac segment should be scanned even when femoral pulses have been palpated because a subclinical stenosis may be present. Duplex scanning can replace indirect studies such as pulsatility indices or high-thigh pressure/pulse volume recordings in the assessment of the aortoiliac segment for hemodynamic abnormalities. Duplex studies of the aortoiliac segment are adequate for interpretation in approximately 80% of patients, with obesity and bowel gas being the major limiting factors.[22] In general, if the velocity waveform in the external iliac and common femoral arteries has a triphasic configuration, the presence of a proximal, pressure-reducing stenosis is unlikely. The use of peak systolic velocity ratios

has been recommended to categorize stenosis severity, particularly in the evaluation of second-order stenoses.[18] Color cross-sectional imaging has also been shown to be helpful in reducing interpretation errors due to slow flow produced by a proximal occlusion or high-grade stenosis.[18,22]

The pressure gradient across primary stenoses in both the aortoiliac and femoropopliteal arterial segments can be estimated from the maximum systolic velocity using a modified Bernoulli equation:

$$\text{Pressure gradient} = 4 \times \text{Maximum velocity (m/sec)}^2 \quad (1)$$

This determination has a specificity of 93% for grading iliac stenoses as compared to pull-through pressures done at the time of angiography.[22] This information can also be used to alert the interventional radiologist that special views are required or to perform pull-through pressures with and without pharmacologic vasodilatation (e.g., prescoline, papaverine). Cossman et al[5] found that a peak systolic velocity greater than 1.8 to 2 m/sec was also an accurate predictor of a hemodynamically significant stenosis. In general, PTA is recommended for patients displaying symptoms who have stenoses with duplex-derived peak systolic velocities of this magnitude or greater. The angiogram can then be planned as an interventional procedure and the patient should be advised in advance of the risks and benefits of PTA. The duplex study can also guide the radiologist to the side, site, and direction of catheter placement. This approach avoids the unfortunate situation of finding a lesion amenable to PTA but having to reschedule the patient for a second angiographic study because of a disadvantageous access site.

If a lesion demonstrates imaging and velocity criteria of a stenosis less than 50%, it is unlikely that this lesion has clinical significance unless located downstream of an occlusion or high-grade stenosis. When the duplex study is equivocal for a stenosis exceeding 50%, reactive hyperemia or measurement of basal and hyperemic pressure gradients at the time of arteriography is indicated to determine the significance of the lesion. If resting and vasodilated peak systolic pressure gradients are greater than 15 and 30 mm Hg, respectively, the lesion should be considered significant and PTA should be offered as a treatment option.

Occlusions are generally easy to identify by the absence

Table 58-3. Preoperative diagnoses derived from color duplex scanning and possible interventions

Color duplex diagnosis	Possible intervention
Focal aortic stenosis	Aortic endarterectomy
Unilateral discrete iliac lesion	PTA
Bilateral discrete iliac lesions	Bilateral PTA
Diffuse unilateral iliac lesion	Femorofemoral bypass
Diffuse bilateral iliac lesions	Aortobifemoral bypass
Discrete common femoral lesion	Femoral endarterectomy
Discrete superficial femoral lesions	Femoral atherectomy
Diffuse femoral-popliteal lesions	Femoropopliteal bypass
Isolated profunda femoris lesion	Profundaplasty
Vein graft stenosis	Vein angioplasty
Anastomotic stenosis	Patch angioplasty
Arteriovenous fistulas	Ligation
Femoral, popliteal aneurysms	Aneursymorrhaphy
Pseudoaneurysms	Repair

PTA, Percutaneous transluminal angioplasty.

of color-coded flow within the lumen and the presence of exit collaterals. Duplex scanning has a sensitivity of 92% to 95% and a specificity of 99% in detection of occlusions and, on the basis of reconstitution of flow via reentry collaterals, can accurately predict occlusion length within 4 cm.[5,18,22] Vessel misidentification, wall calcification, and low flow are causes of diagnostic error. Jets of flow from collateral vessels that are not parallel to the vessel lumen can be erroneously interpreted as stenoses.

Management algorithm based on duplex imaging

The options for intervention vary, depending on the findings of color duplex scanning, such as bilateral versus unilateral iliac disease, focal occlusive lesions versus diffuse disease, and the arterial segment involved (Table 58-3). If unilateral but diffuse iliac disease is confirmed by color Doppler imaging, the patient is best treated by femorofem-

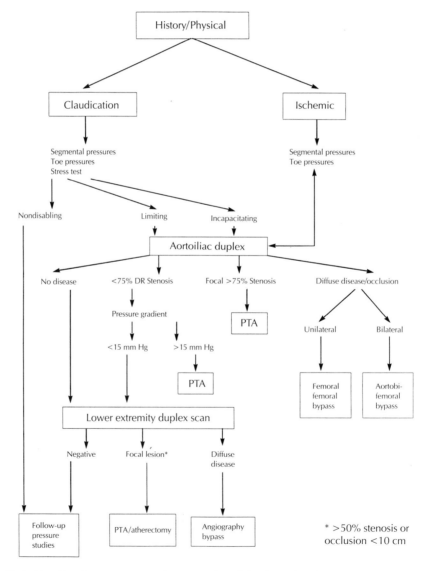

Fig. 58-1. Algorithm for management of patient with multilevel peripheral vascular occlusive disease.

oral bypass grafting. Preintervention angiography is tailored to confirm adequacy of the aortoiliac inflow segment and to visualize the distal runoff arteries. Preliminary duplex imaging permits directed angiographic studies, which require less time and less contrast media. A complete duplex study from the abdominal aorta to the popliteal arteries bilaterally can be performed in less than 1 hour, with unilateral studies or limited examinations requiring 15 to 30 minutes. Examination of the iliac arteries, particularly if there is turbulent flow, accounts for more than one third of the study time. When the aortoiliac segment is found to be normal or minimally diseased by duplex scanning, a similar algorithm can be developed for lesions in the femoropopliteal arterial segment. Depending on presenting signs and duration of symptoms, focal lesions can usually be treated by endovascular techniques. In contrast, bypass grafting is indicated when diffuse stenotic disease is present in the superficial femoral artery (SFA) or a long (greater than 20 cm) occlusion is identified. The length of occlusion in the SFA is determined by imaging flow in the lumen and identifying stem and reentry collateral vessels. Cossman et al[5] documented an accuracy of 90% for color Doppler imaging in predicting SFA occlusion within 4 cm of the angiography results.

Color duplex imaging has a less well defined but still important role in the evaluation of patients with critical limb ischemia. In this patient group, candidates for PTA are identified in less than 20% of cases. Most patients will demonstrate multilevel segmental occlusions or diffuse stenotic disease. Preoperative color duplex is primarily used to distinguish SFA patency from occlusion, assess the aortoiliac segment, and image the popliteal and tibial arteries for continuous patency to the ankle. Patients with a proven isolated aortic or iliac stenosis can be managed in a staged fashion with proximal PTA performed during the diagnostic arteriographic study several days before distal lower extremity bypass.[2]

A small subgroup of patients with lifestyle-limiting rather than disabling claudication may be appropriate for an endovascular procedure. This patient population can be identified by screening with duplex scanning. If an appropriate lesion is detected, the patient can be advised to undergo selective angiography and concomitant PTA as a single therapeutic procedure.[3] Formerly, this group would have been managed without intervention because the only method to adequately localize a treatable lesion would have been arteriography, which had not been previously recommended to patients with this degree of limb ischemia. This diagnostic algorithm is shown in Fig. 58-1. Based on the findings with color duplex imaging, an appropriate endovascular or surgical intervention can be recommended (see Table 58-3).

PERIPHERAL ANEURYSMAL DISEASE

Diagnosis and quantitation of aneurysmal disease has previously been limited to physical examination and plain film radiology. Arteriography only displays the intraluminal aspect of an aneurysm, which is frequently filled with thrombus, and may give an impression of a relatively nondiseased vessel. Thus duplex imaging has emerged as the standard method for diagnosis and preoperative evaluation of patients with suspected aneurysmal disease. Patients older than 60 years of age with known atherosclerosis should be screened for abdominal aortic aneurysmal disease. Even small (less than 4 cm diameter) abdominal aortic aneurysms have a propensity for rupture. The accuracy of ultrasound to measure these malformations has been documented in several studies.[1,13,25,27] The size of the lesions as determined by ultrasound appears to be within 0.3 to 0.4 cm of the actual size. (The diagnosis of aortic aneurysmal disease is covered in greater depth in Chapter 76.)

When duplex scanning is applied to the diagnosis of peripheral artery aneurysms, all the advantages but few of the limitations are apparent. False-positive studies are a rarity, and both the extent and size of aneurysms are readily determined. Preoperative evaluation of femoral and popliteal aneurysms by duplex scanning has several advantages compared with abdominal imaging. If pedal pulses are present, arteriography is not usually required, and thus the inherent complications and costs of invasive diagnostic testing can be avoided. Ultrasound measurements of the extraluminal dimension of peripheral aneurysms are accurate, and identification of mural thrombus is facilitated by color Doppler imaging. The high diagnostic accuracy is partly due to the superficial location of the involved vessels. This characteristic also permits imaging with higher-frequency transducers, thus resulting in improved gray-scale resolution. Virtually all patients can be studied, the cost is less than computed tomography, and no ionizing radiation is used.

A recent natural history study of popliteal aneurysms followed by ultrasound imaging reported complications in approximately 75% of patients when followed for up to 5 years without repair.[7] This study also demonstrated a 32% incidence of aneurysms developing at other locations. Up to 50% of patients who had popliteal aneurysm repair developed an aneurysm at a second location during a 10-year follow-up. An initial presentation with multiple aneurysms was a significant predictor of recurrence of the disease.

Color duplex imaging can facilitate the evaluation of patients with aneurysmal disease at the popliteal level by demonstrating the presence of luminal thrombus and the patency status of the tibial vessels. In many patients, therapeutic intervention can be recommended on the basis of the duplex study alone. Several studies have confirmed the malignant course of popliteal aneurysms, regardless of size, and thus prophylactic repair has been recommended.[15,35] Patients with femoral or popliteal aneurysms should undergo complete bilateral peripheral arterial duplex scanning, including the examination of the infrarenal aorta and tibial vessels. Important surgical features can be identified, including aneurysmal changes of the superficial femoral artery, diseased inflow, or runoff vessels that are occluded due to chronic embolization. Such a thorough arterial assessment is justified due to the diffuse nature of atherosclerosis and aneurysms in these patients. When patients with popliteal aneurysms were studied, 78% had a second aneurysm, 64% had an aortoiliac aneurysm, and 47% had bilateral popliteal artery aneurysms.[8] When focal aneurysmal disease is diagnosed without concomitant occlusive lesions, surgical repair can proceed without an arteriographic study. If duplex scanning reveals disease of the inflow or outflow vessels, selective arteriography should be performed before repair. This approach avoids the risks of routine aortography. These principles are also valid for aneurysms at the femoral level: 95% of patients with a common femoral aneurysm had a second aneurysm, 92% had an aortoiliac aneurysm, and 59% had bilateral femoral aneurysms.[8]

IATROGENIC VASCULAR LESIONS

The increasing use of angioplasty catheters, thrombolytic therapy, and extended heparinization in interventional cardiology and radiology has resulted in an exponential rise in iatrogenic femoral artery injuries.[10,21] The incidence of these injuries of up to 9% has been reported after femoral percutaneous transluminal coronary angioplasties.[21] The most common complication is femoral artery pseudoaneurysm, followed by arteriovenous fistula, hematoma, thrombosis, embolization, and mesenteric ischemia. Asymptomatic intimal flaps and dissections have also been identified but are rare. Precise noninvasive diagnosis of the majority of these conditions can be made by color duplex imaging.[14,24,28,31] Ultrasound imaging can quickly and accurately distinguish a surgically treatable lesion (e.g., expanding pseudoaneurysm, vessel thrombosis) from one in which expectant therapy may be preferable (e.g., hematoma, small pseudoaneurysm). A prospective, natural history study of iatrogenic femoral injuries observed that all pseudoaneurysms having an initial extravascular cavity of less than 3.5 cm in diameter and a well-formed wall (as determined by color Doppler imaging) thrombosed within 4 weeks.[21] However, the same study noted that all iatrogenic arteriovenous fistulas persisted and repair was recommended.

Color duplex scanning can thus stratify patients directly into either an operative or a nonoperative group. The operative group includes patients with pseudoaneurysms that are large, expanding, symptomatic, or associated with a large hematoma. Arteriovenous fistulas also require operative repair, particularly if associated with high flow and venous hypertension. Vessel thrombosis also warrants intervention; however, this can be achieved with surgical or thrombolytic therapy. If thrombolytic therapy is chosen, color duplex can be used to follow thrombolysis and facilitate catheter advancement to help decrease trips to the radiology suite and reduce contrast volume.

The nonoperative group would include small pseudoaneurysms, hematomas, and slow flow arteriovenous fistulas.[20] Ultrasound-guided compression of the femoral puncture site with the duplex probe head has been reported to be successful in up to 90% of all cases in which compression

was technically feasible.[10] Thus the duplex scanner probe itself has become a therapeutic tool in the preintervention study of iatrogenic femoral artery injuries.

CONCLUSION

Color duplex imaging has the capability of providing anatomic and hemodynamic information from the abdominal aorta to the plantar arteries. The categorization of peripheral vascular arterial disease by duplex scanning has been shown to have the anatomic accuracy of arteriography while providing direct hemodynamic information previously unobtainable by noninvasive methods. Selective integration of color duplex imaging as an adjunct to the history, physical, and indirect tests can provide precise information demonstrating the morphology (e.g., stenosis versus occlusion) and location of occlusive arterial lesions. This information can then be used to plan subsequent arteriography or interventional procedures. The information generated is reliable, cost effective, and accurate enough in many cases to allow intervention without confirmatory arteriography. Evaluation of localized peripheral aneurysms and iatrogenic femoral artery injury allows surgical correction based on the duplex scan results.

Color duplex imaging provides enough precise information to obviate the need for arteriography in certain instances and permits more selective use in others. Preoperatively, disease stratification and diagnosis are accurate enough in many cases to proceed with the needed intervention after the duplex scan is performed. Although duplex scanning will never completely replace arteriography, it has assumed an important initial role in preangioplasty and preoperative evaluation.

REFERENCES

1. Bernstein EF, ed: *Noninvasive diagnostic techniques in vascular disease,* St Louis, 1978, Mosby.
2. Blair JK, Bandyk DF: Real-time color Doppler in arterial imaging. In Yao JST, Pearce Wh, eds: *Technologies in vascular surgery,* Philadelphia, 1992, WB Saunders.
3. Collier P et al: Improved patient selection for angioplasty utilizing color Doppler imaging, *Am J Surg* 160:171-174, 1990.
4. Comerota AJ, Cranley JJ, Cook SE: Real-time B-mode carotid imaging in diagnosis of cerebrovascular disease, *Surgery* 89:718, 1981.
5. Cossman DV et al: Comparison of contrast arteriography to arterial mapping with color-flow duplex imaging in the lower extremities, *J Vasc Surg* 10:522-529, 1989.
6. Cranley JJ et al: Near parity in the final diagnosis of deep venous thrombosis by duplex scanning and phlebology, *Phlebology* 4:71-74, 1989.
7. Dawson I et al: Popliteal artery aneurysms: long-term follow-up of aneurysmal disease and results of surgical treatment, *J Vasc Surg* 13:398-407, 1991.
8. Dent TL et al: Multiple arteriosclerotic arterial aneurysms, *Arch Surg* 105:338, 1972.
9. Edwards JM et al: The role of duplex scanning on the selection of patients for transluminal angioplasty, *J Vasc Surg* 13:69-74, 1991.
10. Fellmeth BD et al: Postangiographic femoral artery injuries: nonsurgical repair with US-guided compression, *Radiology* 178:671-675, 1991.
11. Flanigan DP et al: Prebypass operative arteriography, *Surgery* 92:627-633, 1982.
12. Flanigan DP et al: Utility of wide and narrow blood pressure cuffs in the hemodynamic assessment of aorto-iliac occlusive disease, *Surgery* 92:16-20, 1982.

13. Hertzer NR, Beven EG: Ultrasound measurements and elective aneurysmectomy, *JAMA* 240:1966, 1978.

14. Igidbashian VN et al: Iatrogenic femoral arteriovenous fistula: diagnosis with color Doppler imaging, *Radiology* 170:749-752, 1989.

15. Inahara T, Toledo AC: Complications and treatment of popliteal aneurysms, *Surgery* 84:775-783, 1978.

16. Kerr TM et al: Analysis of 1084 consecutive lower extremities involved with acute venous thrombosis diagnosed by duplex scanning, *Surgery* 108:520-527, 1990.

17. Kerr TM et al: Upper extremity venous thrombosis diagnosed by duplex scanning, *Am J Surg* 160:202-206, 1990.

18. Kohler TR et al: Duplex scanning for diagnosis of aortoiliac and femoropopliteal disease: a prospective study, *Circulation* 76(5):1074-1080, 1987.

19. Kohler TR et al: Can duplex scanning replace arteriography for lower extremity arterial disease? *Ann Vasc Surg* 4:280-282, 1990.

20. Kotval PS et al: Doppler sonographic demonstration of the progressive spontaneous thrombosis of pseudoaneurysms, *J Ultrasound Med* 9:185-190, 1990.

21. Kresowik TF et al: A prospective study of the incidence and natural history of femoral vascular complication after percutaneous transluminal coronary angioplasty, *J Vasc Surg* 13:328-336, 1991.

22. Langsfeld M et al: The use of deep duplex scanning to predict hemodynamically significant aortoiliac stenosis, *J Vasc Surg* 7:395-399, 1988.

23. Mattos MA et al: Color-flow duplex scanning for the surveillance and diagnosis of acute deep venous thrombosis, *J Vasc Surg* 15:366-376, 1992.

24. Mitchell DG et al: Femoral artery pseudoaneurysm: diagnosis with conventional duplex and color Doppler US, *Radiology* 165:687-690, 1987.

25. Moloney JD: Ultrasound evaluation of abdominal aortic aneurysms, *Circulation* 56(suppl II):1180, 1977.

26. Moneta GL et al: Accuracy of lower extremity arterial duplex mapping, *J Vasc Surg* 15:275-284, 1992.

27. Nusbaum JW, Freimanis AK, Thomford NR: Echography in the diagnosis of abdominal aortic aneurysm, *Arch Surg* 102:385, 1971.

28. Oweida SW et al: Postcatheterization vascular complications associated with percutaneous transluminal coronary angioplasty, *J Vasc Surg* 12:310-315, 1990.

29. Patel KR, Semel L, Claus RH: Extended reconstruction rate for limb salvage with intraoperative prereconstruction angiography, *J Vasc Surg* 7:531-537, 1988.

30. Rutherford RB et al: Suggested standards for reports dealing with lower extremity ischemia, *J Vasc Surg* 4:80-94, 1986.

31. Sheikh KH et al: Utility of Doppler color flow imaging for identification of femoral arterial complications of cardiac catheterization, *Am Heart J* 117:623-628, 1989.

32. Slot HB, Strijbosch L, Greep JM: Interobserver variability in single plane aortography, *Surgery* 90:497-503, 1981.

33. Thiele BL, Strandness DE: Accuracy of angiographic quantification of peripheral atherosclerosis, *Prog Cardiovasc Dis* 26:223-226, 1983.

34. Thiele BL, Bandyk DF, Zieler RE: A systemic approach to the assessment of aortoiliac disease, *Arch Surg* 118:447-450, 1983.

35. Whitehouse WM et al: Limb-threatening potential of arteriosclerotic popliteal artery aneurysms, *Surgery* 93:694-699, 1983.

CHAPTER 59

The pulse volume recorder in peripheral arterial disease

JEFFREY K. RAINES

Recent advances in electronics, a more complete understanding of peripheral hemodynamics, and the vigorous development of clinical criteria have made the use of quantitative segmental plethysmography an important component in the routine evaluation of peripheral vascular disease.

After years of instrumentation development in the Fluid Mechanics Laboratory at the Massachusetts Institute of Technology[10-12] and clinical trials in the Vascular Laboratory, Massachusetts General Hospital,[2,5,13] the pulse volume recorder (PVR)* has emerged. The PVR is basically a quantitative segmental plethysmograph that has been designed for high sensitivity and oriented toward clinical use (Fig. 59-1).

In the operation of the PVR, appropriate blood pressure cuffs are placed on the extremity or digit, and a measured quantity of air is injected until a preset pressure is reached. This procedure ensures that at a given pressure the cuff volume surrounding the limb is constant from reading to reading. The PVR electronic package measures and records instantaneous pressure changes in the segmental monitoring cuff. Cuff pressure change reflects alteration in cuff volume, which in turn reflects momentary changes in limb volume. PVR units are calibrated so that a 1 mm Hg pressure change in the cuff provides a 20 mm chart deflection.

During the design phase, the frequency response of the complete device (cuff/electronic system) was tested. The system has a flat response to 20 Hz, which is sufficient to evaluate the higher frequency components of the human arterial pressure pulse contour. Additional experiments were performed to verify that linearity is maintained over the full range of clinical interest. For arterial studies the output of the PVR electronics is AC coupled with a 1-second time constant.

Simultaneous PVR traces were compared with direct intraarterial pressure recordings taken at the same location to determine how closely the volume pulse contour resembles the pressure pulse contour. Fig. 59-2 shows a typical comparison in which mean cuff pressures were adjusted between 30 and 80 mm Hg in 10 mm Hg increments. The cuff pressure must be sufficiently high to allow adequate contact

between the cuff bladder and the limb segment. Since the cuff pressure will by necessity reduce the transmural pressure in the underlying arteries, distortion of the recorded pulse contour will result at higher cuff pressures. In clinical practice a cuff pressure of 65 mm Hg gives excellent pneumatic gain and surface contact and maintains the important contour characteristics.

PVR INDICES
PVR amplitude

In clinical trials extending over 8 years, PVR amplitudes were found to remain highly reproducible in the same patient if constant cuff volumes and pressures were used.[5] For example, the presence of limb edema does not influence the height or contour of the PVR recording. Significant changes were consistently correlated with alterations in the underlying vasculature. There were variations in amplitudes from patient to patient. Amplitude can be affected by ventricular stroke volume, blood pressure, vasomotor tone, and volume.

Pulse volume amplitudes, however, are universally affected by exercise. In normal subjects the amplitude increases following standard exercise tests. On the other hand, patients with occlusive arterial disease uniformly show a diminution in pulse volume at the ankle following exercise. In addition, there is a definite relationship between the degree of ischemia as determined by the maximum walking time and the relative fall in pulse volume amplitude. In some cases the recovery time required to establish preexercise pulse amplitudes is useful.

PVR contour

Indications of occlusive arterial disease as demonstrated by the PVR contour include (1) decrease in the rise of the anacrotic limb, (2) rounding and delay in the pulse crest, (3) decreased rate of fall of the catacrotic limb, and (4) absence of the reflected diastolic wave.

The reflected diastolic wave is of particular diagnostic significance; it is generally not seen in the presence of demonstrable occlusive disease. The hemodynamic principles of this phenomenon at rest and after exercise are described in detail by Raines.[10] Examples of normal and abnormal PVR contours are shown in Fig. 59-3.

---

*Life Sciences, Inc, Greenwich, Conn.

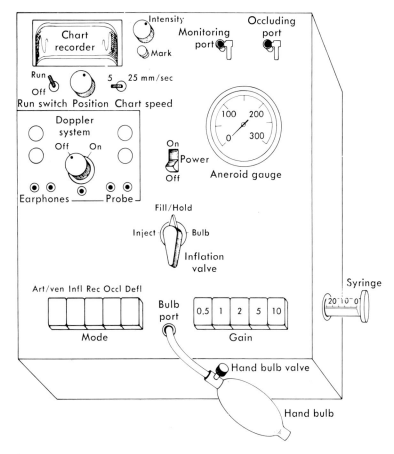

Fig. 59-1. Pulse volume recorder (PVR).

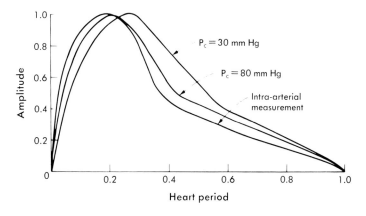

Fig. 59-2. PVR contours at different cuff pressures (P_c) compared with intraarterial measurement in the femoral artery.

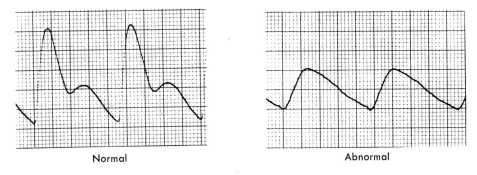

Fig. 59-3. Normal and abnormal pulse volume recordings taken at the ankle level. Cuff pressure, 65 mm Hg; cuff volume, 75 ml.

Limb pressures

In most cases the Doppler velocity detector can be used to measure limb systolic pressures. In addition, the PVR can be used to measure limb or digit systolic and diastolic pressures by placement of the occlusion cuff proximal to the monitoring cuff. Pressures are determined at the site of the occlusion cuff when its pressure obliterates the PVR recording in the distal monitoring cuff. As pressure is lowered in the occluding cuff, oscillations in the monitoring device increase in amplitude, with the maximum excursions occurring at the diastolic level. This method is reliable even at low pressures and does not require specific positioning over an artery, as does the Doppler ultrasonic velocity detector. This method may be the only applicable procedure to obtain a limb pressure when no Doppler signals are obtainable. The systolic and diastolic pressures obtained by the PVR have been compared with intraarterial pressures obtained by radial and femoral artery cannulation. The agreement is excellent for systolic pressure and always within 10 mm Hg for diastolic pressure determinations.

It has been shown that arterial occlusions or high-grade stenoses produce pressure differences in the limb at rest.[5,10,14,16] However, less significant degrees of stenosis, particularly at the aortoiliac level, may not. The hemodynamic significance of such minor degrees of arterial narrowing and the functional capacity of the collateral circulation are best evaluated by resting PVR tracings and the response of PVR amplitudes and pressures after measured exercise.

The remainder of this chapter deals with procedures, techniques, and clinical criteria used in conjunction with the PVR.

EVALUATING ARTERIAL HEMODYNAMICS IN THE LOWER EXTREMITIES

Lower limb vascular laboratory examinations may be performed both before and after exercise and in the resting state. Examples of such examinations in the lower limbs at rest are PVR recordings and systolic pressure measurements at the thighs, calves, and ankles of both legs; Doppler velocity detection in the feet; documentation of pulses and bruits; and brachial blood pressure. Exercise testing is performed when history, clinical examination, and symptoms indicate the procedure to be necessary.

PVR cuffs are placed snugly around both thighs, calves, and ankles (six cuffs in all). The thigh cuff bladders are 36×18 cm, whereas the bladders in the cuffs for the calves and ankles are 22×12 cm.

Each recording is taken separately. The thigh cuff may be inflated using the hand bulb to a pressure of 65 mm Hg (air volume $\approx$ 400 ml). For the calf and ankle level the cuff pressure should also be 65 mm Hg with an injected volume of 75 ± 10 ml using the syringe. If this criterion is not met, the cuff must be reapplied at a slightly different tension. With practice, reapplication is rarely necessary. The PVR or the Doppler velocity detector may be used to obtain

Table 59-1. Definition of PVR categories

	Chart deflection (mm)	
PVR category	Thigh and ankle	Calf
1	>15*	>20*
2	>15†	>20†
3	5 to 15	5 to 20
4	<5	<5
5	Flat	Flat

From Raines JK et al: *Surgery* 79:21, 1976.
*With reflected wave.
†No reflected wave.

systolic pressure at the thigh, calf, and ankle of a lower extremity.

After completion of resting studies, exercise testing is performed and maximum walking time determined. If minimal or no symptoms occur, a 5-minute standard walking time is selected. Immediately after exercise, PVR recordings and pressures are measured at the ankle level and compared with resting values. In addition, postexercise brachial blood pressure is recorded.

When it is desirable to evaluate perfusion at the transmetatarsal or digital level, PVR recordings can be obtained. For transmetatarsal tracings a pediatric cuff (12×7 cm bladder) is used. The bladder is placed in contact with the anterior portion of the foot; 65 mm Hg is the desired cuff pressure, with an injected volume of 50 ± 10 ml.

For digital tracings, specifically designed cuffs[9] are used (7×2 cm and 9×3 cm bladders); 40 mm Hg is the recommended cuff pressure, with an injected volume of approximately 5 ml.

PVR recordings are classified into five categories, as listed in Table 59-1, and are combined with pressure data to define various clinical states. The information given in Tables 59-1 to 59-6 was developed at the Vascular Laboratory of the Massachusetts General Hospital and represents experience gained from 4500 examinations.[13] These tables establish objective criteria useful for the clinical management of peripheral vascular disease.

Rest pain

Table 59-2 summarizes data gathered to provide objective criteria for evaluation of patients with a complaint of rest pain.

Diabetics have significantly elevated ankle pressure, since they often have medical calcinosis of peripheral vessels. This has the effect of artificially elevating the measured ankle pressure.[15] In fact, in at least 5% to 10% of patients with diabetes mellitus, ankle pressures cannot be determined at all because of incompressible vessels. In these patients the PVR tracings are the only measurable parameter, and it is especially important to be able to differentiate between primary neuropathic pain and primary ischemic pain.

Table 59-2. Vascular laboratory criteria for evaluation of rest pain

	Unlikely	Probable	Likely
Ankle pressure (mm Hg)			
Nondiabetic	>55	35-55	<35
Diabetic	>80	55-80	<55
Ankle PVR category			
Nondiabetic and diabetic	1,2,3	3,4	4,5

From Raines JK et al: *Surgery* 79:21, 1976.

Table 59-4. Vascular laboratory criteria for the primary healing of below-knee amputation

	Unlikely	Probable	Likely
Pressure (mm Hg)			
Calf	>65	>65	>65
Ankle	>30	>30	>30
PVR category			
Calf	4,5	4	1,2,3
Ankle	5	4	1,2,3,4

From Raines JK et al: *Surgery* 79:21, 1976.

Table 59-3. Vascular laboratory criteria for the prediction of lesion healing

	Unlikely	Probable	Likely
Ankle pressure (mm Hg)			
Nondiabetic	<55	55-65	>65
Diabetic	<80	80-90	>90
Ankle PVR category			
Nondiabetic and diabetic	4,5	3	1,2,3

From Raines JK et al: *Surgery* 79:21, 1976.

Foot lesions

Table 59-3 provides objective criteria for the evaluation of patients with foot lesions. In a recent study, patients with diabetes mellitus represented only 15% of patients in the rest pain group; 54% of those with necrosis had the disease. This emphasizes the clinically recognized fact that these patients are far more prone to develop traumatic lesions, perhaps because of the frequent incidence of peripheral neuropathy. They also frequently have artificially elevated pressures as a result of calcified vessels; this pressure difference is approximately 25 mm Hg. Furthermore, because of more distal small vessel involvement, a digital or forefoot lesion may develop or progress at a higher ankle pressure than in patients who do not have diabetes.

In predicting healing of foot lesions, determination of ankle pressure and PVR recordings at the ankle, transmetatarsal, and digital levels are again the most important measurements.

Below-knee amputation healing

In the patient with advanced arteriosclerotic peripheral vascular disease in whom arterial reconstruction is not possible and who comes to amputation, it is generally agreed that a below-knee amputation is preferable from the standpoint of rehabilitation. However, it is also recognized that significant morbidity and mortality are present in this group of patients, particularly those in whom a more distal amputation fails and who therefore require a second procedure.

Since the prediction of successful healing of a below-knee amputation on the basis of clinical or arteriographic information is often a difficult task requiring considerable experience, easily obtained and objective vascular laboratory measurements that prove helpful in this regard have been sought.

Table 59-4 summarizes current criteria developed to predict the chances of successful below-knee amputation. Similar criteria for transmetatarsal and digital amputations are also being derived. In these instances, distal PVR recordings play an important role. In fact, in the absence of sepsis and osteomyelitis a toe amputation will heal if a pulsatile PVR tracing is found at the base of the digit in question. In addition, for the same clinical presentation a transmetatarsal amputation will heal if a pulsatile PVR tracing is present at the transmetatarsal level.

Evaluation of claudication

In the patient with lower extremity pain or exertion, it is of utmost importance to distinguish symptoms caused by neurologic or orthopedic processes from those produced by vascular insufficiency. Both entities may coexist. If true claudication is present, it is also important to determine accurately the patient's degree of disability and to establish a quantitative baseline with which medical or surgical therapy can be compared. However, it is often difficult to accomplish this by history and physical examination alone; a vascular laboratory examination including treadmill exercise should be routine in the workup of such patients.

In evaluating the presence or absence of true claudication, the most important parameters are ankle pressure and ankle PVR recording after measured treadmill exercise. Patients are exercised until significant symptoms are produced. The treadmill time at which this level of pain is reached is the maximum walking time, which occurs sometime between the onset of symptoms and the point at which the patient develops disabling pain. The endpoint of the maximum walking time has been shown to be the most reliable.

Table 59-5 provides simple criteria for the laboratory evaluation of limiting claudication.

It should be pointed out that for maximum use of these tables, PVR and pressure measurements *must complement* each other; pressures are not always obtainable and, taken alone, may be misleading. PVR recordings are rarely misleading and are enhanced by pressure measurements. However, when pressures cannot be measured accurately, PVR recordings may be used alone to form sound impressions.

Anatomic localization

Anatomic localization of hemodynamically significant peripheral vascular lesions by noninvasive means is another important contribution to patient management. Table 59-6 is given here as a simple guide for localization. It is important to note that laboratory findings and physical findings must be combined to produce accurate localization. Looking at one parameter is generally not sufficient. The case of combined disease is by far the most challenging; in 5% to 10% of patients with combined disease, noninvasive analysis, although it may define the hemodynamics, cannot accurately localize the major contributing lesion. In these cases an invasive femoral artery pressure study may be indicated.[1] A study is currently in progress at the Miami Heart Institute

to define the accuracy and limitations of noninvasive testing in anatomic localization.

EVALUATING ARTERIAL HEMODYNAMICS IN THE UPPER EXTREMITIES

Occlusive arterial disease of the arteries supplying the upper extremities is rare when compared with the frequency of the disease in the lower extremities. However, arterial trauma and thrombosis following cardiac catheterization result in patients requiring evaluation of upper extremity arterial hemodynamics.

PVR cuffs (22 × 12 cm bladder) are placed snugly around the upper arm and forearm, and 100 ± 15 ml of air is injected with the syringe system into the upper cuff to produce a pressure of 65 mm Hg. This procedure is repeated for the forearm.

When the PVR is used to measure pressures, distal monitoring is obtained at the digital level using a digital cuff.

The upper extremity workup is completed by evaluating digital perfusion. This is done by taking PVR recordings at the base and tip of each digit, as well as digital systolic pressures. The larger digital cuff (9 × 3 cm bladder) is placed at the base of the digit and the smaller digital cuff (7 × 2 cm bladder) at the tip. PVR recordings are taken at these locations at a cuff pressure of 40 mm Hg; approximately 5 ml of atmospheric air is injected.

Systolic pressure at the base of the digits may be measured by using the PVR occlusion technique previously described.

EVALUATING VASOSPASTIC DISEASE

It is often important to differentiate digital small vessel disease from vasospastic disease. Vasospasm is character-

Table 59-5. Vascular laboratory criteria for limiting claudication

	Unlikely	Probable	Likely
Postexercise ankle pressure (mm Hg)	>50	>50	>50
Postexercise ankle PVR category	2,3	4	4,5

From Raines JK et al: *Surgery* 79:21, 1976.

Table 59-6. Anatomic localization

	ΔP$_s$			PVR			Postexercise		Exercise symptoms
	Arm-thigh	Thigh-calf	Calf-ankle	Thigh	Calf	Ankle	P$_s$ ankle† (mm Hg)	PVR category	
AI stenosis ODS	Yes	No	No	Abn	Abn	Abn	<50	5 (quick recovery)	Calf, thigh, buttocks
AI occlusion ODS	Yes	No	No	Abn	Abn	Abn	<20	5	Calf, thigh, buttocks
SFA occlusion (low) No AI disease*	No	Yes	Yes	Nor	Abn	Abn	20-50	4	Calf
SFA occlusion (high) No AI disease*	Yes	Yes	Yes	Abn	Abn	Abn	20-50	4	Calf, lower thigh
Combined disease AI + SFA	Yes	Yes	Yes	Abn	Abn	Abn	<10	5	Calf, thigh, buttocks
Tibial vessel disease	No	No	Yes	Nor	Nor	Abn	30-70	4	Foot, ankle, calf
Small vessel disease	No	No	No	Nor	Nor	Nor‡	—	—	—

AI, Aortoiliac; *ODS*, open distal system; *SFA*, superficial femoral artery; *ΔP$_s$*, systolic pressure difference; *Abn*, abnormal; *Nor*, normal; *P$_s$*, systolic pressure.
*No hemodynamically significant AI disease present.
†Values quoted are not absolute and are given as a guide.
‡PVR recordings at transmetatarsal region and/or digits reduced.

ized by loss of reflected wave, blunting, and reduced amplitude in the PVR recordings. When vasospasm first occurs, digital hemodynamics may be abnormal only when the patient is stressed, such as with cold or tension. Therefore such a patient should be studied at room temperature (a constant temperature room is not required) and also after digital immersion in iced water for 2 minutes. If the patient does not have nearly normal digital tip PVR recordings after 5 minutes at room temperature, vasospasm is probable.

In patients with more advanced vasospastic phenomena, abnormal PVR recordings will be present at room temperature at the digit tip level with near normal digital bases. With disease progression, the digit bases show abnormal recordings and systolic pressures.

In the further differentiation of vasospastic disease from occlusive disease and in predicting the effect of dorsal or lumbar sympathectomy, the study of digital perfusion with the PVR before and after nerve block has proved useful. If studies remain unchanged, sympathectomy may be of little help, and occlusive disease is suggested as a prime factor in the process. If perfusion is improved after block, the contribution resulting from vasospasm may be estimated and a basis for continued therapy established. Serial digital PVR studies also serve as a monitor for medical therapy.[8] The chances of lesion healing are good if pulsatile PVR recordings can be determined at the tip level under normal conditions. This obviously is modified if sepsis is present.

EVALUATING COMPRESSION SYNDROMES

The PVR can be helpful in thoracic outlet syndromes and popliteal artery entrapment.[3,6] Most researchers believe the pain associated with thoracic outlet syndromes is neurologic, secondary to nerve compression at the lowest trunk of the brachial plexus by a cervical or first rib. Since the subclavian artery and the lower trunk of the brachial plexus are in close proximity, the artery also undergoes compression that may be monitored by the PVR.

The patient is first asked to sit erect off the side of the examining table. A PVR monitoring cuff is placed on the upper arm to be evaluated and is inflated to 65 mm Hg. Recordings are taken in the following positions:

1. Erect, with hands in lap
2. Erect, with arm at a 90-degree angle in the same plane as the torso
3. Erect, with arm at a 120-degree angle in the same plane as the torso
4. Erect, with arm at a 90-degree angle in the same plane as the torso and with shoulders in extended military-type brace
5. Same position as in 4 but with head turned sharply toward the monitored arm
6. Same position as in 4 but with head turned sharply away from the monitored arm

In general, PVR amplitudes increase as the arm is elevated. Arterial compression is present if the PVR amplitude goes flat in any of the standard positions. Since the syndrome is often bilateral, the other arm should always be studied. It should be noted that many individuals without symptoms (25% is a good estimate) compress arteries supplying the arm in some of the positions outlined. Therefore it is important to base therapy on symptoms, physical findings, history, and ulnar nerve conduction in addition to vascular laboratory data.

Ischemic pain with exercise may occur because of intermittent compression or entrapment of the popliteal artery by the medial head of the gastrocnemius muscle. In such instances the popliteal artery passes medial to or through fibers of the medial head of the gastrocnemius muscle, which may have an anomalous origin on the femur either cephalad or lateral to its normal position on the posterior face of the medial femoral condyle. Regardless of the anatomic or embryologic anomaly, however, the result is an episodic and functional occlusion of the popliteal artery that occurs with each plantar flexion. The significance of early detection and treatment of this abnormality is related to observations that progressive structural changes may occur in the arterial wall as a result of chronic and recurring trauma ultimately resulting in aneurysm formation, thrombosis, and loss of limb vitality. Less than 30 documented cases of the popliteal entrapment syndrome have been noted. Current review suggests that the syndrome may be characterized by (1) history of unilateral intermittent claudication in young men, (2) laboratory findings of diminution of ankle PVR recordings with sustained plantar flexion and/or passive dorsiflexion of the foot, and (3) angiographic findings of medial deviation of the popliteal artery.

In cases of suspected popliteal artery entrapment, it is extremely important to perform a standard lower extremity examination as well as PVR recordings at the ankle with sustained active plantar flexion and with passive dorsiflexion of the foot. Compression during any of these maneuvers is easily recognized.

With regard to entrapment in other clinical situations, the finding of normal PVR recordings in response to acute hip flexion and knee bending has been of help in advising patients who have had extraordinary, makeshift bypass grafts carried out for the treatment of sepsis or related problems. In many of these patients the grafts have been implanted lateral to the inguinal ligament, across the pubis, deep or superficial to muscle bellies and fascial bands, or around bony prominences at the knee. In such patients it is reassuring to know that the graft does not kink or become entrapped in varying limb positions.[5]

EVALUATING VASCULAR MALFORMATIONS

Pulse volume recordings taken on an extremity or digit over an area of suspected vascular malformation are helpful in differentiating the type of malformation and its extent. Doppler velocity detection over areas of suspected vascular malformation is also useful. Table 59-7 is presented as a simple guide.

In venous malformations, arterial hemodynamics are not

Table 59-7. Malformations

| Malformation | Local PVR | | Doppler abnormal superficial signals |
	Amplitude	Reflected wave	
Venous	Normal	Present	Absent
Arteriovenous	Increased	Absent	Present

significantly affected. Therefore venous pressure remains within normal limits, and pulse volume is not increased. In addition, peripheral resistance is normal, and arterial reflected waves recorded by the PVR are present. In arteriovenous malformation the compliant venous conduits undergo abnormal pulsatile pressure transmitted through the malformation from the arterial system, resulting in increased pulse volume. Decreased local peripheral resistance results in loss of reflected wave.

INTRAOPERATIVE MONITORING

The PVR has been used extensively to monitor the results of reconstructive arterial surgery.[5] It is acknowledged that experienced surgeons performing proximal arterial reconstructions in the presence of patent distal vessels can get a qualitative estimate of the excellence of revascularization by restoration of pedal pulses. However, pulses are not always restored and may be very difficult to appreciate in the operating room. The time to appreciate any operative misadventure is while in the operating room with the vessels exposed and not following a few hours of observation in the recovery room. Intraoperative monitoring is particularly valuable in the teaching setting and provides immediate objective evidence of technical success.

Intraoperative monitoring is essential in patients undergoing proximal arterial reconstruction in the presence of distal occlusive disease. This group of patients includes those with combined aortoiliac and femoropopliteal disease and those with femoropopliteal disease and associated tibial involvement. Absence of definable PVR amplitude in the limb segment immediately distal to the arterial reconstruction has invariably led to a successful search for a cause, whether an anastomotic stenosis, clamp injury, thrombosis, or embolus.

The PVR recording measured immediately following revascularization may be somewhat decreased. This is particularly true if the ankle is monitored following aortoiliac reconstruction in patients with known femoropopliteal occlusive disease. This may reflect several factors, including vasoconstriction, hypotension, and hypovolemia. Therefore with such patients, limb monitoring should be carried out as proximally as possible; the calf is ideal. In no recorded instance has there been a flat trace at the calf if the proximal reconstruction has been adequate. In cases where the pulse amplitude has not returned to more than 50% of its preoperative level, measurement of calf and ankle pressures

has been used to complement the PVR measurements and verify the adequacy of the reconstruction. In patients with patent distal vessels the initial response following clamp removal has been immediate return of the PVR amplitude, usually to normal.

Technical errors during femoropopliteal bypass procedures may account for 6% to 15% of early and 15% to 30% of late failures.[4] Improperly constructed distal anastomoses with obstruction of the outflow tract, valvular or torsion defects with the vein graft, and distal thrombosis caused by intraoperative emboli are the principal causes of graft failure. Intraoperative arteriography has been suggested as a means of detection of these abnormalities. However, intraoperative arteriography is time-consuming, usually visualizes only one plane, and provides no physiologic information about the graft and distal runoff. In addition, the various angiographic techniques employed may lead to complications in themselves. The PVR provides physiologic information on (1) the distal runoff before insertion of the graft, (2) the condition and function of the distal and proximal anastomoses, and (3) the alignment of the saphenous vein.

Simulated pulse volume as monitored by the PVR has allowed correction of technical errors in the operating room, thus avoiding a repeat procedure. In this technique the PVR is connected to a monitoring cuff placed at the ankle; heparinized saline solution is "pulsed" by hand at the rate of ≈ 5 ml/sec at two stages: (1) through the popliteal arteriotomy by means of a Marx needle and (2) through the upper end of the graft following completion of distal anastomosis. After the proximal anastomosis is complete, the initial pulsatile blood flow propelled by the heart is also monitored. If abnormalities are found at any stage, reasons for hemodynamic defects are investigated.

RECOVERY ROOM MONITORING

Following peripheral arterial reconstruction in the presence of known distal occlusive disease, peripheral pulses may not be easily discernible, particularly in the early postoperative course. In addition, palpable pulses may disappear because of lower extremity edema later in the postoperative course. Noninvasive studies using the PVR have been of considerable value in following patients during this period.[5] Nursing personnel are able to monitor arterial reconstructions in the recovery area effectively despite the absence of palpable pulses. By detecting failure early, the surgeon is often able to correct problems, thus salvaging the reconstruction.

In practice the recovery room nurses take PVR recordings at set intervals. PVR amplitudes invariably remain stable or increase during the early postoperative period in the presence of a successful reconstruction. Failing PVR amplitudes, often but not always associated with diminution of the ankle/brachial systolic pressure ratio, invariably mean a failing arterial reconstruction in our experience. These findings should prompt early reexploration of the arterial reconstruction.

CONCLUSION

Function is the most important consideration in evaluating lower extremity occlusive arterial disease. Evaluation such as described in this chapter can be done by means of non-invasive hemodynamic studies more precisely than by clinical examination or angiography. The overall functional accuracy of Tables 59-2 through 59-5 is greater than 95% when the clinical course is used as the standard. If disease is confined to a single level, these studies can anatomically localize (Table 59-6) the lesion in virtually 100% of cases. With bilevel disease, accuracy drops into a range of 90% to 95%.

The PVR (venous mode) in combination with its built-in Doppler system can perform lower and upper extremity noninvasive deep venous tree evaluations. This technique produces approximately 5% false-positive and 2% false-negative results.

Because of the flexibility of the transducer system in the PVR, it has been possible to build a simple attachment to the PVR for the measurement of ophthalmic artery pressure (ocular pneumoplethysmography—OPG*).[7] The attachment is available in both unilateral and bilateral models. This measurement in combination with carotid audiofrequency analysis and cerebral Doppler evaluation has an overall accuracy of 94%.

Newest instrumentation

A small group of vascular laboratory directors, vascular surgeons, electrical engineers, mechanical design engineers, and computer software and hardware engineers combined their skills to produce the automated procedures laboratory (PVR/APL).* The overall system is best described when its two major components are considered.

Measurement unit. The measurement unit (MU) (Fig. 59-4) provides the interface between the operator and the patient. In keeping with basic and validated systems, the MU contains menu-driven automated versions of the PVR, an advanced zero-crossing continuous wave Doppler system (3.5 to 9.2 MHz), a dual-channel OPG (OPG II/500), and a digital carotid phonoangiograph (CPA II). The probes and cuffs are conveniently stored in the MU for use in the vascular laboratory, in the operating room, or at the bedside. The unit has a minimum of buttons and controls, has the same floor space requirement as the current PVR, and is slightly taller. Its mobility also compares favorably.

The operator is prompted by a menu that appears on the cathode-ray tube (CRT) screen. Protocols for all standard vascular laboratory procedures are built in. The operator has control over the various steps in the protocols and may repeat any sequence as desired, such as the data stored (PVR tracings, limb pressures, ophthalmic artery pressures, or carotid phonoangiographic [CBA] data) and cuff inflation/deflation. To perform these functions, the operator uses a controller that fits in the palm of one hand and has one

*Life Sciences, Inc, Greenwich, Conn.

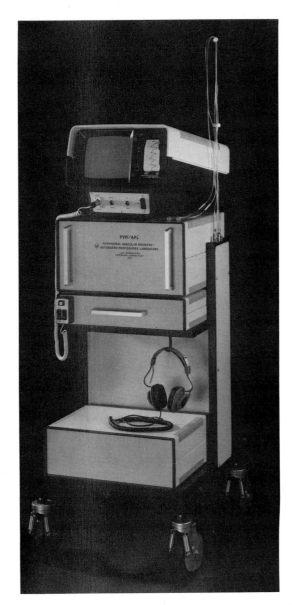

Fig. 59-4. Measurement unit (MU). (From Raines J: *Vasc Lab Rev* 1:10, 1983.)

button and two rocker switches. Patient data are stored on a floppy disk in the MU. At the completion of the tests the patient disk is removed for use in the analysis unit (AU).

Besides being able to perform the standard lower extremity arterial, extracranial arterial, and lower extremity venous evaluations in combination with the AU, the MU can perform these studies independently. It also has a built-in strip-chart recorder for independent hard copy. Capabilities for digital studies, penile studies, femoral artery studies, lesion healing prediction, and amputation healing predictions are also included.

The MU used with the AU also has a built-in teaching program that outlines step by step all the required procedures. Actual patient data are displayed for immediate comparison by the student.

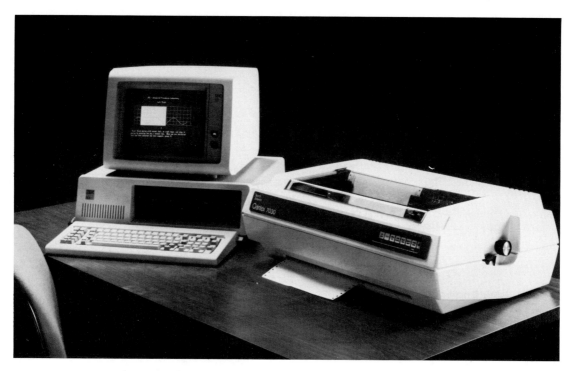

Fig. 59-5. Analysis unit (AU). (From Raines J: *Vasc Lab Rev* 1:10, 1983.)

Analysis unit. The AU (Fig. 59-5) is a combination of the most advanced, supported microcomputer, specifically designed software (an interface that allows the operator to communicate with the computer), and an advanced dot-matrix printer.

Patient data taken from the MU in disk form are displayed by the AU for analysis and final report printings. Reports may be generated after each patient examination or at another convenient time. The patient data are displayed on the CRT, and a menu-driven AU protocol guides the operator in entering the data. Final verification of the data is prepared by the operator with the help of the computer. When the patient data are complete, a quantitative interpretation is presented on the screen. This provides a firm diagnosis based on thousands of cases. The word processing capability of the system allows the operator or laboratory director to alter this interpretation. The operator can then instruct the AU to print the final clinical report. This report includes the history and physical examination information, the data that were measured including all tracings (PVR, OPG, and CPA), interpretation of the data, and a graphic display indicating the anatomic lesions of interest. Patient data are automatically stored on floppy disks in laboratory archives and entered into the peripheral vascular registry, which will be described.

Since the AU is also a powerful computer, a comprehensive office management system has been written for this equipment. The system generates patient logs, has complete office accounting files, includes automated billing, and prints insurance forms. In addition, IBM software for word processing, electronic spread sheet analysis, statistical analysis, and BASIC language is compatible. There are also more than 2000 software packages written for this system by independent programming firms.

Peripheral vascular registry. A peripheral vascular registry is desirable for a number of reasons. The registry can improve patient management by reviewing previous experiences, new certification requirements, regional vascular societies, and surgical/medical results and can generate interest in more automated research. This component has been built into the automated peripheral laboratory. It has been carefully designed to answer the maximum number of potential questions with the minimum of data entry and storage. In addition, most of the data obtained from the vascular laboratory studies are automatically placed in the registry. Extensive sorting, classification, and retrieval routines have been programmed into this system. This allows rapid clinical research on large patient populations. The hard disk in the IBM PC/XT can easily store more than 12,000 registry records for review. Since the registry is completely in software form, changes can be made easily at minimal cost. Nine files can be accessed by this registry as follows:

1. Census data, history, and physical findings
2. Lower extremity arterial laboratory data
3. Cerebral laboratory data
4. Lower extremity venous data
5. Lower extremity arteriography
6. Cerebral arteriography
7. Lower extremity venography
8. Compact surgical record
9. Complete follow-up record

The peripheral vascular registry allows the maximal use of measured noninvasive data in temporal management of patients, as well as in clinical research and natural history studies.

REFERENCES

1. Brener BJ et al: Measurement of systolic femoral arterial pressure during reactive hyperemia, *Circulation* 50(suppl):259, 1974.
2. Buckley CJ, Darling RC, Raines JK: Instrumentation and examination procedures for a clinical vascular laboratory, *Med Instrum* 9:181, 1975.
3. Dale WA, Lewis MR: Management of thoracic outlet syndrome, *Ann Surg* 181:575, 1975.
4. Darling RC, Linton RR: Durability of femoropopliteal reconstructions, *Am J Surg* 123:472, 1972.
5. Darling RC et al: Quantitative segmental pulse volume recorder: a clinical tool, *Surgery* 72:873, 1972.
6. Darling RC et al: Intermittent claudication in young athletes: popliteal artery entrapment syndrome, *J Trauma* 14:543, 1974.
7. Gee W et al: Ocular pneumoplethysmography in carotid artery disease, *Med Instrum* 8:244, 1974.
8. Gifford RW: *The arteriospastic diseases: clinical significance and management*. In Brest AN, ed: *Peripheral vascular disease: cardiovascular clinics,* Philadelphia, 1971, FA Davis.
9. Gundersen J: Segmental measurements of systolic blood pressure in the extremities including the thumb and the great toe, *Acta Chir Scand* 462(suppl):1, 1972.
10. Raines JK: *Diagnosis and analysis of arteriosclerosis in the lower limbs from the arterial pressure pulse,* doctoral thesis, Massachusetts Institute of Technology, 1972, Cambridge, Mass.
11. Raines JK, Jaffrin MY, Rao S: A noninvasive pressure pulse recorder: development and rationale, *Med Instrum* 7:245, 1973.
12. Raines JK, Jaffrin MY, Shapiro AH: A computer simulation of arterial dynamics in the human leg, *J Biochem* 7:77, 1974.
13. Raines JK et al: Vascular laboratory criteria for the management of peripheral vascular disease of the lower extremities, *Surgery* 79:21, 1976.
14. Strandness DE Jr: *Peripheral arterial disease,* Boston, 1969, Little, Brown & Co.
15. Taguchi JT, Suwangool P: Pipe-stem brachial arteries: a cause of pseudohypertension, *JAMA* 228:733, 1974.
16. Yao JST: Haemodynamic studies in peripheral arterial disease, *Br J Surg* 57:761, 1970.

CHAPTER 60

Quantitative air-plethysmography in the management of arterial ischemia

ANDREW N. NICOLAIDES, NIKOS LABROPOULOS, NICOS VOLTEAS,
MIGUEL LEON, and DIMITRIS CHRISTOPOULOS

The ability to measure arterial inflow to the leg in absolute units (millimeters per minute) with a high reproducibility (coefficient of variation 3.2% to 7.6%) using air-plethysmography (APG)[1] has yielded new information in patients with lower limb ischemia that can then be used for planning clinical management. Leg blood flow in 20 normal limbs was found to range from 50 to 120 ml/min, depending on the size of the leg. APG has also been used to assess changes in leg blood flow after vascular surgical intervention and medical treatment in patients with intermittent claudication and ischemic rest pain. Leg blood flow was measured using a commercially available air-plethysmograph (APG-1000; ACI Medical). The technique and its calibration are described in detail in Chapter 23.

EFFECTS OF PERCUTANEOUS TRANSLUMINAL ANGIOPLASTY ON LEG BLOOD FLOW

Leg blood flow was measured before and 1 day after percutaneous transluminal angioplasty (PTA) was performed in 18 patients with intermittent claudication affecting one limb. Lesions were found in the superficial femoral artery in 17 and in the iliac artery in 1, and all cases were documented by both duplex scanning and angiography.

A total of 8 patients had extended occlusion in the superficial femoral artery; in 6, the occlusion was less than 5 cm in length and, in 2, it was more than 5 cm. All the other patients had one or more stenoses in the superficial femoral or iliac arteries with a diameter reduction of greater than 50%.

The mean ankle-brachial index before PTA was 0.55 ± 0.19. PTA was successful in 17 of the 18 patients and failed in 1 patient with a superficial femoral artery occlusion less than 5 cm. PTA increased the leg blood flow (Fig. 60-1) significantly ($p < 0.001$); the ankle-brachial index also showed a significant increase to a mean value of 0.76 ± 0.14 ($p < 0.001$). The walking distance was improved in all patients whose PTA was successful.

EFFECTS OF GRAFT INSERTION ON LEG BLOOD FLOW

In another study consisting of 24 patients, leg blood flow was measured before and 7 days after graft insertion in 17 patients with ischemic rest pain and 7 patients with disabling intermittent claudication. Of the total, 17 of the bypasses were femoro-popliteal (4 above-knee, 13 below-knee), and 7 were femorocrural. A polytetrafluoroethylene (PTFE) graft was used in 8 patients, a reversed arm vein in 3, and an in situ vein in 13. Before the operation, leg blood flow ranged from 30 to 75 ml/min (mean, 50 ml/min), with a mean ankle-brachial index of 0.39 ± 0.10. A total of 7 days after the operation, there was a significant increase in the leg blood flow ($p < 0.001$) to a range of 85 to 159 ml/min (mean, 123 ml/min) (Fig. 60-2), which was associated with a marked increase in the ankle-brachial index of 0.9 ± 0.12 ($p < 0.001$).

In the study, 10 of these patients have been examined every 3 months for 1 year. The leg blood flow after operation was markedly increased and then decreased gradually in the first 3 to 6 months until the leg blood flow stabilized (Fig. 60-3).

EFFECTS OF ILOPROST ON PATIENTS WITH ISCHEMIC REST PAIN

A total of 34 patients with stable ischemic rest pain affecting 42 limbs with ankle pressures equal to or less than 50 mg Hg were treated with synthetic prostacyclin (Iloprost), administered intravenously. None of the patients had gangrenous or pregangrenous changes in the foot or any toe. All patients underwent angiography to establish the presence and extent of the arterial disease because they were also potential candidates for vascular reconstruction. Any patients with moderate to severe aortoiliac disease who were candidates for aortoiliac reconstruction were not considered for Iloprost therapy and thus are not among the 34 patients described here. Leg blood flow was measured using APG before the start of Iloprost therapy and then every 2 days

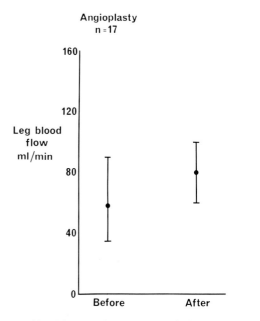

Fig. 60-1. Calf blood flow (median 95% range) before and 1 day after angioplasty (*p* < 0.001; Wilcoxon signed ranks test).

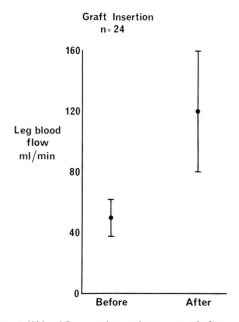

Fig. 60-2. Calf blood flow (median and 95% range) before and 7 days after graft insertion (*p* < 0.001; Wilcoxon signed ranks test).

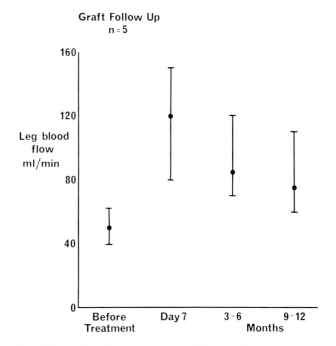

Fig. 60-3. Leg blood flow (median and 95% range) before and during 1 year follow-up.

during therapy up to the eighth day when Iloprost therapy was stopped. The initial infusion rate was 0.5 ng/kg/min, and this was gradually increased during the first 2 days in increments of 0.25 ng/kg/min to a maximum tolerated dose of 2.0 ng/kg/min. The duration of the infusion was 8 hours

every day. The maximum dose used on day 2 of therapy was also the dose given on days 3 to 8.

At the end of the Iloprost therapy, 23 of the 42 limbs became free of pain. In 7 limbs, pain was experienced only when the limb was elevated or during the nighttime, and no improvement was noticed in 12 limbs. The 42 limbs were classified into three groups according to the pretreatment baseline leg blood flow:

Group A: ≥40 ml/min (n = 22)
Group B: 30 to 39 ml/min (n = 11)
Group C: ≤30 ml/min (n = 9)

Iloprost infusion brought about increased leg blood flow in all patients except those with zero-vessel runoff. This increase was 32%, 46%, and 54% for limbs with one-, two-, and three-vessel runoff, respectively (Fig. 60-4). The median and 90% tolerance levels (90% range) of the leg blood flow for the three groups are shown in Fig. 60-5. The increase in flow was statistically significant in all three groups on days 4 to 8 of therapy (*p* < 0.01; Wilcoxon signed ranks test). The median increase in flow was 15 ml/min (range, 5 to 33 ml/min) in group A, 14 ml/min (range, 4 to 45 ml/min) in group B, and 15 ml/min (range, 0 to 25 ml/min) in group C.

The flow on day 8 was related to the flow that was noted before therapy, and this pretreatment blood flow was a good predictor of the effectiveness of therapy (Table 60-1). A total of 20 of 22 limbs with a pretreatment flow of 40 ml/min or less became asymptomatic. There was complete relief of symptoms in 24 (92%) limbs with a final flow that exceeded 50 ml/min, but only 1 of 16 limbs with a final

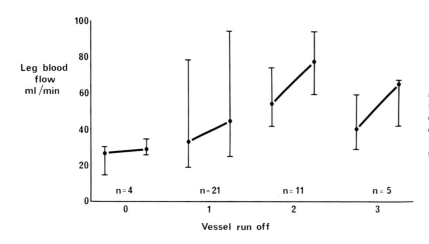

Fig. 60-4. Leg blood flow (median and 95% range) in relation to the number of vessel runoff before and 8 days after Iloprost infusion. The increase in flow on days 4 and 8 was statistically significant in groups with 1, 2, and 3 vessel runoff ($p < 0.001$; Wilcoxon signed ranks test).

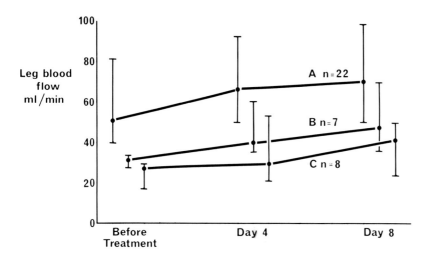

Fig. 60-5. Leg blood flow (median and 95% ranges) in the three groups of patients before and 4 and 8 days after Iloprost infusion.

Table 60-1. Results of Iloprost therapy in relation to pretreatment leg blood flow

Leg blood flow before therapy (ml/min)	No rest pain	Improved	No change	Total
≥40	20 (91%)	1 (4%)	1 (47%)	22
30-39	2 (18%)	5 (45%)	4 (36%)	11
<30	1 (11%)	1 (11%)	7 (78%)	9
TOTAL	23	7	12	42

Table 60-2. Results of Iloprost therapy in relation to final leg blood flow

Leg blood flow on day 8 (ml/min)	No rest pain	Improved	No change	Total
>50	24 (92%)	2 (8%)	0	26
<50	1 (6%)	7 (44%)	8 (50%)	16
TOTAL	25	9	8	42

flow of less than 50 ml/min had complete relief (Table 60-2).

This study was not designed to study the long-term effects of Iloprost therapy, and thus no blood flow measurements were obtained after the last day of therapy. These preliminary results suggest that a randomized placebo-controlled, double-blind study is warranted to test the effectiveness of Iloprost therapy, with blood flow measurements obtained not only during the period of therapy, but also in the long term.

CONCLUSION

The studies described in this chapter show how leg arterial blood flow measurements obtained with APG can be applied in the clinical setting and demonstrate the potential for future practical clinical applications.

REFERENCE

1. Christopoulos D et al: Venous hypertensive microangiopathy in relation to clinical severity and effect of elastic compression, *J Dermatol Surg Oncol* 17:809-813, 1991.

CHAPTER 61

Exercise ankle pressure measurements in arterial disease

D. EUGENE STRANDNESS, Jr., and R. EUGENE ZIERLER

The most common complaint of patients with chronic arterial occlusion is intermittent claudication. It is secondary to the inadequacy of the collateral circulation in fulfilling the metabolic requirements of the exercising muscle. Interestingly, numerous studies have confirmed that even with extensive multilevel occlusive disease, resting blood flows are maintained in the normal range because of the relatively low blood flow requirements at rest and the compensatory decrease in resistance that occurs distal to the areas of occlusion.

Exercise as a method of assessing the degree of disability associated with atherosclerosis is useful for the following reasons: (1) exercise is the specific activity that produces the symptoms, (2) the severity of pain, its localization, and the walking pattern can be simply assessed, (3) it is possible to determine the degree to which the collateral circulation can maintain distal perfusion pressure in response to a near maximal ischemic stimulus, (4) the recovery time (i.e., the period of postexercise hyperemia) can be accurately determined, (5) exercise can be valuable in distinguishing true claudication from the neurospinal conditions that mimic the pain of muscular ischemia, and (6) exercise may be the most sensitive method of assessing both disease progression and improvement.

Before considering the clinical application and usefulness of this type of testing, it is necessary to briefly review the current understanding of the normal physiologic response to exercise.

NORMAL PHYSIOLOGY
Limb blood flow

Blood flow is primarily distributed to the two major components of the limb: skin and muscle. Because of its important role in thermal regulation, skin blood flow does vary widely depending on the ambient conditions. The proportion of skin to muscle in the limbs varies greatly by location, with progressively less muscle mass proceeding distally. The total blood flow to the leg is distributed to the major components: skin, muscle, bone, and fat. The level of resting flow to bone depends on the relative proportions of cancellous and noncancellous bone and is difficult to assess, particularly in terms of the redistribution that may occur in response to exercise.

Under resting conditions, the average blood flow in the normal leg is in the range of 300 to 500 ml/min.[23] Grimby et al[8] and Lassen and Kampp[13] measured resting flows in muscle by the xenon clearance method and found that in general, flows vary between 1.8 and 2.5 ml/100 g/min in the muscle groups tested. At moderate levels of exercise, total leg blood flow increases by a factor of 5 to 10, while muscle blood flow rises to approximately 30 ml/100 g/min (Fig. 61-1). Muscle blood flow may reach 70 ml/100 g/min during strenuous exercise. After the cessation of exercise, limb blood flow returns to resting values within 1 to 5 minutes.

Skin blood flow is extremely sensitive to changes in ambient temperature, and any value expressed must take this into account. Flows to the skin of the hand are much more variable than those to the foot, even with similar changes in temperature. For example, Allwood and Burry[1] found foot blood flow to range from 0.2 ml/100 ml/min at 15° C to 16.5 ml/100 ml/min at 44° C. Corresponding temperature increases produce much higher blood flows to the hand. Although there is no doubt that muscle flow can also respond to changes in temperature, it is much less variable than blood flow to skin and subcutaneous tissue.

Reactive hyperemia. One of the remarkable features of limb blood flow is the phenomenon commonly referred to as *reactive hyperemia*. A poorly understood aspect of this change is the fact that even a few seconds of arterial occlusion will produce an increase in flow even though the duration of occlusion is not sufficient to produce significant ischemia. The actual flow changes that are defined as reactive hyperemia are confined to those situations in which arterial flow has been occluded by a pneumatic tourniquet, whereas the changes that accompany walking represent the period of postexercise hyperemia.

Because flows to skin and muscle have not been measured simultaneously to assess the exact partition that occurs between these tissues, the precise distribution of reactive hyperemic flow is unclear. However, with reactive hyperemia the early marked increase in flow is largely confined to skin.

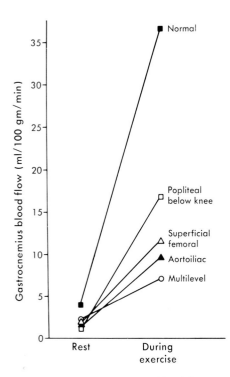

Fig. 61-1. Magnitude of the increase in blood flow to muscle that occurs in normal subjects and in patients with varying degrees of occlusive arterial disease.

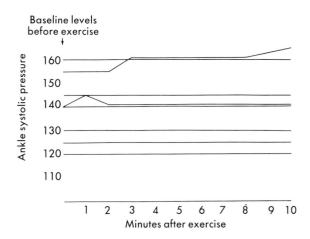

Fig. 61-2. Ankle systolic pressure values of eight normal subjects after walking on a treadmill for 5 minutes at 2 mph on a 12% grade. In every case, the pressure either remained at the preexercise level or increased slightly. (From Strandness DE Jr: *Surgery* 59:325, 1966.)

During exercise, the great demands for blood are in the muscle and there may be a transient reduction in blood flow to skin and, in particular, to the distal foot. Thus with arterial occlusion, there may be a transient but dramatic reduction in foot blood flow, the magnitude of which is related to the severity of the arterial disease.

Limb blood pressure

The limb blood pressure response to stress has been studied most frequently by indirect measurements of ankle systolic blood pressure. This information is most useful when expressed as the ratio of ankle systolic pressure to brachial systolic pressure. The ankle-to-arm pressure index has a mean value of 1.11 ± 0.10 in normal individuals at rest.[28] The following simple analogy to Ohm's law can be made:

$$P_1 - P_2 = RQ$$

where $P_1 - P_2$ is the pressure drop across the segment being evaluated, R is the resistance to flow, and Q is the volume flow. As predicted by this analogy, there should be an increased pressure drop across an arterial segment as flow is increased with either exercise or reactive hyperemia. However, Strandness and Bell[22] demonstrated little or no fall in systolic pressure at the ankle after exercise in normal subjects walking at 2 mph on a 12% grade. Stahler and Strandness[18] were also able to show that as the work load increased above this level, there was a slight decrease in the ankle pressure immediately after exercise with some

delay in recovery related to the level of the work load. Nevertheless, the work loads required to bring about this pressure fall were much more strenuous than those used in evaluating patients with intermittent claudication. Thus for practical purposes, the response of a normal leg to moderate exercise consists of little or no drop in the ankle systolic pressure (Fig. 61-2).

EXERCISE PHYSIOLOGY WITH CHRONIC ARTERIAL OCCLUSION

The development of arterial stenoses or occlusions results in diversion of flow through the collateral channels, which because of the very small size of the midzone components, are high-resistance conduits. Thus even under resting conditions, there is an abnormal pressure drop across the collateral bed that reduces the perfusion pressure to both the muscle and skin distal to the site of involvement.

Although collateral resistance is relatively high and fixed, the resistance of a peripheral runoff bed such as the calf is quite variable. The muscular arterioles are primarily responsible for regulating peripheral resistance and controlling the distribution of flow to various capillary beds. One common example is of a limb with an occluded superficial femoral artery. In this situation, the resistance offered by the profunda-geniculate collateral system is high, but a compensatory decrease in the peripheral calf resistance permits resting blood flow to remain in the normal range.[25] During exercise, the resistance of the proximal collateral bed remains high while the peripheral resistance continues to decrease. Since the ability of the peripheral vessels to compensate for the high proximal resistance is limited, exercise blood flow will be less than normal and there will be a further pressure drop across the diseased arterial segment. The clinical result of this physiologic response is calf muscle ischemia with claudication.

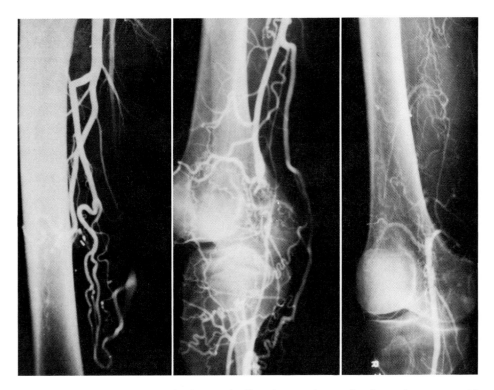

Fig. 61-3. Marked differences in the degree of collateralization that can be observed in patients with disease of the femoropopliteal segment.

In a normal patient, exercise at even moderate work loads produces a large increase in the blood flow to muscle. Although resting limb blood flow in patients with claudication is not significantly different from that in normal subjects, the same degree of exercise in patients with chronic arterial occlusion results in a much smaller increase in flow (Fig. 61-1). Thus limb blood flow can dramatically increase in the normal patient immediately when exposed to stress, in contrast to patients whose maximal limb blood flow is limited by the high-resistance collateral channels. This abnormal response is most easily demonstrated by recording the changes in ankle systolic pressure that follow treadmill exercise to the point of claudication.

As a patient walks, the pressures generated by the contracting muscles in the limb are in opposition to the intraarterial pressure. Therefore depending on the extent of the pressure drop across the collateral bed, the pressure produced by each contraction may exceed that available for perfusion of the muscle. The situation is further complicated by the fact that the resistance vessels in skeletal muscle dilate rapidly in response to the ischemic stimulus. This marked vasodilatation results in a further increase in the pressure available to maintain flow. Thus a vicious cycle is created that can only be reversed by cessation of the exercise.

From a clinical standpoint, it is clear that there is no single pressure-flow response that can be applied to every patient. The reasons for this are the wide variability of (1)

the anatomic patterns of arterial occlusion, (2) the availability and response of the collateral circulation, which also depends on the location of occlusions, duration of disease, degree of exercise maintained by the patient, and age (Fig. 61-3), (3) body weight, (4) systemic blood pressure, and (5) myocardial performance. Thus all of these factors contribute to the degree of disability and the physiologic changes that accompany the disease. However, the advantage of exercise testing is that patients can, in a sense, serve as their own control. The physiologic changes can then be measured and used for long-term studies of the natural history of the disease with or without therapy.[17,19,20]

Observed clinical patterns

As already discussed, the patterns that occur in normal patients are well characterized and, when observed, are adequate indices of normality, particularly if the level of stress is well documented. There are three general patterns of ankle pressure–calf blood flow responses that reflect the level and extent of disease and thus indirectly the collateral potential. These are best discussed in terms of single-segment and multisegment occlusive disease. Single-segment disease refers to isolated occlusions in either the aortoiliac area or superficial femoropopliteal segment. When both segments are occluded, the term *multisegment* is applied.

A brief mention should be made of the medium-sized arteries distal to the popliteal artery (i.e., the tibial and peroneal vessels). Disease confined solely to these arteries does not usually produce claudication but can produce problems involving perfusion of the foot. This is particularly true when distal occlusions are combined with disease at more proximal levels.

It must be emphasized that the resistance to flow offered by collateral arteries becomes greater as successive collateral channels are added; that is, serial resistances are additive. This in large part explains why patients with multisegment disease and multiple collateral pathways always have the most severe symptoms.

Exercise testing for patients with vascular disease is generally carried out on a treadmill set for 2 mph on a 12% grade. This work load is easy for most patients, even elderly ones, and is sufficient to characterize the pressure-flow response that accompanies their disability. Sumner and Strandness[24] in a study of patients with claudication found the following three basic pressure-flow patterns (Fig. 61-4):

1. The calf blood flow increased immediately after exercise as the ankle pressure fell, and the period of postexercise hyperemia was characterized by a lower than normal peak flow and a prolonged recovery time.
2. There was a marked delay before the calf blood flow reached its lower than normal peak value.
3. The calf blood flow fell below even resting levels immediately after exercise, requiring prolonged periods of time for recovery.

An important observation resulting from these studies was that when simultaneous measurements were made of the ankle systolic pressure changes, there was an excellent correlation with the flow measurements (Fig. 61-5).

Some other important clinical observations regarding the response to exercise were as follows: (1) there is an inverse relationship between calf blood flow and ankle systolic pressure, (2) the ankle systolic pressure response can be used alone as an index of the ischemia that occurs, rather than calf blood flow, which is much more difficult to measure, and (3) the degree of fall in pressure and its recovery time can be used as indicators of the severity of the hemodynamic abnormality.

CLINICAL APPLICATIONS OF EXERCISE TESTING

There is little doubt that resting systolic ankle pressures and ankle-to-arm indices are usually sufficient to establish the diagnosis of occlusive disease and its severity. For example, it is known that if the ankle-to-arm pressure index is greater than 0.5, single-segment disease is likely, whereas a lower pressure index is observed most commonly with multi-segment disease. Furthermore, both the amount of improvement and the progression of disease can be documented in most cases by the resting pressures. It must therefore be determined what other factors justify the added testing.

Carter[4] has shown that patients with mild arterial occlusive disease and normal ankle systolic pressures at rest may have their lesions "unmasked" by exercise testing. In these cases, the collateral circulation provides adequate resting flow with little or no reduction in ankle pressure. However, because the capacity to increase flow is limited, pressure gradients may be accentuated when flow rates are increased by exercise. Thus exercise testing provides a method for detecting less severe degrees of arterial occlusive disease.

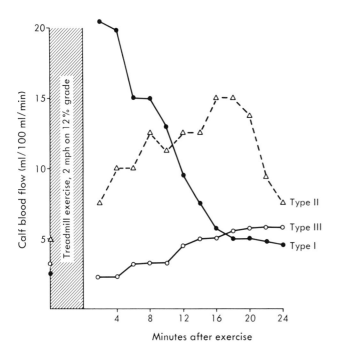

Fig. 61-4. Three patterns of calf blood flow observed in patients with intermittent claudication. See text for explanation. (From Strandness DE Jr: *Cardiovasc Clin* 3:53, 1971.)

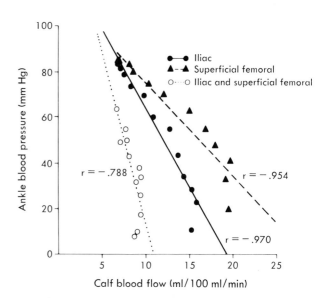

Fig. 61-5. The relationship between ankle blood pressure and calf blood flow in patients with varying degrees of arterial occlusion. (From Sumner DS, Strandness DE Jr: *Surgery* 65:783, 1969.)

Patient testimony is highly subjective and is only sufficient for documenting the qualitative changes that have occurred. These pitfalls must be recognized by all clinicians who evaluate patients with claudication. The treadmill exercise test provides the following objective information: (1) the walking time at a constant work load, (2) the location, time of onset, and severity of pain, (3) the walking pattern as symptoms appear, (4) the critically important relationship between the ankle pressure response and walking time, (5) the degree of improvement following arterial surgery, and (6) the changes in the capacity of the collateral circulation.[17] In addition, walking on a treadmill simulates the activity that produces the patient's symptoms and determines the degree of disability under strictly controlled conditions. A variety of nonvascular factors may affect performance and can also be evaluated during treadmill exercise. These include musculoskeletal or cardiopulmonary disease, level of effort, patient motivation, and pain tolerance.

Walking on the treadmill is continued for 5 minutes or until symptoms force the patient to stop. The two most significant components of the response to exercise are (1) the magnitude of the immediate drop in ankle systolic pressure and (2) the time required for recovery to resting pressures. Changes in both of these parameters are proportional to the severity of the arterial occlusive disease. Extended treadmill testing beyond the onset of claudication does not provide any additional diagnostic information.[14]

In general, the postexercise pressure changes in patients with arterial occlusive disease can be divided into three groups.[24] Ankle pressures that fall to low or unrecordable levels immediately after exercise and then return to resting values in 2 to 6 minutes suggest single-segment occlusive disease. Multisegment occlusive disease is usually associated with ankle pressures that remain low or unrecordable for up to 12 minutes. In patients with severe ischemia and rest pain, postexercise ankle pressures may be unrecordable for 15 minutes or more.

The obvious goal of any form of therapy is to improve the ability of the patient to walk. If the treadmill test is used in the same manner each time, the increase in walking time alone is one index of improvement. However, walking time can be increased on the treadmill even when the disease is unchanged or occasionally is worse. Patients can accomplish this in several ways. First, they may grab the support bar of the treadmill, thus taking some of the weight off their legs. Second, they may walk with one leg slightly externally rotated to minimize the work required by the calf muscles. Both of these problems can be avoided by careful instruction and observation of the patient during walking. It is also possible to detect patients who want to give the impression of improvement by pushing themselves beyond the point at which they would usually stop.

Differential diagnosis of leg pain

In recent years it has been recognized that there are patients with neurospinal disorders and degenerative joint disease who experience pain with walking that may mimic intermittent claudication. Although it is true that a carefully taken history will identify most of these patients, a normal treadmill test is further confirmation. A patient who develops leg pain on the basis of ischemia will *always* experience a drop in ankle pressure to an abnormal degree when exercised to the point of pain. If a normal exercise response is noted, some other cause for the symptoms must be sought.

Documenting results of treatment

The natural course of intermittent claudication is relatively benign, with only 1% to 2% of patients requiring amputation per year of follow-up.[2,10] Thus in the majority of patients, the degree of disability either remains stable or improves spontaneously. This improvement probably results from an increase in collateral flow occurring in response to the large pressure gradients produced in the leg during walking.[27] It is also possible that muscle cells are able to improve their function by undergoing some metabolic adaptation to chronic ischemia.[5] These observations provide the rationale for exercise therapy in patients with intermittent claudication.[12,16,17] Although an exercise program does increase the walking distance of many patients, the degree of clinical improvement that can be documented by treadmill testing is usually modest. The capacity of the collateral circulation to compensate for a major arterial occlusion is clearly limited, even during maximal ischemic and hemodynamic stress.

The response of the ankle systolic pressure to treadmill exercise provides an ideal method for assessing the results of direct arterial surgery.[19,26] Patients who are improved by surgery but still not normal can easily have their condition documented. For example, a patient who can walk on the treadmill for only 2 minutes before an operation and after the procedure can double the walking time but still has the same abnormal hemodynamic response is definitely improved; the difference is that because of the increase in flow, it has simply taken longer to reach the same level of ischemia. Thus one of the great advantages of exercise testing is that it is possible to document the actual degree of improvement in physiologic terms (Fig. 61-6).

In patients with single-segment disease who undergo operation, the ankle pressure response to exercise should return to normal. If it does, the exercise response indicates that all disease that is hemodynamically significant under the degree of stress applied has been eliminated. When the response is improved but remains abnormal, there is either residual uncorrected disease or problems related to the reconstruction itself that continue to pose an abnormal amount of resistance to flow. Thus it is possible to use the response to exercise as an objective indicator of the degree of improvement, the extent of residual disease, and most importantly, the changes that may occur over time.[18,22,26]

Exercise testing has also been used to assess the results of pharmacologic therapy for occlusive arterial disease.[15,21] Clinical studies of vasodilator drugs have failed to show

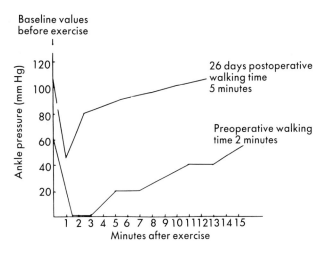

Fig. 61-6. Treadmill exercise test before and after successful femoropopliteal bypass graft with the saphenous vein. Although the walking time was increased to 5 minutes without symptoms, the ankle pressure response remains abnormal. (From Strandness DE Jr: *Surgery* 59:325, 1966.)

any objective benefit in patients with intermittent claudication or ischemic rest pain.[6,21] Furthermore, there is no evidence that vasodilators can increase flow through either collateral vessels or exercising muscle. Treadmill exercise testing was used to evaluate the rheologic agent pentoxifylline in a multicenter clinical trial.[15] Pentoxifylline inhibits platelet aggregation and reduces blood viscosity by altering the membrane flexibility of red blood cells. In this double-blind, placebo-controlled study, the distance walked before the onset of claudication increased in both the pentoxifylline and placebo groups; however, a significantly greater degree of improvement was observed in the patients receiving pentoxifylline. The effect of this drug on the natural course of arterial occlusive disease in not known.

Exercise versus reactive hyperemia testing

As previously mentioned, reactive hyperemia is an alternative to treadmill exercise for stressing the peripheral circulation. Inflating a pneumatic thigh cuff to suprasystolic pressure for 3 to 5 minutes will produce ischemia and vasodilatation in the distal tissues. When the cuff occlusion is released, the changes in the ankle systolic pressure are qualitatively similar to those observed following exercise. However, there are several important differences between reactive hyperemia and postexercise hyperemia. Although normal subjects do not show a drop in ankle systolic pressure after treadmill exercise, a transient but definite drop is observed with reactive hyperemia.[9,11] This mean drop in ankle pressure is in the range of 17% to 34%. In patients with arterial occlusive disease, the response to reactive hyperemia is usually more prominent and there is a good correlation between the maximum pressure drop with reactive hyperemia and the maximum pressure drop after treadmill exercise. There may be considerable overlap, however, in

the ankle pressure response to reactive hyperemia among normal subjects and patients with arterial disease.[11] Furthermore, there is no correlation between reactive hyperemia and treadmill exercise with regard to the time for recovery to resting pressure. In general, patients with single-segment arterial disease show less than a 50% drop in ankle pressure with reactive hyperemia, whereas patients with multisegment arterial disease show a pressure drop greater than 50%.[9]

The reactive hyperemia test is simple and rapid to perform, and it is particularly useful for those patients who are unable to walk on the treadmill because of amputations or other physical disabilities. Although the use of cuff arterial occlusion has not been associated with thrombotic or embolic complications, it is not currently recommended for the evaluation of patients after arterial reconstructions of the leg. The primary advantage of the treadmill exercise test is that it stresses the peripheral circulation in a physiologic manner and reproduces a patient's ischemic symptoms. Which stress test is used in a specific clinical situation depends on individual patient characteristics, the time allotted for testing, and the equipment available.

CONCLUSION

One of the major limitations of treadmill exercise testing is the fact that when the patient has bilateral disease, the degree of disability is rarely the same for both limbs, so the exercise response will reflect functional impairment in the worse limb. Furthermore, it is not possible to predict on the basis of the test results alone the degree of disability that will remain when the flow to the most symptomatic limb has been corrected. For example, if a patient is stopped at 2 minutes with claudication involving one limb, correction of this side will increase the walking distance only to the extent that the other leg is involved.

The level of exercise used in most centers to evaluate peripheral arterial insufficiency involves a much lower work load than is commonly used to detect myocardial ischemia. There is increasing evidence that concomitant ECG monitoring may also provide useful data concerning the presence of coronary artery disease. In a series of 100 consecutive patients with peripheral arterial disease, Cutler et al[7] identified 46 patients who developed ventricular dysrhythmias, ischemia, or both, usually unassociated with symptoms. In this study, the unmasking of coexisting cardiac disease was a useful predictor of postoperative complications. There were 16 patients with abnormal ECGs who were subjected to direct arterial surgery; six had postoperative myocardial infarctions, two of which were fatal. Carroll et al[3] presented similar findings: of 46 consecutive patients, 23% demonstrated serious ECG abnormalities at this minimal work load. These studies clearly indicate that if such surveillance is used, a significant number of patients with myocardial ischemia will also be discovered. As noted in the series by Cutler et al[7] the tests were also useful in predicting the potential for postoperative myocardial infarction.

All patients who are being considered for major arterial reconstructions should have a comprehensive cardiology evaluation. One factor to consider is the medicolegal issue of whether exercise testing at this low work load requires simultaneous ECG monitoring as a standard part of practice. If this requirement is added to the usual testing for peripheral arterial disease, the procedure would have to be monitored by a physician familiar with those ECG changes associated with myocardial ischemia. Avoiding the need for ECG monitoring is therefore one of the potential advantages of reactive hyperemia testing.

REFERENCES

1. Allwood MJ, Burry HS: The effect of local temperature of blood flow in the human foot, *J Physiol (Lond)* 124:345, 1954.
2. Boyd AM: The natural course of arteriosclerosis of the lower extremities, *Proc R Soc Med* 55:591, 1962.
3. Carroll R et al: Cardiac arrhythmias associated with standard 5-minute treadmill claudication testing, In *Proceedings of the Symposium on Noninvasive Diagnostic Techniques in Vascular Disease,* San Diego, Sept 10-14, 1979, University of California at San Diego.
4. Carter SA: Response to ankle systolic pressure to leg exercise in mild or questionable arterial disease, *N Engl J Med* 287:578, 1972.
5. Clyne CAC et al: Ultrastructural and capillary adaption of gastrocnemius muscle to occlusive vascular disease, *Surgery* 92:434, 1982.
6. Coffman JD: Vasodilator drugs in peripheral vascular disease, *N Engl J Med* 300:713, 1979.
7. Cutler BS et al: Assessment of operative risk with electrocardiographic exercise testing in patients with peripheral arterial disease, *Am J Surg* 137:484, 1979.
8. Grimby G, Haggendac E, Saltin B: Local xenon-133 clearance from the quadriceps muscle during exercise in man, *J Appl Physiol* 22:305, 1967.
9. Hummell BW et al: Reactive hyperemia vs. treadmill exercise testing in arterial disease, *Arch Surg* 113:95, 1978.
10. Imparato AM et al: Intermittent claudication—its natural course, *Surgery* 78:795, 1975.
11. Keagy BA et al: Comparison of reactive hyperemia and treadmill tests in the evaluation of peripheral vascular disease, *Am J Surg* 142:158, 1981.
12. Larsen OA, Lassen NA: Effect of daily muscular exercise on patients with intermittent claudication, *Lancet* 2:1093, 1966.
13. Lassen NA, Kampp M: Calf muscle blood flow during walking studied by the Xe 133 method in normals and in patients with intermittent claudication, *Scand J Clin Lab Invest* 17:447, 1965.
14. Mahler DK et al: Treadmill testing in peripheral arterial disease—what can be learned from extended testing? *Bruit* 6:21, 1982.
15. Porter JM et al: Pentoxifylline efficacy in the treatment of intermittent claudication—multicenter controlled double-blind trial with objective assessment of chronic occlusive arterial disease patients, *Am Heart J* 104:66, 1982.
16. Skinner JS, Strandness DE, Jr: Exercise and intermittent claudication. I. Effect of repetition and intensity of exercise, *Circulation* 36:15, 1967.
17. Skinner JS, Strandness DE, Jr: Exercise and intermittent claudication. II. Effect of physical training, *Circulation* 36:23, 1967.
18. Stahler C, Strandness DE, Jr: Ankle blood pressure response to graded treadmill exercise, *Angiology* 18:237, 1967.
19. Strandness DE, Jr: Abnormal exercise responses after successful reconstructive arterial surgery, *Surgery* 59:325, 1966.
20. Strandness DE, Jr: Exercise testing in the evaluation of patients undergoing direct arterial surgery, *J Cardiovasc Surg* 11:192, 1970.
21. Strandness DE, Jr: Ineffectiveness of isoxsuprine on intermittent claudication, *JAMA* 213:86, 1970.
22. Strandness DE, Jr, Bell JW: Peripheral vascular disease: diagnosis and objective evaluation using a mercury strain gauge, *Ann Surg* 161(suppl):1, 1965.
23. Strandness DE, Jr, Sumner DS: *Hemodynamics for surgeons,* New York, 1975, Grune & Stratton.
24. Sumner DS, Strandness DE, Jr: The relationship between calf blood flow and ankle blood pressure in patients with intermittent claudication, *Surgery* 65:763, 1969.
25. Sumner DS, Strandness DE, Jr: The effect of exercise on resistance to blood flow in limbs with an occluded superficial femoral artery, *Vasc Surg* 4:229, 1970.
26. Sumner DS, Strandness DE, Jr: Hemodynamic studies before and after extended bypass grafts to the tibial and peroneal arteries, *Surgery* 86:442, 1979.
27. Winblad JN et al: Etiologic mechanisms in the development of collateral circulation, *Surgery* 45:105, 1959.
28. Yao JST: Hemodynamic studies in peripheral arterial disease, *Br J Surg* 57:761, 1970.

CHAPTER 62

Postocclusive reactive hyperemia in the testing of the peripheral arterial system: pressure, velocity, and pulse reappearance time

ARNOST FRONEK and EUGENE F. BERNSTEIN

The importance of pressure and velocity determinations in the diagnosis of peripheral arterial occlusive disease (PAOD) was discussed in Chapters 53, 55, and 56. These techniques are limited under resting conditions, especially in cases of borderline results. A logical step to increase the sensitivity of these tests is to stress the peripheral circulation in the hope that an increased blood flow induced by standardized local ischemia will (1) help to quantitate the vasodilatory response and (2) exaggerate the pressure drop across the stenotic lesion. Such stress testing is particularly important in those cases in which resting pressure and velocity results do not establish the diagnosis of PAOD unequivocally.

As Strandness has pointed out (see Chapter 61), exercise has been one of the most widely used types of stress for this purpose because it is so clearly related to intermittent claudication. There are, however, several circumstances that limit the application of this otherwise highly sensitive and specific diagnostic technique: (1) the activity of the exercising subject precludes using some of the existing continuous monitoring techniques (e.g., velocity, pulse volume), (2) varying pain thresholds in different patients[20,40] may lower the standardization value of the test, (3) although the risk is small, a large percentage of patients with PAOD also suffer from coronary disease (in a clinical or subclinical form) and therefore ECG monitoring throughout the test may be advisable,[9,39] (4) there are a number of patients who are unable to undergo treadmill exercise (e.g., amputees, arthritics, patients with severe ischemia of the contralateral limb, cardiopulmonary limitation, neurologic disorders), and (5) the expense and bulkiness of the treadmill may limit its application, especially if bedside use is considered. For all of these reasons, postocclusive reactive hyperemia (PORH) has been considered by a number of investigators as an alternative stress procedure to increase the sensitivity and specificity of their respective tests.

Blood flow in the examined limb has been studied using venous occlusion plethysmography either with water or air as the communicating medium or with the mercury-in-rubber (Whitney) gauge.* The introduction of a simple electric calibration[8,22] may lead to wider use of the technique. Despite the well-established reliability of this approach, it has not found wide acceptance for routine clinical diagnostic studies, probably because (1) venous occlusion must be performed intermittently, so no continuous readout is possible and therefore the detection of the peak response may be missed and (2) the evaluation is rather time consuming because the volume increase must be calculated separately for each run (although this last step can be automated).[16]

There are, however, three additional ways to use the transient increase in blood flow induced by temporary inflow compression: (1) the PORH ankle pressure response, (2) the ultrasonically monitored PORH flow velocity response, and (3) the peripherally monitored pulse reappearance time (PRT).

PORH ANKLE PRESSURE RESPONSE

Dornhorst and Sharpey-Schafer[14] described the significance of PORH as a standardized form of stress with ankle pressure measurements, and their results were confirmed by a number of additional investigators.[11,25,31] Johnson[25] observed full pressure recovery in normal subjects within 1 minute, whereas patients with various degrees of arterial occlusive disease showed a significant delay in pressure recovery, with the pressure drop and delay related to the severity of the disease.

Several groups compared the efficiency of PORH with that of different exercise tests[3,23,39] and concluded that the drop in blood pressure is very similar when the 30-second PORH pressure response is compared with the 1-minute treadmill exercise response. The ankle flexion stress,[10] although very convenient and simple, led to a significantly smaller drop than the treadmill and PORH stress tests.[3,39]

---

*References 1, 2, 4-6, 13, 16, 21, 24, 26, 29, 32-35, 38, 41.

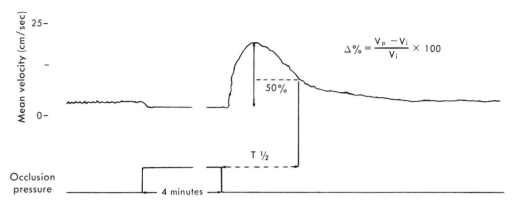

Fig. 62-1. Normal PORH femoral velocity response. The upper tracing is the mean femoral artery flow velocity; the lower tracing is the occlusion pressure.

ULTRASONOGRAPHICALLY MONITORED PORH VELOCITY RESPONSE

The PORH response following a transient flow obstruction can be recorded ultrasonographically.[18] The patient is placed in the supine position and a standard pressure cuff is placed *below* the knee. (Suprasystolic inflation of a cuff placed *above* the knee may sometimes be unpleasant and may cause artifacts by exerting a pull on the ultrasonic probe.) A transcutaneous ultrasonic velocity meter is used, and the probe is placed at the level of the femoral artery with the tip aimed cephalad after the suitable angle and position (maximum output) have been identified. The probe is then held in position by a self-locking magnetic clamp.* A resistance-capacitance filter with a time constant of 1 second may be added to the output stage of the original instrument (if not already built in) to obtain the mean flow velocity.

After a steady-state period has been reached, the cuff is inflated to the suprasystolic pressure. After 4 minutes, the cuff is suddenly deflated and the PORH response is continuously recorded until the velocity value returns to the control level. The response is evaluated in the following two ways (Fig. 62-1):

1. The percentage increase:

$$\frac{(\text{Peak velocity} - \text{Initial velocity})}{\text{Initial velocity}} \times 100$$

2. The recovery half-time ($T_{1/2}$), or the time for the mean velocity to return to 50% of its peak response

Control studies performed on 50 lower extremities in 25 healthy subjects helped establish the normal response: a 226% increase in femoral artery flow velocity (± 16.2 SEM) and above the preocclusion value and a 25-second (± 1.5 SEM) $T_{1/2}$.

In contrast, patients with angiographically documented PAOD in the aortoiliac or femoropopliteal segments had a significantly lower peak response (55% $\pm$ 6.2 SEM) and a significantly longer recovery half-time (47.1 seconds $\pm$ 1.5 SEM). To date, more than 3000 patients have been studied with this technique, and for 400 of them, careful correlations have been made with their angiographic patterns. Based on this experience, a peak velocity response of less than an 80% increase over the control mean velocity and a $T_{1/2}$ longer than 35 seconds may be indicative of a pathologic condition. Fig. 62-2 shows a PORH velocity response before and after successful vascular reconstruction, as also recently reported by Myhre.[30]

PERIPHERALLY MONITORED PULSE REAPPEARANCE TIME

The technique of monitoring the PRT is based on clinical experience with the postexercise[12] disappearance of pedal pulses[15,27] and the significant decrease in distal arterial blood pressure seen in the presence of PAOD.[7,36,37] After a qualitative similarity between the PORH and the postexercise reactive hyperemia response is established,[28] the PORH test is extended to include measuring the change in toe pulse volume induced by a 4-minute calf occlusion. The toe pulse volume can be recorded with a variety of suitable transducers. In the original study,[17] a closed-loop mercury-in-rubber (Whitney) gauge was connected to a low-resistance bridge amplifier* with the output fed into an AC amplifier (band width, 1 to 10 Hz) and recorded simultaneously with the PORH femoral arterial velocity response. After the 4-minute occlusion, the cuff pressure was suddenly released and the reappearance of the toe pulse was continuously recorded (Fig. 62-3).

---

*Flex-O-Post Indicator Holder with Magnetic Base; Starrett Co, Athol, Mass.

---

*Model 270 plethysmograph; Parks Electronics, Beaverton, Ore, or SPG-16 Strain Gauge Plethysmograph; Medsonics, Mountain View, Calif, or EC-4 Plethysmograph; Hokanson, Issaquah, Wash.

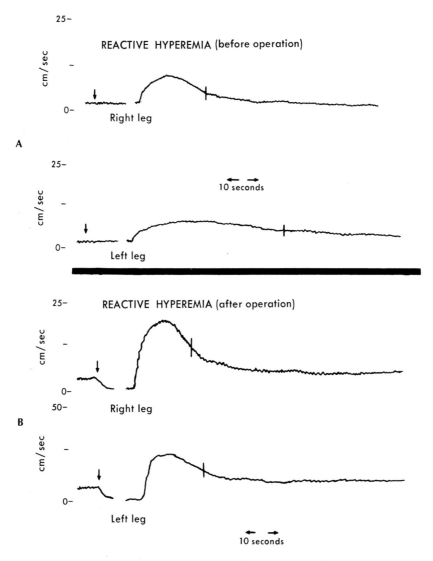

Fig. 62-2. PORH femoral artery velocity response. **A,** Right and left leg before operation. **B,** Right and left leg after operation.

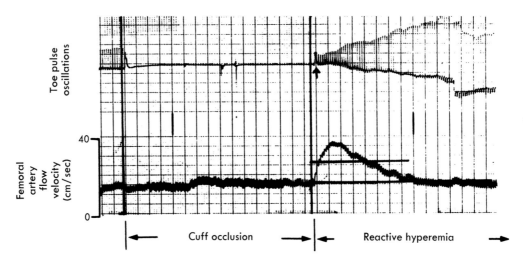

Fig. 62-3. Combined normal PORH femoral artery velocity and PRT/2 response.

Control values were established in 22 healthy subjects (44 limbs), in whom the average time for the toe pulse volume to return to 50% of its control amplitude (PRT/2) was 3.4 seconds ± 0.8 SEM. Fig. 62-3 depicts a normal toe PRT response recorded simultaneously with the ultrasonographically monitored PORH femoral artery velocity response. The very first volume pulse after the cuff release is already higher than 50% of the preocclusion control amplitude. In addition, a typical overshoot response is demonstrated.

The PRT/2 has been correlated with angiographically documented disease in 58 patients (110 limbs). The average PRT/2 in patients with multilevel occlusive disease was 71.2 seconds (±5.5 SEM), whereas the average PRT/2 in three other groups (isolated aortoiliac, femoropopliteal, and trifurcation occlusion) was around 25 seconds. Based on overall experience, a PRT/2 longer than 6 seconds may indicate a pathologic condition. These results were recently confirmed by Gutierrez and Gage[19] using a photoplethysmographic sensor.

DIAGNOSTIC VALUE OF THE PORH ANKLE PRESSURE, VELOCITY, AND PRT/2 RESPONSE

These three tests are closely related and represent three different indices of a common denominator—the hemodynamic response to transient tissue ischemia. Each test, however, documents a different aspect of the response.

The PORH ankle pressure and PRT/2 response are closest as to their genesis. As depicted in Fig. 62-4, the peak PORH response is associated with a transient pressure drop

of 80 mm Hg, compared to a previous resting pressure drop of only 20 mm Hg. This increased pressure drop was induced by the transient increase in blood flow (from 100 to 400 ml/min) and therefore:

$$\Delta P = \frac{0.2}{R} \times \frac{400}{F} = 80 \text{ mm Hg}$$

where ΔP is the pressure drop across the stenosis, R is the resistance (expressed in relative units), and F is the flow at peak PORH response. With a declining flow response, the pressure drop decreases proportionally while the pressure increases by the same amount.

The same mechanism is also responsible for the PRT/2 response, but only the oscillatory component is recorded. The advantage of the PRT/2, however, is its ability to continuously monitor the pulse volume changes. It can be assumed that the PRT/2 value represents an index of overall perfusion, especially when monitored at the toe. Studies currently under way will demonstrate whether the two techniques (PORH ankle pressure and PRT/2 monitoring) yield results of comparable importance.

In contrast to these two methods, PORH velocity monitoring predominantly reflects the response at the femoral artery level and is highly sensitive to stenoses in the superficial femoral artery. The combination of these tests therefore has substantial advantage. For instance, a reduced PORH velocity response combined with a normal PRT/2 response suggests the presence of significant femoral artery occlusive disease with a well-developed collateral circulation. Similarly, in patients who have undergone a bypass

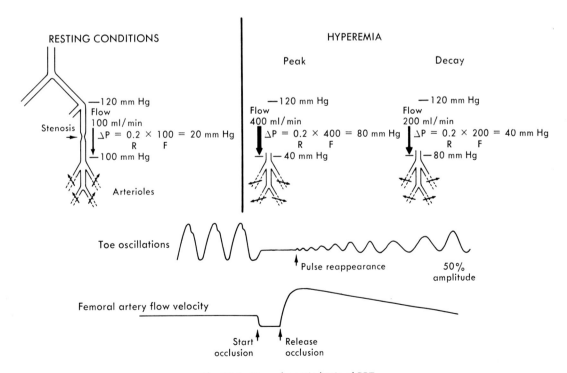

Fig. 62-4. Hemodynamic basis of PRT.

operation without improvement in their femoral artery velocity PORH response but with significant improvement in the PRT/2, benefit from the operation is based on an increase in the overall perfusion of the limb. In such cases, the low PORH velocity response can be attributed to the topography of the bypassing vessel, or prosthesis, or to a local increase in vessel diameter at the site of suture, or from endarterectomy if the velocity probe incidentally monitored this site. Fig. 62-5 depicts changes in PORH and PRT/2 before and after vascular reconstruction.

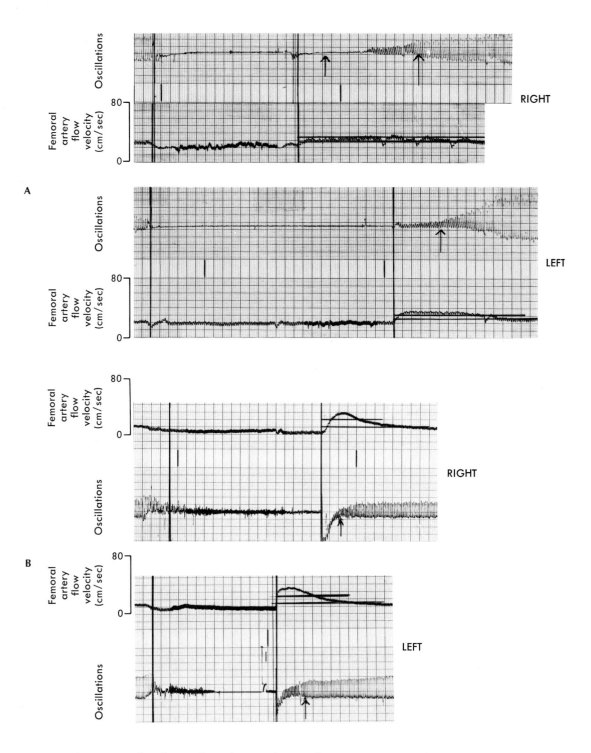

Fig. 62-5. Combined PORH femoral artery velocity and PRT/2 response. *A,* Before vascular reconstruction. The first arrow is the reappearance of the first pulse; the second arrow is the reappearance of 50% amplitude. *B,* After vascular reconstruction.

All three techniques (PORH ankle pressure, PORH velocity response, and PRT/2) are useful adjunct diagnostic procedures, especially in cases when the results of other noninvasive laboratory tests are equivocal. Depression and delay of the PORH velocity response, as well as delay in the PRT/2 response, indicate the presence of femoral artery occlusive disease and impairment of overall leg blood supply, respectively. Dissociation of these results, low PORH and normal PRT/2, generally indicates good collateral circulation, reducing the sequelae of arterial stenosis. On the other hand, normal segmental pressures (not only ankle pressures) in the presence of borderline symptomatology represent a strong indication for performing a stress test to measure the PORH response.

POSTEXERCISE VERSUS POSTOCCLUSIVE REACTIVE HYPEREMIA STRESS
Comparison of diagnostic value

As described in the preceding paragraphs and in Chapter 61, both methods have advantages and disadvantages that are complex. In view of currently available information and experience, the following conclusions can be drawn:

1. The postexercise reactive hyperemia (PERH) induces the most profound hemodynamic changes, reflected mainly in pressure drop and recovery time.

2. There are some limitations specific to the exercise test, especially when the treadmill is used. As mentioned earlier, constant ECG monitoring may be advisable in view of frequent concomitant coronary artery disease.[9,39] There are cases of limited mobility (amputees or other cases of skeletomuscular or neurologic origin) that may distort the results because of difficulty in performing the study.

3. On the other hand, the PORH response leads to smaller hemodynamic changes, but these are standardized and applicable to every patient. The disadvantage of the shorter recovery time may be outweighed by the ease of recording the earliest poststress hemodynamic changes because the patient remains in the supine position and no time is lost in readjusting the instrumentation.

More investigations and experience with different types of stressors are needed for a definitive answer. The ideal dynamic test will have to be highly sensitive and specific and, at the same time, have a negligible effect on the overall cardiovascular system and be applicable to every patient, disregarding concomitant cardiopulmonary, neurologic, or musculoskeletal handicaps.

CONCLUSION

Additional noninvasive diagnostic tests are desirable in cases with equivocal results based on resting peripheral circulatory hemodynamics. PORH measurement has some advantages when compared with PERH, since it permits continuous monitoring of the femoral artery velocity and the pulse volume response. It shows practically the same pressure drop as is seen during the postexercise response, although of shorter duration. The simplicity, absence of risk to the patient, and very good overall patient acceptance represent additional favorable factors.

Generally, a 4-minute period of ischemia is normally followed (1) by a return of ankle blood pressure to the control value within 60 seconds, (2) by an increase in femoral artery velocity of at least 100% above control levels, and (3) by a PRT/2 of 6 seconds or less. Conversely, a delayed return of ankle blood pressure of more than 120 seconds, an increase in femoral artery flow velocity less than 80% above control, and a delay of PRT/2 longer than 10 seconds indicate the presence of hemodynamically significant obstruction of the arterial system in the lower extremity.

Diagnostic implications of the described tests are discussed in light of their common hemodynamic basis: (1) a decrease in PORH velocity response with a normal PRT/2 response suggests the presence of significant femoral artery occlusive disease with a well-developed collateral circulation, (2) a decrease in PORH velocity response combined with a delayed PRT/2 response indicates the presence of femoral artery occlusive disease with an inadequate collateral circulation, and (3) a borderline segmental pressure can be conveniently clarified by repeating the pressure measurement during the PORH response.

REFERENCES

1. Abramson DJ: *Circulation in the extremities*, New York, 1967, Academic Press.
2. Abramson DJ, Katzenstein KH, Ferris EG, Jr: Observations on reactive hyperaemia in various portions of the extremities, *Am J Surg* 22:329, 1941.
3. Baker JD: Post stress Doppler ankle pressures, *Arch Surg* 113:1171, 1978.
4. Bentley TH: Muscle blood flow in patients with arteriosclerosis obliterans, *Am J Surg* 96:193, 1958.
5. Bollinger A: Bedeutung der Venenverschlussplethysmographie in der angiologischen Diagnostik, *Schweiz Med Wochenschr* 95:1357, 1969.
6. Bollinger A: *Durchblutungsmessungen in der klinischen Angiologie*, Bern, Switzerland, 1969, Hans Huber.
7. Bollinger A et al: Measurement of systolic ankle blood pressure with Doppler ultrasound at rest and after exercise in patients with leg artery occlusions, *Scand J Clin Lab Invest* 31(suppl 128):123, 1973.
8. Brakkee AJ, Vendrik AJ: Strain gauge plethysmography: theoretical and practical notes on a new design, *J Appl Physiol* 21:701, 1966.
9. Carroll R et al: *Cardiac arrhythmias associated with standard 5-minute treadmill claudication testing*, Paper presented at the Symposium on Noninvasive Diagnostic Techniques in Vascular Disease, San Diego, Sept 10-14, 1979.
10. Carter SA: Response of ankle systolic pressure to leg exercise in mild or questionable arterial disease, *N Engl J Med* 287:578, 1972.
11. Delius W: Hämodynamische Untersuchungen über den systolischen Blutdruck und die arterielle Durchblutung distal von arteriellen Gefässeverschlussen an den unteren Extremitäten, *Z Kreis* 58:319, 1969.
12. DeWeese JA: Pedal pulses disappearing with exercise: a test for intermittent claudication, *N Engl J Med* 262:1214, 1960.
13. Dohn K: On clinical use of venous occlusion plethysmography of calf. II. Results in patients with arterial disease, *Acta Med Scand* 130:61, 1965.
14. Dornhorst AC, Sharpey-Schafer EP: Collateral resistance in limbs with arterial obstruction: spontaneous changes and effects of sympathectomy, *Clin Sci* 10:371, 1951.
15. Edwards EA, Cohen NR, Kaplan MM: Effect of exercise in peripheral pulses, *N Engl J Med* 160:738, 1959.

16. Ehringer H: *Die reaktive Hyperämie nach arterieller Sperre*. In Bollinger A, Brunner U, eds: *Messmethoden bei arteriellen Durchblutungsstorungen*, Bern, Switzerland, 1971, Hans Huber.

17. Fronek A, Coel M, Bernstein EF: The pulse-reappearance time: an index of over-all blood flow impairment in the ischemic extremity, *Surgery* 81:376, 1977.

18. Fronek A et al: Ultrasonographically monitored postocclusive reactive hyperemia in the diagnosis of peripheral arterial occlusive disease, *Circulation* 43:149, 1973.

19. Gutierrez JZ, Gage AA: *Toe pulse study (using the photopulse photoplethysmograph) in the diagnosis and evaluation of the severity of ischemic arterial disease of the lower extremities*, Paper presented at Symposium on Noninvasive Diagnostic Techniques in Vascular Disease, San Diego, Sept 10-14, 1979.

20. Hillestad LK: The peripheral blood flow in intermittent claudication. IV. The significance of the claudication distance, *Acta Med Scand* 173:467, 1963.

21. Hillestad LK: The peripheral blood flow in intermittent claudication. V. Plethysmographic studies, *Acta Med Scand* 174:23, 1963.

22. Hokanson DE, Sumner DS, Strandness DE, Jr: An electrically calibrated plethysmograph for direct measurement of limb blood flow, *IEEE Trans Biomed Eng* 22:25, 1975.

23. Hummel BW, et al: Reactive hyperemia vs. treadmill exercise testing in arterial disease, *Arch Surg* 113:95, 1978.

24. Hyman C, Winsor T: Blood flow redistribution in the human extremity, *Am J Cardiol* 4:566, 1959.

25. Johnson WC: Doppler ankle pressure and reactive hyperemia in the diagnosis of arterial insufficiency, *J Surg Res* 18:177, 1975.

26. Lewis T, Grant R: Observations upon reactive hyperemia in man, *Heart* 12:73, 1925.

27. Mackereth M, Lennihan R: Ultrasound as an aid in the diagnosis and management of intermittent claudication, *Angiology* 21:704, 1970.

28. Mahler F et al: Postocclusion and postexercise flow velocity and ankle pressures in normals and marathon runners, *Angiology* 27:721, 1976.

29. Myers K: The investigation of peripheral arterial disease by strain gauge plethysmography, *Angiology* 15:293, 1964.

30. Myhre HO: Reactive hyperemia of the human lower limb. Measurement of postischaemic blood flow velocity in controls and in patients with lower limb artherosclerosis, *Vasa* 2:145, 1975.

31. Myhre HO: Reactive hyperemia of the human lower limb. A comparison between systolic pressure at the ankle after timed circulatory arrest and after exercise in controls and in patients with atherosclerosis, *Vasa* 4:227, 1975.

32. Siggaard-Anderson J: Obliterative vascular disease, classification by means of the Dohn plethysmograph, *Acta Chir Scand* 130:190, 1965.

33. Snell ES, Eastcott HH, Hamilton M: Circulation in lower limb before and after reconstruction of obstructed main artery, *Lancet* 1:242, 1960.

34. Storen G: Post-ischemic calf volume recording in functional evaluation of patients with intermittent claudication, *Scand J Clin Lab Invest* 23:339, 1969.

35. Strandell T, Wahren J: Circulation in the calf at rest, after arterial occlusion, and after exercise in normal subjects and in patients with intermittent claudication, *Acta Med Scand* 173:99, 1963.

36. Strandness DE, Jr, Bell JW: An evaluation of the hemodynamic response of the claudicating extremity to exercise, *Surg Gynecol Obstet* 119:1237, 1964.

37. Sumner DS, Strandness DE, Jr: The relationship between calf blood flow and ankle blood pressure in patients with intermittent claudication, *Surgery* 65:763, 1971.

38. Whitney RJ: The measurement of volume changes in human limbs, *J Physiol (Lond)* 121:1, 1953.

39. Wilbur BG, Olcott C: *A comparison of three modes of stress on Doppler ankle pressures*. In Diethrich EB, ed: *Noninvasive cardiovascular diagnosis*, Baltimore, 1977, University Park Press.

40. Yao ST, et al: A comparative study of strain-gauge plethysmography and Doppler ultrasound in the assessment of occlusive arterial disease of the lower extremities, *Surgery* 71:4, 1972.

41. Zelis R, et al: Effects of hyperlipoproteinemias and their treatment of the peripheral circulation, *J Clin Invest* 49:1007, 1970.

CHAPTER 63

The predictive value of laser Doppler measurements in diabetic microangiopathy and foot ulcers

GIOVANNI BELCARO and ANDREW N. NICOLAIDES

Microcirculatory disturbances in diabetic patients are a common complication and are responsible for high rates of morbidity and mortality. Although the correlation between the metabolic control of diabetes and the development or aggravation of diabetic microangiography is still unclear, good metabolic control may partially reverse the early microcirculatory changes caused by diabetes. In later stages, however, even good metabolic control seems to have only minimal influence on the evolution of microangiopathy.

The detection, characterization, and quantification of diabetic microangiography should form part of the routine assessment of vascular disease. In addition, both the natural history and results of interventional measures need to be interpreted in terms of objective measurements.

The term *diabetic microangiopathy* refers to the functional microcirculatory disturbances that cause the loss of microcirculatory autoregulation and impair the reaction to minimal local injuries. These functional disturbances augment fluid and protein leakage from the capillaries and the formation of edema in the tissues. The long-term pericapillary accumulation of proteins produces permanent capillary alterations, particularly capillary wall thickening, that further impair the autoregulatory mechanisms of the microcirculation. Diabetic microangiopathy is clinically evident only in the late stages of the disease, often when neuropathy is also present. Subclinical microcirculatory changes, however, may be observed early in the peripheral skin circulation of most diabetic patients.

The evolution of diabetic microangiopathy may cause the development of skin lesions, which eventually necessitates limb amputation, often in the absence of occlusive peripheral arterial disease, and this serious outcome has promoted much research in the field. This research has been aided by the recent introduction of laser Doppler flowmetry. The blood flow in peripheral skin, such as the distal dorsum of the foot (better defined as flux when referring to laser Doppler flowmetry), is typically increased and the venoarteriolar response (VAR) is impaired in diabetics. The VAR is the vasoconstrictive response of the skin microcirculation observed when subjects change from the supine to standing position or when lowering the leg below the heart level (Fig. 63-1). When the venous pressure is increased by at least 25 mm Hg by lowering the foot below the heart level, the increase in hydrostatic pressure elicits the VAR, which causes an increase in precapillary resistance. This vasoconstriction is mediated by a sympathetic axon reflex, as described by Hendricksen.[10] The presumed mechanism underlying the VAR includes receptors in the small veins. An increase in venous pressure and stretching triggers impulses that are transmitted antidromically to activate the effector. This autonomic reflex response can be easily documented and quantified by laser Doppler flowmetry.

The increase in skin flux and the impairment of the VAR are more pronounced in patients with diabetic neuropathy. They also exhibit different degrees of response to arterial occlusion, and the reactive hyperemia curves differ depending on the degree of diabetic microangiopathy and neuropathy. Although diabetic microangiopathy cannot be easily defined, with criteria derived from microcirculation studies, it has been possible to characterize it as an impairment in autonomic nervous function and an early increase in capillary permeability and filtration.[6,11] The resulting microcirculatory changes are generally manifested and may be observed in the foot microcirculation using noninvasive methods.[5,7,9,12,13] The following guidelines may be used in a vascular laboratory to diagnose diabetic microangiopathy and quantify its severity:

1. Increased skin blood flux (perfusion) at rest, as shown by laser Doppler flowmetry
2. Decreased VAR
3. Decreased reactive hyperemia
4. Decreased response to local thermal stimulation
5. Increased transcutaneous Pco_2 level and decreased Po_2 level (only in late stages of diabetic microangiopathy)
6. Increased capillary filtration and permeability

Neuropathic ulcers develop in many patients with diabetic microangiopathy, and they are a frequent primary indication

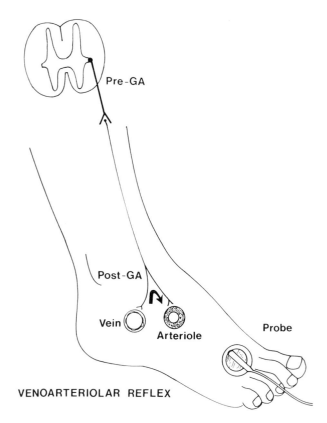

Fig. 63-1. The pathway of the venoarteriolar response. *Pre-GA,* Preganglionic axon; *Post-GA,* postganglionic sympathetic axon.

for amputation. After peripheral arterial occlusive disease that might be causing the significant distal decrease in arterial pressure and perfusion has been ruled out, it is important to then evaluate and quantify the microangiopathy. Early detection and careful noninvasive monitoring of diabetic microangiopathy, along with the institution of appropriate treatment, may circumvent the need for amputation.

Laser Doppler flowmetry may be used to detect early changes as well as to quantify changes in response to therapy.[2] Furthermore, it provides reliable information concerning local microcirculatory conditions that can be used to determine the need for amputation.

Laser Doppler uses a low-power laser in conjunction with state-of-the-art fiberoptics and signal-processing technology. It noninvasively detects the velocities and concentrations of red blood cells in the skin microcirculation and determines the local perfusion in a small (approximately 1 mm³) region of tissue. The perfusion measurement is usually rendered in flux or perfusion units, which are linearly related to the perfusion obtained by isotopic methods. (The principles of laser Doppler are discussed in Chapter 30.) Unfortunately, no standardization has yet been achieved for this method, and the different instruments on the market use different flux units or output measures. Despite this, the basic characteristics of microcirculatory disturbances are comparable and reproducible.

Compared to laser Doppler flowmetry, other microcirculatory techniques, such as capillaroscopy and intravital fluorescence videomicroscopy, are more time consuming, expensive, and difficult to use and are not widely available. Therefore they cannot be used as practical routine screening tests to evaluate the progression of diabetic microangiopathy in a large number of patients. In addition, many postural or dynamic microcirculatory responses can be assessed more easily by laser Doppler flowmetry.

PRACTICAL EVALUATION OF DIABETIC MICROANGIOPATHY

The equipment needed for the evaluation of diabetic microangiopathy includes a laser Doppler flowmeter and a temperature-control module. This chapter presents simple tests based on laser Doppler flowmetry that can yield five measurements. These five measurements can then be used as part of a scoring system that serves as a basis for diagnosing diabetic microangiopathy and for planning appropriate treatment.

All tests should be performed at a stable room temperature (22° C ± 2° C) after the patient has been allowed 30 minutes of acclimatization while resting in the supine position. The fiberoptic probe head is placed on the dorsum of the foot, as shown in Fig. 63-2, using double-sided adhesive rings, or it can be placed on the pulp of the toe but with some loss of stability. It is important to allow at least 5 minutes after placement of the probe before recording any perfusion measurements to ensure a stable flux measurement. The supine resting flux is measured as the average flux in 5 minutes of measurement.

Test 1: the venoarteriolar response

As mentioned previously, the VAR is a sympathetic axon reflex that normally triggers vasoconstriction when the foot is lowered below the heart level.[10] It is particularly evident when a subject moves from the supine to standing position because of the large increase in hydrostatic pressure within the foot. This reflex response is reduced in diabetics with microangiopathy but without neuropathy and is almost abolished in diabetics with microangiopathy and neuropathy (Fig. 63-3).[5,12,13]

The VAR may be evaluated with the leg and foot in different positions. However, a reproducible response is obtained either when changing from the supine to the standing position or when lowering the foot 45 degrees below the heart level. Having the patient lower the foot while remaining supine reduces motion artifacts in the tracing but yields a proportionally weaker response.

The VAR measurement procedure can be summarized as follows. With the patient supine and relaxed, the average resting flux *(RF)* over a 2-minute period is recorded. The patient is then asked to stand upright on both feet while holding onto an orthopedic frame to avoid motion artifact.

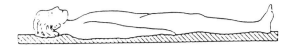

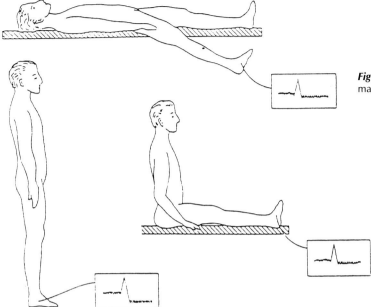

Fig. 63-2. Position of the probe on the dorsum of the foot. The maximum venoarteriolar response is elicited by standing.

There will be a temporary increase in skin perfusion followed by a decrease, as illustrated in Fig. 63-3. After 2 minutes, the standing flux *(SF)* (average flux reading over 2 minutes) is obtained. The VAR is calculated using the following formula:

$$VAR = \frac{RF - SF}{RF} \times 100$$

The microangiopathy index *(MI)* is calculated as follows:

$$MI = \frac{VAR}{RF}$$

The microangiopathy index is useful for differentiating patients with diabetic microangiopathy and neuropathy from normal subjects and even (with some overlapping) from patients with diabetic microangiopathy without neuropathy.

Test 2: reactive hyperemia

A reactive hyperemia response is obtained after a period of tissue ischemia caused by occlusion of the blood supply to the foot. Using the technique described by Franzeck,[9] the reactive hyperemia procedure is performed as follows:

1. The system is set up to record the flow output on a trend recorder. In some flowmeters, the front panel display in the graphic display mode can be used as well.
2. A baseline flux level is obtained over 2 minutes.

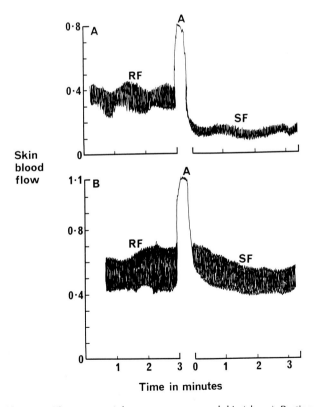

Fig. 63-3. The venoarteriolar response on normal skin (above). Resting flux *(RF)* in the horizontal position shows vasomotor activity; on standing, the standing flux *(SF)* is lower. *A*, Motion artifact. In the skin of a diabetic with microangiopathy (below), there is a high RF with altered vasomotor activity, and on standing, there is no significant or reduced decrease in flux.

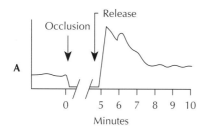

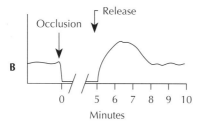

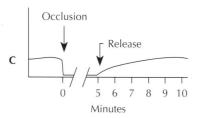

Fig. 63-4. Examples of the three patterns of reactive hyperemia according to the model described by Franzeck.[9] Response of normal skin **(A)**, moderate diabetic microangiopathy **(B)**, and severe diabetic microangiopathy with plantar foot ulceration **(C)**.

3. A standard blood pressure ankle cuff is applied to the limb under study and inflated to a suprasystolic pressure (150 to 200 mm Hg) for 5 minutes.

4. The cuff pressure is quickly released and the characteristics of the hyperemic blood flux curve are observed and recorded continuously for the following 10 minutes.

5. According to Franzeck,[9] the reactive hyperemia response curve is classified into four types. However, to simplify the evaluation system, the response may be classified as either A, B, or C curves using the method shown in Fig. 63-4.

Test 3: the thermal stimulation response

Increasing local skin temperature produces a large increase in skin blood flow and local perfusion in normal skin. This type of localized response is less evident in diabetics and can be greatly reduced or almost abolished in diabetics with neuropathy. This thus provides an effective method to assess the presence of microcirculatory alterations and diabetic microangiopathy.[7] The procedure for measuring the thermal stimulation response is as follows. With the patient acclimatized, the skin temperature control module, which is placed around the laser Doppler flowmeter probe, is set

Table 63-1. Criteria for determining diabetic microangiopathy measurement scores

Variables*	Normal	Abnormal	Severe microangiopathy
RF	0.5-1.0	1.0-1.4	>1.4
VAR	30-100	10-30	0-10
MI	50-100	30-50	0-30
RH	Pattern A (biphasic)	Pattern B (monophasic)	Pattern C (flat)
TSI	400-600 or more	200-400	<100

RF, Resting flux; *VAR,* venoarteriolar response; *MI,* microangiopathy index; *RH,* reactive hyperemia; *TSI,* thermal stimulation response.
*Score assigned for each variable as determined by the pertinent range: 0, normal; 2, abnormal; 4, severe microangiopathy.

at 36° C. After 5 minutes at 36° C, the average skin flux reading over a 1-minute period ($F_{36°}$) is obtained. The skin temperature control is then increased to 45° C and maintained for 10 minutes. The average flow reading at 45° C over a 1-minute period ($F_{45°}$) is then recorded. The thermal stimulation index *(TSI)* is calculated as follows:

$$TSI = \frac{F_{45°}}{F_{36°}} \times 100$$

Other qualitative measurements may also be evaluated using this method, including vasomotion and the presence of rhythmic flow variations caused by sympathetic activity. However, these measurements may require frequency analysis of the signal, and because of the complex instrumentation and time required for the analysis of these data, this method cannot be recommended as part of a routine evaluation.

Scoring

The five variables are scored according to the criteria given in Table 63-1. After each variable is scored, the five scores are totaled to obtain the diabetic microangiopathy score, which is compared to the ranges observed for various conditions, shown in Table 63-2. This scoring system is based on the results of tests performed in 500 patients with diabetic microangiopathy. It can discriminate between groups of patients and has shown a good degree of correlation with the findings from electromyography and vibration sensory threshold testing.[7,14]

The data contained in Table 63-2 are useful for detecting diabetic microangiopathy, determining the prognosis in diabetic patients with microangiopathy, and planning the most appropriate therapy. The diabetic microangiopathy score also appears useful for predicting the risk of foot ulcerations.

DIABETIC FOOT LESIONS AND AMPUTATIONS

Foot lesions pose a major problem in the management of diabetic patients and they are the most frequent reason for amputation. In patients with soft tissue lesions who do not

Table 63-2. Patient scores and classifications for various disease stages

Class	Patient score	Condition	Recommendation
A	0-5	Normal	None
B	6-10	Some increase in capillary permeability, moderate perfusion alteration	Elastic compression, drugs; annual examinations
C	8-12	Serious increase in capillary permeability, obvious perfusion alterations	As above, only more aggressive; antiplatelet agents
D	12-14	As above, with neuropathy; low likelihood of ulceration	Pressure relief on the foot, careful strict metabolic control, 3-month examinations
E	14-20	As above, with high likelihood of ulceration	As above, with ulceration treatment and antibiotics as required, along with frequent examinations to assess healing potential

have significant arterial occlusive disease, laser Doppler flowmetry can be used to assess the healing potential of the ulcerative lesion, and thus unnecessary amputations can be avoided.

To evaluate skin flux in patients with diabetic foot lesions, a flat or right-angle probe is placed on the dorsum of the foot and also on the edge of the ulceration (on intact skin) after the patient is fully acclimatized and supine at a stable room temperature of 22° C. No thermal stimulation is usually applied because the inflammatory response produces a local vasodilatation and skin flux can only be marginally increased by local thermal stimulation.

A resting flux reading is recorded for skin in the area surrounding the lesion, followed, if possible, by another RF reading obtained from intact skin on the same foot.

The resting flux values for the lesion and control site are then compared to obtain a healing potential index (HPI), calculated as follows:

$$HPI = \frac{RF \text{ (lesion)}}{RF \text{ (control area)}} \times 100$$

In the 1-year clinical follow-up of 500 patients with 535 foot ulcerations (average size, 1.48 cm²; range, 0.8 to 18 cm²), an HPI greater than 100 is a positive sign for healing potential. In another prospective study of 185 foot ulcerations in patients with neuropathy and diabetic microangiopathy, the lesions in 98% of those with an HPI greater than 120 healed within 12 months (93% within 6 months) simply by relieving pressure,[2] cleaning the wound regularly, and protecting the area. Only 2% of those with an HPI less than 100 showed healing within 12 months.

Toe lesions are evaluated in the same way, although they are generally associated with a worse prognosis. In a study that included 86 cases of toe lesions, 57% with an HPI greater than 120 healed within 12 months (43% within 6 months). Only 2% of the toe lesions with an HPI less than 100 healed within 12 months (1% within 6 months).

The tracings of the reactive hyperemia response and the variability in the baseline flow curves can yield additional qualitative information. The reactive hyperemia depicted by

pattern C (Fig. 63-4) has been associated with a very poor healing prognosis. Both a flat reactive hyperemia curve and resting flux curve, either with or without poor rhythmic variations due to vasomotion, also appear to indicate a very low healing potential. Information on the precise value of these observations is still limited, however.

When considering microcirculatory factors, the clinical appearance of the lesion is frequently quite irrelevant because an ulceration can often appear serious but skin perfusion may be adequate, and the lesion may actually be due to infection rather than to inadequate perfusion. On the other hand, some small distal lesions may have extremely poor perfusion and very limited healing potential. Therefore it appears that a stable high-resting flux tracing in conjunction with poor vasomotion can indicate severe diabetic microangiopathy.

The microvascular response to skin trauma in subjects with diabetic microangiopathy also appears to be altered, as shown by Rayman et al.[12,13] The response to skin trauma (e.g., needle injection) is not related to the degree of metabolic diabetic control and is not easily explicable in terms of a reduction in superficial skin capillary density. This alteration in the hyperemic response after microtraumas may be an important factor in the development of diabetic ulcerations following minor skin traumas or repeated pressure exerted in limited weight-bearing areas.

LOW- AND HIGH-PERFUSION MICROANGIOPATHY

Two major types of microangiopathy may be defined by laser Doppler flowmetry. The first type, low-perfusion microangiopathy, is present in subjects with severe peripheral vascular disease, Raynaud's phenomenon, and essential hypertension.[8] This microangiopathy is characterized by a severe decrease in skin flux and VAR, low capillary filtration, and low transcutaneous Po_2 and Pco_2.

The second type, high-perfusion microangiopathy, is characterized by elevated skin flux, decreased VAR, marked increase in capillary filtration and permeability,[6,11] and often a marked increase in the transcutaneous Pco_2. High-perfusion microangiopathy is specifically observed in patients

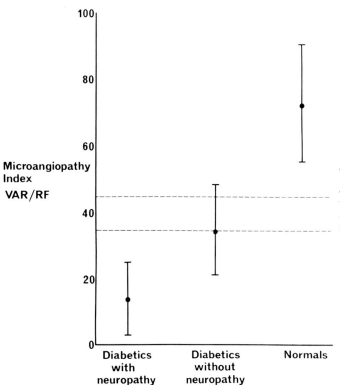

Fig. 63-5. Different distribution of the microangiopathy index (mean ± 2 SD) in normal subjects, diabetic patients without neuropathy, and diabetic patients with neuropathy. The lower dotted line is the limit for foot edema (present), and the line above is for absence of edema associated with microangiopathy. Within the dotted lines, 50% of subjects had foot edema.

Fig. 63-6. A model of the microcirculatory events causing and/or precipitating diabetic microangiopahy. The increased capillary filtration causing microedema in early microangiopathy is associated with increased skin flow and decreased venoarteriolar response. Increased skin flux is associated with an increased filtration rate. Increased local edema may further impair local nerve conduction. The mechanisms are self-aggravating.

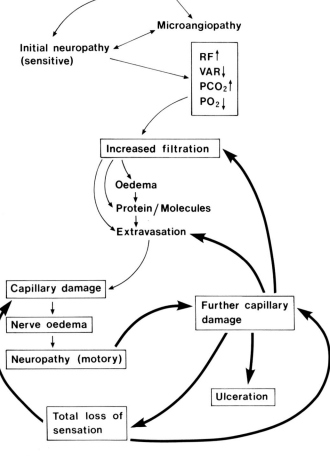

with either diabetic microangiopathy or venous hypertensive microangiopathy leading to liposclerosis and venous ulcerations.[1,4] Both low- and high-perfusion microangiopathies lead to skin and tissue necrosis but through the influence of different mechanisms.

In high-perfusion microangiopathy, the increased capillary filtration and edema, possibly as a consequence of the increase in skin flux, lead to compression and obstruction of the nutrient capillaries.[1,4,6,11] In addition, the edema present in the interstitial tissue may inhibit the diffusion of nutrients and gases in the affected areas. The correlation between RF, VAR, and foot edema is observed in Fig. 63-5. This figure shows the microangiopathy in 50 diabetics with neuropathy, 50 without neuropathy, and 50 normal subjects. The dashed lines indicate the distribution of edema at the level of the foot in these three groups of subjects. No edema was clinically observed in subjects with an MI value higher than the upper dashed line. All subjects with an MI lower than the level indicated by the lower dashed line had edema. A total of 50% of subjects with an MI value between the two horizontal dashed lines had edema. In low-perfusion microangiopathy, the total skin flux detected by laser Doppler flowmetry does not always represent the nutritional flow, which is more superficial and includes only 5% to 10% of the total skin blood flow.[3] Therefore, it is sometimes difficult to evaluate this condition by laser Doppler flowmetry alone. The changes induced in the skin by drugs or other treatments may also change the deeper, nonnutritional flow more than the flux within the nutritional superficial layer. This differs from high-perfusion microangiopathy in which measurements of skin flux and the VAR may be successfully used to monitor the efficacy of treatment, especially in groups of patients.[4] Fig. 63-6 is a diagram of the microcirculatory events that can be anticipated in patients with diabetic microangiopathy.

Increased capillary filtration is observed very early in diabetic patients.[6,11] An increase in skin flux is a common finding in patients with subclinical diabetic microangiopathy[7] and seems to be related to altered thermoregulatory control, which is also observed very early.[12,13]

The flux values presented in this chapter were obtained with a first generation Laserflo (TSI, St. Paul, Minnesota) laser Doppler flowmeter. The data obtained with different laser Dopler flowmeters may be completely different, since no standard of measurements exists at the moment among different instruments. In addition, data from flowmeters of different generations from the same producer may differ because technology in the field is rapidly changing. However, relative measurements with the same flowmeter and venoarteriolar response, reactive hyperemia, thermal stimulation, microangiopathy index, vasomotion and vasomotor responses, and other parameters are broadly comparable with all instruments. It is recommended that each vascular/ microcirculation laboratory establish standard normal values in standard environmental conditions.

CONCLUSION

Recent studies have demonstrated that laser Doppler flowmetry is a practical and effective method for evaluating diabetic microangiopathy. It may be effective for detecting diabetic microangiopathy. Laser Doppler flowmetry may also be used to study the natural history and monitor the results of treatment. The HPI can predict the outcome of most diabetic ulcerations.

REFERENCES

1. Belcaro G, Christopoulos D, Nicolaides AN: Skin flow and swelling in post-phlebitic limbs, *Vasa* 18:136-139, 1989.
2. Belcaro G, Christopoulos A, Nicolaides AN: Diabetic microangiopathy treated with elastic compression: a microcirculatory evaluation using laser-Doppler flowmetry, transcutaneous Po_2/Pco_2 and capillary permeability measurements, *Vasa* 19:247, 1990.
3. Belcaro G, Nicolaides AN: The venoarteriolar response in diabetics, *Angiology* 42:827-835, 1991.
4. Belcaro G, Renton S, Nicolaides AN: Elastic compression in diabetic microangiopathy, *Clin Exp* (suppl 1):89, 1990.
5. Belcaro G et al: Evaluation of skin blood flow and venoarteriolar response in patients with diabetes and peripheral vascular disease by laser-Doppler flowmetry, *Angiology* 40:953-957, 1989.
6. Bollinger A et al: Patterns of diffusion through skin capillaries in patients with long-term diabetes, *N Engl J Med* 307:1305-1310, 1982.
7. Cesarone MR et al: *Studio della microangiopatia diabetica con metodiche non-invasive (flussimetria laser Doppler, misurazione transcutanea di Po_2-Pco_2 termometria: elaborazione di un modello microcircolatorio per valutare l'evoluzione e l'effetto di terapie sulla microangiopatia diabetica. In Belcaro G, ed: Flussimetria laser-Doppler e. microcircolazione, Torino, Italy, 1989, Edizioni Minerva Medica.*
8. Fagrell B et al: *Combination of laser-Doppler flowmetry and capillary microscopy for evaluating the dynamics of skin microcirculation. In Mahler F, Messmer K, Hammersen F, eds: Techniques in clinical capillary microscopy,* vol II (Progress in Applied Microcirculation), Basel, Switzerland, 1987, Karger.
9. Franzeck UK et al: Cutaneous reactive hyperemia in short term and long term type I diabetes—continuous monitoring by a combined laser Doppler and transcutaneous oxygen probe, *Vasa* 19:8-15, 1990.
10. Hendricksen O: Local sympathetic reflex mechanism in regulation of blood flow in subcutaneous adipose tissue, *Acta Physiol Scand* (suppl 450):1977.
11. Parving HH: Microvascular permeability to plasma proteins in hypertension and diabetes mellitus in man—on the pathogenesis of hypertensive and diabetic microangiopathy, *Dan Med Bull* 22:217-233, 1975.
12. Rayman G, Hassan A, Tooke J: Blood flow in the skin of the foot related to posture in diabetes mellitus, *Br Med J* 292:87-90, 1986.
13. Rayman G et al: Impaired microvascular hyperaemic response to minor skin trauma in type I diabetes, *Br Med J* 292:1295-1298, 1986.
14. Sozenko JM et al: Comparison of quantitative sensory-threshold measures for their association with foot ulceration in diabetic patient, *Diabetes Care* 13:1057-1061, 1990.

CHAPTER 64

Amputation level determination techniques

JAMES M. MALONE and JEFFREY L. BALLARD

The patient requiring lower extremity amputation due to vascular occlusive disease poses a challenging problem for the surgeon. Correct choice of amputation level can make the difference between successful prosthetic rehabilitation and a bed-and-wheelchair existence. This chapter focuses on the value of quantitative techniques for selecting the amputation level. The data yielded can precisely identify the lowest level at which an amputation can be carried out and yet afford good primary healing. Armed with such information, the surgeon can perform an amputation at a level that provides maximum length for optimal prosthetic rehabilitation, knowing that blood flow will most likely be sufficient for healing.

MAGNITUDE OF THE AMPUTATION PROBLEM

There are conflicting data as to whether the number of lower limb amputations has decreased, increased, or remained the same, despite a large upsurge in the number of limb salvage vascular surgical procedures. These data notwithstanding, there are approximately 50,000 lower extremity amputations performed each year in the United States. Two thirds are required for the care of diabetics with peripheral vascular disease, with or without infection, and the remainder are done for patients suffering from peripheral vascular disease alone, trauma, or other causes. The amputation level selected by the surgeon has far-reaching implications for the patient with respect to morbidity, mortality, and the likelihood of prosthetic rehabilitation. The problem with the patient who requires amputation for vascular disease is that the amputation level adequately encompassing the gangrenous or infectious process may not possess a sufficient blood supply to promote healing. The presence of viable, intact skin at the proposed amputation level is no assurance that the blood flow can support healing of the surgical incision because healing requires considerably greater blood flow than does the maintenance of intact skin. The ideal test for determining amputation level is one that identifies the most distal level that possesses adequate blood flow to guarantee primary skin healing. The ultimate method for amputation level selection must be quantitative, and it must have a significantly strict end point so that an undue number of healing failures can be avoided in those patients with flow

rates that fall near the lower end of the "safe" scale. Such an end point will also discourage surgeons from selecting the next higher amputation level in those patients with blood flow near the low end of the safe scale, as this would rule out a successful conservative amputation in many patients with healing potential at the lower level.

The general requirements of a lower limb amputation are the following: (1) the amputation must remove all necrotic, painful, or infected tissue, (2) it must be possible to fit the amputation stump with a functional and easily applied prosthesis; and (3) the blood supply at the level of the proposed amputation must be sufficient to allow primary skin healing. Appropriate selection of amputation level is therefore of critical importance. A too proximal amputation, such as a midthigh amputation, deprives the patient of the opportunity for subsequent ambulation under most circumstances, even though the amputation wound might heal without difficulty. On the other hand, if a distal amputation site is selected and the blood supply is inadequate for amputation healing, this will necessitate further surgery to achieve healing at a higher level. This then increases the likelihood of morbidity and mortality and may ultimately result in rehabilitation failure.

The inherent advantages of a below-knee as opposed to above-knee amputation are obvious. It is simply easier to ambulate on a below-knee prosthesis, a consideration that is extremely important in geriatric patients. In most series, geriatric patients who undergo unilateral below-knee amputation show a greater than 90% success rate of rehabilitation to ambulation. On the other hand, the success rate for a similar group of above-knee amputees is 30% or less. A unilateral below-knee amputee requires an approximate 40% increase in energy expenditure for ambulation compared with that needed for walking with an intact extremity. In contrast, the energy expenditure required of a unilateral above-knee amputee is approximately double that of a unilateral below-knee amputee. Crutch walking without a lower extremity prosthesis uses approximately the same amount of energy as an above-knee amputee with a prosthesis, whereas wheelchair use necessitates only a 9% increase in energy expenditure. It is therefore easy to see why elderly patients, many of whom have severe coronary artery disease or severe chronic obstructive pulmonary disease, may be physically unable to provide the additional energy required for ambulation on an above-knee prosthesis.

It is usually possible for the surgeon to decide on an amputation level that will remove necrotic, painful, or infected tissue as well as provide an amputation stump that can be fitted with a prosthesis. However, determining the adequacy of blood flow at the proposed amputation level has been one of the most difficult problems facing the amputation surgeon.

CONVENTIONAL METHODS OF AMPUTATION LEVEL DETERMINATION

The earliest attempts at amputation level selection fall into two general categories: those based on objective evidence obtained from the physical examination and those based on an empiric or "favorite" amputation level.

The presence of pulses in the affected extremity, noninstrumentally assessed measurement of skin temperature, and clinical judgment do not yield information with consistent enough correlation to amputation healing to serve as a sound basis for clinical decision making. Robbs and Ray[37] retrospectively analyzed the morbidity, mortality, and rates of healing in 214 patients who underwent lower limb amputation in which the amputation level was determined by such subjective criteria. The failure rates for above-knee and below-knee amputation were 8.9% and 25%, respectively. These authors concluded that skin flap viability could not be predicted by the extent of the ischemic lesion in relation to the ankle joint, the popliteal pulse status, or lower limb angiographic findings. These comments regarding the value of angiography have been challenged by the findings of a recent study published by Van den Broek et al,[45] in which 53 patients undergoing amputations of the lower limb were evaluated in terms of clinical criteria, pulse volume recordings, Doppler pressures, photoplethysmographic skin perfusion pressures, and angiography. Although not as reliable as photoplethysmographic skin perfusion pressures, angiographic findings correlated significantly with the success of healing. One physical finding that has some value in identifying proposed amputation levels is the presence of dependent rubor. Skin that develops dependent rubor is clearly ischemic, and hence skin with dependent rubor, like gangrenous tissue, is an absolute contraindication to amputation at that level. However, the absence of dependent rubor does not necessarily ensure healing ability.

Although performing an amputation at the level immediately below the most distal palpable pulse generally results in a high rate of amputation healing, many patients who have healing potential at a more conservative level are thus denied the benefits of an optimum amputation. Historically, many surgeons concerned about healing complications and possible prolonged hospitalization in the vascular impaired amputee advocated the routine performance of above-knee amputations despite the poor rehabilitation results to promote a greater chance of healing. In the 1960s, Lim et al[27] reported their findings in a series of below-knee amputations

for arterial occlusive disease born at this site regardless of the patient's pulse status. More than 70% of these amputations healed primarily, and 83% ultimately healed primarily or secondarily. However, use of an empiric below-knee amputation selection technique, although an improvement over empiric above-knee amputation, then denies some patients who might have healed with a more distal amputation, such as a transmetatarsal or Syme's amputation, the rehabilitation advantages afforded by these lower levels. In addition, the inability to identify those 20% to 30% of patients whose below-knee amputations are doomed to failure means that such patients will have to undergo one or more additional surgical procedures to achieve amputation healing. In the final analysis, none of the methods based on clinical judgment or the results of physical examination have a consistent enough correlation with amputation healing to provide a sound basis for clinical decision making.

NONINVASIVE METHODS OF AMPUTATION LEVEL SELECTION

The need for more sensitive and objective measurements for selecting preoperative amputation levels has led to the development of numerous noninvasive techniques, including sophisticated skin temperature evaluation,[15] Doppler ankle and calf systolic blood pressure measurement with or without pulse volume recordings,* xenon-133 skin blood flow studies,† digital or transmetatarsal photoplethysmographic pressures,[38] transcutaneous oxygen determination,‡ skin fluorescence after the intravenous infusion of fluorescent dye,[16,31,40-42] laser Doppler skin blood flow,[19,21] pertechnetate skin blood pressure studies,[11,22,24] and photoelectrically measured skin color changes.[44] The various selection criteria for the prediction of healing of lower limb amputations are summarized in Tables 64-1 to 64-4. Data from Table 64-1 suggest that preoperative amputation level selection techniques correctly predicted primary healing in 96 of 99 (97%) toe amputations. Similar data in Table 64-2 indicate primary healing was correctly predicted in 120 of 135 (89%) forefoot amputations. The data in Table 64-3, representing a variety of selection criteria (with variable interpretation cut-off points), suggest that primary healing was correctly predicted in 616 of 653 (94%) below-knee amputations, and the data in Table 64-4 show that healing was correctly predicted in 34 of 39 (87%) above-knee amputations. Clearly, objective amputation level selection techniques can not only predict the healing potential of a more distal level of amputation but also accurately assess the healing potential of a below-knee compared with an above-knee amputation. Therefore elective lower extremity amputations should not be performed without some type of objective preoperative testing to ensure primary healing of the most distal amputation possible.

---

*References 1-4, 14, 35, 38, 46, 48.
†References 6, 18, 20, 26, 29, 33, 39.
‡References 5, 7, 8, 12, 17, 25, 28, 30, 32, 36, 39, 47.

Table 64-1. Toe amputation selection criteria

Selection criteria	Reference	Healing
Photoplethysmographic or TMA pressure >20 mm Hg	38	20/20 (100%)
Doppler systolic pressure		
Ankle >35 mm Hg	46	44/46 (96%)
Toe >15 mm Hg	45	20/21 (95%)
Fiberoptic fluorometry DFI >44	42	12/12 (100%)
TOTAL		96/99 (97%)

TMA, Transmetatarsal amputation; *DFI,* dye fluorescence index.

Table 64-2. Forefoot amputation selection criteria

Selection criteria	Reference	Healing
Doppler ankle systolic pressure		
>80 mm Hg	45	27/31 (87%)
>70 mm Hg	2	38/44 (86%)
Fiberoptic fluorometry DFI >42	41, 42	29/31 (94%)
TcPo$_2$ >20 mm Hg	30, 47	26/29 (90%)
TOTAL		120/135 (89%)

DFI, Dye fluorescence index; *TcPo$_2$,* transcutaneous oxygen pressure.

Table 64-3. Below-knee amputation selection criteria

Selection criteria	Reference	Healing
Doppler calf or thigh systolic pressure*	3, 35, 48	95/95 (100%)
Fluorescein dye/fiberoptic fluorometry*	31, 49	53/59 (90%)
Skin blood pressure	23	24/26 (92%)
Photoelectric skin pressure	34, 44	60/71 (84%)
TcPo$_2$ >20 mm Hg	5, 7, 12, 13, 25, 30, 36, 47	312/325 (96%)
Xenon-133 skin clearance*	6, 20, 26, 29	72/77 (94%)
TOTAL		616/653 (94%)

TcPo$_2$, Transcutaneous oxygen pressure.
*Variable criteria.

Table 64-4. Below-knee amputation selection criteria

Selection criteria	Reference	Healing
TcPo$_2$		
>20 mm Hg	7	12/14 (86%)
>30 mm Hg	47	12/15 (80%)
Fiberoptic fluorometry DFI >42	42	10/10 (100%)
TOTAL		34/39 (87%)

TcPo$_2$, Transcutaneous oxygen pressure; *DFI,* dye fluorescence index.

Skin temperature

One of the earliest noninvasive methods of evaluating skin blood flow was the measurement of skin temperature. In this method, a surface thermometer was placed on the skin at the proposed level of amputation, and the temperature, which could be recorded in tenths of a degree, was compared with temperatures at other levels on the ipsilateral limb or with those on the contralateral limb. Unfortunately, the temperature difference between skin with blood flow that was adequate for healing and skin with blood flow not adequate for healing was not broad enough to identify a clear end point for level selection. More recent data obtained by Golbranson et al[15] using improved methods of skin temperature measurement indicated a high degree of accuracy (90%) for selecting below-knee versus above-knee amputation levels. In addition, Spence and Walker[43] have demonstrated a clear correlation between three different temperature isotherms (1.8° C separation) and isotopically derived skin blood flow ($p < 0.001$). Both of these reports have indicated that this method is relatively reliable for differentiating between above-knee and below-knee amputation levels. However, the ultimate role of skin temperature measurement for selecting amputation level in the performance of Syme's, transmetatarsal, or toe amputation awaits further evaluation.

Doppler systolic pressure determinations

Techniques for using ankle, calf, and popliteal Doppler systolic blood pressure determinations in selecting amputation levels have been well described.[2-4,14,35,46,48] Similarly, the use of photoplethysmographic data for the determination of digit and transmetatarsal blood pressures was well described by Schwartz et al[38] and more recently by Lee et al.[28] Both Doppler systolic pressure and photoplethysmographic measurements are relatively simple, inexpensive, and totally noninvasive. However, because blood pressure less than a predetermined level does not necessarily guarantee failure of amputation healing at that level, this limits the value of both approaches. The problem can be summarized as follows: a high Doppler ankle pressure does not ensure the likelihood of successful healing, but a low Doppler ankle pressure does not necessarily rule out the potential for primary healing. Both Gibbons et al[14] and Raines et al[35] suggested the ancillary use of pulse volume recordings to increase the accuracy of Doppler ankle pressures. Although Raines et al[35] quoted 100% successful healing in 27 patients undergoing below-knee amputations whose Doppler ankle pressures were greater than 30 mm Hg, calf pressure in these patients exceeded 65 mm Hg and there was a pulsatile pulse volume recorded in the foot. Gibbons et al[14] were unable to duplicate these results and concluded that they could "find no consistent criteria which are more accurate and reliable than clinical judgement and no ankle pressure above which primary healing was guaranteed." In addition, systolic pressure measurements in patients with diabetes may be falsely elevated because of medial calcinosis of the popliteal and tibial vessels.

A recent paper by Apelqvist et al[1] on the value of systolic ankle and toe blood pressure measurements in predicting healing in patients with diabetic foot ulcers presents data for both patients who underwent amputation and those who did not. Primary healing was achieved in 139 of 164 (85%) patients with a toe pressure greater than 45 mm Hg, whereas 43 of 117 (36%) patients with toe pressures less than 45 mm Hg experienced healing without amputation. In contrast, below-ankle amputations in 27 of 31 patients with ankle pressures in excess of 80 mm Hg were associated with healing, and 20 of 21 of these patients who underwent amputation had toe pressures in excess of 50 mm Hg. These authors concluded that "different pressure levels have to be used to predict primary healing for [diabetic ulcers] compared to healing after minor amputation."

Skin fluorescence

The measurement of skin fluorescence for determining amputation level holds significant promise as a minimally invasive objective test. Initial studies measured skin fluorescence with a Wood's ultraviolet light after the intravenous injection of fluorescein. Although this technique is somewhat more invasive then Doppler ankle systolic pressure measurements or pulse volume recordings, it is less complicated and less invasive than xenon-133 skin blood flow or pertechnetate skin perfusion measurements. New fluorometers that can provide objective numerical readings quickly without the need for a Wood's lamp have enhanced the value of this technique.

McFarland and Lawrence[31] originally reported an accuracy rate of 80% for skin fluorescence compared to 33% for Doppler popliteal systolic blood pressure (50 mm Hg) in predicting healing of below-knee amputations. In addition, they found that when skin fluorescence and Doppler pressure disagreed in indicating the level of amputation, the fluorescein method always predicted a more distal level.

Silverman et al[41] reported their updated data on the use of fiberoptic fluorometry for selecting digital, transmetatarsal, Syme's, below-knee, and above-knee amputation levels. In 86 cases with cellulitis at the site of amputation, preoperative fluorometry clearly distinguished between healing and nonhealing sites. The amputation healed in all but one patient whose dye fluorescence index (OFI) was greater than 42. The technique maintained its high accuracy in patients with diabetes. These authors pointed out, however, that DFI values between 38 and 42 constitute a transitional zone in which the precision of fluorometric determinations is unclear.

Fluorometry may be advantageous in the context of marginal limb perfusion because it facilitates easy assessment at multiple sites on the same limb. Techniques such as laser Doppler perfusion and transcutaneous oximetry are less suited for the evaluation of multiple sites. The primary problem with the use of fluorescence for amputation level selection has to do with its safety. In the most recent Silverman study,[42] in which fluorescein was administered slowly, there was only a 1.6% incidence of nausea, which is lower than

the incidence previously reported after the bolus injection of fluorescein for the performance of retinal angiography. In addition, there was no evidence of major cardiac or pulmonary complications or of significant changes in blood pressure. Fluorescein can be associated with anaphylactic reactions, and therefore the exact safety and efficacy of its intravenous administration are unknown, although clearly slow injection is safer.

Laser Doppler

Since it is noninvasive and measures capillary blood flow, this would appear to make laser Doppler an ideal tool for skin blood flow determination. However, preliminary data obtained by Holloway et al[18,20,21] and Matsen[32] suggest that although there is a linear correlation among techniques (i.e., Doppler blood flow microspheres, electromagnetic blood flow probes, and xenon-133 clearance), there is also considerable variance. These same groups have noted that the use of local skin heating (44° C) enhances the accuracy of the laser Doppler and makes it a more valuable test for amputation level selection. In a previous publication, Holloway and Burgess[19] reported their experience with laser-Doppler velocimetry in 20 lower extremity amputations. Accuracy rates for foot and forefoot, below-knee, and above-knee amputations were 33%, 100%, and 100%, respectively. These preliminary data are promising but remain to be validated by further studies.

Xenon-133 skin clearance

There have been extensive amounts of literature on the use of xenon-133 skin clearance for amputation level selection,[9,10,29,33] and the techniques that use it have been well described. One of the major difficulties with this method for amputation level selection, even at the time of the publications of Moore,[33] Malone et al,[29] and Daly and Henry,[9] is the lack of reproducibility of results by other investigators. Holloway and Burgess[20] were not able to document a clear-cut end point above which all amputations healed. On the other hand, Silberstein et al[39] found it predicted excellent healing in 38 of 39 patients, although the ability to predict healing failure was not as precise. An additional problem is that xenon-133 in the form of gas dissolved in saline is no longer produced by a reliable supplier. The product must now be manufactured by local nuclear medicine departments, and such local production probably accounts for the variability of published results. However, despite previously published excellent results, some no longer use xenon-133 skin clearance for amputation level selection. In part, this change stemmed from the difficulties already enumerated, but more importantly, the results of a previously published study showed xenon-133 skin clearance is not statistically reliable as a selection method for amputation level determination.[30]

A recent publication by Dwars et al[11] describing a modified scintigraphic technique for amputation level selection in diabetics is of interest with respect to the xenon "controversy." In a collected series of papers published by

Moore,[33] Malone et al,[29] and others,[9,39] the cut-off point for successful healing for the xenon-133 method was a skin blood flow of 2.4 to 2.8 ml/min/100 g of tissue. In the recent study by Dwars et al,[11] who used a modified iodine-123–antipyrine cutaneous washout technique, the lowest skin blood flow value found in the group of patients with healed amputations was 2.78 ml/min/100 g of tissue. This article points out that there were broad overlaps in skin blood flow values between healing and nonhealing cases, and that it was difficult to pick a strict cut-off point.

Skin perfusion pressure

Using the disappearance of intradermal ^{99m}Tc-pertechnetate, Na[131]I, ^{131}I-antipyrine, or xenon-133 in the presence of external pressure as the basis for amputation level selection, Holstein[22] and Holstein and Lassen[23] reported data that were comparable to the blood flow data obtained with the xenon-133 method reported by Moore,[33] Daly and Henry,[9] and Malone et al.[29] At the time the data were published, this was of interest because xenon-133 is trapped in subcutaneous fat and there are solid theoretical issues supporting the use of an isotope other than xenon-133 for the measurement of skin blood flow. The important distinction among the various studies is, however, that Holstein's group[22,23] was measuring skin perfusion pressure rather than skin blood flow. They documented no significant differences among Na[131]I, ^{131}I-antipyrine, or ^{99m}Tc-pertechnetate for the measurement of skin perfusion pressure.[24] In the previously mentioned paper by Dwars et al,[11] ^{123}I-antipyrine disappearance showed an excellent cut-off point for the prediction of amputation healing; all amputations healed when the skin perfusion pressure exceeded 20 mm Hg.

Stockel et al[44] and Ovesen and Stockel[34] reported preliminary data on the use of a photodetector and plethysmography for amputation level selection that correlated well with the results of xenon-133 skin perfusion pressure techniques reported by Holstein et al.[22,24] In this technique, a blood pressure cuff is placed over a photoelectric detector that is connected to a plethysmograph and this measures the minimum external pressure required to prevent skin reddening after blanching. Although not as reliable as other noninvasive methods (85% accuracy), the test is relatively noninvasive and inexpensive.

Transcutaneous oxygen pressure

The results of excellent studies have been published by multiple authors on the use of transcutaneous oxygen pressure (TcPo$_2$) measurement for determining amputation level.* One of the initial papers was by Franzeck et al.[12] In this study, the mean TcPo$_2$ in patients who experienced primary healing of a lower extremity amputation was compared with those values in patients who failed to heal. The respective values for healing and nonhealing were 36.5 ± 17.5 and less than 0.3 mm Hg, respectively. However, three

of nine patients healed primarily whose TcPo$_2$ was less than 10 mm Hg.

In a study of below-knee amputations, Burgess et al.[5] noted that all 15 amputations that were associated with a TcPo$_2$ greater then 40 mm Hg healed, 17 of 19 healed with a TcPo$_2$ between 1 and 40 mm Hg, but none of the three with a TcPo$_2$ of 0 mm Hg healed. Katsamouris et al[25] reported that the lower extremity amputations healed in all 17 of their patients with a TcPo$_2$ greater than 38 mm Hg or a Po$_2$ index (chest wall control site) greater than 0.59. Ratliff et al[36] reported that the below-knee amputations healed in 18 patients with a Po$_2$ greater than 35 mm Hg, whereas healing failed in 10 of 15 with a Po$_2$ less than 35 mm Hg. In a study of 42 lower extremity amputations (28 below-knee and 14 above-knee), Christiansen and Klarke[7] found that 27 of 31 patients with a TcPo$_2$ greater than 30 mm Hg healed primarily; seven patients with values between 20 and 30 mm Hg healed, although four patients had delayed healing, and the stumps in all four patients with a value below 20 mm Hg failed to heal because of skin necrosis.

All investigators have reported that healing can occur in some patients with a low TcPo$_2$ value. This may be partially explained by the nonlinear relationship between TcPo$_2$ and cutaneous blood flow. Matsen et al[32] have reported that TcPo$_2$ measurements are mostly dependent on arterial-venous gradients and cutaneous vascular resistance. In essence, there can be nutritive blood flow with a TcPo$_2$ of 0 mm Hg.

Techniques to improve the accuracy of TcPo$_2$ measurement include local probe heating (44° C), which minimizes local vascular resistance and makes TcPo$_2$ more linear with respect to cutaneous blood flow, measurements performed before and after oxygen administration, oxygen isobar extremity mapping, and transcutaneous oxygen recovery halftime. Wyss et al[47] have subsequently published the results of a follow-up study on TcPo$_2$ as a predictor of success after amputation. This study analyzed 162 patients who had 206 lower extremity amputations. These authors concluded that TcPo$_2$ is one of the most reliable indicators of local ischemia and is the best available method for predicting the failure of amputation healing due to ischemia. However, there are two theoretical inadequacies that must be considered when using TcPo$_2$ measurements. First, the measurement of TcPo$_2$ is quite localized, and one value may not be representative of the overall degree of limb ischemia. Second, as previously mentioned, there may still be some nutritive flow to the skin despite a TcPo$_2$ of 0 mm Hg. Although a TcPo$_2$ of 0 mm Hg at the proposed site of amputation does not always indicate ischemia that precludes healing, a TcPo$_2$ of 20 mm Hg or less clearly indicates severe ischemia. In the Wyss study,[47] a TcPo$_2$ of 20 mm Hg or less was associated with a rate of failure for amputations distal to the knee that was more than ten times the 4% rate of failure in patients that had a TcPo$_2$ of more than 20 mm Hg.

These data from Wyss et al[47] are comparable to those yielded by a prospective study evaluating multiple tests for

---

*References 5, 12, 13, 25, 30, 36.

amputation level selection. In this study, TcPO$_2$, transcutaneous carbon dioxide pressure, transcutaneous oxygen-to-carbon dioxide pressure, foot-to-chest transcutaneous oxygen pressure, the intradermal xenon-133 clearance level, the ankle brachial index, and the absolute popliteal artery pressure were all assessed prospectively for their accuracy in amputation level selection. All metabolic variables exhibited a high degree of statistical accuracy in predicting amputation healing, but none of the other tests showed statistical reliability. All amputations in this study (transmetatarsal, below-knee, and above-knee) showed primary healing when the TcPO$_2$ was greater than 20 mm Hg, and there was no incidence of false-positive or false-negative results.[30] It was also noted that the successful prediction of amputation healing for any of the metabolic parameters was not affected by the presence of diabetes mellitus. This agrees with the observations of Wyss et al.[47]

Because of the potential technical difficulties with measuring TcPO$_2$ and because these measurements are time consuming, the results of a recent study comparing TcPO$_2$ and photoplethysmography findings reported by Lee et al[28] are of interest. Peak-to-peak photoplethysmographic voltages were compared with TcPO$_2$ values. Although the two methods are intrinsically different and measure two different physiologic variables, linear regression analysis showed a correlation of 0.60. The anatomic location did not affect the photoplethysmographic readings or the TcPO$_2$ measurements. This study should encourage further investigation of photoplethysmography for amputation level selection. In addition to photoplethysmography, such a study should prospectively assess several other techniques such as TcPO$_2$ measurement and fiberoptic fluorometry.

CONCLUSION

Elective lower extremity amputation should not be performed without objective testing to ensure selection of the most distal amputation site that will heal primarily yet allow removal of infected, painful, or ischemic tissue. A variety of techniques are available to achieve this, but which technique is chosen depends on the equipment available, the amputation level under consideration, and the accuracy rates for the reported techniques. TcPO$_2$ measurement currently appears to be the most reliable technique; however, it is not suitable for limb mapping. Fiberoptic fluorometry may have some advantages due to its ability to measure multiple sites simultaneously, although the risk associated with the intravenous administration of fluorescein must be considered.

The ultimate role of any method for measuring the severity of limb ischemia is to inform the surgeon of the quantitative risk of nonhealing at proposed amputation levels. The level of amputation can then be decided on the basis of these findings in conjunction with the surgeons' clinical judgment and the patients' physical findings. For example, a surgeon might perform an amputation distal to the knee through a site with a very low TcPO$_2$ in a patient who is well motivated, relatively young, and healthy. Such an amputation would almost certainly be ruled out in a fragile elderly person who faces a limited prospect for successful rehabilitation.

REFERENCES

1. Apelqvist J et al: Prognostic value of systolic ankle and toe blood pressure levels in outcome of diabetic foot ulcer, *Diabetes Care* 12:373-377, 1989.
2. Baker WH, Barnes RW: Minor forefoot amputation in patients with low ankle pressure, *Am J Surg* 133:331-332, 1977.
3. Barnes RW, Shanik GO, Slaymaker EE: An index of healing in below-knee amputation: leg blood pressure by Doppler ultrasound, *Surgery* 79:13-20, 1976.
4. Bernstein EF: *The noninvasive vascular diagnostic laboratory*. In Najarian JS, Delaney JP, eds: *Vascular surgery,* Miami, 1978, Symposia Specialists–Stratton Intercontinental.
5. Burgess EM et al: Segmental transcutaneous measurements of PO$_2$ in patients requiring below the knee amputations for peripheral vascular insufficiency, *J Bone Joint Surg [Am]* 64:378-392, 1982.
6. Cheng EY: Lower extremity amputation level: selection using noninvasive hemodynamic methods of evaluation, *Arch Phys Med Rehabil* 63:475-479, 1982.
7. Christensen KS, Klarke M: Transcutaneous oxygen measurement in peripheral occlusive disease: an indicator of wound healing in leg amputation, *J Bone Joint Surg* [Br] 68:423-426, 1986.
8. Clyne CAC et al: Oxygen tension on the skin of ischemic legs, *Am J Surg* 143:315-318, 1982.
9. Daly MJ, Henry RE: Quantitative measurement of skin perfusion with xenon-133, *J Nucl Med* 21:156-160, 1980.
10. Durham JR, Anderson GG, Malone JM: *Methods of preoperative selection of amputation level*. In Flanigam P, ed: *Modern methods of perioperative assessment in peripheral vascular surgery,* New York, 1986, Marcel Decker.
11. Dwars BJ et al: A modified scintigraphic technique for amputation level selection in diabetics, *Eur J Nucl Med* 15:38-41, 1989.
12. Franzeck UK et al: Transcutaneous PO$_2$ measurement in health on peripheral arterial occlusive disease, *Surgery* 91:156-163, 1982.
13. Friedmann LW: The prosthesis—immediate or delayed fitting? *Angiology* 23:513-524, 1972.
14. Gibbons GW et al: Noninvasive prediction of amputation level in diabetic patients, *Arch Surg* 114:1253-1257, 1979.
15. Golbranson FL, Yu EC, Gelberman HH: The use of skin temperature determination in lower extremity amputation level selection, *Foot Ankle* 3:170-172, 1982.
16. Graham BH et al: Surface quantification of injection fluorescein as a predictor of flap viability, *Plast Reconstr Surg* 71:826-833, 1983.
17. Harward TRS et al: Oxygen inhalation induced transcutaneous PO$_2$ changes as a predictor of amputation level, *J Vasc Surg* 2:220-227, 1985.
18. Holloway GA Jr: Cutaneous blood flow responses to infection trauma measured by laser Doppler velocimetry, *J Invest Dermatol* 74:1-4, 1980.
19. Holloway GA Jr, Burgess EM: Preliminary experiences with laser Doppler velocimetry for the determination of amputation levels, *Prosthet Orthot Int* 7:63-66, 1983.
20. Holloway GA Jr, Burgess EM: Cutaneous blood flow and its relation to healing of below knee amputation, *Surg Gynecol Obstet* 146:750-756, 1978.
21. Holloway GA Jr, Watkins BW: Laser Doppler measurement of cutaneous blood flow, *J Invest Dermatol* 69:300-309, 1977.
22. Holstein P: Level selection in leg amputation for arterial occlusive disease: a comparison of clinical evaluation and skin perfusion pressure, *Acta Orthop Scand* 53:821-831, 1982.
23. Holstein P, Lassen NA: *Assessment of safe level of amputation by measurement of skin blood pressure*. In Rutherford R et al, eds: *Vascular surgery,* Philadelphia, 1977, Saunders.
24. Holstein P et al: Skin perfusion pressure measured by isotope wash out in legs with arterial occlusive disease, *Clin Physiol* 3:313-324, 1983.
25. Katsamouris A et al: Transcutaneous oxygen tension in selection of amputation level, *Am J Surg* 147:510-516, 1984.

26. Kostuik JP et al: Measurement of skin blood flow in peripheral vascular disease by the epicutaneous application of xenon-133, *J Bone Joint Surg* 58:833-837, 1964.

27. Lim RC Sr et al: Below knee amputation for ischemic gangrene, *Surg Gynecol Obstet* 125:493-501, 1967.

28. Lee TQ et al: Potential application of photoplethysmography technique in evaluating microcirculatory status of STAMP patients: preliminary report, *J Rehabil Red Dev* 27:363-368, 1990.

29. Malone JM et al: The "gold standard" for amputation level selection: xenon-133 clearance, *J Surg Res* 30:449-455, 1981.

30. Malone JM et al: Prospective comparison of noninvasive techniques for amputation level selection, *Am J Surg* 154:179-184, 1987.

31. McFarland DC, Lawrence FF: Skin fluorescence: a method to predict amputation site healing, *J Surg Res* 32:410-415, 1982.

32. Matsen FA et al: The relationship of transcutaneous Po_2 and laser Doppler measurements in human model of local arterial insufficiency, *Surg Gynecol Obstet* 159:418-422, 1984.

33. Moore WS: Determination of amputation level: measurement of skin blood flow with xenon-133, *Arch Surg* 107:798-802, 1973.

34. Ovesen J, Stockel M: Measurement of skin perfusion pressure by photoelectric technique: aid to amputation level selection in arteriosclerotic disease, *Prosthet Orthot Int* 8:39-41, 1984.

35. Raines JK et al: Vascular laboratory criteria for the management of peripheral vascular disease of the lower extremities, *Surgery* 79:21-29, 1976.

36. Ratliff DA et al: Prediction of amputation healing: the role of transcutaneous Po_2 assessment, *Br J Surg* 71:219-222, 1984.

37. Robbs JV, Ray R: Clinical predictors of below-knee stump healing following amputation for ischemia, *South Afr J Surg* 20:305-310, 1982.

38. Schwartz JA et al: Predictive value of distal perfusion pressure in the healing of amputation of the digits and the forefoot, *Surg Gynecol Obstet* 154:865-869, 1982.

39. Silberstein EB et al: Predictive value of intracutaneous xenon clearance for healing of amputation and cutaneous ulcer sites, *Radiology* 147:227-229, 1983.

40. Silverman DG et al: Quantification of fluorescein distribution to strangulated reticulum, *J Surg Res* 34:179-186, 1983.

41. Silverman DG et al: Fluorometric prediction of successful amputation level in the ischemic limb, *J Rehabil Res Dev* 22:29-34, 1985.

42. Silverman DG et al: Fluorometric quantification of low-dose fluorescein delivery to predict amputation site healing, *Surgery* 101:335-341, 1987.

43. Spence VA, Walker WF: The relationship between temperature isotherms and skin blood flow in the ischemic limb, *J Surg Res* 36:278-281, 1984.

44. Stockel M et al: Standardized photoelectric techniques as routine method for selection of amputation level, *Acta Orthop Scand* 53:875-878, 1982.

45. Van Den Broek TAA et al: A multivariate analysis of determinants of wound healing in patients after amputation for peripheral vascular disease, *Eur J Vasc Surg* 4:291-295, 1990.

46. Verta MJ et al: Forefoot perfusion pressure and minor amputation surgery, *Surgery* 80:792-734, 1976.

47. Wyss CR et al: Transcutaneous oxygen tension as a predictor of success after an amputation, *J Bone Joint Surg [Am]* 70:203-207, 1988.

48. Yao JST, Bergan JJ: Application of ultrasound to arterial and venous diagnosis, *Surg Clin North Am* 54:23-38, 1974.

CHAPTER 65

Evaluation of vascular trauma

KAJ JOHANSEN

Vascular emergencies require rapid diagnosis because acute arterial insufficiency or exsanguinating hemorrhage needs definitive management within a time span that may not permit a conventional history taking, physical examination, and the performance of diagnostic techniques. Thus the availability of accurate yet expeditious diagnostic modalities for use in the emergency setting might significantly improve patient care. This chapter presents the initial experiences in the acute situation using various noninvasive diagnostic techniques that have been previously validated for use in patients with chronic arterial and venous disease.

VASCULAR TRAUMA

Vascular trauma confronts the clinician with two different dilemmas. First, in the patient with clear evidence of vascular injury, such as an ischemic leg after multiple gunshot wounds, or a nonfunctioning kidney after blunt abdominal trauma, definitive management may only be successful if it is performed immediately. The delay created while precise anatomic localization of the injury is being carried out may result in an unacceptable risk of uncontrollable hemorrhage or irreversible tissue or organ ischemia.

A second and more common dilemma arises in the victim of blunt or penetrating trauma who does not manifest symptoms or signs of a vascular injury but whose mechanism of injury or wound location heightens clinical suspicion. For example, a stab or gunshot wound to the groin or a "suspicious" chest roentgenogram in the victim of a deceleration motor vehicle accident are situations in which the prudent clinician should rule out a silent but potentially catastrophic vascular injury.

Routine vessel exploration in the trauma victim with a worrisome wound, although practiced extensively in the past, was ultimately found to be ineffective because its diagnostic yield was too low.[19] Although the accuracy and utility of performing serial physical examinations have recently been reemphasized,[5] it is clear that physical examination alone may not be adequately sensitive to the presence of significant vascular injuries.[15] Accordingly, formal contrast angiography has become the diagnostic "gold standard" for imaging acute arterial and venous injuries.[2] It is highly accurate in demonstrating vascular occlusion, pseudoaneurysm, intimal flap, thrombus, extrinsic compression, vessel displacement, and collateral blood supply.

In the emergency setting, however, angiograms may be impractical. For example, angiography consumes too much time in the patient with an obvious vascular injury who requires immediate diagnosis (diagnostic arteriography required a mean of 2.4 hours in a series of 100 extremity injuries[10]). Furthermore, extremity injuries may not exist in isolation; a patient with an ischemic limb associated with a femur fracture who is hypotensive because of a ruptured spleen needs a laparotomy and will not tolerate either the diagnostic delay required by arteriography or the risk inherent in attempting resuscitation in the radiology suite.

In the larger group of trauma victims who do not have solid evidence of vascular injury but in whom there is a clinical suspicion of occult arterial injury, "exclusion" or "screening" arteriography has been widely used.[20] However, arteriography is not only time consuming in this setting but also invasive, potentially toxic, and very costly. In the study mentioned previously,[10] arteriography cost an average of $850 per patient; hospital charges for such studies may be even higher in other metropolitan trauma centers.

Although, as previously noted, contrast arteriography is highly accurate for defining intraluminal lesions, radiologists' interpretations can sometimes "overread" arteriographic detail such that at least 2% of the readings are false-positive.[17] Such findings can lead to unproductive and costly vessel explorations in the operating room. Even more significantly, recent data have suggested that a substantial number of lesions producing arteriographic abnormalities in the trauma patient actually follow a relatively benign course. Frykberg et al[6] and Stain et al[21] have demonstrated that most posttraumatic intimal flaps, pseudoaneurysms, and arteriovenous fistulas do not result in complications over time but heal uneventfully. Perhaps, therefore, these lesions do not need to be detected. Thus, besides arteriography's invasiveness, potential toxicity, cost, and requisite time, it may be both too sensitive and inadequately specific for use in the trauma setting.

The optimal adjunctive diagnostic tool in the emergency setting would therefore be rapid, simple, noninvasive, portable, and accurate in confirming or excluding significant vascular injuries. Several novel approaches that use currently available noninvasive diagnostic modalities show promise for this purpose.

DOPPLER PRESSURE MEASUREMENTS

Introduced in the 1970s, Doppler arterial pressure measurement and the calculation of pressure indices have become widely used for quantitating chronic arterial occlusive disease. Doppler arterial pressures were tested in 93 consecutive trauma victims with a total of 100 injured limbs using arteriography as a control.[10] An arterial pressure index (systolic arterial pressure in the injured limb/systolic arterial pressure in a normal arm) of greater than 0.90 was considered normal. Compared with arteriographic findings, Doppler arterial pressure indices showed a sensitivity of 87% and a specificity of 97% for detecting arterial injury; the overall accuracy was 95%. Of the total, 2 of the 100 contrast arteriograms were falsely positive in that subsequent vessel exploration and intraoperative arteriography demonstrated no abnormalities: in both of these cases, Doppler arterial pressures had been normal. The sensitivity and specificity of Doppler arterial pressure measurement rose to 95% and 97.5%, respectively, and accuracy to 97% when recalculated against the ultimate clinical outcome, thereby offsetting the effects of the two false-positive arteriographic studies.

The single false-negative Doppler arterial pressure study in this series occurred in a patient with a gunshot wound to the left thigh that resulted in a small pseudoaneurysm of a secondary profunda femoris artery branch that was ultimately detected by arteriography. This patient had an arterial pressure index greater than 0.90. In one victim of a gunshot wound to the left thigh, the Doppler arterial pressure index and arteriogram were both normal initially, but the patient was later found to have a popliteal artery pseudoaneurysm. This emphasizes the importance of clinical follow-up in these patients.

Armed with this arteriographically confirmed evidence for the high sensitivity, specificity, and accuracy of Doppler arterial pressure measurement in extremity trauma, a new management algorithm can be proposed (Fig. 65-1).[7,10] Patients with extremity trauma and an obvious arterial injury undergo either immediate operation or arteriography. Those without "hard" evidence of vascular disruption but who need to have such injury ruled out undergo Doppler arterial pressure measurement and pressure index calculation. Patients with an arterial pressure index of less than 0.90 undergo arteriography, whereas those with a normal index may be discharged and their course monitored. During the 7-month period of clinical testing of this diagnostic algorithm, no major vascular disruptions were missed among 100 consecutive injuries so evaluated; contrast arteriography was required in only 17 patients, and the savings in time (181.7 hours) and hospital charges ($65,175) were substantial. Arteriograms performed to rule out occult extremity arterial injury, as a proportion of all arteriograms performed, fell

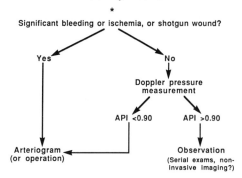

A Possible Diagnostic Algorithm for Extremity Trauma

Fig. 65-1. Proposed diagnostic algorithm for extremity trauma, with Doppler arterial pressure measurement as a screening technique.

from 14% to 5.5% ($p < 0.01$, χ^2) at the trauma center involved.[7]

The findings from these two studies clearly suggest that Doppler arterial pressure measurement may be a rapid, cost-effective, and accurate technique for evaluating extremity arterial injury in the emergency room setting. Its limitations have subsequently become clear as well: it cannot be used where massive wounds, dressings, or splints prevent placement of a proximal cuff; it may not detect non–flow-limiting lesions or damage to nonaxial arteries; and it cannot distinguish between arterial spasm and vessel occlusion. Doppler pressure measurement is not accurate for assessing arterial injuries of the trunk, such as penetrating trauma to the iliac or subclavian regions, and should be used only when potential vascular injuries are distal to the axillary or inguinal crease. Although Doppler pressure measurements are used routinely in some trauma centers, as indicated in Fig. 65-1, other centers have reported a mixed experience with the technique.[1]

DUPLEX SCANNING

Duplex sonography, which is the melding of pulsed wave Doppler with high-resolution B-mode ultrasound, has become increasingly popular for the assessment of atherosclerosis of the carotid bifurcation and other peripheral arteries[9,22] as well as for evaluating various venous conditions.[16] Its ability to provide useful physiologic data from imaging of the vessel in question has led some investigators to suggest that the technique might be substituted for contrast arteriography in certain circumstances.[9,12]

Meissner et al[11] used duplex scanning to evaluate 89 trauma patients who mostly had injuries to their extremities. No major arterial injuries were missed, as confirmed either by follow-up arteriography or by clinical follow-up. Numerous cases of arterial pseudoaneurysm, occlusion, intimal flap, and arteriovenous fistula were diagnosed (Fig. 65-2). Similarly, Bynoe et al[3] used duplex sonography to evaluate 198 trauma victims with 319 actual or potential vascular injuries: 42 vessels (13%) were found to have major or minor

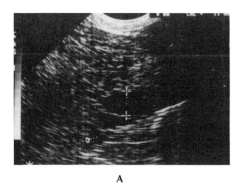 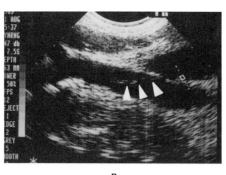 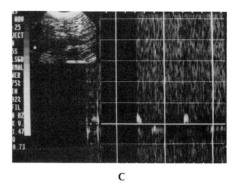

A B C

Fig. 65-2. Duplex scanning in cases of occult arterial trauma revealed a radial artery pseudoaneurysm *(A)*, a carotid artery intimal flap *(B)*, and spectral waveform evidence for arterial occlusion *(C)*.

abnormalities that were further documented by arteriography or surgical exploration. Duplex sonography showed a sensitivity, specificity, and overall accuracy of 95%, 99%, and 98%, respectively, values equivalent to those of exclusion arteriography and at a cost reduction of 60% to 73%.

Injuries that threaten the extracranial carotid and vertebral arteries pose a particular dilemma for the clinician. In the event of penetrating trauma to zone II of the neck, either surgical exploration or a diagnostic protocol including arteriography is required to rule out occult injury to the extracranial cerebral arteries. In patients who have suffered blunt trauma to the neck, cranium, cervical spine, or face, a small but unpredictable proportion have also incurred silent extracranial vascular injury, occasionally leading to serious complications such as carotid occlusion, transient ischemia, or stroke. Park et al[14] performed duplex scanning in 24 patients with blunt or penetrating trauma that threatened the cervical arteries and found seven arterial lesions (four vessel occlusions, three intimal flaps). No missed injuries were identified by follow-up arteriography or at postmortem examination, which led them to suggest that screening with duplex scanning may solve the diagnostic dilemma in such patients.

Panetta et al[13] carried out an arteriographically controlled experimental study of duplex scanning of different types of arterial injury in a canine model; injuries produced included arterial occlusion, laceration, intimal flap, hematoma, and arteriovenous fistula. The study found that duplex scanning was significantly more sensitive than arteriography overall ($p < 0.01$) and was much more accurate than arteriography in detecting arterial lacerations ($p < 0.01$). Duplex sonography's ability to examine arterial wall morphology was particularly advantageous in this situation. These researchers concluded that duplex scanning is highly accurate in evaluating arterial trauma. It could also provide unique data regarding the arterial wall and might be especially useful for performing serial examinations of various posttraumatic lesions to determine their natural history.

Duplex scanning clearly can provide important diagnostic data in trauma victims. Its capabilities to a certain extent complement those of Doppler pressure measurement, since it is able to define non–flow-reducing lesions, potentially detect disruptions in nonaxial arteries, and perhaps diagnose injuries to truncal vessels. The technique is operator dependent and cannot be used to evaluate arteries obscured by extensive dressings, splints, or casts; however, it is portable and noninvasive, and the time and cost of performing it are less than one fifth of those for arteriography.[11]

EMERGENCY ABDOMINAL ULTRASOUND

In elderly patients who suffer sudden cardiovascular collapse, timely and accurate diagnosis is of paramount importance if resuscitation and definitive therapy are to be successful. Although a number of diagnoses may be entertained in such patients, the vast majority have suffered either a myocardial infarction or a ruptured abdominal aortic aneurysm (AAA). This distinction is obviously crucial: transfer to the coronary care unit will likely be lethal for the patient with a ruptured AAA, whereas urgent laparotomy in a hypotensive patient who is actually in cardiogenic shock may be equally catastrophic.

In the Seattle metropolitan area, all elderly patients suffering from cardiovascular collapse are brought to a single institution by the paramedics of the Seattle Medic 1 system.[4] Emergency abdominal ultrasound examinations are performed in such patients within the first 5 minutes of their admission to the emergency department.[18] The rapidity with which AAA can be detected, with line insertion and volume resuscitation carried out at the same time, has contributed substantially to an average emergency department stay of 12 minutes in such patients.[8]

Since 1980 the ultrasonographic diagnosis of ruptured AAA recorded by the emergency department has been made in more than 200 patients and was later confirmed in all cases of operation or postmortem examination. During the past decade, a ruptured AAA was not missed in a single patient admitted to the institution; no patients later found to have a ruptured AAA were incorrectly transferred to the coronary care unit. Two patients thought to have a ruptured AAA underwent emergency laparotomy with negative findings, though both patients were found to have an unruptured AAA. One patient's collapse had actually been occasioned by the perforation of a duodenal ulcer, and the other patient had a ruptured thoracic aortic aneurysm. The abdominal aortas in approximately 2% of patients cannot be imaged due to bowel gas, massive obesity, or ascites. The technique is not accurate for delineating AAA rupture itself, as borne out by the fact that extraaortic blood or fluid has been imaged in only approximately 50% of ruptured aneurysm patients.[18]

NOVEL APPLICATIONS IN EMERGENCY VASCULAR DIAGNOSIS

As outlined in this chapter, the rapidity, portability, and noninvasiveness of several commonly used diagnostic techniques have facilitated the identification of several important life- or limb-threatening conditions in the emergency setting. Several other conditions, most notably thoracic aortic tear after deceleration trauma or various types of aortic dissection, continue to require emergency aortography for definitive diagnosis. The possibility that various novel noninvasive or minimally invasive diagnostic techniques, such as computerized tomographic or magnetic resonance imaging, transesophageal echo, or duplex scanning, might be substituted for arteriography in these circumstances deserves further exploration. For the successful treatment of patients with these conditions, as well as acute arterial disruption, time is essential, and the efficiency and accuracy of various noninvasive vascular diagnostic modalities may contribute toward reducing the substantial morbidity and mortality associated with diagnostic delay.

REFERENCES

1. Anderson RJ et al: Reduced dependency on arteriography for penetrating extremity trauma: influence of wound location and non-invasive vascular studies, *J Trauma* 30:1059-1065, 1990.
2. Ben-Menachem Y: Vascular injuries of the extremities: hazards of unnecessary delays in diagnoses, *Orthopedics* 9:333-338, 1986.
3. Bynoe RP et al: Non-invasive diagnosis of vascular trauma by duplex ultrasonography, *J Vasc Surg* 14:346-352, 1991.
4. Cobb LA, Alvarez H, Copass MK: A rapid response system for out-of-hospital cardiac emergencies, *Med Clin North Am* 60:283-289, 1976.
5. Francis H et al: Vascular proximity: is it a valid indication for arteriography in the asymptomatic patient? *J Trauma* 31:512-514, 1991.
6. Frykberg ER et al: A reassessment of the role of arteriography in penetrating proximity extremity trauma: a prospective study, *J Trauma* 29:1041-1052, 1989.
7. Johansen K et al: Non-invasive vascular tests reliably exclude occult arterial trauma in injured extremities, *J Trauma* 31:515-522, 1991.
8. Johansen K et al: Ruptured abdominal aortic aneurysm: the Harborview experience, *J Vasc Surg* 13:240-247, 1991.
9. Kohler TR et al: Can duplex scanning replace arteriography for lower extremity arterial disease? *Ann Vasc Surg* 4:280-287, 1990.
10. Lynch K, Johansen K: Can Doppler pressure measurement replace "exclusion" arteriography in the diagnosis of occult extremity arterial trauma? *Ann Surg* 214:737, 1991.
11. Meissner M, Paun M, Johansen K: Duplex scanning for arterial trauma, *Am J Surg* 161:552-555, 1991.
12. Moore WS et al: Can clinical evaluation and non-invasive testing substitute for arteriography in the evaluation of carotid artery disease? *Ann Surg* 208:91-94, 1988.
13. Panetta T et al: Duplex scanning and arteriography for the diagnosis of arterial injury: an experimental study, *J Trauma* 33:627-663, 1992.
14. Park S, Paun M, Johansen K: Duplex scanning for extracranial carotid artery trauma, *Ann Vasc Surg* (in press).
15. Perry MO, Thal ER, Shires GT: Management of arterial injuries, *Ann Surg* 173:403-408, 1971.
16. Raghavendra BN et al: Deep venous thrombosis: detection by high-resolution real-time ultrasonography, *Radiology* 152:789-793, 1984.
17. Rose SC, Moore EE: Trauma angiography: the use of clinical findings to improve patient selection and care preparation, *J Trauma* 28:240-245, 1988.
18. Shuman WP et al: Suspected leaking abdominal aortic aneurysm: use of sonography in the emergency room, *Radiology* 168:117-119, 1988.
19. Sirinek K et al: Reassessment of the role of routine operative exploration in vascular trauma, *J Trauma* 21:339-344, 1981.
20. Snyder WH et al: The validity of normal arteriography in penetrating trauma, *Arch Surg* 113:424-428, 1978.
21. Stain SC et al: Selective management of non-occlusive arterial injuries, *Arch Surg* 124:1136-1141, 1989.
22. Strandness DE Jr: Duplex scanning: past, present, and future, *Semin Vasc Surg* 1:2-8, 1988.

CHAPTER 66

Monitoring during and after distal arterial reconstruction

DENNIS F. BANDYK

Vascular laboratory surveillance of infrainguinal bypass grafts to verify technical adequacy and hemodynamic function has become an accepted part of arterial reconstructive surgery. Despite a careful operative technique, however, a spectrum of lesions (box) can occur that are not recognized after the completion of endarterectomy or bypass grafting procedures and thus lead to thrombosis or embolization. Most surgeons rely on physical examination findings, Doppler-derived ankle systolic pressures, and arteriography to monitor distal arterial reconstructions during the immediate postbypass period and after the patient's discharge from the hospital. Although a number of retrospective[1,12,20,22] and prospective* studies have confirmed improved assisted primary patency (i.e., patency when a stenosis has been repaired before occlusion) when a graft surveillance protocol that uses duplex scanning is implemented, many vascular surgeons and internists remain reluctant to recommend such intense graft monitoring in their patients. Detection of the "hemodynamically failing" but patent graft is particularly important after autologous vein bypass, since graft salvage is often not possible after thrombosis. The reluctance to institute a formal graft surveillance protocol appears to stem from several concerns, including the efficacy of graft revision in an asymptomatic patient, reimbursement for vascular testing, and increased vascular laboratory workload. Barnes et al[6] questioned the value of graft surveillance when no benefit was demonstrated in postoperative patients in whom the ankle–brachial systolic pressure index (ABI) was used as an end point for monitoring changes. Graft failure rates were similar (approximately 60%) in patients with both stable and recently decreased (greater than 0.2) ABIs. The concerns regarding the value of graft surveillance can only be addressed by a randomized, prospective clinical trial.[5] Unfortunately, the logistics of conducting such a clinical trial are significant and practically beyond the scope of a single institution. Thus at present, each surgeon must ascertain the merits of graft surveillance and institute a program based on the resources available.

The goal of postoperative monitoring is not only to detect lesions that may precipitate graft thrombosis but also to provide surgeons with guidelines for identifying those grafts at highest risk that should be revised in a secondary procedure. Depending on the graft type (autologous vein or prosthetic) and status of runoff arteries, graft failure rates in excess of 30% at 5 years are common. There is convincing evidence that autologous vein graft strictures detected by both angiography and duplex scanning are associated with a significantly increased risk of graft occlusion compared to normal grafts. Grigg et al[13] and Moody et al[18] observed a 21% to 23% incidence of graft thrombosis in stenotic bypasses when a conservative (no revision) policy was adopted. In a recent report published by Idu et al,[14] occlusion occurred in all vein grafts found to have a greater than 70% diameter reduction stenosis, compared with 10% in grafts with similar lesions that underwent revision ($p < 0.004$). Mattos et al[16] also recently reported that they had found infrainguinal grafts identified by color duplex scanning to have stenosis that exhibited a significantly lower 4-year patency of 57%, compared with 83% in normal grafts.

Revision of a stenotic graft without interruption in patency is most important for autologous vein conduits because most will not remain patent after thrombectomy and thrombolysis either alone or with vein patch angioplasty. There have been 5-year graft patencies in the range of 30% to 50% observed after secondary procedures performed on thrombosed grafts, as compared with assisted primary patencies of 82% to 93% after stenosis repair in patent by-

---

*References 4, 9, 10, 15, 17, 21.

LESIONS THAT PRECIPITATE GRAFT FAILURE

Technical errors	Postimplantation lesions
Retained or scarred valve cusps	Myointimal hyperplasia
Errors in graft tunneling (graft entrapment)	Atherosclerosis
Injured vein segments	Aneurysmal degeneration
Sclerosed veins	
Runoff artery thrombosis	
Platelet aggregation	
Anastomotic stricture	
Intimal flaps	

passes.[8,11] On the basis of available clinical data, it appears that graft surveillance is beneficial and associated with a 10% to 15% increase in assisted primary patency rates. At present, graft surveillance protocols should be considered to be in an evolutionary phase, but it is possible to make some recommendations regarding testing methods, intervals, and diagnostic criteria based on the known temporal patterns and mechanisms of graft failure. The best surveillance program has not been validated, and most investigators have adopted a policy of "selective" secondary intervention when a graft stenosis is identified by changes in the ABI, duplex scanning, or arteriography. The rationale for graft surveillance is based on the hypothesis that careful monitoring of graft and limb hemodynamics can bring about a decrease in the observed steady decline in the patency of arterial grafts by identifying those grafts that harbor lesions and should thus undergo elective revision. Those practitioners advocating graft surveillance must remain cognizant of the costs induced and develop protocols that minimize the frequency of testing but yield positive results.

MECHANISMS OF GRAFT FAILURE

Graft failure can occur as the result of three mechanisms: occlusion by thrombosis, hemodynamic failure, and structural failure (e.g., aneurysmal degeneration). After operation, the frequency of graft failure is highest within the first several days (4% to 10%), decreases to approximately 1% per month (12% during the first year), and then remains at approximately 2% to 4% per year thereafter. The timing of graft failure usually predicts the underlying mechanism. Perioperative (within 30 days) failure is most commonly due to technical errors in bypass construction, including suture stenosis, intimal flaps, retained thrombus, graft entrapment/torsion, and retained valve cusps. The incidence of early graft failure can be minimized by careful intraoperative assessment, but uncommon mechanisms such as congenital or acquired hypercoagulable states, the use of marginal sclerotic venous conduits, low cardiac output, and poor outflow tracts can be responsible for sporadic early graft thrombosis despite a technically perfect reconstruction. Infrainguinal bypasses, especially those using prosthetic grafts, with poor runoff can demonstrate a blood flow velocity near the "thrombotic threshold velocity" of the conduit and are thus prone to thrombosis when there are slight decreases in blood flow.

A number of abnormalities can persist after infrainguinal vein bypass grafting, especially when the in situ saphenous vein grafting technique has been used. Retained valve cusps, errors in tunneling, vein conduit injury, and partial anastomotic occlusion can reduce graft flow to abnormally low levels and precipitate thrombosis. These lesions can also be the foci for the subsequent development of myointimal hyperplasia during the first 2 years after operation. Postimplantation lesions have been identified in 11% to 33% of saphenous vein grafts either by angiography or duplex scanning, with approximately 75% developing within the first postoperative year.[8,14,15,21,22]

Atherosclerosis can also develop de novo in vein grafts or progress in adjacent native arteries and cause late graft failure. This type of failure tends to occur after the second postoperative year in patients with autologous vein bypasses but has been observed earlier after the occurrence of polytetrafluoroethylene (PTFE) bypass grafting thrombosis, typically with involvement of the distal artery tree. Structural failure is an uncommon source of late graft thrombosis and is usually manifested as aneurysmal degeneration. The mechanism of graft thrombosis involves the accumulation of mural thrombus within the aneurysmal segment, and this leads to occlusion or distal embolization. This mode of failure should be suspected when thrombosis occurs despite normal findings in graft surveillance studies. Occlusive lesions, such as those due to technical errors, acquired myointimal graft stenosis, or atherosclerotic disease progression may precipitate graft thrombosis by decreasing blood flow velocity below a minimum level at which thrombus formation can ensue.

MEASUREMENT TECHNIQUES

By providing objective data on hemodynamics, duplex scanning can identify that subgroup of grafts with low-flow hemodynamics. Grafts with abnormal hemodynamics appear to be at increased risk for thrombus formation. Green et al[12] reported their findings in a retrospective comparison of graft surveillance techniques and noted that grafts harboring lesions decreasing the ABI by 10% or greater, in conjunction with an abnormal duplex scan (low graft flow and/or stenosis), exhibited a 66% incidence of thrombosis within 3 months, compared with a 14% risk of failure if only the ABI was abnormal and a 4% risk of failure if only the duplex scan was abnormal.

Color duplex imaging, a powerful diagnostic imaging technique similar to arteriography, is capable of identifying a spectrum of lesions that place the graft at risk for sudden thrombosis. High-resolution graft and vessel imaging is possible, and this permits the morphology of the vascular defect

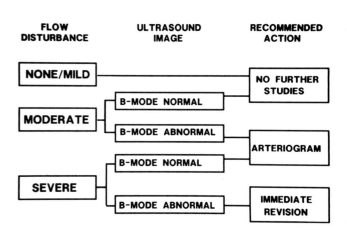

Fig. 66-1. Diagnostic algorithm using duplex scanning for intraoperative assessment of infrainguinal vein bypasses. The recommended action is based on the severity of the flow disturbance and abnormality on real-time B-mode imaging.

to be determined in a region of disturbed, turbulent flow. The technique is appropriate for intraoperative and postoperative diagnostic studies. An algorithm based on the severity of flow disturbance and abnormalites in the color-coded B-mode image (Fig. 66-1) provides the information necessary to assess the technical adequacy of the graft or to determine the need for immediate revision of the reconstruction.

The relationship between the degree of stenosis detected by duplex scanning and arteriography after distal arterial reconstruction and the risk of graft thrombosis requires further study. Recent studies indicate that high-grade (exceeding 70% diameter reduction) stenoses with an end-diastolic velocity greater than 100 cm/sec or a velocity ratio across the stenosis of greater than 3.5 are highly correlated with graft thrombosis. However, use of a single criterion to identify unexpected graft thrombosis, such as a peak systolic velocity of less than 45 cm/sec in a normal graft segment or a decrease in the ABI, is associated with a low positive predictive value. Prospective studies of graft surveillance programs have confirmed that the development of a low-flow graft state, particularly if prior testing demonstrated normal graft flow velocity, is a harbinger of thrombosis and should prompt complete imaging of the lower limb arterial circulation to delineate sites of stenosis.[1,4,17] Color duplex imaging, if available, is the best initial technique for imaging the bypass site, although incomplete evaluation of inflow and runoff vessels limits its effectiveness in some patients. In selected patients (i.e., those with a high-grade stenosis identified in the main body of the graft or at an anastomosis and low graft flow velocity/ABI), duplex scanning can supplant arteriography for deciding the need for graft revision. Serial evaluation of graft hemodynamics offers several advantages: it gauges initial technical success, identifies deterioration in graft functional patency at a time when developing occlusive lesions may be managed easily by either

Table 66-1. Peak systolic flow velocity measured in mid- or distal segments of femoropopliteal and femorotibial saphenous vein and PTFE grafts

Graft type	No.	Velocity (cm/sec)
In-situ saphenous vein		
Femoropopliteal	65	76±12
Femorotibial	95	72±16
Femoropopliteal, isolated segment	10	62±15
Reversed saphenous vein		
Femoropopliteal	20	80±16
Femorotibial	12	69±14
Cephalic vein		
Femoropopliteal/tibial	8	52±14
PTFE, 6 mm diameter		
Femoropopliteal	28	76±12
Femorotibial	26	63±12
PTFE, 5 mm diameter		
Femorotibial	5	77±11

Blood flow velocity calculated 1 to 3 months after surgery. Flow velocities are means ± standard deviation. *PTFE*, Polytetrafluorothylene.

elective surgical revision or percutaneous transluminal angioplasty, and equally important, documents the hemodynamic benefit of graft revision (i.e., normalization of graft flow velocity).[3]

A wide range of duplex scanning–derived blood flow velocities have been measured in infrainguinal grafts after successful bypass grafting (Table 66-1).[2] In general, peak systolic velocity in the middistal graft segments exceeds 40 to 45 cm/sec unless the conduit diameter is greater than 6 mm or the graft runoff is limited (isolated tibial artery segment or dorsalis pedis artery bypass). Belkin et al[7] demonstrated that peak systolic velocity differs with varying luminal diameter and recommended the performance of duplex surveillance scans of vein grafts using diameter-specific criteria. Of note, these authors found graft flow velocity was lower ($p < 0.04$) in inframalleolar grafts (59 cm/sec) than in tibial (77 cm/sec) or popliteal (71 cm/sec) grafts. Only 4 of 72 grafts, all anastomosed to inframalleolar arteries, had a peak systolic velocity below 45 cm/sec. Use of arm vein (cephalic, basilic) or varicose saphenous segments is also associated with low graft conduit flow velocity, but this hemodynamic finding by itself does not indicate impending thrombosis, though it may serve as an indication for implementing postoperative anticoagulation. When normal-sized (3- to 6-mm diameter) venous conduits are used, identification of a graft flow velocity below 40 to 45 cm/sec is uncommon during or after operation, and this finding has correlated with a residual graft lesion if encountered in the perioperative period or with an acquired lesion if found during follow-up. Low graft flow velocity due to poor runoff is an infrequent finding and, when it occurs, is usually obvious, based on angiographic assessment of the runoff vessels and the presence of low systolic and diastolic flow despite severe foot ischemia. When a low-flow state is identified, a prompt and thorough graft evaluation should be undertaken, especially if the ABI is also abnormal (less than 0.9). Management of low-flow grafts due to poor runoff is controversial, but options include anticoagulation, sequential bypass grafting, or adjunctive distal arteriovenous fistula; the last two modalities are intended to augment graft flow.

The velocity spectra used to monitor vascular grafts can be classified into two normal and three abnormal categories (Table 66-2). In limbs that undergo revascularization because of critical ischemia, a hyperemic flow pattern is normally recorded from the graft in the perioperative period (Fig. 66-2). Antegrade flow throughout the pulse cycle indicates low peripheral vascular resistance and correlates with signs of revascularization hyperemia (skin warmth, vasodilatation). Within days to several weeks, this hyperemic graft flow dissipates and the velocity waveform evolves to a triphasic configuration, typically of normal peripheral artery flow and associated with normalization of the ABI.

Transformation of the normal triphasic graft velocity waveform to a biphasic or monophasic configuration coupled with a decrease in peak systolic velocity implies the existence of a remote occlusive lesion. Three waveform

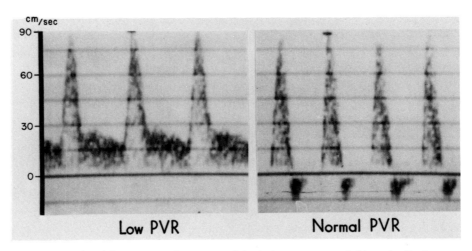

Fig. 66-2. Normal graft flow patterns. Shown are serial velocity spectra recorded from the distal segment of a femorotibial in situ saphenous vein (3.5 mm diameter) graft. The hyperemic flow pattern *(left)* recorded 1 day after surgery evolved by 4 weeks to a triphasic configuration *(right)*. The change in the waveform was due to an increase in the peripheral vascular resistance *(PVR)*. Note that the peak systolic velocity remained constant during this time interval.

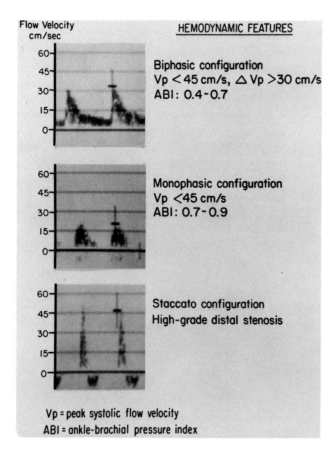

Fig. 66-3. Velocity spectra and hemodynamic characteristics of three abnormal graft flow patterns observed with the development of graft stenosis are shown. *Delta Vp*, Decrease in peak systolic velocity between 3-month serial studies.

Table 66-2. Categories of graft blood flow patterns

Duplex category	Velocity spectra (waveform) characteristics
Normal	
Normal PVR	Triphasic configuration, Vp >45 cm/sec at mid or distal graft recording site; applicable for vein diameter 3-5 mm
Low PVR	Biphasic configuration, end-diastolic flow velocity >0, Vp >45 cm/sec; an expected waveform at operation and in early postoperative period
Abnormal, low-flow velocity	
High PVR	Monophasic configuration, no diastolic forward flow, Vp <45 cm/sec; ABI typically between 0.7 and 0.9
	Staccato Doppler signal with flow reversal during diastole, Vp <45 cm/sec; minimum antegrade flow due to high-grade distal stenosis
Low PVR	Biphasic waveform with Vp <45 cm/sec or decrease of >30 cm/sec compared to prior level; compensatory diastolic flow due to abnormal ABI (0.4-0.7)

PVR, Peripheral vascular resistance; *Vp,* peak systolic velocity; *ABI,* ankle-brachial systolic pressure index.

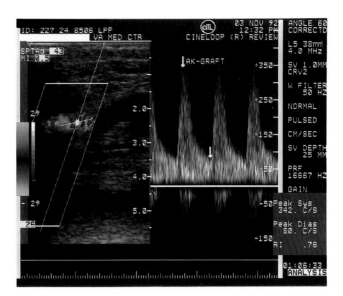

Fig. 66-4. Color flow image and velocity spectra of a vein conduit stenosis are shown. The localized increase in Doppler frequency shift and spectral broadening was due to a retained valve leaflet after in situ saphenous vein bypass grafting.

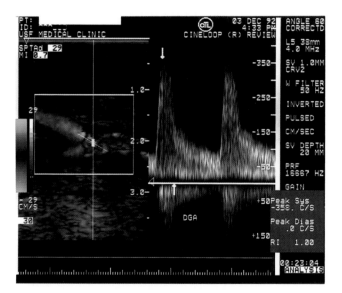

Fig. 66-5. Color duplex image of distal anastomosis of a femoral posterior tibial in situ saphenous vein bypass recorded 6 months postoperative showing a greater than 75% diameter reduction stenosis (end-diastolic velocity of 100 cm/sec). Proximal graft velocity had decreased from 100 to 50 cm/sec. The graft was revised by interposition grafting.

configurations have been observed with the development of a graft stenosis that is both pressure and flow reducing (Fig. 66-3). All these are associated with a low (less than 45 cm/sec) or decreased (more than 30 cm/sec compared to prior level) peak systolic flow velocity. The most common abnormal graft waveform, present in approximately one half of the cases, is biphasic and associated with a resting ABI of 0.4 to 0.7. The forward diastolic flow occurs in response

to compensatory arteriolar dilatation, and the site of graft stenosis may be proximal or distal to the recording site. A monophasic waveform with low peak systolic flow velocity has been observed in approximately 40% of grafts with stenosis (Fig. 66-4). All such patients are asymptomatic and have a resting ABI of between 0.7 and 0.9. Typically, the stenosis is classified in the 50% to 75% diameter reduction category based on both duplex scanning and arteriographic findings (Fig. 66-5). An uncommon (6% of abnormal grafts) but ominous waveform manifests a staccato-velocity spectra representing a to-and-fro motion of the blood within the compliant venous conduit with each pulse cycle. This waveform is always associated with a high-grade distal graft stenosis and is a harbinger of graft thrombosis. The minimal antegrade flow in these grafts complicates angiographic visualization of the distal graft and anastomosis, which is sometimes termed *pseudoocclusion graft occlusion*. Grading the severity of graft stenosis or classifying functional patency is best performed using duplex scanning–derived velocity criteria in combination with waveform analysis and calculation of the resting ABI.

ESSENTIALS OF GRAFT SURVEILLANCE
Intraoperative monitoring

Color duplex systems greatly facilitate intraoperative decision making, particularly of in situ saphenous vein bypass and extended profunda femoris endarterectomy procedures, and are superior to the use of handheld continuous wave Doppler probes, conventional duplex scanners, or arteriography. The superficial position of the graft and anastomotic sites within the surgical wound allows the entire reconstruction to be imaged after restoration of flow. Use of a water-impregnated standoff on the transducer and placement within a sterile plastic sleeve containing acoustic gel are necessary to accomplish acoustic coupling and near-field imaging of the vessels and surrounding tissue. A linear array transducer with an imaging frequency of 7 to 10 MHz provides high-resolution B-mode color-coded images, and electronic steering of the Doppler beam enables blood flow patterns to be imaged at insonation angles of 65° or less. A uniform color-coded flow field during systole and the absence of anatomic defects in the B-mode image are features of a normal study. Identification of an occlusive lesion (stenosis) by color duplex scanning is determined by the following flow features: jetting at the stenosis, complexing color-coded flow mixing within and distal to the stenosis, and large flow reversals along the wall downstream from the stenosis. The spectral criteria of a significant lesion include focal increases in peak systolic velocities to greater than 150 cm/sec and spectral broadening with simultaneous reversed-flow components throughout systole. Identification of a severe flow disturbance within a graft segment or anastomosis, particularly if associated with lumen reduction, is highly diagnostic of a residual defect that warrants immediate correction or further assessment by arteriography if color duplex findings are judged equivocal.

Color duplex imaging has been used at operation in 50 consecutive patients after femorotibial ($n = 34$) or femoropopliteal ($n = 16$) in situ saphenous vein bypass grafting. Color flow imaging accurately identified the presence, location, and hemodynamic significance of residual arteriovenous fistulae, the adequacy of the valve cusp incision, anastomotic and runoff artery patency, and the presence of adequate graft blood flow velocity (peak systolic velocity greater than 40 cm/sec and antegrade diastolic flow). The entire arterial bypass, including proximal and distal anastomoses, was imaged in all but one patient, with scan times ranging from 10 to 15 minutes, including the acquisition and processing of hard-copy data. No complications (e.g., repair disruption or postoperative wound infection) occurred that were related to the examination. Of the total, 8 (16%) of the 50 intraoperative scans were abnormal, and this prompted immediate graft revisions. Six abnormal valve sites were identified by characteristic abrupt stenotic flow, and two graft segments containing platelet aggregates were demonstrated in both the color-coded B-mode image and centerstream velocity spectra. Completion arteriography (used in 40 cases) demonstrated no abnormality in grafts judged normal by color duplex imaging. All vein bypasses remained patent after operation, with a 30-day and 3-month patency of 100%, but one graft, modified at the primary operation, required revision at 4 months because of a focal myointimal graft stenosis.

Postoperative monitoring

The need for graft surveillance depends on the graft type, status of runoff, and the likelihood of residual postimplantation lesions, as well as whether limb pressures (e.g., pedal pulses, ABI) have normalized. The hemodynamics and failure rate of infrainguinal bypass grafts mandate surveillance of a developing low-flow graft state, which suggests the existence of residual or acquired graft stenosis and frequently precedes graft thrombosis.

Most patients whose grafts become stenosed are asymptomatic, and physical examination is incapable of detecting the subtle signs of the hemodynamically failing but patent graft. Less than one quarter of these patients have unequivocal evidence of graft stenosis on the basis of decreased pulses or recurrence of limb ischemia.[11,19,21,22] Angiographic screening of patients is not warranted because of the insensitivity and expense of such serial evaluations. Although measurement of the resting ABI is well established for the diagnosis of arterial occlusive disease of the lower limb, it has low diagnostic sensitivity and specificity in detecting graft stenosis or predicting graft failure.[1,5,6] Barnes et al[6] found that a decrease in the ABI of greater than 0.2 occurred with equal frequency in both failed and patent grafts. Many other investigators have also confirmed a low positive predictive value in the range of 12% to 34% when ABI alone was used to predict the presence of graft stenosis. In prospective studies that used both duplex scanning and Doppler-derived ABI measurements, it was observed that graft thrombosis may occur despite normalization of the ABI after

operation, and an abnormal ABI in the perioperative period does not reliably identify grafts requiring revision.[10,17] After infrainguinal saphenous vein bypass grafting, serial measurements of resting ankle systolic pressure did not identify 20 (36%) of 56 graft stenoses because of an insignificant change in the ABI (less than 0.15) or because the tibial arteries were incompressible, making pressure measurements unreliable. In contrast, all patients had abnormal duplex scan findings, based on changes in the magnitude and configuration of the graft velocity waveform. Graft stenosis was suspected when a low-flow graft state was detected, and this finding then prompted complete duplex imaging of the arterial bypass. The location and severity of stenosis were ascertained in 85% of the patients examined. Two thirds of the patients were asymptomatic despite a decrease in their ABI to a mean of 0.62. Most investigators have observed that once patients exhibit recurrent symptoms of limb ischemia, the graft has occluded. Similarly, although a decrease in the ABI indicates a reduction in overall limb perfusion, resting ankle pressures do not always distinguish between functionally normal, low-flow, and occluded grafts.

The combination of Doppler-derived ABIs and color flow duplex imaging of the graft with duplex-derived velocity determination can be used for monitoring vascular grafts. Accurate graft imaging requires the examiner to be knowledgeable in a number of areas (box). At sites of stenosis, color flow imaging typically demonstrates aliasing of the color map and a color-coded flow jet, a hemodynamic characteristic of lesions with a greater than 50% diameter reduction (see Fig. 66-3). Peak systolic velocities exceeding 150 to 180 cm/sec, spectral broadening throughout the pulse cycle including reversed-flow components in systole, and a velocity ratio greater than 2 are accepted duplex scanning findings indicating stenosis with a greater than 50% diameter reduction. The instrumentation, scanning technique, and diagnostic criteria are similar for monitoring saphenous vein (in situ and reversed), autologous vein, prosthetic, and composite arterial bypasses.

ESSENTIALS OF GRAFT SURVEILLANCE

Color duplex instrumentation
　　Time-gain compensation
　　Color-coding algorithm
　　Color maps
Pitfalls of color duplex imaging
　　Aliasing
　　Doppler angle correction
Arterial and bypass graft anatomy
Normal arterial and graft flow patterns
Measurement of duplex-derived blood flow velocities
Velocity spectral criteria for grading stenosis
Recognition of graft lesions
　　Arteriovenous fistulae
　　Graft entrapment
　　Anastomotic, vein graft aneurysms

POSTOPERATIVE SCANNING PROTOCOL

The following protocol is observed for the postoperative scanning of patients. Patients are placed in the supine position with the pertinent lower limb rotated externally and the knee bent slightly. This position affords complete visualization of the arterial system from the aorta to the tibial arteries. The examiner (either a vascular technologist or physician) should have available a complete description of the bypass graft procedure, the type and location of the conduit, the sites of anastomoses, and any technical difficulties encountered during the primary operation. The bypass graft is visualized in the upper thigh and then traced cephalad to the proximal anastomosis, typically the common femoral artery. The presence of a triphasic waveform in the femoral artery indicates a hemodynamically normal aortoiliac segment. In the presence of a patent infrainguinal bypass, a pulsatility index greater than 4.0 also confirms the absence of inflow occlusive disease.[16] In questionable cases, the aortoiliac segment can be imaged directly for determining plaque formation that reduces the diameter of the lumen and also for identifying any flow abnormalities indicative of stenosis. After assessment of graft inflow, all anastomotic sites and the graft conduit are mapped to reveal any structural abnormalities (e.g., stenosis, aneurysmal dilation, intraluminal defect) and sites of flow disturbance. In situ vein bypasses lie superficial to the muscle fascia and are imaged easily throughout their length. When the saphenous vein is left in situ, the bypass conduit presents a tapered appearance, with the largest diameter located in the thigh. Abrupt reductions in venous diameter typically occur at branch points and in duplicated venous segments. Reversed and prosthetic grafts are commonly placed through deeper tunnels adjacent to the native vessels. Graft anastomoses to the below-knee popliteal artery are best imaged from a posterior approach with the patient in a prone position. Anastomotic sites to the peroneal artery are the most difficult to examine because of their deeper location. A distal graft anastomosis is typically made to the native artery in an end-to-side fashion, thereby permitting blood to flow in both caudal and cephalad directions. When such distal anastomotic sites cannot be imaged directly for analysis of the flow pattern, the functional resistance to flow (arterial impedance) of the anastomosis and outflow vessels can be determined based on the magnitude and configuration of the velocity waveform in the distal graft.

After the graft is imaged, centerstream velocity waveforms are recorded from several above- and below-knee graft segments, where the diameter does not vary and accurate assignment of the Doppler beam angle is possible. The magnitude and configuration of the velocity waveform are compared with those obtained in previous studies performed at the same recording site. It is not necessary to image the entire arterial system of the lower limb and the entire graft at each postoperative examination. Only grafts that develop a low-flow state, indicated by a peak systolic flow velocity of less than 45 cm/sec or a decrease of more than 30 cm/sec in bloodflow velocity, require complete duplex mapping. When velocity measurements are used to categorized graft hemodynamics as low or normal, the highest blood flow velocity (Vp) measured within the graft is used as the recorded value. For in situ bypasses, this corresponds to blood flow velocity in the distal graft segment, whereas for reversed vein bypasses, the proximal graft segment should have the highest blood flow velocity. Sites of flow disturbance are examined in detail to delineate the morphology of the lesion and to assess their hemodynamic significance on the basis of changes in peak velocity and spectral content compared with the findings in normal proximal arterial segments.

Graft monitoring should be repeated before the patient is discharged from the hospital and should include complete duplex mapping of the arterial bypass plus measurement of graft blood flow velocity and resting limb pressures (ABI and toe systolic pressure). Wound edema, hematoma, and incisional tenderness may preclude detailed assessment of anastomotic sites in approximately 20% of patients for 2 to 3 weeks after surgery. After the patient is discharged from the hospital, graft surveillance should be carried out first at 6 weeks and next at 3-month intervals for 2 years and then every 6 months thereafter. This protocol appears adequate for detecting the occasional rapid development of myointimal lesions at valvular and anastomotic sites possessing moderate residual (less than 50% diameter reduction stenosis) flow or anatomic abnormalities. A normal duplex scan at 3 months is a good predictor for a low incidence of subsequent graft stenosis. In a series consisting of 120 consecutive distal saphenous vein bypasses, duplex imaging was normal in 115 grafts at 3 months, and no graft occluded or developed a high-grade (greater than 70%), flow-reducing stenosis during the subsequent 6 months of surveillance. However, further confirmation of this observation is required before the intervals between graft surveillance can be lengthened in this group of patients. In general, graft surveillance can be carried out by well-trained vascular laboratory personnel, and only when abnormalities are identified is a physician-supervised evaluation necessary.

CATEGORIES OF GRAFT STENOSIS

A localized increase in blood flow velocity and spectral broadening on duplex scanning can identify the site of a stenosis. On the basis of the velocity spectra obtained both distal and proximal to a stenotic vessel segment, the severity can be classified into four categories: wall irregularity with less than 20% diameter reduction, 20% to 49% diameter reduction, 50% to 75% diameter reduction, and greater than 75% diameter reduction. In the last two categories, a pressure gradient will exist across the lesion at resting flow, and a reduction in ankle pressure is found. This finding of a lesion with a greater than 50% diameter reduction has been uniformly associated with an angiographically detected lesion that warranted surgical correction. The only exception has been the identification of a residual valve cusp or cusps after in situ bypass during the perioperative period. Angiographically demonstrated lesions that show mild to moderate disruption in flow (stenosis less than 50%) on duplex scanning can be safely observed for progression. At present, it appears that moderate stenoses (peak systolic velocity of 180 to 250 cm/sec) require only clinical observation if graft flow velocity is normal and the ABI is greater than 0.9. High-grade stenoses (peak systolic velocity, greater than 250 cm/sec; velocity ratio, greater than 3.5; end-diastolic velocity, greater than 100 cm/sec) should be corrected surgically. The method of secondary graft revision will vary from percutaneous transluminal angioplasty to direct surgical repair by patch angioplasty or interposition graft depending on the location and length of the lesion.

OUTCOME OF GRAFT SURVEILLANCE

The ability of duplex ultrasonography to identify graft lesions in their preocclusive phase, coupled with a low potential for complication and high frequency of interpretable studies, makes it the preferred technique for monitoring the outcome of distal arterial reconstructions. The development of the color Doppler technique and the availability of suitable probes and standoffs minimize many of the cumbersome aspects of intraoperative imaging. A carefully conducted surveillance program should identify bypasses at risk for thrombosis, clarify the mechanism of graft failure, and thereby reduce the incidence of unexpected infrainguinal vein bypass failure to less than 2% per year. The institution of a vein graft surveillance program led to a cumulative assisted primary patency of 96% at 1 year and 85% at 5 years in patients who underwent in situ saphenous vein femorodistal bypass grafting.[4] These results were superior to the 3-year secondary patency of 47% observed in cases of vein graft revision performed because of an acutely thrombosed in situ vein bypass. Thus waiting for symptomatic limb ischemia to occur should not serve as the requisite criterion for deciding to perform graft revision. Because graft type, luminal diameter, configuration, and runoff vary widely, the surveillance protocol should not be based on rigid criteria but rather designed to detect changes in baseline graft (peak systolic and end-diastolic velocity) and limb (ABI and toe systolic pressure) hemodynamics, determined either at operation or in the perioperative period once a successful bypass is apparent. Interpreters of graft surveillance studies must keep in mind the magnitude and configuration of the graft velocity waveform, which depends on several factors, including the recording site, the time interval after operation, and the outflow resistance of the runoff vessels. No single velocity criterion can be used to predict the likelihood of graft thrombosis. However, in the setting of serial testing, an increased failure rate was observed, especially for prosthetic grafts, when the maximum (measured from the smallest-diameter but normal graft segment) graft systolic velocity was less than 40 cm/sec and there was no forward diastolic flow.

The basis for recommending graft revision has not been defined clearly, except when patients have recurrent symptoms of claudication or ischemic lesions develop. Recurrent limb ischemia has been observed in only one third of patients in the study despite conclusive vascular laboratory studies indicating a hemodynamically failing bypass graft. Graft revision is recommended to asymptomatic patients when a correctable lesion is identified by duplex scanning or arteriography, a low-flow state has developed in the graft, and the ABI decreases by more than 0.15. The majority (approximately 60%) of graft stenoses repaired have had velocity spectra indicating a diameter reduction stenosis exceeding 75%.

An effective graft surveillance protocol must be applicable for all patients; practical in terms of time, effort, and cost; and reliable and must be able to detect, grade, and assess the progression of postimplantation lesions. The combination of Doppler-derived pressure measurements and color duplex imaging is currently the most accurate method for monitoring distal arterial reconstructions. The accuracy of duplex scanning for the detection of occlusive and aneurysmal lesions is comparable to that of arteriography, and graft revision can be recommended and implemented based on the findings of noninvasive testing alone. The ultimate fate of a distal arterial reconstruction depends not just on graft and patient risk factors but also on the philosophy and commitment of the surgeon to carrying out graft surveillance. Such a program can be expected to bring about an excellent late graft patency rate (85% at 5 years after revision). Procedures that excise the postimplantation lesion, use autologous vein reconstruction, and restore hemodynamics in the limb and bypass to normal are associated with the lowest incidence of restenosis and late graft failure. In bypasses with low flow but no correctable abnormality, especially those using prosthetic grafts, oral anticoagulation with sodium warfarin may decrease the incidence of graft thrombosis.

REFERENCES

1. Bandyk DF, Cato RF, Towne JB: A low flow velocity predicts failure of femoropopliteal and femorotibial bypass, *Surgery* 98:799-802, 1985.
2. Bandyk DF et al: Hemodynamics of in situ saphenous vein arterial bypass, *Arch Surg* 123:477, 1988.
3. Bandyk DF et al: Hemodynamics of vein graft stenosis, *J Vasc Surg* 8:688-695, 1988.
4. Bandyk DF et al: Monitoring functional patency of in situ saphenous vein bypasses: the impact of a surveillance protocol and elective revision, *J Vasc Surg* 9:284-296, 1989.
5. Bandyk DF et al: Clinical research trials using noninvasive vascular testing, *J Vasc Surg* 15:897-901, 1992.
6. Barnes RW et al: Serial noninvasive studies do not herald postoperative failure of femoropopliteal or femorotibial bypass grafts, *Ann Surg* 210:486-494, 1989.
7. Belkin M et al: The variation in vein graft flow velocity with luminal diamter and outflow level, *J Vasc Surg* 15:991-999, 1992.
8. Bergamini TM et al: Experience with in situ saphenous vein bypasses during 1981 to 1989: determinant factors of long-term patency, *J Vasc Surg* 13:137-149, 1991.
9. Buth J et al: Color-flow duplex criteria for grading stenosis in infrainguinal vein grafts, *J Vasc Surg* 14:716-728, 1991.
10. Disselhoff B, Buth J, Jakimowicz J: Early detection of stenosis of femoro-distal grafts: a surveillance study using color-duplex scanning, *Eur J Vasc Surg* 3:43-48, 1989.

11. Donaldson MC, Mannick JA, Whittemore AD: Causes of primary graft failure after in situ saphenous vein bypass grafting, *J Vasc Surg* 15:113-120, 1992.
12. Green RM et al: Comparison of infrainguinal graft surveillance techniques, *J Vasc Surg* 11:207-215, 1990.
13. Grigg MJ, Nicolaides AN, Wolfe JHN: Femorodistal vein graft stenoses, *Br J Surg* 75:737-740, 1988.
14. Idu MM et al: Impact of a color-flow duplex surveillance program on infrainguinal vein graft patency: a five-year experience, *J Vasc Surg* 17:42-53, 1993.
15. Londrey GL et al: Initial experience with color-flow duplex scanning of infrainguinal bypass grafts, *J Vasc Surg* 12:284-290, 1990.
16. Mattos MA et al: Does correction of stenoses identified with color duplex scanning improve infrainguinal graft patency? *J Vasc Surg* 17:59-66, 1993.
17. Mills JL et al: The importance of routine surveillance of distal bypass grafts with duplex scanning: a study of 379 reversed vein grafts, *J Vasc Surg* 12:379-389, 1990.
18. Moody AP, Gould DA, Harris PL: Vein graft surveillance improves patency in femoropopliteal bypass, *Eur J Vasc Surg* 4:117-121, 1990.
19. Sauvage LR et al: Current arterial prostheses, *Arch Surg* 114:687-692, 1979.
20. Sladen JD, Gilmour JL: Vein graft stenosis: characteristics and effect of treatment, *Am J Surg* 141:549-551, 1981.
21. Sladen JG, Reid JDS, Cooperberg PL: Color flow duplex screening of infrainguinal grafts combining low- and high-velocity criteria, *Am J Surg* 158:107-112, 1989.
22. Turnipseed WD, Acher CW: Postoperative surveillance: an effective means of detecting correctable lesions that threaten graft patency, *Arch Surg* 120:324-326, 1985.

CHAPTER 67

Arteriography, angioscopy, or B-mode imaging for completion monitoring in peripheral arterial disease

RALPH B. DILLEY

Operations for peripheral arterial disease are among those most commonly performed by vascular surgeons. In addition to the standard aortofemoral bypass, which is performed for aortoiliac disease, there are increasing numbers of operations done for femoral, popliteal, and tibial occlusive disease. Inflow vessels include the common femoral, superficial femoral, and popliteal arteries, and outflow vessels consist of the popliteal, tibial, and paramalleolar or pedal vessels. Conduits include the reversed saphenous vein, in situ saphenous vein, arm veins, and occasionally prosthetic materials. In many cases, the anastomosis is located in vessels 1.5 to 3 mm in diameter, and conduits are often quite long and tortuous. Consequently, the chance for technical error is high, and because these errors may lead to early graft thrombosis, intraoperative assessment of the technical result of operation is critically important.

Technical problems that must be identified intraoperatively include anastomotic stenoses, disease distal to the anastomosis in the native vessel that went unrecognized preoperatively, intraluminal thrombus (native vessel or conduit), residual valve obstruction in the in situ vein graft, stricture of the vein graft at side branches, and kinks in the conduit caused by tunneling. Completion arteriography is generally regarded as the gold standard for identifying an intraoperative technical problem, but recently, intraoperative angioscopy and B-mode ultrasonography have been evaluated for this purpose.

INTRAOPERATIVE ARTERIOGRAPHY

Intraoperative arteriography is considered the standard technique for assessing the technical result of vascular reconstruction.[1,2] It has not been universally accepted for a number of reasons, however. The technique is cumbersome, requires the presence of an x-ray technician and a portable x-ray unit in the operating room, may expose operating room personnel to radiation, and requires the development and interpretation of the film once it is exposed. In addition, the film shows the operative segment in only one plane and may thus miss a significant lesion. Despite these limitations, intraoperative arteriography remains the most useful method

to determine the technical adequacy of the operation, and if performed with care, complications are rare.

There are two ways to perform intraoperative arteriography. First, a bolus of contrast material is injected into the artery either distal to an arterial clamp or within the flowing stream, and a single film is exposed. This is the most widely used technique, but it possesses a potential for error because the density of contrast material is high and small technical defects may be missed. Fig. 67-1 shows a completion arteriogram of an above-knee femoropopliteal bypass obtained in this way. The anastomosis is clearly seen and the runoff vessels are adequately demonstrated, yet the density of the contrast agent is high because it was injected distal to an occluding clamp. The use of a proximal clamp avoids the problem of timing the exposure, which is common when contrast material is injected into a flowing stream.

To overcome the deficiencies of single-shot arteriograms, the second technique for intraoperative arteriography uses a portable C-arm unit with digital subtraction capability. This markedly improves the rapidity with which completion studies can be obtained. Contrast material is injected into the flowing stream and the images are summated by the digital subtraction process. This instant image is projected onto a monitor and can be reproduced on either x-ray film or paper to furnish a permanent record. Because the portable digital subtraction unit has road-mapping capabilities, this technique can also be used to treat isolated arterial lesions by balloon angioplasty, atherectomy, or stent placement, as depicted in Fig. 67-2. Its main disadvantage is that only a small field can be visualized during a single injection; however, replay of the results permits assessment of flow that is not possible with static arteriography and allows a better estimate of the physiologic significance of minor defects. Once familiarity is achieved with the various techniques for intraoperative arteriography, its use adds only a few minutes to the surgical procedure.

ANGIOSCOPY

A newer approach to the intraoperative assessment of vascular reconstruction is angioscopy. This method has gained

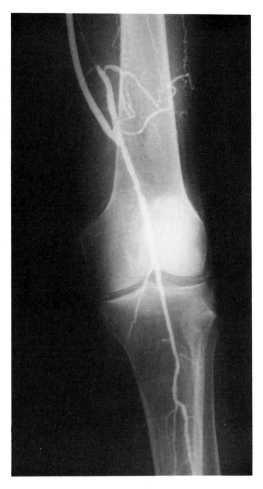

Fig. 67-1. Intraoperative arteriogram obtained by injecting contrast distal to an occluding clamp. No defects are seen in this femoral popliteal bypass, but note the high density of the contrast medium.

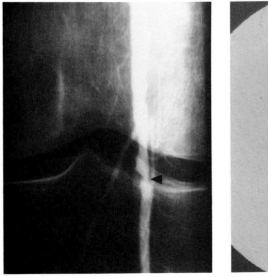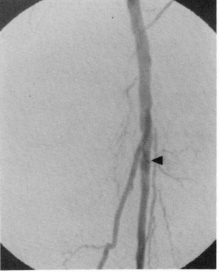

Fig. 67-2. Intraoperative arteriograms that were obtained with C-arm and digital subtraction capability. The contrast was injected into the flowing stream. In this case an intraoperative atherectomy was carried out. Preintervention film is on left and completion study is on right at arrow.

wide acceptance since Vollmar et al[14] reported visualization of the arterial lumen with an angioscope in 1969. The technology has been dramatically improved with the development of very small fiberoptic scopes (1.4 to 2.8 mm), as shown in Fig. 67-3. In addition, the angioscopes are coupled to a video camera that transmits a high-resolution color image to a monitor. A most important aspect of intraoperative angioscopy is the maintenance of a blood-free field. Because a small quantity of blood within the arterial lumen obscures the image, the recent development of a pump irrigation system through which crystalloid can be rapidly infused has measurably improved the operator's ability to visualize the arterial lumen. The small, 1.4-mm scope (Fig. 67-3, *left*) requires an external sheath through which the angioscope is advanced, and fluid is infused into this sheath. The larger scopes (Fig. 67-3, *right*) have an infusion channel in the angioscope.

For assessing the technical result of an infrainguinal bypass, the angioscope is introduced into the most proximal portion of the vein after completion of the distal anastomosis. Particular attention should be paid to valve sites in an in situ bypass, possible kinking of the graft, and sites of side branches. Both the outflow vessel and the anastomosis should be examined.[11] The examination is best accomplished by passing the angioscope through the entire course of the graft and as far as possible into the outflow vessel; the scope is then slowly withdrawn while each part of the bypass is examined. The use of a high-flow crystalloid infusion allows excellent assessment of the conduit and native vessel distal to the anastomosis.

A logical further application of angioscopy in the assessment of an infrainguinal bypass is for identifying and confirming the immediate destruction of venous valves in an in situ vein conduit. In this method, the saphenous vein is exposed at the groin and the angioscope is introduced through the cut end of the saphenous vein or through a large branch. The vein is then distended with irrigating solution, and as a valve is approached, it is cut under direct vision using a flexible valvulotome introduced through the distal end of the saphenous vein. Besides making possible a precise valve incision, the angioscope can be used to identify side branches, sites of which can be marked on the skin for later clipping or division. In these cases, angioscopy is used for therapeutic rather than diagnostic purposes, and data are accumulating in support of its effectiveness in this setting.

The chief disadvantage of angioscopy is its potential for damaging the intima of a vein graft or native vessel. Care must be taken not to force the angioscope against the wall or to use an angioscope that is too large. Most often, the 1.4-mm angioscope is used for the evaluation of an in situ saphenous vein and for identification of valves before cutting. This system is expensive and fragile and requires dedicated personnel to maintain the angioscope and ensure that the fiberoptic bundles are not broken. There is a learning curve in the performance of angioscopy that embraces use of the equipment, avoidance of complications, and use of the information acquired. For instance, numerous abnormalities are seen, many of which are not clinically important, and a substantial amount of time is needed to decide which technical problems require attention. Most angio-

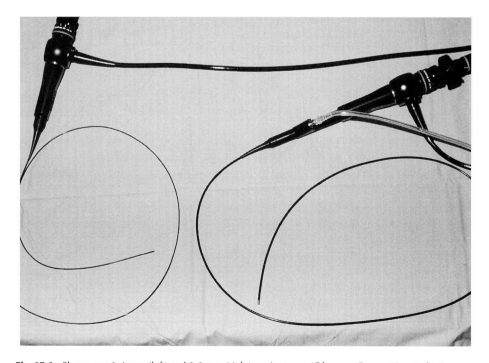

Fig. 67-3. Shown are 1.4 mm *(left)* and 2.8 mm *(right)* angioscopes (Olympus Corporation, Lake Success, NY). Note that the larger angioscope has an indwelling port for infusion of the crystalloid.

scopes can only be passed a short distance beyond the distal anastomosis, and therefore the information obtained about the more distal native vessel outflow is quite limited. Finally, the operator must be cautious about the volume of irrigating solution infused and keep the anesthesiologist fully informed of this. Approximately 500 ml of fluid is used during the preparation of an in situ vein graft as a bypass conduit.

B-MODE IMAGING

High-resolution B-mode imaging has also been used as a completion examination. The experimental basis for this technique was developed by Coelho et al,[3,4] who showed that the imaging of exposed vessels in experimental animals could be performed with the same sensitive resolution potential of high-frequency scanners. Their findings suggested that flaps as small as 1 mm could be identified in exposed vessels and that this technique was much more sensitive than intraoperative arteriography in the detection of vascular thrombi and reduction in vessel diameter.

Transducer frequencies of 7.5 to 10 MHz are required, and transducer probe design has been the limiting factor in making this examination easily applicable. Many of the early probes were bulky and difficult to position over the exposed vessel because of anatomic constraints. Recently, much smaller probes with custom-designed angles and shapes have been developed, which makes the application of this technique more feasible. Acoustic coupling is achieved by flooding the operative field with saline and holding the probe just above the vessel. Because the distal anastomoses are small, they are difficult to evaluate by ultrasound alone, and arteriography may be required in conjunction with real-time B-mode imaging. On the other hand, B-mode imaging allows the vessel to be interrogated from multiple directions, and this yields three-dimensional information that cannot be obtained with arteriography.

COMPARISON OF TECHNIQUES

The three techniques described in this chapter all provide useful anatomic information. Arteriography provides data in one plane, but use of a C-arm digital subtraction unit yields several views. This is also the case with real-time B-mode imaging in which it is possible to move the probe around the vessel and characterize defects from different angles. Angioscopy provides a three-dimensional view from the interior of the vessel and furnishes the most direct view of potential technical defects. Each of these three techniques is somewhat different, and studies that compare them are few. Thus whether ultrasound or angioscopy will replace intraoperative arteriography or whether they are complementary is still uncertain.

Arteriography has traditionally been the method used by most surgeons in assessing the results of infrainguinal bypass. Stept et al[13] reviewed arteriograms obtained in 617 cases of femorodistal bypass. Of these, 587 arteriograms were satisfactory and 30 were unsatisfactory. In those patients with satisfactory studies, early graft failure occurred

in 57, but only 6 cases were due to a technical defect. Likewise, of the 30 unsatisfactory arteriograms (4.9% of the total), graft failure developed in 16 cases because of a technical problem. These data yield a specificity of 90% for arteriography but a rather low sensitivity of 76%. Consequently, when the arteriogram is normal, it is highly unlikely the graft will fail for technical reasons.

Miller et al[9,10] studied 259 infrainguinal bypass grafts using angioscopy alone and noted that 124 clinical or surgical decisions were based on the findings. Valve destruction in this group of patients was not guided by angioscopy, and the angioscope was used only for completion assessment of the technical results. There was a high rate of technical defects (47%) found, and defects included residual competent valve leaflets, unligated tributaries, inadequate graft tunneling, and graft torsion. In addition, narrowed fibrotic vein segments that required resection and a small percentage of distal anastomotic problems were recognized.

In a series of 20 in situ infrainguinal bypasses, Gilbertson et al[6] evaluated the results of operation by randomly using arteriography, duplex scanning, or angioscopy to search for residual uncut valve cusps, unligated vein side branches, and distal anastomotic stenoses with greater than 30% diameter reduction. In none of these cases was angioscopy used to guide the valve cutting process. Angioscopy proved 100% sensitive in diagnosing uncut valve leaflets, whereas angiography showed only a 22% sensitivity. In this study, a total of 63 critical graft defects were suggested in the 20 grafts, and 41 were confirmed by direct inspection.

In a comparison of the angioscopy and arteriography carried out in 66 patients, Flinn et al[5] encountered 13 (19%) abnormal arteriograms that were confirmed by angioscopy in 10 cases. A total of 53 patients had normal completion arteriograms, but major abnormalities were subsequently discovered by angioscopy in 3. This yields a sensitivity of 94% and a specificity of 77% for angioscopy when compared with arteriography. Only 15 of these patients had an in situ bypass, however, which may explain the lower overall incidence of abnormal findings in the completion study.

When angioscopy is used to direct the incision of venous valves and identify side branches, the number of technical imperfections subsequently discovered during intraoperative assessment is much less. Mehigan et al[8] studied 55 patients, all of whom also had postoperative arteriograms; angioscopy had been used to guide valve cutting and assess the technical result of operation in these patients. A retained valve leaflet was found in 1 patient and three residual branch lesions were found in 2 patients. There was a 30-day patency rate of 98%. Similar results were reported by Pearce et al.[12]

Less experience has been reported with real-time B-mode imaging for the intraoperative assessment of infrainguinal bypasses. Machi et al[7] studied 218 patients with B-mode ultrasound as a completion assessment alternative and compared these findings with those obtained by intraoperative arteriography. They found B-mode imaging had a high sensitivity and specificity, with an overall accuracy of 97%

compared to arteriography. On the other hand, because B-mode imaging identified anastomotic areas only with difficulty, completion arteriograms were regularly obtained.

CONCLUSION

Most investigators agree that the intraoperative assessment of the technical results of an infrainguinal bypass is essential. Although arteriography has been the most commonly used technique for this purpose, its sensitivity is low. Angioscopy is more sensitive, particularly for identifying persistent valve cusps and side branches. B-mode imaging, which exhibits both high sensitivity and specificity, is not as good for evaluating anastomotic areas and continues to be cumbersome to perform in the operating room.

Studies to date have not generated sufficient findings to allow a recommendation regarding the routine use of angioscopy by surgeons who have excellent results with arteriography, which is highly specific but less sensitive. It may be that angioscopy will evolve as the best technique for directing valve destruction, but this is a therapeutic rather than an intraoperative diagnostic application. Clearly, more investigation is needed before firm conclusions can be reached as to which modality is most valuable in assessing the technical result of peripheral arterial operations.

REFERENCES

1. Blaisdell FW, Lim R Jr, Hall AD: Technical result of carotid endarterectomy: arteriographic assessment, *Am J Surg* 114:239, 1967.
2. Bowald S, Eriksson E, Faberberg S: Intraoperative angiography in arterial surgery, *Acta Chir Scand* 144:463, 1978.
3. Coelho JCU et al: Detection of arterial defects by real-time ultrasound scanning during vascular surgery: an experimental study, *J Surg Res* 30:535, 1981.
4. Coelho JCU et al: An experimental evaluation of arteriography and imaging ultrasonography in detecting arterial defects at operation, *J Surg Res* 32:130, 1982.
5. Flinn WR et al: *A comparative study of angioscopy and completion arteriography after infrainguinal bypass.* In Yao JST, Pearce WH, eds: *Technologies in vascular surgery,* Philadelphia, 1992, Saunders.
6. Gilbertson JJ et al: A blinded comparison of angiography, angioscopy and duplex scanning in intraoperative evaluation of in situ saphenous vein bypass grafts, *J Vasc Surg* 15:121, 1992.
7. Machi J, Sigel B, Roberts AB: *Intraoperative use of B-mode and color Doppler imaging.* In Yao JST, Pearce WH, eds: *Technologies in vascular surgery,* Philadelphia, 1992, Saunders.
8. Mehigan JT, Schell WW: *Angioscopic control of in situ saphenous vein arterial bypass.* In Moore WS, Ahn SS, eds: *Endovascular surgery,* Philadelphia, 1989, Saunders.
9. Miller A et al: Routine intraoperative angioscopy in lower extremity revascularization, *Arch Surg* 124:604, 1989.
10. Miller A, et al: Continued experience with intraoperative angioscopy for monitoring infrainguinal bypass grafting, *Surgery* 109:286, 1991.
11. Olcott C: *Angioscopic inspection of an anastomosis: indications and technique.* In Moore WS, Ahn SS, eds: *Endovascular surgery,* Philadelphia, 1989, Saunders.
12. Pearce WH et al: *The use of angioscopy in the saphenous vein bypass graft.* In Yao JST, Pearce WH, eds: *Technologies in vascular surgery,* Philadelphia, 1992, Saunders.
13. Stept LL et al: Technical defects as a cause of early graft failure after femorodistal bypass, *Arch Surg* 122:599, 1987.
14. Vollmar JF, Junghanns K: Die Arterioskopie, eine neue Moglichkeit der intraoperativen Erfolgsbeurteilung bei rekonstrukiven Gefasseingriffen (Farbfilm), *Langenbecks Arch Klin Chir* 325:1201, 1969.

CHAPTER 68

Alternative approaches to postoperative surveillance in peripheral bypass

ANDREW N. NICOLAIDES and PETER TAYLOR

There are three main reasons for femorodistal graft failure: (1) thrombosis during the first postoperative month, which is due to either errors in judgment or surgical technique; (2) the development of stenoses within the conduit or adjacent to the anastomoses producing thrombosis from 1 month to 1 year postoperatively; and (3) progression of the underlying atheromatous disease after the first year.[5,6,9] The reported results of salvage procedures undertaken to treat graft thrombosis are markedly inferior to those obtained when the procedure is performed with the graft still patent.[2,10] It is therefore necessary to identify grafts that are hemodynamically compromised before thrombosis occurs.

A Doppler-derived peak systolic velocity of less than 45 cm/sec within the graft has been advocated as the criterion for identifying grafts at risk for occlusion (see Chapter 66). However, the peak systolic velocity does not always reveal the existence of a severe stenosis (e.g., in a hypertensive patient), and this variable will differ with changes in cardiac output and peripheral resistance. Another method, which uses duplex scanning, consists of detecting localized changes in velocity at a point of narrowing in the graft. If V1 denotes the velocity in a nonstenosed part of the graft within 2 cm of the stenosed V2 locality, a velocity ratio (V2/V1) of 2.0 or greater indicates a stenosis causing a greater than 50% reduction in diameter. This method can detect all angiographically demonstrable graft stenoses.[3,4] However, the changes in velocity (V2/V1 ratio) in the graft would not be expected to detect stenoses in the native arteries either proximal or distal to the graft, even though these may also result in graft thrombosis.

The V2/V1 ratio method is time consuming because it requires sampling of the Doppler velocity along the whole length of the graft. However, the use of color flow imaging can speed up the examination. Color flow imaging provides a road map for accurate and quick positioning of the sample volume to record peak velocity.

The aim of this chapter is to demonstrate how the sensitivity, specificity, and speed of duplex scanning for detecting stenotic graft lesions can be improved using color flow imaging in conjunction with the application of the following two criteria: peak systolic velocity less than 45 cm/sec and a V2/V1 ratio equal to or greater than 2.

PATIENTS AND METHODS

A total of 74 consecutive patients with either femoropopliteal or more distal vein grafts were prospectively studied at 6 weeks and at 3, 6, 9, and 12 months by intravenous digital subtraction angiography (IVDSA) and color flow imaging. The peak systolic velocity was measured at 2-cm intervals along the whole length of the graft. The color flow image was used as a road map for positioning the sample volume in the axial stream. Stenoses were identified by the finding of a local increase in peak systolic velocity in the graft. The IVDSA was independently interpreted by radiologists who looked for stenoses both in the graft and in the proximal and distal native arteries. Although many centers consider IVDSA to lack in quality, only 5% of IVDSA investigations need to be repeated and only 1% to 2% require an intraarterial injection of contrast material. No attempt was made to identify stenoses distal to the graft based on localized increases in velocity, and the technique described here was used for both femoropopliteal and femorocrural grafts.

RESULTS

IV-DSA detected stenoses (greater than 50% reduction in diameter) in 19 grafts (26%); 4 patients were also found to have stenoses in the native vessel beyond the distal anastomosis. No stenoses were detected in the proximal native artery. The V2/V1 ratio was greater than 2.0 in 19 (83%) of the 23 limbs with stenosis (Table 68-1). It detected all stenoses in the grafts but not the 4 in the distal native artery. The peak systolic velocity was less than 45 cm/sec in 14 (61%) of the 23 limbs with a stenosis. It detected all 4 stenoses in the distal native artery but not 9 of the stenoses in the graft itself (Table 68-2).

By combining the two criteria (peak systolic velocity of less than 45 cm/sec and a V2/V1 ratio of at least 2.0), the sensitivity for detecting a stenosis, irrespective of whether it was in the graft or the native artery, increased to 100%,

Table 68-1. V2/V1 ratio determined by color flow imaging related to angiographically detected stenoses*

	No stenosis (V2/V1 < 2.0)	Stenosis (V2/V1 ≥ 2.0)	Total
No angiographic stenosis	51	0	51
Angiographic stenosis†	4	19	23
TOTAL	55	19	74

*Sensitivity, 83%; specificity, 100%.
†Stenosis, >50% reduction in lumen diameter in distal native artery.

Table 68-2. Peak systolic velocity detected by color flow imaging related to angiographically detected stenoses*

	Peak systolic velocity		
	≥45 cm/sec	<45 cm/sec	Total
No angiographic stenosis	50	1	51
Angiographic stenosis†	9‡	14	23
TOTAL	59	15	74

*Sensitivity, 61%; specificity, 98%.
†Stenosis, >50% reduction in lumen diameter in distal native artery.
‡All were in the graft itself.

Table 68-3. Both V2/V1 ratio and peak systolic velocity related to angiographically detected stenoses*

	Combined criteria		
	V2/V2 <2.0 and peak velocity ≥45 cm/sec	V2/V1 ≥2.0 and/or peak velocity <45 cm/sec	Total
No angiographic stenosis	50	1†	51
Angiographic stenosis‡	0	23	23
TOTAL	50	24	74

*Sensitivity, 100%; specificity, 98%.
†V2/V1 = 1; peak velocity = 30 cm/sec (see Fig. 68-1).
‡Stenosis, >50% reduction in lumen diameter in distal native artery.

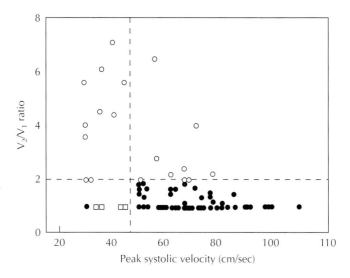

Fig. 68-1. V2/V1 ratio plotted against peak systolic velocity, showing the distribution of the points representing graft stenosis. ●, No stenosis; ○, graft stenosis; □, native artery stenosis.

DISCUSSION

In this series, the incidence of stenosis as detected by IVDSA was 26%, and this is similar to that reported by others. This confirms the view that stenoses, a correctable cause of graft failure within the first 2 years after operation, are common. Previously reported findings have shown that duplex-derived measurements of localized changes in peak systolic velocity (V2/V1 ratio) within a graft are indicative of a stenosis.[3,7,11] Furthermore, there has been a good correlation between the V2/V1 ratio and the degree of stenosis shown by IVDSA. Some authors have suggested that grafts at risk of occlusion can be identified by the finding of an average blood flow velocity of less than 45 cm/sec.[1] If this criterion alone had been used in this study, 9 graft stenoses would have been missed. If the V2/V1 ratio alone had been used, all stenoses within the graft would have been predicted but stenoses in the native artery distal to the graft would have been missed in 4 patients.

The results confirm that color flow imaging used in conjunction with average peak velocity and V2/V1 criteria can accurately indicate the presence or absence of stenoses in both the graft and native vessels. In addition, a number of other practical points have emerged. Color flow imaging is useful in assessing difficult areas such as the region of the knee, where the depth and direction of the graft can make identification difficult using conventional duplex scanning. Using the color flow image as a road map, the graft can be followed to the site of the anastomosis. Areas of stenosis are particularly well seen with color flow imaging since turbulence caused by the disturbance in flow is readily identified by a mixed-color pattern. After the rapid localization of a stenosis by color flow imaging, conventional measurements of peak systolic velocity permit an objective assessment of the degree of stenosis. This represents an advantage

which was at the expense of a slightly lower specificity (98%) (Table 68-3).

The results of the combined criteria are shown in Fig. 68-1, in which the V2/V1 ratio was plotted against the average peak systolic blood flow velocity. A total of 19 grafts had V2/V1 ratios greater than 2.0. Of these, 10 had a peak velocity less than 45 cm/sec and 9 had a velocity of more than 45 cm/sec or more; 55 grafts had no evidence of stenosis based on the V2/V1 ratio, but 5 of these had a peak velocity less than 45 cm/sec. The mean time required for scanning a graft with color flow imaging was 14 minutes (range, 10 to 24 minutes).

over conventional duplex scanning, which requires the measurement of velocity throughout the length of the graft.

The results suggest that if both criteria (V2/V1 ratio equal to or greater than 2.0 and peak velocity less than 45 cm/sec) are used to select patients for angiography, all stenotic lesions that may lead to graft occlusion can be identified.[8] The combination of both criteria can also be applied in the setting of conventional duplex scanning, but color flow imaging adds speed without sacrificing accuracy.

REFERENCES

1. Bandyk DF, Cato RF, Towne JB: A low flow velocity predicts failure of femoropopliteal and femorotibial bypass grafts, *Surgery* 98:799, 1985.
2. Cohen JR et al: Recognition and management of impending vein-graft failure, *Arch Surg* 121:758, 1986.
3. Grigg MJ, Nicolaides AN, Wolfe JHN: Femorodistal vein bypass graft stenoses, *Br J Surg* 75:737, 1988.
4. Grigg MJ, Nicolaides AN, Wolfe JHN: Detection and grading of femorodistal vein graft stenoses: duplex velocity measurements compared with angiography, *J Vasc Surg* 8:661, 1988.
5. Harris PL, Jones D, How T: A prospective randomised clinical trial to compare in situ and reversed vein grafts for femoropopliteal bypass, *Br J Surg* 74:252, 1987.
6. Rutherford RB et al: Factors affecting the patency of infrainguinal bypass, *J Vasc Surg* 8:236, 1988.
7. Taylor PR et al: Graft stenosis: justification for 1-year surveillance, *Br J Surg* 77:1125, 1990.
8. Taylor PR et al: Colour flow imaging in the detection of femorodistal graft and native artery stenosis: improved criteria, *Eur J Vasc Surg* 6:232, 1992.
9. Veith FJ et al: Six-year prospective multicentre randomized comparison of autologous saphenous vein and expanded polytetrafluoroethylene grafts in infrainguinal arterial reconstructions, *J Vasc Surg* 3:104, 1986.
10. Whittemore AD et al: Secondary femoropopliteal reconstruction, *Ann Surg* 193:35, 1981.
11. Wolfe JHN et al: Early diagnosis of femorodistal graft stenoses, *Br J Surg* 74:268, 1987.

CHAPTER 69

How much postoperative screening is appropriate after arterial reconstruction?

ROBERT W. BARNES

During the past decade, noninvasive techniques have been applied increasingly in the surveillance of infrainguinal bypass grafts in the early and late postoperative period. The objectives of such monitoring include documentation of the hemodynamic success of operation, early identification of atherosclerotic disease progression, and evaluation of patients with recurrent symptoms of vascular disease. Most important, however, has been the ability of noninvasive surveillance to detect technical or degenerative defects in the bypass graft or its anastomoses, often before symptoms develop. Most investigators believe that prophylactic correction of these asymptomatic lesions reduces the risk of subsequent graft thrombosis and leads to improved secondary patency rates of bypass grafts. Recently, this concept has been challenged.[2] This chapter reviews the published data addressing the role of postoperative surveillance of infrainguinal arterial reconstruction for identifying stenotic lesions implicated in the setting of failing bypass grafts.

PATIENTS AND METHODS

Between January 1981 and December 1991, 48 papers were published on the topic of postoperative surveillance of femoropopliteal or femorotibial bypass using prosthetic or vein grafts. In 21 of these publications, a separate series of patients was reported, which avoided duplication of data and outcomes.[1-21] The design of the study was prospective in 14 reports* and retrospective in 7.† Infrainguinal bypasses were surveyed in 3165 extremities of 3068 patients. Femoropopliteal bypasses constituted 60% of the procedures, and the remainder were femorotibial reconstructions. The principal method of graft surveillance in 7 studies was the ankle–brachial pressure index (ABI),[2-5,7,16,20] duplex scanning (real-time B-mode ultrasonic imaging/Doppler) was used in 10 studies,[1,6,8-14,17] and digital or conventional arteriography was used in 4 investigations.[15,18,19,21]

*References 1, 4, 6-9, 11, 13-15, 17-19, 21.
†References 2, 3, 5, 10, 12, 16, 20.

RESULTS

Incidence of lesions

The incidence of postoperative stenosis detectable by the surveillance protocol was reported in 18 of the 21 studies.[1,2,4-15,17-19,21] Stenosis was detected in 650 (21.6%) of the 3003 extremities undergoing infrainguinal bypass. These lesions were located in the graft or its anastomoses in 519 extremities and in the native artery in 131 limbs, which consisted of arterial inflow in 77 and outflow in 54 extremities. The high proportion of stenoses detected in the graft or its anastomoses may be a reflection of the surveillance protocol that was designed to study the bypass graft instead of the native circulation.

Incidence by surveillance technique

The method of postoperative graft surveillance was found to influence the ultimate incidence of stenoses detected. Lesions were identified in 226 (18.8%) of 1200 extremities assessed by ABI.[2,4,5,7] Stenoses were detected in 341 (22.9%) of 1491 limbs evaluated by duplex scanning.[1,6,8-14,17] Significant (greater than 50% diameter reduction) stenoses were visualized in 83 (26.6%) of 312 extremities that underwent routine postoperative arteriography.[15,18,19,21]

Incidence by vein graft technique

In 10 studies, the influence of the technique of vein bypass grafting on the incidence of postoperative stenosis could be determined.* Postoperative stenosis was detected in 186 (22.8%) of 816 extremities that underwent in situ vein bypass grafts. Stenosis occurred in 218 (17.3%) of 1261 limbs undergoing bypass with reversed veins.

Management of detected lesions

The indications for intervention when stenoses were detected during postoperative surveillance differed among the published series. Routine prophylactic repair, regardless of

*References 2, 5-9, 11, 12, 14, 15.

the presence or absence of symptoms, was the practice in 18 of the 21 reports.[1,3-9,11-14,16-21] Therapeutic intervention, either radiologic or surgical, was reserved for the treatment of recurrent disabling claudication or limb-threatening ischemia in only 3 studies.[2,10,15]

Cumulative graft patency

Despite the importance of reporting surgical results using life-table methods, only 7 (33%) of the 21 studies[1,2,5,8-11] presented data about cumulative graft patency (Table 69-1). Of these, cumulative patency rates for a follow-up period of greater than 2 years were furnished in only 4 publications.[1,2,5,10] The primary graft patency in these 4 studies varied between 60% and 66%, and the secondary patency rates, after prophylactic or therapeutic intervention for detected stenoses, ranged between 72% and 85%. The secondary graft patency of 80% cited in the study of Green et al,[10] in which intervention was reserved for patients with recurrent symptoms or signs of limb ischemia, did not significantly differ from the secondary patency rates (72% and 85%) in the two studies[1,5] in which routine prophylactic intervention was carried out for all detected graft stenoses.

Cumulative limb salvage

Only two reports[2,8] cited data about cumulative limb salvage. The limb salvage rate (80% at 2 years) in the one study[8] employing routine prophylactic repair of postoperative graft stenoses was similar to the limb salvage rate (82% at 5 years) observed in the study[2] consisting of patients who did not undergo prophylactic repair of such lesions.

Cumulative patient survival

Two studies[1,2] provided data about cumulative patient survival. Once again, the survival rate was similar both for the series of patients undergoing routine prophylactic repair of lesions detected postoperatively[1] (65% at 4 years) and for patients[2] in whom prophylactic repair was not the practice (63% survival at 5 years).

Mean follow-up

The average period of patient follow-up was stated in six studies* and ranged between 12 and 24 months. The total duration of patient follow-up ranged between 2 and 180 months.

DISCUSSION

The reported primary patency rates for infrainguinal bypass grafts vary between 60% and 70% at 5 years. The secondary cumulative graft patency after intervention because of thrombosis or detected stenosis ranges between 70% and 85% at 5 years. The success of such secondary intervention is acknowledged to be much better if carried out before graft thrombosis occurs. For this reason, the majority of vascular surgeons recommend the use of serial postoperative graft

---

*References 2, 4, 9, 11, 14, 19.

Table 69-1. Cumulative graft patency

Author	Year	No. of limbs	Primary patency (%)	Secondary patency (%)	Maximum follow-up (yr)
Cullen et al[8]	1986	49	69	80	2
Grigg et al[11]	1988	75	78	85	1
Bandyk et al[1]	1989	250	62	85	4
Barnes et al[2]	1989	232	60	—	5
Berkowitz et al[5]	1989	521	62	72	5
Disselhoff et al[9]	1989	77	63	79	2
Green et al[0]	1990	177	66	80	5

surveillance, usually with noninvasive techniques, to detect hemodynamically significant stenoses that threaten graft patency. Most surgeons recommend prophylactic intervention using either radiologic or surgical methods to eliminate such lesions that allegedly contribute to failing grafts, even if they are not responsible for recurrent symptoms. The resultant improved secondary graft patency is assumed to justify this practice.

Unfortunately, such an aggressive approach to postoperative graft or host vessel stenoses discovered by a routine surveillance protocol has limited the understanding of the natural history of these lesions. To date, there has not been a randomized clinical trial to validate the practice of routine prophylactic repair for detected stenoses to prevent early or late postoperative graft thrombosis.

A report in 1989[2] was the first to suggest that patients who manifested a significant drop in their ABI after infrainguinal bypass were at no greater risk of graft failure than those whose ABI remained stable throughout the postoperative period. Of significance was the fact that no patient underwent prophylactic intervention merely on the basis of a deteriorating ABI. In a retrospective case-control study, the outcomes in 232 patients undergoing femoropopliteal or femorotibial bypass were reviewed over a 5-year period. A significant postoperative drop in ABI was defined as a sustained decrement of 0.20 or greater below the maximum value recorded after operation, but to a value no lower than 0.20 or more above the preoperative index. The 40 patients who manifested such hemodynamic signs of failing grafts had a cumulative 5-year graft patency rate of 62%, which was essentially the same as the 60% 5-year patency seen in the 192 patients who had a stable ABI throughout the postoperative period. This study was criticized for using ABI as the method of postoperative graft surveillance because it is admittedly a less sensitive method than duplex scanning, which is currently employed by most laboratories. However, the rationale for using a more sensitive technique is unclear if there is no significant difference in graft outcomes in patients screened by ABI. A recognized limitation of ABI is its inability to distinguish between a graft and native arterial obstruction as the cause of an abnormal index. Both ABI and duplex scanning are currently being used for the postoperative surveillance of patients with infrainguinal bypass grafts, and intervention is limited to those patients with detected lesions who exhibit recurrence of disabling claudication or limb-threatening ischemia. The patient sample is too small to draw any definitive conclusions from, but to date adverse patient outcomes that would justify a change in this therapeutic policy have not been observed.

Green et al[10] reported their findings in a prospective study of 177 patients monitored by both ABI and duplex scanning after infrainguinal bypass grafting. The incidence of hemodynamically significant graft stenosis detected after operation was 30% for duplex scanning and 15% for ABI. Most important in this study was the fact that therapeutic intervention was instituted only in patients when graft thrombosis or recurrent disabling symptoms developed. The 5-year cumulative primary and secondary graft patency rates, 66% and 80%, respectively, were similar to those reported in the other 5 studies in which prophylactic repair of the identified stenoses was the standard practice.[1,5,8,9,11]

CONCLUSION

This overview of publications addressing the role of postoperative graft surveillance after infrainguinal bypass allows several conclusions to be drawn based on the experience of the past decade. First, noninvasive diagnostic techniques are assuming an increasingly important role in documenting the success of treatment in peripheral vascular disease. Second, such routine postoperative hemodynamic monitoring identifies a significant incidence (22% in this review) of stenosis in infrainguinal bypass grafts, their anastomoses, or the native inflow or outflow arteries. The incidence of such lesions is higher if more sensitive techniques such as duplex scanning or angiography are used instead of ABI. Third, postoperative stenoses are found with nearly equal frequency in both reversed and in situ vein grafts. In addition, in situ vein grafts may harbor lesions, a problem unique to this popular method of grafting. Namely, these lesions consist of retained competent valve cusps and arteriovenous fistulas, which may compromise graft function. Fourth, most surgeons (85%) consider such lesions to be a threat to longitudinal graft patency and thus prophylactically intervene using radiologic or surgical methods.[1,3-9,11-14,16-21] Fifth, this practice of carrying out routine prophylactic intervention in lesions detected by postoperative graft surveillance limits the understanding of the natural history of these stenoses. Sixth, the few studies limiting therapeutic intervention to those patients with recurrent disabling symptoms report primary and secondary patency rates similar to those cited in studies employing routine prophylactic repair of stenoses detected postoperatively. Finally, there have been no randomized clinical trials documenting the efficacy of prophylactic intervention for asymptomatic stenosis in preventing late graft thrombosis.

The observations gleaned from this overview suggest that noninvasive techniques can detect significant graft or host vessel stenosis in patients who have undergone infrainguinal bypass. Whether such lesions should be repaired prophylactically remains unproven. This therapeutic dilemma is analogous to that attending asymptomatic carotid artery stenosis. The management of this latter lesion will be defined by the ongoing multicenter randomized trials. The most effective approach for treating stenoses in femorodistal bypass grafts will hopefully be similarly resolved.

REFERENCES

1. Bandyk DF et al: Monitoring functional patency of in situ saphenous vein bypasses: the impact of a surveillance protocol and elective revision, *J Vasc Surg* 9:286-296, 1989.
2. Barnes RW et al: Serial noninvasive studies do not herald postoperative failure of femoropopliteal or femorotibial bypass grafts, *Ann Surg* 210:486-493, 1989.
3. Bartlett ST et al: The reoperative potential of infrainguinal bypass: long-term limb and patient survival, *J Vasc Surg* 5:170-179, 1987.
4. Benveniste GL et al: The detection of early femorodistal vein graft stenosis by treadmill exercise testing, *J Cardiovasc Surg* 29:723-726, 1988.
5. Berkowitz HD et al: Late failure of reversed vein bypass grafts, *Ann Surg* 210:782-786, 1989.
6. Chang BB et al: Hemodynamic characteristics of failing infrainguinal in situ vein bypass, *J Vasc Surg* 12:596-600, 1990.
7. Cohen JR et al: Recognition and management of impending vein-graft failure, *Arch Surg* 121:758-759, 1986.
8. Cullen PJ, et al: The influence of duplex scanning on early patency rates of in situ bypass to the tibial vessels, *Ann Vasc Surg* 1:340-346, 1986.
9. Disselhoff B, Buth J, Jakimowicz J: Early detection of stenosis of femorodistal grafts: a surveillance study using colour-duplex scanning, *Eur J Vasc Surg* 3:43-48, 1989.
10. Green RM et al: Comparison of infrainguinal graft surveillance techniques, *J Vasc Surg* 11:207-215, 1990.
11. Grigg MJ, Nicolaides AN, Wolfe JHN: Detection and grading of femorodistal vein graft stenosis: duplex velocity measurements compared with angiography, *J Vasc Surg* 8:661-666, 1988.
12. Killewich LA, Fisher C, Bartlett ST: Surveillance of in situ infrainguinal bypass grafts: conventional vs. color flow duplex ultrasonography, *J Cardiovasc Surg* 31:662-667, 1990.
13. Londrey GL et al: Initial experience with color-flow duplex scanning of infrainguinal bypass grafts, *J Vasc Surg* 12:284-290, 1990.
14. Mills JL et al: The importance of routine surveillance of distal bypass grafts with duplex scanning: a study of 379 reversed vein grafts, *J Vasc Surg* 12:379-389, 1990.
15. Moody P et al: Asymptomatic strictures in femoro-popliteal vein grafts, *Eur Vasc Surg* 3:389-392, 1989.
16. Perler BA et al: Balloon dilatation versus surgical revision of infrainguinal autogenous vein graft stenoses: long term follow-up, *J Cardiovasc Surg* 31:656-661, 1990.
17. Robison JG, Elliott BM: Does postoperative surveillance with duplex scanning identify the failing distal bypass?, *Ann Vasc Surg* 5:182-185, 1991.
18. Sladen JG et al: Color flow duplex screening of infrainguinal grafts combining low- and high-velocity criteria, *Am J Surg* 158:107-112, 1989.
19. Turnipseed WD, Acher CW: Postoperative surveillance: an effective means of detecting correctable lesions that threaten graft patency, *Arch Surg* 120:324-328, 1985.
20. Veith FJ et al: Diagnosis and management of failing lower extremity arterial reconstructions prior to graft occlusion, *J Cardiovasc Surg* 25:381-384, 1984.
21. Wolfe JHN et al: Early diagnosis of femorodistal graft stenoses, *Br J Surg* 74:268-270, 1987.

CHAPTER 70

Duplex scanning of hemodialysis access operations

JAN H. M. TORDOIR

Vascular access for hemodialysis is usually achieved by creating an arteriovenous (AV) anastomosis between any adequate artery and vein in the upper extremity. The resulting low peripheral venous resistance and the large pressure drop over the AV anastomosis result in acceleration of blood flow velocity, an increase in blood flow volume, and a subsequent dilatation of the forearm veins that then become accessible for puncture.

Most clinical symptoms and signs of AV fistulas are attributable to a low-resistance leak that forms between the high arterial and low venous pressures of the circulation. Hemodynamic alterations can cause general or local circulatory changes, such as distal ischemia and venous hypertension. Depending on the amount of flow volume in the fistula and the type of fistula, systemic effects such as high-output cardiac failure can also develop. Because of local high velocities at the site of the anastomoses, intimal hyperplasia can often cause significant stenoses. These stenoses may jeopardize fistula flow with subsequent thrombotic occlusion. This is the most common source of failure and is responsible in 30% to 50% of cases, including all types of AV fistulas. In addition, the frequently performed punctures can spawn infection, pseudoaneurysm formation, and hematoma.

Correct diagnosis and treatment of hemodialysis access complications may therefore contribute to better durability and patency of these AV fistulas. Besides invasive angiographic techniques, several noninvasive diagnostic methods that can be used for this purpose have been developed in recent years.[14,16,18] This chapter summarizes the applicability of duplex ultrasound scanning for evaluating the results of hemodialysis access operations.

DUPLEX SCANNING FOR THE DIAGNOSIS OF AV FISTULA STENOSES

Duplex ultrasound scanning has recently been introduced for the evaluation of hemodialysis access operations.[6,10,20,23] The duplex approach combines two methods: B-mode sonography and pulsed Doppler examination. In this technique, arteries and veins are detected by B-mode sonography, and then each vascular segment with a known sample volume size and angle of insonation undergoes Doppler spectrum analysis. The low venous resistance and high flow in AV fistulas result in increased systolic and end-diastolic velocities as well as turbulence that produces spectral broadening. Stenotic lesions further elevate blood flow velocity with marked turbulence occurring beyond the stenosis. These changes can be characterized by Doppler scanning (Fig. 70-1).

Technique of duplex scanning

Duplex scanning is performed with the patient in the supine position before dialysis is done. Doppler signals are obtained by a handheld probe incorporating a 5-MHz pulsed Doppler system combined with a 10-MHz B-mode imager. B-mode vessel imaging is carried out from the distal brachial artery to the artery-to-graft anastomosis in graft interposition fistulas or to the AV anastomosis in Brescia-Cimino (BC) fistulas. For graft fistulas, the arterial anastomosis, graft, venous anastomosis, and efferent vein are all examined. For BC fistulas, a selective insonation and spectral analysis of proximal and distal arterial and venous segments are obtained (Fig. 70-2). After this, the efferent vein is screened from the forearm to the shoulder.

Vascular segments

For the purpose of comparing the Doppler spectra with angiographic data in the different types of AV fistulas, a number of specific segments are defined: the anastomotic segments in BC fistulas, the anastomoses and graft itself in the graft fistulas, and the efferent vein in both BC and graft fistulas (Fig. 70-3).

Quantification of Doppler spectra

Doppler spectral analysis is carried out for each segment with measurement of peak systolic and end-diastolic velocities, and the resistance index is calculated according to the following formula:

$$RI = 1 - \frac{EDV}{PSV}$$

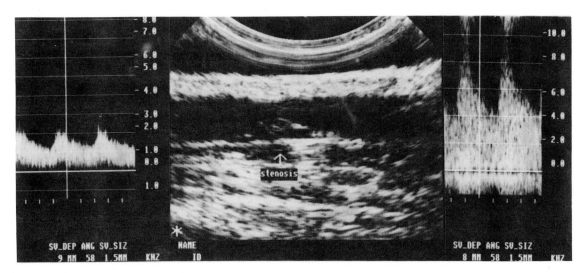

Fig. 70-1. B-mode image and Doppler spectral analysis of a significant stenosis in the efferent vein. Notice the increased velocities in the stenosis *(right)* and normal velocities *(left)* just before the stenosis.

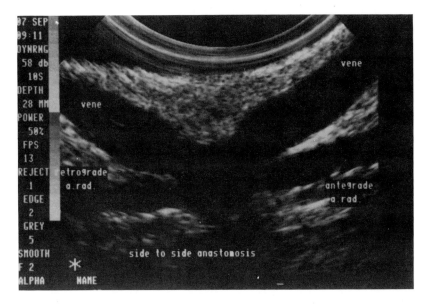

Fig. 70-2. B-mode image of a side-to-side AV anastomosis between the radial artery and cephalic vein at the wrist; the proximal and distal vessels are clearly visible.

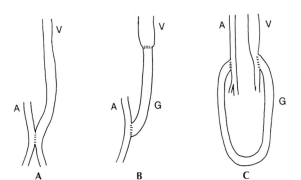

Fig. 70-3. The different types of AV fistulas for hemodialysis. *A,* Brescia/Cimino fistula. *B,* Straight graft interposition. *C,* Loop graft interposition. *A,* Afferent artery; *G,* graft interposition; *V,* efferent vein.

Accuracy of duplex scanning

Peak systolic and end-diastolic velocities are significantly higher in stenotic segments (50% or more diameter reduction) of BC and graft AV fistulas and in the efferent vein area, compared to the velocities in nonstenotic segments (Table 70-1). The best criterion for the diagnosis of stenosis appears to be the peak systolic velocity (Fig. 70-4). With a cutoff value of 375 cm/sec, the accuracy of duplex scanning for the detection of stenoses in BC fistulas is 81%, with a sensitivity of 79% and a specificity of 84%. For graft AV fistulas, its accuracy is 86%, with a cutoff value of 310

cm/sec. Duplex scanning can identify efferent vein stenoses and shows an accuracy of 96%. The end-diastolic velocity and resistance index are of no additional value for determining the degree of stenosis.

The best results yielded by duplex scanning for the detection of stenoses of 50% or more diameter reduction are obtained in graft AV fistulas and in the efferent vein area (Table 70-2). The detection of stenoses at the AV anastomosis of BC fistulas is less accurate. Difficulties in the recognition of fistula anatomy and the high velocities in the anastomosis itself may account for these relatively poor results. Further experience with duplex scanning and the application of color-coded Doppler systems may improve the diagnostic accuracy of the noninvasive assessment of hemodialysis AV fistulas.

THE VALUE OF DUPLEX SCANNING FOR THE PREDICTION OF COMPLICATIONS IN HEMODIALYSIS ACCESS FISTULAS

The detection of AV fistulas at risk for the development of complications may be of great value. Early diagnosis of a complication, followed by surgical or radiologic intervention, may preserve the access site. Usually, clinical symptoms and difficulties with dialysis will point to the existence of stenoses in the afferent arteries or efferent veins. Noninvasive assessment can detect and determine the influences of these stenoses on the development of complications.

In a surveillance study of 90 patients on long-term hemodialysis treatment, AV fistulas were evaluated every 3 months by duplex scanning.[21] The number and location of significant stenoses (50% or more diameter reduction) in the afferent artery, anastomotic vessels, and efferent vein were determined and correlated with the development of thrombotic occlusion, venous hypertension, or ischemia. In addition, brachial artery Doppler spectral analysis was performed with an open and closed fistula circuit. The results showed that the brachial artery peak systolic and end-diastolic velocities, the velocity ratio (peak systolic velocity with open fistula/peak systolic velocity with closed fistula), and the total number of stenoses were significant predictors of thrombotic occlusion ($p < 0.005$). The number of stenoses in the efferent vein was significantly greater ($p < 0.01$) in fistulas that developed venous hypertension (Table 70-3). Stepwise multiple regression analysis showed that brachial artery peak systolic velocity and the number of venous stenoses were the most important independent

Table 70-1. Mean values ($\pm$ SEM) of PSV and EDV for stenotic and nonstenotic segments*

Velocity (cm/sec)	Stenosis	No stenosis	p value
PSV			
BC fistulas	419 ± 17	266 ± 17	<0.001
Graft fistulas	419 ± 15	186 ± 11	<0.001
Efferent vein	375 ± 32	104 ± 5	<0.001
EDV			
BC fistulas	307 ± 17	173 ± 14	<0.001
Graft fistulas	291 ± 21	115 ± 8	<0.001
Efferent vein	243 ± 34	65 ± 4	<0.001

PSV, Peak systolic velocity; *EDV*, end-diastolic velocity; *BC*, Brescia-Cimino.
*Stenosis is defined as a 50% or greater reduction in lumen diameter.

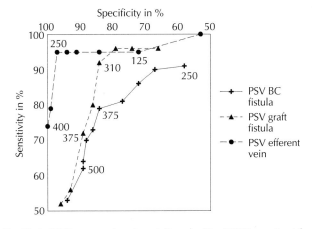

Fig. 70-4. ROC curves of peak systolic velocities (PSV in cm/sec) for the diagnosis of stenoses (≥50%) in BC fistulas, graft fistulas, and the efferent vein.

Table 70-2. Comparative results from duplex scanning

Site	PSV (cm/sec)	Accuracy	Sensitivity	Specificity	PPV	NPV
BC fistulas	375	81%	79%	84%	86%	76%
Graft fistulas	310	86%	92%	84%	66%	97%
Efferent vein	250	96%	95%	97%	82%	99%

PSV, Peak systolic velocity; *PPV*, positive predictive value; *NPV*, negative predictive value; *BC*, Brescia-Cimino.

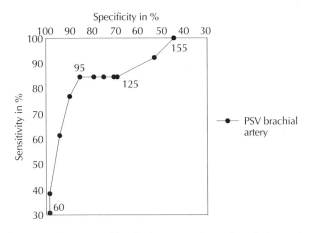

Fig. 70-5. ROC curve of brachial artery peak systolic velocities (PSV in cm/sec) in AV fistulas that developed thrombotic occlusion.

Table 70-3. Duplex scanning data (mean ± SEM) for the various fistulas by complication

| | Complications | | |
Site	None	Thrombosis	Venous hypertension
Brachial artery PSV (cm/sec)	143 ± 6	77 ± 9	158 ± 22
Brachial artery EDV (cm/sec)	71 ± 6	34 ± 9	81 ± 16
Brachial artery PSV ratio	2.32 ± 0.12	1.57 ± 0.17	2.29 ± 0.18
Total number of stenoses	1.38 ± 0.71	2.38 ± 1.12	1.90 ± 0.30
Afferent artery stenoses	0.07 ± 0.02	0.15 ± 0.06	0.10 ± 0.04
Anastomotic stenoses	1.00 ± 0.19	1.69 ± 0.38	0.80 ± 0.20
Efferent vein stenoses	0.31 ± 0.06	0.54 ± 0.18	1.00 ± 0.21

PSV, Peak systolic velocity; *EDV,* end-diastolic velocity.

predictors of complications. Fig. 70-5 shows the receiver-operating characteristic curve for different threshold values of brachial artery peak systolic velocity as a predictor of fistula occlusion. With a cutoff value of 95 cm/sec, the sensitivity and specificity are 85%. Duplex ultrasound scanning therefore has the ability to identify patients at risk for complications and is of value for observing the course of AV fistulas.

HEMODYNAMIC ASSESSMENT OF AV FISTULAS

In the presence of AV fistulas, blood shunting from the arterial into the venous system may produce local or general hemodynamic changes.[8] Arterial insufficiency and venous hypertension of the hand are well-known complications of dialysis fistulas.[14,16,18] These problems can be ascribed to a steal of blood from the hand arteries or to excessive shunting in the AV fistula.[3,19] Patients with diabetes mellitus and

Table 70-4. Grading of steal phenomenon in the distal radial artery versus thumb blood pressure and T/B indices

Blood flow status	No.	Thumb pressure (mm Hg; mean ± SD)	T/B index (mean ± SD)
Antegrade flow	2	169 ± 41	0.77 ± 0.10
Transient steal	4	162 ± 20	0.80 ± 0.06
Permanent steal	36	100 ± 35	0.67 ± 0.22
Occlusion	7	137 ± 49	0.83 ± 0.26

T/B, Thumb/brachial blood pressure.

peripheral arterial disease have a higher risk of hand ischemia.[4] The type of fistula can also be relevant to the development of ischemia.[12]

Various invasive and noninvasive methods have been used to diagnose ischemia (arterial steal phenomenon) and quantify the function of AV fistulas.[2,5,7] Duplex scanning can be performed for the investigation of hemodynamic changes in the upper extremity after the creation of an AV fistula. To assess this application, 59 patients on maintenance hemodialysis were examined noninvasively. A total of 4 had clinical evidence of arterial insufficiency with symptoms of pain, coldness, and discoloration; 5 had diabetes mellitus. The technique of duplex scanning was similar to that described for the diagnosis of stenosis. However, special attention was paid to brachial artery flow and the direction and quantity of flow in the radial artery, distal to the AV anastomosis of BC fistulas. The direction of flow in this artery was described as antegrade or permanent retrograde or as transiently alternating with the heart cycle (Fig. 70-6). The results of duplex scanning were then correlated with the thumb blood pressure measurements. The correlation between flow direction in the distal radial artery and the thumb blood pressure and thumb/brachial blood pressure index (T/B index) is shown in Table 70-4. Patients with a permanent radial steal syndrome showed significantly lower T/B indices compared to patients with a transient steal syndrome. The T/B indices in patients with a permanent steal syndrome were also lower than those in patients with only antegrade flow or radial artery occlusion. However, these differences were not statistically significant.

Fistula function was indirectly evaluated by means of Doppler spectral analysis of the brachial artery in which the peak systolic velocities were determined with and without digital compression of the fistula. Increased brachial artery Doppler velocities correlated with a decrease in the thumb blood pressure and T/B indices. Brachial artery peak systolic velocity ratios correlated significantly with T/B indices (Fig. 70-7). The influences of severe stenoses located in the radial artery proximal and distal to the AV anastomosis and in the efferent vein on digital blood pressures are shown in Table 70-5. No significant differences in T/B indices could be determined between patients with and without proximal or distal radial artery stenoses. In addition, the presence of efferent vein stenoses showed no effect on the thumb blood

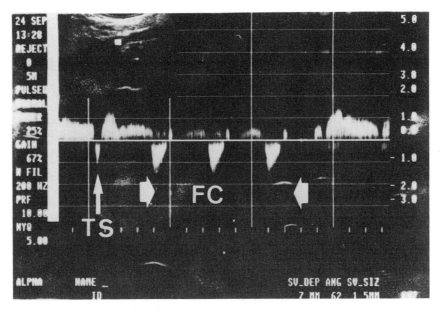

Fig. 70-6. Doppler spectrum from the distal radial artery in a patient with a Brescia/Cimino fistula. A transient steal *(TS)* is present with retrograde flow during systole and antegrade flow at the end of diastole *(small arrow).* Permanent antegrade flow occurs during compression of the fistula *(FC; big arrows).*

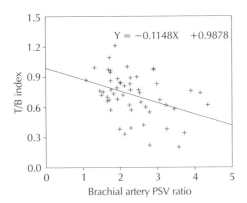

Fig. 70-7. Scattergram of brachial artery peak systolic velocity (PSV) ratios versus T/B indices (r = −0.3926).

Table 70-5. Proximal radial artery stenosis, distal radial artery stenosis, and efferent vein stenosis versus thumb pressure and T/B indices

Site	No.	Thumb pressure (mm Hg; mean ± SD)	T/B index (mean ± SD)
Proximal radial artery			
No stenosis	26	116 ± 49	0.68 ± 0.20
Stenosis	20	112 ± 32	0.71 ± 0.16
Occlusion	3	100 ± 52	0.57 ± 0.27
Distal radial artery			
No stenosis	32	112 ± 41	0.68 ± 0.18
Stenosis	10	99 ± 38	0.64 ± 0.20
Occlusion	7	137 ± 49	0.77 ± 0.22
Efferent vein			
No stenosis	13	111 ± 48	0.65 ± 0.25
Stenosis	30	115 ± 40	0.70 ± 0.17
Occlusion	6	109 ± 49	0.71 ± 0.13

T/B, Thumb/brachial pressure.

pressure. These studies show that duplex scanning seems to be a valuable method for assessing hemodynamic changes in the upper extremity stemming from AV fistulas formed for hemodialysis access.

PREOPERATIVE SCREENING OF THE UPPER EXTREMITY FOR ACCESS SURGERY

About 10% of BC fistulas fail within 1 month of creation.[11,17] Inadequate arteries in diabetic patients or thrombosed veins after previous intravenous infusions are usually the causes for failure. Women are more susceptible to fistula occlusion than men because of their smaller veins. Patients who have undergone access operations that failed may have atherosclerosis or defects in the superficial venous system. Therefore a careful preoperative arterial and venous evaluation is very important and noninvasive methods may eventually replace arteriography and phlebography in this setting.

Duplex scanning can be used for this purpose and involves selective scanning of the arm arteries from the axillary artery down to the radial and ulnar arteries at the wrist. A special standoff device is used for obtaining good-quality images (Fig. 70-8). Doppler spectral analysis is

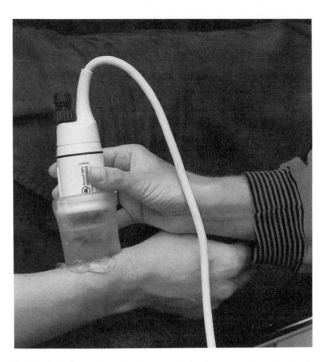

Fig. 70-8. Preoperative duplex scan of the forearm veins. Notice the special stand-off device.

Table 70-6. Results of duplex scanning of the upper extremity arteries and veins compared to operative findings

| | Agreement | | Specificity |
	+	−	(%)
Arterial vessels	54	4	93
Venous vessels	51	7	88

Table 70-7. Results of duplex scanning of the upper extremity veins versus early postoperative occlusion

Duplex scan findings	No.	Occlusion	Fistula failure
Normal	29	1	2
Abnormal	29	4	8

Table 70-8. Mean diameter (± SD) of arteries and veins used for creating hemodialysis access fistulas

Vessel	Occlusion	No occlusion	p
Artery (mm)	3.7 ± 1.4	3.5 ± 1.5	NS
Vein (mm)	2.9 ± 0.9	3.0 ± 1.0	NS

NS, Not significant.

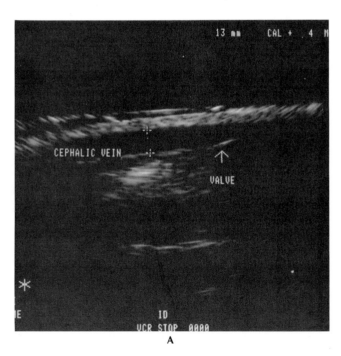

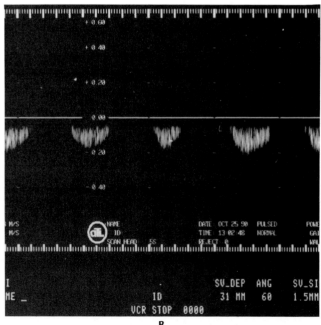

Fig. 70-9. **A,** B-mode image of the cephalic vein with measurement of vein diameter. **B,** Doppler spectral analysis shows normal flow.

performed along the arterial tree, and significant stenoses or occlusions are identified by an increase in peak systolic velocities or the absence of blood flow.

The diameters of arteries and veins can also be measured by B-mode imaging. The patency and continuity of the cephalic vein from the wrist up to the shoulder is determined by Doppler spectral waveform analysis (Fig. 70-9). Finally, the subclavian vein can be insonated to exclude stenosis or occlusion resulting from previously inserted dialysis catheters (Fig. 70-10).

In one vascular laboratory, routine preoperative duplex scanning is performed in all patients who need primary or secondary access operations. In Table 70-6, the results of duplex scanning are compared with the findings noted during surgical exploration in 58 upper extremities. A total of 54 of the arteries were found suitable for an adequate anastomosis, but only 51 of the 58 veins explored were found suitable. This translates into a specificity of 93% for arterial scanning and 88% for venous scanning. The relationship between preoperative venous assessment and early postoperative occlusion (within 30 days) is shown in Table 70-7. The incidence of early occlusion and failure in patients with normal arm veins was significantly lower (3 of 29; 10%) than that in patients with abnormal or occluded superficial veins (12 of 29; 41%; $p < 0.05$). No differences in the mean diameters of the anastomosed vessels were found between patients with and without failed AV fistulas (Table 70-8).

Duplex scanning is therefore a reliable noninvasive method for assessing the status of upper extremity vessels before hemodialysis access operations. The presence of defects in the veins correlates with a higher incidence of early postoperative fistula occlusion. The diameter of the anastomosed vessels has no bearing on the occurrence of postoperative thrombosis.

COLOR FLOW DOPPLER EVALUATION OF HEMODIALYSIS ACCESS FISTULAS

Color flow Doppler scanning may be of particular interest in the investigation of AV fistulas.[22] Flow velocities and directions can be readily estimated by the scale of colors displayed on the screen. Arterial steal and retrograde venous flow are easily visualized, and Doppler spectral analysis can be performed in areas of special interest (Figs. 70-11 and 70-12).

Duplex and color flow Doppler devices may be very helpful in quantifying volume flows in dialysis patients with problems of inadequate flow through the dialysis machine.[16] Hower et al[9] have documented volume flows in BC and graft AV fistulas. By compiling hemodynamic data, it became possible to use changes in flow velocity and volume as indicators of graft function. When flow volumes in polytetrafluoroethylene grafts are less than 400 ml/min and corresponding velocities are below 100 cm/sec, graft failure is imminent. Color flow analysis also allows rapid and accurate differentiation between perigraft fluid collections and graft pseudoaneurysms.

Quantitative color flow Doppler studies are reported to have an accuracy of 84% to 94% for the diagnosis of AV fistula stenoses.[13,15] The results are most reliable in the area

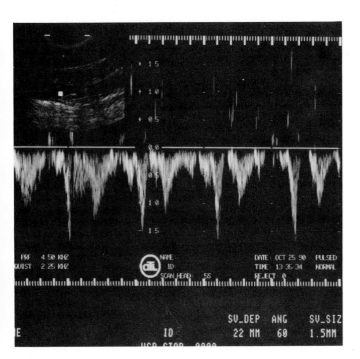

Fig. 70-10. Doppler spectrum of the subclavian vein with normal respiratory waves.

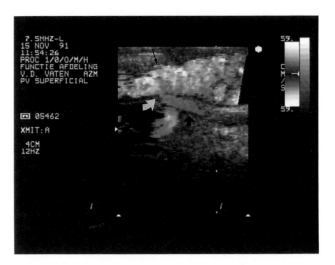

Fig. 70-11. Color flow Doppler scan of the anastomosis of a Brescia/Cimino fistula. Forward flow in the proximal radial artery is shown in red. Permanent steal in the distal artery is outlined in blue colors (black arrow). The anastomosis (white arrow) and cephalic vein (small arrow) are clearly visible.

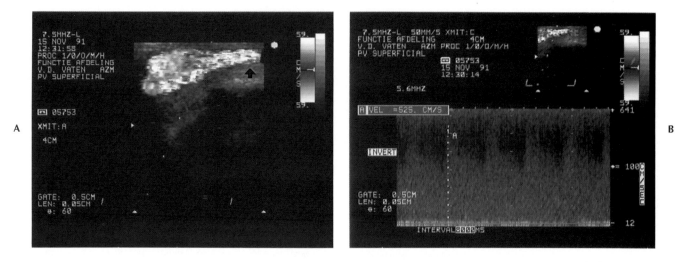

Fig. 70-12. **A,** Efferent vein stenosis detected by color flow Doppler *(arrow).* **B,** Doppler spectral analysis of the stenotic area. The peak systolic and end-diastolic velocities are markedly increased.

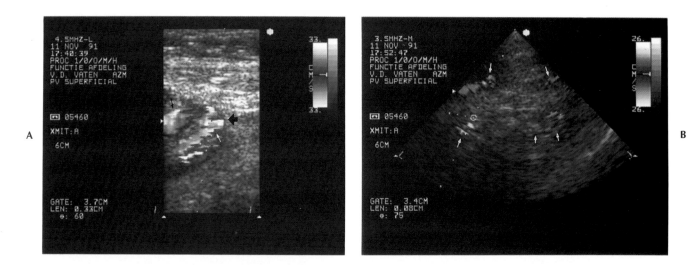

Fig. 70-13. **A,** Color flow Doppler scan of the infraclavicular region in a patient with a subclavian vein occlusion. The confluence of the cephalic vein *(black arrow)* and subclavian vein *(white arrow)* is visible; the proximal subclavian vein is occluded *(big arrow).* **B,** Numerous collateral draining veins are visible *(white arrows).*

of the efferent veins and less so for the detection of anastomotic and subclavian vein stenoses. Conventional duplex scanning may underestimate subclavian vein lesions because of the retroclavicular position of that vein.[7] In contrast, color flow Doppler scanning may identify altered flow patterns and collateral circulation in the neck (Fig. 70-13). Because color flow Doppler represents new technology, its impact on the investigation of hemodialysis access operations is not entirely known. However, it has the potential of becoming the preferred method for the initial evaluation of vascular access function and for predicting impending graft failure.

CONCLUSION

In the past decade, duplex scanning has been successfully used for the diagnosis of carotid artery, aortoiliac, and peripheral vascular disease. It has also assumed an important role in the investigation of hemodialysis access operations. Duplex scanning can be performed for the screening of the upper extremity before access surgery is performed; it can detect stenoses accurately and has a high predictive value for the development of complications. Systemic and local hemodynamic changes caused by the AV fistula can also be determined and quantified. In addition, color flow Doppler devices allow a more accurate diagnosis of stenotic AV fistulas, and their use may be extended to the investigation of the subclavian vein area.

REFERENCES

1. Brady HR et al: Diagnosis and management of subclavian vein thrombosis occurring in association with subclavian cannulation for hemodialysis, *Blood Purif* 7:214-217, 1989.
2. Dally P, Brantigan CO: Plethysmography and the diagnosis of the steal syndrome following placement of arteriovenous fistulas and shunts for hemodialysis access, *J Cardiovasc Surg* 28:200-203, 1987.
3. Duncan H, Ferguson L, Faris I: Incidence of the radial steal syndrome in patients with Brescia fistula for hemodialysis: its clinical significance, *J Vasc Surg* 4:144-147, 1986.
4. Gemert MJC van, Bruyninckx CMA: Simulated hemodynamic comparison of arteriovenous fistulas, *J Vasc Surg* 6:39-44, 1987.
5. Gerwen JA van et al: Noninvasive tests assessing the capacity and hemodynamic sequelae of arteriovenous fistulas for hemodialysis, *Dialysis Transplantation* 15:97-100, 1986.
6. Glickman MH, Clark S, Goodrich V: Determination of outflow stenosis of arteriovenous fistulas for hemodialysis, *Bruit* 9:16-19, 1985.
7. Gundersen J: The systolic finger blood pressure before and after establishment of a Brescia fistula, *Vasa* 9:21-23, 1980.
8. Haimov M et al: Complications of arteriovenous fistulas for hemodialysis, *Arch Surg* 110:708-712, 1975.
9. Hower JF, Villemarette PA, Kornick AL: *Color flow Doppler evaluations of vascular access graft function,* In Tordoir JHM, Kitslaar PJEHM, Kootstra G, eds: *Progress in access surgery,* Maastricht, 1991, Datawyse.
10. Kathrein HP et al: Nicht-invasive morphologische und funktionelle Beurteilung arteriovenöser Fisteln von Dialysepatienten mit der Duplexsonographie, *Ultraschall* 10:33-40, 1989.
11. Kherlakian GM et al: Comparison of autogenous fistula versus expanded polytetrafluoroethylene graft fistula for angioaccess in hemodialysis, *Am J Surg* 152:238-243, 1986.
12. Kinnaert P et al: Intermittent claudication of the hand after creation of an arteriovenous fistula in the forearm, *Am J Surg* 139:838-843, 1980.
13. Landwehr P et al: Wertigkeit der farbkodierten Duplex sonographie des Dialyseshunts, *Fortschr Röntgenstr* 153:185-191, 1988.
14. Mattson WJ: Recognition and treatment of vascular steal secondary to hemodialysis prostheses, *Am J Surg* 154:198-201, 1987.
15. Middleton WD et al: Color Doppler sonography of hemodialysis vascular access: comparison with angiography, *Am J Radiol* 152:633-639, 1989.
16. Oates CP, Williams ED, McHugh MI: The use of a Diasonics DRF400 duplex ultrasound scanner to measure volume flow in arteriovenous fistulae in patients undergoing haemodialysis: an analysis of measurement uncertainties, *Ultrasound Med Biol* 16:571-579, 1990.
17. Reilly DT, Wood RFM, Bell PRF: Prospective study of dialysis fistulas: problem patients and their treatment, *Br J Surg* 69:549-553, 1982.
18. Rittgers SE et al: Noninvasive blood flow measurement in expanded polytetrafluoroethylene grafts for hemodialysis access, *J Vasc Surg* 3:635-642, 1986.
19. Strandness DE, Sumner DS: *Arteriovenous fistulas.* In *Hemodynamics for surgeons,* New York, 1975, Grune & Stratton.
20. Tordoir JHM et al: Duplex ultrasound scanning in the assessment of arteriovenous fistulas created for hemodialysis access: comparison with digital subtraction angiography, *J Vasc Surg* 10:122-128, 1989.
21. Tordoir JHM et al: The correlation between clinical and duplex ultrasound parameters and the development of complications in arteriovenous fistulas for hemodialysis, *Eur J Vasc Surg* 4:179-184, 1990.
22. Vorwerk D et al: Farbkodierte Duplexsonographie (Angiodynographie) in der Beurteilung arteriovenöser Shunts, *Fortschr Röntgenstr* 148:265-268, 1988.
23. Zwicker C et al: Duplex sonographie von Hämodialyse shunts, *Angio* 9:47-52, 1987.

CHAPTER 71

Noninvasive testing in the diagnosis and assessment of arteriovenous fistula

ROBERT B. RUTHERFORD

The diagnosis of an arteriovenous (AV) fistula may be obvious on physical examination by (1) the auscultation of a characteristic bruit, (2) the obliteration of a thrill producing a bradycardic response, (3) the observation of secondary varicosities and cutaneous signs of chronic venous hypertension, or (4) the association of a "birthmark" and limb overgrowth in congenital AV fistulas. Unfortunately, such classic findings are often absent, and the diagnosis may only be suspected.

For example, in one of the largest series of AV malformations,[22] the classic triad of birthmark, varicosities, and limb enlargement was present in only 30% of the patients, with various other combinations of signs present in 38% and 32% of those presenting with only a single physical finding.

Thus there is a need for noninvasive screening tests that confirm or refute such suspicions, as well as for simple and innocuous methods of estimating the magnitude of AV shunt flow in an extremity and practical means of serially monitoring naturally occurring AV fistulas or those created for angioaccess purposes. In addition to a number of invasive diagnostic techniques identifying the presence or absence of hemodynamically significant AV communications, [1,5,8-10,14,15] several noninvasive diagnostic approaches have been published. Changes in blood flow, detected by venous occlusive plethysmography,[23] pulse volume,[2,20] and segmental pressure,[2,8] have been described, as well as changes in flow velocities determined by Doppler velocity measurements.[2,7,12,15] This chapter summarizes some of these techniques.

HEMODYNAMIC BACKGROUND

An understanding of the hemodynamics and pathophysiology of AV fistulas provides the necessary background for their noninvasive diagnosis. Sumner[21] has written a comprehensive and detailed review on this subject. Although increased arterial flow leading into the fistula, decreased resistance and mean arterial pressure in the involved extremity, and increased venous volume and pressure are common and well-recognized features, other hemodynamic changes vary, depending on the size of the fistula and the degree of collateral circulation development. With small fistulas or good collateral development, effects distal to the fistula may be so minor as to be undetectable by current physiologic testing. With large fistulas or poor collateral development, a number of readily detectable hemodynamic disturbances occur that are often described collectively under the term *distal steal*. Systolic as well as mean arterial pressure is decreased distal to the fistula, as is pulsatility, as gauged by volume or pressure measurements. Reversal of flow in the artery distal to the fistula marks the turning point in fistula development. These changes, along with the secondary effect of obstructing flow through the fistula or its afferent or efferent arteries and veins, are the basis for many of the following tests.

SCREENING TESTS FOR EXTREMITY AV FISTULAS

Three noninvasive diagnostic tests that were primarily developed for the detection and localization of peripheral arterial occlusive lesions also constitute an effective screening battery for extremity AV fistulas: (1) segmental limb systolic pressure determinations (SLPs), (2) segmental limb plethysmography or pulse-volume recordings (PVRs), and (3) the analysis of arterial velocity tracings or waveforms (VWFs). The techniques of performing these tests are well established and are described elsewhere in this text (see Chapters 55 to 59). The focus here is on the specific application of the SLP, PVR, and VWF to the diagnosis of extremity AV fistulas, a potential that has not been widely realized. Directional Doppler scans are discussed elsewhere.

Segmental limb systolic pressures

The SLP test is performed exactly as described for the detection and localization of peripheral arterial occlusive lesions. The four-cuff is preferable over the three-cuff method, with two standard-size rather than one large thigh cuff because although the second gives a more accurate estimate of true systolic pressure in the thigh arteries, the first provides better localization of arterial lesions.[7] The reduced peripheral resistance associated with AV fistulas decreases mean arterial pressure in the arterial tree but increases pulse pressure. Therefore proximal to an AV fistula,

SLPs will usually be increased[8] in comparison to those of the contralateral (normal) extremity, whereas distal to the fistula, SLPs may be normal, or if the fistula is "stealing" significantly from distal arterial flow, they may be decreased. This description applies primarily to the situation in which there is a fairly localized and hemodynamically significant AV fistula, whether it be acquired or a congenital macrofistula. However, even in AV fistulas so diffusely located that segmental localization is not possible, the systolic pressure determinations in the involved extremity may be higher than those in the contralateral normal extremity, as long as fistula flow is significantly great.

Segmental limb plethysmography or pulse-volume recording

An AV fistula increases the volume changes normally produced by pulsatile arterial flow. These can be monitored by segmental strain gauge, impedance, or volume plethysmography. Characteristically, these PVRs are greater proximal to the fistula than in the normal contralateral extremity, and they have a sharper systolic peak and a decreased or absent anacrotic notch. Distal to the fistula PVRs are often not changed until the digital level, where they may be decreased. However, this decrease is usually relatively less than the decrease in systolic pressure. As previously observed for SLPs, the magnitude of these plethysmographic changes and their ability to localize an extremity AV fistula depend on the type of fistula and the volume of fistula flow. In the case of multiple, diffuse microfistulas, segmental localization often is not possible, and the presence of the lesion may only be apparent after careful comparison with properly calibrated plethysmographic tracings recorded at equivalent levels on the contralateral extremity.

Arterial velocity tracings or waveforms

Lower extremity arterial flow is normally triphasic, with the major systolic and the minor early diastolic forward components being interrupted by a period of reversed flow. The circulation in a resting extremity is normally in a high-resistance, low-flow state to such a degree that late diastolic flow is negligible.[6,11] For these reasons a VWF recorded by Doppler probe over the major inflow artery to an extremity is normally triphasic and appears to "rest" on the zero velocity baseline. Occlusive arterial lesions upstream and downstream from the monitoring Doppler probe produce characteristic abnormalities that are well known, but the changes produced by distally located AV fistulas are equally striking. Rittenhouse et al[17] have shown that changes in peripheral arterial resistance in an otherwise normal arterial tree modify the VWF in a predictable way. Decreased peripheral resistance eliminates reversed flow and increases forward flow, particularly in diastole. As a result, end-diastolic velocity and therefore the entire VWF are elevated above the zero baseline in direct proportion to the decrease in peripheral resistance. Increases in the magnitude and steepness of the upslope of the systolic peak, as well as irregularities produced by turbulence, are also observed when peripheral resistance is significantly decreased, but these changes are not as striking or as quantifiable as the elevation in the level of end-diastolic velocity.

Hyperemia associated with exercise, the relief of ischemia, artificial warming, vasodilator drugs, inflammation, and sympathectomy all produce changes in the VWF similar to those observed with AV fistulas. However, in the usual clinical situations where the diagnosis of AV fistula is being considered, these other causes of hyperemia are unlikely and easily ruled out. Increased velocity occurs in the jet stream of a high-grade arterial stenosis, and velocity tracings recorded immediately distal to such a lesion are also raised above the zero baseline. However, this characteristically widens the systolic peak and produces more irregularities, particularly on the systolic downslope. Furthermore, stenotic lesions capable of producing such waveform abnormalities should also produce decreases in systolic pressure distally and thus a telltale SLP gradient. The same information can be obtained with a duplex scan, which should also show significantly higher velocities than on the contralateral, normal side.

Comparison of methods

The diagnostic sensitivity of these three tests is the reverse order of their presentation, the most reliable being the VWF. However, as with other noninvasive diagnostic test situations, accuracy improves when they are considered in combination. Microfistulas producing small degrees of AV shunting relative to total limb blood flow (e.g., 3% to 7%) might not be detected by these tests.

These screening tests have their greatest clinical application in the evaluation of patients with congenital AV fistulas, particularly (1) in determining whether a birthmark or hemangioma is associated with an AV fistula, (2) in ruling out AV fistulas as a cause of varicose veins of atypical distribution or early onset, and (3) in screening patients with unequal limb length to rule out the possibility of an underlying AV fistula.[19] Patients with such clinical problems are likely to be children in whom the advantages of avoiding arteriography are even greater. In addition, in approximately 40% of congenital AV malformations, the AV fistulas themselves cannot be visualized angiographically,[22] and diagnosis depends on indirect evidence, such as early venous filling, increase in the size or number of branches of arteries in the region, or rapid clearance of contrast material. In the study by Szilagyi et al,[22] almost 30% of the arteriograms were "normal." These tests do not eliminate the need for arteriography but limit its application to essentially therapeutic indications. Because acquired AV fistulas secondary to trauma are usually more readily diagnosed on the basis of physical examination and because arteriography is not only definitive but necessary, the advantages of screening tests are not as great in this setting. However, the tests may be helpful in differentiating false aneurysm from AV fistula as the cause of pulsation or bruit discovered after extremity trauma.

The major weaknesses with this approach are that it is only applicable to peripheral AV malformations (e.g., not to those of iliac/hypogastric origin), it is qualitative, it provides only crude segmental localization of the site of AV shunting, and it provides no idea of anatomic extent or the specific tissues or anatomic structures involved. Nevertheless, these tests are painless and can be performed with inexpensive equipment in 20 to 30 minutes. They are readily applied to children by using appropriately smaller cuffs for the SLPs and PVRs.

ESTIMATING EXTREMITY AV SHUNT FLOW BY THE LABELED MICROSPHERE METHOD

The percentage of total extremity flow that passes through AV communications may be estimated by comparing the relative levels of pulmonary radioactivity following first an arterial and then a peripheral venous injection of radionuclide-labeled human albumin microspheres.[18,19] This study may be used to confirm or refute the diagnosis of extremity AV fistula if the results of the noninvasive screening tests are equivocal. It also provides a quantitative estimate of AV shunt flow, which may assist in determining the prognosis and in gauging the need for and effectiveness of therapeutic interventions.

Method

A detailed account of the preparation of the microspheres and the methodology employed in establishing and standardizing this test has been published.[7] However, the test has been simplified by the widespread and ready availability of labeled microspheres and gamma cameras. In practice, a suspension of ^{99m}Tc-labeled 35 μ human albumin microspheres* is injected into the major inflow artery of the involved extremity while the lungs are monitored by a gamma camera. The radioactivity incident to the arterial injection of microspheres is compared to that following a subsequent peripheral intravenous injection, 100% of which should be trapped by the lungs. The venous injectate usually contains less radioactivity than the arterial injectate (roughly one fourth to one third) to ensure similar counting efficiencies. The relative radioactivity of the injectates is determined by counting the syringes before and after injection. Therefore it is important that there be no extravasation at the time of injection. The percentage of extremity flow passing through AV shunts is then estimated by multiplying the ratio of pulmonary activity following the arterial injection to that following the venous injection by the ratio of the respective injectates themselves and then multiplying this product by 100. For example, if the ratio of pulmonary radioactivity incident to venous injection is 2.5 times that following arterial injection, even though the venous injectate was only one-fourth as great, the estimate of AV shunt is:

$$\frac{1}{2.5} \times \frac{1}{4} \times \frac{100}{1} = 10\%$$

Normally the level of AV shunting in an extremity of an unanesthetized patient is less than 3%.[18] At the time of this study a perfusion scan of the leg should also be obtained, since the distribution of the arterial injectate may indicate not only the location of a fistula but the degree to which it is "stealing" from the distal vascular bed.

Because the labeled microsphere method of studying AV fistulas supplies more objective and quantitative information than the noninvasive screening tests, it possesses a number of different clinical applications. By estimating the relative magnitude of the AV fistula, the test provides a more precise gauge of its hemodynamic significance and therefore should allow closer prediction of the likelihood of such complications as limb overgrowth, ulceration and secondary skin changes, distal arterial insufficiency secondary to the steal phenomenon, and systemic hemodynamic effects such as forward heart failure. Serial estimates of AV shunting may indicate whether to expect a stable or progressive natural course and may help to determine the need for therapeutic intervention in the form of ablative surgery or palliative embolism, as well as gauge the effectiveness of these efforts. The test can be performed in conjunction with angiography, not only to avoid an additional arterial puncture but also to provide more precise localization, either by multiple injections from different angiographic catheter tip locations or from the same location using sphygmomanometer cuffs at different levels, temporarily inflated above systolic pressure. This test can be performed during angiographic or direct surgical attempts at fistula control to provide a more objective therapeutic end point. However, both general and regional anesthetics increase shunting through naturally occurring AV communications, and this must be controlled either by an additional postinduction baseline determination or by a comparative study of the uninvolved extremity.

This test is particularly useful when noninvasive screening tests are equivocal or normal, and when AV fistulas are still suspected. One of the best applications of this test is in detecting and quantifying microfistulous AV shunt flow or ruling out its existence. Lindenauer[12] has pointed out that a patient can have varicose veins, a birthmark, and limb enlargement without demonstrable AV fistulas (i.e., a Klippel-Trenaunay rather than a Parkes-Weber syndrome), but there is some concern that microfistulous AV fistulas could still be present without being seen angiographically.[15] In the large Henry Ford Hospital experience with congenital AV fistulas, arteriography did not demonstrate AV fistulas in 28% of the cases.[22] The labeled microsphere study eliminates the guesswork. That there may be microfistulous AV fistulas in such cases is clear, but the clinician needs to know this with certainty because if AV fistulas are not present, focus should shift to evaluating the venous system for anomalies.

Venous studies

Patients with congenital vascular malformations may present primarily with venous signs, particularly varicose

---

*3M, St. Paul, Minn.

veins. Some may harbor AV fistulas and have secondary venous insufficiency, whereas others may have no AV fistulas but primarily a venous anomaly (e.g., a Klippel-Trenaunay rather than a Parkes-Weber syndrome). These possibilities can be pursued further by using venous noninvasive studies. Deep venous valvular insufficiency is easily identified by Doppler evaluation of the femoral, popliteal, and posterior tibial veins with compression and Valsalva maneuvers. Doppler interrogation of major veins draining a limb segment containing significant AV fistulas will detect flow that is continuous, often with accentuations synchronous with the cardiac cycle, and not phasic and synchronous with the respirator cycle, which is the normal finding. Chronic dilatation also produces detectable valve insufficiency. By using photoplethysmographic (PPG) monitoring of distal venous volume changes in response to calf pumping action performed against gravity and then seeing if tourniquet application at various levels from upper thigh to distal calf improves the venous refill time, the clinician can not only assess this venous reflux but also localize it to the region of the congenital vascular malformation. If there is a vascular mass or a localized cluster of varicosities, the examiner can focus on this area with B-mode ultrasound or, preferably, a duplex scanner. Cavernous hemangioma or venous angiomata without significant arterial involvement

are evidenced by the characteristic appearance of the vascular spaces and the lack of high flow signals in the spaces that are synchronous with the heart beat. Thus there are secondary venous changes associated with long-standing AV fistulas that are easily recognized by simple venous noninvasive tests, which are confirmatory in that setting. If the screening tests for AV fistulas are negative, these same tests can be used to assess what may be a pure venous malformation. Finally, in both settings, when there is an obvious localized vascular mass, duplex scan (with or without color coding) can be useful in characterizing the lesion.

The varied clinical applications of both the noninvasive test and the labeled microsphere study are illustrated by the following brief case presentations.

1. S.D. (UH No. 596-978). A 10-year-old girl with hemangiomas of the left leg since birth was referred by an orthopedist for evaluation of the possibility that congenital AV fistulas might be producing progressive inequality in leg length (3 cm) and girth (2 cm), even though previous arteriography had been unable to detect them. The left extremity was somewhat warmer than the right, but there were no bruits, varicose veins, or cutaneous stigmata of chronic venous hypertension. Systolic SLPs were 10 mm Hg higher on the left at the calf but equal at other levels. However, the PVRs on the left were clearly greater at all levels, and the femoral artery VWF on the left showed an absence of end-systolic reversal and increased diastolic velocity (Fig. 71-1). Shunt quantitation by the labeled microsphere method estimated 12% of the femoral flow passed through AV communication(s).

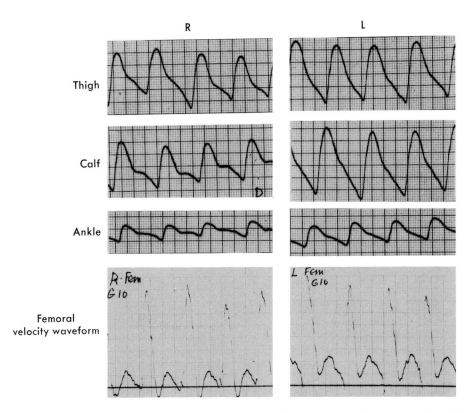

Fig. 71-1. PVRs and *(bottom)* femoral artery VWFs of young girl (S.D.) with 12% shunting through multiple congenital fistulas of the left leg. (From Rutherford RB, Fleming PW, McLeod FD: *Vascular diagnostic methods for evaluating patients with arteriovenous fistulas.* In Diethrich EB, ed: *Noninvasive cardiovascular diagnosis: current concepts,* Baltimore, 1978, University Park Press.)

R. R. 2-1-77

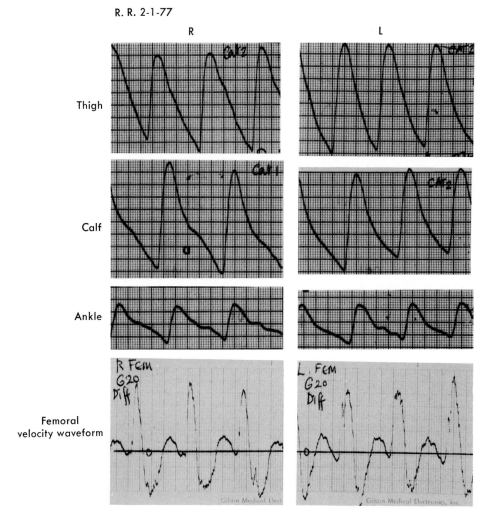

Fig. 71-2. PVRs and VWFs of a 16-year-old boy (R.R.) with extensive, early-onset varicosities and cutaneous capillary hemangiomas who did not have associated AV fistulas (AV shunt, 2.1%). (From Rutherford RB, Fleming PW, McLeod FD: *Vascular diagnostic methods for evaluating patients with arteriovenous fistulas.* In Diethrich EB, ed: *Noninvasive cardiovascular diagnosis: current concepts,* Baltimore, 1978, University Park Press.)

Comment: The diagnosis of congenital AV fistulas as the cause of unequal limb growth was easily established by relatively simple methods in spite of a "negative" arteriogram.

2. R.R. (UH No. 628-314). A 16-year-old boy with bilateral varicose veins of progressing severity since their appearance at age 2 was referred after high ligation and stripping of the left greater saphenous system caused increased discomfort and swelling with an early recurrence of the varicosities. Arteriography, performed before the surgery, "ruled out" the presence of AV fistulas. On examination there were extensive bilateral varicosities as well as purplish port-wine stains over both extremities. Both lower extremities seemed disproportionately large for the patient's size (height 5 feet 9 inches, shoe size 12). The diagnosis of bilateral congenital AV fistulas seemed likely in spite of the arteriogram. Systolic SLPs were equal bilaterally, as were the PVRs, although the dimensions of the latter at the thigh and calf level seemed greater than normal. However, there was no increase in diastolic velocity in either femoral artery. In fact, there was an increased end-systolic reversal (Fig. 71-2). Measurement of shunt flow in the left extremity by the labeled microsphere method estimated it to be only 2.1%. Subsequent venous Doppler study demonstrated severe reflux at the femoropopliteal level bilaterally.

Comment: The clinical suspicion of AV fistula was so great that the lack of increased diastolic velocity was "ignored" and an AV shunt study obtained. Only after this confirmed the absence of significant AV shunt flow was a venous Doppler study performed to demonstrate the existence of extensive deep venous valvular insufficiency.

3. M.B. (UH No. 614-761). This 50-year-old man had a huge congenital AV malformation of the right lower extremity, causing gigantic limb overgrowth, venous "stasis" pigmentation, and brawny edema with periodic ulceration. A surgical attack on the fistulas was abandoned 5 years earlier at another institution after 70 units of blood had been transfused. Transaxillary angiography was performed with injection of both contrast material and labeled microspheres at several locations. The latter indicated 50% AV shunting of right common iliac flow, 65% shunting of right common femoral flow, but no shunting of superficial femoral flow, indicating the AV malformation was essentially limited to the distribution of the deep femoral artery. An arteriogram obtained at the same time demonstrated a major macrofistula at this location (Fig. 71-3).

Comment: The microsphere study indicated a more localized and therefore more treatable fistula than expected from physical examination and even arteriography.

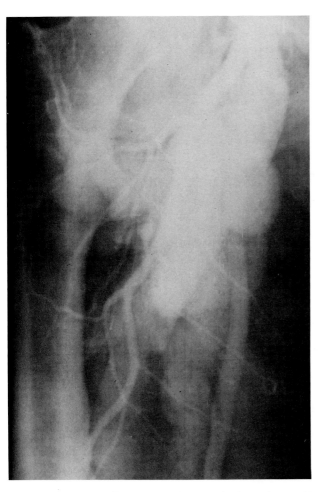

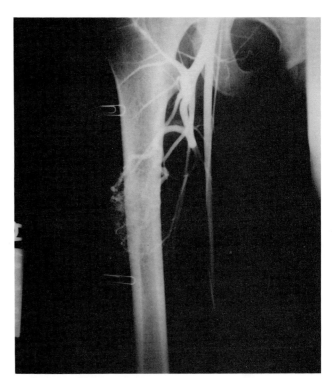

Fig. 71-4. This arteriogram shows an extensive vascular network fed by profunda femoris branches. Early venous filling was seen in later views. (From Sumner DS, Rutherford RB: *Diagnostic evaluation of the arteriovenous fistulas.* In Rutherford RB, ed: *Vascular surgery,* ed 3, Philadelphia, 1989, Saunders.)

Fig. 71-3. Huge AV malformation arising near the femoral artery bifurcation. AV shunting above this level was 65% but negligible more distally in the superficial femoral artery.

MAGNETIC RESONANCE IMAGING

Although a combination of noninvasive tests and a labeled microsphere study will often provide adequate information to allow management decisions to be made for the patient with a congenital vascular malformation, particularly if the condition is primarily a venous anomaly, these diagnostic approaches are only applicable in evaluating peripheral extremity congenital vascular malformations; these approaches give physiologic but not anatomic information. Therefore a third noninvasive approach is necessary in most patients to achieve sufficient information on which to base major clinical decisions. In this situation, magnetic resonance imaging (MRI) is preferred. Before the advent and availability of MRI, contrast-enhanced computed tomography (dynamic CT) scans were used in evaluating congenital vascular malformations. However, MRI avoids contrast medium and irradiation, gives information about flow characteristics of the malformation, gives a better definition of the anatomic extent and the feasibility of surgical resection than CT, and allows multiplanar views. The only relative disadvantages

of the MRI are its current expense and lack of universal availability, but these are less likely to be problems in the future. It also does not give quantifiable flow information, although this too is expected in the future.

The principles of MRI are beyond the scope of this presentation but can be found in the literature, including examples of its applicability to congenital vascular malformations.[13] It can show invasion or involvement of bone or specific muscle groups and the extent of that involvement through longitudinal and cross-sectional images. Since rapidly flowing blood creates "black holes" in MRI images, the high flow AV fistula component of a congenital vascular malformation is easily recognized. Conversely, when the vascular spaces are all white, there is little or no AV shunting, and the clinician may be dealing primarily with a venous malformation. The value of MRI may be best demonstrated by a brief case presentation.

4. A young man was referred for surgical resection of a localized but asymptomatic congenital AV fistula of the right thigh. Previously performed arteriograms (Fig. 71-4) showed the vascular malformation to be fed by large terminal arteries, all emanating from the right profunda femoris artery. Other views showed early venous filling, enlargement, and tortuosity of the profunda femoris and a massive network of small vessels. Noninvasive testing showed a rapid velocity profile in the right common femoral artery but no evidence of distal arterial steal or venous reflux. An MRI was obtained (see Fig. 71-5), which showed an exten-

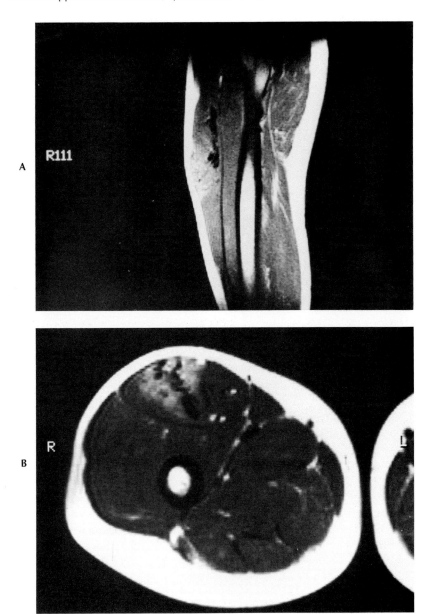

Fig. 71-5. **A,** The longitudinal view shows a high-flow (dark) draining vein and low-flow (light) vascular spaces involving the anterior thigh muscles. (From Anderson BO, Rutherford RB, Szilagyi DE: *Congenital vascular malformations of the extremities.* In Moore WS, ed: *Vascular surgery: comprehensive review,* ed 3, Philadelphia, 1991, Saunders.) **B,** The transverse view shows a vascular mass with high-flow changes involving most of the vastus medialis muscle. (From Sumner DS, Rutherford RB: *Diagnostic evaluation of the arteriovenous fistulas.* In Rutherford RB, ed: *Vascular surgery,* ed 3, Philadelphia, 1989, Saunders.)

sive high flow network of large vessels in a mass that largely replaced the vastus medialis muscle. A microsphere study showed that over a third of common femoral arterial blood was being shunted through the fistula. Because the patient was suffering no disability from this lesion and because surgery would risk injury to the femoral nerve and remove important functioning muscles, interventional therapy was postponed until surgery became the only option. He is still asymptomatic 5 years later.

Rationale for the recommended diagnostic approach

The essential diagnostic goals in dealing with congenital vascular malformations are: (1) establish the presence and type of malformation, (2) define its anatomic extent and the

involvement of adjacent structures, and (3) determine its local, regional, and occasionally systemic hemodynamic effects. Performance of noninvasive tests, a labeled microsphere study, and MRI will furnish this information in the vast majority of patients presenting with congenital vascular malformations. Evaluation of the cardiac effects can also be performed noninvasively.

The management of peripheral congenital vascular malformations can be based largely on the information provided by the recommended diagnostic approach. As shown in the algorithm (Fig. 71-6), using a combination of noninvasive tests and MRI and occasionally the labeled microsphere

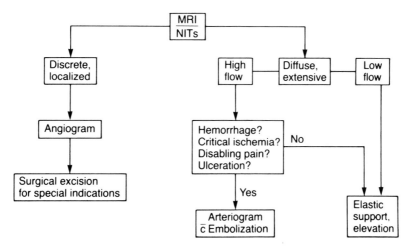

Fig. 71-6. Algorithm showing how noninvasive tests and MRI can direct therapy, determining the ultimate need for arteriography and likely therapeutic intervention. (From Sumner DS, Rutherford RB: *Diagnostic evaluation of the arteriovenous fistulas.* In Rutherford RB, ed: *Vascular surgery,* ed 3, Philadelphia, 1989, Saunders.)

study, the clinician can determine whether the malformation is discrete and localized. Since these are the only lesions that are potentially curable by surgical intervention, the clinician would obtain an angiogram in this subgroup and proceed with excisional surgery as indicated. On the other hand, if this combination of studies showed a diffuse and extensive congenital vascular malformation (e.g., a low-flow lesion), simple elastic support and elevation would be the only treatment offered and required. Finally, if these tests showed an extensive high-flow lesion, the clinician could predict that ultimately the extremity would become symptomatic and intervention would be required. However, because neither surgery nor embolism gives permanent, curative results in diffuse, extensive lesions with multiple AV fistulas, specific indications would be required before intervention became necessary and elastic support and elevation would be used during the interval for palliation and control. Ultimately, intervention would be indicated, probably in the form of therapeutic embolism, with surgery as a last resort. Only then would angiography be required, and the results of therapy could then be monitored by the labeled microsphere method.

APPLICATION OF NONINVASIVE TESTS TO THE MANAGEMENT OF PATIENTS WITH ANGIOACCESS AV FISTULAS
Preoperative monitoring

Most patients undergoing angioaccess surgery receive frequent intravenous infusions, some of which result in venous thrombosis, which may in turn dictate the placement of an AV fistula. One of the accepted indications for these operations is the decreasing availability of patent peripheral veins. Therefore preoperative venous evaluation is important. This may and in certain cases should be accomplished by venography, but a complete study of all the veins of one or more prospective extremities is impractical in most cases.

Venous mapping of superficial veins was originally performed to evaluate lower extremity veins before their use in infrainguinal arterial bypass for limb ischemia. It is now routine in the preoperative evaluations of upper extremity veins before angioaccess surgery. The study is done in the dependent extremity without tourniquet application and, on the average, underestimates vein diameter by at least 1 mm. It is accurate in determining functional patency, although it may miss minor defects or the subtler changes of prior phlebitis that have not resulted in complete luminal obliteration. Venography can therefore be saved for the more complicated minority of cases.

Uremic, diabetic, and arteriosclerotic patients, and particularly patients with previous failed attempts at creation of AV fistulas, may have peripheral arterial occlusive lesions that will influence not only the choice of the "donor" artery but also the likelihood of fistula success. As with venous evaluation, the thoughtful use of noninvasive methods can reduce the need for angiography and aid in its interpretation.

The preoperative evaluation of the arterial system of an extremity that may serve as a potential site for an AV fistula or shunt should include SLPs and PVRs extended distally to include representative digits. PVRs provide important baseline information for postoperative monitoring. In addition, if consideration is being given to using either of the arteries lying parallel in the forearm or leg, the radial or ulnar differential compression maneuvers should also be performed. These are analogous to the Allen patency test as applied to the ulnar and radial arteries but are more informative when carried out using a Doppler probe. Arterial velocity signals are monitored over these arteries using a directional Doppler system and a strip chart recorder, noting

Table 71-1. Testing of parallel arteries with directional Doppler system and collateral compression

Condition	Direction	Form	Collateral compression
Both patent	Forward	Triphasic	Augmentation
Occluded proximally	Reversed	Triphasic	Diminution
Occluded distally	Forward	Triphasic	No response
Occluded collaterally	Forward	Triphasic	No response
Both occluded	Forward	Monophasic	No response
Common inflow occluded	Forward	Monophasic	Augmentation

first if flow is normally triphasic and antegrade. If so, compression of the companion artery should result in an augmented signal. If not, there is probably an occlusive lesion in that vessel or the intervening collateral vessels. If on the other hand the artery being monitored shows retrograde flow diminished by compression of its companion vessel, it must be proximally occluded. Table 71-1 outlines the alternative findings in performing collateral compression testing. If only one of these vessels is patent, normal SLPs and PVRs may be found. However, if an AV fistula is created using this lone artery, the likelihood of a distal steal phenomenon developing is great, as is the likelihood of severe ischemia or gangrene should the fistula undergo thrombosis.

The same test can be applied to the lower extremity arteries, which involves monitoring over the posterior tibial and dorsalis pedis arteries while the companion vessel is compressed proximally. This approach has been shown by Rittenhouse and Brockenbrough[16] to predict the patency of each of the tibial arteries, even beyond a proximal occlusion.

Finally, even if these studies are normal, it is wise to do a stress test, monitoring the response of arm or ankle pressure to induced reactive hyperemia. Fee and Golding[4] have reported a case in which a femoral artery–saphenous vein fistula was created proximal to an unrecognized superficial femoral artery stenosis, causing distal ischemia and requiring reoperation.

Perioperative monitoring

The extremity should be studied noninvasively immediately after the creation of an AV fistula or shunt. In fact, if there is suspicion of a technical mishap, a sterilized Doppler probe can be used intraoperatively. Otherwise digital systolic pressures and plethysmography should be monitored at the end of the operation to rule out the possibility of an unrecognized complication. In addition, the point of maximum thrill or bruit should be localized and marked so that it may be readily monitored during the ensuing days, when regional swelling, hematoma formation, or the need for a bulky dressing may prevent the thrill from being readily palpated. Alternatively, the VWF proximal to the fistula may be recorded. If there is further doubt, a labeled microsphere study may be performed by injecting into the artery proximal to the fistula, settling any question of fistula patency.

Postoperative monitoring

As soon as the wounds have healed sufficiently and before the fistula or shunt is used for dialysis, the preoperative studies should be completely repeated. The level of elevation of the Doppler velocity tracing over the proximal artery may serve as an index of fistula flow, and the monitoring of digital pressures and plethysmographic tracings allows detection of thromboembolic complications or distal steal phenomena. Retesting at the time of development of any pain, color, or temperature changes is recommended.

In this regard it is important to recognize what changes can normally be expected after creation of AV fistulas, as documented by Brenner et al.[3] Fig. 71-7 shows the characteristic change in digital pulse tracing and pressure beyond a radial artery–cephalic vein fistula. There is an increase in the amplitude of the plethysmographic tracing but a decrease in the systolic pressure. However, Brenner showed that every patient with a radial artery–cephalic vein fistula had a drop in digital perfusion pressure, but there was rarely a further drop at the time of dialysis, even though many of the patients complained of discomfort, which was suspected to be ischemic in origin.

After a proximally placed brachial artery–axillary vein interposition AV shunt (Fig. 71-8), digital pressures dropped to an even greater extent. The plethysmographic tracings became almost flat, but with time, pulsatile flow and then pressures were restored by compensatory collateral development. In spite of this greater initial drop in digital pressure, again there was little further drop during dialysis. Thus the pressure and plethysmographic changes monitored distal to these AV fistulas are greatest in the immediate postoperative period and vary in degree with the size and location of the fistula. However, these decreases in distal perfusion improve with time and the development of collateral circulation and usually do not become much worse during dialysis.

The preceding discussion applies to uncomplicated angioaccess fistulas but has even greater application in identifying postoperative complications of AV fistulas. Thrombosis of the fistula itself or one of its limbs can be detected readily, particularly if postoperative baseline studies are available for comparison. This complication and either distal arterial steal or venous hypertension may all produce pain, color, or temperature changes in the hands and fingers and must be differentiated from each other. For such an evaluation, digital pressures and plethysmography should be performed at rest and then with occlusive compression of the fistula, each of its limbs, and the companion artery.[21]

Table 71-2 summarizes the findings in a case of radial artery–cephalic vein fistula that was stealing flow from the distal radial artery. The key observations are that digital

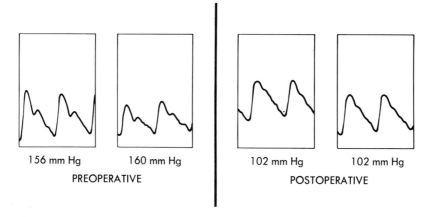

Fig. 71-7. PVRs from digits before and after creation of a radial artery–cephalic vein fistula. (From Brener BJ, Brief DK, Parsonnet AV: *The effect of vascular access procedure on digital hemodynamics.* In Diethrich EB, ed: *Noninvasive cardiovascular diagnosis: current concepts,* Baltimore, 1978, University Park Press.)

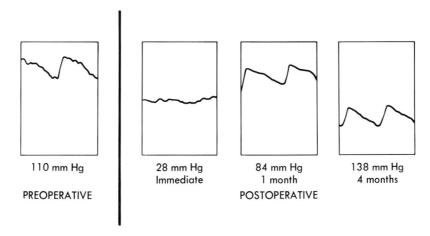

Fig. 71-8. PVRs before and after a brachial artery–axillary vein graft. The plethysmographic changes are similar to the digital pressure changes after insertion of prosthetic grafts. (From Brener BJ, Brief DK, Parsonnet AV: *The effect of vascular access procedure on digital hemodynamics.* In Diethrich EB, ed: *Noninvasive cardiovascular diagnosis: current concepts,* Baltimore, 1978, University Park Press.)

pressure is greatly reduced and is improved significantly by occlusion of either the fistula itself or the radial artery distally, whereas it decreases further with occlusion of the companion artery. This interpretation was corroborated by the effects of ligation of the radial artery distal to the fistula. Thus noninvasive study not only established the diagnosis but ensured that it could be treated by distal arterial ligation without the need to interrupt the fistula.

The findings in a case of distal venous hypertension are recorded in Table 71-3. The increases in digital pressure associated with compression of the fistula and the distal radial artery indicated a distal steal phenomenon, but the resting digital pressure was not low enough to produce isch-

Table 71-2. Radial steal—effect of ligating distal radial artery on blood pressure in the index finger ipsilateral to a radial artery–cephalic vein fistula

Blood pressure	Before ligation (mm Hg)	After ligation (mm Hg)
Brachial	100	100
Index finger		
Fistula open	32	80
Fistula occluded	68	92
Distal artery occluded	60	—
Ulnar artery occluded	0	0

From Sumner DS: *Diagnostic evaluation of arteriovenous fistulas.* In Rutherford RB, ed: *Vascular surgery,* ed 2, Philadelphia, 1984, Saunders.

Table 71-3. Distal venous hypertension—effect of ligating distal vein on blood pressure in the index finger ipsilateral to a radial artery–cephalic vein fistula

Blood pressure	Before ligation (mm Hg)	After ligation (mm Hg)
Brachial	156	160
Index finger		
Fistula open	100	110
Fistula occluded	160	186
Distal artery occluded	140	178
Proximal vein oc-cluded	110	140
Distal vein occluded	152	110

From Sumner DS: *Diagnostic evaluation of arteriovenous fistulas.* In Rutherford RB, ed: *Vascular surgery,* ed 2, Philadelphia, 1984, Saunders.

emic pain. However, the restoration of digital pressure to normal by compression of the distal vein indicated that this was the major venous outflow and was causing painful venous congestion in the hand and, as is commonly the case, in the carpal tunnel. After ligation of the distal vein, venous outflow was primarily through the proximal vein, so its compression now raised digital pressure.

TRANSCUTANEOUS DOPPLER MEASUREMENT OF FISTULA FLOW

Ideally fistula flow would be monitored during the postoperative period because it correlates well with fistula performance and certain flow-related complications. For example, if fistula flow is under 300 ml/min, it is probably not adequate for perfusion; if it is initially less than 150 ml/min or has been higher but is steadily dropping, the fistula will inevitably undergo thrombosis. At the other end of the scale, when fistula flow increases, particularly when greater than 800 ml/min, the likelihood of distal steal is high; when fistula flow is greater than 1000 ml/min, the risk of cardiac embarrassment becomes significant, particularly in older patients.

The principle of measuring flow transcutaneously with Doppler scan is based on the equation:

$$\overline{V} = \frac{\Delta F \times c}{2f(\cos\theta)}$$

where:

$\overline{V}$ = Mean velocity
F = Frequency of incident sound beam
c = Velocity of sound in tissue (1.56×10^5)
θ = Angle of incident sound beam

Flow (Q) can then be calculated as the product of $\overline{V}$ and A, the cross-sectional area. The two essential components are the angle of the probe to the artery and its area. If the vessel is concentric, close, and parallel to the skin, the probe angle can be established with reasonable accuracy and the diameter from a power scan can be used to estimate area.

In practice, a pulsed Doppler probe is scanned across the artery, giving a velocity profile that can be integrated to produce the mean velocity.[19] The same sweep can give both a depth scan and a power scan, and the arterial diameter can be determined by subtending vertical angles from the edge of the velocity profile to the depth scan. The mean velocity recording is produced by using a filter to time average the velocity profile signal. A frequency-to-voltage converter allows a direct calibrated reading of ΔF, and because the other factors of the Doppler equation are constant, mean velocity can be read directly. However, it cannot be applied directly to the fistula because the probe angle cannot be established with certainty and the rapid, turbulent flow produces errors in estimating $\overline{V}$. Instead, flow over the major arterial inflow to the extremity is measured and compared with that of the contralateral normal vessel at the same level, with the difference assumed to represent fistula flow. Obviously such an approach will not accurately estimate flow in an eccentrically narrowed arteriosclerotic vessel whose anatomic course in relation to the skin surface is not determinable. For most, this approach proved too difficult and time consuming, but now it can be more readily applied using the newer prototypes of duplex scanner with appropriate software modifications and appropriate probe selection for the depth of the artery. Cross-sectional areas of normal arteries are rather easily obtained. However, the main source of error will continue to be the angle of incidence of the ultrasound beam, since being a few degrees off greatly affects the estimate of flow. This approach is useful in problem cases but cannot be justified for routine serial examination.

CONCLUSION

Existing noninvasive diagnostic methods, although developed primarily for the detection of arterial and venous occlusive lesions, have practical value in the evaluation and management of AV fistulas, particularly the congenital and angioaccess types. Measurements of relative and absolute fistula flow using radionuclides and advanced Doppler instrumentation add an important quantitative dimension and, with further technical refinement, should establish their place in clinical practice. In congenital vascular malformations, MRI now answers questions of the anatomic extent of the malformation.

REFERENCES

1. Anderson CB et al: Local blood flow characteristics of arteriovenous fistulas in the forearm for dialysis, *Surg Gynecol Obstet* 144:531, 1977.
2. Barnes RW: Non-invasive assessment of arteriovenous fistula, *Angiology* 29:691, 1978.
3. Brener BJ, Brief DK, Parsonnet AV: *The effect of vascular access procedure on digital hemodynamics.* In Diethrich EB, ed: *Noninvasive cardiovascular diagnosis: current concepts,* Baltimore, 1978, University Park Press.
4. Fee HJ, Golding AL: Lower extremity ischemia after femoral arteriovenous bovine shunts, *Ann Surg* 183:42, 1976.
5. Frohlich ED, DeWolfe VG, Vugrincic CF: Unusual arteriovenous communications: arteriographic and hemodynamic studies, *Cleve Clin Q* 38:153, 1971.

6. Gosling RG, King DH: Audio signals in arteriovenous bruits: use in flow monitoring and possible relevance to clotting, *J Appl Physiol* 27:106, 1969.

7. Heitz SE et al: Value of arterial pressure measurements in the proximal and distal part of the thigh in arterial occlusive disease, *Surg Gynecol Obstet* 146:337, 1978.

8. Holman E, ed: *Abnormal arteriovenous communications, peripheral and intra-cardiac acquired and congenital,* ed 2, Springfield, Ill, 1968, Charles C Thomas.

9. Ingebritsen R, Husom O: Local blood pressure in congenital arteriovenous fistulae, *Acta Med Scand* 163:169, 1959.

10. Johnson G Jr, Blythe WB: Hemodynamic effects of arteriovenous shunts used for hemodialysis, *Ann Surg* 171:715, 1970.

11. Lichti EL, Erickson TG: Traumatic arteriovenous fistula: clinical evaluation and intraoperative monitoring with the Doppler ultrasonic flowmeter, *Am J Surg* 127:333, 1974.

12. Lindenauer SM: The Klippel-Trenaunay syndrome: varicosity, hypertrophy and hemangioma with no arteriovenous fistula, *Ann Surg* 162:303-314, 1965.

13. Pearce WH et al: Nuclear magnetic resonance imaging: its diagnostic value in patients with congenital vascular malformations of the limbs, *J Vasc Surg* 8:64-67, 1988.

14. Pisko-Dubienski ZA et al: Identification and successful treatment of congenital microfistulas with the aid of directional Doppler, *Surgery* 78:564, 1975.

15. Rhodes BA et al: Arteriovenous shunt measurements in extremities, *J Nucl Med* 13:357, 1972.

16. Rittenhouse EA, Brockenbrough EC: A method for assessing the circulation distal to a femoral artery obstruction, *Surg Gynecol Obstet* 129:538, 1969.

17. Rittenhouse E et al: Directional arterial flow velocity: a sensitive index of changes in peripheral vascular resistance, *Surgery* 79:350, 1976.

18. Rutherford RB: *Clinical applications of a method of quantitating arteriovenous shunting in extremities.* In Rutherford RB, ed: *Vascular surgery,* Philadelphia, 1977, Saunders.

19. Rutherford RB, Fleming PW, McLeod RD: *Vascular diagnostic methods for evaluating patients with arteriovenous fistulas.* In Diethrich EB, ed: *Noninvasive cardiovascular diagnosis: current concepts,* Baltimore, 1978, University Park Press.

20. Strandness DE Jr, Gibbons GE, Bell JW: Mercury strain gauge plethysmography, *Arch Surg* 85:215, 1962.

21. Sumner DS: *Diagnostic evaluation of arteriovenous fistulas.* In Rutherford RB, ed: *Vascular surgery,* ed 3, Philadelphia, 1989, Saunders.

22. Szilagyi DE et al: Congenital arteriovenous anomalies of the limbs, *Arch Surg* 111:423, 1976.

23. Yao ST et al: Limb blood flow in congenital arteriovenous fistula, *Surgery* 73:80, 1973.

CHAPTER 72

Clinical experience with transcutaneous Po_2 and Pco_2 measurements

ARNOST FRONEK

Transcutaneous Po_2 ($tcPo_2$) and to a lesser degree transcutaneous Pco_2 ($tcPco_2$) have been examined in the last several years to evaluate their clinical usefulness. This effort was stimulated by the noninvasive nature of the methodology as well as by its ease of operation.[29] The attractiveness of this approach is potentiated by the fact that it offers an objective estimate of oxygen delivery to the skin, which is critically important in the widening spectrum of reconstructive vascular surgery. In addition, it offers results independent of the mechanical properties of the arterial wall that can be a source of erroneous pressure measurements, especially in diabetics.

The $tcPo_2$ probe is usually operated under conditions of cutaneous hyperemia achieved by increasing the skin temperature to 43° C to 44° C. Several investigators, however, have evaluated $tcPo_2$ results obtained with minimal skin heating (37° C). These studies demonstrated that the monitored $tcPo_2$ values are drastically reduced (to 2 to 15 mm Hg)[12] and that the reproducibility is also worse than with the more conventional 44° C probe temperature. However, it does permit recordings of reflex changes that are otherwise suppressed with the high skin temperature.[12]

Ewald, Rooth, and Tuvemo[23] demonstrated that with a skin temperature kept at 37° C, it is possible to obtain a postocclusive reactive hyperemia response that is diminished in diabetics, whereas there is no significant difference in the recovery parameters after a transient occlusion if the probe temperature is kept at 44° C.[21] Under the latter conditions there is no transient hyperemic response, probably because the cutaneous vascular bed is already maximally vasodilated. This explains the different results obtained during a variety of tests involving various limb positions, transitional occlusion, and the effects of drugs. It was anticipated that these tests could increase the accuracy of the $tcPo_2$ measurement and reduce the considerable overlap of resting values obtained in normal control subjects and patients with peripheral arterial occlusive disease (PAOD).

LEG POSITION

In normal extremities, $tcPo_2$ values decrease with leg dependency, especially if the skin temperature is maintained at 37° C.[12] In patients with severe PAOD (Fontaine classification IV), an increase is usually observed. The response is different with a 44° C heated probe. The change from a supine to sitting position induced an average increase of 15.1 ± 7.1 mm Hg in control subjects, whereas the increase in patients with PAOD was 28.1 ± 14.2 mm Hg.[27] Leg dependency is recommended by Becker et al[2,3] to improve the classification of patients with PAOD. If forefoot $tcPo_2$ (44° C, in the sitting position) was greater than 40 mm Hg, only 5% of the patients required amputation, whereas those with an increase less than 10 mm Hg had an 85% chance of amputation. Johnson et al[35] arrived at similar conclusions using 44° C skin temperature. They observed a 22 mm Hg increase in $tcPo_2$ if the site of measurement was 36 cm below heart level. Severely diseased patients did not respond at all to leg dependency. These investigators even recommended leg dependency (in combination with oxygen inhalation) as a therapeutic procedure. Leg dependency $tcPo_2$ response can also be used as an indicator of revascularization success. Patients with rest pain showed an average increase of 20 mm Hg with the leg in dependent position, whereas the average postoperative increase was about 70 mm Hg.[52]

TRANSITIONAL OCCLUSION

As mentioned, a relatively low skin temperature is needed to demonstrate a postocclusive reactive hyperemia response. Ewald, Tuvemo, and Rooth[24] found 37° C to be the optimum temperature, although even with this temperature the initial $tcPo_2$ value is rather low (1 to 12 mm Hg). This reduces the value of initial $tcPo_2$ but produces a response in the range of 7.5 to 22.5 mm Hg. The reproducibility of the response (coefficient of variation) was 14%, and day-to-day variation was 19% to 28%.[21] It is interesting to note that children exhibited a greater postocclusive reactive hyperemia response than adults, and females showed higher responses than males.

In most cases, however, the 44° C probe temperature is used. Although the overshoot response is abolished, various indices that reflect the rate of circulatory recovery may be used. Franzeck et al[27] measured the $tcPo_2$ T/2 (the time it takes to reach 50% of the initial tcPo₂ value) after a 4-minute occlusion: in control subjects it was 87.1 ± 27.3 seconds compared with 136.1 ± 73.2 seconds (measured on the dorsum of the foot) in patients with severe PAOD. Similar results were reported by Kram et al,[40] who found a transcutaneous oxygen recovery half-time (TORT) of less than 1.5 minutes in normal subjects; limbs with symptomatic PAOD yielded higher values. These results based on the limb/chest ratio are similar to those observed by Franzeck et al,[27] who used single, nonnormalized limb tcPo₂ values. This is noteworthy for two reasons: (1) it is important to evaluate the significance of normalizing the limb tcPo₂ readings (in analogy to limb segment/arm pressure index) because normalization (chest or arm tcPo₂) requires either an additional apparatus or adds an additional 30 minutes to the examination, and (2) the same authors[40] described an increase in chest tcPo₂ during the occlusion that persisted for several minutes after release of occlusion, which has not been confirmed by other investigators.

The TORT is also a useful index in postoperative evaluation. It is significantly shorter in successful cases, although it usually does not reach normal values, probably due to residual disease. The same group[41] also compared the TORT with the pulse reappearance half-time (PRT/2)[30] and found the TORT to be superior. The lesser discriminating capability of the PRT/2 is mainly because of a large number of pulseless limbs that made the PRT/2 determination impossible. More recently, Lusiani et al[45] and Slagsvold et al[73] analyzed the accuracy of several indices reflecting the postocclusive response. They found the oxygen reappearance time (ORT) more promising than the oxygen recovery time index (ORI), which reflects the slope of the postocclusive recovery curve. All patients had an ORT longer than 20 seconds, but most important, this index (monitored from the dorsum of the foot) was able to differentiate claudicants, normal subjects, and patients with critical ischemia. As a follow-up, Slagsvold et al[72] compared the postischemic tcPo₂ indices with capillary morphology and found good correlation between pathologic ORT, ORI values, and pericapillary edema and hemorrhages as detected by vital microscopy.[25]

EFFECT OF EXERCISE

The inadequate separation between normal subjects and claudicants offered by the resting tcPo₂ values prompted several researchers to use different "sensitizing" methods to improve the diagnostic accuracy. By recognizing the good results observed with the effect of exercise on the ankle/arm pressure index, it was only natural that the same approach was tried with tcPo₂ monitoring. Various types of exercises were tried because the standard treadmill-type exercise test is often too difficult for patients with critical ischemia (Fontaine III or IV). Ohgi et al[60] used the old Ratschow foot exercise test and demonstrated good separation between critical ischemia and normal subjects, but the separation of claudicants was less convincing. Hauser

and Shoemaker[32] and Holdich et al[33] used a standardized treadmill protocol, but the correlation between the tcPo₂ drop and pain-free walking distance was not satisfactory. This can be explained either by the unreliability of the pain-free walking distance determination or by the changes in the protocol imposed by the limitations of exercise performance in older patients. Schmidt et al[70] recently reported good separation of normal subjects from claudicants (Fontaine classification II) on the basis of tcPo₂ drop induced by treadmill exercise at 5 km/hr and an inclination of 10% for 750 meters or until they became symptomatic. Simultaneously recorded tcPco₂ offered less useful information with the exception of recovery time, which was significantly delayed in the patient group (6 minutes versus 2 minutes for controls). Although the exercise-induced tcPo₂ drop and delayed recovery indices seem to be promising, technical difficulties such as probe leakage during exercise and maintaining a standardized protocol make this sensitizing procedure less desirable.

AMPUTATION LEVEL DETERMINATION

Although it was soon recognized that resting tcPo₂ values with a 44° C probe temperature does not offer sufficient accuracy for separating patients with PAOD from normal patients,[15,27,42,45] it became evident that the viability of the skin can be reliably evaluated on the basis of tcPo₂ determination. There is a relatively wide range of critical tcPo₂ values that separates successful from unsuccessful amputation stump healing, and the majority of researchers consider 40 to 30 mm Hg as the critical dividing line.* Malone et al[46] concluded that a tcPo₂ value greater than 20 mm Hg is associated with primary healing of an amputation stump. Kram, Appel, and Shoemaker[39] found that a calf/brachial tcPo₂ ratio greater than 0.20 predicted successful amputation stump healing. Franzeck et al[27] considered 10 mm Hg as a dividing line but found some primary amputation stump healing even below a tcPo₂ of 10 mm Hg. Since then, false-negative findings have also been found by other investigators, and the inhalation of oxygen has been used to increase the accuracy of predicting primary amputation stump healing. Harward et al[31] found that an increase of more than 10 mm Hg after oxygen inhalation predicted successful primary amputation stump healing, even if the initial (preinhalation) tcPo₂ value was below the 10 mm Hg level. This was recently confirmed by Oishi, Franek, and Golbranson,[61] who found that values above 10 mm Hg are reliable predictors of successful amputation stump healing, whether they are measured as an initial value or after oxygen inhalation. This method also proved to be superior to ankle blood pressure, Doppler velocity measurement, and laser Doppler flux determination. McCollum, Spence, and Walker[49] prefer the determination of rate of change of tcPo₂ during oxygen inhalation. They consider less than 9 mm Hg/min as the dividing line.

---

*References 11, 14, 18, 36, 53, 65, 67, 75.

Bongard and Krähenbühl followed an abbreviated natural history of patients with severe PAOD. They found that patients who responded with less than a 10 mm Hg increase to 100% oxygen inhalation had to undergo an amputation within 13 months.

Lantsberg and Goldman[44] reported less encouraging results when resting tcPo$_2$ values were used to predict amputation stump healing. The scatter of values was too big to be meaningful and was inferior to laser Doppler flux results. It should be pointed out, however, that there were no amputation failures reported in this series, which makes it even more difficult to determine a dividing line. Most important, no sensitizing procedures were used in these tcPo$_2$ studies. At present, it is difficult to explain the relatively wide range of critical tcPo$_2$ values predicting amputation stump healing as reported by various investigators. It can be assumed that in addition to different clinical criteria and practices, one of the most important factors may be the differences in electrical specifications of the tcPo$_2$ probes used. Various electrodes have different oxygen consumptions that are negligible under normal oxygen supply conditions. A high oxygen consumption electrode, however, can use up much of the oxygen available under limited supply conditions, thus producing a false-positive result.

POSTOPERATIVE MONITORING

A number of investigators have found tcPo$_2$ useful in monitoring the immediate results of vascular reconstruction. Ohgi et al found a significant increase in a number of parameters (e.g., resting tcPo$_2$, exercise test, oxygen inhalation). Earlier results based on tcPo$_2$ comparison studies were reported by Eickhoff and Engell.[20] Lalka et al[43] found that a tcPo$_2$ less than or equal to 22 mm Hg or foot/chest tcPo$_2$ index less than or equal to 0.53 predicts that revascularization is likely to fail. Kram, Appel, and Shoemaker[38] found the postocclusive recovery time most useful to predict success or failure of femoro-popliteal bypass grafts: foot tcPo$_2$ recovery times of 3.1 ± 1.2 and 4.6 ± 0.9 minutes corresponded to postoperative success and failure, respectively. Osmundson, Rooke, and Hallett[62] combined the initial resting tcPo$_2$ values obtained in the supine position with those obtained after 3 minutes of leg elevation. Patients with critical ischemia had a foot/chest index of 0.30 and a mean elevation-induced index of 0.06, whereas patients with aortoiliac disease and claudication but with neither rest pain nor trophic changes had an index of greater than 0.5 supine and 0.15 with elevation. Both parameters improved significantly after vascular reconstruction. Rooke and Osmundson[68] analyzed the correlation of PAOD severity with foot tcPo$_2$ and the response to leg elevation. On the basis of their results, it can be concluded that the percentage decrease is closely related to the severity of the disease. If Fontaine's classification is applied to their description, the following relationship can be established: Fontaine IIa, IIb, III correspond to ~90%, ~76%, ~61%, respectively. tcPo$_2$ was reduced in diabetics with severely limiting claudication

and rest pain, whereas diabetics with minimal symptoms had normal tcPo$_2$ values. Rhodes and Cogan described islands of ischemia surrounded by well-perfused skin and overall improved tcPo$_2$ values postoperatively, whereas nonhealing foot ulcers after revascularization were encircled by skin areas whose tcPo$_2$ remained unaffected.

Oh, Provan, and Anidi[58] used the increase in tcPo$_2$ induced by standing as a predictor of graft patency. They concluded that an increase of less than 15 mm Hg predicts a poor prognosis for arterial reconstruction, probably reflecting inadequate runoff conditions. Wyss et al[76] pointed out that the usual predictive criteria related to reconstruction do not apply to diabetics. Although a postoperative tcPo$_2$ below 20 mm Hg predicts an unfavorable clinical outcome, they also observed diabetics with postoperative tcPo$_2$ values greater than 20 mm Hg with an unfavorable outcome. Finally, Andersen et al[1] recommend perioperative tcPo$_2$ monitoring during abdominal aortic bypass grafting. The immediate and significant improvement in tcPo$_2$ values after insertion of the vascular prosthesis may contribute to intraoperative quality assurance.

TcPo$_2$ IN VENOUS DISEASE

In contrast to PAOD, tcPo$_2$ determination in patients with suspected venous disease is still within the domain of research. Although most investigators have found tcPo$_2$ to be reduced in extreme cases of venous disease (e.g., in venous ulcers), the diagnostic and pathophysiologic implications are still unclear. Partsch[63] described a decreased tcPo$_2$ in the presence of increased dermal blood flow as documented by increased laser Doppler flux values in the proximity of venous ulcers. Comparing the response to oxygen inhalation of venous ulcers and arterial ulcers, Partsch[63] documented an almost normal tcPo$_2$ increase in the former, but the tcPo$_2$ change in the proximity of arterial ulcers was significantly reduced. The author's explanation that there is maximal vasodilatation is supported by the finding that laser Doppler flux values do not increase if skin temperature is increased to 40° C, although it is increased in control subjects by about 2.5 arbitrary units (AU) (from 0.5).

The reduced tcPo$_2$ values in venous disease, reported by a number of investigators,* can also be explained by the results obtained with a modified tcPo$_2$ electrode that permits simultaneous vital microscopy.[28,34] Significantly decreased tcPo$_2$ values correlated well with areas of reduced capillary density. For example, in patches of atrophic blanche, the tcPo$_2$ value was zero. The heterogeneity of tcPo$_2$ findings was also pointed out by Falanga et al,[26] who confirmed reduced tcPo$_2$ values in legs with venous ulcers but also found a variability of tcPo$_2$ in the skin surrounding the ulcers. Belcaro et al[6] evaluated tcPo$_2$ and tcPco$_2$ in normal subjects and patients with postphlebitic syndrome. Although there was no statistically significant difference in tcPo$_2$ val-

---

*References 8, 16, 37, 47, 48, 57, 71.

ues, they found a significantly higher tcP_{CO_2} in the patient group.

In contrast to these findings, Dodd, Gaylarde, and Sarkany[17] described an increased tcP_{O_2} in liposclerotic skin when using a 37° C heated electrode. (All the studies described were performed with a 44° C heated tcP_{O_2} probe.) The question of tcP_{O_2} values came into the center of attention after Browse and Burnand[10] published their theory regarding the genesis of venous ulceration, incriminating pericapillary fibrinogen deposits with reduced oxygen diffusion. This theory is now being scrutinized more thoroughly in view of the disappointing results with fibrinolytic therapy in lipodermatosclerosis. There are also theoretical reasons that lead researchers to question the "fibrin cuff" theory. A significant disproportionality between the large fibrin and the small oxygen molecule has been cited by Michel.[50] On the other hand, Stacey et al[74] documented reduced tcP_{O_2} readings in apparently normal contralateral limbs where the other limb presented with venous ulceration or a healed ulcer. This would indirectly indicate that there already may be some oxygen diffusion block in the apparently normal limb. This assumption may be strengthened by the reduced postischemic tcP_{O_2} response in patients with severe venous disease.[64] Moosa et al[51] found tcP_{O_2} values significantly reduced in the proximity of venous ulcers, and in addition, the response to oxygen inhalation was found to be reduced when compared with that recorded with the chest electrode. Reduced resting tcP_{O_2} values were found not only in the skin close to venous ulcers but also in the beginning stages of venous disease.[48] Although the significantly lower tcP_{O_2} values in the proximity of venous ulcers could be confirmed by Nemeth, Eaglstein, and Falanga,[54] they had no predictive value because there was no difference between healed and unhealed groups.

EFFECT OF VENOACTIVE DRUGS

Venoactive drugs can increase the tcP_{O_2} and decrease the tcP_{CO_2} values.[5] Similar results were reported by Neumann and van den Brock[56] with the same drug (Venoruton) after 4 weeks and to a lesser extent even after 2 weeks.

Factors influencing tcP_{O_2} in venous disease

Edema. External intermittent compression reduces edema in ulcerated limbs, but this procedure has no effect on the tcP_{O_2} values.[55] This would indicate that edema has no significant effect on tcP_{O_2} values, a conclusion that has still to be verified because it contradicts the results reported by Kolari, Pakanmäki, and Pohjola,[37] who found an increase in tcP_{O_2} accompanied by decreased edema. The effect of 4 weeks of 4 hours/day intermittent compression was evaluated in patients with severe venous disease.[13] Although some changes in xenon-133 clearance and laser Doppler flux have been observed, there were no changes in tcP_{O_2} values.

Elastic compression. Rooke et al[69] described an interesting method to estimate a so-called venomotor index by com-

paring the tcP_{O_2} values obtained with two different temperatures, 42° C and 45° C; the index is the ratio of these two values. They found a decreased tcP_{O_2} and decreased venomotor index in stasis dermatitis, which improved with elastic compression.

EFFECT OF EXERCISE AND LEG DEPENDENCY

Normal control subjects as well as patients with mild degrees of venous disease (varicose veins) showed no difference in the initial tcP_{O_2}, although there was a significant increase in both groups after 20 minutes in a standing position.[16] Remarkably, no change was observed in a group of patients with severe venous disease (skin changes or ulceration), although the initial tcP_{O_2} values were significantly lower than those in the normal control group.

Seemingly contradictory results were reported by Dodd et al,[17] who observed a decrease in tcP_{O_2} on standing in controls as well as in patients with venous insufficiency. The difference can be explained, however, by the lower tcP_{O_2} probe temperature (37° C) used in these studies, if it can be assumed that the higher probe temperature (44° C) used in the former studies suppressed the vasoconstrictor reflex responsible for the tcP_{O_2} drop. It is interesting to note that exercise (e.g., plantar dorsiflexion) used by the same group yielded similar results as those reported by Clyne et al[16] despite the fact that there was a difference in probe temperature. In patients with significant venous valvular insufficiency, there was no tcP_{O_2} change after exercise, probably because exercise did not lead to the significant drop in venous pressure that would occur under normal hemodynamic conditions and that removes the stimulus for reflex vasoconstriction. In patients, however, venous pressure remains high during exercise, and it can be assumed that reflex vasoconstriction persists. Dodd et al[17] concluded that although normal legs are protected by a rise in skin oxygenation during exercise, this does not occur in patients with venous insufficiency and that the sustained low skin oxygen tension in the upright position even during exercise is responsible for leg ulcer development.

CONCLUSION

The application of tcP_{O_2} value determination to clinical practice has emphasized the importance of the microcirculation in diagnostic decision making. After many studies that have systematically examined the capabilities of this new diagnostic tool, some areas are already firmly delineated but others need additional investigation. Currently, it seems that tcP_{O_2} determination has its prime area of application in the field of arterial occlusive disease, mainly in the quantification of disease severity and specifically in the determination of optimal amputation level.

Although the lower probe temperature (37° C) seems to fulfill physiologic requirements, considerable uncertainties accompany the very low skin P_{O_2} recorded with a 37° C heated probe. It seems that the main areas of application of this low temperature probe are studies in which reflex responses are the prime interest. In all other studies, the 44° C heated probe is preferred, despite the maximum hyperemia induced by this temperature.

In view of the rather poor separation capability of resting tcPo$_2$ values, a number of ancillary sensitizing procedures have been tested, and it seems that transitional ischemia, oxygen exposure, and leg position changes are the more useful tests; the technical difficulties often associated with exercise make it less satisfactory as an ancillary sensitizing method.

The application of tcPo$_2$ in the evaluation of venous disease is not yet clearly defined, although it seems established that it helps to quantify the impaired skin viability in severe venous disease and thus may help in evaluating therapeutic procedures.

Although the preliminary results with tcPco$_2$ are disappointing, there is not enough experience and information for a definitive conclusion. Considering various well-known physiologic and pathophysiologic facts related to increased Pco$_2$, systematic research in this area must continue.

REFERENCES

1. Andersen PT et al: Lower limb transcutaneous oxygen tension during aortic bypass grafting, *Thorac Cardiovasc Surg* 35:342-344, 1987.
2. Becker F et al: Predictive value of tcPo$_2$ in chronic severe ischemia of the lower limbs, *Intl J Microcirc Clin Exp* 7:261-271, 1988.
3. Becker F et al: *Transcutaneous oxygen pressure and chronic peripheral arterial occlusive disease.* In Messer K, ed: *Ischemic diseases and the microcirculation,* Munich, 1989, Zuckschwerdt.
4. Belcaro G, Rulo A, Candiam C: An evaluation of the microcirculatory effects of Venoruton in patients with chronic venous hypertension by laser Doppler flowmetry, transcutaneous Po$_2$ and Pco$_2$ measurements, leg volumetry and ambulatory venous pressure measurements, *VASA* 18:146-151, 1989.
5. Belcaro G, Rulo A, Candiam C: An evaluation of the microcirculatory effects of Venouton in patients with chronic venous hypertension by laser Doppler flowmetry, transcutaneous Po$_2$ and Pco$_2$ measurements, leg volumetry and ambulatory venous pressure measurements, *Phlebology* 4:23-29, 1989.
6. Belcaro G, et al: Combined evaluation of postphlebitic limbs by laser Doppler flowmetry and transcutaneous Po$_2$/Pco$_2$ measurements, *VASA* 17:259-261, 1988.
7. Bongard O, Krähenbühl B: Predicting amputation in severe ischaemia: the value of transcutaneous Po$_2$ measurement, *Br J Bone Joint Surg* 70-B:465-467, 1988.
8. Borzykowski J, Krähenbühl B: Measurement of pedal transcutaneous oxygen tension to follow up lower limb arterial occlusive disease, *VASA* 10:37-40, 1981.
9. Borzykowski J, Krähenbühl B: Mésure non invasive de l'oxyénation cutanée en cas d'ulcères chroniques des membres inférieurs, *Schw Med Wchsch* 111:1972-1974, 1981.
10. Browse NL, Burnand KG: The cause of venous ulceration, *Lancet* II:243-245, 1982.
11. Burgess EM et al: Segmental transcutaneous measurements of Po$_2$ in patients requiring BK amputation for peripheral vascular insufficiency, *J Bone Joint Surg* 64-A:378-382, 1982.
12. Caspary L, Creutzig A, Alexander K: *Comparison of laser-Doppler-flux and tcPo$_2$, in healthy probands and patients with arterial ischemia.* In Huch A, Huch R, Rooth G, eds: *Continuous transcutaneous monitoring (advances in experimental medicine and biology 220),* New York, 1987, Plenum Press.
13. Cheatle TR et al: Three tests of microcirculatory function in the evaluation of treatment for chronic venous insufficiency, *Phlebology* 5:165-172, 1990.
14. Cina C, Katsamouris A, Megerman J: Utility of transcutaneous oxygen tension measurements in peripheral arterial occlusive disease, *J Vasc Surg* 1:362-371, 1989.
15. Clyne CAC, et al: Oxygen tension on the skin of ischemic legs, *Am J Surg* 143:315-318, 1982.
16. Clyne CAC et al: Oxygen tension on the skin of the gaiter area of limbs with venous disease, *Brit J Surg* 72:644-647, 1985.
17. Dodd HJ, Gaylarde PM, Sarkany J: Skin oxygen tension in venous insufficiency of the lower leg, *J Royal Soc Med* 78:373-376, 1985.
18. Dowd GSE, Linge K, Bentley G: The effect of age and sex in normal volunteers upon the transcutaneous oxygen tension in the lower limb, *Clin Phys Physiol Meas* 4:65-68, 1983.
19. Dowd GSE, Linge K, Beutler G: Measurement of transcutaneous oxygen pressure in normal and ischaemic skin, *Br J Bone Joint Surg* 65:79-83, 1983.
20. Eikhoff JH, Engell HC: Transcutaneous oxygen tension (tcPo$_2$) measurements on the foot in normal subjects and in patients with peripheral artery disease admitted for vascular surgery, *Scand J Clin Lab Invest* 41:743-748, 1981.
21. Ewald U: Evaluation of the transcutaneous oxygen method used at 37° C for measurement of reactive hyperemia in the skin, *Clin Physiol* 4:413-423, 1984.
22. Ewald U, Huch A, Huch R: *Skin reactive hyperemia recorded by a combined tcPo$_2$ and laser Doppler sensor.* In Huch A, Huch R, Rooth G, eds: *Continuous transcutaneous monitoring (advances in experimental medicine and biology 220),* New York, 1987, Plenum Press.
23. Ewald U, Rooth G, Tuvemo T: Postischaemic hyperaemia studied with a transcutaneous oxygen electrode used at 33-37° C, *Scand J Clin Lab Invest* 41:641-645, 1981.
24. Ewald U, Tuvemo T, Rooth G: Early reduction of vascular reactivity in diabetic children detected by transcutaneous oxygen electrode, *Lancet* I:1287-1288, 1981.
25. Fagrell B, Lundberg G: A simplified evaluation of vital capillary microscopy for predicting skin viability with severe arterial insufficiency, *Clin Phys* 4:403-411, 1984.
26. Falanga V, McKenzie A, Eaglstein WH: Heterogeneity in oxygen diffusion around venous ulcers, *J Dermatol Surg Oncol* 17:336-339, 1991.
27. Franzeck UK et al: Transcutaneous Po$_2$ measurements in health and peripheral arterial occlusive disease, *Surgery* 91:156-163, 1982.
28. Franzeck UK et al: Transcutaneous oxygen tension and capillary morphologic characteristics and density in patients with chronic venous incompetence, *Circulation* 70:806-811, 1984.
29. Fronek A: *Noninvasive diagnostics of vascular disease,* New York, 1989, McGraw-Hill.
30. Fronek A, Coel M, Bernstein EF: The pulse-reappearance time: an index of overall blood flow impairment in the ischemic extremity, *Surgery* 81:376-381, 1977.
31. Harward TRS et al: Oxygen inhalation-induced transcutaneous Po$_2$ changes as a predictor of amputation level, *J Vasc Surg* 2:220-227, 1985.
32. Hauser JH, Shoemaker WC: Use of transcutaneous Po$_2$ regional perfusion index to quantify tissue perfusion in peripheral vascular disease, *Ann Surg* 197:337-343, 1983.
33. Holdich TAH et al: Transcutaneous oxygen tension during exercise in patients with claudication, *Brit Med J* 292:1625-1628, 1986.
34. Huch A et al: A transparent transcutaneous oxygen electrode for simultaneous studies of skin capillary morphology flow dynamics and oxygenation, *Intl J Microcirc Clin Exp* 2:103-108, 1983.
35. Johnson WC et al: Supplemental oxygen and dependent positioning as adjunctive measures to improve forefoot tissue oxygenation, *Arch Surg* 123:1227-1230, 1988.
36. Katsamouris A et al: Transcutaneous oxygen tension in selection of amputation level, *Am J Surg* 147:510-517, 1984.
37. Kolari PJ, Pakanmäki K, Pohjola RT: Transcutaneous oxygen tension in patients with post-thrombitic leg ulcers: treatment with intermittent pneumatic compression, *Cardiovasc Res* 22:138-141, 1988.
38. Kram HB, Appel PL, Shoemaker WC: Comparison of transcutaneous oximetry, vascular hemodynamic measurements, angiography, and clinical findings to predict the success of peripheral vascular reconstruction, *Am J Surg* 155:551-558, 1988.
39. Kram HB, Appel PL, Shoemaker WC: Multisensor transcutaneous oximetric mapping to predict below-knee amputation wound healing: use of a critical Po$_2$, *J Vasc Surg* 9:796-800, 1989.
40. Kram HB et al: Assessment of peripheral vascular disease by post-occlusive transcutaneous oxygen recovery time, *J Vasc Surg* 1:628-634, 1984.

41. Kram HB et al: Transcutaneous oxygen recovery and toe pulse reappearance time in the assessment of peripheral vascular disease, *Circulation* 72:1022-1027, 1985.
42. Kvernebo K et al: Response of skin photoplethysmography, laser Doppler flowmetry and transcutaneous oxygen tensiometry to stenosis-induced reduction in limb blood flow, *Eur J Vasc Surg* 2:1-8, 1988.
43. Lalka SG et al: Transcutaneous oxygen and carbon dioxide pressure monitoring to determine severity of limb ischemia and to predict surgical outcome, *J Vasc Surg* 7:507-514, 1988.
44. Lantsberg L, Goldman M: Laser Doppler flowmetry transcutaneous oxygen tension measurements and Doppler pressure compared in patients undergoing amputation, *Eur J Vasc Surg* 5:195-197, 1991.
45. Lusiani L et al: Transcutaneous oxygen tension (tcPo₂) measurement as a diagnostic tool in patients with peripheral vascular disease, *Angiology* 39:873-880, 1988.
46. Malone JM et al: Prospective comparison of noninvasive techniques for amputation level section, *Am J Surg* 154:179-184, 1987.
47. Mani R, Gorman FW, White JE: Transcutaneous measurements of oxygen tension at edges of leg ulcers: preliminary communication, *J Royal Soc Med* 79:650-654, 1986.
48. Mannarino E et al: Chronic venous incompetence and transcutaneous oxygen pressure: a controlled study, *VASA* 17:159, 1988.
49. McCollum PT, Spence VA, Walker WF: Oxygen inhalation induced changes in the skin as measured by transcutaneous oxymetry, *Br J Surg* 73:882-885, 1986.
50. Michel CC: Aetiology of venous ulceration, *Brit J Surg* 77:1071, 1990.
51. Moosa HH et al: Oxygen diffusion in chronic venous ulceration, *J Cardiovasc Surg* 28:464-467, 1987.
52. Moosa HH et al: Transcutaneous oxygen measurements in lower extremity ischemia: effects of position, oxygen inhalation and arterial reconstruction, *Surgery* 103:193-198, 1988.
53. Mustapha NM et al: Transcutaneous partial oxygen pressure assessment of the ischaemic lower limb, *Surg Gynecol Obstet* 156:582-584, 1983.
54. Nemeth AJ, Eaglstein WH, Falanga V: Clinical parameters and transcutaneous oxygen measurements for the prognosis of venous ulcers, *J Am Acad Dermatol* 20:186-190, 1989.
55. Nemeth AJ et al: Ulcerated edematosis limbs: effect of edema removal on transcutaneous oxygen measurements, *J Am Acad Dermatol* 20:191-197, 1989.
56. Neumann HAM, van den Brock MJTB: Evaluation of O-(β-hydroxyethyl)-rutosides in chronic venous insufficiency by means of non-invasive techniques, *Phlebology* 5(suppl 1):13-20, 1990.
57. Neumann HAM et al: Transcutaneous oxygen tension in chronic venous insufficiency syndrome, *VASA* 13:213-219, 1984.
58. Oh PI, Provan JL, Anidi FM: The predictability of success of arterial reconstruction by means of transcutaneous oxygen tension measurement, *J Vasc Surg* 5:356-362, 1987.
59. Ohgi S, Ho K, Mori T: *Quantitative evaluation of ischemic legs before and after arterial reconstruction by transcutaneous Po₂ measurement.* In Huch R, Huch A, eds: *Continuous transcutaneous blood gas monitoring,* New York, 1983, Dekker.
60. Ohgi S et al: Continuous measurement of transcutaneous oxygen tension on stress test in claudicants and normals, *Angiology* 37:27-35, 1986.
61. Oishi C, Fronek A, Golbranson FL: The role of non-invasive vascular studies in determining levels of amputation, *Am J Bone Joint Surg* 70:1520-1530, 1988.
62. Osmundson PJ, Rooke TW, Hallett JW: Effect of arterial revascularization transcutaneous oxygen tension of the ischemic extremity, *Mayo Clin Proc* 63:897-902, 1988.
63. Partsch H: Hypraemic hypoxia in venous ulceration, *Brit J Derm* 110:249-251, 1984.
64. Quigley FG, Faris IB: Transcutaneous oxygen potentials in venous disease, *Austr NZ J Surg* 59:165-168, 1989.
65. Ratliff DA, Chant ADB, Webster JHH: Prediction of amputation wound healing: the role of transcutaneous Po₂ assessment, *Brit J Surg* 71:219-222, 1984.
66. Rhodes GR, Cogan F: "Islands of ischemia." Transcutaneous Ptco₂ documentation of pedal malperfusion following lower limb revascularization, *Am J Surg* 51:407-413, 1985.
67. Rhodes GR, Skudder P: Salvage of ischemic diabetic feet: role of tcPo₂ mapping and multiple configurations of in-situ bypass, *Am J Surg* 152:165-171, 1986.
68. Rooke TW, Osmundson PJ: The influence of age, sex, smoking and diabetes on lower limb transcutaneous oxygen tension in patients with arterial occlusive disease, *Arch Int Med* 150:129-132, 1990.
69. Rooke TW et al: The effect of elastic compression on tcPo₂ in limbs with venous stasis, *Phlebology* 2:23-28, 1987.
70. Schmidt JA et al: Transcutaneous measurement of oxygen and carbon dioxide tension (tcPo₂ and tPco₂) during treadmill exercise in patients with arterial occlusive disease (AOD stages I and II), *Angiology* 41:547, 1990.
71. Sindrup JH et al: Transcutaneous Po₂ and laser Doppler blood flow measurements in 40 patients with venous leg ulcers, *Acta Dermatol Venerol (Stockholm)* 67:160-163, 1987.
72. Slagsvold CE, Rosen L, Stranden E: The relation between changes in capillary morphology induced by ischemia and the post-ischemic transcutaneous Po₂ response, *Intl J Microcirc Clin Exp* 10:117-125, 1991.
73. Slagsvold CE et al: Postischemic transcutaneous oxygen tension response in assessment of peripheral atherosclerosis, *Vasc Surg* 22:102-109, 1988.
74. Stacey MC et al: Changes in the apparently normal limb in unilateral venous ulceration, *Brit J Surg* 74:936-939, 1987.
75. White RA et al: Noninvasive evaluation of peripheral vascular disease using transcutaneous oxygen tension, *Am J Surg* 144:68-72, 1982.
76. Wyss CR et al: Relationship between transcutaneous oxygen tension, ankle blood pressure and clinical outcome of vascular surgery in diabetic and nondiabetic patients, *Surgery* 101:56-62, 1987.

CHAPTER 73

Clinical value of laser Doppler fluxmetering

ARNOST FRONEK

Since the introduction of laser Doppler fluxmetering (LDF) devices, various attempts have been made to find an appropriate place for this methodology in routine vascular diagnostic practice. Several features of the instrumentation promised rapid acceptance. These include noninvasiveness, ease of operation, and continuous monitoring capability. At the same time, however, several disadvantages reduced this initial enthusiasm, and efforts in the last several years have focused on overcoming technical problems such as lack of calibration capability, measurement reproducibility, and motion sensitivity.

Recently, clinical investigation has been centered around the significance of vasomotion, or flow motion. Two different flow phenomena have been identified, the higher one observed under conditions of compromised blood flow but ultimately disappearing completely under conditions of critical ischemia.

In view of questionable temporal and spatial reproducibility, this review emphasizes the evaluation of responses to standardized sensitizing methods. Postocclusive reactive hyperemia response has become the preferred method because it relies on measurement of relative changes and does not require calibration. Equally important are LDF responses induced by temperature changes and changes in leg position (effect of hydrostatics). The disappearance of the venoarteriolar reflex under conditions of ischemia and venous hypertension opens some specific diagnostic avenues. Finally, the usefulness of LDF monitoring is discussed as a tool in the evaluation of vasoactive drugs.

Although the LDF methodology has yet to find a niche in the armamentarium of the vascular laboratory, several promising avenues are being developed, and there is hope that LDF methodology will introduce clinical microcirculation into the daily consideration of peripheral vascular diagnostics.

REPRODUCIBILITY

Significant flux variations (spatial and temporal) were found by several investigators,[21,31] with coefficients of variation from 4% to 25%. These variations are largely caused by a highly responsive cutaneous vasculature and significant regional differences in anatomy and function. For example,

Sundberg[29] found that the forehead yielded the lowest coefficient of variation, but for continuous monitoring (e.g., physiologic testing, drug evaluation), even the forearm skin can serve as a suitable testing site. Studying hour-to-hour and day-to-day variations, no significant tendencies could be measured, although the lowest values were identified around noon. Unfortunately, there was no information as to whether these measurements were taken before or after food intake. Kvernebo, Slagsvold, and Gjoberg[13] demonstrated that although median values are satisfactorily reproducible for a given group of control subjects, this did not hold true for individual subjects. These investigators also determined that the highest LDF output was obtained from the pulp of the toe. This is most likely due to a high concentration of arteriovenous shunts, a fact to be considered when nutritional flow conditions are the focus of an investigation.

CALIBRATION

The output from currently available systems is usually the root mean square of the averaged spectrum of recorded frequencies that corresponds to the product of blood flow velocity and hematocrit.[28] Recently, a new processing mode of the Doppler-shifted signals has been employed resulting in an output that primarily reflects flow velocity changes and is less sensitive to changes in hematocrit.[15] The application of a rotating disk carrying a blood smear of known hematocrit also makes it possible to calibrate and standardize the whole system, including the probe.

VASOMOTION

Rhythmical variations of flux within the skin have been recognized, which are independent of the central nervous system, as documented by the observation that anesthetic block of the nerve innervating the examined region had no effect on the LDF output.[21,32] Considerable differences in vasomotion temporal patterns have been described.[5,26,27] The low frequency (LF) (2 cycles/min) waves that were usually seen in normal subjects can be distinguished from the high frequency (HF) ($\approx$ 9 cycles/min) waves that were found more often in patients with severe ischemia. Because of the diagnostic potential, more sophisticated analytical methods have been applied to extract both the flux amplitudes and the frequencies of these spontaneous flow velocity fluctuations. Hoffmann et al[10] described a digital filter system that yields a frequency histogram. This approach is more suitable for the detection of low amplitude contents than systems using the fast Fourier algorithm, which is more amplitude dependent.[22–24] HF waves were seen more often in patients with severe limb ischemia, and the amplitudes diminished with increasing severity of disease. Hoffmann, Schneider, and Bollinger[9] demonstrated the sensitivity of this method in an analysis of vasomotion patterns before and after transluminal angioplasty. After successful treatment, prevalence of HF waves decreased but the number remained unchanged after failed procedures. The prevalence of LF waves was not affected by the procedure. Similar results have been reported by Moneta et al[16] from the same laboratory comparing the LDF results with ankle pressure measurements. There was no correlation, which raises the question of small versus large artery disease; ankle pressure primarily reflecting the latter abnormality. However, vasomotion patterns seem to correlate well if ankle pressure is at least 80 mm Hg. Schmidt et al[25] recently found a 12% prevalence of slow waves in patients with mild peripheral arterial occlusive disease (PAOD) (Fontaine I and II), whereas the incidence increased to 84% in patients in the Fontaine III and IV group.

Based on microcirculatory experiments and these pathophysiologic observations, it can be concluded that vasomotion patterns are an expression of the arteriolar autoregulatory mechanism. Vasomotion is accentuated under conditions of reduced perfusion but diminishes with severe ischemia, a condition during which LDF-monitored vasomotion also disappears.

LDF-INDUCED RESPONSES

Several investigators have concluded that the scatter of LDF resting values is too large to permit separation of patients with ischemic peripheral vasculature from normal control subjects. Various sensitizing maneuvers have been evaluated to improve sensitivity, including: postocclusive reactive hyperemia, increased temperature, and leg position (hydrostatics).

POSTOCCLUSIVE REACTIVE HYPEREMIA

Vasodilatation of the terminal vasculature in response to transient ischemia is a well-known physiologic phenomenon and has been frequently used to sensitize a diagnostic procedure.[8] Although a standardized and highly reproducible postocclusive reactive hyperemia response has been demonstrated,[17] the LDF response to postocclusive reactive hyperemia (PDRH) depends on the initial perfusion conditions among other factors. The extent to which the LDF response can be used to quantify the degree of arterial occlusive disease has not been clearly determined. Kvernebo, Slagsvold, and Stranden[14] analyzed the PORH response in several groups of patients and control subjects. They found that the delay between tourniquet deflation and the first increase in recorded flux (T_1) was the most sensitive index for sepa-

rating normal subjects, claudicants, and patients with severe ischemia (Fontaine III and IV classification).

In a previous study, Pabst et al[19] used the peak PORH response and found significant differences between controls and severely ischemic patients but less significant differences between those groups and claudicants. In an earlier study, Karanfilian et al[11] identified vascular beds with a relatively high LDF output (e.g., finger, toe, forehead) and those with significantly lower signals (e.g., plantar and dorsal aspect of the foot). They also found significant differences in resting baseline values between control subjects and patients with peripheral arterial disease; however, this latter group consisted primarily of patients with severe ischemia. A better separation was obtained by using the PORH response, and the most sensitive index was found to be the time to maximal response (18 seconds in the control group versus 150 seconds in the patient group). The observations of Del Guercio, Leonardo, and Arpaia[7] were even more encouraging because they studied patients in Fontaine group II (claudicants) without signs or symptoms of severe ischemia. From a qualitative viewpoint, they found a significant vasomotion response superimposed on the postocclusive reaction in about 80% of normal subjects, whereas only 35% of the patient group demonstrated this phenomenon. They also compared the PORH response induced by thigh cuff occlusion with that resulting from ankle cuff occlusion. The most pronounced difference was in the latency time between the end of occlusion and the subsequent resumption of cutaneous blood flow. Most encouraging was the difference in latency time when thigh compression was used; practically no overlap with the control group was seen, but there was some overlap of values if ankle compression was applied. Differences in the site of the occlusive disease may have been responsible for this overlap.

A less reliable separation was obtained by Seifert, Jäger, and Bollinger,[27] who found a significant reduction of PORH response in patients with severe ischemia but could not separate claudicants (Fontaine II classification) from the control group.

EFFECT OF TEMPERATURE

A number of phenomena related to smooth muscle activity have a temperature optimum. The built-in heating element available with some of the LDF systems makes it impossible to investigate the effect of temperature changes on resting flux as well as on induced responses.[18] It has been shown that by setting the thermostat at 40° C, a flux increase of about 70% can be achieved in normal subjects. Surprisingly, during the 10-minute heating period, the flux starts to decline after about the sixth minute and stabilizes thereafter at about 31% above the initial preheating value. The most plausible explanation for this is the autoregulatory response of the microvasculature. From a practical point of view, it is important to consider the inverse exponential relationship between the initial flux and the heat-induced response: the higher the initial flux, the smaller the response.[18] Creutzig et al[6] found 37° C to be the optimum temperature for LDF studies performed on the foot. Vasomotion activity was clearly higher at 37° C (skin temperature), but patients (Fontaine IIb with severe claudication) had lower frequencies than the control group. Change in skin temperature was also used by Sundberg and Castrén[30] to demonstrate vasomotor activity of dermal vasculature.

EFFECT OF LEG POSITION

Using the venoarteriolar reflex, Sundberg and Castrén[30] also examined the effect of increased venous pressure by occluding venous outflow with a 40 mm Hg cuff. They found a decrease of LDF in both healthy subjects and patients. Leg elevation caused an increase in LDF in both groups. The response to leg dependency was more informative, with a decrease in LDF in control subjects and an increase in patients. However, these results require some additional qualification because the significant increase occurred at 37° C, which may have influenced the venoarteriolar reflex, although the same temperature did not influence the response in the normal control group. These results are somewhat contradictory to those reported by Seifert, Jäger, and Bollinger,[27] who found a decrease in LDF values in the sitting position in patients as well as control subjects. It is possible that a lower thermostat setting (32° C) may be the explanation. Belcaro and Nicolaides[3] studied the effect of orthostatics on LDF in normal subjects, diabetics, claudicants, and patients with severe ischemia without altering the skin temperature. They found a significant reduction of LDF on standing in all normal volunteers, whereas there was no significant flux reduction in the patient group. It is of interest that after 1 week of nifedipine administration, the venoarteriolar response improved but was still below the normal range (greater than 25% of resting flux in normal subjects, on standing).

LDF AND EVALUATION OF VASOACTIVE SUBSTANCES

The ease of application and noninvasive character of the LDF method makes it potentially useful for investigating the efficacy of vasoactive drugs. In view of the variability of the method,[21,31] it is not yet clear whether long-term studies could yield reliable results with drugs that induce borderline vasoactive effects. The use of LDF to monitor short-term effects, however, was clearly documented by Sundberg,[29] who found a rapid and transient increase in LDF after administration of 0.5 mg of sublingual nitroglycerin. Sundberg and Castrén[30] demonstrated the vasoactive effects of a variety of drugs, including that of a transdermal nitroglycerine patch. Similarly, reliable results can be expected after intravenous or intraarterial administration of vasoactive substances, such as the infusion of prostaglandin E or energy-rich phosphates.[6] More recently Belcaro and Nicolaides[4] demonstrated a significant increase in resting flux after oral administration of nifedipine for 1 week.

APPLICATION OF LDF IN VENOUS DISEASE

LDF has been used in two areas: skin viability with venous ulcers and the efficacy of the venoarteriolar reflex (VAR). Partsch[20] pointed out that the initial resting dermal flux in the area surrounding a venous ulcer is increased when compared to normal skin. In addition, a 40° C thermostat setting, which usually induces a significant increase in flux,[18] had practically no effect on perfusion. The reduced VAR response was described by Belcaro[1] in patients with a severe degree of venous valvular insufficiency (refilling time of less than 6 seconds). A similar reduction in VAR response was found in patients with postphlebitic syndrome.[4] The sensitivity of the VAR response was documented in two other studies by the same group in which venoactive drugs had improved the response in patients with venous hypertension.[2,3]

In conclusion, LDF has not yet found its permanent niche in the vascular diagnostic laboratory, but it can be expected to eventually play a role, especially in the quantitative evaluation of skin perfusion in patients with different degrees of arterial ischemia and in pharmacologic research.

REFERENCES

1. Belcaro G: *Evaluation of the venivasomotor response by a laser-Doppler flowmeter in patients with varicose ulcers due to chronic venous hypertension.* In Negas D, Jantet G, eds: *Phlebology 85,* London, 1986, J. Libby.
2. Belcaro G: Microvasculature evaluation by laser-Doppler flowmetry of the effects of Centellase in the treatment of severe venous hypertension and leg ulcers, *Phlebology* 2:61-67, 1987.
3. Belcaro G, Nicolaides AN: Microvascular evaluation of the effects of Nifedipine in vascular patients by laser-Doppler flowmetry, *Angiology* 40:689-694, 1989.
4. Belcaro G, Christopoulous D, Nicolaides AN: Skin flow and swelling in postphlebitic limbs, *VASA* 18:136-139, 1989.
5. Bollinger A, Hoffmann U, Seifert H: *Flux motion in peripheral ischemia.* In Intaglietta M, ed: *Vasomotion and flow modulation in the microcirculation,* Basel, Switzerland, 1989, Karger.
6. Creutzig A, et al: Temperature-dependent laser Doppler fluxmetry in healthy and patients with peripheral arterial disease, *Int J Microcirc Clin Exp* 6:381-390, 1987.
7. Del Guercia R, Leonardo G, Arpaia MR: Evaluation of postischemic hyperemia on the skin using laser Doppler velocimetry: study on patients with claudicatio intermittens, *Microvasc Res* 32:289-299, 1986.
8. Fronek A: *Noninvasive diagnostics in vascular disease,* New York, 1989, McGraw-Hill.
9. Hoffman U, Schneider E, Bollinger A: Flow motion waves with high and low frequency in severe ischemia before and after percutaneous transluminal angioplasty, *Cardiovasc Res* 24:711-718, 1990.
10. Hoffmann U et al: The frequency histogram—a new method for the evaluation of laser Doppler flux motion, *Microvasc Res* 40:293-301, 1990.
11. Karanfilian RG et al: The assessment of skin blood flow in peripheral vascular disease by laser Doppler velocimetry, *Am J Surg* 50:641-644, 1984.
12. Kvernebo K: Laser Doppler flowmetry in evaluation of lower limb atherosclerosis, *J Oslo City Hosp* 38:127-136, 1988.
13. Kvernebo K, Slagsvold CE, Gjoberg T: Laser Doppler flow reappearance time (FRT) in patients with lower limb atherosclerosis and healthy controls, *Eur J Vasc Surg* 2:171-176, 1988.
14. Kvernebo K, Slagsvold CE, Stranden E: Laser Doppler flowmetry in evaluation of skin post-ischemic reactive hyperemia, *J Cardiovasc Surg* 30:70-75, 1989.

15. Ledbetter-Nelepovitz CC, Rao VD, Fronek A: Determination of in vitro simulated blood cell velocity by laser-Doppler with state space methods, *Microvasc Res* 41:164-172, 1991.
16. Moneta GL et al: Laser Doppler flux and vaosmotion in patients before and after transluminal angioplasty for limb salvage, *VASA* 17:26-31, 1988.
17. Ninet J, Fronek A: Cutaneous post-occlusive reactive hyperemia monitored by laser Doppler flux metering and skin temperature, *Microvasc Res* 30:125-132, 1985.
18. Ninet J, Fronek A: Laser flux monitored cutaneous response to local cooling and heating, *VASA* 14:38-43, 1985.
19. Pabst TS et al: Evaluation of the ischemic limb by pressure and flow measurements of the skin microcirculation as determined by laser Doppler velocimetry, *Curr Surg* 42:29-31, 1985.
20. Partsch H: Hyperaemic hypoxia in venous ulceration, *Br J Dermat* 110:249-251, 1984.
21. Salerud EG et al: Rhythmical variations in human skin blood flow, *Int J Microcirc Clin Exp* 2:91-102, 1983.
22. Scheffler A, Rieger H: A microcomputer system for evaluation of laser Doppler blood flux measurement, *Int J Microcirc Clin Exp* 9:357-368, 1990.
23. Scheffler A, Mussler K, Rieger H: Computed-unterstutzte Erfassung, Answertung und Dokumentation von Messungen des lokalen Blut-fluxes mit der laser-Doppler-Flowmetrie, *VASA* (suppl 20):394-396, 1987.
24. Schmid-Schönbein H et al: Analysis of rhythmic variation in blood content and RBC-motion: differentiation between active and passive determination of perfusion, *Int J Microcirc Clin Exp* Aug 1988, p 92.
25. Schmidt JA et al: Vasomotion as a flow dependent phenomenon, *Int J Microcirc Clin Exp* 71(suppl):92, 1988 (abstract).
26. Seifert H, Jäger K, Bollinger A: *Laser-Doppler probes for the evaluation of arterial ischemia.* In Huch A, Huch R, Rooth G, eds: *Continuous transcutaneous monitoring,* New York, 1987, Plenum Press.
27. Seifert H, Jäger K, Bollinger A: Analysis of flow motion by the laser Doppler technique in patients with peripheral arterial occlusive disease, *Int J Microcirc Clin Exp* 7:223-236, 1988.
28. Stern MD et al: Continuous measurement of tissue blood flow by laser-Doppler spectroscopy, *Am J Physiol* 232:441-448, 1977.
29. Sundberg A: Acute effects and long-term variations in skin blood flow measured with laser Doppler flowmetry, *Scand J Clin Lab Invest* 44:341-345, 1984.
30. Sundberg S, Castrén M: Drug- and temperature-induced changes in peripheral circulation measured by laser-Doppler flowmetry and digital-pulse plethysmography, *Scand J Clin Lab Invest* 46:359-365, 1986.
31. Tenland T et al: Spatial and temporal variations in human skin blood flow, *Int J Microcirc* 2:81-90, 1983.
32. Tooke J, Östergren J, Fagrell B: Synchronous assessment of human skin microcirculation by laser Doppler flowmetry and dynamic capillaroscopy, *Int J Microcirc Clin Exp* 2:277-284, 1983.

CHAPTER 74

Evaluation of upper extremity ischemia

JAMES M. EDWARDS and JOHN M. PORTER

Only 5% to 10% of patients with symptomatic limb ischemia have primary upper extremity involvement. Because of the small number of patients seen at any single institution, the relative frequency of the various categories of upper extremity arterial ischemia is not known with certainty. During the past 20 years, researchers at the Oregon Health Sciences University have prospectively evaluated and followed over 1000 patients with symptomatic vasospastic or arterial occlusive disease of the upper extremity. It is most useful to classify patients with upper extremity ischemia into three groups: large artery occlusive disease proximal to the wrist, small artery occlusive disease of the hands and fingers, and vasospastic disease primarily involving the hands and fingers. In this chapter, the noninvasive vascular laboratory techniques that are used in the evaluation of upper extremity ischemia and the differential diagnoses are reviewed.

BACKGROUND

Patients with upper extremity ischemia may present with fixed or intermittent symptoms of acute or chronic ischemia of the arm or hand. Patients with small artery occlusive disease or vasospastic disease usually have symptoms limited to the hand, which may include Raynaud's syndrome or ischemic digital ulceration, whereas those with large artery occlusive disease usually have ischemic symptoms involving the arm and the hand.

RAYNAUD'S SYNDROME

Raynaud's syndrome is defined as episodic digital ischemia occurring in response to cold or emotional stress. Classically, the attacks consist of intense pallor of the distal extremities followed by cyanosis and rubor on rewarming, with full recovery requiring 15 to 45 minutes after resolution of the stress. Patients with Raynaud's syndrome often present with variations from this typical presentation and may develop only pallor, rubor, or cyanosis during the attacks. It is now clear that the classic tricolor attack occurs only in a small proportion of patients. A number of patients complain only of cold hands without digital color changes and have abnormal arteriographic and blood flow findings identical to patients with classic digital color changes; therefore digital color change may not be essential for diagnosis.

In the past, patients with Raynaud's syndrome without any recognized associated disease process were diagnosed as having *Raynaud's disease,* whereas those with an associated disease were said to have *Raynaud's phenomenon.* There is little justification in attempting a rigid separation of Raynaud's disease from Raynaud's phenomenon, because patients with presumed Raynaud's disease continue to evolve symptoms of associated diseases for years after their initial presentation. It seems most reasonable to refer to the condition as *Raynaud's syndrome* and to recognize that all patients with this condition have an increased, life-long risk for the development of associated disease processes, especially autoimmune disease.[8]

Patients with Raynaud's syndrome can be divided into two distinct pathophysiologic groups; obstructive and spastic.[43,51,59] Patients with obstructive Raynaud's syndrome have significant fixed obstruction of the palmar and digital arteries caused by one of a variety of diseases that will be described in detail later. To experience a Raynaud's attack, the patient must have sufficiently severe arterial obstruction to cause significant reduction in resting digital artery pressure, a condition that requires obstruction of both arteries of a single digit. The quantitative relationship between arterial obstruction and Raynaud's attacks has been described in a series of detailed studies by Hirai.[31] Available evidence suggests that in such patients, a normal vasoconstrictive response to cold is sufficient to overcome the diminished intraluminal distending pressure and cause arterial closure. This theory predicts that all patients with sufficient arterial obstruction to cause resting digital hypotension will experience cold-induced Raynaud's attacks. Digital ulcers occur only in patients with fixed arterial occlusions and never result from vasospasm alone (Fig. 74-1).

Patients with primary or vasospastic Raynaud's syndrome do not have significant palmar-digital artery obstruction and therefore have normal digital artery pressure at room temperature. Arterial closure in these patients appears to be caused by a markedly increased degree of cold-induced arterial spasm (Figs. 74-2 and 74-3). An angiogram of a patient with obstructive Raynaud's syndrome for comparison is shown in Fig. 74-4. Thus individual patients may have both an obstructive and a vasospastic component responsible for their Raynaud's syndrome.

A 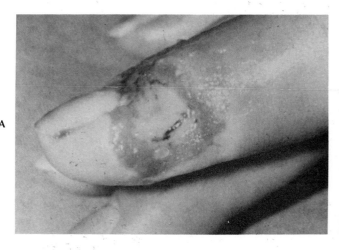 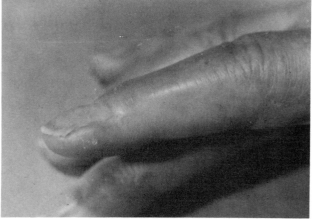 B

Fig. 74-1. *A,* Digital ulceration in a patient with scleroderma and digital artery occlusion. *B,* Healing of the ulcer after several months of conservative therapy.

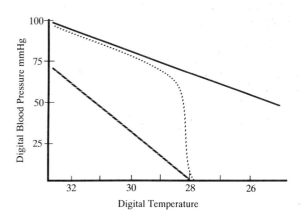

Fig. 74-2. Response of digital blood pressure to cold exposure in normal subjects *(solid line),* patients with vasospastic Raynaud's syndrome *(dotted line),* and patients with obstructive Raynaud's syndrome *(dashed line).*

LARGE ARTERY OCCLUSIVE DISEASE

Patients with large artery occlusive disease are most likely to have atherosclerosis involving the origin of the left subclavian artery, but a variety of other conditions may also affect the arteries of the upper extremity proximal to the wrist.[65] Takayasu's disease and giant cell arteritis are autoimmune disorders involving the arteries of the head, neck, and arms that are characterized by long segment stenoses or occlusions.[22] A total of 10% to 20% of cardiac emboli lodge in the upper extremity, and approximately 70% of upper extremity emboli originate in the heart.[1,23] Radiation arteritis is known to involve the subclavian and axillary arteries and has led to critical limb ischemia in a small group of patients.[13,37,41] Traumatic injuries to the upper extremity arteries may be of a blunt, penetrating, or avulsion type.[9] Fibromuscular dysplasia has been reported as a cause of upper extremity ischemia.[20,42] Thoracic outlet syndrome may also cause subclavian artery occlusion or aneurysm and lead to upper extremity ischemia.[57]

The most useful diagnostic test for localizing large artery occlusive disease is the segmental arm pressure measurement with a three cuff system (brachial/above elbow, below elbow, above wrist), with Doppler arterial signal detection at the wrist. Duplex scanning may also be quite helpful.

The measurement of digital pressure in addition to segmental arm pressure frequently permits differentiation of hand and finger ischemia caused by only proximal disease from that caused by proximal disease and distal embolization. In the latter case, the digital pressure is considerably lower than wrist pressure. The initial evaluation of patients with upper extremity large artery occlusive disease should include a plain chest film to detect bony abnormalities of the thoracic outlet, sedimentation rate to rule out arteritis, segmental arm pressures, digital pressures and waveforms, and an upper extremity arterial duplex examination in selected patients. Transesophageal echocardiography is emerging as the diagnostic test of choice if cardiac embolic disease is suspected.

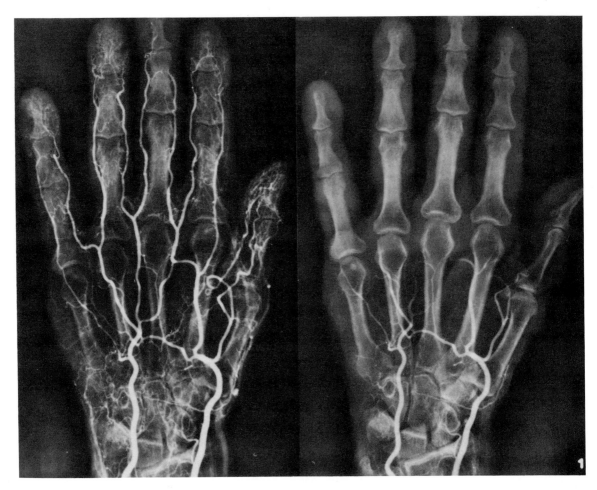

Fig. 74-3. Angiogram of a patient with vasospastic Raynaud's syndrome revealing normal palmar and digital arteries on the left, with marked vasospasm after cold exposure on the right.

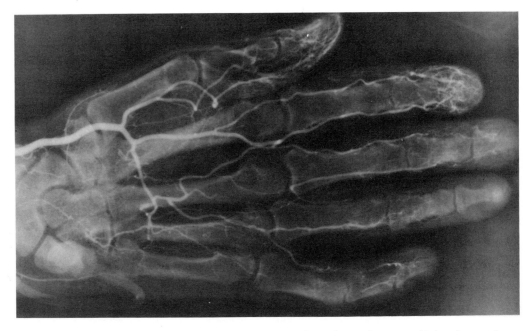

Fig. 74-4. Angiogram of a patient with obstructive Raynaud's syndrome showing multiple palmar and digital artery occlusions.

DUPLEX SCANNING

Duplex scanning of the upper extremity is performed with the same techniques used in studying the carotid or lower extremity arteries. The arteries of the upper extremity are fairly constant in location and are not far below the surface.

A 3- or 5-MHz probe is used to examine the origin of the subclavian artery. The axillary, brachial, ulnar, radial, and palmar and digital arteries are superficial and are best scanned with a higher frequency probe (7.5 or 10 MHz). A gel standoff or mound of acoustical gel is often necessary to visualize the smaller subcutaneous vessels clearly without compressing them. Color duplex scanners facilitate identification of the vessels as they do in the lower extremities.

The subclavian artery (Fig. 74-5) may be visualized via

a supraclavicular, infraclavicular, or sternal notch approach and should be scanned from its origin distally to where it crosses under the clavicle and over the first rib and becomes the axillary artery. It is often necessary to scan the subclavian artery from several approaches (e.g., sternal notch, infraclavicular, supraclavicular) to completely visualize the artery.

The axillary artery (Fig. 74-6) lies behind the pectoralis major and minor muscles and may be scanned from an anterior or axillary approach. The axillary artery becomes progressively more superficial as it courses distally and becomes the brachial artery at the point where it crosses the teres major muscle. The brachial artery (Fig. 74-7) is located in a groove between the biceps and triceps muscles. The brachial artery spirals anteriorly around the humerus and, in its midportion, gives off the profunda brachii (deep brachial) artery, which is the source of most collateral flow around the elbow.

The radial and ulnar arteries can be visualized from the bifurcation of the brachial artery in the antecubital fossa to the wrist. The location of the ulnar artery is constant at the wrist as it emerges laterally from behind the flexor carpi ulnaris tendon and passes over the pisiform bone and under the hook of the hamate. This area is very important, since traumatic aneurysms of the ulnar artery are often located here. The radial artery (Fig. 74-8) is easily found by palpation at the wrist or can be reliably located between the flexor carpi radialis tendon and the head of the radius.

Although the number of articles on the use of duplex scanning in the diagnosis of upper extremity arterial disease is limited, use of this method has been reported in the diagnosis of atherosclerosis,[2,26] Takayasu's disease,[55] ulnar artery aneurysms,[36] thoracic outlet syndrome,[27] pseudoaneurysms of the brachial or axillary artery after catheterization,[61] and congenital arterial abnormalities.[44]

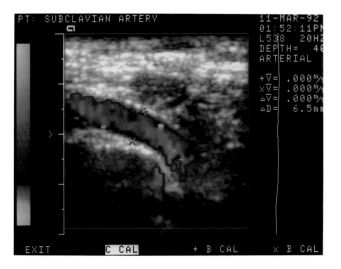

Fig. 74-5. Color duplex scan of the origin of the left subclavian artery.

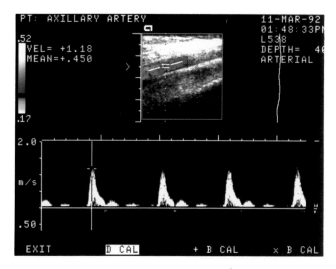

Fig. 74-6. Color duplex scan of the axillary artery and the Doppler spectrum. Note the characteristic triphasic waveform.

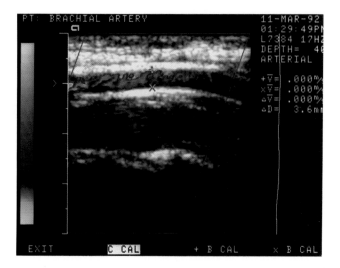

Fig. 74-7. Color duplex scan of the brachial artery in the antecubital fossa.

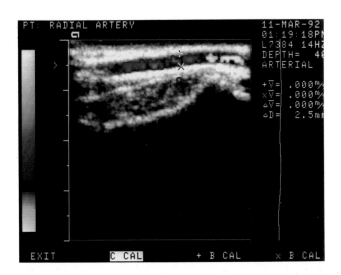

Fig. 74-8. Color duplex scan of the radial artery just proximal to the wrist.

Upper extremity arterial repairs may easily be followed for postoperative stenosis or occlusion with duplex scanning.[16,36,64] The examination techniques for postoperative surveillance are similar to those for lower extremity arteries.

As in other arteries, stenoses in upper extremity arteries result in high velocity jets, poststenotic turbulence, and dampened distal waveforms. At present there are no specific frequency or velocity criteria with which to gauge the severity of stenoses comparable to those for carotid or lower extremity arteries.[34]

Waveforms in the upper extremity arteries are normally triphasic, but hemodynamic resistance in the arm may decrease markedly with arm exercise or warming of the hand; the resulting flow pattern may become monophasic and continuous throughout diastole. With cooling, the amplitude of the velocity waveform decreases drastically, although the triphasic pattern generally persists. Normal peak systolic velocities range from 100 to 150 cm/sec in the proximal subclavian artery to about 20 cm/sec in the radial artery leading to a cool hand.

SMALL ARTERY OCCLUSIVE DISEASE AND VASOSPASM

Upper extremity small artery occlusive disease involves the palmar and digital arteries. As previously noted, many of the patients suffer from associated vasospasm, which is frequently the presenting clinical symptom. Many disorders that cause upper extremity small artery occlusive disease may also produce upper extremity vasospasm in the absence of arterial occlusion. Thus the differential diagnosis of these two conditions must be considered together, with emphasis on the vascular laboratory differentiation of small artery occlusive disease from primary vasospasm in the absence of fixed arterial obstruction.

In the past, patients with upper extremity vasospastic symptoms were divided into two groups depending on the presence or absence of an associated disease process. In 1901, Hutchinson[33] accurately noted that Raynaud's phenomenon may be caused by vasospasm, such as chillblains in children, or by arterial obstruction, such as senile gangrene in the elderly associated with progressive calcification of the arteries, but he made no effort to subdivide patients by disease process. In the early 1930s, Allen and Brown[4-6] proposed strict criteria for the diagnosis of Raynaud's disease, which they considered a benign idiopathic form of intermittent digital ischemia, and Raynaud's phenomenon, a similar condition seen in association with systemic diseases. Of 204 cases seen at the Mayo Clinic between 1920 and 1931, 147 (72%) patients had no associated disease, whereas the remaining 57 (28%) patients had an associated disease, frequently scleroderma or arthritis.

In 1934, Lewis and Pickering[39] interviewed 60 men and 62 women and found prevalence of episodic color changes after exposure to cold in 27% of this group. Although they clearly recognized that many conditions such as scleroderma, trauma, and cervical ribs may be associated with Raynaud's syndrome, they did not describe the relative number of patients with and without associated diseases. In 1945, Hines and Christensen[30] reported their experience with 847 patients diagnosed as having Raynaud's disease, including 198 (23%) males. They obtained follow-up on 100 of these patients and found that 16 (16%) eventually developed a disease associated with the Raynaud's symptoms. Gifford and Hines reviewed female patients with a diagnosis of Raynaud's disease at the Mayo Clinic from 1920 to 1945.[25] Of the 756 diagnosed patients, they were able to obtain sufficient information on 418 to adequately evaluate the presence or absence of an associated disease. An associated disease process was found in 74 (18%) patients.

A much higher prevalence of associated diseases in patients with Raynaud's syndrome has been noted consistently by investigators since 1950. Blain, Coller, and Carver[7] at the University of Michigan reported their experience with 238 patients with Raynaud's syndrome treated between 1934 and 1946. They found that 119 of these patients (50%) met the Allen and Brown criteria for Raynaud's disease, whereas the other 119 had another disease process in association with their episodic digital ischemic symptoms. A total of 100 of these patients had been followed for more than 5 years, which permitted evaluation of symptoms over a long period. Of these, 69% remained the same or improved, 6% had moderate progression of symptoms, and 25% had severe progression of symptoms.

Allen and Brown proposed that primary Raynaud's disease may be confidently diagnosed if 2 years pass after the onset of vasospastic symptoms without diagnosis of an associated disease, but this conclusion was challenged by de Takats and Fowler in 1962.[17] They accurately noted that many years may elapse after the onset of vasospastic symptoms before the signs and symptoms of an associated autoimmune disease become clinically evident. In 1970, Velayos et al[63] reviewed the records of 137 hospitalized patients with Raynaud's symptoms and found only 28 patients (20%) with no associated disease. Of the remaining patients, 57 (42%) had a connective tissue disease and 52 (38%) had one or more of a variety of disease processes in association with the Raynaud's attacks, including such conditions as atherosclerosis and nerve injury. Porter et al,[53] reported their experience with the long-term follow-up of 73 patients in 1976. They found that 81% of these patients had an associated disease process. Vayssairat, Fiessinger, and Housset[62] reported their experience with 100 patients hospitalized with Raynaud's symptoms; they found that only 18 (18%) patients had no associated disease process. The associated diseases included connective tissue disease in 50 patients, usually scleroderma (37 patients), as well as a miscellaneous group of conditions including arteritis, trauma, and atherosclerosis. In 1980, Kellenberg, Wauda, and Hauw The[35] evaluated 91 patients with Raynaud's syndrome for clinical or laboratory evidence of an autoimmune disease. They were able to demonstrate abnormalities in 59 (65%) patients. They also noted that the severity of Raynaud's syndrome generally correlated with the severity of the underlying disorder. Harper et al[28] followed 91 patients with Raynaud's attacks for an average of 28 months. At entry 49 (54%) patients had no apparent associated disease, 22 (24%) patients had undifferentiated connective tissue disease, and 20 (22%) patients had scleroderma. At the completion of their study, 46 patients had no apparent associated disease, 26 patients had scleroderma, 16 patients had undifferentiated connective tissue disease, and 1 patient had systemic lupus erythematosus.

An important study was published by Priollet, Vayssairat, and Housset[54] in 1987. They previously had classified 240 patients with Raynaud's syndrome: 70 patients were diagnosed as having primary Raynaud's syndrome (no disease states found); suspected secondary Raynaud's syndrome was diagnosed in 26 (11%) patients (abnormality of one or more immunologic tests but not meeting American Rheumatism Association criteria), and secondary Raynaud's syndrome was diagnosed in 144 (60%) patients. The 96 patients diagnosed as having either primary or suspected secondary Raynaud's were followed for a mean of 4.7 years. At the time of final evaluation, the data from 49 patients originally diagnosed as primary Raynaud's syndrome and 24 patients originally considered suspected secondary Raynaud's syndrome were available for classification. After the evaluation, 1 of the 49 patients thought to have primary Raynaud's was reclassified as suspected secondary Raynaud's, 14 of the 24 patients with suspected secondary Raynaud's developed an immunologic disease, and the remainder of the patients were again classified as suspected secondary Raynaud's syndrome. The researchers concluded that patients who had totally normal initial examinations could be reliably diagnosed as having primary Raynaud's, but those with one or more laboratory abnormalities should be followed closely because many of these patients would later develop an associated disease.

Why patients with autoimmune diseases develop arteritis that for the most part is limited to the palmar and digital arteries without involvement of the feet or the rest of the body remains a mystery. It is known that various autoimmune diseases may cause palmar and digital arterial occlusive disease of differing degrees. Patients with Sjögren's syndrome, scleroderma, and undifferentiated connective tissue disease have the most severe problems with hand ischemia and ulceration, whereas patients with mixed connective tissue disease, rheumatoid arthritis, or systemic lupus erythematosus frequently have less difficulty.

Disorders other than the autoimmune diseases may be associated with Raynaud's syndrome. A partial list includes atherosclerosis, Buerger's disease, cancer, hypersensitivity angiitis, cold injury (frostbite), chronic exposure to vibrating tools, proximal or distal aneurysmal disease, carpal tunnel syndrome, disorders of thyroid function, hematologic abnormalities, and trauma.[29,45,53,60] Individually, these conditions are less likely to be found in patients presenting for evaluation of Raynaud's syndrome, but as a group, they form a small but significant proportion of associated diseases. The nonautoimmune-associated diseases also produce Raynaud's syndrome through obstruction of the digital arteries.

The relative incidence of associated nonautoimmune diseases in patients with Raynaud's syndrome has not been established. There are numerous studies on vibration-associated Raynaud's syndrome, but all patients in these studies are workers who have vibration exposure. Similarly, most studies of patients with digital ischemia of diverse causes have not specifically sought the incidence of Raynaud's syndrome in association with digital ischemia. Velayos et al[63] reported that 38% of their patients had a nonautoimmune-associated disease, a number that was nearly equal to the 42% who had an autoimmune disease. Vayssairat, Fiessinger, and Housset[62] found that 32% of their patients hospitalized with Raynaud's syndrome had a nonautoimmune associated disease, which was a lower proportion than those with associated autoimmune diseases (50%).

At the Oregon Health Sciences University, a regular weekly clinic devoted to Raynaud's syndrome patients has been held for 20 years. To date, over 1000 patients with digital ischemia have been evaluated. The relative incidence of associated diseases has decreased from 81% in 1976 to 46% in 1989.[8,19,49,53,56] In the most recent report, 27% of patients had an autoimmune disease, which was scleroderma in over half (56%). No associated disease has been recognized to date in 54% of patients in the study. The remaining 19% have a variety of other associated diseases, the most common of which has been atherosclerosis. Of the patients who have presented with ischemic finger ulceration (100 patients), 56 have been diagnosed as having an autoimmune disease with associated hand artery occlusions, and the remaining 44 have been diagnosed as having one of a variety of conditions.[46]

Remarkably, the incidence of vasospastic disease in the general population is unknown. It has been estimated that 20% to 25% of people in cool, damp climates such as Scandinavia and the Pacific Northwest are affected by Raynaud's syndrome to some degree.[48,50] Many theories have been proposed to explain the hyperreactivity of the digital arteries in response to environmental cold exposure, including deficiencies or excesses of α-adrenoceptors, β-adrenoceptors, endothelin, and most recently, calcitonin gene-related peptide.[11,12,21,40,66] The pathophysiology of vasospastic Raynaud's syndrome remains the subject of investigation in a number of laboratories.

Evaluation of small artery disease and vasospasm

The vascular laboratory is of great help in objectively establishing the diagnosis of upper extremity ischemia and permits a separation of spastic from obstructive Raynaud's syndrome. The available tests can be separated into several groups. Digital pressure measurements and the analysis of digital waveforms are used to separate obstruction from vasospasm. Cold challenge tests and specialized tests of sympathetic function are used to detect cold-induced vasospasm and thermal vasomotion abnormalities.

At the Oregon Health Sciences University, basic evaluation of the patient presenting with Raynaud's syndrome consists of a history and physical examination; measurement of digital pressure; evaluation of digital waveforms; a digital hypothermic challenge test; a radiograph of the hand to detect the presence of tuft resorption, calcinosis, or arthritis; and a basic immunology screen consisting of a sedimentation rate, complete blood count, antinuclear antibody (ANA), and rheumatoid factor.

Digital pressures and waveforms. The measurement of digital blood pressures and analysis of photoplethysmographic (PPG) digital waveforms permits an objective measurement of the severity of ischemia and is the primary test for the differentiation of obstructive Raynaud's syndrome from vasospastic Raynaud's syndrome. Digital blood pressure determination with PPG waveform analysis is as accurate as arteriography in the detection of significant digital artery obstruction.[32] Blood pressure cuffs specifically designed for this purpose are used.*

The finding of an obstructive digital plethysmographic waveform and a digital pressure of more than 20 torr below brachial pressure establishes the diagnosis of significant digital artery obstruction. This technique is extremely simple to perform by attaching the probe with double-sided tape and moving it from finger to finger. In addition to determining digital pressure, this technique provides digital artery waveforms. The finding of a peaked pulse on the PPG digital waveform has been associated with the presence of vasospastic Raynaud's syndrome.[59] The presence of a peaked pulse in at least one digital PPG waveform tracing

*Medasonics, Mountain View, Calif; and D.E. Hokanson, Bellevue, Wash.

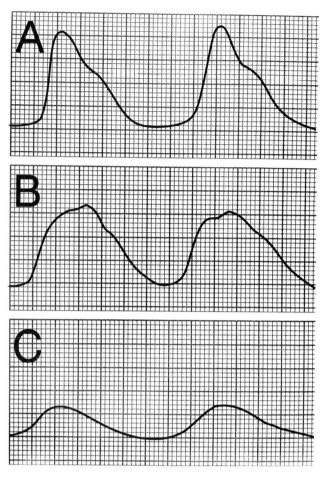

Fig. 74-9. Digital PPG waveform. **A**, Normal. **B**, Peaked pulse associated with vasospastic Raynaud's syndrome. **C**, Obstructive.

has been reported to identify the presence of Raynaud's syndrome with a specificity of 100% and a sensitivity of 66%.[3] Representative tracings of normal, obstructive, and peaked digital waveforms are shown in Fig. 74-9. An important caveat in performing this test is that the patients and their hands must be allowed to equilibrate to room temperature to avoid false-positive results.

Cold challenge testing. The change in digital blood pressure caused by a change in finger temperature is shown in Fig. 74-2 for three groups: normal individuals, patients with vasospastic Raynaud's syndrome, and patients with significant digital artery obstruction. Normal individuals show only a modest digital pressure drop with decreasing temperature, usually not exceeding 20%.[14,15] Patients with vasospastic Raynaud's syndrome show a similar curve to normal subjects until a critical temperature is reached, at which time abrupt arterial closure occurs. Patients with severe arterial obstruction parallel normal subjects but at a much lower pressure, with closure occurring at about 20 to 30 torr.

The first vascular laboratory test widely used for objective diagnosis of Raynaud's syndrome was the measurement

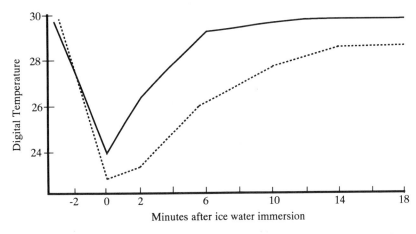

Fig. 74-10. Recovery of finger temperature after immersion in ice water. Patients with Raynaud's syndrome *(dotted line)* have prolonged recovery when compared to normal subjects *(solid line).*

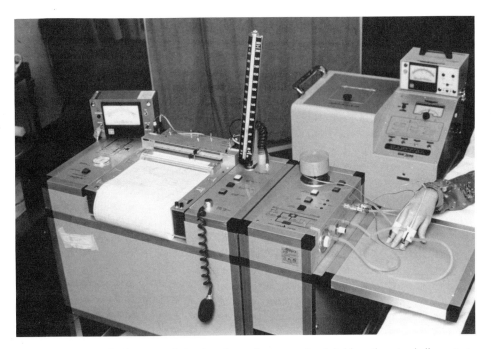

Fig. 74-11. Test and reference cuffs in place for performance of a digital hypothermic challenge test.

of fingertip temperature recovery time after digital ice water exposure (Fig. 74-10).[52] Although normal individuals and patients with Raynaud's syndrome usually have similar resting digital temperatures and similar digital temperature drops after ice water exposure, the time required for return of digital temperature to normal averages 5 to 10 minutes in normal individuals and is prolonged to more than 20 minutes in most Raynaud's patients. Increasing experience has revealed that although this test is 100% specific, it is only about 50% sensitive and thus is insufficiently accurate for clinical use.

In recent years the digital blood pressure response to 5 minutes of digital occlusive hypothermia as described by

Nielsen and Lassen[47] has proved to be quite accurate in the vascular laboratory diagnosis of Raynaud's syndrome. This test is performed by a machine especially designed for this purpose—Medimatic model SP2 strain gauge plethysmograph with digit cooling system.* A double-inlet cuff that allows temperature-controlled cooling of a digit is placed around the test finger (second digit), and a single-inlet cuff is place around the reference digit (fourth finger) (Fig. 74-11). Mercury-in-silastic strain gauges are then placed around the fingertips of the two fingers. Both cuffs are inflated for

_____

*Medimatic, Medasonics, Mountain View, Calif.

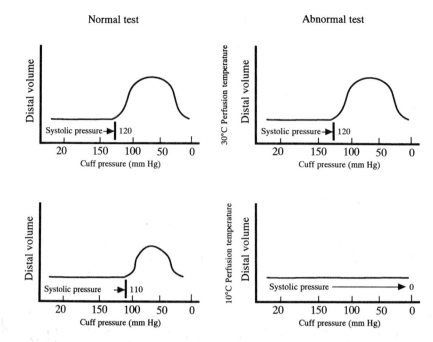

Fig. 74-12. Normal *(left)* and a positive test *(right)* for vasospasm with the digital hypothermic challenge test.

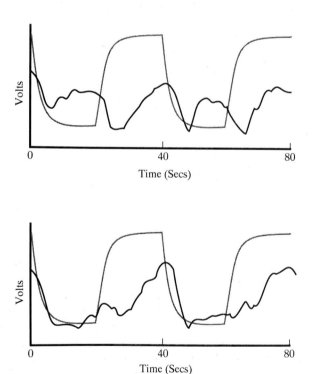

Fig. 74-13. Normal response *(top)* to thermal entrainment and the response of a patient with Raynaud's syndrome *(bottom)* to thermal entrainment. The patient with Raynaud's syndrome has a blunted response to temperature change, which can be quantified by calculating the power spectrum of the PPG waveform. The gray line represents the bath temperature and the solid line represents the PPG tracing.

5 minutes, during which time the test finger cuff is perfused with water at 30° C, 15° C, and 10° C during successive tests. After each 5-minute period, the cuff pressure is slowly decreased and the systolic blood pressure is measured by the return of pulsatile flow recorded by the strain gauge. A decrease in pressure of the test finger of greater than 20% over that seen in the reference finger is considered a positive test (Fig. 74-12). Whole body cooling may also be added as a systemic cold challenge. In an evaluation of 100 patients, the test was found to be 87% specific and 90% sensitive when compared with the clinical diagnosis yielding an overall accuracy of 92%.[24] This is presently the vascular laboratory diagnostic test of choice to document objectively the presence of Raynaud's syndrome. The use of such an objective test is most helpful in specific patient groups, including those in whom the diagnosis is in doubt, epidemiologic study groups, and those with pending litigation in whom historical accuracy is uncertain.

Several variations of this method have recently been reported. In one test, an A-mode ultrasound scan was used to determine the diameter of the digital arteries.[58] The decrease in digital artery diameter with decreasing temperature is measured and is much greater in those patients with Raynaud's syndrome than in normal subjects. The other cold challenge test that has recently been described uses laser Doppler.[10] A 1 cm² patch of skin on the volar surface of the forearm is cooled to 4° C to 6° C for 2 minutes. The cooling device is removed and the laser Doppler probe is placed over the skin. Normal patients will display reactive hyperemia easily detected as a spike on the laser Doppler output. This spike is absent or attenuated in patients with Raynaud's syndrome. Both of these tests must be considered experimental until the results are replicated in other laboratories.

Thermal entrainment. Although the sympathetic nervous system has been implicated in the pathogenesis of Raynaud's syndrome for almost a century, its role remains unclear. In a series of papers by Lafferty et al,[18,38] abnormalities of the thermoregulatory response in patients with Raynaud's syndrome have been demonstrated by means of a test termed *thermal entrainment*. In this test, the blood flow patterns in one hand are measured while the contralateral hand is alternately dipped in baths of hot and cold water. There are clear differences in blood flow responses demonstrable between normal subjects and Raynaud's patients (Fig. 74-13). The obvious way to account for contralateral changes in blood flow is an alteration of the function of the sympathetic nervous system, although no research has been done to prove or disprove this hypothesis. This test is currently available in only one or two vascular laboratories.

CONCLUSION

It is useful to classify patients with upper extremity ischemia into three groups: large artery obstructive disease, small artery obstructive disease, and vasospastic disease, although all three may coexist. This classification can be achieved from the history, physical examination (including pulse status), and vascular laboratory tests. These tests include blood pressure measurements at the level of the brachial artery, wrist, and digits; analysis of digital waveforms; and cold challenge testing. This evaluation permits the diagnosis of large artery occlusive disease (with or without digital emboli), small artery occlusive disease, and vasospasm. Accurate, early classification is clearly important because it has both therapeutic and prognostic implications.

REFERENCES

1. Abbot WM et al: Arterial embolism: A 44 year perspective, *Am J Surg* 143:460, 1982.
2. Ackerstaff RGA et al: Ultrasonic duplex scanning in atherosclerotic disease of the innominate, subclavian, and vertebral arteries: a comparative study with angiography, *Ultrasound Med Biol* 10:409-418, 1984.
3. Alexander S et al: Usefulness of digital peaked pulse for diagnosis of Raynaud's syndrome, *J Vasc Technol* 12:71-75, 1988.
4. Allen E, Brown G: Raynaud's disease: a clinical study of 147 cases, *JAMA* 99:1472-1478, 1932.
5. Allen E, Brown G: Raynaud's disease: a critical review of minimal requisites for diagnosis, *Am J Med Sci* 83:187-200, 1932.
6. Allen E, Brown G: Raynaud's disease affecting men, *Ann Int Med* 5:1384-1386, 1932.
7. Blain A, Coller F, Carver G: Raynaud's disease: a study of criteria for prognosis, *Surg* 29:387-397, 1951.
8. Blunt RJ, Porter JM: Raynaud's syndrome, *Sem Arth Rheumatism* 10:282-308, 1981.
9. Borman KR, Snyder WH II, Weigelt JA: Civilian arterial trauma of the upper extremity: an 11 year experience in 267 patients, *Am J Surg* 148:796, 1985.
10. Brain SD et al: Cutaneous blood flow responses in the forearms of Raynaud's patients induced by local cooling and intradermal injections of CGRP and histamine, *Br J Clin Pharmacol* 30:853-859, 1990.
11. Brotzu G et al: The role of presynaptic beta-receptors in Raynaud's disease, *Artery* 13(2):77-86, 1985.
12. Bunker CB et al: Deficiency of calcitonin gene-related peptide in Raynaud's phenomenon, *Lancet* 336:1530-1533, 1990.
13. Butler MS, Lane RHS, Webster JHH: Irradiation injury to large arteries, *Br J Surg* 67:341-343, 1980.
14. Carter SA: The effect of cooling on toe systolic pressures in subjects with and without Raynaud's syndrome in the lower extremities, *Clin Physiol* 11:253-262, 1991.
15. Carter SA, Dean E, Kroeger EA: Apparent finger systolic pressures during cooling in patients with Raynaud's syndrome, *Circulation* 77:988-996, 1988.
16. Cormier JM et al: Arterial complications of the thoracic outlet syndrome: fifty-five operative cases, *J Vasc Surg* 9:778-787, 1989.
17. de Takats G, Fowler E: Raynaud's phenomenon, *JAMA* 179:99-105, 1962.
18. de Trafford JC et al: Modeling of the human thermal vasomotor control system and its application to the investigation of arterial disease, *Proc IEEE* 129:A646-A650, 1982.
19. Edwards JM, Porter JM: Associated diseases. In Cooke ED, Nicoliades AN, Porter JM, *Raynaud's syndrome*, London, 1991, Med Orion.
20. Edwards JM, Antonius JI, Porter JM: Critical and ischemia caused by forearm fibromuscular dysplasia, *J Vasc Surg* 2:459-463, 1985.
21. Edwards JM et al: Alpha-2 adrenoreceptor differences in vasospastic and obstructive Raynaud's syndrome, *J Vasc Surg* 5:38-45, 1987.
22. Fauci AS, Haynes BF, Katz P: The spectrum of vasculitis: clinical, pathologic, immunologic, and therapeutic considerations, *Ann Intern Med* 89:660, 1978.
23. Forgarty TJ et al: Experience with balloon catheter technic for arterial embolectomy, *Am J Surg* 122:231, 1971.
24. Gates KH et al: The non-invasive quantification of digital vasospasm, *Bruit* 8:34, 1984.
25. Gifford R, Hines E: Raynaud's disease among women and girls, *Circulation* 16:1012-1021, 1957.
26. Grosveld WJHM et al: Clinical and hemodynamic significance of innominate artery lesions evaluated by ultrasonography and digital angiography, *Stroke* 19:958-962, 1988.
27. Guzzetti A, Bellotti R: Usefulness of Doppler echocardiography in the diagnosis of upper thoracic outlet syndrome, *Chir Ital* 40:152-155, 1988.
28. Harper F et al: A prospective study of Raynaud phenomenon and early connective tissue disease, *Am J Med* 72:883-888, 1982.
29. Harris EJ, Edwards JM, Porter JM: *Vibration associated arterial disease*. In Flanigan P, ed: *Civilian vascular trauma*, 1992 (in press).
30. Hines E, Christensen N: Raynaud's disease among men, *JAMA* 129:1-4, 1945.
31. Hirai M: Cold sensitivity of the hand in arterial occlusive disease, *Surgery* 85:140, 1979.
32. Holmgren K, Baur GM, Porter JM: The role of digital photoplethysmography in the evaluation of Raynaud's syndrome, *Bruit* 5:19, 1981.
33. Hutchinson J: Raynaud's phenomena, *Med Press Circular* 128:403-405, 1901.
34. Jager KA et al: Noninvasive mapping of lower limb arterial lesions, *Ultrasound Med Biol* 11:515-521, 1985.
35. Kallenberg C, Wouda A, Hauw The T: Systemic involvement and immunologic findings in patients presenting with Raynaud's phenomenon, *Am J Med* 69:675-680, 1980.
36. Koman LA et al: Evaluation of upper extremity vasculature with high resolution ultrasound, *J Hand Surg* 10A;249-255, 1985.
37. Kretscher G et al: Irradiation-induced changes in the subclavian and axillary arteries after radiotherapy for carcinoma of the breast, *Surgery* 99:658-663, 1986.
38. Lafferty K et al: Raynaud's phenomenon and thermal entrainment: an objective test, *Br Med J* 286:90-92, 1983.
39. Lewis T, Pickering G: Observations upon maladies in which the blood supply to the digits ceases intermittently or permanently and upon bilateral gangrene of the digits: observations relevant to so-called "Raynaud's disease," *Clin Sci* 1:327-366, 1934.
40. MacKiewisz A, Piskorz A: Raynaud's phenomenon following long-term repeated action of great differences of temperature, *J Cardiovasc Surg* 18:151, 1977.
41. McCallion WA, Barros D'Sa AAB: Management of critical upper extremity ischemia long after irradiation injury of the subclavian and axillary arteries, *Br J Surg* 78:1136-1138, 1991.

42. McCready RA et al: Fibromuscular dysplasia of the right subclavian artery, *Arch Surg* 117:1243-1245, 1982.

43. Mendlowitz M, Naftchi N: The digital circulation of Raynaud's disease, *Am J Cardiol* 4:580, 1959.

44. Merlob P et al: Real-time echo-Doppler duplex scanner in the evaluation of patients with Poland sequence, *Eur J Obstet Gyn Repro Bio* 32:103-108, 1989.

45. Mills JL, Taylor LM Jr, Porter JM: Buerger's disease in the modern era, *Am J Surg* 154:123-129, 1987.

46. Mills JL et al: Upper extremity ischemia caused by small artery disease, *Ann Surg* 206:521-528, 1987.

47. Neilsen SL, Lassen NA: Measurement of digital blood pressure after local cooling, *J Appl Physiol* 43:907, 1977.

48. Olsen N, Nielsen SL: Prevalence of primary Raynaud's phenomenon in young females, *Scand J Clin Lab Invest* 37:761, 1978.

49. Porter JM: *Raynaud's syndrome.* In Rutherford RB, ed: *Vascular surgery,* ed 2, New York, 1984, Saunders.

50. Porter JM: Unpublished data, 1984.

51. Porter JM, Rivers SP, Anderson CJ: Evaluation and management of patients with Raynaud's syndrome, *Am J Surg* 142:183, 1981.

52. Porter JM et al: The diagnosis and treatment of Raynaud's phenomenon, *Surgery* 77:11, 1975.

53. Porter JM: The clinical significance of Raynaud's syndrome, *Surgery* 80:756-764, 1976.

54. Priollet P, Vayssairat M, Housset B: How to classify Raynaud's phenomenon: long-term follow-up study of 73 cases, *Am J Med* 83:494-498, 1987.

55. Reed AJ, Fincher RME, Nichols FT: Case report: Takayasu arteritis in a middle aged caucasian woman: clinical course correlated with duplex ultrasonography and angiography, *Am J Med Sci* 298:324-327, 1989.

56. Rivers SP, Porter JM: *Raynaud's syndrome.* In Najarian JS, Delaney JP, eds: *Advances in vascular surgery,* New York, 1983, Grune & Stratton.

57. Robb CG, Standeven A: Arterial occlusion complicating thoracic outlet compression syndrome, *Br Med J* 2:709-712, 1958.

58. Singh S et al: Digital artery calibre measurement—a new technique of assessing Raynaud's phenomenon, *Eur J Vasc Surg* 5:199-203, 1991.

59. Sumner DS, Strandness DE: An abnormal finger pulse associated with cold sensitivity, *Ann Surg* 175:294, 1972.

60. Taylor LM Jr et al: Digital ischemia as a manifestation of malignancy, *Ann Surg* 206:62-68, 1987.

61. Thomas VC, Roder HU, Moser GH: Diagnostiche wertigkeit der Angiodynographie bei pulsierenden Raumforderungen, *Fortschr Rontgenstr* 150:454-457, 1989.

62. Vayssairat M, Fiessinger J, Housset E: Phenomene de Raynaud: etude prospective de 100 cas, *Nouvelle Presse Medicale* 26:2177-2180, 1979.

63. Velayos E et al: Clinical correlation analysis of 137 patients with Raynaud's phenomenon, *Am J Med Sci* 262:347-356, 1970.

64. White RA et al: Initial human evaluation of argon laser-assisted vascular anastomoses, *J Vasc Surg* 9:542-547, 1989.

65. Williams SJ: Chronic upper extremity ischemia: current concepts in management, *Surg Clin North Am* 66:355, 1986.

66. Zamora MR et al: Serum endothelin-1 concentrations and cold provocation in primary Raynaud's phenomenon, *Lancet* 336:1144-1147, 1990.

CHAPTER 75

Quantitative diagnosis of stenosis and cross-sectional area from Doppler information

PRAVIN M. SHAH

BACKGROUND

In 1842, Christian Johann Doppler, an Austrian physicist, first described the principle that bears his name in a paper entitled, "On the Coloured Light of Double Stars and Some Other Heavenly Bodies." He observed that stars emit blue or red color depending on whether they are moving toward or away from the earth. This principle, termed the *Doppler effect,* states that a change in the observed frequency of a wave is produced by relative motion between the observer and the wavefront. This may apply to any wave, including sound waves. Satomura[8] applied the Doppler principle to detect blood velocity on the basis of backscattered ultrasound from moving red blood cells.

Blood flow in large caliber vessels is generally described as laminar or as having relatively uniform velocities. Stenosis or obstruction results in disruption of normal laminar flow, creating whirls and eddies of differing velocities and directions. This disturbed or turbulent flow generally characterizes flow across stenosis.

The two basic types of Doppler ultrasound are pulsed and continuous wave Doppler. Pulsed Doppler uses a single piezoelectric crystal that transmits a burst of ultrasound and then receives the reflected signal. The Doppler shift is derived by subtraction of the transmitted ultrasound frequency from the reflected ultrasound frequency. The time interval between transmission and reception of a pulse determines the depth of the sample volume from which the Doppler shift is obtained. The location of the sample volume can be adjusted by the operator. Using a two dimensional B-mode image, the operator may place the sample volume at anatomically defined locations in the cardiovascular system. The ability to obtain a range-gated Doppler shift is an important advantage of the pulsed Doppler approach. There is, however, one important limitation relating to the maximum velocities that can be displayed. The maximum frequency shift that can be measured accurately by a pulsed Doppler is the Nyquist limit and is equal to one half of the pulse repetition frequency (PRF):

$$\text{Nyquist limit} = \frac{\text{PRF}}{2}$$

Flow velocities with Doppler shifts exceeding the Nyquist limit cause aliasing in which the higher velocities appear as flow in the opposite direction. This Doppler artifact is a major limitation in measurement of the high velocities that often occur in the region of a stenosis.

A continuous wave Doppler uses two ultrasound crystals to provide continuous transmission and reception of the reflected ultrasound signal. A major advantage of this system is the absence of aliasing due to extremely high PRFs. Thus higher velocities can be recorded without ambiguity. A disadvantage of this approach is the absence of range gating or localization of the source of the velocities. The highest velocities recorded by continuous wave Doppler are simply the highest velocities encountered in any location along the path of the transmitted ultrasound beam. The current practice of Doppler imaging combines both the pulsed and continuous wave approaches for maximal diagnostic advantage.

Velocity calculations for blood flow are based on the Doppler equation:

$$V = \frac{C(F_r - F_t)}{2\,F_o\,\cos\theta}$$

where:

V = Flow velocity
F_t = Transmitted frequency
F_r = Received frequency
$F_r - F_t$ = Doppler shift
C/F_o = Wavelength of ultrasound
θ = Angle between transmitted ultrasound beam and direction of blood flow

This equation permits calculation of flow velocity by using current instrumentation. Since the velocity obtained is inversely related to cosine θ, a maximum Doppler shift occurs when the angle is zero (cosine of $\theta = 1$). As the angle approaches 90°, progressive decrease of the Doppler shift is observed ($\cos 90 = o_t$). For an angle θ of 20°, the velocity measured is within 94% of the actual axial velocity vector. Thus a degree of freedom of nearly 20° is permissive for clinical accuracy.

641

Doppler instrumentation has been successfully used to assess the degree of pressure drop across stenotic cardiac valves.[1,3,9] This approach has been validated in careful in vitro studies as well as in correlative clinical studies. Furthermore, the continuity principle has been validated to derive the cross-sectional area of stenotic valves. This chapter deals primarily with the approaches currently in use to assess intracardiac valve stenosis, with a hope that similar approaches may be feasible for peripheral vascular stenoses as well.

ASSESSMENT OF PRESSURE GRADIENTS ACROSS STENOSES

The ability to measure pressure gradients on the basis of Doppler echocardiographics is based on the Bernoulli equation.[11] Daniel Bernoulli, a Dutch mathematician, showed a relationship between pressure and flow velocity in 1738. The complete equation is:

$$P_1 - P_2 = \tfrac{1}{2}\rho(V_2^2 - V_1^2) + \rho\int_1^2 \frac{dv}{dt} \times ds + R(v)$$

$$\underset{\text{drop}}{\text{Pressure}} = \underset{\text{acceleration}}{\text{Corrective}} + \underset{\text{acceleration}}{\text{Flow}} + \underset{\text{friction}}{\text{Viscous}}$$

The contributions of flow acceleration and viscous friction are negligible for most cardiovascular applications, and hence the Bernoulli equation is simplified as:

$$P_1 - P_2 = \tfrac{1}{2}P(V_2^2 - V_1^2)$$

where:

P_1 = Upstream pressure (i.e., proximal to stenosis)
P_2 = Downstream pressure (i.e., distal to stenosis)
V_1 = Upstream flow velocity
V_2 = Downstream flow velocity
ρ = Mass density of blood

The proximal velocity (V_1) is generally less than 1 m/sec and may be ignored, and for blood, $\tfrac{1}{2}P$ is approximately 4. Thus the simplified Bernoulli equation can be stated as:

$$P_1 - P_2 = 4V_2^2$$

This simplified equation permits ready and accurate assessment of pressure gradients across native and prosthetic valves and congenital defects.

Wong et al[11] examined the relationship of pressure gradient and flow velocity using Doppler recording during in vitro mode studies. The accurate assessment of pressure gradients in a simulated pulsatile flow system could be made at multiple points along the flow velocity profile with the simplified Bernoulli equation. The pressure gradient profile derived from the flow velocity profile accurately predicted the directly recorded pressure gradient profile.

The mean pressure gradient can therefore be estimated by averaging a number of instantaneous pressure drops. Hence mean pressure gradient = $4(Va^2) + 4(Vb^2) + \ldots 4(Vn^2)$ divided by n, with n representing the number of observations. Estimated mean pressure gradients corre-

late well with planimetered mean pressure gradients from simultaneously recorded pressures by using high-fidelity catheter systems.

ASSESSMENT OF VALVE ORIFICE AREA

A relationship between flow volume (Q), cross-sectional area (CSA), and velocity can be expressed as:

$$Q = CSA \times \text{Velocity integral}$$

Thus flow across the left ventricular outflow tract equals the cross-sectional area of left ventricular outflow tract (LVOT) times the velocity integral.

Flow volume during each beat is nearly equal across each of the four intracardiac valves, since the heart valves are interposed between chambers representing a closed system in series. Hence cardiac output measured across each valve in the absence of valve incompetence would be nearly equal. This information permits estimation of the cross-sectional area of a stenotic valve from the velocity integral and the flow volume derived from a normal valve.

Therefore flow across the tricuspid valve equals flow across the pulmonic valve equals flow across the mitral valve equals flow across the aortic valve. In other words, flow across the tricuspid or pulmonic valve equals the cross-sectional area of stenotic mitral valve times the velocity integral across the mitral valve. Thus mitral valve area equals Q/velocity integral across the mitral valve. This approach is called the *continuity principle* and requires the absence of valve regurgitation.

In deriving the aortic valve area in patients with aortic valve stenosis, the LVOT is used because the presence of valve regurgitation becomes immaterial. All of systolic flow across the LVOT must cross the stenotic aortic valve.

Thus the aortic valve area times the velocity across the aortic valve equals the LVOT area times the velocity integral across the LVOT. In practice, the clinician obtains the LVOT diameter using a parasternal long axis view and a cross-sectional area derived as $\pi\gamma^2$ assuming a circular configuration. The LVOT velocity is obtained with pulsed wave Doppler by positioning the sample volume across the LVOT using the apical five-chamber cross section. The aortic stenosis velocity is obtained by continuous wave Doppler to provide a clearly outlined signal with maximum velocity. The aortic valve area so derived correlates closely with that determined at cardiac catheterization using the Gorlin formula.[1,2,9,10,12]

The assessment of mitral valve area in mitral stenosis may be made by using the continuity principle and flow across another valve so long as neither is incompetent. More commonly, a hemodynamic principle that relates pressure half-time to the valve area is used. With cardiac catheterization data, the Libanoff and Rodbard demonstration[6a] that the pressure half-time across the stenotic mitral valve (defined as the time for the peak transvalvar gradient to reach half its maximum value) is directly related to the severity of stenosis and is independent of flow and heart rate was first exploited by Hatle et al[3,4] using the Doppler-derived gradients. They demonstrated that:

$$MVA = \frac{220}{Pressure\ half\text{-}time}$$

where MVA is the mitral valve area. Since the pressure gradient is related to velocity squared, a simple approach is to designate peak velocity as point E. Then the peak velocity is divided by 1.4 and the value obtained is marked on the mitral stenosis velocity profile. The time taken from point E to the point of peak velocity divided by 1.4 is the pressure half-time in milliseconds. Since mitral valves with an area of 1 cm^2 had an average pressure half-time of 220 m/sec, this formula can be applied to derive the mitral valve area. This valve area also correlates well with that derived at cardiac catheterization by using the Gorlin formula.

POTENTIAL APPLICATIONS FOR CROSS-SECTIONAL AREA ACROSS LARGER-CALIBER BLOOD VESSELS

The continuity principle should be able to be applied for assessing stenosis severity in the aorta and the major arteries, provided that the lesion does not occur at a major branching site. The cross-sectional area of the normal proximal segment and the peak velocity can be obtained by pulsed Doppler and B-mode imaging. An angle correction may be required, with its potential for error. The velocity across the stenotic segment may be obtained by pulsed or continuous wave Doppler, depending on its magnitude and ease of access requiring a narrow (less than 20°) angle θ. These approaches must be validated with quantitative angiography or anatomic measurements. Successful applications of these principles to large artery stenoses have already been published by Kohler et al[5] and Langsfeld et al.[6]

REFERENCES

1. Currie PJ et al: Continuous wave Doppler echocardiographic assessment of severity of calcific aortic stenosis: a simultaneous Doppler-catheter correlative study in 100 adult patients, *Circulation* 71:1162-1169, 1986.
2. Galan A, Zoghbi WA, Quinones MA: Determination of severity of valvular aortic stenosis by Doppler echocardiography and relation of findings to clinical outcome and agreement with hemodynamic measurements determined at cardiac catheterization, *Am J Cardiol* 67:1007-1012, 1991.
3. Hatle L: Noninvasive assessment and differentiation of left ventricular outflow obstruction with Doppler ultrasound, *Circulation* 64:381-387, 1981.
4. Hatle L, Angelsen B, Tromsdal A: Noninvasive assessment of atrioventricular pressure half-time by Doppler ultrasound, *Circulation* 60:1097-1104, 1979.
5. Kohler TR et al: Assessment of pressure gradient by Doppler ultrasound: experimental and clinical observations, *J Vasc Surg* 6:460-469, 1987.
6. Langsfeld M et al: The use of deep duplex scanning to predict hemodynamically significant aortoiliac stenoses, *J Vasc Surg* 7:395-399, 1988.
6a. Libanoff A, Rodbard S: Atrioventricular pressure half-time, measure of mitral valve orifice area, *Circulation* 38:144-150,1968.
7. Nishimura RA et al: Doppler echocardiography: theory, instrumentation, technique, and application, *Mayo Clin Proc* 60:321-343, 1985.
8. Satomura S: A study on examining the heart with ultrasonics. I. Principles. II. Instrumentation, *Jap Circ J* 20:227, 1956.
9. Shah PM, Graham BM: Management of aortic stenosis: is cardiac catheterization necessary? *Am J Cardiol* 67:1031-1032, 1991.
10. Skjaerpe T, Hegrenaes L, Hatle L: Noninvasive estimation of valve area in patients with aortic stenosis by Doppler ultrasound and two-dimensional echocardiography, *Circulation* 72:810-818, 1985.
11. Wong M et al: In vitro study of the pressure-velocity relation across stenotic orifices, *Am J Cardiol* 56:465-469, 1985.
12. Zoghbi WA et al: Accurate noninvasive quantification of stenotic aortic valve area by Doppler echocardiography, *Circulation* 73:452-459, 1986.

Introduction

CHRISTOPHER R. B. MERRITT and EDWARD G. GRANT

Although Doppler ultrasound has played an important role in the evaluation of peripheral vascular disease for many years, the role of Doppler in the abdomen is only beginning to be appreciated. Until recently, abdominal ultrasonography has relied primarily on evaluation of morphologic changes in organ size, shape, position, contour, and parenchymal patterns and relatively little attention has been directed to the evaluation of abdominal blood flow. With real-time, large vessels such as the aorta, the inferior vena cava, and the mesenteric, portal, splenic, hepatic, and renal vessels are routinely imaged. Although major vessels are shown with real-time, little information about flow is provided, and significant pathology related to vascular thrombosis, narrowing, or changes in flow direction of dynamics may be overlooked. The ability of Doppler ultrasound to detect and quantify blood flow provides a valuable adjunct to imaging in the abdomen and pelvis and has had a profound impact on the sonographic evaluation of the abdomen.

Currently, the most important abdominal applications of Doppler are to aid in the identification of vessels, determine the direction of blood flow, evaluate vessel narrowing or occlusion, and aid in the characterization of flow to organs and tumors. Large vessel changes, such as flow reversal in the portal vein, the presence of portosystemic collaterals, the occlusion of portal, splenic, or renal veins, and stenosis of mesenteric or renal arteries, are all readily identifiable when using Doppler ultrasonographic methods. Analysis of the Doppler shift frequency obtained from vessels may be used to infer both stenosis at the sample site and changes in distal vascular impedance. Changes in tissue function are often associated with changes in blood flow, and Doppler ultrasound, with its ability to display such changes, is leading closer to the goal of noninvasive tissue characterization. The use of Doppler in the inference of abnormalities in the peripheral vascular bed of an organ or tissue is of particular interest. Doppler patterns may be important in the early identification of rejection of transplanted organs, parenchy-

mal dysfunction, and fetal compromise due to intrauterine growth retardation. Characteristic Doppler signals have also been described that may eventually aid in differentiation of benign from malignant masses.

Quality ultrasonography, whether it is imaging, duplex Doppler, or color flow imaging, demands special skills in the operation of equipment as well as in training and experience in the interpretation of the results. Successful interpretation requires an understanding of the basic principles and of the unique nature of the Doppler information, as well as knowledge of the techniques and instrumentation necessary to ensure the generation of high-quality data. A knowledge of the patterns of normal and abnormal flow necessary to establish a diagnosis is also necessary. Finally, the operator must differentiate real and clinically important findings from artifact. This is particularly true in the abdomen and pelvis in which greater examination depths result in the potential for artifacts and technical errors not usually encountered in peripheral vascular applications. Pitfalls await the careless or poorly trained user. No matter how sophisticated the machine is, the success or failure of the investigation is ultimately determined by the clinical, technical, and interpretive skill of the user.

Abdominal applications of Doppler are becoming increasingly important as familiarity with Doppler principles and instruments grows. New duplex and color flow imaging instruments specifically adapted for use in the abdomen and pelvis have stimulated interest in the use of Doppler techniques as a complement to imaging. Although the simultaneous display of tissue and flow information has enhanced the ease of evaluation of vascular abnormalities and increased diagnostic confidence, the role of abdominal Doppler is continuing to evolve. Since blood flow is a fundamental factor in health and disease, it seems likely that the new information provided by Doppler evaluation of the abdomen will continue to advance the role of ultrasound as a primary diagnostic method.

CHAPTER 76

Screening for abdominal aortic aneurysm in the vascular laboratory

YEHUDA G. WOLF, SHIRLEY M. OTIS, and EUGENE F. BERNSTEIN

Abdominal aortic aneurysm (AAA) is a chronic, progressive disease that is usually asymptomatic and may present initially with the catastrophic complication of rupture. When diagnosed before rupture, AAA may be treated with elective surgery with a very low mortality. These characteristics favor asymptomatic screening. However, AAA has relatively low prevalence in the general population, occurring mostly in the elderly. In addition, elective surgical treatment is expensive. These issues raise the question of social justification for a screening program aimed at discovering asymptomatic AAA compared with the cost of such screening to the expected gain in life.[6]

PREVALENCE OF DISEASE

The reported frequency of AAA in autopsies is 2% in the general population,[23] 6.6% in male veterans in the United States,[4] and 3% in the United Kingdom.[67] The apparent incidence of AAA in a population-based study in Rochester, Minnesota, increased over three decades and was 36.5 per 100,000 person-years between 1971 and 1980.[48] The incidence of rupture of AAA was 6 per 100,000 in Sweden and 7 to 17 per 100,000 in the United Kingdom.[25,36,39] In the United States, rupture of AAA is the cause of 1.2% of male deaths and 0.6% of female deaths in people over the age of 65[69] and is the thirteenth leading cause of death.[32] AAA is the cause of 1.25% of all deaths in England and Wales.[49] In Canada, AAA is associated with standard mortality rates of 9 per 100,000 males and 2.8 per 100,000 females.[14] A population-based study in Australia reported an increasing age-standardized mortality rate for AAA that was 46 per 100,000 for men over 55 years of age and 11 for women over 55 years of age in 1986 to 1988.[52]

DETECTION

Screening for AAA may be performed by a variety of modalities, including physical examination and abdominal x-ray, ultrasound, computed tomographic scan, and magnetic resonance imaging. Angiography is too insensitive, invasive, expensive, and morbid to be used as a screening test.

Physical examination may identify large aneurysms in thin and normal subjects (abdominal girth of less than 100 cm) and usually results in reliable diagnosis when findings are defined as "definitely positive" by experienced examiners.[41,57] However, physical examination is not sensitive or specific enough to serve as a screening test for smaller aneurysms. In several studies the sensitivity for detection of AAA by physical examination was 22%, 50%, and 69%, and the positive predictive value was 15%, 17%, 35%, and 77%.[2,5,41,57]

Plain abdominal radiography relies on the presence of sufficient calcium in the aneurysm wall. This method has a reported sensitivity of 56%, 60%, and 77% but is more commonly positive in larger aneurysms and is occasionally interpreted as false-positive because of a calcified tortuous aorta.[35,45,57]

B-mode ultrasound is a highly practical and reliable test for AAA screening. Early reports documented that ultrasound could estimate the size of an AAA within 1.0 cm of the size measured at operation in 92% of cases, and the average difference was 0.42 cm in the transverse diameter and 0.29 cm in the anteroposterior diameter.[35,45] In another study, measurement of the anteroposterior diameter was highly accurate[12] and was within 0.3 cm of the measurement at operation.[31] Modern gray-scale units with real-time capability have even better definition than earlier models. In a recent study, ultrasound measurement of aneurysm size had a sensitivity and positive predictive value of 100% as verified by computed tomographic scan or surgery.[41] Aortic diameter was highly reproducible in serial ultrasound examinations,[8] and in comparing aneurysm size measured by ultrasound, computed tomography, and magnetic resonance imaging, discrepancies were less than 0.2 cm.[3]

Computed tomography and magnetic resonance imaging are highly accurate in defining the presence and the size of aortic aneurysms as well as their anatomic relations.[3,30] However, the associated cost, time, and logistic difficulty make these tests less practical for routine screening.

Of the various modalities, ultrasound is clearly the most useful for screening. Imprecise definition of the retroperi-

Table 76-1. Screening for abdominal aortic aneurysms by ultrasound

Author	Year	Country	N	Population screened	Prevalence* >3 cm/>4 cm
Cabellon[13]	1983	United States	73	PVD or CAD	9.5%†
Twomey[68]	1984	United Kingdom	84	Males >50 yr, HTN	10.7%†
Lindholm[43]	1985	Sweden	245	50-69 yr, HTN	0.4%†
Thurmond[65]	1986	United States	120	>50 yr, cardiology clinic patients	23.0%/5.0%
Allen[2]	1987	United Kingdom	168	>65 yr	1.7%/0.6%
Allardice[1]	1988	United Kingdom	100	PVD	10.0%/5.0%
Lederle[41]	1988	United States	201	Males 60-76 yr, HTN or CAD	9.0%/5.0%
Collin[17]	1988	United Kingdom	746	Males 65-74 yr	4.2%/2.0%
O'Kelly[53]	1989	United Kingdom	906	Males 65-74 yr	5.0%/1.5%‡
Berridge[10]	1989	United Kingdom	104	PVD	6.7%/5.7%
Shapira[61]	1990	Israel	101	PVD	4.0%/2.0%
Bengstsson[7]	1991	Sweden	375	Males 74 yr	7.6%/3.3%
Scott[60]	1991	United Kingdom	4237	65-80 yr	4.3%/1.3%
This study	1992	United States	341	PVD	5.3%/2.6%

PVD, Peripheral vascular disease; *CAD,* coronary artery disease; *HTN,* hypertension.
*The prevalence rate was calculated as the fraction of those visualized and was corrected for the definition of size where possible.
†Size of AAA not specified.
‡Numbers reported for aortic diameter >2.5 cm (7.8%) and >4.0 cm (1.5%)

toneal relations of the aneurysm is unimportant in this application and is outweighed by the advantage of simplicity and low cost.

PREVIOUS SCREENING PROJECTS

A total of 13 prior reports on screening for AAA by means of ultrasound have been published (Table 76-1).* Of these studies, 7 were performed in the United Kingdom where the three largest studies were carried out, screening 746, 906, and 4237 elderly people from the general population.[17,53,60] The other studies examined 73 to 375 patients and were performed in the United States, Sweden, and Israel. The prevalence of AAA, defined as a localized dilatation measuring at least 3 cm, was 4.3% in a large study screening the general population over 65 years of age.[60] In males 65 to 74 years old, aneurysm prevalence was 4.2%,[17,53] and in a cohort of males 74 years old, it was 7.4%.[7] In one Swedish study, 245 hypertensive patients between the ages of 50 and 69 years were screened, and only one patient with AAA was detected (prevalence— 0.4%), a result clearly different from the other studies.[43] Patients with heart disease or hypertension had a prevalence rate of 4.0% to 23.0% and a mean prevalence rate of 10%.† Patients with peripheral arterial disease are known to have an increased prevalence of AAA.[4] The visit of such patients to the vascular laboratory, where the required instrumentation and the expertise are available, presents an excellent opportunity to screen for the presence of AAA.

METHODS AND MATERIALS

Over a period of 17 months, 341 patients who were initially referred with peripheral arterial occlusive disease were screened at Scripps Clinic and Research Foundation. The

patients were prepared with overnight fasting, and after lower extremity or carotid artery examination in the vascular laboratory, the abdominal aorta was scanned with B-mode ultrasound. The aorta was adequately visualized in 303 (89%) patients. Aortic aneurysms (greater than 3.0 cm) were detected in 16 patients (4.7%, 5.3% of those visualized), and all were confined to the infrarenal aorta. The maximum transverse diameter was 3.0 to 3.9 cm in 8 patients, 4.0 to 4.9 cm in 5 patients, and over 5.0 cm in 3 patients. All aneurysms were found in males and 15 of those in males over 60 years of age with a positive smoking history. This group constituted only 35% of the screened population yet included 94% of the aneurysms; the prevalence rate in this group was 13%. The number of patients detected by screening was substantial and constituted 18% of the number of patients seen in consultation with a diagnosis of AAA at the hospital during the same time period. The prevalence of abdominal aneurysms in the study is lower than the previously reported prevalence in patients with peripheral arterial disease.[1,4] However, screening in the vascular laboratory in conjunction with arterial examination is rapid and inexpensive and, in this setting, may be cost effective.

HIGH-RISK GROUPS

In targeting a population for screening, the definition of high-risk groups is essential. AAA is clearly associated with aging: a postmortem study found an aneurysm prevalence of 1% in people younger than 55 years, increasing to a prevalence of 13% in people over 75 years.[4] In males, AAAs are about five times more prevalent and five times more frequent as a cause of death.[60] With increasing age, the difference between the sexes diminishes, and beyond 85 years, the prevalence and the related mortality rates are equal in males and females. In at least some cases, AAAs are familial, and the risk for AAA is increased 11.6-fold in a first-degree relative of a diagnosed patient.[37,66] AAA is

---

*References 1, 2, 7, 10, 13, 17, 41, 43, 53, 60, 61, 65, 68.
†References 1, 10, 13, 41, 61, 65, 68.

Table 76-2. Cost of elective and urgent repair of AAAs

Author	City	Years	Elective repair	Urgent repair	Urgent repair survival >24 hr
Pasch[55]	Rochester, NY	1980-1981	$10,114	$18,223	$27,144
Breckwoldt[11]	Boston, Mass	1986-1989	$24,642	$49,787	
Johansen[38]	Seattle, Wash	1985-1989	$14,555	$23,145	$38,627

strongly related to smoking, as shown in the screening study, and was eight times more common in heavy smokers at autopsy.[4] Peripheral arterial disease and coronary artery disease are associated with an aneurysm prevalence of about 10%, compared with 5% in the general population. Hypertension was associated with a prevalence rate of 10% in one study,[68] but there was no increase in prevalence in two others[7,43] nor in the study done at Scripps Clinic and Research Foundation.

NATURAL HISTORY

The mean diameter of the normal infrarenal aorta is 2.1 cm, and it tends to be larger in males and with increasing age.[54] Aneurysms in the infrarenal location are commonly defined as a localized aortic dilatation with a diameter exceeding 3.0 cm.

Most aneurysms expand gradually at a rate that appears to relate to the size of the aneurysm.[18,33,42] It is 0.22 cm annually for AAAs smaller than 4.0 cm and 0.4 cm per year in AAAs smaller than 6.0 cm.[8] The mean annual expansion rate varies in different reports from 0.21 to 0.79 cm[44,51] and appears to be lower in population-based studies compared with a referral patient population. Individual AAA expansion rates vary over time.[22]

Rupture has been reported to occur in one third of patients with AAA,[63] and 25% of AAAs in one autopsy study were found to be ruptured.[23] The incidence of rupture for all AAAs was 6% at 5 years and 8% after 10 years in one study[51] and 12% after 5 years in another study.[28] The annual rupture rate of 6% in patients with aneurysms was similar to the mortality rate from other causes.[21] The frequency of rupture is clearly related to AAA size[64] and has been reported to be more common in patients with chronic obstructive lung disease and in the presence of diastolic hypertension.[21] For AAAs larger than 5 cm, the 5- to 6-year rupture rate was 20% to 25%.[33,51] Rupture of AAAs less than 5 cm is uncommon, but rupture of AAAs less than 4 cm has been reported.[23,33,54] Once rupture has occurred, 47% to 64% of patients die before reaching the hospital.[24,25,47]

INTERVENTION

Elective surgical repair of AAAs in modern series from major centers carries a mortality rate of 2% or less.[15] These results have been achieved by aggressive preoperative screening for cardiac disease and improved perioperative care.[29] After repair, survival rates approach those of the general age-matched population.[62] These observations re-

garding the safety of the procedure and its long-term results extend to patients over the age of 70 years as well.[9]

In contrast, results of surgery for ruptured AAAs are poor. The impact of surgical intervention is limited by the high mortality rates (47% to 64%) before reaching the hospital. Of those patients arriving at the hospital alive, short-term survival rates of 30%, 36%, 67%,[34,38,46] and 77% in Crawford's personal series[20] have been reported. The overall survival rate after rupture is therefore 11% to 36%. After recovery, however, the long-term survival rate and quality of life after a ruptured AAA are no different from after elective repair and are comparable to those of the general age- and sex-matched population.[26,58]

Elective and urgent repair of AAAs differs markedly in cost (Table 76-2). The ratio of the cost of a ruptured AAA to the cost of elective repair in several reports varied from 1.56 to 2.02.[11,19,38,55] The ratio of the treatment costs of patients with ruptured AAA surviving 24 hours to the cost of elective repair was 2.65 and 2.68 in two reports.[11,38]

COST-BENEFIT ANALYSIS

On the basis of the foregoing data, an estimate of the cost and the impact on the mortality rate of an ultrasound screening project of 100,000 people has been performed. The assumptions are the following:

- The sensitivity and specificity of ultrasound is 100%.
- The prevalence rate of AAAs greater than 4 cm is one-third the rate of AAAs greater than 3 cm.
- Surgical repair is recommended to all patients with AAAs larger than 4 cm.
- For patients in whom operation is recommended, 80% will ultimately undergo surgical repair.
- Patients with AAAs 3 to 4 cm are reevaluated at 3-year intervals until the AAA is greater than 4 cm or rupture or death occurs (three times on average).
- A total of 50% of AAAs 3 to 4 cm will remain stable and 50% will expand beyond 4 cm.
- Of patients with undiagnosed AAAs, 25% of the AAAs will ultimately rupture.
- Of patients with known, untreated AAAs, 5% of the AAAs will rupture.
- No rupture occurs in AAAs less than 4 cm.
- In an unscreened population, 25% of the AAAs are detected.
- After rupture, 50% of patients die before reaching the hospital.
- The overall mortality rate after rupture is 85%.

- The mortality rate of elective repair of AAAs is 2%.
- The total cost of screening is $100 per examination.
- The cost of elective repair of AAAs is $25,000.
- The cost of a ruptured AAA is $43,500.

Direct screening-related expenses are presented in Table 76-3. The cost of diagnosing one AAA greater than 4 cm is $1450 to 3630. This cost is inversely related to the prevalence rate in the screened population and may be reduced by focusing on high-risk groups. Another controllable variable is the cost of examination, which may be lowered by linking the test to another study, such as a peripheral arterial or cerebrovascular examination, as in the study done at Scripps Clinic and Research Foundation. Direct screening costs are, however, only a minor component of the expense related to the whole screening project, decreasing from 14% to 6% with increasing aneurysm prevalence.

The total expenditure is primarily the cost of elective repair and the savings resulting from prevention of rupture (Table 76-4). Screening for AAAs will result in a savings of 422 to 1410 lives per 100,000 people screened at a cost of $87,800 to 118,750 per life saved. Two analyses performed in the United States resulted in similar or higher cost estimates,[27,56] whereas European estimates were significantly lower (Table 76-5).

The analysis presented here is only an approximation. Many of the assumptions on which it is based cannot be defined with accuracy. This is true for the rates related to the natural history of the disease and, as a result, for the size at which surgical repair should be recommended, which is still controversial. The estimate includes reevaluation of AAAs measuring 3 to 4 cm but does not address the issue of rescreening of those people without AAAs, a study that appears to be much less cost efficient.[27]

The expenses associated with screening for AAAs compare favorably with an accepted screening modality—mammography for early detection of breast cancer. The cost for detection of one aneurysm greater than 4 cm is $1450 to $3630 compared to $23,400 for detection of one breast cancer.[50] The cost per death averted is $87,800 to $118,500 for AAA screening and $123,400 for breast cancer in general and $60,000 for women at the age of 60 years.[50] Analysis of cost per quality life-years saved also showed a lower rate for AAA screening compared with a breast cancer screening program.[59]

Definition of the population to be screened is clearly important in determining the cost-benefit ratio of the project. This ratio is expected to be lowest for a screening program directed at men over 60 years with a positive smoking history and evidence of peripheral or coronary artery disease. Although women have lower prevalence rates, screening costs per life-year saved are only slightly higher than in men due to their longer life expectancy.

The ultimate merit of a screening project for AAA will be determined only by a clinical trial that includes treatment outcome. Even then, problems of interpretation may exist. The labeling of patients with the diagnosis of AAA may have a direct psychological effect on the patient or on the physician. In addition, as in other "sniper diseases" that may remain undiagnosed even after causing death, AAA may be recognized more frequently as a cause of death in the screened group as compared with the unscreened group, in which death from AAA may be erroneously ascribed to another disease.[40]

CONCLUSION

The mortality resulting from rupture of a AAA may be reduced by early detection by screening the elderly population with ultrasound. In patients being evaluated for peripheral arterial disease, a visit to the vascular laboratory provides an excellent, low-cost opportunity to screen for the presence of AAA. In the elderly population, such a screening project coupled with surgical therapy would be expected to save 422 to 1410 lives per 100,000 people screened at a cost of $87,800 to $118,500 per life saved. Whether this represents a justified and desirable investment will ultimately be a societal judgment.

Table 76-3. Cost of screening 100,000 people for AAAs

	AAA prevalence >3 cm—4.5%; >4 cm—1.5%			AAA prevalence >3 cm—15.0%; >4 cm—5.0%		
	Cost (× $1000)	Number of aneurysms found		Cost (× $1000)	Number of aneurysms found	
		AAAs 3-4 cm*	AAAs >4 cm†		AAAs 3-4 cm*	AAAs >4 cm†
Initial scan	10,000	3000 ↓	1500	10,000	10,000 ↓	5000
Repeat scans of AAAs 3-4 cm	900	1500	1500	3000	5000	5000
TOTAL	10,900	1500	3000	13,000	5000	10,000
Cost per AAA >4 cm	3.63			1.30		
(= total cost/ no. AAAs >4 cm)						

*To be followed and scanned at 3-year intervals, three times on average—$300/patient.
†AAAs >4 cm referred for elective repair.

Table 76-4. Consequences of screening 100,000 people for AAAs

Prevalence AAAs >4 cm/AAAs >3 cm	Population	Screening* cost (× $1000)	Elective repair		Ruptured AAAs		Total		Cost per life saved (× $1000)
			Mortality† (deaths/el ops)	Cost‡ (× $1000)	Mortality§ (deaths/ruptures)	Cost‖	Mortality (no.)	Cost (× $1000)	
1.5%/4.5%	Screened	10,900	48/2400	60,000	26/30	6525	74	77,425	
	Unscreened		12/600	15,000	484/570	12,397	496	27,397	
	Difference	10,900	36	45,000	−458	−5872	−422	50,023	119
5.0%/15.0%	Screened	13,000	160/8000	200,000	85/100	2175	245	215,175	
	Unscreened		40/2000	50,000	1615/1900	41,325	1655	91,325	
	Difference	13,000	120	150,000	−1530	−39,150	−1410	123,850	88

El ops, Elective operations.

*Total cost derived from Table 76-3.

†Calculated at 2% of those acutally operated on times 80% of those referred for elective surgery.

‡Estimated at $25,000 per elective operation.

§Based on mortality rate of 85% for ruptured AAAs. Rupture rate — 5% for known and 25% for undiagnosed AAAs.

‖Based on a 50% operation rate for ruptured AAAs at a cost of $43,500.

Table 76-5. Cost-benefit estimates of screening for AAAs

Author	Country	Year	Cost per life saved	Cost per life year
Collin[16]	United Kingdom	1985	$15,300	$1530*
Bengtsson[6]	Sweden	1989	$6984	$698*
Quill[56]	United States	1989	$78,000-108,000	$7800-10,800*
Russell[59]	United Kingdom	1990	$7480-25,670*	$748-2567
Frame[27]	United States	1991	$470,000*	$47,000†
Present estimate	United States	1992	$88,000-119,000	$8780-11,850*

*Calculated for an average prolongation of life by 10 years.

†The most probable result within a range of $14,000 to $249,000.

REFERENCES

1. Allardice JT et al: High prevalence of abdominal aortic aneurysm in men with peripheral vascular disease: screening by ultrasonography, *Br J Surg* 75:240-242, 1988.

2. Allen PIM et al: Population screening for aortic aneurysms, *Lancet* 2:736-737, 1987.

3. Amparo EG et al: Comparison of magnetic resonance imaging and ultrasonography in the evaluation of abdominal aortic aneurysms, *Radiology* 154:451-456, 1985.

4. Auerbach O, Garfinkel L: Atherosclerosis and aneurysm of aorta in relation to smoking habits and age, *Chest* 78:805-809, 1980.

5. Beede SD et al: Positive predictive value of clinical suspicion of abdominal aortic aneurysm, *Arch Intern Med* 150:549-551, 1990.

6. Bengtsson H et al: Ultrasonographic screening for abdominal aortic aneurysm: analysis of surgical decisions for cost-effectiveness, *World J Surg* 13:266-271, 1989.

7. Bengtsson H et al: A population-based screening of abdominal aortic aneurysms, *Eur J Vasc Surg* 5:53-57, 1991.

8. Bernstein EF, Chan EL: Abdominal aortic aneurysm in high risk patients, *Ann Surg* 200:255-263, 1984.

9. Bernstein EF, Dilley RB, Randolph HF: The improving long-term outlook for patients over 70 years of age with abdominal aortic aneurysms, *Ann Surg* 207:318-322, 1988.

10. Berridge DC et al: Screening for clinically unsuspected abdominal aortic aneurysms in patients with peripheral vascular disease, *Eur J Vasc Surg* 3:421-422, 1989.

11. Breckwoldt WL, Mackey WC, O'Donnell TF: The economic implications of high-risk abdominal aortic aneurysms, *J Vasc Surg* 13:798-804, 1991.

12. Brewster DC et al: Assessment of abdominal aortic aneurysm size, *Circulation* 56(suppl II):164-169, 1977.

13. Cabellon S et al: Incidence of abdominal aortic aneurysm in patients with atheromatous arterial disease, *Am J Surg* 146:575-576, 1983.

14. Canadian Task Force on Periodic Health Examination: *Periodic health examination, 1991 update: 5. Screening for abdominal aortic aneurysm*, Ottawa, Ontario, 1991, Health Services Directorate, Department of National Health and Welfare.

15. Clark ET et al: Current results of elective aortic reconstruction for aneurysmal and occlusive disease, *J Cardiovasc Surg* 31:438-441, 1990.

16. Collin J: Screening for abdominal aortic aneurysms, *Br J Surg* 72:851-852, 1985.

17. Collin J, Araujo L, Walton J: A community detection program for abdominal aortic aneurysm, *Angiology* 41:53-58, 1990.

18. Collin J, Heather B, Walton J: Growth rates of subclinical abdominal aortic aneurysms—implication for review and rescreening programmes, *Eur J Vasc Surg* 5:141-144, 1991.

19. Cooley DA, Carmichael MJ: Abdominal aortic aneurysm, *Circulation* 70(suppl I):5-6, 1984.

20. Crawford ES: Ruptured abdominal aortic aneurysm: an editorial, *J Vasc Surg* 13:348-350, 1991.

21. Cronenwett JL et al: Actuarial analysis of variables associated with rupture of small abdominal aortic aneurysms, *Surgery* 98:472-483, 1985.

22. Cronenwett JL et al: Variables that affect the expansion rate and outcome of small abdominal aortic aneurysms, *J Vasc Surg* 11:260-269, 1990.

23. Darling CR et al: Autopsy study of unoperated abdominal aortic aneurysms, *Circulation* 56(suppl II):161-164, 1977.

24. Dent A, Kent SJS, Young TW: Ruptured abdominal aortic aneurysm: what is the true mortality? *Br J Surg* 73:318, 1986.

25. Drott C et al: Age-standardized incidence of ruptured aortic aneurysm in a defined Swedish population between 1952 and 1988: mortality rate and operative results, *Br J Surg* 79:175-179, 1992.

26. Fielding JWL et al: Diagnosis and management of 528 abdominal aortic aneurysms, *Br Med J* 283:355-359, 1981.

27. Frame PS: *Screening for abdominal aortic aneurysm: a commentary on the Canadian task force on the periodic health examination*, Nov 1991, US Preventive Services Task Force.

28. Glimaker H et al: Natural history of patients with abdominal aortic aneurysms, *Eur J Vasc Surg* 5:125-130, 1991.

29. Golden MA et al: Selective evaluation and management of coronary artery disease in patients undergoing repair of abdominal aortic aneurysms, *Ann Surg* 212:415-423, 1990.

30. Gomes MN, Wallace RB: Present status of abdominal aorta imaging by computed tomography, *J Cardiovasc Surg* 26:1-6, 1985.

31. Graeve AH et al: Discordance in sizing of abdominal aortic aneurysm and its significance, *Am J Surg* 144:627-634, 1982.

32. Grove RD, Hetzel AM: Vital statistics in the United States, 1940-1960, Washington, 1968, US Government Printing Office.

33. Guirguis EM, Barber GG: The natural history of abdominal aortic aneurysms, *Am J Surg* 162:481-483, 1991.

34. Harris LM et al: Ruptured abdominal aortic aneurysms: factors affecting mortality rates, *J Vasc Surg* 14:812-820, 1991.

35. Hertzer NR, Beven EG: Ultrasound measurement and elective aneurysmectomy, *JAMA* 140:1966-1968, 1978.

36. Ingolby CJH, Wujanto R, Mitchell JE: Impact of vascular surgery on community mortality from ruptured aortic aneurysms, *Br J Surg* 73:551-553, 1986.

37. Johansen K, Koepsell T: Familial tendency for abdominal aortic aneurysms, *JAMA* 256:1934-1936, 1986.

38. Johansen K et al: Ruptured abdominal aortic aneurysm: the Harborview experience, *J Vasc Surg* 13:240-247, 1991.

39. Johansson G, Swedenborg J: Ruptured abdominal aortic aneurysms: a study of incidence and mortality, *Br J Surg* 73:101-103, 1986.

40. Lederle FA: Screening for snipers: the burden of proof, *J Clin Epidemiol* 43:101-104, 1990.

41. Lederle FA, Walker JM, Reinke DB: Selective screening for abdominal aortic aneurysms with physical examination and ultrasound, *Arch Intern Med* 148:1753-1756, 1988.

42. Limet R, Sakalihassan N, Albert A: Determination of the expansion rate and incidence of rupture of abdominal aortic aneurysms, *J Vasc Surg* 14:540-548, 1991.

43. Lindholm L et al: Low prevalence of abdominal aortic aneurysm in hypertensive patients, *Acta Med Scand* 218:305-310, 1985.

44. Littooy FN et al: Use of sequential B-mode ultrasonography to manage abdominal aortic aneurysms, *Arch Surg* 124:419-421, 1989.

45. Maloney JD et al: Ultrasound evaluation of abdominal aortic aneurysms, *Circulation* 56(suppl II):80-85, 1977.

46. Martin RS et al: Ruptured abdominal aortic aneurysm: a 25-year experience and analysis of recent cases, *Am J Surg* 54:539-543, 1988.

47. Mealy K, Salman A: The true incidence of ruptured abdominal aortic aneurysms, *Eur J Vasc Surg* 2:405-408, 1988.

48. Melton LJ et al: Changing incidence of abdominal aortic aneurysms: a population-based study, *Am J Epidemiol* 120:379-386, 1984.

49. Mortality Statistics, England and Wales, Series DH2, 12, HMSO, London, 1985, Office of Population Censuses and Surveys.

50. Moskowitz M: Costs of screening for breast cancer, *Radiol Clin North Am* 25:1031-1037, 1987.

51. Nevitt MP, Ballard DJ, Hallett JW: Prognosis of abdominal aortic aneurysms, *N Engl J Med* 321:1009-1014, 1989.

52. Norman PE, Castleden WM, Hockey RL: Prevalence of abdominal aortic aneurysm in Western Australia, *Br J Surg* 78:1118-1121, 1991.

53. O'Kelly TJ, Heather BP: General practice-based population screening for abdominal aortic aneurysms: a pilot study, *Br J Surg* 76:479-480, 1989.

54. Ouriel K et al: An evaluation of new methods of expressing aneurysm size: relationship to rupture, *J Vasc Surg* 15:12-20, 1992.

55. Pasch AR et al: Abdominal aortic aneurysm: the case for elective resection, *Circulation* 70(suppl I):1-4, 1984.

56. Quill DS, Colgan MP, Sumner DS: Ultrasonic screening for the detection of abdominal aortic aneurysms, *Surg Clin North Am* 69:713-720, 1989.

57. Robiscek F: The diagnosis of abdominal aneurysms, *Surgery* 89:275-276, 1981.

58. Rohrer MJ, Cutler BS, Wheeler B: Long-term survival and quality of life following ruptured abdominal aortic aneurysm, *Arch Surg* 123:1213-1217, 1988.

59. Russell JGB: Is screening for abdominal aortic aneurysm worthwhile? *Clin Radiol* 41:182-184, 1990.

60. Scott RAP, Ashton HA, Kay DN: Abdominal aortic aneurysm in 4237 screened patients: prevalence, development and management over 6 years, *Br J Surg* 78:1121-1125, 1991.

61. Shapira OM et al: Ultrasound screening for abdominal aortic aneurysms in patients with atherosclerotic peripheral vascular disease, *J Cardiovasc Surg* 31:170-172, 1990.

62. Soreide O et al: Abdominal aortic aneurysms: survival analysis of four hundred thirty-four patients, *Surgery* 91:188-193, 1982.

63. Szilagyi DE, Elliott JP, Smith RF: Clinical fate of the patient with asymptomatic abdominal aortic aneurysm and unfit for surgical treatment, *Arch Surg* 104:600-606, 1972.

64. Szilagyi DE et al: Contribution of abdominal aortic aneurysmectomy to prolongation of life, *Ann Surg* 164:678-699, 1966.

65. Thurmond AS, Semler HJ: Abdominal aortic aneurysm: incidence in a population at risk, *J Cardiovasc Surg* 27:457-460, 1986.

66. Tilson DM, Seashore MR: Human genetics of abdominal aortic aneurysm, *Surg Gynecol Obstet* 158:129-132, 1984.

67. Turk KAD: The postmortem incidence of abdominal aortic aneurysm, *Proc R Soc Med* 58:869-870, 1965.

68. Twomey A et al: Unrecognized aneurysmal disease in male hypertensive patients, *Br J Surg* 71:307-308, 1984.

69. US Department of Health and Human Services: *Vital statistics of the United States, 1985, vol II, mortality part A,* Hyattsville, Md, 1988, National Center for Health Statistics.

CHAPTER 77

Evaluation of renal artery stenosis

MARK H. MEISSNER and D. EUGENE STRANDNESS, Jr.

RENOVASCULAR DISEASE

Renovascular disease can be defined as the presence of stenotic lesions of the main renal artery or its branches.[22,32] However, such an anatomic definition implies little regarding the hemodynamic or physiologic significance of these lesions. Hemodynamically, a critical stenosis occurs at the point where further small reductions in luminal area produce large changes in pressure and flow. In the renal arteries, activation of the renin-angiotensin system presumably occurs at this point. Hamovici and Zinicola[11] defined such critical lesions in the canine renal artery and reported that stenoses up to 50% resulted in no pressure gradient and no effect on renal function whereas lesions greater than 60% produced both a pressure drop and an absent nephrogram on urography. Physiologically, two clinical syndromes—renovascular hypertension and ischemic nephropathy—may be associated with a hemodynamically significant stenosis. When such a lesion leads to activation of the renin-angiotensin system, renovascular hypertension may result. With bilateral flow-reducing lesions, ischemic renal failure may be the outcome. The important problem clinically is to identify those patients with anatomic renovascular disease and to determine which anatomic lesions are physiologically significant.

Since renal artery stenosis may be correctable, identification of patients with hemodynamically significant renovascular disease becomes critically important. End organ damage in patients with atherosclerotic renovascular hypertension has been reported to be more common than in patients with essential hypertension.[22] Although advances in the medical management of hypertension may reduce the incidence of cardiovascular complications, progressive loss of renal function may occur despite acceptable blood pressure control.[6] Failure to identify a renovascular origin of hypertension also commits the patient to a lifetime of medical therapy, which may be poorly tolerated in this elderly population.

Epidemiology

Hypertension is estimated to affect approximately 60 million people in the United States.[33] Among secondary causes of hypertension, renovascular hypertension is most com-

mon. The true prevalence of renovascular hypertension is unknown and varies with the population studied. This lack of epidemiologic data reflects the absence of widely available, sensitive, noninvasive screening tests. In clinically screened populations, the incidence of renovascular hypertension ranges from 16.7% to 32%[27,33] and may be as high as 45% in patients with both uncontrollable hypertension and renal failure.[16] Although this may reflect the incidence in tertiary referral centers, the prevalence among nonselected populations of hypertensive patients is estimated to be less than 2% to 3%.[3,8,16,32,33]

Etiology

Atherosclerosis and fibromuscular dysplasia are the most common causes of renovascular hypertension in the United States. Atherosclerosis represents two thirds of all renovascular lesions and is the most common cause of renovascular hypertension in patients over age 50. Renovascular disease in this setting is most commonly caused by atherosclerosis affecting multiple arterial beds, although isolated renal lesions may be found in 15% to 20% of patients.[33] Men are affected twice as frequently as women, and lesions are frequently bilateral. Atherosclerotic lesions characteristically involve the origin and proximal 2 cm of the renal artery, are frequently eccentric, and may be accompanied by poststenotic dilatation.[17,33] In contrast, fibromuscular disease most commonly affects patients under age 40 and is almost exclusively a disease of women. Several pathologic variants, including intimal fibroplasia, medial fibroplasia, medial hyperplasia, paramedial fibroplasia, medial dissection, and periarterial fibroplasia, have been recognized.[15] A thorough discussion of all recognized variants, differing in anatomy and clinical course, is beyond the scope of this text. However, the most common variant, medial fibroplasia, characteristically consists of a series of circumferential stenoses, predominantly affecting the distal two thirds of the artery.[15,31] Rare causes of renovascular disease include Takayasu's disease, renal artery thrombosis or embolism, extrinsic renal artery compression by cysts or tumors, abdominal aortic coarctation, and congenital vascular lesions.[31,33]

SCREENING FOR RENOVASCULAR DISEASE
Indications for screening

Identification of hypertensive subpopulations likely to have physiologically significant renovascular disease is important for several reasons. When used for screening a large population for an uncommon disease, any diagnostic test with less than perfect specificity will result in a significant number of false-positive studies. Appropriate clinical screening reduces the number of false-positive tests, thereby reducing the number of patients subjected to the expense and small but definite risk of arteriography, the gold standard of diagnosis. Additionally, the coincident occurrence of hemodynamically insignificant renovascular disease and essential hypertension is probably more common than true renovascular hypertension.[32] Because only the latter will benefit from interventional therapy, precise identification of those with symptomatic renovascular disease is crucial.

Unfortunately, no clinical features reliably distinguish renovascular hypertension from essential hypertension.[22,24] However, certain aspects of the hypertensive patient's presentation may increase the diagnostic yield of further evaluation. Clinical criteria suggestive of a renovascular origin of hypertension include onset of hypertension at an early (younger than 30 years) or late (older than 50 years) age, abrupt onset of hypertension at any age, accelerated hypertension, malignant hypertension, hypertension refractory to optimal management with three or more drugs, azotemia, and the presence of a flank bruit.[27,33] An episode of acute renal failure related to antihypertensive therapy, particularly angiotensin-converting enzyme (ACE) inhibitors, has also been suggested as an indication for further evaluation.[18] Patients with these findings constitute a subpopulation with a significantly higher prevalence of renovascular disease.[27,33]

Screening tests

The diagnosis of renovascular hypertension requires three elements.[26] An anatomic lesion of one or both renal arteries must be found, the hemodynamic significance of such a lesion must be inferred, and the clinical presentation must be compatible with renovascular hypertension. Since renovascular disease may coexist with other causes of hypertension, the recognition of lesions that are hemodynamically significant becomes critically important in determining further management. Only those lesions that produce a reduction in distal renal artery pressure sufficient to activate the renin-angiotensin system are clinically significant. In some instances, proof of the relationship between a stenosis and hypertension can be assessed only after correction of the lesion. In theory, renovascular hypertension should be cured or improved after correction of the stenosis. Although diagnostic percutaneous transluminal angioplasty has been proposed by some,[32] exposing patients to the potential morbidity of this procedure before a thorough evaluation is not justified.

Any proposed screening test should have a high sensitivity so that all patients with renovascular hypertension are identified and afforded further evaluation. However, high specificity is also desirable so that few patients with hypertension due to other causes are subjected to the expense and potential morbidity of arteriography. It must be appreciated that most screening tests have been validated in populations with a high prevalence of disease. In the case of an uncommon disease such as renovascular hypertension, small decreases in specificity translate into large numbers of false-positive studies when applied to all patients with hypertension. Because essential hypertension is substantially more common than renovascular hypertension, even very sensitive tests will not reliably distinguish between the two groups if specificity is lacking.[22] Additionally, the positive and negative predictive values of such tests, which depend on disease prevalence, cannot be extrapolated to the general hypertensive population.

Renal arteriography is the only diagnostic test for renovascular hypertension that has withstood the test of time. However, arteriography provides only anatomic information regarding the extent of renovascular disease. On the basis of the canine model of Hamovici and Zinicola,[11] lesions reducing luminal diameter by more than 60% are presumed to produce distal reduction of pressure and flow. Arteriography may be misleading if oblique views are not obtained, and it provides no direct information regarding the hemodynamic significance of a stenotic lesion. Additionally, the expense and small but definite risk of complications make it an unsuitable screening test.

Many screening tests have been developed to identify those patients who would benefit from further arteriographic evaluation. Hypertensive urography was the first widely available test used for this purpose. Abnormal urograms have been reported in 77% to 78% of patients with significant renovascular disease, with corresponding specificities ranging from 66% to 98%.[10,22] However, diagnostic findings such as a delayed nephrogram, delayed contrast excretion, and a discrepancy in renal length depend on the presence of a unilateral stenosis. The inadequacy of urography in bilateral and segmental disease and its limited sensitivity and specificity make it an inadequate screening test.[8,27] Additionally, no features of the urogram reliably predict improvement after surgery or angioplasty.[22] Radionuclide renography suffers from similar deficiencies. Although the sensitivity may be better than urography, false-positive studies with unilateral parenchymal disease significantly reduce the specificity.[23,31] Such lesions may be more common than renovascular disease among hypertensive patients.[23] ACE inhibitors selectively decrease the glomerular filtration rate in kidneys with renal artery stenosis and may improve the accuracy of radionuclide studies. However, even after premedication with ACE inhibitors, sensitivities of renographic differential glomerular filtration rate and effective renal plasma flow have been prospectively reported to be 91% and 80% with corresponding specificities of only 50% and 42%, respectively.[27] Plasma renin activity has also been advocated as an easily performed test to screen for renovascular hypertension. However, plasma renin activities in essential and renovascular hypertension may overlap significantly.[24] Even after pretreatment with ACE inhibitors, prospective sensitivities and specificities of only 39% to 73% and 72% to 96%, respectively, have been reported.[24,27] Plasma renin activity is also significantly influenced by sodium balance, posture, and chronic illnesses, such as diabetes, congestive heart failure, and cirrhosis.[31] Furthermore, the study requires discontinuing antihypertensive medication 2 weeks before the test, which may be unwise in many patients.[10,24] Intravenous digital subtraction arteriography has been enthusiastically recommended by others.[27] However, this technique is limited by the high doses of contrast material required, inadequate renal artery visualization in patients with cardiac dysfunction, inadequate visualization of branch vessels, and difficulty in identifying fibromuscular lesions.[8,33] In general, all of these screening tests are associated with significant false-negative rates and may yield positive results with diseases other than renovascular hypertension. For maximizing sensitivity, the performance of multiple screening tests has been proposed.[10,22] Although such an approach may improve accuracy, it points out the inadequacy of the individual screening tests.

The combination of B-mode ultrasound imaging with pulsed Doppler technology was first applied to the carotid bifurcation and is now a well-established diagnostic modality. However, evaluation of the renal and visceral arteries has become feasible only with the introduction of low-frequency transducers and improved signal processing.[19] Ultrasonic duplex scanning is unique in that it provides information regarding the location of a stenosis as well as a measure of its hemodynamic significance. In addition, it can be performed concurrent with antihypertensive therapy as well as in the presence of renal failure and hypertensive crisis.[16]

RENAL DUPLEX
The renal spectral waveform

Greene at al[9] first use duplex sonography to characterize normal and pathologic renal artery flow in humans. Their initial work involved study of the luminal anatomy with the B-mode image, measurement of renal artery flow rates, and a description of the renal artery velocity waveform. Although use of the B-mode image and measurement of volume flow rates are currently of limited clinical utility, their initial characterization of the renal artery waveform has been validated by others.[19]

The spectral waveform of the renal arteries is characteristic of arteries supplying low resistance vascular beds. Such arteries include the internal carotid, hepatic, and mesenteric arteries in the postprandial state. These arteries are characterized by forward flow during both systole and diastole, with no diastolic flow reversal, a sharp systolic peak with gradual systolic deceleration, and high end diastolic flow (Fig. 77-1).[19,25] A clear window beneath the systolic peak may be present, but this is obscured when the pulsed Dopp-

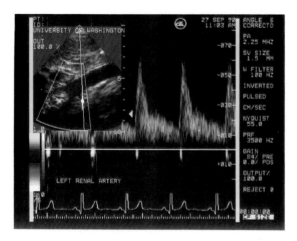

Fig. 77-1. Normal renal artery spectral waveform. The normal renal velocity waveform is characterized by forward flow during both systole and diastole, a sharp systolic peak with gradual deceleration, and high end diastolic flow.

ler sample volume is large with respect to the arterial diameter.[26] Peak systolic velocity is currently the most clinically useful component of the Doppler spectral waveform. The peak systolic velocity in normal renal arteries averages 104 ± 25 cm/sec,[16] although an upper limit of 125 to 150 cm/sec may be more useful clinically.[4] Flow velocities have been shown to be independent of body surface area,[9] although aortic flow velocity and consequently renal artery flow velocity have been documented to decrease with age.[19]

Characteristic changes in the renal artery velocity waveform with progressive stenosis have been described by several authors. In a canine model of graded renal artery stenosis, Rittgers, Norris, and Barnes[25] demonstrated disturbances of the velocity waveform before significant reductions in blood flow. Significant stenoses have been noted to be associated with an irregular waveform, a blunted systolic peak, and loss of the systolic window.[25] With progressive diameter reduction, there is a focal increase in peak systolic velocity with an abrupt velocity decrease distal to the lesion (Fig. 77-2).

Conduct of the examination

Perhaps the greatest limitation of duplex sonography as a screening exam for renovascular hypertension is the expertise required to perform the study. Considerable knowledge, patience, and persistence by the technologist are required to obtain a satisfactory exam. Even in experienced laboratories, satisfactory studies may be unobtainable in 4% to 16% of patients because of obesity, bowel gas, or recent abdominal surgery.[1,14,16,19,29]

The examination should be performed in the morning after an overnight fast to minimize the effects of bowel gas. A low-frequency transducer capable of penetrating to depths of 3 to 17 cm is required.[1] A 3.0-MHz mechanical sector probe or a 2.25-MHz phased array probe for color imaging

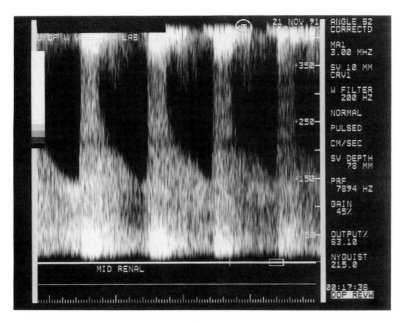

Fig. 77-2. Hemodynamically significant renal artery stenosis secondary to fibromuscular dysplasia. The peak systolic velocity increases with progressive diameter reduction.

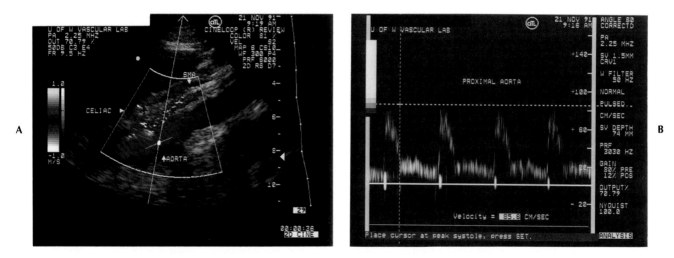

Fig. 77-3. A, The color flow image illustrates a long axis view of the aorta at the level of the celiac and superior mesenteric arteries *(SMA).* For determining the renal aortic ratio, centerstream peak aortic velocity is recorded at the level of the superior mesenteric artery. **B,** The spectral display illustrates the centerstream aortic velocity waveform with a peak systolic velocity of 85.6 cm/sec.

has been found to be acceptable for this purpose. The abdominal aorta is imaged from the anterior midline, with the head of the patient's bed elevated 30°. From a long axis view of the aorta, a centerstream peak aortic velocity is obtained at the level of the superior mesenteric artery (Fig. 77-3). The scan head is then rotated 90° to image the aorta in cross section, and the origins of both renal arteries are identified by using the left renal vein as a landmark. The renal arteries are identified by their B-mode image as well as by their characteristic Doppler velocity waveform (see Fig. 77-1). A large sample volume approximating the arterial diameter may be initially useful in allowing flow to be monitored throughout the respiratory cycle. Artifacts produced by respiratory movement can be further minimized by breath holding during velocity measurements. The angle of insonation is maintained at 60° or less as velocity signals are interrogated from the origin of the renal artery to the hilum on each side. Velocity waveforms are recorded from the renal artery origin and proximal, mid, and distal sites, with the angle of insonation noted at each site (Fig. 77-4).

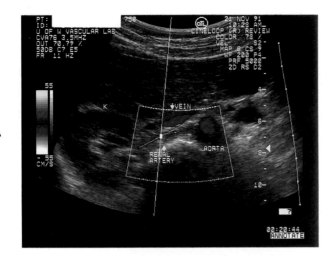

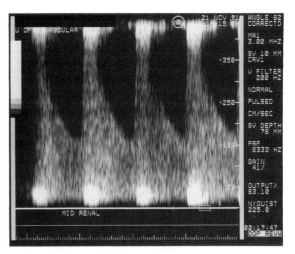

Fig. 77-4. A, The color Doppler display demonstrates placement of the pulsed Doppler sample volume within the midrenal artery. The Doppler angle is maintained at 60° or less. Velocity signals are similarly recorded from the origin as well as the proximal and distal renal artery. **B,** The spectral display illustrates the focal velocity increase within a hemodynamically significant stenosis. The degree of luminal narrowing is derived from the ratio of peak renal artery systolic velocity to that from the abdominal aorta.

The highest velocity signals proximal to, within, and distal to any detected stenotic lesions are also recorded. The patient is then moved into a decubitus position, and parenchymal abnormalities are evaluated from a flank approach with the B-mode image. Velocity waveforms from the distal renal artery are again evaluated by this approach. This is particularly important if the distal renal artery is inadequately visualized from an anterior approach and should serve to validate these measurements. Velocity signals from the hila, interlobar, and arcuate arteries are then obtained with a large (10 mm) sample volume and 0° angle of insonation. Color Doppler is used selectively throughout the exam to facilitate location of the renal arteries.

Diagnostic criteria

Duplex sonography provides both anatomic information with the B-mode image and flow information with the pulsed Doppler. Although initial studies attempted to characterize the cross-sectional anatomy of the renal arteries by using B-mode ultrasound,[9] this has not proved to be useful in identifying renal artery stenosis. Renal size as determined from the B-mode image may be helpful in documenting both renal artery occlusion and the progression of renovascular disease.[30] When combined with the spectral waveform, the B-mode image is also useful in accurately localizing lesions to the origin, proximal, mid, or distal renal artery.[16] However, the actual diagnosis of renal artery stenosis is currently based exclusively on velocity changes along the course of the renal artery. The B-mode image is primarily used to guide placement of the sample volume. Other characteristics of the spectral waveform, particularly spectral broadening, that have been useful in documenting nonlaminar flow in the carotid system have limited utility in as-

Table 77-1. Renal duplex diagnostic criteria

Criteria	Normal	<60%	>60%	Occluded
Renal/aortic ratio	<3.5	<3.5	≥3.5	N/A
Velocity	<180 cm/ sec	>180 cm/ sec	>180 cm/ sec	No flow Kidney <9 cm/sec Parenchyma <10 cm/sec

sessment of the renal arteries. The large sample volume required in minimizing the effects of respiration, as well as the small caliber of the renal arteries, precludes the use of spectral broadening as a diagnostic criterion.

As a result of these limitations, classifying the degree of renal artery diameter reduction in small increments is not possible at this time. However, the goal of identifying those high-grade stenoses associated with the clinical syndromes of renovascular hypertension and ischemic nephropathy is achievable.[26] Both renal ischemia and activation of the renin-angiotensin system presumably occur at the point of critical stenosis, where further small reductions in luminal area produce large changes in pressure and flow. Theoretically, development of such a critical stenosis depends both on flow velocity and the area ratio between stenotic and nonstenotic segments of the artery.[2] With arteriography, distal pressure reduction and activation of the renin-angiotensin system are inferred from the presence of a greater than 60% diameter-reducing lesion. In contrast, the duplex diagnosis of such a lesion depends on demonstration of a localized increase in

Table 77-2. Renal duplex scanning

Author	Year	Patients*	Inadequate	Sensitivity	Specificity	Criteria
Avasthi[1]	1984	26(52)	16%	89%	73%	Velocity
Rittgers[25]	1985	42(84)	10%	83%	97%	Velocity
Kohler[19]	1986	22(43)	10%	91%	95%	RAR
Taylor[29]	1988	29(58)	12.4%	84%	97%	RAR
Hansen[14]	1990	74(142)	4%	88%	99%	RAR
Hoffman[16]	1991	41(85)	13%	92%	62%†	RAR

RAR, Renal aortic ratio.
*Number of renal arteries studied in parentheses.
†See text for explanation.

systolic velocity, with associated poststenotic turbulence, rather than strictly anatomic criteria. It is currently possible to define four diagnostic categories by duplex criteria: normal, less than 60% diameter-reducing lesions, greater than 60% diameter-reducing lesions, and occlusion (Table 77-1).

Different criteria for the identification of greater than 60% diameter-reducing stenoses have been proposed. Based on initial characterization of normal renal artery flow, Avasthi, Voyles, and Greene[1] proposed criteria including a peak systolic velocity greater than 100 cm/sec (one standard deviation above a series of normal controls), absence of diastolic flow, absence of any detectable flow secondary to occlusion, and spectral broadening due to turbulence. However, with increased experience, it has become apparent that a velocity of 100 cm/sec is too low to be clinically useful.[14,16] The absence of diastolic flow is also affected by parameters such as intrinsic renal disease, and spectral broadening may be difficult to interpret. The renal aortic ratio, which is defined as the ratio of the angle-adjusted peak renal systolic velocity to the centerstream peak aortic velocity, has been proposed as a more accurate measure of a hemodynamically significant stenosis.[19,25] This ratio may compensate for variations in systemic hemodynamics and aortic velocity while avoiding the use of absolute velocity measurements. In a retrospective series by Kohler et al,[19] a renal aortic ratio of greater than 3.5 provided a sensitivity of 91% and specificity of 95% in identifying diameter-reducing lesions of greater than 60%. These criteria have subsequently been validated in several prospective series, with sensitivities of 84% to 92% (Table 77-2).* With the exception of one study, specificities of 95% to 99% have been equally good. In the single study[16] reporting a marginal specificity (62%) for the detection of greater than 60% stenoses, duplex scanning and arteriography disagreed as to the magnitude of narrowing rather than the presence or absence of a lesion in 9 of 10 false-positive studies.

More recently, it has been suggested that velocity measurements may be useful in detecting subcritical renovascular lesions. Because the functional significance of a lesion

may be difficult to predict on the basis of either duplex sonography or arteriography, identification of less than 60% diameter-reducing lesions may be important. Hoffman et al[16] noted that a peak systolic velocity of greater than 180 cm/sec reliably discerns normal from diseased arteries with a sensitivity of 95% and specificity of 91%. This measure may prove useful in identifying patients with an appropriate clinical picture of renovascular hypertension who warrant further workup despite a renal aortic ratio of less than 3.5.

The diagnosis of renal artery occlusion depends on demonstration of no detectable flow signal within an adequately visualized vessel. The diagnosis may be supported by additional findings such as a low-amplitude parenchymal velocity signal (less than 10 cm/sec) and a renal length less than 9 cm. Although these parameters have been shown to be 91% to 100% sensitive for the detection of renal artery occlusion,[14,16] false-negative studies of occluded arteries may occasionally result from interrogation of collateral arteries.[25]

Several other criteria have been proposed to identify hemodynamically significant renal artery lesions. However, only the renal aortic ratio and peak systolic velocity have been proved to have an acceptable sensitivity and specificity. It is notable that although the sensitivity of renal duplex scanning is not 100%, the overall agreement between duplex scanning and arteriography is similar to the agreement between two radiologists reviewing the same films.[16,29] Renal duplex sonography also has the advantage of providing information regarding the hemodynamic significance of a lesion.

Predicting the response to revascularization

Although renovascular disease can be effectively demonstrated by either arteriography or duplex scanning, a diagnosis of renovascular hypertension can often be conclusively established only in retrospect, that is, after anatomic correction of the lesion results in clinical improvement. Since many patients with renovascular disease have other causes of hypertension, several functional tests have been proposed as predictors of the response to revascularization. These include measurements of plasma renin activity, renal vein renin ratios, and split renal function tests. The renal

*References 1, 14, 16, 19, 25, 29.

vein renin ratio, defined as the ratio of renin levels between the affected and unaffected kidney, has been most widely used for this purpose. A lateralizing ratio of 1.4 to 2.4 has been suggested as a marker of a favorable response to intervention, with a ratio of 1.5 most commonly used.[20,28] Although an elevated renal vein renin ratio may indeed predict a favorable response in 92% to 93% of patients with high renin levels from one kidney, 51% to 65% of patients with nonlateralizing ratios may also respond to surgery or angioplasty.[20,32] Hemodynamically significant bilateral and segmental renovascular lesions may also fail to produce lateralizing ratios. Split renal function tests suffer from a similar lack of accuracy, as well as being invasive studies that are difficult to perform.

More recently, the severity of underlying parenchymal disease has been proposed as a parameter for selection of patients unlikely to respond to intervention.[12,19] Advanced ischemic parenchymal changes may preclude the salvage of renal function by revascularization. Long-standing renovascular hypertension may similarly become unresponsive to correction.[5] Hypertension in such instances may be renin independent and related to structural changes in the kidney. Essential hypertension may also be associated with characteristic renal structural changes resulting in increased parenchymal vascular resistance.[12] In this capacity, duplex scanning may be useful in assessing renal parenchymal vascular resistance as an index of underlying parenchymal disease. Several measures of parenchymal resistance have been proposed, including resistive index, systolic to diastolic ratio,[12] and end diastolic ratio (EDR).[19] All reflect the tendency of renal artery diastolic velocity to decrease with increasing vascular resistance. However, the renal artery EDR, defined as the end diastolic velocity or frequency divided by peak systolic velocity or frequency, has been the most thoroughly investigated in this regard. As resistance to flow increases, end diastolic velocity and the EDR should decrease.[19] An EDR of 0.33 or less is currently used as a marker of abnormally high resistance to flow. Although several investigators have confirmed a progressive decrease in EDR with increasing serum creatinine, the clinical application of the EDR in this situation has been limited.[12,19] Hansen et al[14] found no relationship between EDR and blood pressure or renal response to intervention. Further work in this area is needed to define the relationship between EDR and response to therapy.

Limitations of renal duplex scanning

Several limitations of renal duplex scanning have become apparent with wider application of the technology. The examination itself is time consuming (1 to 3 hrs) and requires a skilled and dedicated technologist. A significantly diminished sensitivity of duplex in some series[4,7] may have partly resulted from time limitation of the examination. Even in experienced laboratories, 4% to 16% of examinations may be inadequate due to bowel gas, obesity, recent abdominal

surgery,* or calcified renal vessels.[13] However, adequate studies on such patients may frequently be obtained by having them return for a second examination. From a technologic standpoint, B-mode resolution is limited by the low-frequency transducers required. Use of a large sample volume to overcome respiratory movement may cause mistaken interrogation of collateral vessels and produce spectral broadening in the velocity waveform. Errors may also result from inaccurate estimation of the angle of insonation. Multiple renal arteries constitute the greatest anatomic limitation of duplex sonography. Accessory renal arteries, occurring in 5% to 22% of kidneys,[4,14,21,29,30] are not currently detectable with duplex scanning. Diseased polar arteries may clearly cause renovascular hypertension and may be a source of false-negative studies.[14,16] Although the sensitivity of detecting multiple renal arteries may be improved with color flow imaging, preliminary reports are discouraging.[4,7,14]

NEW DIRECTIONS
Renal hilar duplex scanning

Despite the proven accuracy of renal duplex scanning, the complexity of the examination and technical problems imaging the renal arteries have presented some limitation to its widespread acceptance. A more limited examination of the renal hilar arteries from a flank or translumbar approach has been advocated to circumvent these problems. Such techniques depend on detecting the hemodynamic changes distal to a significant stenosis. Advantages of such an approach include a technically simplified examination, reduction of the examination time to approximately 30 minutes, and a lower incidence of inadequate studies in comparison with the transabdominal approach.[12,13,21]

Similar to the transabdominal approach, a low-frequency

---

*References 1, 14, 16, 19, 25, 29.

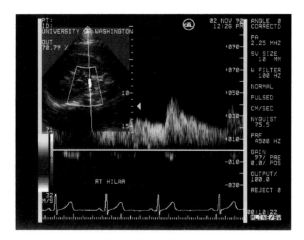

Fig. 77-5. Velocity signals from the renal hilum are recorded from the flank by using a 0° angle of insonation. Acceleration index and time are calculated from the spectral display.

2.5- to 3.0-MHz probe is used with a large sample volume. However, the kidney is imaged from either the flank[21] or paravertebral region.[12,13] A cross-sectional view of the kidney facilitates the examination because the distal renal artery is visualized in long axis. By using color-flow imaging, the distal renal arteries and interlobar branches are identified by their pulsations within the hilum. Doppler spectra are then recorded as for the transabdominal approach. All velocity spectra are recorded with a Doppler angle of 0° (Fig. 77-5).

Several algorithms have been proposed based on the hemodynamic changes observed distal to a significant stenosis. These changes include dampening of the parenchymal velocity waveform and a delay of the systolic upstroke.[21] Parameters proposed for detection of proximal stenoses include the *acceleration index,* defined as the tangential slope of the systolic upstroke (kHz/sec) divided by the transmitted frequency; the *acceleration time,* defined as the time interval between the onset of systole and the initial peak; and the *acceleration time ratio,* defined as the ratio of the renal to aortic acceleration time (Fig. 77-6). Handa et al[13] reviewed all three parameters and found an acceleration index of less than 3.78 (kHz/sec/MHz) to be most accurate (95%), with a sensitivity and specificity of 100% and 93%, respectively. The acceleration index was also found to significantly correlate with the percentage of stenosis determined arteriographically. In contrast, Martin et al[21] found an acceleration time of greater than 0.100 sec to be superior to the acceleration index in detecting hemodynamically significant stenoses, with a sensitivity of 86.5% and specificity of 98.4%. It must be noted that acceleration time was specifically defined in this study as the time interval between the onset of systole and the *initial systolic* or *compliance peak,* which may not coincide with the peak systolic frequency.

Although the technical simplicity of hilar duplex is attractive, some limitations have been noted. No anatomic information regarding the location of a stenosis is provided by this technique. In addition, difficulties in discerning high-grade stenosis from occlusion with collateral flow have been noted.[21] An abnormal acceleration time and index may be normalized by concomitant parenchymal disease,[21] and acceleration time may be significantly influenced by peak velocity.[13] At present, further prospective studies are needed to validate this technique. Although hilar examination is not

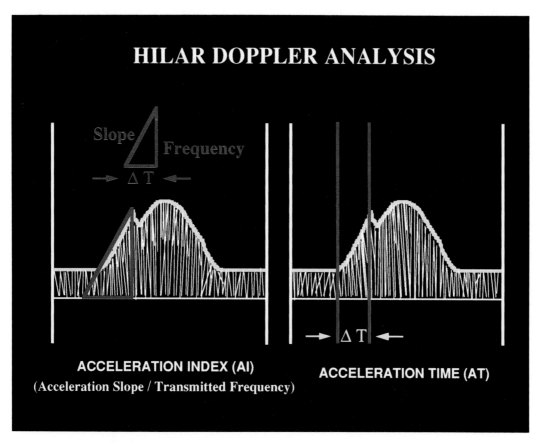

Fig. 77-6. Acceleration index and acceleration time. Calculation of both parameters is based on the initial systolic or compliance peak, which may not coincide with peak systolic velocity. In calculation of acceleration index, the acceleration slope (kHz/sec) is divided by transducer frequency (MHz). Acceleration time is calculated from the onset of systole to the initial systolic peak.

a substitute for complete transabdominal duplex scanning, it may play some role when the conventional examination is difficult or impossible to complete.

Color flow Doppler

The addition of color to duplex technology allows Doppler information to be added to the real-time B-mode display. Although theoretically this technology could be useful in identifying the site and degree of flow-reducing lesions, its application in abdominal scanning is somewhat limited. The greatest potential of color flow imaging may be in aiding visualization of the renal arteries, facilitating placement of the pulsed Doppler sample volume, and permitting more accurate measurement of the angle of insonation. Color flow imaging aided identification of the renal arteries in 52% of cases in one early study.[4] A role in the detection of accessory renal arteries is also attractive, since an inability to identify these vessels is a well-recognized limitation of renal duplex scanning. Unfortunately, preliminary evaluation has not confirmed improved detection of accessory renal arteries with this technique,[4,7] which makes further evaluation necessary to define its role in renal duplex scanning.

RELATED APPLICATIONS

Although the primary utility of renal duplex scanning may be in screening for hemodynamically significant renovascular disease, several related applications have been proposed. As a diagnostic modality, duplex scanning may be better than arteriography in defining fibromuscular lesions.

The hemodynamic significance of such sequential, subcritical lesions may be impossible to determine by arteriography. The ability of duplex sonography to anatomically localize sites of significant disease allows its use in planning intervention at the time of initial arteriography. The potential usefulness of duplex scanning in predicting response to therapy has been discussed. In addition, it provides a modality for the noninvasive follow-up of transluminal angioplasty, aorto-renal bypass grafts, and renal transplants. Efficacy in this regard has been documented by several investigators.[12,13,30] Such follow-up is particularly important to exclude technical problems in patients not responding to intervention. A high rate of graft thrombosis has been reported in this population.[22] Finally, duplex sonography provides a noninvasive means for following the natural history of atherosclerotic renovascular disease, which has been reported to progress in 36% to 63% of patients over 5 years.[31]

CONCLUSION

Although renovascular lesions are the cause of hypertension in less than 5% of patients, their identification has important therapeutic implications. The lesion not only is correctable in appropriately selected patients but may also contribute to progressive renal failure despite optimal medical management. Unfortunately, identification of these patients has been limited by lack of an accurate, reproducible, noninvasive, and widely available screening test. Several screening tests, including hypertensive urography, isotope renography, intravenous digital subtraction arteriography, and

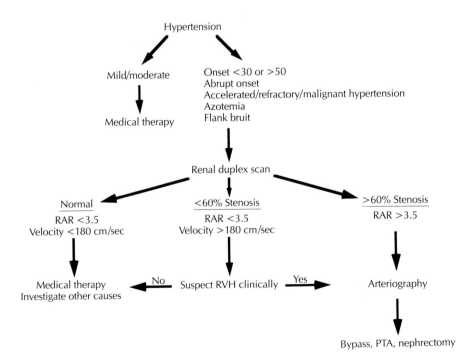

Fig. 77-7. Diagnostic algorithm for renovascular hypertension. (From Taylor DC et al: *J Vasc Surg* 7:363, 1988.)

plasma renin activity, have been proposed. However, after initial enthusiasm, each has been marked by unacceptably high false-positive and false-negative rates.

Renal artery stenosis presents a unique diagnostic challenge in that it requires not only a demonstration of an anatomic lesion but also proof of its functional significance. Duplex sonography is theoretically ideal in this regard, providing both anatomic and hemodynamic information. Although limitations do exist, duplex scanning has been shown to be a suitable screening test by laboratories experienced in its use. By using absolute velocity criteria and the ratio of peak systolic velocity in the renal artery to the aorta, it is possible to identify patients with clinically significant renal artery stenosis. With these criteria, sensitivities of 84% to 92% may be expected for the identification of greater than 60% diameter-reducing lesions. On the basis of velocity and the renal aortic ratio as diagnostic criteria, a screening algorithm such as shown in Fig. 77-7 can be proposed. The role of hilar and parenchymal scanning remains to be fully defined, however. It may have implications regarding therapy and the natural history of renovascular disease.

REFERENCES

1. Avasthi PS, Voyles WF, Greene ER: Noninvasive diagnosis of renal artery stenosis by echo-Doppler velocimetry, *Kidney Int* 25:824-829, 1984.
2. Bergeur R, Hwang NHC: Critical arterial stenosis: a theoretical and experimental solution, *Ann Surg* 180(1):39-50, 1974.
3. Berglund G, Andersson O, Wilhelmensen L: Prevalence of primary and secondary hypertension: studies in a random population sample, *Br Med J* 2:554-556, 1976.
4. Berland LL et al: Renal artery stenosis: prospective evaluation of diagnosis with color duplex US compared with angiography, *Radiology* 174:421-423, 1990.
5. Brown JJ et al: Mechanism of renal hypertension, *Lancet* 1:1219-1221, 1976.
6. Dean RH et al: Renovascular hypertension: anatomic and renal function changes during drug therapy, *Arch Surg* 116:1408-1415, 1981.
7. Desberg AL et al: Renal artery stenosis: evaluation with color Doppler flow imaging, *Radiology* 177:749-753, 1990.
8. Dunnick NR, Sfakianakis GN: Screening for renovascular hypertension, *Radiol Clin North Am* 29(3):497-510, 1991.
9. Greene ER et al: Noninvasive characterization of renal artery blood flow, *Kidney Int* 20:523-529, 1981.
10. Grim CE et al: Sensitivity and specificity of screening tests for renal vascular hypertension, *Ann Int Med* 91(4):617-622, 1979.
11. Hamovici H, Zinicola N: Experimental renal-artery stenosis, diagnostic significance of arterial hemodynamics, *J Cardiovasc Surg* 3:259-262, 1962.
12. Handa N et al: Echo-Doppler velocimeter in the diagnosis of hypertensive patients: the renal artery Doppler technique, *Ultrasound Med Biol* 12(12):945-952, 1986.
13. Handa N et al: Efficacy of echo-Doppler examination for the evaluation of renovascular disease, *Ultrasound Med Biol* 14(1):1-5, 1988.
14. Hansen KJ et al: Renal duplex sonography: evaluation of clinical utility, *J Vasc Surg* 12(3):227-236, 1990.
15. Harrison EG, McCormack LJ: Pathological classification of renal artery disease in renovascular hypertension, *Mayo Clin Proc* 46:161-167, 1971.
16. Hoffman U et al: Role of duplex scanning for the detection of atherosclerotic renal artery disease, *Kidney Int* 39:1232-1239, 1991.
17. Holley KE et al: Renal artery stenosis: a clinical-pathological study in normotensive and hypertensive patients, *Am J Med* 37:14-22, 1964.
18. Jacobsen HR: Ischemic nephropathy: an overlooked clinical entity, *Kidney Int* 34:729-743, 1988.
19. Kohler TR et al: Noninvasive diagnosis of renal artery stenosis by ultrasonic duplex scanning, *J Vasc Surg* 4(5):450-456, 1986.
20. Marks LS, Maxwell MH: Renal vein renin: value and limitations in the prediction of operative results, *Urol Clin North Am* 2(2):311-325, 1975.
21. Martin RL et al: Renal hilar Doppler analysis in the detection of renal artery stenosis, *J Vasc Technol* 15(4):173-180, 1991.
22. Maxwell MH: Cooperative study of renovascular hypertension: current status, *Kidney Int* 8:S-153–S-160, 1975.
23. McAfee JG et al: Diagnosis of angiotensinogenic hypertension: the complementary roles of renal scintigraphy and the saralasin infusion test, *J Nucl Med* 18(7):669-675, 1977.
24. Postma CT et al: The captopril test in detection of renovascular disease in hypertensive patients, *Arch Intern Med* 150:625-628, 1990.
25. Rittgers SE, Norris CS, Barnes RW: Detection of renal artery stenosis: experimental and clinical analysis of velocity waveforms, *Ultrasound Med Biol* 11(3):523-531, 1985.
26. Strandness DE: *Duplex scanning in vascular disorders,* New York, 1990, Raven Press.
27. Svetkey LP et al: Prospective analysis of strategies for diagnosing renovascular hypertension, *Hypertension* 14(3):247-257, 1989.
28. Swales JD: Blood pressure and the kidney, *J Clin Pathol* 34:1233-1240, 1981.
29. Taylor DC et al: Duplex ultrasound scanning in the diagnosis of renal artery stenosis: a prospective evaluation, *J Vasc Surg* 7(2):363-369, 1988.
30. Taylor DC et al: Follow-up of renal artery stenosis by duplex ultrasound, *J Vasc Surg* 9(3):410-415, 1989.
31. Treadway KK, Slater EE: Renovascular hypertension, *Ann Rev Med* 665-692, 1984.
32. van Bockel JH et al: Renovascular hypertension, *Surg Gynecol Obstet* 169:467-478, 1989.
33. Working group on renovascular hypertension: Detection, evaluation, and treatment of renovascular hypertension, *Arch Intern Med* 147:820-829, 1987.

CHAPTER 78

Pitfalls in duplex ultrasonography of the renal arteries

BRIAN L. THIELE, MARSHA M. NEUMYER, DEAN A. HEALY, and
MICHAEL J. SCHINA, Jr.

Duplex ultrasonography of the renal arteries is being used increasingly in a variety of patients. This latest application is now frequently used in patients with suspected renovascular hypertension. A number of studies have reported a high statistical correlation between duplex ultrasonography and arteriography.[2,6,7] Despite these reports, this technique has not been widely adopted, partly because of the demanding nature of the study and the difficulties encountered in obtaining results comparable with those reported in the literature. The purpose of this chapter is to address the problems encountered during the performance and interpretation of this study in the hope that it will improve the quality of these examinations.

To appreciate the pitfalls encountered with renal artery duplex ultrasonography, clinicians must be familiar with the anatomy, technical features, and interpretation of the normal examination. After this is accomplished, variables inherent in the examination technique and their interpretation are more easily understood. First, examiners must master the normal examination by having a thorough understanding of the relevant anatomy. This is particularly important because many patients will exhibit variations from the normal that if not recognized, will contribute to examination difficulties or errors.

ANATOMY

The transpyloric plane is the topographic transverse plane on the upper abdomen, halfway between the suprasternal notch and the upper border of the symphysis pubis. This line cuts through the pylorus, the tips of the ninth costal cartilages, and the lower border of the first lumbar vertebrae. The renal arteries are located 2 cm below the transpyloric plane, and recognition of this important surface anatomic landmark provides the initial identification of the area to be examined.

The renal arteries arise at right angles from the respective posterolateral aspects of the aorta at the level of the upper border of the second lumbar vertebrae immediately inferior to the origin of the superior mesenteric artery. The right renal artery, which is longer than the left, passes posterior to the inferior vena cava and the right renal vein. The left renal artery, which usually arises from the aorta somewhat more cephalad than the right, passes posterior to the left renal vein and is crossed by the inferior mesenteric vein. Each artery divides into two to five branches before reaching the hilum of the kidney. These are generally arranged in an anterior and posterior distribution to supply the various segments of the kidney.

One or two accessory renal arteries are present in approximately 10% to 20% of patients, and they are seen more often on the left than the right. They usually arise from the aorta below the main renal artery and pass directly to the surface of the kidney instead of entering the kidney at the hilum. Less commonly, they originate from the common iliac and, rarely, the internal iliac artery. Before entering the kidney, the renal artery divides into a large anterior and a smaller posterior branch. Further subdivisions occur that result in the formation of the interlobar, arcuate, and interlobular arteries within the renal parenchyma.

The renal veins are located anterior to the renal arteries. The left is longer than the right and passes anterior to the aorta just below the origin of the superior mesenteric artery. This latter relationship is an important one to recognize during the initial part of the examination. The renal veins terminate in the respective sides of the inferior vena cava. The left renal vein is retroaortic in from 2% to 5% of patients, and it is important to be aware of this variant because the left renal vein is also used as a major landmark in locating the renal arteries.

PATIENT PREPARATION

Adequate patient preparation is of paramount importance for satisfactory duplex ultrasonography of the renal arteries. The examination is preferably performed in the morning to avoid accumulation of bowel gas during the day that will preclude satisfactory imaging of the renal arteries. The patients should have nothing by mouth after midnight to minimize abdominal gas accumulation before the examination. This includes avoiding gum chewing and smoking. It is possible, however, for a small number of oral medications to be taken by the patient.

BACKGROUND

Duplex ultrasonography of the renal arteries is performed by using mechanical sector, phased, or curved array transducers ranging in frequency from 2.25 to 5.0 MHz. Color flow images derived from Doppler information at multiple sites, which is color encoded and superimposed on a real-time B-mode gray-scale image, facilitate identification of anatomic landmarks and visualization of vessels. The presence of a flow-reducing stenosis is confirmed by interpretation of Doppler velocity spectral waveform data and cannot be made on the basis of a distorted Doppler color flow pattern.

Kohler et al[2] have reported that a ratio of peak systolic frequency in the renal artery to peak systolic frequency in the abdominal aorta greater than 3.5 indicates the presence of a hemodynamically significant stenosis of the renal artery. In studies conducted in the laboratory at the Pennsylvania State University using this parameter, an overall accuracy of 93% has been documented for determining hemodynamically significant renal artery stenosis with a sensitivity of 92% and a specificity of 95%.[3]

Intrinsic renal pathology results in edema and interstitial cellular infiltrates that cause an increase in renovascular resistance. Arima et al[1] and Norris et al[5] have shown that as renovascular resistance increases, the end diastolic velocity of the Doppler spectral waveform decreases. Other investigations have indicated that parenchymal Doppler signals with diastolic flow velocities less than 20% of the peak systolic velocity (resistive index of 0.8 or more) are consistent with renal parenchymal disease.[4] On the basis of duplex ultrasonography, therefore, renal artery stenosis can be differentiated from renal parenchymal disease in many patients.

EXAMINATION TECHNIQUE

The abdominal aorta is initially imaged longitudinally immediately below the aorta with the patient in the supine position using a left paramedian scan plane. A centerstream Doppler velocity waveform is obtained from the juxtarenal aorta with an angle of 60° or less and a sample volume size of 1.5 mm. The peak systolic velocity is noted for later use in calculating the renal aortic ratio. Aneurysmal or atherosclerotic disease of the aorta in this area should be noted.

After the celiac and superior mesenteric arteries and the left renal vein in the longitudinal plane have been identified, the aorta is imaged in the transverse plane at this level and the origin of the renal arteries is identified (Fig. 78-1). It may be difficult to identify the vessels in this location with this window, and it may be more appropriate to initially evaluate the distal renal artery, which is more easily scanned with the patient in the lateral decubitus position. Doppler velocity spectral waveforms should be obtained from the proximal, mid, and distal renal arteries bilaterally at an angle <60° by using a variable sample volume size ranging from 1.5 to 3 mm. Atherosclerotic disease of the renal artery usually involves the proximal vessel (Fig. 78-2). Mid and

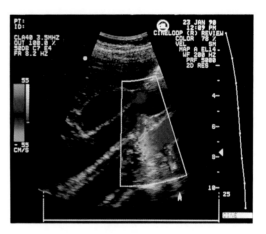

Fig. 78-1. Color duplex ultrasonography of the determined aorta and both renal arteries in the same exposure. It should be emphasized that this is the exception rather than the rule.

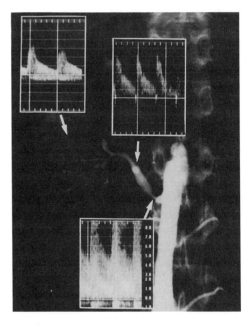

Fig. 78-2. Arteriogram of a patient with a high-grade stenosis of the proximal renal artery and the corresponding spectra obtained immediately distal to the lesion.

distal renal artery disease may be encountered in patients with fibromuscular dysplasia (Fig. 78-3), emphasizing the need to scan the entire length of both renal arteries. The highest peak systolic velocity obtained from each renal artery is noted for later use in calculating the renal aortic ratio for that side.

The kidneys are imaged with the patient in the left and right lateral decubitus positions by using the lateral axillary approach to obtain a coronal and long axis view of the

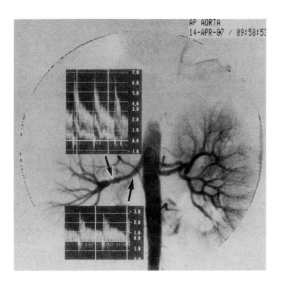

Fig. 78-3. Arteriogram of a patient with fibromuscular dysplasia of the right renal artery and the spectra obtained from the proximal renal artery and the distal renal artery. Note that the proximal waveform is relatively normal and it is only the distal artery yielding the diagnostic information.

kidney. The pole-to-pole length of each kidney is measured and the sample volume size is increased to a 3-mm axial length; pulse Doppler signals are obtained throughout the interlobar and arcuate renal arteries. Because discrete vessels are not well visualized, the Doppler sample volume is passed throughout the renal parenchyma to identify the highest peak systolic and end diastolic shifted frequencies.

INTERPRETATION
Renal artery signals

The Doppler velocity spectral waveform from the juxtarenal aorta is normally triphasic or biphasic with a peak systolic velocity of at least 60 cm/sec and little spectral broadening. The Doppler velocity spectral waveform from the normal renal artery demonstrates a high diastolic forward flow component because of the low resistance of the renovascular bed. In renal artery stenosis, there is a marked increase in systolic velocity as well as spectral broadening, but diastolic blood flow remains antegrade unless the stenosis exceeds 80%, at which point a marked reduction in systolic velocity may occur.

Because of its frequent tortuosity, a higher systolic velocity may be obtained from the proximal right renal artery compared to its mid and distal segments or in comparison to the proximal left renal artery. A spectral waveform from the proximal right renal artery with high systolic velocity and distal turbulence is suggestive of disease. A renal-to-aortic peak systolic velocity ratio greater than 3.5 is diagnostic of the presence of a flow-reducing stenosis (greater than 60% diameter reduction) of the renal artery. Turbulence is usually present and identified by spectral broadening of the Doppler velocity signal. Absence of flow in a visualized renal artery with low-amplitude, low-frequency Doppler signals documented in the renal parenchyma is highly suggestive of occlusion of the renal artery. This pattern may also be seen in preocclusive lesions (Fig. 78-4).

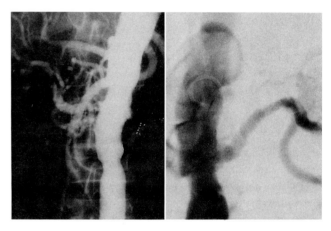

Fig. 78-4. Arteriogram of a patient with hypertension and occlusion of the left renal artery. No distal renal arteries are visualized. Duplex ultrasonography confirmed no signal in the renal artery but parenchymal signals of good quality were identified. The arteriogram obtained after reconstruction confirmed normal parenchymal vascularization.

Parenchymal signals

In the normal kidney, the Doppler velocity spectral waveform demonstrates continuous high diastolic flow from all regions of the organ. As renovascular resistance increases, the impedance to arterial inflow to the kidney is reflected in reduction of diastolic flow and increased pulsatility of the Doppler waveform. In cases of marked renovascular resistance, the diastolic component approaches zero or reverses. Diastolic flow velocities less than 20% of the peak systolic velocity (resistive index of 0.8 or more) are consistent with renal parenchymal disease.

With a good understanding of the anatomy, examination technique, and the basis for interpretation, it is appropriate to consider the problems that may be encountered during duplex ultrasonography of the renal arteries.

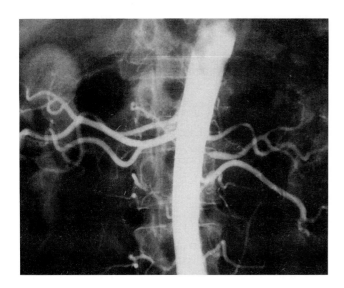

Fig. 78-5. Arteriogram of a patient with three renal arteries on the left side and two on the right. This is one of the variants of the renal anatomy.

PITFALLS IN THE STUDIES
Patient-related factors

The most common difficulty encountered in this area relates to inadequate patient preparation that may result in the accumulation of large amounts of bowel gas interfering with ultrasound transmission to the renal arteries. In an occasional patient, useful information may be obtained by altering the acoustic window being used and relying on a flank approach. Although this may give excellent information about the renal parenchymal blood flow patterns, it is not usually possible to adequately evaluate the whole length of the renal arteries from origin to the renal hilum. This does slightly limit the use of duplex ultrasonography in emergency situations in patients who cannot be prepared, but fortunately, these cases are rare. A sudden onset of anuria may raise the question of renal artery occlusion, and this can sometimes be inferred by identifying lower amplitude parenchymal signals from the flank approach. The presence of normal parenchymal signals excludes this diagnosis.

Adequate studies are frequently impossible in obese patients because of the signal attenuation associated with increased distance from the transducer head to the renal arteries. The presence of fat itself is not a problem and is usually beneficial in the perinephric area and somewhat enhances visualization of the kidney.

Although these studies can occasionally be performed in a short time, they frequently require that the patient lie quietly and be capable of some cooperative effort for 45 to 60 minutes. This degree of cooperation may be particularly important to control respiratory activity so that good quality Doppler signals can be obtained from stationary renal arteries. Occasionally, patients may not be able to cooperate adequately for the duration of the study.

Anatomic factors

One major difficulty currently encountered is recognition that a patient has multiple renal arteries on one or both sides. This anatomic variation from the normal has a number of important features of which the examiner must be aware. The first is to recognize that in many kidneys there is an accessory renal artery usually originating from the infrarenal abdominal aorta and coursing to the lower pole. It is usually seen on the left side. When single, accessory renal arteries rarely supply the upper pole. In this situation, the main renal artery is of normal caliber and not difficult to identify.

The second pattern encountered is that of multiple renal arteries, which is a less common situation. These patients usually have three arteries but there may be more. They may not have a renal artery that is markedly dominant, and consequently the examiner may ignore all the vessels. It is uncommon to find more than three renal arteries in this variant (Fig. 78-5).

There is no way to ensure that multiple renal arteries have not been missed, but it is important when performing the study to scan along the paraaortic plane to attempt to locate these arteries. Accessory renal arteries are more likely to be missed because of their small size, although kidneys with multiple renal arteries are also difficult to examine adequately for the same reason.

Retroaortic renal veins occur in 1% to 5% of the population and may cause the unwary some confusion during the early part of the study because this vein is used as an important landmark. Identification of the renal vein serves as a means of deciding where to scan in the paraaortic area for the renal arteries; the two are usually closely related with the vein lying anterior to the artery. Knowledge of this variability enables the examiner to scan posterior to the aorta if the vein is not located anteriorly and then identify the renal arteries.

Finally, a rare anatomic variant is that of a horseshoe kidney, which is always associated with multiple renal arteries. In these patients, the two kidneys are joined across the lower poles by an isthmus of renal parenchyma, which is usually located anterior to the distal abdominal aorta. Although this anomaly is rare, it emphasizes the importance of a complete examination in all these patients, including the infrarenal abdominal aorta. The echoic mass of the isthmus is usually readily identified.

Examination factors

The renal arteries are relatively small (3 mm to 5 mm), originate from the posterolateral aspect of the abdominal aorta, and course through the retroperitoneum to the hilar regions of the kidney. They are frequently tortuous, particularly when the patient is supine, and move in a cephalad to caudad direction during respiration. In contrast, the carotid arteries are located subcutaneously in the neck, are of moderate size, do not move appreciably with respiration, and are never duplicated. This comparison is important because it serves to emphasize the great differences involved in the examination of these two sets of vessels, with all the advantages being associated with examination of the carotid arteries.

First, the examiner must be able to reliably identify the renal arteries. Depending primarily on body habitus, it may be necessary to use a range of frequencies from 2.25 MHz to 5.0 MHz. It may also be important to increase the sample volume to facilitate scanning of the retroaortic area. If difficulties are encountered with image quality during the study, the examiner should switch to a transducer with a different frequency. Color-coded Doppler instruments have reduced the time required to identify these arteries; with gray-scale registering systems, the detection of the renal arteries is primarily based on an auditory interpretation. With color technology, they may now actually be visualized.

The most successful approach is to start scanning in the longitudinal plane immediately distal to the xiphoid and to identify the abdominal aorta. The transducer can then be traversed distally until the characteristic origins of the celiac and superior mesenteric artery are visualized. The left renal vein is then located wedged between the superior mesenteric artery and the aorta. At this point, the scan plane is converted to a transverse one, the sample volume of the Doppler is opened, and the paraaortic regions are swept through while the examiner looks for the color-coded arterial signal and listens for the characteristic renal artery signal. During this part of the study, it is important to ask the patient to adopt a shallow breathing technique and when the vessels are located, to hold in peak inspiration while the Doppler signals are recorded. It is frequently only possible to record three to five satisfactory velocity spectra before the patient movement recommences and the signal is lost.

It is also important to sweep the Doppler sample volume through the aorta and into the proximal renal artery to identify major frequency shifts. Atherosclerotic disease of the renal arteries commonly occurs at the orifice and may be missed if the signal for interpretation is obtained too far distally. After obtaining appropriate spectra from the aorta just above the renal arteries and spectra from the orificial zone of the renal artery, the examiner must scan the remaining artery and the renal parenchyma. This is best accomplished by widening the sample volume and traversing the more lateral zone from the aorta. When the appropriate signal is identified, the sample volume can be reduced and the diagnostic spectra can be recorded for later interpretation. Signals should be obtained from the proximal, mid, and distal renal arteries because of the patterns of disease that are seen in the renal artery.

Pathologic factors

Atherosclerotic lesions. Primary atherosclerotic disease of the renal artery usually involves the proximal portion and midportion of the renal arteries while sparing the distal vessel. This disease distribution is the one most easily identified because the lesions tend to have some length and flow disturbances are frequently propagated for long distances along the artery.

The more difficult lesions occur primarily in the wall of the aorta around the orifice of the renal artery and are usually focal, with the result that flow disturbances are not propagated for long distances distally. They are also frequently difficult to assess on arteriography for the same reason. A second feature of these lesions contributing to examination difficulties is that they are often calcified and no Doppler signal will be registered in the throat of the stenosis. An awareness of these disease patterns is important in tailoring the examination to the patient for the best results.

FIBROMUSCULAR DYSPLASIA

The most common and characteristic types of fibromuscular dysplasia are those affecting the media. This process affects the mid and distal portions of the renal artery and may also extend into the parenchymal vessels. In patients with this condition, the proximal renal artery is usually normal and the spectra obtained are also normal, although the examiner may identify a low-amplitude signal, particularly in severe cases. An awareness that this disease occurs primarily in young women and in an age group not affected by atherosclerosis is also important in detecting this abnormality. An intimal variety, more common in males, usually produces a focal stenosis in the mid or distal renal artery (Fig. 78-6).

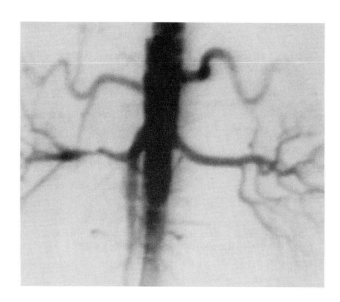

Fig. 78-6. Arteriogram of a patient with the intimal variety of fibromuscular dysplasia. This lesion is more common in males.

RENAL ARTERY OCCLUSION

As in occlusion of other arteries, identification of this abnormality with duplex ultrasonography is frequently difficult. Surgically, it is important to know if the distal renal artery is patent and if the renal parenchyma is viable. Whenever no renal arteries can be identified, the examiner should reverse the examination and insonate the kidneys. If the kidneys are of normal length and the parenchymal signals are normal, the examiner should consider the possibility of multiple renal arteries. Normally, an occluded renal artery is associated with a major reduction in the pole-to-pole length of the kidney, and if a small kidney is detected on one side, renal artery occlusion should be suspected. Parenchymal signals should be sought and an attempt also should be made to detect flow in the distal renal artery.

INTERPRETATION

Accurate diagnosis of vascular disease with duplex ultrasonography depends on obtaining appropriate information under circumstances in which the important technical variables are controlled. Evaluation of the renal arteries is the most difficult of all the arteries examined because information is obtained at the limit of the technical capability of the instrumentation. Because of this technical factor and of the anatomic difficulties, it is not possible to achieve the same degree of examination technical control as in other studies. Awareness of the potential problems is an important first step in minimizing these difficulties.

The determination that a significant renal artery lesion is

present is made by evaluating the ratio of peak systolic frequency or velocity in the renal artery compared with the abdominal aortic signal. Although it is not common to find severe disease in the aorta producing high-velocity signals, sampling too close to the wall may yield a lower amplitude signal and be responsible for false-positive results. The best quality signal from the abdominal aorta should be identified, recorded, and used for determination of the renal/aortic ratio.

The numerator in this equation, peak systolic frequency of the renal artery signal, is the one most likely to be incorrectly recorded. This is influenced by the technical factors described earlier but may also be affected by the difficulty in controlling the insonating angle. This is the most challenging aspect of the study and one of the reasons why the renal aortic ratio is relatively high. If the examiner has to err from the ideal angle of 60°, it is best to obtain a signal between 40° and 60°, rather than between 60° and 80°. Finally, it is of utmost importance that the most representative signal be used from the renal artery. Very focal lesions may be missed if the examiner does not carefully sweep through the whole course of the renal artery listening for major frequency shifts.

CONCLUSION

Duplex sonography of the renal arteries is a demanding study to perform. It is important that the examiner be aware of the many difficulties and poor results that may be encountered initially. Careful and thoughtful attention is necessary when learning how to perform this examination. The development and application of a troubleshooting list (Table 78-1) is helpful for improving results. Attention to the details of the wide range of factors discussed in this chapter should result in better quality studies and greater examiner satisfaction.

Table 78-1. Troubleshooting list

Problem	Solution
Excessive bowel gas	Reschedule
Poor definition of aorta	Reduce transmitting frequency
No renal vein identified	Insonate posterior to aorta
Renal arteries not identified	Increase sample volume size, sweep along side of aorta
Renal arteries mobile	Examine at full inspiration
Low-amplitude signals	Look at renal size, suspect occlusion/parenchymal disease
Young patient	Suspect fibromuscular disease
Old patient	Suspect bilateral disease

REFERENCES

1. Arima M et al: Analysis of the arterial blood flow patterns of normal and allografted kidneys by the directional ultrasonic Doppler technique, *J Urol* 122:587-591, 1979.
2. Kohler ER et al: Noninvasive diagnosis of renal artery stenosis by ultrasonic duplex scanning, *J Vasc Surg* 4:450-456, 1986.
3. Neumyer M, Thiele BL: *Accuracy of duplex ultrasonography in the diagnosis of renal artery stenosis,* Paper presented at the annual meeting of the Royal Australian College of Surgeons, Canberra, Australia, May 1992.
4. Neumyer MM et al: The differentiation of renal artery stenosis from renal parenchymal disease by duplex ultrasonography, *J Vasc Tech* 13:205-211, 1989.
5. Norris CS et al: Noninvasive evaluation of renal artery stenosis and renovascular resistance, *J Vasc Surg* 1:192-201, 1984.
6. Taylor DL, Moneta GL, Strandness DE: Follow-up of renal artery stenosis by duplex ultrasound, *J Vasc Surg* 9:410-415, 1989.
7. Taylor DC et al: Duplex ultrasound in the diagnosis of renal artery stenosis: a prospective evaluation, *J Vasc Surg* 7:363-366, 1988.

CHAPTER 79

Natural history of renal artery stenosis

R. EUGENE ZIERLER

Natural history studies are designed to provide detailed information on the course of a disease without any specific treatment. The characteristic feature of a natural history study is serial follow-up of patients to document both the initial severity of their disease and any subsequent changes that occur. Such data are essential for evaluating the efficacy of therapeutic interventions, particularly in cases of asymptomatic disease. Only in this manner is it possible to determine whether a particular treatment results in a better clinical outcome than no treatment at all.

Since natural history studies typically involve repeated evaluations of relatively large numbers of patients, many of whom have minimal or no symptoms, the risks and costs of the testing methods used are of critical importance. For example, standard contrast arteriography would not be considered an acceptable method for screening and follow-up of patients with asymptomatic carotid stenosis. Similarly, clinicians have been reluctant to use arteriography as a screening test for renal artery stenosis in patients with suspected renovascular hypertension. Noninvasive testing methods are ideally suited for the screening and follow-up examinations that are necessary in natural history studies. The most important requirement of a noninvasive method is that it be sufficiently accurate to provide meaningful clinical data.

Duplex scanning is a noninvasive test that has been successfully used to follow the natural history of asymptomatic carotid artery disease. In one such study, correlation of stenosis severity with neurologic events showed a significantly higher incidence of ipsilateral transient ischemic attack, stroke, and carotid occlusion in patients with internal carotid stenosis of 80% or greater diameter reduction.[8] Subsequent experience also suggested that clinical outcome can be improved in this patient population by prophylactic carotid endarterectomy.[7] In patients with renal artery disease, the value of renal revascularization for renovascular hypertension and ischemic renal failure is generally accepted; however, the role of intervention for renal artery stenosis that is not associated with uncontrollable hypertension or decreased renal function has not been established. Prophylactic intervention for asymptomatic renal artery stenosis can only be justified on the basis of data that include the incidence and rate of disease progression in the renal arteries and the resulting changes in blood pressure and renal function. This chapter reviews the available information on the natural history of renal artery stenosis and discusses the role of duplex scanning in further studies of this important clinical problem.

CLINICAL APPLICATIONS OF RENAL DUPLEX SCANNING

In most segments of the arterial system, both indirect and direct noninvasive diagnostic tests can be used. Indirect methods include the periorbital Doppler examination and oculoplethysmography for carotid bifurcation disease, ankle pressure measurement by pneumatic cuff and Doppler for lower extremity arterial occlusive disease, and impedance plethysmography for lower extremity deep vein thrombosis.[14] However, even in these areas, the direct approach of duplex scanning has become the preferred noninvasive diagnostic method. Because none of the indirect techniques are capable of detecting renal artery stenosis, it was not until the development of abdominal duplex scanning that such lesions could be reliably identified by noninvasive means.[3,5,11] (A detailed discussion of renal artery duplex scanning is presented in Chapter 77.)

The clinical applications of renal duplex scanning include screening of selected patients with hypertension, screening of selected patients with renal failure, follow-up of renal revascularization (percutaneous transluminal angioplasty or surgical bypass), evaluation of renal transplants, and natural history studies. In addition to measurement of renal length and estimation of renovascular resistance, the degree of renal artery narrowing can be classified into one of four categories based on the peak systolic velocity (PSV) in the renal artery and the renal to aortic velocity ratio (RAR) (Table 79-1). In a recent validation study, a PSV of at least 180 cm/sec on duplex scanning discriminated between normal and diseased renal arteries with a sensitivity of 95% and a specificity of 90%.[3] A RAR of 3.5 or more identified renal artery stenoses of 60% or greater diameter reduction with a sensitivity of 92% and a specificity of 62%. This relatively low specificity was due to a large number of borderline lesions that were interpreted as being in the range of 50% to 60% diameter reduction by arteriography. Renal artery occlusion was correctly identified by duplex scanning in 10 of 11 cases.

Table 79-1. Diagnostic criteria for renal duplex scanning

Renal artery diameter reduction	Renal artery PSV	RAR
Normal	<180 cm/sec	<3.5
<60%	≥180 cm/sec	<3.5
≥60%	< or ≥180 cm/sec	≥3.5
Occlusion	No signal	No signal

PSV, Peak systolic velocity; *RAR,* renal aortic ratio (ratio of peak systolic velocity in the renal artery to the peak systolic velocity in the aorta).

RETROSPECTIVE STUDIES OF RENAL ARTERY STENOSIS

Published data on the prevalence of renal artery stenosis have been derived primarily from autopsy studies and selected patients undergoing arteriography. Moderate or severe renal artery stenosis was found at autopsy in 53% of 295 patients, including 49% of 256 patients who were normotensive and 77% of 39 patients with a history of hypertension.[4] Severe renal artery stenosis was rare in patients less than 50 years old but became more frequent with increasing age. In a series of 500 patients undergoing arteriography for a variety of vascular problems, renal artery abnormalities were observed in 219 (44%).[2] These lesions were present in 32% of 304 normotensive patients and 62% of 196 patients with hypertension. Another arteriographic study documented renal artery stenoses in 22% of patients with abdominal aortic aneurysms.[1]

Most reports on the natural history of renal artery stenosis are based on serial arteriography; however, since these studies include only patients requiring multiple arteriograms, it is likely that the incidence of disease progression has been overestimated. In a review of 39 patients with atherosclerotic renal artery lesions who underwent serial arteriography at intervals ranging from 6 months to 10 years, an increase in stenosis severity was noted in 10 and renal artery thrombosis occurred in 4, giving an overall progression rate of 36%.[6] A similar study that followed 30 patients for a mean period of 42 months found progression in 50% of the renal artery lesions.[13] Follow-up of 85 patients for a mean period of 52 months with serial arteriograms revealed progressive atherosclerotic renal artery stenosis in 37 (44%) patients, including 14 patients who developed total renal artery occlusion.[9] The risk of progression to occlusion was particularly high in renal arteries with more than 75% stenosis on the initial arteriogram. In the last two studies, impairment of renal function and a decrease in renal size were both more common in patients showing progression of renal artery disease compared with those patients in whom the renal artery lesions remained stable.

A more recent study reviewed 48 patients with atherosclerotic renal artery stenosis who underwent serial arteriography for aortic disease but did not have repair of the renal artery lesions.[12] All patients had a minimum of two arteriograms at least 1 year apart and were followed for a mean period of 7.3 years. Of the 79 renal artery lesions identified, progression of stenosis was noted in 42 (53%)

patients. The overall rate of stenosis progression was 4.6% per year. Seven lesions (9%) progressed to total occlusion, and all seven had stenoses averaging 80% diameter reduction on the arteriogram immediately before the one documenting the occlusion. No renal artery stenoses of less than 60% diameter reduction on the preceding arteriogram progressed to occlusion. A variety of factors, including smoking, diabetes, serum cholesterol level, changes in blood pressure, and serum creatinine level did not correlate with the severity or rate of renal artery stenosis progression. Although renal size varied inversely with stenosis severity, it did not serve as a significant predictor for progression to occlusion.

PROSPECTIVE EVALUATION OF RENAL ARTERY STENOSIS

Since the studies reviewed are all retrospective and based on highly selected patient groups, they may not accurately represent the true prevalence and progression rate of renal artery stenosis in the general population. These data can only be obtained by prospective follow-up of a large, unselected patient population. To make informed clinical decisions, clinicians need to know not only the rate of disease progression in stenotic renal arteries but also the risk factors associated with progression and the incidence of renal artery occlusion.

In one prospective study, duplex scanning was used to follow 27 patients with 35 renal artery stenoses of 60% to 99% diameter reduction.[10] A total of 19 stenoses were observed without intervention for a mean of 13 months. Although all 19 stenotic renal arteries remained patent during the follow-up period, renal length decreased by a mean of −1.0 cm, a significant change ($p < 0.01$). There was also a trend toward an increase in serum creatinine level that did not reach statistical significance (mean change in serum creatinine level +1.0 mg/dl, $p = 0.08$). In those patients with unilateral renal artery stenosis, there was no significant change in renal length for kidneys with nonstenotic renal arteries.

In the same study, 16 renal artery stenoses were followed after therapeutic interventions. Percutaneous transluminal angioplasty (PTA) was performed on 6 arteries in 5 patients, and 10 arteries in 7 patients were treated by surgical bypass. The PTA group was followed for a mean of 6.5 months. Duplex scanning documented relief of renal artery stenosis in 2 patients whose hypertension improved after PTA and persistent stenosis in 3 patients whose hypertension did not improve. Follow-up of the surgical bypass group for a mean of 9 months showed 8 patent and 2 occluded grafts.

Based on the experience with duplex scanning for follow-up of renal artery disease, a prospective study has been initiated in the vascular research laboratory at the University of Washington. The study population consists of patients with renal artery disease identified by duplex scanning who do not require immediate intervention. Eligible patients must have at least one renal artery with a PSV of at least 180 cm/sec or a RAR of at least 3.5 (Table 79-1) and be willing to participate in a 5-year follow-up protocol. Patients were initially evaluated at 6-month intervals; however, a 12-

month follow-up interval is now being used to facilitate the growing number of patient evaluations required by the study. At the baseline and each subsequent follow-up visit, a detailed questionnaire on general health status and cardiovascular risk factors is completed. A renal duplex scan is then performed, along with a carotid artery duplex scan and a noninvasive evaluation of the lower extremity arterial circulation. The last tests are being done to assess the prevalence and progression rate of atherosclerosis in other segments of the arterial circulation. Blood is also obtained for determination of renal function and lipid levels.

Disease progression in the renal artery is defined as an increase in stenosis severity on serial duplex examinations according to the criteria given in Table 79-1. Renal arteries that are normal at the baseline visit show disease progression if they fall in any disease category on a subsequent evaluation. Those arteries with less than 60% stenosis at baseline may progress to either at least 60% stenosis or occlusion; renal arteries with at least 60% stenosis at baseline can only progress to occlusion. If a renal artery is occluded at the baseline visit, no further disease progression is possible.

Initial baseline and follow-up data are currently available on the first 70 patients enrolled in the study protocol. The patient group includes 30 males and 40 females with a mean age of 61 years (range 36 to 83 years). Most of these patients were originally referred for renal artery screening because of hypertension or decreased renal function. At the baseline visit, 40% of the patients had coronary artery disease, 39% had lower extremity arterial disease, 40% had extracranial carotid artery disease, and 11% had diabetes mellitus. The status of the 140 renal arteries, as determined by the baseline duplex scan, was normal in 35, less than 60% stenosis in 33, at least 60% stenosis in 62, occluded in 9, and indeterminate in 1. The majority of these lesions were located at the origin or within the proximal segment of the renal artery. During follow-up, 11 renal artery stenoses required therapeutic interventions: 9 underwent PTA, 1 had a renal artery endarterectomy, and 1 had a nephrectomy. In addition, 2 patients have initiated hemodialysis for progressive renal failure. A total of 3 patients have died, and 3 patients have been lost to follow-up.

Preliminary data on renal artery disease progression are now available on 82 arteries followed for 6 months, 62 arteries followed for 12 months, and 40 arteries followed for 18 months (Table 79-2). The overall rates of renal artery disease progression are 10% at 6 months, 24% at 12 months, and 20% at 18 months. No consistent relationship has been observed in this patient population between progression of renal artery disease and changes in renal length or function.

CONCLUSION

The reported prevalence of renal artery stenosis in selected patient populations is in the range of 20% to 50%. Retrospective studies indicate that progression of renal artery stenosis occurs in 30% to 50% of patients followed for mean periods of up to 7 years. Preliminary data from a prospective study at the University of Washington show disease progression in 20% of stenotic renal arteries after 18 months of follow-up. These observations are consistent with data from natural history studies of internal carotid artery disease, including the tendency for progression of severe stenoses to total occlusion.

Progression of renal artery stenosis to occlusion is particularly disturbing, since the value of revascularizing a kidney after the renal artery has occluded appears to be limited. At present, the available data suggest that selected patients with very severe renal artery stenoses could benefit from repair of the lesions, particularly those with solitary kidneys or bilateral renal artery stenoses. However, more information on the natural history of these lesions is needed to identify better clinical markers for renal artery disease progression. Furthermore, the response to renal revascularization, both in terms of blood pressure control and preservation of renal function, needs to be documented before intervention can be strongly recommended.

REFERENCES

1. Brewster DC et al: Angiography in the management of aneurysms of the abdominal aorta—its value and safety, *N Engl J Med* 292:822, 1975.
2. Eyler WR et al: Angiography of the renal areas including a comparative study of renal arterial stenoses in patients with and without hypertension, *Radiology* 78:879, 1962.
3. Hoffmann U et al: Role of duplex scanning for the detection of atherosclerotic renal artery disease, *Kidney Int* 39:1232, 1991.
4. Holley KE et al: Renal artery stenosis—a clinical-pathologic study in normotensive and hypertensive patients, *Am J Med* 37:14, 1964.
5. Kohler TR et al: Noninvasive diagnosis of renal artery stenosis by ultrasonic duplex scanning, *J Vasc Surg* 4:450, 1986.
6. Meaney TF, Dustan HP, McCormack LJ: Natural history of renal arterial disease, *Radiology* 91:881, 1968.
7. Moneta GL et al: Operative versus nonoperative management of asymptomatic high-grade internal carotid artery stenosis: improved results with endarterectomy, *Stroke* 18:1005, 1987.
8. Roederer GO et al: The natural history of carotid arterial disease in asymptomatic patients with cervical bruits, *Stroke* 15:605, 1984.
9. Schreiber MJ, Pohl MA, Novick AC: The natural history of atherosclerotic and fibrous renal artery disease, *Urol Clin North Am* 11:383, 1984.
10. Taylor DC, Moneta GL, Strandness DE Jr: Follow-up of renal artery stenosis by duplex ultrasound, *J Vasc Surg* 9:410, 1989.
11. Taylor DC et al: Duplex ultrasound in the diagnosis of renal artery stenosis—a prospective evaluation, *J Vasc Surg* 7:363, 1988.
12. Tollefson DF, Ernst CB: Natural history of atherosclerotic renal artery stenosis associated with aortic disease, *J Vasc Surg* 14:327, 1991.
13. Wollenweber J, Sheps SG, Davis GD: Clinical course of atherosclerotic renovascular disease, *Am J Cardiol* 21:60, 1968.
14. Zierler RE: The role of the vascular laboratory in clinical decision-making, *Semin Roentgenol* 28:63, 1992.

Table 79-2. Preliminary data on renal artery disease progression*

Baseline duplex†	6 mo	12 mo	18 mo
Normal	3/27	7/20	4/14
<60%	4/20	6/16	3/8
≥60%	1/35	2/26	1/18
TOTAL	8/82	15/62	8/40

*Numerator is the number of renal arteries showing disease progression at selected follow-up interval; denominator is the number of renal arteries at indicated duplex category at baseline.
†Baseline occlusions omitted.

CHAPTER 80

Doppler evaluation of the renal parenchyma

CHRISTOPHER R.B. MERRITT

In contrast to the routine use of Doppler in the evaluation of renal transplants, the use of duplex Doppler and Doppler color imaging (DCI) to evaluate the native kidney is still evolving. The highly vascular nature of the kidney and the importance of renal perfusion in the maintenance of renal function, as well as in the pathogenesis of hypertension, make the noninvasive assessment of blood flow to the native kidney provided by ultrasound especially attractive. Potential applications for Doppler in renal evaluation are summarized in the box.[15] The combination of DCI and duplex Doppler is increasing the usefulness of Doppler imaging in the assessment of renal flow. Doppler ultrasound makes it possible to confirm renal arterial and venous patency and to noninvasively diagnose vascular anomalies such as aneurysms, pseudoaneurysms, and arteriovenous fistulas. Analysis of renal arterial impedance aids in the detection and characterization of obstruction and certain parenchymal abnormalities. Finally, Doppler findings may aid in the differentiation of benign and malignant renal masses. In this chapter, a review and overview of the most promising applications of Doppler in renal evaluation are provided. For a discussion of renal artery stenosis and renal transplantation, the reader is referred to Chapters 76, 77, 79, and 91.

EXAMINATION TECHNIQUE

The preparation required for performing renal ultrasound is minimal. Having the patient fast before the examination helps minimize the amount of intestinal gas overlying the renal areas. Imaging and Doppler evaluation are also improved if the patient is well hydrated, and therefore good fluid intake up to about 4 hours before examination should be encouraged. Scanning is best performed with transducers small enough to gain access to the kidneys using acoustic windows between the ribs as well as through the flank and anterior abdomen. Sector scanners with mechanically steered single-element or annular array transducers provide excellent image quality and are preferred to linear arrays. Curved arrays with a medium radius of curvature (4 cm) and phased array sector scanners are also well suited for the evaluation of the native kidneys. Imaging frequencies of from 2.25 to 5.0 MHz are used, with the lower frequencies reserved for use in large or obese patients. In infants, frequencies as high as 7.5 to 10.0 MHz are suitable. Doppler frequencies of 3.0 to 5.0 MHz are those typically employed. Examinations using pulsed Doppler for spectral analysis should be performed with wall filter settings as low as possible (50 to 100 Hz) to avoid removal of low-velocity components from the waveform that may affect calculation of the resistive index (RI). Sample volume sizes may vary, depending on the vessel being examined, but usually range from 2 to 8 mm. Because of the depth from which the Doppler data are sampled, relatively low pulse repetition frequencies (PRFs) of 1000 to 1500 Hz may be required, increasing the likelihood of aliasing (see Chapters 10 and 11). Because of kidney movement during respiration, Doppler sampling is usually performed with the patient in a state of suspended respiration.

The imaging examination of the kidneys should include longitudinal and transverse views of each kidney along with measurement of the craniocaudal, anteroposterior, and transverse diameters of each kidney. The normal renal length varies from 9 to 12 cm in adults and tends to decrease with age. The renal cortex is moderately echogenic in contrast to the less echogenic medullary pyramids, and the renal sinus is highly echogenic with strong echoes arising from the renal sinus fat, vessels, and renal pelvis (Fig. 80-1). With gray-scale imaging, the normal renal vessels entering the renal sinus are generally not seen; however, with DCI these vessels are routinely imaged (Fig. 80-2). Differentiation of pyelocalicectasis from normal renal vessels is occasionally a problem in fetuses and infants, and DCI is

---

USES OF DOPPLER IN RENAL EVALUATION

Diagnosis of renal artery occlusion
Diagnosis of renal vein occlusion
Detection of hemodynamically significant renal artery stenosis
Differentiation of obstructive from nonobstructive calicectasis
Identification of renal parenchymal abnormality (e.g., acute tubular necrosis)
Characterization of renal masses—diagnosis of renal carcinoma
Diagnosis of aneurysm and pseudoaneurysm
Diagnosis of arteriovenous fistulas and malformations
Intraoperative monitoring of renal artery reconstruction
Evaluation of renal transplant dysfunction

---

useful for differentiating the renal collecting system from prominent hilar blood vessels. In the fetus and infant, sonolucent areas measuring 2 mm or greater in the antero-posterior dimension are unlikely to represent renal vasculature.[1]

In the absence of renal disease, the corticomedullary junction is usually visible and serves as a landmark for placement of the Doppler sample volume, indicating the position of the arcuate arteries, which lie over the pyramids and separate them from the renal cortex (Fig. 80-3). The interlobar arteries lie along the sides of the medullary pyramids. In the presence of renal parenchymal disease, cortical echogenicity often increases. Chronic medical renal disease leads to thinning of the cortex and reduced renal size, resulting in the characteristic sonographic pattern of end-stage renal parenchymal disease (Fig. 80-4).

In the Doppler evaluation of the kidneys, the main renal vessels as well as the segmental, interlobar, and interlobular arteries should be examined. In most patients, the main renal arteries arise from the aorta approximately 1 cm caudal to the origin of the superior mesenteric artery (SMA). This is nearly level with the upper border of the second lumbar vertebra. The renal arteries pass transversely across the crura of the diaphragm and upper portions of the psoas muscles to enter the kidneys. The right renal artery passes posterior

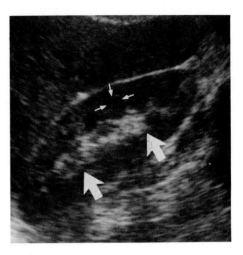

Fig. 80-1. Normal right kidney. Longitudinal real-time image shows normal cortex and medulla. The medullary pyramids *(small arrows)* are normally less echogenic than the renal cortex. The strong central renal sinus echo complex *(large arrows)* arises from the fat, vessels, and the pelvocalyceal system.

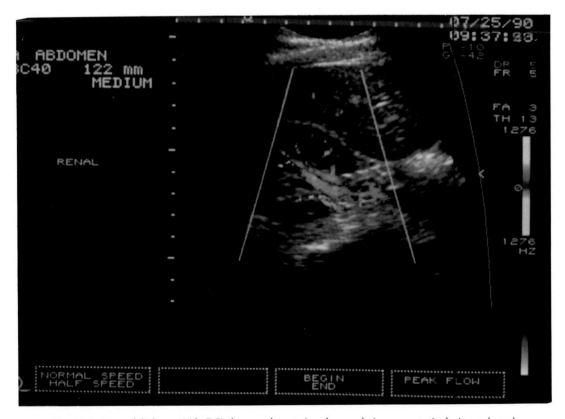

Fig. 80-2. Normal kidney. With DCI the vessels entering the renal sinus are routinely imaged, and prominent vessels may be easily differentiated from mild degrees of pyelocalyceal dilatation.

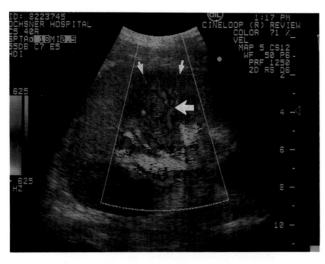

A

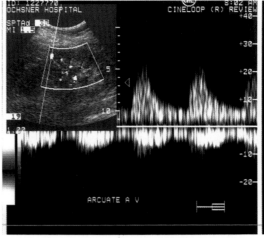

B

Fig. 80-3. Normal intrarenal vessels. *A,* DCI reveals flow in the arcuate arteries *(small arrows),* which lie between the renal cortex and medulla, and interlobar arteries *(large arrow),* which lie along the sides of the medullary pyramids. *B,* DCI aids in selecting sites for Doppler spectral analysis. The waveform shows normal flow in an arcuate artery.

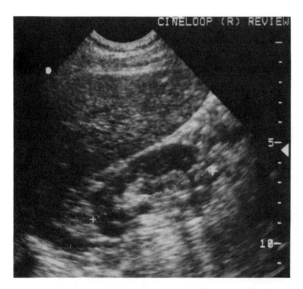

Fig. 80-4. Chronic renal parenchymal disease. Real-time image shows thinning of the renal cortex, small renal size, and increased cortical echogenicity. The overall length of the kidney is only 7.1 cm. These findings are the hallmarks of chronic renal parenchymal disease.

to the inferior vena cava (IVC) and is often visible in this location with ultrasound, particularly in parasagittal imaging planes (Fig. 80-5). The level where the right renal artery passes posterior to the IVC is usually within 1 or 2 cm of the level where the portal vein crosses anterior to the IVC. The portal vein, along with the SMA, serves as a useful landmark when beginning a search for the renal arteries. The right renal artery passes posterior to the head of the pancreas and the second portion of the duodenum, and the left renal artery passes behind the pancreas and the left renal and splenic veins. A problem in the evaluation of renal

arteries arises from the common occurrence of accessory arteries. These are reported to occur in approximately 23% of the population. Accessory arteries are more common on the left side and tend to supply the inferior pole. Accessory renal arteries may also originate from the iliac and other abdominal vessels.[28] The renal veins lie anterior to the renal arteries. The right renal vein is relatively short and empties directly into the IVC. The left renal vein is considerably longer than the right, passing anterior to the aorta and posterior to the pancreas, splenic vein, and superior mesenteric artery and vein. Ultrasound will commonly reveal some dilatation of the left renal vein as a result of compression in the base of the mesentery as it passes between the aorta and the proximal SMA (Fig. 80-6).

When performing Doppler sampling of the renal arteries, the examiner must be constantly aware of the Doppler angle, keeping the angle of insonation to the direction of flow as small as possible to maximize detection of the returning signal. If direct sampling of the arteries through the anterior abdomen is unsuccessful, scanning through the flank to evaluate the renal artery as it enters the renal sinus may be helpful, with DCI used as a guide. This approach also results in a small Doppler angle, thus improving the detectability of flow. If all else fails, a posterior approach may be used. Because of the greater attenuation of the back muscles, lower scanning frequencies may be required to obtain adequate imaging and Doppler data.

Within the kidney, the main renal arteries split into anterior and posterior segmental branches that then divide into a number of interlobar branches to supply apical, upper anterior, middle anterior, lower, and posterior segments of the kidney (Fig. 80-7). Each of the five segments of the kidney is supplied by its own branch of the interlobar artery, and no collateral circulation exists between the segments.

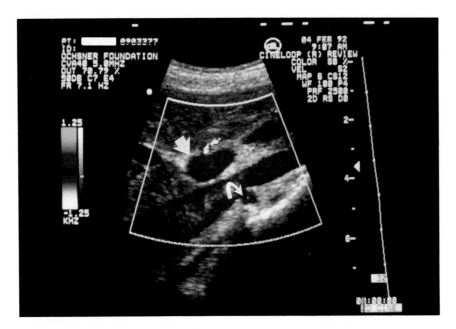

Fig. 80-5. Right renal artery. Longitudinal DCI image slightly to the right of midline shows a single right renal artery *(curved arrow)* as it passes posterior to the inferior vena cava. Note that the level at which the right renal artery passes posterior to the inferior vena cava is approximately the same level that the portal vein *(large arrow)* passes anterior to the inferior vena cava.

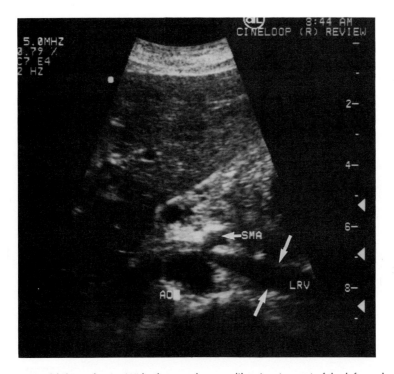

Fig. 80-6. Normal left renal vein. With ultrasound, some dilatation *(arrows)* of the left renal vein *(LRV)* is commonly seen as a result of compression in the base of the mesentery as it passes between the aorta *(AO)* and the proximal superior mesenteric artery *(SMA)*.

The relatively constant segmental distribution of the branches of the interlobar branches is important in the evaluation of intrarenal blood flow with DCI, since flow to individual segments of the kidney may be interrupted with obstruction of these branches and DCI may identify resulting areas of segmental hypoperfusion. Within the kidneys, the interlobar vessels pass between the medullary columns and give rise to the arcuate arteries at the corticomedullary junction. Small intralobular arteries arise from the arcuate arteries and penetrate the cortex. These vessels are routinely imaged with DCI in renal transplants and are also visible in native kidneys using the newer and more sensitive DCI scanners.

In the native kidney, imaging of the main renal arteries is often possible, provided a suitable acoustic window is found. Both supine and decubitus transabdominal as well as prone translumbar approaches may be helpful in achieving DCI in visualization of the extrarenal segment of the renal arteries. Usually the renal arteries are imaged in the axial plane at the level of the SMA and the left renal vein (Fig. 80-8). In sagittal scan planes, identification of the right renal artery as it passes posterior to the IVC may be helpful. The acoustic window provided by the liver and IVC makes it easier to evaluate the right renal vessels than the left. In the presence of an enlarged spleen, access to the left kidney is improved. For examinations of adults, satisfactory penetration and flow sensitivity usually require the use of 2.5- to 3.5-MHz transducers, with higher frequencies reserved for small patients and children.

Measurement of peak velocity in the renal artery can be used to evaluate the renal arteries for stenosis. Velocity measurements in the main renal artery are normally less than 100 cm/sec; however, values as high as 180 cm/sec have been reported.[11] (For further discussion of renal artery stenosis, see Chapter 77.) In the assessment of hydronephrosis and medical renal disease, in which downstream

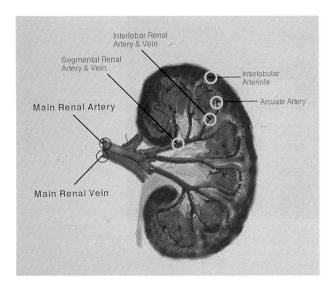

Fig. 80-7. Renal vasculature. Within the kidney, the main renal artery splits into anterior and posterior segmental branches that then divide into a number of interlobar branches. These give rise to arcuate and interlobular arteries. The veins follow a similar pattern. With DCI the main, segmental, and interlobar vessels are routinely imaged. (From Merritt CRB: *Abdomen.* In Merritt CRB, ed: *Doppler color imaging,* New York, 1992, Churchill Livingstone.)

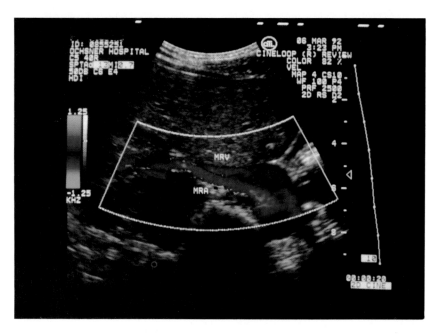

Fig. 80-8. Normal main renal artery and vein. Axial DCI image at the level of the SMA shows the normal right renal artery (red) and vein (blue). Note that the artery lies posterior to the renal vein as the vein joins the inferior vena cava.

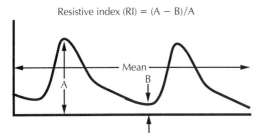

Resistive index (RI) = (A − B)/A

Mean

A

B

A, Peak systolic frequency (velocity).
B, Minimum or end-diastolic frequency (velocity).

Fig. 80-9. The RI is calculated by dividing the difference in the maximum *(A)* and minimum *(B)* heights of the Doppler waveform by the maximum height *(A)*.

Table 80-1. Normal renal artery resistive index values

Author and year	Resistive index	Comment
Platt et al,[21] 1989	0.64 ± 0.04	—
Platt et al,[19] 1991	0.61 ± 0.07	Renal transplant
Gottlieb et al,[8] 1989	0.58 ± 0.04	—
Dodd et al,[6] 1991	0.65 ± 0.05	Dog kidneys
Palmer et al,[17] 1991	0.67	Infants

vascular changes are of interest, the RI of Pourcelot is calculated by dividing the difference in the maximum *(S)* and minimum *(D)* heights of the Doppler waveform by the maximum height *(S)*: RI = (S − D)/S (Fig. 80-9). When waveform analysis using RI measurement is done, it is advisable to use an average value calculated over three to five waveforms to correct for variations related to slight variations in the angle of insonation stemming from transducer or vessel movement. Analysis of renal artery RI reveals a relatively high renal artery resistance at birth, which decreases with time.[14] In normal adults, the RI in the main renal artery as well as in the segmental and interlobar arteries is typically less than 0.7 (Table 80-1). As a result, the spectral waveform obtained from the main renal artery and its branches exhibits a pattern typical of a low-resistance vessel with high-flow velocity persisting throughout diastole (Fig. 80-10). Although the segmental, interlobar, and arcuate arteries of the native kidney are not visible with conventional real-time imaging, they may be detected with DCI (Fig. 80-3). DCI thus aids in locating these vessels for spectral sampling and in obtaining a suitable Doppler angle. Even though DCI currently cannot quantify renal arterial resistance, variations in flow throughout the cardiac cycle in the normal renal artery may be imaged, provided the instrument settings have not been adjusted to limit the display of lower-frequency shifts present in diastole. DCI can depict venous flow within the kidney as well as the main renal veins, and the identification of normal and symmetric venous flow from the kidneys may be useful in ruling out the possibility of main renal vein thrombosis.

OBSTRUCTION

Differentiation of obstructive dilatation of the renal collecting system from nonobstructive dilatation poses a common and important clinical dilemma that cannot be readily resolved by ultrasound imaging alone. Renal obstruction has been shown to increase renal vascular resistance in experimental animals, leading to abnormal RI values, and there is evidence that this also occurs in humans (Fig. 80-11). The results of several attempts to use Doppler to differentiate obstructive hydronephrosis from nonobstructive dilatation of the renal collecting system have been reported. The duplex Doppler measurements of renal artery RI typically differ significantly for obstructed and nonobstructed kidneys (Table 80-2). In 1989, Platt et al[21] reported the results of duplex Doppler evaluation of 14 obstructed and 7 nonobstructed kidneys immediately before percutaneous nephrostomy was performed. Doppler waveforms obtained from the arcuate or cortical arteries were then used to determine the RI, and values were correlated with manometric measurements of pressure within the collecting system obtained at the time of nephrostomy. A statistically significant ($p < 0.001$) difference was found in the mean RI of obstructed kidneys (0.77 ± 0.04) compared to nonobstructed kidneys (RI = 0.64 ± 0.04). On the basis of these findings, an RI of 0.70 was suggested as an appropriate threshold for the identification of significant renal obstruction, and this showed a sensitivity of 93% and a specificity of 100%. These authors also noted a significant reduction in renal artery RI after decompression of the obstruction by nephrostomy, with a drop in the mean RI from 0.77 to 0.63 (±0.03) from 2 to 9 days after treatment. A larger study by Platt et al,[20] involving 133 patients (229 kidneys), extended their initial observations. Normal kidneys were found to have RI values of from 0.50 to 0.67, dilated, nonobstructed collecting systems had RI values of from 0.50 to 0.74, and dilated, obstructed kidneys had RI values of 0.60 to 0.90 or more. Receiver-operating characteristics (ROC) analysis confirmed that an RI of 0.70 is optimal for distinguishing renal obstruction from nonobstructive dilatation, showing a sensitivity of 92%, specificity of 88%, and accuracy of 90%. The only false-positive and false-negative cases encountered with the use of this value were in a small number of patients with RI measurements in the range of 0.69 to 0.72.

Similar results were obtained by Gottlieb et al,[8] who determined a mean RI of 0.58 from normal kidneys (maximum value, 0.66). In four obstructed kidneys, the mean interlobar artery RI was 0.75 and the lowest value was 0.71. Bude et al[3] have also reported that this method successfully differentiated obstructive from nonobstructive hydronephrosis in two patients with ileal loop urinary diversions. Using duplex Doppler to evaluate flow in segmental renal arteries, they found an RI of 0.88 in a patient with acute ureteral obstruction due to calculus, whereas another patient

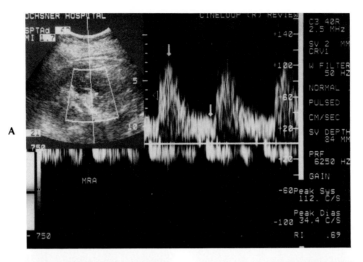

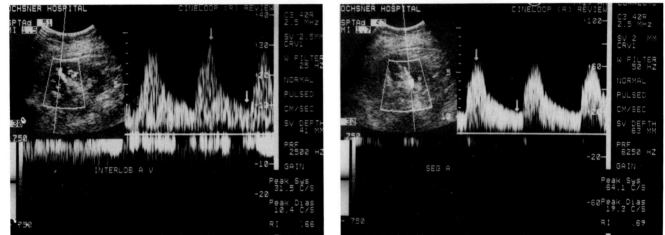

Fig. 80-10. Normal renal artery waveforms. Doppler spectra from the main renal artery *(A)*, a segmental renal artery *(B)*, and an interlobar artery *(C)* all show low-impedance waveforms with a resistive index of 0.60 to 0.69. The peak systolic velocity in the main renal artery is normal (112 cm/sec).

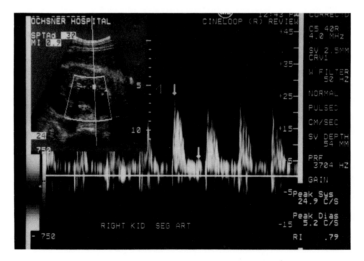

Fig. 80-11. Increased impedance. In a patient with urinary tract obstruction, there is diminished diastolic flow. Increased renal artery impedance is indicated by an elevated resistive index *(RI)* of 0.79 compared to a normal of less than 0.70.

Table 80-2. Renal artery resistive index in identifying obstruction

Author and year	Condition	Resistive index	No. of patients studied
Platt et al,[21] 1989	Nonobstructed	0.64 ± 0.04	14
	Obstructed	0.77 ± 0.04	7
	Treated obstruction	0.63 ± 0.04	10
Platt et al,[20] 1989	Normal	0.58 ± 0.05	109
	Obstructed	0.77 ± 0.05	38
	Nonobstructed	0.63 ± 0.06	32
Platt et al,[19] 1991	Normal transplant	0.61 ± 0.07	9
	Obstruction only	0.82 ± 0.06	7
	Obstruction and leak	0.72 ± 0.04	3
Gottlieb et al,[8] 1989	Normal	0.58 ± 0.04	15
	Obstructed	0.75	4
	Nonobstructed	0.60	4
Dodd et al,[6] 1991*	Unobstructed	0.65 ± 0.05	6
	Ureteral obstruction	0.77 ± 0.06	5
Palmer et al,[17] 1991†	Nonobstructed	0.67 (0.67)‡	8
	Unilateral obstruction	0.72 (0.78)‡	3
	Bilateral obstruction	0.76 (0.81)‡	4
Bude et al,[3] 1991	Obstructed	0.88	1
	Nonobstructed	0.66	1

*Data obtained in dogs.
†Data obtained in infants.
‡Values in parentheses are measurements obtained 10 minutes after diuretic administration (see text).

with passive dilatation of the renal collecting system had a normal segmental artery RI of 0.66. Obstruction is also recognized as an important cause of RI elevation in transplanted kidneys.[19] After transplantation, a normal RI is strong evidence against obstruction unless a ureteral leak is also present.

In infants, the Doppler criteria for the diagnosis of obstruction differ from those used in adults, reflecting the higher RI values observed in the renal arteries of neonates and infants. Palmer et al[17] determined the renal RI in 12 children with a median age of 8 months who were undergoing other standard diagnostic studies to evaluate hydronephrosis. In this study, measurement of renal RI was influenced by prior placement of a bladder catheter, oral hydration, and administration of 1 mg/kg of furosemide after baseline measurements were obtained. Renal RI was measured 10 and 30 minutes after administration of the diuretic. This study showed diuretic administration had no measurable influence in 10 nonobstructed kidneys. In these kidneys, the mean RI before diuretic administration was 0.667; 10 and 30 minutes after diuretic administration, the mean RI was unchanged (0.669 at 10 minutes and 0.684 at 30 minutes). The baseline RI values were higher in the group with obstructed kidneys than in the nonobstructed group, but this difference was not significant. RI measurements obtained 10 minutes after diuretic administration were significantly higher ($p < 0.001$) in the obstructed kidneys (mean RI, 0.798) than in the nonobstructed kidneys (mean RI, 0.669). In addition, the RI values after diuretic administration were higher in the presence of bilateral obstruction than unilateral obstruction. These authors noted that al-

though an unmodified RI in excess of 0.75 probably indicates obstruction in children, challenge with a diuretic and elimination of back pressure from the bladder by catheterization are important in identifying obstruction in neonates, whose normal RI values tend to be higher than those later in life. After 1 month of age, the finding of a 10-minute postdiuretic RI of 0.75 or greater indicates functional obstruction, and this criterion possesses a specificity of 100%. In children with only one obstructed kidney, an increase of 15% from the baseline RI after diuretic administration is suggested as another criterion of obstruction.

Using a dog model, Dodd et al[6] investigated the temporal relationship of the alteration in the Doppler spectrum to the onset of urinary obstruction. Duplex Doppler examination identified a statistically significant difference ($p < 0.05$) in the Doppler-derived RI value between the obstructed and nonobstructed kidneys of dogs on days 1, 2, 4, and 28 after ureteral ligation. When an RI of greater than 0.7 was used as a discriminatory threshold for obstruction, this yielded a sensitivity of 74% and a specificity of 77%. Based on their findings, the authors concluded that renal arterial duplex Doppler sonography can detect a change in renal perfusion caused by urinary obstruction as early as 24 hours after obstruction, although with limited sensitivity and specificity.

From these data, it is clear that Doppler measurements are most promising in aiding the differentiation of obstructive from nonobstructive calicectasis. Although the mechanism responsible for increasing the RI in the presence of obstruction has not been fully defined, it seems likely that increased pressure on the renal vessels precipitates increased resistance to flow, which then causes the elevation of the

RI. The use of DCI in conjunction with waveform analysis improves the ease with which intrarenal blood flow can be evaluated. In addition, examination time is reduced and optimum Doppler angles can be obtained.

MEDICAL RENAL DISEASE

Ultrasound imaging is commonly used in the evaluation of acute and chronic renal parenchymal diseases. Chronic end-stage renal disease is typically manifested by small (less than 9 cm) kidneys, whereas more acute parenchymal disease is usually manifested by changes in renal size, cortical echogenicity, and altered corticomedullary boundaries. Although changes in renal size and echogenicity often exist in patients with acute glomerulonephritis, acute tubular necrosis (ATN), acute cortical necrosis, and interstitial nephritis, these findings are nonspecific and vary in sensitivity. Doppler-detected abnormalities have been reported in association with a variety of renal parenchymal abnormalities and may improve both the sensitivity and specificity of standard ultrasound imaging (Table 80-3).

In the evaluation of acute renal failure (ARF), Doppler is helpful in differentiating ATN from other causes. Platt et al[22] recently looked for changes in the Doppler waveform associated with ARF to determine whether Doppler can provide information not available with ultrasound imaging. The RI in the arcuate or interlobar arteries was measured in 91 adult patients with ARF using duplex Doppler. In the presence of ATN, significant elevation of the RI was found. A total of 46 patients had ATN and the mean RI in this group was 0.85 ± 0.06; 91% of these patients had RI values exceeding 0.75. In 30 patients with prerenal ARF, the mean RI was significantly less (0.67 ± 0.09). A total of 15 patients with ARF not due to ATN had a mean RI of 0.74 ± 0.13. An elevated RI (greater than or equal to 0.75) was recorded in only 20% of patients with prerenal azotemia. Using ROC analysis, these investigators found that an RI of 0.75 was optimal for discriminating ATN from prerenal failure. When they studied the relationship of the Doppler findings to the cause of ATN, no significant differences were discerned. Most of the elevated RIs were noted in the patients with prerenal ARF who had severe liver disease (hepatorenal syndrome), and this resembled the findings in the ATN group. Patients with prerenal ARF not related to hepatic disease had normal RIs (mean, 0.64).

In this study, imaging abnormalities such as increased cortical echogenicity were discovered in only 11% of the patients with ARF. This study also revealed that patients with prolonged renal failure had higher RIs than did patients with reversible ARF. There was a poor correlation between RI measurements and serum creatinine levels. The mechanism responsible for the Doppler changes seen in ATN is uncertain but probably involves increased vascular resistance caused by arteriolar vasoconstriction triggered by humoral or neurogenic factors. If 0.70 is accepted as the upper limit of normal for RI in the adult, 96% of patients with ARF due to ATN may be expected to have abnormal RI values. This study demonstrates that intrarenal Doppler ultrasound far more often detects the changes associated with ARF than does standard ultrasound. More important, Doppler ultrasound may be helpful in distinguishing ATN from prerenal azotemia, using an RI of 0.75 as the discriminating value.

Further evidence for the value of Doppler ultrasound in the assessment of renal disease comes from studies performed in children with hemolytic-uremic syndrome.[18] In these patients, there was either no intrarenal arterial flow or absent, reversed, or markedly reduced diastolic flow, with RIs in excess of 0.90 in 12 of 14 children with anuria or oliguria compared to normal RIs of less than 0.70. Within 24 to 48 hours after diastolic Doppler shifts returned to normal, diuresis occurred, allowing serial measurements of renal artery impedance to predict the likelihood of recovery and allow dialysis treatment to be abbreviated or, in some cases, canceled.

Not all reports addressing the use of Doppler in medical and renal disease have been enthusiastic. In contrast to reports endorsing its use in evaluating patients with ARF, Mostbeck et al[16] reported a poor correlation of renal artery RI measurements in patients with glomerulonephritis, interstitial nephritis, nephroangiosclerosis, ATN, and idiopathic glomerular minimal change disease. This study consisted of 34 adult patients with histopathologic changes of renal parenchymal diseases. Most of the patients (*n* = 21) had glomerulonephritis and small numbers of patients were in the other disease categories. RI measurements from the segmental, interlobar, and arcuate arteries obtained immediately before percutaneous renal biopsy was performed ranged from 0.48 to 1.0, with a mean of 0.67. In 70% of the patients, the RI values were less than 0.70. The RI

Table 80-3. Renal artery resistive index in medical renal disease

Author and year	Condition	Resistive index	No. of patients studied
Platt et al,[20] 1989	Renal disease	0.71 ± 0.10	50
Platt et al,[22] 1991	ATN	0.85 ± 0.06	46
	Prerenal ARF	0.67 ± 0.09	30
	Intrinsic (non-ATN)	0.74 ± 0.13	15
Patriquin et al,[18] 1989	Hemolytic-uremic syndrome	>0.90	17
Mostbeck et al,[16] 1991	Glomerulonephritis	0.67	21

ATN, Acute tubular necrosis; *ARF,* acute renal failure.

values did not differentiate among the causes of renal disease, but there was a positive correlation between RI values and histopathologic findings of arteriolosclerosis, glomerular sclerosis, arteriosclerosis, edema, and focal interstitial fibrosis, and a significant positive correlation of RI with blood urea nitrogen levels, but not with serum creatinine. This report provided no data regarding RI measurements in normal subjects.

Measurement of the renal artery diastolic-to-systolic (D/S) ratio has recently been proposed as another approach to the evaluation of renal function.[29] The ratio of the peak diastolic waveform (D) to the peak systolic value (S) in the segmental renal arteries was correlated with the status of renal function in healthy subjects and 76 patients with varying degrees of impaired renal function. The ratio of the peak diastolic to systolic velocity also correlated well with both p-aminohippurate clearance ($r = 0.61$) and creatinine clearance ($r = 0.85$). The D/S ratio also showed good correlation with the split renal glomerular filtration rate ($r = 0.81$ to 0.83).

Finally, in the pediatric population, it has been suggested that Doppler ultrasound may be valuable in identifying alterations in renal blood flow secondary to medication use[27] and in assessing a multicystic dysplastic kidney.[10]

RENAL CARCINOMA

As in the liver, the vascular changes associated with malignant tumors may be demonstrated by Doppler ultrasound (Fig. 80-12).[7,13] Using a Doppler frequency shift in excess of 2.5 kHz (for 3.0-MHz insonating frequency) as the criterion for diagnosis, tumor signals have been reported in up to 83% of the cases of untreated renal cell carcinomas and in 75% of the cases of both Wilms' tumors and metastases to the kidney but not in association with benign renal masses.[23] Correlation with angiographic findings suggests

that the high-frequency shifted Doppler signals are indicative of arteriovenous shunts. The sensitivity of Doppler in identifying malignant tumors of the kidney is reported to be 70%, with a specificity of 94%.[12] Doppler ultrasound adds useful information to the study of renal masses and the detection of high-velocity signals can aid in the differential diagnosis of renal masses. DCI has also been reported to reveal changes associated with renal carcinoma.[24] Increased vascularity is often seen in the presence of hypervascular renal carcinoma, and DCI can aid in the selection of sampling sites to obtain the characteristic spectral abnormalities described previously. These methods are, however, limited in their ability to detect avascular tumors.

OTHER CONDITIONS

In addition to the identification and quantification of renal artery stenosis, duplex and color Doppler may aid in the noninvasive diagnosis of renal artery and vein occlusion, as well as the detection of renal artery aneurysms and arteriovenous fistulas. Renal artery occlusion is manifested by the absence of renal hilar and intrarenal arterial and venous waveforms. Collateral vessels supplying blood to a kidney with renal artery occlusion may be a source of confusion, and the use of DCI is theoretically helpful in this setting. Although experience with Doppler ultrasonography in the evaluation of renal vein thrombosis is limited, experience using DCI has been encouraging in patients when size and the presence of gas do not prevent assessment. The demonstration of renal vein distention without evidence of flow using duplex Doppler or DCI is a reliable indicator of renal vein thrombosis. DCI is also useful for confirming tumor invasion of the renal veins when real-time imaging findings are equivocal.

The global Doppler sampling provided with DCI aids in identifying renal pseudoaneurysms and arteriovenous mal-

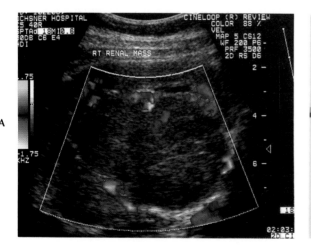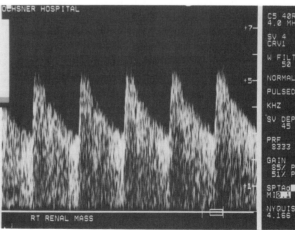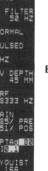

Fig. 80-12. Renal carcinoma. ***A,*** DCI shows a hypervascular mass arising from the upper pole of the kidney. Vessels are increased in number and size and do not follow normal anatomic patterns. ***B,*** Spectral Doppler shows high-velocity, low-impedance flow, a pattern commonly associated with tumor neovascularity.

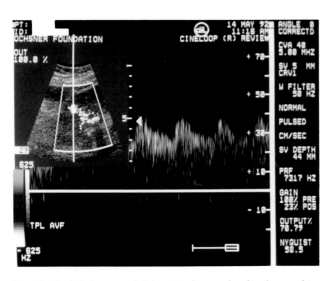

Fig. 80-13. Arteriovenous fistula. DCI shows a localized area of increased vascularity and tissue vibration at the site of a prior renal biopsy. Spectral analysis of flow in the renal vein shows pulsatile flow, confirming arteriovenous shunting through an iatrogenic arteriovenous fistula.

formations, including lesions not observed with ultrasound imaging or computed tomography.[25] Color Doppler findings associated with arteriovenous fistulas include a visible bruit, which is manifested as a mosaic of color superimposed over the soft tissues adjacent to the lesion. Spectral analysis shows high peak systolic frequencies resulting from high-flow states and low RIs resulting from the arteriovenous shunting. Spectral analysis of veins draining the arteriovenous malformation also reveals typical arterialized signals (Fig. 80-13). Renal pseudoaneurysms possess characteristics similar to those noted in pseudoaneurysms elsewhere in the body, including bidirectional swirling blood flow. Other conditions for which Doppler ultrasound has been recommended as an ancillary imaging method are renal vein varix[26] and true aneurysm of the renal artery.[2,4] Intraoperative Doppler may aid in the performance of renal artery reconstruction. The identification of major surgical defects with Doppler, leading to immediate operative revision, has been reported in 11% of vessels undergoing surgical reconstruction.[9]

A current drawback to Doppler methods is their limited ability to directly assess tissue perfusion. This problem is likely to be addressed in the near future once ultrasound contrast agents become available for clinical use. Perfluorooctylbromide (PFOB), when administered intravenously, permits DCI identification of perfusion defects due to renal infarction in rabbits.[5] By enhancing signals from renal vessels, PFOB facilitates the detection of truncated embolized vessels by DCI. Other recently developed agents containing microbubbles suitable for intravenous injection are in the early stages of clinical testing and are also likely to find their way in the evaluation of renal and other organ perfusion.

CONCLUSION

Doppler ultrasound, aided by DCI and coupled with continuing improvements in the sensitivity of instrumentation, has begun to provide clinically useful data in patients with renal disease. Although the criteria for diagnosis based on Doppler indices are still evolving, Doppler is currently useful for distinguishing obstructive from nonobstructive calicectasis and in the differential diagnosis of ARF. The abnormal vascular patterns it can reveal also aid in the differentiation of benign and malignant lesions. In the near future, the introduction of ultrasound contrast agents will likely expand the clinical usefulness of ultrasonography in the evaluation of renal disorders.

REFERENCES

1. Betz BW et al: Mild fetal renal pelviectasis: differentiation from hilar vascularity using color Doppler sonography, *J Ultrasound Med* 10:243-245, 1991.
2. Brondum V, Fiirgaard B: Renal artery aneurysm detected by pulsed Doppler ultrasound, *Rontgenblatter* 43:510-511, 1990.
3. Bude RO et al: Dilated renal collecting systems: differentiating obstructive from nonobstructive dilation using duplex Doppler ultrasound, *Urology* 37:123-125, 1991.
4. Bunchman TE et al: Sonographic evaluation of renal artery aneurysm in childhood, *Pediatr Radiol* 21:312-313, 1991.
5. Coley BD et al: Potential role of PFOB enhanced sonography of the kidney. II. Detection of partial infarction, *Kidney Int* 39:740-745, 1991.
6. Dodd GD III, Kaufman PN, Bracken RB: Renal arterial duplex Doppler ultrasound in dogs with urinary obstruction, *J Urol* 145:644-646, 1991.
7. Dubbins PA, Wells I: Renal carcinoma: duplex Doppler evaluation, *Br J Radiol* 59:231-236, 1986.
8. Gottlieb RH, Luhmann K 4th, Oates RP: Duplex ultrasound evaluation of normal native kidneys and native kidneys with urinary tract obstruction, *J Ultrasound Med* 8:609-611, 1989
9. Hansen KJ et al: Intraoperative duplex sonography during renal artery reconstruction, *J Vasc Surg* 14:364-374, 1991.
10. Hendry PJ, Hendry GM: Observations on the use of Doppler ultrasound in multicystic dysplastic kidney, *Pediatr Radiol* 21:203-204, 1991.
11. Hoffman U et al: The role of duplex scanning for the detection of atherosclerotic renal artery disease, *Kidney Int* 39:1232-1239, 1991.
12. Kier R et al: Renal masses: characterization with Doppler US, *Radiology* 176:703-707, 1990.
13. Kuijpers D, Jaspers R: Renal masses: differential diagnosis with pulsed Doppler US, *Radiology* 170:59-60, 1989.
14. Lamont AC et al: Doppler ultrasound studies in renal arteries of normal newborn babies, *Br J Radiol* 64:413-416, 1991.
15. Merritt CRB: Abdomen. In Merritt CRB, ed: *Doppler color imaging*, New York, 1992, Churchill-Livingstone.
16. Mostbeck GH et al: Duplex Doppler sonography in renal parenchymal disease: histopathologic correlation, *J Ultrasound Med* 10:189-194, 1991.
17. Palmer JM et al: Diuretic Doppler sonography in postnatal hydronephrosis, *J Urol* 146:605-608, 1991.
18. Patriquin HB et al: Hemolytic-uremic syndrome: intrarenal arterial Doppler patterns as a useful guide to therapy, *Radiology* 172:625-628, 1989.
19. Platt JF, Ellis JH, Rubin JM: Renal transplant pyelocaliectasis: role of duplex Doppler US in evaluation, *Radiology* 179:425-428, 1991.
20. Platt JF, Rubin JM, Ellis JH: Distinction between obstructive and nonobstructive pyelocaliectasis with duplex Doppler sonography, *AJR* 153:997-1000, 1989.
21. Platt JF, Rubin JM, Ellis JH: Duplex Doppler US of the kidney: differentiation of obstructive from nonobstructive dilatation, *Radiology* 171:515-517, 1989.
22. Platt JF, Rubin JM, Ellis JH: Acute renal failure: possible role of duplex Doppler US in distinction between acute prerenal failure and acute tubular necrosis, *Radiology* 179:419-423, 1991.

23. Ramos IM et al: Tumor vascular signals in renal masses: detection with Doppler US, *Radiology* 168:633-637, 1988.

24. Shimamoto K et al: Intratumoral blood flow: evaluation with color Doppler echography, *Radiology* 165:683-685, 1987.

25. Sullivan RR et al: Color Doppler sonographic findings in renal vascular lesions, *J Ultrasound Med* 10:161-165, 1991.

26. Sussman SK et al: Cross-sectional imaging of idiopathic solitary renal vein varix: report of two cases, *Urol Radiol* 13:98-102, 1991.

27. van Bel F et al: Indomethacin-induced changes in renal blood flow velocity waveform in premature infants investigated with color Doppler imaging, *J Pediatr* 118:621-626, 1991.

28. Woodburne RT: *Essentials of human anatomy,* New York, 1961, Oxford University Press.

29. Yura T et al: Total and split renal function assessed by ultrasound Doppler techniques, *Nephron* 58:37-41, 1991.

CHAPTER 81

The evaluation of renal transplant dysfunction with duplex ultrasonography and Doppler color flow imaging

MARSHA M. NEUMYER, HAROLD C. YANG, ROBERT R. M. GIFFORD, and BRIAN L. THIELE

.

Kidney transplantation has evolved from the stage of tentative experimentation to become the procedure of choice for treating the majority of patients with terminal renal failure. Advances in surgical technique and the use of immunosuppressive agents, most notably cyclosporin A, have combined to bring about a remarkable improvement in allograft survival rates. Multiple causes of posttransplant renal failure still exist, and the list of potential causes for deterioration in renal function after transplantation consists of acute tubular necrosis (ATN), acute rejection, stenosis of the transplant renal artery, and vascular technical error resulting in thrombosis of the transplant renal artery or vein. Additional complications may include obstruction of the collecting system, technical problems with the ureteral anastomosis to the bladder, infection, and cyclosporin A toxicity.

Therapeutic decision making depends on accurate differentiation of these entities, but clinically this may be quite difficult. The standard diagnostic approach has included the performance of DTPA (diethylene-triamine-pentaacetic acid) technetium 99m scans to identify acute tubular necrosis[31] and cortical needle biopsy with histologic examination for the characteristics of cellular rejection.[4,12] Standard contrast arteriography is performed to evaluate the vascular anastomoses.[1-6] These procedures may necessitate the patient's hospitalization and have a known associated low morbidity.[13,16] In addition, DTPA scanning has demonstrated low sensitivity for distinguishing resolving ATN from allograft rejection.

Ideally, B-mode ultrasound examination of the transplanted organ would reveal those features consistent with allograft deterioration. The sonographic criteria that have been used to define acute transplant rejection include increased renal volume, decreased renal sinus fat, pyramidal enlargement, indistinct corticomedullary boundaries, increased echogenicity of the renal cortex, decreased echogenicity of the renal parenchyma, and pelvic thickening.[4,12,14,24] Using ultrasound in a prospective evaluation, Griffin et al[10] discovered its findings correlated poorly with renal biopsy results and it accurately detected failure in only

52% of the histologically abnormal kidneys. Other investigators have evaluated the feasibility of using duplex ultrasonography and the quantitation of the Doppler velocity spectral waveforms to detect and differentiate the causes of allograft failure. The accuracy reported for such an approach has varied widely, and in general, it is neither sensitive nor specific for the differential diagnosis of transplant dysfunction.*

BACKGROUND

The decrease in blood flow to the cortex of the transplanted kidney undergoing acute rejection was demonstrated by Sampson et al[30] in 1969 using continuous-wave Doppler velocimetry. Since that time, ultrasound has been used by many investigators to study the alterations in blood flow patterns in the transplanted renal artery and parenchyma that occur with deterioration in organ function.† These studies demonstrated that the degree of vascular resistance of the transplanted kidney was reflected by the Doppler velocity waveform recorded from the renal, segmental, interlobar, and arcuate arteries of the allograft. In 1982, using duplex technology, Berland et al[4] represented the resistance to arterial inflow to the kidney by calculating a resistive index derived from the pulsed Doppler velocity waveform.

Using a ratio of the end-diastolic to systolic frequencies of the Doppler waveform recorded in native renal arteries, Norris et al[22] defined both normal waveform patterns and those associated with renal artery stenosis and increased parenchymal resistance. These investigators noted that increased renal vascular resistance was characterized by a concomitant decrease in the end-diastolic frequency of the Doppler signal recorded from the renal artery. Since that time, several methods for quantitating transplant vascular resistance have been reported.

---

*References 1, 2, 7, 9, 13, 15, 16, 26-29, 35.
†References 4, 8, 21-23, 26-28, 32.

PULSATILITY INDEX

Using a pulsatility index calculated from the formula:

$$\frac{\text{Peak systolic velocity} - \text{Minimum end-diastolic velocity}}{\text{Mean velocity}}$$

Rigsby et al[28] documented successful identification of acute renal allograft rejection using an index of 1.5 as the threshold value.

POURCELOT RESISTIVE INDEX

The most commonly used quantitative method is the Pourcelot resistive index, which is derived from the following equation:

$$\frac{\text{Peak systolic velocity} - \text{Minimum diastolic velocity}}{\text{Peak systolic velocity}}$$

Rifkin et al[26] reported a specificity of 100% when an index value greater than 0.9 was used to identify acute transplant rejection. However, these authors noted that the resistive index varies within the kidney, depending on the sampling location, but did not confirm the reports of others who described a significant reduction in the diastolic flow component of the spectral waveforms from allografts with acute tubular necrosis or cyclosporin A toxicity.*

DIASTOLIC-TO-SYSTOLIC RATIO

Buckley et al[5] attempted to differentiate acute transplant rejection and cyclosporine nephrotoxicity using Doppler waveform quantitation. These investigators successfully identified acute transplant rejection using a diastolic-to-systolic ratio less than 0.2 in 89% of the histologically confirmed cases.

Other investigators have challenged the use of the resistive indices for the identification of acute allograft rejection, pointing out that vascular resistance may increase in the transplanted organ for numerous reasons other than allograft rejection.[8,21,23]

In view of the fact that the pathophysiologic characteristics vary for the different types of allograft dysfunction, the blood flow patterns may also vary, thus yielding clues to the differential diagnosis. A combined retrospective and prospective analysis of the pulsed Doppler velocity spectral waveforms recorded from normal transplants and those with acute rejection, ATN, renal artery stenosis, vascular occlusion, arteriovenous fistulas, and cyclosporine toxicity was performed.

RENAL TRANSPLANT EXAMINATION TECHNIQUE

The renal allograft is evaluated with duplex ultrasonography in conjunction with Doppler color flow imaging. The real-time B-mode image facilitates identification of perinephric fluid collections, hydronephrosis, and parenchymal acoustic changes. Doppler color flow imaging assists in locating vessels, detecting areas of disorganized flow, and confirming arteriovenous communications and areas of infarcted

*References 3, 5, 8, 23, 26, 35.

tissue. Abnormal flow patterns are identified using pulsed-Doppler velocity spectral analysis.*

The transplanted kidney lies superficially within the pelvis, and this location facilitates ultrasound interrogation. Unlike the native kidney, there are no loops of bowel interposed between the skin and the transplant. The allograft is examined in both the longitudinal and transverse planes using a 3- or 5-MHz transducer. The region of the allograft is evaluated and the presence of perigraft fluid collections or hydronephrosis is noted. The pole-to-pole length of the kidney is also measured (Fig. 81-1).

The external iliac artery is examined proximal and distal to the anastomosis of the transplant renal artery. The Doppler velocity signal is recorded throughout the length of the imaged vessel using a small sample volume size (1.5 mm) and an angle of insonation of less than 60° with respect to the blood flow vector. The velocity signal should be triphasic with a sharp reverse diastolic flow component characteristic of a normal peripheral artery. Care must be taken to avoid recording the Doppler signal from the internal iliac artery (hypogastric). The signature Doppler waveform from this vessel resembles that of the transplant renal artery, since it may also be characterized by forward diastolic flow.

The region where the transplant renal artery is anastomosed to the external iliac artery is identified and the anastomotic flow patterns are evaluated with Doppler color flow imaging and spectral analysis. Particular attention is paid to the presence of high-velocity signals, perivascular color artifacts, and disorganized flow that may signify transplant renal artery stenosis. The entire length of the transplant artery, from the anastomosis to the hilum of the allograft, is interrogated with Doppler ultrasound.

The transplant medulla and cortex are evaluated using color flow imaging to facilitate visualization of the interlobar and arcuate vessels (Fig. 81-2). The sample volume size is enlarged to 3 mm and swept throughout the medullary and cortical regions, recording those arterial Doppler waveforms demonstrating the highest peak systolic and end-diastolic frequency shifts. Because of the arteriovenous network that exists in the renal cortex and the small parenchymal arteries relative to the sample volume size, venous signals may be recorded concomitantly throughout the cortical region.

NORMAL EXAMINATION

Flow disturbance, without a significant increase in the peak systolic velocity, is normally associated with end-to-side anastomosis. The Doppler color flow image and spectral patterns are recorded as the region of the iliac-renal artery anastomosis is traversed (Fig. 81-3). High velocities and turbulent flow denote luminal narrowing and anastomotic stenosis.

The classic flow patterns of a vessel feeding a low-resistance end organ are recorded throughout the length of the transplant renal artery. Normally, diastolic velocity is ap-

*References 4-9, 11, 12, 17-23, 25-29, 32-36.

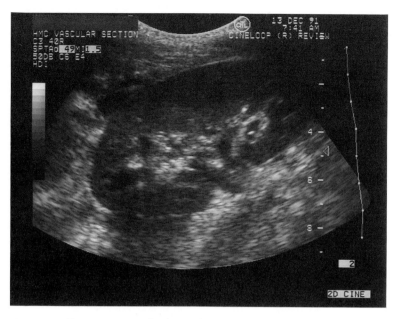

Fig. 81-1. Longitudinal B-mode image of a renal allograft.

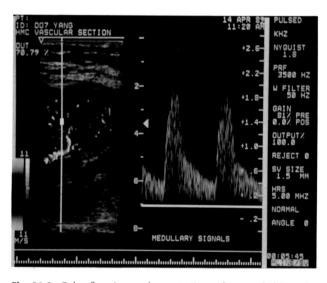

Fig. 81-2. Color flow image demonstrating color-encoded Doppler shifts in the intersegmental and arcuate vessels of the renal transplant, medulla, and cortex. Doppler time velocity waveforms from medullary arteries.

proximately half the peak systolic velocity. The velocity variables decrease proportionately in the distal artery. Although vessel length, tortuosity, and extrinsic compression may affect the diastolic-to-systolic ratio, a diastolic flow of zero is never seen in the normal vessel.

The Doppler velocity waveforms obtained from the medullary segmental and interlobar arteries and those recorded throughout the cortex of the allograft will be quasi-steady, demonstrating forward flow throughout the diastolic phase.

Such signals reflect the low vascular resistance of the renal parenchyma. There is a further reduction in the velocity values as the sample volume is moved from the medullary vessels to the cortical region of the transplant (Fig. 81-4).

Spontaneous respiratory phasicity and a retrograde flow pattern characterize the velocity signal obtained from the transplant renal vein. In contrast, the venous signals recorded within the medulla and cortex of the organ exhibit minimal phasicity. High-velocity venous signals may be recorded in the presence of edema, extrinsic compression, or arteriovenous fistulas.

The primary features consistent with normal blood flow patterns are found in the shape of the spectral envelope and the magnitude of the diastolic forward flow component recorded in the transplant renal artery and the segmental, interlobar, and arcuate vessels. This last feature should be prominent in all signals from a normal study.

ACUTE TRANSPLANT REJECTION

Based on histologic findings, two types of acute transplant rejection have been recognized: cellular and vascular. Frequently, both types occur together. Acute cellular rejection is associated with cellular infiltrate and fluid within the interstitium. The arteries and arterioles usually remain normal. Acute vascular rejection is accompanied by a proliferative endovasculitis that results in intimal thickening with varying degrees of luminal obliteration. Platelet-fibrin aggregates form, and this may lead to thrombosis of the parenchymal vessels.

As the arteriolar diameter decreases, arterial inflow to the allograft is further impeded. This increased vascular resistance is expressed as a decrease in diastolic flow

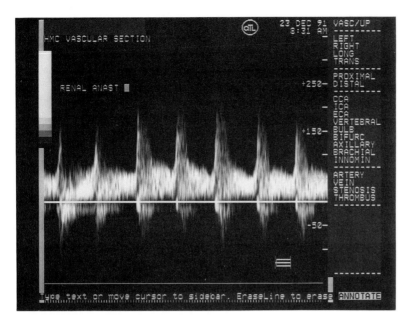

Fig. 81-3. Time velocity spectral waveforms recorded from the region of the anastomosis of the transplant renal artery and the external iliac artery. Note the disturbed flow pattern.

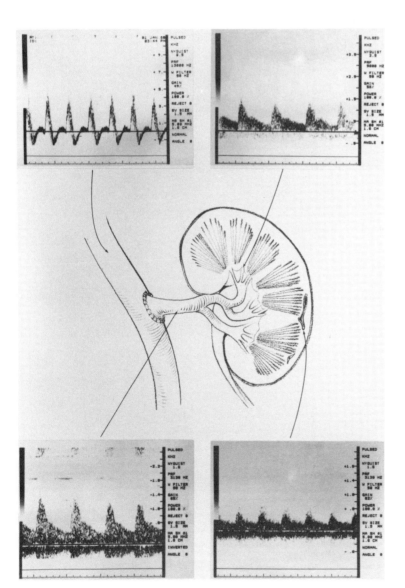

Fig. 81-4. Montage of Doppler velocity spectral waveforms from a normal renal transplant. Note the forward diastolic flow in the signals recorded from the transplant renal artery, medulla, and cortex.

throughout the medulla and cortex of the allograft and may also be reflected in increased pulsatility of the Doppler time-velocity waveform recorded from the transplant renal artery (Fig. 81-5). As the rejection episode becomes more severe, the diastolic flow approaches zero, reverses, or in critical cases, may be absent. The edema associated with acute cellular rejection also augments renovascular resistance, and pulsatility of the Doppler velocity waveform is seen in all of the parenchymal samples.

Doppler color flow imaging demonstrates continuous flow during systole and no significant diastolic flow, reflecting the increased vascular resistance in the allograft. Diagnosis cannot be based on the color flow image alone because the color patterns depict only increased resistance to flow and do not reveal its cause.

If the Doppler spectral waveforms are sequentially evaluated throughout the rejection episode, the response to immunosuppressive therapy can be monitored. A decrease in the renovascular resistance with resolving rejection will be reflected in the reappearance of the diastolic flow component of the Doppler velocity waveform. Continued loss of diastolic flow, despite the administration of steroids and anti-lymphocyte globulin, most often indicates a poor prognosis for the transplanted organ.

ACUTE TUBULAR NECROSIS

The ability to distinguish acute renal transplant rejection from ATN on the basis of Doppler velocity waveform analysis remains controversial. Most frequently, investigators have relied on the calculated resistive index of the Doppler waveform in conjunction with the clinical presentation to judge the existence of acute rejection.

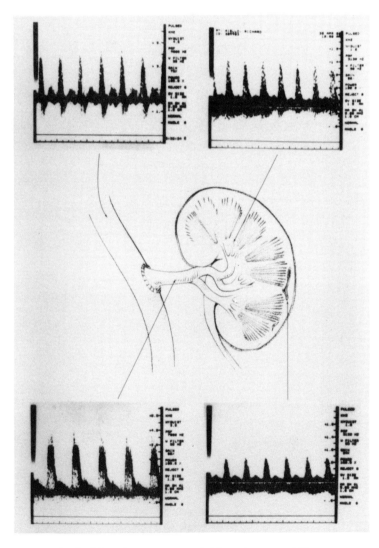

Fig. 81-5. Montage of pulsed Doppler spectra recorded from the external iliac artery, transplant renal artery, and the medullary and cortical vessels of a transplant undergoing acute rejection. Note the decreased diastolic flow component of the Doppler spectral waveforms.

Mild ATN is associated with prominent antegrade diastolic flow (Fig. 81-6), which is thought to be the result of medullary shunting known to occur in such cases. Moderate to severe ATN is accompanied by tubular and interstitial edema, extraneous features that result in increased resistance to arterial flow to the kidney. As the necrosis worsens, the diastolic flow component of the velocity waveform decreases and the spectral waveform exhibits remarkable pulsatility. Rapid systolic deceleration, decreased diastolic flow, and a reduction in the amplitude and descent of the diastolic flow component are apparent in the waveforms recorded from the cortex, medulla, and transplant renal artery in cases of severe ATN. As the diastolic flow decreases, the resulting waveform may become indistinguishable from that associated with severe acute rejection. An important

feature in difficult cases is the information that may be obtained from serial studies.

There is a continuum of waveform pulsatility as the necrosis worsens, and attempts to quantify the waveform and use this information to differentiate moderate to severe ATN from acute rejection have failed. Clinical impressions and sequential monitoring of the Doppler spectral waveform to document the return of diastolic flow have been most helpful in the management of these oliguric patients.

CYCLOSPORINE TOXICITY

Nephrotoxic reactions to the immunosuppressive agent cyclosporin A occur infrequently, but when they arise, may jeopardize allograft function. Previous investigators have noted that there is little change in renovascular resistance

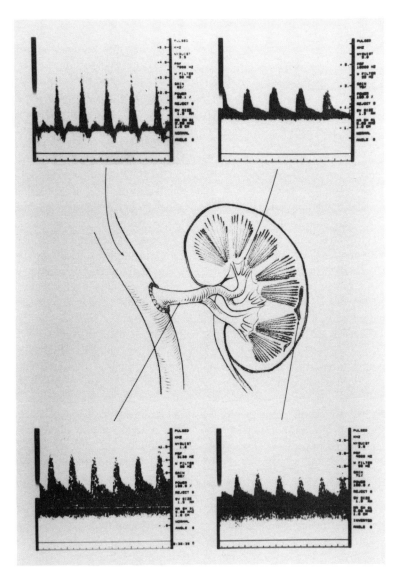

Fig. 81-6. Montage of pulsed Doppler velocity spectra from a renal allograft with mild acute tubular necrosis. Note the rapid systolic deceleration and forward diastolic flow demonstrated in the signals from the transplant renal artery, medulla, and cortex of the allograft.

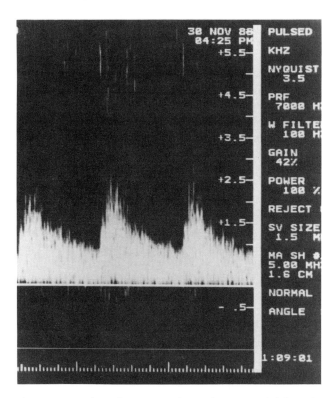

Fig. 81-7. Doppler velocity spectral waveforms recorded from the cortex of a renal allograft with cyclosporin A toxicity. Note the shagginess in the spectral envelope.

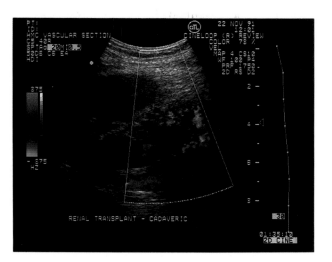

Fig. 81-8. Doppler color flow image of a transplant renal artery demonstrating disordered blood flow patterns resulting from vessel tortuosity.

with cyclosporine toxicity, even though vasculopathy may be present in severe cases.[6] Six cases of histologically confirmed nephrotoxicity to cyclosporine were evaluated and normal resistive indices were found in all. A unique spectral pattern, however, has been recorded in each examination. Flow disturbance, which has a "shaggy" quality, is evident in the outer envelope of the Doppler spectral waveform (Fig. 81-7). This feature is noted earliest in the cortical signals but may be propagated throughout the medulla in severe cases.

Pathologic studies have demonstrated dystrophic microcalcifications and vacuoles within the tubular cells of patients suffering from cyclosporine toxicity but fail to offer a satisfactory explanation for this waveform feature. Current investigations are directed toward determining if such Doppler signal characteristics can be used to detect cyclosporine nephrotoxicity.

TRANSPLANT RENAL ARTERY STENOSIS

Hypertension, often in association with allograft dysfunction, may indicate stenosis of the transplant renal artery. Such stenotic lesions are thought to occur in as many as 1% to 12% of transplanted organs.[4-8,33] Two types of luminal narrowing have been described. The first is a postoperative stenosis that is confined to the anastomotic site. This lesion may be associated with acute angulation of the transplant renal artery at the anastomosis. The other type is thought to be caused by compression or reduction of the arterial lumen produced by ischemic stricture or disease progression and will usually be along the proximal course of the transplant renal artery. Predisposing factors may include graft injury incurred during harvesting, atherosclerotic disease of the donor or recipient vessels, chronic rejection, and intimal hyperplasia.[33]

In 1982, Reinitz et al[25] evaluated 11 transplant recipients and identified 5 patients who were thought to have renal artery stenosis based on the findings of elevated peak systolic frequency shifts, spectral broadening, and disorganized flow patterns. Taylor et al[34] established a peak systolic frequency shift greater than 7.5 kHz and poststenotic turbulence as the criteria to identify flow-reducing transplant renal artery stenosis. Needleman and Kurtz[19] documented elevated frequency shifts at the stenotic site and turbulent but dampened distal peak frequencies. Furthermore, they believed a frequency shift of 4 to 5 kHz may indicate a stenotic lesion.

Such diagnostic guidelines may depend on the carrier frequency of the transducer and the angle of insonation with respect to the path of blood flow, which is rarely axial. If the flow information is obtained in the form of frequency-shifted data, the angle of insonation will not severely affect the peak frequency values, as long as the Doppler signals are collected at an angle less than 60°. However, with some instrumentation, the angle at which the transducer is held relative to the skin and the transplant renal artery may alter the recorded peak frequency shift. If peak velocity is being measured, knowledge of the angle of insonation with respect to the blood flow vector is crucial for making accurate velocity determinations. Because of the orientation of the transplant renal artery, inadequate visualization of the vessel may rule out accurate velocity determination. Doppler color flow imaging may facilitate definition of the renal artery and measurement of the Doppler angle (Fig. 81-8).

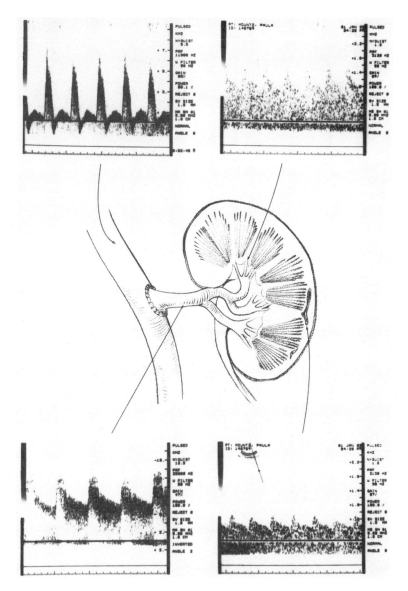

Fig. 81-9. Montage of spectral waveforms recorded from a renal allograft with transplant renal artery stenosis. Note the propagation of high-velocity disturbed flow into the vascular tree of the renal medulla and cortex.

Because ratios are independent of the insonation angle, a ratio of the peak systolic renal artery velocity or frequency shift to the peak systolic iliac artery velocity or frequency shift may be used. A ratio of greater than 3.0 indicates flow-reducing transplant renal artery stenosis. Although this method has not been successfully used to differentiate primary transplant renal artery stenosis from kinking of the transplant renal artery beyond the anastomosis, there is a 98% accuracy for identification of hemodynamically significant transplant renal artery stenosis, as confirmed by angiographic findings.

The entire course of the transplant renal artery must be interrogated with Doppler and color flow imaging to ensure accurate identification of stenotic areas. In the event of short-segment stenosis, the poststenotic frequencies may be quite

normal and disturbed flow may be propagated for only a short distance downstream. In the presence of severe stenosis, turbulent flow patterns may be recorded throughout the length of the transplant renal artery and are often propagated into the hilum of the allograft (Fig. 81-9). Doppler color flow imaging may be used to help establish the location, severity, and length of the stenotic segment. A perivascular color artifact may be noted if a bruit is associated with a stenotic lesion.

A total of 8 of 10 cases of angiographically confirmed stenosis of the transplant renal artery caused by kinking of the proximal segment of the vessel beyond the anastomosis have been sequentially monitored. In all cases, the medullary and cortical flow patterns have remained normal without evidence of increased renovascular resistance. In ad-

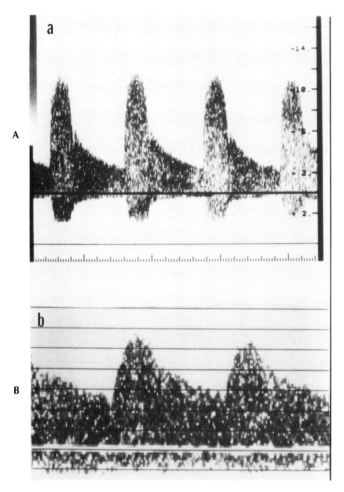

Fig. 81-10. *A,* Pulsed Doppler waveforms recorded distal to a transplant renal artery stenosis. Note the elevated peak systolic frequency shifts. *B,* Doppler spectral waveforms recorded from the transplant renal artery demonstrated in *(A)* postangioplasty. Note the decrease in peak systolic frequency shifts and normalization of the blood flow pattern.

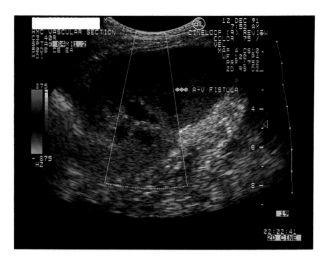

Fig. 81-11. Doppler color flow image of a renal transplant demonstrating an arteriovenous fistula within the medulla of the kidney. Note the disordered venous and arterial flow patterns.

dition, there has been no significant elevation in the serum creatinine levels in any of these patients during a mean follow-up of 32 months. One patient underwent percutaneous transluminal dilatation of an anastomotic stenosis. Postdilatation duplex evaluation demonstrated high-velocity Doppler signals consistent with recurrent transplant renal artery stenosis (Fig. 81-10). Vein patch angioplasty was performed and normalization of renal artery Doppler velocity signals was confirmed intraoperatively. During postoperative follow-up, a renal-to-iliac velocity ratio of 1.8 was demonstrated.

ARTERIOVENOUS FISTULAS

Acute renal transplant rejection is usually confirmed by the histologic examination of tissue obtained by percutaneous cortical needle biopsy. However, the development of arteriovenous fistulas after biopsy has been documented by several authors.[17,18,34] Doppler color flow imaging can facilitate localization of the arteriovenous communication and determination of the fistula's size[17,18] (Fig. 81-11). Doppler velocity waveform analysis can confirm the high-pressure gradients in the feeding vessels as well as the extent of the arteriovenous communication.

TRANSPLANT ARTERIAL OR VENOUS OCCLUSION

Thrombosis of the transplant renal artery or vein may result from surgical technical error or from the intravascular accumulation of platelet-fibrin aggregates stemming from severe vascular rejection of the allograft. Immediate surgical, or lytic, intervention is usually required to salvage the transplanted organ. The existence of transplant renal vein thrombosis is suggested by the absence of a Doppler signal in the visualized vessel. In addition, the Doppler velocity waveforms recorded from the medulla and cortex of the allograft may exhibit low systolic frequency shifts and reverse flow during diastole. These waveform characteristics reflect the increased vascular resistance, which permits only antegrade flow during systole.

The absence of Doppler signals within the renal parenchyma or the visualized transplant renal artery may indicate arterial occlusion. Because low-amplitude, low-velocity signals may be encountered, it is advisable to increase the axial length of the Doppler sample volume, lower the wall filter to at least 50 Hz, and increase the color sensitivity to low-velocity flow.

Occasionally segmental infarction of the transplanted organ is encountered. This entity may present as hyperechoic regions throughout the gray-scale image of the ischemic tissue. Doppler color-flow imaging may confirm perfusion defects within the corticomedullary regions of the allograft and the absence of Doppler signals in the thrombosed vessels.

Table 81-1. Comparison of the quantitative anaylsis of pulsed-Doppler spectral waveforms with the qualitative assessment of waveform pulsatility using subjective spectral pattern recognition

Method	Sensitivity	Specificity	Accuracy
DSR	38% (20/52)	63% (12/19)	45% (32/71)
PI	56% (29/52)	58% (11/19)	54% (38/71)
SPR	93% (42/45)	89% (17/19)	92% (59/64)*

DSR, Diastolic-to-systolic ratio; PI, pulsatility index; SPR, subjective spectral pattern recognition

*$p < 0.005$. By chi-square analysis, SPR was statistically better than either DSR or PI in determining the sensitivity, specificity, and accuracy of renal allograft rejection by duplex examination.

SIGNAL ANALYSIS

The Doppler velocity waveforms from 275 transplants were analyzed using the pulsatility index, diastolic-to-systolic ratio, and subjective spectral pattern recognition to determine the most sensitive method for differentiating acute renal transplant rejection from other complications that may jeopardize allograft survival (Table 81-1). The pulsatility index and diastolic-to-systolic ratio were calculated in all cases for the transplant renal artery, medulla, and cortex using the velocity signals with the highest frequencies. Acute rejection was diagnosed if the calculated values from two of the three locations within each transplant agreed. The relative pulsatility of the Doppler velocity waveforms recorded from the renal artery, medulla, and cortex was considered collectively for the purpose of spectral pattern recognition analysis. This subjective evaluation required review of the real-time image data and spectral information either from videotape copy or at the time of the examination. All patients underwent percutaneous renal transplant biopsy so that pathologic diagnosis could be established.

In many cases, the calculated pulsatility index or diastolic-to-systolic ratio from the transplant renal artery indicated increased vascular resistance and acute rejection even though normal values were obtained from the segmental, interlobar, and arcuate vessels of the kidney. Doppler color flow imaging ruled out tortuosity of the renal artery as a cause for this increased pulsatility of the waveform. In several cases, the calculated pulsatility index or diastolic-to-systolic ratio from the medulla and cortex of the same transplant yielded different results. Extraneous factors that may elevate the resistance indices have already been discussed.

The use of spectral pattern recognition can demonstrate the variation in pulsatility that occurs in Doppler waveforms recorded from the main transplant renal artery, medulla, and cortex of the allograft. In this method, the examiner obtains a global appreciation of the degree of vascular resistance reflected in the Doppler waveforms. This method requires extensive examiner experience and sequential monitoring of the allograft flow patterns. Although subjective, it has

shown excellent sensitivity and specificity for the identification of acute renal transplant rejection (Table 81-1).

CONCLUSION

The traditional methods used for the investigation of renal transplant dysfunction are not ideal because they lack sensitivity and specificity or because they carry a risk of morbidity. However, the different therapeutic approaches required to reverse failure necessitate a clear diagnosis of its cause.

Ultrasound evaluations of the transplanted kidney have focused on the acoustic properties of the parenchymal tissues, renal size, pyramidal prominence, and possible thickening of the pelvic-infundibular region.[14] Duplex ultrasonography complemented by Doppler color flow imaging of the vasculature of the allograft has proved valuable in the assessment of a transplanted organ. Sonographic imaging and the quantitation of Doppler velocity spectral waveforms have shown wide variations in accuracy for differentiating the causes of transplant dysfunction. Thus there is considerable controversy concerning the diagnostic value of these tests.

Diagnostic approaches using the calculation of resistive indices to quantify the degree of renovascular impedance have failed to accurately identify acute transplant rejection for a number of reasons. Extraneous factors can be responsible for elevating the resistive index by causing increased impedance to arterial inflow to the kidney. The most commonly implicated causes of increased renovascular resistance include renal vein thrombosis, severe ATN, extrinsic compression of the allograft, pyelonephritis, and hypotension.[6,24,36]

Using the subjective evaluation of Doppler velocity spectral waveforms obtained from the renal artery, medullary, and cortical vessels has been successful in identifying acute renal transplant rejection. Additionally, it is possible for an experienced examiner to recognize spectral patterns associated with ATN, transplant renal artery stenosis, arteriovenous fistulas, and vascular occlusion. Research continues on the use of spectral pattern recognition for the identification of cyclosporine toxicity.

Renal transplant duplex ultrasonography complemented by Doppler color flow imaging is evolving into an accurate diagnostic modality for the evaluation of allograft dysfunction. Although the quantitation of Doppler velocity waveforms for the identification of transplant rejection has been shown to be both insensitive and nonspecific, promising results have been documented for the use of subjective assessment of the velocity spectral patterns from the renal artery and parenchyma of the allograft. The accuracy of this technique depends on the sequential monitoring of transplant blood flow patterns and technical experience and is diminished by interobserver variability.

Duplex examination with spectral pattern recognition may assume an important role in the diagnostic algorithm for renal transplant dysfunction. It is currently used to guide clinical management, monitor the therapeutic response, and evaluate blood flow patterns after dilatation or revascularization of the transplant renal artery.

REFERENCES

1. Arima M et al: Analysis of the arterial blood flow patterns of normal and allografted kidneys by the directional ultrasonic Doppler technique, *J Urol* 122:587-591, 1979.
2. Arima M et al: Predictability of renal allograft prognosis during rejection crisis by ultrasonic Doppler technique, *Urology* 19:389-394, 1982.
3. Bergren CT et al: The role of ultrasound in the diagnosis of cyclosporine toxicity in renal transplantation, *Bol Assoc Med PR* 78:50-53, 1986.
4. Berland LN et al: Evaluation of renal transplants with pulsed Doppler duplex sonography, *J Ultrasound Med* 1:215-222, 1982.
5. Buckley AR et al: The distinction between acute renal transplant rejection and cyclosporine nephrotoxicity: value of duplex sonography, *AJR* 149:521-525, 1987.
6. Don S et al: Duplex Doppler US of renal allografts: causes of elevated resistive index, *Radiology* 171:709-712, 1989.
7. Fleisher AC et al: Duplex Doppler sonography of renal transplants: correlation with histopathology, *J Ultrasound Med* 8:89-94, 1989.
8. Genkins SM, Sanfilippo FP, Carroll BA: Duplex Doppler sonography of renal transplants: lack of sensitivity and specificity in establishing pathologic diagnosis, *AJR* 152:535-540, 1989.
9. Grenier N et al: Detection of vascular complications in renal allografts with color Doppler flow imaging, *Radiology* 178:217-223, 1991.
10. Griffin JF et al: Diagnosis of disease in renal allografts: correlation between ultrasound and histology, *Clin Radiol* 37:59-62, 1986.
11. Grigat KP et al: Monitoring of renal allografts by duplex ultrasound, *Transplant Int* 2:102-107, 1989.
12. Hricak H et al: Acute post-transplantation renal failure: differential diagnosis by ultrasound, *Radiology* 139:441-449, 1981.
13. Kaude JV, Hawkins IF: Angiography of the renal transplant, *Radiol Clin North Am* 14:295-308, 1976.
14. Kelcz F et al: Pyramidal appearance and resistive index: insensitive and nonspecific indicators of renal transplant rejection, *AJR* 155:531-535, 1990.
15. Marchioro TL, Strandness DE Jr, Krugmire RB Jr: The ultrasonic velocity detector for determining vascular patency in renal homografts, *Transplantation* 8:296-298, 1969.
16. Matas A et al: Value of needle renal allograft biopsy. I. A retrospective study of biopsies performed during putative rejection episodes, *Ann Surg* 197:226-237, 1983.
17. Middleton WD et al: Postbiopsy renal transplant arteriovenous fistulas: color Doppler US characteristics, *Radiology* 171:253-257, 1989.
18. Mostbeck G et al: Comparison of duplex sonography and color Doppler imaging in renal allograft evaluation: prospective study, *Radiology* 169:355, 1988 (abstract).
19. Needleman L, Kurtz AB: Doppler evaluation of the renal transplant, *J Clin Ultrasound* 15:661-673, 1987.
20. Neumyer MM, Thiele BL, Gifford RRM: Duplex ultrasound evaluation of renal transplant dysfunction, *Dynamic Cardiovasc Imaging* 2(1):39-42, 1989.
21. Neumyer MM et al: Identification of early rejection in renal allografts with duplex ultrasonography, *J Vasc Tech* 12:19-25, 1988.
22. Norris CS et al: Noninvasive evaluation of renal artery stenosis and renovascular resistance, *J Vasc Surg* 1:192-201, 1984.
23. Perella RR et al: Evaluation of renal transplant dysfunction by duplex Doppler sonography: a prospective study and review of the literature, *Am J Kid Dis* 15:544-550, 1990.
24. Pozniak MA et al: Extraneous factors affecting resistive index, *Invest Radiol* 23:899-904, 1988.
25. Reinitz ER et al: Evaluation of transplant renal artery blood flow by Doppler sound-spectrum analysis, *Arch Surg* 118:415-419, 1983.
26. Rifkin MD et al: Evaluation of renal transplant rejection by duplex Doppler examination: value of the resistive index, *AJR* 148:759-762, 1987.
27. Rigsby CM et al: Renal allografts in acute rejection: evaluation using duplex ultrasonography, *Radiology* 158:375-378, 1986.
28. Rigsby CM et al: Doppler signal quantitation in renal allografts: comparison in normal and rejecting transplants with pathologic correlation, *Radiology* 162:39-42, 1987.
29. Rosenfield AT et al: Experimental acute tubular necrosis: US appearance, *Radiology* 157:771-774, 1985.
30. Sampson D: Ultrasonic method for detecting rejection of human renal allotransplants, *Lancet* 2:976-978, 1969.
31. Shanahan WS, Klingensmith WC III, Weil R: Technetium-99m DTPA renal studies for acute tubular necrosis: specificity of dissociation between perfusion and clearance, *AJR* 1346:249-253, 1981.
32. Skotnicki SH et al: Evaluation of renal allograft function by Doppler spectrum analysis, *Transplant Int* 2:167-172, 1989.
33. Snider JF et al: Transplant renal artery stenosis: evaluation with duplex sonography, *Radiology* 172:1027-1030, 1989.
34. Taylor KJW et al: Vascular complications in renal allografts: detection with duplex Doppler US, *Radiology* 162:31-38, 1987.
35. Townsend RR et al: Combined Doppler and morphologic sonographic evaluation of renal transplant rejection, *J Ultrasound Med* 9:199-206, 1990.
36. Warshauer DM et al: Unusual causes of increased vascular impedance in renal transplants: duplex Doppler evaluation, *Radiology* 169:367-370, 1988.

CHAPTER 82

Noninvasive assessment of mesenteric and celiac artery blood flow

WILLIAM R. FLINN, MICHAEL P. LILLY, ROBERT J. RIZZO, and GAIL P. SANDAGER

MESENTERIC ARTERY DISEASE

Arterial occlusive disease of the major mesenteric vessels, the celiac artery (CA) and the superior mesenteric artery (SMA), is rare and has been a challenge to diagnose accurately. Acute thrombosis or mesenteric embolization may produce intraabdominal catastrophes that require emergency surgical treatment and allow little time for elective diagnostic maneuvers. However, chronic atherosclerotic mesenteric arterial occlusions can develop insidiously. These lesions may initially be asymptomatic, but when they become clinically significant, patients most frequently manifest symptoms of chronic epigastric pain ("abdominal angina") and marked weight loss. When pain and weight loss occur in patients in their fifties or sixties, who are considered prime atherosclerotic patients, an undiagnosed malignancy is frequently presumed to be the cause. Typical symptoms of postprandial pain and disorders of gastrointestinal motility in patients with chronic mesenteric ischemia often lead to the performance of repeated gastrointestinal radiographic and endoscopic examinations. Far too often, severe mesenteric occlusive lesions progress to thrombosis with bowel infarction, and the diagnosis of mesenteric ischemia is then confirmed only at laparotomy, when successful treatment is rarely possible and attendant mortality may exceed 50% to 75%. To avoid this catastrophic complication, there is a clear need for an effective diagnostic strategy for the evaluation of patients with suspected visceral ischemic syndromes.

Until recently, the accurate diagnosis of mesenteric arterial occlusive lesions required arteriography, which was often not considered or was deferred until all other diagnostic maneuvers had been done. Concerns about patient risk and the discomfort of arteriography, coupled with the low prevalence of the disease, were responsible for a reported delay in the diagnosis of chronic mesenteric ischemia that averaged 18 months in one report.[7] Difficulty with the clinical diagnosis of chronic mesenteric ischemia together with the unacceptable morbidity of gastrointestinal infarc-

tion have long indicated the need for a less invasive method for identifying patients with mesenteric arterial lesions.

Duplex ultrasound scanning has been perfected for the evaluation of carotid artery disease, a method confirmed by innumerable arteriograms. The combination of real-time B-mode arterial imaging and image-directed pulsed Doppler physiologic flow measurements has since been applied to almost every area of noninvasive vascular diagnosis. The application of duplex scanning to visceral (renal and mesenteric) arterial disease is more recent because significant technologic modifications in the ultrasound scan heads were necessary so that routine deep abdominal scanning could be achieved. Nevertheless, the most dramatic impact of duplex scanning may ultimately lie in its ability to evaluate visceral vessels, which has not been possible with any other noninvasive technique. Clearly this is an exciting area of evolving research.

MESENTERIC DUPLEX SCANNING
Technique

All patients undergoing mesenteric duplex scans are requested to fast overnight, which is usually adequate preparation. Intestinal gas reduces the likelihood of technical success, but simethicone-containing compounds may be helpful in alleviating this problem in mild cases. Hospitalized patients may receive mild cathartics or enemas to facilitate difficult examinations if such measures do not compromise their general medical condition. The ileus associated with *acute* mesenteric ischemia or other intraabdominal inflammatory processes unfortunately limits the application of ultrasonic testing in cases of abdominal apoplexy. When mesenteric ischemia is suspected in emergency surgical conditions, arteriography clearly remains the examination of choice.

Mesenteric duplex scanning is performed with the patient supine and the head slightly elevated. A midline sagittal scan of the aorta (Fig. 82-1) can usually identify the origins of the CA and SMA as they course ventrally (Fig. 82-2).

695

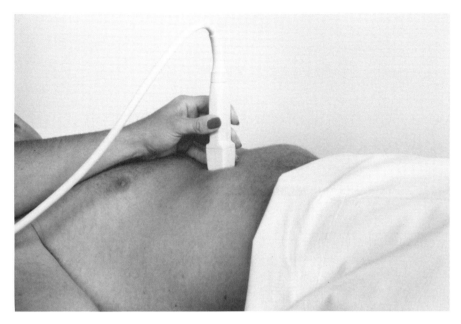

Fig. 82-1. A standard subxiphoid midline approach is used initially for imaging the origins of the celiac and superior mesenteric arteries as they course ventrally from the suprarenal aorta. In most patients, with satisfactory preparation, a sagittal scan of the aorta will allow identification of these vessels.

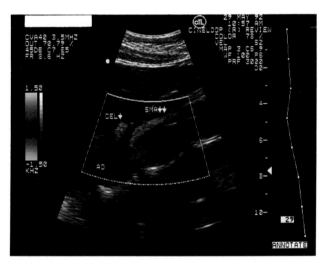

Fig. 82-2. Sagittal B-mode scan of the suprarenal aorta demonstrates the origins of the CA and SMA. Most occlusive lesions of these vessels occur at or near their origin, and flow disturbances are most often identified in those regions. The use of color flow duplex may aid initial visual identification of color "mosaics" in the area of significant stenosis.

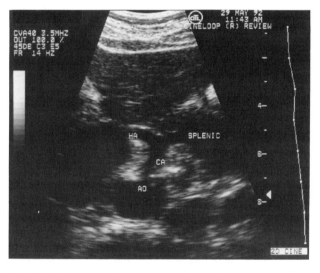

Fig. 82-3. A transverse B-mode image of the celiac axis demonstrates the origins of the common hepatic and splenic arteries that branch from the relatively short celiac trunk. This "rabbit ears" appearance is quite characteristic and explains why rapid changes in arterial flow direction make pulsed Doppler sampling in these vessels challenging in many cases.

The main trunk of the SMA continues caudad and roughly parallels the abdominal aorta, so identification and pulsed Doppler sampling is somewhat easier than that in the CA. Most atherosclerotic occlusive lesions in the CA and SMA are at or near the origins of the vessels; therefore insonation of the first few centimeters usually suffices for diagnosis.

A lower-frequency imaging scan head (usually 2.25 MHz for color imaging and 3 MHz for gray-scale analysis) with a 3-MHz pulsed Doppler frequency is used. Peak systolic and end-diastolic arterial flow velocities are recorded using a 1.5-mm sample volume.

Accurate interrogation of the celiac trunk remains a challenge. The celiac trunk itself is rarely longer than 1 to 2 cm, and the anatomy of its branches (common hepatic, splenic, and left gastric arteries) may be extremely variable. Although flow in the origin of the CA roughly parallels that in the SMA, ventral from the aorta, early branching of the CA results in rapid changes in the direction of arterial flow at almost 90° angles to both the right (hepatic) and left (splenic) of the main trunk. These anatomic relationships can often be appreciated with a transverse B-mode scan of the CA and have been termed the *rabbit-ear* appearance (Fig. 82-3).

This description helps clarify some of the remaining technologic difficulties that can be encountered in the field of mesenteric scanning. Rizzo et al[6] observed that reliable pulsed Doppler arterial flow velocities from the mesenteric vessels *must be measured at angles of insonation less than 60°*. Because the anatomy of the vessels themselves may be responsible for producing sudden changes in vessel direction, it is incumbent on the technologist to be as certain as possible about the location and angle of the sample.

The evolution of color flow duplex scanning has had an impact on mesenteric scanning, as it has on all duplex applications. Color flow scanning often allows more rapid identification of the origins of the CA and SMA and detection of focal areas of flow disturbance that require further interrogation. This will often reduce the time required for an examination. However, because color assignment is based solely on the direction of flow, the anatomic variations discussed can produce confusing color flow patterns beyond the origins of these vessels because of the sudden changes in flow direction.

Feasibility

Mesenteric duplex scanning was initially investigated in healthy young normal volunteers to assess the feasibility and reproducibility of the examination technique. With minimal preparation, the origins of the CA and SMA could be visualized on standard sagittal B-mode scans of the abdominal aorta (Fig. 82-2). In addition, the fasting Doppler flow-velocity waveforms from the CA and SMA were discovered to be recognizably different in normal subjects. Normal fasting celiac waveforms are characteristic of vascular beds with low-outflow resistance, with continuous forward flow throughout systole and diastole, similar to the waveforms from the internal carotid artery. The normal SMA waveform exhibits a triphasic pattern typical of higher-outflow resistance and more elastic arteries: flow reversal is seen in early diastole with return of forward flow in later diastole.

Because the symptoms of chronic mesenteric ischemia are induced by the ingestion of food, it seemed logical to determine the normal response of the major mesenteric vessels to feeding. Normal subjects have characteristic changes in mesenteric arterial blood flow after eating standardized balanced caloric supplements.[2,3] These changes include predictable alterations in the flow velocity waveforms in the SMA, with a loss of the reversed flow component in early

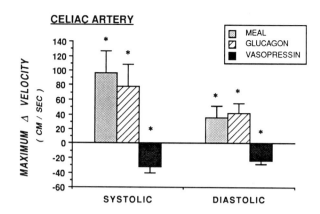

CELIAC ARTERY

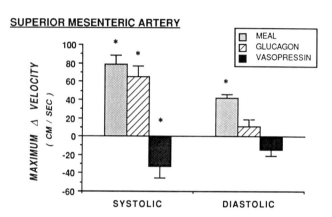

SUPERIOR MESENTERIC ARTERY

Fig. 82-4. Reproducible, characteristic changes in systolic and diastolic flow velocities in the CA and SMA of normal subjects can be induced by physiologic (meal) or pharmacologic (glucagon, pitressin) stimuli. (From Lilly et al: *J Vasc Surg* 9:18-25, 1989.)

diastole, suggesting splanchnic vasodilatation in response to eating. Additionally, there are increased flow velocities in the CA and SMA during systole and diastole. Lilly et al[4] demonstrated that these postprandial changes in peak systolic and end-diastolic flow velocities in the CA and SMA could be exaggerated by increasing the volume and caloric content of the test meal. Others have noted that the postprandial changes in mesenteric flow velocities may be altered by the composition of the test meal—fat, protein, or carbohydrate. Lilly et al[4] also demonstrated that velocity changes similar to those observed postprandially in normal volunteers could be induced in these same subjects by the intravenous infusion of glucagon, a potent splanchnic vasodilator. They further demonstrated that a significant reduction in CA and SMA flow velocities could be induced by the infusion of the splanchnic vasoconstrictor, vasopressin (Fig. 82-4).

Diagnostic applications

The findings yielded by these initial investigations in normal subjects suggested that mesenteric duplex scanning could become useful for the evaluation of patients with suspected mesenteric ischemia, allowing rational selection of those patients who might benefit from more invasive evaluation with arteriography. Its usefulness also remained to be demonstrated in patients with atherosclerotic disease. Because atherosclerotic occlusions of the visceral vessels most frequently occur at the ostia, this is the site that needed to be most accessible to duplex examination. In addition because the clinical symptoms of chronic mesenteric ischemia usually only appear in the presence of severe disease (high-grade stenosis or occlusion) of both the CA and SMA, the demands on this testing modality to detect and clarify lesser degrees of disease are reduced. However, the relative rarity of this condition has slowed the formulation of strict diagnostic criteria, such as those that have evolved in carotid disease for which extensive arteriographic correlation has been available.

Moneta et al[5] retrospectively compared the results of mesenteric duplex scanning to arteriographic findings in 34 patients with known advanced atherosclerosis. Some patients were suspected of having visceral ischemia and others required arteriography to assess lower extremity ischemic symptoms. An elevated peak systolic flow velocity above 275 cm/sec in the SMA (normal, 125 to 163 cm/sec) predicted a severe SMA stenosis (greater than 70%), and this criterion showed a sensitivity and specificity of 92%. A similar diagnostic accuracy was observed when peak systolic flow velocities exceeded 200 cm/sec in the CA. Total occlusions of the CA and SMA were also accurately diagnosed by duplex scanning. This retrospective study failed to confirm the usefulness of a mesenteric-aortic systolic velocity ratio to predict the presence of severe stenosis in the CA or SMA, as has been reported for duplex scanning of the renal arteries. Moneta's group is currently involved in a prospective evaluation of these diagnostic criteria.

The usefulness and accuracy of mesenteric duplex scanning for the diagnosis of significant CA and SMA lesions was further confirmed by Bowersox et al,[1] who compared mesenteric duplex scanning and arteriographic findings in 25 patients, most of whom were suspected of having visceral ischemia. They found that a stenosis of the SMA that exceeded a 50% diameter reduction was best predicted by an end-diastolic velocity of greater than 45 cm/sec or a fasting

peak systolic velocity of more than 300 cm/sec. This latter figure is nearly identical to that observed independently by Moneta's group. Bowersox's team of investigators had difficulty establishing reliable duplex scan velocity criteria for identifying CA stenosis; however, they noted that the anatomy of the CA and its branches may compromise precise insonation, as described previously in this chapter. In a study of only 25 patients, therefore, it is possible that anatomic and collateral variants account for these observed differences. Thus there is a continued need for prospective studies that include arteriographic comparison.

CONCLUSION

Deep abdominal duplex scanning, including mesenteric scanning and renal, portal vein, and vena caval duplex scanning, is more technologically demanding than studies conducted on more superficial vessels and extremity grafts. In the past, virtually no other noninvasive techniques have existed for assessment of these intraabdominal vessels in humans. Ultrasound permits the study of both normal physiologic responses and the diagnosis of specific pathologic states. Solid investigative groundwork has already been laid in this area, and precise diagnostic guidelines are being rigorously developed. On the basis of this evolving experience, mesenteric duplex scanning will likely become a routine noninvasive diagnostic modality for the evaluation of patients with suspected visceral ischemia and perhaps other functional visceral disorders.

REFERENCES

1. Bowersox JC et al: Duplex ultrasonography in the diagnosis of celiac and mesenteric artery occlusive disease, *J Vasc Surg* 14:780-788, 1991.
2. Flinn WR et al: *Duplex scan of celiac and mesenteric arteries*. In Bergan JJ, Yao JST, eds: *Arterial surgery: new diagnosis and operative techniques*, Orlando, Fla, 1988, Grune & Stratton.
3. Flinn WR et al: *Measurement of mesenteric blood flow*. In Bernstein EF, ed: *Recent advances in noninvasive diagnostic techniques in vascular disease*, St Louis, 1990, Mosby.
4. Lilly MP et al: Duplex ultrasound measurement of changes in mesenteric flow velocities with pharmacologic and physiologic alteration of intestinal blood flow in man, *J Vasc Surg* 9:18-25, 1989.
5. Moneta GL et al: Duplex ultrasound criteria for the diagnosis of splanchnic artery stenosis or occlusion, *J Vasc Surg* 14:519, 1991.
6. Rizzo RJ et al: Mesenteric flow velocity variations as a function of angle of insonation, *J Vasc Surg* 11:688-694, 1990.
7. Stony RJ: Duplex ultrasound criteria for the diagnosis of splanchnic artery stenosis or occlusion, *J Vasc Surg* 14:519, 1991.

CHAPTER 83

Pitfalls in mesenteric and celiac sonography

DEAN A. HEALY, MARSHA M. NEUMYER, and BRIAN L. THIELE

Duplex ultrasonography has been used successfully to diagnose disease in the carotid arteries,[8] renal arteries,[14] and lower extremity veins.[2] The use of duplex scanning for the assessment of visceral artery occlusive disease was first suggested by Jager et al[5] in 1984, but its clinical role in the diagnosis of intestinal angina is still being defined. Despite the accuracy of duplex ultrasonography in visualizing other vascular beds, some of its pitfalls in the mesenteric circulation may limit its clinical utility.

An appreciation of some of the difficulties likely to be encountered during mesenteric duplex studies is enhanced by a thorough understanding of the procedures followed in a normal study. Proper technique cannot be overemphasized. Patients should be studied early in the morning after a strict overnight fast, and beverage consumption and cigarette smoking must be avoided before examinations. Cathartics are not routinely administered but may be helpful in selected cases.

The patient is placed supine with the head slightly elevated so that gravity pulls the viscera to an inferior position within the abdomen. The abdominal aorta is located in a longitudinal scan plane with the celiac and superior mesenteric arteries on its anterior surface. The origins of the two vessels may be quite close or they may have a common origin. It is usually possible to visualize the superior mesenteric artery in the long axis over the course of several centimeters. Although it is sometimes difficult to insonate the origin of the superior mesenteric artery, an angle of 60° or less is usually attainable beyond the first 1 to 2 cm. A good technique is to try to "sweep through" the artery while maintaining an acceptable Doppler angle.

The evaluation of the celiac trunk is usually more difficult. The early branching pattern of this artery makes it possible for only a relatively short segment to be insonated, and because the vessel is short, flow disturbance originating from the aortic ostium may frequently be present despite the absence of stenotic lesions.

Usually a 2.5- to 3.5-MHz mechanical sector, curved array, or phased array scan head with a range-gated pulsed Doppler is used. Color Doppler assists in vessel location and may image areas of disturbed flow associated with stenosis, but the examiner should rely on Doppler spectral changes when interpreting a study.

PITFALLS INHERENT IN ALL DUPLEX APPLICATIONS

Duplex scanning has revolutionized the noninvasive approach to vascular diagnosis and has proved to be a valuable clinical tool. Nevertheless, it is not an infallible technology, and it is important to understand the limitations and pitfalls involved in duplex scanning, particularly those that can be controlled by the sonographer.

Doppler angle

Accurate knowledge of the Doppler angle used is mandatory with any duplex application. Although visceral arteries are usually readily identified, imaging the vessel in a long axis view can sometimes be difficult. This is particularly true for the celiac artery because early branching and tortuosity can lead to error in estimating the Doppler angle.

Use of a Doppler angle greater than 60° increases the risk of error in determining the velocity (Table 83-1). For example, although a 5° error in estimating the Doppler angle at 30° will cause only a 5.4% error in velocity determination, at 60° this error becomes 12%, and at 70° 19%.[6] Therefore an angle of insonation of 60° or less should always be used.

Whether to report duplex results in terms of frequency rather than velocity continues to be a matter of controversy. If the arterial flow velocity vector was always parallel to the long axis of the vessel, results could be reported in either frequency or velocity because they are proportionally related by the Doppler equation. In fact, if this were true, there

Table 83-1. Percent velocity error for 2° and 5° angle errors

True angle (degrees)	Percent velocity error for 2° angle error	Percent velocity error for 5° angle error
0	0.06	0.38
10	0.68	1.9
20	1.3	3.6
30	2.0	5.4
40	3.0	7.7
50	3.9	9.1
60	5.6	12
70	8.7	19
80	16	33

From Kremkau FW: *Doppler ultrasound: principles and instruments*, Philadelphia, 1990, Saunders.

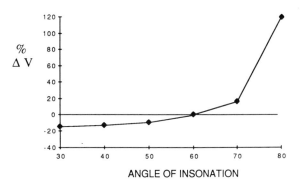

Fig. 83-1. The effect of the angle of insonation on the percentage change in peak systolic velocity measured at 60°. (From Rizzo RJ et al: *J Vasc Surg* 11:688, 1990.)

would be an advantage to reporting in units of velocity because data collected at different Doppler angles could then be normalized. The calculated velocity would be the true blood velocity and thus blood flow could also be determined.

However, arterial flow is not always parallel to the long axis of a vessel, and for this reason, there has been a plea to report Doppler results in terms of frequency.[11] It is well known that nonaxial flow exists in several vascular beds, including the extracranial carotid circulation.[7] In such vessels, there are helical flow patterns in which the angle between the axis of flowing blood and the ultrasound beam cannot be known. Because of this, the true blood velocity cannot be calculated. Therefore it can be argued that with current Doppler technology, (1) blood velocity cannot be accurately determined, (2) volume flow cannot be accurately calculated, and (3) angle correction cannot be used to "normalize" data collected at different Doppler angles. Furthermore, if standard published criteria are used to report degrees of stenosis, Doppler data should be obtained using the same incident frequency and Doppler angle as those used in the laboratories where the criteria were developed. If this rule is adhered to, it does not matter whether the data are reported in terms of frequency or velocity as long as the examiner realizes that the reported velocity does not necessarily reflect the true velocity. When angle correction is used over a range of Doppler angles, the calculated velocities have shown wide variations in both the carotid and mesenteric circulations (Fig. 83-1).[12]

Calcification

Extensive calcification caused by atherosclerosis may limit duplex scanning because ultrasound cannot penetrate calcific vascular walls. Theoretically, such vessels are identifiable, but no Doppler signal can be obtained, leading to the false assumption that the vessel is occluded. Whether this is of frequent clinical relevance in the mesenteric circulation is unknown.

Sample volume placement

Accurate sample volume placement is crucial to accurate duplex testing. Ideally the Doppler sample volume should be placed at the origin of a given artery and then swept through the entire vessel. This will permit focal increases in frequency shift or systolic velocity to be identified, findings that suggest arterial stenosis. Failure to investigate a vessel in this manner may lead to false-negative results because stenotic lesions can be missed.

PARTICULAR FEATURES OF THE MESENTERIC CIRCULATION
Vessel identification and anomalies

Proper vessel identification is of obvious importance to any duplex application. Although a patent superior mesenteric artery is usually easily identified, the celiac trunk can pose problems because of anatomic variations. The celiac trunk contains all three branches (left gastric, splenic, and hepatic arteries) in 85% of people, with the most frequent anomaly a separate origin of one of these vessels.[4] Because the celiac trunk may be as short as 1 cm, insonation at an appropriate angle can be difficult. Tortuosity and acute angulation of the vessel can also impede examination and lead to errors in estimating the Doppler angle (Fig. 83-2).

Although considered a significant contributor to the visceral circulation, the inferior mesenteric artery is infrequently identified during duplex scanning. Some surgeons believe that knowledge of the hemodynamic and anatomic status of this vessel is critical in clinical decision making, information not always yielded by duplex scanning.

One common anomaly of the mesenteric circulation is the replaced right hepatic artery. In this variant, which may occur as often as 20% of the time, the right hepatic artery originates from the superior mesenteric artery. Normally a high-resistance vessel in the fasting state, the superior mesenteric artery may assume some of the characteristics of the celiac trunk when it supplies the right hepatic artery. Forward diastolic flow is usually minimal in the superior mesenteric artery but is occasionally increased in patients with a replaced right hepatic artery. It appears that the continuous flow demands of the liver provide a low-resistance pathway for its feeding arteries.

Celiac compression syndrome

Extrinsic compression of the celiac trunk by the median arcuate ligament can significantly impinge on the arterial lumen, thus increasing focal velocity. Although such compression can cause a true stenosis, the obstruction may be intermittent. In the event of celiac compression, high-velocity signals are obtained during normal respiration (Fig. 83-3, *A*), with deep inspiration leading to normalization (Fig. 83-3, *B*).[13] The functional significance of the celiac compression syndrome is controversial but the sonographer must be able to differentiate such extrinsic compression from atherosclerotic stenosis. The celiac trunk should always be

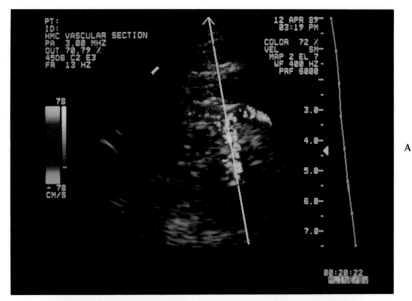

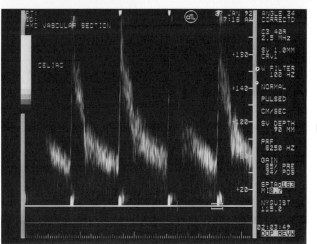

Fig. 83-2. **A,** Color Doppler image of the celiac artery with the aorta in transverse section. There appears to be a stenosis in the midportion of the celiac artery. This vessel was found to be tortuous, and the velocity increase represented acute angulation rather than stenosis. **B,** Spectral waveform from the area of the velocity increase shown in **A.** Although peak systolic velocity is increased, the spectal window remains clear. This finding supports a velocity increase that is caused by tortuosity rather than stenosis.

interrogated during both inspiration and expiration to distinguish extrinsic compression from intrinsic vascular disease.

Ostial stenosis

Because duplex ultrasonography depends on placement of the Doppler sample volume within a stenosis, narrowings at the ostium of a branch of the aorta can be difficult to investigate. Often such stenoses constitute extensive aortic atherosclerosis rather than primary disease in a visceral or renal artery. Unless the sonographer is able to identify a jet beyond the stenosis, a significant narrowing in this location can be missed.

Occlusions and collateral vessels

Proximal occlusions of visceral arteries may go undetected when the collateral blood supply is abundant. The examiner might expect there to be no Doppler signal beyond such an occlusion, but in fact the collateral circulation between the superior mesenteric artery and celiac artery usually reconstitutes the obstructed vessel. This phenomenon may also apply to high-grade stenoses in that such lesions may go undetected if the distal vessel is well collateralized.

Collateral flow can also be the source of error when a vessel that provides flow to an occluded artery is insonated (Fig. 83-4). Flow in the superior mesenteric artery may be increased to compensate for a critical stenosis or occlusion

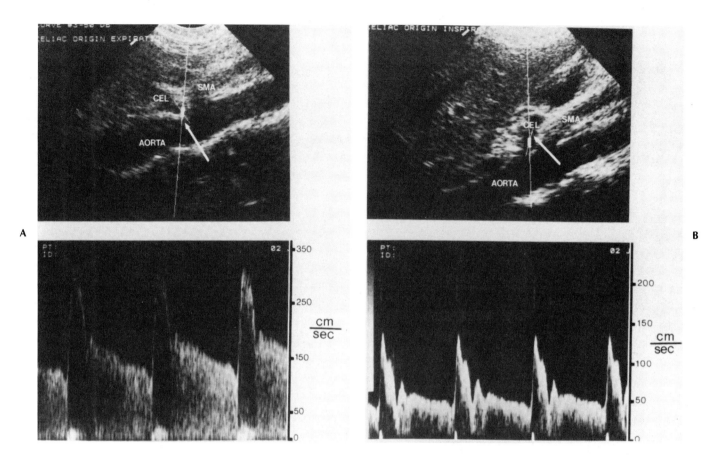

Fig. 83-3. *A,* Duplex examination of the celiac artery during normal respiration. The high peak systolic velocity (290 cm/sec) at the origin of the celiac axis was also associated with poststenotic turbulence. There also appears to be extrinsic compression *(arrow)* at the origin of the vessel causing it to be directed cephalad. *B,* Repeat duplex examination of the same patient's celiac artery during deep inspiration. Note the normalization of the spectral waveform with decreased peak systolic velocity (100 cm/sec) and the downward displacement of the vessel away from the median arcuate ligament of the diaphragm *(arrow).* (From Taylor DC et al: *J Vasc Tech* XI:236, 1987.)

in the celiac trunk. Doppler-determined velocity will therefore be increased in the superior mesenteric artery, suggesting an occlusive lesion in this normal artery. This concept is supported by the finding that celiac and superior mesenteric artery velocities are both increased in patients with visceral atherosclerosis, indicating that flow increases in one vessel to compensate for a stenosis in the companion artery.[3]

Diagnostic accuracy

Diagnostic criteria have been developed for the interpretation of duplex findings in the superior mesenteric artery and celiac trunk. Moneta et al[10] have prospectively evaluated mesenteric duplex scanning results in patients who have undergone lateral aortography and found that a peak systolic velocity in excess of 275 cm/sec in the superior mesenteric artery is associated with stenosis exceeding a 70% diameter reduction (Fig. 83-5, *A*). In the celiac trunk, a peak systolic velocity greater than 200 cm/sec correlated with a similar degree of stenosis (Fig. 83-5, *B*). These criteria proved to be both sensitive and specific. Others have confirmed the accuracy of the systolic velocity criteria used for identifying stenosis of the superior mesenteric artery but had highly variable results for celiac artery stenosis.[1] Duplex criteria for diagnosing occlusion or stenosis of the mesenteric vessels will have to be verified prospectively, since other groups have found a poor correlation between duplex-derived peak systolic velocities and angiographic results.[3]

Focal increases in peak systolic velocity associated with disturbed flow are the general criteria used for the detection of arterial stenosis, and at present, it seems prudent to apply such criteria to visceral artery duplex evaluations as well. The normal duplex-derived velocities at a 60° Doppler angle are approximately 125 ± 20 cm/sec in both the superior mesenteric artery and the celiac trunk. Color scanners may display a variegated pattern in a region of disturbed flow (Fig. 83-6, *A*). Disturbed flow can be detected on spectral displays by the presence of spectral broadening and, when

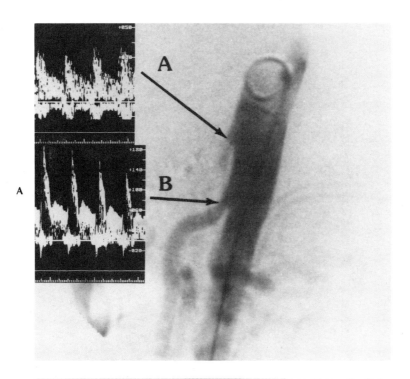

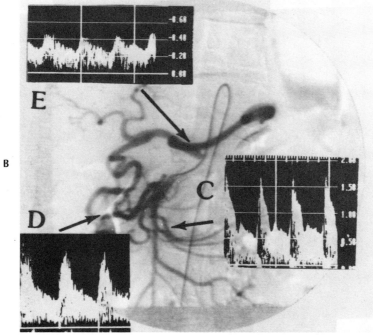

Fig. 83-4. A, Lateral aortogram from a patient with mesenteric vascular disease. *A* identifies a preocclusive stenosis in the celiac artery. The accompanying Doppler spectral waveform shows marked attenuation of peak systolic velocity (35 cm/sec, normal is 125 ± 20 cm/sec). *B* identifies the normal superior mesenteric artery. Despite the normal angiographic appearance, the spectral waveform exhibits an increase in peak systolic velocity (180 cm/sec, normal is 125 ± 20 cm/sec). This is probably related to increased flow in the superior mesenteric artery and not to stenosis. ***B,*** Anteroposterior aortogram from the same patient. *C* demonstrates the superior mesenteric artery, and *D* is a collateral between the superior mesenteric artery and celiac artery. *E* shows the celiac artery filling from the collateral. This supports the notion that the superior mesenteric artery can have increased flow velocity in the absence of hemodynamically significant stenosis. (From Healy DA et al: *J Ultrasound Med* 11:481-485, 1992.)

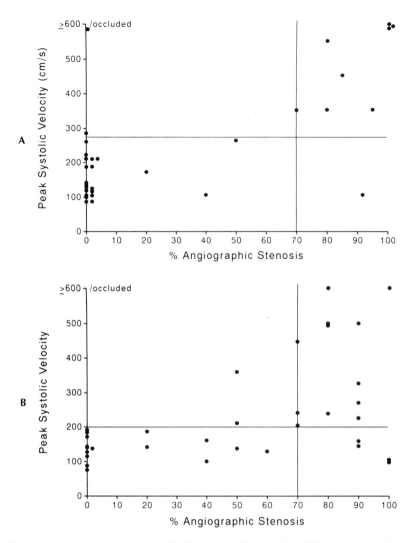

Fig. 83-5. A, Superior mesenteric artery *(SMA)* peak systolic velocities *(PSV)* as a function of angiographic stenosis in patients with visualization of their superior mesenteric artery by both angiography and duplex scanning (r = 0.68, *p* = 0.0001 for angiographically patent superior mesenteric arteries). Note that the angiographic occlusions successfully identified by duplex scanning are positioned at the extreme upper right. The horizontal line indicates the proposed PSV (275 cm/sec) for detecting an angiographic stenosis of at least 70% (vertical line). **B,** Celiac artery *(CA)* peak systolic velocities *(PSV)* as a function of angiographic stenosis (r = 0.59, *p* = 0.006 for angiographically patent celiac arteries). Note that the angiographic occlusion successfully identified by duplex scanning is positioned in the extreme upper right. The horizontal line indicates the proposed PSV (200 cm/sec) for detecting an angiographic stenosis of at least 70%. (vertical line). (From Moneta GL et al: *J Vasc Surg* 14:511, 1991.)

more severe, by high-velocity forward- and reverse-flow patterns (Fig. 83-6, *B*) that are propagated several centimeters from the lesion (Fig. 83-6, *C*). Such findings suggest disordered flow and the presence of multiple velocity vectors typically seen with arterial stenoses.

After a meal, blood flow in the splanchnic circulation increases and such changes can be detected by duplex ultrasound.[9] Performing both fasting and postprandial examinations might therefore enhance the reliability of duplex ultrasound in detecting mesenteric arterial stenosis and may provide insight into the functional significance of such le-

sions. Such postprandial studies can be likened to the exercise treadmill testing done to evaluate the lower extremities for claudication. However, none of these hypotheses has been validated yet.

CONCLUSION

Duplex ultrasonography has proved to be of great value in the noninvasive diagnosis of arterial and venous disease. Recently this technology has been applied to the mesenteric circulation, and specific criteria for diagnosing mesenteric arterial stenosis may be forthcoming. However, there are

A

B

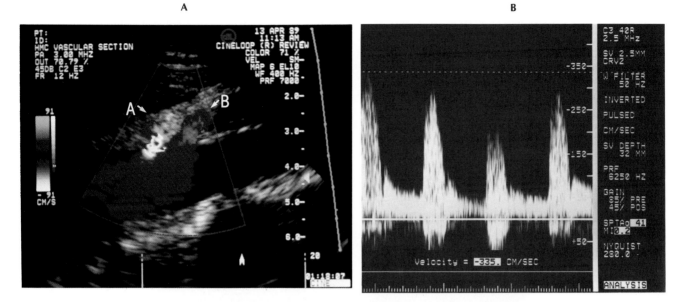

C

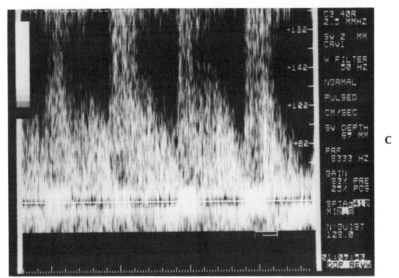

Fig. 83-6. A, Longitudinal color Doppler image of the suprarenal abdominal aorta from a patient with celiac artery stenosis. A velocity increase is suggested in the celiac artery (arrow *A*), whereas the superior mesenteric artery (arrow *B*) is normal. ***B,*** Spectral waveform obtained from the proximal celiac artery shown in Fig. 83-5, *A.* The high peak systolic velocity (250 cm/sec) and associated spectral broadening confirm the suspicion of stenosis from the color Doppler image. ***C,*** Spectral waveform obtained from the distal celiac artery shown in Fig. 83-5, *A.* Peak systolic velocity has fallen (160 cm/sec) but is still abnormal, and spectral broadening persists. The poststenotic pattern helps confirm the presence of an upstream lesion. If the spectral pattern from the proximal artery were due to an angle problem alone, the examiner would not expect to see a poststenotic signal in the distal artery.

several general limitations to duplex scanning, including problems with vessel identification, tortuosity, anatomic variations, and vessel calcification. The sonographer should strive to perform examinations at a consistent angle relative to the long axis of the vessel and maintain this angle at less than or equal to 60°.

The celiac trunk should be insonated during both inspiration and expiration to detect extrinsic compression exerted by the median arcuate ligament. In the mesenteric circulation, the abundant collateral circulation may confound the detection of occlusions and critical stenoses. Such collaterals may be fed by the nonobstructed companion artery that carries increased flow. This increased flow may be associated with an increase in the peak systolic velocity, which can be mistaken to indicate a stenosis. Interrogating as much of the vessel as possible should minimize such errors. The examiner should attempt to sweep through the vessel with the Doppler sample volume to detect focal increases in peak systolic velocity and identify poststenotic flow disturbances.

REFERENCES

1. Bowersox JC et al: Duplex ultrasonography in the diagnosis of celiac and mesenteric artery occlusive disease, *J Vasc Surg* 14:780-788, 1991.
2. Camerota AJ et al: Venous duplex imaging: should it replace hemodynamic tests for deep venous thrombosis? *J Vasc Surg* 11:53, 1990.
3. Healy DA et al: Evaluation of celiac and mesenteric vascular disease with duplex ultrasonography, *J Ultrasound Med* 11:481-485, 1992.
4. Hollinshead WH: *Textbook of anatomy,* ed 3, Hagerstown, Md, 1974, Harper & Row.
5. Jager KA et al: Noninvasive diagnosis of intestinal angina, *J Clin Ultrasound* 12:588, 1984.
6. Kremkau FW: *Doppler ultrasound: principles and instruments,* Philadelphia, 1990, Saunders.
7. Ku DN et al: Hemodynamics of the normal human carotid bifurcation: in vitro and in vivo studies, *Ultrasound Med Biol* 11:13-26, 1985.
8. Langlois Y et al: Evaluating carotid artery disease: the concordance between pulsed Doppler/spectrum analysis and angiography, *Ultrasound Med Biol* 9:51, 1983.
9. Moneta GL et al: Duplex ultrasound measurement of postprandial intestinal blood flow: effect of meal composition, *Gastroenterology* 95:1294, 1988.
10. Moneta GL et al: Mesenteric duplex scanning: a blinded prospective study, *J Vasc Surg* 17:79-86, 1993.
11. Phillips DJ et al: Should results of ultrasound Doppler studies be reported in units of frequency or velocity? *Ultrasound Med Biol* 15:205-212, 1989.
12. Rizzo RJ et al: Mesenteric flow velocity variations as a function of angle of insonation, *J Vasc Surg* 11:688-694, 1990.
13. Taylor DC et al: Extrinsic compression of the celiac artery by the median arcuate ligament of the diaphragm: diagnosis by duplex ultrasound, *J Vasc Tech* 11:236-238, 1987.
14. Taylor DC et al: Duplex ultrasound scanning in the diagnosis of renal artery stenosis: a prospective evaluation, *J Vasc Surg* 7:363, 1988.

CHAPTER 84

Operative assessment of intestinal viability

ROBERT W. HOBSON II and THOMAS G. LYNCH

The need for the intraoperative determination of intestinal viability in cases of potential bowel ischemia has stimulated the evaluation of techniques to supplement clinical criteria, such as the presence or absence of a mesenteric pulse and the color and peristaltic activity of the bowel. Several reports published over the past 15 years have emphasized that no one method has proved acceptable in all clinical settings. The use of technetium 99m-labeled albumin microspheres,[13,19] electromyography,[10] Doppler ultrasound,[4,9,18] fluorescein fluorescence patterns,[1] quantitative perfusion fluorometry,[17] helium-neon laser Doppler ultrasound,[16] and photoplethysmography[15] has been suggested by various authors. More recently, pulse oximetry[5,7] has been proposed as a technique for assessing intestinal viability. Many of these methods, however, require highly specialized equipment, and this has limited their routine clinical application. Ideally, such a technique should be accurate and not excessively cumbersome to perform and should not require expensive equipment or sophisticated monitoring for interpretation. So far, no technique has met all these criteria.

Those techniques that tend to be more readily interpretable and have found some place in clinical practice include Doppler ultrasound[9,14] and fluorescein fluorescence pattern recognition.[2] In addition, semiquantitative techniques that have been investigated in both the research laboratory and the clinical setting include helium-neon laser–Doppler ultrasound[16] perfusion fluorometry,[17] photoplethysmography,[15] and pulse oximetry.[5,7] Whether these more quantitative and investigative methods find an application in surgical practice will require further clinical evaluation.

QUALITATIVE TECHNIQUES FOR SURGICAL DETERMINATION OF BOWEL VIABILITY

Traditional physical findings are useful in the determination of intestinal viability, and their accuracy has ranged between 75% and 80%.[2] However, reliance on physical findings alone can sometimes lead to inaccurate conclusions regarding intestinal viability. Initially the surgeon should carefully examine the bowel mesentery for the presence of visible or palpable pulses and hemorrhage within the mesentery and over the serosal surface of the bowel. Hemorrhage may alter serosal color and appearance and thus obscure the true status

of intestinal viability. Finally, the presence of peristalsis in response to bowel stimulation is a further indication of viability. Some clinicians[9,18] have had extensive experience with the use of qualitative Doppler ultrasound as an adjunct technique. The occurrence of Doppler flow signals over the mesentery, mesentery-bowel junction, and serosal surface of the bowel is an important indication of viability (Fig. 84-1), and an absent Doppler signal has correlated well with nonviability. The accuracy of the technique for the determination of intestinal viability in both experimental and surgical settings has been the subject of literature.[9,18]

Doppler ultrasound has also been employed to detect left colonic ischemia[8] following aortic reconstruction (Fig. 84-2), supplementing the measurement of back pressure in the inferior mesenteric artery.[6] In addition, the Doppler technique has been used to assess viability following colon bypass.[11] The latter indication, however, also illustrates one of the weaknesses of qualitative Doppler ultrasound shared with other methods. Although a Doppler arterial signal recorded over the serosal surface of the bowel correlates with intestinal viability, this does not rule out subsequent venous obstruction and ultimate nonviability of the segment.

Cooperman et al[4] confirmed the accuracy of the Doppler method by correlating Doppler arterial flow with the histologic findings in intestinal biopsy specimens. These investigators identified the point of the last audible Doppler flow on the antimesenteric border of the bowel that had been devascularized 1, 2, and 3 cm from the point of investigation. They found that the incidence of mucosal and subsequent transmural infarction and perforation increased as the distance between the site of biopsy and the point of the last Doppler flow signal increased. The findings from similar experiments have confirmed the value of the technique in predicting the viability of end-to-end small bowel anastomosis. This pathologic confirmation of the usefulness of the Doppler technique promoted its application in clinical practice.

Some investigators[2] have reported difficulty in applying the technique and have instead recommended use of qualitative fluorescein fluorescence patterns to determine intestinal viability. Bulkley et al[1] compared Doppler ultrasound findings and fluorescein fluorescence patterns seen with an

707

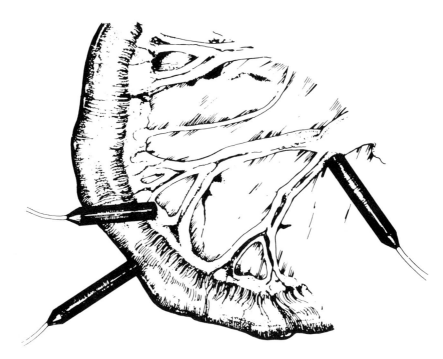

Fig. 84-1. Application of the Doppler ultrasound device to the mesenteric vessels, mesentery bowel junction, and antimesenteric bowel surface to detect flow after experimental intestinal ischemia. (From Wright CB, Hobson RW: *Am J Surg* 129:642, 1975.)

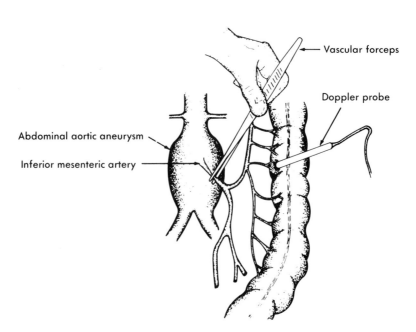

Fig. 84-2. Application of the sterile Doppler probe during temporary occlusion of the inferior mesenteric artery (IMA). Detectable collateral arterial blood flow during IMA occlusion predicted colonic viability. (From Hobson RW et al: *J Surg Res* 20:231, 1976.)

ultraviolet (Wood's) light after the intravenous administration of fluorescein in a feline model of intestinal ischemia. These investigators reported a 100% sensitivity for this method, whereas Doppler ultrasound showed a sensitivity of only 33%. In a subsequent clinical trial,[2] these authors reported a 100% sensitivity for fluorescence pattern recognition, a 78% sensitivity for clinical judgment only, and a 63% sensitivity for Doppler ultrasound. However, other authors have been unable to duplicate the remarkable sensitivity data claimed for fluorescein fluorescence pattern recognition.

Silverman et al[17] found that the pattern recognition method showed a sensitivity of only 40% and thus questioned its application in the clinical setting. These investigators went on to introduce a method of quantitative perfusion fluorometry possessing better sensitivity and specificity than those of fluorescence patterns.

Although Bulkley et al[2] suggested that the fluorescein fluorescence patterns were readily applicable to clinical practice, Silverman et al[17] noted five quantitative fluorescence time-distribution curves in the bowel, two of which were associated with viable bowel. In the first pattern, fluorescence peaked within 2 minutes, decreased rapidly for several minutes, and then decreased more slowly. In the second pattern, which was associated with postischemic hyperemia, the rise in fluorescence was greater and the initial decline more rapid than that in normal bowel. The three remaining patterns were associated with bowel necrosis. In the first, dye uptake was normal; however, the dye did not clear because elimination was impaired. In the second and third patterns, initial uptake was impaired: in one, uptake continued gradually but with no elimination, and in the other, there was only minimal uptake. From this, it is reasonable to conclude that the qualitative pattern methodology has an associated complexity that perhaps limits its general clinical application.

Because of these conflicting reports, surgeons have continued to rely on physical findings for assessing intestinal viability. However, in instances when these findings are ambiguous Doppler ultrasound has enjoyed some success because of its simplicity and ready availability in the operating room, and because it does not require the intravenous injection of contrast material. Clearly, it is not a technique that should be used to the exclusion of physical diagnostic criteria; however, it can be a useful supplement to the surgical determination of intestinal viability.

QUANTITATIVE TECHNIQUES FOR DETERMINING INTESTINAL VIABILITY

Several newer techniques that offer quantitative assessment beyond the qualitative data yielded by Doppler ultrasound or fluorescein fluorescence pattern recognition have been evaluated in the laboratory. Silverman et al[17] proposed that an uptake 2 minutes after fluorescein injection of less than 75% (relative to a reference control) was abnormal and indicated necrosis. If the 2-minute uptake was greater than

75% of the control value, a second reading was taken at 10 minutes, and if this dye fluorescence index (DFI) was greater than that at 2 minutes, necrosis was predicted. Using the data obtained at 2 minutes, they found the method showed a sensitivity of 82% in detecting nonviable bowel; combining this with a subsequent observation at 10 minutes, they found the sensitivity was 97%. These observations were made in a rat model employing reversible bowel strangulation and were subsequently corroborated in a canine model.[3] Lynch et al[12] recently compared the qualitative Doppler method with quantitative perfusion fluorometry, as recommended by Silverman, in a canine model of intestinal ischemia. They cited a 95% sensitivity for fluorometry and an 83% to 86% sensitivity for Doppler ultrasound. These observations confirmed the authors' impression that the fluorescein fluorescence method requires quantitative assessment before intestinal viability can be accurately predicted.

In an effort to use a more quantitative Doppler method, the use of laser Doppler velocimetry has been investigated.[12] Rotering et al[16] were the first to suggest that a helium-neon laser Doppler velocimeter could be used to determine viability in canine ischemic small intestine. These investigators used the laser Doppler to estimate the last site of antimesenteric serosal and mucosal perfusion. Comparing these results with those from Doppler ultrasound, they concluded that the laser Doppler was more accurate in identifying the point of transmural necrosis. The average distance from the loss of the Doppler signal to the point of total necrosis was 5.0 ± 2.6 cm with Doppler ultrasound, 1.9 ± 1.5 cm with mucosal laser Doppler, and 0.4 ± 1.4 cm with serosal laser Doppler flow velocimetry. Both laser Doppler estimates, however, were obtained within a zone of partial necrosis.

Pearce et al[15] have used photoplethysmography to assess viability in an ischemic canine bowel model. Photoplethysmography can monitor changes in tissue blood flow by detecting alterations in the reflected infrared light as a function of absorption by hemoglobin. When an intestinal photoplethysmographic waveform of less than 50% of the reference value, recorded from the stomach, was used as the threshold value, the method showed a 100% sensitivity for detecting an ischemic intestine. If the last pulsatile waveform was used as the end point, however, the sensitivity decreased to 50%.

In a recent comparison of Doppler ultrasound, laser Doppler, and quantitative perfusion fluorometry,[12] the data yielded were used to evaluate the various methods' sensitivity to and quantitation of ischemia. The sensitivities calculated for each of the techniques were 86% for Doppler ultrasound, 85% for laser Doppler flow velocity, 94% for the laser-Doppler index, and 95% for the DFI (less than 75%) (Table 84-1). Although the sensitivity of Doppler ultrasound was significantly less than that of both perfusion fluorometry and LDI, this is expected, since the last two techniques are more quantitative than the qualitative Doppler ultrasound. Although graded decrease in perfusion was reported for fluorometry and laser Doppler velocimetry in

Table 84-1. Sensitivity of techniques

	Technique	No.	Sensitivity (%)
A.	Dye fluorescence index (<75%)	289/305	95
B.	Laser-Doppler velocity (<531 mV)	258/302	85
C.	Laser-Doppler index (<75%)	210/224	94
D.	Doppler ultrasound (≥3)	250/302	83
E.	Doppler ultrasound (≥2)	261/302	86

From Lynch TG et al: Doppler ultrasound, laser Doppler, and perfusion fluorometry in bowel ischemia, *Arch Surg* 123:483, 1988.
For A versus B, A versus D, A versus E, C versus D, and C versus E, $p < 0.05$.
For A versus C and D versus E, $p > 0.05$.

this experimental model, scattered segments distal to the most proximal necrotic segment demonstrated apparent viability. Despite the viability predicted, these segments were necrotic because for these segments to remain viable, flow across nonviable segments would have had to exist. Thus the sensitivities of Doppler ultrasound, laser-Doppler flow velocity, the laser-Doppler index, and the DFI were also evaluated relative to the most proximal point of ischemia, and this yielded values of 90%, 91%, 97%, and 97%, respectively. These investigators concluded that Doppler ultrasound was not as sensitive to the subtle variations in flow made apparent by perfusion fluorometry and laser Doppler velocimetry. Nonetheless, in a clinical sense, its sensitivity to subsequent necrosis does compare favorably with that of the last two techniques. The low cost and relative simplicity of performing intraoperative Doppler ultrasound make it an ideal technique for most patients. Perfusion fluorometry and laser Doppler velocimetry, however, provide valuable adjunctive data and the opportunity to quantitate the ischemia as well as to evaluate the influence of therapeutic and pharmacologic manipulations.

More recently, pulse oximetry has been recommended for the assessment of intestinal viability. Ferrara et al[7] reported that pulse oximetry was superior to the use of traditional clinical criteria and Doppler ultrasound in a model of canine intestinal ischemia. DeNobile et al[5] reported on the oxygen saturation measurements obtained simultaneously from beneath the tongue and at the antimesenteric border of the small bowel in a canine model of intestinal ischemia. Once an initial measurement was obtained from a normal-appearing segment of the bowel, the probe was moved slowly toward the ischemic area. At the site where oxygen saturation was significantly lower than the tongue oxygen saturation, pathologic findings from intestinal biopsy specimens correlated well with the presence of intestinal ischemia.[5] The increasing availability of pulse oximetry devices in the operating room may make this technique readily available and acceptable to surgeons in the future.

REFERENCES

1. Bulkley GB et al: Assessment of small intestinal recovery from ischemic injury after segmental, arterial, venous, and arteriovenous occlusion, *Surg Forum* 30:210-213, 1979.
2. Bulkley GB et al: Intraoperative determination of small intestinal viability following ischemic surgery, *Ann Surg* 193:628-637, 1981.
3. Carter MS et al: Qualitative and quantitative fluorescein fluorescence in determining intestinal viability, *Am J Surg* 147:117-123, 1984.
4. Cooperman M et al: Determination of viability of ischemic intestine by Doppler ultrasound, *Surgery* 83:705-710, 1978.
5. DeNobile J, Guzzetta P, Patterson K: Pulse oximetry as a means of assessing bowel viability, *J Surg Res* 48:21-23, 1990.
6. Ernst CB et al: Inferior mesenteric artery stump pressure: a reliable index for safe IMA ligation during abdominal aneurysmectomy, *Ann Surg* 187:641-646, 1978.
7. Ferrara JJ et al: Surface oximetry: a new method to evaluate intestinal perfusion, *Am Surg* 54:10-54, 1988.
8. Hobson RW et al: Assessment of colonic ischemia during aortic surgery by Doppler ultrasound, *J Surg Res* 20:231-235, 1976.
9. Hobson RW et al: Determination of intestinal viability by Doppler ultrasound, *Arch Surg* 114:165-168, 1979.
10. Katz S et al: New parameters of viability in ischemic bowel disease, *Am J Surg* 127:136-141, 1974.
11. Kurstin RD et al: Ultrasonic blood flow assessment in colon esophageal bypass procedures, *Arch Surg* 112:270-272, 1977.
12. Lynch TG et al: Doppler ultrasound, laser Doppler, and perfusion fluorometry in bowel ischemia, *Arch Surg* 123:483-486, 1988.
13. Mossa AF et al: Assessment of bowel viability using 99m technetium tagged albumin microspheres, *J Surg Res* 16:466-472, 1974.
14. O'Donnell JA, Hobson RW: Operative confirmation of Doppler ultrasound in evaluation of intestinal ischemia, *Surgery* 87:109-112, 1979.
15. Pearce WH et al: The use of infrared photoplethysmography in identifying early intestinal ischemia, *Arch Surg* 122:308-310, 1987.
16. Rotering RH et al: A comparison of the He Ne laser and ultrasound Doppler systems in the determination of viability of ischemic canine intestine, *Ann Surg* 196:705-707, 1982.
17. Silverman DG et al: Quantification of fluorescein distribution to strangulated rat ileum, *J Surg Res* 34:179-186, 1983.
18. Wright CB, Hobson RW: Prediction of intestinal viability using Doppler ultrasound technics, *Am J Surg* 129:642-645, 1975.
19. Zarins CK et al: Predictions of the viability of revascularized intestine with radioactive microspheres, *Surg Gynecol Obstet* 138:576-580, 1974.

CHAPTER 85

Noninvasive imaging of the liver: the role of color and duplex Doppler

EDWARD G. GRANT

Recent advances in sonographic technology have made color and duplex imaging of the abdominal organs possible. The difficulties involved in constructing such equipment are considerable, but most modern scanners are capable of penetrating to the required depths without unacceptably compromising such parameters as frame rate, resolution, or field of view. In the abdomen, color Doppler technology has had a particular impact on the noninvasive evaluation of the liver and its vasculature. The liver is a relatively easy target for sonographic imaging and essentially provides its own acoustic window. In addition, the main hepatic and portal veins are large and the spectral patterns of each of the major vascular systems in the liver (hepatic artery, hepatic veins, and portal vein) are unique.[32]

TECHNIQUE

Doppler evaluation of the hepatic vasculature should be performed only after real-time sonography has been used to thoroughly examine the parenchyma of the liver. Rarely, if ever, can the examination be directed solely at the hepatic vessels. Parenchymal processes often underlie vascular abnormalities, and primary vascular diseases almost invariably have a significant effect on the parenchyma. Transducers with a sector format are best for upper abdominal scanning. The small area of contact facilitates positioning of the transducer and intracostal access, both of which are essential if adequate Doppler angles are to be maintained. For most adults, a Doppler transducer with a 3.5-MHz frequency or less should be used for hepatic vascular imaging. In many cases, in fact, lower-frequency transducers than would normally be used for real-time imaging (2 to 2.25 MHz) are preferable and permit a considerable increase in Doppler sensitivity with little effect on resolution. Depending on the equipment used, optimum real-time imaging may require use of a different transducer from that used for the Doppler examination. A wide array of transducer types may be necessary for a complete evaluation.

Positioning of the transducer will vary with the vessel that is being examined, and specific details about techniques unique to individual vessels are discussed in the appropriate section. As previously noted, however, an optimum Doppler angle should be maintained whenever possible. Although relatively simple to accomplish in the carotid arteries of the leg veins, a Doppler angle of less than 60° may be difficult to achieve in the upper abdomen because vessels are often perpendicular to the Doppler beam and access is limited. The examiner must often scan from several vantage points in an effort to decrease the Doppler angle and to optimize signal reception.

Having the patient fast is not essential when specifically evaluating the intrahepatic vasculature and may actually be detrimental when studying the portal vein. A recent investigation has shown portal vein velocity is increased postprandially; this phenomenon may heighten the visibility of small portal veins or those with a very slow flow.[18] Obviously an empty stomach is essential when evaluating extrahepatic vessels, such as the splenic or superior mesenteric veins or the hepatic artery between the porta hepatis and the celiac axis.

Although color Doppler imaging is the focus of this chapter, it should be noted that spectral analysis is of continued importance in the differentiation of hepatic vessels and the characterization of abnormal flow patterns. The three major hepatic vascular systems are anatomically and physiologically distinct, and each has a characteristic spectral waveform.[32] The hepatic artery exhibits a typical low-resistance pattern with flow throughout diastole. The portal venous system, on the other hand, is an isolated vascular unit with no significant source of pulsatility; flow in the portal vein is nonphasic. Finally, the hepatic veins are in direct communication with the inferior vena cava and right atrium. The strongly pulsatile nature of the right atrium is reflected in a complex triphasic flow pattern found in all central systemic veins. The hepatic veins have two periods of forward flow, with each cardiac cycle corresponding to the two phases of right atrial filling. Right heart contraction produces a brief period of transient normal flow reversal (Fig. 85-1).

THE HEPATIC ARTERY

In most patients, the hepatic artery originates as one of two major branches of the celiac axis. The normal hepatic artery initially courses over the anterosuperior edge of the pancreas

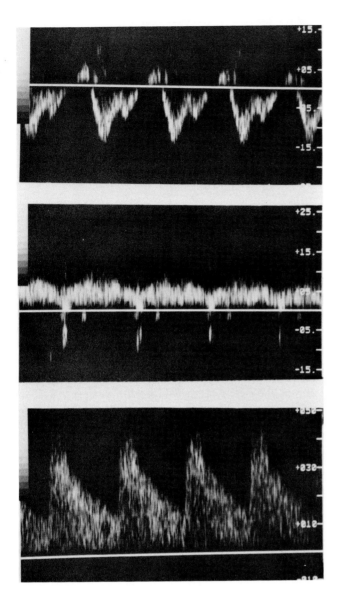

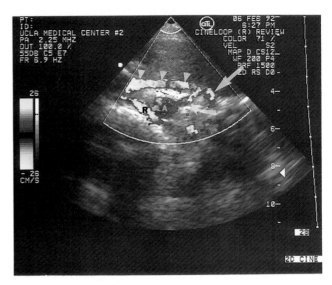

Fig. 85-2. Normal hepatic artery origin. The hepatic artery *(arrowheads)* and splenic artery *(arrow)* arise from the celiac axis *(curved arrow),* which is the first major branch of the abdominal aorta *(A).* The color in the hepatic artery changes from red to blue as flow is directed toward and then away from the Doppler beam. Note the presence of a retrocaval left renal vein *(R).*

Fig. 85-1. Spectral analysis. *Top:* Hepatic vein shows a "choppy" triphasic signal with two forward phases of flow (below the baseline) corresponding to two phases of right atrial filling. Note periodic flow reversal with right atrial contraction. *Middle:* Portal vein flow is relatively nonphasic. Changes secondary to cardiac activity or respiratory motion are minimal. *Bottom:* Hepatic artery exhibits typical low-resistance flow observed in arteries supplying parenchymal organs.

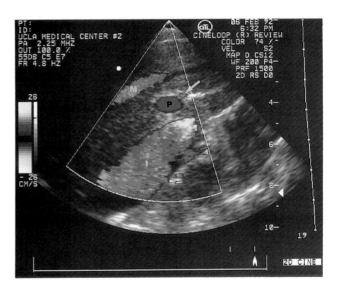

Fig. 85-3. Major hepatic vessels. A longitudinal intercostal section through the right lobe of the liver demonstrates the portal vein *(P),* hepatic artery *(arrow),* middle hepatic vein *(M),* and IVC *(I).* Note the yellow color assignment in the hepatic artery, whereas portal vein is red, indicating higher-velocity flow in the artery.

and, after the gastroduodenal artery branches off, runs cephalad with the portal vein and common bile duct into the porta hepatis. The extrahepatic portions of the artery are often best visualized by identifying the celiac axis anterior to the aorta and following the branch that runs to the right (Fig. 85-2). Although significant atherosclerotic disease rarely affects the hepatic artery itself (and would probably be of no significance if it did), stenosis of the celiac artery origin may contribute to the development of mesenteric ischemia when the superior mesenteric artery is compromised. In the porta hepatis, the common hepatic artery is generally easily visualized lying anterior to the portal vein when scan-

ning from an oblique intercostal approach (Fig. 85-3). Inside the liver, the hepatic artery branches follow their attendant portal veins and should be visible well into the periphery if the color technique is optimized. Pulsatility, higher velocity (often displayed in a different shade of color), and the smaller size of the hepatic artery help dif-

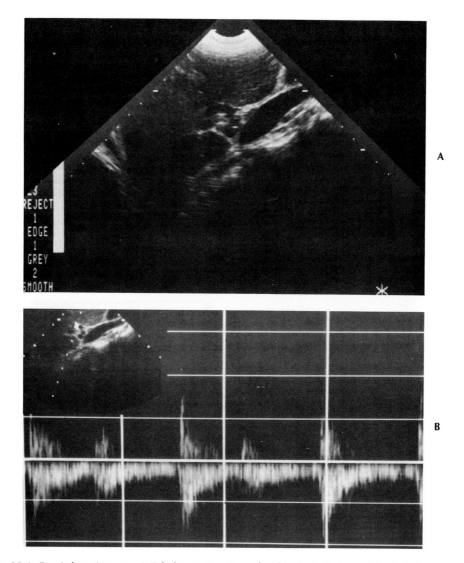

Fig. 85-4. Ectatic hepatic artery. *A,* Tubular structure *(arrowheads)* anterior to the portal vein in the porta hepatis could represent either an ectatic hepatic artery or a mildly dilated common bile duct. *B,* Spectral Doppler applied to the structure clearly defines its vascular nature.

ferentiate it from the adjacent vein. However, spectral analysis should be used for absolute differentiation between the two vessels or when confirmation of hepatic artery patency is necessary.

The liver is unique because the hepatic artery is subordinate to the portal vein in parenchymal oxygenation. Overall, the portal vein supplies 70% to 75% of incoming blood.[30] This dual blood supply makes hepatic infarction rare in the native liver. The oxygen-rich portal venous blood is usually sufficient to promote normal hepatic function even in the face of complete hepatic artery thrombosis. Altered arterial flow to the liver is rarely, if ever, a primary cause of hepatic disease. Enlargement of the hepatic artery, increased flow, and a tortuous "corkscrew" appearance,[28] however, are commonly observed in patients with cirrhosis and portal hypertension. Undoubtedly, the decrease in portal venous flow leads to increased dependence on the arterial

system for oxygenation. In such patients, color Doppler may more easily identify the hepatic artery than the portal vein. This may be a particularly troublesome situation when encountered in pre–liver transplant evaluations because a well-defined patent portal vein is essential in this setting. In addition, the ectatic hepatic arteries of cirrhotic patients may be difficult to distinguish from dilated intrahepatic biliary radicals when using real-time sonography.[36] This problem is easily solved using color or duplex Doppler because bile ducts produce no Doppler signal[29] (Fig. 85-4).

Although not associated with intrinsic hepatic disease, the splenic and hepatic arteries may be affected by pseudoaneurysms. These lesions typically arise in association with trauma or pancreatitis and may appear as a complex or cystic mass on routine real-time examination.[9] The Doppler characteristics of pseudoaneurysms anywhere in the body should be sufficiently specific to allow a definitive diagnosis.

THE PORTAL VENOUS SYSTEM

The portal vein and its major branches should be easily visualized in all patients by means of an anterior, right, oblique, intercostal approach (see Fig. 85-3). From this vantage point, flow in the main and left portal veins is invariably directed toward the transducer and displayed in red, assuming that a red–toward and blue–away color scheme is used. Flow in the posterior branch of the right portal vein, however, is directed away from the transducer and should not be confused with that of the nearby right hepatic vein (also typically displayed in blue). If a question exists, the vessel may be followed to its origin or evaluated with spectral Doppler.

Most significant abnormalities of the portal venous system are readily characterized with duplex and color Doppler imaging. Anatomic abnormalities are relatively unusual, but duplication, several normal variants, and aneurysms have all been described.[17,35] In addition, fistulas may affect the portal venous system and can involve either the hepatic artery or the hepatic veins. Communications between the hepatic artery and portal vein tend to be symptomatic, since the high pressure in the artery delivers large quantities of blood to the portal system and causes severe portal hypertension. Most hepatic vein–portal vein fistulas, on the other hand, are asymptomatic unless they are large enough to divert most of the portal flow and cause hepatic ischemia. Such patients occasionally are seen because of encephalopathy. The results of color Doppler imaging should be definitive for both types of fistula. In patients with hepatic artery–portal vein communications, markedly dilated portal venous structures with abundant collateral formation are typical.[8] Turbulent, high-velocity, low-resistance arterial flow with a color-Doppler "bruit" (i.e., random color assignment outside the region of an actual vessel[23]) may be present and portal signals may be arterialized. Portal vein flow is almost always reversed. In the presence of portal vein–hepatic vein fistulas, large cystic spaces may be seen within the liver in the area of the communication. Color Doppler confirms the diagnosis by identifying flow in the "cysts" and should be able to define the attendant vascular connections.[2] In cases of hepatic vein–portal vein fistulas, the communication between the systemic and portal venous systems causes the triphasic spectral pattern of the hepatic veins to be reflected back into the portal vein. This produces an unusual pattern of portal vein pulsatility (Fig. 85-5).

Thrombosis may also affect the portal vein. The symptoms are relatively nonspecific and include the new onset or worsening of ascites and abdominal pain or distention. Hepatomegaly is not a typical finding. Considering the nonspecific nature of the clinical presentation of portal vein thrombosis (PVT), an effective screening technique would be of considerable value. One recent study of color Doppler in diagnosing PVT showed color Doppler performs well in this role.[34] The high negative predictive value (0.98) implies that a normal color Doppler study effectively excludes the diagnosis of thrombosis. On the other hand, severe portal

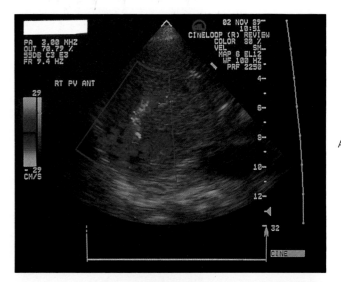

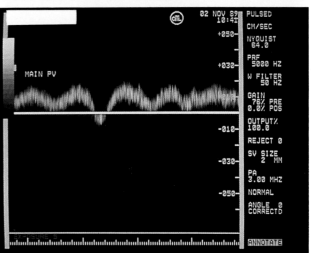

Fig. 85-5. Hepatic vein/portal vein fistula. *A,* The patient was referred for biopsy of several "hypoechoic" masses beneath the dome of the liver. Color Doppler evaluation revealed swirling flow internally *(arrowheads).* Lesions could be connected easily to the portal vein *(P)* and hepatic veins (not shown). These findings are typical of hepatic vein–portal vein fistula. *B,* Spectral analysis of the portal vein reveals marked pulsatility. A pulsatile portal vein is to be expected secondary to portosystemic communication.

hypertension may reduce flow to such an extent that Doppler signals are not returned. In such cases, the diagnosis of PVT would be suggested, but unless an obvious hypoechoic clot expands the lumen (Fig. 85-6), an alternative imaging modality (magnetic resonance imaging [MRI] or preferably angiography) should be considered for confirmation. Fortunately such patients are unusual in the general population (Fig. 85-7).

In the evaluation of patients for PVT, the complexity of the color Doppler examination should not be underestimated. Machine settings and the Doppler angle must be optimized, and scanning should be performed with a max-

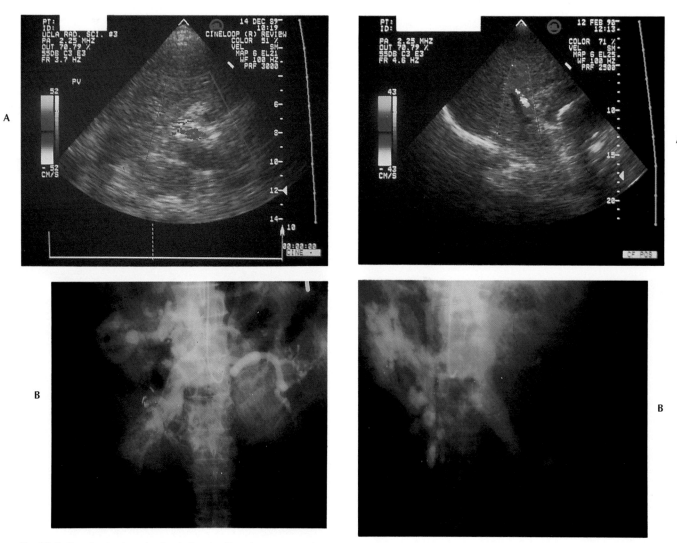

Fig. 85-6. Portal vein thrombosis. **A,** A color Doppler sonogram in a patient with hepatoma reveals a dilated, thrombus-filled portal vein *(T).* Note the accentuated hepatic arterial flow anteriorly *(arrowhead).* **B,** Late phase of superior mesenteric arteriogram confirms sonographic findings.

Fig. 85-7. False-positive sonogram. **A,** Despite optimization of scan technique, flow could not be demonstrated in the portal vein *(V).* The hepatic artery flow was accentuated *(arrowheads).* The patient had a history of severe portal hypertension. **B,** Late phase of mesenteric angiogram shows a patent portal vein *(P).* Note the presence of an extensive collateral bed that facilitated reduction of portal vein flow.

imal sensitivity to low flow. High wall-filter settings are particularly effective in eliminating low-velocity signals of the portal vein and should be minimized. A postprandial scan should be considered in patients who show no flow. Suspected thrombosis is best confirmed with spectral analysis.

Although color Doppler seems useful in identifying PVT, its role in assessing portal hypertension remains undefined. The noninvasive diagnosis of portal hypertension is rendered difficult by the complexity of the vascular dynamics involved. Certainly the ability of Doppler to yield directional information allows a definitive diagnosis to be made when reversed flow is identified in the portal vein (Fig. 85-8). Unfortunately, patients with reversed flow represent a rel-

atively small portion of the total patient population with the disease. Several studies have evaluated a decrease in velocity as an indicator of portal hypertension.[25,27] Although this method was successful in selected patients, the normal velocity of the portal vein is extremely variable, and the main collateral pathway largely dictates the flow dynamics of the portal vein. For example, a recanalized umbilical vein (Fig. 85-9) may actually cause an increase in portal flow despite the presence of severe liver disease. The evaluation of the portal vein alone, therefore, seems inadequate when diagnosing portal hypertension. The most important contribution of color Doppler may be its superior identification and characterization of portal vein collaterals (Fig. 85-10). Color Doppler will often identify vessels that are otherwise in-

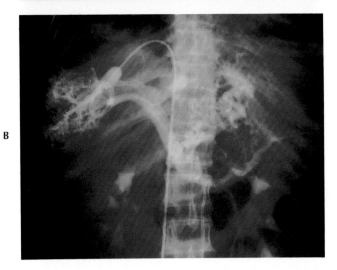

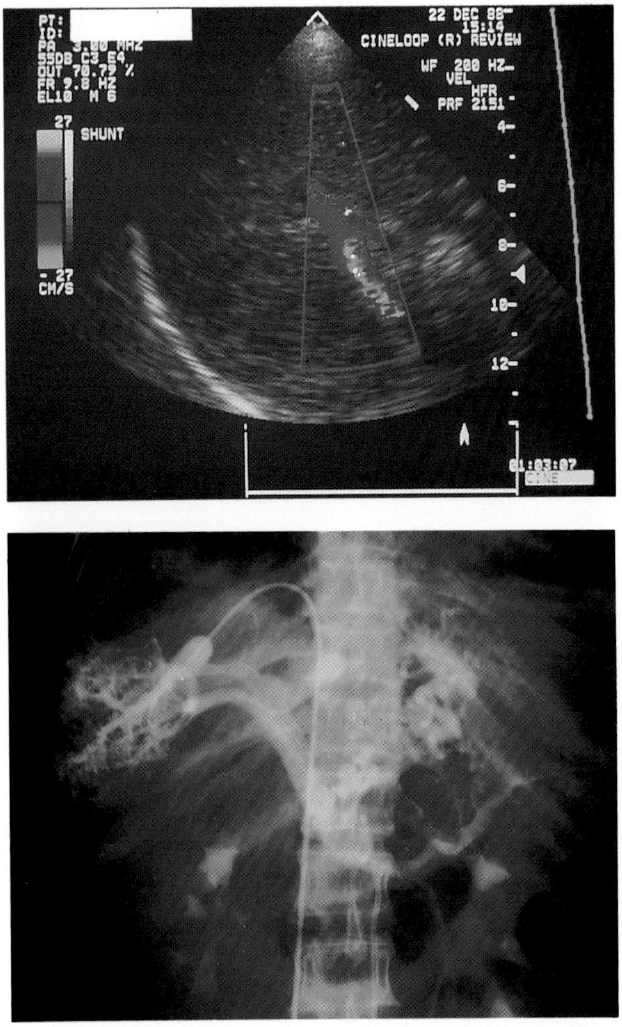

Fig. 85-8. Reversed portal vein flow. **A,** Reversal of portal vein flow is indicated by the blue color in the vessel. Note the prominence of arterial flow, which is directed normally (displayed in red). **B,** Portal vein *(V)* was unable to be visualized by usual arterial injection. Reversal of flow was confirmed with wedged hepatic venography.

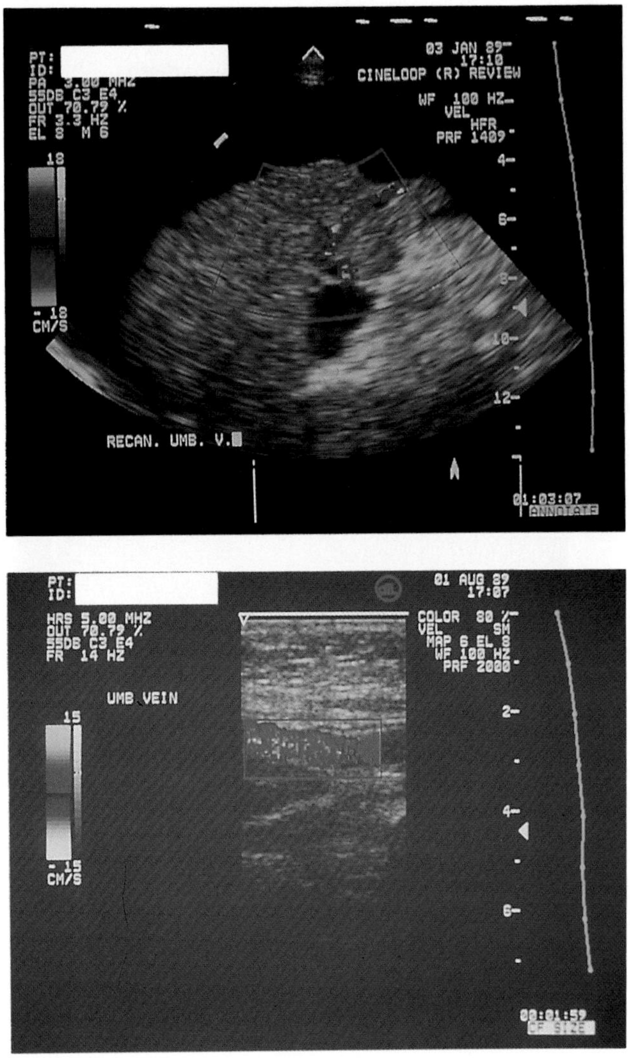

Fig. 85-9. Umbilical vein collaterals. **A,** The umbilical (or paraumbilical) vein serves as a common collateral pathway in patients with portal hypertension. Flow is displayed in red and directed away from the liver. The recanalized umbilical vein serves as an intrahepatic shunt and may actually increase or normalize flow velocity in the main portal vein. **B,** By scanning beneath the anterior abdominal wall, superficial portions of the umbilical vein can be followed as they course toward the umbilicus.

visible in the real-time examination because they are shrouded by bowel gas.

The major clinical complications of portal hypertension are ascites and variceal hemorrhage. Although ascites can often be controlled with diuretic therapy, gastrointestinal hemorrhage in patients with portal hypertension remains a major cause of mortality and morbidity. Sclerotherapy is currently used as a palliative measure, but patients with repeated bouts of hemorrhage or intractable ascites may require construction of a portosystemic shunt. Three main types of shunts are used: portocaval, mesocaval, and splenorenal. A new fourth option is an intrahepatic catheter that is percutaneously placed between the hepatic and portal veins. The most commonly used shunt has been the relatively simple portocaval shunt. Such shunts may be con-

structed in an end-to-side or side-to-side manner and should be easily imaged in most patients by means of color Doppler technology (Fig. 85-11). The few patients with extremely small cirrhotic livers or those who have undergone surgical removal of the right lobe may be difficult to scan because the usual acoustic window provided by the right lobe of liver is absent.

Although the simplest to construct and easiest to examine sonographically, portocaval shunts are now performed less frequently as orthotopic transplantation becomes an accepted form of treatment in patients with end-stage liver disease. An intact portal vein is desirable when performing a transplant, and any form of disturbance, such as the con-

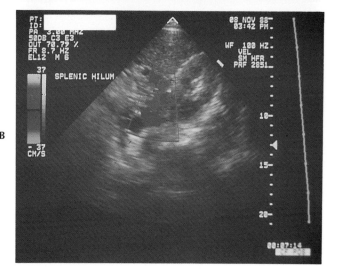

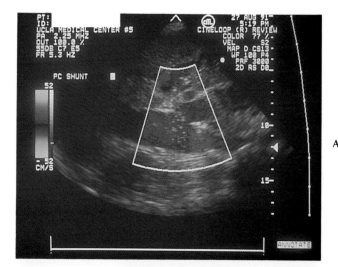

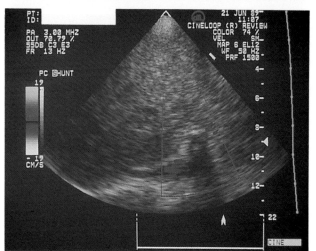

Fig. 85-10. Collaterals in portal hypertension. *A,* A large crescentic vessel thought to represent a dilated coronary vein is identified cephalad to a smaller, normal splenic vein (not shown). The vessel could be followed across the upper abdomen to the region of the stomach and esophagus. *B,* Splenorenal collaterals. An extensive network of left upper quadrant collaterals may be encountered as shown. These naturally occurring pathways serve a similar function to a surgically created splenorenal shunt and help to alleviate portal hypertension.

Fig. 85-11. Portacaval shunt. *A,* Patency is confirmed by demonstrating anastomosis. Note the flow in the splenic/portal vein *(P)* and IVC *(C). B,* With thrombosis, flow is absent in the region of the shunt *(arrowheads);* flow in the IVC *(arrow)* persists.

struction of a portocaval shunt, should therefore be avoided. In addition, so-called selective shunts (mesocaval and splenorenal) are considered advantageous because they do not divert all the blood supply from the portal vein, which can contribute to the development of hepatic encephalopathy.

A mesocaval shunt is typically an H-type synthetic graft placed between the mid–superior mesenteric vein and the inferior vena cava (IVC). These shunts are located deep in the midabdomen and may be difficult to identify because they tend to be covered by bowel gas and mesentery. Experience with color Doppler sonography in patients with these shunts, however, shows that persistence yields good results.[13] In general, real-time scanning is done initially in an effort to identify the characteristic serrated walls of the Gortex graft.* Once flow is identified among the surrounding bowel gas and mesentery, either duplex or color Doppler may be used to confirm it (Fig. 85-12). Alternatively, color Doppler may be used to follow the IVC either proximally or distally until flow enters from a large vessel below the level of the renal veins. Because no other native vessels enter the IVC in this area, flow can be taken as presumptive evidence that the junction between the graft and the IVC has been found and that the shunt is patent. Gentle continued pressure will often be sufficient to part the bowel gas and allow at least a portion of the graft to be identified. Iden-

---

*W.L. Gore & Associates, Prescott, Ariz.

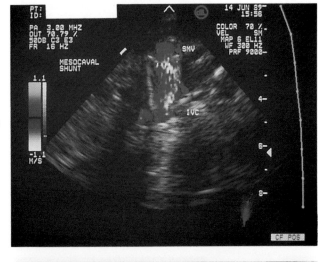

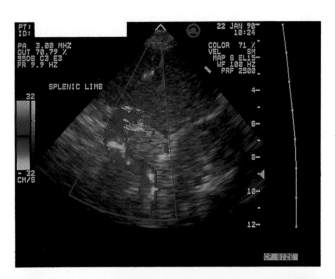

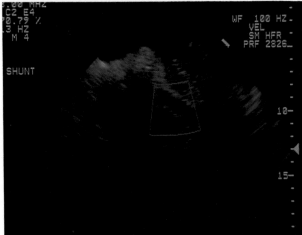

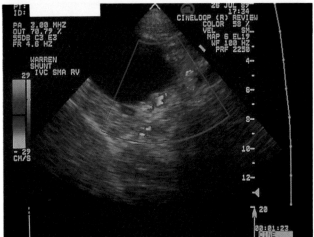

Fig. 85-12. Mesocaval shunt. *A,* The shunt diverts blood from the mid to distal superior mesenteric vein to the adjacent IVC via a Gortex graft *(arrowheads).* The walls of such grafts are brightly echogenic; color confirms patency. *B,* A patient with thrombosed mesocaval shunt *(M)* has no flow in the graft. Mesocaval shunts may be difficult to evaluate because the graft is frequently surrounded by bowel gas. In cases where the shunt cannot be identified, reversed flow in the superior mesenteric vein may be used to imply patency.

Fig. 85-13. Distal splenorenal (Warren) shunt. *A,* The splenic limb of the shunt is most optimally visualized from an anterior approach through the spleen. Note the large single vessel with flow running from the splenic hilum toward the left kidney. *B,* A patient with a pseudocyst *(P)* and recurrent esophageal hemorrhage has numerous venous structures in the left upper quadrant *(arrowheads).* Singular splenic and renal limbs were not identified; thrombosis was suspected and confirmed by arteriography.

tification of flow in any one portion of the mesocaval graft should be sufficient to imply patency.

Distal splenorenal or Warren shunts are a third alternative and involve severing the distal splenic vein and anastomosing it to the left renal vein. Portal hypertension is theoretically reduced by diverting splenic blood flow; oxygenated blood from the gut continues to reach the liver. Splenorenal shunts are the most difficult to image sonographically. The anastomosis usually lies deep in the left upper quadrant and the walls of this native vein–to–native vein graft are invisible sonographically. In an older study by Foley et al,[11] duplex sonography was found unacceptable,

and a more recent study corroborated this.[13] However, color Doppler was found to be quite successful in evaluating distal splenorenal shunts. The limbs of these shunts typically lie perpendicular to each other, and Doppler signals are optimally received from two different vantage points. The splenic limb is often best imaged from an anterior approach because the vessel is usually oriented vertically. The renal vein runs in a horizontal plane, and reception of Doppler signals is optimized by scanning from the posterior flank. The anastomosis itself may be difficult to define in one plane, but its identification is not essential; appropriately directed flow in well-defined splenic and renal limbs can be used to imply patency. The thrombus itself is difficult to define because flow is the only factor that generates Doppler signals and color images. The identification of multiple left upper quadrant collaterals instead of single, well-defined splenic and renal limbs should suggest thrombosis or at least physiologic compromise (i.e., possible narrowing of the proximal left renal vein). In any case in which a question exists, further studies are warranted (Fig. 85-13).

Any discussion of the portal vein must also consider portal pulsatility. Such pulsatility is best characterized by spectral Doppler, but severe cases may be evident on the color examination when an alternating red and blue pattern is noted. As mentioned previously, portal vein flow is typically nonphasic, with relatively minor fluctuations secondary to cardiac and respiratory motion. Occasionally, however, pulsatile flow may be identified in the portal vein. Some degree of portal pulsatility may be observed in normal patients, but a greater than two-thirds change from the peak to minimum velocity should be viewed with suspicion.[7] As previously discussed, any anatomic communication between the systemic and portal veins, including surgically created portocaval shunts or hepatic vein–portal vein fistulas, may result in a pulsatile portal vein. More commonly, however, significant portal vein pulsatility is secondary to right heart failure (e.g., increased right atrial pressure) or tricuspid regurgitation, or both.[1,7] If patients have no history of heart disease, they should be referred for a cardiac evaluation that includes a detailed echocardiogram with specific attention to the tricuspid valve.

THE HEPATIC VEINS

The hepatic veins are anatomically distinct from the portal system and are normally the only route of egress of blood from the liver. There are normally three main hepatic veins (left, middle, and right) that join the IVC immediately inferior to the diaphragm and openly communicate with the right atrium. Unlike the portal circulation, a significant disorder affecting the hepatic veins is almost invariably associated with some form of obstruction. The resultant symptoms are typically hepatomegaly, ascites, and upper abdominal pain. Together, this set of abnormalities is termed *Budd-Chiari syndrome*.

Compromise of hepatic venous outflow may be caused by a lesion located anywhere between the IVC and the hepatic venules, and because symptoms are not specific, a method for both adequately screening and characterizing the blockage would be desirable. Experience with color Doppler imaging has been quite encouraging, and the initial reported results in five patients[12] have been borne out in a much larger group. Color Doppler can effectively be used as the first radiographic examination in any patient with suspected Budd-Chiari syndrome.

Several investigators have considered the use of real-time or duplex sonography in the diagnosis of Budd-Chiari syndrome[16,31]; the hepatic veins should be quite obvious on real-time images in all normal patients. Hepatomegaly and

cirrhosis (the former existing in numerous acute forms of hepatic disorders, including Budd-Chiari syndrome), however, will often compress these vessels and render them invisible to the real-time examination. In such cases, duplex sonography is also inadequate for revealing the nature of the problem because the Doppler cursor cannot be properly positioned. The potential of duplex sonography in diagnosing Budd-Chiari syndrome is further reduced by the propensity for pulsations from the left atrium to be transmitted throughout much of the left lobe of the liver. Doppler signals can literally be obtained almost anywhere in the parenchyma. Color Doppler lessens these problems and allows visualization of compressed but patent hepatic veins even when they are not clearly visible on the real-time examination. The anatomic display yielded by color Doppler can also differentiate the vessel from the background flash of cardiac motion. Admittedly, color imaging of the hepatic veins is more difficult in patients with severely shrunken, cirrhotic livers, but acute Budd-Chiari syndrome is quite unusual in this population. In addition, patients with cirrhosis secondary to long-standing Budd-Chiari syndrome should have specific and readily identifiable abnormalities.

Acute Budd-Chiari syndrome is diagnosed when color Doppler shows a lack of flow in the hepatic veins. Depending on the cause, the actual thrombus may or may not be seen with real-time imaging. Three patent hepatic veins must be identified to exclude the diagnosis, since all of the vessels may not be involved. The veins of the caudate lobe drain directly into the IVC and are frequently spared, although the main hepatic veins are always compromised. A large patent caudate vein should not be confused with a patent middle hepatic vein. In patients receiving thrombolytic therapy for acute hepatic vein thrombosis, color Doppler is useful for monitoring the effect of treatment. Color Doppler can also be used to guide angioplasty and observe the course of patients with caval webs.[19]

After an acute thrombotic episode, collateral pathways open rapidly in and about the liver. Many of these pathways are unique to Budd-Chiari syndrome and constitute definitive features for diagnosis with color Doppler. The identification of a bicolored hepatic vein is pathognomonic and indicates a proximal blockage. In fact, any intrahepatic collateral except for a recanalized umbilical vein should suggest Budd-Chiari syndrome because the portal hypertension diverts blood around and not through the liver (Fig. 85-14). In patients with evidence of Budd-Chiari syndrome, the portal vein should be evaluated for concurrent thrombosis, which is claimed to occur in 20% of such patients.[26]

The tendency for caval compromise is also considerable in Budd-Chiari syndrome (greater than 50%), and this may be part of the primary underlying problem (e.g., extension of thrombus or neoplasm from the IVC, congenital web) or secondary to extrinsic compression exerted by an enlarged caudate lobe (a common feature of Budd-Chiari syndrome) or a hepatic mass (Fig. 85-15). Evaluation of the IVC is essential because its status dictates the procedure chosen in

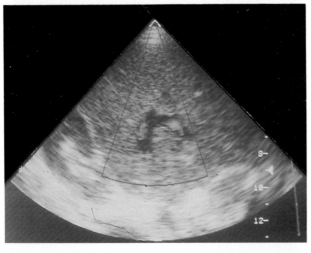

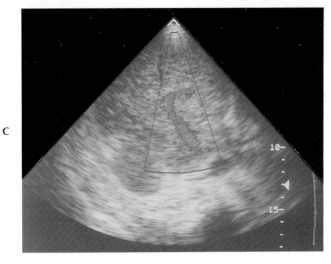

patients who are being considered for surgical decompression. Conversion of the portal vein to an outflow tract can adequately decompress the hepatic congestion and actually halt the progression of parenchymal damage.[3] Unfortunately, caval compromise precludes simple decompression of the portal vein via the IVC and necessitates the construction of a far more complex mesoatrial shunt in which the mid–superior mesenteric vein is anastomosed directly to the right atrium. Mesoatrial shunts have a high propensity for thrombosis and thus require frequent imaging. Patency can be implied by the finding of reverse flow in the portal vein, but the shunt itself is usually easily visualized directly be-

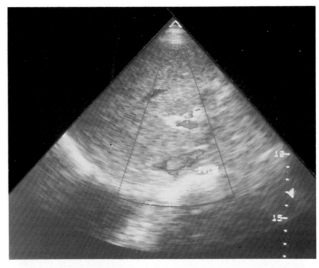

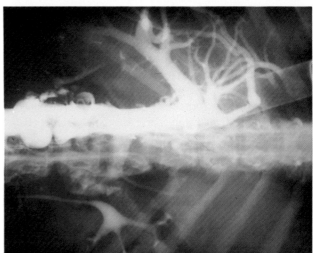

Fig. 85-14. Intrahepatic collaterals in Budd-Chiari syndrome. *A,* Color Doppler evaluation revealed bicolor hepatic vein bifurcation. The flow in one branch was directed normally and displayed in blue. The flow in the adjacent branch was toward the periphery of the liver and displayed in red. *B,* Another image from the same patient demonstrated a large intrahepatic collateral. *C,* The patient had a large, patent right hepatic vein *(V).* All three hepatic veins may not be involved in the thrombotic process.

Fig. 85-15. Budd-Chiari syndrome. *A,* Further evaluation of the patient shown in Fig. 85-14 reveals complete occlusion of the proximal IVC *(arrowheads).* Note the portal vein *(arrow)* is patent and appropriately directed. *B,* Inferior vena cavagram on the same patient confirms findings in Figs. 85-14 and 85-15. Note the complete occlusion of the proximal IVC *(arrows),* numerous intrahepatic collaterals, and the large patent right hepatic vein *(R).* The large cylindrical structure is the mesoatrial shunt *(arrowheads).*

neath the anterior abdominal wall in the right upper quadrant. Similar to mesocaval grafts, appropriately directed flow in any part of the mesoatrial shunt should imply patency.

ULTRASOUND IN LIVER TRANSPLANTATION

Sonography plays a major role in the preoperative and postoperative evaluation of candidates for hepatic transplantation. Preoperatively, duplex and color sonography is the pivotal screening examination and is performed in almost all potential recipients. The main purpose of this examination is to evaluate the portal vein. A preoperative knowledge of size and patency is essential, since a small or thrombosed vessel will render the surgery more difficult or exclude the patient as an operative candidate.[21,24,33] A normal ultrasound of the portal vein should be sufficient to rule out any significant abnormality.[34] If the ultrasound image of the portal anatomy is not entirely normal, the patient must undergo MRI or angiography. The hepatic artery, hepatic veins, and IVC should also be assessed. The hepatic parenchyma must be carefully evaluated to identify hepatic masses because the incidence of hepatoma is increased in this usually cirrhotic population. Finally, biliary dilatation and the presence of portosystemic collaterals should be noted as well. Besides evaluating the liver and upper abdominal vasculature, assessment of splenic size and both kidneys is an essential part of all pretransplant evaluations.

Postoperatively, hepatic artery thrombosis is the most serious complication that can arise in the early posttransplant period and occurs most frequently in the first weeks. The incidence of hepatic artery thrombosis has been reported to be 3% to 12% in adults and 11% to 42% in children.[24] Thrombosis is particularly common in pediatric patients with small arteries or in patients who have required complex surgical procedures.

Combined duplex and color evaluation of the hepatic artery is usually begun in the region of the porta hepatis. In this location, the hepatic artery is large and easily visualized; the vessel also maintains a relatively constant relationship with the portal vein if an unusual arterial reconstruction has not been necessary. In most situations, a well-defined low-resistance arterial signal in the region of the porta hepatis is considered to confirm vascular patency. An absent hepatic arterial signal implies thrombosis of the hepatic artery. This is a poor prognostic sign and almost invariably dictates the need for retransplantation (Fig. 85-16). Unlike the normal liver, collateral pathways are absent and do not form for a considerable time, if at all. Compromise of the hepatic arterial circulation is typically associated with parenchymal infarction or ischemic damage to the biliary tree. The former produces focal hypoechoic lesions, whereas the latter causes segmental intrahepatic strictures. According to the study conducted by Worzney et al,[37] the incidence of hepatic artery thrombosis is 86% in patients with such lesions.

At some institutions, routine Doppler evaluation of the

hepatic artery is performed on specific postoperative days. As the experience in some centers has increased, the rate of vascular complication has declined enough that routine ultrasound is no longer performed in adults but reserved for patients with evidence of hepatic dysfunction. In addition, hepatic artery compromise is strongly suspected in any patient with imaging evidence of abscess, infarction, delayed biliary leak, or massive hepatic necrosis, and such patients should undergo Doppler evaluation.[37] In fact, patients with focal abnormalities or intrahepatic biliary dilatation are so likely to have hepatic artery compromise that arteriography should be considered even if the ultrasound reveals intrahepatic arterial signals. The Doppler study should be quite accurate in most cases, however; Flint et al[10] reported it showed a 92% accuracy in identifying hepatic artery thrombosis.

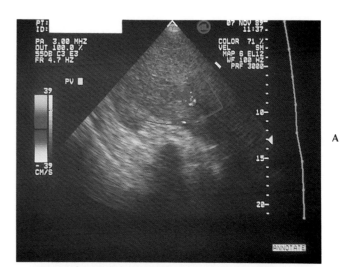

A

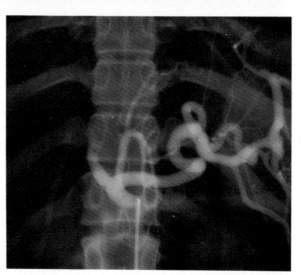

B

Fig. 85-16. Hepatic artery thrombosis. *A,* The patient 3 weeks after orthotopic liver transplantation with increasingly abnormal liver function tests. Color Doppler imaging shows normal flow in the portal vein. Hepatic artery signals are not identified in porta or elsewhere in the liver. *B,* A selective celiac arteriogram confirms hepatic artery thrombosis.

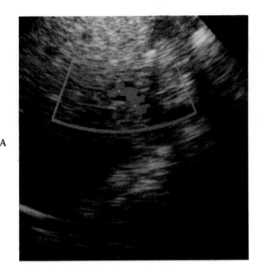

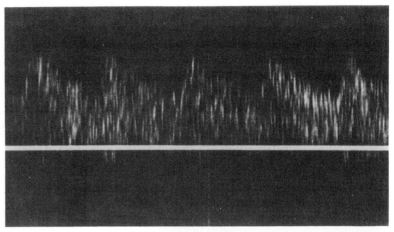

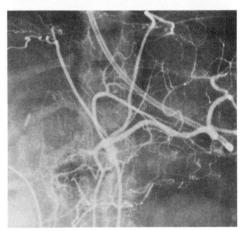

Fig. 85-17. Arterial collateral circulation in a pediatric liver transplant recipient with thrombosis of the hepatic artery. *A,* Color flow Doppler examination of the porta hepatis clearly shows flow in the transplanted liver. *B,* Analysis of spectral display from the anterior vessel confirms the presence of arterial blood flow in the porta (calculated resistive index is 0.4). *C,* A subsequent arteriogram shows thrombosis of the hepatic artery and several tiny collateral vessels. Additional small collaterals were seen with injection of the superior mesenteric artery (not shown).

The ability to form collateral vessels is limited after transplantation but may occur in children. (Collaterals have only been rarely identified in adults.) Flint et al,[10] however, concluded that flow in children with collaterals is sufficiently reduced such that Doppler signals should remain undetectable. Others have had the opposite experience,[14] and hepatic arterial signals have clearly been identified within the livers of some children (Fig. 85-17). Although arterial collateralization brings blood to the liver, the supply is insufficient and ischemia remains. Therefore these children are typically troubled by recurrent bouts of sepsis and persistent intrahepatic biliary dilatation. Arteriography should be considered in pediatric patients with evidence of hepatic artery ischemia, even if arterial signals are found. A review of the spectral tracings from these children shows that in general, the resistive index of the hepatic artery is low when a collateral bed is being sampled. Children with hepatic artery thrombosis and collateral formation may survive for long periods without retransplantation despite ischemic damage.[14,15]

Another potential problem affecting the hepatic artery is the development of anastomotic stenoses. Although relatively uncommon, this complication is yet another cause of ischemia and can produce findings similar to those of acute or chronic thrombosis. Patients with parenchymal abnormalities or bile duct strictures should be thoroughly evaluated with color Doppler to identify any potential area of hepatic artery stenosis because following the entire length of the hepatic artery may be difficult with duplex sonography alone. As expected, turbulent high-velocity flow is typical of focal hepatic artery stenosis.[4] Unfortunately, abnormal constricted hepatic arteries without stenosis may generate similar signals. Although ultrasound findings may not be specific, arteriography is indicated in either situation so that an unnecessary invasive procedure is not performed. Early identification of hepatic artery stenosis is essential to prevent complete thrombosis and extensive parenchymal damage. Once identified, hepatic artery stenosis can be treated successfully by angioplasty, thereby avoiding a surgical procedure.

Several investigators have analyzed hepatic arterial waveforms in an effort to diagnose transplant rejection. It is common to find instances in which there is little or no diastolic flow in this normally low-resistance artery (Fig. 85-18). Nevertheless, the studies of Longley et al[20] and Marder et al[22] have shown no correlation between absent diastolic flow and rejection. The reasons for the wide variations in the hepatic arterial flow patterns remain unclear;

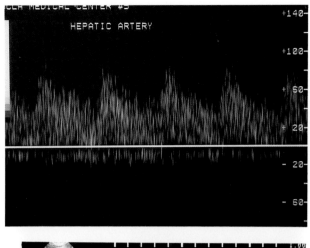

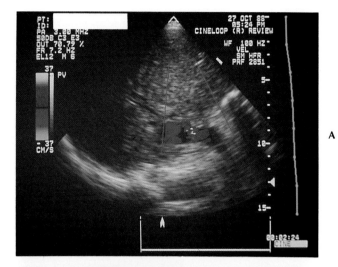

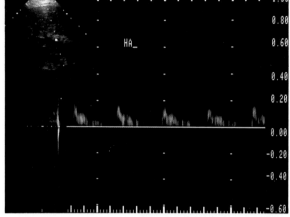

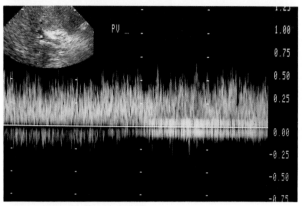

Fig. 85-18. Hepatic artery spectral patterns. *A,* A normal hepatic artery exhibits a low-resistance waveform with flow throughout diastole. *B,* A patient scanned portably 24 hours after transplant fails to show diastolic flow in the hepatic artery. The significance of loss of diastolic flow is uncertain but does not correlate with the presence of rejection.

Fig. 85-19. Normal portal vein. *A,* Color Doppler imaging reveals a narrow waist in the region of the vascular anastomosis *(arrowheads).* Note the mild postanastomotic dilatation. *B,* Spectral Doppler tracings reveal a spiked appearance, likely secondary to turbulence created by the anastomotic narrowing.

however, it was the conclusion in both studies that decreased diastolic flow has no apparent clinical significance.

PVT may also occur after transplantation. According to some authors, PVT is unusual, although Dalen et al[6] reported a frequency of 7.1%. Like hepatic arterial thrombosis, PVT is a devastating vascular complication, usually requiring retransplantation. As is true in the native liver, duplex or color Doppler should identify the vast majority of these thromboses.[34] The large normal portal vein is easily visualized in all transplants. A narrow waist with perivascular echogenic foci is produced by surgical clips and is frequently noted in the region of the anastomosis; moderate postanastomotic dilatation may also exist. Unusual spectral patterns that have an almost gurgling sound are common in patients after transplantation and are most likely due to turbulence originating in the region of the anastomosis (Fig.

85-19). Anastomotic narrowing may occasionally be severe enough to cause high-velocity flow, implying the existence of significant stenosis. The clinical implications of such stenoses, however, remain uncertain, but these cases do not appear to progress to frank thrombosis. In general, any patient who does not have a clearly patent portal vein identified by ultrasound should undergo angiography or at least MRI for further evaluation.

Air in the portal vein is also a frequent occurrence after transplantation. Although the exact cause is uncertain in this setting, it should not be considered a grave prognostic sign in transplant patients.[5] Moving, brightly echogenic foci within the portal vein and a bubbly sound on spectral Doppler analysis connote the presence of air in the portal vein (Fig. 85-20).

Although hepatic artery and portal vein thromboses are

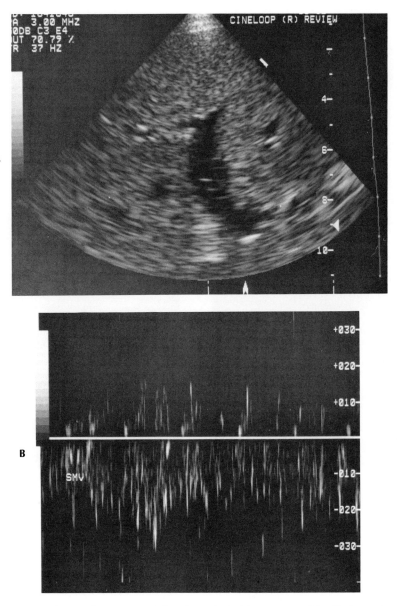

Fig. 85-20. Air in the portal vein. **A,** Brightly echogenic foci *(arrows)* were identified coursing through the portal vein in a patient 7 weeks after liver transplantation. **B,** Spectral Doppler from the portal vein and superior mesenteric vein revealed an unusual "pinging" sound; note the spikelike spectral tracing. These findings are typical of air in the portal vein.

the most clinically significant vascular abnormalities after transplantation, compromise of the IVC is far more common.[6] Moderate narrowing of the proximal IVC in the region of the surgical anastomosis has been sufficiently common that it is not now usually considered clinically significant (Fig. 85-21). Even complete thrombosis can be followed expectantly, and patients seem to do relatively well. Patients who have undergone retransplantation almost invariably suffer considerable compromise of the IVC and exhibit minor or no symptoms. Although compromise or thrombosis of

the IVC is common after transplantation, hepatic vein thrombosis is unusual. Three patent hepatic veins, however, should be visible in all transplant recipients to rule out thrombosis. Color Doppler may be required to define flow, since minor degrees of swelling can compress the vessels and render them invisible on real-time examination. Rarely, one or more (usually the middle and left) veins may be compromised at their junction with the IVC. Such focal narrowing of the hepatic veins is probably mechanical in origin and is usually seen in patients with a relatively small cavity who received a large liver.

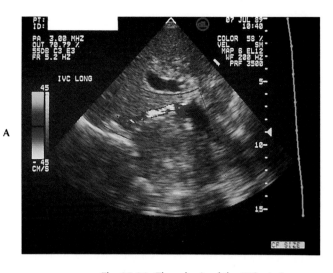
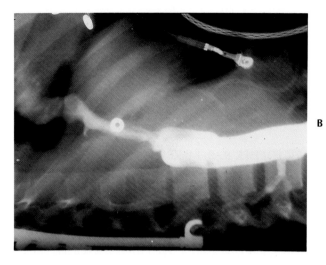

Fig. 85-21. Thrombosis of the IVC. *A,* Sonogram of a patient who has undergone a second transplant reveals marked narrowing of the proximal IVC *(arrows).* Note the large amount of thrombus posteriorly. *B,* An inferior vena cavagram confirmed the sonographic findings. Although such patients were initially a cause for concern, experience has shown that the majority of these cases do well.

REFERENCES

1. Abu-Yousef MM, Milam SG, Farner RM: Pulsatile portal vein flow: a sign of tricuspid regurgitation on duplex Doppler sonography, *AJR* 155:785-788, 1990.
2. Bezzi M et al: Iatrogenic aneurysmal portal-hepatic venous fistula: diagnosis by color Doppler imaging, *J Ultrasound Med* 7:457-459, 1988.
3. Cameron JL, Kadir S, Pierce WS: Mesoatrial shunt: a prosthesis modification, *Surgery* 96:114-116, 1984.
4. Cantarero JM et al: Hepatic artery anastomotic stenosis after transplantation: detection with duplex Doppler US, *J Ultrasound Med* 9:S26, 1990.
5. Chezmar JL, Nelson RC, Bernardino ME: Portal venous gas after hepatic transplantation: sonographic detection and clinical significance, *AJR* 153:1203-1205, 1989.
6. Dalen K et al: Imaging of vascular complications after hepatic transplantation, *AJR* 150:1285-1290, 1988.
7. Duerinckx A et al: The pulsatile portal vein: correlation of duplex Doppler with right atrial pressures, *Radiology* 176:655-658, 1990.
8. Endress C, Kling GA, Medrazo BL: Diagnosis of hepatic artery aneurysm with portal vein fistula using image-directed Doppler ultrasound, *J Clin Ultrasound* 17:206-208, 1989.
9. Falkoff GE, Taylor KJW, Morse S: Hepatic artery pseudoaneurysm: diagnosis with real-time and pulsed Doppler US, *Radiology* 158:55-56, 1986.
10. Flint EW et al: Duplex sonography of hepatic artery thrombosis after liver transplantation, *AJR* 151:481-483, 1988.
11. Foley WD et al: Dynamic computed tomography and pulsed Doppler ultrasonography in the evaluation of splenorenal shunt patency, *J Comput Assist Tomogr* 7:106-112, 1983.
12. Grant EG et al: Budd-Chiari syndrome: the results of duplex and color Doppler imaging, *AJR* 152:377-381, 1989.
13. Grant EG et al: Color Doppler imaging of portosystemic shunts, *AJR* 154:393-397, 1990.
14. Hall TR et al: False-negative duplex Doppler studies in children with hepatic artery thrombosis after liver transplantation, *AJR* 154:573-575, 1990.
15. Hoffer FA et al: Infected bilomas and hepatic artery thrombosis in infant recipients of liver transplants: interventional radiology and medical therapy as an alternative to retransplantation, *Radiology* 169:435-438, 1988.
16. Hosoki T et al: Hepatic venous outflow obstruction: evaluation with pulsed duplex sonography, *Radiology* 170:733-737, 1989.
17. Huey H, Cooperberg PL, Bogoch A: Diagnosis of giant varix of the coronary vein by pulsed-Doppler sonography, *AJR* 143:77-78, 1984.
18. Linberg B: *Diagnosis of portal hypertension by duplex sonography.* Paper presented at the 35th meeting of the American Institute of Ultrasound in Medicine, Atlanta, Ga, 1991.
19. Lois JF et al: Budd-Chiari syndrome: treatment with percutaneous transhepatic recanalization and dilation, *Radiology* 170:791-793, 1989.
20. Longley DG, Skolnick ML, Sheahan DG: Acute allograph rejection in liver transplant recipients: lack of correlation with loss of hepatic artery diastolic flow, *Radiology* 169:417-420, 1988.
21. Longley DG et al: Duplex Doppler sonography in the evaluation of adult patients before and after liver transplantation, *AJR* 151:687-696, 1988.
22. Marder DM et al: Liver transplant rejection: value of the resistive index in Doppler US of hepatic arteries, *Radiology* 173:127-129, 1989.
23. Middleton WD, Erickson S, Melson GL: Perivascular color artifact: pathologic significance and appearance on color Doppler US images, *Radiology* 171:647-652, 1989.
24. Morton MJ et al: Applications of duplex ultrasonography in the liver transplant patient, *Mayo Clin Proc* 65:360-363, 1990.
25. Nelson RC et al: Comparison of pulsed Doppler sonography and angiography in patients with portal hypertension, *AJR* 149:77-81, 1987.
26. Parker RGF: Occlusion of the hepatic veins in man, *Medicine* 38:369-402, 1959.
27. Patriquin H et al: The duplex Doppler examination in portal hypertension: technique and anatomy, *AJR* 149:71-76, 1987.
28. Ralls PW: Color Doppler sonography of the hepatic artery and portal venous system, *AJR* 155:522-525, 1990.
29. Ralls PW et al: The use of color Doppler sonography to distinguish dilated intrahepatic ducts from vascular structures, *AJR* 152:291-292, 1989.
30. Shenk WG et al: Direct measurement of hepatic blood flow in surgical patients, *Ann Surg* 156:463-467, 1962.
31. Sukigara M, Kimura S, Adachi H: Primary Budd-Chiari syndrome: demonstration by real-time two dimensional Doppler echography, *J Clin Ultrasound* 17:615-618, 1989.
32. Taylor KJW et al: Blood flow in deep abdominal and pelvic vessels: ultrasonic pulsed-Doppler analysis, *Radiology* 154:487-493, 1985.
33. Taylor KJW et al: Liver transplant recipients: portable duplex US with correlative angiography, *Radiology* 159:357-363, 1986.
34. Tessler FT et al: Diagnosis of portal vein thrombosis: value of color Doppler imaging, *AJR* 157:293-296, 1991.
35. Vine HS et al: Portal vein aneurysm, *AJR* 132:557-558, 1979.
36. Wing VW et al: Sonographic differentiation of enlarged hepatic arteries from dilated intrahepatic bile ducts, *AJR* 145:57-60, 1985.
37. Worzney P et al: Vascular complications after liver transplantation: a 5-year experience, *AJR* 147:657-663, 1986.

CHAPTER 86

Ultrasound of the pancreas, pancreatic transplant, and spleen

CHRISTOPHER R. B. MERRITT

Ultrasound is one of several imaging methods currently used to evaluate the pancreas and spleen. When not limited by the presence of excessive bowel gas, ultrasound has demonstrated good sensitivity and specificity in the identification of tumors, inflammatory conditions, and cysts. Although computed tomography (CT) and magnetic resonance imaging (MRI) are generally used for the primary imaging of suspected disease, ultrasonography remains an important complementary imaging method because the equipment is portable and, when used in conjunction with Doppler, is capable of evaluating flow. Ultrasound is also important as an aid in the localization of masses for aspiration or biopsy. Duplex Doppler ultrasound and Doppler color imaging (DCI) add to the specificity of ultrasound and have improved the diagnosis of the relatively uncommon vascular abnormalities that arise in the pancreas and spleen. In addition, ultrasound methods have become indispensable in the postoperative management of patients after pancreatic transplantation.

EXAMINATION TECHNIQUE

The primary impediment to successful sonographic examination of the pancreas is the presence of gas within the stomach and bowel. This is less a problem for splenic ultrasound and the evaluation of pancreatic transplant recipients. Having patients fast before ultrasound examination is helpful in reducing the amount of bowel gas. Patients should also be encouraged not to smoke or chew gum before examination because this may cause the ingestion of large quantities of air. Positioning the patient in an erect, semierect, or decubitus position occasionally enhances visualization of the pancreas by shifting the position of bowel gas. Similarly, scanning with the patient in suspended inspiration may permit the left lobe of the liver to be used as an acoustic window by displacing gastric contents inferiorly and laterally. If the pancreas is not clearly seen using these maneuvers, it may be helpful to partially fill the stomach with water or other noncarbonated liquid and use the fluid path created as an acoustic window into the area of interest. In most patients, satisfactory imaging of the head and body of the pancreas is possible using these techniques. Imaging of the pancreatic tail is more difficult and occasionally is

made possible by using prone views through the upper pole of the left kidney. The spleen is more easily evaluated than the pancreas. For splenic imaging, it is desirable to use a transducer face small enough to permit scanning through the lower intercostal spaces. Coronal and axial imaging planes are used to evaluate splenic size and contour when scanning through the left lower rib cage. Subcostal imaging is possible if the spleen extends below the costal margin. Most pancreatic transplants are placed in the iliac fossa and are readily accessible for imaging.

Imaging is generally performed using 3.5- to 5.0-MHz sector scanners or curved arrays. In very large patients, transducers operating at lower frequencies may be helpful. Frequencies as high as 7.5 MHz may be used to examine superficial pancreatic transplants in thin patients. In general, the examination should be conducted using the highest imaging frequency that permits complete visualization of the pertinent structures. Duplex Doppler and DCI usually require frequencies in the range of 2.25 to 5.0 MHz so that penetration is achieved to sample deep abdominal vessels. When using Doppler, it is important to remember that the low pulse-repetition frequency required to investigate deep vessels may result in aliasing, particularly at higher Doppler frequencies.

Routine examination of the pancreas should include axial and longitudinal views of the pancreas and the splenic, mesenteric, and portal vessels, as well as the common bile duct and inferior vena cava. Each of these structures is intimately related to the pancreas and serves as a landmark for the delineation of pancreatic anatomy. Duplex Doppler and DCI are indicated in patients with hepatic disease and masses related to the pancreas or spleen. In patients with portal hypertension, color-Doppler evaluation of the splenic hilum and retroperitoneum in the vicinity of the left kidney and left renal vein should be performed to identify portosystemic collateral veins that commonly form in this location. The presence and direction of flow in the splenic artery and vein should be determined along with the existence of any collateral veins.

The major sonographic landmarks for delineating the pancreas include the aorta, the superior mesenteric artery and vein, the portal and splenic veins, and the inferior vena cava. The left adrenal gland and upper pole of the left kidney lie posterior to the tail of the pancreas. The splenic and mesenteric vessels as well as the inferior vena cava constitute the most visible landmarks for sonographic examination of the pancreas (Fig. 86-1). The head of the pancreas lies anterior to the inferior vena cava just caudal to the level of the main portal vein. In axial and longitudinal images, the common bile duct is often visible as it descends along the posterolateral margin of the head of the pancreas. With the application of high-quality imaging or DCI, the gastroduodenal artery can be seen from its origin at the hepatic artery and then as it descends along the anterolateral margin of the pancreatic head. Starting from the head of the pancreas, the uncinate process extends medially to the left and then lies posterior to the superior mesenteric vein. The main portal vein and the confluence of the splenic and superior mesenteric veins, which forms the portal vein, lie posterior to the neck of the pancreas. The superior and posterior borders of the body and tail of the pancreas are delineated by the splenic artery and vein, with the artery lying superior to the vein. These vessels are usually visible with real-time imaging. The pancreas is normally imaged in transverse (axial) planes as well as in parasagittal longitudinal planes. Inspection of the pancreas includes evaluation of its size, parenchymal echogenicity, and the presence of masses or vascular abnormalities. The usual vascular abnormalities seen in the native pancreas include venous and, less often, arterial occlusion stemming from invasion by pancreatic carcinoma or occlusion related to pancreatitis.

The spleen is a homogeneous organ with an echogenicity similar to that of the liver and is normally less than 12 cm in greatest diameter. Accessory splenic tissue is common, and small masses near the splenic hilum or splenic border are frequently observed with ultrasound and must be differentiated from enlarged lymph nodes. The splenic hilum and major divisions of the splenic vein and artery are regularly imaged with real-time ultrasound, and secondary and tertiary branches of these vessels are demonstrable with DCI. Splenic artery aneurysms due to arteriosclerosis or secondary to vascular damage caused by pancreatitis are also demonstrable with ultrasound. Transverse images in the epigastrium are usually best for demonstrating the splenic artery and vein in the region of the pancreatic body. The more distal portions of the splenic vessels are best shown by scanning in axial or oblique planes through the spleen, using the homogeneous splenic tissue as an acoustic window.

PANCREAS

Pancreatitis and pancreatic carcinoma are the most important pancreatic abnormalities in which ultrasonography plays a role. The diagnosis of acute pancreatitis is usually based on clinical and laboratory findings. CT and ultrasound are used to identify complications, including phlegmon, hemorrhage, abscess, necrosis, and pseudocyst. Vascular complications of pancreatitis include splenic and portal vein thrombosis and aneurysm formation. A potentially life-threatening complication of pancreatitis is the development of splenic artery pseudoaneurysm. Rupture of such vascular lesions may cause recurrent bleeding or rapid exsanguination. Doppler ultrasound, particularly in conjunction with DCI, permits the rapid and simple evaluation of sonolucent masses associated with pancreatitis, confirmation of splenic artery and vein patency, and differentiation of cystic masses from aneurysm, pseudoaneurysm, portosystemic collateral veins, and arteriovenous fistulas.[4,12]

A continuing challenge in abdominal imaging is the early diagnosis of pancreatic carcinoma and the differentiation of benign pancreatic conditions, particularly pancreatitis, from pancreatic carcinoma. Most pancreatic cancers are identified at a stage when successful treatment is impossible, and the long-term survival rate of patients with pancreatic carcinoma has not improved over the past 25 years, despite the advent of ultrasound, CT, and MRI. In skilled hands, ultrasound imaging is comparable to or better than CT in the diagnosis of pancreatic cancer, provided the examination permits imaging of the entire pancreas.[3] When portions of the pancreas are obscured, ultrasound is less reliable than CT. CT is also preferred over ultrasonography in demonstrating changes stemming from direct extension of tumors into the retroperitoneal fat.

Differentiating focal pancreatitis or focal masses associated with chronic pancreatitis from pancreatic cancer may be difficult because the clinical presentation may be similar and CT and ultrasound imaging findings are relatively nonspecific. Histologic examination of biopsy material is currently the only reliable method for distinguishing pancreatic

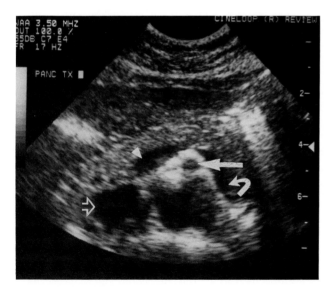

Fig. 86-1. The normal pancreas. This transverse real-time image at the level of the superior mesenteric artery shows the splenic vein *(curved arrow)*, superior mesenteric artery *(straight arrow)*, superior mesenteric vein *(arrowhead)*, and inferior vena cava *(open arrow)*. These vessels delineate the posterior border of the body of the pancreas.

cancer from chronic pancreatitis. Doppler ultrasound has the potential to improve the specificity of pancreatic ultrasonography. Tumor neovascularity has been reported to be a useful finding in differentiating benign inflammatory and malignant conditions at numerous sites in the abdomen and pelvis. Continuous-wave Doppler as well as Doppler spectral analysis and DCI display characteristic patterns useful in the differentiation of benign and malignant pancreatic lesions.[9,18] Taylor et al[18] have shown that frequency shifts in excess of 3 kHz (3.0-MHz insonating frequency) are associated with pancreatic carcinoma as well as a variety of hepatic and renal lesions. DCI has been reported to show abnormal blood flow patterns in patients with pancreatic carcinoma as well as other tumors.[9]

New approaches to the evaluation of the pancreas and surrounding retroperitoneum include the use of endoscopic scanning techniques. Using high-frequency transducers, these devices may be able to detect much smaller lesions than transabdominal scanners and eliminate many of the restrictions to examination posed by bowel gas and large patient size. The sensitivity and specificity of endoscopic ultrasonography in pancreatic tumor diagnosis are significantly higher than those of transabdominal ultrasound and CT but equal to those of endoscopic retrograde cholangiopancreatography, although endoscopic ultrasonography cannot reliably differentiate malignant from inflammatory pancreatic masses.[7,17] The possibility of adding endoscopic Doppler to the imaging assessment has not been investigated. With the higher Doppler sensitivity permitted by this approach, increased specificity of ultrasound diagnosis might be achieved.

Another area in which ultrasound has shown considerable success is in the intraoperative evaluation of patients with functional pancreatic tumors, such as insulinomas.[14,19] Although new methods such as transhepatic venous sampling have aided in confirming the presence of insulinomas in the pancreas, they do not provide the precise localization needed for surgical removal. Intraoperative ultrasound is the single best method for identifying occult functional pancreatic tumors. Because functional tumors may be highly vascular, there is a potential for improving detection using Doppler methods; however, the possible contributions of Doppler ultrasound and DCI to intraoperative imaging remain to be investigated.

PANCREATIC TRANSPLANTATION

Since 1966, when the first segmental pancreatic transplantation was performed, this therapy has become an increasingly important option for the management of type I diabetes mellitus. Although early efforts were frustrated by technical failure and organ rejection, resulting in high graft failure rates and recipient mortality, recent improvements in immunosuppression and higher technical success rates have spawned a sharp increase in the number of patients undergoing transplantation. With better control of rejection, graft ischemia due to arterial or venous thrombosis or stenosis

has become the major cause of transplant failure in the early posttransplant period. As in renal and hepatic transplant patients, the integrity of the arterial and venous supply is critical in pancreatic transplant recipients, and duplex and color Doppler are now commonly used to monitor postoperative blood flow to the pancreas.[1,15,20]

The transplanted pancreas, like the kidney, is located superficially, making it well suited for ultrasound examination. Imaging with high-frequency transducers (5.0 to 7.5 MHz) is possible, and major vessels are readily accessible for duplex or color Doppler interrogation. The arterial supply of the pancreatic allograft comes from the celiac and superior mesenteric arteries. These vessels are anastomosed to the iliac artery (Fig. 86-2). The portal vein is anastomosed to the external iliac vein to provide venous drainage. Drainage of pancreatic secretions is achieved by a variety of procedures, frequently by duodenocystostomy.

Common complications of pancreatic transplantation are vascular thrombosis, intraabdominal infection, rejection, anastomotic leaks, and pancreatitis. Biochemical abnormalities may accompany these complications but are not specific. Imaging techniques, including CT, ultrasound imaging, Doppler ultrasonography, and radionuclide imaging, may aid in the diagnosis of these complications. Scintigraphy using ^{99m}Tc-DTPA perfusion scanning is a sensitive method for confirming normal function; however, abnormal results may be due to a variety of causes. Sonography, using both imaging and flow assessment, is the procedure of choice for detecting fluid collections and identifying pancreatitis, vascular thrombosis, pancreatic duct malfunction, and to some extent organ rejection.

Postoperative evaluation of the pancreas transplant patient should include careful inspection of the pancreas, the transplant vessels, and surrounding structures. The normal pancreatic transplant appears sonographically as a homogeneous structure possessing low to moderate echogenicity and lying medial to the iliac vessels. The normal anteroposterior dimension of the pancreatic allograft ranges from 1.5 to 2.0 cm. Changes in size are not specific, and pancreatic enlargement may accompany pancreatitis, acute rejection, infection, or venous thrombosis. Similarly, changes in the echogenicity of the pancreas may accompany infarction, pancreatitis, and rejection.[11] Peritransplant fluid collections of varying size are noted in over 50% of patients after transplantation.[2] These collections may indicate the presence of pseudocyst, abscess, hematoma, seroma, or lymphocele; aspiration and examination of the fluid are required to establish the diagnosis.[16] Doppler ultrasound characterizes arterial flow to the transplant as a low-resistance waveform with flow continuing throughout diastole.

Doppler ultrasound aids in the early identification of technical problems with arterial and venous anastomoses and is increasingly important in transplant evaluation (Fig. 86-3). Imaging and Doppler evaluation of the pancreas transplant are complementary, in that each component of the examination provides unique information useful in patient man-

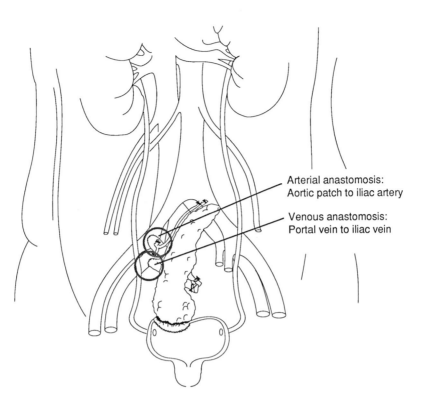

Fig. 86-2. Common vascular anastomoses used in pancreatic transplantation. The arterial supply of the pancreatic allograft is from the celiac and superior mesenteric arteries. These vessels are anastomosed to the iliac artery. The portal vein is anastomosed to the external iliac vein to provide venous drainage. Pancreatic secretions are drained by a variety of procedures, frequently by duodenocystostomy.

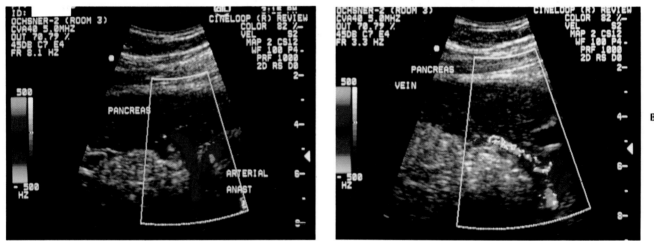

Fig. 86-3. A normal pancreatic allograft. DCI clearly shows the main arterial **(A)** and venous **(B)** anastomoses of the pancreatic allograft as well as intrapancreatic arterial and venous branches.

agement. The iliac artery and vein are examined to identify the anastomoses of the celiac and superior mesenteric arteries and the portal vein. It is easy to confirm flow within the body of the pancreas by visualizing the splenic artery and vein along the posterior aspect of the allograft. Thrombosis of the veins draining the pancreatic transplant is a particularly important cause of graft loss.[8] Venous thrombosis is reported to be most common in the first week after transplantation and, if untreated, results in rapid infarction of the transplant. Combined with scintigraphy, ultrasound has permitted the early identification of transplant vein thrombosis and ultimate salvage of the organ.[1] Duplex

Doppler findings associated with venous thrombosis include absence of demonstrable flow in the transplant vein and abnormalities in the transplant celiac and splenic arteries with a blunted systolic peak and reversal of flow in diastole. This waveform indicates high vascular resistance and suggests the existence of venous outflow obstruction.

In contrast to the clear value of ultrasound for identifying technical complications of transplantation, the role of ultrasound in the diagnosis of transplant rejection is clouded by the lack of large studies that properly evaluate its sensitivity and specificity. Changes in the echogenicity of the transplant organ have been observed in association with rejection but appear to be nonspecific. The Doppler patterns in patients with transplant dysfunction have also been inconsistent. Kubota et al[10] have reported the results of duplex Doppler evaluation in nine insulin-dependent type I diabetics undergoing pancreatic transplantation. The transplant arterial resistive index (RI) determined with Doppler was correlated with the findings from biochemical and pathologic assessment of rejection. A relatively high RI (0.72) was found in the immediate posttransplant period (3 days). In normal transplant recipients, the RI later declined, and the mean RI was 0.64 in patients who showed no signs of rejection. In the event of acute rejection, the RI was slightly elevated, but the difference was not useful for diagnosing rejection. Absence of arterial pulsation was noted in one patient with arterial thrombosis. Other studies using color and duplex Doppler[13] noted a mean normal arterial RI of 0.71 ± 0.12 but revealed that RI calculations alone were not helpful in diagnosing graft rejection. In contrast to these reports, some investigators have noted an association between acute rejection and high RI values (greater than 0.8). In a study of 22 patients in which duplex ultrasonography was used, Patel, Wolverson, and Mahanta[15] noted an RI of 0.70 or less in the parenchymal vessels of normal transplant recipients and values greater than 0.70 obtained during seven of eight clinical episodes of rejection (87.5%). In all studies performed during these eight cases of rejection, the positive predictive value of an RI exceeding 0.70 was 100%. The negative predictive value of an RI less than 0.70 for excluding rejection was 90%. High RI values were not found in the content of isolated episodes of cyclosporine toxicity, pancreatitis, peripancreatic hemorrhage, or infection. Gilabert et al[5] also reported low-impedance arterial waveforms in five patients with normally functioning grafts and abnormal waveforms in cases of rejection and venous thrombosis, in which Doppler showed increased arterial impedance. Despite these findings, when rejection is suspected, biopsy is usually necessary. Ultrasound is helpful in guiding biopsy, and if DCI is used, major transplant vessels can be visualized, thus reducing the risk of inadvertent vascular damage.

SPLEEN

Ultrasound, CT, and MRI are primary methods for evaluating the spleen. Because it is extremely homogeneous, the spleen is well suited for sonographic examination. Although ultrasound constitutes an accurate and noninvasive method for examining the splenic vasculature, Doppler currently has a relatively minor role in this setting. DCI or duplex Doppler ultrasound can be used to confirm splenic artery and vein patency and aid in the diagnosis of splenic vascular abnormalities such as splenic artery aneurysms and portosystemic collaterals.

The splenic artery is the largest branch of the celiac trunk, arising distal to the left gastric artery. It is normally visible at its origin and as it courses laterally along the posterior and superior margin of the pancreas (see Fig. 86-1). At the hilum of the spleen, the artery branches into six or more main divisions. The splenic artery has a low-resistance waveform characterized by continuous diastolic flow (Fig. 86-4). The splenic vein passes medially posterior to the pancreas. Here it is readily distinguished from the splenic artery by its more caudal location and a diameter roughly twice that of the artery. Although the spleen is located intraperitoneally, the splenorenal ligament, which contains the splenic artery and vein, is situated retroperitoneally. In most persons, a portion of the splenic capsule is fused with the dorsal mesentery anterior to the upper pole of the left kidney. In this area, vascular communications from the spleen to systemic veins, including the left renal vein, may develop in patients with portal hypertension. Paraumbilical, gastroesophageal, pancreaticoduodenal, retroperitoneal, splenorenal, and gastrorenal collaterals have all been found in patients with portal hypertension examined with duplex Doppler or DCI. Portosystemic shunts may develop spontaneously through collateral vessels or may be created surgically to treat symptomatic portal hypertension. DCI is valuable in demonstrating both natural splenorenal shunts and the patency of surgically created portosystemic shunts extending from the splenic vein to the renal vein (distal splenorenal or Warren shunts). In the case of splenorenal shunts, patency is established by demonstration of flow in both the splenic and renal veins in appropriate directions. Grant et al[6] have reported the successful identification of shunt patency or thrombosis in 100% of 22 portosystemic shunts and found DCI to be clearly superior for such purposes. In these patients, scanning through the spleen usually allows good visualization of the pertinent vessels. DCI often indicates the presence of more extensive collaterals than does gray-scale imaging alone (Fig. 86-5).

Ultrasound examination of the spleen can reveal changes stemming from a variety of abnormalities, but in many cases the abnormalities are not specific. Diffuse diseases, including infection, neoplasm, infiltration, metabolic disease, hematologic disease, and portal hypertension, may all precipitate splenomegaly but are not characterized by specific sonographic patterns. Focal splenic lesions can result from infection, neoplasm, trauma, and other conditions, but most of these are not vascular enough to be detected by Doppler ultrasound. Splenic infarction produces characteristic peripheral wedge-shaped hypoechoic lesions on ultrasound imaging, but vascular changes have not been described.

Congenital anomalies of the spleen include accessory

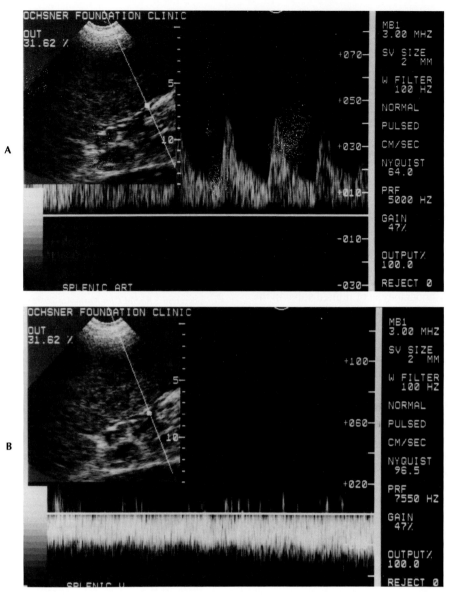

Fig. 86-4. Normal splenic vessels. Splenic arterial *(A)* and venous *(B)* waveforms are shown.

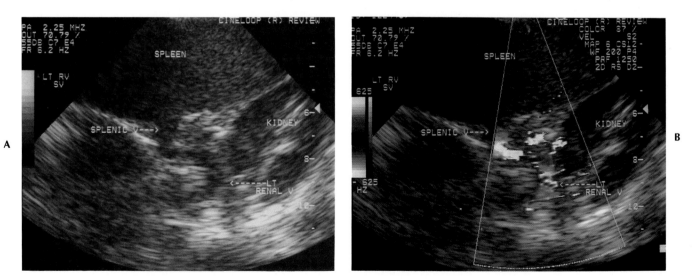

Fig. 86-5. Splenorenal shunt. *A,* Real-time gray-scale image of the retroperitoneum adjacent to the splenic vein in a patient with portal hypertension fails to clearly indicate vascular abnormality. *B,* With DCI, however, a spontaneous splenorenal shunt is seen. Flow is from the splenic vein through retroperitoneal collaterals into the left renal vein. DCI is valuable in demonstrating natural splenorenal shunts as well as the patency of surgically created portosystemic shunts.

spleens, and in some cases, Doppler may aid in differentiating an accessory spleen from enlarged lymph nodes by showing their vascular supply. If the spleen develops with a long, mobile mesentery, it may undergo torsion and cause acute abdominal pain. Doppler may be helpful in identifying this by showing abnormal blood flow. Splenic abnormalities may also be seen in asplenia and polysplenia syndromes. In these disorders, it is important to determine the location of the liver and spleen and the arrangement of the abdominal vasculature. Because biliary atresia is associated with polysplenia and its attendant vascular abnormalities, it is important to recognize this problem in patients being considered for liver transplantation to treat biliary atresia.

CONCLUSION

Although Doppler ultrasonography is of limited value in the examination of the pancreas and spleen, it is a useful adjunct to real-time imaging, CT, and MRI in selected patients. This is especially true when an aneurysm, pseudoaneurysm, or arteriovenous fistula is suspected. Doppler investigation is also valuable in the identification and mapping of portosystemic collaterals, the diagnosis of vein occlusion, and the characterization of masses as vascular or avascular. Although Doppler is currently an ancillary procedure in the examination of the native pancreas, it is an essential component in the postoperative management of pancreatic transplant recipients, aiding in the early recognition of technical problems associated with vascular anastomoses. Doppler is currently less useful for identifying pancreatic transplant rejection. Intraoperative, endoscopic, and contrast-enhanced applications may offer new opportunities for pancreatic and splenic ultrasound in the near future.

REFERENCES

1. Boiskin I et al: Acute venous thrombosis after pancreas transplantation: diagnosis with duplex Doppler sonography and scintigraphy, *AJR* 154:529-531, 1990.
2. Crass JR et al: Radiology of the human segmental pancreatic transplant, *Gastrointest Radiol* 7:153-158, 1982.
3. DelMaschio A et al: Pancreatic cancer versus chronic pancreatitis: diagnosis with CA 19-9 assessment, US, CT, and CT-guided fine-needle biopsy, *Radiology* 178:95-99, 1991.
4. Falkoff GE, Taylor KJ, Morse S: Hepatic artery pseudoaneurysm: diagnosis with real-time and pulsed Doppler US, *Radiology* 158:55-56, 1986.
5. Gilabert R et al: Duplex-Doppler ultrasonography in monitoring clinical pancreas transplantation, *Transpl Int* 1:172-177, 1988.
6. Grant EG et al: Color Doppler imaging of portosystemic shunts, *AJR* 154:393-397, 1990.
7. Grimm H, Maydeo A, Soehendra N: Endoluminal ultrasound for the diagnosis and staging of pancreatic cancer, *Baillieres Clin Gastroenterol* 4:869-888, 1990.
8. Hanto DW, Sutherland DER: Pancreas transplantation: clinical considerations, *Radiol Clin North Am* 25:333-343, 1987.
9. Itoh K et al: Evaluation of blood flow in tumor masses by using 2D-Doppler color flow mapping—case reports, *Angiology* 38:705-711, 1987.
10. Kubota K et al: Duplex-Doppler ultrasonography for evaluating pancreatic grafts, *Transplant Proc* 22:183, 1990.
11. Letourneau JG et al: Ultrasound and computed tomography in the evaluation of pancreatic transplantation, *Radiol Clin North Am* 25:345-355, 1987.
12. Merritt CRB: *Vascular accidents: aneurysms and thrombosis of the hepatic, splenic and portal vessels.* In Serafini AN, Guter M, eds: *Medical imaging of the liver and spleen,* Norwalk, Conn, 1983, Appleton-Lange.
13. Milner LN et al: Ultrasound imaging of pancreaticoduodenal transplants, *J Clin Gastroenterol* 13:570-574, 1991.
14. Norton JA: Localization and surgical treatment of occult insulinomas, *Ann Surg* 212:615-620, 1990.
15. Patel B, Wolverson MK, Mahanta B: Pancreatic transplant rejection: assessment with duplex US, *Radiology* 173:131-135, 1989.
16. Patel BK et al: Fluid collections developing after pancreatic transplantation: radiologic evaluation and intervention, *Radiology* 181(1):215-220, 1991.
17. Rosch T et al: Endoscopic ultrasound in pancreatic tumor diagnosis, *Gastrointest Endosc* 37:347-352, 1991.
18. Taylor KJ et al: Correlation of Doppler US tumor signals with neovascular morphologic features, *Radiology* 166:57-62, 1988.
19. Wilms G et al: Percutaneous transhepatic venous sampling of the pancreas in localizing insulinomas, *J Belge Radiol* 73:453-457, 1990.
20. Yang HC et al: Evaluation of pancreatic allograft circulation using color Doppler ultrasonography, *Transplant Proc* 22:609-611, 1990.

CHAPTER 87

Intraoperative ultrasonic evaluation: hepatic anatomy

TREVOR LEESE and HENRI BISMUTH

Intraoperative ultrasonography is now a firmly established procedure in hepatic surgery. It has made the liver "transparent"—an advance that is proving as important for hepatic surgery as the introduction of intraoperative cholangiography in biliary surgery some 50 years ago. In this chapter, the technical aspects, methodology, and applications of intraoperative sonography in hepatic surgery are described and examples from the experience at Paul Brousse Hospital over the past 6 years with more than 1000 patients who had abdominal surgery are given.

INTRAOPERATIVE ULTRASONOGRAPHY

Intraoperative ultrasonography was introduced in the 1960s in both urologic[23] and biliary surgery. The applications were considerably limited by the poor images obtained with A-mode ultrasound.

The development of the new generation of real-time B-mode ultrasound machines has resulted in images possessing a quality that corresponds closely to anatomic reality. Much information can be obtained as to the nature, exact position, and vascularization of lesions. Once again, major applications for this new technique are in urologic and biliary surgery, but its use has been extended to other domains, including pancreatic[5] and hepatic surgery.[19]

The ultrasound signal used in the abdomen has a frequency of 2 to 10 MHz. These frequencies provide good definition and permit study of an adequate depth of parenchyma. One of the great advantages of intraoperative ultrasound is that the transducer, which alternatively emits and receives the signal, can be placed directly in contact with the organ. Thus the depth to be explored is reduced in comparison with percutaneous examination in which the thickness of the abdominal wall must be added. Because no energy is lost by passage of the ultrasound signal through the abdominal wall, higher frequencies can be used to obtain better definition. Another advantage of it is that the liver can be mobilized at the time of surgery, allowing multiple images to be taken without interference from intervening ribs or gas-filled loops of bowel.

At Paul Brousse Hospital, a real-time B-mode ultrasound machine with a linear rather than a sectoral array is used. The linear array deforms the image less, and the structure to be studied can be situated in the direct axis of the beam. The machines used at first were the Scanel 300 and 500* and the Aloka SSD-256,† but other good machines are also available. These machines were not designed specifically for intraoperative use. Ideally, the machine should be small and mobile for ease of movement between one operating room and another and should be simple to use. The gain and the focus should be the only adjustments required on a daily basis.

The probe is the element that is specific to intraoperative use, and the choice is important. It must be waterproof and totally sterilizable, including the attachment to the machine. The cable must be sufficiently long (approximately 2.5 m) and supple to enable the maneuvers necessary for a thorough exploration. Most important is the sound itself: 5-MHz probes 7 × 2 × 1.5 cm for the Aloka machine (UST 582 I 5 and UST 582 T 5) are used and 5- and 7.5-MHz probes 7 × 2 × 0.5 cm for the Scanel (slot 5 and slot 7.5). For the liver, a T-shaped probe is the most useful because it can be placed parallel to the portal bifurcation (Fig. 87-1) and can be moved easily between the liver and the diaphragm. A 5-MHz sound permits a maximum depth of exploration of 10 to 15 cm, which is sufficient for the liver. For the extrahepatic bile ducts and pancreas, a straight probe is easier to manipulate, and 7.5 MHz or even 10 MHz can be used because the depth of tissue to be explored is less.

Immediately beneath the probe is a zone that is inexplorable. The size of the zone varies according to the probe being used, but it is often about 0.5 cm. To overcome this, a water-filled bag can be placed between the probe and the organ being examined. This moves the probe back 1 to 2 cm while conserving good ultrasonographic contact. The wall of the bag must be thin and the liquid must be free of air bubbles to avoid attenuation of the signal. A water-filled rubber preservative is also suitable and inexpensive. For liver ultrasound, the probe is usually placed directly on the surface of the liver without the use of a water bag. It is not necessary to use contact gel because the natural humidity of the organ is usually enough to obtain a good contact.

*CGR Ultrasonic, 77102 Meaux, France.
†Aloka Co, Ltd., Japan.

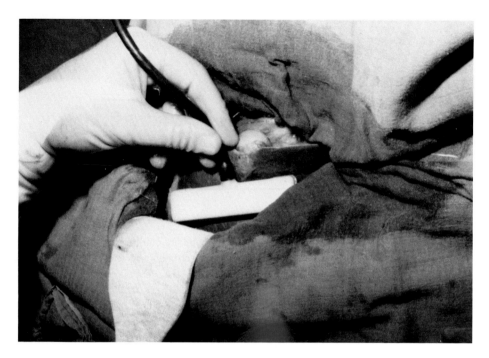

Fig. 87-1. The T-shaped Scanel beam placed directly on the surface of the liver.

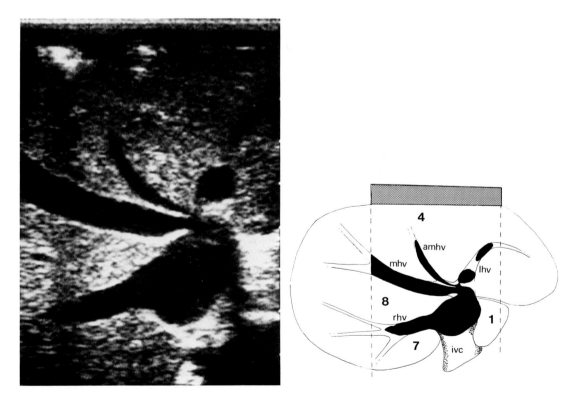

Fig. 87-2. The union of the hepatic veins with the inferior vena cava *(ivc)*. This patient has an accessory middle hepatic vein *(amhv)* joining the confluence of the left hepatic vein *(lhv)* and the middle hepatic vein *(mhv)*. *rhv,* Right hepatic vein.

The water-filled bag is used principally in the exploration of the extrahepatic bile ducts and pancreas.

SURGICAL ANATOMY OF THE LIVER

A thorough ultrasound examination of the liver requires the division of any adhesions and mobilization of the liver so that one hand and the probe can be placed between the diaphragm and the liver. The examination can be made through most abdominal incisions, but a right subcostal or upper median or paramedian incision is the easiest to use. The examination can be performed through a small preliminary incision to determine if there are any formal contraindications to continuing the operation. The probe should be held against the surface of the liver with gentle pressure that is sufficient to obtain good contact but not enough to distort the intrahepatic vascular structures, particularly the hepatic veins. The probe is moved gently in different directions, creating small rotatory movements about its axis and a sweep in depth that allows the real volume of structures to be recognized.

A systematic examination of the liver starts with a study of the three hepatic veins at their points of entry into the inferior vena cava. This is achieved by placing the probe on the anterior surface of the liver and angling the plane of examination obliquely upward (Fig. 87-2). By inclining the probe to the right and left, it is possible to follow the hepatic veins into the liver parenchyma and to their branches of origin, even down to branches of 2 or 3 mm in diameter.

The examination continues with a study of the portal pedicles, surrounded by their echo-dense prolongations of Glisson's capsule. Once again the sound probe is placed horizontally on the anterior surface of the liver, slightly lower than the position used for the study of the hepatic veins. To the left, the recess of Rex is readily identified (Fig. 87-3) continuing into the round ligament. The left portal branch can be followed back to the hilum and to the right portal branch, which divides into anterior and posterior pedicles.

Next, the liver parenchyma of each segment must be explored meticulously and, finally, the gallbladder and he-

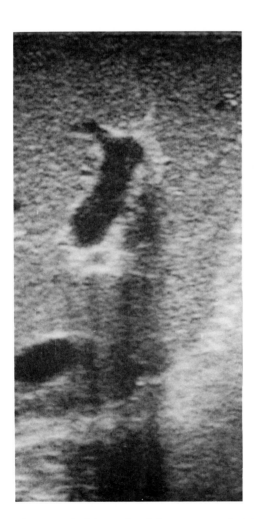
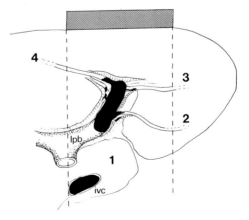

Fig. 87-3. The left portal pedicle, comprising the left portal branch *(lpb)* surrounded by its covering of Glisson's capsule. The branches to segments 2, 3, and 4 are seen. *ivc,* Inferior vena cava.

patic pedicle. The last is explored in part transhepatically and in part directly by using the water bag.

The inferior vena cava and hepatic veins

The inferior vena cava runs longitudinally to the right of the midline. It appears as an echo-free band with a thin wall that is quite posterior in relation to the liver. Its diameter alters slightly with respiration. The confluence of the three hepatic veins and the inferior vena cava is relatively easy to locate. The hepatic veins have no covering of Glisson's capsule and thus appear in the liver parenchyma as echo-free linear bands. Their walls are not visible or appear only as a fine margin echo. The hepatic veins also can be recognized by transmitted heartbeats and by the presence of flux of blood, visible as moving acoustic shadows.

Usually (86% of subjects[2]), the left and middle hepatic veins have a common opening into the inferior vena cava. More rarely, they open separately. The left hepatic vein is formed by several venous tributaries, most often (67%) by a large posterior trunk and several small anterior veins. The main left hepatic vein is 2 to 3 cm long.

The middle hepatic vein is formed by the union of two anterior tributaries from segments 4 and 5 (Fig. 87-4). The main trunk of the vein is 3 to 5 cm long and often receives a branch draining the upper part of segment 4 (53%); in 7% of cases, it receives a branch from segment 8, which may enter the inferior vena cava independently.

The confluence of the right hepatic vein with the right side of the inferior vena cava is slightly lower than that of the other hepatic veins. Usually there is a single large right hepatic vein, but in 13% of cases, an accessory inferior right hepatic vein drains directly into the inferior vena cava at a similar level to that of the liver hilum[9,19] (Fig 87-5).

The hepatic veins draining segment 1 are small and independent. They are difficult to see on ultrasound, but there are usually three or four and they drain directly into the left border of the inferior vena cava.

The portal pedicles

The branches of the portal vein, the hepatic artery, and the bile ducts are surrounded by a fibrous capsule that is a prolongation of Glisson's capsule. This is thick in the hilar region (hilar plaque) but progressively diminishes as the branches of the portal pedicle penetrate the liver parenchyma. This covering provides a thick hyperechogenic line that is much greater than the line that occasionally may be seen around the hepatic veins and thus enables the two entities to be distinguished easily. Within the portal triad, the portal vein is the major element and can be followed far into the liver parenchyma. The smaller arterial and biliary elements are readily discernible in the hilar region only; the arterial branches can be made out by their visible pulsations.

In the liver hilum, the extrahepatic portal bifurcation is easily recognizable on a horizontal cut centered over the

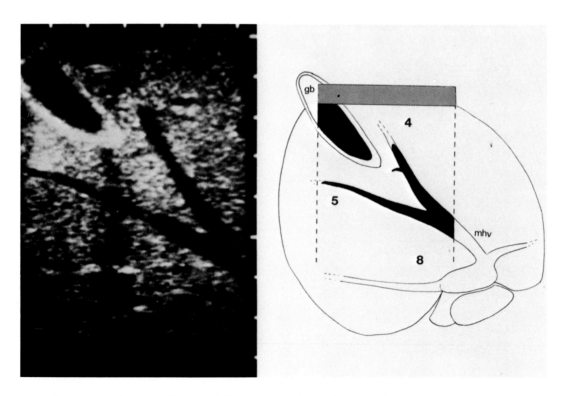

Fig. 87-4. The formation of the middle hepatic vein *(mhv)* by the union of two veins from the anterior parts of segments 4 and 5. *gb,* Gallbladder.

hilum passing through the hepatic parenchyma. The bile ducts are anterior and superior to the vein, and the arterial branches are found between the two. The arteries tend to be difficult to visualize on the same cut as the portal and biliary branches; the arterial bifurcation is lower, so the direction of the arteries is slightly different from that of the other elements.

In the same plane, the left portal pedicle can be followed and small branches passing posteriorly into segment 1 may be seen by moving the probe to the left. The left branch turns forward to terminate in the recess of Rex. Here the round ligament joins it, appearing as a well-defined hyper-echogenic band in the continuation of the line of the left portal branch. At the level of the forward angulation of the left portal pedicle, the branch to segment 2 arises. At the recess of Rex, the portal pedicle divides in a plane that is almost horizontal, giving off a branch to the right for segment 4 and a branch to the left for segment 3.

The right portal branch passes in a slightly oblique upward direction from the hilum and after only about 2 cm divides into two trunks: an anterior trunk for the anterior sector of the right side of the liver that has branches to segments 5 and 8, passing between the middle and right hepatic veins, and a posterior trunk that divides into several branches for segments 6 and 7. Often two or three branches pass superiorly into segment 7, and three or four branches pass inferiorly into segment 6.

The segmental anatomy of the liver

Intraoperative ultrasonography permits visualization of the major hepatic vasculature, and the vessels can be followed far into the liver parenchyma. Thus the liver is made transparent, and the routes of the vessels can be mapped accurately on the liver's surface. This facilitates anatomic liver resections based on a precise knowledge of its natural lines of division.

The liver, as it appears at laparotomy, is divided by the umbilical fissure and the teres and falciform ligaments into two lobes: the left lobe and the larger right lobe (Fig. 87-6). On the inferior surface of the right lobe is the transverse hilar fissure. The part of the right lobe located anterior to this fissure is called the *quadrate lobe;* it is limited on the left by the umbilical fissure and on the right by the gallbladder fossa. Posterior to the hilar fissure is a fourth lobe, the caudate lobe. Thus the liver has two main lobes and two accessory lobes, which are demarcated by easily visible fissures. These correspond to the true definition of a lobe as part of the parenchyma limited by fissures or grooves.

This morphologic description is inadequate to guide the surgeon in performing anatomic liver resections, and a functional description has now been superimposed.[1] This second method was reported first by Cantlie in 1898[7] and was followed by the works of McIndoe and Counseller,[22] Hjorsjo,[12] Ton That Tung,[25] Couinaud,[9] and Goldsmith and Woodburne.[10] Couinaud's description is relied on principally here.

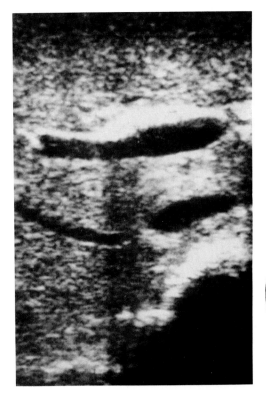

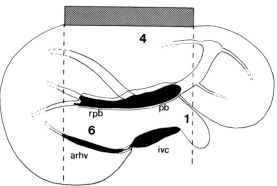

Fig. 87-5. Accessory right hepatic vein *(arhv)* draining into the right border of the inferior vena cava *(ivc)* at the level of the liver hilum. *pb,* Portal bifurcation; *rpb,* right portal branch (posterior division).

A study of the functional anatomy of the liver permits the description of a hepatic segmentation based on the location of the hepatic veins and the distribution of the portal pedicles (Fig. 87-7). The three main hepatic veins divide the liver into four sectors, each of which receives a portal pedicle. The hepatic veins are contained in the portal scissuras dividing the four portal sectors.

According to this functional description, the liver is separated into two hemilivers by the main portal scissura, also called *Cantilie's line*. It is preferable to call these two parts the right and left livers rather than right or left lobes to avoid confusion with the morphologic lobes; it would also be erroneous because there are no visible markers that permit the division between the hemilivers. The main portal scissura runs approximately from the middle of the gallbladder fossa anteriorly to the left side of the inferior vena cava posteriorly, describing an angle of 75° with the horizontal plane (Fig. 87-8). Intraoperative ultrasound enables study of the middle hepatic vein so that the scissura can be marked accurately on the liver capsule. The right and left livers are independent as regards the portal and arterial vascularization and biliary drainage.

The right and left livers are themselves divided into two parts by other portal scissuras. These subdivisions may be called *sectors*, although they are often called *segments* in the Anglo-Saxon nomenclature.[13]

The right portal scissura, containing the right hepatic vein, divides the right liver into a right posterolateral sector, posterior to the right hepatic vein and containing segments 6 and 7, and a right anteromedial sector, between the right and middle hepatic veins and containing segments 5 and 8. The scissura is inclined at 45° to the right (Fig. 87-8). Its exact location is not well defined because it has no external landmarks. According to Couinaud,[9] it extends from the midpoint between the right angle of the liver and the right side of the gallbladder fossa on the anterior border of the liver to the confluence of the inferior vena cava and right hepatic vein posteriorly. According to Ton That Tung,[26] the scissura follows a line parallel to the right lateral border of

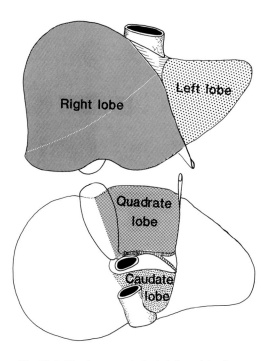

Fig. 87-6. The four morphologic lobes of the liver.

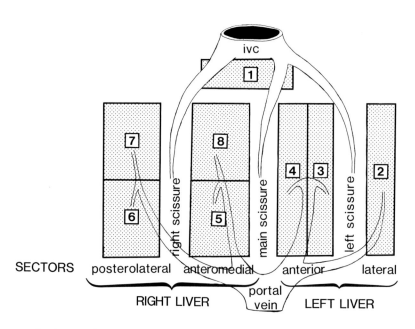

Fig. 87-7. The functional anatomy of the liver. The three main hepatic veins divide the liver into four sectors, each receiving a portal pedicle. *ivc*, Inferior vena cava.

the liver, three finger breadths more anteriorly. Once again, the exact location of the scissura is easily determined using intraoperative ultrasound to identify the right hepatic vein.

The left portal scissura, containing the left hepatic vein, divides the left liver into a left anterior sector, between the middle and left hepatic veins and containing segments 3 and 4, and a left lateral sector, posterolateral to the left hepatic vein and containing segment 2. This left scissura is not the umbilical fissure, which is a hepatic scissura containing a portal pedicle. The left portal scissura is posterior to the ligamentum teres in the left lobe of the liver. Thus the anterior sector of the left liver is composed of the part of the right lobe that is to the left of the main portal scissura (segment 4) and the anterior part of the left lobe (segment 3).

The subdivision of the sectors of the liver into individual segments (Fig. 87-9) is rendered by the major branchings of the portal pedicles. The only contraindication to this scheme is the division of the anterior sector of the left liver into segments 3 and 4, since for convenience, the line of division passes along the umbilical fissure, which is a hepatic rather than a portal scissura. The segments of Couinaud correspond approximately to the subsegments described by Goldsmith and Woodburne.[10] Each of the two sectors of the right liver is divided into two segments: the posterolateral sector into segment 6 inferiorly and segment 7 superiorly and the anteromedial sector into segment 5 inferiorly and segment 8 superiorly. The anterior sector of the left liver is divided by the umbilical fissure into segments 4 and 3. The lateral sector of the left liver is composed of only one segment, segment 2, which is the posterior part of the left lobe. The caudate lobe (or segment 1) must be considered from a functional point of view as an autonomous segment because its vascularization is independent of the portal divisions and of the three main hepatic veins. It receives its blood from branches of the left and right portal veins and arteries, and its hepatic veins drain directly into the inferior vena cava.

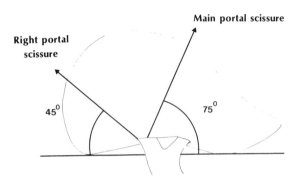

Fig. 87-8. The obliquity of the middle and right portal scissuras.

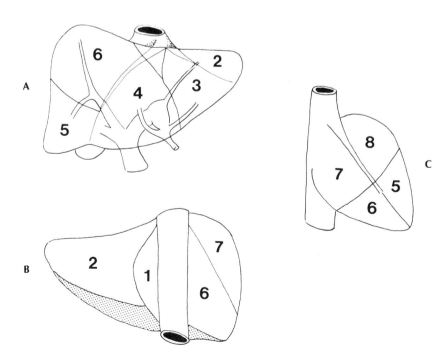

Fig. 87-9. The segmental classification of liver anatomy shown in anterior *(A)*, posterior *(B)*, and right lateral *(C)* views. The segments are numbered accordingly.

APPLICATIONS OF INTRAOPERATIVE ULTRASOUND IN HEPATIC SURGERY
Diagnosis

Despite great improvement in the diagnostic accuracy of preoperative morphologic examinations such as ultrasound, computed tomography (CT), selective arteriography, and magnetic resonance imaging, tumor recognition is the first and most important application of intraoperative ultrasound. Careful visual inspection and manual palpation are still important in detecting intrahepatic and extrahepatic disease not identified by preoperative investigations, but intraoperative ultrasound has added a new dimension to diagnosis. In addition to accurately defining the segmental anatomy of known lesions, a careful ultrasound examination of the liver will often reveal daughter nodules or other metastases not demonstrated preoperatively. Even though some of these lesions, particularly if they are near the surface of the liver, are palpable or even visible to the naked eye, many of the smaller, deep-seated lesions would otherwise be overlooked. This is particularly important in the cirrhotic liver in which the accuracy of manual palpation is considerably reduced.

In a study by Sheu et al,[24] 46% of hepatocellular carcinomas smaller than 3 cm in diameter and 14% of lesions 3 to 5 cm in diameter were detected by intraoperative ultrasound but were impalpable and invisible to the surgeon. In a prospective study,[8] it was found that intraoperative ultrasound was more sensitive than preoperative ultrasound, CT scanning, selective arteriography, and intraoperative palpation in identifying liver tumors, particularly in the detection of tumors less than 1 cm in diameter. A total of 13 (32%) of 40 tumors less than 1 cm in diameter were detected by intraoperative ultrasound only. In contrast, only 1 of 60 tumors greater than 3 cm in diameter was detected by intraoperative ultrasound only.

Accurate intraoperative ultrasound-guided needle biopsies of individual lesions can be performed even when these lesions are deep within the liver. At the same time, major vessels can be avoided. For example, an automatic Menghini needle (18 or 20 gauge) can be used. For experienced hepatobiliary pathologists, such as are found in a specialist center, a positive diagnosis can usually be made while the patient is still under general anesthesia in the operating room. With this additional information, definitive treatment can be planned. The findings at intraoperative sonography provide supplementary information in one third of the patients undergoing surgery for primary liver tumors and result in modification of the intended surgical procedure in 27%.[3] Preoperative investigations may suggest that surgical resection of the lesion is possible, but intraoperative ultrasonography may reveal diffuse, infiltrating, inoperable lesions or satellite nodules and vascular invasion, indicating that a more extensive resection is required. The information may obviate trial dissections and inappropriate resection of tumors that would be better treated by nonsurgical means. Alternatively, ultrasonography often enables more precise and limited resections of lesions shown to be operable by

revealing that adequate clearance of tumor can be obtained without the systematic performance of major liver resections.[5] Blind radical resection for inaccessible lesions, some of which will be benign, can thus be avoided.

Anatomic liver resections

Intraoperative ultrasound is mandatory for performing accurate segmental liver surgery, particularly when lesser resections of one or two segments are required. The branches of the hepatic veins can be marked accurately on the surface of the liver by using a diathermy needle to make small incisions in Glisson's capsule. This is particularly important in the presence of large lesions or segmental liver hypertrophy or atrophy, often associated with cirrhosis, which may distort the vascular anatomy considerably. In addition to accurately locating space-occupying lesions and thus helping the surgeon plan the resection, intraoperative ultrasound is useful in monitoring the progress of a resection, ensuring that adequate margins of resection are maintained and checking the relationship of major vascular structures to the resection. In this way, the risks of major intraoperative hemorrhage and the inadvertent devascularization of hepatic parenchyma adjacent to the resection are reduced.

The principal anatomic hepatectomies are the left and right hepatectomies, in which the line of transection is the main portal scissura, and the right and left lobectomies, in which the line of transection is the umbilical fissure (Fig. 87-10). In Couinaud's nomenclature, the right lobectomy corresponds to a right hepatectomy extended to include segment 4 and sometimes also segment 1, and the left lobectomy corresponds to a bisegmentectomy of segments 2 and 3.

The lesser typical resections are theoretically numerous; indeed, all the individual or associated segmentectomies can be described. In practice the number is more limited, and they are described in detail elsewhere.[4,5] One of the main advantages of liver segmentectomy and bisegmentectomy is that they permit the anatomic resection of lesions without the removal of large amounts of functional hepatic parenchyma. This is particularly important in the cirrhotic liver in which the reserves of hepatic function and the regenerative powers are considerably limited.

Hepatectomies classically can be approached either by preliminary vascular control[18] or primary parenchymatous transection.[26] Another technique (Fig. 87-11) combines the advantages of both techniques while seeking to avoid the disadvantages.[1] The principle is to begin with hilar dissection to control the portal elements to the liver to be resected. These elements are clamped without ligation. The liver parenchyma is then opened along the chosen anatomic scissuras, and the portal elements are located by a superior approach within the hepatic parenchyma; thus ligation of these vessels is performed distal to the clamps. At the end of the liver transection, the hepatic vein is ligated inside the liver. This technique has the advantage of proceeding with control of the vessels before liver transection and thus

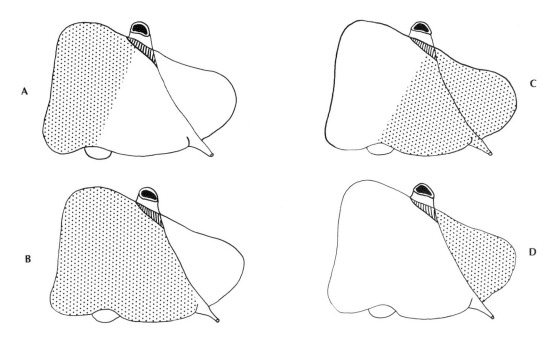

Fig. 87-10. The four common hepatectomies. *A* and *B,* The right and left hepatectomies according to the main portal scissura. *C* and *D,* The right and left lobectomies according to the umbilical fissure, which in Couinaud's nomenclature are the right extended hepatectomy and bisegmentectomy 2 and 3, respectively.

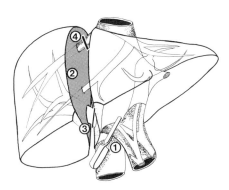

Fig. 87-11. The stages of liver resection according to Bismuth[18] for right hepatectomy. *1,* Clamping of the portal elements to the liver to be resected. *2,* Opening of the liver parenchyma along the main scissura. *3,* Division of the portal elements within the liver parenchyma. *4,* Ligation of the right hepatic vein.

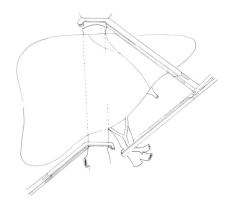

Fig. 87-12. Complete vascular exclusion of the liver.

reducing intraoperative blood loss, as in the Lortat-Jacob technique, and of dividing the vessels within the parenchyma safe from anatomic anomalies that might make adjacent liver ischemic, as in the Ton That Tung technique. Complete vascular exclusion of the liver is a useful supplementary technique for some centrally located tumors[11] (Fig. 87-12).

The liver substance itself can be divided using the classic finger-fracture technique described by Lin et al.[17] A Kelly arterial clamp can also be used to fraction the liver parenchyma, and this method isolates the vascular structures, which are more resistant, for individual ligation and section. An ultrasonic dissector can then be used (e.g., Cavitron Ultrasonic Aspirator*).

Over the past 20 years, up to September 1987, 324 typical hepatic resections based on the segmental anatomy of the liver have been performed at Paul Brousse Hospital (Table 87-1). Of these, 44% were major, defined as the resection of three or more segments; the remaining 56% were lesser

---

*CUSA, Stamford, Conn.

Table 87-1. Anatomic liver resections performed at Paul Brousse Hospital, 1967-1987

Operation	No.*	
MAJOR HEPATECTOMIES	142	(8)
Right hepatectomy	73	(6)
Right extended hepatectomy	30	(1)
Left hepatectomy	18	(1)
Left extended hepatectomy	12	(0)
Trisegmentectomy	9	(0)
LESSER HEPATECTOMIES	182	(9)
Bisegmentectomy 2 and 3 (left lobectomy)	84	(4)
Other bisegmentectomies	34	(1)
Unisegmentectomy	38	(3)
Subsegmentectomy	26	(1)
TOTAL	324	(17)

*Numbers in parentheses are number of deaths that occurred within 2 months of surgery.

Table 87-2. Indications for anatomic liver resections performed at Paul Brousse Hospital, 1967-1987

Indication	No.*	
MALIGNANT DISEASE	226	(12)
Primary hepatocellular carcinoma	92	(10)
With cirrhosis	53	(7)
Without cirrhosis	39	(3)
Other primary liver tumors	25	(0)
Direct invasion of adjacent tumor (including gallbladder)	13	(0)
Metastatic tumors	96	(2)
Colorectal	54	(0)
Others	42	(2)
BENIGN DISEASE	98	(5)
Benign liver tumors	38	(1)
Intrahepatic lithiasis	14	(0)
Hydatid cysts	12	(0)
Liver abscesses	5	(0)
Liver trauma	29	(4)
TOTAL	324	(17)

*Numbers in parentheses are number of deaths that occurred within 2 months of surgery.

hepatectomies in which one or two segments were resected (including bisegmentectomy of segments 2 and 3 or left lobectomy). A total of 70% were performed for malignant disease, principally hepatocellular carcinoma and liver metastases. Resections for nonmalignant disease were principally for benign liver tumors and liver trauma (Table 87-2).

The mortality within 2 months of surgery was 5.2%; most of the deaths occurred after resections for liver trauma or in patients with cirrhosis. The mortality for nontraumatic noncirrhotic resections was 2.5%. The results have improved steadily during the study period, and in the past 5 years the mortality after hepatectomy has been 0% for benign lesions and 3.5% for malignant lesions.

The accuracy of intraoperative ultrasound-guided anatomic resections undoubtedly has contributed to the low morbidity and mortality that are now being seen. Perioperative blood loss has been reduced considerably, and necrotic liver parenchyma adjacent to resection margins is avoided, as are unduly radical resections.

In addition to its usefulness in anatomic liver resection, intraoperative ultrasound may also result in therapeutic advances in that it provides a means of visualizing and gaining access to the vascular and biliary trees of the liver. The many therapeutic options made possible by transhepatic access to the biliary tree are beyond the scope of this chapter, but transhepatic access to the portal venous radicles is of particular value in the segmental and subsegmental surgical excision of hepatocellular carcinoma in the cirrhotic liver.

Hepatectomies of the cirrhotic liver must conserve more of the hepatic parenchyma because the reserves of hepatic function are minimal and postoperative compensatory hypertrophy is virtually absent.[6] Surgical techniques of liver segmentectomy and subsegmentectomy are mandatory. The principal method of dissemination of hepatocellular carcinoma is via the portal venous route.[14] Portal vessels may be invaded by the tumor itself or by a tumor thrombus that propagates along the lumen toward the portal trunk in a retrograde fashion. Small fragments of tumor can become detached and embolize at a portal bifurcation into adjacent venous tributaries and segments (Fig. 87-13). All susceptible portal territory, comprising all the portal branches distal to the apex of the tumor thrombus, must be resected beyond the first noninvolved junction to attempt a complete tumor excision. An overextensive resection, however, may precipitate hepatocellular failure.

Intraoperative ultrasound permits clear definition of the invaded portal branches and indicates whether resection is feasible. It is useful for limiting the extent of hepatic resection, a technique developed in the Far East.[13,20] Using ultrasound guidance, the apex of the tumor thrombus within the portal vein can be identified and a 7-French triple-lumen balloon catheter can be introduced transhepatically into the first noninvolved junction using the Seldinger technique (Fig. 87-13). The balloon is then inflated, thus arresting portal venous flow to that segment, and methylene blue is injected into the occluded segment behind the balloon while the central lumen is perfused with saline-containing heparin. This demarcates the segment or subsegment to be resected on the liver surface (Fig. 87-14). By clamping the appropriate branch of the hepatic artery at the hilum of the liver, a limited yet oncologically sound resection can be performed under relatively avascular conditions. This technique increases the number of cirrhotic patients who can tolerate hepatic resection.[3,17]

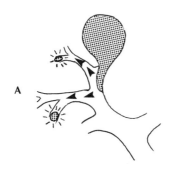
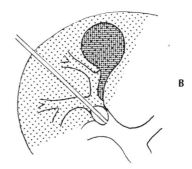

Fig. 87-13. A, Tumor spread by embolization of tumor thrombus to adjacent portal branches. *B,* Subsegmental portal venous occlusion by a balloon catheter passed transhepatically under ultrasound guidance into the portal branch beyond the apex of the tumor thrombus.

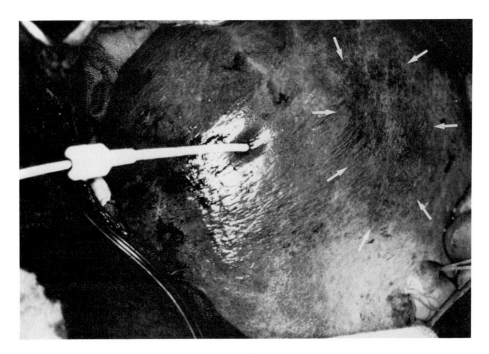

Fig. 87-14. The triple-lumen catheter in position. The subsegment of susceptible portal venous territory is demarcated on the liver surface *(arrows)* by the injection of methylene blue behind the occluding balloon.

CONCLUSION

Intraoperative sonography can be considered an extension of the surgeons' hands and eyes. It allows them to "see" inside an organ whose volume and nature traditionally have made surgical exploration difficult. It allows the discovery and positive identification of small tumors at a time when resection appears to offer real hope of improved survival. It also clearly demonstrates the vascular anatomy within the liver and thus facilitates appropriate anatomically based liver resections.

REFERENCES

1. Bismuth H: Surgical anatomy and anatomical surgery of the liver, *World J Surg* 6:3, 1982.
2. Bismuth H, Castaing D: *Echographie per-opératoire du foie et des voies biliaires,* Paris, 1985, Flammarion Médecine-Sciences.
3. Bismuth H, Castaing D, Garden OJ: The use of operative ultrasound in surgery of primary liver tumours, *World J Surg* 11:610, 1987.
4. Bismuth H, Castaing D, Garden OJ: Segmental surgery of the liver, *Surg Annu* 20:291, 1988.
5. Bismuth H, Castaing D: Major and minor segmentectomies 'réglées' in liver surgery, *World J Surg* 6:10, 1982.
6. Bismuth H et al: Liver resections in cirrhotic patients: a Western experience, *World J Surg* 10:311, 1986.

7. Cantlie J: On a new arrangement of the right and left lobes of the liver, *Proc Anat Soc Great Britain Ireland* 32:4, 1898.

8. Castaing D et al: Utility of operative ultrasound in the surgical management of liver tumours, *Ann Surg* 204:600, 1986.

9. Couinaud C: *Le foie: études anatomiques et chirurgicales*, Paris, 1957, Masson.

10. Goldsmith NA, Woodburne RT: Surgical anatomy pertaining to liver resection, *Surg Gynecol Obstet* 195:310, 1957.

11. Heaney JP, Jacobson A: Simplified control of upper abdominal hemorrhage from the vena cava, *Surgery* 78:138, 1975.

12. Hjorstjo CH: The topography of the intrahepatic duct system, *Acta Anat* 11:599, 1931.

13. Kanematsu T et al: Limited hepatic resection for selected cirrhotic patients with primary liver cancer, *Ann Surg* 199:51, 1984.

14. Kishi K et al: Hepatocellular carcinoma: a clinical and pathologic analysis of 57 hepatectomy cases, *Cancer* 51:542, 1983.

15. Knight PR, Newell JA: Operative use of ultrasonics in cholelithiasis, *Lancet* 1:1023, 1963.

16. Lane RJ, Glazer G: Intraoperative B-mode ultrasound scanning of the extrahepatic biliary tree and pancreas, *Lancet* 1:334, 1980.

17. Lin TY et al: Study on lobectomy of the liver: a new technical suggestion on hepatectomy and reports of three cases of primary hepatoma treated with left lobectomy of the liver, *Formosan Med Assoc* 57:742, 1958.

18. Lortat-Jacob JL, Robert HG, Henry C: Un cas d'hépatectomie droite réglée, *Mem Acad Chir* 78:244, 1952.

19. Makuuchi M, Hasegawa H, Yamazaki S: Intraoperative ultrasonic examination for hepatectomy, *Jpn J Clin Oncol* 11:367, 1981.

20. Makuuchi M, Hasegawa H, Yamazaki S: Ultrasonically guided subsegmentectomy, *Surg Gynecol Obstet* 161:346, 1985.

21. Makuuchi M et al: The inferior right hepatic vein: ultrasonic demonstration, *Radiology* 148:213, 1983.

22. McIndoe AH, Counseller VS: A report of the bilaterality of the liver, *Arch Surg* 15:589, 1927.

23. Schlebel JO, Diggdon P, Cuellar J: The use of ultrasound for localizing renal calculi, *J Urol* 86:367, 1961.

24. Sheu JC et al: Intraoperative hepatic ultrasonography: an indispensable procedure in resection of small hepatocellular carcinoma, *Surgery* 97:97, 1985.

25. Ton That Tung: *La vascularisation veineuse du foie et ses applications aux résections hépatiques*, Hanoi, 1939, University of Hanoi (doctoral dissertation).

26. Ton That Tung: *Les résections majeures et mineures du foie*, Paris, 1979, Masson.

CHAPTER 88

Doppler studies of tumor neovascularity

KENNETH J. W. TAYLOR

The process of angiogenesis involved in neovascularization is attracting increased attention from biologists and pathologists. Angiogenesis is fundamental to a number of physiologic responses as well as pathologic states. It is involved in ovulation, placentation, and embryonic development and is an important contributing factor in the evolution of many diseases, including psoriasis, osteoarthritis, diabetic retinopathy, retrolental fibroplasia, and autoimmune diseases. It is also a prerequisite for the development of the malignant propensity by tumors. In a landmark paper published in 1972, Folkman et al[8] recognized that tumors had to develop vascularity to supply their nutritional needs before they could grow much beyond a millimeter in diameter. These investigators hypothesized that angiogenesis in the host tissues surrounding the tumor was induced by a substance secreted by the tumor (tumor angiogenic factor). Since that time, many other angiogenic agents have been isolated, including the fibroblastic growth factors, angiotensin, heparin, transforming growth factors, prostaglandins, urokinase, and copper.[7,21]

The findings from many morphologic and angiographic studies have been used to define the characteristics of these tumor vessels (Fig. 88-1).[23] Such vessels are abnormal and frequently show arteriovenous shunts, which spawn high velocities that can be detected by current Doppler techniques. Tumor vessels also tend to have less smooth muscle in their walls, resulting in lower impedance to flow because most of the normal vascular impedance resides in the arteriolar muscle. Taylor et al[26] recognized a small number of tumors in which the impedance was very low, with little or no systolic and diastolic variation, and correlated the presence of such signals with the existence of thin-walled sinusoids (Fig. 88-2). They hypothesized that arterial inflow into tumor sinusoids or lakes could explain this very low impedance.

Malignant tumors are characterized by local growth and distant metastases. Nutrients from an adequate blood supply are therefore essential for local growth, and access to the host circulation is important for distant spread. Thus neovascularization is a critical stage in the evolution of malignant behavior and has given rise to the concept that avascular tumors may remain dormant for many years and only exhibit a malignant propensity once they become vascularized.

Based on this finding, Folkman[6] recognized the potential for controlling tumor growth by inhibiting the angiogenic factors.

It may also be hypothesized that the most vascular tumors are the most malignant. Data on breast tumors support this concept, as discussed later in this chapter. It is also possible that the localization of neovascularization may be used to guide the biopsy needle into tumors while avoiding the inflammatory or desmoplastic area surrounding the tumor. The demonstration of tumor vascularity by color flow Doppler could also be used to guide alcohol injection into tumors, monitor the successful treatment of tumors through the abolition of neovascularity, and detect early recurrence through the reappearance of neovascularity.

BREAST

In 1977 Wells et al[28] were the first to detect vascularity using continuous wave (CW) Doppler ultrasound in breast tumors. The results of several other small series were subsequently published and documented similar findings. The first systematic study of a large group of patients was reported in 1982 by Burns et al,[3] who studied 350 breast masses, of which 52 proved to be cancerous. Using a 10-MHz CW

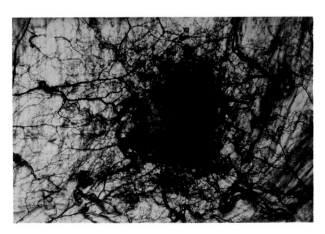

Fig. 88-1. Vascular injection of experimental tumor. A bizarre neovascularity is seen surrounding a Walker 256 tumor. Note the abnormal morphology of the vessels.

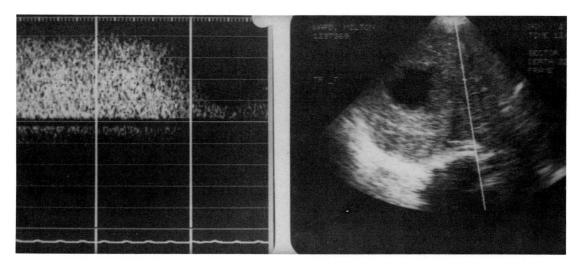

Fig. 88-2. Ultrasound scan shows a metastasis in the right lobe of the liver. Central necrosis is seen and abnormal signals are elicited around the periphery of the tumor. A continuous waveform is seen, lacking systolic/diastolic variation, at a high velocity, giving a Doppler frequency shift of around 4 kHz (corresponding to approximately 100 cm/sec).

probe, these researchers compared the Doppler shift around the palpable mass with the Doppler shift in the mirror image of the other breast. Using a difference of 2 kHz as a criterion for determining abnormality yielded a sensitivity of 90% for the prediction of cancer, with only 4% false-positive rate in cases of fibroadenomas.[3] Schoenberger, Sutherland, and Robinson[19] demonstrated an even higher sensitivity of 100% in 12 cases of breast cancer and a specificity of 100% in 26 cases of benign lesions. Other authors have not confirmed such a high sensitivity or specificity using the same criterion; in our series, a 71% sensitivity was noted for the prediction of breast cancer and there was a significant incidence (15%) of false-positive results in patients with fibroadenomas. These false-positives occurred in an inordinate number of cases of juvenile cellular fibroadenoma. Although these figures appear rather low, conventional mammography has a specificity of only approximately 30%, so three biopsies are usually required to confirm every positive case of breast cancer. Furthermore, the sensitivity and specificity of color Doppler differentiation between benign and malignant tumors need to be established with the high-resolution linear arrays now available.

Other investigators[20] have also hypothesized that the presence of neovascularity in breast tumors, as detected by current CW Doppler techniques, might predict the biologic behavior of the tumor. Therefore the presence of Doppler signals has been correlated with multiple known predictors of prognosis. The results of this study showed that Doppler detected neovascularity in 93% of the patients whose tumor exceeded 2 cm in diameter, 97% of the patients with advanced disease at presentation, all patients with residual disease after surgery, 96% of patients with positive lymph nodes, and all patients whose cancer subsequently recurred.

In contrast, the absence of Doppler-detected signals correlated with the presence of a small tumor, noninvolved lymph nodes, complete resection at surgery, and lack of recurrence. Clearly, more work is needed in a larger series of patients to establish the true merits of this technique.

LIVER TUMORS

Considerable clinical concern may be raised and imaging expense incurred by the discovery of an incidental mass in the liver during routine sonography for an unrelated cause. In our population, hemangiomas are found in approximately 2% of the patients. Focal fatty infiltration is common and may produce an echogenic lesion on sonograms that resembles a hemangioma. In addition, many metastases are echogenic, 90% of hepatocellular carcinomas are echogenic, and several other benign masses have similar appearances, including focal nodular hyperplasia and liver cell adenoma. Duplex and color flow Doppler makes a modest contribution in differentiating among these various processes, particularly between benign and malignant growths. However, a negative finding has no value because most benign masses and many metastases are relatively avascular.

Going from a high-frequency CW probe for the investigation of superficial lesions to a 3-MHz, pulsed and color Doppler probe for the examination of deep abdominal tumors demands a greatly improved signal-to-noise ratio. Adequate color machines are only now becoming available for this purpose.

Results based on 68 cases of confirmed liver tumors examined by duplex Doppler techniques have been published,[25] and this investigation has now been extended to 198 cases of confirmed liver tumors.[9] The method that is now applied clinically includes a color flow examination,

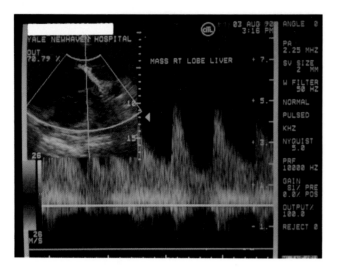

Fig. 88-3. Ultrasound color flow shows neovascularity in the right lobe of the liver. Doppler interrogation revealed a Doppler shift of 5 kHz corresponding to velocities in excess of 100 cm/sec. Biopsy revealed a hepatocellular carcinoma.

which expedites the localization of a vascular area for further quantitation by pulse Doppler. When a space-occupying mass is disclosed by gray-scale sonography, color flow is then used to search for peripherally situated neovascularization. Such areas are then interrogated by pulsed Doppler using angle correction (Fig. 88-3).

These results showed the Doppler signals in cases of hepatocellular carcinoma markedly differed from those obtained in benign masses (mainly hemangiomas). Using an insonating frequency of 3 MHz, 32 of 46 hepatomas and 4 metastases showed a Doppler shift greater than 4.5 kHz and yielded a 70% sensitivity, 95% specificity, and 89% positive predictive value for differentiating hepatomas from metastatic lesions. The mean kilohertz shifts ($\pm$ SD) for the various tumors assessed were the following: hepatomas, 4.7 ± 1.74; metastases, 2.04 ± 1.65; hemangiomas, 0.33 ± 0.77; and other benign masses, 0.34 ± 0.77. There were significant differences between hepatomas and metastases ($p < 0.001$) and between metastases and benign lesions ($p < 0.001$).

A recent study employing receiver-operator curve (ROC) analysis examined the optimum cutoff velocity for diagnosing neovascularity in a diverse group of tumors, including hepatocellular carcinoma.[5] These authors reported that 40 cm/sec was the optimum cutoff value. Several other authors[24] have reported finding neovascularization in cases of hepatocellular carcinoma when the mass exceeds 3 cm in diameter but have not noted the higher velocities that others have reported.[24] However, this appears to reflect differences in equipment sensitivity, since the author's group is also unable to detect such high velocities when using the same type of equipment as that used by these other researchers. From a practical point of view, hemangiomas in adults should not exhibit high velocities. Thus further in-

vestigation is warranted if high velocities are detected in a focal liver lesion. This is not true for neonatal liver masses. Hemangiomas and hemangioendotheliomas in the neonatal group may show massive shunting, and these patients may present with heart failure.

The anatomic source of the high velocities is probably arteriovenous shunting, which is often made apparent on angiography by the presence of early venous filling and is considered to exist pathologically in all cases of hepatocellular carcinoma. Another mechanism for arteriovenous shunting in such tumors stems from its propensity to invade the branches of the portal vein. This arterialized tumor may then undergo necrosis and then produce arterioportal shunting. Due to invasion of the portal vein, portal vein thrombosis is a well-recognized complication of hepatocellular carcinoma. Color flow Doppler has recently been recommended as useful for differentiating between bland thrombus and tumor thrombus. The former is avascular whereas the latter is arterialized and generates hepatofugal flow.[16]

Skepticism about the value of detecting neovascularization in the liver has been expressed by the Michigan group, who noted the existence of arteriovenous shunting in cirrhotic livers in the absence of tumor involvement.[14] They reported that 27% of such cirrhotic livers have arteriovenous shunting in the same range as that detected in hepatocellular carcinoma. Superficially, these results appear to cast great doubt on the validity of the technique. However, these arteriovenous shunts in cases of cirrhosis are not associated with a mass, as disclosed by sonography. Further, such shunting is unusual in the well-compensated cirrhotic liver of patients who are being screened for hepatocellular cancer. The high prevalence of arteriovenous shunting in the population studied in Michigan was based on a group of end-stage cirrhotics being evaluated as candidates for liver transplantation.

LYMPH NODES

High velocities in lymph nodes occur most commonly because of lymphadenitis and not tumor involvement. Such marked hypervascularity is common in patients with AIDS or AIDs-related complex (ARC) (Fig. 88-4).

KIDNEY

Computed tomography (CT) and sonography have improved the detection rate of small renal masses.[22] However, differentiating these masses from pseudotumors due to columns of Bertin poses more of a problem in terms of tissue characterization. Fine-needle aspiration of renal masses guided by ultrasound or CT has yielded low sensitivities of between 20% and 62%.[1] Although there was early enthusiasm about the ability to stage renal cancers with magnetic resonance imaging,[17] this has proved to be of relatively limited value.[15]

Neovascularity in the kidney is relatively easy to detect by Doppler (Fig. 88-5).[18] Two of the early studies demonstrated abnormal Doppler-shift frequencies in 78% to 83% of the patients with renal-cell carcinomas.[11,12]

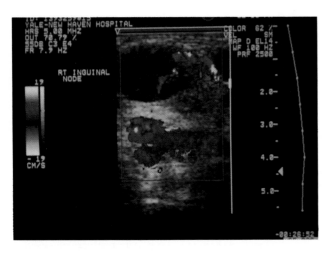

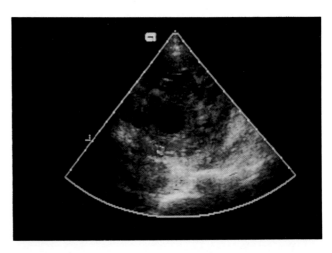

Fig. 88-4. Ultrasound scan of right inguinal lymph nodes demonstrating afferent and efferent vessels at the hilum. Such marked hypervascularity is most commonly seen in lymphadenitis especially when associated with AIDS or manifestations of AIDS-related complex.

Fig. 88-5. Ultrasound color flow of renal cell cancer showing peripheral hypervascularity.

In a prospective study consisting of 70 patients who were examined with duplex ultrasound, 37 patients had malignant lesions and 33 had benign lesions.[26] The peak systolic frequency shifts were significantly different between the two groups; benign lesions showed a mean shift of 0.91 ± 0.95 kHz and malignant lesions showed a mean shift of 3.57 ± 2.41 kHz ($p = 0.0003$). The end-diastolic frequency shifts were also significantly different.[11] To develop a ratio that could be applied in individual patients, the author's team compared the peak systolic frequency shift in the tumor with that in the main renal artery. The mean $\pm$ SD for benign lesions was 0.52 ± 0.57 kHz and that for malignant lesions was 3.47 ± 2.17 kHz ($p = 0.0002$). The Pourcelot index (resistive index) showed no significant difference: that for benign lesions was 0.71 ± 0.1 and that for malignant lesions, 0.70 ± 0.2. A cutoff of 2.5 kHz was used to discriminate between benign and malignant processes, and the sensitivity of this criterion was 75% and the specificity was 92%, with an overall accuracy of 83%.

This study concluded that the addition of duplex and color flow examination in the assessment of renal tumors was helpful for evaluating indeterminate renal masses and, in particular, for differentiating between a pseudotumor and a malignancy.[26] A positive result consisting of a Doppler shift exceeding 2.5 kHz (using a carrier frequency of 3 MHz) should prompt further evaluation. There were only two false-positives and these were encountered in cases of renal abscess, in which neovascularization is expected (Fig. 88-6). This caused no confusion in the clinical management of these patients because urosepsis was already apparent from the clinical and bacteriologic results.

CARCINOMA OF THE OVARY

The ability to detect carcinoma of the ovary has not improved in the last century. Approximately 70% of these

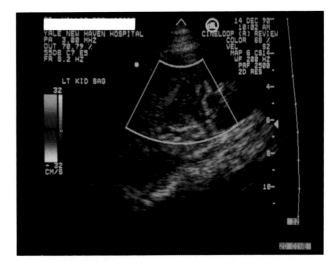

Fig. 88-6. Ultrasound color flow of renal abscess demonstrating peripheral neovascularization associated with chronic infection. The cause of this abnormality was apparent from the patient's symptoms and bacteriologic examination of the urine.

tumors present in stage III or IV when there is only a 20% chance of a 5-year survival.[10] This appalling prognosis has not been changed by the use of routine pelvic examinations. The incidence of the disease is highest in the upper and professional classes whose compliance with regular gynecologic surveillance is optimal. A major problem for screening is the relatively low prevalence of the disease, and this translates into a lack of cost efficacy. Campbell et al[4] performed 16,000 scans on 5000 women and detected only five cases of primary ovarian malignancy. Assuming that there is a combined professional and technical charge of $250 for the ultrasound examination, this means a cost of $800,000 per case of ovarian cancer detected. Despite this lack of

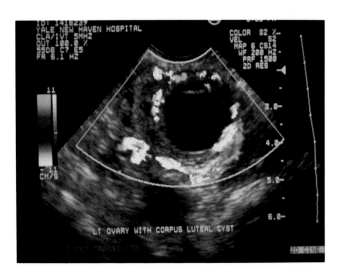

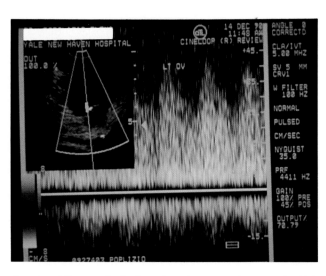

Fig. 88-7. Ultrasound color flow showing neovascularization around a corpus luteal cyst. These appearances are indistinguishable from those of ovarian cancer except that the luteal flow is cyclic.

Fig. 88-8. Ultrasound color flow of ovarian cancer demonstrating high peak systolic shifts and high diastolic shift giving a low impedance characteristic of ovarian cancer.

proven cost efficacy, the Kings College group in London is advocating a screening examination for women at normal risk to be performed every 18 months.

The introduction of endovaginal color flow ultrasound (EVCF) represents a major improvement in high-resolution imaging, and this method provides superb scans of the ovaries. The addition of color flow imaging allows the detection of neovascularity. Bourne et al[2] have applied the technique in a small group of women with ovarian masses and established a cutoff resistive index of 0.5 for the diagnosis of malignancy. Kurjack et al,[13] reporting from Zagreb, have cited similar findings. In postmenopausal women, the detection of such low-impedance flow within the ovary, especially when accompanied by a mass effect, must be considered a strong indication for surgery.

There is a problem in applying the same criterion to the diagnosis of ovarian cancer in premenopausal women because neovascularization also occurs in the corpus luteum and manifests flow characteristics indistinguishable from those of ovarian cancer (Figs. 88-7 and 88-8). At present, the only way the two can be distinguished is through repeat examinations, since luteal flow is cyclic. Several groups have tried to overcome this difficulty by timing the examination within the first 7 days of the menstrual cycle.[4,13] However, as the machines become more sensitive, low-amplitude, low-impedance flow is still frequently seen even in the first week of the menstrual cycle and probably represents residual activity from the previous cycle. Repeat scans then become necessary and this adds to the expense of the technique.

Because of these difficulties, it is impractical to scan women with only an average risk of ovarian cancer. Instead, clinicians should concentrate on three groups of women:

1. Those with a family history of ovarian cancer
2. Those with a pelvic mass detected on physical examination
3. Those with elevated serum Ca 125 levels

Ca 125 is a tumor marker for ovarian cancer. Elevated levels have a specificity of approximately 85% in postmenopausal women but only about 15% in premenopausal women.[27] False-positives are common and are due to ovarian cysts, pregnancy, endometriosis, and fibroids, all much more common conditions than ovarian cancer.[27] The sensitivity of the tumor marker for stage IA ovarian cancer is reported to be 33% to 50%. Thus most premenopausal women with elevated Ca 125 levels are affected by benign causes. Endovaginal sonography can be used to diagnose such benign causes, and this also makes it possible to reassure the patient.

To date, 200 women with a family history of ovarian cancer have been examined, and no ovarian cancers detected in this group. However, using this method, it has also been possible to reassure patients that an ovarian cyst detected on physical examination exhibited cyclic flow and was therefore a physiologic luteal cyst. In patients with a pelvic mass, 26 underwent operation and the following was found: 2 bilateral ovarian cancers, 2 stage I cancers, 1 borderline ovarian cancer, 2 carcinomas of the endometrium, 1 fallopian tube carcinoma, 2 bladder cancers, and 16 benign masses. Among 30 patients with elevated serum Ca 125 levels (greater than 30 U/ml), there was 1 ovarian cancer, 1 bladder cancer, 1 endometrial cancer, 9 fibroids, 2 endometriomas, and 1 pregnancy. No definite cause for the abnormal tumor marker was identified in half of the patients.

Pedunculated fibroids are a serious potential pitfall when examining patients for ovarian cancer. This entity simulates

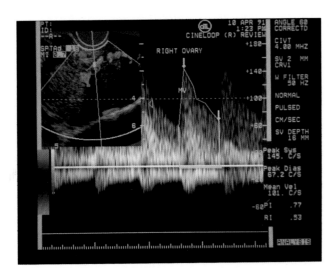

Fig. 88-9. Ultrasound color flow of the pelvis showing hypervascularity in a right adnexal mass. Doppler examination demonstrated high velocities and low impedance similar to that seen in ovarian cancer. Surgery revealed a pedunculated fibroid.

an ovarian mass on both pelvic examination and ultrasound imaging. Doppler may show high vascularity in these benign tumors, and fibroids may also cause elevated serum Ca 125 levels. Such a false-positive appearance, which can lead to unnecessary surgery, is shown in Fig. 88-9.

CONCLUSION

Despite the wide publicity in the medical and lay press about the possibility of screening for ovarian cancer, no cost-effective program currently exists for patients at normal risk. In those patients at higher risk of the disease because of family history, the cost per case detected is around $30,000, which is comparable to the cost of mammography. The main hope for the future is that a combination of tumor markers will become available that possess sufficient sensitivity and specificity to allow endovaginal color Doppler to be cost effective in this setting. Despite the enthusiastic reports from London and Zagreb about the discriminant ability of a 0.5 resistive index, this overlaps completely with luteal flow. In addition, resistive indices have not proved to be discriminatory for any other type of tumor, and it is likely that a peak systolic velocity or other quantitative differences in the waveform shape may prove more helpful. Such discriminants are currently under investigation.

Tumor vascularity can be detected by pulse and color flow in a wide variety of tumor types, but the practical clinical application of these techniques for diagnosis and therapy is only just beginning. Further improvements in the sensitivity of Doppler equipment will enhance the value of these techniques.

REFERENCES

1. Amendola MA et al: Small renal carcinoma: resolving a diagnostic dilemma, *Radiology* 166:637, 1988.
2. Bourne TH et al: Transvaginal color flow imaging: a new screening technique for ovarian cancer, *Brit Med J* 299:1367, 1989.
3. Burns PN et al: Ultrasonic Doppler studies of the breast, *Ultrasound Med Biol* 8:127, 1982.
4. Campbell S et al: Transabdominal ultrasound screening for early ovarian cancer, *Brit Med J* 299:1363, 1989.
5. Dock W et al: Tumor vascularization: assessment with duplex sonography, *Radiology* 181:241, 1991.
6. Folkman J: Antiangiogenesis: new concept for therapy of tumors, *Ann Surg* 175:409, 1972.
7. Folkman J, Klagsburn M: Angiogenic factors, *Science* 235:442, 1987.
8. Folkman J et al: Isolation of a tumor factor responsible for angiogenesis, *J Exp Med* 133:275, 1971.
9. Hammers L et al: Pulse Doppler US of focal liver masses, *Radiology* 181:225, 1991.
10. Katz ME et al: Epithelial carcinoma of the ovary: current strategies, *Ann Intern Med* 95:98, 1981.
11. Kier R et al: Renal masses: characterization with Doppler US, *Radiology* 176:703, 1990.
12. Kuijpers D, Jasper SR: Renal masses: differential diagnosis with pulse Doppler US, *Radiology* 270:59, 1989.
13. Kurjack A et al: The assessment of abnormal blood flow by transvaginal color and pulse Doppler ultrasound, *Med Biol* 16:437, 1990.
14. Marn CS et al: Arteriovenous shunts in cirrhosis: pitfalls in the Doppler evaluation of focal hepatic lesions, *Radiology* 177:156, 1990.
15. Marotti M et al: Complex and simple renal cysts: comparative evaluation with MR imaging, *Radiology* 162:697, 1987.
16. Pozniak M, Baus KM: Hepatofugal arterial signal in the main portal vein: an indicator of intravascular tumor spread, *Radiology* 108:663, 1991.
17. Quint LE et al: In vivo and in vitro MR imaging of renal tumors: histopathologic correlation and pulse sequence optimization, *Radiology* 169:359, 1988.
18. Ramos IM et al: Tumor vascular signals in renal mass: detection with Doppler US, *Radiology* 168:633, 1988.
19. Schoenberger SG, Sutherland CM, Robinson AE: Breast neoplasms: duplex sonographic imaging as an adjunct to diagnosis, *Radiology* 168:665, 1988.
20. Scoutt IM et al: Correlation of Doppler detected neovascularity with histologic predictors of breast cancer behavior, *Radiology* 177:287, 1990.
21. Shor AM, Shor GL: Tumor angiogenesis, *J Pathol* 141:385, 1983.
22. Smith SJ et al: Renal cell carcinoma: earlier discovery and increased detection, *Radiology* 170:699, 1989.
23. Strickland B: The value of arteriography in the diagnosis of bone tumors, *Br J Radiol* 32:705, 1959.
24. Tanaka S et al: Color Doppler flow imaging of liver tumors, *AJR* 154:509, 1990.
25. Taylor KJW et al: Focal liver masses: differential diagnosis with pulsed Doppler US, *Radiology* 164:643, 1987.
26. Taylor KJW et al: Correlation of Doppler US tumor signals with neovascular morphologic features, *Radiology* 166:57, 1988.
27. Vasilev SA et al: Serum Ca 125 levels in preoperative evaluation of pelvic masses, *Obstet Gynecol* 71:751, 1987.
28. Wells PNT et al: Tumor detection by ultrasonic Doppler blood flow signals, *Ultrasonics* 15:231, 1977.

CHAPTER 89

Intraoperative evaluation of renal and visceral artery reconstruction

RONALD J. STONEY and STEVEN P. OKUHN

Technical imperfections are a threat to the success of any vascular reconstruction, and arterial repairs involving all vascular beds and types of methods are susceptible to technical failure. Endarterectomy is particularly vulnerable because it demands a precise technique to avoid creating defects that are certain to lead to reconstruction failure. Acute (early) failures are virtually all due to technical problems with the revascularization itself, and many chronic (late) failures can also be traced to an intraoperative problem. There are numerous older reports citing technical factors that contribute to failures in revascularization,[1-3,6-9] and these authors emphasized the necessity of intraoperative assessment.

Early attempts to intraoperatively assess the results of revascularization procedures were crude. Palpation of the pulsatile quality of a repair could identify the presence, absence, or reduction in pulse volume; frequently a thrill appeared, signifying turbulence. However, this method could not quantify flow or detect intraluminal defects. The electromagnetic flowmeter was introduced to provide quantitative flow data, but the information it yielded was imprecise, systemic hemodynamic variables could not be reliably controlled, and it could not localize a suspected defect. Intraoperative arteriography, the gold standard for preoperative imaging of the cardiovascular system, has a number of disadvantages when applied intraoperatively. These include exposure to radiation, the nephrotoxicity of contrast materials, hypersensitivity reactions, arterial trauma, embolization during the introduction or manipulation of the catheter, the need for an additional arterial cross-clamp, the limitations of films obtained in a single plane at a single point in time, and anatomic restrictions that prevent optimal viewing of some reconstructions.

It became apparent that a more reliable, universally applicable, safe, and noninvasive method for the intraoperative assessment of vascular reconstruction was needed, and duplex ultrasonography was the logical choice. Duplex scanning is rapid and provides a dynamic real-time B-mode image in multiple planes. Doppler flow spectral analysis provides functional hemodynamic information that helps to confirm an adequate reconstruction or reveal technical problems. The 7.5- and 10.0-MHz probes have a superior imaging resolution not achieved with lower-frequency probes, and gated Doppler scanning leaves no doubt that the sample volume is truly in the center of the flow stream.

Intraoperative duplex assessment of vascular repairs can detect those defects that if not corrected, will cause ultimate reconstruction failure and distinguish these from minor, nonthreatening lesions that do not warrant intraoperative correction. This technology provides information that allows not only the identification and repair of specific defective reconstructions but also the performance of reconstructions free of even minor technical defects.

The vascular bed and the major artery supplying it are both important factors in the accurate intraoperative assessment of an arterial reconstruction. If the vascular bed (end organ) is not directly accessible or visible and its ischemic tolerance is low, the importance of obtaining a technically flawless arterial repair is magnified. Furthermore, arterial reconstruction sites that are within body cavities and thus less accessible for direct evaluation postoperatively should be examined at the time of operation. A reconstruction of any part of the renal or visceral vessels merits intraoperative assessment because renal and visceral ischemia may be fatal and acute perioperative failure of these types of reconstructions may go undetected for an extended interval, during which irreversible organ ischemia can develop.

This chapter reviews the initial experience with duplex scanning of renal and visceral reconstructions at the University of California, San Francisco Medical Center.[5] Since publication of the earlier report, additional confirmatory experience has been gained.

The study population consisted of 62 patients who underwent ultrasound assessment of 122 renal and visceral arteries. Of the 96 arteries that were operated on, 83 were renal and 13 were visceral. Of the 26 arteries that were not operated on, 14 were visceral and 12 were renal. Transaortic thromboendarterectomies were performed in 79% of the cases and bypasses in 18%.

A duplex scanner combining a high-resolution B-mode imager with pulsed Doppler ultrasonography (Hoffrel system 518; Hoffrel Instrument Co, South Norwalk, Conn.) was used for all studies. Insonation was performed in more than 96% of the cases using the 7.5-MHz probe. The probe, which had a 0.5-cm focus, was placed inside a sterile glove and sleeve. B-mode images were obtained in sagittal and transverse planes, and stereo Doppler signals were analyzed in real-time. Defects were graded on the basis of appearance and morphology, location, and percentage of luminal narrowing. Occlusion was presumed to exist when flow signals were absent or there was a characteristic "tom-tom" signal proximal to the obstruction.

Data were recorded on videotape (VHF) for offline fast-Fourier spectral analysis to allow calculation of the peak systolic and mean velocities. Spectral broadening was correlated with the percentage of the systolic window and graded as follows: 0, greater than 75% window; 1, 50% to 75% window; and 2, less than 50% window.

RESULTS

All studies were technically satisfactory and completed in a mean time of 8 minutes, with no complications. Two-thirds of the reconstructed arteries appeared normal, and among the 36 in which the studies were abnormal, only 4 had a major defect. These consisted of three cases of vessel occlusion and one case of an intraoperative luminal thrombus with audibly abnormal flow. All these arteries were reexplored and repaired, and the findings of the intraoperative study were confirmed.

The 32 minor defects were analyzed, and all had audibly normal flow signals. The defects consisted of a proximally based flap (20% luminal narrowing or less, $n = 13$), residual orifice lesion (20% luminal narrowing or less, $n = 6$), residual stenosis (20% luminal narrowing or less, $n = 11$), proximally based flap (50% luminal narrowing or less, $n = 1$), and residual stenosis (50% luminal narrowing or less, $n = 1$).

Of the total, 14 of the 26 nonreconstructed vessels appeared normal. The remaining 12 exhibited a variety of heterogeneous (atherosclerotic) lesions. Review of spectral analysis data demonstrated a difference between reconstructed and nonreconstructed (normal) renal arteries but not between reconstructed and nonreconstructed visceral arteries. The more normal renal arteries had higher velocities

and less spectral broadening. When flow data were compared with the B-mode images, *only* spectral broadening correlated with an abnormal B-mode result. Comparison of intraoperative duplex scanning with postoperative studies done to confirm the status of the renal and visceral arteries (e.g., direct inspection, intravenous and arterial digital subtraction angiography, renal scan, pathologic examination) revealed two false-negatives (sensitivity, 89%) and 17 false-positives (specificity, 77%); all were minor defects.

The 17 false-positives represented minor defects that were identified intraoperatively but not seen 7 to 14 days later on a confirmatory study. Most of these defects were probably the consequence of the thromboendarterectomy technique and simply healed during the early postoperative period. Furthermore, the techniques used for most confirmatory studies are much less sensitive than the intraoperative duplex scan, so some small defects may have been overlooked.

The importance of a sensitive technique for the intraoperative assessment of these reconstructions is obvious if the goal is to prevent an acute failure after visceral or renal revascularization. An 11% false-negative rate cannot be ignored; however, in this protocol, there is a variable interval between the intraoperative scan and confirmatory study, and false-negative scans are therefore not eliminated because these reconstruction failures may reflect increased thrombogenicity of the repaired vessel and *not* a missed technical defect.[5] Perhaps the proved patency rate at the time of discharge observed in this study (82 of 83 vessels) is a better overall indication of the superiority of the duplex scanner as a reliable technique for intraoperative assessment. This 99% patency rate at discharge exceeds that achieved at the University of California, San Francisco Medical Center for similar operations when intraoperative arteriography was the method used to assess the revascularizations.

These results have subsequently been confirmed by Hansen et al.[4] Using intraoperative duplex sonography, these investigators found a comparable number of major defects (6/57, 11%) that were repaired and minor defects (7/57, 12%) that were monitored during follow-up. They compared the results of intraoperative duplex scanning with those obtained postoperatively from confirmatory surface duplex scans and found that intraoperative duplex scanning showed a sensitivity of 86%. In contrast, Hansen et al.[4] noted that Doppler spectra with focal increases in peak systolic velocity greater than 2 m/sec helped to define major defects that required immediate revision.

CONCLUSION

Duplex ultrasonography is a rapid, safe, and sensitive technique for the intraoperative assessment of renal and visceral reconstructions. Doppler ultrasound clearly enhances B-mode imaging in the detection of major defects that require repair, and the findings from a recent study suggest that spectral analysis may add further information to the B-mode image and audible Doppler signal. The highly accurate results have persuaded many clinicians to use duplex scanning for the intraoperative arterial assessment in virtually all major arterial reconstructions.

REFERENCES

1. Anderson CA, Collins GJ, Rich NM: Routine operative arteriography during carotid endarterectomy: a reassessment, *Surgery* 83:67, 1978.
2. Blaisdell RW, Lim R, Hall AD: Technical result of carotid endarterectomy: arteriographic assessment, *Am J Surg* 114:239, 1967.
3. Dardik II et al: Routine intraoperative angiography: an essential adjunct in vascular surgery, *Arch Surg* 110:184, 1975.
4. Hansen KJ et al: Intraoperative duplex sonography during renal artery reconstruction, *J Vasc Surg* 14:364, 1991.
5. Okuhn SP et al: Intraoperative assessment of renal and visceral artery reconstruction: the role of duplex scanning and spectral analysis, *J Vasc Surg* 5:137, 1987.
6. Plecha FR, Pories WJ: Intraoperative angiography in the immediate assessment of arterial reconstruction, *Arch Surg* 105:902, 1972.
7. Renwick S, Royle JP, Martin P: Operative angiography after femoropopliteal artery reconstruction: its influence on early failure rate, *Br J Surg* 55:134, 1968.
8. Rosental JJ, Gaspar MR, Movius HJ: Intraoperative arteriography in carotid thromboendarterectomy, *Arch Surg* 106:806, 1973.
9. Stoney RJ, James DR, Wylie EJ: Surgery for femoropopliteal atherosclerosis: a reappraisal, *Arch Surg* 103:548, 1971.

CHAPTER 90

Penile ultrasound

E. MEREDITH JAMES

High-resolution ultrasound imaging of the penis, combined with color and spectral Doppler analysis, provides a useful noninvasive means of evaluating both morphologic and hemodynamic penile abnormalities. It can be successfully used in the investigation of congenital anomalies, masses, Peyronie's disease, and trauma-related abnormalities. Most of the recent work in this field has focused on the use of duplex sonography in the diagnostic evaluation of patients with impotence. The ability to identify both the arterial and venous causes of impotence makes duplex sonography an attractive potential screening method. The combined use of color and spectral Doppler analysis helps the examiner define the vascular anatomy, detect small vessels, demonstrate dynamic changes in blood flow, and make accurate velocity measurements.

ANATOMY

A thorough understanding of the anatomy of the penis is vital to the proper performance of a duplex ultrasound examination. The penis is made up of three corporal bodies: two corpora cavernosa, which lie in the dorsal two thirds of the penis, and a single corpus spongiosum, which lies in the ventral one third (Fig. 90-1). The urethra travels through the center of the corpus spongiosum. These corpora are surrounded by a thick fascial layer called the *tunica albuginea*. The two corpora cavernosa are the main erectile bodies of the penis. They contain multiple sinusoidal cavities that are lined by smooth muscle and endothelium and that distend with blood during an erection. A septum divides both corpora cavernosa, but it contains many fenestrations that serve as multiple anastomotic connections between the sinusoidal spaces of both corpora.

The blood supply of the penis is derived primarily from the internal pudendal arteries, which are branches of the internal iliac arteries. Each internal pudendal artery gives off a perineal branch, a bulbar artery, and a small urethral artery before continuing as the artery of the penis. The penile arteries enter the base of the penis and branch into a deep cavernosal artery and a dorsal artery. The cavernosal artery travels near the center of the corpus cavernosum, sending off small helicine branches that communicate directly with the sinusoidal spaces. The cavernosal arteries are the pri-

mary source of blood flow to the erectile tissue of the penis. The two dorsal penile arteries lie outside the tunica albuginea and primarily supply blood to the skin and glans of the penis. Multiple small anastomotic channels connect the cavernosal arteries with the dorsal arteries.

The venous drainage of the erectile tissue of the penis takes place primarily via emissary veins that drain the corpora cavernosa. These veins perforate the thick tunica albuginea and empty into circumflex veins, which ultimately drain into the deep dorsal vein of the penis. The deep dorsal vein, which is normally flanked on each side by the dorsal penile arteries, empties into the retropubic venous plexus. The corpora cavernosa also drain to some extent directly into the cavernosal and crural veins at the base of the penis. The superficial dorsal vein, which varies in location, drains the glans and skin of the penis.

PHYSIOLOGY

Penile erection results from the relaxation of the smooth muscle that lines the walls of the sinusoids and the helicine and cavernosal arteries of the corpora cavernosa.[3,13,22,33] The subsequent increased arterial flow fills the sinusoidal spaces and produces the penile tumescence. As the sinusoids become more distended, the intracavernosal pressure increases, and this causes the emissary veins draining the corpora cavernosa to be squeezed against the inner margin of the rigid tunica albuginea (Fig. 90-2). This venoocclusive phenomenon prevents venous outflow, thus maintaining sinusoidal distention and resulting in penile rigidity. When the psychoerotic stimulus subsides, the smooth muscle relaxation and dilatation of the blood vessels supplying the penis diminish. The sinusoids then shrink, easing the compression from the emissary veins, and allowing unimpeded venous outflow to resume. The penis then becomes flaccid.

The actions of the neurochemical mediators of sinusoidal relaxation are poorly understood. Adrenergic activity appears to inhibit smooth muscle relaxation and thus serves to maintain the penis in a flaccid state. Parasympathetic activity, which is mediated by acetylcholine, increases with psychoerotic stimulation and triggers suppression of the baseline adrenergic activity, thus allowing for smooth muscle relaxation. Other substances, such as endothelium-de-

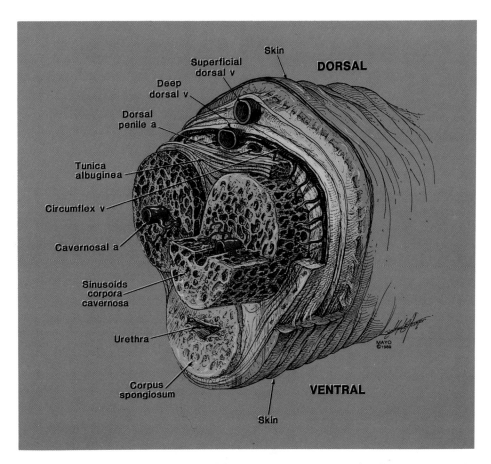

Fig. 90-1. Cross section of the anatomy of the penis. (From Quam JP et al: *AJR* 153:1141, 1989.)

rived relaxing factor, may act as cellular mediators and may be necessary for normal erectile function.[33]

IMPOTENCE

In the past, psychologic factors were considered responsible for most cases of erectile dysfunction. In recent years, however, physiologic and anatomic studies have revealed that the cause of impotence in most patients is organic. Today, vasculogenic erectile failure is regarded as one of the most common sources of organic impotence.[19,27,35] It may be due to either poor arterial flow into the penis (arteriogenic impotence) or excessive venous leakage of blood from the penis (venogenic impotence). In some patients, both mechanisms operate. It has recently been suggested that as yet poorly understood local factors within the helicine arteries or the endothelium lining the sinusoidal spaces may account for a significant number of cases of impotence.[6]

Arteriography with selective internal iliac artery injection is considered the gold standard for the evaluation of arteriogenic impotence.[5,7,15] This technique is invasive, however, and not suitable as a screening method. Traditionally, cavernosometry and cavernosography have been used to diagnose venogenic impotence,[11,20,21,25,26] but these examinations are also invasive and not ideally suited for screening purposes.

Several noninvasive techniques have been used to evaluate men with impotence; these include measuring the penile-brachial blood pressure index and monitoring the patient in a sleep laboratory to assess the status of nocturnal erections.[1,2,9,17] More recently, many patients with suspected vasculogenic impotence have undergone direct intracavernosal injection of a vasodilating agent such as papaverine, phentolamine, or prostaglandin E_1.[1,8,36,38] The injection bypasses the psychoerotic and neurologic pathways that normally induce an erection. If the patient develops a full erection after the injection, this indicates adequate arterial inflow and an intact venoocclusive mechanism and rules out vasculogenic causes. Conversely, a poor or absent response to injection implies a vascular cause. However, this technique cannot differentiate arteriogenic from venogenic impotence, which is an important distinction because the current treatment options (mainly surgical) for each type of impotence are different. Today, duplex sonography in conjunction with color Doppler imaging is being used increasingly as the initial screening method for evaluating impotent men, particularly in the selection of patients who would benefit from further evaluation with the more invasive studies.*

---

*References 4, 10, 14, 16, 18, 23, 24, 28, 29, 30-32, 34, 37.

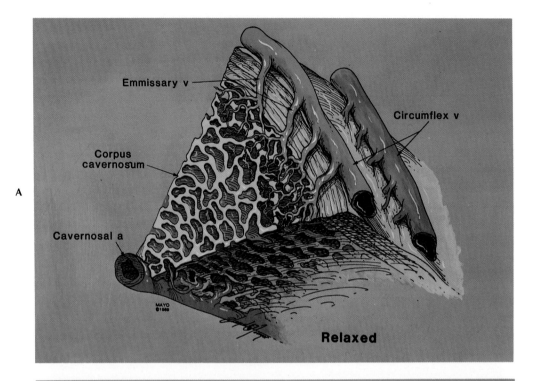

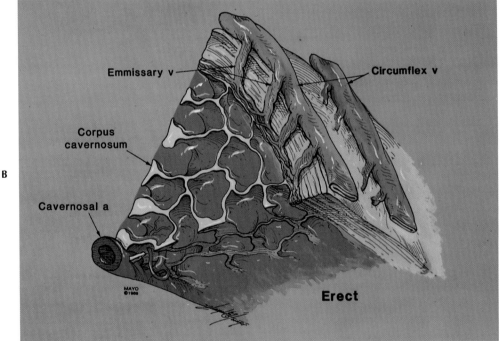

Fig. 90-2. *A,* A wedge transverse section of the corpus cavernosum in the relaxed or flaccid state shows the collapsed sinusoidal spaces and their draining emissary and circumflex veins. *B,* In the erect state, the sinusoids are distended, resulting in compression of the emissary veins against the rigid tunica albuginea. (From Lewis RW: *Int J Impotence Res* 2:1, 1990.)

ULTRASOUND EXAMINATION TECHNIQUE

Ultrasound examination of the penis is best performed with a high-frequency (7.5-MHz) electronically focused linear transducer. The patient lies supine with the penis in the anatomic position, resting on the anterior abdominal wall (Fig. 90-3). No special patient preparation is needed for the study. The transducer is placed on the ventral surface, and the penis is examined in both longitudinal and transverse planes from the glans to the base. The two corpora cavernosa are seen on transverse images as adjacent circular structures separated by the septum penis. The corpus spongiosum is often compressed and difficult for the examiner to visualize when scanning from the ventral surface but may be visualized by applying generous amounts of acoustic gel and exerting minimal pressure with the transducer (Fig. 90-4). The echo texture of the corpora cavernosa is homogeneous and consists of medium-level echoes. The septum penis is seen as a prominent hypoechoic band with some associated acoustic shadowing.

The cavernosal arteries are located near the central and medial aspects of the corpora cavernosa and may be seen with gray-scale imaging alone but are virtually always identified by color Doppler imaging. Occasionally color Doppler imaging demonstrates collateral vessels crossing the septum penis from one cavernosal artery to another or from the dorsal penile artery to the cavernosal artery. The two dorsal penile arteries are smaller than the cavernosal arteries and may be visualized when scanning is performed from a dorsal approach.

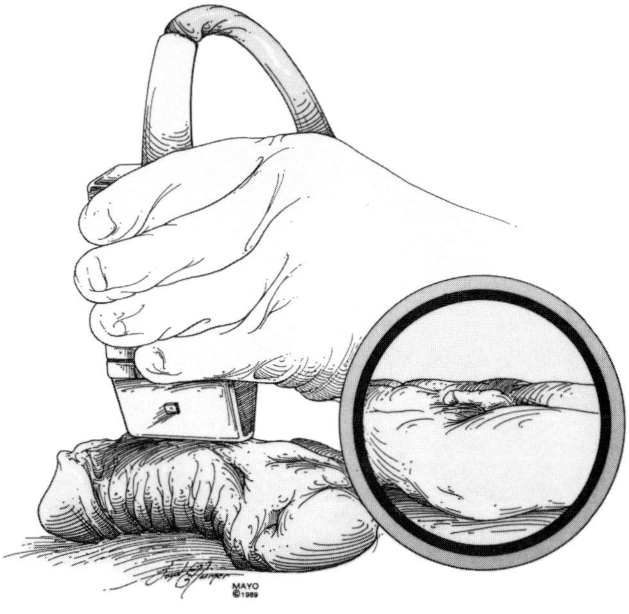

The examination begins with an anatomic survey. This is performed in both longitudinal and transverse planes to detect possible echogenic fibrous or calcific plaque or other anatomic abnormalities (Fig. 90-5), as well as to identify and measure the diameters of the cavernosal arteries (Fig. 90-6).

After this initial survey, a vasodilating agent (or a combination of agents) is injected directly into the corpus cav-

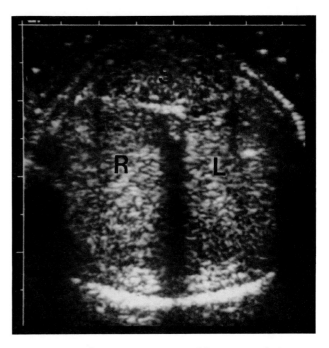

Fig. 90-4. Normal transverse sonogram of the penis. With the transducer on the ventral surface, the larger right *(R)* and left *(L)* corpora cavernosa are seen dorsally, and the smaller corpus spongiosum *(S)* is seen ventrally. Applying a copious amount of acoustic gel permits visualization of the curving ventral surface of the penis.

Fig. 90-3. The positioning of the penis for duplex ultrasound examination. The penis is placed in the anatomic position, with the transducer on the ventral aspect. (From Quam JP et al: *AJR* 153:1141, 1989.)

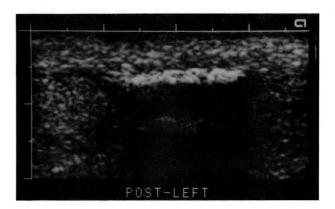

Fig. 90-5. Penile plaque. Longitudinal sonogram of the left corpus cavernosum shows a linear echogenic plaque with distal acoustic shadow. This is the typical lesion of Peyronie's disease.

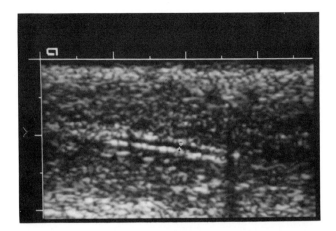

Fig. 90-6. Longitudinal sonogram of the right corpus cavernosum shows the cavernosal artery running centrally. Electronic calipers are placed on the inner walls to measure the luminal diameter. Before injection, this measurement is often less than 0.5 mm.

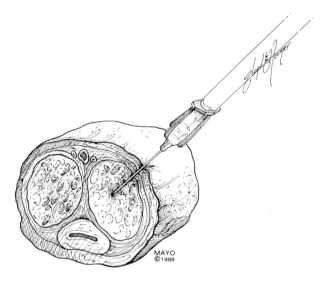

Fig. 90-7. Cross section of the penis shows proper needle position within the corpus cavernosum during injection of vasoactive agents. (From King BF Jr et al: *Semin Intervent Radiol* 7:215, 1990.)

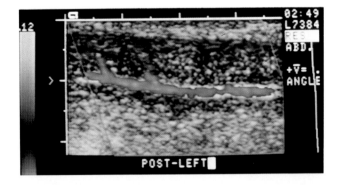

Fig. 90-8. Longitudinal color Doppler image of the left cavernosal artery after intracorporal injection of vasoactive agents. Color Doppler imaging allows rapid identification of the cavernosal arteries.

ernosum (Fig. 90-7). For example, 10 μg of prostaglandin E$_1$ in a 0.5-ml volume can be used. The vasodilating agent diffuses rapidly across the many fenestrations in the septum to enter the opposite corpus cavernosum. One must be careful not to inject the vasodilating agent into the corpus spongiosum or the subcutaneous tissues.

The major potential complication of this method is priapism, which may occur in up to 10% of the patients.[12] Prolonged rigid erection (lasting more than 1 to 3 hours) can cause ischemic necrosis and ultimately fibrosis of the cavernosal tissue. Therefore all patients should be told to contact the referring physician or go directly to the emergency room for proper management if a painful erection occurs or if the erection does not subside after 1 hour.

Priapism is more likely in patients with sickle cell disease or sickle cell trait, leukemia, or multiple myeloma, as well as in heparinized patients, and therefore intracavernosal injection should not be performed in these patients.

After the injection, the diameters of the cavernosal arteries are measured again and velocity measurements are obtained using spectral Doppler analysis. The optimal times when these measurements should be made is disputed. The maximal effect of the vasodilating agents is reached 5 to 20 minutes after injection, and the effects begin to subside at 20 to 30 minutes. Therefore velocity measurements in the cavernosal arteries should commence approximately 5 minutes after injection. Because the time when the highest peak systolic velocity is reached varies, it is important to obtain serial measurements. For example, peak systolic and end-diastolic velocities in both cavernosal arteries can be measured 5, 10, 15, and 20 minutes after the injection. Cavernosal artery diameters are measured at approximately 20 minutes.

Color Doppler imaging is a sensitive means of detecting cavernosal artery blood flow, thus permitting more rapid identification of these vessels (Fig. 90-8). Color Doppler imaging may also identify collateral vessels in some patients. When velocities within the cavernosal artery are measured, it is important to accurately align the angle-correction cursor with the direction of flow. Color Doppler imaging can aid in establishing the correct axis of blood flow, thus making accurate angle correction possible. Angle-corrected velocity measurements are most accurate when the Doppler angles are small. Sampling at a site near the base of the penis where the cavernosal artery changes from an anterior to a cephalad direction usually provides an optimum shallow Doppler angle.

SPECTRAL WAVEFORM ANALYSIS

Schwartz et al[34] have reported that the Doppler spectral pattern of cavernosal arteries has five phases in normal patients without impotence (Fig. 90-9). In the first minutes after the injection of a vasodilator, blood velocity increases and the spectral waveform exhibits a rounded systolic peak with prominent diastolic flow; this reflects low-flow resistance within the sinusoidal spaces. As intracavernosal pressure increases, the systolic peak becomes sharper while the diastolic flow diminishes and ultimately ceases. As the veno-occlusive mechanism engages, intracavernosal pressure exceeds the diastolic arterial pressure, causing the blood flow to reverse during diastole. Finally, once full rigidity is reached, diastolic flow again ceases and there is dampening of the systolic peak. All normal phases in patients with vasculogenic impotence may not be completed because of abnormal arterial inflow or excessive venous leakage. Because of the dynamic nature of the velocity profile, the appearance of the spectral waveform must be correlated with the status of the erection (i.e., flaccid, tumescent, rigid), as well as with the time when the waveform is obtained after injection.

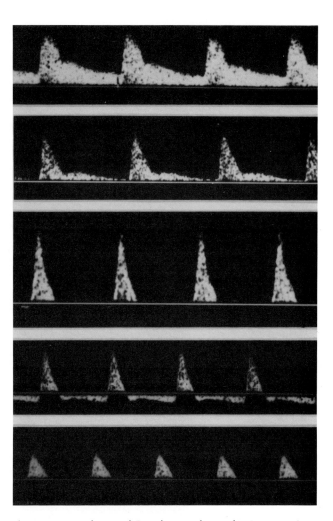

Fig. 90-9. Normal spectral Doppler waveforms after injection. Soon after injection the spectral waveform has a low-resistance pattern, with prominent diastolic flow. Thereafter, as intracorporal pressure increases, diastolic flow diminishes and, ultimately, reverses. With a full, rigid erection, systolic peaks are dampened and there is no diastolic flow.

ARTERIOGENIC IMPOTENCE

Arterial flow is a function of both the blood velocity and the cross-sectional area of the vessel lumen. Some investigators have therefore studied the change in diameter of the cavernosal arteries after intracavernosal injection of a vasodilating agent and have found that a 75% increase in vessel diameter correlates with a good anatomic response and indicates adequate arterial inflow.[24] The small size of the artery, however, makes accurate diameter measurements difficult and the attendant potential error may be significant. Therefore cavernosal artery diameter measurement should probably remain a secondary diagnostic method for identifying patients with arteriogenic impotence.

Measurement of peak systolic velocities in the cavernosal arteries after intracavernosal injection currently appears to be the best ultrasound approach for evaluating patients with suspected arteriogenic impotence.[4,28,29,34] Because the time

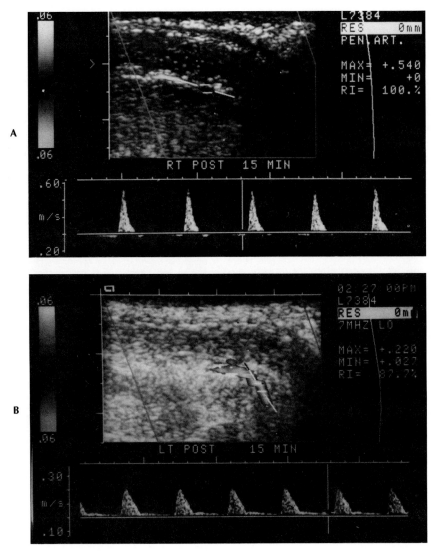

Fig. 90-10. Unilateral arterial disease. **A,** Peak systolic velocity of the right cavernosal artery is 54 cm/ sec. **B,** Peak systolic velocity of the left cavernosal artery is 22 cm/sec. Although the average of these two measurements is normal (greater than 30 cm/sec), the marked disparity from right to left suggests a significant arterial lesion on the left.

when the highest peak systolic velocity is reached after intracavernosal injection varies among individuals, it is important to obtain serial measurements. These velocities may occur 5, 10, 15, or 20 minutes after injection, with a nearly equal distribution.

The velocity criteria reported for distinguishing normal from abnormal arterial flow have varied. Schwartz et al[34] found that the normal average (i.e., mean right and left) peak systolic velocity after intracavernosal injection of a vasodilating agent is 30 to 40 cm/sec. Lue et al[24] found that most patients who show a moderate to good clinical response to papaverine injection have peak systolic velocities of 25 cm/sec or greater. More recently, Benson and Vickers[4] concluded that a velocity of 40 cm/sec or greater should be considered normal. In a series of 12 patients with

suspected arteriogenic impotence who underwent pelvic arteriography, all 5 patients with abnormal arteriograms had average peak systolic velocities of less than 25 cm/sec.[29]

Despite the variability in the velocity criteria used to judge arterial responses, it is generally agreed that a mean peak systolic velocity in the cavernosal arteries of less than 25 cm/sec indicates arterial insufficiency and should prompt a more definitive evaluation with selective arteriography. For some clinicians, values between 25 and 30 cm/sec are also considered abnormal, and those greater than 30 cm/ sec are regarded as normal. Occasionally there is a marked discrepancy between the velocities of the two cavernosal arteries (more than 10 cm/sec) despite an average value that is normal (Fig. 90-10). This may indicate the existence of unilateral arterial disease. Although a single cavernosal

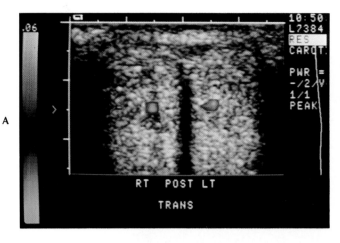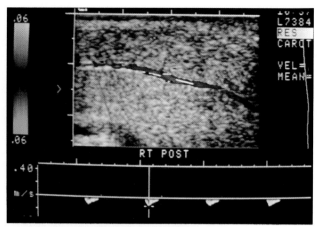

Fig. 90-11. Arterial flow reversal. **A,** Transverse color Doppler image shows the right and left cavernosal arteries in cross section, with flow in opposite directions (red versus blue). **B,** Longitudinal color/spectral Doppler image of the right cavernosal artery shows reversed flow direction (i.e., toward the base of the penis). This finding should indicate high-grade stenosis or occlusion proximally on the right with retrograde filling of the cavernosal artery by collateral flow.

artery may provide sufficient blood flow for adequate erection to be achieved, unilateral arterial disease may be significant in some individuals, and arteriography is necessary for definitive evaluation.

As mentioned previously, it is a normal phenomenon for blood flow to reverse during diastole as intracavernosal pressures increase. Indeed, the finding of diastolic flow reversal on duplex examination has proved to be a reliable indicator of adequate arterial inflow and an intact venoocclusive mechanism, thus eliminating the need for more invasive studies. Although not frequently encountered, reversed flow during systole is always an abnormal finding (Fig. 90-11). It is apparently due to proximal penile artery occlusion with retrograde collateral flow into the affected cavernosal artery. Collateral vessels that travel from one cavernosal artery to the other or from the dorsal penile artery to the cavernosal artery may be normal variants but may also indicate proximal vessel disease. These collateral vessels can often be seen with color Doppler imaging.

Arterial-sinusoidal or arteriovenous fistulas within the corporal tissue are usually the result of penile trauma and can cause partial priapism. Color Doppler evaluation can identify the location of such fistulas. In this setting, spectral Doppler shows increased velocities with prominent diastolic flow due to high arterial inflow into the low-resistance vascular bed.

VENOGENIC IMPOTENCE

Vasculogenic impotence may also be due to excessive venous leakage from the corpora cavernosa. Although the exact cause of this venous leakage is unknown, most likely it is secondary to stretching of the tunica albuginea, which prevents adequate compression of the emissary veins draining the cavernosal sinusoids. Thus venous outflow from the corporal bodies continues and a rigid erection can never be achieved.

In a normal patient, there is an increase in both systolic and diastolic velocities soon after intracavernosal injection of vasodilating agents. During sinusoidal filling, resistance in the cavernosal and helicine arteries diminishes and diastolic flow is prominent. As the sinusoids become maximally distended and the venoocclusive mechanism engages, vascular resistance increases and diastolic flow ceases or even reverses. If the venoocclusive mechanism is not intact, excessive venous flow will persist and the intracavernosal pressures will remain low. Therefore the Doppler spectral waveform in patients with venous leakage continues to exhibit prominent diastolic flow well after the injection, and this indicates a low-resistance vascular bed (Fig. 90-12).

Because elevated diastolic velocities are normally seen in the early minutes after intracavernosal injection, the determination of abnormal diastolic flow should be based on velocity measurements made 15 or 20 minutes after injection. For example, venous incompetence is suspected in patients with end-diastolic velocities of 3 cm/sec or greater despite normal arterial inflow (peak systolic velocities greater than 30 cm/sec), and cavernosometry with cavernosography is recommended to establish diagnosis. When the ultrasound results have been compared with those from cavernosometry and cavernosography, this criterion has shown a sensitivity of 94% and a specificity of 69% for identifying or ruling out venous leakage. When peak systolic velocities are abnormal (less than 30 cm/sec), however, persistent forward flow at end diastole does not necessarily indicate venous leakage because the venoocclusive mechanism may not engage fully when arterial inflow is inadequate. Alternatively, as noted earlier, the development of diastolic flow reversal after injection is a reliable indicator of venous competence.

Some investigators have recommended the velocity measurement of the deep dorsal penile vein as a means of de-

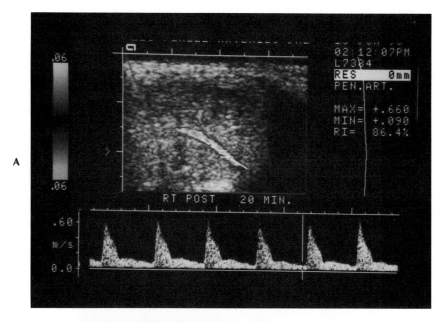

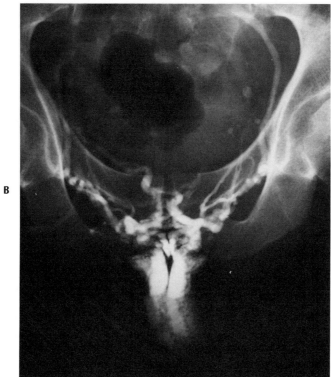

Fig. 90-12. Venogenic impotence. *A,* Spectral Doppler tracing of the right cavernosal artery, obtained 20 minutes after injection, shows prominent diastolic flow, with an end-diastolic velocity of 9 cm/sec. This prolonged low-resistance pattern indicates probable venous leakage. A peak systolic velocity of 66 cm/sec is normal. *B,* Cavernosography shows marked venous leakage from the corpora cavernosa with filling of the retropubic venous plexus and internal pudendal veins.

tecting venous leakage, since this vein carries most of the venous outflow from the corpora cavernosa. Some results indicate, however, that many patients with venous leakage do have measurable flow in the deep dorsal vein but so do many normal patients, thus making this an unacceptable criterion for diagnosing venogenic impotence. In addition, cavernosometry and cavernosography have shown that sometimes the leakage occurs primarily via the crural veins near the base of the penis and not via the deep dorsal penile vein.

CONCLUSION

Duplex and color Doppler ultrasonography are playing increasingly important roles in the noninvasive evaluation of patients with suspected vasculogenic impotence. Cavernosal arterial peak systolic and end-diastolic velocities appear to provide useful information that may differentiate arterial from venous causes of impotence and thus help in the appropriate selection of more invasive diagnostic procedures. Further refinements in the sonographic criteria can be anticipated as ultrasound findings are correlated with the results of arteriography and cavernosometry.

REFERENCES

1. Abber JC et al: Diagnostic tests for impotence: a comparison of papaverine injection with the penile-brachial index and nocturnal penile tumescence monitoring, *J Urol* 135:923, 1986.
2. Abelson D: Diagnostic value of the penile pulse and blood pressure: a Doppler study of impotence in diabetics, *J Urol* 113:636, 1975.
3. Aboseif SR, Lue TF: Hemodynamics of penile erection, *Urol Clin North Am* 15:1, 1988.
4. Benson CB, Vickers MA: Sexual impotence caused by vascular disease: diagnosis with duplex sonography, *AJR* 153:1149, 1989.
5. Bookstein JJ: Penile vascular catheterization in the diagnosis and treatment of impotence, *Cardiovasc Intervent Radiol* 11:183, 1988.
6. Bookstein JJ, Valji K: The arteriolar component in impotence: a possible paradigm shift, *AJR* 157:932, 1991.
7. Bookstein JJ et al: Pharmacoarteriography in the evaluation of impotence, *J Urol* 137:333, 1987.
8. Buvat J et al: Is intracavernous injection of papaverine a reliable screening test for vascular impotence? *J Urol* 135:476, 1986.
9. Chiu RC-J, Lidstone D, Blundell PE: Predictive power of penile/brachial index in diagnosing male sexual impotence, *J Vasc Surg* 4:251, 1986.
10. Collins JP, Lewandowski BJ: Experience with intracorporeal injection of papaverine and duplex ultrasound scanning for assessment of arteriogenic impotence, *Br J Urol* 59:84, 1987.
11. Delcour C et al: Impotence: evaluation with cavernosography, *Radiology* 161:803, 1986.
12. Dilworth JP, Lewis RW, Hattery RR: 1991 (unpublished data).
13. Fujita T, Shirai M: Mechanism of erection, *J Clin Exp Med* 148:249, 1989.
14. Gall H et al: Diagnostic accuracy of Doppler ultrasound technique of the penile arteries in correlation to selective arteriography, *Cardiovasc Intervent Radiol* 11:225, 1988.
15. Gray RR et al: Investigation of impotence by internal pudendal angiography: experience with 73 cases, *Radiology* 144:773, 1982.
16. Hattery RR et al: Vasculogenic impotence: duplex and color Doppler imaging, *Radiol Clin North Am* 29:629, 1991.
17. Karacan I, Salis PJ, Williams RL: *The role of the sleep laboratory in diagnosis and treatment of impotence*. In William RL, Karacan I, Frazier SH, eds: *Sleep disorders: diagnosis and treatment*, New York, 1978, John Wiley & Sons.
18. King BF Jr et al: Duplex sonography in the evaluation of impotence: current techniques, *Semin Intervent Radiol* 7:215, 1990.
19. Krane RJ, Goldstein I, Saenz de Tejada I: Impotence, *N Engl J Med* 321:1648, 1989.
20. Lewis RW: This month in investigative urology: venous impotence, *J Urol* 140:1560, 1988.
21. Lewis RW: Venous ligation surgery for venous leakage, *Int J Impotence Res* 2:1, 1990.
22. Lue TF, Tanagho EA: Physiology of erection and pharmacological management of impotence, *J Urol* 137:829, 1987.
23. Lue TF et al: Evaluation of arteriogenic impotence with intracorporeal injection of papaverine and the duplex ultrasound scanner, *Semin Urol* 3:43, 1985.
24. Lue TF et al: Vasculogenic impotence evaluated by high-resolution ultrasonography and pulsed Doppler spectrum analysis, *Radiology* 155:777, 1985.
25. Lue TF et al: Functional evaluation of penile veins by cavernosography in papaverine-induced erection, *J Urol* 135:479, 1986.
26. Malhotra CM et al: Cavernosography in conjunction with artificial erection for evaluation of venous leakage in impotent men, *Radiology* 161:799, 1986.
27. Mueller SC, Lue TF: Evaluation of vasculogenic impotence, *Urol Clin North Am* 15:65, 1988.
28. Paushter DM: Role of duplex sonography in the evaluation of sexual impotence, *AJR* 153:1161, 1989.
29. Quam JP et al: Duplex and color Doppler sonographic evaluation of vasculogenic impotence, *AJR* 153:1141, 1989.
30. Rajfer J et al: Correlation between penile angiography and duplex scanning of cavernous arteries in impotent men, *J Urol* 143:1128, 1990.
31. Robinson LQ, Woodcock JP, Stephenson TP: Duplex scanning in suspected vasculogenic impotence: a worthwhile exercise? *Br J Urol* 63:432, 1989.
32. Rosen MP et al: Radiologic assessment of impotence: angiography, sonography, cavernosography, and scintigraphy, *AJR* 157:923, 1991.
33. Saenz de Tejada I, Goldstein I, Krane RJ: Local control of penile erection: nerves, smooth muscle, and endothelium, *Urol Clin North Am* 15:9, 1988.
34. Schwartz AN et al: Evaluation of normal erectile function with color flow Doppler sonography, *AJR* 153:1155, 1989.
35. Shabsigh R, Fishman IJ, Scott FB: Evaluation of erectile impotence, *Urology* 32:83, 1988.
36. Stackl W, Hasun R, Marberger M: Intracavernous injection of prostaglandin E1 in impotent men, *J Urol* 140:66, 1988.
37. Vickers M, Benson C, Richie J: High resolution ultrasonography and pulsed wave Doppler for detection of corporovenous incompetence in erectile dysfunction, *J Urol* 143:1125, 1990.
38. Virag R et al: Intracavernous injection of papaverine as a diagnostic and therapeutic method in erectile failure, *Angiology* 35:79, 1984.

CHAPTER 91

The female pelvis

KENNETH J. W. TAYLOR

The recently introduced method of endovaginal color flow can yield dramatic images of the pelvic vasculature that have enabled confirmation of many of the cyclic variations in ovarian and uterine flow earlier observed by transabdominal pulsed Doppler techniques.[9,11,14] Endovaginal ultrasound has several striking advantages over the transabdominal approach. First, the proximity between the endovaginal transducer and the pelvic organs allows the use of higher frequencies in the range of 5 to 7.5 MHz, and this greatly improves resolution. The image quality is also improved because of the absence of subcutaneous fat, which can cause severe artifact formation. This is especially important in obese patients for whom both pelvic examination and transabdominal sonography are very limited. In addition to the dramatic images of pelvic vasculature furnished by color flow ultrasound, pulsed Doppler allows quantitative time-varying parameters to be derived. However, one disadvantage of endovaginal color flow imaging is that the field of view is limited, making orientation extremely difficult. Thus the learning curve for optimal operator use is in terms of years rather than weeks. The limited depth of the field due to the higher frequency also means that ovarian tumors or ectopic pregnancies may be missed if they are displaced out of the pelvis and lie above the uterus. Nevertheless, overall endovaginal color flow imaging represents a dramatic improvement in ultrasound technology.

NORMAL ANATOMY

In color flow images, the most obvious structures on the side walls of the pelvis are the iliac veins. The external iliac vein is always clearly seen and, with deeper penetration, the common iliac vein and its bifurcation (Fig. 91-1). The application of pulsed Doppler analysis demonstrates the normal venous waveform with its physiologic phasicity (Fig. 91-2). The adjacent internal and external iliac arteries are smaller vessels but can be easily noted and the waveform elicited. The normal triphasic waveform is observed in the common and external iliac arteries (Fig. 91-3). In contrast, the internal iliac artery exhibits continuous forward flow in diastole (Fig. 91-4).

The uterine vasculature is apparent in every patient. The main uterine arteries can be seen as they approach the cervix, then travel on either side of the lateral aspect of the body of the uterus to send the arcuate branches around the uterine body that pierce the myometrium (Fig. 91-5). The uterine waveform in the nongravid woman and during the first trimester of pregnancy is characteristic and consists of rather high-impedance flow with a typical notch during diastole (Fig. 91-6, A). During the early second trimester, this high-impedance flow changes to a very low-impedance flow (Fig. 91-6, B) because between the twelfth and eighteenth weeks of pregnancy, there is a secondary invasion of the trophoblast that destroys the elastic lamina of the spiral arteries and converts the fetal and maternal interface into a low-impedance shunt. This brings about the increased blood flow necessary for the fetal growth spurt that occurs during the second trimester. It has also been demonstrated that if this does not take place, it can precipitate complications such as intrauterine growth retardation.[4]

The position of the ovary varies widely, particularly in patients who have undergone a hysterectomy. However, the most common position is between the iliac vein laterally and the uterine vascularity in the region of the cornua medially (Fig. 91-7). The ovary has a specific though variable

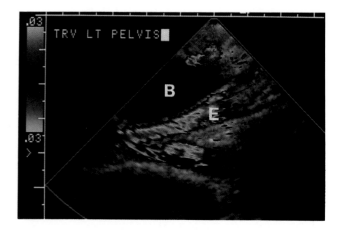

Fig. 91-1. Color flow scan showing bladder *(B)* with the internal and external iliac veins *(E)* on the side wall of the pelvis. (From Taylor KJW et al: *Obstetric and gynecologic applications.* In *Clinics in diagnostic ultrasound,* vol 27, New York, 1992, Churchill Livingstone.)

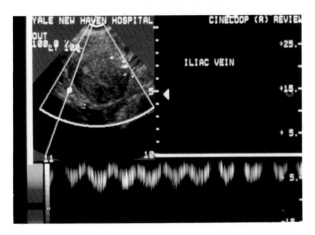

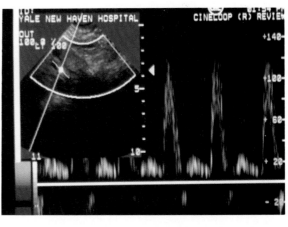

Fig. 91-2. Endovaginal ultrasound showing color flow of iliac vein and corresponding pulse Doppler spectrum with the typical physiologic variations. (From Taylor KJW et al: *Obstetric and gynecologic applications.* In *Clinics in diagnostic ultrasound,* vol 27, New York, 1992, Churchill Livingstone.)

Fig. 91-3. Doppler waveform of external iliac artery. Note the normal triphasic waveform with reversal of flow in early diastole and antegrade flow in mid-diastole. (From Taylor KJW et al: *Obstetric and gynecologic applications.* In *Clinics in diagnostic ultrasound,* vol 27, New York, 1992, Churchill Livingstone.)

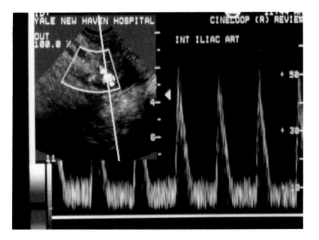

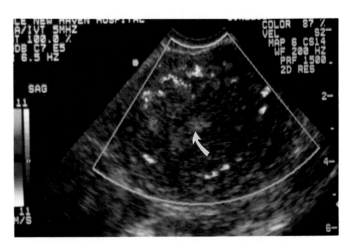

Fig. 91-4. Pulse and color endovaginal ultrasound of pelvic side wall demonstrating waveform in the internal iliac artery. Notice that there is continuous flow during diastole. (From Taylor KJW et al: *Obstetric and gynecologic applications.* In *Clinics in diagnostic ultrasound,* vol 27, New York, 1992, Churchill Livingstone.)

Fig. 91-5. Endovaginal ultrasound of uterus in sagittal plane. Note the endometrial stripe *(arrow)* and the uterine arteries and arcuate branches in color. (From Taylor KJW et al: *Obstetric and gynecologic applications.* In *Clinics in diagnostic ultrasound,* vol 27, New York, 1992, Churchill Livingstone.)

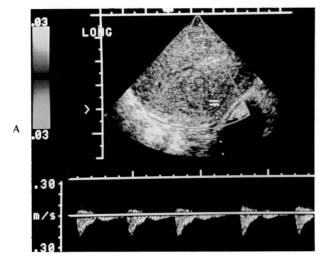

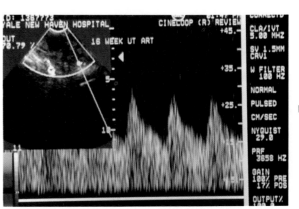

Fig. 91-6. *A,* Sagittal scan of the uterus demonstrating the echogenic endometrial stripe and branches of the uterine artery, which are clearly seen traversing the myometrium. A pulse Doppler spectrum demonstrates the typical uterine waveform with a diastolic notch. ***B,*** Uterine blood flow in a fetus at 16 weeks gestation demonstrating low-impedance flow. Compare this waveform to that in ***A.*** (From Taylor KJW et al: *Obstetric and gynecologic applications.* In *Clinics in diagnostic ultrasound,* vol 27, New York, 1992, Churchill Livingstone.)

morphology during the reproductive years. Ovarian follicles are always seen in fertile women, and follicular or luteal cysts of various sizes are also seen depending on the time in the menstrual cycle. Taylor et al[11] were the first to demonstrate the change in functional flow in the ovary associated with ovulation and the function of the corpus luteum. These functional changes in the ovary convert the high-impedance ovarian flow to the low-impedance luteal pattern (Fig. 91-8). Such low-impedance luteal flow is seen in the first trimester of every normal pregnancy and in 90% of ectopic pregnancies.[13] The presence of this low-impedance flow has been correlated with a greater likelihood of successful fertilization in patients undergoing ovulation stimulation.[2] However, it is very important that the characteristics of luteal flow be recognized, since they can be confused with the neovascular flow associated with ovarian cancer. Thus when screened for ovarian cancer, the patient must be scanned early in the cycle before luteal flow is established. Even then, persistent luteal flow from the preceding cycle is not infrequent, and repeat scanning may be necessary to establish whether the low-impedance flow is cyclic or permanent. A functional tumor should exhibit noncyclic, low-impedance flow, as demonstrated in a patient who had a hilar cell tumor (arrhenoblastoma).[2]

Relatively high-velocity, low-impedance flow is also characteristic of ectopic pregnancies (vide infra), and this makes it important to differentiate between luteal flow and a tubal vascular structure due to an ectopic pregnancy.

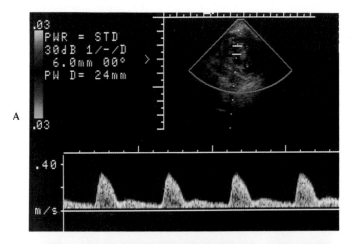

Fig. 91-7. Endovaginal ultrasound of the left adnexa. The typical ovarian morphology is seen with the iliac vein *(open arrow)* below the ovary and the uterine artery branches near the cornuum *(closed arrow)* above the ovary. (From Taylor KJW et al: *Obstetric and gynecologic applications.* In *Clinics in diagnostic ultrasound,* vol 27, New York, 1992, Churchill Livingstone.)

A

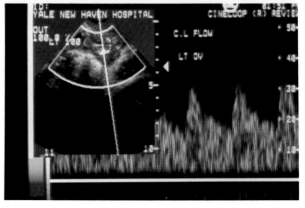

C

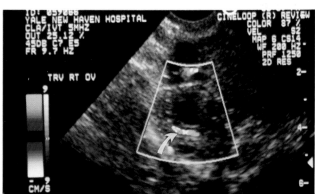

B

Fig. 91-8. *A,* Duplex and color transvaginal ultrasound on day 7 shows a relatively avascular ovary with high impedance flow (resistance index, 0.87). *B,* Endovaginal ultrasound of the ovary showing the normal follicular morphology seen in women of reproductive age. Color represents vascularization of the functioning corpus luteum *(arrow).* *C,* Pulse and color endovaginal ultrasound demonstrates vascularization of the corpus luteum with low-impedance flow (resistance index, 0.56). (From Taylor KJW et al: *Obstetric and gynecologic applications.* In *Clinics in diagnostic ultrasound,* vol 27, New York, 1992, Churchill Livingstone.)

NORMAL FIRST TRIMESTER OF PREGNANCY

As previously stated, the normal uterine waveform in the first trimester of pregnancy shows a high-impedance low-diastolic flow. However, a low-impedance area appears in the endometrium approximately 36 to 50 days after the last menstrual period, and this represents the increased vascularity associated with placentation (Fig. 91-9). This vascularity is obvious on color flow images in the first trimester of pregnancy, and pulsed Doppler demonstrates the high velocities (peak systolic velocity ranging from 21 to 100 cm/sec) with low impedance (resistance index, 0.504 ± 0.2).[4,8] These physiologic findings can be explained in terms of the anatomy and hemodynamics of the fetomaternal junction. The high peak velocities indicate flow across a pressure gradient such as an arteriovenous shunt. In fact, the mean pressure in the maternal spiral arteries is 70 mm Hg at the fetomaternal junction, whereas that in the intervillous space is 10 mm, yielding a pressure gradient of 60 mm Hg. There is therefore a good physiologic reason for these high velocities. The fetomaternal junction also demonstrates low-impedance flow. Most of the impedance in arteries exists in the smooth muscle of the arteriolar walls, so a very low impedance suggests the absence of arteriolar muscle tone. Indeed, it has been shown that the low impedance in tumors is associated with flow into sinusoids or tumor lakes that often have no muscle in their walls but are lined only with endothelium.[12] A similar situation exists within the placenta. Because maternal arterial flow from the spiral arteries goes into the intervillous space that has no muscle in its walls, the low impedance is observed there.

There is still some concern about the risk of biohazard from insonation.[1,6] In clinical terms, there has never been more insonation performed in early pregnancies because so many women are undergoing ovulation induction therapy, which first involves multiple endovaginal ultrasound examinations to monitor follicular size and growth and then further multiple examinations to demonstrate the presence of the gestational sac. In this regard, color flow involves similar amounts of exposure as gray-scale ultrasound. However, pulsed Doppler tends to employ higher intensities, and therefore exposure of the fetus should be minimized. In one study, all of the data regarding normal first trimesters were accrued from patients undergoing therapeutic abortions.[6] Women in normal first trimester pregnancies should not undergo pulsed Doppler ultrasound unless it is medically indicated for the benefit of the mother or fetus. The most common indication for doing so is to differentiate among an abnormal first trimester of pregnancy such as a blighted ovum, an incomplete abortion with contained products of conception, and the pseudosac associated with an ectopic pregnancy.

INCOMPLETE ABORTION OR BLIGHTED OVUM

By using morphologic criteria alone, there may be considerable confusion between the appearances of an abnormal first trimester gestational sac and a pseudosac associated with an ectopic pregnancy. A normal first trimester gestation can be recognized by the double decidual sac,[3] but this feature is not present in most abnormal first trimester gestational sacs. In this situation, which is difficult to diagnose and frequently encountered, the specific perfusion characteristics of placentation are extremely helpful in recognizing placental (peritrophoblastic) flow (Fig. 91-10). Because the flow results from placentation, it is independent of the fetus.

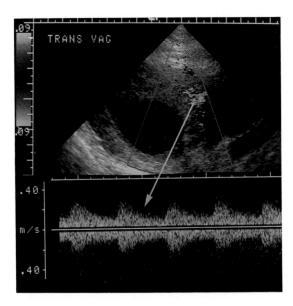

Fig. 91-9. Montage of pulse and color EVUS showing well-developed placental flow on color with typical low-impedance flow on pulsed Doppler. (From Taylor KJW et al: *Obstetric and gynecologic applications.* In *Clinics in diagnostic ultrasound,* vol 27, New York, 1992, Churchill Livingstone.)

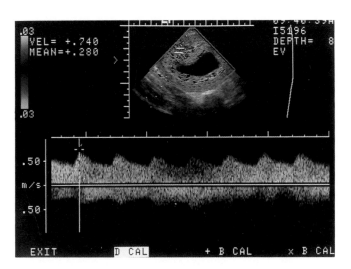

Fig. 91-10. Endovaginal ultrasound of a blighted ovum. Typical low-impedance and high-velocity placental flow is seen. (From Taylor KJW et al: *Obstetric and gynecologic applications.* In *Clinics in diagnostic ultrasound,* vol 27, New York, 1992, Churchill Livingstone.)

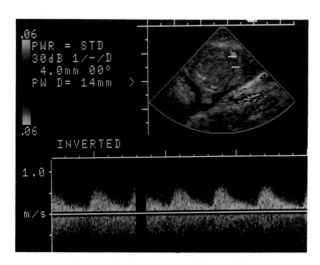

Fig. 91-11. Color and pulse endovaginal ultrasound of an ectopic pregnancy. A nonspecific mass is seen on gray-scale imaging, with peripheral flow seen on color Doppler flow. Interrogation with pulsed Doppler demonstrates a high velocity (exceeding 50 cm/sec) with comparatively low-impedance flow consistent with an ectopic pregnancy. (From Taylor KJW et al: *Obstetric and gynecologic applications.* In *Clinics in diagnostic ultrasound,* vol 27, New York, 1992, Churchill Livingstone.)

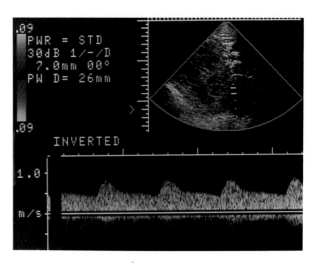

Fig. 91-12. Pulse and color Doppler endovaginal ultrasound. Molar material is seen within the uterus on imaging and is noted to be highly vascular. Pulsed Doppler evaluation demonstrates peak velocities of almost 1 m/sec and low impedance (resistance index, 0.5). (From Taylor KJW et al: *Obstetric and gynecologic applications.* In *Clinics in diagnostic ultrasound,* vol 27, New York, 1992, Churchill Livingstone.)

Therefore, it can be used to detect the small amounts of peritrophoblastic flow associated with an incomplete abortion. Dillon, Feycock, and Taylor[5] demonstrated that using a peak systolic velocity of greater than 21 cm/sec to identify a normal pregnancy correctly classified 26 of 31 intrauterine pregnancies (84%) and all 9 pseudosacs (specificity, 100%) in their study.

ECTOPIC PREGNANCY

Ectopic pregnancy continues to be a major problem for diagnosis and a major source of medicolegal litigation. During the past 20 years, its incidence has increased fivefold. A decade ago most patients with ectopic pregnancies presented acutely with rupture, but ectopic pregnancy is now diagnosed much earlier and few patients are ruptured at the time of presentation.

Many of these patients are found to have lower than normal increases in their serum levels of hCG (beta subunit of the human chorionic gonadotropin). Others exhibit symptoms, usually unilateral pelvic pain. For every three patients evaluated because of a clinical suspicion of ectopic pregnancy, one has the condition. Thus the specificity of any test is also very important and the ability to discriminate between an intrauterine pseudosac, which is associated with an ectopic pregnancy, and an incomplete abortion is essential.

The specific perfusion characteristics of placentation can be used to aid in the difficult diagnosis of ectopic pregnancy. The typical high-velocity, low-impedance flow is seen medial to the ovary within the fallopian tube (Fig. 91-11). In 90% of ectopic pregnancies, the luteal flow is found on the same side as the ectopic pregnancy. The addition of color flow has been observed to improve the sensitivity of endovaginal ultrasound in the diagnosis of ectopic pregnancy, increasing 84% using morphologic criteria alone to 98% when color flow is added.[7]

GESTATION TROPHOBLASTIC NEOPLASIA

Like ectopic pregnancy, practitioners are being called upon to diagnose molar disease at ever earlier stages. It is now relatively seldom to see the classic presentation of an enlarged uterus full of large vesicles caused by hydropic degeneration of the chorionic villi. The serum hCG levels in such patients are usually markedly elevated (greater than 100,000 U/ml), and endovaginal ultrasound reveals varying amounts of echogenic material due to the existence of microvesicles. With the addition of color flow, the typical high-velocity, low-impedance trophoblastic flow can be demonstrated (Fig. 91-12).[10]

CONCLUSION

The advent of endovaginal color flow has introduced new diagnostic potential, ranging from the simplistic, such as improved visualization of the iliac vessels, to the exciting, such as the ability to evaluate ovarian function. It is an extraordinarily valuable technique for evaluating the whole spectrum of complications of the first trimester. The next decade is likely to witness major new applications for this technology, especially as an era of improved quantitation of Doppler signals is entered.

REFERENCES

1. American Institute of Ultrasound in Medicine, Bioeffects Committee: Bioeffects considerations for the safety of diagnostic ultrasound, *J Ultrasound Med* 7(suppl):54, 1988.
2. Baber RJ et al: Transvaginal pulsed Doppler ultrasound assessment of blood flow to the corpus luteum in IVF patients following embryo transfer, *Br J Obstet Gynaecol* 95:1226, 1988.
3. Bradley W, Fiske C, Filly R: The double sac sign of early intrauterine pregnancy: use in exclusion of ectopic pregnancy, *Radiology* 143:223, 1982.
4. Campbell S et al: New Doppler technique for assessing uteroplacental blood flow, *Lancet* 1:675, 1983.
5. Dillon E, Feyock AL, Taylor KJW: Pseudogestational sacs: Doppler US differentiation from normal or abnormal intrauterine pregnancies, *Radiology* 176:359-364, 1990.
6. Dillon EH et al: Endovaginal pulsed and color Doppler of the normal first trimester pregnancy (in press).
7. Pellerito J et al: Endovaginal color flow Doppler imaging in the evaluation of ectopic pregnancy, *Radiology* 183:407-411, 1992.
8. Russell JB et al: Androgen-producing hilus cell tumor of the ovary: detection in a postmenopausal woman by duplex Doppler scanning, *JAMA* 257:7, 1987.
9. Schulman H et al: Development of uterine artery compliance in pregnancy as detected by Doppler ultrasound, *Am J Obstet Gynecol* 155:1031, 1986.
10. Taylor KJW, Schwartz PE, Kohorn EI: Gestational trophoblastic neoplasia: diagnosis with Doppler US, *Radiology* 165:445-448, 1987.
10a. Taylor KJW, Strandness DE Jr, eds: *Duplex Doppler ultrasound,* 1990.
11. Taylor KJW et al: Doppler flow studies of the ovarian and uterine arteries, *Br J Obstet Gynaecol* 92:240, 1985.
12. Taylor KJW et al: Correlation of Doppler US tumor signals with neovascular morphologic features, *Radiology* 166:57-62, 1988.
13. Taylor KJW et al: Ectopic pregnancy: duplex Doppler evaluation, *Radiology* 173:93-97, 1989.
14. Taylor KJW et al: *Obstetric and gynecologic applications.* In *Clinics in diagnostic ultrasound*, vol 27, New York, 1992, Churchill Livingstone.

Introduction

ANDREW N. NICOLAIDES

The aim of venous investigations is to detect the presence and extent of deep vein thrombosis (DVT) and chronic venous insufficiency and their respective effect on the skin microcirculation.

DEEP VEIN THROMBOSIS

Because the symptoms and signs of DVT are not unique to the disorder, any patient with leg pain, swelling, or tenderness should undergo objective testing that can either confirm or exclude the diagnosis. Reliance on clinical signs alone will only lead to large numbers of patients being treated unnecessarily with anticoagulants, which are both expensive and associated with occasional significant complications.

In the past, venography has been the gold standard in the evaluation of such patients because it could detect both the presence and the extent of the thrombus and whether it was fresh or old. Indirect tests such as phleborheography, impedance plethysmography, and strain-gauge plethysmography have a high sensitivity and specificity for identifying a DVT proximal to the calf but not in the calf. In contrast, duplex scanning has a high sensitivity and specificity for identifying all thrombi. The addition of color flow imaging to the new generation of scanners has made the examination quicker and the detection of calf thrombosis more accurate. Thus duplex scanning has become the test of choice in most centers, and venography is now rarely performed.

Because of the time constraints placed on duplex scanning, in that only a finite number of patients can be studied a day, some groups have explored the possibility of preceding duplex examination with other screening tests. Liquid-crystal thermography (LCT) is relatively inexpensive and has proved to have a negative predictive value of 95% for this purpose. Thus if LCT is used as the first test and the result is negative, DVT can be confidently ruled out, thus avoiding the need for duplex scanning. If the results of both impedance (IPG) and air (APG) plethysmography are positive, it means that there is extensive DVT and treatment is mandatory. Again, duplex scanning can be avoided in this instance. Using this approach, a smaller number of patients will need a duplex scan (those with positive LCT results and negative IPG or APG findings), thus freeing up the duplex scanner for other patients. Screening for DVT in asymptomatic patients such as medical or surgical hospital populations is not cost effective and not recommended.

Accurate screening tests are required for research pur-poses in clinical studies assessing the efficacy of prophylactic measures. In the 1970s and 1980s, the [^{125}I]fibrinogen test was the most useful method for studying the incidence of DVT in hospital populations, and it was instrumental in the development of the various prophylactic regimens available today. The need for a noninvasive screening test that could accurately detect not only proximal disease but also calf thrombosis is being met by the new generation of duplex scanners with color flow imaging. It is essential to detect calf thrombi because without adequate treatment, 20% extend proximal to the calf, giving rise to clinical pulmonary emboli and destroying the popliteal or more proximal valves, leading to chronic venous hypertension and eventually the postthrombotic syndrome.

CHRONIC VENOUS INSUFFICIENCY

Chronic venous insufficiency is caused by malfunction of the venous system associated with chronic venous hypertension. When the venous system is normal, exercise such as walking activates the calf muscle pump, reducing the venous pressure in the foot from 90 mm Hg on standing to 20 to 30 mm Hg during walking. With every thigh and calf muscle contraction, blood is expelled out of the leg. During muscle relaxation, the competent valves prevent reflux. The venous pressure remains low because of slow filling from arterial inflow. Obstruction to venous outflow or reflux due to valve damage interferes with this normal mechanism and results in high ambulatory venous pressure during exercise. In such individuals, the mean venous pressure is high throughout the day. The microcirculation is damaged and there is subsequent chronic edema, pain, and skin changes.

Chronic venous insufficiency can be primary or it can be due to acute venous thrombosis. Primary insufficiency commonly affects the superficial venous system. Reflux (deep to superficial) can occur at five key sites: the saphenofemoral junction, the junction of the short saphenous vein to the popliteal vein, high incompetent perforating veins, incompetent perforating veins in the calf, and the deep veins. In the past, reflux in the deep veins was thought to result from valvular damage caused by thrombosis. However, it is now clear that in 25% to 30% of patients with reflux in the popliteal and more proximal veins, the reflux is due to primary venous dilatation and floppy valve cusps. Such floppy valves can be repaired surgically. In the remaining patients, the valves are absent or destroyed and the venous walls are irregular as a result of recanalization after thrombosis. Blood refluxing down the deep veins usually exits via the incompetent perforating veins.

Failure of the veins to recanalize after DVT precipitates chronic obstruction, which is often a major source of venous hypertension. Compensatory collateral circulation tends to develop, but in the absence of adequate therapy or because of thrombosis, thrombi may extend into the collateral circulation, making the obstruction worse.

The objectives of investigating a patient with chronic venous insufficiency are to determine whether there is obstruction or reflux and the sites affected, as well as to measure its severity. All this can now be done noninvasively.

Quantitation of obstruction or reflux can be achieved using APG. Other methods, such as photoplethysmography, foot volumetry, and ambulatory venous pressure, can quantitatively measure the net effect of both obstruction and reflux.

Finally, a number of new noninvasive tests can now determine the effect of chronic venous hypertension on the skin microcirculation. These include laser Doppler, transcutaneous Po_2 and Pco_2, and tests that measure the rate of capillary leakage. So far, these tests have offered insight into the pathophysiologic nature of skin changes and ulceration, but their place in the routine clinical investigation is still unknown.

CHAPTER 92

The clinical spectrum of venous disease

D. EUGENE STRANDNESS, Jr.

The role of the noninvasive vascular laboratory in the diagnosis of acute and chronic venous disorders has become increasingly important during the past 20 years. The diagnosis of acute deep vein thrombosis (DVT) must be established by an objective test to remove the uncertainty raised by the observations made during the bedside evaluation.[2,10] Once this was recognized, a variety of noninvasive tests were implemented that have provided valuable insights into the nature of the problem and its prompt identification. The major diagnostic methods in use are described in this section of the book.

The diagnostic techniques now used range from the simple continuous-wave Doppler to the sophisticated ultrasonic duplex scanning methods that are currently the most commonly and successfully used for screening purposes. The indirect plethysmographic methods, although superseded to some extent by duplex scanning, continue to play an important role in the study of the physiologic changes that result from both acute and chronic venous insufficiency. Because the proper use of these methods depends on the conditions being studied and the information that is desired, the several areas in which noninvasive testing can be applied are briefly reviewed.

Those areas that are of special importance include DVT, superficial thrombophlebitis, recurrent DVT, varicose veins, the postthrombotic syndrome, and pulmonary embolism. The pathophysiologic characteristics, clinical importance, and clinical relevance to noninvasive testing procedures are also summarized.

ACUTE DEEP VEIN THROMBOSIS

Acute DVT of the lower limb remains a common and difficult clinical problem. There is little evidence that it is becoming less common, and it may actually be on the rise, given the ability to keep patients alive longer in a hospital setting where the risk factors responsible for its development persist. Although prophylactic measures for its prevention are in more common use, no data are yet available that show their impact on the incidence of the disease.

The labeled fibrinogen studies yielded a great deal of information about the natural history of the disease in the hospitalized patient.[14] Acute DVT is now known to be most common in patients who undergo major general, thoracic, or orthopedic procedures that require confinement to bed for prolonged periods.[15] It is also common in medically treated patients and the victims of malignant disease.

It appears to arise in specific sites from which the early thrombi may propagate to involve other segments of the venous system. The soleal sinuses and the sinuses of the venous valves are the most common sites.[25] When the process remains confined to these areas, few problems develop and the patient remains asymptomatic. However, in up to 20% of patients, the thrombi may propagate, leading to the appearance of symptoms either in the limb or secondary to pulmonary embolism.[14] Because calf vein thrombosis was frequently discovered by the labeled fibrinogen studies, most if not all thrombi are believed to originate there, with involvement of the proximal venous segments occurring by direct extension. However, many proximal thrombi appear to develop de novo, and it is likely that some of the proximal thrombi may start in the sinus of a venous valve and extend from that point. Another important consideration is the frequent involvement of the left common iliac vein,[7] and compression by the right common iliac artery may be responsible for this.

Pathophysiology

Although the development of acute venous thrombosis may be an entirely benign process that never becomes apparent to the patient or the treating physician, it often poses a serious clinical problem with a variety of consequences. When the thrombi remain confined to the soleal sinuses and the sinuses of the venous valves, little trouble results and the patient is not usually aware of a problem. The process itself incites very little in the way of inflammation. This also underscores the fact that the term *thrombophlebitis* is a misnomer and should not be used when referring to involvement of the deep venous system. This is not true for the superficial veins, a subject that will be discussed shortly.

The thrombus can progress in two major ways, each of which may have different consequences. In most instances, the thrombus will totally occlude the involved venous segments, forcing the blood to find alternate collateral pathways back to the right heart and lungs. In this setting, edema is likely to develop, depending on the location of the occlusion.[17] If the occlusion extends above the inguinal ligament, pronounced leg swelling will often occur. This scenario is commonly referred to as *iliofemoral thrombosis*. When the DVT also involves the major veins proximal to the inguinal ligament, the most severe form of the process may arise. This is called *phlegmasia cerulea dolens* and is one of the few instances in which the clinical presentation is easily recognized at the bedside. The massive leg swelling, severe pain, deep cyanosis, and decrease in limb temperature are not mimicked by any other clinical problem. In its most malignant form, venous gangrene can develop.

Although less common, partial venous occlusion can occur and this is particularly treacherous because it may not be recognized in the absence of limb swelling. It is seen in about 19% of cases. Although difficult to prove, it may be in this setting that sudden and totally unexpected pulmonary emboli develop.

Until ultrasonic duplex scanning became widely used, the fate of thrombi after their initial formation was poorly understood.[17] Although spontaneous lysis was known to occur, there was little prospective data about the natural history of acute DVT. Such knowledge is particularly valuable because lysis not only tends to restore patency but may also play a role in the preservation of venous valve function. The findings from long-term studies have now documented that thrombolysis occurs rapidly in many patients, thus restoring venous patency.[23] Apparently, the process is progressive and results in restoration of the lumen in nearly 100% of involved segments by the end of the third year.

Although clot lysis restores flow through the involved segment, the fate of the valves in these segments is even more important. The postthrombotic syndrome will develop in up to 60% of the patients with occluded proximal venous segments (popliteal to the inferior vena cava). The remaining 40% will have no difficulty, indicating that venous function has normalized.

Although the pathophysiologic events underlying venous valve injury and recovery are not well understood, the rate of lysis may have a beneficial effect on the preservation of valve function. The earlier and the faster the lysis, the more likely is the maintenance of valve function. This may explain the observation made by Browse, Burnand, and Thomas[4,5] that the extent of venous thrombosis seen at the time of the initial event may not predict the subsequent outcome. Duplex scanning may bring to light many aspects of the long-term outcome.

Clinical manifestations

As already noted, the only clinical presentation secondary to DVT that can be recognized easily at the bedside is phlegmasia cerulea dolens, with a presentation so dramatic and unique that it should not be missed. Although the symptoms and signs of acute deep venous occlusion include pain and edema, these are not specific enough for making a certain diagnosis.[2,10] This has led to the development and

application of noninvasive testing procedures. When duplex scanning has been used to screen patients with suspected DVT, only 25% are found to have DVT.[24] Thus, the 75% who are found free of disease are spared anticoagulant treatment, which is not only costly but potentially dangerous.

Diagnostic approaches

The gold standard for establishing the diagnosis of DVT has been contrast venography.[1] With the injection of dye into the veins on the dorsum of the foot, it is possible to opacify most of the deep veins of the lower limbs, but there are some areas that pose difficulty. Up to one half of the deep femoral veins cannot be seen. In addition, up to 20% of the iliac veins may not be adequately visualized because of the dilution of the contrast material, and up to 10% of patients may incur a contrast-induced phlebitis that will require therapy. Allergy to the contrast material can also be a serious problem.

The desirability of a noninvasive objective test that could replace venography was obvious, and several methods have been extensively tested against venography and found to be satisfactory, as long as their shortcomings are understood. The earliest ultrasonic method was continuous wave Doppler, which can interrogate the deep veins from the level of the external iliac vein to the posterior veins at the level of the ankle.[30] The major disadvantage of this method is that the user must have considerable experience. A well-performed test can establish or rule out the diagnosis of DVT, but this method has been made obsolete, particularly by ultrasonic duplex scanning.

Other indirect methods that have been widely tested are the plethysmographic techniques,[8,11] including the mercury strain gauge, impedance, and phleborheography. These methods are satisfactory for screening purposes, and a positive or negative result is sufficient for directing the physician to the most appropriate form of therapy.

Despite some dispute, it is clear that the most suitable noninvasive test available today is ultrasonic duplex scanning.[17] This method combines imaging with Doppler and, besides its diagnostic capability, can be used to follow the natural history of the disease, which is not feasible with any of the other noninvasive methods.[18-20,22-24]

Therapy

The therapy for acute DVT is fairly standardized. During the acute phase, intravenous heparin is administered, followed later by a course of the oral anticoagulant coumadin. Although the duration of therapy has routinely been for up to 6 months in patients with involvement of the major proximal veins, this has been undergoing reevaluation, so practitioners must keep abreast of changes in this policy.[12]

The use of fibrinolytic agents constitutes an area of great interest and potential importance[21] because rapid lysis of offending thrombi may not only restore patency but may also be very helpful in preserving valve function. Although the role of thrombolysis on the arterial side of the circulation is better understood, it is very difficult to identify patients who are candidates for therapy on the venous side because most such patients have contraindications to the therapy. It appears that less than 10% of the patients with acute DVT can safely receive the drug.[21]

Prognosis

The goals of therapy are first to eliminate the risk of pulmonary embolism and second to reduce the threat of the postthrombotic syndrome. In one study, 9% of patients presenting to the vascular laboratory for duplex scanning had pulmonary embolism.[24] The administration of heparin can reduce this incidence by at least fivefold.

In recent years, increasing attention has been given to the role of underlying contributing factors that lead to the development of acute DVT. Although uncommon, protein C, protein S, and antithrombin III deficiencies must be considered, particularly when the patient has a strong family history and evidence of repeat episodes of DVT without obvious underlying causes.[28] It is important to uncover these cases because they will require life-long therapy with coumadin.

RECURRENT DEEP VEIN THROMBOSIS

Once an episode of DVT occurs, the likelihood of recurrence is in the range of 10%. Short of some underlying hematologic cause, this recurrence most often follows a traumatic injury, which is frequently minimal. Treatment of recurrence is the same as that for the initial event. Lifelong therapy is not necessary unless a protein C, protein S, or antithrombin III deficiency is found to be the major contributing factor.

Diagnosis and verification of the new episode may be difficult unless the results of previous diagnostic tests are available for comparison. Even venography may not be definitive in this setting unless the dye can form a "sleeve" around the fresh thrombosis. If the diagnosis in more of these patients is established by duplex scanning, it will be a simpler problem to contend with in the future.

Unfortunately, because a certain diagnosis of recurrent venous thrombosis will remain impossible to establish in a large number of patients, physicians will be forced to treat patients based on the clinical presentation and the degree to which the diagnosis appears likely. Although this is not an entirely satisfactory approach, there is no other ready solution offered by any of the accepted diagnostic methods.

SUPERFICIAL THROMBOPHLEBITIS

It is commonly believed that thrombosis of the deep and superficial venous systems represents the same process. However, there does not appear to be any evidence to support it. The terminology describing this entity is appropriate because it is truly an inflammatory process.

Contributing factors

The most common cause of superficial thrombophlebitis is intravenous infusions that inflict a chemical injury on the vein wall that leads to inflammation and then inevitably thrombosis of the involved vein, or veins. In the lower limb, superficial thrombophlebitis most commonly occurs in varicose veins. This commonly follows trauma, which need not be severe. The development of migratory superficial phlebitis may be the first sign of an underlying malignancy (Trousseau's sign) and has also been associated with Buerger's disease (thromboangiitis obliterans).

Clinical manifestations

The clinical presentation of superficial thrombophlebitis consists of severe pain, redness, inflammation, swelling, and pyrexia. This is evident simply on examination of the involved area, and because the process leads to the development of thrombosis, a palpable cord is commonly seen.

Differential diagnosis

The most common entities that can be confused with superficial thrombophlebitis are lymphangitis and cellulitis. In most cases, the differential diagnosis is not too difficult, particularly if the examiner realizes that cellulitis and lymphangitis do not typically lead to thrombosis of the superficial veins.

Diagnostic approach

Because superficial thrombophlebitis leads to thrombosis of the involved veins, continuous-wave Doppler is the ideal method for establishing diagnosis. The finding of a patent vein in the area of inflammation rules out phlebitis.[3] In the lower limb, if there is any concern over the extent of the thrombosis, particularly whether it involves the deep venous system, it is important to use duplex scanning to depict both the thrombus and its extent.

Therapy

For most cases, the treatment of superficial thrombophlebitis consists of heat, analgesics, and especially, antiinflammatory therapy. Anticoagulants are rarely needed unless the thrombus appears to extend to the deep venous system. In the lower limb, this most commonly occurs when the phlebitis involves the greater saphenous vein close to its junction with the common femoral vein.

Some investigators also recommend aggressive surgical therapy when this entity involves the superficial veins of the lower limb.[13,19] In this setting, some consider ligation and stripping the treatment of choice.

VARICOSE VEINS

By far the most common venous problem is the presence of dilated and tortuous greater and lesser saphenous veins and their tributaries. When this is all that exists and the deep veins are not involved, the diagnosis is usually primary varicose veins.[9] Other clues to primary varicose veins include a positive family history and a lack of the skin changes commonly found in patients with the postthrombotic syndrome. Many of these patients are actually free of symptoms with the exception of some cosmetic deformity.

However, varicosities can develop in the lower limb in response to disease of the deep veins, with consequential loss of valvular competence in these vessels as well as the perforating veins that connect the two major venous systems. The frequent finding of edema, pigmentation, and ulceration strongly implicates the postthrombotic syndrome as the primary cause of such varicose veins.[31] Other factors that can precipitate varicose veins include arteriovenous fistulas, which may be either congenital or acquired.

Pathophysiology

In the normal limb, flow is directed from the superficial veins to the deep system.[20] This is augmented by the communicating veins, each of which is protected by a valve that permits only unidirectional flow. With loss of the venous valves in the superficial system and the subsequent dilatation, the normal cyclic drainage is disrupted. In fact, during walking, flow in the superficial veins will tend to oscillate, with forward and reverse-flow components often yielding little net forward flow.[31]

One of the remarkable aspects of primary varicose veins is that they may become large and tortuous yet cause little in the way of symptoms and signs. This attests to the importance of a patent and competent deep venous system and its network of communicating veins. Unless the deep system is also involved, it is unlikely that such patients will have significant problems in the way of either symptoms or skin changes.

Diagnosis

The diagnosis of primary varicose veins is suggested by a positive family history, the presence of varicosities, and a lack of advanced skin changes. Most patients will not have severe symptoms but may complain of some mild swelling and dull pain, which is immediately relieved by either elevation of the leg or the use of elastic compression stockings. The greater saphenous vein along with its tributaries is the most commonly involved. Although the lesser saphenous vein can also be affected, this is much less common.

To confirm the clinical impression of primary varicose veins, duplex scanning may be used to assess the patency and competence of the venous valves in the deep venous system.[22,23] Although this may seem an unnecessary application of the technology, it can be of great help, particularly if some form of intervention is being contemplated. For example, it is possible to determine the extent of saphenous vein involvement. In addition, it can determine the location of the secondary varices and the status of their drainage into the saphenous system. This affords more complete planning of treatment, whether it be surgery or sclerotherapy.

Therapy

Of all the venous disorders, primary varicose veins is the most benign. Because it is rarely associated with the development of serious symptoms or signs, most patients never require any direct form of therapy. In fact, all of its symptoms can usually be relieved by the wearing of elastic compression hose. These stockings need not have the high pressures required for patients with the postthrombotic syndrome and are also useful from a cosmetic standpoint.

When therapy is required, there are three approaches. The first is only to recommend the use of elastic support stockings. This treatment is successful in most patients. The second form of therapy is sclerotherapy and this is being carried out with increasing frequency. It is best used for secondary varicosities and not in patients with incompetent greater and lesser saphenous veins compromised in their upper extent where they enter the deep venous system. The third form of therapy is a combination of ligation, stripping, and removal of branch vessels through small incisions. The proper combination of interventional procedures can be successful for the treatment of primary varicose veins. The cosmetic results are good, and the recurrence rate can be kept low.

THE POSTTHROMBOTIC SYNDROME

Once an episode of acute DVT has occurred, the subsequent outcome is unpredictable and depends primarily on the status of the venous valves in the deep system.[29] As noted earlier, the extent to which valve function is preserved depends on the rate and extent of subsequent thrombolysis. Other entities that can cause venous valvular incompetence include arteriovenous fistulas, which can either be congenital or acquired.

Pathophysiology

Venous valves are located at all levels of the venous system. Although they are found in the iliac and common femoral veins, they are not as regularly seen because these locations are distal to the junction of the common femoral with the superficial femoral vein. In fact, the numbers and concentrations of valves increase toward the lower leg. This is of great importance in understanding the function of the calf muscle pump and the communicating veins and their collective role in the development of the skin changes commonly associated with the postthrombotic syndrome.

The activation of the calf muscle pump triggers several changes that are important for optimizing the return of venous flow. With muscle contraction, flow is forced toward the heart, with the valves distal to the muscle group, or groups, closing to prevent reflux of venous blood. The valves in the communicating veins also close, thus preventing the blood reflux (the high-pressure leak) that has been implicated as one of the factors responsible for the development of hyperpigmentation and ultimately ulceration.

The valves below the knee are the most critical for the protection of the skin in the gaiter area. Despite some disagreement, it is unlikely that valve incompetence in the proximal veins plays any role in the development of the most common complications of the postthrombotic syndrome. One recently recognized factor is the frequent association of deep vein with greater and lesser saphenous vein valvular incompetence in patients who develop ulceration sometime after an episode of DVT. In contrast, the greater or lesser saphenous veins of patients who are free of ulceration do not exhibit incompetence, although the deep veins may be incompetent, even below the knee.

Clinical manifestations

Patients with the postthrombotic syndrome will commonly exhibit edema, pain, stasis dermatitis, and in the late stages, ulceration.[29] In its full-blown form, this scenario is unmistakable.

An unusual symptom of the postthrombotic syndrome is venous claudication.[16] Such patients will give a history of bursting pain, usually in the thigh, which is brought on by exercise and relieved only by rest. Some patients find that the pain can be relieved only by elevation. This unusual complication is secondary to chronic venous outflow obstruction and not to valvular incompetence.

Diagnosis

The constellation of pain, swelling, hyperpigmentation, and ulceration is easily recognized and consistent with the diagnosis of the postthrombotic syndrome. When the patient has had a previous episode of acute DVT, there is little else that can be the cause. It is interesting, however, that up to one half of patients with far advanced leg changes may deny a history of previous DVT. In these cases, either the previous episode of venous thrombosis was silent or other causes of the symptoms should be sought.

Although uncommon, congenital arteriovenous fistulas can manifest all of the complications associated with damage of the venous system secondary to DVT,[4] because venous dilatation and accompanying valve incompetence can result from the large volumes of blood shunted to the venous system under higher than usual pressures.

The application of ultrasonic duplex scanning can now easily establish the diagnosis of deep venous incompetence in terms of both its location and extent. This is best carried out with the patient in the upright position and with the use of pneumatic cuffs.[32] The cuffs are placed at the level of the thigh, upper and lower calf, and foot. When the cuffs are inflated, the veins below it are emptied. When the cuffs are suddenly deflated, the collapsed venous segments fill by either antegrade inflow or reflux if the valves within that region or proximal to that level are incompetent. The great advantage of this method is that it can be used to study both the superficial and deep venous systems. The time it takes for the valves to close upon sudden reversal of the transvalvular pressure gradient is less than 0.5 seconds in normal subjects.

When there are skin changes, it is likely that the valvular incompetence noted by duplex scanning is below the knee. Popliteal vein valve incompetence is also frequently observed. The presence of ulceration secondary to the postthrombotic syndrome is almost always associated with incompetence of the greater saphenous vein.

Treatment

Because the valves of the deep system are damaged, it is not feasible to repair or replace them. Although surgical repair or replacement has been undertaken for the superficial femoral and popliteal veins, it has not been attempted for the valves below the knee. This is the site where valvular incompetence has its greatest impact on long-term cutaneous integrity. Unfortunately, the valves in this region cannot yet be replaced or repaired from a surgical standpoint.

The mainstay of therapy for most cases of the postthrombotic syndrome is long-term compression using pressure-gradient stockings.[5] The compression used in most cases is in the 30 to 50 mm Hg range. This will prevent edema, relieve the pain, and protect the skin from the long-term effects of reverse flow through the communicating veins.

If the disease progresses, an ulcer may form, usually in the gaiter area along the medial side of the lower leg, together with marked stasis hyperpigmentation surrounding the area of skin breakdown. For over 90% of these patients, successful treatment can be achieved by the use of a semirigid medicated bandage Gelocast Unna's boot,* if treatment is continued long enough. The dressing appears to work by compressing the stagnant superficial veins and minimizing edema, which is known to interfere with wound healing. The dressing should be changed once a week. This form of therapy has several advantages: it is inexpensive compared with hospitalization and the patient may remain ambulatory during therapy.

If the compressive bandage therapy is unsuccessful, other more direct forms of treatment may be required. Skin grafting may be offered to such patients, since this offers hope for complete coverage. However, even if grafting is successful, pressure-gradient stockings must be worn to prevent a recurrence after discharge from the hospital.

Other methods of therapy have included venous ligation and stripping, as well as subfascial interruption of the perforating veins of the lower leg.[5] Because valvular incompetence is responsible for the problem, this therapy should be definitive. Although this approach is still widely used, it should rarely be necessary, given the success of the more conservative forms of treatment.

PULMONARY EMBOLISM

During the acute phase of DVT, the danger of breakup of the thrombus and pulmonary embolism is of greatest concern. Although pulmonary emboli can originate from sites other than the limbs, most attention is focused on the legs and pelvis.

---

*Beiersdorf, Inc., Norwalk, Conn.

Risk factors

The major risk factors for the development of pulmonary emboli are the same as those for the development of DVT.[24] Once a thrombus forms in the lower leg, the patient is always at risk and the magnitude appears to depend on the location and extent of the thrombosis. For example, thrombi that are confined to the veins below the knee rarely become serious pulmonary emboli. On the other hand, thrombi that involve the iliofemoral system are the most dangerous. Because of their size, it is thought that emboli from these veins are the ones most likely to be fatal.

Pathophysiology

When pulmonary embolism develops, patients exhibit a broad range of symptoms and signs related to the magnitude of the arterial obstruction. The clinical presentation ranges from no symptoms to sudden death. In patients with clinically significant emboli, the most common symptoms include chest pain, shortness of breath, anxiety, tachycardia, and hyperventilation.[27] Although arterial oxygen tension is commonly elevated during the acute phase, this finding is of little diagnostic value.

Clinical manifestations

Patients with acute pulmonary arterial obstruction may have symptoms and signs, but as in DVT, the clinical presentation is nonspecific and may be the end result of many other conditions. The major point to remember is that once the diagnosis is suspected, its resolution must be pursued with vigor.[26]

Diagnostic methods

The most commonly used test is the ventilation-perfusion scan. If the ventilation scan and chest x-ray study are normal but a pulmonary perfusion defect is noted, the diagnosis of pulmonary embolism is almost certain. Short of this combination, the clinician should not place too much trust in the results of these studies. Whenever the diagnosis is in doubt, it is important to obtain a pulmonary arteriogram because it will provide the necessary anatomic confirmation regarding the presence or absence of pulmonary emboli. This diagnostic test is not applied as often as it should be to settle this important issue.

Another important finding in patients with suspected pulmonary embolism is the presence of DVT.[24] When DVT is present, it is usually not necessary to pursue the diagnosis of pulmonary embolism, since the treatment would be the same.

Therapy

In general terms, the treatment of pulmonary embolism is the same as that for proximal DVT. The best therapy is intravenous heparin followed by approximately 6 months of coumadin treatment. There may also be circumstances in which thrombolytic therapy is helpful for rapidly clearing emboli to augment perfusion. Thrombolysis may greatly improve the patient's condition during the acute phase and reduce the later risk of pulmonary hypertension.

There will be situations in which anticoagulant therapy is contraindicated because of a bleeding risk. In this setting, it is necessary to install a filter in the inferior vena cava. Because of the development of smaller catheters, this can now be done percutaneously. These methods are effective in reducing the likelihood of a fatal embolic event. There has also been a very low incidence of late occlusion of the inferior vena cava with thrombosis of the filter.

REFERENCES

1. Athanasoulis CA: *Phlebography for the diagnosis of deep vein thrombosis.* In *Prophylactic therapy of deep vein thrombosis and pulmonary embolism,* Washington, DC, 1975, DHEW Publication (NIH) 76:866.
2. Barnes RW, Wu KK, Hoak JC: Fallibility of the clinical diagnosis of venous thrombosis, *JAMA* 234:605, 1975.
3. Barnes RW, Wu KK, Hoak JC: Differentiation of superficial thrombophlebitis from lymphangitis by Doppler ultrasound, *Surg Gynecol Obstet* 143:23, 1976.
4. Browse NL, Burnand KG, Thomas ML: *Venous ulceration: diagnosis.* In *Diseases of the veins: pathology, diagnosis and treatment,* London, 1988, Edward Arnold.
5. Browse NL, Burnand KG, Thomas ML: *Venous ulceration: natural history and treatment.* In *Diseases of the veins: pathology, diagnosis and treatment,* London, 1988, Edward Arnold.
6. Cockett FB, Elgan Jones DE: The ankle blow-out syndrome: a new approach to the varicose ulcer problem, *Lancet* 1:17, 1953.
7. Cockett FB, Thomas ML: The iliac compression syndrome, *Br J Surg* 52:816, 1965.
8. Cranley JJ et al: A plethysmographic technique for the diagnosis of deep venous thrombosis of the lower extremities, *Surg Gynecol Obstet* 136:385, 1973.
9. Gunderson J, Gauge M: Hereditary factors in venous insufficiency, *Angiology* 20:346, 1969.
10. Haeger K: Problems of acute deep venous thrombosis. I. The interpretation of signs and symptoms, *Angiology* 20:2199, 1969.
11. Hull R et al: Impedance plethysmography using the occlusive cuff technique in the diagnosis of venous thrombosis, *Circulation* 53:696, 1976.
12. Hull R et al: Different intensities of oral anticoagulant therapy in the treatment of proximal-vein thrombosis, *N Engl J Med* 307:1676, 1982.
13. Husni EA, Williams WA: Superficial thrombophlebitis of lower limbs, *Surgery* 91:70, 1982.
14. Kakkar VV et al: Natural history of deep vein thrombosis, *Lancet* 2:230, 1969.
15. Kakkar VV et al: Efficacy of low doses of heparin in the prevention of deep vein thrombosis after major surgery: a double-blind, randomized trial, *Lancet* 2:101, 1972.
16. Killewich L et al: The pathophysiology of venous claudication, *J Vasc Surg* 4:507, 1984.
17. Killewich LA et al: Diagnosis of deep venous thrombosis: a prospective study comparing duplex scanning to contrast venography, *Circulation* 79:810, 1989.
18. Killewich LA et al: Spontaneous lysis of deep venous thrombosis: rate and outcome, *J Vasc Surg* 9:89, 1989.
19. Lofgren EP, Lofgren KA: The surgical treatment of superficial thrombophlebitis, *Surgery* 90:49, 1981.
20. Ludbrook J: Functional aspects of the veins of the leg, *Am Heart J* 64:796, 1962.
21. Markel R, Manzo, Strandness DE Jr: The potential role of thrombolytic therapy in venous thrombosis, *Arch Intern Med* 152:1265, 1992.
22. Markel A et al: Pattern and distribution of thrombi in acute venous thrombosis, *Arch Surg* 127:305, 1992.
23. Markel A et al: Valvular reflux after deep vein thrombosis: incidence and time of occurrence, *J Vasc Surg* 15:377, 1992.
24. Markel A et al: Acute deep vein thrombosis: diagnosis, localization, risk factors, *J Vasc Med Biol* (in press).
25. Nicolaides AN, Kakkar VV, Renney JTG: Soleal sinuses and stasis, *Br J Surg* 58:307, 1971.

26. Robin ED: Overdiagnosis and overtreatment of pulmonary embolism: the emperor may have no clothes, *Ann Intern Med* 87:775, 1977.

27. Sasahara AA et al: Pulmonary thromboembolism: diagnosis and treatment, *Clin Cardiol* 249:2945, 1983.

28. Stead RB: *The hypercoagulable state*. In Goldhaber SZ, ed: *Pulmonary embolism and deep venous thrombosis*, Philadelphia, 1985, Saunders.

29. Strandness DE et al: Long-term sequelae of acute venous thrombosis, *JAMA* 250:1289, 1983.

30. Strandness DE Jr, Sumner DS: Ultrasonic velocity detector in the diagnosis of thrombophlebitis, *Arch Surg* 104:180, 1972.

31. Strandness DE Jr, Thiele BL: *Postthrombotic venous insufficiency*. In Strandness DE Jr, Thiele BL, eds: *Selected topics in venous disorders: pathophysiology, diagnosis and treatment*, Mount Kisco, NY, 1981, Futura.

32. Van Bemmelen PS et al: Quantitative segmental evaluation of venous valvular reflux with duplex ultrasound scanning, *J Vasc Surg* 10:425, 1989.

CHAPTER 93

Natural history of minimal calf deep vein thrombosis

JACK HIRSH and ANTHONIE W. A. LENSING

Calf vein thrombosis is usually asymptomatic, and the term *minimal calf vein thrombi* refers to small asymptomatic thrombi. Minimal calf vein thrombi are encountered regularly in hospitalized patients undergoing radioactive fibrinogen leg scanning[9,22] and in asymptomatic postoperative orthopedic patients who undergo venography before discharge from the hospital.[7] Because these two diagnostic maneuvers are only used for research purposes to evaluate new methods of prophylaxis, the management of minimal calf vein thrombosis is of greater theoretical than practical importance. Nevertheless, the basis for making management decisions in patients with minimal calf vein thrombosis is of interest because it is relevant to the management of symptomatic calf vein thrombosis, which is of considerable practical importance.

Symptomatic thrombi are usually located in the proximal veins but can also occur as isolated calf vein thrombi.* These symptomatic calf thrombi are usually larger than asymptomatic ones and are important because they occur in 10% to 45% of symptomatic patients with proven venous thrombosis.* They may also not be detected by routine noninvasive diagnostic testing.[13-15,18]

Studies in the late 1960s revealed a surprisingly high incidence of venous thrombi is postoperative patients undergoing routine screening with leg scanning.[9,21,22] Because clinically obvious venous thrombosis or pulmonary embolism was uncommon in these patients,[9,21] the observation was met with skepticism by many authorities who considered these leg scan–detected thrombi clinically irrelevant. Two decades later, the clinical relevance of minimal calf vein thrombosis remains uncertain.

It is now clear that calf vein thrombi are common in high-risk hospitalized patients but that they are usually small, asymptomatic, and clinically unimportant, provided they remain confined to the calf.[9,21,22] Most of these thrombi form at or soon after operation, but many disappear because they either undergo spontaneous lysis[21] or embolize into the pulmonary circulation where they undergo spontaneous lysis. Contrary to popular opinion, calf vein thrombi are associated with a pulmonary embolism that is detected postoperatively by pulmonary perfusion scanning in 20% to 30% of asymptomatic patients who have a positive leg scan.[4,8] These emboli are small, almost always asymptomatic, and clinically unimportant. An even higher frequency of pulmonary embolism is seen in association with symptomatic calf vein thrombosis.[25]

The incidence of leg scan–detected calf vein thrombi varies widely depending on the patient groups. The following rates have been reported: postpartum, less than 5%; simple hysterectomy in young women, less than 3%; major abdominal surgery, between 10% and 30%, depending on the type of surgery and the presence of other risk factors; neurosurgery, 25%; paralytic stroke, 50% and greater; nonparalytic stroke, less than 10%; major knee surgery, 60% to 70%; and hip surgery, 40%.[28] Most of these calf vein thrombi are asymptomatic and almost all are clinically unimportant, as long as they remain in the calf. They rarely if ever lead to clinically evident pulmonary embolism.

Calf vein thrombi become clinically important if they extend into the proximal venous system. In one small study, Kakkar et al[21] observed that approximately 20% of asymptomatic calf vein thrombi detected by radioactive fibrinogen leg scanning extended into the popliteal vein and were then associated with a substantial risk of clinically symptomatic pulmonary embolism. The risk of such extension in ambulant orthopedic patients who undergo routine venography just before hospital discharge is unknown, but it is likely to be similar to that encountered in patients with asymptomatic calf vein thrombi detected by leg scanning. When calf vein thrombi extend into the proximal veins, they are usually asymptomatic. If they go untreated, these proximal vein thrombi may become clinically important pulmonary emboli that can be fatal. The exact frequency of these complicating emboli in asymptomatic patients with proximal vein thrombi is unknown, but there is evidence that untreated symptomatic proximal vein thrombosis is associated with pulmonary embolism, as detected by perfusion lung scanning in 50% of cases.[8]

The long-term consequences of asymptomatic calf vein thrombosis are unknown but may not be entirely benign. Thus a number of studies have examined this problem and identified a history of hospital admission over the preceding

---

*References 6, 12, 17, 25, 26, 29.

6 months as a major risk factor for the occurrence of venous thrombosis and pulmonary embolism in ambulatory patients who are seen at the emergency department with confirmed symptomatic venous thromboembolism.[1] It is possible that some of these patients have asymptomatic calf vein thrombosis when discharged from the hospital that then extends and becomes symptomatic during convalescence at home.

Whether untreated venous thrombi detected by leg scanning predispose to the postphlebitic syndrome is also debated. Lindhagen, Bergqvist, and Hallbook[24] examined patients who had undergone a surgical procedure 3 to 5 years previously and were screened at that time for evidence of venous thrombosis. They found no evidence of an increased incidence of the postphlebitic syndrome between patients who had a positive leg scan at their prior hospital admission and those who did not. Browse and Clemenson[3] reported that patients who had mild calf symptoms when calf vein thrombi were diagnosed by leg scanning had persistent pain 3 to 4 years later, but leg symptoms were also common in patients with negative leg scan results. Francis et al[10] reported that abnormal venous function was detected during follow-up in patients with a previous history of asymptomatic deep vein thrombosis. More recently, Anderson and Willie-Jorgensen[2] used plethysmography to assess venous function 5 to 8 years after operation in patients who had undergone postoperative radioactive fibrinogen leg scanning. The prevalence of impaired venous function was significantly higher in those patients who had asymptomatic venous thrombosis than in those who were free of thrombosis.

The management of asymptomatic minimal calf vein thrombosis is problematic. Three different approaches can be used: (1) no treatment, (2) treatment with anticoagulants for 6 weeks, and (3) surveillance using either impedance plethysmography or B-mode imaging to detect extension.

The natural history of untreated minimal calf vein thrombosis has not been carefully studied, but an estimate of the complication rate can be pieced together from composite sources. In one small study composed of 45 patients with leg scan–detected calf vein thrombosis, 9 (20%) of the thrombi extended into the proximal venous segment and were left untreated; symptoms of pulmonary embolism developed in 4 of these patients.[21] If all 4 patients truly had pulmonary embolism, then symptomatic pulmonary embolism would be expected to develop in approximately 9% of patients with a positive leg scan. The postoperative incidence of a positive leg scan in moderate-risk patients undergoing general surgery (e.g., cholecystectomy) is between 10% and 15%.[28] On the basis of the above calculations, the projected postoperative incidence of symptomatic pulmonary embolism in moderate-risk general surgical patients would be approximately 1%. The calculated risk of symptomatic pulmonary embolism is approximately 2% to 3% for high-risk patients (e.g., colectomy for carcinoma of the colon), 30% of whom have positive leg scans.

The clinically important complications of venous thrombosis are fatal pulmonary embolism, the postthrombotic syndrome, and the inconvenience and side effects associated with anticoagulant therapy. The incidence of fatal embolism when calf vein thrombosis is left untreated can also be estimated from composite sources. The postoperative incidence of fatal embolism is approximately 0.2% for moderate-risk patients and 0.7% for high-risk general surgical patients.[5,20,23,27] Because these fatal emboli most likely arise from calf vein thrombi that have extended into the proximal venous segment, the following calculations can be made: For moderate-risk patients, a 10% incidence of leg scan–detected calf vein thrombosis is associated with a 0.2% incidence of fatal pulmonary embolism; therefore the risk of fatal embolism from an untreated minimal calf vein thrombosis is approximately 2%. For high-risk patients, a 30% to 40% incidence of leg scan–detected calf vein thrombosis is associated with a 0.7% incidence of fatal pulmonary embolism; therefore the risk of fatal pulmonary embolism from an untreated minimal calf vein thrombosis is approximately 2%. The incidence of asymptomatic calf vein thrombosis can be reduced by 70% through the use of safe and effective prophylactic agents.

It is likely that minimal calf vein thrombosis does not precipitate the postthrombotic syndrome unless the thrombus extends into the large axial calf veins or into the proximal venous segment. The incidence of the postthrombotic syndrome at 5 years after an episode of symptomatic proximal vein thrombosis is approximately 60%. Its incidence in the presence of an asymptomatic proximal vein thrombosis is unknown but is likely to be lower because asymptomatic thrombi are usually smaller than symptomatic thrombi. If the incidence of the postthrombotic syndrome after asymptomatic proximal vein thrombosis is 20%, the risk of the postthrombotic syndrome resulting from untreated minimal calf vein thrombosis would be approximately 4%, based on a 20% rate of extension of calf vein thrombosis.

Thus an untreated minimal calf vein thrombosis that is detected by leg scanning might be complicated by fatal pulmonary embolism in 2% of bedridden patients and by the postthrombotic syndrome in 4%. The risk of these complications in ambulatory orthopedic patients who have asymptomatic calf vein thrombi detected by routine predischarge venography is unknown but is likely to be lower than that in bedridden patients. Based on the findings from the two studies carried out in patients with symptomatic calf vein thrombosis,[16,23] it is likely that a treatment protocol consisting of heparin followed by warfarin is very effective for preventing extension of calf vein thrombi and therefore for preventing fatal pulmonary embolism and postthrombotic syndrome. The risk of major bleeding has been found to be less than 5% and the risk of fatal bleeding, less than 1%, when the following treatment regimen is followed: heparin and warfarin started at the same time, with heparin discontinued after 4 days and less-intense warfarin (international normalized ratio [INR] = 2.0 to 3.0) continued for 6 weeks.[11,19] Thus the net benefits of treatment are likely to outweigh those of no treatment.

Fatal pulmonary embolism is likely to be prevented and the risk of the postthrombotic syndrome reduced if such patients are just observed using impedance plethysmography or B-mode imaging for 7 to 10 days (or longer if the patient remains bedridden), with treatment reserved for those thrombi that extend to the popliteal vein, which will prevent further extension.[13,15,18] Thus surveillance is a reasonable alternative to anticoagulant therapy. Routine anticoagulant therapy with heparin and warfarin is not only costly but also inconvenient, especially in patients whose asymptomatic calf vein thrombus is detected just before hospital discharge, since the heparin therapy will delay discharge. If the thrombus is small, it is reasonable to discharge the patient and treat the thrombus with one or two injections of high-dose subcutaneous heparin and 6 weeks of oral anticoagulants.

A 29% rate of symptomatic extension or recurrence has been reported for patients with symptomatic calf vein thrombosis if treated with an inadequate course of anticoagulants.[23] This recurrence rate was prevented by a 3-month course of anticoagulant therapy.[23] Therefore patients with symptomatic calf vein thrombosis should be treated with heparin for at least 4 days and oral anticoagulants for 6 weeks to 3 months.

REFERENCES

1. Anderson FA Jr et al: A population-based perspective on the incidence and case-fatality rates of venous thrombosis and pulmonary embolism: the Worcester DVT Study, *Arch Intern Med* 151:933-938, 1991.
2. Anderson M, Willie-Jorgensen P: Late venous function after asymptomatic deep venous thrombosis, *Thromb Haemost* 62(1):336, 1989 (abstract).
3. Browse NL, Clemenson C: Sequelae of an ^{125}I-fibrinogen detected thrombus, *Br Med J* 2:468-470, 1974.
4. Browse NL, Thomas M: Source of non-lethal pulmonary emboli, *Lancet* 1:258, 1974.
5. Collins R et al: Reduction in fatal pulmonary embolism and venous thrombosis by perioperative administration of subcutaneous heparin, *N Engl J Med* 318:1162-1173, 1988.
6. Cranley JJ, Canos AJ, Sull WJ: The diagnosis of deep vein thrombosis: fallibility of clinical signs and symptoms, *Arch Surg* 111:34-36, 1976.
7. Cruickshank MK et al: An evaluation of impedance plethysmography and 125-I fibrinogen leg scanning in patients following hip surgery, *Thromb Haemost* 62:830-834, 1989.
8. Doyle DJ et al: Adjusted subcutaneous heparin or continuous intravenous heparin in patients with acute deep vein thrombosis, *Ann Intern Med* 107:441-445, 1987.
9. Flanc C et al: The detection of venous thrombosis of the legs using 125-I fibrinogen, *Br J Surg* 55:742-747, 1968.
10. Francis CW et al: Long-term clinical observations and venous functional abnormalities after asymptomatic venous thrombosis following total hip or knee arthroplasty, *Clin Related Res Orthoped* 232:271-278, 1988.
11. Gallus AS et al: Safety and efficacy of warfarin started early after submassive venous thrombosis or pulmonary embolism, *Lancet* 2:1293-1296, 1986.
12. Haeger K: Problems of acute deep venous thrombosis. I. Interpretation of signs and symptoms, *Angiology* 20:219-223, 1969.
13. Heijboer H et al: Efficacy of real-time B-mode ultrasonography versus impedance plethysmography in the diagnosis of deep vein thrombosis in symptomatic outpatients, *Thromb Haemost* 1991 65(6):804 (abstract).
14. Hirsh J: Reliability of noninvasive tests for the diagnosis of clinically suspected deep vein thrombosis, *Thromb Haemost* 65:221-222, 1991.
15. Huisman MV et al: Serial impedance plethysmography for suspected deep venous thrombosis in outpatients: the Amsterdam General Practitioner Study, *N Engl J Med* 314:823-826, 1986.
16. Hull R et al: Warfarin sodium versus low-dose heparin in the long-term treatment of venous thrombosis, *N Engl J Med* 302:855-858, 1979.
17. Hull RD, Secker-Walker RH, Hirsh J: *Diagnosis of deep vein thrombosis.* In Colman RW et al, eds: *Hemostasis and thrombosis*, Philadelphia, 1987, Lippincott.
18. Hull RD et al: Diagnostic efficacy of impedance plethysmography for clinically suspected deep-vein thrombosis: a randomized trial, *Ann Intern Med* 102:21-26, 1985.
19. Hull RD et al: Heparin for 5 days as compared with 10 days in the initial treatment of proximal venous thrombosis, *N Engl J Med* 322:1260-1264, 1990.
20. Kakkar VV, Corrigan TP, Fossard DP: Prevention of fatal postoperative pulmonary embolism by low doses of heparin: an international multicentre trial, *Lancet* 2:375-379, 1975.
21. Kakkar VV et al: Natural history of postoperative deep-vein thrombosis, *Lancet* 2:230-231, 1969.
22. Kakkar VV et al: Deep vein thrombosis of the leg: is there a "high-risk" group? *Am J Surg* 120:527-530, 1970.
23. Lagerstedt CI et al: Need for long-term anticoagulant treatment in symptomatic calf-vein thrombosis, *Lancet* 2:515-518, 1985.
24. Lindhagen A, Bergqvist D, Hallbook T: Deep venous insufficiency after postoperative thrombosis diagnosed with ^{125}I-labelled fibrinogen uptake test, *Br J Surg* 71:511-515, 1984.
25. Moreno-Cabral R, Kistner RL, Nodyke RA: Importance of calf vein thrombophlebitis, *Surgery* 80:735-742, 1976.
26. O'Donnell TF et al: Diagnosis of deep vein thrombosis in the outpatient by venography, *Surg Gyn Obstet* 150:69-74, 1980.
27. Pezzuoli G et al: Prophylaxis of fatal pulmonary embolism in general surgery using low molecular weight heparin CY216: a multicentre, double-blind, randomized, controlled, clinical trial versus placebo (STEP), *Int Surg* 74:205-210, 1989.
28. Salzman EW, Hirsh J: *Prevention of venous thromboembolism.* In Coleman RW et al, eds: *Hemostasis and thrombosis*, Philadelphia, 1987, Lippincott.
29. Stamatakis JD et al: The origin of thrombi in the deep veins of the lower limb: a venographic study, *Br J Surg* 65:449-451, 1978.

CHAPTER 94

Basic aspects of peripheral venous testing

ANDREW N. NICOLAIDES

Acute deep vein thrombosis (DVT) and chronic venous insufficiency can be suspected on clinical grounds, but it is now well established that the diagnosis and extent of disease cannot be correctly determined solely on the basis of the history and clinical findings.

ACUTE DEEP VEIN THROMBOSIS

The advent of the [^{125}I]fibrinogen test in the mid-1960s and early 1970s and its use in surgical patients brought to light the fact that the actual incidence of postoperative DVT is much higher than suspected: 25% to 30% in general surgical patients, 50% to 75% in orthopedic patients, and 80% in patients paralyzed as a result of stroke or spinal injury. It was also discovered that only 5% of calf thrombi and 40% of thrombi proximal to the calf ever produce clinical symptoms. Because of these findings, it became routine to institute prophylaxis in hospitalized patients. Similarly, the use of venography in the 1960s and 1970s in patients with symptoms and signs of DVT revealed that only 50% actually have DVT and that there are many other causes of pain, swelling, and tenderness. Thus if the clinical findings were relied on, half the patients would be unnecessarily treated with anticoagulants, which are expensive and can cause some serious complications. These facts were an important incentive for the development of noninvasive tests for the diagnosis of DVT.

Continuous wave Doppler ultrasound was first developed in the early 1970s and exhibited an 83% sensitivity and 88% specificity for detecting thrombi proximal to the calf. Its main defects were its inability to detect calf thrombi and the need to be performed by an experienced operator.[2] Strain-gauge plethysmography was developed in the late 1970s and had a reported sensitivity greater than 90% and a specificity greater than 80%. It appeared to be less dependent on the skill of the technologist than did continuous wave Doppler (see Chapter 97).[2] Phleborheography and impedance plethysmography were developed at about the same time (see Chapters 96 and 98). Impedance plethysmography showed a sensitivity of 92% and specificity of 88% for detecting proximal DVT, but none of these tests was able to accurately detect calf DVT.

The detection of calf DVT is now considered important because 20% of such thrombi extend proximally (see Chapter 93). This problem has been overcome by the use of duplex scanning. In the past few years, duplex scanning has become the method of choice for establishing the diagnosis of DVT in symptomatic patients (see Chapter 95). For identifying thrombi proximal to the calf, both the sensitivity and specificity of this method exceed 95%; for detecting calf thrombi, they both exceed 80%. Because of this, few patients now undergo venography, and it is reserved for only a small number of patients, such as those with a tender leg wound or in a cast and others who may be unsuitable for duplex scanning.

For many years, the screening of asymptomatic patients was performed with [^{125}I]fibrinogen scanning. This was an important research tool that was used in the 1970s and 1980s to determine the incidence of DVT in different hospital populations so that effective methods of prevention could be developed. With the increase in AIDS, however, this test, which requires pooled blood, became impractical for use and there is now a great need for a new test to replace it. Fortunately, the prophylactic methods now available are not only clinically effective but also cost effective, and there is little need for a routine screening test except for research purposes. The early reports of the results of duplex scanning in asymptomatic patients (see Chapter 95) were disappointing, with sensitivities for detecting all types of thrombi ranging from 26% to 89%. For calf DVT, the reported sensitivities ranged from 5% to 67%. However, with the introduction of color flow imaging, increased operator experience, and determination of better criteria for identifying DVT, its sensitivity for detecting above-knee thrombi has risen to 100% and for below-knee thrombi, to 79% (Chapter 95). It appears that the current high-resolution images of color duplex scanners have the potential for achieving the necessary accuracy, but this must be substantiated by several independent studies before the method can be used in clinical trials to replace venography or [^{125}I]fibrinogen scanning.

CHRONIC VENOUS INSUFFICIENCY

Varicose veins, pain, ankle or leg edema, skin irritation, pigmentation, and ulceration are common findings in patients with chronic venous disease. A careful clinical history and physical examination will usually confirm that the patient has a venous problem. However, the clinical findings will not always indicate the location and extent of the underlying disorder. The aim of subsequent investigations is to elucidate the nature of the underlying abnormalities (obstruction and/or reflux) in the venous system and to determine their severity by quantitative measurements so that the clinician can form a rational plan of management.

The symptoms of chronic venous insufficiency are produced by venous hypertension, which is itself the result of obstruction or reflux, or both. Venous hypertension results in dilatation of the capillaries with an increased leakage of plasma, plasma proteins, and red cells. Pericapillary fibrin deposits then impair oxygen transport, with eventual hypoxia, local ischemia, fat necrosis, skin pigmentation, and ulceration.[1]

Outflow obstruction is found in patients with DVT who have experienced inadequate subsequent recanalization and poor development of collateral circulation. Less frequently, it is the result of extramural venous compression. Reflux occurs when the valves are damaged, due either to venous thrombosis followed by recanalization or to dilatation of the vein that prevents the valve cusps from making contact with each other.

Varicose veins are often associated with deep to superficial reflux because of valvular incompetence of the superficial or communicating system, usually resulting from venous dilatation without previous thrombosis (primary varicose veins). Less often this stems from valvular damage caused by thrombosis and recanalization, which produces incompetent deep and perforating veins (secondary varicose veins).

Reflux in the deep veins is often the result of venous thrombosis and recanalization, with attendant destruction of the venous valves, but it may also be idiopathic. In recent years, routine descending venography has demonstrated that there is no evidence of previous DVT in approximately 30% of limbs with deep venous reflux, the reflux actually resulting from floppy valve cusps.

Two compensatory physiologic mechanisms exist that tend to ameliorate the effects of venous hypertension. These are lymphatic drainage and the body's natural fibrinolytic activity. The rate of lymphatic drainage in postthrombotic limbs may be increased up to ten times and the fibrinolytic activity that removes the pericapillary fibrin markedly varies between individuals. The development of edema, skin changes, and ulceration is now believed to be the result of a delicate balance between the severity of venous hypertension and the operation of compensatory mechanisms.

Clinical examination performed using the classic Trendelenburg and Perthes tourniquet tests can yield misleading results or be impossible to perform when varicose veins are not prominent and may offer relatively little information about the true state of the deep veins (obstruction or reflux). In extreme cases in which there is a history of pain on walking (venous claudication), severe swelling, and prom-

inent veins over the lower abdominal wall, the diagnosis is obvious. In some patients, symptoms become worse after operations on varicose veins, which were acting as collaterals in the presence of undiagnosed and unsuspected deep venous obstruction (often in the superficial femoral vein). In addition, a large number of "recurrent" varicose veins are actually the result of unsuspected incompetent short saphenous veins. To deal with this problematic diagnosis, a number of methods have been developed during the past few years. They can furnish qualitative and quantitative information and provide answers to most questions posed in a clinical practice. The difficulty is in deciding when to use these methods and how to interpret the results.

The use of continuous wave Doppler ultrasound will confirm the presence of obstruction or reflux, indicating the site (obstruction, femoropopliteal or iliofemoral; reflux, saphenofemoral junction, saphenopopliteal, incompetent thigh-perforating veins, or popliteal) in 90% of outpatients. The remaining 10% of patients will be complicated cases, many of whom had a previous operation on their veins or whose Doppler ultrasound results are not clear. In a small group of patients suspected to have incompetent calf-perforating veins, confirmation is required. In most of these patients, the answer will be provided by one of the following tests: maximal venous outflow measurements (strain gauge), photoplethysmography, duplex scanning, or air-plethysmography.

Localization of obstruction or reflux

The accurate localization of a venous obstruction in preparation for surgery necessitates a venogram, although duplex scanning is proving equally helpful in this regard, particularly for lesions distal to the common femoral vein. Until recently, accurate localization of the sites of deep to superficial reflux (e.g., saphenofemoral, saphenopopliteal, incompetent thigh-perforating veins, calf-perforating veins) and reflux in the deep veins (femoral, popliteal, tibial) was only possible with venography. Duplex scanning is proving to be a simpler and functionally more accurate method, so ascending functional or descending venography is now rarely performed. The main indication for venography is to detect floppy valves in the deep veins. Duplex scanning is the method of choice for identifying the site of incompetent perforating veins and the junction of the short saphenous with the popliteal vein.

The information yielded by the tests described herein about the status of obstruction and reflux suffices for planning a rational plan of management.

Quantitative measurements of obstruction or reflux

Quantitative measurements of outflow obstruction or reflux are needed for research purposes, particularly for studying the natural history of different forms of chronic venous insufficiency and for assessing established and new methods of treatment. These quantitative measurements have now opened up new avenues that have led to a better scientific basis for the management of patients. Until recently, the measurement of ambulatory venous pressure was the only quantitative test. Although invasive, it could indicate the severity of venous hypertension. It was a measure of the end-result of both outflow obstruction and reflux. However, the new tests, particularly duplex scanning (see Chapter 111) and air-plethysmography (see Chapter 112), can distinguish the relative contribution of different abnormalities, such as venous obstruction or reflux in the superficial or deep veins, as well as assess the function of the calf muscle pump and whether an abnormality is the result of intrinsic venous disease, a musculoskeletal disorder, or both.

REFERENCES

1. Browse NL, Burnand KG: The cause of venous ulceration, *Lancet* 2:243, 1982.
2. Nicolaides AN, Sumner DS: *Investigation of patients with deep vein thrombosis and chronic venous insufficiency,* London, Los Angeles, Nicosia, 1991, Med-Orion.

CHAPTER 95

Diagnosis of deep vein thrombosis with real-time color and duplex scanning

DAVID S. SUMNER and MARK A. MATTOS

Over the past decade, the noninvasive diagnosis of deep vein thrombosis (DVT) has witnessed a transformation that almost qualifies as revolutionary. Before 1983, when Talbot[67] demonstrated that B-mode ultrasound could be applied to the diagnosis of DVT, clinicians had been forced to rely on handheld Doppler surveys and plethysmographic studies. Although these physiologic tests are widely applicable, inexpensive, relatively simple to perform, and reasonably accurate for detecting occlusions of above-knee veins, they are severely limited in their ability to diagnose thrombi in below-knee veins, often fail to detect nonocclusive clots, overlook thrombi in duplicated veins, provide little information about the location or extent of the thrombotic process, and detect asymptomatic thrombi developing in the calves of high-risk patients only when there is clot propagating into the thigh.

It is little wonder, therefore, that B-mode scanning attracted a great deal of interest and was rapidly embraced by many noninvasive laboratories.[8,11,16] The technique also appealed to radiologists, who found physiologic methods foreign to their discipline but were comfortable with ultrasound. With B-mode scanning, veins could be visualized and individually identified, both occlusive and nonocclusive clots could be seen and their extent determined, and under favorable conditions, below-knee thrombi could be detected. Extensive investigations conducted by Flanagan, Sullivan, and Cranley[17] established the essential diagnostic criteria and, in the process, identified the limitations and potential sources of error. Among the most vexing problems has been the difficulty in detecting hypoechogenic thrombi. The presence of these thrombi requires indirect confirmation by the time-consuming and tedious process of obtaining serial cross-sectional views centimeter by centimeter along the entire length of the vein and, at each site, observing the effect of externally applied pressure on the venous lumen. Other problem areas include the iliac veins, which are often poorly visualized, and the veins of the calf, which, because of their small size, are hard to identify and distinguish from neighboring arteries.[26,77]

By supplementing B-mode imaging with Doppler flow detection, the duplex scanner has overcome many of these deficits. Questions regarding the presence of a hypoechogenic thrombus or the identity of a vascular structure seen on a B-mode image can be resolved by interrogating the vessel with Doppler ultrasound. Moreover, distortion of the Doppler flow signal can be used to verify the presence of thrombi in areas beyond the scope of the B-mode image. In turn, the B-mode image facilitates the selection and identification of veins to be interrogated with the Doppler method. Some drawbacks remain, however. Although duplex scanning reduces the potential for error, examination of the entire limb continues to be a demanding and protracted exercise, requiring evaluation of venous compressibility or multiple sampling of venous flow patterns along the course of each of many veins potentially subject to thrombosis. Surveys of small paired infrapopliteal veins—where clots are frequently nonocclusive and often isolated and may be confined to a short segment of vein—pose the greatest challenge. Rather than meeting this challenge, many laboratories restrict examination to the above-knee veins, justifying this abbreviated approach on the grounds that infrapopliteal thrombi are of dubious clinical significance.

The introduction of color flow duplex imaging in the late 1980s radically changed the complexion of noninvasive venous evaluation. These technologically advanced instruments superimpose a real-time color flow map on the conventional duplex image, providing instantaneous flow information over an extended segment of vein. Color flow imaging not only immediately identifies vascular structures and discriminates veins from arteries, but also decreases the need to assess audible or recorded Doppler signals and venous compressibility. Thus it facilitates longitudinal tracking of veins, graphically displays flow patterns, demonstrates partial occlusions by revealing encroachment on the flow image, and establishes the presence of total occlusion by confirming the absence of blood flow. These advantages translate into an accurate, less demanding, and less time-consuming examination, features that are especially important to the novice operator, who may be intimidated by the complexity of conventional duplex scanning. Finally, color flow imaging makes routine scanning of calf veins feasible and brings the possible surveillance of high-risk patients closer to reality.

This chapter describes the use of duplex and color flow scanning for diagnosing acute DVT of the lower extremity, compares the accuracy of both modalities, and discusses their application in clinical practice.

SCANNING TECHNIQUE

The fundamentals of scanning for DVT are similar whether the examiner uses a conventional or color duplex device.[17,42,66] To ensure venous filling, patients lie supine on a bed or examination table tilted to a 20° to 30° reversed-Trendelenburg position. The legs are slightly separated and externally rotated. It is important that the patient be comfortable and relaxed to avoid venous compression by tense muscles. Reassuring the patient that the procedure is painless and entirely noninvasive will do much to alleviate muscle tension and random motion.

Scanning is begun at the groin with the common femoral vein and its tributaries and proceeds down the limb along the anteromedial thigh (just posterior to the quadriceps femoris muscle) to the level of the adductor hiatus. Within this segment, the superficial femoral vein, lying in Hunter's canal, is readily visualized. Because the popliteal veins are deeply situated in relation to the medial surface of the limb, they must be approached posteriorly. Ideally, the examination is conducted with the patient prone and the feet supported on a pillow to flex the knee about 30°. This position relaxes the tissues, prevents venous compression, and provides ready access to the entire popliteal space, both above and below the knee. Alternatively, the patient can be turned to the lateral decubitus position so that the leg undergoing examination is uppermost. Flexing the thigh and knee places the upper leg in front of the extended lower leg and allows the knee to rest comfortably on the bed. Unfortunately, many patients in whom DVT is suspected are on respirators, in casts or traction, recovering from a major operation, seriously ill, or morbidly obese and cannot assume these positions. In such cases, it may be possible to carry out the examination with the patient supine, provided the knee can be flexed enough to provide access to the popliteal space.

Tributaries of the popliteal vein (including the cephalic portions of the posterior tibial and peroneal veins, the gastrocnemial and soleal veins, and the termination of the lesser saphenous vein) are also studied from the posterior approach as an extension of the popliteal examination. Farther down the leg, the peroneal veins may be visualized when the patient is prone by placing the probe 1 to 2 cm medial to the edge of the fibula. It is convenient to survey other portions of the infrapopliteal veins with the patient supine and the knee slightly flexed to relax the calf muscles. Studies are begun at the ankle and continued up the leg. To visualize the paired posterior tibial veins, the probe is placed along the medial calf just behind the tibia and directed laterally and slightly anteriorly. Anterior tibial venae comitantes are examined with the probe placed over the anterior compartment and oriented to cast the sound beam posteriorly and medially. From both of these approaches, the peroneal veins may be seen lying deep to the posterior tibial veins or deep to the anterior tibial veins, just beyond the interosseous membrane. Adjustments of the probe angle will usually be required because these vessels may lie in different planes. Some investigators prefer to study infrapopliteal veins with the patient sitting with the foot resting on a low stool or on the examiner's knee. However, for reasons already stated, many patients cannot assume this position.

To complete the examination, the greater saphenous vein is traced along its course from its origin anterior to the medial malleolus, up the medial calf, behind the femoral condyle, and to the groin, where it enters the common femoral vein.

CONVENTIONAL DUPLEX SCANNING

Vascular structures are identified on the B-mode image by the greater echogenicity of their walls compared with that of their lumens, which normally are relatively devoid of reflections.[17] Deep veins lie adjacent to arteries bearing the same name and may be distinguished from arteries by their anatomic position, by the ease with which they collapse in response to externally applied pressure, and by their lack of pulsation. If doubt remains, pulsed Doppler interrogation of their flow characteristics will decide their identity. After cross-sectional (short-axis) views have been used to locate the vessel, longitudinal (long-axis) views may be obtained. Superficial veins are best examined with high-frequency probes (7.5 to 8.0 MHz), and more deeply located veins are optimally studied with lower-frequency probes (3.5 to 5.0 MHz).

Visualization of iliac veins is often inadequate because of their relatively deep location and the presence of overlying bowel gas. At the groin, the common femoral and all of its tributaries, including the greater saphenous, superficial femoral, and profunda femoris veins, are easily seen, albeit not in the same examination plane. Problems may also be encountered in the adductor canal region. Although the tibial veins are ordinarily not hard to image with high-resolution scanners, their assessment is rendered difficult by their small diameters, complicated anatomy, and multiplicity.

Actual visualization of clot within the venous lumen is the most specific indicator of DVT.[16,17] Fresh thrombi, however, may have an acoustic density only slightly greater than that of blood and thus may escape detection. Shortly after a clot is formed, there is a period of decreasing echogenicity, after which the clot becomes progressively more reflective.[48,53] Acute thrombi may have a tail that remains unattached to the vessel wall and can be observed waving about in the bloodstream.[6,17] A clot seen in a transverse view should also be perceptible in a longitudinal plane.

Because clot visualization is often imperfect, determination of venous compressibility is considered a most important part of the examination. Indeed, some authors rely almost exclusively on this maneuver.[4,12,51] Studies are conducted in the transverse view, since veins tend to roll away from the plane of visualization when they are examined longitudinally, leading to false-positive interpretations. Normal veins collapse completely when subjected to minimal probe pressure (10^4 dynes/cm^2, or about 8 mm Hg).[12] As the anterior and posterior walls coapt, the vein appears to "wink" at the observer. Veins that are completely filled with thrombus remain distended despite firm application of the probe. Partially occluded veins exhibit incomplete compressibility. Because a clot may be confined to a relatively short venous segment, it is necessary to repeat the compression maneuver every few centimeters along the course of the vein. Unfortunately, the profunda femoris vein and the superficial femoral vein in the adductor hiatus are relatively resistant to compression. Positive findings in these veins must therefore be interpreted cautiously. Although the infrapopliteal veins are readily compressible, their small diameters may make assessment of complete or partial collapse difficult.

Pulsed Doppler interrogation of the vein resolves most of these problems by demonstrating the presence or absence of blood flow. Investigators at the University of Washington[26] have concluded that flow assessment with the Doppler is the most accurate portion of the duplex examination. The diagnostic criteria are identical to those developed for the continuous wave Doppler evaluation.[63] Spontaneous flow, which is phasic with respiration, is indicative of venous patency both at the site of examination and above; continuous, nonphasic flow suggests outflow obstruction; and absent or impaired augmentation with distal limb compression implies the presence of an intervening venous occlusion. Use of the Doppler feature is particularly important for evaluating the patency of veins that are difficult to image or compress. For example, patency of the iliac veins can be assessed indirectly by examining the flow patterns in the common femoral vein. In most cases of iliac vein obstruction, the common femoral vein is also involved and little or no flow will be detected. Even if there are no clots in the common femoral vein, the presence of continuous flow strongly suggests iliac vein obstruction. Similarly, altered flow patterns or impaired augmentation may be indicative of obstructions concealed in the adductor canal. Finding increased flow velocity in superficial veins is an excellent, though indirect, method of confirming the presence of acute DVT.[63]

Occasionally other tests or observations may be helpful if considered in the context of the total examination. These include Valsalva maneuver, visible blood flow, and valve motion. Dilatation of the common femoral vein in response to increased venous pressure generated by a Valsalva maneuver has been used to indicate patency of the common femoral and iliac veins.[4,17] The accuracy of this test, however, is highly dependent on patient cooperation and may be compromised by the presence of a more centrally located competent valve.[2] Ultrasound may be reflected from slowly

Table 95-1. Criteria for distinguishing acute from chronic venous thrombosis

Characteristic	Acute	Chronic
Echogenicity	Slight	Marked
Texture	Homogeneous	Heterogeneous
Surface	Smooth	Irregular
Diameter	Often dilated	May be constricted
Compressibility	Soft, easily compressed	Firm, difficult to compress
Attachment	May be free floating	Adherent
Collaterals	Few	Well developed

Modified from Flanagan LD, Sullivan ED, Cranley JJ: *Venous imaging of the extremities using real-time B-mode ultrasound.* In Bergan JJ, Yao JST, eds: *Surgery of the veins,* Orlando, Fla, 1985, Grune & Stratton.

moving blood, generating echoes that make flow visible on the B-mode scan. (Although this phenomenon has been attributed to rouleaux formation,[60] there is no proof that erythrocytes aggregate in this way outside of the microcirculation.) Although flow observed throughout the lumen implies total patency, stagnant blood may resemble a fresh clot, perhaps leading to a false-positive interpretation. Slowed flow is frequently seen in pregnant women but disappears when the patient turns on her side.[68] Valve cusps, moving in response to changes in flow, are often observed in normal veins using high-resolution scanners.[17] "Fixed" valves imply a previous inflammatory response and sluggish motion suggests the presence of small clots.

Certain duplex scan characteristic are said to distinguish between acute and chronic venous thrombosis (Table 95-1).[17] Acute thrombi are slightly echogenic, have a homogeneous appearance and a smooth surface, and may be "free-floating," whereas chronic thrombi are more densely echogenic, have a heterogeneous appearance and an irregular surface, and tend to be tightly attached to the venous wall.[43,53] In fact, veins that have been occluded for a long time may be so echogenic that they blend in with the surrounding tissues and may be difficult to identify. Fresh clots may distend the venous lumen, but older organized clots may result in contraction of the lumen. Moreover, the configuration of acute thrombi can be altered with external probe pressure, giving the appearance of moderate compressibility. Chronic thrombi, on the other hand, are resistant to compression. Extensive collateral development and frozen or contracted valves are also indicative of chronicity. All of these criteria, however, are relatively imprecise.

COLOR FLOW SCANNING

Descriptions of color flow instruments are to be found elsewhere in this book and will not be repeated here. Color designation is assigned so that centrally directed flow is blue and peripherally directed flow is red to correspond to the predominant direction of flow in veins and arteries, respectively. Color expedites the identification of vessels and provides a rapid method for distinguishing arteries from veins. Unless there is arterial obstruction, flow is almost always spontaneously visible in all named arteries of the leg. The initial step at each level of the venous examination consists of locating the corresponding artery. This is especially important in areas where there are multiple veins and the anatomy is complex, a situation common below the knee. By tilting the probe and shifting its longitudinal orientation, the examiner brings the venous structures into the field of view. The probe is then further manipulated to optimize the venous flow image. Although flow is usually "spontaneously" visible in the popliteal and femoral veins, augmentation may be necessary to visualize flow in the infrapopliteal veins. Gentle manual compression of the foot or calf below the site of the probe or compression and release of the calf above the probe is sufficient to produce a visible flow image in normal tibioperoneal veins.

With the color mode "off," the gain control is adjusted so that the arterial lumen is echo free and appears black. At this setting, when the color mode is "on," the lumens of large veins, such as the common and superficial femoral, should be completely filled with blue pixels. Phasic variations in flow coinciding with respiration are clearly evident in normal veins. When flow velocity is augmented by manual compression of the leg, the venous lumen expands and color shifts from a darker to lighter shade of blue. If venous valves cephalad to the probe are incompetent, the color changes from blue to red in response to proximal limb compression or a Valsalva maneuver, indicating reversal of flow direction. Effects of probe pressure can be observed directly on the flow image or with the color mode "off" on the B-mode image.

At the groin, where the examination begins, flow images of the common femoral, superficial femoral, profunda femoris, and saphenous veins are easily seen when the probe angle is properly adjusted (Fig. 95-1). In some patients, the confluence of all four veins may be visualized simultaneously. Longitudinal tracking of veins is greatly facilitated by color because the flow image is easily followed. As the examination proceeds down the leg, tissue planes on both sides of the artery should be interrogated to avoid missing duplicate channels, which frequently exist in the superficial femoral and popliteal areas. Although serial cross-sectional views need not be obtained, it is advisable to check the cross-sectional anatomy periodically, again to avoid overlooking a parallel vein. Behind the knee, the junction of the lesser saphenous and popliteal veins is usually seen without difficulty (Fig. 95-2).

Color makes it feasible to examine infrapopliteal veins as part of the routine venous examination. Even so, this area continues to be the most technically demanding region of the leg. Because clots may involve only one of the two venae comitantes that parallel the tibioperoneal arteries, both must be visualized throughout their entire extent to absolutely exclude the existence of an isolated thrombus (Fig. 95-3). Augmentation is often required to obtain a color

image, although "slow-flow" software incorporated in some instruments makes spontaneous flow detection possible. With this feature, frequency shifts as low as 33 Hz or velocities less than 1.0 cm/sec can be detected. In a study focusing on deep veins of the calf, Polak, Cutler, and

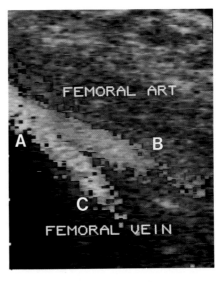

Fig. 95-1. Color duplex scan of normal groin veins showing the common femoral *(A)*, superficial femoral *(B)*, and profunda femoris veins *(C)*. A short segment of the adjacent common femoral artery is also depicted. (In this and the following figures, the head is to the left and the skin surface is at the top.) (From Sumner DS et al: *Study of deep venous thrombosis in high-risk patients with color flow Doppler.* In Bergan JJ, Yao JST, eds: *Venous disorders,* Philadelphia, 1991, Saunders.)

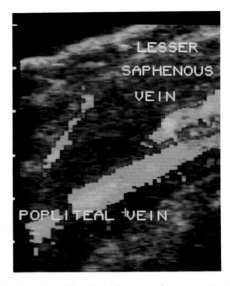

Fig. 95-2. Normal popliteal and lesser saphenous veins. A few red pixels are visible in the popliteal artery, which was imaged in diastole. (From Sumner DS et al: *Study of deep venous thrombosis in high-risk patients with color flow Doppler.* In Bergan JJ, Yao JST, eds: *Venous disorders,* Philadelphia, 1991, Saunders.)

O'Leary[50] found that augmentation produced color flow images of all normal peroneal and posterior tibial veins but only 55% of the anterior tibial veins were visualized. Because clots are seldom isolated to the anterior tibial veins, failure to image these veins may not be a serious indictment of the test. On the other hand, van Bemmelen, Bedford, and Strandness[70] were able to image all paired calf veins from the ankle to the knee in a series of 30 normal subjects.

With the aid of color, it is more often possible to obtain satisfactory images of the iliac veins and inferior vena cava than it is with conventional duplex scanning.[55] There is less need to rely on compression, since the color image itself provides confirmation of either patency or partial or complete occlusion (Fig. 95-4).

Interpretation

All of the observations that can be made with conventional duplex scanning are also possible with color flow imaging.[42,66] There are observations peculiar to color, however, that change the emphasis of the examination. The flow image markedly reduces (but does not entirely obviate) the need to employ venous compression or to sample flow with the pulsed Doppler. Absence of visible flow in the major veins immediately suggests the presence of an occlusive thrombus, and when no color appears with augmentation, the diagnosis is virtually established (Figs. 95-5 to 95-7). Thus fresh hypoechogenic thrombi are less likely to escape detection. Providing the gain settings are correct, a filling defect seen in the flow image is indicative of a partially occluding thrombus (Fig. 95-8). This diagnosis can therefore be made without resorting to probe compression. When the thrombus is "free floating," its tail may be seen waving about in the flow stream even if the B-mode image is difficult to perceive (Fig. 95-9).

Color flow scans can be classified into one of three categories[66]: negative, positive, and equivocal.

In a negative scan, no thrombus is visualized, flow is either spontaneous or easily augmented, and the color image fills the entire lumen. In most cases, the vein collapses completely with probe pressure (Figs. 95-1 to 95-3).

A scan is positive if flow is absent with augmentation or

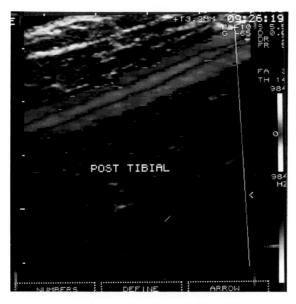

Fig. 95-3. Posterior tibial artery and normal paired venae comitantes.

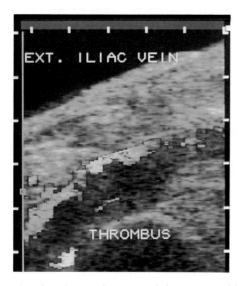

Fig. 95-4. Partial occlusion of an external iliac vein. A phlebogram of the same region showed an identical picture. (From Sumner DS et al: *Study of deep venous thrombosis in high-risk patients with color flow Doppler.* In Bergan JJ, Yao JST, eds: *Venous disorders,* Philadelphia, 1991, Saunders.)

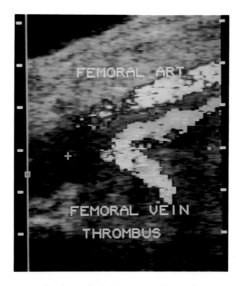

Fig. 95-5. Completely occluded common femoral vein (+). Flow is seen in the profunda femoris vein and in a partially thrombosed superficial femoral vein. (From Sumner DS et al: *Clinical application of color Doppler in venous problems.* In Yao JST, Pearce WH, eds: *Technologies in vascular surgery,* Philadelphia, 1992, Saunders.)

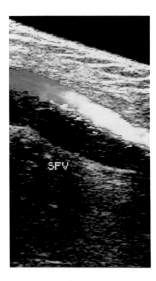

Fig. 95-6. Hypoechogenic thrombus in completely occluded superficial femoral vein *(SFV).* The adjacent superficial femoral artery is shown in red.

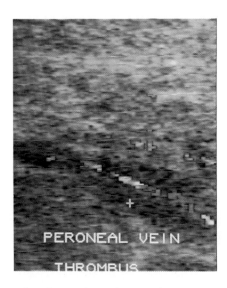

Fig. 95-7. Total occlusion of paired peroneal venae comitantes. Red pixels identify the peroneal artery lying between the thrombosed veins. (From Sumner DS et al: *Study of deep venous thrombosis in high-risk patients with color flow Doppler.* In Bergan JJ, Yao JST, eds: *Venous disorders,* Philadelphia, 1991, Saunders.)

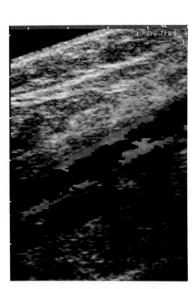

Fig. 95-8. Hypoechogenic thrombus in a partially occluded popliteal vein.

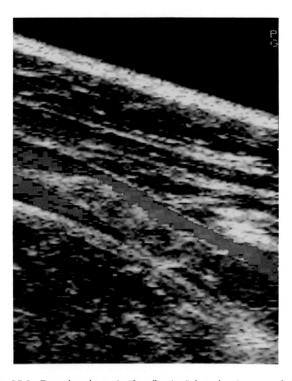

Fig. 95-9. Densely echogenic "free floating" thrombus in a superficial femoral vein.

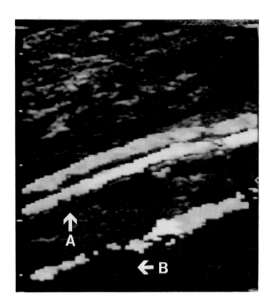

Fig. 95-10. Absence of flow in one posterior tibial vein *(A)* and non-confluent flow pattern in a peroneal vein *(B)*. A patent posterior tibial vein and artery are also shown. (From Mattos MA et al: Color-flow duplex scanning for the surveillance and diagnosis of acute deep venous thrombosis, *J Vasc Surg* 15:366, 1992.)

there is definite encroachment on the flow image. Depending on their echogenicity, thrombi may or may not be visualized and venous compressibility is usually absent or incomplete (Figs. 95-4 to 95-9).

Scan findings are equivocal if, despite the absence of thrombus, spontaneous or augmented flow patterns are abnormal. The flow image may appear nonconfluent or there may be time-dependent or spatially dependent irregularities of the image without consistent areas of encroachment (Figs. 95-10 and 95-11). Results in larger veins (femoral and popliteal) seldom fall into this category. Most equivocal findings arise in the examination of calf veins. Retrospective review of clinical material suggests that most equivocal studies are in fact positive for the existence of small, isolated, nonocclusive thrombi.

The technologists in the laboratory at the Southern Illinois University School of Medicine record their observations for each of the following venous segments: common femoral, profunda femoris, superficial femoral, popliteal, anterior tibial, posterior tibial, peroneal, greater saphenous (both above and below the knee), and lesser saphenous. Clots visualized in the gastrocnemial or sural veins are also noted. Survey of the veins above the inguinal ligament is routinely attempted, but it is frequently necessary to rely on indirect Doppler assessment of flow in the common femoral vein to evaluate the iliac venous system. As mentioned previously, pulsed Doppler information is also used in the interpretation of flow patterns in superficial or collateral veins and in poorly visualized venous segments (such as the superficial femoral in the adductor canal). The physician reviewing videotapes recorded by the technologist makes the final interpretation.

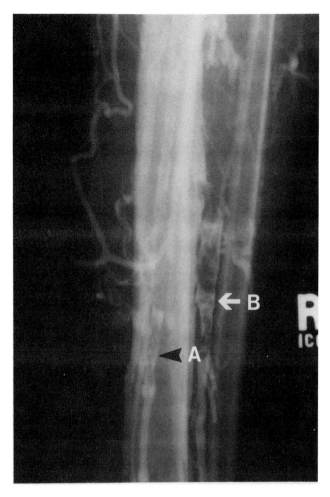

Fig. 95-11. Phlebogram of the same area shown in Fig. 95-10. The deeper posterior tibial vein *(A)* and the peroneal vein *(B)* are partially occluded. (From Mattos MA et al: Color-flow duplex scanning for the surveillance and diagnosis of acute deep venous thrombosis, *J Vasc Surg* 15:366, 1992.)

OTHER CAUSES OF LIMB SWELLING OR PAIN

Hematomas and popliteal cysts are often found in patients with symptoms suggesting DVT, occasionally in association with venous thrombi.[2,5,14,35] Hematomas appear as ellipsoidal, hypoechogenic areas surrounded by muscle or adipose tissue.[5] Layering of a clot may be observed. Aneurysms, which have a similar appearance, can be distinguished from hematomas by their expansile pulsation and by the presence of Doppler flow signals. Popliteal cysts are sharply defined, echolucent, oblong structures that usually lie medial to the vascular bundle.[5,35] Other causes of venous obstruction, such as enlarged lymph nodes and tumor masses, are also easily recognized. Color is an especially valuable adjunct because it clearly differentiates between aneurysms and hematomas and between vascular and nonvascular structures.

ACCURACY

Phlebography remains the most appropriate, albeit somewhat tarnished, gold standard for evaluating the accuracy of noninvasive tests designed to detect DVT. Ascending phlebography seldom visualizes the profunda femoris vein, often opacifies the iliac system inadequately, and may not reveal many of the deep veins of the calf. One or more venous segments may not be demonstrated in 10% to 30% of the phlebograms.[73] Even trained observers disagree about the presence of a thrombus in as many as 10% of the examinations.[56] In a postmortem study, phlebography proved to be 89% sensitive and 97% specific.[32] It is likely, therefore, that some of the false-positive and false-negative results attributed to duplex or color flow scanning actually represent phlebographic errors.

Because of the low but real risk of complications and the discomfort associated with phlebography, physicians are often reluctant to obtain x-ray studies when noninvasive tests have been performed, especially when the diagnosis of DVT seems unlikely. Consequently, the number of patients undergoing both examinations tends to be restricted, and the number of positive results in the population being studied tends to be disproportionally large. Few prospective studies have been undertaken. Further compounding the problem is the hubris of some ultrasonographers, who believe that B-mode or duplex scanning in their hands is inherently accurate and findings require no phlebographic confirmation. In other words, the scan becomes its own gold standard. Although there is some justification for this attitude, it can hardly be termed scientific. Finally, there is a tendency for only the best results to reach the literature. It follows that the published figures for the accuracy of duplex or color flow scanning (or any other noninvasive test for DVT) must be viewed with some skepticism and with the realization that they may not represent the results in a true cross section of symptomatic patients.

Duplex and color flow scanning must be held to a higher standard of excellence than that set by physiologically based tests for DVT. Although the most that can be expected of handheld Doppler surveys and plethysmographic tests is the accurate diagnosis of occlusive thrombi in above-knee veins, ultrasonic scans should also be able to detect nonocclusive clots, locate thrombi and define their extent, and evaluate below-knee veins for the presence of thrombi. In considering the accuracy of ultrasonic scans, it is imperative that a distinction be made between those studies conducted on symptomatic patients and those carried out on high-risk "surveillance" patients, since the diagnosis of DVT in the latter group is an order of magnitude more difficult than that in the former group.

Conventional duplex scanning for clinically suspected DVT

Table 95-2 summarizes the findings from 20 reports comparing the results of conventional duplex scanning with those of phlebography in almost 3000 limbs (or venous segments) of symptomatic patients. For all parameters of accuracy, the cumulative, median, and mean values hovered around 95%. In 14 (70%) of the reports, both the sensitivity and specificity exceeded 90%, and all cited an overall accuracy greater than 90%. In 7 papers, a sensitivity and negative predictive value of 100% was reported for the detection or exclusion of proximal vein thrombi.* Less than half of the studies were prospective, however. Therefore excluding prospective studies and two with incomplete data, only 6.5% (629 of 9582) of limbs undergoing duplex examination also underwent phlebography.† In most studies, the decision to obtain a confirmatory phlebogram was left to the discretion of the referring physician. Because the cumulative prevalence of venous thrombosis in these reports was quite high (43%; 1257 of 2912), it appears that the decision to obtain a phlebogram was prompted either by positive duplex scan findings or by a strong clinical suspicion of DVT. The remarkably good positive predictive value (96.5%) of duplex scanning in part reflects the high prevalence of disease in the study populations.

Despite methodologic defects in these studies, there seems little doubt that the accuracy of duplex scanning for identifying symptomatic DVT exceeds that of physiologic testing.[64] Most series documenting the accuracy of physiologic testing suffer from the same problems. Two studies in which duplex scanning results were compared to physiologic findings in the same patients clearly demonstrate the superiority of the former (Table 95-3).[11,46]

Although most of the studies listed in Table 95-2 included infrapopliteal vein thrombosis in their data analysis, few directly addressed the issue of accuracy in this area. In fact, many laboratories considered calf vein scanning an unproductive exercise and restricted their studies to the popliteal and more proximal veins.[4,30,51,71,72] As a result, there is relatively little concrete data concerning the accuracy of duplex scanning below the knee.

It is generally acknowledged that calf veins are difficult to scan. In several series, failure to detect infrapopliteal thrombi accounted for all false-negative errors.[26,40,77] A literature review by Wright et al[77] disclosed 65 erroneous or equivocal duplex scans, of which 23 (35%) could be attributed to difficulty in diagnosing isolated calf vein thrombosis. A few authors, however, report remarkably good results. Rollins et al[53] examined 319 individual veins in 46 symptomatic limbs and found that the location and extent of thrombi detected with B-mode scanning corresponded within approximately 1.5 cm to that observed on the phlebogram in 84% of anterior tibial, 86% of posterior tibial, and 93% of peroneal veins. In another study conducted by the same group, Semrow et al[59] scanned 203 individual calf vein segments in 36 limbs with clinically suspected DVT. Clots were detected in 127 of 130 veins in which phlebography demonstrated acute or chronic thrombosis (sensitivity, 98%). There were only 6 false-positive scans, yielding a specificity of 92% (67 of 73). A similar accuracy was cited by Elias et al,[16] but others report somewhat less favorable

---

*References 11, 16, 18, 30, 40, 51, 77.
†References 12, 25, 26, 37, 44, 46, 51, 53.

Table 95-2. Accuracy of B-mode and duplex imaging for diagnosing deep vein thrombosis

Author	Number of extremities	Sensitivity (%)	Specificity (%)	Positive predictive value (%)	Negative predictive value (%)	Overall accuracy (%)
Oliver (1985)[44]	28	88 (7/8)	95 (19/20)	88 (7/8)	95 (19/20)	93 (26/28)
Raghavendra et al (1986)[51]	20*	100 (14/14)	100 (6/6)	100 (14/14)	100 (6/6)	100 (20/20)
Dauzat et al (1986)[14]	145	94 (94/100)	100 (45/45)	100 (94/94)	88 (45/51)	96 (139/145)
Appelman et al (1987)[4]	110*†	96 (48/50)	97 (58/60)	96 (48/50)	97 (58/60)	96 (106/110)
Cronan et al (1987)[13]	51*†	89 (25/28)	100 (23/23)	100 (25/25)	88 (23/26)	94 (48/51)
Aitken and Godden (1987)[2]	42*†	94 (15/16)	100 (26/26)	100 (15/15)	96 (26/27)	98 (41/42)
Elias et al (1987)[16]	847†	98 (325/333)	94 (483/514)	91 (325/356)	98 (483/491)	95 (808/847)
Vogel et al (1987)[72]	53*†	95 (19/20)	100 (33/33)	100 (19/19)	97 (33/34)	98 (52/53)
Karkow et al (1987)[25]	75	96 (44/46)	90 (26/29)	94 (44/47)	93 (26/28)	93 (70/75)
Rollins et al (1988)[53]	46	100 (40/40)	100 (6/6)	100 (40/40)	100 (6/6)	100 (46/46)
Cronan et al (1988)[12]	62	95 (42/44)	89 (16/18)	95 (42/44)	89 (16/18)	94 (58/62)
Killewich et al (1989)[26]	50	92 (35/38)	92 (11/12)	97 (35/36)	79 (11/14)	92 (46/50)
Patterson et al (1989)[46]	64	89 (24/27)	92 (34/37)	89 (24/27)	92 (34/37)	91 (58/64)
Lensing et al (1989)[30]	220†	91 (70/77)	99 (142/143)	99 (70/71)	95 (142/149)	96 (212/220)
Montefusco et al (1989)[37]	698‡	100 (224/224)	99 (470/474)	98 (224/228)	100 (470/470)	99 (694/698)
Mussurakis et al (1990)[40]	94†	83 (30/36)	100 (58/58)	100 (30/30)	91 (58/64)	94 (88/94)
Fletcher et al (1990)[18]	44*†	100 (14/14)	97 (29/30)	93 (14/15)	100 (29/29)	98 (43/44)
Comerota et al (1990)[11]	72	98 (43/44)	86 (24/28)	92 (43/47)	96 (24/25)	93 (67/72)
Wright et al (1990)[77]	71	91 (31/34)	95 (35/37)	94 (31/33)	92 (35/38)	93 (66/71)
van Ramshorst et al (1991)[71]	120*†	91 (58/64)	95 (53/56)	95 (58/61)	90 (53/59)	93 (111/120)
CUMULATIVE	2912	96 (1202/1257)	96 (1597/1655)	95 (1202/1260)	97 (1597/1652)	96 (2799/2912)
RANGE	20-847	83-110	86-100	88-100	79-100	91-100
MEDIAN	67.5	94.5	97.0	96.5	95.0	94.5
MEAN ± SD	146 ± 221	94 ± 5	96 ± 4	96 ± 4	94 ± 5	95 ± 3

*Infrapopliteal veins not studied or not included in analysis.
†Prospective studies.
‡Individual veins, 139 limbs.

Table 95-3. Comparative accuracy of duplex imaging and physiologic tests for diagnosing DVT

Author	Modality	Sensitivity (%)	Specificity (%)	Positive predictive value (%)	Negative predictive value (%)	Overall accuracy (%)
Patterson et al (1989)[46]	Duplex	89 (24/27)	92 (34/37)	89 (24/27)	92 (34/37)	91 (58/64)
	IPG	75 (15/20)	45 (13/29)	48 (15/31)	72 (13/18)	57 (28/49)
Comerota et al (1990)[11]	Duplex	98 (43/44)	86 (24/28)	92 (43/47)	96 (24/25)	93 (67/72)
	PRG	61 (27/44)	79 (22/28)	82 (27/33)	56 (22/39)	68 (49/72)

IPG, Impedance plethysmography; *PRG,* phleborheography.

results (Table 95-4). The findings from this brief survey of the literature therefore suggest that unless duplex examinations are meticulously performed, the accuracy for detecting and excluding infrapopliteal thrombi will be disappointing and a high degree of accuracy is more likely to be the exception rather than the rule.

Color-coded duplex scanning for clinically suspected DVT

The accuracy of color flow scanning in 77 symptomatic limbs of 75 patients is shown in Table 95-5.[34] Scan findings were positive at one or more anatomic sites in all 40 limbs with phlebographically demonstrated thrombi (sensitivity, 100%). All clots in superficial femoral veins were detected, and only 1 of 18 thrombi in the common femoral veins were missed. Although 4 of 27 popliteal thrombi were overlooked

(mostly because of duplicated veins), all but 2 of 33 tibioperoneal thrombi were identified, giving an overall below-knee sensitivity of 94%. This high sensitivity can be ascribed to the extensive nature of the thrombotic process. Totally occluding clots accounted for 58% of the cases, and 73% involved both above-knee and below-knee veins.

There was one false-positive study in a superficial femoral vein, for an above-knee specificity of 98%. Below the knee, however, there were a number of false-positive scans: four in popliteal veins and eight in tibioperoneal veins. Thus for the limb as a whole, the specificity was only 80%, reflecting a below-knee specificity of 75%. Classifying equivocal studies in below-knee veins as positive probably accounts for the low specificity in this area.

Because of the high sensitivity of the test, negative pre-

Table 95-4. Accuracy of B-mode and duplex imaging for diagnosing symptomatic calf vein thrombosis

Author	Modality	Sensitivity (%)	Specificity (%)	Positive predictive value (%)	Negative predictive value (%)
Dauzat et al (1986)[14]	B-mode	63 (5/8)	100 (45/45)	100 (5/5)	94 (45/48)
Elias et al (1987)[16]	Duplex	91 (84/92)	96 (483/501)	82 (84/102)	98 (483/491)
Fletcher et al (1990)[18]	Duplex	85 (11/13)	83 (25/30)	69 (11/16)	93 (25/27)
Comerota et al (1990)[11]	Duplex	86 (6/7)	—	—	96 (24/25)
Mitchell et al (1991)[36]	Duplex	81 (17/21)	89 (25/28)	85 (17/20)	86 (25/29)

—, Information not available.

Table 95-5. Accuracy of color-coded duplex imaging for diagnosing symptomatic DVT

Anatomic site	Number	Sensitivity (%)	Specificity (%)	Positive predictive value (%)	Negative predictive value (%)	Overall accuracy (%)
Total limb	77	100 (40/40)	73 (27/37)	80 (40/50)	100 (27/27)	87 (67/77)
Above knee	77	100 (32/32)	98 (44/45)	97 (32/33)	100 (44/44)	99 (76/77)
Common femoral	77	94 (17/18)	100 (59/59)	100 (17/17)	98 (59/60)	99 (76/77)
Superficial femoral	77	100 (32/32)	98 (44/45)	97 (32/33)	100 (44/44)	99 (76/77)
Below knee	75	94 (33/35)	75 (30/40)	77 (33/43)	94 (30/32)	84 (63/75)
Popliteal	75	85 (23/27)	92 (44/48)	85 (23/27)	92 (34/36)	89 (67/75)
Tibioperoneal	75	94 (31/33)	81 (34/42)	80 (31/39)	94 (34/36)	87 (65/75)

Data from Mattos MA et al: *J Vasc Surg* 15:366, 1992.

Table 95-6. Accuracy of color-coded duplex imaging for diagnosing symptomatic DVT in femoropopliteal veins

Author	Number of extremities	Sensitivity (%)	Specificity (%)	Positive predictive value (%)	Negative predictive value (%)	Overall accuracy (%)
Persson et al (1989)[47]	23	100 (15/15)	100 (8/8)	100 (15/15)	100 (8/8)	100 (23/23)
Foley et al (1989)[19]	47*	89 (17/19)	100 (28/28)	100 (17/17)	93 (28/30)	96 (45/47)
Schindler et al (1990)[57]	94	98 (54/55)	100 (39/39)	100 (54/54)	98 (39/40)	99 (93/94)
Rose et al (1990)[54]	75	96 (25/26)	100 (49/49)	100 (25/25)	98 (49/50)	99 (74/75)
Mattos et al (1992)[34]	77†	100 (32/32)	98 (44/45)	97 (32/33)	100 (44/44)	99 (76/77)

*100% accuracy for femoral vein segment.
†Above-knee popliteal vein only.

Table 95-7. Accuracy of color-coded duplex imaging for diagnosing symptomatic DVT in tibioperoneal veins

Author	Number of extremities	Sensitivity (%)	Specificity (%)	Positive predictive value (%)	Negative predictive value (%)	Overall accuracy (%)
Foley et al (1989)[19]	16	100 (4/4)	100 (12/12)	100 (4/4)	100 (12/12)	100 (16/16)
Mattos et al (1992)[34]	75	94 (31/33)	81 (34/42)	80 (31/39)	94 (34/36)	87 (65/75)
Rose et al (1990)[54]	74	73 (22/30)	86 (38/44)	79 (22/28)	83 (38/46)	81 (60/74)
Technically adequate*	44	95 (19/20)	100 (24/24)	100 (19/19)	96 (24/25)	98 (43/44)
Inadequate	30	30 (3/10)	70 (14/20)	33 (3/9)	67 (14/21)	57 (17/30)
Extent, not isolated	25	86 (18/21)	75 (3/4)	95 (18/19)	50 (3/6)	84 (21/25)
Isolated†	49	44 (4/9)	88 (35/40)	44 (4/9)	88 (35/40)	80 (39/49)

*Tibioperoneal trunk and all portions of the posterior tibial and peroneal veins visualized.
†Clots confined to calf veins (no above-knee thrombus).

dictive values at all levels were quite good (100% for the limb as a whole). Likewise, positive predictive values were good above the knee but were only about 80% reliable for below-knee thrombi.

A review of the still rather scant literature suggests that color flow imaging is at least as accurate as conventional duplex scanning for diagnosing DVT in proximal veins of symptomatic patients (Table 95-6). For below-knee applications, the accuracy of color flow scanning equals that of the best studies employing conventional duplex scanning (see Tables 95-4 and 95-7). As Rose et al[54] have shown, the results of color flow scanning of tibioperoneal veins are heavily influenced by the adequacy of the study and by the extent of the thrombotic process (Table 95-7). When examinations were deemed technically adequate (i.e., complete visualization of the tibioperoneal veins), all parameters of accuracy exceeded 95%. In contrast, poor visualization of the veins translated into a striking decrease in sensitivity and a marked reduction in specificity. The sensitivity of color flow scanning for detecting clots isolated to the tibioperoneal veins was only half that attained when more proximal veins were also involved. Moreover, color imaging detected only 50% of those clots that were less than 3 cm long.

Surveillance of high-risk asymptomatic patients

Table 95-8 summarizes findings from several reports documenting the accuracy of B-mode and conventional duplex scanning in surveillance studies of patients after total hip or knee arthroplasties[7,9-11,21,76] or fractures of the hip[20] or pelvis.[75] For above-knee studies, the sensitivity of duplex scanning ranged from 52% to 100% and the specificity equaled or exceeded 94%. Although investigators who used compression assessment alone[9,10,21] reported a lower sensitivity, their specificity was as good. In view of the relatively low prevalence of thrombosis (14%; 111 of 779), positive predictive values were remarkably good—all but two laboratories[7,21] reported values in excess of 80% and three laboratories reported values of 100%. Of equal importance, most negative predictive values were well above 90%. In contrast, physiologic testing, which is quite accurate for above-knee evaluations in symptomatic patients, fared far less well than ultrasonic imaging in surveillance studies.[1,21] In a series of 38 postarthroplasty limbs studied by Comerota et al,[11] duplex scanning detected all 7 phlebographically confirmed above-knee thrombi (sensitivity, 100%); phlebo-rheography identified only 2 (sensitivity, 29%).

Only a few laboratories have investigated the accuracy

Table 95-8. Accuracy of B-mode and duplex imaging for diagnosing asymptomatic DVT in postoperative surveillance studies of high-risk patients

Author	Number of extremities	Sensitivity (%)	Specificity (%)	Positive predictive value (%)	Negative predictive value (%)	Overall accuracy (%)
TOTAL LIMB						
Barnes et al (1989)[7]	153*	34 (10/29)	95 (118/124)	63 (10/16)	86 (118/137)	84 (128/153)
Woolson et al (1990)[76]	150*	63 (17/27)	100 (123/123)	100 (17/17)	92 (123/133)	93 (140/150)
Comerota et al (1990)[11]	38	89 (8/9)	100 (29/29)	100 (8/8)	97 (29/30)	97 (37/38)
Borris et al (1989)[9]	60†	54 (15/28)	91 (29/32)	83 (15/18)	69 (29/42)	73 (44/60)
Borris et al (1990)[10]	61†	71 (10/14)	94 (44/47)	77 (10/13)	92 (44/48)	89 (54/61)
Ginsberg et al (1991)[21]	247‡	26 (16/61)	99 (184/186)	89 (16/18)	80 (184/229)	81 (200/247)
ABOVE KNEE						
Barnes et al (1989)[7]	153	83 (10/12)	96 (135/141)	63 (10/16)	99 (135/137)	95 (145/153)
Froehlich et al (1989)[20]	40	100 (5/5)	97 (34/35)	83 (5/6)	100 (34/34)	98 (39/40)
Woolson et al (1990)[76]	150	89 (17/19)	100 (131/131)	100 (17/17)	97 (131/133)	99 (148/150)
Comerota et al (1990)[11]	36	100 (7/7)	100 (29/29)	100 (7/7)	100 (29/29)	100 (36/36)
White et al (1990)[75]	32	92 (11/12)	100 (20/20)	100 (11/11)	95 (20/21)	97 (31/32)
Borris et al (1989)[9]	60†	63 (15/24)	94 (34/36)	88 (15/17)	79 (34/43)	82 (49/60)
Borris et al (1990)[10]	61†	73 (8/11)	96 (48/50)	80 (8/10)	94 (48/51)	92 (56/61)
Ginsberg et al (1991)[21]	247‡	52 (11/21)	97 (219/226)	61 (11/18)	96 (219/229)	93 (230/247)
BELOW KNEE						
Comerota et al (1990)[11]	31	50 (1/2)	100 (29/29)	100 (1/1)	97 (29/30)	97 (30/31)
Borris et al (1989)[9]	60†	29 (4/14)	—	—	—	—
Borris et al (1990)[10]	61†	67 (2/3)	—	—	—	—
Ginsberg et al (1991)[21]	223‡§	5 (2/37)	99 (184/186)	50 (2/4)	84 (184/219)	83 (186/223)

*Calf veins not studied.
†B-mode scans.
‡Compression studies only.
§Isolated calf veins only.

of ultrasonic imaging for detecting isolated calf vein thromboses in asymptomatic high-risk patients. As indicated in Table 95-8, the reported sensitivity of studies performed in this area is distinctly inferior to that in the proximal veins. Its sensitivity for detecting infrapopliteal venous clots in surveillance patients is also inferior to that reported in symptomatic patients, in whom the thrombotic process is more extensive and clots are less likely to be isolated to the calf veins (see Tables 95-4 and 95-8). Consequently, a number of investigators have restricted venous surveys to the femoropopliteal segment, purposely neglecting the tibioperoneal veins. As a result, the sensitivity for detecting thrombi in the limb as a whole suffers (Table 95-8). For example, in the series of patients studied by Barnes et al,[7] clots were isolated to the calf veins in 17 (59%) of 29 limbs in which thrombi were demonstrated phlebographically. Because only proximal veins were studied, the sensitivity for the limb as a whole was only 34%. Similarly, isolated calf vein thrombi were found in only 8 (30%) of 27 phlebographically positive limbs in Woolsen's series.[76] Again, failure to study the infrapopliteal veins reduced the "total limb" sensitivity to 63%.

Results from color duplex scanning in the postoperative surveillance of 190 limbs of 99 patients who underwent total joint arthroplasty are detailed in Table 95-9.[34] This appears to be the only published report concerning the use of color duplex imaging for surveillance purposes. In this series, 93% of the clots were confined to below-knee veins and 89% were nonoccluding. Initially, the low sensitivity (25%) for detecting clots in the limb as a whole was discouraging,[65] but in the later half of the study, as the technologists became more skillful, the interpreters gained experience, and the instrumentation was improved to include slow-flow capabilities, the sensitivity rose to 79%. In the last 50 patients, 78% of the tibioperoneal clots were detected. This improvement in sensitivity occurred without sacrificing specificity, which remained high (greater than 96%) throughout the study. "Total limb" positive and negative predictive values rose from an initial low of about 84% to 90% or better in the last group of patients. A comparison of the data in Tables 95-8 and 95-9 suggests that the use of color confers an advantage in surveys of below-knee veins in postarthroplasty patients. Because of the paucity of above-knee thrombi in this series, little can be said concerning the accuracy of color duplex in this area, but there is no reason to suspect that the addition of color would be detrimental.

Sources of error

Inexperience on the part of the technologist or interpreter is undoubtedly a major source of error, and the results with the surveillance studies (Table 95-9) bear this out.[34] The improvement seen in the latter half of the study was in part due to learning from the errors committed in the first half. Even though some investigators assume that duplex or B-mode images are self-substantiating, there is no substitute for comparing ultrasound findings with the results of a well-performed phlebogram.

Table 95-9. Accuracy of color-coded duplex imaging for diagnosing asymptomatic high-risk patients undergoing surveillance for DVT after total hip or knee arthroplasty*

Anatomic site	Sensitivity (%)	Specificity (%)	Positive predictive value (%)	Negative predictive value (%)	Overall accuracy (%)
TOTAL GROUP (n = 190 limbs)					
Total limb	55 (24/44)	98 (143/146)	89 (24/27)	88 (143/163)	88 (167/190)
Above knee	67 (2/3)	100 (187/187)	100 (2/2)	99 (187/188)	99 (189/190)
Common femoral	0 (0/1)	100 (189/189)	—	99 (189/190)	99 (189/190)
Superficial femoral	67 (2/3)	100 (187/187)	100 (2/2)	99 (189/190)	99 (189/190)
Below knee	56 (24/43)	98 (144/147)	89 (24/27)	88 (144/163)	88 (168/190)
Popliteal	33 (3/9)	99 (180/181)	75 (3/4)	97 (180/186)	96 (183/190)
Tibioperoneal	56 (23/41)	97 (145/149)	85 (23/27)	89 (145/163)	88 (168/190)
FIRST 49 PATIENTS (n = 98 limbs)					
Total limb	25 (5/20)	99 (77/78)	83 (5/6)	84 (77/92)	84 (82/98)
Above knee	0 (0/1)	100 (97/97)	—	99 (97/98)	99 (97/98)
Below knee	26 (5/19)	99 (78/79)	83 (5/6)	85 (78/92)	85 (83/98)
Tibioperoneal	28 (5/18)	99 (79/80)	83 (5/6)	86 (79/92)	86 (84/98)
SECOND 50 PATIENTS (n = 92 limbs)					
Total limb	79 (19/24)	97 (66/68)	90 (19/21)	93 (66/71)	92 (85/92)
Above knee	100 (2/2)	100 (90/90)	100 (2/2)	100 (90/90)	100 (92/92)
Below knee	79 (19/24)	97 (66/68)	90 (19/21)	93 (66/71)	92 (85/92)
Tibioperoneal	78 (18/23)	96 (66/69)	86 (18/21)	93 (66/71)	91 (84/92)

Data from Mattos MA et al: *J Vasc Surg* 15:366, 1992.

The major problem areas have already been mentioned. Visualization of the deeply situated iliac veins is often impaired by overlying bowel gas. Having the patient fast overnight may diminish this impediment, but many elderly patients are chronically flatulent and any opinion regarding the patency of the iliac veins must then be based on the observations gleaned from indirect flow studies in the common femoral veins. Continuous, nonphasic flow in a patent common femoral vein, together with poor augmentation, implies obstruction of the iliac vein or vena cava. Demonstration of collateral venous channels with increased flow velocity in the groin or lower abdomen is highly suggestive of proximal venous obstruction. Fortunately, obstruction of the iliac vein often occurs in conjunction with thrombosis of the common femoral vein, thus establishing the diagnosis. Color, which facilitates imaging of the iliac veins, reduces the need to rely on indirect methods of assessment.[55]

False-positive errors have been made in pregnant patients, owing to the obstructive flow pattern produced by uterine compression and to the reduced compressibility of the common femoral vein. Turning the patient onto her side will usually resolve this problem.[29]

Another problem area is the superficial femoral vein in the adductor canal region. Not only is this segment of vein deep and difficult to visualize, it is also resistant to compression. If the vein in the adductor canal is not completely compressed, a false-positive interpretation may result. Indirect assessment of patency can be based on the pattern of blood flow in the superficial femoral vein above and the popliteal vein below. Problems may also be encountered in the upper calf where the tibial and peroneal veins join to form the popliteal vein. In this area, the large number of veins, their depth, and their complex anatomy complicate assessment. Duplication of veins in the popliteal or superficial femoral regions is a well-recognized source of false-negative errors. Obtaining cross-sectional views at frequent intervals decreases the likelihood that a parallel channel (which may contain a thrombus) will be overlooked.

As previously emphasized, evaluation of the infrapopliteal veins continues to challenge the expertise of even the most astute sonographer. Although the paired tibial and peroneal veins are usually easily traced throughout most of their length in normal limbs, it may prove difficult to exclude thrombi isolated to one of the venae comitantes. The examination is complicated by the large number of deep and relatively long veins with small diameters that carry blood at low velocities. In addition, perforating veins and the soleal and gastrocnemial sinusoids, all potential sites of venous thrombi, must be studied to avoid the risk of false-negative errors when the tibioperoneal veins are free of clots. Many clots in the infrapopliteal area are nonocclusive (especially in surveillance patients) and are often only a few centimeters long, adding to the frustration. Moreover, the results of compression studies are often difficult to interpret, especially when they are obtained from the smaller venous segments.

Finally, there are some factors beyond the control of the examiner that also determine the adequacy of the examination. Obesity, excessive edema, and collateral veins impair visualization; small veins may be difficult to locate and follow; and apprehension, pain, muscle tension, excessive motion, agitation, and combativeness on the part of the patient always hinder the process. Surgical wounds, casts, traction, and braces may interfere with access to large areas of the limb, particularly in surveillance studies, and positioning of the postarthroplasty patient to obtain optimal access to veins is frequently limited by the patient's pain or fear that movement of the limb might cause joint dislocation. When one or more of these confounding factors exist, the examiner and interpreter should note any attendant uncertainty on the final report.

CLINICAL APPLICATION

Inasmuch as the ideal test for the presence of DVT has yet to be developed, factors unique to each must be considered when deciding which to employ in a given clinical or research setting. Although accuracy is paramount, other considerations, such as ease of use, patient discomfort and safety, availability, repeatability, and expense, must be weighed against the risk of a false-positive or false-negative result. Requirements differ, depending on whether the test is to be used to diagnose acute DVT, detect clots forming after a surgical procedure, or accumulate information concerning the prevalence and natural history of venous thrombi. In many situations, duplex scanning emerges as the method of choice.

Symptomatic patients

Almost all proximal thrombi in symptomatic patients can be detected by skillfully performed duplex and color flow imaging (and also by physiologic tests such as impedance plethysmography or continuous wave Doppler surveys). Thus a positive above-knee duplex scan is sufficiently reliable to justify the institution of anticoagulant therapy (Fig. 95-12). Similarly, a negative above- and below-knee scan (especially one obtained with color imaging) effectively excludes the existence of significant DVT anywhere in the limb, allowing treatment to be withheld. Because approximately 20% to 40% of the thrombi developing in symptomatic patients are confined to the infrapopliteal veins[28,34,41,52] (70% in one series[24]), restricting the study to the above-knee veins (as is the practice in some laboratories) fails to identify an appreciable number of clots. Although these clots may be insignificant clinically (vide infra), it seems prudent, now that the technology is available, to take the extra time required to perform a complete venous survey. By doing so, the need for serial examinations of all patients with negative above-knee studies is avoided.

A problem arises, however, when the scan is negative above the knee but positive below the knee (Fig. 95-12). Unfortunately, most authors calculate the positive predictive value for below-knee thrombi based on the total number of

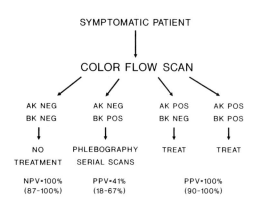

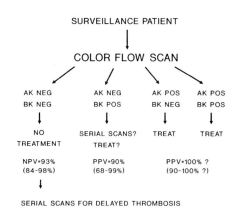

Fig. 95-12. Algorithm showing approach to the diagnosis and management of symptomatic patients with suspected DVT based on the results of color duplex scanning. Negative *(NPV)* and positive *(PPV)* predictive values and 95% confidence intervals (in parentheses) are derived from Mattos et al.[34]

Fig. 95-13. Algorithm showing approach to the diagnosis and management of DVT in asymptomatic high-risk patients after total hip or knee arthroplasty. NPV, PPV, and 95% confidence limits for the "AK NEG" scans are based on data from the last 50 surveillance patients reported by Mattos et al.[34] PPV for the "AK POS" group is estimated from other reports and from data obtained from symptomatic patients.[34]

limbs with below-knee thrombi, 80% of which are quite extensive and involve the above-knee veins as well. The positive predictive value for isolated below-knee clots is seldom clearly distinguished from that for all below-knee clots. In the initial experience of some investigators,[34,54] the color duplex diagnosis of isolated infrapopliteal thrombi was confirmed phlebographically in only about 40% of the cases. It is good practice, therefore, to recommend phlebography or serial scanning in patients whose color duplex findings above the knee are negative but positive below the knee, unless the scan is unequivocally positive. Nonetheless, routine examination of the below-knee veins, although plagued with false-positive findings, does reduce by about two-thirds the number of patients considered for serial scanning. With improvements in technology and increasing experience, it is anticipated that the incidence of false-positive studies will decrease and the number of patients requiring serial scans further lowered.

As mentioned earlier in this chapter, duplex scanning readily identifies hematomas, popliteal cysts, enlarged lymph nodes, tumor masses, and aneurysms—structures that may also cause pain and swelling or impinge on the venous lumen and be confused with acute DVT.

Surveillance of asymptomatic patients

In some early studies, color duplex scanning of asymptomatic postoperative patients suffered from a high incidence of false-negative studies.[65] Current results are much more acceptable (Table 95-9).[34,66] Provided the examination encompasses both the above- and below-knee veins and is not compromised by technical problems, a negative color duplex scan affords reasonable assurance that the limb is free of clots (negative predictive value, approximately 90%). Negative results therefore reduce the need for serial studies to detect clot propagation but do not preclude the possibility of thrombus formation in the days or weeks after

the study is completed (Fig. 95-13).[69,75] Although negative findings limited to the proximal veins effectively exclude the threat of more dangerous proximal venous thrombi, this does not rule out the existence of clots in the infrapopliteal veins. Because 30% to 90% of thrombi developing in postoperative patients are confined to the calf veins,[7,34,76] serial scanning must be considered in all high-risk patients with negative above-knee studies when the infrapopliteal veins have not been examined.

A positive duplex scan above the knee can be accepted as strong evidence for the presence of thrombus (Table 95-8), allowing appropriate treatment to be instituted without the need for other examinations (Fig. 95-13). When color duplex scans are negative above the knee but positive below the knee, the likelihood of a thrombus in the calf veins or elsewhere in the limb approaches 90%. Depending on the philosophy of the clinician, these patients can be either treated or observed with serial scans to detect any proximal propagation (Fig. 95-13).

Despite the proved capability of duplex scanning to detect or exclude thrombi in postoperative patients, the role of surveillance studies remains unclear.[10] Surveillance studies are expensive, time consuming, and labor intensive, especially when serial scans are necessary. To arrive at a conclusion, the cost of duplex scanning must be weighed against the cost and efficacy of routine perioperative prophylaxis.[45] Although the incidence of thrombi forming after abdominal operations can be appreciably reduced using prophylactic measures, this approach is not as effective after orthopedic procedures.[15] In one study of patients undergoing total joint arthroplasty, thrombi developed in 40% even though all received some form of prophylaxis.[34] Clearly, therefore, prophylaxis is not the complete answer, and perhaps the time will come when surveillance studies are accepted as part of the overall management of certain high-risk patient groups.[3]

Calf vein thrombi

One of the advantages of duplex scanning and especially color-coded duplex scanning over other noninvasive methods is its ability to identify a high percentage of calf vein thrombi. There is considerable debate, however, concerning the importance of clots confined to this area (see Chapter 93).[31,49] Is the extra effort required to survey the calf justified? Although pulmonary emboli have been reported in patients with isolated calf vein thrombi,[39] most investigators agree that significant embolization rarely occurs unless there is propagation into the popliteal or more proximal veins.[49] Retrospective reviews of untreated symptomatic patients with negative plethysmographic test results have shown that limiting the examination to above-knee veins poses little hazard, even though an appreciable number of calf vein thrombi are missed.[61,74] Serial testing of symptomatic patients whose initial above-knee findings were negative has been strongly advocated for detecting potentially dangerous propagation. Prospective follow-up studies have shown that pulmonary emboli rarely occur in patients who have run the gantlet of tests, with consistently negative results.[22,23] However, this more cautious approach requires serial testing of a large number of patients, yields few positive results (2.6% in one series[23]), and is unlikely to be cost effective. Even if the clinician elects not to treat isolated below-knee thrombi, color duplex scanning of the calf veins permits serial testing to be restricted to those patients with positive findings; patients with negative above- and below-knee findings require no further testing.

There is also some evidence that calf vein thrombi may be responsible for chronic venous insufficiency.[24,38,58,62] Thus the threat of calf vein thrombi may transcend that of their immediate embolic potential. The detection and treatment of clots isolated to this area may decrease the risk of lipodermatosclerosis and stasis ulceration.

CONCLUSION

The evidence presented in this chapter supports the conclusion that duplex scanning is the best noninvasive method for diagnosing symptomatic DVT, detecting calf vein thrombi, and monitoring the course of postoperative patients. Unlike other noninvasive techniques, duplex scanning not only establishes the diagnosis of DVT but also defines the location and extent of the clot. No other method is better adapted to natural history studies.[27,28,31,33] The addition of a color flow map has the extra advantage of facilitating the identification of veins and decreasing the time and effort required to conduct a thorough examination.[66]

REFERENCES

1. Agnelli G et al: Impedance plethysmography in the diagnosis of asymptomatic deep vein thrombosis in hip surgery: a venograph-controlled study, *Arch Intern Med* 151:2167, 1991.
2. Aitken AGF, Godden DJ: Real-time ultrasound diagnosis of deep vein thrombosis: a comparison with venography, *Clin Radiol* 38:309, 1987.
3. Anderson FA Jr: Duplex ultrasound surveillance for asymptomatic DVT, *J Vasc Technol* 15:15, 1991.
4. Appelman PT, De Jong TE, Lampmann LE: Deep venous thrombosis of the leg: US findings, *Radiology* 163:743, 1987.
5. Aronen HJ et al: Sonography in differential diagnosis of deep venous thrombosis of the leg, *Acta Radiol* 28:457, 1987.
6. Baldridge ED, Martin MA, Welling RE: Clinical significance of free-floating venous thrombi, *J Vasc Surg* 11:62, 1990.
7. Barnes RW et al: Perioperative asymptomatic venous thrombosis: role of duplex scanning versus venography, *J Vasc Surg* 9:251, 1989.
8. Becker DM, Philbrick JT, Abbitt PL: Real-time ultrasonography for the diagnosis of lower extremity deep venous thrombosis: the wave of the future? *Arch Intern Med* 149:1731, 1989.
9. Borris LC et al: Comparison of real-time B-mode ultrasonography and bilateral ascending phlebography for detection of post operative deep vein thrombosis following elective hip surgery, *Thromb Haemost* 61:363, 1989.
10. Borris LC et al: Real-time B-mode ultrasonography in the diagnosis of postoperative deep vein thrombosis in non-symptomatic high-risk patients, *Eur J Vasc Surg* 4:473, 1990.
11. Comerota AJ et al: Venous duplex imaging: should it replace hemodynamic tests for deep venous thrombosis, *J Vasc Surg* 11:53, 1990.
12. Cronan JJ, Dorfman GS, Grusmark J: Lower-extremity deep venous thrombosis: further experience with and refinements of US assessment, *Radiology* 168:101, 1988.
13. Cronan JJ et al: Deep venous thrombosis: US assessment using vein compression, *Radiology* 162:191, 1987.
14. Dauzat MM et al: Real-time B-mode ultrasonography for better specificity in the noninvasive diagnosis of deep venous thrombosis, *J Ultrasound Med* 5:625, 1986.
15. Dorfman GS: Lower-extremity venous thrombosis in patients with acute hip fractures: determination of anatomic location and time of onset with compression sonography, *AJR* 154:851, 1990.
16. Elias A et al: Value of real-time B-mode ultrasound imaging in the diagnosis of deep vein thrombosis of the lower limbs, *Inter Angio* 6:175, 1987.
17. Flanagan LD, Sullivan ED, Cranley JJ: *Venous imaging of the extremities using real-time B-mode ultrasound.* In Bergan JJ, Yao JST, eds: *Surgery of the veins,* Orlando, Fla, 1985, Grune & Stratton.
18. Fletcher JP et al: Ultrasound diagnosis of lower limb deep venous thrombosis, *Med J Aust* 153:453, 1990.
19. Foley WD et al: Color Doppler ultrasound imaging of lower-extremity venous disease, *AJR* 152:371, 1989.
20. Froehlich JA et al: Compression ultrasonography for the detection of deep venous thrombosis in patients who have a fracture of the hip: a prospective study, *J Bone Joint Surg* [Am] 71:249, 1989.
21. Ginsberg JS et al: Venous thrombosis in patients who have undergone major hip or knee surgery: detection with compression US and impedance plethysmography, *Radiology* 181:651, 1991.
22. Huisman MV et al: Serial impedance plethysmography for suspected deep venous thrombosis in outpatients: the Amsterdam General Practitioner Study, *N Engl J Med* 314:823, 1986.
23. Hull RD et al: Diagnostic efficacy of impedance plethysmography for clinically suspected deep-vein thrombosis: a randomized trial, *Ann Intern Med* 102:21, 1985.
24. Kakkar VV, Lawrence D: Hemodynamic and clinical assessment after therapy for acute deep vein thrombosis, *Am J Surg* 150(4A):54, 1985.
25. Karkow WS, Ruoff BA, Cranley JJ: *B-mode venous imaging.* In Kempczinski RE, Yao JST, eds: *Practical noninvasive diagnosis,* ed 2, Chicago, 1987, Mosby.
26. Killewich LA et al: Diagnosis of deep venous thrombosis: a prospective study comparing duplex scanning to contrast venography, *Circulation* 79:810, 1989.
27. Killewich LA et al: Spontaneous lysis of deep venous thrombi: rate and outcome, *J Vasc Surg* 9:89, 1989.
28. Krupski WC et al: Propagation of deep venous thrombosis identified by duplex ultrasonography, *J Vasc Surg* 12:467, 1990.
29. Langsfeld M et al: Real-time venous imaging in pregnancy: a case report illustrating the potential pitfalls in diagnosing deep venous thrombosis, *Bruit* 10:244, 1986.
30. Lensing AWA et al: Detection of deep-vein thrombosis by real-time B-mode ultrasonography, *N Engl J Med* 320:342, 1989.
31. Lohr JM et al: Lower extremity calf thrombosis: to treat or not to treat, *J Vasc Surg* 14:618, 1991.
32. Lund F, Diener L, Ericsson J: Postmortem interosseous phlebography as an aid in studies of venous thromboembolism, *Angiology* 20:155, 1969.

33. Mantoni M: Deep venous thrombosis: longitudinal study with duplex US, *Radiology* 179:271, 1991.

34. Mattos MA et al: Color-flow duplex scanning for the surveillance and diagnosis of acute deep venous thrombosis, *J Vasc Surg* 15:366, 1992.

35. Meibers DJ et al: B-mode scan characteristics of Baker's cysts, *J Vasc Technol* 11:125, 1987.

36. Mitchell DC et al: Comparison of duplex ultrasonography and venography in the diagnosis of deep venous thrombosis, *Br J Surg* 78:611, 1991.

37. Montefusco CM et al: *Duplex ultrasonographic venography: the definitive diagnostic tool for thrombophlebitis.* In Veith FJ, ed: *Current critical problems in vascular surgery,* St Louis, 1989, Quality Medical.

38. Moore DJ, Himmel PD, Sumner DS: Distribution of venous valvular incompetence in patients with the postphlebitic syndrome, *J Vasc Surg* 3:49, 1986.

39. Moreno-Cabral R, Kistner RL, Nordyke RA: Importance of calf vein thrombophlebitis, *Surgery* 80:735, 1976.

40. Mussurakis S et al: Compression ultrasonography as a reliable imaging monitor in deep venous thrombosis, *Surg Gynecol Obstet* 171:233, 1990.

41. Nicolaides AN, O'Connell JD: *Origin and distribution of thrombi in patients presenting with clinical venous thrombosis.* In Nicolaides AN, ed: *Thromboembolism: etiology, advances in prevention and management,* Baltimore, 1975, University Park Press.

42. Nix ML, Troillett RD: The use of color in venous duplex examination, *J Vasc Technol* 15:123, 1991.

43. Ohgi S et al: Echogenic types of venous thrombi in the common femoral vein by ultrasonic B-mode imaging, *Vasc Surg* 25:253, 1991.

44. Oliver MA: Duplex scanning in venous disease, *Bruit* 9:206, 1985.

45. Paiement GD, Wessinger JJ, Harris WH: Cost-effectiveness of prophylaxis in total hip replacement, *Am J Surg* 161:519, 1991.

46. Patterson RB et al: The limitations of impedance plethysmography in the diagnosis of acute deep venous thrombosis, *J Vasc Surg* 9:725, 1989.

47. Persson AV et al: Use of triplex scanner in diagnosis of deep venous thrombosis, *Arch Surg* 124:593, 1989.

48. Peter DJ, Flanagan LD, Cranley JJ: Analysis of blood clot echogenicity, *J Clin Ultrasound* 14:111, 1986.

49. Philbrick JT, Becker DM: Calf deep venous thrombosis: a wolf in sheep's clothing? *Arch Intern Med* 148:2131, 1988.

50. Polak JF, Culter SS, O'Leary DH: Deep veins of the calf: assessment with color Doppler flow imaging, *Radiology* 171:481, 1989.

51. Raghavendra BN et al: Deep venous thrombosis: detection by probe compression of veins, *J Ultrasound Med* 5:89, 1986.

52. Rollins DL et al: Origin of deep vein thrombosis in an ambulatory population, *Am J Surg* 156:122, 1988.

53. Rollins DL et al: Progress in the diagnosis of deep venous thrombosis: the efficacy of real-time B-mode ultrasonic scanning, *J Vasc Surg* 7:638, 1988.

54. Rose SC et al: Symptomatic lower extremity deep venous thrombosis: accuracy, limitations, and role of color duplex flow imaging in diagnosis, *Radiology* 175:639, 1990.

55. Sarpa MS et al: Reliability of venous duplex scanning to image the iliac veins and to diagnose iliac vein thrombosis in patients suspected of having acute deep venous thrombosis, *J Vasc Technol* 15:299, 1991.

56. Sauerbrei E et al: Observer variation in lower limb venography, *J Can Assoc Radiol* 31:28, 1981.

57. Schindler JM et al: Colour coded duplex sonography in suspected deep vein thrombosis of the leg, *Br Med J* 301:1369, 1990.

58. Schulman S et al: Long-term sequelae of calf vein thrombosis treated with heparin or low-dose streptokinase, *Acta Med Scand* 219:349, 1986.

59. Semrow CM et al: The efficacy of ultrasonic venography in the detection of calf vein thrombosis, *J Vasc Technol* 12:240, 1988.

60. Sigel B et al: Red cell aggregation as a cause of blood flow echogenicity, *Radiology* 148:799, 1983.

61. Stallworth JM, Plonk GW Jr, Horne JB: Negative phleborheography: clinical follow-up in 593 patients, *Arch Surg* 116:795, 1981.

62. Strandness DE et al: Long-term sequelae of acute venous thrombosis, *JAMA* 250:1289, 1983.

63. Sumner DS: *Diagnosis of venous thrombosis by Doppler ultrasound.* In Bergan JJ, Yao JST, eds: *Venous problems,* Chicago, 1978, Mosby.

64. Sumner DS: *Diagnosis of deep venous thrombosis.* In Rutherford RB, ed: *Vascular surgery,* ed 3, Philadelphia, 1989, Saunders.

65. Sumner DS et al: *Study of deep venous thrombosis in high-risk patients using color flow Doppler.* In Bergan JJ, Yao JST, eds: *Venous disorders,* Philadelphia, 1991, Saunders.

66. Sumner DS et al: *Clinical application of color Doppler in venous problems.* In Yao JST, Pearce WH, eds: *Technologies in vascular surgery,* Philadelphia, 1992, Saunders.

67. Talbot SR: Use of real-time imaging in identifying deep venous obstruction: a preliminary report, *Bruit* 6:41, 1982.

68. Talbot SR: *B-mode evaluation of peripheral arteries and veins.* In Zwiebel WJ, ed: *Introduction to vascular ultrasonography,* ed 2, Orlando, Fla, 1986, Grune & Stratton.

69. Tremaine MD, Choroszy CJ, Menking SA: Deep vein thrombosis in the total hip arthroplasty patient after hospital discharge, *J Vasc Technol* 16:23, 1992.

70. van Bemmelen PS, Bedford G, Strandness DE: Visualization of calf veins by color flow imaging, *Ultrasound Med Biol* 16:15, 1990.

71. van Ramshorst B et al: Duplex scanning in the diagnosis of acute deep vein thrombosis of the lower extremity, *Eur J Vasc Surg* 5:255, 1991.

72. Vogel P et al: Deep venous thrombosis of the lower extremity: US evaluation, *Radiology* 163:747, 1987.

73. Wheeler HB, Anderson FA Jr: Diagnostic approaches for deep vein thrombosis, *Chest* 89(suppl):407, 1986.

74. Wheeler HB et al: Suspected deep vein thrombosis: management by impedance plethysmography, *Arch Surg* 117:1206, 1982.

75. White RH et al: Deep-vein thrombosis after fracture of the pelvis: assessment with serial duplex-ultrasound screening, *J Bone Joint Surg* [Am] 72:495, 1990.

76. Woolson ST et al: B-mode ultrasound scanning in the detection of proximal venous thrombosis after total hip replacement, *J Bone Joint Surg* [Am] 72:983, 1990.

77. Wright DJ et al: Pitfalls in lower extremity venous duplex scanning, *J Vasc Surg* 11:675, 1990.

CHAPTER 96

Diagnosis of deep vein thrombosis by phleborheography

JOHN J. CRANLEY

In collaboration with Larry D. Flanagan, M.D., and Eugene D. Sullivan, M.D.*

Phleborheography is a plethysmographic technique originally introduced for the noninvasive diagnosis of deep vein thrombosis (DVT) of the lower extremities.[5-14] It consists of tracing of flowing currents within veins. The original concepts of the nature of DVT and phleborheographic instrumentation have been confirmed, modified, and broadened in the years since the modality was introduced. The understanding of venous blood flow was altered by the realization that blood flow may be substantially arrested by the extended knee, the flexed thigh, the gravid uterus, bulky movable tumors, and the position of the extremities and torso. From the beginning, it was recognized that the method could not detect clots outside the mainstream (e.g., in the saphenous veins, the soleal veins, the deep femoral vein, the hypogastric veins). This limitation did not prove to be the drawback that was anticipated because there is evidence that thrombi in the soleal or tibial veins frequently do not become major thrombi and that most lethal emboli are large or the type that would occlude an entire segment of the femoral vein or the iliac system. Furthermore, it is probable that most small emboli are lysed in the lung without clinical sequelae.

The original phleborheograph was designed for the detection of DVT of the lower extremity and was a simplified version of the standard research polygraph. Now many of the features of the standard polygraph have been incorporated into the equipment, making it virtually a minipolygraph and allowing its application beyond the detection of obstruction in the deep veins of the extremities. The current model is useful not only for the analysis of venous physiology, but also for the study of other physiologic variables. This model may be used as a recorder for analysis of arterial pulse waves in the extremities and for assessing the colonic circulation in the rectum. In addition, it can be used along with other input signals, such as the photoelectric cell, various strain gauges, the Doppler ultrasound flow detector, and the electrocardiograph.

Phleborheography was the mainstay of noninvasive diagnosis of DVT in Good Samaritan Hospital in Cincinnati, Ohio, for 10 years (approximately 30,000 limbs tested) until it was replaced by duplex scanning. It is still used in an affiliated clinic located in a rural community and in other units that do not have access to scanning techniques. It has successfully detected acute mainstream thrombi from the popliteal vein to the vena cava, and the decision to hospitalize for treatment has been influenced by the results of this test.

PRINCIPLES
Reduction of respiratory waves in deep venous thrombosis

Normal breathing produces a rhythmic increase and decrease in the volume of the lower extremity, which is transmitted to the phleborheograph and recorded as an oscillation on the tracing that is synchronous with the wave produced by a recording cuff placed around the chest. Called *respiratory waves,* these oscillations are present in all normal extremities. Acute DVT obliterates or significantly reduces the size of the respiratory waves. With the development of collateral circulation, waves that have been absent usually reappear, and those that have been smaller become larger. The change is noticeable in approximately 2 weeks. However, although these respiratory waves are now present or have become larger, they may differ from normal waves in being relatively small and more rounded. In a patient with femoroiliac thrombophlebitis, the respiratory waves may be visible in tracings from the leg if the veins of the leg are patent, despite the absence of waves in the thigh, probably because the respiratory influence travels down the limb through the collateral veins. Respiratory waves in the lower extremity are usually larger in amplitude when the patient lies on the left side than when the patient is supine. This is thought to be a result of moving the weight of the intraabdominal viscera from the inferior vena cava and the iliac veins. Occasionally, however, the respiratory waves are larger when the patient lies on the right rather than the left side. There is no explanation for this phenomenon.

---

*Good Samaritan Hospital, Cincinnati, Ohio.

Interference with blood outflow from the extremity

DVT interferes with the normal outflow of blood from the extremity in response to rhythmic compression. Similar to the active muscle contraction that occurs on walking, intermittent compression of the extremity propels blood proximally. A recording cuff proximal to the site of compression detects the momentary damming up of blood when venous thrombosis or extraluminal compression blocks its exit. Indicative of the blockage, there is a rise in baseline of the volume recorder. However, if compression is applied to the normal extremity when there is no impediment to venous outflow, the baseline remains level. This phenomenon localizes the site of thrombosis. If the thigh tracing shows a stepwise rise while the calf is being compressed, the level of obstruction to the deep veins is located above the thigh cuff. Rarely, external compression is to blame; generally, intraluminal thrombosis is present.

Similarly, if there is obstruction at or above the recording cuffs, compression of the foot causes a rise in the baseline of the phleborheographic tracings from the leg, which is unequivocal evidence of venous obstruction.

Compression of the calf

Compression of the calf has two effects: blood is propelled up the unobstructed extremity, and blood is siphoned out of the normal foot. When the calf is compressed, a recording cuff on the foot shows a fall in the baseline. Absent or less than normal foot emptying in the presence

of a rise in the baseline and absent respiratory waves are indicative of acute DVT. More susceptible to artifacts than other maneuvers, this procedure nevertheless permits detection of a normal tracing at a glance.

TECHNIQUE

The patient lies quietly in bed with the lower extremities placed approximately 10° below the heart level. The first four cuffs of the phleborheograph are used for recording purposes only. Cuff 1 is placed around the thorax, cuff 2 at the midthigh, cuffs 3, 4, and 5 at the upper calf in close approximation to each other, and cuff 6 on the foot. Cuffs 5 and 6 are used to both record transmitted impulses and apply compression (Fig. 96-1). There are three operational modes, run A, run B_1, and run B_2. In run A, all cuffs on the thigh and leg record the response to compression of the foot by applying pressure to the foot cuff. In run B_1, pressure is applied to the midcalf (cuff 5). All other cuffs record the response, including the cuff on the foot (cuff 6), which records changes in pedal volume. In run B_2, cuff 5 is moved to the ankle level and used to apply compression. The remaining cuffs are used for recording.

Run A: foot compression

In run A, the recording cuffs are automatically inflated to 10 mm Hg. The chart speed is 2.5 mm/sec. Calibration is performed by adjusting the amplification so that the 0.2-ml volume calibrator causes a 2-cm pen deflection. Res-

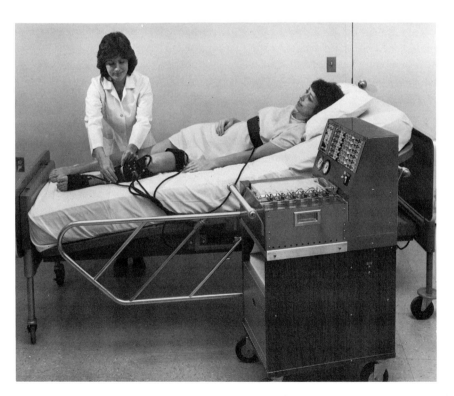

Fig. 96-1. In preparation for phleborheography of the lower extremities, the patient lies quietly with the legs below heart level and six cuffs applied.

piratory waves are observed first. Following this, the compress control is operated and three short bursts of 100 mm Hg each are delivered to the foot cuff (cuff 6); these are 0.5 second in duration and delivered at 0.5-second intervals. About 40% of the pressure is expended in inflating the cuff, so only about 60 mm Hg of pressure is actually exerted on the foot.

Although the recording pen may move erratically with the application of pressure, the baseline remains level in a normal extremity (Fig. 96-2). If there is interference with the outflow of blood from the extremity, the baseline rises with each successive compression as the extremity swells. Time is allowed for venous refilling of the lower leg to occur before the next compression. This usually takes 20 seconds. This maneuver is repeated at least three times, but if there is any interference with the tracing, pressure may be applied as often as necessary.

If the respiratory waves appear to be smaller than usual, the patient is turned on the left side with both knees slightly flexed and the right leg lying behind the left. This maneuver increases the size of the respiratory waves; however, in a patient with acute DVT, changing the position usually does not restore the obliterated waves. If the baseline continues to show a rise with each compression or if the respiratory waves remain smaller than usual, minor positional changes may be tried in an attempt to minimize the effect of compressions on the respiratory waves. Prone or near-prone positions should not be used because these positions tend to

produce a normal tracing in the presence of deep vein obstruction for reasons that are unclear.

Run B_1: calf compression

In run B_1, the recording cuff on the lower part of the calf becomes a compression cuff (cuff 5) and the cuff on the foot (cuff 6) is converted to a recording cuff. In this run, operating the compress control automatically causes 50 mm Hg of pressure to compress the cuff on the calf three times, similar to compression of the foot in run A. Again, about 40% of this pressure is expended in inflating the cuff, so only about 30 mm Hg is actually exerted on the calf.

Emptying of the foot is observed. This decrease in volume of the foot is demonstrated in the tracing (cuff 6) by a fall in baseline. This test is repeated at least three times. Time must be allowed for the pen to return to its baseline before the next application of pressure. In a fully normal extremity, the pen baseline falls at least 3 cm, corresponding to a 0.3-ml volume change under the cuff, the dimensions of which are 9×17 cm. The return to baseline is gradual rather than abrupt.

As the lower part of the calf is compressed, the recording from the midcalf normally falls somewhat, mimicking the fall in the baseline of the foot. This is thought to be an artifact caused by the proximity of cuffs 4 and 5. Meanwhile, the baseline of the tracing from the upper part of the calf and lower part of the thigh remains level. However, if any obstruction to the deep venous system exists above the

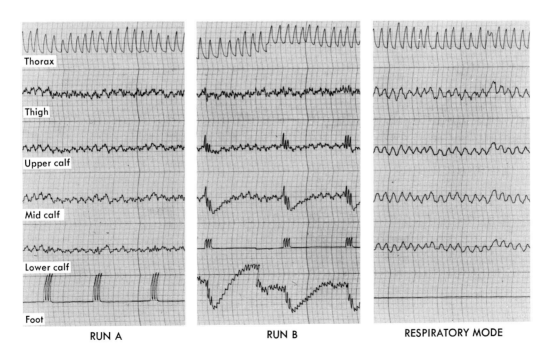

Fig. 96-2. Normal tracing. There are good respiratory waves throughout run A (foot cuff used as a compression cuff) and run B (lower calf cuff used as a compression cuff). Note the absence of a baseline shift when either the foot or lower cuff is compressed. Note also the good foot emptying in run B. The respiratory mode shows good respiratory waves after the arterial pulses have been filtered.

recording cuff, a rise in the baseline occurs that is progressive with each compression. In the presence of extensive thrombophlebitis, this may be a sharp, abrupt rise; on the other hand, a stepwise rise of greater than 1 mm is significant (Fig. 96-3).

Run B_2: ankle compression

In run B_2, the midcalf cuff (cuff 5) is moved to the ankle level and is used to deliver compressions. Cuffs 1 through 4 and cuff 6 are used for recording as in run B_1. Compressions are identical to those used in run B_1 with regard to timing, duration, and pressure.

Once again, emptying of the foot is observed, as in run B_1. Unlike run B_1, however, the midcalf recording does not usually fall. The baseline of this recording cuff and the others remains level. If there is obstruction to venous outflow, a rise in baseline occurs. In addition, foot emptying may be reduced or absent.

Interpretation

Interpretation of the tracing is based on the physiologic principles previously described. Strict adherence to criteria derived from over 27,000 phleborheograms (PRGs) and 748 phlebographic correlations is required.

In tracings of the lower extremities, it is necessary to obtain nine normal compressions, three each in run A, run B_1, and run B_2. Each set of three must be obtained without changing the position of the patient; however, sets need not be consecutive. The positions used for runs A, B_1, and B_2 may differ. Only three normal compressions are required in the upper extremity, all obtained in the same position.

The characteristics of a normal compression have been precisely outlined.[5] They include the following: (1) a normal respiratory wave amplitude averaging 50% or more of the amplitude of waves in the opposite extremity, (2) no absolute baseline rise, and (3) no dynamic baseline rise with compression. The absolute baseline is a plot of points connecting the minimum volume of each respiratory wave. The dynamic baseline is a plot of points representing the normal volume of the extremity expected at any point in the respiratory cycle. A rise greater than 1 mm in either the absolute or dynamic baseline is considered significant. Fig. 96-4 portrays tracings that illustrate abnormalities in these parameters.

Baseline evaluation and respiratory waves are considered major criteria and must be normal, as defined, for a compression to be considered normal. The minor criteria of pulsatility and foot emptying are less important. Pulsatility refers to the amplitude of the superimposed arterial waves that are seen in the respiratory waves of every tracing. When compared to the opposite leg, increased pulsatility suggests the presence of either deep vein obstruction (usually acute) or a popliteal arterial aneurysm. Bilateral increased pulsatility may be seen in patients with congestive heart failure and tricuspid insufficiency. Foot emptying has already been described. Abnormal foot emptying and increased pulsatility

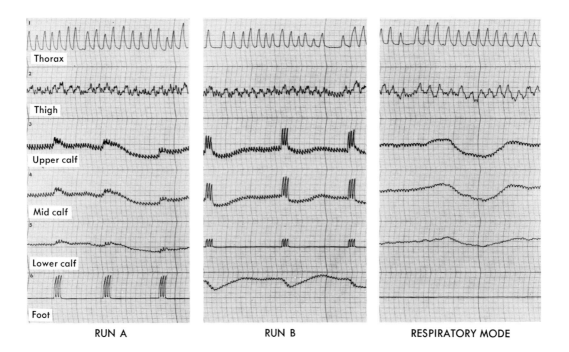

Thorax

Thigh

Upper calf

Mid calf

Lower calf

Foot

RUN A   RUN B   RESPIRATORY MODE

Fig. 96-3. Acute popliteal thrombosis. Note the normal respiratory waves and the absence of any baseline rise in the thigh; however, there is obliteration of the respiratory waves in the calf and baseline evaluation secondary to the foot (run A) and calf (run B) compression, indicating deep venous obstruction. Note the total absence of respiratory waves distal to the thigh on the respiratory mode trace, indicating deep venous obstruction at the popliteal level.

are merely suggestive, however, and not diagnostic of deep vein obstruction. Their major usefulness is to clarify an equivocal tracing.

Further consideration of a particular tracing may allow a diagnosis of acute versus chronic or complete versus partial obstruction. For example, a persistent baseline rise (dynamic or absolute) coupled with absent respiratory waves suggests acute complete obstruction. A baseline rise with near-normal respiratory waves suggests partial acute obstruction or complete obstruction with recanalization or collateralization (chronic versus early acute) (Fig. 96-5). The level of obstruction can frequently be ascertained by careful scrutiny of the changes occurring in each cuff with compression.

Serial tracings can show the gradual transition from acute occlusion to the chronic state or to dissolution of the thrombi. Caution and clinical judgment must be used in diagnosing the chronic process. For example, a tracing will show obstruction and large respiratory waves, indicating excellent collateral circulation, the day after ligation of the femoral vein (not for venous thrombosis). Thus the test reflects the actual state (i.e., obstruction and good collateral circulation), although it is obviously not long term. Another pitfall is a thrombus that only partially occludes a small segment of a vein, such as the popliteal or femoral, and that may cause the test to show a rise in baseline but with normal respiratory waves. Instead of a chronic occlusion, this connotes an early acute lesion. When the test is repeated

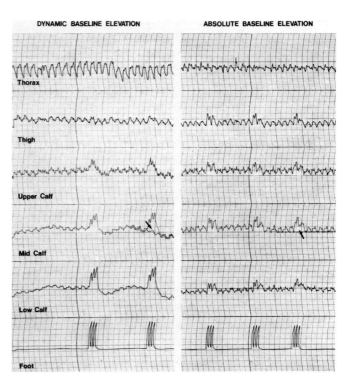

Fig. 96-4. Abnormality of a dynamic baseline rise and an absolute baseline rise.

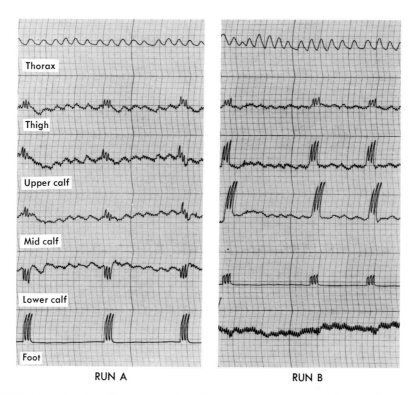

RUN A   RUN B

Fig. 96-5. A baseline rise with near normal respiratory waves suggests a partial acute obstruction with recanalization or collateralization (chronic versus early acute).

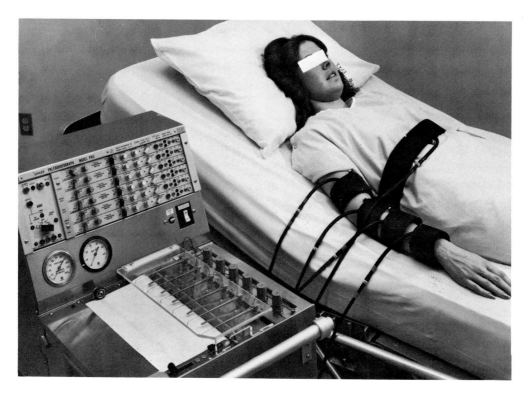

Fig. 96-6. A modified technique for upper extremity diagnosis showing the recording cuffs around the thorax, upper arm, and middle and lower forearm with the compression cuff on the wrist.

in a day or two, respiratory waves may be absent. In other words, the partially occluding thrombus has now propagated.

UPPER EXTREMITY TECHNIQUE

Certain modifications are necessary for carrying out the upper extremity technique.[18] Recording cuffs are placed around the thorax, upper arm, and upper and middle forearm, along with a compression cuff on the wrist (Fig. 96-6). The mode selector is turned to run B and the wrist cuff is rapidly inflated to 50 mm Hg, producing compressions that pump the blood proximally. The proximal arm cuffs record any changes in volume that occur at rest or in response to these volume challenges. In the upper extremity, respiratory waves can persist despite complete venous occlusion, probably because of the rich venous collaterals around the shoulder. Therefore a diagnosis of upper extremity deep vein occlusion is usually based on the presence of a baseline rise alone.[15] However, one study has shown two tracings interpreted as normal that exhibited a 50% decrease in respiratory wave amplitude compared to the opposite side and that had no baseline rise, yet phlebography showed a clot in the deep vein system in these patients.

RESULTS

Results are shown in Table 96-1. To assess the efficacy of the method, a subgroup of 748 lower extremities with phle-

Table 96-1. Phlebographic–phleborheographic correlations: 748 lower extremities

False negatives	
Equivocal	2/290 (0.7%)
Interpretive error	7/290 (2.4%)
True miss	15/290 (5.2%)
TOTAL	24/290 (8.3%)
False positives	
Equivocal	3/458 (0.7%)
Technical error	5/458 (1.1%)
Interpretive error	4/458 (0.9%)
True miss	11/458 (2.4%)
TOTAL	23/458 (5%)

bographic confirmation was studied. An equivocal tracing is usually resolved by repeating the tracing in 24 hours. At times, vein imaging using the B-mode scanner makes it possible to confirm to refute the phleborheographic findings immediately. Errors in interpretation have been determined by a review of the tracing after a phlebogram has been obtained. The technical errors have been almost completely eliminated. The percentage of inherent false negatives has remained at approximately 5% throughout the period of the instrument's availability. These false negatives have usually stemmed from small clots below the knee. In a group of 60

Table 96-2. Phlebographic–phleborheographic correlations: 25 upper extremities

False negatives	
Equivocal	0/10
Interpretive error	0/10
True miss	2/10 (20%)
TOTAL	2/10 (20%)
False positives	
Equivocal	0/15
Technical error	0/15
Interpretive error	0/15
True miss	1/15 (7%)
TOTAL	1/15 (7%)

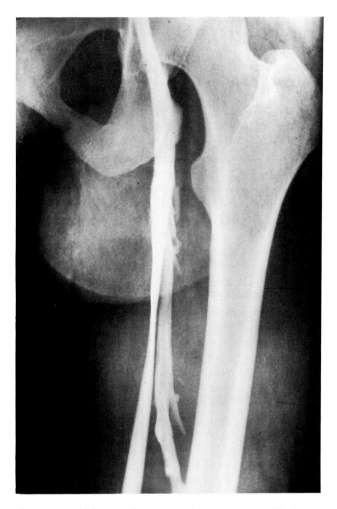

Fig. 96-7. A phlebogram showing significant narrowing of the lumen of the femoral vein in the thigh of a young patient with a positive PRG with normal respiratory waves. PRG accurately showed an obstruction to blood flow.

patients with clots limited to the infrapopliteal area, 15 (25%) false-negative results have occurred.

False positives are more difficult to explain; thus studying these patients has augmented knowledge of venous physiology. Results of upper extremity studies are shown in Table 96-2.

Venous compression

Extrinsic compression of a vein obstructs the flow of venous blood and is indicated by a rise in baseline. This is particularly true of the extended rise.[1] The laboratory at Good Samaritan Hospital has noted 10 patients with venous compression without DVT. Inclusion of these cases as errors is debatable, inasmuch as the test did detect the true status, namely, obstruction of venous blood flow.

In addition to the previously mentioned physiologic obstruction of venous blood flow, false-positive tracings were re-encountered in several young, nervous, otherwise healthy individuals. Almost invariably, the false-positive tracing becomes normal after the administration of a sedative or on repeat testing. Recently, the laboratory has seen two phlebograms from young patients with a positive PRG that showed quite obvious narrowing of the femoral vein in the thigh, causing what appeared to be a significant constriction of the lumen (Fig. 96-7). This phenomenon cannot be explained, but is reemphasizes the accuracy of the PRG showing abnormal respiratory waves, indicating obstruction to the flow of blood. It also stresses the difficulty of judging whether this is a false-positive tracing.

Results of other investigators

The findings from the published reports of other investigators are shown in Table 96-3. At first glance, Bynum et al[2] appear to be reporting a negative experience. However, analysis of their data[8] shows that in 6 (54%) of the 11 extremities with clots below the knee, the thrombi were in the veins of the soleus-gastrocnemius muscles. In only one of these six "errors" was the clot in a named vein below the knee, which is actually a false-negative result. In earlier publications, it has been emphasized that phleborheography

cannot detect clots that are not in the mainstream, thus excluding thrombi in veins of the soleus muscle and in the deep femoral, hypogastric, and saphenous veins. Therefore the data from Bynum et al have been adjusted in the totals.

Of the four false-negative results in the femoropopliteal system, three occurred in patients with duplications of the popliteal vein. This has been the observation of others, most often in patients with chronic venous disease. Interestingly, for one of three patients in the study of Bynum et al who had thrombosis in one of the duplicated veins, the test result was positive. The fourth patient in their series with thrombi in the venous mainstream not detected by the test had Cheyne-Stokes respiration. This is a recognized source of error, a fact stressed in earlier publications. Usually if respiratory waves are present when the patient is actually breathing, the major venous trunks are probably not completely occluded.

Table 96-3. Phlebographic–phleborheographic correlations of the lower extremities

Investigator	No. of extremities	False negatives		Sensitivity		False positives		Specificity		Overall accuracy	
Sull[17] (1978)	24	1/10	(10%)	9/10	(90%)	0/14	(0%)	14/14	(100%)	23/24	(96%)
Collins et al[4] (1979)	64	0/41	(0%)	41/41	(100%)	3/23	(13%)	19/23	(83%)	61/64	(95%)
Bynum et al[2] (1978)	59	11/35	(31%)	24/35	(69%)	0/24	(0%)	24/24	(100%)	35/59	(59%)*
Data adjusted (see text)	59	4/28	(14%)	24/28	(86%)	0/24	(0%)	24/24	(100%)	48/59	(81%)
Elliott et al[15] (1980)	216	6/41	(15%)	35/41	(85%)	24/175	(14%)	151/175	(86%)	192/216	(89%)
Stallworth et al[16] (1981)	39	1/13	(8%)	12/13	(92%)	1/24	(4.6%)	23/24	(96%)	35/39	(89.7%)
Classen et al[3] (1982)	90	4/24	(17%)	20/24	(83%)	2/66	(97%)	64/66	(97%)	84/90	(93%)
Cranley et al (1983)	748	24/290	(8.3%)	266/290	(92%)	23/458	(5.1%)	435/458	(93%)	701/748	(94%)
TOTALS	1240	40/447	(9%)	407/447	(91%)	53/784	(6.6%)	730/784	(93%)	1144/1240	(92%)

*Data include thrombi not detectable by this technique.

DISCUSSION

Phleborheography is noninvasive and painless and involves physiologic principles. Most patients can be examined in 30 to 45 minutes, although studies in acutely ill, disabled, or less cooperative patients may take longer. Interpretation must be learned by each physician, and the principles previously outlined must be applied.

Nonocclusive thrombi

A thrombus that is attached to a vein wall but does not actually, or at least nearly, obstruct the flow of blood is not detected by phleborheography. As the clot occludes more venous flow, there may be a slight rise in the baseline, but respiratory waves are still present. When the clot totally occludes the vein, the respiratory waves disappear. A thrombus attached to the vein wall over which blood continues to flow will usually lyse.

Acute and chronic deep vein thrombosis

An area of acute DVT may develop in an extremity with the postphlebitic syndrome. This new episode, when superimposed on chronic disease, poses some difficulties in diagnosis in the early stage. In the postphlebitic limb, the respiratory waves are so large that even when reduced as a result of obstruction by fresh thrombus they may still appear to be within normal limits. An exacerbation of existing symptoms or the onset of new ones in such a chronically insufficient limb may be indicative of acute thrombosis, and the physician should follow the patient's clinical course.

CHRONIC OCCLUSION OF MAJOR VEINS

A negative tracing in a patient with an acute obstruction of the popliteal or femoral vein has not been encountered; however, tracings from limbs with chronic occlusion of these vessels have been negative at times. Chronicity can be detected radiologically by the presence of a large number of collateral veins around the obstruction, by clot retraction, or by irregularity (tree-barking) of the walls of the veins. Occasionally the patient's clinical history will also indicate a chronic occlusion.

PULMONARY EMBOLISM FOLLOWING A NEGATIVE PRG

Four instances of a pulmonary embolism arising after a negative PRG have been observed and four other cases have been reported. In five, the interval between the negative phleborheogram and the pulmonary embolism ranged between 8 and 12 days. It was 6 days in two patients. In one instance, reported in 1991, it was 2 days. This was a postpartum patient who was taking hormones to relieve breast engorgement and who had been on heparin that was abruptly discontinued. It is believed that DVT may propagate rapidly at times, which it did in this instance.

There is a 25% rate of false-negative PRGs in patients with clots limited to veins below the knee. Usually such thrombi are small and probably do not propagate, but they can potentially progress to involve the popliteal vein and then become lethal. Accordingly, there may be a policy of deferring diagnosis whenever the PRG is normal in a patient with a tender calf; instead repeat tests are obtained at 2-day intervals until the clinical symptoms clear or the findings become positive, indicating that propagation to the popliteal area has taken place. In this event, treatment for DVT is initiated.

A small occlusive acute clot, which is a potential source of later pulmonary embolism, may be interpreted as a "chronic occlusion." The terms *acute* and *chronic* are clinical judgments. The PRG is merely capable of recording the presence or absence of obstruction and either large or small respiratory waves. Usually an obstruction in the absence of collateral circulation represents an acute obstruction, and the presence of large respiratory waves connotes a chronic obstruction. However, as already pointed out, the day after a femoral vein ligation (not for venous thrombosis), a PRG tracing in that patient will indicate obstruction with normal respiratory waves. This could be interpreted as "chronic occlusion" if the clinical history were not known. Similarly, a small clot occluding a very short segment of the femoral or iliac vein might be interpreted as chronic occlusion, with the tracing showing a rising baseline combined with large respiratory waves. For this reason, tracings are now reported as either normal or abnormal. If they are abnormal because of a rise in baseline and the absence of respiratory waves, this is interpreted as indicative of typical acute DVT. A rise in baseline and normal-appearing or larger than normal respiratory waves are interpreted as abnormal, consistent with early acute or chronic disease. If the symptoms are acute, the patient should be followed with repeat tests at 2- to 3-day intervals.

Finally, retrospective analysis has shown that some patients have the pulmonary embolus before the PRG is obtained. If a large clot breaks off totally, leaving an empty vein behind, the PRG would be normal. This problem has not been solved. However, proved clots in the lung may occur in the patient whose phlebogram shows a patent venous tree from the ankles to the vena cava.

SOURCES OF ERROR IN INTERPRETATION

Most false-positive test findings are probably a result of temporary physiologic obstruction of the venous tree. Many normal patients have a segment of their tracing that appears to be positive; then, simply by having them flex the knee or straighten the thigh or shifting them from one side to the other, the tracing becomes totally normal. This has been demonstrated by phlebography.[1] At first it was difficult to believe this could be true, but the frequency of such occurrences plus the occasional patient in whom it was possible to document these facts has confirmed the existence of this physiologic phenomenon.

Other difficulties in the statistical analysis of the accuracy of these tests stem from the fact that phlebography, the diagnostic standard, is frequently incomplete or subject to error. The likelihood of obtaining 100 consecutive excellent phlebograms is virtually impossible. However, this is a requirement if it is to be used as a standard. The most common drawback is that the pelvic veins are not visualized. Classen, Richardson, and Koontz[3] reported two false-positive tracings in the same patient. Visualization of the iliac veins was not obtained and possible filling defects were thus noted. Bi-plane films are at times essential for accurate interpretation because the presence or absence of clots in the veins below the knee is frequently subject to contrary interpretations by different radiologists. Skill and experience in reading the PRG tracings are important.

EQUIPMENT

Calibration of the phleborheograph is performed by removing precisely 0.2 cc of air from each cuff. Thus the actual size of the respiratory waves can be compared from day to day in the same patient or from patient to patient. Since it is basically an amplifier and direct-writing recorder that uses a low-pressure transducer, the equipment is highly versatile. (For further uses of the phleborheograph refer to Chapter 23.)

The single greatest problem in the development of this system is that the technique is new and must be learned. Interpretation of the tracing is not always easy. In most instances, however, a physician can learn to interpret the tracings accurately within approximately 5 days of study. The test is technologist sensitive, and thus the technologist must be highly trained, which usually requires 3 weeks. The technologist learns to recognize abnormal patterns and then maneuver the patient to various positions to see if the tracing reverts to normal. If it does, it is considered normal. On the other hand, if the tracing is positive, this means it is impossible to make it become normal by any maneuvering of the patient's position. The most common artifact encountered is compression of the popliteal vein by the extended knee, as previously discussed.[1] Similarly, flexing the thigh in some patients may obstruct the femoral vein in the inguinal area. In young athletic adults, compression of the veins by a muscle mass may result in a false-positive tracing. Many times, there is no explanation for compression of the veins in a particular position. When the test result appears to be positive, the technologist turns the patient first on the left side; if the result remains abnormal, the patient is turned on the right side. Occasionally, a positive PRG then becomes normal. The reason for this phenomenon is not known, but it is likely that the transmission is an accurate reflection of the physiologic status of the venous tree at the moment of recording and that the PRG is revealing some previously unrecognized physiologic state. The technologist must be aware of these hemodynamic vagaries.

Phleborheography has provided physicians with a highly practical, useful modality for detecting DVT, which has great value in the clinical setting. A negative PRG in a patient with a hugely swollen lower extremity indicates that the swelling is not caused by DVT. There is no exception to this. The patient with a positive PRG with or without clinical symptoms is admitted to the hospital for anticoagulant therapy. The patient with calf tenderness whose PRG is negative is instructed to return for a repeat test in 2 or 3 days if the clinical symptoms persist.

Phleborheography's rate of successful detection is keyed to certain limitations of the physiologic transmission of hydraulic impulses. Although not perfect, it is the most accurate functional test for diagnosing acute DVT. Phleborheography has been replaced by duplex scanning, which is both functional and anatomic, in many laboratories, but it is still used in hospitals and clinics in which a duplex scanner is not available.

REFERENCES

1. Arkoff RS, Gilfillan RS, Burhenne HJ: A simple method for lower extremity phlebography: pseudoobstruction of the popliteal vein, *Radiology* 90:66, 1968.
2. Bynum LJ et al: Noninvasive diagnosis of deep venous thrombosis by phleborheography, *Ann Intern Med* 89:162, 1978.
3. Classen JN, Richardson JR, Koontz C: A three-year experience with phleborheography, *Ann Surg* 195:800, 1982.
4. Collins GJ et al: Phleborheographic diagnosis of venous obstruction, *Ann Surg* 189:25, 1979.
5. Comerota AJ et al: Phleborheography: results of a ten-year experience, *Surgery* 91:573, 1982.
6. Cranley JJ: Phleborheography, *RI Med J* 58:111, 1975.
7. Cranley JJ: *Vascular surgery*, vol 2, *Peripheral venous diseases*, Hagerstown, Md, 1975, Harper & Row.

8. Cranley JJ: Phleborheography for thrombosis, *Ann Intern Med* 89:1006, 1978 (letter to editor).
9. Cranley JJ: *Phleborheography.* In Kempczinski RF, Yao JST, eds: *Practical noninvasive vascular diagnosis,* Chicago, 1982, Mosby.
10. Cranley JJ, Canos AJ, Mahalingam K: *Noninvasive diagnosis and prophylaxis of deep venous thrombosis.* In Madden JL, Hume M, eds: *Venous thromboembolism: prevention and treatment,* New York, 1976, Appleton-Lange.
11. Cranley JJ, Canos AJ, Mahalingam K: *Diagnosis of deep venous thrombosis by phleborheography.* In Gross W et al, eds: *Symposium on venous problems in honour of Geza de Takats,* Chicago, 1977, Mosby.
12. Cranley JJ, Canos AJ, Sull WJ: Diagnosis of deep venous thrombosis: fallibility of clinical symptoms and signs, *Arch Surg* 111:34, 1976.
13. Cranley JJ et al: A plethysmographic technique for the diagnosis of deep venous thrombosis of the lower extremities, *Surg Gynecol Obstet* 136:385, 1973.
14. Cranley JJ et al: Phleborheographic technique for diagnosing deep venous thrombosis of the lower extremities, *Surg Gynecol Obstet* 141:331, 1975.
15. Elliott JP et al: Phleborheography: a correlative study with venography, *Henry Ford Hosp Med J* 28:189, 1980.
16. Stallworth JM, Plonk GW Jr, Horne JB: Negative phleborheography: clinical follow-up in 593 patients, *Arch Surg* 116:795, 1981.
17. Sull WJ: Diagnosis of thrombophlebitis in the lower extremity, *Mo Med* 75:552, 1978.
18. Sullivan ED, Reece CI, Cranley JJ: Phleborheography of the upper extremity, *Arch Surg* 118:1134, 1983.

CHAPTER 97

Diagnosis of deep vein thrombosis by strain-gauge plethysmography

DAVID S. SUMNER

Acute deep vein thrombosis (DVT) can be diagnosed by plethysmographic methods. Any of the various types of plethysmographs are suitable for this purpose, including the impedance, air-filled, water-filled, and strain-gauge varieties, and all yield essentially the same information. This chapter deals only with the strain-gauge plethysmograph, since the other modalities are discussed elsewhere in this book. The strain-gauge plethysmograph has some advantages when compared to the other methods: it is far less cumbersome than the water-filled type but approaches it in accuracy, and although it may be more difficult to use than the air-filled or impedance plethysmograph, it is more sensitive, more easily calibrated, and probably more reliable.

Basically, the tests include (1) measurement of calf volume expansion in response to a standardized venous congesting pressure and (2) measurement of the rate at which blood flows out of the leg after the congesting pressure has been released.

CALF VOLUME EXPANSION AND VENOUS OUTFLOW

Calf volume expansion and venous outflow tests are performed with the patient in a supine position. To minimize the volume of blood in the calf and to avoid obstructing the veins in the popliteal fossa, the leg is elevated well above the level of the left atrium, and the knee is slightly flexed. In practice, this position can be achieved by placing a low pillow beneath the thigh and by supporting the foot on a foam block or pillow 20 to 30 cm high. A pneumatic cuff is applied to the thigh above the knee (Fig. 97-1). To obtain optimum venous occlusion at low pressures, the bladder of this cuff should encircle the limb completely and its width should be at least 1.2 times the diameter of the limb. A contoured cuff measuring 22 × 71 cm fulfills these requirements in most cases. In addition, the tubes leading to the cuff must have a large diameter (internal diameter, 1 cm) to permit rapid inflation and deflation.[27]

Although a large reservoir of air can be used for accurate inflation and the cuff evacuated directly to the atmosphere, it is much easier to employ one of the solenoid-controlled inflation-deflation devices that are commercially available. These instruments, which can be set to deliver a given pressure almost instantly, are pressurized by a compressed air source or a pump. It is merely necessary to throw a switch to inflate the cuff and reverse the switch to deflate it.

Changes in calf volume are measured with a mercury-in-silicone strain gauge wrapped around the calf at its widest point. The length of the unstretched gauge should be about 90% of the circumference of the limb. When stretched to completely encircle the calf, the gauge should exert enough tension to secure good contact with the skin but should not compress the underlying veins. Depending on the type of gauge selected, it can be applied as a single or double strand. Although it is possible to use gauges so long that they exceed the circumference, it may be necessary to apply correction factors to obtain valid results in such cases.[19] Electrically calibrated plethysmographs[13] are commercially available and greatly simplify the calculations and procedure by eliminating the need to quantify the stretch mechanically (see Chapter 20).

Procedure

When the pneumatic cuff around the thigh is inflated to a pressure exceeding that in the underlying vein (50 to 80 mm Hg), the calf begins to expand, at first rapidly and then more slowly as the capacitance vessels are filled. After approximately 2 minutes, a new equilibrium is attained with venous outflow again equaling the arterial inflow. At this point, the venous pressure distal to the cuff equals that in the cuff (Fig. 97-2). Because of the increased capillary pressure, fluid will continue to be lost into the interstitial spaces, resulting in a slow increase in calf volume. There may also be some continued stretch relaxation of the venous walls. Therefore, a stable volume is never really reached.[24]

Calf volume expansion (sometimes called *venous volume, maximal incremental venous volume,* or *venous capacitance*) is measured by comparing the rise of the curve from the baseline with a standard stretch of the gauge (as

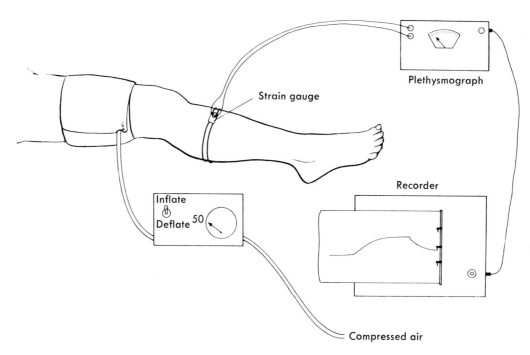

Fig. 97-1. Apparatus used for measuring calf volume expansion and venous outflow. As discussed in the text but not shown in this figure, the heel should be elevated by about 20 cm and the thigh supported on a pillow. (From Barnes RW et al: *Surgery* 72:971, 1972.)

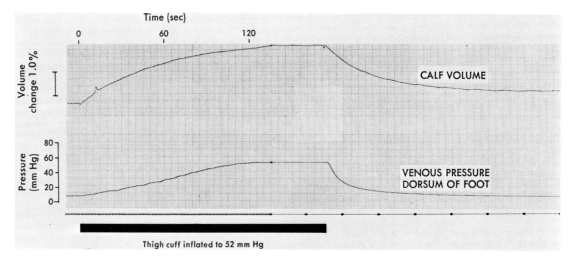

Fig. 97-2. The response of the calf volume and venous pressure to inflation of a pneumatic cuff placed around the thigh. Although the venous pressure rises to equal the pressure in the thigh cuff in about 2 minutes, the calf volume continues to increase, albeit at a much reduced rate. (From Strandness DE Jr, Sumner DS: *Hemodynamics for surgeons,* New York, 1975, Grune & Stratton.)

described in Chapter 22) or against an electrical standard that indicates a 1% rise in volume (Fig. 97-3). With the electrically calibrated device, calculations are simple:

$$\frac{\text{Div rise}}{\text{Div}/1\% \text{ vol change}} = \% \text{ Vol increase} \qquad (1)$$

where *div* indicates a division on the recording paper.

The results are expressed as a percent volume increase or as ml/100 ml of calf volume.

After a relatively stable calf volume has been achieved in response to a standard congesting pressure, the cuff is suddenly deflated.[3,9,11] The rate at which the calf volume decreases can be obtained by drawing a tangent to the initial part of the downslope. This gives the maximum venous

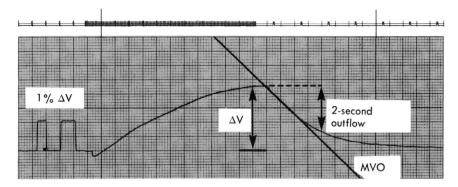

Fig. 97-3. Recording of the calf volume expansion (ΔV), slope of MVO, and 2-second outflow. The paper speed in seconds is indicated at the top of the tracing. A 1% volume change (electrical calibration) equals 10.5 divisions. Calf volume expansion: 23 div/10.5 = 2.2 ml/100 ml; MVO: 564 div/min/10.5 = 54 ml/100 ml/min; 2-second outflow: (16 div × 30)/10.5 = 46 ml/100 ml/min.

outflow (MVO).[3] Another method, which yields lower values but equally consistent results, is to measure the extent of the volume decrease after an arbitrary period of 2 seconds following cuff deflation.[5] (Techniques based on the volume decrease between two time periods have also been suggested.[8]) As shown in Fig. 97-3, the MVO can be calculated as follows, provided an electrical calibration is available:

$$\text{MVO (ml/100 ml/min)} = \frac{\text{Slope (div/min)}}{\text{Calibration (div/1\% vol change)}} \quad (2)$$

The 2-second venous outflow is calculated from the following:

2-second venous outflow (ml/100 ml/min)

$$= \frac{\text{Div fall} \times 30}{\text{Div/1\% vol change}} \quad (3)$$

If electrical calibration is not available, the circumference of the calf must be measured and the slope compared to a standard deflection produced by a known stretch of the gauge (see Chapter 22).

Calf volume expansion: interpretation of data

Normal values for calf volume expansion vary with the congesting pressure and with the time allowed before the measurement is made (usually 2 or 3 minutes from the time of cuff inflation). At a congesting pressure of 50 mm Hg, the calf volume increase approximates 2% to 3% in normal limbs.[4] In limbs with acute phlebitis, expansion of the calf is limited, usually less than 2%.[11] The reduced expansion is probably related to the following two factors: (1) fewer veins are available for inflation, since some are occupied by thrombi, and (2) increased venous pressure distal to a proximal obstructing thrombus will have already resulted in partial venous distention. Little further expansion is possible because the veins are already in the stiff portion of the venous compliance curve (Fig. 97-4).[24]

There are several potential sources of error in the measurement of calf expansion. First, the veins of the calf even

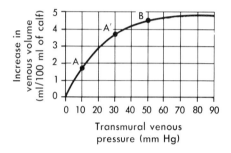

Fig. 97-4. The relationship between the venous volume and the transmural venous pressure. A indicates the venous pressure and the corresponding venous volume in the limbs of a normal supine subject. A' indicates the venous pressure and volume in a limb with acute phlebitis. B indicates the venous pressure and volume in a normal or phlebitic limb after the thigh cuff has been inflated to 50 mm Hg. Note that the venous wall becomes less compliant at higher pressures.

in the normal extremity may not be completely empty before the cuff is inflated. When this occurs, venous expansion in response to a given congesting pressure will be reduced. Therefore a standard elevation of the heel (one that ensures venous collapse) should be employed.[27] Second, unless the calf veins have undergone preliminary stretching, repeat determinations of calf expansion may show a progressively increasing calf volume change at the same congesting pressure.[14] (Two or three preliminary 45-second cuff inflations before the definitive measurement will stretch the calf veins, reduce the effects of venous tone, and provide more consistent results.[27]) Third, failure to use a standard congesting pressure or to ensure that the design and application of the thigh cuff are adequate to transmit the pressure will result in inconsistent measurements.

As shown in Table 97-1, most investigators have found statistically significant differences between the mean values for calf volume expansion obtained from normal limbs and those obtained from limbs with acute phlebitis. The differences are also sometimes significant in postphlebitic limbs but not in every study. Limbs with varicose veins appear to have the largest venous volume. In view of the many factors influencing the extent of calf volume expansion, it is not surprising that there is considerable overlap between the values obtained from normal limbs and those obtained from limbs with venous thrombosis (Fig. 97-5). This same over-

lap has been observed in similar studies performed with the impedance plethysmograph (see Chapter 98).

For these reasons, calf volume expansion has not proved to be sufficiently reliable as a diagnostic method when used alone.[22]

Venous outflow: interpretation of data

The rate of venous outflow (Q) is directly proportional to the pressure gradient propelling blood from the calf veins (P_{cv}) to the inferior vena cava (P_{ivc}) and inversely proportional to the resistance of the venous channels lying between (R):

$$Q = \frac{P_{cv} - P_{ivc}}{R} \qquad (4)$$

Because the cuff provides a consistent congesting pressure and because the central venous pressure is quite low, the rate of venous outflow would be expected to be decreased in the presence of acute venous thrombosis. That this is indeed the case is shown by the mean values in Table 97-2. As Barnes et al[3] have observed, there is a good but not complete separation between normal and abnormal studies (Fig. 97-6). When an MVO of 25 ml/100 ml/min was selected as the dividing line between normal and abnormal, the test proved to be 95% sensitive for detecting acute DVT and 82% specific for ruling it out. Other investigators have reported comparable figures (Table 97-3).

Using the 2-second outflow method, Barnes et al[5] found mean values of 45 ± 18 ml/100 ml/min in normal volunteers, with a range of 20 to 91 ml/100 ml/min. Mean outflows for limbs with acute venous thrombosis were as follows: iliofemoral, 13 ± 7 ml/100 ml/min; femoropopliteal, 11 ± 4 ml/100 ml/min; and calf vein, 20 ± 16 ml/100 ml/min. When 20 ml/100 ml/min was used as the dividing line, the sensitivity of the 2-second method was 90% for thrombi detected above the knee and 66% for thrombi isolated to veins below the knee. The specificity for excluding venous thrombosis was 81% at all levels. In this study, 13 of the 16 false-negative errors were in limbs with calf vein thrombi. Similar results were reported by Pini et al.[22] Although they found the sensitivity of strain-gauge plethysmography for detecting acute proximal venous

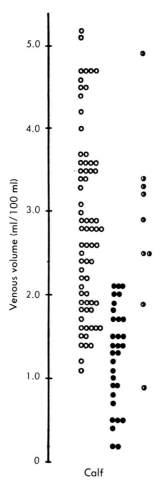

Fig. 97-5. Calf volume expansion in response to a congesting pressure of 50 mm Hg. Open circles indicate normal legs; closed circles, limbs with acute phlebitis; and half-closed circles, postphlebitic limbs. (Modified from Hallböök T, Göthlin J: *Acta Chir Scand* 137:37, 1971.)

Table 97-1. Calf volume expansion (ml/100 ml of calf)*

Investigator	Cuff pressure (mm Hg)	Normal	Limbs with varicose veins	Limbs with acute DVT	Postphlebitic limbs
Dahn and Eiriksson (1968)[9]	50	3.5 ± 0.6	5.1 ± 1.5†	2.4 ± 0.7†	2.7 ± 0.9†
Hallböök and Göthlin (1971)[11]	50	2.9 ± 1.1	—	1.3 ± 0.6†	2.8 ± 1.1
Sakaguchi et al (1972)[23]	80	2.1 ± 0.6	2.4 ± 1.0	1.1 ± 0.6†	1.5 ± 0.6†
Barnes et al (1973)[4]	50	2.1 ± 0.5	—	—	1.9 ± 0.7
Thulesius et al (1978)[25]	60	2.7 ± 0.6	4.9 ± 1.2 †	1.7 ± 0.8†	—
Pini et al (1984)[22]	55	3.3 ± 1.1	—	1.5 ± 0.8	—
Doko et al (1991)[10]	—	3.6 ± 0.6	—	1.4 ± 0.8	—

*Mean ± standard deviation.
†Statistically significant compared with normal values.

thrombosis was 97%, it was only 60% for thrombi in the calf veins.

The venous outflow method is subject to a number of errors.[12] Acute venous thrombosis cannot be distinguished from other causes of increased venous resistance. These include the following: severe residual obstruction in the postphlebitic extremity and extrinsic pressure from tumors, hematomas, and Baker's cysts. In addition, false-negative studies may result when the thrombus is nonocclusive and does not seriously interfere with venous outflow. When the distal superficial femoral and popliteal veins are paired, as they frequently are, clots confined to one channel of these veins may escape detection. As already mentioned, calf vein thrombi cannot be diagnosed reliably.

Zetterquist et al[29] have called attention to a biphasic pattern of the venous outflow curve that appears to occur in limbs with thrombi isolated to the iliac level when the calf and thigh veins are completely patent. In these limbs, the initial outflow slope may be quite steep (giving a normal MVO), but the second phase of the outflow slope suddenly becomes much slower. The breaking point between the two slopes always begins within 1.5 seconds of the time of cuff deflation. If the initial slope were taken as representative of the outflow, the study would be falsely interpreted as being negative when, in fact, there would be a thrombus lying in the iliac system. Use of the 2-second outflow method might avoid some of these errors.

The explanation offered for the biphasic curve is as follows: first, the inflated thigh cuff serves to empty the normal thigh veins; then when the cuff pressure is released, the blood trapped in the calf flows rapidly up the leg to fill the space in the thigh, thus accounting for the initial rapid phase of venous emptying. Once the thigh veins are filled, the proximal obstruction in the pelvic veins impedes the further outflow of blood, producing the second more gradual slope. Similar curves have been observed in patients with increased central venous pressure caused by right ventricular heart

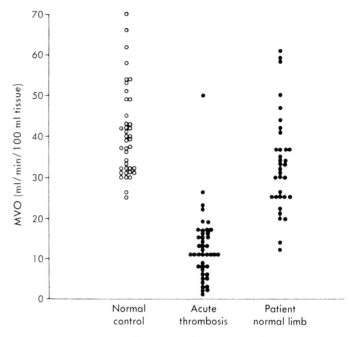

Fig. 97-6. MVO in normal patients and in patients with acute DVT. (From Barnes RW et al: *Surgery* 72:971, 1972.)

Table 97-2. Maximum venous outflow (ml/100 ml/min)*

Investigator	Cuff pressure (mm Hg)	Normal	Limbs with varicose veins	Limbs with acute DVT	Postphlebitic limbs
Dahn and Eiriksson (1968)[9]	50	82 ± 24	168 ± 48†	16	58
Hallböök and Göthlin (1971)[11]	50	78 ± 22	—	23 ± 8†	64 ± 21
Sakaguchi et al (1972)[23]	80	87 ± 14	110 ± 46†	32 ± 17†	55 ± 44†
Barnes et al (1972, 1973)[3,4]	50	41 ± 11	—	12 ± 8†	34 ± 15†
Thulesius et al (1978)[25]	60	58 ± 18	96 ± 23†	17 ± 9†	—
Pini et al (1984)[22]	55	64 ± 18	—	21 ± 13	—
Doko et al (1991)[10]	—	74 ± 19	—	19 ± 19	—

*Mean ± standard deviation.
†Statistically significant compared with normal values.

Table 97-3. Accuracy of MVO for detecting acute DVT

Investigator	Cuff pressure (mm Hg)	Dividing line (ml/100 ml/min)	Sens (%)	Spec (%)	PPV (%)	NPV (%)
Barnes et al (1972)[3]	50	20	91	88	91	88
	50	25	95	82	87	93
AbuRahma and Osborne (1984)[1]	50	20	96	99	98	97
Pini et al (1984)[22]	55	37.5	91	91	94	92

MVO, Maximum venous outflow; *DVT*, deep vein thrombosis; *Sens*, sensitivity; *Spec*, specificity; *PPV*, positive predictive value; *NPV*, negative predictive value.

failure. The examiner should be aware of these pitfalls when a biphasic outflow curve is obtained.

There are also a number of methodologic errors that must be avoided. Because the rate of venous outflow is a function of the calf vein pressure (P_{cv} in equation 4), it follows that the MVO (or 2-second outflow) will increase with increasing cuff pressure and that a standard congesting pressure must be used.[28] Less obvious, perhaps, is the direct relationship between leg elevation and the rate of venous outflow.[27,28] Given a constant congesting pressure, the increasing MVO as the heel is raised may be due to the increased gravitational potential energy of blood in the elevated calf, more complete evacuation of the thigh veins that act as a flow sink, or an increased capacitance of the calf veins, which plays a role in determining venous outflow. To maintain consistent results, the foot should always be supported at the same level. As Tripolitis et al[27] have shown, the rate at which the congesting cuff is deflated also determines the rate of venous outflow. If the cuff pressure drops slowly, the pressure gradient in the numerator of equation 4 is no longer the difference between the pressure in the calf veins (P_{cv}) and that in the inferior vena cava (P_{ivc}), but rather it is the much smaller difference between the calf venous pressure and the pressure in the cuff. Therefore if the cuff is deflated slowly, the rate at which blood leaves the calf will be decreased. To avoid this problem, the tubes that evacuate the congesting cuff must have a diameter large enough to ensure practically instantaneous decompression.

RELATIONSHIP BETWEEN VENOUS OUTFLOW AND CALF VOLUME EXPANSION

Many investigators have noted a direct relationship between the rate of venous outflow and the magnitude of calf volume expansion (Fig. 97-7).* In particular, those using impedance methods have combined these measurements to enhance the overall accuracy of the technique, either by calculating venous outflow/venous expansion ratios or by plotting the outflow versus the calf volume expansion on a graph. A discriminate analysis line that slopes upward from left to right on a graph with venous outflow on the ordinate and venous expansion on the abscissa serves to separate normal values, which lie above the line, from abnormal values, which lie below the line (see Chapter 98).[7,15]

Inspection of the tracing in Fig. 97-3 reveals that the venous outflow curve is not straight but decreases in slope as the calf volume decreases.[24] Several factors are responsible for this. First, the pressure driving blood out of the leg (P_{cv}) falls rapidly following cuff deflation (equation 4). The rate at which the pressure declines is proportional to the decrease in blood volume within the veins, which in turn depends on the resistance to venous outflow (R) and to the elastic modulus of the venous wall (E). If E is assumed to be the ratio of the venous transmural pressure (P) to the

---

*References 6, 7, 10, 16, 17, 25.

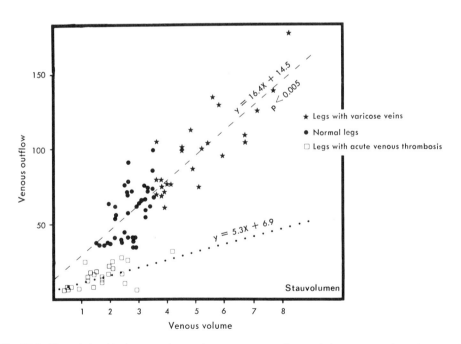

Fig. 97-7. The relationship between the maximum venous outflow and the venous volume in normal legs, legs with varicose veins, and legs with acute venous thrombosis. (From Thulesius O et al: *Diagnostik bei akuter Venethrombose der unteren Extremitaten.* In Kriessman A, Bollinger A, eds: *Ultraschall-Doppler-Diagnostik in der Angiologie,* Stuttgart, 1978, Georg Thieme Verlag.)

venous volume (V), then the quantity of blood remaining at any time after cuff release *(V_t)* is:

$$V_t = V_o e^{-(E/R)t} \qquad (5)$$

and the rate of venous outflow *(Q_t)* at that time is:

$$Q_t = \frac{E}{R} V_o e^{-(E/R)t} \qquad (6)$$

where:

$$E = P/V$$
$$V_o = \text{Maximum extent of calf expansion}$$
$$R = \text{Venous resistance}$$
$$t = \text{Time in seconds after cuff release}$$

These equations are analogous to those used in the analysis of electrical circuits to describe the discharge of a capacitor through a resistance.

At the point of cuff release, when *t* equals zero, equation 6 reduces to the following:

$$Q_o = \text{MVO} = \frac{E}{R} V_o = \frac{P_o}{R} \qquad (7)$$

which is the same as equation 4, the formula for the MVO.

It can be seen from equation 7 that MVO increases as the stiffness of the veins (E) and the calf volume expansion (V_o) increase. Therefore MVO is not totally dependent on venous resistance, which is the factor that is being measured. In fact, equation 7 can be rearranged as follows to justify the use of venous outflow/venous expansion ratios or graphic methods for assessing venous resistance:

$$R = E \frac{V_o}{Q_o} \qquad (8)$$

In other words, given a certain venous expansion (V_o), the greater the venous outflow (Q_o), the less the resistance (R) and the less likely is the limb to be the site of venous thrombosis (Fig. 97-7). Less evident is the fact that given a certain venous outflow (Q_o), the greater the venous expansion (V_o), the more likely the limb is to harbor a significant venous clot (Fig. 97-7).

Equation 7 also accounts for the different slopes of the MVO-venous capacitance regression lines applied to normal limbs and to those with major venous thrombosis.[16,25] Since the ratio E/R represents the slope of the line, the greater the resistance (R), the lower the slope. Thus points describing limbs with venous thrombosis have a lower slope than the line that fits the values for normal limbs (see Figs. 98-1, 98-2, and 97-7).

The second factor that complicates the interpretation of the venous outflow curve is the venous elasticity (E), which is the reciprocal of the venous compliance. Venous elasticity varies, not only from limb to limb, but also throughout the course of the venous decompression that follows release of the thigh cuff. As shown in Fig. 97-4, E is high at higher pressures where the venous wall is quite stiff but becomes low at low pressure ranges where the wall is compliant. In Fig. 97-8, a family of curves is plotted, based on equation

5, in which the congesting (cuff) pressure, the MVO, and the venous resistance (R) all remain constant. Various values of E yield correspondingly different values of venous expansion. Although an accurately drawn tangent to the initial part of each curve would give identical MVOs of 60 ml/min, the 2- or 3-second outflows would differ greatly. Thus it is possible to have the same venous resistance and yet measure widely varying venous outflows. Again, from this graph the correlation of venous expansion with the 2- or 3-second venous outflow can be seen.

Clearly, the 2- or 3-second venous outflows and even the MVO are complex functions that do not solely reflect changes in venous resistance. Although the discrimination provided by venous outflow studies when used alone has been good, accuracy should be improved by incorporating volume expansion into the final analysis.[7]

Tripolitis et al[26] reported that after a few days of bed rest, the venous outflow consistently decreased in patients who had undergone various operations. Because there was no evidence of venous thrombosis in these patients, it is likely that the changes in venous outflow were not caused by an increase in venous resistance but rather by a change in

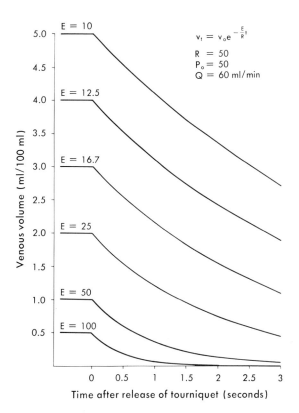

Fig. 97-8. Theoretic venous outflow curves based on equation 5. In all curves, congesting (cuff) pressure *(PO)* is 50 mm Hg, and outflow resistance *(R)* is 50 mm Hg/ml^{-1}/min. Elastic modulus *(E)* is the ratio of the venous transmural pressure to the venous volume. Q, Flow. (From Strandness DE Jr, Sumner DS: *Hemodynamics for surgeons*, New York, 1975, Grune & Stratton.)

venous elasticity. This is another argument for considering both venous capacitance and venous outflow when assessing patients for DVT.

APPLICATIONS OF THE OUTFLOW/COMPLIANCE RELATIONSHIP

Cramer, Beach, and Strandness[7] at the University of Washington have devised a discriminant line that distinguishes limbs with acute venous thrombosis from normal limbs and have reported a sensitivity of 100% and specificity of 92% for this criterion (Fig. 97-9). Venous volume expansion (in ml/100 ml) measured at 2 minutes after cuff inflation is plotted on the horizontal axis, and venous outflow (in ml/100 ml/min) measured at 0.5 ($VO_{0.5}$) and 2.0 ($VO_{2.0}$) seconds after cuff release is plotted on the vertical axis. The outflow parameter ($VO_{0.5-2.0}$) is calculated as follows:

$$VO_{0.5-2.0} = \left(\frac{4}{3}\right)VO_{2.0} - \left(\frac{1}{3}\right)VO_{0.5} \qquad (9)$$

Based on their observations, they concluded that this outflow parameter provided more consistent results and was less prone to error than measurement of the MVO, which is subject to cuff artifacts and may be spuriously high in limbs with large proximal collateral beds.[8] This method does not appear to have been evaluated independently.

Besides providing a means of incorporating both compliance and resistance information, the use of discriminant lines has another important advantage. Because both venous volume expansion and venous outflow are measured with the same strain gauge, any error in calibrating the gauge will have the same relative effect on both measurements. Therefore the length of the gauge is less critical than it is when interpretations are based on absolute values; this permits the same gauge to be used on limbs with different circumferences without diminishing diagnostic accuracy.

Methods other than the discriminant line approach that incorporate both outflow and capacitance data have been advocated. Recognizing the difficulty sometimes encountered in measuring the initial slope of the outflow curve, Lundgren and Thulesius[20] adapted equation 5 to permit calculation of the MVO based on the elapsed time between the point of cuff deflation and the point at which the tracing falls to one half of the maximum level achieved during cuff inflation ($V_o/2$). This time interval ($T_{1/2}$) is quite easily measured. By substituting $V_o/2$ for V_t, $T_{1/2}$ for t, and MVO/V_o for E/R (see equation 7) in equation 5, the following is obtained:

$$\frac{V_o}{2} = V_o e^{-\frac{MVO}{V_o}T_{1/2}}$$

which can be restated in logarithmic form as:

$$MVO = V_o\frac{\ln 2}{T_{1/2}} \qquad (10)$$

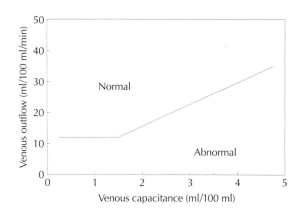

Fig. 97-9. Outflow/capacitance discriminant line. See text for explanation. (Modified from Cramer et al: *Bruit* 7:17, 1983.)

If V_o is measured in ml/100 ml/min and $T_{1/2}$ in seconds, equation 9 becomes:

$$MVO = 41.6\left(\frac{V_o}{T_{1/2}}\right) \qquad (11)$$

since the natural logarithm of 2×60 sec/min = 41.6.

Thus only two simple measurements are required to obtain the MVO. Although equation 10 is based on the rather questionable assumption that the elastic modulus (E) remains constant throughout the outflow curve, Lundgren and Thulesius[20] found that the calculated and measured MVO values were highly correlated ($r = 0.94$)—an observation that substantiates the validity of equations 5 and 6. Even more important, this method, at least theoretically, eliminates the obfuscating effect that variations in venous compliance can have on measurements of venous outflow.

Åkesson et al[2] have proposed a somewhat different method for using the information in equations 5 and 6. They calculate the time constant ($k = E/R$) of these two equations by dividing the MVO, rendered in ml/100 ml/min, by the maximum calf volume expansion (V_o), rendered in ml/100 ml, and then divide the result by 60 to obtain k in sec^{-1} (equation 7). (A simpler method, requiring only one measurement, would be to use the half emptying time [$T_{1/2}$] because k = $\ln 2/T_{1/2}$ [equations 9 and 10].) In normal limbs, k averages 0.37 sec^{-1}, with a 95% tolerance range of 0.21 to 0.65 sec^{-1}. A k value less than 0.21 sec^{-1} is considered abnormal. Because k incorporates both venous compliance and outflow resistance, these investigators have found it particularly useful for evaluating legs with a high venous capacitance, in which the MVOs may be within normal limits despite the presence of a venous obstruction. When the diagnosis of venous obstruction was based on both k and *MVO*, sensitivity improved, with little accompanying drop in specificity.[2]

CONCLUSION

In the United States, impedance plethysmography has been more popular than strain-gauge plethysmography for the diagnosis of deep venous disease. In part the preference for impedance plethysmography may be attributed to the perception that strain gauges are delicate and difficult to use. Mercury strain gauges are extremely sensitive, making them responsive to the slightest movement. Therefore unless the patient is quiet and cooperative, the tracings are apt to be erratic. In addition, it is necessary to have a battery of gauges of various lengths to fit the calves of different individuals. Furthermore, the gauges are difficult to calibrate when the mechanical method is used. The gauge must be stretched precisely with a micrometer-controlled device, and the girth of the calf must also be measured accurately. Finally, the gauges are delicate and have a tendency to deteriorate because of oxidation of the mercury column.

Newer developments have overcome many of these problems. Electrical calibration, which is available on several plethysmographs, is rapid and accurate and simplifies calculations.[13] Backing the gauges with Velcro has greatly simplified their application to the calf. Because of the way in which these new gauges contact the skin, the same gauge may be used for a variety of different calf sizes without appreciably affecting the diagnostic accuracy (provided the discriminant line approach is used). The substitution of an indium-gallium alloy for mercury promises to extend the shelf life of the gauges.

These technologic improvements, coupled with the obvious advantages of the strain gauge (e.g., high sensitivity, linearity, accuracy), make it ideally suited for physiologic studies of venous disease. Although duplex and color flow scanning are rapidly replacing all plethysmographic methods as the primary noninvasive technique for diagnosing acute DVT, images and isolated flow measurements do not permit quantification of the degree of obstruction or the reduction in calf vein compliance. The ability to numerically define the extent of the functional deficit has proved valuable to clinical investigators wishing to document the natural history of venous disease.[2,18,21] Strain-gauge plethysmography also affords the surgeon an objective method for evaluating the effects of therapeutic intervention on venous physiology.

REFERENCES

1. AbuRahma AF, Osborne L: A combined study of the strain gauge plethysmography and I-125 fibrinogen leg scan in the differentiation of deep vein thrombosis and postphlebitic syndrome, *Am Surg* 50:585, 1984.
2. Åkesson H et al: Physiological evaluation of venous obstruction in the post thrombotic leg, *Phlebology* 4:3, 1989.
3. Barnes RW et al: Noninvasive quantitation of maximum venous outflow in acute thrombophlebitis, *Surgery* 72:971, 1972.
4. Barnes RW et al: Noninvasive quantitation of venous hemodynamics in postphlebitic syndrome, *Arch Surg* 107:807, 1973.
5. Barnes RW et al: Detection of deep vein thrombosis with an automatic electrically calibrated strain gauge plethysmograph, *Surgery* 82:219, 1977.
6. Bygdeman S, Aschberg S, Hindmarsh T: Venous plethysmography in the diagnosis of chronic venous insufficiency, *Acta Chir Scand* 137:423, 1971.
7. Cramer M, Beach KW, Strandness DE Jr: The detection of proximal deep venous thrombosis by strain gauge plethysmography through the use of an outflow/capacitance discriminant line, *Bruit* 7:17, 1983.
8. Cramer M et al: Standardization of venous outflow measurement by strain gauge plethysmography in normal subjects, *Bruit* 7:33, 1983.
9. Dahn I, Eiriksson E: Plethysmographic diagnosis of deep venous thrombosis of the leg, *Acta Chir Scand* 398[suppl]:33, 1968.
10. Doko S et al: Maximum venous outflow and development of deep vein thrombosis, *Jpn Circ J* 55:185, 1991.
11. Hallböök T, Göthlin J: Strain-gauge plethysmography and phlebography in diagnosis of deep venous thrombosis, *Acta Chir Scand* 137:37, 1971.
12. Hallböök T, Ling L: Pitfalls in plethysmographic diagnosis of acute deep venous thrombosis, *J Cardiovasc Surg* 14:427, 1973.
13. Hokanson DE, Sumner DS, Strandness DE Jr: An electrically calibrated plethysmograph for direct measurement of limb blood flow, *IEEE Trans Biomed Eng* 22(1):25, 1975.
14. Hollenberg NK, Boreus LO: The influence of rate of filling on apparent venous distensibility in man, *Can J Physiol Pharmacol* 50:310, 1972.
15. Hull R et al: Impedance plethysmography using the occlusive cuff technique in the diagnosis of venous thrombosis, *Circulation* 53:696, 1976.
16. Hull R et al: Impedance plethysmography: the relationship between venous filling and sensitivity and specificity for proximal vein thrombosis, *Circulation* 58:898, 1978.
17. Johnston KW, Kakkar VV: Plethysmographic diagnosis of deep vein thrombosis, *Surg Gynecol Obstet* 138:41, 1974.
18. Killewich LA et al: Pathophysiology of venous claudication, *J Vasc Surg* 1:507, 1984.
19. Knox R et al: Pitfalls of venous occlusion plethysmography, *Angiology* 33:268, 1982.
20. Lundgren PO, Thulesius O: Maximal venous outflow in the diagnosis of deep venous thrombosis, new principles for its determination, *Vasa* 14:346, 1985.
21. Mahler DK et al: Follow-up of old deep venous thrombosis by Doppler ultrasound and strain gauge plethysmography, *Bruit* 6:30, 1982.
22. Pini M et al: Accuracy of strain-gauge plethysmography as a diagnostic test in clinically suspected deep venous thrombosis, *Thromb Res* 35:149, 1984.
23. Sakaguchi S, Ishitobi K, Kameda T: Functional segmental plethysmography with mercury strain gauge, *Angiology* 23:127, 1972.
24. Strandness DE Jr, Sumner DS: *Hemodynamics for surgeons*, New York, 1975, Grune & Stratton.
25. Thulesius O et al: *Diagnostik bei akuter Venethrombose der unteren Extremitäten*. In Kriessman A, Bollinger A, eds: *Ultraschall-Doppler-Diagnostik in der Angiologie*, Stuttgart, 1978, Georg Thieme.
26. Tripolitis AJ et al: Venous capacitance and outflow in the postoperative patient, *Ann Surg* 190:634, 1979.
27. Tripolitis AJ et al: The influence of limb elevation, examination technique, and outflow system design on venous plethysmography, *Angiology* 31:154, 1980.
28. Voorhoeve R, Berends ERJ: Venous outflow measurement in the diagnosis of deep vein thrombosis—principles and practice, *Neth J Surg* 38-I:6, 1986.
29. Zetterquist S, Ericsson K, Volpe V: The clinical significance of biphasic venous emptying curves from the lower limb in venous occlusion plethysmography, *Scand J Clin Lab Invest* 35:497, 1975.

CHAPTER 98

Diagnosis of deep vein thrombosis by impedance plethysmography

H. BROWNELL WHEELER and FREDERICK A. ANDERSON, Jr.

Impedance plethysmography (IPG) is a widely used non-invasive method for the diagnosis of deep vein thrombosis (DVT). The method is based on measurement of the changes in blood volume produced by temporary venous obstruction. Venous thrombosis alters this response dramatically. This chapter describes the background of the method and the current role for IPG in the diagnosis of DVT.

When IPG was first introduced for the diagnosis of DVT, temporary venous occlusion was produced by deep inspiration or a Valsalva maneuver. Good results with this technique were obtained by several investigators,* but others reported less accurate results.[16,50] The necessity for the patient to increase intraabdominal pressure sufficiently to obstruct venous return proved to be a major limitation in terms of both the accuracy and usefulness of the method. Some patients were too sick or uncooperative to be tested. In evaluating the result obtained, the observer always had to take into account the response of the patient. The reliability of the test depended in large part on the experience, knowledge, and patience of the examiner.

To yield consistent results that could be reproduced by the average hospital technician, an objective and standardized method of producing temporary venous occlusion was necessary. Venous occlusion plethysmography (VOP) was developed for this purpose.[14] The details of the testing procedure, the instrumentation, and the method of interpretation were all made simple and objective. Minimal patient cooperation was required, and the possibility of operator error was greatly reduced. This revised VOP technique of IPG has now been studied in many laboratories† and has proved much more satisfactory than the original respiratory test.

RATIONALE

The rationale for measuring blood volume changes indirectly through changes in electrical resistance is based on

Ohm's law (voltage = current × resistance). Blood is a good conductor of electricity. The more blood present in the body segment being studied, the lower the resistance to passage of an electrical current. Measurement of the resistance (or impedance) to passage of a weak, high-frequency current through the lower leg provides a convenient and safe way to measure changes in venous blood volume. (The theoretic basis and experimental verification of IPG are explained in more detail in Chapter 21.)

The physiologic basis for IPG is simple and straightforward. In normal individuals, temporary venous obstruction with continuing arterial inflow results in a marked increase in venous volume, followed by a rapid venous outflow when the obstruction is released. If thrombi are present in the major veins draining the lower leg, the venous outflow rate is diminished, often dramatically so. The initial volume increase is usually reduced as well. The outflow depends to some extent on the amount of blood dammed up following venous obstruction, and therefore results are more accurately evaluated when the venous outflow is expressed as a function of the venous volume increase (Figs. 98-1 and 98-2).

IPG may be thought of as a "stress test" of the venous system, which is challenged to carry away a large volume of blood within a short period of time. Normally, the large-caliber veins of the leg can carry large quantities of blood rapidly, reflecting their low fluid resistance. Consequently, the normal venous system is able to respond to an increasing volume challenge with a proportionately greater outflow rate. The amount of blood dammed up behind the thigh occlusion cuff will determine the venous outflow in the first few seconds after release of the cuff. However, when thrombosis is present in any of the major veins draining the lower leg, there is a marked reduction in the maximum rate of venous outflow, irrespective of the amount of blood dammed up behind the thigh occlusion cuff. An obstructed venous system will respond with an outflow rate proportional to the degree of obstruction but largely independent of the magnitude of the venous volume challenge (Fig. 98-3).

---

*References 42, 43, 49, 55, 58, 59.

†References 9, 12, 18-22, 26-28, 30, 31, 36, 37, 39, 47, 48, 51, 52, 54, 56, 57, 60-62.

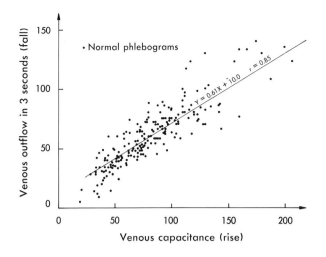

Fig. 98-1. In patients with normal venograms (phlebograms), occlusive IPG shows a progressive increase in the venous outflow as the venous capacitance improves.

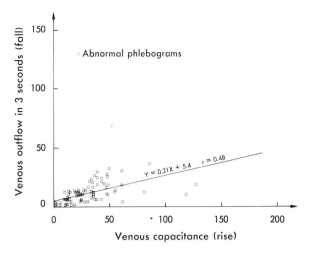

Fig. 98-2. In patients whose venograms (phlebograms) show thrombosis in major veins, IPG indicates that the venous outflow is low. As the venous capacitance increases, the venous outflow does not increase proportionally, as occurs in normal subjects.

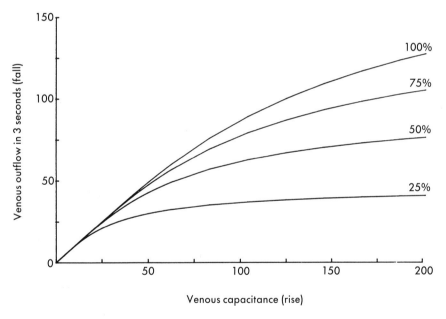

Fig. 98-3. Relationship between the venous capacitance and outflow with varying degrees of venous outflow obstruction. Percentages are minimum venous outflow lumen diameter, referred to as the venous diameter index (VDI). A VDI of 100% indicates no outflow obstruction. A VDI of 25% indicates that approximately 75% of the lumen diameter is obstructed. (From Anderson FA, Jr: *Quantification of the degree of venous obstruction from venous occlusion plethysmography,* Worcester, Mass, Worcester Polytechnic Institute, 1984 [dissertation].)

METHOD

The IPG test is carried out with the subject in the supine position. The leg is elevated sufficiently to facilitate venous drainage, and the calf should be slightly above heart level. Usually this is best accomplished by placing the leg on a pillow and elevating the foot of the bed about 20 degrees.

It is important that the patient is comfortable and the leg muscles relaxed.

A pneumatic cuff is placed around the thigh. The cuff should not be applied tightly, or it may inadvertently act as a venous tourniquet. Circumferential electrodes are then placed around the calf (Fig. 98-4).

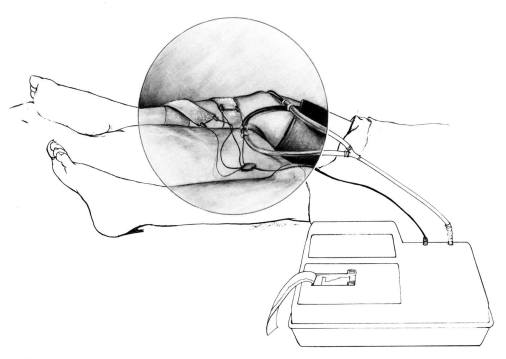

Fig. 98-4. Position for IPG. The leg is slightly elevated. The electrode bands encircle the calf, and the pneumatic cuff is wrapped around the thigh. The electrodes and cuff are connected to the IPG.

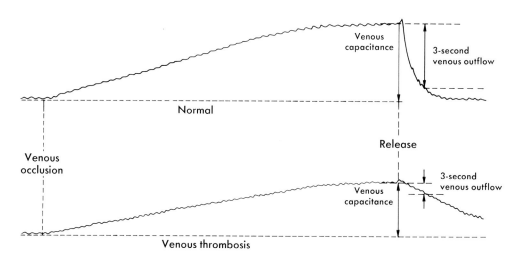

Fig. 98-5. Interpretation is based on measurement of (1) the increase in blood volume that follows inflation of the pneumatic cuff (venous capacitance) and (2) the decrease in blood volume that follows the release of cuff pressure (3-second venous outflow).

The electrodes are connected to an IPG (current frequency, 22 kHz; current strength, 1 mA). The pneumatic cuff is connected to an air pressure system that allows rapid deflation and is then inflated to 70 cm H_2O (about 50 mm Hg)—above venous pressure but well under arterial pressure. This pressure is maintained until the tracing "levels off," which usually occurs within 1 to 2 minutes. There is no need to time venous occlusion precisely. The thigh cuff pressure should be maintained until the venous volume has reached maximum, as shown by the tracing reaching a pla-

teau (Fig. 98-5). This may take anywhere from 15 seconds to 3 minutes or more, depending on the arterial inflow, the degree of venous obstruction, and the baseline venous pressure.

It should be emphasized that the key to obtaining accurate results is maximum filling of the venous system. Prolonging the occlusion time has been demonstrated to improve venous filling.[28] Other methods of improving venous filling include increasing the occlusion pressure, repetitive testing at the same pressure, active or passive movement of the calf mus-

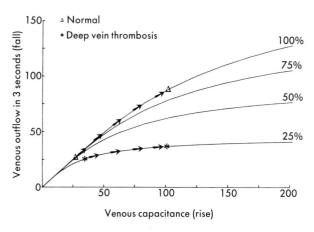

Fig. 98-6. Test points that are equivocal on initial testing are often clearly resolved by test repetition, prolonged occlusion, or other maneuvers that improve venous filling. (From Anderson FA Jr: *Quantification of the degree of venous outflow obstruction from venous occlusion plethysmography,* Worcester, Mass, Worcester Polytechnic Institute, 1984 [dissertation].)

cles, locally applied heat, and vasodilating drugs. Repetitive testing and prolonged occlusion times are now standard methods of increasing venous filling. Borderline test results have then usually resolved into clearly normal or abnormal findings (Fig. 98-6).

After the tracing has leveled off and it is clear that maximum venous filling has been obtained, cuff pressure is rapidly released. The cuff must deflate promptly, since any mechanical delay in deflation might simulate a decrease in venous outflow caused by venous thrombosis.

The increase in venous volume following inflation of the cuff and the decrease in venous volume during the first 3 seconds following release of the cuff are measured from the strip-chart recording (Fig. 98-5). These two variables, termed *venous capacitance* and *venous outflow,* respectively, are then plotted on a scoring graph. Whenever a clearly normal result is obtained, the test can be terminated. However, if the result is equivocal or abnormal, the test should be repeated either until a normal result has been obtained or until the examiner is sure that optimum venous filling has been achieved and there is no technical reason for the poor tracing, such as calf muscle tension or a tourniquet effect from tight clothing, bandages, or the thigh cuff.[4] This usually requires multiple test repetitions. Others originally advocated repeating the test five times, with occlusion times of 2 minutes' duration for two of the five tests.[26-28] The later "stop-line" concept reduced the IPG testing time by demonstrating that it is safe to terminate the IPG procedure whenever a clearly normal result has been obtained.[51]

FACTORS AFFECTING THE IPG RESPONSE

Although abnormal findings are usually the result of DVT, several pathophysiologic conditions may influence the re-

sults obtained. In a normal subject, there is a marked increase in venous volume following temporary venous obstruction. However, the rate of this increase may vary considerably, even in the same individual. The initial rate of venous pooling is a reflection of peripheral blood flow. It is influenced by cardiac output, the patency of the major arteries, the degree of peripheral vasoconstriction, and the initial venous pressure. Many pathophysiologic conditions affect these variables. Important clinical considerations are myocardial function, chronic obstructive pulmonary disease, hypovolemia, occlusive arterial disease, and peripheral vasoconstriction. Even healthy individuals exhibit peripheral vasospasm caused by apprehension, pain, or cold.

Often improved venous capacitance is observed with test repetition, particularly when the venous tourniquet is maintained in place until the tracing reaches a plateau. This probably represents the effect of compliance changes in the vein wall.

Extravascular compression

Infrequently, venous outflow may be obstructed by extravascular compression of major veins. This has been observed with cancer of the pelvis, hematomas, Baker's cysts, and other extrinsic masses that compress the venous system. Extravascular compression can also be produced by tight bandages or clothing.

A subtle but more common cause of extravascular compression is calf muscle tension. Radiologists have long been familiar with the squeezing of the calf veins that can be produced by muscle contraction during venography. For this reason, it is important to be sure that the calf muscles are relaxed during IPG.

The possibility of extravascular compression of major veins is usually apparent from a careful history or physical examination. It has rarely been a problem in the interpretation of IPG results, with the exception of calf muscle tension, which may be transient and therefore difficult to recognize.

Decreased peripheral blood flow

Whenever arterial inflow is impaired, the early phase of the venous capacitance curve is reduced. This reduction in venous capacitance causes a corresponding reduction in the venous outflow. Reduced venous capacitance has often been observed in hypovolemic states, myocardial infarction, and congestive heart failure. It may also result from reduced arterial inflow caused by occlusive arterial disease or peripheral vasoconstriction. However, the outflow response will often be normal if the period of venous obstruction is prolonged, allowing a larger venous volume to dam up slowly behind the tourniquet.

Increased vasoconstriction may change the compliance of the venous system, as well as reduce peripheral blood flow, resulting in a diminished volume response to a given occlusion pressure. Increased vasomotor tone is often observed in patients who are apprehensive, cold, in pain, or suffering from hypovolemia or low cardiac output. With correction of the underlying cause of venoconstriction, the plethysmographic response usually reverts to normal. Dramatic improvement in venous capacitance is often seen after reactive hyperemia, application of local heat, peripheral vasodilator administration, or sympathetic blockade.

Interpretation of tests is often facilitated by a knowledge of concurrent physiologic conditions that may influence peripheral hemodynamics.

INTERPRETATION OF RESULTS

VOP has been performed for the detection of DVT using a variety of plethysmographic instruments, many of which are described elsewhere in this book. The tracings obtained are qualitatively similar to the IPG curves shown in Fig. 98-5. From inspection of the VOP curves, it is obvious that the most dramatic difference between normal limbs and those with DVT is found in the venous outflow portion of the tracing. Most investigators have based interpretation of VOP results on some measure of venous outflow. A variety of criteria have been used, which makes it difficult to compare results between publications, even when the same instrument and test procedure have been employed (see Table 105-7).

Common indices of venous outflow used to interpret VOP tracings include the maximum venous outflow (MVO) slope and measurements of the venous outflow in a fixed time interval following the release of occlusion pressure. Based on an empiric analysis of VOP data, one study found that the venous outflow volume in 3 seconds (VO_3) discriminates between normal limbs and those with DVT better than MVO or venous outflow volume at other time intervals.[5] This empiric analysis was subsequently verified experimentally.[3] Calculation of the difference in venous outflow volume versus time for an average normal and abnormal VOP curve demonstrates that the maximum difference occurs 3 seconds after cuff release (Fig. 98-7). This provides objective evidence that 3 seconds is the optimal time at which to measure venous outflow differences for the detection of DVT.[3]

The accuracy of IPG results is further improved by expressing the 3-second venous outflow as a function of the amount of venous filling. IPG results are conveniently displayed on a graph in which venous filling is plotted against 3-second outflow.

There is surprisingly good discrimination between patients with normal venograms and those with recent thrombosis, as shown in Figs. 98-1 and 98-2. In earlier publications,[60,61] interpretation of results was based on where a given test fell in relation to overall zones of normal and abnormal, as defined by previous experience. With this method, an overall accuracy of 96% was obtained in differentiating normal patients from those with recent thrombosis of major veins.

Most commonly, interpretation has been based on a discriminant analysis line developed at McMaster University Medical Center (Fig. 98-8). This diagonal line slopes up-

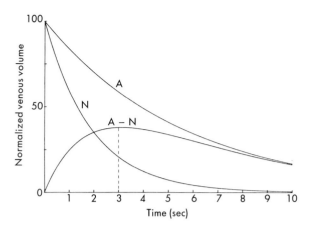

Fig. 98-7. The maximum difference between average normal *(N)* and abnormal *(A)* IPG outflow curves occurs at a point approximately 3 seconds from release of venous occlusion. (From Anderson FA Jr: *Quantification of the degree of venous outflow obstruction from venous occlusion plethysmography,* Worcester, Mass, Worcester Polytechnic Institute, 1984 [dissertation].)

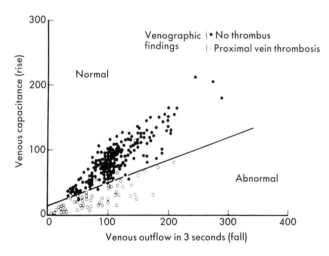

Fig. 98-8. IPG interpretation using the discriminant line as developed by Hull et al.[26]

ward from left to right on a graph of venous capacitance versus venous outflow. Points that fall above the line are reported as normal. Points that fall below the line are considered abnormal. This simple classification of results provided 97% specificity and 93% sensitivity in the prospective screening of mainly asymptomatic patients[25] and 95% specificity and 98% sensitivity for symptomatic patients.[27]

The aggregate results of all studies in which venographic correlation has been obtained routinely for validation of IPG show a 94% specificity and a 93% sensitivity in nonorthopedic patients (2724 venograms; see Chapter 105). The majority of these patients had symptoms suggesting DVT.

There was a 97% specificity but only a 29% sensitivity in patients undergoing total hip replacement (2405 venograms; see Chapter 105). The majority of these patients were entirely asymptomatic with respect to DVT. Lower accuracy has also been reported when only a small percentage of patients undergoing IPG testing have had venography, probably reflecting a selection bias favoring venography in problem patients.[46]

Both these methods of interpretation provide excellent results but suffer from being too simplistic. The results are "black or white" and do not give the full spectrum of information available from the tracings. Common sense dictates that points close to the dividing line between normal and abnormal should be considered less reliable than those some distance away. Treatment based on borderline results may be less valid than treatment based on results that fall clearly in the normal or abnormal zones. The possibility of inadvertent mismanagement of patients is therefore increased by these methods of data reporting.

What is the ideal way to express the results of an IPG tracing? It seems obvious that the reporting method should be simple and easy for a clinician to understand. The report should also give some indication of the reliability of the result. These objectives are best accomplished by reporting the IPG results in the same way that other laboratory results are reported—by expressing them as a number with a defined range of normal. An individual test result can then be weighed by the clinician in relation to where the specific value falls with respect to the range of normal.

IPG results can also be expressed as a percentage of predicted normal, much as some tests of cardiac or pulmonary function are currently reported. In this method of interpretation, normality relates to the anticipated lumen diameter of the proximal veins. The percentage of predicted lumen diameter is referred to as the *venous diameter index (VDI)*. A normal individual is expected to have a VDI of 75% or greater. Patients with DVT usually have a VDI of 0% to 40%. This method of interpretation is based on firm theoretic grounds and convincing experimental data.[3,6] Equally important, it is easily understood by clinicians.

The rationale rests on actual measurements of venous diameter carried out in 100 normal extremities (using ultrasonic imaging) and in 33 limbs with DVT (using venograms). The results of VOP tracings in all limbs were correlated with the minimum venous diameter measured in the proximal veins. For a given degree of venous outflow obstruction, the time constant of venous outflow (τ) was found to vary with the amount of venous filling (VC). In mathematical terms, $\tau / VC = $ constant.* For convenience, τ / VC is referred to as F. In any given patient, the F value is constant, regardless of the degree of venous filling, and reflects the degree of venous outflow obstruction. In addition to studies in patients and normal volunteers, this observation

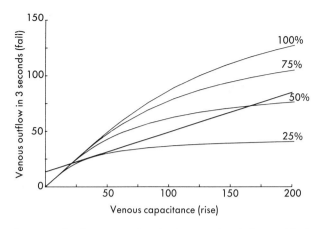

Fig. 98-9. The discriminant line divides normal and abnormal limbs at about 50% of normal venous outflow capacity. (From Anderson FA Jr: *Quantification of the degree of venous outflow obstruction from venous occlusion plethysmography,* Worcester, Mass, Worcester Polytechnic Institute, 1984 [dissertation].)

has also been confirmed in a laboratory model of the venous system of the leg under widely varying conditions.[3,6]

In 100 normal legs, the mean F value was 0.63 ± 0.16. An F value of 0.63 was therefore taken as 100% of predicted venous diameter. An inverse relationship was found between VDI and F. Thus VDI $= 63/F$. VDI in the 100 normal limbs varied from 63% to 188%, whereas the VDI in 33 limbs with DVT varied from 1% to 38%.

Precise calculation of VDI from F values is facilitated by a computer. However, it is also possible simply to plot VO_3 and VC on a routine scoring graph to which curves approximating VDI values of 100%, 75%, 50%, and 25% have been added (Fig. 98-9). The approximate VDI can then be estimated from the graph.

CLINICAL USES OF IPG
Evaluation of symptomatic patients

The most common use for IPG is to evaluate a patient with clinically suspected DVT. Patients often complain of minor signs or symptoms suggesting the possibility of DVT. Many times the clinical suspicion is so slight that the physician hesitates to order a venogram with its attendant discomfort, inconvenience, and expense. Duplex scanning may also be used, but it is expensive and may not be available in small hospitals.[2] However, physicians are also well aware that patients can harbor life-threatening thrombi in the deep veins, even though they may have minimal signs or symptoms. Therefore clinicians need a simple, readily available noninvasive test that assesses the patient's present risk of significant thromboembolism. With a clearly normal IPG test result, the clinician can be confident that the patient does not have sufficient venous thrombosis to pose the threat of major pulmonary embolism (see Chapter 105).

Even when the clinical diagnosis of DVT has been made on an apparently firm basis, IPG is useful in confirming the diagnosis. In the past, such patients have often been sub-

---

*The potential value of this ratio in interpretation of VOP tracings was first suggested by Frank Ingle, Ph.D.

jected to prolonged anticoagulant treatment on the strength of the clinical diagnosis alone. Many studies have now demonstrated the fallibility of the clinical diagnosis of DVT,[8,11,17,41] even when the signs and symptoms appear to be typical. Before a patient is treated on clinical grounds alone, the diagnosis of DVT must be confirmed with some objective diagnostic method.

Prospective clinical trials have demonstrated the usefulness of IPG in the management of outpatients with symptoms suggestive of DVT.[24,25,32,34] In the context of a normal IPG, the incidence of subsequent DVT or pulmonary embolism in these patients is no higher than that in similar patients who have normal venograms.[29] Thus even patients with clinical symptoms that strongly suggest DVT can be managed safely as outpatients without further testing or treatment if they have normal IPG findings, provided follow-up IPG testing is carried out according to a standard protocol.[24,25,32,34]

Screening of asymptomatic patients

The value of IPG for screening asymptomatic patients at risk depends on the expected incidence of DVT. When low-dose heparin or other prophylactic measures are employed, the occurrence of DVT is so infrequent in some patient groups that routine screening is not justified.[7] However, in patients in whom such prophylaxis is contraindicated or in patients who are at unusually high risk for DVT, IPG is a useful screening technique (Fig. 98-10).

Some investigators have questioned the use of IPG for screening asymptomatic patients because of its low sensitivity in the diagnosis of calf vein thrombi. Since the calf contains many veins in parallel, there is usually no detectable impairment in venous outflow until several veins are obstructed. However, the likelihood of major pulmonary embolism is extremely low in patients with normal impedance test results.[24,34,35,62]

In one study, no fatal pulmonary emboli were observed in 1074 patients with normal IPG tests; in only 1% of these patients was there even a suspicion of nonfatal pulmonary embolism.[62] A similar low incidence of thromboembolic complications has been reported in patients with normal noninvasive test results of other types (see Chapter 105).

It should be emphasized that normal IPG findings do *not* guarantee the patient will not suffer major venous thrombosis at a later date. When patients have continuing risk factors, repeat testing should be done every 48 hours for as long as the patient remains at high risk.[25,34]

IPG has been advocated for screening patients after total hip replacement in combination with the radiolabeled fibrinogen uptake test,[22,27] but because radiolabeled fibrinogen is no longer commercially available in the United States, this approach is now obsolete. By itself, IPG is not a satisfactory end point for screening this group of patients because recent studies have shown that a false-negative IPG finding may occur in the presence of an asymptomatic, nonocclusive thrombus proximal to the knee.[1,10,13,45] Duplex

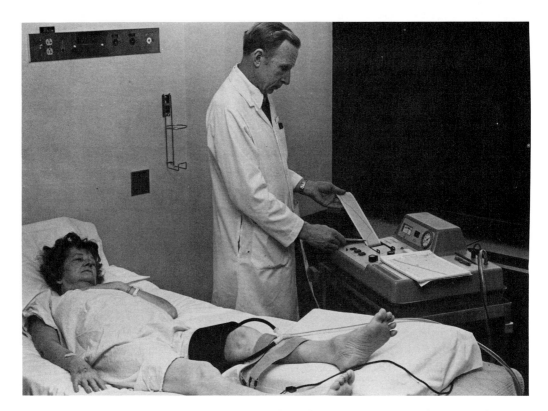

Fig. 98-10. Screening a patient 4 days after aortofemoral reconstruction. A normal tracing excludes thrombosis in the major veins with 99% certainty.

scanning, venography, or both may be more appropriate screening methods after total hip replacement.[53]

Evaluation of suspected pulmonary embolism

IPG is also useful in the evaluation of suspected pulmonary embolism, since practically all pulmonary emboli are associated with thrombosis of the leg veins. The finding of normal IPG results in a patient with suspected pulmonary embolism casts doubt on this diagnosis.[48]

A common diagnostic approach for suspected pulmonary embolism is to combine IPG and radionuclide lung scanning. When both test results are negative, clinically significant pulmonary embolism is virtually ruled out. When both are positive, this establishes the diagnosis of pulmonary embolism. When the results of IPG and the lung scan disagree, a pulmonary angiogram may be required to establish the diagnosis. Results of a recent randomized prospective study have shown that it is safe to withhold anticoagulant treatment in patients with clinically suspected pulmonary embolism and a negative IPG, even when the lung scan suggests a low probability of embolism.[35]

Long-term management of DVT

Recent thrombosis in the popliteal, femoral, or iliac vein typically provides a marked delay in venous outflow following release of the thigh cuff. There is usually an impairment of venous capacitance as well. However, as days go by, the venous capacitance improves and often returns to normal. The venous outflow rate improves more gradually but may also return to normal as collateral pathways develop.[38] (It is sometimes useful in patients with abnormal venous outflow and a history of old DVT to place the leg slightly dependent and look for respiratory venous excursions. These are typically seen in cases of old DVT but have not been observed in fresh venous thrombosis.) If recanalization of the vein occurs as a result of lysis, the IPG result reverts to normal. Sequential IPG results thus give the clinician an objective assessment of the extent of venous outflow obstruction.[23,24,33] Sometimes significant outflow obstruction persists in patients who no longer exhibit any clinical signs or symptoms to suggest DVT. Such patients should be continued on anticoagulant therapy, even though they may appear to have recovered completely according to clinical criteria.

IPG has been used in this fashion to help determine the appropriate duration of anticoagulant treatment. Although most patients with proved thrombosis are maintained on oral anticoagulants for 6 months, some patients are difficult to manage on an outpatient basis. Continued anticoagulant therapy poses a risk. Under these circumstances, the physician may consider discontinuing anticoagulant therapy if the IPG findings have reverted to normal.

When the IPG test continues to show significant venous outflow obstruction, the risk of recurrent thrombophlebitis is higher. Since venous stasis is well recognized as one of the major factors predisposing to recurrence, physicians may

be reluctant to discontinue anticoagulation therapy in such patients. Recurrent thrombophlebitis is rare in patients with normal IPG tests in whom anticoagulant medication is discontinued.

In the future, IPG may be used to evaluate other pathophysiologic states in which peripheral hemodynamics are altered. The striking influence of peripheral vasoconstriction and reduced blood flow on venous capacitance offers promise for clinical usefulness once these parameters have been more fully studied.

PRELIMINARY SCREENING BEFORE VENOGRAPHY OR DUPLEX SCANNING

In some hospitals, venography remains the gold standard for establishing the diagnosis of DVT, but its invasive character, inconvenience, discomfort, and cost limit its widespread use. Low-cost screening techniques, such as IPG or the handheld Doppler flowmeter, have proved useful for initial screening or long-term follow-up in combination with the selective use of venography to provide anatomic visualization and to confirm a questionable IPG diagnosis. Because of the lower cost of IPG, as compared to duplex scanning or venography, such an approach is highly cost effective. Patients with normal IPG results are at low risk for suffering clinically important DVT or pulmonary embolism, and venography can be limited to selected patients with abnormal IPG findings.

During the 1980s, high-resolution B-mode ultrasonic scanning revolutionized the management of DVT. Like IPG, ultrasonic scanning is noninvasive and readily accepted by patients, even for repeat examinations. If necessary, it can be performed at the bedside. It can directly visualize the venous system and occasionally a thrombus. In many hospitals, B-mode or duplex ultrasonography has replaced venography as the gold standard in the anatomic diagnosis of DVT.[15] However, the high cost of ultrasonic equipment, competing demands for the ultrasonic imaging system, and the need for a highly skilled technologist or sonographer to perform the test have resulted in IPG's continued use in many institutions. Even where duplex scanning is readily available, IPG has been used as a convenient low-cost screening method, reserving duplex scanning for those patients with abnormal IPG findings or patients with special problems.

COST-BENEFIT ANALYSIS OF IPG

In proposing any new medical test, the proponent must be sensitive to the cost of the procedure and its potential effect on the already overwhelming cost of medical care. The public and third-party payers rightfully wish to know that new technology and new test procedures will not add further to this cost burden without providing corresponding benefits. Fortunately, with respect to IPG, the case for cost benefit seems as compelling as the case for medical benefit (see Chapter 107).[20,29,30,44]

The cost of IPG in most hospitals is roughly equivalent

to that of an electrocardiogram, usually $50 to $100. This is a relatively low charge in view of the large saving made possible by eliminating unnecessary or delayed treatment. Based on the findings from studies examining the accuracy of the clinical diagnosis of venous thrombosis,[8,11,41] the likelihood of preventing unnecessary treatment appears to be 40% or more. Avoiding an unnecessary hospitalization for the treatment of DVT translates into considerable cost saving and eliminates the risks of anticoagulant treatment and time lost from work.

In 1991, the Medicare reimbursement for treatment of pulmonary embolism was $5286 (DGR 078). Even occasionally eliminating the cost of such hospitalizations would justify a great many test procedures. In addition, under a provider-at-risk reimbursement system, any cost savings will directly benefit hospitals by allowing them to keep their costs low. The cost-conscious environment created by DGRs and other forms of prospective payment may lead to reexamination of the merits of low-cost screening methods that have demonstrated high accuracy and yielded excellent patient outcomes.

The cost benefit of IPG is greatest in symptomatic patients, approximately two thirds of whom will have normal IPG results, making venography or anticoagulant therapy unnecessary.[24,25,32,34] Duplex ultrasonic scanning can also be employed for screening such patients but is much more expensive. Typical hospital and professional charges for duplex venous scanning range between $300 and $600 (3 to 12 times the typical charge for IPG testing). Venography is even more expensive, besides being invasive. In asymptomatic patients, the cost effectiveness of IPG depends on the expected incidence of DVT in the patient group being studied. IPG is not cost effective when applied randomly because of the low incidence of DVT in a general hospital population. It is cost effective when used selectively in patients at high risk, such as in the late follow-up of patients undergoing total hip reconstruction.[30,40]

IPG often leads to a firm diagnosis of venous thrombosis earlier in the patient's hospital course than might otherwise have been the case. The duration of treatment also seems likely to be shorter and the medical complications less serious under these circumstances. Cost savings should be significant, although they are difficult to document.

The low cost of IPG, coupled with the frequent errors in clinical diagnosis (both false positive and false negative), makes a strong case for the cost effectiveness of this diagnostic procedure.[20,30]

CONCLUSION

The accuracy of IPG has now been thoroughly documented in the literature, with an aggregate 93% sensitivity and 94% specificity in all reported series (see Table 105-6). The accuracy is even higher in symptomatic patients. It is widely employed in major medical centers and community hospitals. It is a simple, safe procedure that is free of discomfort or inconvenience and provides immediate and reliable re-sults at the bedside or in the clinic. It is particularly useful for outpatient evaluation, which eliminates many unnecessary hospital admissions and is highly cost effective.

The principal liability of the method has been false-positive or equivocal results in patients with pathophysiologic conditions other than DVT that also affect the peripheral circulation. Severe peripheral vasoconstriction, congestive heart failure, hypotension, and severe pulmonary disease may all elicit abnormal findings as a result of reduced compliance of the venous system. The incidence of false-positive results in such patients is markedly reduced by multiple repetitions of the test procedure or by prolonging the duration of cuff occlusion.

Quantitative methods for interpreting IPG results have recently been developed. Reporting test results quantitatively with an established range of normal for reference purposes makes IPG results more understandable to clinicians and promises to further increase the usefulness of this common diagnostic test.

REFERENCES

1. Agnelli G et al: Impedance plethysmography in the diagnosis of asymptomatic deep vein thrombosis in hip surgery: a venography-controlled study, *Arch Intern Med* 151:2167, 1991.
2. Ahola SJ et al: Effects of physician education on the evaluation of deep venous thrombosis in a small community hospital, *Conn Med* 47:392, 1983.
3. Anderson FA Jr: *Quantification of the degree of venous outflow obstruction from venous occlusion plethysmography*, Worcester, Mass, 1984, Worcester Polytechnic Institute, (doctoral dissertation).
4. Anderson FA Jr, Cardullo PC: Problems commonly encountered in IPG testing and their solution, *Bruit* 4:21, 1980.
5. Anderson FA Jr, Wheeler HB: Venous occusion plethysmography for the detection of venous thrombosis, *Med Instrum* 13:350, 1979.
6. Anderson FA Jr et al: *Non-invasive quantification of the degree of venous outflow obstruction in the extremities by means of venous occlusion plethysmography*. In Bartel DL, ed: *1983 Advances in bioengineering*, New York, 1983, American Society of Mechanical Engineers.
7. Anderson FA Jr et al: A population-based perspective of the hospital incidence and case-fatality rates of venous thrombosis and pulmonary embolism: the Worcester DVT study, *Arch Intern Med* 151:933, 1991.
8. Browse N: Deep vein thrombosis—diagnosis, *Br Med J* 4:676, 1969.
9. Clarke-Pearson DL, Creasman WT: Diagnosis of deep venous thrombosis in obstetrics and gynecology by impedance phlebography, *Obstet Gynecol* 58:52, 1981.
10. Comerota AJ et al: The comparative value of noninvasive testing for diagnosis and surveillance of deep vein thrombosis, *J Vasc Surg* 7:40, 1988.
11. Coon WW, Coller FA: Clinicopathologic correlation in thromboembolism, *Surg Gynecol Obstet* 109:259, 1959.
12. Cooperman M et al: Detection of deep venous thrombosis by impedance plethysmography, *Am J Surg* 137:252, 1979.
13. Cruickshank ML et al: An evaluation of impedance plethysmography and ^{125}I-fibrinogen leg scanning in patients following hip surgery, *Thromb Haemost* 62:830, 1989.
14. Dahn I, Eriksson E: Plethysmographic diagnosis of deep vein thrombosis of the leg, *Acta Chir Scand* [Suppl] 398:33, 1968.
15. de Valois JC et al: Contrast venography: from gold standard to 'golden backup' in clinically suspected deep vein thrombosis, *Eur J Radiol* 11:131, 1990.
16. Dmochowski JR, Adams DF, Couch NP: Impedance measurement in the diagnosis of deep vein thrombosis, *Arch Surg* 104:170, 1972.
17. Flanc C, Kakkar VV, Clarke MB: The detection of venous thrombosis of the legs using ^{125}I-labelled fibrinogen, *Br J Surg* 55:742, 1968.
18. Flanigan DP et al: Vascular-laboratory diagnosis of clinically suspected acute deep-vein thrombosis, *Lancet* 2:331, 1978.

19. Foti ME, Gurewich V: Fibrin degradation products and impedance plethysmography: measurements in the diagnosis of acute deep vein thrombosis, *Arch Intern Med* 140:903, 1980.
20. Gross WS, Burney RE: Therapeutic and economic implications of emergency department evaluation for venous thrombosis, *J Am Coll Emer Physicians* 8:110, 1979.
21. Gross WS et al: *Role of the vascular laboratory in the diagnosis of venous thrombosis.* In Bergan JJ, Yao JST, eds: *Venous problems,* Chicago, 1978, Mosby.
22. Harris WH et al: Cuff-impedance phlebography and ^{125}I-fibrinogen scanning versus roentgenographic phlebography for diagnosis of thrombophlebitis following hip surgery, *J Bone Joint Surg* [Am] 58:939, 1976.
23. Hirsh J: Clinical ability of impedance plethysmography in the diagnosis of recurrent deep-vein thrombosis, *Arch Intern Med* 148:519, 1988.
24. Huisman MV, Buller HR, ten Cate JW: Utility of impedance plethysmography in the diagnosis of recurrent deep-vein thrombosis, *Arch Intern Med* 148:681, 1988.
25. Huisman MV et al: Serial impedance plethysmography for suspected deep venous thrombosis in outpatients: the Amsterdam general practitioner study, *N Engl J Med* 314:823, 1986.
26. Hull R et al: Impedance plethysmography using the occlusive cuff technique in the diagnosis of venous thrombosis, *Circulation* 53:696, 1976.
27. Hull R et al: Combined use of leg scanning and impedance plethysmography in suspected venous thrombosis: an alternative to venography, *N Engl J Med* 296:1497, 1977.
28. Hull R et al: Impedance plethysmography: the relationship between venous filling and sensitivity and specificity for proximal vein thrombosis, *Circulation* 58:898, 1978.
29. Hull R et al: Clinical validity of a negative venogram in patients with clinically suspected venous thrombosis, *Circulation* 64:622, 1981.
30. Hull R et al: Cost effectiveness of clinical diagnosis, venography and noninvasive testing in patients with symptomatic deep-vein thrombosis, *N Engl J Med* 304:1561, 1981.
31. Hull R et al: Replacement of venography in suspected venous thrombosis by impedance plethysmography and ^{125}I-fibrinogen leg scanning: a less invasive approach, *Ann Intern Med* 94:12, 1981.
32. Hull RD, Raskob GE, Carter CJ: Serial impedance plethysmography in pregnant patients with clinically suspected deep-vein thrombosis, *Ann Intern Med* 112:663, 1990.
33. Hull RD et al: The diagnosis of acute, recurrent deep-vein thrombosis: a diagnostic challenge, *Circulation* 67:901, 1983.
34. Hull RD et al: Diagnostic efficacy of impedance plethysmography for clinically suspected deep-vein thrombosis: a randomized trial, *Ann Intern Med* 102:21, 1985.
35. Hull RD et al: A new noninvasive management strategy for patients with suspected pulmonary embolism, *Arch Intern Med* 149:2549, 1989.
36. Hume M et al: Extent of leg vein thrombosis determined by impedance and ^{125}I-fibrinogen, *Am J Surg* 129:455, 1975.
37. Hume M et al: Venous thrombosis after total hip replacement: combined monitoring as a guide for prophylaxis and treatment, *J Bone Joint Surg* [Am] 58:933, 1976.
38. Jay R et al: Outcome of abnormal impedance plethysmography results in patients with proximal-vein thrombosis: frequency of return to normal, *Thromb Res* 36:259, 1984.
39. Johnston KW, Kakkar VV: Plethysmographic diagnosis of deep vein thrombosis, *Surg Gynecol Obstet* 139:41, 1974.
40. Mallory TH et al: Impedance plethysmography for surveillance of deep venous thrombosis following early discharge of total joint replacement patients, *Orthopedics* 13:1347, 1990.
41. McLachlin J, Richard T, Paterson JC: An evaluation of clinical signs in the diagnosis of deep venous thrombosis, *Arch Surg* 85:738, 1962.
42. Mullick SC, Wheeler HB, Songster GF: Diagnosis of deep vein thrombosis by measurement of electrical impedance, *Am J Surg* 119:417, 1970.
43. Nadeau JE et al: Impedance phlebography: accuracy of diagnosis in deep vein thrombosis, *Can J Surg* 18:219, 1975.
44. O'Donnell TF Jr et al: The socioeconomic effects of an iliofemoral venous thrombosis, *J Surg Res* 22:483, 1977.
45. Paiement G et al: Surveillance of deep vein thrombosis in asymptomatic total hip replacement patients: impedance phlebography and fibrinogen scanning versus roentgenographic phlebography, *Am J Surg* 155:400, 1988.
46. Patterson RB et al: The limitations of impedance plethysmography in the diagnosis of acute deep vein thrombosis, *J Vasc Surg* 9:725, 1989.
47. Richards KL et al: Noninvasive diagnosis of deep venous thrombosis, *Arch Intern Med* 136:1091, 1976.
48. Sasahara AA: Current problems in pulmonary embolism: introduction, *Prog Cardiovasc Dis* 17:161, 1974.
49. Seeber JJ: Impedance plethysmography: a useful method in the diagnosis of deep vein thrombophlebitis in the lower extremity, *Arch Phys Med Rehabil* 55:170, 1974.
50. Steer ML et al: Limitations of impedance plethysmography for diagnosis of venous thrombosis, *Arch Surg* 106:44, 1973.
51. Taylor DW et al: Simplification of the sequential impedance plethysmograph technique without loss of accuracy, *Thromb Res* 17:561, 1980.
52. Toy PCTY, Schrier SL: Occlusive impedance plethysmography, *West J Med* 90:89, 1978.
53. Wheeler HB: Diagnosis of deep vein thrombosis: using the right test for the right purpose, *Arch Intern Med* 151:2145, 1991.
54. Wheeler HB, Anderson FA Jr: *Impedance plethysmography.* In Yao SJT, Kempcninski RF, eds: *Practical noninvasive vascular diagnosis,* Chicago, 1987, Mosby.
55. Wheeler HB, Mullick SC: Detection of venous obstruction in the leg by measurement of electrical impedance, *Ann NY Acad Sci* 170:804, 1970.
56. Wheeler HB, Patwardhan NA: *Evaluation of venous thrombosis by impedance plethysmography.* In Madden JL, Hume M, eds: *Venous thromboembolism: prevention and treatment,* New York, 1976, Appleton-Lange.
57. Wheeler HB, Patwardhan NA, Anderson FA Jr: *The place of occlusive impedance plethysmography in the diagnosis of venous thrombosis.* In Bergan JJ, Yao JST, eds: *Venous problems,* Chicago, 1978, Mosby.
58. Wheeler HB et al: Diagnosis of occult deep vein thrombosis by a noninvasive bedside technique, *Surgery* 70:20, 1971.
59. Wheeler HB et al: Impedance phlebography: technique, interpretation and results, *Arch Surg* 104:164, 1972.
60. Wheeler HB et al: Bedside screening for venous thrombosis using occlusive impedance phlebography, *Angiology* 26:199, 1975.
61. Wheeler HB et al: Occlusive impedance phlebography: a diagnostic procedure for venous thrombosis and pulmonary embolism, *Prog Cardiovasc Dis* 17:199, 1974.
62. Wheeler HB et al: Suspected deep vein thrombosis: management by impedance plethysmography, *Arch Surg* 117:1206, 1982.

CHAPTER 99

Diagnosis of deep vein thrombosis by air-plethysmography

ANDREW N. NICOLAIDES, EVI KALODIKI, DIMITRIS CHRISTOPOULOS,
MIGUEL LEON, and NICOS VOLTEAS

The use of segmental plethysmographic methods such as strain-gauge and impedance plethysmography to diagnose deep vein thrombosis (DVT) is based on the observation that the ratio of venous outflow to venous volume decreases in the presence of thrombosis in the major veins (see Chapters 96, 97, and 98). In normal limbs, temporary venous obstruction provided by a thigh pneumatic cuff causes a marked increase in venous volume followed by a rapid venous outflow when the cuff is deflated. If there is a thrombus in the major axial deep veins, the initial volume increase is reduced because the veins are already distended to a certain extent and the venous outflow rate is decreased, often dramatically.

Quantitative air-plethysmography (APG), which can measure volume changes in the whole leg in absolute units (milliliters) (see Chapter 23), arterial inflow in milliliters per minute (see Chapter 60), and venous reflux in milliliters per second (see Chapter 112), can also be used in the detection of DVT. APG has three advantages over segmental plethysmography: it assesses the whole leg, volume changes can be expressed in absolute units, and because it encloses all tissues from knee to ankle, the tissue shifts inherent to segmental plethysmography are avoided, resulting in higher reproducibility.

METHOD

The patient is examined in the supine position, with the knee of the affected leg slightly flexed and elevated and the heel supported 15 cm above the horizontal. The air chamber is inflated to 6 mm Hg, which is the lowest pressure that ensures good contact between the air chamber and the limb but with minimum compression of the veins (see Chapter 23). To calibrate the equipment, the plunger of the syringe (Fig. 99-1) is depressed; this compresses the air in the APG (air chamber and tubing), reducing its volume by 100 ml, and the corresponding pressure change is observed. After calibration, the plunger is pulled back to its original position once the pressure in the air chamber returns to 6 mm Hg.

An 11-cm-wide pneumatic tourniquet with a 40-cm-long

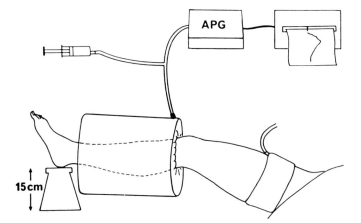

Fig. 99-1. Position of the leg and APG for recording volume changes in the diagnosis of DVT.

bladder is placed on the proximal thigh. When a stable leg-air-chamber-room temperature gradient has been reached, 10 minutes after the air chamber is inflated, the tourniquet is inflated to 70 mm Hg and maintained at this pressure until maximum filling is obtained, as shown by a plateau on the recorder (Fig. 99-2). This usually takes 2 to 3 minutes. The long saphenous vein at the medial aspect of the knee is compressed digitally or by using a specially designed wedge* attached to a band with a Velcro strip, and the tourniquet is deflated rapidly. Rapid deflation is essential and is achieved by the wide tubing (1-cm internal diameter) and a large valve.† The venous volume and the 1-second venous outflow (in milliliters) are obtained from the recording (Fig. 99-2) and plotted on a graph with a discriminant line that distinguishes normal from abnormal results (Fig. 99-3).

---

*ACI Medical, Sun Valley, Calif.
†D. E. Hokanson, Bellevue, Wash.

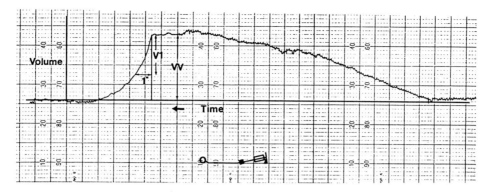

Fig. 99-2. Recording of the venous volume after inflation of the thigh cuff and outflow curve during rapid deflation. V_I, 1-second outflow in ml; VV, venous volume in ml.

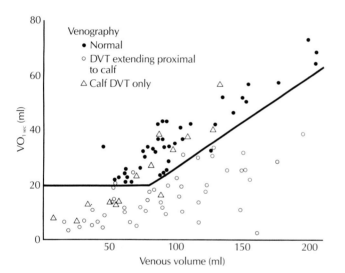

Fig. 99-3. This plot shows the 1-second venous outflow (VO_1) against venous volume and the discriminant line.

Table 99-1. Air-plethysmography compared with venography*

| | Air-plethysmography | | |
Venography	Positive	Negative	Total
Proximal DVT	45 (94%)	3	48
Isolated calf DVT	7 (50%)	7	14
Normal venogram	1	39 (97.5%)	40

*Sensitivity for proximal DVT, 94%; sensitivity for calf DVT, 50%; specificity, 97.5%.

RESULTS

The APG findings from a series of 102 patients who presented with clinical symptoms and signs of DVT are shown in Fig. 99-3. Venography was performed in all. The venogram was normal in 40, isolated calf thrombi were four in 14, and thrombosis extending proximal to the calf (popliteal, femoral, and iliac) was noted in 48. The results are summarized in Table 99-1. The sensitivity of APG for detecting thrombosis proximal to the calf was 94%, and its specificity was 97.5%. As with other plethysmographic tests, its sensitivity for identifying calf DVT is poor.

CLINICAL APPLICATION

The results just presented are encouraging but need to be validated by further studies. The effect of increasing the arterial inflow by gentle active plantar flexion and dorsiflexion of the foot just before repeating the test in borderline cases should also be investigated to determine whether it can improve the test's discrimination. Combining APG with liquid-crystal thermography (LCT) may improve the accuracy for detecting all DVTs. A negative APG result may miss the presence of calf DVT and proximal partially occluding DVT. However, a negative LCT finding (see Chapter 102) plus a negative APG result will reliably exclude all thrombi. This combination of APG and LCT is practical for use in a busy department where the time available on a duplex scanner is limited. A positive thermogram but negative APG result suggests the existence of a calf or partially occluding proximal DVT, and such patients should be further tested with duplex scanning.

A positive APG indicates the existence of proximal DVT, and treatment may then be instituted with or without duplex confirmation. However, if the APG result is positive, the duplex examination will be much faster because the examiner can then concentrate on confirming the presence of thrombosis in the proximal veins.

The use of APG and LCT for the diagnosis of DVT may at first appear to represent a backward step for the 1990s, which is the era of duplex scanning. When looked at in a different light, however, the considerations mentioned constitute possible ways to save time and money in busy noninvasive laboratories and hospitals where there is also a limit on the fees that can be charged for a duplex scan. Such alternatives offer the possibility of greater cost effectiveness without a sacrifice in standards or diagnostic accuracy.

CHAPTER 100

Significance of a negative duplex scan for deep vein thrombosis

LOUIS M. MESSINA and LAZAR J. GREENFIELD

Acute deep vein thrombosis (DVT) is a common vascular disorder that is diagnosed in up to 800,000 new patients per year, with acute pulmonary embolism developing in approximately 5% of these patients. In addition, the post-thrombotic syndrome will develop in up to 35%, resulting in long-term disability. Because the diagnosis of DVT cannot be made reliably on the basis of clinical signs and symptoms, some objective diagnostic study is necessary for this purpose.[2] Until recently, contrast venography had been the only modality available for the accurate diagnosis of DVT. Because it is associated with a significant incidence of serious complications and its practical limitations prevent serial examinations, a number of alternative noninvasive diagnostic methods have been evaluated over the past two decades. One of these, duplex ultrasonography, shows a high degree of sensitivity and specificity in the diagnosis of acute DVT and is readily repeatable. Consequently, it is rapidly supplanting contrast venography as the most widely used diagnostic test in the initial evaluation of patients with suspected acute DVT.[1,4,5-7,9,12-13]

A number of important issues concerning the role of venous duplex ultrasonography in the diagnosis of DVT remain unresolved, however. Considerable variability exists in the criteria used for diagnosing DVT as well as in the anatomic extent studied by the venous duplex examination.[4,8,11,13] Despite these concerns, a positive venous duplex scan is increasingly accepted as sufficient evidence of DVT. It is less certain to what extent and when a negative scan fits into the algorithm of the evaluation of the patients with suspected acute DVT. A false-negative study represents a serious error because it leaves the patient at risk for life-threatening pulmonary embolism. To address this problem, a clinical study[10] was conducted that asked the following questions: Is a negative venous scan sufficiently accurate to exclude the diagnosis of DVT, thus precluding the need for venography? What is the risk of withholding anticoagulation from patients with suspected acute DVT on the sole basis of a negative duplex scan?

To find the answers to these questions, a retrospective review was done of the hospital records, duplex scan results, and follow-up data in 570 consecutive patients who were referred to the diagnostic vascular laboratory at the Uni-versity of Michigan to be examined for DVT. The patients' presenting signs and symptoms and the results of venous duplex scanning were compiled. In addition, for those patients in whom there was persistent clinical suspicion of DVT despite the results of duplex scanning, the results of any follow-up venogram or repeat duplex scan were obtained. Because this study was done at a time when referring physicians were still becoming familiar with venous duplex scanning, a significant number of patients underwent venography after the duplex scanning. The results of venous duplex scanning and venography in these patients were correlated so that the specificity (true negative/true positive plus false-negative) of a negative duplex scan could be calculated. This study population should represent a worst case scenario for calculating the specificity of a negative scan because the patients were identified clinically as those most likely to have a positive study.

All patients underwent bilateral venous duplex scanning with color flow imaging using a 7.5-MHz ultrasound probe, and this included imaging of the common femoral, superficial femoral, popliteal, and posterior tibial veins. The effect of a Valsalva's maneuver on the Doppler flow signal in the common femoral vein was used as an indirect test for the presence of thrombus in the iliac veins. The criteria used to diagnose acute DVT were incompressibility of the vein during light probe pressure; abnormal Doppler flow signals, including absence of spontaneous flow or loss of phasicity of flow with respiration; and failure to increase flow velocity with distal augmentation (Fig. 100-1). Frequently, the presence of an intraluminal clot was noted by its echogenecity. DVT was also usually associated with a more dilated vein than that on the contralateral normal side. The study obtained from a venous segment was considered "adequate" when the aforementioned duplex criteria could be assessed satisfactorily. The criteria for determining a normal venous duplex scan consisted of complete compressibility of the vein with light probe pressure, no evidence of intraluminal thrombus, visualization of good blood flow throughout the vein, and normal Doppler signals. Follow-up was obtained in all patients with a negative duplex scan to ascertain whether signs and symptoms of either recurrent DVT or pulmonary embolism occurred after the negative

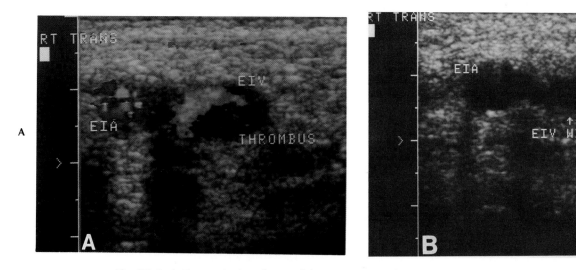

Fig. 100-1. ***A,*** Transverse view of external iliac artery *(EIA)* and vein *(EIV)* by color-flow duplex scanning that shows partially occluding thrombus. ***B,*** Noncolor flow ultrasound image of the same vessels that shows incompressibility of the external iliac vein due to presence of thrombus. Incompressibility of a vein due to thrombus is the primary diagnostic criterion of duplex scanning for acute venous thrombus.

duplex scan studies. If a patient died during the follow-up period, the specific cause of death was identified.

Of the 570 consecutive patients, the duplex scans were negative in 431. The presenting signs and symptoms in all were typical of suspected acute DVT. Lower extremity swelling, found in 230 patients, was the most common presenting sign. There was pain in the affected extremity in 160 of the patients. Of the 22 patients who were seen because of shortness of breath, 9 were deemed to have a high probability of pulmonary embolism based on a ventilation-perfusion scan. A total of 9 patients underwent duplex scanning to identify the source of a pulmonary embolism previously identified on angiography. Finally, 9 patients had experienced an acute exacerbation or worsening of signs and symptoms of chronic venous disease.

After venous duplex scanning, 66 patients were referred for venography because of a persistent clinical suspicion of DVT despite a negative venous duplex scan. All of these venograms were performed within 48 hours of the venous duplex scan. The specificity of a negative venous duplex scan in the subgroup of patients who had a negative venous duplex scan was found to be 95%; acute DVT was ruled out by venography in 56 of the 59 patients with negative scans. The three false-negative venous duplex scans were in patients who had isolated peroneal vein thrombi detected by venography. At the time of this study, only the posterior tibial veins in the calf were routinely imaged, and no effort was made to detect isolated peroneal vein thrombi. More recently venous duplex scanning has been extended to include the iliac veins as well as all three sets of calf veins.[11] In 10 of the 431 patients, the venous duplex scan was interpreted to indicate chronic DVT and was specifically considered to rule out acute DVT. Chronic DVT was diagnosed

on the basis of a highly echogenic thrombus surrounding the lumen of a recanalized vein, usually associated with veins of smaller diameter. In all of these patients with chronic DVT diagnosed by venous duplex scans, there was a 100% correlation with the results of venography. Follow-up information was obtained in all 431 patients with negative duplex scans for a mean period of 8 months after they underwent scanning; any untoward outcome of a negative venous duplex scan would occur during this interval. During this period, there were two deaths, one due to cancer and another due to renal failure. There were no episodes of pulmonary embolism nor was there any clinical evidence of recurrent or acute DVT in the remaining 429 patients.

These results demonstrate that a negative venous duplex scan can accurately exclude the existence of acute DVT in the lower extremity and rule out the need for routine venography. The specificity of 95% for a true-negative venous duplex scan found in our study is similar to that found by other investigators.[5,12] The follow-up results also indicate that withholding anticoagulation on the basis of a negative venous duplex scan is a safe and reasonable strategy.

Despite the findings of this study, there are limitations to the use of venous duplex imaging in patients with suspected acute DVT. It is not always possible to image all segments of the venous system from the common iliac veins to the level of the calf veins. Under such circumstances, it is best to perform venography if indicated clinically or, alternatively, to repeat the scan 24 to 48 hours later. The most common reason for difficulty in imaging the venous system is the presence of significant edema or obesity. When there is severe leg edema, most such patients have thromboses in other areas of the venous system, usually in the more proximal veins. Thus venous duplex scanning can facilitate determining the appropriate therapeutic approach even though not every segment of the venous system, particularly calf veins, may be imaged. By recognizing the limitations of venous duplex imaging in a particular patient with suspected acute DVT the overall value of duplex scanning as a diagnostic modality is enhanced.

Another consideration when evaluating the role of venous duplex scanning in the diagnosis of DVT is that it requires a high degree of skill and is initially associated with a learning curve. Frequent venographic confirmation of the duplex scan is essential when the operator is gaining initial experience with this modality. Similarly, any laboratory performing this study must maintain a rigorous quality assurance program to ensure the accuracy and consistency of results. Some of the criticisms of venous duplex scanning are directed at the nonrigorous manner of its application and not at the technique itself. However, many of the limitations of venous duplex scanning just discussed, including the frequency of equivocal studies, are shared by contrast venography.[7] Often these limitations are not recognized by clinicians. In a recent large prospective study, ascending venography was considered to be technically inadequate in 10% of the patients.[3] Under most circumstances, venographic imaging of the iliac veins requires skill and special techniques to obtain a complete study.[13] Up to 25% of the patients who require venography cannot have the test done because of technical reasons or have a study that is not interpretable.[1] In addition, there is considerable interobserver variability in the accuracy of interpreting venograms, with diagnostic errors in 10% of patients.[9] Perhaps most significantly, 2% to 3% of patients undergoing venography experience adverse reactions to the contrast material. In some patients, these reactions can result in life-threatening complications. Venography and venous duplex scanning can be viewed as complementary. Although venography is and will remain an essential study in the evaluation of all forms of venous disease, a carefully performed and critically analyzed venous duplex scan should be the initial diagnostic test in patients with suspected acute DVT. A negative duplex scan in such a patient can constitute sufficient reason for withholding anticoagulation and not performing venography.

REFERENCES

1. Aitken AGF, Godden DJ: Real-time ultrasound diagnosis of deep vein thrombosis: a comparison of venography, *Clin Radiol* 38:309-313, 1987.
2. Haeger K: Problems of acute deep venous thrombosis, *Angiology* 209:219-223, 1969.
3. Hull R et al: Replacement of venography in suspected venous thrombosis by impedance plethysmography and I-fibrinogen leg scanning, *Ann Intern Med* 94:12-15, 1981.
4. Killewich LA et al: Diagnosis of deep venous thrombosis: a prospective study comparing duplex scanning to contrast venography, *Circulation* 79:810-814, 1989.
5. Langsfeld M et al: Duplex B-mode imaging for the diagnosis of deep venous thrombosis, *Arch Surg* 122:587-591, 1987.
6. Lensing AWA et al: Detection of deep-vein thrombosis by real-time B-mode ultrasonography, *N Engl J Med* 320:342-345, 1989.
7. Naidich JB et al: Contrast venography: reassessment of its role, *Radiology* 168:97-100, 1988.
8. Nix ML et al: Duplex venous scanning: image vs Doppler accuracy, *J Vasc Tech* 12:121-126, 1989.
9. Redman HC: Deep venous thrombosis: is contrast venography still the diagnostic "gold standard?" *Radiology* 168:277-278, 1988.
10. Sarpa MS et al: Significance of a negative duplex scan in patients suspected of having acute deep vein thrombosis of the lower extremity, *J Vasc Tech* 13:224-226, 1989.
11. Sarpa MS et al: Reliability of venous duplex scanning to image the iliac veins and to diagnose iliac vein thrombosis in patients suspected of having acute deep venous thrombosis, *J Vasc Tech* 15:299-302, 1991.
12. Vogel P et al: Deep venous thrombosis of the lower extremity: US evaluation, *Radiology* 163:747-751, 1987.
13. White RJ et al: Diagnosis of deep-vein thrombosis using duplex ultrasound, *Ann Intern Med* 111:297-304, 1989.

CHAPTER 101

[^{125}I]fibrinogen leg scanning

RUSSELL D. HULL, GARY E. RASKOB, and JACK HIRSH

BACKGROUND AND PRINCIPLES OF USE

[^{125}I]fibrinogen leg scanning has been a useful research technique that has provided important information about the natural history, epidemiology, pathogenesis, and therapy for venous thrombosis. Leg scanning has also been useful as a diagnostic test when combined with impedance plethysmography in the assessment of symptomatic patients. Now, however, [^{125}I]fibrinogen leg scanning is mainly of historical interest for two reasons. First, clinical trials have established the safety of withholding anticoagulant therapy in symptomatic patients whose repeated impedance plethysmography or B-mode venous ultrasound results remain negative (see Chapter 104). Serial testing with either impedance plethysmography or B-mode ultrasound has thus replaced the combined approach of impedance plethysmography and leg scanning in symptomatic patients. Second, the concern about the possible transmission of HIV infection through the use of fibrinogen has led to the withdrawal of commercially prepared [^{125}I]fibrinogen from clinical use.

The diagnosis of venous thrombosis by radioiodine-labeled fibrinogen scanning depends on incorporation of circulating labeled fibrinogen into a developing or existing thrombus; this fibrinogen is then detected by measuring the increase of overlying surface radioactivity with an isotope detector. The feasibility of this technique was demonstrated in animals and humans[5] in the early 1960s; the method was then extensively evaluated over the ensuing decade.[17]

The equipment used initially for external scanning was cumbersome, but in more recent years, portable, convenient, and sensitive equipment has become available so that the test can be performed at the patient's bedside in approximately 15 minutes. Fibrinogen leg scanning is a sensitive method for detecting calf vein thrombosis and is relatively sensitive to thrombi in the midthigh and lower thigh. However, its accuracy is limited in the upper thigh, and it is totally insensitive to thrombi in the pelvis.[2,12] The insensitivity to thrombi in the pelvic veins occurs because [^{125}I]fibrinogen is a relatively low-energy gamma emitter, and its unreliability in the upper thigh is caused by high background counts as a result of radioactive urine in the bladder and circulating [^{125}I]fibrinogen in large veins and arteries.

DOSAGE, SIDE EFFECTS, AND PRECAUTIONS

The use of radioactive fibrinogen carries a theoretic risk of transmission of serum hepatitis, but this risk has been eliminated for practical purposes by preparing fibrinogen from a small number of carefully selected donors who have not transmitted hepatitis during years of frequent blood donation and who are free of hepatitis-associated antigen. However, as previously mentioned, of greater concern is the possibility that the use of [^{125}I]fibrinogen prepared from donors could transmit HIV infection. This risk could be eliminated if [^{125}I]fibrinogen were prepared from autologous plasma, and leg scanning using autologous radiolabeled fibrinogen could have potential applications in clinical trials of new prophylactic approaches.

^{125}I crosses the placenta, and a small amount enters the fetal circulation.[13] The radioactivity also appears in the breast milk of lactating women.[13] For these reasons, [^{125}I]fibrinogen scanning is contraindicated during pregnancy and lactation and should not be used in young patients unless very definite indications exist, since radioiodine accumulates in the thyroid gland.

Following the injection of 100 μCi of [^{125}I]fibrinogen, approximately 200 mrem is delivered to the blood, 20 mrem to tissues, and 5 mrem to the kidneys.[13] This is less than the acceptable annual total absorbed radiation dose (500 mrad/yr) recommended for the general population by the British National Council for Radiation Protection.[13]

SCANNING TECHNIQUE

Patients are scanned via a lightly shielded isotope detector probe with their legs elevated 15 degrees above horizontal to minimize venous pooling in the calf veins. Readings are taken over both legs and recorded as a percentage of the surface radioactivity measured over the heart. The surface radioactivity is measured over the femoral vein at 7- to 8-cm intervals starting just below the inguinal ligament and then at similar intervals over the medial and posterior aspects of the popliteal region and calf. The criteria for a positive leg scan have been established by a number of researchers. Venous thrombosis is suspected if there is an increase in the radioactive reading of more than 20% at any point compared with readings over adjacent points of the same leg, over the same point on a previous day, and at the corresponding point on the opposite leg. Venous thrombosis is diagnosed if the scan remains abnormal for more than 24 hours after repeated examination. The technique is simple and rapid, and up to 15 to 20 patients may be screened each day by one technician. Scanning time is limited by the in vivo survival of fibrinogen, so after a single injection of 100 μCi, counting is possible for about 7 days. The thyroid gland is blocked by a daily 100-mg dose of potassium iodide given orally for 14 days to prevent excessive uptake of radioiodine. If the patient is still at risk for developing venous thrombosis after 7 days, the injection can be repeated at intervals to extend the scanning time for the high-risk period.

USES AND LIMITATIONS OF [¹²⁵I]FIBRINOGEN LEG SCANNING

It is important to recognize that leg scanning has certain limitations. Its major limitations are its inability to detect venous thrombi above the inguinal ligament and its relative unreliability for detecting thrombi in the upper thigh.[3,12] High levels of surface radioactivity in the absence of venous thrombosis are seen in patients with superficial thrombophlebitis, hematoma, cellulitis, cutaneous vasculitis, and arthritis. High counts are also seen over surgical wounds in the legs, an important limitation in patients having leg or hip surgery. Finally, if used diagnostically in patients with clinically suspected venous thrombosis, the leg scan result may not become positive for hours and sometimes even for days after injection of the isotope.

The practical indications for using [¹²⁵I]fibrinogen leg scanning are as follows:
1. Screening certain high-risk patient groups in whom prophylaxis is either contraindicated or ineffective
2. As an adjunct to impedance plethysmography or Doppler ultrasound in the diagnosis of clinically suspected venous thrombosis
3. As a diagnostic test in patients with clinically suspected acute recurrent venous thrombosis
4. Screening patients who develop calf vein thrombosis when there are relative or absolute contraindications to anticoagulant therapy

Screening high-risk patients

Although screening high-risk patients by [¹²⁵I]fibrinogen leg scanning to detect and treat thrombi early in their development is one approach for preventing major venous thromboembolism, it is expensive and relatively inefficient.[9] Primary prophylaxis with small doses of heparin, intermittent calf compression, or in certain circumstances, dextran or oral anticoagulant prophylaxis is much more cost-effective and is the preferred approach in most patient groups.[9]

The cost effectiveness of primary prophylaxis versus secondary prevention by screening is illustrated by the findings from a cost-effectiveness analysis carried out in high-risk general surgical patients.[9] These findings are summarized in Table 101-1. Primary prophylaxis is clearly preferred to

Table 101-1. Total cost per 1000 patients of alternative approaches for the prevention of fatal pulmonary embolism in high-risk general surgical patients (1982)*

Strategy	Cost ($)
SUBCUTANEOUS ADMINISTRATION OF HEPARIN IN LOW DOSES	
Administration for 7 days in 1000 patients	20,000
Ascending venography in 10 patients	880
Lung scanning in 10 patients	1170
Treatment of venous thromboembolism in 8 patients	17,682
TOTAL	39,722
INTERMITTENT PNEUMATIC COMPRESSION OF THE LEGS	
Use for 7 days in 1000 patients	33,000
Venography in 10 patients	880
Lung scanning in 10 patients	1170
Treatment of venous thromboembolism in 8 patients	17,672
TOTAL	52,722
INTRAVENOUS ADMINISTRATION OF DEXTRAN	
Administration for 4 days to 1000 patients	103,000
Venography in 20 patients	1760
Lung scanning in 10 patients	1170
Treatment of venous thromboembolism in 13 patients	28,717
TOTAL	134,647
LEG SCANNING WITH [¹²⁵I]FIBRINOGEN	
Scanning for 7 days in 1000 patients	85,000
Venography in 135 patients	11,880
Lung scanning in 15 patients	1755
TOTAL	350,461
TRADITIONAL (NO PROGRAM) APPROACH	
Venography in 40 patients	3520
Lung scanning in 30 patients	3510
Treatment of venous thromboembolism in 33 patients	72,897
TOTAL	79,927

*Although the actual costs may have changed because of inflation, the rankings of the alternate approaches should remain the same.

screening. Leg scanning is the most expensive of the alternative approaches and necessitates full-dose anticoagulant treatment of large numbers of patients with subclinical venous thrombi. It should therefore be reserved for patients in whom primary prophylaxis is either contraindicated or unavailable. Leg scanning may occasionally be used in addition to primary prophylaxis in extremely high-risk patients, for example, those with a recent history of venous thrombosis who require surgery.

A number of researchers have compared results of expectant scanning and venography in general surgical and medical patients and have reported an accuracy for leg scanning of 90%.* As mentioned, leg scanning has special limitations when used to screen patients for thrombosis after

---

*References 1, 3, 5, 12, 15, 16.

leg surgery.[4] This is because extravascular isotope accumulation in the hematoma and the healing wound invariably leads to scanning abnormalities at the site of surgery, so thrombi near the wound cannot be detected. This is a major limitation in patients having hip surgery, since up to 20% of all thrombi (in about 10% of all patients) are isolated in the femoral vein close to the surgical wound.[4]

Harris et al[4] reported on the accuracy of [^{125}I]fibrinogen leg scanning in 83 patients who underwent leg scanning following elective hip surgery. All patients had venograms performed regardless of the result of the leg scan, and leg scanning was compared with venography in 142 limbs. The leg scan was positive in 85% of patients who had thrombi located venographically outside the area of surgery. However, because a large number of thrombi were isolated to the femoral vein close to the site of surgery, the overall accuracy was only 50%.

The positive predictive value of [^{125}I]fibrinogen leg scanning for the detection of venous thrombosis in high-risk patients has been evaluated.[7] Leg scanning was performed in 630 patients who had general surgical procedures and 385 patients who had hip surgery. Venography was performed if the leg scan was positive, and the positive predictive value was determined. This was 79% for general surgical patients and 86% for hip surgery patients. The patients were also screened with impedance plethysmography (IPG) to determine the value of adding this screening test to [^{125}I]fibrinogen leg scanning in high-risk patients.[7] In general surgical patients, this identified only 1 additional patient with proximal vein thrombosis (0.2%), whereas in hip surgery patients, it identified 25 additional patients with proximal vein thrombosis (6%). Thus the addition of IPG to leg scanning was not useful as a screening test among general surgical patients but was of substantial clinical value in hip surgery patients.

The results of this study were consistent with previous findings, which suggested that the majority of venous thrombi that occur in general surgical patients arise in the calf and so can be detected by leg scanning, whereas a considerable number of thrombi in hip surgery patients arise in the femoral vein and may occur as isolated events.

Natural history of the positive leg scan in asymptomatic patients. Approximately 50% of patients who develop thrombi detected by [^{125}I]fibrinogen leg scanning postoperatively also develop new asymptomatic abnormalities in the lung scan (ventilation-perfusion mismatch). The abnormalities incur a high risk for pulmonary emboli, indicating that approximately 50% of leg scan–detected thrombi embolize. If the thrombi are confined to the calf, the emboli are small and rarely clinically significant. However, if the calf vein thrombi are large or if the patient has a compromised cardiac or respiratory system, even emboli that arise from a calf vein thrombus could be clinically dangerous.

Untreated, approximately 20% of silent calf vein thrombi in bedridden patients extend into the popliteal or more proximal veins. When this occurs, it is associated with a much

higher risk of clinically significant thromboemboli, and in the one small study[14] in which the silent proximal vein thrombi detected by leg scanning remained untreated, the frequency of symptomatic pulmonary emboli was reported to be approximately 50%. Most thrombi that form in surgical patients undergoing general abdominal surgical procedures or that occur in medical patients arise in the calf veins, and when proximal vein thrombosis occurs, it is almost always associated with calf vein thrombosis. The site of origin of venous thrombi is different in patients who have hip and pelvic surgery.[7] In these patients, isolated proximal vein thrombosis occurs more frequently, and it is possible that in some cases of calf and proximal vein thrombosis the proximal vein thrombi precede calf vein thrombi by a number of days and therefore may not be detected by leg scanning until distal extension to the calf occurs.

Clinical management of the positive leg scan in asymptomatic patients. The approach to the patient who develops a positive leg scan is controversial. Management can include venography, with therapeutic decisions based on the results of venography. There are two major reasons for this approach. First, between 10% and 20% of patients with positive leg scans do not have venous thrombosis shown by venography and these patients do not require treatment with anticoagulants. Second, the size of the venous thrombus may not be accurately reflected by the extent of positivity of the leg scan. Thus scanning may only be positive in the calf in patients who have thrombosis in the calf and in the proximal femoral or iliofemoral segment.

If contraindications to anticoagulants do not exist and the venogram confirms the presence of venous thrombosis, patients are treated with anticoagulants to prevent extension of the thrombosis. If contraindications to anticoagulant therapy exist and the thrombus is relatively small and confined to calf veins, the patients' courses can be followed by leg scanning and IPG since extension does not occur in about 80% of these patients. If the contraindication to anticoagulant therapy is transient (e.g., only in the early postoperative period), treatment with anticoagulants can be started when the contraindication is no longer present. However, if the contraindication to anticoagulants is permanent (e.g., in patients with subarachnoid hemorrhage or recent neurosurgery), leg scanning can be continued for a prolonged period if the thrombus remains confined to the calf. If anticoagulant therapy is contraindicated and the venogram shows a large calf vein or proximal vein thrombus or if the thrombus extends, a venous interruption procedure should be considered.

Adjunct to impedance plethysmography in the diagnosis of clinically suspected venous thrombosis

Leg scanning should never be used as the only diagnostic test in patients with clinically suspected venous thrombosis. This is because it fails to detect approximately 30% of thrombi in these patients (many of which are in the femoral or iliac veins) and because there may be a delay of hours or even days before a sufficient amount of fibrinogen accumulates in the thrombus to make the test positive. The [^{125}I]fibrinogen leg scanning test is most useful for the diagnosis of clinically suspected venous thrombosis when it is used to complement IPG.[6,8] In the majority of patients with acute venous thrombosis, the leg scan becomes positive within 24 hours of injection with [^{125}I]fibrinogen, but in some patients with symptomatic acute venous thrombosis, it may take 48 or even 72 hours for enough radioactivity to accumulate in the thrombus to allow a positive diagnosis to be made.

The combined use of [^{125}I]fibrinogen leg scanning and IPG in patients with clinically suspected venous thrombosis has been evaluated.[6] In this study, patients were injected with [^{125}I]fibrinogen and had IPG performed on the day of referral. Patients then had leg scanning and IPG performed daily for the next 3 days. All patients underwent bilateral ascending venography, which was scheduled to be performed on the third day if the tests were negative or earlier if either of the tests became positive. Either leg scanning or IPG was positive in 81 of 86 patients with positive venograms (sensitivity, 94%), and both tests were negative in 104 of 114 patients who had negative venograms (specificity, 91%). These two tests detected all 60 patients with proximal vein thrombosis and 21 of 26 patients with calf vein thrombosis. A total of 21 of the 26 patients with calf vein thrombosis had symptoms for less than a week, and leg scanning was positive in 20 of these. The results of this study have now been confirmed in a second study of an additional 300 patients.[8]

The combined approach of IPG and leg scanning provides an alternative to venography in patients with clinically suspected deep vein thrombosis,[6,8] and it is safe to withhold anticoagulant therapy in patients who remain negative.[8]

However, the use of serial testing with either IPG or real-time B-mode ultrasound has now replaced the combined approach of IPG plus leg scanning in patients with their first episode of venous thromboembolism.[10] Leg scanning combined with IPG remains a useful approach in selected patients with suspected acute recurrent venous thrombosis.[11] (The approach of serial IPG alone [or serial B-mode ultrasound] for the diagnosis of suspected venous thrombosis in patients with their first episode of venous thromboembolism and the use of leg scanning in the diagnosis of suspected acute recurrent venous thrombosis are outlined in detail in Chapter 104.)

Management of the positive [^{125}I]fibrinogen leg scan in patients with clinically suspected venous thrombosis. [^{125}I]fibrinogen is only injected into patients with clinically suspected venous thrombosis if the IPG is negative. Approximately 10% to 15% of patients with clinically suspected venous thrombosis had a negative IPG and a positive leg scan. If cellulitis, previous knee surgery or trauma, arthritis of the knee, superficial phlebitis, or muscle injury can be excluded, a diagnosis of deep vein thrombosis can be made with over 95% confidence. It would therefore be

reasonable to base treatment on the leg scan result. If, however, the patient has clinical features that are recognized to cause a false-positive leg scan, the result of this test should be confirmed by venography before initiating anticoagulant therapy.

Diagnostic test in patients with clinically suspected acute recurrent venous thrombosis

When a patient reports symptoms of pain, tenderness, or swelling in a leg that has been the site of previous venous thrombosis, it may be difficult to distinguish between acute recurrent venous thrombosis and a nonthrombotic complication of chronic venous insufficiency. The clinical features may be localized to either the calf or the thigh and may appear either as an acute exacerbation against a background of long-standing, less severe pain or swelling or as repeated subacute exacerbations against a background of long-standing chronic venous insufficiency. The latter is much more frequently caused by a nonthrombotic complication of the postphlebitic syndrome and usually does not require further investigation, whereas the former may or may not result from acute venous thrombosis complicating venous insufficiency.

The approach to these patients depends on the nature of their clinical presentation, on their symptoms and signs, and on the presence of documented evidence of previous venous thrombosis. Venography alone is of limited diagnostic value in these patients unless the results can be compared with a previous venogram and unless a new filling defect is demonstrated. IPG may be falsely positive because of persistent venous outflow obstruction resulting from a previous episode of venous thrombosis or falsely negative because of large collateral channels that have developed consequent to the first episode. Leg scanning is useful for detecting active calf and distal thigh vein thrombi but is relatively insensitive in the upper thigh and cannot detect external and common iliac vein thrombi. In combination, however, the approach of IPG and leg scanning plus venography has high clinical utility in the diagnosis of patients with clinically suspected acute recurrent deep vein thrombosis.[11] A cohort analytic study[11] has recently been completed that incorporated the long-term follow-up data in 270 patients with symptoms and signs of acute recurrent deep vein thrombosis who were evaluated by combined IPG and leg scanning plus venography. The results of this study are presented in detail in Chapter 104 and provide the basis for the recommended practical approach to the diagnosis of clinically suspected acute recurrent deep vein thrombosis.

Screening patients who develop calf vein thrombosis where there are relative or absolute contraindications to anticoagulant therapy

In addition to the use of leg scanning as a screening test in high-risk patients, a further indication for leg scanning arises in the patient who has leg pain in the early postoperative period. If venography confirms the presence of a small calf vein thrombus and anticoagulant therapy is contraindicated, [^{125}I]fibrinogen can be injected and the patient followed by leg scanning and impedance plethysmography for 10 to 14 days. If extension does not occur, anticoagulant therapy can be delayed until the risk of postoperative hemorrhage has been considerably diminished.

REFERENCES

1. Becker J: The diagnosis of venous thrombosis in the legs using I-labelled fibrinogen: an experimental and clinical study, *Acta Chir Scand* 138:667, 1972.
2. Browse NL: The ^{125}I-fibrinogen uptake test, *Arch Surg* 104:160, 1971.
3. Gallus AS, Hirsh J: *^{125}I-fibrinogen leg scanning*. In Fratatoni J, Wessler S, eds: *Prophylactic therapy for deep venous thrombosis and pulmonary embolism,* DHEW Publication No (NIH) 76-866, Washington, DC, 1975, US Government Printing Office.
4. Harris WH et al: Comparison of ^{125}I-fibrinogen count scanning with phlebography for detection of venous thrombi after elective hip surgery, *N Engl J Med* 292:665, 1975.
5. Hobbs JT, Davies JWL: Detection of venous thrombosis with ^{131}I-labelled fibrinogen in the rabbit, *Lancet* 2:134, 1960.
6. Hull R et al: Combined use of leg scanning and impedance plethysmography in suspected venous thrombosis: an alternative to venography, *N Engl J Med* 296:1497, 1977.
7. Hull R et al: The value of adding impedance plethysmography to ^{125}I-fibrinogen leg scanning for the detection of deep vein thrombosis in high risk surgical patients: a comparative study between patients undergoing general surgery and hip surgery, *Thromb Res* 15:227, 1979.
8. Hull R et al: Replacement of venography in suspected venous thrombosis by impedance plethysmography and ^{125}I-fibrinogen leg scanning: a less invasive alternative, *Ann Intern Med* 94:12, 1981.
9. Hull R et al: Cost effectiveness of primary and secondary prevention of fatal pulmonary embolism in high-risk surgical patients, *Can Med Assoc J* 127:990, 1982.
10. Hull R et al: A randomized trial of diagnostic strategies for symptomatic deep vein thrombosis, *Thromb Haemost* 50:160a, 1983.
11. Hull R et al: The diagnosis of acute, recurrent deep-vein thrombosis: a diagnostic challenge, *Circulation* 67:901, 1983.
12. Kakkar VV: The diagnosis of deep-vein thrombosis using the ^{125}I-fibrinogen test, *Arch Surg* 104:152, 1972.
13. Kakkar VV: Fibrinogen uptake test for detection of deep vein thrombosis: a review of current practice, *Semin Nucl Med* 7:229, 1977.
14. Kakkar VV et al: Natural history of postoperative deep vein thrombosis, *Lancet* 2:230, 1969.
15. Lambie JM et al: Diagnostic accuracy in venous thrombosis, *Br Med J* 2:142, 1970.
16. Milne RM et al: Postoperative deep venous thrombosis: a comparison of diagnostic techniques, *Lancet* 2:445, 1971.
17. Palko PD, Nanson EM, Fedoruk SO: The early detection of deep venous thrombosis using ^{131}I-tagged human fibrinogen, *Can J Surg* 7:215, 1964.

CHAPTER 102

The value of liquid crystal thermography in the diagnosis of deep vein thrombosis

ANDREW N. NICOLAIDES and EVI KALODIKI

Thermography is a noninvasive method that can detect temperature differences on the surface of the human body. The principle underlying use of the test for the diagnosis of deep vein thrombosis (DVT) is based on the observation that the skin temperature of limbs with DVT is frequently increased.[15] A temperature difference between two legs is more readily observed after a short period of leg elevation and exposure to room temperature because there is a delay in cooling of the limb affected with DVT.

A temperature difference of greater than 0.7° C between limbs is considered abnormal, and because a temperature difference of less than 2° C cannot always be detected by an examiner's hand, sensitive thermographic devices were developed for this purpose.

EQUIPMENT AND METHODS

Early thermographic devices consisted of an infrared telecamera that could produce gray-scale images of lower limbs with a thermal resolution of 0.2° C. The darkest gray tones represented cooler areas and the lighter tones, warmer areas. Images were obtained with the patient in the supine position at the level of the calves, knees, thighs, and the groin. The device was bulky and expensive and had to be placed in a special room maintained at 20° C.[17]

In recent years, liquid crystal thermography (LCT) overcame these limitations. The equipment now consists of latex sheets impregnated with cholesterol crystals* that change color with increasing temperature, from brown (cool) to yellow, green, and finally blue (warm). The latex sheets are approximately 30 by 40 cm and are packaged in special boxes with a Perspex viewing face. Eight types of detectors (sheets) are available, which are calibrated to cover temperature ranges of 2° C above and below a mean temperature of 22° C, 24° C, 26° C, 28° C, 30° C, 32° C, 34° C, and 36° C. A frame is used to hold the thermographic detector to a Polaroid camera containing a flash unit so that a color photograph of each thermographic image can be taken. After the patient's legs have been exposed to room temperature

for 10 minutes, the patient lies prone on a bed or couch and the detector is placed over the calves (Fig. 102-1). After 20 to 30 seconds, an image is formed that shows the temperature patterns of both lower limbs. The image can be assessed immediately and photographed, if necessary. The procedure can be repeated with the patient supine and the thermographic detectors placed on the shins and thighs.[13]

The presence of a homogeneous area showing a temperature rise of more than 0.7° C in the symptomatic limb compared with the similar area of the asymptomatic limb constitutes a positive thermographic diagnostic finding (Figs. 102-2 and 102-3), except when the temperature change is caused by varicose veins, which should be checked for during the clinical examination.[2,3,5,14,20] The thermograph is considered negative if the temperature distribution is similar in both limbs.

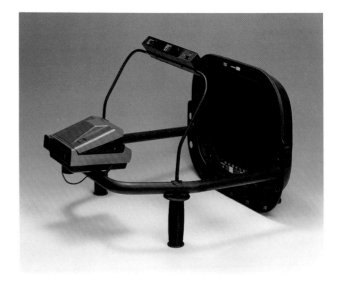

Fig. 102-1. The liquid crystal thermographic detector with electronic flash and Polaroid camera, which is placed over the legs.

---

*Novamedix Ltd, Andover, United Kingdom.

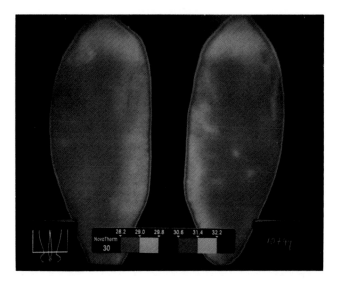

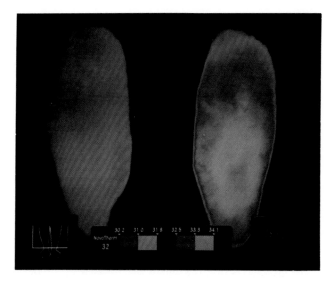

Fig. 102-2. A thermogram recorded on Polaroid film indicating similar patterns of skin temperature in both legs.

Fig. 102-3. A thermogram indicating an obvious skin temperature difference of at least 2° C between the two legs.

Table 102-1. Thermography compared with venography in symptomatic patients

Author and year	Instrumentation	Specificity correctly identified as normal	Sensitivity correctly identified as proximal DVT
Cooke and Pilcher,[5] 1974	TC	49/49 (100%)	51/53 (96%)
Leiviska & Perttala,[12] 1975	TC	17/17 (100%)	34/38 (89%)
Bergqvist et al,[2] 1977	TC	22/32 (69%)	75/77 (97%)
Bystrom et al,[3] 1977	TC	22/25 (88%)	26/26 (100%)
Nilsson et al,[14] 1979	RT	7/14 (50%)	35/37 (95%)
Watz & Bygdeman,[20] 1979	TC	27/35 (77%)	19/20 (95%)
Ricthie et al,[17] 1979	TC	113/139 (81%)	53/72 (74%)
Aronen et al,[1] 1981	TC	81/100 (81%)	38/41 (93%)
Pochaczersky et al,[16] 1982	LCT	15/18 (83%)	12/12 (100%)
Jacobsson et al,[10] 1983	RT	33/70 (47%)	123/130 (95%)
Sandler & Martin,[18] 1985	LCT	28/45 (62%)	34/35 (97%)
TOTAL		414/544 (76%)	595/637 (92%)

TC, Thermographic camera; *LCT,* liquid crystal thermography; *RT,* radiation thermometry.

ACCURACY

A number of studies have assessed the value of thermography in the diagnosis of DVT by comparing its findings to the results of ascending venography in symptomatic patients (Table 102-1). In the most recent study, LCT showed a sensitivity of 97%, but a specificity of only 62%.[18] Ruptured Baker's cysts, cellulitis, muscular or joint trauma, and superficial thrombophlebitis are the main conditions responsible for false-positive results and hence the relatively poor specificity of thermography. False-negative thermograms may occur when the thrombosis is older than a week or when the thrombi are small (less than 2 cm) and limited to a compartment not close to the skin surface.[1,18]

The value of thermography lies in the fact that when the test is normal, the likelihood of DVT is less than 5%. Thus

it is a good screening test that can be performed at the bedside and that requires minimal training on the part of the medical, paramedical, and nursing staff. However, if the test is positive, this is merely an indication for further investigation, since there are many conditions other than DVT that can produce a warm skin.

THERMOGRAPHY COMBINED WITH DUPLEX SCANNING

Because duplex scanning has shown both a sensitivity and specificity in excess of 95% in the detection of acute DVT (see Chapter 95), this has spawned a marked decrease in the number of venographic examinations performed to diagnose this condition. In addition, because duplex scanning is more cost effective than venography, the demand for this method has increased to such an extent that the availability of scanning time has become a limiting factor. This, together with the restrictions on the reimbursement for duplex scanning imposed in some countries, has highlighted the need for an even more simple and inexpensive screening method that could rule out DVT in limbs and avoid the need for duplex scanning. LCT was identified as having the potential to meet these criteria, and this was confirmed by a recently published study.[11]

LCT, DUPLEX SCANNING, AND VENOGRAPHY

To assess the merits of LCT, a study was conducted that consisted of 100 patients with clinically suspected acute DVT. A total of 22 patients were referred from the accident and emergency department, 22 by general practitioners, 26 from medical wards, and 30 from surgical wards. All were tested with LCT and duplex scanning, and ascending venography was performed within the subsequent 12 to 48 hours. Interpretation of the noninvasive and venographic results was done blindly.

Of the 100 patients, 55 were male and 45 were female, and their mean age was 53.3 years (range, 20 to 90 years). DVT was demonstrated by venography in 47 patients: 30 (64%) of the thromboses were in the left leg and 17 (36%) were in the right. In addition, 12 (26%) of the thrombi were confined to the calf and 34 (74%) extended to or arose from the popliteal or more proximal veins.

The results of LCT are compared with the venographic findings in Table 102-2. One patient had had one leg amputated and another had a plaster of paris cast, so LCT could be performed in only 98 patients. LCT showed an overall accuracy of 83% and a negative predictive value of 93%. Of 41 patients with a negative LCT, 38 had a normal venogram. The remaining 3 had false-negative thermograms: 1 patient had a small thrombus in the left peroneal vein and the remaining 2 had a history of DVT that was 10 and 21 days old; venography demonstrated soleal vein thrombosis in one and calf, popliteal, and femoral vein thrombi in the other, respectively. Symptoms and signs suggestive of DVT

had lasted less than 1 week in 39 of the 41 patients with a negative LCT. Thermograms were falsely positive in 15 patients (Table 102-2). Of these, 4 had arthritis, 2 had had a recent operation, 2 had a history of muscular strain, 1 had short saphenous vein thrombosis, and 1 had a hematoma. There was no apparent reason for the increase in temperature in 5 of the patients.

The comparison of the duplex scan findings with the results of venography is shown in Table 102-3, and duplex scanning showed an overall accuracy of 92%, a sensitivity of 93%, and a specificity of 91%. There were three false-negative duplex scans: two were in patients who had extremely tense and tender edematous legs that made examination difficult, and femoral thrombi were found in both. The third patient had a small (less than 2-cm-long) peroneal DVT. This case was the one also missed by LCT. There were five false-positive duplex scans. Two of these patients had undergone a recent operation (iliofemoral and femoro-popliteal bypass) and the affected leg was edematous, which made compression of the femoral veins very difficult. In the remaining three patients, duplex scanning falsely showed calf vein thrombosis.

The results of LCT in the study just described are similar to those reported by others.[5,18] The negative predictive value of 93% means that a negative thermogram indicates a small likelihood of DVT. Few conditions produce false-negative thermograms, but this may occur when the signs and symptoms of thrombosis have lasted more than 1 week, when the thrombi are small (less than 2 cm in length) and are limited to a compartment not closely related to the skin surface, or when there is peripheral neuropathy.[1,5] For the study just discussed, if the two patients with a history of DVT longer than 1 week had been excluded, because thermography would have been an inappropriate test under these circumstances (Table 102-2), and if it had been the practice to neither proceed to other tests nor treat any of the remaining 39 patients whose thermograms were negative, then one calf DVT would have been missed, yielding a negative predictive value of 97%.

Table 102-2. Comparison of results of liquid crystal thermography and venography*

	Liquid crystal thermography		
	Positive	**Negative**	**Total**
Venography			
DVT	42 (93%)	3†	45
No DVT	15	38 (72%)	53
TOTAL	57	41	98

DVT, Deep vein thrombosis.
*Sensitivity, 93%; specificity, 72%; positive predictive value, 74% (42/57); negative predictive value, 93% (38/41); overall accuracy, 83%.
†Two patients had symptoms suggestive of DVT for more than 1 week (venography demonstrated calf DVT in one and proximal DVT in the other); the third patient had peroneal DVT found on venography only.

Table 102-3. Comparison of the results of duplex scanning and venography*

	Duplex scanning		
	DVT	**No DVT**	**Total**
Venography			
DVT	43 (93%)	3†	46
No DVT	5‡	49 (91%)	54
TOTAL	48	52	100

DVT, Deep vein thrombosis.
*Sensitivity, 93%; specificity, 91%; positive predictive value, 89% (43/48); negative predictive value, 94% (49/52); overall accuracy, 92%.
†Two patients with femoral DVT (tense and tender edematous thighs); one patient with peroneal (less than 2-cm-long) DVT.
‡Two falsely diagnosed as femoral DVT (groin and thigh wounds); three falsely diagnosed as calf DVT.

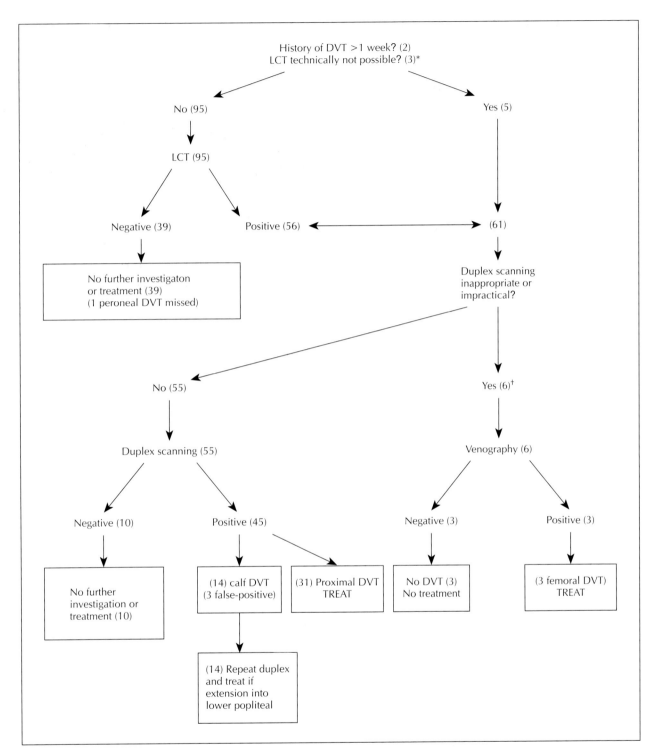

Fig. 102-4. The suggested policy for investigating patients with clinically suspected DVT. Numbers in brackets indicate the number of patients from the study that would have passed through the various points of the algorithm. *One amputee, one patient in plaster of Paris cast, and one patient with leprosy. †Very edematous, tense tender legs with a surgical wound in four patients.

The results of duplex scanning in this study are also similar to those of others.[4,6,7] The sensitivity of 93% indicates that this method can detect most thrombi, and previous studies have indicated that such missed thrombi are usually in the calf.[4,6,7] In the presence of severe edema, tenderness, or surgical wounds, compression of the veins cannot be adequately achieved, rendering this test inappropriate. If the duplex examination is inadequate or inapplicable because of such conditions, venography may be the only method for making the diagnosis. In another series of 100 patients, six limbs fell into this category.[11]

If it had been the practice to exclude patients with such limbs from duplex scanning and use venography only, the sensitivity and specificity of duplex scanning would rise to 97% (43/44) and 94% (47/50), respectively. As already mentioned, one small (less than 2-cm-long) peroneal DVT would have been missed (also missed by LCT), and three calf DVT would have been falsely diagnosed. The safety of withholding treatment in patients with suspected DVT that is confined to the calf has been demonstrated by the results of several studies.[8,9,19]

FORMULATION OF NEW POLICY

On the basis of these observations, a new policy for the investigation of patients with clinically suspected DVT has been formulated (Fig. 102-4). In this policy, LCT is the first diagnostic test performed unless it is deemed inappropriate (i.e., symptoms suggestive of DVT longer than 1 week) or technically impossible. If LCT is negative, no further investigation or treatment is necessary. If LCT is inappropriate, technically impossible, or positive, duplex scanning should be performed unless a surgical wound or severe tenderness and edema make such a test difficult, in which case a venogram should be obtained instead. Had this been the policy in the 100 patients in the study described, DVT would have been ruled out and no treatment instituted in 49 patients: in 39 because of a negative thermogram and in 10 because of a negative duplex scan.[11] As a result, DVT in the calf would have been missed in one patient. In the same way, 34 patients with thrombosis in veins proximal to the calf would have been hospitalized and treated: 31 on the basis of a positive duplex scan and 3 on the basis of a positive venogram. Duplex scanning would have diagnosed DVT that was confined to the calf in 14 patients (11 true positive; 3 false positive) (see Fig. 102-4). If ambulant, these patients would have been rescanned every 2 days until they were found to be free of symptoms and to ensure that there was no proximal extension into the popliteal vein. On the basis of this proposed policy (Fig. 102-4), only six venograms would have been performed. Although this policy is rational, it should be validated prospectively, with follow-up of all patients for at least 1 year to determine whether any of the untreated patients suffer further DVT or pulmonary embolism.

Cost effectiveness of the new policy

Three policies have been analyzed for cost effectiveness[11]: policy A, consisting of venography in all patients, which is still practiced in some countries; policy B, which involves duplex scanning in all patients; and policy C, which is the protocol outlined in Fig. 102-4. It has been found that policy C would result in a 60% reduction in cost compared to policy A and 20% compared to policy B. In addition, policy C would lead to a 39% reduction in the number of duplex scanning sessions. This would free up the facility for the performance of other useful tests, such as the detection and grading of carotid stenosis.

REFERENCES

1. Aronen HJ, Suorant HT, Taaritsainen MJ: Thermography in deep venous thrombosis of the leg, *AJR* 137:1179, 1981.
2. Bergqvist D, Efsing HO, Hallbook TL: Thermography: a noninvasive method for diagnosis of deep venous thrombosis, *Arch Surg* 122:600, 1977.
3. Bystrom LG et al: The value of thermography and the determination of fibrin-fibrinogen degradation products in the diagnosis of deep venous thombosis, *Acta Med Scand* 202:319, 1977.
4. Comerota AJ et al: Venous duplex imaging: should it replace hemodynamic tests for deep venous thrombosis? *J Vasc Surg* 11:53, 1990.
5. Cooke ED, Pilcher MF: Deep vein thrombosis: preclinical diagnosis by thermography, *Br J Surg* 61:971, 1974.
6. Cranley JJ et al: Near parity in the final diagnosis of deep venous thrombosis by duplex scan and phlebography, *Phlebology* 4:71, 1989.
7. Elias E et al: Value of real-time B-mode ultrasound imaging in the diagnosis of deep vein thrombosis of the lower limbs, *Int Angiol* 6:175, 1987.
8. Huisman M et al: Serial impedance plethysmography for suspected deep venous thrombosis in outpatients: the Amsterdam general practitioner's study, *N Engl J Med* 314:823, 1986.
9. Hull RD et al: Diagnostic efficacy of impedance plethysmography for clinically suspected deep vein thrombosis, *Ann Intern Med* 102:21, 1985.
10. Jacobsson H et al: Standardised leg temperature profiles in the diagnosis of acute deep venous thrombosis, *Vasc Diagn Ther* 4:55, 1983.
11. Kalodiki E et al: The combination of liquid crystal thermography and duplex scanning in DVT diagnosis, *Eur J Vasc Surg* 6:310-316, 1992.
12. Leiviska T, Perttala Y: Thermography in diagnosing deep venous thrombosis of the lower limb, *Radiol Clin* 44:417, 1975.
13. Nicolaides AN, Sumner DS, eds: *Investigation of patients with deep vein thrombosis and chronic venous insufficiency*, London, Calif, Nicosia, 1991, Med Orion Publishing Company.
14. Nilsson E, Sunden P, Zetterquist S: Leg temperature profiles with a simplified thermographic technique in the diagnosis of acute venous thrombosis, *Scand J Clin Lab Invest* 9:171, 1979.
15. Pilcher R: Postoperative thrombosis and embolism, *Lancet* 2:629, 1939.
16. Pochaczersky R, Pillari G, Feldman F: Liquid crystal contact thermography on deep venous thrombosis, *Am J Radiol* 138:717, 1982.
17. Ritchie WGM, Lapayowker MC, Soulon RL: Thermographic diagnosis of deep venous thrombosis: anatomically based diagnostic criteria, *Radiology* 132:321, 1979.
18. Sandler DA, Martin JF: Liquid crystal thermography as a screening test for deep vein thrombosis, *Lancet* 1:665, 1985.
19. Stallworth JM, Plong CW Jr, Horne JB: Negative phlebography: clinical follow-up in 593 patients, *Arch Surg* 116:795, 1981.
20. Watz R, Bygdeman S: Noninvasive diagnosis of acute deep vein thrombosis, *Acta Med Scand* 206:463, 1979.

CHAPTER 103

Significance of free-floating venous thrombi

LAZAR J. GREENFIELD

On December 7, 1937, Dr. John Homans addressed the Boston Surgical Society in connection with a demonstration by Dr. C. N. Best concerning the use of heparin to prevent the clotting of blood in glass tubes. In his presentation, Homans described the pathogenesis of a clinical deep vein thrombus (DVT) as follows[7]:

> Should it grow into a current, it may become so soft and flimsy that finally it can hardly be distinguished from normal blood. Insofar as this friable portion builds itself away from the heart it merely blocks more and more of the peripheral venous tree, but if it grows toward the heart, unfixed in the vein and waving in the current of an entering branch, fragile and ready to break from the body, it is a potential embolus—a serious threat to life.

As heparin gained widespread use, its effectiveness in the management of DVT and prevention of pulmonary thromboembolism (PE) became well accepted. Clinical studies, such as that of Coon, Willis, and Symons[5] consisting of a 20-year experience at the University of Michigan, showed that 99% of 639 patients presenting with a single PE were protected by anticoagulation against a fatal recurrence. However, the combined rate of nonfatal and fatal recurrent PE for patients on anticoagulant therapy remains around 10%. Although this means that 90% of patients are protected by anticoagulation, obviously it would be most helpful for clinicians to know, on the basis of specific risk factors, whether a patient was likely to fall into the 10% category of those not adequately protected by anticoagulation. Therefore the studies that have attempted to define those patients at higher risk for recurrent thromboembolism are reviewed.

CLINICAL STUDIES

It was retrograde venous angiography that allowed visualization of the characteristics of the proximal end of a venous thrombus (Fig. 103-1). The recognition of a free-floating tail on the thrombus has always been a source of concern to the clinician, prompting treatment that varied from immediate anticoagulation to thrombectomy. Thrombectomy remains popular in Russia, and anticoagulation or venous interruption is reserved for those patients unable to tolerate thrombectomy. The results of this policy were reported by Savelyev et al[10] for a series of 353 patients with either DVT

or PE. Retrograde iliocavography showed floating thrombi in 37.5% of cases. Thrombectomy of the inferior vena cava or iliac veins using temporary balloon occlusion of the vena cava was performed in 59 patients. Venous plication, accomplished by sutures, clips, or staples, was used in 10 patients and a vena caval filter was inserted in 44. The vena cava was ligated in 3 patients and combined procedures were performed in 57. The incidence of postoperative pulmonary embolism was 1.5%, but the postoperative mortality rate was 9.2%. In a group of 11 patients with floating thrombi who did not undergo thrombectomy, there were 4 deaths (36%) stemming from massive PE. Because this was a retrospective study in which all patients with floating thrombi were considered candidates for operative intervention, it is difficult to judge the risk of PE in patients receiving anticoagulant treatment alone.

In 1985, Norris, Greenfield, and Herrmann[8] reported on a study of 78 patients with iliofemoral DVT, all of whom were treated by standard anticoagulation with heparin. Venograms showed that 73 (94%) of the thrombi were occlusive, and 5 (6%) had a floating tail at least 5 cm long. The overall incidence of PE within 10 days of diagnosis, which was confirmed by a high-probability lung scan, was 9% (n = 7). However, the PE rate in the 73 patients with adherent thrombi was 5.5% (n = 4), and it was 60% (n = 3) in the 5 patients with a free-floating tail ($p < 0.05$).

Although there was a small number of patients in this series with floating thrombi, the findings from a subsequent study, reported in 1986, documented the risk of recurrent PE in patients who showed residual DVT that was detected by noninvasive venous studies.[2] In this report by Alexander et al,[2] 10 patients who suffered recurrent PE while on anticoagulant therapy were compared with 31 patients who did not sustain recurrent PE. The risk factors were the same for both groups, but they differed dramatically in terms of the evidence of residual DVT in their lower extremities. Combined Doppler and phleborheography (PRG) was positive for DVT in all 10 patients who had recurrent PE while on treatment with heparin (8), warfarin (1), or the two agents combined (1). Recurrent PE was documented angiographically in each case. In contrast, combined Doppler and PRG

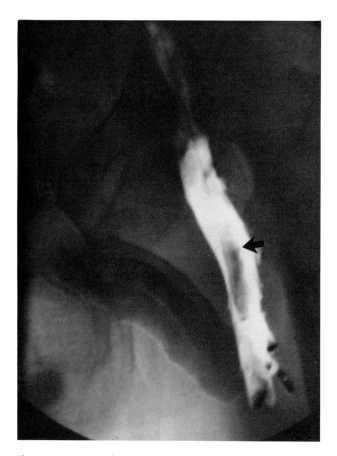

Fig. 103-1. Retrograde venogram showing a free-floating thrombus within the vein *(arrow)* that extends proximally and distally. Such a thrombus is susceptible to detachment in spite of anticoagulation treatment.

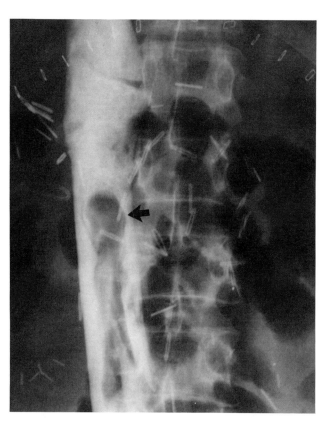

Fig. 103-2. Contrast venacavogram showing a large free-floating thrombus *(arrow)* extending upward from the occluded left iliac vein.

showed residual DVT in only 2 of the 31 (6%) patients treated successfully with anticoagulation but without recurrence ($p < 0.001$). Although it was not specified whether the residual DVT was adherent or free floating, the data indicated that noninvasive venous studies could be used to identify those patients with PE who remain at high risk for recurrence despite anticoagulation. Browse et al[4] also reported that 38% of their patients with PE demonstrated residual free-floating thrombi. Because the standard indication for insertion of the Greenfield filter into the vena cava to treat recurrence requires that the recurrence be documented, the authors[2] suggest that their criteria will identify in advance those patients most likely to sustain recurrent PE, thus justifying prophylactic filter placement. However, such a conclusion should be validated by a prospective randomized trial.

The risk of PE from free-floating thrombi in the inferior vena cava (Fig. 103-2) was studied by Radomski et al.[9] In a series of 39 patients, 26 (67%) had thrombi in the vena cava characterized as free floating by venography. In patients with free-floating thrombi, the incidence of PE as the presenting symptom was 50% (13 of 26 patients) as compared

to 15% (2 of 13 patients) in those with adherent thrombi ($p < 0.05$). The incidence of recurrent PE after anticoagulation was initiated was 27% (7 of 26 patients) in the group with free-floating thrombi compared to 12% (1 of 8 patients) in those with adherent thrombi ($p > 0.05$). An additional group of five patients with thrombotic occlusion of the vena cava did not exhibit PE on presentation or after heparin treatment. The authors conclude that it is mandatory to define the proximal extent of any DVT occurring in the lower extremity, using venocavography if necessary. When a free-floating vena caval thrombus is demonstrated, meticulous anticoagulation is required, and there should be a low threshold for indicating insertion of a Greenfield filter. A similar approach has been advocated by Akers, Musto, and Marinco.[1] Inability to visualize the proximal portion of the thrombus by duplex scanning may be an indication for retrograde venography.

The role of thrombolytic therapy is difficult to define in the setting of a free-floating thrombus. Of particular concern is the risk of lysis of the thrombus attachment, which would lead to massive embolism. This fatal outcome has been documented by Goldsmith, Loller, and Hoak.[6] An alternative approach that has been successful is to place a Greenfield filter above the level of the thrombus or occluded vena cava via the jugular vein and then pass a catheter through the filter and into the thrombus to achieve selective thrombolysis. It has been possible to open an obstructed vena cava in four patients in this fashion; some fragments of thrombus were found to be temporarily trapped in the filter and subsequently lysed.

The results of interesting serial studies using duplex ultrasound were reported by Voet and Afschrift,[11] who documented floating thrombi in 44 of 76 patients with above-knee DVT. By 3 months, 87% of the floating segments had disappeared. In 33%, PE was documented by ventilation-perfusion lung scans (11), pulmonary angiography (1), and autopsy (1). The iliofemoral segment was the site of 67% of the floating thrombi. A malignant tumor was diagnosed in 28% of the patients with floating thrombi.

A different conclusion was reached in a report on the significance of free-floating thrombi. Baldridge, Martin, and Welling[3] reviewed the outcome in 73 patients with DVT that was diagnosed by duplex scan as free floating, representing approximately 10% of their DVT cases. The incidence of PE was 14%, with most (78%) occurring before duplex scanning. On follow-up scans in 33 (45%) of the patients, 18 (55%) showed attachment of the thrombus, 8 (24%) showed a decrease in the size or disappearance of the thrombus, 4 (12%) showed persistent (unchanged) thrombus, and 3 (9%) showed enlargement of the tail. These authors concluded that most free-floating thrombi either become attached to the vein wall or resolve. This study has several limitations: less than half of the patients underwent follow-up duplex scanning, the characterization of free floating was accomplished by ultrasound rather than venography, and the thrombi were all infrainguinal. Despite these limitations, the incidence of PE in patients with floating thrombi in the superficial femoral vein was 30%. Defining the risk of pulmonary embolism in the presence of free-floating thrombi and the appropriate treatment for these patients will require well-designed prospective studies.

CONCLUSION

Anticoagulation affords protection against PE in 90% of patients with DVT. The 10% incidence of PE despite anticoagulation appears to correlate with the incidence of thrombi with a proximal free-floating tail. Although the actual risk of PE represented by a free-floating thrombus at the femoral level (30%) is controversial, several retrospective studies suggest that a free-floating thrombus at the level of the iliac veins carries a 36% to 60% risk of PE in spite of anticoagulation. For patients with a floating thrombus in the vena cava, the risk of PE is 50% at the time of presentation and remains 27% after anticoagulation. A danger posed by lytic therapy is that it may cause detachment of the floating thrombus. Therefore patients with free-floating thrombi in major veins are least likely to be protected by anticoagulation and should be considered for Greenfield filter placement. Anticoagulation should be used whenever possible to control the underlying thrombotic disorder and limit distal propagation. Further prospective studies are needed to clarify the relationship between the configuration of the proximal thrombus and the risk of pulmonary thromboembolism.

REFERENCES

1. Akers S, Musto S, Marinco PL: Altered therapy of suspected pulmonary embolism using leg venography, *Chest* 92:1105-1106, 1987.
2. Alexander JJ et al: New criteria for placement of a prophylactic vena cava filter, *Surg Gynecol Obstet* 163:405-409, 1986.
3. Baldridge ED, Martin MA, Welling RE: Clinical significance of free-floating venous thrombi, *J Vasc Surg* 11:62-69, 1990.
4. Browse NL et al: Prevention of recurrent pulmonary embolism, *Br Med J* 3:382-386, 1969.
5. Coon WW, Willis PE, Symons MJ: Assessment of anticoagulant treatment of venous thromboembolism, *Am Surg* 170:559, 1969.
6. Goldsmith JC, Loller P, Hoak JC: Massive fatal pulmonary embolism with fibrinolytic therapy, *Circulation* 64:1068-1069, 1982.
7. Homans J: Thrombophlebitis in the legs, *N Engl J Med* 218:594-599, 1938.
8. Norris CS, Greenfield LJ, Herrmann JB: Free-floating iliofemoral thrombus. A risk of pulmonary embolism, *Arch Surg* 120:806-808, 1985.
9. Radomski JS et al: Risk of pulmonary embolus with inferior vena caval thrombosis, *Am Surg* 53:97-101, 1987.
10. Savelyev VS et al: Surgical prevention of pulmonary embolism, *World J Surg* 4:709-716, 1980.
11. Voet D, Afschrift M: Floating thrombi: diagnosis and follow-up by duplex ultrasound, *Br J Radiol* 64:1010-1014, 1991.

CHAPTER 104

Comparative value of tests for the diagnosis of venous thrombosis

RUSSELL D. HULL, GARY E. RASKOB, and JACK HIRSH

It is now widely accepted that it is risky to diagnose venous thrombosis on the basis of clinical findings because of their low sensitivity and specificity.[19,22,38,53,62] This low sensitivity arises from the fact that many potentially dangerous venous thrombi are nonobstructive and not associated with inflammation of the vessel wall or of the surrounding perivascular tissues and consequently have no detectable clinical manifestations. Clinical findings are nonspecific because none of the symptoms or signs of venous thrombosis are unique to this condition and all can be caused by nonthrombotic disorders. The exception is phlegmasia cerulea dolens, in which massive iliofemoral thrombosis is clinically obvious and usually requires no further investigation. This syndrome constitutes less than 1% of the cases of clinically suspected venous thrombosis, however. In the vast majority of patients, the symptoms and signs are less overt, and the clinical suspicion is not confirmed by objective tests in more than 50% of these patients.[19,22,38,60,61] Patients with relatively minor symptoms and signs may have extensive venous thrombi, whereas patients with marked symptoms and signs of deep vein thrombosis (DVT) frequently may exhibit no objective evidence of venous thrombosis. Therefore because of the nonspecificity of clinical findings, they should not be used as the basis for management decisions in patients with suspected venous thrombosis.

The potential disadvantages of investigating all patients with clinically suspected venous thrombosis using objective testing are the expense, the inconvenience to the patient, and the possible morbidity caused by the test. However, all of these potential disadvantages are outweighed by the test's advantages. Considered in a different light, the cost of objective testing is substantially less than the cost of a prolonged hospital stay and, in the instance of an incorrect diagnosis, of unnecessary anticoagulant therapy.[39] The same is true for the inconvenience of objective testing. Although there is some morbidity associated with venography,[7] there is virtually none associated with the alternative noninvasive tests. Furthermore, even the morbidity associated with venography is much less than that associated with anticoagulant therapy.

VENOGRAPHY

Venography is accepted as the reference standard objective method for the diagnosis of venous thrombosis.[38,56,69] Although venography has been used for more than 30 years,[4] its widespread application was delayed because the fallibility of clinical diagnosis has been accepted only relatively recently.

Because venography is not readily repeatable, it is not suitable for screening subclinical venous thrombosis. A number of methods for performing venography have been described.[56,69] With good technique, ascending venography outlines the deep venous system of the legs in most patients, including the external and common iliac veins. However, common femoral or iliac venography may be needed if the external and common iliac veins are not properly visualized or if the inferior vena cava needs to be outlined.

Ascending venography. The aim of ascending venography is to inject radiopaque contrast medium into a dorsal foot vein so that the deep venous system of the leg is clearly outlined. A number of venography techniques have been described, but in all, the goal is to clearly opacify the deep veins of the leg.[56,69] The quality of venography can be maximized and the frequency of artifacts caused by nonfilling of venous segments minimized by injecting a large volume of dye and using careful technique. Filling of the calf veins is improved if the patient is examined with the table tilted 40° from horizontal and if weight bearing on the affected leg is avoided. The use of fluoroscopic monitoring during injection makes it possible to identify suspicious areas, which can then be examined more closely, and this reduces the likelihood of confusing a flow defect with a filling defect. These flow defects arise when opacified blood in the major venous channels is mixed with nonopacified blood coming from a tributary. Such an artifact can often be distinguished from an intraluminal defect by performing a Valsalva maneuver while the dye is being injected under fluoroscopic guidance.

The use of an ankle tourniquet to obstruct the superficial veins and thus promote filling of the deep venous system is controversial. Some authorities believe that it may prevent adequate filling of the deep veins and that it is unecessary when a tilt table is used. However, some patients may have extensive superficial vein varicosities that overlap and obscure the deep veins, and an ankle tourniquet may be helpful in the examination of these patients. The deep femoral vein and the internal iliac veins are usually not adequately visualized by ascending venography even when a Valsalva maneuver is performed.

Iliac venography. Visualization of the external and common iliac veins and the inferior vena cava can be achieved by direct injection of the contrast medium into the common femoral vein,[57] by intraosseous injection,[57] or by retrograde injection through a catheter passed via the right atrium and inferior vena cava.[15] The simplest of these techniques is femoral vein puncture. This is usually performed by entering the femoral vein on the nonaffected side and passing a catheter into the common iliac vein of the affected side using a Seldinger technique. The intraosseous technique is very painful, requires a general anesthetic, and has been reported to produce fatal fat embolism.[58] Retrograde catheterization is more complex than femoral vein puncture but allows examination of the internal iliac system and may be combined with pulmonary angiography.

In practice, ascending venography combined with a meticulous technique can adequately image the deep veins of the calf, the popliteal vein, and the femoral vein, as well as the external and common iliac veins. Occasionally, it is necessary to perform a direct puncture of the femoral vein to clarify the nature of a suspicious defect in the common femoral or iliac veins.

Normal anatomy of the venous system

Accurate interpretation of venographic findings requires a knowledge of both the normal and variant anatomy of the venous system. The venous system in the leg consists of three pairs of deep calf veins (the posterior tibial, the peroneal, and the anterior tibial), plus the soleal and gastrocnemius plexus of the veins and the superficial venous system. The soleal plexus drains into the posterior tibial vein, the gastrocnemius plexus drains into the peroneal veins, and the three pairs of deep calf veins converge to form the popliteal vein. The popliteal vein becomes the superficial femoral vein at the junction of the proximal part of the popliteal fossa and the adductor canal in the thigh. The superficial femoral vein is joined by the deep femoral vein in the upper thigh to form the common femoral vein, which becomes the external iliac vein at the level of the inguinal ligament. The external iliac vein is joined by the internal iliac vein in the pelvis to form the common iliac vein, and the common iliac veins converge to form the inferior vena cava. The superficial venous system consists of two major veins, the long and short saphenous veins, which drain into the common femoral and popliteal veins, respectively. The superficial system is connected with the deep venous system by communicating veins, which contain valves that direct flow from the superficial into the deep system. Several vari-

ations of the deep venous system are recognized, the most common being accessory popliteal veins, bifid superficial femoral veins, and an abnormally high or low origin of the popliteal vein.

Criteria for the diagnosis of venous thrombosis

A number of venographic characteristics have been established as criteria for the diagnosis of acute deep vein thrombosis.[56,65,69] The most reliable criterion is the presence of an intraluminal filling defect that is seen in all films and in a number of projections. Other, less reliable, criteria include: (1) nonfilling of a segment of the deep venous system with abrupt termination of contrast medium at a constant site below the segment and reappearance of the contrast medium at a constant site above the segment and (2) nonfilling of the deep venous system above the knee despite a careful venographic technique. The likelihood that these appearances are due to venous thrombosis is increased if abnormal collateral vessels are also seen. A constant intraluminal filling defect usually represents acute venous thrombosis, whereas the other two abnormalities or variations thereof may be caused by old venous thrombi, or they may be due to artifacts caused by incomplete mixing of the contrast medium with blood, external compression of a vein, or injection of the contrast medium too far proximally in the foot.

Pitfalls of venography

Venography is difficult to perform well and requires considerable experience to execute adequately. It is also difficult to interpret results accurately. Unless care is taken to inject the contrast dye distally into a dorsal foot vein, there may be nonfilling of the calf veins, which may be incorrectly interpreted either as stemming from a thrombus (because the vein is not filled) or as normal because a filling defect is not seen. Adequate filling of the common femoral, external iliac, and common iliac veins may not be accomplished by ascending venography, and frequently an incorrect diagnosis is rendered as a result. There are two common errors that can occur when trying to interpret the results of an inadequate venogram. The first is to miss even a large nonobstructive thrombus in the common femoral region because flow into the external iliac or common iliac vein appears to be adequate, even though filling of the common femoral vein is suboptimal. The second is to incorrectly diagnose venous thrombosis because of a streaming effect in the common femoral or iliac veins caused by inadequate opacification. Misinterpreting an inadequate venogram (usually a false-positive diagnosis of venous thrombosis) has become a serious problem, since the use of venography has increased in centers without a special interest or expertise in the technique. This problem can be prevented if radiologists and clinicians are sensitive to the pitfalls of venography and either repeat the venogram when the results of the test are inadequate or equivocal or instead base the diagnosis on the results of noninvasive tests.

Side effects of venography

Venography is an invasive procedure that may produce pain in the foot while the dye is being injected or pain in the calf 1 or 2 days after injection.[7] The radiopaque medium has been shown to damage endothelial cells, and both the early and delayed pain are probably due to this.[7] This insult may lead to superficial phlebitis and even deep vein thrombosis in a small percentage of patients who have normal venograms. In one study, a positive fibrinogen leg scan develops in 3% to 4% of the patients who initially have negative venograms, and clinically significant venous thrombosis develops in about 1% to 2%.[38] Others have reported a higher frequency of positive postphlebographic fibrinogen leg scans,[1] but these differences could be due to differences in venographic technique or in the patient population under study. It is possible, for example, that the frequency of positive postvenographic leg scans is higher in patients who remain immobilized after venography because the thrombogenic effects of venous damage produced by the radiopaque contrast medium are compounded by venous stasis.

Other less common complications of venography include hypersensitivity reactions to the radiopaque dye and local skin and tissue necrosis caused by extravasation of dye at the site of injection.[7] Many of these side effects can be prevented by careful attention to detail. It is important that the needle is firmly implanted in the vein and that the dye is not injected under pressure. Local pain can be reduced if lidocaine is mixed with the radiopaque material, and the likelihood of postvenographic phlebitis can be minimized if the leg is elevated after venography and the dye washed out with an infusion of 150 to 250 ml of normal or heparinized saline solution. Hypersensitivity reactions and necrosis can also be prevented by the use of isotonic radiopaque contrast medium, but the preparations currently available are very expensive. Patients with a history of hypersensitivity to radiopaque dye should not undergo venography.

NONINVASIVE TESTS FOR THE DIAGNOSIS OF VENOUS THROMBOSIS

A number of noninvasive or less invasive techniques for the diagnosis of venous thrombosis have been developed.[2,6,55,63] Of these, four have been carefully evaluated: [^{125}I]fibrinogen leg scanning,* impedance plethysmography (IPG),[33,49,50,74,75] Doppler ultrasonography,[16,28,61,70-72] and real-time B-mode ultrasound.[5,10,20,60,76] Details of the methodology of these techniques are presented elsewhere in this volume. Each of the tests has different applications, depending on whether the patient has clinically suspected venous thrombosis or has a high risk of developing venous thrombosis. A number of other diagnostic techniques, including other forms of plethysmography,[3] thermography,[13] and various isotopic methods,[26,48,59] have been evaluated to a limited extent. Sensitive blood tests that can detect intravascular fibrin for-

mation and lysis are also undergoing clinical evaluation[9,77,78] and may be of future value.

[^{125}I]fibrinogen leg scanning

Principles. The principle underlying the use of radioiodine-labeled [^{125}I]fibrinogen scanning to diagnose venous thrombosis is that circulating labeled fibrinogen is incorporated into a thrombus, and the attendant increase in the overlying surface radioactivity is then detected by an isotope detector. The feasibility of this technique was first demonstrated in animals[27] and humans[66] in the early 1960s, and the method has been extensively evaluated since then. The equipment initially used for external scanning was cumbersome, but in later years, portable, convenient, and accurate equipment became available that allowed the test to be performed at the patient's bedside. Leg scanning is now mainly of historical interest and has been withdrawn from clinical practice because of the risk of HIV transmission from donor fibrinogen.

Fibrinogen scanning can be used expectantly for screening medical and surgical patients who are at high risk of developing venous thrombosis. It can also be used to complement IPG to confirm or exclude the diagnosis of venous thrombosis.

[^{125}I]fibrinogen leg scanning detects thrombi in the calf vein and the distal half of the thigh that are actively accreting fibrin at the time of [^{125}I]fibrinogen injection. Fibrinogen leg scanning detects over 90% of the cases of acute calf vein thrombi,[17,23,52,54] but only between 60% and 80% of patients with proximal vein thrombi, depending on the location. Leg scanning is relatively insensitive for evaluating the upper thigh and very insensitive to the presence of venous thrombi in the pelvis.[23,51]

Potential limitations. [^{125}I]fibrinogen scanning cannot detect thrombi in the pelvic veins[23,52] because ^{125}I is a relatively low-energy gamma emitter. Test findings are unreliable in the upper thigh because of its proximity to the bladder, which frequently contains radioactive urine, and the presence of large veins and arteries, which produce an increase in the background count. [^{125}I]fibrinogen scanning is contraindicated in women during pregnancy and lactation and should not be used in young patients unless very definite indications exist.

[^{125}I]fibrinogen leg scanning should never be used as the only diagnostic test in patients with clinically suspected venous thrombosis because it cannot detect many high proximal vein thrombi and because it may take hours or even days before enough fibrinogen accumulates in the thrombus to make the test positive. For practical purposes, these problems are overcome when [^{125}I]fibrinogen leg scanning is used to complement IPG in patients with clinically suspected venous thrombosis.[34]

Causes of discrepancy between the results of leg scanning and venography. An abnormal leg scan but normal venogram may be the result of hematoma, inflammation, uptake into a surgical wound, or nonvisualization of thrombus by the

---

*References 11, 12, 17, 18, 54, 64, 67.

venogram. A false-negative scan may occur when the venous thrombus is old and no longer taking up fibrinogen, forming after most of the radioactive fibrinogen has been cleared from the circulation, is too small to be detected, or is isolated in the common femoral or iliac vein.

Impedance plethysmography

Principles. Plethysmography is a noninvasive method that detects volume changes in the leg. Several plethysmographic techniques have been used, including IPG,[33,50,75] strain-gauge plethysmography,[3,29] and air cuff plethysmography,[14] but IPG has been the most thoroughly evaluated.

IPG is sensitive and specific for identifying thrombosis of the popliteal, femoral, or iliac veins (proximal veins) but is relatively insensitive for detecting calf vein thrombosis. The underlying principle of the method is that blood volume changes in the calf, which are produced by maximal respiratory effort or by the inflation or deflation of a pneumatic thigh cuff, cause changes in electrical resistance (impedance). These changes are reduced in patients with thrombosis of the popliteal or more proximal veins. The original method,[74] which entailed maximal respiratory effort, had shortcomings because sick patients were frequently unable to cooperate sufficiently for the test results to be reliable. The test was therefore modified and a pneumatic cuff used to temporarily occlude the venous outflow (occlusive IPG).[75] This modified test is sensitive and specific for detecting proximal vein thrombosis.[33,75]

Occlusive cuff IPG is performed with patients supine and the affected lower limb elevated 25° to 30°. The knee is flexed 10° to 20°, and the ankle is placed 8 to 15 cm higher than the knee. A pneumatic cuff, 15 cm in width, is applied to the midthigh and inflated to 45 cm H_2O, thereby occluding venous return. After a predetermined period, the cuff is rapidly deflated. The changes in electrical resistance (impedance) resulting from alterations in blood volume distal to the cuff are detected by circumferential calf electrodes. Both the total rise during cuff inflation and the fall in the first 3 seconds of deflation are plotted on a two-way IPG graph. The graph includes a "discriminant line," which was developed by discriminant function analysis to optimally distinguish normal results from abnormal results indicating proximal vein thrombosis (Fig. 104-1).[33]

The accuracy of IPG is critically dependent on the degree of venous filling during cuff occlusion.[35] The occlusive cuff test, as originally performed, used a 45-second occlusion time. However, it was found that venous filling was frequently suboptimal, and this compromised the accuracy of the test. Thus the period of cuff occlusion was increased to 2 minutes and this ensured that maximum venous filling occurred in all patients for each test. Repeated sequential testing was also introduced because this brought about an increase in venous capacitance by promoting stress relaxation of the vessel wall. These maneuvers increase both venous filling and the sensitivity and specificity of the test. It was also noted that in normal legs, if venous filling in-

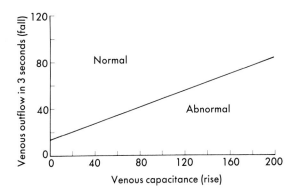

Fig. 104-1. IPG scoring graph with discriminant line. The numbers on the horizontal and vertical axes refer to impedance units.

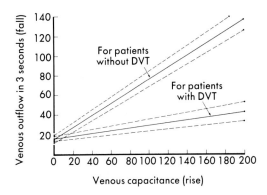

Fig. 104-2. Relationship between venous filling (IPG rise) and venous emptying (IPG fall) in patients with and without proximal deep vein thrombosis *(DVT)*. As venous filling improves, regression lines expressing the relationship between venous filling and emptying diverge and are significantly different for patients with and without proximal vein thrombosis (p < 0.001). Broken lines indicate 95% confidence limits. (From Hull R et al: *Circulation* 58:898, 1978.)

creased, there was a corresponding increase in venous emptying, but this was not the case in legs with proximal vein thrombosis; therefore the regression lines relating venous filling and emptying (Fig. 104-2) in normal and abnormal legs diverged significantly (p < 0.001). Thus by increasing venous filling, the separation between normal and abnormal IPG results was more distinct and this enhanced the accuracy of the test.

Four patterns of IPG response are observed on sequential tests (Fig. 104-3). In 76% of legs that are normal according to venography, the initial result falls above the discriminant line, as do all subsequent results. However, in 20% of such legs, the initial result recorded after only 45 seconds of occlusion falls below the discriminant line; when venous filling is improved by prolonging the cuff occlusion time and performing sequential tests, subsequent results fall above the discriminant line. In 82% of legs shown to have proximal vein thrombosis by venography, the initial and all subsequent results fall below the discriminant line. However, in 10%, the initial result after 45 seconds of occlusion falls above the discriminant line, but as venous filling is improved, it is not accompanied by a corresponding improvement in venous emptying and the results fall below the discriminant line. This last pattern is sometimes seen in patients with nonobstructive proximal vein thrombi.

In a prospective study consisting of 324 patients, it was found that if only a single result was obtained after a 45-second occlusion, specificity deteriorated to 20% and sensitivity to 10%. Because sequential testing is time consuming, an additional study was performed to determine whether the sequential approach could be simplified without loss of

accuracy. By analyzing those cases with an abnormal IPG result and venographically shown proximal vein thrombosis it was possible to establish a "stop line" parallel to the discriminant line. This allowed the multiple test sequence to be terminated early without loss of accuracy when any result in the sequence fell above this line (Fig. 104-4). Using this approach, it was found that the IPG test sequence can be terminated without loss of accuracy in 44% of normal patients after one test, in 59% after two tests, and in 80% after three tests.

Causes of discrepancy between IPG and venographic results. IPG only detects thrombi that obstruct venous outflow. Therefore it will not disclose most calf vein thrombi, since they do not obstruct the main outflow tract, and it may not detect small nonocclusive thrombi in proximal veins. Findings may also be negative when proximal vein thrombosis is associated with well-developed collateral vessels.

IPG does not distinguish between thrombotic and non-thrombotic obstruction to venous outflow. Thus false-positive results may be obtained if (1) a patient is positioned incorrectly or inadequately relaxed, because this may result in venous constriction due to contracted leg muscles; (2) the vein is compressed by an extravascular mass; (3) venous outflow is impaired because of raised central venous pressure; or (4) arterial inflow to the limb is reduced because of severe obstructive arterial disease, also leading to reduced outflow.

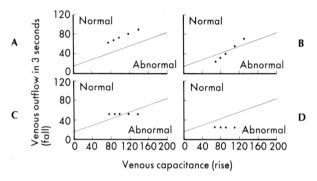

Fig. 104-3. Four patterns of IPG response observed in patients with and without proximal DVT using occlusive cuff IPG technique with sequential testing and prolonged cuff occlusion. In 76% of legs found normal by venography, the initial tests fall above the discriminant line, as do all subsequent tests **(A).** In 20% of legs found normal by venography, the initial tests fall below the discriminant line **(B),** but subsequent tests, including the test with the highest rise and greatest fall, land in the normal zone above the line. In 10% of legs with proximal DVT, the initial tests fall above the line **(C).** However, subsequent tests, including the test with the highest rise and greatest fall, lie below the line in the abnormal zone. This pattern of improved venous filling without corresponding improvement in venous emptying is commonly seen in patients with obstructive proximal venous thrombosis, resulting in fixed venous outflow. In 82% of legs with proximal DVT, the initial tests and all subsequent tests fall below the discriminant line **(D).**

Unrecognized contraction of leg muscles in either nervous patients or after surgery, particularly in patients with postoperative pain, is an acknowledged cause of false-positive IPG results. The inexperienced technician and, on occasion, the experienced technician may have difficulty distinguishing an abnormal IPG result caused by venous thrombosis from that caused by isometric muscle contraction. Because isometric muscle contraction can be measured directly by electromyography, the potential clinical value of this method to detect leg muscle contraction that would

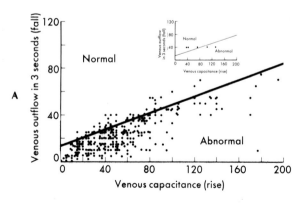

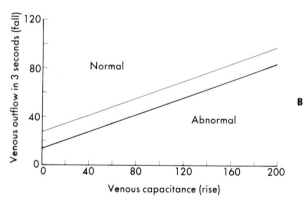

Fig. 104-4. **A,** Many of the points of the tests early in the IPG sequence of patients with proximal vein thrombosis fall above the discriminant line. **B,** The second line (stop line) was drawn above and parallel to the discriminant line so that it enclosed these points. The validity of this stop line was then confirmed prospectively.

interfere with the IPG result was investigated.[8] Voluntarily induced leg muscle contraction that altered the IPG tracing for venous filling or emptying could always be detected when the electrodes were placed both laterally and medially over the distal thigh and a ground electrode was placed over the patella. This approach detected a threshold of isometric muscle contraction below which false-positive IPG results

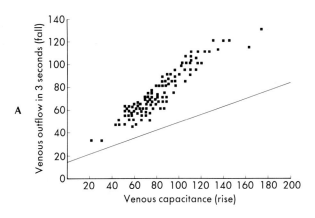

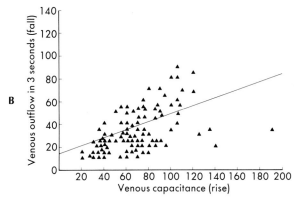

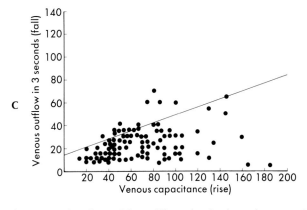

Fig. 104-5. The effects of three different levels of muscle contraction on the IPG result in 100 legs with normal baseline IPG results. Test results above the discriminant line are in the normal zone, whereas those below the line are in abnormal zone. *A,* Electromyographic readings between 0 and 25 units (mild leg muscle tension)—all IPG results are in the normal zone. *B,* Electromyographic readings between 25 and 50 units (moderate leg muscle tension)—65% of IPG results are in the abnormal zone. *C,* Electromyographic readings above 50 units (severe leg muscle tension)—89% of IPG results are in the abnormal zone. (From Biland L et al: *Thromb Res* 14:811, 1979.)

did not occur and above which there was a very high frequency of false-positive IPG results (Fig. 104-5). It proved to be clinically feasible to attach the electromyograph to the IPG machine, and it took only 5 more minutes to apply the skin electrodes.

Doppler ultrasonography

Principles. The Doppler ultrasound flowmeter examination is a noninvasive method that has been evaluated as a diagnostic test in patients with clinically suspected deep vein thrombosis.[70-72] In expert hands, Doppler ultrasound is a sensitive method for detecting occluding thrombi in the popliteal and more proximal veins but less sensitive for identifying calf vein thrombi and nonocclusive proximal thrombi. Obstruction to venous outflow may cause (1) loss of phasicity of the venous signal, producing a continuous venous signal because the normal respiratory fluctuation is lacking, and/or (2) diminished or absent augmentation of the venous signal that normally occurs when the limb distal to the probe is compressed or compression proximal to the probe is released; this augmentation may also be high pitched and of short duration.

Causes of discrepancy between Doppler ultrasound and venography. The Doppler flowmeter method has many of the same limitations as IPG: It is relatively insensitive for identifying calf vein thrombosis and may not detect small, partly occluding proximal vein thrombi. The technique is simple and rapid, but interpretation of results depends much more on the experience of the examiner than is the case with IPG. Recently, an objective Doppler method has been developed that overcomes the limitation imposed by the subjective interpretation.[61] This method has proved both sensitive and specific for identifying proximal vein thrombosis in symptomatic patients.

False-positive results may be obtained under two circumstances: (1) if the underlying vein is compressed with the transducer or the femoral vein or calf is compressed when the limb is drained of blood and (2) if the patient is incorrectly positioned, since this can eliminate or decrease the augmentation sound.

Real-time B-mode ultrasonography and duplex scanning

Principles. The availability of high-resolution, real-time ultrasound probes has led to the application of ultrasound imaging in the diagnosis of DVT.[5,10,20,60,76] Duplex ultrasound combines real-time ultrasound imaging with Doppler ultrasound.[76] Real-time imaging directly visualizes the major deep veins, whereas the Doppler component assesses venous flow. Because of recent technologic advances, the Doppler signal generated by moving blood can now be converted into a color image, so-called color flow Doppler or color imaging.[76]

Real-time B-mode ultrasound is highly sensitive and specific for detecting proximal vein thrombosis in symptomatic patients but, like other methods, is relatively insensitive for disclosing isolated calf vein thrombosis.[5,60,76] A recent prospective study[60] has shown that the single criterion of vein compressibility has high sensitivity and specificity for identifying proximal vein thrombosis (100% and 99%, respectively). Other criteria are less useful. This includes visualization of an echogenic band, which is highly sensitive for revealing proximal vein thrombosis but has a specificity of only 50%.[60] The percentage of change in venous diameter during a Valsalva maneuver is both insensitive (55%) and relatively nonspecific (67%).[60]

The specificity of real-time B-mode ultrasound is potentially better than that of hemodynamic tests such as IPG in patients with raised central venous pressure (e.g., due to congestive cardiac failure, which may produce false-positive IPG findings). In addition, venous imaging may identify patients with extrinsic venous compression (e.g., from a Baker's cyst).

Causes of discrepancies between B-mode ultrasonography and venographic results. Real-time B-mode ultrasonography is insensitive for identifying calf-vein thrombosis[76] and may not detect isolated iliac vein thrombi.[21,76] In a recent prospective study[60] carried out in symptomatic outpatients, the areas of scanning were confined to the common femoral vein in the groin and the popliteal vein, for the reason that isolated iliac vein thrombosis is rare in symptomatic outpatients, and when thrombosis occurs, it almost always involves either the common femoral vein or the popliteal vein. This approach has shown a sensitivity of 100% and specificity of 99% for demonstrating proximal vein thrombosis. Its inability to detect isolated iliac vein thrombi, however, may limit its use in patient groups in whom isolated iliac vein thrombosis is more common (such as pregnant women with clinically suspected venous thrombosis).

Other noninvasive techniques for the diagnosis of venous thrombosis

A number of other techniques have been less extensively evaluated for the diagnosis of venous thrombosis, including phleborheography (air cuff plethysmography),[14] strain-gauge plethysmography,[3,29] thermography,[13] radioisotope venography,[26,48] and blood tests that detect intravascular fibrin formation and fibrin proteolysis.[9,77,78] Both phleborheography and strain-gauge plethysmography can identify proximal vein thrombosis, although strain-gauge plethysmography was shown to be less sensitive than IPG.[29] Phleborheography requires the subjective interpretation of results, and this is a disadvantage. Thermography has shown promise, but further studies are required before its value and limitations can be adequately known. Radioisotope venography has also been evaluated[48,59] and, in a recent prospective study,[59] was shown to be significantly less specific than IPG in the evaluation of symptomatic patients. Sensitive and specific blood tests that can detect intravascular fibrin formation and fibrin proteolysis have been developed but are not yet available for routine use because they are technically cumbersome to perform. These tests, which include the radioimmunoassay fibrinopeptide A,[77] fragment E,[78] or fragment D-dimer of fibrin,[9] are sensitive in the context of acute venous thrombosis but by their nature are nonspecific.

APPLICATION OF NONINVASIVE TESTS FOR THE DIAGNOSIS OF CLINICALLY SUSPECTED VENOUS THROMBOSIS

Two types of prospective studies are required to adequately define the role of noninvasive tests in the diagnosis of clinically suspected venous thrombosis: (1) those in which the *accuracy* of noninvasive testing is evaluated by direct comparison with venography and (2) those that incorporate long-term follow-up to evaluate the *clinical outcome* in patients whose treatment has been based on the findings of noninvasive testing. The accuracy of four such noninvasive tests has been extensively evaluated: [125I]fibrinogen leg scanning,[51,52] IPG,[33-35] Doppler ultrasonography,[61,70,72] and real-time B-mode ultrasonography.[5,60,76] None of these tests when used alone is as accurate as venography in the diagnosis of symptomatic venous thrombosis; leg scanning cannot detect thrombi in the proximal thigh, and IPG, Doppler ultrasonography, and real-time B-mode ultrasound are all relatively insensitive for identifying isolated calf vein thrombosis. However, clinical trials performed over the past decade have brought to light two important findings: (1) combining [125I]fibrinogen leg scanning with IPG is essentially as accurate as venography in diagnosing symptomatic patients[34,40] and (2) it is safe to withhold anticoagulant therapy in symptomatic patients when the results of serial testing with either IPG[25,30,32,44,45] or real-time ultrasonography[25] remain negative. This latter observation is particularly important because, as mentioned earlier, [125I]fibrinogen leg scanning is no longer performed because of the risk of HIV transmission. Therefore serial testing with either IPG or real-time ultrasonography is now the preferred noninvasive approach in patients with clinically suspected venous thrombosis, and the thinking that underlies this approach is that calf vein thrombi, which are not detected by IPG or real-time ultrasonography, do not precipitate a clinically important pulmonary embolism unless they extend into the proximal veins. This has now been confirmed by clinical observations made in multiple studies.[25,30,32,44,45] Repeated examinations with IPG or real-time ultrasonography will identify those patients who develop proximal extension of calf vein thrombosis. To date, the effectiveness and safety of serial Doppler ultrasonography has not been prospectively evaluated in terms of clinical outcome during long-term follow-up (this applies to both the subjective interpretation of results and the more recently developed objective technique). Therefore either IPG or real-time B-mode ultrasonography remains the preferred approach.

Real-time ultrasound imaging equipment is widely available at hospitals, and this technique potentially represents the "wave of the future" for the noninvasive testing of venous thrombosis. IPG is a highly effective, low-cost technology that continues to play an important role in centers where it is available. The equipment for real-time B-mode ultrasonography is considerably more expensive than that for IPG. This is an important issue in the current health care environment, particularly because IPG is a highly effective diagnostic tool. It could be argued that the increased cost of real-time ultrasound equipment over IPG can only be justified if the method confers some important added clinical benefit; this matter should be resolved by the results of clinical trials released over the next few years. Preliminary data comparing the two approaches are already coming available.[25] This matter may also be resolved if the cost of real-time ultrasound equipment is considerably reduced. Another important issue is the relative value of IPG and B-mode ultrasonography in the diagnosis of acute recurrent venous thrombosis because real-time ultrasonography has some potentially important limitations in this context[76] (see p. 857). The comparative roles of real-time ultrasonography, IPG, and other noninvasive tests will be further clarified by the results of clinical trials becoming available over the next few years.

The findings from studies evaluating both the accuracy and long-term clinical outcome associated with IPG, Doppler ultrasonography, and real-time ultrasonography are summarized in the following sections. Although [125I]fibrinogen leg scanning is no longer used for clinical purposes, the combined approach of leg scanning and IPG is discussed for historical interest and because this information provides an important perspective on the relative effectiveness of serial IPG and venography.

Impedance plethysmography

A number of studies have evaluated the accuracy of IPG in patients with clinically suspected venous thromboembolism.* Wheeler et al[75] compared the results of IPG and venography in 168 legs. The results of both IPG and venography were normal in 106 of 108 legs and the IPG findings were abnormal in 40 of 41 legs with venographically demonstrated recent thrombi of the popliteal, femoral, or iliac veins (proximal vein thrombosis). However, IPG identified only 3 of 19 calf vein thrombi detected by venography. In an investigation conducted by Johnston and Kakkar,[49] who used a similar technique, all 20 proximal vein thrombi were detected by IPG. IPG results were normal in 40 of 44 legs without thrombosis and abnormal in only 5 of 15 legs with calf vein thrombi.

In a study carried out in 346 patients with suspected venous thrombosis,[33] the IPG result was abnormal in 124 of 133 limbs with venographically confirmed proximal vein thrombosis, yielding a sensitivity of 93%. IPG results were normal in 73 of 88 limbs with calf vein thrombosis. The IPG result was falsely positive in 11 of 397 legs, most of which had clearly recognizable clinical conditions known to produce such results. Thus in patients with clinically

suspected venous thrombosis, a positive IPG result can be used to determine therapeutic decisions when there are no clinical conditions known to produce false-positive results (e.g., congestive cardiac failure, severe peripheral vascular disease, local leg muscle tension). A normal result essentially rules out proximal vein thrombosis but does not exclude the possibility of calf vein thrombosis or a small nonocclusive proximal vein thrombus. As collateral vessels form or as partial recanalization of the vessel occurs, the IPG result may become normal.

IPG and [125I]fibrinogen leg scanning. As discussed earlier, IPG may not detect calf vein thrombosis. Therefore the combined use of IPG and [125I]fibrinogen leg scanning was evaluated in 200 patients with clinically suspected venous thrombosis.[34] On the day of referral, each patient was injected with [125I]fibrinogen and leg scanning was carried out daily for the next 3 days. IPG was also performed on the day of referral and then daily for the next 3 days. In addition, all patients underwent bilateral ascending venography, which was performed on the third day if the test results were negative or earlier if either of the results became positive. Either IPG or leg scanning was positive in 81 of 86 patients with positive venograms (sensitivity, 94%), and both tests were negative in 104 of 114 patients who had negative venograms (specificity, 91%). These two tests identified all 60 patients with proximal vein thrombosis, 21 of 26 patients with calf vein thrombosis, and 20 of 21 patients with calf vein thrombosis who had had symptoms for less than 1 week. The findings of this study have been confirmed by a more recent study consisting of 274 additional symptomatic patients.[40] The results of either IPG or leg scanning were positive in 103 of 114 patients with positive venograms (sensitivity, 90%) and results of both tests were negative in 152 of 160 patients who had negative venograms (specificity, 93%).[40] This approach identified all 78 patients with proximal vein thrombosis, 25 of 36 patients with calf vein thrombosis, and 16 of 17 patients with calf vein thrombosis who had had symptoms for less than 1 week.[40]

These results therefore confirm the findings of the previous study and indicate that the combined use of IPG and leg scanning offers an alternative to venography in patients with clinically suspected acute deep vein thrombosis. However, as already mentioned, because of possible HIV transmission, serial IPG has now replaced this combined approach.[44]

Doppler ultrasonography

There have been several carefully performed studies that compared the results of the Doppler flowmeter examination with the venographic findings in patients with clinically suspected venous thrombosis. The results of these studies show that this technique is sensitive for detecting proximal vein thrombosis but not calf vein thrombosis.[60,70,72] A positive Doppler finding when the probe is placed over the thigh is highly specific for indicating acute proximal vein thrombosis. However, if the Doppler result is only positive

---

*References 34, 35, 39, 49, 50, 75.

when the probe is placed over the posterior tibial vein, venographic confirmation should be obtained, since the Doppler results are relatively nonspecific at this site.[79]

The Doppler ultrasound examination can be performed more conveniently and rapidly and is less expensive than IPG. Until recently, its major disadvantage was that the results were interpreted subjectively, and this required considerable skill and experience. More recently, an objective Doppler method has been introduced that eliminates this problem, and this new method is both sensitive and specific for detecting proximal vein thrombosis in symptomatic patients. Doppler ultrasound is more reliable than IPG for detecting proximal vein thrombosis in patients with raised central venous pressure or arterial insufficiency and can be used in patients with legs in plaster casts or in traction.

Real-time B-mode ultrasonography or duplex scanning

The accuracy of venous imaging and duplex scanning have been evaluated by multiple studies[5,60,76] in patients with clinically suspected venous thrombosis. The findings indicate that these approaches are highly sensitive and specific for diagnosing proximal vein thrombosis, but like IPG and the Doppler ultrasound flowmeter examination, real-time ultrasonography cannot detect isolated calf vein thrombosis. In a prospective study of 220 consecutive outpatients with suspected venous thrombosis, Lensing et al[60] compared the results of real-time B-mode ultrasonography with those of contrast venography. The common femoral and popliteal veins were assessed for the presence of full compressibility (no thrombosis) or noncompressibility (thrombosis). This technique identified all 66 patients with proximal vein thrombosis, for a sensitivity of 100%, and both veins were fully compressible in 142 of the 143 patients with normal venograms, for a specificity of 99%. A second examiner, who was unaware of the results of the first test, repeated the compression ultrasound test in a subset of 45 consecutive patients. These second results agreed with the first ones in all patients. Several other studies consisting of smaller numbers of patients have revealed a similar high sensitivity and specificity for the diagnosis of proximal vein thrombosis using real-time ultrasonography.[5,76]

Repeated examination with IPG, Doppler ultrasound, or real-time B-mode ultrasonography

The rationale for repeated testing using one of the tests described is based on the concept that calf vein thrombi are only clinically important when they extend into the proximal veins, at which point detection with IPG or with Doppler or real-time ultrasound is possible. Therefore repeated examinations using one of these tests should identify those patients with extending calf vein thrombosis and appropriate treatment then instituted. Because extension occurs only in a minority of such patients (about 20%), treatment is confined to those who will best benefit. An alternative approach is to detect and treat all calf vein thrombi, but this may do more harm than good because the potential benefits of anticoagulant therapy may be outweighed by the risk of bleeding.

The effectiveness and safety of serial testing with IPG or real-time B-mode ultrasonography has been evaluated by prospective studies,[25,30,32,44,45] but the use of serial Doppler ultrasound alone has not been formally evaluated.

In a randomized clinical trial, the results of combined IPG and leg scanning (which is essentially as accurate a method as venography) were compared with the results of serial IPG alone in the diagnosis of clinically suspected venous thrombosis.[44] IPG was performed on the day of referral and, if results were negative, again on the following day, the fifth to seventh day, the tenth day, and the fourteenth day. It was found that this method is as effective as the combination of IPG and leg scanning. Furthermore, the long-term clinical outcomes indicate that is it safe to withhold anticoagulant therapy in patients whose serial IPG results remain negative for 14 days.[44] None of the 303 patients so treated died from pulmonary embolism, and only 6 (2%) returned with clinically evident venous thromboembolism documented by objective testing. This prognosis for patients with negative serial IPG results is similar to that observed for symptomatic patients with negative venograms.[38] The findings of this randomized trial have been confirmed by four subsequent prospective studies,[25,30,32,45] including a recent study conducted in pregnant women with clinically suspected venous thrombosis.[45] The findings from a recent randomized trial also indicate that serial real-time B-mode ultrasonography is as effective and safe as serial IPG.[25]

The long-term clinical outcomes seen in symptomatic patients who remain negative by serial IPG or B-mode ultrasonography are in striking contrast to the findings observed using a modified form of IPG, computerized impedance plethysmography (CIP). In CIP, a modified device is used to measure impedance, and it responds differently to the increased venous filling achieved by prolonged cuff occlusion and sequential testing. Importantly, the line discriminating normal from abnormal results differs from that for standard IPG. Prandoni et al[68] recently published their observations in a prospective study evaluating the safety of withholding anticoagulant therapy in symptomatic patients with repeatedly normal CIP findings. This study was prematurely terminated by the safety monitoring committee because of an unacceptably high incidence of fatal pulmonary embolism (4 of 311 patients, or 1.3%). This experience is strikingly different from that with standard IPG, as demonstrated by four prospective studies. These studies documented no episodes of fatal pulmonary embolism in 870 patients with repeatedly normal IPG results (95% confidence interval, 0% to 0.4%). CIP therefore cannot be regarded as safe for evaluating patients with clinically suspected venous thrombosis, and the results with the CIP should not be generalized to standard IPG, which is both effective and safe in symptomatic patients.

Tests that measure fibrin formation or its lysis in plasma or serum

The presence of intravascular fibrin can be determined by measuring the level of fibrinopeptide A in the plasma or fibrin degradation products in the serum. The fibrinopeptide A assay result is only positive if the test is performed while the thrombus is being laid down, whereas fibrin degradation products may be detected for days after the thrombotic process has been arrested. The standard tests for fibrin degradation products, such as the latex agglutination test, tagged red cell hemagglutination inhibition assay, and staphylococcal clumping, are not sufficiently sensitive to be of clinical value in patients with acute venous thrombosis. However, a recently developed radioimmunoassay for fragment E has proved useful for excluding a diagnosis of acute venous thrombosis.[78] Because both the fibrinopeptide A assay[77] and the radioimmunoassay for fibrin degradation products detect only intravascular fibrin formation, they are not specific for diagnosing acute venous thrombosis. Either of these tests might be useful in combination with some of the other noninvasive diagnostic tests, but the real merit of this approach has not yet been determined. The major current drawbacks of these tests are that they are technically difficult to carry out and not readily available; they also take a number of hours to perform. However, if they were simplified, they would be a potentially valuable addition to the objective assessment of venous thrombosis.

PRACTICAL APPROACH TO THE DIAGNOSIS OF CLINICALLY SUSPECTED VENOUS THROMBOSIS USING NONINVASIVE TESTS

An algorithm for the noninvasive diagnosis of clinically suspected venous thrombosis is presented in Fig. 104-6. In this protocol, IPG (or B-mode ultrasonography) is performed immediately; if it is positive and the patient has no clinical conditions that are known to produce false-positive results, venous thrombosis is diagnosed and the patient is treated accordingly. If the result of the initial IPG or B-mode evaluation is negative, anticoagulant therapy is withheld and the test is repeated on the following day and again on the third day, the fifth to seventh day, the tenth day, and the fourteenth day. If the result becomes positive during this time, venous thrombosis is diagnosed and anticoagulant therapy is commenced. A positive IPG in the context of conditions known to produce a false-positive result (e.g., congestive cardiac failure) should be confirmed by venography. If noninvasive tests for the diagnosis of venous thrombosis are not available, ascending venography should be performed to objectively confirm or exclude the diagnosis.

DIFFERENTIAL DIAGNOSIS OF SUSPECTED DEEP VEIN THROMBOSIS

The differential diagnosis in patients with clinically suspected venous thrombosis includes muscle strain (usually

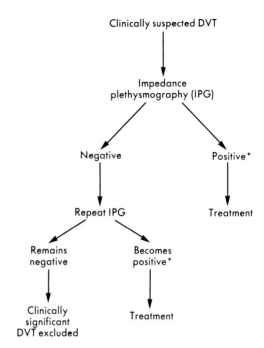

Fig. 104-6. Practical noninvasive approach for diagnosis of clinically suspected DVT using serial IPG. *Indicates absence of conditions known to produce false-positive IPG result (e.g., congestive cardiac failure). Recent data[25] indicate that real-time B-mode ultrasonography can be substituted for IPG in this algorithm.

associated with unaccustomed exercise), direct twisting injury to the leg, vasomotor changes in a paralyzed leg, venous reflux, lymphangitis, lymphatic obstruction, muscle tear, Baker's cyst, cellulitis, internal derangement of a knee hematoma, heart failure, and the postphlebitic syndrome.[38] It is frequently not possible to establish an alternate diagnosis at the time of referral, but without objective testing, it is also not possible to rule out venous thrombosis.[38] Often, however, the cause of symptoms can be determined during careful follow-up once venous thrombosis has been ruled out.[38] In some patients, the cause of pain, tenderness, and swelling remains uncertain even after careful follow-up and is presumably due to inflammation of other soft tissues of the leg.[38]

DIAGNOSIS OF ACUTE RECURRENT VENOUS THROMBOSIS

When patients have pain, tenderness, or swelling in a leg site where previous venous thrombosis has been confirmed or suspected, it may be difficult to distinguish between acute recurrent thrombosis and the nonthrombotic complications of chronic venous insufficiency.

Patients with clinically suspected recurrent DVT pose a diagnostic challenge because the clinical diagnosis of recurrent DVT is highly nonspecific and because each of the objective tests for diagnosing this disorder has potential limitations in this context. Recurrent leg symptoms after DVT may be due to acute recurrent DVT, the postphlebitic syndrome, or a variety of nonthrombotic disorders. Differentiation among these three causes of recurrent symptoms is important because anticoagulant therapy is only necessary in patients with recurrent thrombosis.

A drawback of venography alone is that the diagnostic hallmark, a constant intraluminal filling defect, may be masked by obliteration and recanalization. Consequently, the venographic findings may be inconclusive in patients who have had previous disease. IPG findings may be falsely positive if there is persistent venous outflow obstruction resulting from a previous episode of venous thrombosis, or they may be falsely negative if large collateral channels have formed after the first episode. Abnormal B-mode ultrasonography findings (e.g., noncompressible vessels) may persist for months to years after an episode of proximal vein thrombosis. [125I]fibrinogen leg scanning can detect active calf and distal thigh vein thrombi but is relatively insensitive in the upper thigh and cannot detect external and common iliac vein thrombi.

Evaluation of objective testing for suspected recurrent deep vein thrombosis

A cohort analytic study[43] has been completed that incorporated the long-term findings in 270 patients with symptoms and signs of acute recurrent DVT who were evaluated by combined IPG and [125I]fibrinogen leg scanning plus venography. Previously it had not been possible to use conventional methods to assess the accuracy of this diagnostic approach because there was no acceptable reference standard for the diagnosis of acute recurrent venous thrombosis. The problem was overcome in this study by establishing prior diagnostic criteria for the presence or absence of acute recurrence and then determining the validity of the criteria by the results of long-term follow-up. At the onset of the study, the decision was made to withhold anticoagulant therapy in patients with negative IPG and leg scanning results, regardless of the severity or extent of the clinical findings.

The diagnostic protocol used in the study is outlined in Fig. 104-7. IPG was performed immediately on referral; if the results were negative, the patient was injected with [125I]fibrinogen and leg scanning was performed 1 and 3 days later, at which time IPG was also repeated. Anticoagulant therapy was withheld in all patients whose test results remained negative. If the initial IPG result was positive, venography was performed. Anticoagulant therapy was begun in all such patients if venography also detected a constant intraluminal filling defect. If the venographic findings were negative, the patient was injected with [125I]fibrinogen and underwent leg scanning 1 and 3 days later. Anticoagulant therapy was begun if the [125I]fibrinogen

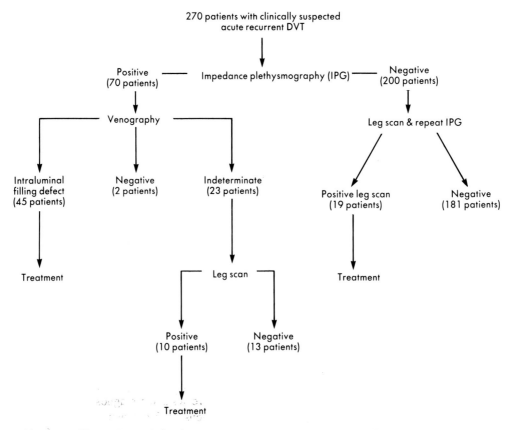

Fig. 104-7. Diagnostic process and outcome on entry in 270 patients with clinically suspected acute recurrent DVT.

scan result was positive. All patients were then evaluated at 3 and 12 months.

Of the total 270 patients in the study, 181 (67%) had negative IPG and leg scan results (Fig. 104-7); 89 (33%) patients had positive IPG and leg scan results.[43] Anticoagulant therapy was withheld in all 181 patients with the negative results. During long-term follow-up, none died as the result of pulmonary embolism and only 3 (1.7%) returned with objectively documented recurrence. In contrast, 18 (20%) of the 89 patients with positive IPG or leg scan results (who were treated) suffered new episodes of objectively documented venous thromboembolism, and this included 4 deaths (4.5%) due to massive pulmonary embolism (*p* < 0.001). The long-term results indicate that the combination of noninvasive testing and venography can be used to separate such patients into two groups: a negative cohort in whom it is safe to withhold anticoagulant therapy[43] and a positive cohort who requires anticoagulant therapy.[37,43]

Differential diagnosis. Once acute recurrent DVT has been ruled out by objective means, the differential diagnosis in patients with recurrent leg symptoms includes the postphlebitic syndrome and a variety of nonthrombotic causes. Postphlebitic syndrome is suggested by the presence of venous insufficiency, and the incompetence of the valves of the deep veins that leads to this can be demonstrated by Doppler ultrasound or by a variety of plethysmographic techniques. Nonthrombotic causes for leg symptoms should be considered when both recurrent DVT and the postphlebitic syndrome have been ruled out. The nonthrombotic causes of recurrent leg symptoms are essentially the same as those for a first episode of clinically suspected DVT. In many such patients, however, a cause for leg symptoms is not identified, and when this happens, a diagnosis of thromboneurosis should be considered.

Thromboneurosis is a common but poorly recognized clinical syndrome that may simulate acute recurrent venous thrombosis. It is seen most frequently in patients with a morbid fear of the complications of venous thromboembolism and especially those who have had a previous episode of objectively documented venous thrombosis or who were originally misdiagnosed with false-positive results.

The clinical presentation of thromboneurosis includes leg pain and tenderness, and in its most severe form, the patient may be totally incapacitated by the fear of recurrent venous thromboembolism, limb loss, and even death.

Patients with thromboneurosis frequently have a history of multiple hospital admissions for the treatment of "recurrent venous thrombosis." Because of the recurrent nature of these episodes, many patients are maintained on long-term anticoagulant therapy, and some have even undergone vena caval interruption. Because thromboneurosis is often iatrogenic and the patient's fear of recurrence is only reinforced by hospital admission and treatment based purely on clinical suspicion, it can best be prevented by ensuring that a clinical suspicion of acute venous thrombosis is always confirmed or excluded by objective testing.

PRACTICAL APPROACH TO THE DIAGNOSIS OF ACUTE RECURRENT VENOUS THROMBOSIS

Acute recurrent venous thrombosis can be diagnosed by IPG if the test result was negative before presentation and is positive at the time of presentation. This finding can greatly simplify the practical diagnostic approach in such patients.

It is rare for venous thromboembolism to recur in patients on adequate anticoagulant therapy (less than 5%),[37,41,42] and most recurrences take place 3 months after anticoagulant therapy has been stopped. Prospective studies indicate that 60% to 70% of patients with their first episode of extensive proximal DVT have a normal IPG result when anticoagulant therapy is discontinued at 3 months.[31,47] For this reason, a baseline IPG evaluation can be an effective approach in all such patients when long-term anticoagulant therapy is terminated.

The algorithm for the diagnosis of clinically suspected recurrent DVT is shown in Fig. 104-8. The approach is based on the use of IPG because the value of B-mode ultrasonography in this context is uncertain and because it has not yet been adequately evaluated by prospective studies.

Since completion of the 1983 study,[43] two developments have occurred that have influenced the approach to the diagnosis of suspected acute recurrent DVT. First, serial testing with IPG has proved as effective as the combined approach of IPG and leg scanning,[44] and second, [¹²⁵I]fibrinogen is no longer used in clinical practice. This latter development has necessitated a modified approach to the diagnosis of suspected acute recurrent venous thrombosis. In such patients with initially negative IPG or B-mode ultrasonography findings, it would appear reasonable to perform serial testing with either of these tests, since the effectiveness and safety of this approach has been documented in patients with a first episode of suspected venous thrombosis.[25,32,44] On the basis of the data shown in Fig. 104-7, serial testing with IPG is sufficient in about 75% of the cases of clinically suspected acute recurrent DVT. For example, in the study previously disclosed, 200 of 270 patients had negative IPG results at the initial presentation.[43]

If the IPG result is positive at the time of referral, management is determined by whether the IPG result was previously negative or was previously abnormal or unknown, as shown in Fig. 104-8. A positive IPG finding in a patient with a previously negative IPG is highly predictive of acute recurrent venous thrombosis,[43] and in the absence of conditions known to produce false-positive results, the patient can be treated accordingly.

Venography should be performed in patients with positive IPG findings at referral whose previous results were abnormal or unknown (Fig. 104-8). The diagnosis of acute recurrent venous thrombosis is definitively established if venography documents new intraluminal filling defects. Patients with indeterminate venographic findings (because of unfilled venous segments or persistent intraluminal filling defects) pose a diagnostic dilemma. In these patients, it may

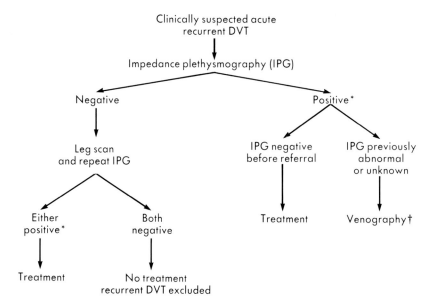

Fig. 104-8. Practical diagnostic approach in patients with clinically suspected acute recurrent DVT. *Indicates absence of conditions known to produce false-positive test result. †See text for discussion of management of venographic findings.

be prudent to err on the side of treatment, rather than risk death from massive pulmonary embolism. Data suggest that by using IPG and venography in combination, a definitive decision to institute or withhold anticoagulant therapy can be made in more than 90% of patients with clinically suspected acute recurrent DVT.[43]

THE USE OF NONINVASIVE TESTS FOR SCREENING HIGH-RISK PATIENTS

The use of noninvasive tests for screening asymptomatic patients at high risk for developing venous thrombosis has now been evaluated in multiple studies.* This has been most extensively evaluated in patients undergoing major orthopedic surgery of the lower limb.* In contrast to symptomatic patients, the findings indicate that the use of IPG or real-time B-mode ultrasonography for screening asymptomatic patients at high risk for venous thrombosis because of recent hip or knee surgery has major limitations. These tests fail to detect 40% to 60% of proximal vein thrombi (and most calf vein thrombi).[10,20] Therefore venography is required for the optimal detection of thrombosis after such procedures.

---

*References 2, 6, 10, 20, 23, 24, 36, 46, 51, 55, 67, 73.

REFERENCES

1. Albrechtsson V, Olsson CB: Thrombotic side effects of lower limb phlebography, *Lancet* 1:723, 1976.
2. Atkins P, Hawkins LA: Detection of venous thrombosis in the legs, *Lancet* 2:1217, 1965.
3. Barnes RW et al: Noninvasive quantitation of maximum venous outflow in acute thrombophlebitis, *Surgery* 72:971, 1972.
4. Bauer G: A venographic study of thromboembolic problems, *Acta Chir Scand* 84(suppl 161):1, 1940.
5. Becker DM et al: Real-time ultrasonography for the diagnosis of lower extremity deep venous thrombosis: the wave of the future? *Arch Intern Med* 149:1731, 1989.
6. Becker J: The diagnosis of venous thrombosis in the legs using I-labelled fibrinogen: an experimental and clinical study, *Acta Chir Scand* 138:667, 1972.
7. Bettman MA, Paulin S: Leg phlebography: the incidence, nature and modification of undesirable side effects, *Radiology* 122:101, 1977.
8. Biland L et al: The use of electromyography to detect muscle contraction responsible for falsely positive impedance plethysmographic results, *Thromb Res* 14:811, 1979.
9. Boneu B et al: D-dimers, thrombin antithrombin III complexes and prothrombin fragments 1 + 2: diagnostic value in clinically suspected deep vein thrombosis, *Thromb Haemost* 65:28, 1991.
10. Boris LC et al: Comparison of real-time B-mode ultrasonography and bilateral ascending phlebography for detection of postoperative deep vein thrombosis following elective hip surgery, *Thromb Haemost* 61:363, 1989.
11. Browse NL: The ¹²⁵I-fibrinogen uptake test, *Arch Surg* 104:160, 1972.
12. Browse NL et al: Diagnosis of established deep vein thrombosis with the ¹²⁵I-fibrinogen uptake test, *Br Med J* 4:325, 1971.
13. Cooke Ed, Pilcher MF: Deep vein thrombosis: a preclinical diagnosis by thermography, *Br J Surg* 61:971, 1974.
14. Cranley JJ et al: A plethysmographic technique for the diagnosis of deep venous thrombosis of the lower extremities, *Surg Gynecol Obstet* 136:385, 1973.
15. Dow JD: Retrograde phlebography in major pulmonary embolism, *Lancet* 2:407, 1973.
16. Evans DS: The early diagnosis of thromboembolism by ultrasound, *Ann R Coll Surg Engl* 49:225, 1971.
17. Flanc C, Kakkar VV, Clarke MB: The detection of venous thrombosis of the legs using ¹²⁵I-labelled fibrinogen, *Br J Surg* 55:742, 1968.
18. Gallus AS, Hirsh J: ¹²⁵I-labelled fibrinogen leg scanning. In Frantantoni J, Wessler S, eds: *Prophylactic therapy for deep venous thrombosis and pulmonary embolism*, DHEW Pub No (NIH) 76-866, Washington, DC, 1975, US Government Printing Office.
19. Gallus AS et al: Diagnosis of venous thromboembolism, *Semin Thromb Hemost* 2:203, 1976.
20. Ginsberg JS et al: Venous thrombosis in patients who have undergone major hip or knee surgery: detection with compression US and impedance plethysmography, *Radiology* 181:651, 1991.
21. Gocke JE et al: Detection of deep-vein thrombosis by B-mode ultrasonography, *N Engl J Med* 321:613, 1989.

22. Haeger K: Problems of acute deep venous thrombosis. I. The interpretation of signs and symptoms, *Angiology* 20:219, 1969.

23. Harris WH et al: Comparison of ^{125}I-fibrinogen count scanning with phlebography for detection of venous thrombi after elective hip surgery, *N Engl J Med* 292:665, 1975.

24. Harris WH et al: Cuff-impedance phlebography and ^{125}I-fibrinogen scanning versus roentgenographic phlebography for diagnosis of thrombophlebitis following hip surgery, *J Bone Joint Surg [Am]* 58:939, 1976.

25. Heijboer H et al: Efficacy of real-time B-mode ultrasonography versus impedance plethysmography in the diagnosis of deep-vein thrombosis in symptomatic outpatients, *Thromb Haemost* 65:804, 1991.

26. Highman JH, O'Sullivan E, Thomas E: Isotope venography, *Br J Surg* 60:52, 1973.

27. Hobbs JT, Davies JWL: Detection of venous thrombosis with ^{131}I-labelled fibrinogen in the rabbit, *Lancet* 2:134, 1960.

28. Holmes MCG: Deep venous thrombosis of the lower limbs diagnosed by ultrasound, *Med J Aust* 1:427, 1973.

29. Huismann MV et al: A comparison of impedance plethysmography and strain gauge plethysmography in the diagnosis of deep venous thrombosis in symptomatic outpatients, *Thromb Res* 40:533, 1985.

30. Huismann MV et al: Serial impedance plethysmography for suspected deep-venous thrombosis in outpatients: the Amsterdam General Practitioner Study, *N Engl J Med* 314:823, 1986.

31. Huismann MV et al: Utility of impedance plethysmography in the diagnosis of recurrent deep-vein thrombosis, *Arch Intern Med* 148:681, 1988.

32. Huismann MV et al: Management of clinically suspected acute venous thrombosis in outpatients with serial impedance plethysmography in a community hospital setting, *Arch Intern Med* 149:511, 1989.

33. Hull R et al: Impedance plethysmography using the occlusive cuff technique in the diagnosis of venous thrombosis, *Circulation* 53:696, 1976.

34. Hull R et al: Combined use of leg scanning and impedance plethysmography in suspected venous thrombosis: an alternative to venography, *N Engl J Med* 296:1497, 1977.

35. Hull R et al: Impedance plethysmography: the relationship between venous filling and sensitivity and specificity for proximal vein thrombosis, *Circulation* 58:898, 1978.

36. Hull R et al: The value of adding impedance plethysmography to ^{125}I-fibrinogen leg scanning for the detection of deep vein thrombosis in high-risk surgical patients: a comparative study between patients undergoing general surgery and hip surgery, *Thromb Res* 15:227, 1979.

37. Hull R et al: Warfarin sodium versus low-dose heparin in the long-term treatment of venous thrombosis, *N Engl J Med* 301:855, 1979.

38. Hull R et al: Clinical validity of a negative venogram in patients with clinically suspected venous thrombosis, *Circulation* 64(3):622, 1981.

39. Hull R et al: Cost effectiveness of clinical diagnosis, venography, and noninvasive testing in patients with symptomatic deep-vein thrombosis, *N Engl J Med* 304:1561, 1981.

40. Hull R et al: Replacement of venography in suspected venous thrombosis by impedance plethysmography and ^{125}I-fibrinogen leg scanning: a less invasive approach, *Ann Intern Med* 94:12, 1981.

41. Hull R et al: Adjusted subcutaneous heparin versus warfarin sodium in the long-term treatment of venous thrombosis, *N Engl J Med* 306:189, 1982.

42. Hull R et al: Different intensities of oral anticoagulant therapy in the treatment of proximal vein thrombosis, *N Engl J Med* 307:1676, 1982.

43. Hull R et al: The diagnosis of acute, recurrent, deep vein thrombosis: a diagnostic challenge, *Circulation* 67(4):901, 1983.

44. Hull R et al: Diagnostic efficacy of impedance plethysmography for clinically suspected deep-vein thrombosis: a randomized trial, *Ann Intern Med* 102:21, 1985.

45. Hull R et al: Serial impedance plethysmography in pregnant patients with clinically suspected deep-vein thrombosis: clinical validity of negative findings, *Ann Intern Med* 112:663, 1991.

46. Hume M et al: Extent of leg vein thrombosis determined by impedance and ^{125}I-fibrinogen, *Am J Surg* 129:455, 1975.

47. Jay R et al: Outcome of abnormal impedance plethysmography results in patients with proximal vein thrombosis: frequency of return to normal, *Thromb Haemost* 50:152a, 1983.

48. Johnson WC et al: Technetium 99[m] isotope venography, *Am J Surg* 127:424, 1974.

49. Johnston KW, Kakkar VV: Plethysmographic diagnosis of deep-vein thrombosis, *Surg Gynecol Obstet* 139:41, 1974.

50. Johnston KW et al: A simple method for detecting deep vein thrombosis: an improved electrical impedance technique, *Am J Surg* 127:349, 1974.

51. Kakkar VV: The diagnosis of deep vein thrombosis using the ^{125}I-fibrinogen test, *Arch Surg* 104:152, 1972.

52. Kakkar VV: Fibrinogen uptake test for detection of deep vein thrombosis: a review of current practice, *Semin Nucl Med* 7:229, 1977.

53. Kakkar VV et al: Natural history of postoperative deep vein thrombosis, *Lancet* 2:230, 1969.

54. Kakkar VV et al: ^{125}I-labelled fibrinogen test adapted for routine screening for deep vein thrombosis, *Lancet* 1:540, 1972.

55. Lambie JM et al: Diagnostic accuracy in venous thrombosis, *Br Med J* 2:142, 1970.

56. Lea Thomas M: Phlebography, *Arch Surg* 104:145, 1972.

57. Lea Thomas M, Fletcher EWL: The techniques of pelvic phlebography, *Clin Radiol* 18:399, 1967.

58. Lea Thomas M, Tighe JR: Death from fat embolism as a complication of intraosseous phlebography, *Lancet* 2:1415, 1973.

59. Leclerc JR et al: Technetium-99 in red blood cell venography in patients with clinically suspected deep-vein thrombosis: a prospective study, *J Nucl Med* 29:1498, 1988.

60. Lensing AWA et al: Detection of deep-vein thrombosis by real-time ultrasonography, *N Engl J Med* 320:342, 1989.

61. Lensing AWA et al: Diagnosis of deep-vein thrombosis using an objective Doppler method, *Ann Intern Med* 113:9, 1990.

62. McLachlin J, Richard T, Paterson JD: An evaluation of clinical signs in the diagnosis of venous thrombosis, *Arch Surg* 85:738, 1962.

63. Milne RM et al: Postoperative deep venous thrombosis: a comparison of diagnostic techniques, *Lancet* 2:445, 1971.

64. Negus D et al: ^{125}I-labelled fibrinogen in the diagnosis of deep vein thrombosis and its correlation with phlebography, *Br J Surg* 55:835, 1968.

65. Nicolaides AN et al: The origin of deep vein thrombosis: a venographic study, *Br J Radiol* 44:653, 1971.

66. Palko PD, Nanson EM, Fedoruk SP: The early detection of deep venous thrombosis using I[131]-tagged human fibrinogen, *Can J Surg* 7:215, 1964.

67. Partsch H, Lofferer O, Mostbeck A: Diagnosis of established deep vein thrombosis in the leg using ^{131}I-fibrinogen, *Angiology* 25:719, 1974.

68. Prandoni P et al: Failure of computerized impedance plethysmography in the diagnostic management of patients with clinically suspected deep-vein thrombosis, *Thromb Haemost* 65:233, 1991.

69. Rabinov K, Paulin S: Roentgen diagnosis of venous thrombosis in the leg, *Arch Surg* 104:134, 1972.

70. Sigel B et al: Diagnosis of lower limb venous thrombosis by Doppler ultrasound technique, *Arch Surg* 104:174, 1972.

71. Strandness DE: Postoperative deep venous thrombosis: comparison of diagnostic techniques, *Lancet* 2:763, 1971.

72. Strandness DE, Sumner DS: Ultrasonic velocity detector in the diagnosis of thrombophlebitis, *Arch Surg* 104:180, 1972.

73. Tsapogas MJ et al: Postoperative venous thrombosis and the effectiveness of prophylactic measures, *Arch Surg* 103:561, 1971.

74. Wheeler HG et al: Impedance phlebography: technique, interpretation, and results, *Arch Surg* 104:164, 1972.

75. Wheeler HB et al: Bedside screening for venous thrombosis using occlusive impedance phlebography, *Angiology* 26:199, 1975.

76. White RH: Diagnosis of deep-vein thrombosis using duplex ultrasound, *Ann Intern Med* 111:297, 1989.

77. Yudelman IM et al: Plasma fibrinopeptide A levels in symptomatic venous thromboembolism, *Blood* 51:1189, 1978.

78. Zielinsky A et al: Evaluation of radioimmunoassay for fragment E in the diagnosis of venous thrombosis, *Thromb Haemost* 42:28, 1979.

79. Zielinsky A et al: Doppler ultrasonography in patients with clinically suspected deep-vein thrombosis: improved sensitivity by inclusion of the posterior tibial vein examination site, *Thromb Haemost* 50:153a, 1983.

CHAPTER 105

Use of noninvasive tests as the basis for treatment of deep vein thrombosis

H. BROWNELL WHEELER and FREDERICK A. ANDERSON, Jr.

Because the clinical diagnosis of deep vein thrombosis (DVT) is known to be unreliable, confirmatory diagnostic tests are necessary before treatment can be instituted. Some investigators have stated that venography should be done in every patient before treatment, but there are important practical limitations to this policy. Simpler and less expensive noninvasive tests are now available for the diagnosis of DVT. This chapter describes their use as a basis for the treatment of DVT.

Although venography has traditionally been regarded as the gold standard for the diagnosis of DVT, until the 1960s, it was widely considered unreliable and even dangerous. With advances in technique and extensive clinical experience, venography became much more accurate and safe. Even so, a 10% error rate has been reported when the same venograms are reviewed by independent and equally experienced observers.[116] The procedure is available in most major medical centers but not in many community hospitals across the country. Even if available in these hospitals, the accuracy and safety of this procedure cannot be assumed to be as good as that reported by major medical centers.

Venography requires the transportation of sometimes critically ill patients to the radiology department. Patients frequently experience pain at the injection site and occasionally complain of nausea, faintness, and other systemic side effects caused by the large amount of contrast material that must be injected. Although the occurrence of clinically apparent DVT as a result of venography is relatively rare in patients with normal venograms, there is a disturbingly high incidence of [125I]fibrinogen "hot spots" and frequent superficial thrombophlebitis at the injection site, clearly indicating that ionic contrast material is irritating to the intima and potentially thrombogenic. After injection of contrast material into an obstructed deep venous system, it seems likely that thrombosis may sometimes propagate distally. Another limitation of venography is the need for a skilled radiologist and sophisticated x-ray equipment, inevitably entailing considerable expense. Finally, because of the many reasons listed, venography is not a procedure that is easily and frequently repeatable.

These limitations in venography have led to widespread efforts to develop noninvasive tests of comparable accuracy. Many such tests have been proposed for the diagnosis of DVT, and a few have progressed from research status to widespread clinical use. Recent experience in community hospitals as well as in research laboratories has clarified the overall place of these tests in patient management. Prospective clinical trials have demonstrated that in selected patient groups, noninvasive test results can be used safely as the basis for treatment of DVT.

METHODS

Of the many noninvasive tests proposed for detecting DVT in recent years, only a few have gained broad acceptance. These include ultrasound imaging, radioisotope scanning, Doppler blood flow evaluation, and plethysmography. Other diagnostic tests also show promise and may eventually become better established. Such tests include examination of the peripheral blood for breakdown products of the thrombus, especially fibrin split products. This chapter deals primarily with those tests that are generally available and widely employed. A more detailed description of these techniques can be found elsewhere in this book.

Of the various radioisotopic methods, the most popular and extensively employed has been [125I] labeled fibrinogen. This tracer is incorporated into a developing thrombus, causing a local hot spot that can be detected by external scintillation counting. Use of radiolabeled fibrinogen was first described by Hobbs and Davis,[59] subsequently popularized by Kakkar et al,[77-79] and has now been studied by many investigators (Tables 105-1 to 105-3). It is the most sensitive of all noninvasive diagnostic procedures for detecting early DVT and the only one that will reliably detect small calf vein thrombi (Table 105-1). It has been invaluable in defining the prevalence and natural history of DVT as well as in identifying risk factors and evaluating methods of prophylaxis. It is best used for prospective screening, where the tracer can be administered to the patient before the period of risk. For example, it is well suited for preoperative administration in patients scheduled to undergo surgery that

Table 105-1. [^{125}I]fibrinogen—correlation with 718 venograms (expectant studies)

Investigator	Year	Correlation with normal venograms (specificity)	Correlation with recent DVT (sensitivity)	Location of thrombi
Negus et al[96]	1968	60% (3/5)	100% (24/24)	Below-knee
Lambie et al[81]	1970	90% (18/20)	90% (38/42)	Mainly below-knee
Milne et al[91]	1971	71% (12/17)	100% (18/18)	Below-knee
Tsapogas et al[131]	1971	100% (178/178)	92% (11/12)	Below-knee
Kakkar[78]	1972	93% (50/54)	94% (32/34)	Mainly below-knee
Becker[10]	1972	100% (74/74)	88% (15/17)	Below-knee
Walsh et al[135]	1974	80% (12/15)	100% (50/50)	Below-knee
Hirsh and Hull[58]	1978	—	69% (37/54)	Proximal to knee
Hirsh and Hull[58]	1978	—	92% (96/104)	Below-knee
TOTALS		96% (347/363)	90% (321/355)	

OVERALL ACCURACY = 93% (668/718)

Table 105-2. [^{125}I]fibrinogen—correlation with 654 venograms in symptomatic limbs

Investigator	Year	Correlation with normal venograms (specificity)	Correlation with recent DVT (sensitivity)
Browse et al[19]	1971	91% (91/100)	78% (66/85)
Kakkar[78]	1972	54% (15/28)	85% (63/74)
Browse[17]	1972	85% (104/123)	64% (46/72)
Walker[134]	1972	85% (46/54)	19% (22/118)
TOTALS		84% (256/305)	56% (197/349)

OVERALL ACCURACY = 69% (453/654)

Table 105-3. [^{125}I]fibrinogen—correlation with 1418 venograms in hip surgery

Investigator	Year	Correlation with normal venograms (specificity)	Correlation with recent DVT (sensitivity)
Pinto[106]	1970	60% (3/5)	100% (20/20)
Field et al[45]	1972	78% (25/32)	94% (29/31)
Harris et al[53]	1975	86% (25/29)	49% (25/51)
Gallus and Hirsh[48]	1975	83% (24/29)	93% (38/41)
Hirsh and Hull[58]	1978	—	64% (53/83)
Sautter et al[117]	1979	70% (67/96)	58% (29/50)
Cruickshank et al[35]	1989	95% (737/776)	45% (78/175)
TOTALS		91% (881/967)	60% (272/451)

OVERALL ACCURACY = 81% (1153/1418)

is known to be associated with a high risk of postoperative DVT. On the other hand, for the evaluation of patients with clinically suspected DVT, the [^{125}I]fibrinogen method is less accurate (Table 105-2). A delay of 48 hours before the test findings can be assumed negative is a serious disadvantage. False-negative results have been reported to be more frequent in patients undergoing anticoagulant therapy. False-positive results may be caused by an inflammatory or infectious process in the leg. Perhaps the most serious drawback to the use of the [^{125}I]fibrinogen test is the high background radiation from the trunk that renders the test unreliable in detection of clots that originate in the groin or pelvis. Although isolated proximal thrombi are uncommon

in the absence of more distal disease, they are nevertheless worrisome because of their high potential for major pulmonary embolism. For these reasons, as well as the expense of the commercially available [^{125}I]fibrinogen preparations, this method is less useful in routine clinical practice than for prospective studies. Its clinical application has been chiefly in combination with plethysmography or a Doppler system. Unfortunately, [^{125}I]fibrinogen is no longer commercially available in the United States and its use is now limited to research centers able to make their own radioisotope tracers.

At about the same time that the [^{125}I]fibrinogen technique was introduced, *ultrasonic blood flow detectors* based on

Table 105-4. Doppler ultrasound—correlation with 2462 venograms

Investigator	Year	Correlation with normal venograms (specificity)	Correlation with recent proximal DVT (sensitivity)	Patient group
Evans[44]	1970	100% (110/110)	95% (57/60)	50% asymptomatic
Milne et al[91]	1971	41% (7/17)	No venographically demonstrated proximal DVT	Asymptomatic
Sigel et al[121]	1972	92% (150/165)	84% (46/55)	Symptomatic
Strandness and Sumner[124]	1972	83% (10/12)	100% (38/38)	Symptomatic
Holmes[61]	1973	94% (51/54)	100% (17/17)	Symptomatic
Johnson[76]	1974	94% (15/16)	40% (4/10)	Mainly symptomatic
Yao et al[146]	1974	87% (27/31)	82% (104/127)	Symptomatic
Bolton and Hoffman[14]	1975	82% (32/39)	93% (13/14)	Symptomatic
Meadway et al[90]	1975	72% (55/76)	91% (86/94)	Symptomatic
Richards et al[110]	1976	88% (79/90)	73% (27/37)	Symptomatic
Flanigan et al[46]	1978	96% (94/98)	65% (35/54)	Symptomatic
Nicholas et al[97]	1977	70% (21/30)	89% (17/19)	Mainly symptomatic
Dosick and Blakemore[41]	1978	93% (100/108)	96% (50/52)	Symptomatic
Maryniak and Nicholson[88]	1979	90% (26/29)	100% (11/11)	Symptomatic
Sumner and Lambeth[127]	1979	90% (35/39)	94% (34/36)	Mainly symptomatic
Holden et al[60]	1981	91% (87/96)	73% (22/30)	Mainly symptomatic
Hanel et al[52]	1981	91% (118/130)	92% (49/53)	69% symptomatic
Schroeder and Dunn[118]	1982	73% (36/49)	70% (19/27)	Mainly symptomatic
Bounameaux et al[15]	1982	62% (20/33)	83% (33/40)	Mainly symptomatic
Bendick et al[11]	1983	90% (85/94)	73% (22/30)	Symptomatic
Zielinsky et al[149]	1983	76% (117/153)	95% (20/21)	Symptomatic
Voorhoeve et al[133]	1984	87% (34/39)	92% (34/37)	Symptomatic
Lensing et al[83]	1990	99% (106/107)	91% (41/45)	Symptomatic
TOTALS		88% (1415/1615)	85% (722/847)	

OVERALL ACCURACY = 87% (2137/2462)

the Doppler principle became available and were employed for the diagnosis of DVT by Sigel et al,[120] Strandness and Sumner,[124] Yao et al,[145] and many others. This method had great initial appeal because the equipment was relatively inexpensive and the results of the test were immediately available. Although it was inaccurate in the detection of calf DVT, excellent sensitivity and specificity for iliac and femoral thrombosis were reported by several investigators (Table 105-4). Interpretation was subjective, based on the flow sounds heard over the venous system in response to various maneuvers designed to stimulate or impede venous flow. A number of examiners were unable to repeat the excellent results of the originators of the method, and the technique earned a possibly undeserved reputation for poor reliability. Barnes et al[6] refined the technique and its interpretation and also developed a training program for those interested in its use. Through careful training and experience, users of the Doppler method can achieve excellent results in the detection of proximal thrombi. However, the interpretation, which remains subjective, is highly dependent on the skill and experience of the examiner. Several months of supervised patient testing may be necessary before a new vascular technologist is able to perform the Doppler venous test with an accuracy comparable to that reported in Table 105-4.

The Doppler method has the great advantage of using equipment that is inexpensive and portable. Even if its accuracy is somewhat less than that of competing methods, it may prove to be the only technique possible for laboratories with serious budgetary limitations. In addition, Doppler testing may be a useful adjunct to plethysmography, particularly in patients with severe congestive heart failure, chronic obstructive pulmonary disease, or vasospasm.

The use of plethysmography for the diagnosis of DVT was given its original impetus in this country by early reports describing *impedance plethysmography (IPG)*. Used to monitor changes in venous blood volume, the original IPG technique relied on the measurement of respiration-induced changes in venous volume. Excellent results were obtained by several investigators,* but as in the case of Doppler examination, other investigators had less satisfactory results.[40,123]

Subsequently, using a six-channel pneumatic plethysmograph, Cranley[30-33] also studied respiration-induced changes in venous volume and added the observation of volume changes proximal and distal to an inflated pneumatic cuff. This technique, known as *phleborheography (PRG),* was more complex than the original IPG technique but also provided the examiner with more information and a slightly greater accuracy (Table 105-5).

In the meantime, the inconsistencies originally encountered with the IPG technique had been identified as the result

---
*References 94, 95, 119, 138, 140, 141.

Table 105-5. Phleborheography—correlation with 886 venograms

Investigator	Year	Correlation with normal venograms (specificity)	Correlation with recent proximal DVT (sensitivity)
Collins et al[23]	1979	87% (20/23)	100% (41/41)
Nolan et al[99]	1982	100% (21/21)	87% (13/15)
Comerota et al[24]	1982	95% (418/441)	96% (247/256)
Classen et al[22]	1982	87% (20/23)	97% (64/66)
TOTALS		94% (479/508)	97% (365/378)
OVERALL ACCURACY = 95% (844/886)			

Table 105-6. Occlusive impedance plethysmography—correlation with 5129 venograms

Investigator	Year	Correlation with normal venograms (specificity)	Correlation with recent proximal DVT (sensitivity)	Patient group
CORRELATION OF IPG WITH VENOGRAPHY IN MAINLY SYMPTOMATIC INPATIENTS AND OUTPATIENTS				
Wheeler and Anderson[142]	1974	92% (191/208)	98% (88/90)	Mainly symptomatic
Todd et al[129]	1976	100% (11/11)	100% (11/11)	Spinal cord injury
Hull et al[65]	1976	97% (386/397)	93% (124/133)	24% asymptomatic
Hull et al[66]	1977	95% (108/114)	98% (59/60)	Symptomatic
Toy and Schrier[130]	1978	100% (9/9)	94% (15/16)	Symptomatic
Flanigan et al[46]	1978	95% (93/98)	96% (52/54)	Symptomatic
Hull et al[67]	1978	96% (304/317)	92% (155/169)	40% asymptomatic
Gross and Burney[50]	1979	94% (32/34)	100% (9/9)	Symptomatic (emergency room)
Cooperman et al[28]	1979	96% (72/75)	87% (20/23)	Symptomatic
Liapis et al[85]	1980	90% (219/243)	91% (43/47)	Symptomatic
Foti and Gurewich[47]	1980	79% (19/24)	90% (19/21)	Symptomatic
Hull et al[70]	1981	98% (157/160)	95% (74/78)	Symptomatic
Harris et al[55]	1981	88% (36/41)	100% (2/2)	Hip surgery (DVT/pulmonary emboli history)
Clarke-Pearson and Creasman[21]	1981	40% (2/5)	100% (10/10)	Symptomatic pregnant
Peters et al[105]	1982	93% (115/124)	92% (36/39)	Symptomatic
TOTALS		94% (1819/1930)	93% (741/794)	
OVERALL ACCURACY = 94% (2560/2724)				
CORRELATION OF IPG WITH VENOGRAPHY IN ASYMPTOMATIC INPATIENTS FOLLOWING HIP REPLACEMENT SURGERY				
Hume et al[74]	1975	100% (10/10)	77% (17/22)	
Harris et al[54]	1976	92% (55/60)	70% (7/10)	
Cruickshank et al[35]	1989	98% (767/784)	29% (14/49)	
Comerota et al[25]	1988	90% (53/59)	32% (11/34)	
Paiement et al[103]	1988	99% (856/864)	12% (9/73)	
Agnelli et al[1]	1991	90% (337/373)	24% (16/67)	
TOTALS		97% (2078/2150)	29% (74/255)	
OVERALL ACCURACY = 89% (2152/2405)				

of variable patient effort in respiratory maneuvers and the necessity for the examiner to evaluate the patient effort subjectively when considering the results. Accordingly, a more dependable method of producing venous outflow obstruction was developed to make the method simpler to perform and more objective to interpret. A pneumatic cuff, placed around the thigh and inflated to slightly above venous pressure but well below arterial pressure, satisfied this need quite well. Following release of the occlusion cuff, the venous outflow rate was shown to be markedly impaired by DVT. The venous outflow in the first few seconds after release of the thigh occlusion cuff also increased with the amount of blood dammed up behind the cuff in normal subjects but not in those with venous thrombosis.[137,139,142,143] Measurements of venous filling (after cuff occlusion) and venous emptying (after cuff release) provided a simple and objective basis for the diagnosis of DVT. This "occlusive" IPG method has now been widely used and has proved highly satisfactory in community hospitals, as well as medical centers (Table 105-6).

Several other plethysmographic techniques based on venous occlusion and measurement of venous outflow after release of the occlusion have now been described[126] (Table 105-7). In general, the results have been good to excellent,

Table 105-7. Review of various nonstandard methods based on venous occlusion plethysmography

Investigator	Year	Method of interpretation	Correlation with normal venograms (specificity)	Correlation with recent proximal DVT (sensitivity)
WATER-FILLED PLETHYSMOGRAPHY				
Dahn and Eiriksson[36]	1968	VC vs. MVO	100% (2/2)	100% (6/6)
STRAIN-GAUGE PLETHYSMOGRAPHY				
Barnes et al[7]	1972	MVO = 25%/min	82% (28/34)	95% (41/43)
Hallböök and Ling[51]	1974	MVO = 35%/min	100% (70/70)	100% (31/31)
Barnes et al[8]	1977	MVO = 20%/min	No venograms	90% (28/31)
Boccalon et al[13]	1981	VC vs. MVO	96% (27/28)	100% (26/26)
Bounameaux et al[15]	1982	VO_3 = 1.0%	63% (21/33)	95% (35/37)
Cramer et al[29]	1983	VC vs. $VO_{0.5-2}$	92% (11/12)	100% (12/12)
IMPEDANCE PLETHYSMOGRAPHY				
Johnston and Kakkar[77]	1974	VO_2/VC = 0.70	92% (35/38)	100% (13/13)
Yao et al[146]	1974	MVO = 1.0%/sec	81% (22/27)	91% (84/92)
Richards et al[110]	1976	VC vs. VO_3	87% (78/90)	83% (30/36)
Moser et al[93]	1977	VO_{10} = 0.2%	100% (19/19)	100% (14/14)
Salles-Cunha et al[114]	1978	VC, τ, Doppler	74% (54/73)	94% (49/52)
Lepore et al[84]	1978	VO_2/VC = 0.65	86% (71/83)	92% (48/52)
Young et al[147]	1978	VC vs. MVO	100% (7/7)	60% (12/20)
O'Donnell et al[100]	1983	VC vs. VO_3	93% (53/57)	100% (23/23)
PNEUMATIC PLETHYSMOGRAPHY				
Nicholas et al[97]	1977	VO_2/VC = 0.50	78% (36/46)	91% (21/23)
Hanel et al[52]	1981	VC vs. MVO	62% (81/130)	77% (41/53)
Holden et al[60]	1981	VO_2/VC = 0.70	96% (60/63)	38% (6/16)
Sufian et al[125]	1981	VC, MVO, Doppler	98% (40/41)	83% (20/24)
McBride et al[89]	1981	VC, MVO, MVO/VC	73% (?)	83% (?)
Schroeder and Dunn[118]	1982	VC, MVO, Doppler	84% (21/25)	66% (21/32)

VC, Venous capacitance; *MVO,* maximum rate of venous outflow, *VOₙ,* venous outflow volume in *n* seconds following release of venous occlusion pressure.

Table 105-8. Thermography—correlation with 1164 venograms in symptomatic limbs

Investigator	Year	Correlation with normal venograms (specificity)	Correlation with recent proximal DVT (sensitivity)
Cooke and Pilcher[27]	1974	100% (49/49)	96% (51/53)
Leiviskä and Perttala[82]	1975	100% (17/17)	89% (34/38)
Bergqvist et al[12]	1977	69% (22/32)	97% (75/77)
Bystrom et al[20]	1977	88% (22/25)	100% (26/26)
Nilsson et al[98]	1979	50% (7/14)	95% (35/37)
Watz and Bygdeman[136]	1979	77% (27/35)	95% (19/20)
Ritchie et al[111]	1979	81% (113/139)	74% (53/72)
Aronen et al[4]	1981	81% (81/100)	93% (38/41)
Lockner et al[86]	1981	49% (31/63)	99% (95/96)
Pochaczevsky et al[107]	1982	83% (15/18)	100% (12/12)
Jacobsson et al[75]	1983	47% (33/70)	95% (123/130)
TOTALS		74% (417/562)	93% (561/602)

OVERALL ACCURACY = 84% (978/1164)

Table 105-9. Fibrinopepetide A or fragment D-dimer (ELISA)—correlation with 418 venograms in symptomatic patients

Investigator	Year	Specificity	Sensitivity	Test
Yudelman et al[148]	1978	85% (29/34)	89% (42/47)	FPA
Heaton et al[56]	1987	47% (16/34)	100% (26/26)	D-dimer
Rowbotham et al[113]	1987	54% (32/59)	100% (45/45)	D-dimer
Declerck et al[39]	1987	—	92% (11/12)	D-dimer
Ott et al[102]	1988	65% (45/69)	97% (38/39)	D-dimer
Bounameaux et al[16]	1989	31% (10/32)	100% (21/21)	D-dimer
de Boer et al[38]	1991	48% (10/21)	100% (12/12)	D-dimer
TOTAL		58% (132/228)	96% (183/190)	
OVERALL ACCURACY = 75% (315/418)				

FPA, Fibrinopeptide.

corroborating the underlying premise of this method of diagnosis. However, none of these venous occlusion techniques has been as thoroughly evaluated as either IPG or PRG.

Thermography was first evaluated as a method for the noninvasive diagnosis of DVT in 1973 by Cooke and Pilcher.[26,27] A highly sensitive instrument must be used for temperature measurement, since the typical change in the surface temperature of the leg as a result of acute DVT is only 1° C. Most investigators use an infrared camera to produce thermographic images on a television monitor. Unfortunately, this equipment is fragile, expensive, and somewhat cumbersome. Simpler techniques using liquid crystal thermography[107] or a portable noncontact infrared radiation transducer[75,139] have been reported. These techniques are less expensive and more portable than an infrared camera. To obtain valid data, thermography must be performed after exposing the lower half of the body to room air for at least 15 minutes. This allows the skin temperature to achieve thermal equilibrium. As presented in Table 105-8, the sensitivity reported for thermography has been quite good; however, the specificity has not been as good. This is not surprising, since numerous conditions unrelated to DVT might raise the skin temperature of the legs. It is therefore necessary to combine thermography with other noninvasive methods that have demonstrated a high specificity to avoid false-positive results.[75]

Hematologists have long sought a blood test that could accurately detect the presence of DVT. Assays of fibrin breakdown products, particularly the *D-dimer assay,* have achieved nearly 100% sensitivity in research settings. Unfortunately, this high sensitivity is associated with a low specificity, which averages only 58% (see Table 105-9). Accordingly, although a patient with a negative D-dimer assay almost certainly does not have DVT, a patient with a positive D-dimer assay requires further studies to confirm the diagnosis. Currently, for methodologic reasons, use of D-dimer assays is confined primarily to research centers.

In recent years, *ultrasound imaging* has revolutionized the diagnostic approaches to DVT.[128] It provides anatomic visualization of the deep veins and can noninvasively define

Table 105-10. Ultrasonic imaging—correlation with recent proximal DVT based on 1928 venograms in symptomatic patients

Investigator	Year	Specificity	Sensitivity for proximal DVT
B-MODE ULTRASONOGRAPHY WITH PROBE COMPRESSION			
Effeney et al[42]	1984	86% (12/14)	83% (19/23)
Raghavendra et al[109]	1984	100% (5/5)	100% (6/6)
Dauzat et al[37]	1986	100% (45/45)	97% (89/92)
Raghavendra et al[108]	1986	100% (6/6)	100% (14/14)
Aitken and Godden[2]	1987	100% (26/26)	94% (15/16)
Appleman et al[3]	1987	97% (58/60)	96% (48/50)
Cronan et al[34]	1987	100% (24/24)	93% (25/27)
Rosner and Doris[112]	1988	100% (22/22)	90% (9/10)
Lensing et al[83]	1989	99% (142/143)	100% (66/66)
Pedersen et al[104]	1991	97% (74/76)	89% (101/113)
SUBTOTAL		98% (414/421)	94% (392/417)
DUPLEX SCANNING			
Elias et al[43]	1987	94% (483/514)	100% (241/241)
George et al[49]	1987	100% (26/26)	92% (22/24)
Vogel et al[132]	1987	100% (33/33)	95% (19/20)
O'Leary et al[101]	1988	96% (24/25)	92% (23/25)
Mantoni et al[87]	1989	96% (48/50)	97% (34/35)
Baxter et al[9]	1990	100% (26/26)	93% (13/14)
Mitchell et al[92]	1991	85% (28/33)	96% (23/24)
SUBTOTAL		94% (668/707)	98% (375/383)
OVERALL RESULTS = 96% (1849/1928)			

the anatomic extent and location of thrombi. Its use is readily accepted by patients, even for repeat examinations, and if necessary, it can be performed at the bedside. A high degree of accuracy has been demonstrated through comparison with venography (see Table 105-10). Because of this accuracy, as well as its noninvasive nature, ultrasound imaging has now replaced venography as the anatomic standard for the diagnosis of DVT in some hospitals.

Selection of a noninvasive test for the management of DVT is now generally considered to be a choice of Doppler ultrasound, IPG, or ultrasound imaging. Since these tests have different strengths and weaknesses, some laboratories consider the methods complementary and use more than one.

CLINICAL EXPERIENCE

Extensive retrospective studies have yielded favorable findings from the use of noninvasive tests for the management of suspected DVT (Fig. 105-1). In hospitals with established reliability in the noninvasive evaluation of DVT, it is safe and cost effective to stop a diagnostic workup when normal results are obtained. In one study, no fatal pulmonary emboli were observed in 1074 patients with bilaterally normal IPG results.[144] In only 1% of these patients was there a suspicion of nonfatal pulmonary emboli. Similarly, in 593 patients with negative PRG tests, Stallworth et al[122] found a 0.7% incidence of thromboembolic complications. Only one pulmonary embolism was reported in an aggregate of 1351 patients with negative [^{125}I]fibrinogen leg scans.[18] Similarly, Hull et al[22] reported no major pulmonary emboli in patients with suspected pulmonary embolism in whom a low-probability lung scan was associated with a normal IPG.

An extremely low incidence of thromboembolic complications has also been reported in patients with normal findings from Doppler examinations[5] or thermography.[75] Thus the risk of *not* treating patients with normal results of noninvasive tests appears to be appreciably less than the complications of anticoagulant treatment, perhaps less than the risk of venography. In addition, the cost savings are considerable.[69]

Even more impressive are the findings from prospective clinical trials in which treatment has been based on the results of noninvasive tests. Hull et al[71] reported only a 1% to 2% incidence of thromboembolic complications in outpatients with symptoms suggesting DVT who had normal IPG results and were followed on an outpatient basis without receiving anticoagulant treatment. There were no major or life-threatening pulmonary emboli. This low incidence of thromboembolic complications is comparable to that observed in similar patients with normal venograms.[68] Huisman et al[62] obtained similar results in a prospective study conducted in a group of outpatients with symptoms suggesting DVT but who had normal IPG results. Their findings were replicated in a community hospital setting, indicating that such results could be obtained outside a major academic center with significant research interest in venous thromboembolic disease.[63] Similar studies with ultrasound imaging have not been reported on to date, but in view of the high accuracy reported for the procedure, it seems probable that comparable results will be obtained.

Relying on abnormal results of noninvasive tests as an indication to start treatment for DVT is associated with more risk. False-positive results can be obtained with all noninvasive techniques, and anticoagulant treatment has an incidence of major complications variously reported from 1% to 20%.[115] It is a matter of clinical judgment and local laboratory accuracy as to whether venography should be obtained before starting anticoagulant treatment. It may be

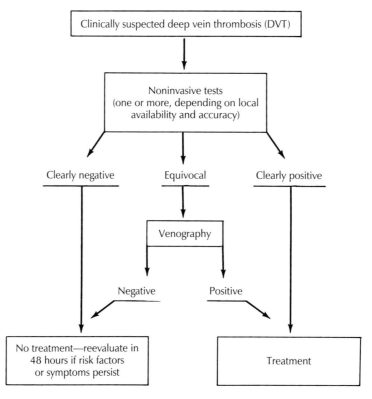

Fig. 105-1. Diagnostic approach for management of clinically suspected DVT.

the policy to rely on noninvasive test results when there is no clinical reason to suspect a false-positive examination and particularly on ultrasound imaging when a thrombus can be visualized.

Use of noninvasive tests has been especially beneficial in the emergency room and outpatient clinics when ruling out the need for venography or hospitalization. Over 90% of these patients do not have DVT; 323 patients were evaluated by IPG and 302 proved normal.[144] Some of these patients were admitted to the hospital for other reasons, but 284 were discharged after undergoing no further study or treatment. There were no pulmonary emboli, and only 1 patient (0.3%) developed DVT during further follow-up. By comparison, of 160 patients with negative venograms, 2 (1.25%) developed DVT during follow-up, perhaps as a result of the venography.[68]

Other prospective clinical trials carried out in symptomatic outpatients have demonstrated that roughly two thirds of such patients have normal IPG results and can be followed safely on an outpatient basis without receiving treatment.[63,71]

DISCUSSION

As in the use of diagnostic tests for other disease states, the intelligent application of diagnostic tests for DVT requires an understanding of both the disease process and the test used. There is no test that is universally applicable to all patients. To rely on noninvasive tests as the basis for treatment in a particular patient, the clinician must take into account certain underlying principles that will be considered in the following discussion.

Natural history of DVT

There is a widespread spectrum of severity in DVT that ranges from clinically insignificant to life threatening. The minor forms of DVT are extremely prevalent in patients who are bedridden for any great length of time. The more serious stages of the disease are fortunately much less common. The overwhelming majority of pulmonary emboli originate in the iliac or femoral veins, but a small number may originate in the hypogastric veins or the heart. Detection of DVT in these last locations remains an unsolved problem. In selecting which noninvasive test (or combination of tests) to use, clinicians must determine the relative importance of thrombi detected in different anatomic areas. However, no test, including venography, can detect all thrombi capable of causing pulmonary emboli.

The relative importance of detecting calf vein thrombosis, or the lack thereof, has been the source of considerable confusion. The widespread prevalence of calf vein thrombi disclosed by [125I]fibrinogen studies at first amazed many clinicians. They simply could not understand the disparity between the very large number of patients with DVT documented by this extremely sensitive technique and the very small number of patients who exhibited any clinical ill effects of the disease. The implicit assumption of most physicians had been that whenever DVT existed, at whatever

stage, it posed a potentially serious threat to the patient and required aggressive treatment. DVT, like pregnancy or cancer, was simplistically regarded as an all-or-nothing phenomenon. The patient either had DVT or did not, and if DVT was present, treatment was mandatory. However, with the high sensitivity of the [125I]fibrinogen technique and the ability to diagnose small calf thrombi, physicians were confronted with the decision of whether to treat the earliest stages of the disease, which proved to be much more frequent and much more benign than had previously been suspected. The surgeon, for example, was suddenly faced with the prospect of having to prescribe anticoagulants for up to 30% of all postoperative patients over the age of 40. The risk of serious bleeding complications from such treatment is sufficiently great that such a course seemed unthinkable to most surgeons—or at least seemed riskier than leaving the patients untreated, just as they had always been left untreated before the use of [125I]fibrinogen testing. Dilemmas such as this raised obvious questions about the treatment of DVT. Does DVT in its earliest stages need to be treated at all? Is there not a group of patients with such minimal disease that the risk of treatment outweighs the risk of nontreatment? If so, is it really of any practical importance to detect these early stages of the disease?

There is still disagreement on these questions. However, certain facts have become well established. Thrombosis confined solely to the calf veins is extremely common in hospitalized patients. Even if left untreated, the overwhelming majority of such patients never have any untoward clinical sequelae. The risk of life-threatening pulmonary embolism from DVT confined to one or two calf veins alone is less than the risk of anticoagulant treatment. A few calf thrombi—perhaps 20% at most—will propagate to the popliteal vein if untreated.[80] In this small percentage of patients, the risk of pulmonary embolism is substantially increased. Accurate detection of popliteal vein thrombosis is therefore an important prerequisite of any noninvasive test for DVT.

Lethal pulmonary emboli are usually very large thrombi, essentially "casts" of the iliac or femoral veins. Any noninvasive test that serves as a basis for treatment of DVT must be extremely reliable in the detection of these large thrombi in major veins.

Patients with acute DVT, reflected by signs and symptoms in the leg, usually have extensive disease. Swelling does not occur until major venous obstruction exists and is not caused by isolated calf vein thrombosis. Symptomatic patients are easily evaluated by plethysmographic or Doppler methods.

For several years, the policy of some investigators has been merely to observe patients with small calf thrombi who do not have major continuing risk factors and to treat those patients who have either extensive calf DVT or less severe calf DVT but also major continuing risk factors, particularly prolonged bed rest. There have been no adverse clinical consequences as the result of this approach. However, *all* patients with calf vein thrombosis or with major risk factors leaving them vulnerable to DVT are placed on continuing surveillance with noninvasive tests or given prophylactic treatment for as long as they remain at risk. If major risk factors are expected to persist indefinitely, long-term anticoagulation has often been instituted.

Finally, when managing patients on the basis of noninvasive tests, it is important to understand that venous thrombosis is a dynamic disease that can change appreciably from day to day, resulting both from lysis of existing thrombus and from development of further thrombosis.[73] Such changes can occur within a few hours, but the time span is usually a few days. In choosing a suitable diagnostic test to assess the extent of venous thrombosis, the clinician should ensure that the test be easily repeatable.

Patient considerations

In selecting a diagnostic test, the physician must first know its sensitivity and specificity for the patient group in question. Generalizations about overall accuracy, involving all stages of DVT and all types of patients, are meaningless with respect to the usefulness of the test in a specific patient. A test that has little use in one patient group may be the procedure of choice in another.

Patients with symptoms caused by DVT almost invariably have involvement of the popliteal, femoral, or iliac veins or else have extensive calf vein disease. Often the symptoms in suspected cases of DVT are the result of other conditions, and the venous system is completely normal. Symptomatic patients can be accurately assessed by plethysmographic methods, Doppler flowmeter study if performed by an experienced observer, or ultrasonic imaging. The results of these tests are immediately available, unlike the results of [^{125}I]fibrinogen testing. These methods are particularly well suited for patients who present with symptoms suggesting DVT. On the other hand, if the clinician wishes to detect asymptomatic calf vein thrombi, nonocclusive mural thrombi, or fresh thrombus in a patient with postphlebitic syndrome, [^{125}I]fibrinogen testing is currently the most reliable noninvasive method and venography is still required for most such patients.

How accurate must a test be to be relied on clinically? Realistically, a 100% sensitivity and specificity under all circumstances is not achievable by any test. Even venography is not 100% accurate. It is considered the gold standard partly because it gives the most detailed anatomic picture of the extent of disease and partly because there is nothing known to be more reliable with which to compare it. However, venography has its own errors. Ascending venography may fail to demonstrate thrombi in the iliac veins and also fail to visualize uniformly all of the calf veins. Such problems are frequent, especially in the hands of an inexperienced radiologist. Sometimes thrombi in the iliac veins have not been visualized by conventional ascending venography, even after they were suspected on the basis of noninvasive test results. Their presence was subsequently confirmed only by percutaneous femoral venography.

Medical practice will always be an imprecise science.

The physician must decide for each patient whether a given degree of diagnostic accuracy is an adequate basis for determining treatment. As in much of medical practice, clinical judgment is essential. Consideration must be given to individual circumstances when deciding to treat DVT on the basis of noninvasive test results.

In considering how high a degree of diagnostic accuracy is necessary before test results can be used as the basis for treatment of DVT, physicians must consider the consequences of an inaccurate diagnosis. From a clinical point of view, failure to detect isolated calf vein thrombi is relatively unimportant, provided the patient continues under surveillance for the period of risk so that significant propagation of thrombus can be detected. On the other hand, failure to detect large clots in the femoral or iliac veins may be life threatening, not to mention the greater likelihood of postphlebitic syndrome with any delay in treatment. In the selection of a diagnostic test, it is therefore critical that the procedure be highly accurate in detecting main vessel thrombi of sufficient size to pose a threat of significant pulmonary embolism. It is less important whether the procedure can detect small calf thrombi, which pose little immediate threat to the patient. All noninvasive tests are currently less accurate than venography in detecting small thrombi, especially in the calf veins, but prospective studies of clinical outcome have failed to show any adverse effects in patients in whom such small thrombi may have been overlooked, provided that the patient's course is observed appropriately with repeated noninvasive tests.[62-64,71,72]

Deciding when a diagnosis is sufficiently well established to undertake treatment is ultimately a matter of clinical judgment that is based on all available clinical and laboratory information, with each patient's circumstances considered individually. There is a small but inevitable element of uncertainty in the diagnosis of many diseases, just as there is with DVT. If venography is done in every patient, an absolute diagnosis can be established in the majority. On the other hand, an element of uncertainty will remain in some patients despite the venographic findings. Furthermore, even if a venogram is apparently negative, DVT may be present 72 hours later, possibly even as a result of the venogram.

Now that noninvasive tests are consistently achieving overall diagnostic correlations with venography as high as 95% and even higher in certain patient groups, it is reasonable to use the findings yielded by such tests as the primary basis for treatment. For a patient with a typical clinical picture of DVT and an abnormal result from a noninvasive test that is at least 95% accurate, it seems unnecessary to subject the patient to the inconvenience, discomfort, risk, and expense of venography.

Selection of diagnostic tests

The prime consideration in selecting any diagnostic test is the sensitivity and specificity demonstrated for a given patient group. Another consideration is the long-term patient outcome following negative diagnostic tests, if such information is available from prospective studies. Other factors that must be considered include the convenience and acceptability of the test procedure to the patient, as well as the ability to obtain repeat examinations for as long as the patient remains at risk. The immediate availability of results is often important clinically and may lead physicians to favor certain procedures for this reason, including such tests as ultrasonic imaging, plethysmography, and Doppler examination, rather than choosing procedures in which the results are delayed, such as the [^{125}I]fibrinogen-uptake test.

None of the noninvasive tests involves risk for the patient, and thus potential complications of the procedure are not a factor in test selection. The expense of the various noninvasive procedures should also be considered but usually has not been a major determinant of which tests to use, although this may be a more important factor in the future. None of the noninvasive tests is expensive by comparison with the economic and medical importance of the information obtained in patients with a high risk of DVT.

Several noninvasive methods have now withstood the test of time, and others may establish themselves in the future. [^{125}I]fibrinogen testing has been widely studied and is clearly the most sensitive test for the diagnosis of calf vein thrombosis when it has been performed in the period before the patient is at risk. For more proximal thrombi, which are of much greater clinical importance, Doppler ultrasound is adequate in the hands of skilled examiners, although its subjective nature makes for unacceptable results in the hands of those less experienced in its use. PRG gives excellent results when performed by those with adequate training. IPG has been used by many investigators and has proved consistently reliable for detecting major DVT in symptomatic patients. It is a simpler and more objective test than PRG or Doppler and is also one of the few noninvasive tests that has been proved effective in prospective clinical trials that study patient outcome. Other types of venous outflow plethysmography have been less thoroughly studied but have also shown generally good to excellent results. Thermography and various blood tests, particularly assays of D-dimer or fibrin split products, have shown excellent sensitivity, although their specificity has been disappointing. Any of these techniques (or various combinations of them) can reasonably form a basis for clinical decision making, provided that local accuracy is comparable to results reported in the literature. This is possible with all these techniques but is easier with some than with others.

The usefulness of ultrasound imaging techniques has rapidly expanded in recent years. They are a particularly attractive alternative to venography because they frequently provide anatomic visualization of the thrombus. They have demonstrated an impressive overall sensitivity and specificity, although some authors still recommend venography in the event of a normal duplex examination, especially in total hip replacement patients.[35] Although ultrasonic imaging is more expensive than simpler noninvasive tests and requires an experienced vascular technologist to be done accurately, it is currently the most widely accepted alternative to venography.

No single test is ideal under all circumstances. When using noninvasive tests, clinicians must be aware of those patient groups in which a particular test may have limitations or inaccuracies. Physicians must also know the major risk factors that lead to the development of DVT and be able to identify patients at high risk. They must understand the broad spectrum of the disease, realizing that small clots originating in the calf veins are very common but relatively innocuous—and probably pose less danger to the patient than prolonged anticoagulant therapy. They must also realize that although clots originating in the groin or pelvis are relatively uncommon, they are potentially lethal. Finally, they must consider all aspects of the patient's medical condition and interpret the test results in the context of all the information available.

Cost considerations

Because of the high cost of medical care, increasing concern about the cost/benefit ratio of various noninvasive tests has been expressed by third-party payors. Although the selection of diagnostic tests has traditionally been left up to the physician, cost effectiveness will be an increasing consideration in the future, especially if third-party payors define which tests will be reimbursed and under what circumstances.

Venography is particularly vulnerable because of its high cost. Given the high accuracy of much less expensive noninvasive tests, it is likely that in the future venography may be warranted only under selected circumstances. Ultrasound imaging is an attractive alternative to venography because of its lower cost. Despite the high cost of ultrasonic imaging equipment and the fee for interpretation, the procedure itself remains less expensive to perform than conventional venography.

Noninvasive tests vary widely in the cost of equipment, the amount of technician time required, and the cost of the individual test procedure. By far the least expensive instrument is the pocket Doppler flowmeter. Its accuracy, however, depends on the strict adherence to carefully defined criteria by an experienced observer. The cost of the various plethysmographic instruments is significantly higher, but the short time for technician training and the enhanced accuracy justify the additional expense. Ultrasonic imaging devices are by far the most expensive pieces of noninvasive testing equipment. However, generally, the most expensive instruments provide the most precise definition. They also require the services of a highly experienced vascular technologist. Their ability to provide convincing anatomic visualization of thrombus in the major veins still renders them highly cost effective as a replacement for venography.

CONCLUSION

A competent physician who understands the pathophysiology of DVT should be able to manage the great majority of patients suspected of having this disease on the basis of noninvasive test findings, reserving venography for particularly complex or controversial circumstances.

REFERENCES

1. Agnelli G et al: Impedance plethysmography in the diagnosis of asymptomatic deep vein thrombosis in hip surgery: a venography-controlled study, *Arch Intern Med* 151:2167, 1991.
2. Aitken AGF, Godden DJ: Real-time ultrasound diagnosis of deep vein thrombosis: a comparison with venography, *Clin Radiol* 38:309, 1987.
3. Appelman PT, de Jong TE, Lampman LE: Deep venous thrombosis of the leg: US findings, *Radiology* 163:743, 1987.
4. Aronen HJ et al: Thermography in deep venous thrombosis of the leg, *AJR* 137:1179, 1981.
5. Baker WH, Hayes AC: The normal Doppler venous examination, *Angiology* 34:283, 1983.
6. Barnes RW, Russell HE, Wilson MF: *Doppler ultrasonic evaluation of venous disease, a programmed audiovisual instruction*, ed 2, Iowa City, Iowa, 1975, University of Iowa.
7. Barnes RW et al: Noninvasive quantitation of maximum venous outflow in acute thrombophlebitis, *Surgery* 72:971, 1972.
8. Barnes RW et al: Detection of deep vein thrombosis with an automatic electrically calibrated strain gauge plethysmograph, *Surgery* 82:219, 1977.
9. Baxter GM, McKechnie S, Duffy P: Colour Doppler ultrasound in deep venous thrombosis: a comparison with venography, *Clin Radiol* 42:32, 1990.
10. Becker J: The diagnosis of venous thrombosis in the legs using I-labelled fibrinogen: an experimental and clinical study, *Acta Chir Scand* 138:667, 1972.
11. Bendick PJ et al: Pitfalls of the Doppler examination for venous thrombosis, *Am Surg* 49:320, 1983.
12. Bergqvist D et al: Thermography: a noninvasive method for diagnosis of deep venous thrombosis, *Arch Surg* 112:600, 1977.
13. Boccalon H et al: Venous plethysmography applied in pathologic conditions, *Angiology* 32:822, 1981.
14. Bolton JP, Hoffman VJ: Incidence of early postoperative iliofemoral thrombosis, *Br Med J* 1:247, 1975.
15. Bounameaux H, Krähenbühl B, Vukanovic S: Diagnosis of deep vein thrombosis by combination of Doppler ultrasound flow examination and strain gauge plethysmography: an alternative to venography only in particular conditions despite improved accuracy of the Doppler method, *Thromb Haemost* 47:141, 1982.
16. Bounameaux H et al: Measurement of plasma D-dimer for diagnosis of deep venous thrombosis, *Am J Clin Pathol* 91:82, 1989.
17. Browse NL: The ^{125}I fibrinogen uptake test, *Arch Surg* 104:160, 1972.
18. Browse NL, Thomas ML: Source of nonlethal pulmonary emboli, *Lancet* 1(7845):258, 1974.
19. Browse NL et al: Diagnosis of established deep vein thrombosis with the 125 I-fibrinogen uptake test, *Br Med J* 4:325, 1971.
20. Byström LG et al: The value of thermography and the determination of fibrin-fibrinogen degradation products in the diagnosis of deep vein thrombosis, *Acta Med Scand* 202:319, 1977.
21. Clarke-Pearson DL, Creasman WT: Diagnosis of deep venous thrombosis in obstetrics and gynecology by impedance phlebography, *Obstet Gynecol* 58:52, 1981.
22. Classen JN, Richardson JB, Koontz C: A three-year experience with phleborheography: a noninvasive technique for the diagnosis of deep venous thrombosis, *Ann Surg* 195:800, 1982.
23. Collins GL Jr et al: Phleborheographic diagnosis of venous obstruction, *Ann Surg* 189:25, 1979.
24. Comerota AJ et al: Phleborheography—results of a ten-year experience, *Surgery* 91:573, 1982.
25. Comerota AJ et al: The comparative value of noninvasive testing for diagnosis and surveillance of deep vein thrombosis, *J Vasc Surg* 7:40, 1988.
26. Cooke ED, Pilcher MF: Thermography in diagnosis of deep venous thrombosis, *Br Med J* 2:523, 1973.
27. Cooke ED, Pilcher MF: Deep vein thrombosis: preclinical diagnosis by thermography, *Br J Surg* 61:971, 1974.
28. Cooperman M et al: Detection of deep venous thrombosis by impedance plethysmography, *Am J Surg* 137:252, 1979.
29. Cramer M, Beach KW, Strandness DE Jr: The detection of proximal deep vein thrombosis by strain gauge plethysmography through the use of an outflow/capacitance discriminant line, *Bruit* 7:17, 1983.
30. Cranley JJ, Canos AJ, Mahalingam K: *Noninvasive diagnosis and prophylaxis of deep venous thrombosis of the lower extremity*. In Madden JL, Hume M, eds: *Venous thromboembolism: prevention and treatment*, New York, 1976, Appleton-Lange.
31. Cranley JJ, Canos AJ, Mahalingam K: *Diagnosis of deep venous thrombosis by phleborheography*. In Bergan JJ, Yao JST, eds: *Venous problems*, Chicago, 1978, Mosby.
32. Cranley JJ et al: A plethysmographic technique for the diagnosis of deep venous thrombosis of the lower extremities, *Surg Gynecol Obstet* 136:385, 1973.
33. Cranley JJ et al: Phleborheographic technique for diagnosing deep venous thrombosis of the lower extremities, *Surg Gynecol Obstet* 141:331, 1975.
34. Cronan JJ et al: Deep venous thrombosis: US assessment using vein compressibility, *Radiology* 162:191, 1987.
35. Cruickshank ML et al: An evaluation of impedance plethysmography and ^{125}I-fibrinogen leg scanning in patients following hip surgery, *Thromb Haemost* 62:830, 1989.
36. Dahn I, Eiriksson E: Plethysmographic diagnosis of deep venous thrombosis of the leg, *Acta Chir Scand* [suppl] 398:33, 1968.
37. Dauzat MM et al: Real-time B-mode ultrasonography for better specificity in the noninvasive diagnosis of deep venous thrombosis, *J Ultrasound Med* 5:626, 1986.
38. de Boer WA et al: D-Dimer latex assay as screening method in suspected deep venous thrombosis of the leg: a clinical study and review of the literature, *Neth J Med* 38(1-2):65, 1991.
39. Declerk PJ et al: Fibrinolytic response and fibrin fragment D-dimer levels in patients with deep vein thrombosis, *Thromb Haemost* 58:1024, 1987.
40. Dmochowski JR, Adams DF, Couch NP: Impedance measurement in the diagnosis of deep venous thrombosis, *Arch Surg* 104:170, 1972.
41. Dosick SM, Blakemore WS: The role of Doppler ultrasound in acute deep vein thrombosis, *Am J Surg* 136:265, 1978.
42. Effeney DJ, Friedman MD, Gooding GAW: Iliofemoral venous thrombosis: real-time ultrasound diagnosis, normal criteria, and clinical application, *Radiology* 150:787, 1984.
43. Elias A et al: Value of realtime B-mode ultrasound imaging in the diagnosis of deep vein thrombosis of the lower limbs, *Int Angiol* 6:175, 1987.
44. Evans DS: The early diagnosis of deep-vein thrombosis by ultrasound, *Br J Surg* 57:726, 1970.
45. Field ES et al: Deep vein thrombosis in patients with fractures of the femoral neck, *Br J Surg* 59:377, 1972.
46. Flanigan DP et al: Vascular-laboratory diagnosis of clinically suspected acute deep vein thrombosis, *Lancet* 2(8085):331, 1978.
47. Foti ME, Gurewich V: Fibrin degradation products and impedance plethysmography: measurements in the diagnosis of acute deep vein thrombosis, *Arch Intern Med* 140:903, 1980.
48. Gallus AS, Hirsh J: ^{125}I-Fibrinogen scanning. In Mobin-Uddin K, ed: *Pulmonary thromboembolism*, Springfield, Ill, 1975, Charles C Thomas.
49. George JE, Smith MO, Berry RE: Duplex scanning for the detection of deep venous thrombosis of lower extremities in a community hospital, *Curr Surg* 44:203, 1987.
50. Gross WS, Burney RE: Therapeutic and economic implications of emergency department evaluation for venous thrombosis, *J Am Coll Emer Physicians* 8:110, 1979.
51. Hallböök T, Ling L: Plethysmography in the diagnosis of acute deep vein thrombosis, *Vasa* 3:263, 1974.
52. Hanel KC et al: The role of two noninvasive tests in deep venous thrombosis, *Ann Surg* 194:725, 1981.
53. Harris WH et al: Comparison of ^{125}I fibrinogen count scanning with phlebography for detection of venous thrombi after elective hip surgery, *N Engl J Med* 292:665, 1975.
54. Harris WH et al: Cuff-impedance phlebography and ^{125}I fibrinogen scanning versus roentgenographic phlebography for diagnosis of thrombophlebitis following hip surgery, *J Bone Joint Surg [Am]* 58a:939, 1976.
55. Harris WH et al: The accuracy of the *in vivo* diagnosis of deep vein thrombosis in patients with prior venous thromboembolic disease or severe varicose veins, *Thromb Res* 21:137, 1981.
56. Heaton DC, Billings JD, Hickton CM: Assessment of D-dimer assays for the diagnosis of deep vein thrombosis, *J Lab Clin Med* 110:588, 1987.
57. Henkin RE et al: Radionuclide venography (RNV) in lower extremity venous disease, *J Nucl Med* 15:171, 1974.
58. Hirsh J, Hull RD: *Comparative value of tests for the diagnosis of venous thrombosis*. In Bernstein EF, ed: *Noninvasive diagnostic techniques in vascular disease*, St Louis, 1978, Mosby.

59. Hobbs JT, Davies JWL: Detection of venous thrombosis with 131 I-labeled fibrinogen in the rabbit, *Lancet* 2:134, 1960.
60. Holden RW et al: Efficacy of noninvasive modalities for diagnosis of thrombophlebitis, *Diagn Radiol* 141:63, 1981.
61. Holmes MCG: Deep venous thrombosis of the lower limbs diagnosed by ultrasound, *Med J Aust* 1:427, 1973.
62. Huisman MV et al: Serial impedance plethysmography for suspected deep venous thrombosis in outpatients: the Amsterdam general practitioner study, *N Engl J Med* 314:823, 1986.
63. Huisman MV et al: Management of clinically suspected acute venous thrombosis in outpatients with serial impedance plethysmography in a community hospital setting, *Arch Intern Med* 149:511, 1989.
64. Hull RD, Raskob GE, Carter CJ: Serial impedance plethysmography in pregnant patients with clinically suspected deep-vein thrombosis, *Ann Intern Med* 112:663, 1990.
65. Hull R et al: Impedance plethysmography using the occlusive cuff technique in the diagnosis of venous thrombosis, *Circulation* 53:696, 1976.
66. Hull R et al: Combined use of leg scanning and impedance plethysmography in suspected venous thrombosis: an alternative to therapy, *N Engl J Med* 296:1497, 1977.
67. Hull R et al: Impedance plethysmography: the relationship between venous filling and sensitivity and specificity for proximal vein thrombosis, *Circulation* 58:898, 1978.
68. Hull R et al: Clinical validity of a negative venogram in patients with clinically suspected venous thrombosis, *Circulation* 64:622, 1981.
69. Hull R et al: Cost effectiveness of clinical diagnosis, venography, and noninvasive testing in patients with symptomatic deep-vein thrombosis, *N Engl J Med* 304:1461, 1981.
70. Hull R et al: Replacement of venography in suspected venous thrombosis by impedance plethysmography and ¹²⁵I-fibrinogen leg scanning: a less invasive approach, *Ann Intern Med* 94:12, 1981.
71. Hull RD et al: Diagnostic efficacy of impedance plethysmography for clinically suspected deep-vein thrombosis: a randomized trial, *Ann Intern Med* 102:21, 1985.
72. Hull RD et al: A new noninvasive management strategy for patients with suspected pulmonary embolism, *Arch Intern Med* 149:2549, 1989.
73. Hume M: *Postoperative venous thrombosis—the dynamics of propagation, resolution and embolism*. In Bergan JJ, Yao JST, eds: *Venous problems*, Chicago, 1978, Mosby.
74. Hume M et al: Extent of leg vein thrombosis determined by impedance and ¹²⁵I-fibrinogen, *Am J Surg* 129:455, 1975.
75. Jacobsson H et al: Standardized leg temperature profiles in the diagnosis of acute deep venous thrombosis, *Vasc Diagn Ther* 55, May/June 1983.
76. Johnson WC: Evaluation of newer techniques for the diagnosis of venous thrombosis, *J Surg Res* 16:473, 1974.
77. Johnston KW, Kakkar VV: Plethysmographic diagnosis of deep vein thrombosis, *Surg Gynecol Obstet* 139:41, 1974.
78. Kakkar VV: The diagnosis of deep vein thrombosis using the ¹²⁵I-fibrinogen test, *Arch Surg* 104:152, 1972.
79. Kakkar VV: Fibrinogen uptake test for detection of deep vein thrombosis—a review of clinical practice, *Semin Nucl Med* 7:229, 1977.
80. Kakkar VV et al: Natural history of postoperative deep vein thrombosis, *Lancet* 2:230, 1969.
81. Lambie JM et al: Diagnostic accuracy in venous thrombosis, *Br Med J* 2:142, 1970.
82. Leiviskä T, Perttala Y: Thermography in diagnosing deep venous thrombosis of the lower limb, *Radiol Clin* 44:417, 1975.
83. Lensing AWA, Levi MM, Buller HR: An objective Doppler method for the diagnosis of deep-vein thrombosis, *Ann Intern Med* (in press).
84. Lepore TJ et al: Screening for lower extremity deep venous thrombosis: an improved plethysmographic and Doppler approach, *Am J Surg* 135:529, 1978.
85. Liapis CD et al: Value of impedance plethysmography in suspected venous disease of the lower extremity, *Angiology* 31:522, 1980.
86. Lockner D et al: Thermography in the diagnosis of DVT, *Thromb Haemost* 46:652, 1981.
87. Mantoni M: Diagnosis of deep venous thrombosis by duplex sonography, *Acta Radiol* 30:575, 1989.
88. Maryniak O, Nicholson CG: Doppler ultrasonography for detection of deep vein thrombosis in lower extremities, *Arch Phys Med Rehabil* 60:277, 1979.
89. McBride KJ et al: Venous volume displacement plethysmography: its diagnostic value in deep venous thrombosis as determined by receiver operator characteristic curves, *Bull Texas Heart Inst* 8:499, 1981.
90. Meadway J et al: Value of Doppler ultrasound in diagnosis of clinically suspected deep venous thrombosis, *Br Med J* 4:552, 1975.
91. Milne RM et al: Postoperative deep venous thrombosis: a comparison of diagnostic techniques, *Lancet* 2:445, 1971.
92. Mitchell DC et al: Comparison of duplex ultrasonography and venography in the diagnosis of deep venous thrombosis, *Br J Surg* 78:611, 1991.
93. Moser KM, Brach BB, Dolan GF: Clinically suspected deep venous thrombosis of the lower extremities: a comparison of venography, impedance plethysmography, and radiolabeled fibrinogen, *JAMA* 237:2195, 1977.
94. Mullick SC, Wheeler HB, Songster GF: Diagnosis of deep venous thrombosis by measurement of electrical impedance, *Am J Surg* 119:417, 1970.
95. Nadeau JE et al: Impedance phlebography: accuracy of diagnosis in deep vein thrombosis, *Can J Surg* 18:219, 1975.
96. Negus D et al: ¹²⁵I-labelled fibrinogen in the diagnosis of deep vein thrombosis and its correlation with phlebography, *Br J Surg* 55:835, 1968.
97. Nicholas GG et al: Clinical vascular laboratory diagnosis of deep venous thrombosis, *Ann Surg* 186:213, 1977.
98. Nilsson E, Sundén P, Zetterquist S: Leg temperature profiles with a simplified thermographic technique in the diagnosis of acute venous thrombosis, *Scand J Clin Lab Invest* 39:171, 1979.
99. Nolan TR et al: Diagnostic accuracy of phleborheography in deep venous thrombosis, *Am Surg* 48:77, 1982.
100. O'Donnell JA et al: Impedance plethysmography: noninvasive diagnosis of deep venous thrombosis and arterial insufficiency, *Am Surg* 49:26, 1983.
101. O'Leary DH, Kane RA, Chase BM: A prospective study of the efficacy of B-scan sonography in the detection of deep venous thrombosis in the lower extremities, *J Clin Ultrasound* 16:1, 1988.
102. Ott P et al: Assessment of D-dimer plasma: diagnostic value in suspected deep venous thrombosis of the leg, *Acta Med Scand* 224:263, 1988.
103. Paiement G et al: Surveillance of deep vein thrombosis in asymptomatic total hip replacement patients: impedance phlebography and fibrinogen scanning versus roentgenographic phlebography, *Am J Surg* 155:400, 1988.
104. Pedersen OM et al: Compression ultrasonography in hospitalized patients with suspected deep venous thrombosis, *Arch Intern Med* 151:2217, 1991.
105. Peters SHA et al: Home-diagnosis of deep venous thrombosis with impedance plethysmography, *Thromb Haemost* 48:297, 1982.
106. Pinto DJ: Controlled trial of an anticoagulant (warfarin sodium) in the prevention of venous thrombosis following hip surgery, *Br J Surg* 57:349, 1970.
107. Pochaczevsky R et al: Liquid crystal contact thermography of deep venous thrombosis, *AJR* 138:717, 1982.
108. Raghavendra BN et al: Deep venous thrombosis: detection by high resolution real-time ultrasonography, *Radiology* 152:789, 1984.
109. Ragavendra BN et al: Deep venous thrombosis: detection by probe compression of veins, *J Ultrasound Med* 5:89, 1986.
110. Richards KL et al: Noninvasive diagnosis of deep venous thrombosis, *Arch Intern Med* 136:1091, 1976.
111. Ritchie WG et al: Thermographic diagnosis of deep venous thrombosis, *Radiology* 131:341, 1979.
112. Rosner NH, Doris PE: Diagnosis of femoropopliteal venous thrombosis: comparison of duplex sonography and plethysmography, *AJR* 150:623, 1988.
113. Rowbotham BJ et al: Measurement of crosslinked fibrin derivatives—use in the diagnosis of venous thrombosis, *Thromb Haemost* 57:59, 1987.
114. Salles-Cunha SX, Bernhard VM, Imray TJ: Reliability of Doppler and impedance techniques for the diagnosis of thrombophlebitis, *Med Instrum* 12:117, 1978.
115. Salzman EW, Davies GC: Prophylaxis of venous thromboembolism: analysis of cost effectiveness, *Ann Surg* 191:207, 1980.
116. Sauerbrei E et al: Observer variation in lower limb venography, *J Can Assoc Radiol* 31:28, 1981.

117. Sautter RD et al: The limited utility of fibrinogen I-125 leg scanning, *Arch Intern Med* 139:148, 1979.

118. Schroeder PJ, Dunn E: Mechanical plethysmography and Doppler ultrasound, *Arch Surg* 117:301, 1982.

119. Seeber JJ: Impedance plethysmography: a useful method in the diagnosis of deep vein thrombophlebitis in the lower extremity, *Arch Phys Med Rehabil* 55:170, 1974.

120. Sigel B et al: A Doppler ultrasound method for diagnosing lower extremity venous disease, *Surg Gynecol Obstet* 127:339, 1968.

121. Sigel B et al: Diagnosis of lower limb venous thrombosis by Doppler ultrasound technique, *Arch Surg* 104:174, 1972.

122. Stallworth JM et al: Negative phleborheography, *Arch Surg* 116:175, 1981.

123. Steer ML et al: Limitations of impedance phlebography for diagnosis of venous thrombosis, *Arch Surg* 106:44, 1973.

124. Strandness DE Jr, Sumner DS: Ultrasonic velocity detector in the diagnosis of thrombophlebitis, *Arch Surg* 104:180, 1972.

125. Sufian S: Noninvasive vascular laboratory diagnosis of deep venous thrombosis, *Am Surg* 47:254, 1981.

126. Sumner DS: *The approach to diagnosis and monitoring of venous disease.* In Rutherford RB, ed: *Vascular surgery,* Philadelphia, 1977, Saunders.

127. Sumner DS, Lambeth A: Reliability of Doppler ultrasound in the diagnosis of acute venous thrombosis both above and below the knee, *Am J Surg* 138:205, 1979.

128. Talbot SR: Use of real-time imaging in identifying deep venous obstruction: a preliminary report, *Bruit* 6:41, 1982.

129. Todd JW et al: Deep venous thrombosis in acute spinal cord injury: a comparison of ^{125}I fibrinogen leg scanning and venography, *Paraplegia* 14:50, 1976.

130. Toy PTCY, Schrier SL: Occlusive impedance plethysmography: a noninvasive method of diagnosis of deep vein thrombosis, *West J Med* 129:89, 1978.

131. Tsapogas MJ et al: Postoperative venous thrombosis and the effectiveness of prophylactic measures, *Arch Surg* 103:561, 1971.

132. Vogel P et al: Deep venous thrombosis of the lower extremity: US evaluation, *Radiology* 163:747, 1987.

133. Voorhoeve R et al: The value of Doppler ultrasound studies in the diagnosis of venous thrombosis: results in 100 consecutively studied patients, *Ned Tijdschr Geneeskd* 128:2297, 1984.

134. Walker MG: The natural history of venous thromboembolism, *Br J Surg* 59:753, 1972.

135. Walsh JJ, Bonnar J, Wright FW: A study of pulmonary embolism and deep leg vein thrombosis after major gynaecological surgery using labelled fibrinogen-phlebography and lung scanning, *J Obstet Gynaecol Br Commonw* 81:311, 1974.

136. Watz R et al: Noninvasive diagnosis of acute deep vein thrombosis, *Acta Med Scand* 206:463, 1979.

137. Wheeler HB: *Plethysmographic diagnosis of deep venous thrombosis.* In Rutherford RB, ed: *Vascular surgery,* ed 2, Philadelphia, 1984, Saunders.

138. Wheeler HB, Mullick SC: Detection of venous obstruction in the leg by measurement of electrical impedance, *Ann NY Acad Sci* 170:804, 1970.

139. Wheeler HB, Patwardhan NA, Anderson FA Jr: *The place of occlusive impedance plethysmography in the diagnosis of venous thrombosis.* In Bergan JJ, Yao JST, eds: *Venous problems,* Chicago, 1978, Mosby.

140. Wheeler HB et al: Diagnosis of occult deep vein thrombosis by a noninvasive bedside technique, *Surgery* 70:20, 1971.

141. Wheeler HB et al: Impedance phlebography: technique, interpretation and results, *Arch Surg* 104:164, 1972.

142. Wheeler HB et al: Occlusive impedance phlebography: a diagnostic procedure for venous thrombosis and pulmonary embolism, *Prog Cardiovasc Dis* 17:199, 1974.

143. Wheeler HB et al: Bedside screening for venous thrombosis using occlusive impedance phlebography, *Angiology* 26:199, 1975.

144. Wheeler HB et al: Suspected deep vein thrombosis: management by impedance plethysmography, *Arch Surg* 117:1206, 1982.

145. Yao JST, Gourmos C, Hobbs JT: Detection of proximal vein thrombosis by Doppler ultrasound flow-detection method, *Lancet* 1:1, 1972.

146. Yao JST, Henkin RE, Bergan JJ: Venous thromboembolic disease: evaluation of new methodology in treatment, *Arch Surg* 109:664, 1974.

147. Young AE et al: Impedance plethysmography: its limitations as a substitute for phlebography, *Cardiovasc Radiol* 1:233, 1978.

148. Yudelman IM et al: Plasma fibrinopeptide A levels in symptomatic venous thromboembolism, *Blood* 51:1189, 1978.

149. Zielinsky A et al: Doppler ultrasonography in patients with clinically suspected deep-vein thrombosis: improved sensitivity by inclusion of posterior tibial vein examination site, *Thromb Haemost* 50:153, 1983 (abstract).

CHAPTER 106

Rationale and results of thrombolytic therapy for deep vein thrombosis

ANTHONIE W. A. LENSING and JACK HIRSH

Anticoagulant therapy is generally considered to be effective in preventing death from pulmonary embolism and reducing the short-term morbidity in patients with venous thrombosis.[9,11] Until recently, the evidence that heparin is required for the initial treatment of established venous thrombosis was derived from animal studies and subgroup analysis of prospective cohort studies conducted in patients treated with heparin.[7,12,13] A recent placebo-controlled randomized trial carried out in patients with proximal vein thrombosis has now demonstrated that the incidence of recurrent venous thromboembolism is greatly reduced by an initial course of adjusted-dose intravenous heparin therapy.[3] Although heparin prevents recurrent venous thromboembolism, it may have little effect in preventing the postthrombotic syndrome. Studies comparing thrombus size, as documented by venography, before and after heparin treatment in patients with symptomatic proximal vein thrombosis have revealed that complete lysis is very uncommon and partial lysis occurs in only 20% to 25% of cases.[10] Furthermore, approximately 60% to 70% of patients with symptomatic proximal vein thrombosis who are treated with anticoagulants have been reported to develop the postthrombotic syndrome within 5 years of treatment.[11]

Venographic findings have documented that early thrombolytic therapy for deep vein thrombosis (DVT) produces complete or substantial thrombolysis in between 20% and 70% of patients.[24] It remains uncertain, however, if this size reduction in the acute stage lowers the incidence of recurrent venous thromboembolism or lessens the likelihood of the postthrombotic syndrome. The major shortcoming of thrombolytic therapy is its high potential for precipitating severe bleeding.[18] Thrombolytic agents cause hemorrhage primarily by dissolving fibrin in the hemostatic plug. Contributing factors include plasma proteolysis, with its associated depletion of fibrinogen and other coagulation factors, and the production of fibrinogen degradation products, which interfere with fibrin polymerization. Because the hemorrhagic complications of thrombolytic agents may be life threatening,[1,7,27,30,31] the risk and benefits of thrombolytic therapy must be carefully weighed for patients with acute DVT before the therapy is instituted.

In a critical review of the reported randomized trials that compared thrombolytic therapy with heparin, the following factors were assessed: (1) their relative effectiveness in achieving lysis of venous thrombi, (2) their relative effectiveness in the prevention of recurrent venous thromboembolism, (3) the relative frequency of clinically significant bleeding stemming from their use, and (4) the relative effectiveness of these treatments in preventing the postthrombotic syndrome.

METHODS

Selection and classification of clinical studies

Articles published in the English literature were reviewed that compared the results of thrombolytic therapy with those of standard heparin for the treatment of DVT. An earnest effort was made to identify all such articles. This consisted of a Medline search of the literature, a review of bibliographies of appropriate publications, and a search for recent articles listed in *Current Contents: Clinical Practice* that may not have been included in the Medline database. Because streptokinase (the first thrombolytic agent) has been used for the lysis of thrombosis since 1959,[15] the search was conducted for the period 1959 to 1991.

Evaluation of studies

Only randomized trials that included treatment with streptokinase, urokinase, or tissue plasminogen activator (rt-PA) as well as a heparin-treated group were considered eligible for this review. All studies were carefully examined with particular emphasis on identifying any potential bias and on the appropriateness of the diagnostic methods used. Studies were evaluated if they were duplicate reports or preliminary reports of data later presented in full. Each study was then evaluated to determine whether it possessed the following essential features of study design.[25,26]

1. Objective methods to diagnose deep venous thrombosis: The diagnosis of DVT based on clinical findings is highly nonspecific and therefore represents an unacceptable method of diagnosis. Only studies that used contrast venography to confirm the initial thrombotic episode were included in this review.

2. A clear definition of the patient population: It was determined whether the study cohort consisted of symptomatic patients or asymptomatic postoperative patients. An attempt was made to estimate the age of the thrombus based on the period that elapsed between the onset of symptoms (or day of operation) and the day of treatment.

3. An appropriate method of randomization: To be eligible for inclusion in the analysis, studies had to have used appropriate randomization methods (to eliminate bias). Therefore studies in which treatment allocation was based on odd or even dates of birth or hospital numbers and studies that used alternate, nonrandom allocation or historical controls were excluded.

4. An acceptable method for assessing outcome measures: Studies were included only if they used the following clinically relevant objective outcome measures:

   a. Acceptable criteria for diagnosing recurrent venous thromboembolism: The acceptable criteria for the diagnosis of recurrent DVT were: (1) a new constant intraluminal filling defect not present on the last available venogram or (2) if the venogram was not diagnostic, either a positive [^{125}I]-fibrinogen leg scan or positive noninvasive test result that had been negative before the suspected recurrent episode.[14]

   Pulmonary embolism was considered to exist if the diagnosis was made on the basis of (1) a high-probability perfusion lung scan (segmental defect) and the chest roentgenogram did not show abnormalities in that area, (2) pulmonary angiography, or (3) autopsy findings.

   b. Venographically confirmed lysis of venous thrombi: The primary aim of thrombolytic agents in the treatment of venous thrombosis is to dissolve the clot and maintain normal valve function. Repeat venography using a quantitative method to estimate the change in thrombus size is mandatory for evaluating thrombolysis.

   c. Hemorrhage: Reported hemorrhagic episodes were classified as major or minor. They were major if they were intracranial or retroperitoneal, if they led directly to death, or if they necessitated transfusion, interruption of antithrombotic treatment, or reoperation. All other hemorrhages were classified as minor. In addition, the changes in the hemoglobin level during treatment were compared between both groups.

5. Appropriate criteria to assess the presence and severity of the postthrombotic syndrome: The clinical spectrum of the postthrombotic syndrome varies widely and ranges from minor signs such as pigmentation to more severe manifestations such as chronic pain and swelling, intractable edema, and skin ulceration. An attempt was therefore made to grade the reported clinical manifestations of the postthrombotic syndrome as minimal, moderate, and severe.

6. Blind assessments of study outcomes: Because knowledge of treatment allocation might introduce bias, the studies were assessed to determine whether the outcome measures were evaluated by an investigator blinded to the original treatment regimens.

When possible the 95% confidence intervals of incidence and statistical significance were calculated. The data collected from the different studies were combined and analyzed by the Mantel-Haenszel chi-square test.

RESULTS

A total of 13 potentially eligible studies were identified. Of these, 5 used improper randomization procedures or historical controls and were therefore excluded from this analysis.[1,4,5,19,32] In the 8 remaining reports, the patients evaluated had DVT of the leg documented by contrast venography (Table 106-1).* Most studies included patients whose symptoms appeared within 7 days of treatment. However, Porter et al[20] and Goldhaber et al[8] included patients whose symptoms began within 14 days of treatment. Streptokinase was used in all except two studies, which used rt-PA.[8,29] Urokinase was not used as the thrombolytic agent in any of the randomized studies.

Relative effectiveness for the prevention of symptomatic recurrent venous thromboembolism

In none of the studies was the frequency of symptomatic recurrent venous thromboembolism recorded in a systematic manner using a standardized protocol. Robertson, Nilsson, and Nylander[23] reported clinically suspected pulmonary embolism in 4 (24%) of their 17 patients during the infusion with streptokinase. An objective test was performed in only 1 of these patients, and it confirmed the diagnosis of pulmonary embolism. No symptoms of pulmonary embolism occurred in patients in the heparin group. Kakkar et al[16] observed 1 (10%) fatal case of pulmonary embolism among 10 patients treated with heparin, whereas this occurred among none of the patients treated with streptokinase. Elliot et al[6] screened all patients for asymptomatic pulmonary embolism; a high probability of ventilation-perfusion mismatch was seen in 1 (4%) of the streptokinase-treated patients. In the heparin-treated group, 2 (8%) patients died of pulmonary embolism, proven at autopsy. No information on the incidence of recurrent venous thrombosis or pulmonary embolism was given in the remaining 7 reports.

Relative effectiveness for the lysis of venous thrombus

All reports provided data on the resolution of venous thrombus as determined by comparing a posttreatment venogram with the pretreatment venogram. Robertson, Nilsson, and Nylander,[23] Goldhaber et al,[8] and Turpie et al[29] stated

---

*References 6, 8, 16, 20, 22, 23, 28, 29.

Table 106-1. Summary of thrombolysis regimen

Author	Heparin regimen	Thrombolytic agent	Thrombolytic regimen	Duration of symptoms	Follow-up
Robertson et al,[22] 1968	Day 1: ±50,000 IU Day 2-3: 50,000 IU† Day 4-6: 25,000 IU Day 7-8: 12,500 IU†	Streptokinase	Day 1: 2 × tid* ± 2,250,000 U Day 2-8: as for heparin	<96 hours	No
Kakkar et al,[16] 1969	Day 1: bolus 10,000 IU Day 1-5: 40,000-60,000 IU	Streptokinase	Day 1: bolus 500,000 U Day 1-5: 900,000 6 hr	<4 days	No
Robertson et al,[23] 1970	Day 1-3: ±50,000 IU Day 4-8: 25,000 IU†	Streptokinase	Day 1: 2 × tid* Day 1-3: 2,400,000 U Day 4-8: as for heparin	<96 hours	No
Tsapogas et al,[28] 1973	Day 1: bolus 7,000 IU Day 1-8: APTT 2-2.5	Streptokinase	Day 1: tid Day 1-3: 100,000 U/hr‡ Day 4-8: as for heparin	<5 days	No
Porter et al,[20] 1975	Day 1: 150 IU/kg Day 1-10: APTT 2-2.5	Streptokinase	Day 1: bolus 250,000 U Day 1-3: 100,000 U/hr	<14 days	No
Eliot et al,[6] 1979	Day 1: bolus 10,000 IU Day 1-7: 40,000 IU	Streptokinase	Day 1: bolus 600,000 U Day 1-3: 100,000 U/hr	<8 days	Yes
Goldhaber et al,[8] 1990	Day 1: bolus 100 IU/kg Day 1-10: APTT 1.5-2.5	rt-PA	Day 1: 0.05 mg/kg/hr Day 1-10: as for heparin	<14 days	No
Turpie et al,[29] 1990	Day 1: bolus 5000 IU Day 1-7/10: APTT 1.5-2	rt-PA	Day 1: 0.5 mg/kg/4 hr (one chain) or 0.5 mg/kg/8 hr repeated after 24 hr (two-chain) Day 1-7/10: APTT 1.5-2	<7 days	Yes

rt-PA, Tissue plasminogen activator; *APTT,* activated partial thromboplastin time.
*Titrated dose.
†Subcutaneously.
‡Duration dependent or thrombolysis achieved.

Table 106-2. Quantitative assessment of pretreatment and posttreatment venograms

Author	Heparin (n = 144)			Thrombolytics (n = 188)			Blind assessment of venograms
	None	Moderate	Marked	None	Moderate	Marked	
Robertson et al,[22] 1968	5 (63%)	2 (25%)	1 (13%)	1 (13%)	2 (25%)	5 (63%)	No
Kakkar et al,[16] 1969	5 (56%)	2 (23%)	2 (23%)	2 (23%)	1 (11%)	6 (67%)	No
Robertson et al,[23] 1970	5 (71%)	1 (14%)	1 (14%)	3 (33%)	1 (11%)	5 (56%)	Yes
Tsapogas et al,[28] 1973	14 (93%)	1 (7%)	0	9 (47%)	0	10 (53%)	No
Porter et al,[20] 1975	16 (62%)	2 (8%)	8 (31%)	9 (39%)	2 (9%)	13 (57%)	No
Eliot et al,[6] 1979	25 (100%)	0	0	5 (19%)	4 (15%)	17 (65%)	No
Goldhaber et al,[8] 1990	10 (83%)	2 (17%)	0	24 (45%)	14 (26%)	15 (28%)	Yes
Turpie et al,[29] 1990	33 (79%)	7 (17%)	2 (5%)	18 (45%)	9 (23%)	13 (33%)	Yes
TOTALS	113 (78%)	17 (12%)	14 (10%)	71 (38%)	33 (18%)	84 (45%)	

that the venograms were interpreted by experts who were unaware of the treatment allocation. The remaining studies did not include such an explicit statement to this effect (Table 106-2).

A statistically significant reduction in thrombus size was demonstrated in all studies (chi-square test for combined results, $p < 0.000001$), thus supporting the use of thrombolytic therapy. Moderate or significant thrombolysis was achieved 2.9 times more often in patients treated with thrombolytic agents than in patients treated with heparin (62.2% versus 21.5%; 95% confidence interval, 1.9 to 4.5 times).

Incidence of hemorrhage

Details on the occurrence of minor and major bleeding were furnished in all reports. Overall, the incidence of bleeding was significantly more frequent in patients treated with thrombolytic agents (24.2%) than in those treated with heparin (11.0%; 2.2 times more often; 95% confidence interval, 1.1 to 5.1 times; $p < 0.002$). Major bleeding was observed in 13.2% of patients treated with thrombolytic agents and in 3.5% of patients treated with heparin (3.8 times more often; 95% confidence interval, 1.1 to 15.8 times; $p < 0.004$). Turpie et al[29] reported a significant decrease in the hemoglobin level of more than 2 g/dl without evidence of overt bleeding in 2 (5%) of the 41 rtPa-treated patients and in 1 (2%) of the 42 heparin-treated patients. Goldhaber et al[8] observed a slight (not statistically significant) decrease from baseline in the mean 24-hour hemoglobin levels for both the rt-PA- and heparin-treated groups.

Incidence of the postthrombotic syndrome

The frequency of the postthrombotic syndrome during follow-up was investigated in only two studies.[6,29] Elliot et al[6] evaluated 41 patients at a mean follow-up of 19 months. A total of 21 of the heparin-treated patients were available for follow-up. Of these, only 2 (10%) were asymptomatic and the remaining 19 (90%) had evidence of postthrombotic syndrome; there were severe manifestations in 5 (24%) and moderate manifestations in 14 (67%). Of the 20 streptokinase-treated patients who were available for follow-up, 12 (60%) had no evidence of the postthrombotic syndrome and the other 8 (40%) had clinical evidence of the syndrome; there were severe manifestations in 2 (10%) and moderate manifestations in 6 (30%; $p < 0.0001$).

Turpie et al[29] performed long-term follow-up in 19 heparin-treated and 27 rt-PA–treated patients. Patients were examined 2 to 3 years after treatment by an independent investigator blinded to the original treatment regimens. Patients who complained of persistent (greater than 1 month's duration) pain and swelling of the legs and who had evidence of reflux on Doppler ultrasonograms were considered to have the postthrombotic syndrome. A total of 3 (25%) of the 12 patients in whom greater than 50% lysis was achieved had symptoms of the postthrombotic syndrome, compared with 19 (56%) of the 34 in whom less than 50% or no lysis was achieved.

DISCUSSION

Plasminogen activators, including streptokinase and rt-PA, accelerate lysis of venous and arterial thrombi. Although the clinical benefits of early thrombolysis in patients with coronary artery thrombosis are unequivocal and dramatic, the benefits of early thrombolysis in patients with venous thrombosis are less clear. Compared to heparin treatment, thrombolytic therapy is associated with a fourfold increase in cases of major bleeding and is more expensive. Therefore before thrombolytic therapy can be endorsed in patients with venous thrombosis, there should be clear evidence that it improves the clinical outcome. The clinically important consequences of DVT are fatal pulmonary embolism, recurrent venous thromboembolism, and the postthrombotic syndrome. Heparin administration followed by oral anticoagulant therapy is at least as effective as thrombolytic therapy in preventing fatal pulmonary embolism and recurrent venous thromboembolism and is associated with a much lower rate of major bleeding. However, the postthrombotic syndrome develops in approximately 60% to 70% of patients who are treated with anticoagulants. Although there is ev-

idence that thrombolytic therapy prevents the postthrombotic syndrome, the results are not conclusive. The results of all of the randomized studies included in this analysis showed that streptokinase is more effective than heparin in lysing acute venous thrombi. Although it is reasonable to hypothesize that improved thrombolysis should foster a reduction in the frequency of the postthrombotic syndrome, the evidence supporting this contention is limited to that furnished by only two small studies.[6,29] Therefore additional large clinical trials that include long-term follow-up in a broad spectrum of patients are required before the relative risks and benefits of thrombolytic therapy in patients with acute DVT can be known. Until such studies are performed, it would be reasonable to limit the use of thrombolytic therapy to those patients who do not have contraindications and are most likely to benefit from it. Thrombolytic therapy is contraindicated when there is a risk of serious bleeding. Other contraindications include recent surgery or trauma, malignant disease, recent stroke, active peptic ulcer disease, recent liver or renal biopsy, and recent arterial puncture. Patients who are most likely to benefit from it are those whose onset of venous thrombosis is recent (preferably within 72 hours) and those who are relatively young and active, since the postthrombotic syndrome takes years to develop and is likely to interfere less with the quality of life in immobile or inactive individuals.

Results of a recent study conducted by Brandjes et al[2] indicate that the incidence of the postthrombotic syndrome is reduced by the early use of elastic compression stockings. In this study, patients with symptomatic proximal vein thrombosis were treated with intravenous heparin followed by oral anticoagulants and were randomized to either wear or not wear compression stockings; their clinical course was observed for a mean of 2.6 years. The incidence of the postthrombotic syndrome was 62.3% in the untreated group and 27% in the treated group (risk reduction, 56%; $p < 0.01$). These results are consistent with the findings of a similar prospective cohort study made up of 189 patients with proximal vein thrombosis who were treated with compression stockings.[21] The incidence of postthrombotic syndrome in these patients was 34% after 36 months of follow-up.

CONCLUSION

Although there is good evidence that thrombolytic therapy accelerates the lysis of venous thrombi, the evidence that this approach improves clinical outcome is less certain and more studies are required before its merits are truly known. The incidence of the postthrombotic syndrome can be reduced by the early use of compression stockings, and heparin is very effective in preventing fatal pulmonary embolism and recurrent venous thromboembolism. Therefore thrombolytic therapy should be restricted to that subgroup of patients at low risk of bleeding and, at the same time, most likely to benefit from treatment.

REFERENCES

1. Arnesen H et al: A prospective study of streptokinase and heparin in the treatment of deep vein thrombosis, *Acta Med Scand* 203:457-463, 1978.
2. Brandjes D et al: Comparative trial of heparin and oral anticoagulants in the initial treatment of proximal deep-vein thrombosis, *Thromb Haemost* 65:703, 1991 (abstract).
3. Brandjes D et al: The effect of graded compression stockings on the development of the postthrombotic syndrome in patients with proximal vein thrombosis, *Throm Haemost* 65:1568, 1991.
4. Browse NL, Thomas ML, Pim HP: Streptokinase and deep vein thrombosis, *Br Med J* 3:717-720, 1968.
5. Duckert F et al: Treatment of deep vein thrombosis with streptokinase, *Br Med J* 1:479-481, 1975.
6. Elliot MS et al: A comparative randomized trial of heparin versus streptokinase in the treatment of acute proximal venous thrombosis: an interim report of a prospective trial, *Br J Surg* 66:838-843, 1979.
7. Gitel SN, Wessler S: The antithrombotic effects of warfarin and heparin following infusions of tissue thromboplastin in rabbits: clinical implications, *J Lab Clin Med* 94:481-488, 1979.
8. Goldhaber SZ et al: Randomized controlled trial of tissue plasminogen activator in proximal deep venous thrombosis, *Am J Med* 88:235-240, 1990.
9. Hirsh J: Heparin, *N Engl J Med* 324:1565-1574, 1991.
10. Hirsh J, Levine MN: Low molecular weight heparin, *Blood* 79:1-17, 1992.
11. Hirsh J et al: *Treatment of venous thromboembolism.* In Colman RW et al, eds: *Hemostasis and thrombosis,* ed 2, Philadelphia, 1987, Lippincott.
12. Hull RD, Raskob GE, Hirsh J: Continuous intravenous heparin compared with intermittent subcutaneous heparin in the treatment of proximal-vein thrombosis, *N Engl J Med* 315:1109-1114, 1986.
13. Hull RD, Raskob GE, Hirsh J: Heparin for 5 days as compared with 10 days in the initial treatment of proximal-vein thrombosis, *N Engl J Med* 322:1260-1266, 1990.
14. Hull RD et al: The diagnostic of acute recurrent deep-vein thrombosis: a diagnostic challenge, *Circulation* 67:901-905, 1983.
15. Johnson AJ, McCarty WR: The lysis of artificially induced intravascular clots in man by intravenous infusions of streptokinase, *J Clin Invest* 38:1627-1643, 1959.
16. Kakkar VV et al: Treatment of deep vein thrombosis: a trial of heparin, streptokinase, and arvin, *Br Med J* 1:806-810, 1969.
17. Loscalzo J, Braunwald E: Tissue plasminogen activator, *N Engl J Med* 319:925-931, 1988.
18. Marder VJ, Sherry S: Thrombolytic therapy: current status, *N Engl J Med* 318:1512-1520, 1585-1595, 1988.
19. Marder VJ et al: Quantitative venographic assessment of deep vein thrombosis in the evaluation of streptokinase and heparin therapy, *J Lab Clin Med* 89:1018-1029, 1977.
20. Porter JM et al: Comparison of heparin and streptokinase in the treatment of venous thrombosis, *Am Surgeon* 41:511-519, 1975.
21. Prandoni P et al: Elastic compression stockings and the postphlebitic syndrome: an unknown analysis of a prospective cohort study in patients with proximal vein thrombosis, *Thromb Haemost* 65:1579, 1991.
22. Robertson BR, Nilsson IM, Nylander G: Value of streptokinase and heparin treatment of acute deep venous thrombosis, *Acta Chir Scand* 134:203-208, 1968.
23. Robertson BR, Nilsson IM, Nylander G: Thrombolytic effect of streptokinase as evaluated by phlebography of deep venous thrombi of the leg, *Acta Chir Scand* 136:173-180, 1970.
24. Rogers LQ, Lutcher CL: Streptokinase therapy for deep vein thrombosis: a comprehensive review of the English literature, *Am J Med* 80:389-397, 1990.
25. Sackett DL: Rules of evidence and clinical recommendations on the use of antithrombotic agents, *Chest* 95:2S-4S, 1989.
26. Sackett DL, Haynes RB, Tugwell P: *The interpretation of diagnostic data.* In *Clinical epidemiology: a basic science for clinical medicine,* Boston, 1985, Little, Brown.
27. Tognoni G et al: Thrombolysis in acute myocardial infarction, *Chest* 99:121S-127S, 1991.
28. Tsapogas MJ et al: Controlled study of thrombolytic therapy in deep vein thrombosis, *Surgery* 74:973-984, 1973.
29. Turpie AGG et al: Tissue plasminogen activator (rt-PA) vs heparin in deep vein thrombosis, *Chest* 97:172S-175S, 1990.
30. Urokinase pulmonary embolism trial: phase 1 results, *JAMA* 214:2163-2172, 1970.
31. Urokinase-streptokinase embolism trial: phase 2 results, *JAMA* 229:1606-1613, 1974.
32. Watz R, Savidge GF: Rapid thrombolysis and preservation of valvular venous function in high deep vein thrombosis: a comparative study between streptokinase and heparin therapy, *Acta Med Scand* 205:293-298, 1979.

CHAPTER 107

Cost effectiveness of noninvasive diagnosis of deep vein thrombosis in symptomatic patients

RUSSELL D. HULL, GARY E. RASKOB, and JACK HIRSH

This cost-effectiveness analysis is based to a large extent on data derived from approximately 500 patients with clinically suspected deep vein thrombosis (DVT) studied at McMaster University between 1975 and 1979.[8] All of these patients were carefully assessed clinically by a limited number of competent physicians according to a standard protocol using impedance plethysmography (IPG), [125I]fibrinogen leg scanning, and venography.[8]

Cost-effectiveness analysis is an economic tool that when applied to health care evaluation, ranks alternative approaches to the same health problem to determine which is "best."[17] The best approach in economic terms can be defined as the approach that (1) accomplishes the desired health effect at minimum cost (cost minimization), (2) produces maximal health benefit for a given cost, or (3) carries the maximum effectiveness/cost ratio.

The application of cost-effectiveness analysis to the diagnosis of DVT is readily accomplished using cost minimization.[8] This cost-effectiveness technique makes it possible to rank the diagnostic approaches from "worst" to "best," with the best approach defined as that which accomplishes the desired health effect at minimum cost.

Effectiveness (health benefit) may be defined in this context as the number or proportion of patients with DVT correctly identified by objective testing. The reasons for correctly identifying DVT are (1) to treat patients with DVT in an attempt to prevent fatal pulmonary embolism and (2) to obviate the need for treatment and hospital admission for patients with clinically suspected DVT in whom the diagnosis is not confirmed by objective tests. It is generally accepted that proximal vein thrombosis is much more likely to lead to fatal pulmonary embolism[14,15] than is calf vein thrombosis and that the incidence of fatal pulmonary embolism can be markedly reduced if DVT is treated with heparin. Prevention of fatal pulmonary embolism is therefore used as a major parameter for assessing effectiveness. A second important complication of DVT is the postphlebitic syndrome. However, no reliable information is available on the prevalence of this syndrome in treated versus untreated patients with DVT. Therefore this important complication is not considered further in the cost-effectiveness analysis.

The parameters considered in the cost are the intrinsic costs of the tests, the cost of hospitalization, and the cost of treatment, which are the major costs for which hard data are available.[8] Other costs include the cost of treating side effects of the diagnostic procedure and of patient treatment (bleeding).[8] These costs are relatively minor and not considered in the cost analysis, although they would detract from the effectiveness of any approach with which they were associated. The costs used in this analysis are based on mean conservative figures derived from a number of regions in North America. The costs are based on 1980 U.S. dollars and have been adjusted to reflect 1992 costs using the *U.S. Consumer Price Index for Medical Care*, which indicates that $1 in 1980 equals $2.4 in 1992.

The parameters considered in determining effectiveness are the proportion of patients with proximal vein thrombosis and with calf vein thrombosis correctly identified and the number of patients in whom fatal pulmonary embolism will be prevented by correct identification and treatment of DVT. Hard facts are provided for the proportion of patients with DVT correctly identified by testing, but the proportion of deaths averted by correct identification and treatment of DVT is based in part on hard data and in part on extrapolation from information obtained from (1) the frequency of fatal pulmonary embolism in patients with untreated DVT reported by Zilliacus[19] in the 1940s before anticoagulant therapy was available, (2) studies by Barrit and Jordan[1] and by Kakkar et al,[14] and (3) a number of recent reports in the literature[2,4,16] regarding the effectiveness of heparin therapy for the treatment of objectively documented DVT. In the report by Zilliacus, between 11% and 22% of patients with clinically diagnosed DVT died from major pulmonary embolism. This estimate of mortality for untreated DVT is supported by the findings of more recent studies that show that (1) 50% of patients with proximal vein thrombosis develop clinical pulmonary embolism, (2) 25% of patients with untreated pulmonary embolism suffer a fatal pulmonary embolic event,[1] and (3) more than 50% of patients suffering a fatal pulmonary embolic event do so without premonitory pulmonary embolic episodes.[3] By extrapolation, the two last findings support the more conservative estimate of an 11% fatality rate from pulmonary embolism in patients with untreated clinically suspected DVT.

Heparin therapy followed by orally administered anticoagulant therapy is effective in averting death from pulmonary embolism.[1-4,6,10-12,16] Commencement of anticoagulant therapy at the time of DVT diagnosis is clearly preferable to treating the complicating pulmonary embolic events, since half of the fatal pulmonary embolic events would not be averted by the latter approach.

Methods for diagnosing DVT in symptomatic patients include clinical findings, venography, and one or more noninvasive approaches. The best evaluated of the noninvasive approaches are IPG, Doppler ultrasonography, [^{125}I]fibrinogen leg scanning,[4] and more recently, B-mode venous ultrasound imaging, or duplex ultrasound.[18]

The data that provided the basis for this cost-effectiveness analysis were derived from a study of approximately 500 patients referred to the Hamilton Regional Thromboembolism Programme with a first episode of clinically suspected DVT.[8] All were assessed clinically and then investigated by venography, IPG, and if the IPG was negative, leg scanning, which was carried out for 72 hours. Adequate venograms were obtained in 478 of these patients (Fig. 107-1).[8]

Treatment with heparin for 10 to 14 days plus orally administered anticoagulants for 3 months was given to patients in whom a positive diagnosis of acute DVT was made.

None of the patients in this study died from pulmonary embolism, and there were no fatal bleeding episodes in patients receiving anticoagulant therapy.[8]

Because all patients with negative IPG results underwent leg scanning, the effectiveness of serial IPG evaluations (used alone) could not be directly determined from this study.[4] A randomized clinical trial has recently been completed that compares combined IPG and [^{125}I]fibrinogen leg scanning with serial IPG alone for the diagnosis of clinically suspected venous thrombosis.[13] The results of this randomized trial provide relevant new data enabling the cost effectiveness of serial IPG alone to be accurately evaluated. Doppler ultrasonography was not formally evaluated in the study and therefore is not discussed here, but the cost effectiveness of Doppler ultrasound can be approximated by interchanging the anticipated results obtained by Doppler ultrasound with those obtained by IPG. It should be noted, however, that the safety of withholding anticoagulant therapy on the basis of Doppler ultrasonographic findings has not been formally evaluated.[4] B-mode venous ultrasound imaging is highly sensitive and specific for detecting proximal vein thrombosis in symptomatic patients[18] but, like IPG, is relatively insensitive for identifying calf vein thrombosis; therefore serial testing is required in this instance. The cost effectiveness of serial B-mode ultrasound has not been formally evaluated, although this approach has been found to be as effective as serial IPG in detecting thrombosis (see Chapter 104).

The simplified economic analysis of the results are dis-

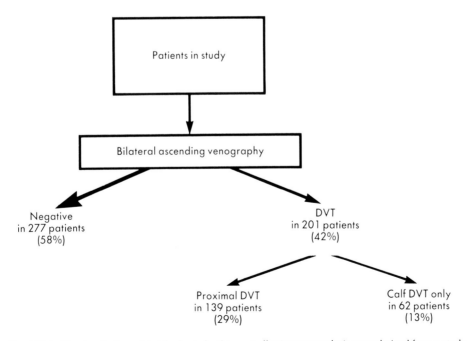

Fig. 107-1. The data that provided the basis for this cost-effectiveness analysis were derived from a study consisting of 478 patients with first episodes of clinically suspected DVT, all of whom underwent bilateral ascending venography and noninvasive testing.

played in two ways: (1) as though the patient had no co-morbid condition requiring hospitalization and (2) as though the patient had co-morbid conditions requiring hospital care.

COST EFFECTIVENESS OF DIAGNOSTIC APPROACHES FOR DVT IN PATIENTS WITHOUT CO-MORBID CONDITIONS REQUIRING HOSPITAL ADMISSION
Clinical diagnosis

Of the 478 patients with clinically suspected DVT, the diagnosis was not confirmed by venography in 277 (58%). This figure for false-positive results is remarkably similar to that obtained in a number of other studies evaluating the specificity of clinical diagnosis.[5] Thus if admission to the hospital and treatment were based on clinical diagnosis, over 50% of patients would have been inappropriately admitted to the hospital and exposed to hazards of short- and long-term anticoagulant therapy, to say nothing of the psychologic effects of an incorrect diagnosis of DVT.

An alternative approach to treatment in all patients with clinically suspected DVT would be to subselect patients for treatment who have severe symptoms. However, further analysis of the symptoms and signs suggesting a clinical diagnosis of DVT revealed that no clinical findings alone or in combination had sufficiently high predictive power to appreciably lessen this false-positive rate. Furthermore, many patients with extensive proximal vein thrombosis did not have florid symptoms or signs of DVT, and many with "severe" clinical features did not have DVT. Thus selection of patients on clinical grounds alone not only would expose patients without DVT to inappropriate admission to the hospital and treatment but would deny treatment in a large proportion of patients with extensive DVT.

Obviously, selecting patients for anticoagulant therapy on clinical grounds alone subjects untreated patients to the risk of massive or fatal pulmonary embolism. It therefore follows that if clinical diagnosis is not combined with objective tests, all patients with clinically suspected DVT would have to receive treatment so that pulmonary embolic deaths could be reduced to a minimum.

The most important complication of anticoagulant therapy is major bleeding. This occurs in approximately 7% of such patients. This is thus an undesirable and needless risk in patients who do not actually have DVT. However, because the cost of this complication is relatively low compared with other costs and because death caused by bleeding is rare, neither the cost nor the impact of this side effect is formally evaluated in this analysis.[8]

It can be estimated from the information given previously that the mortality from pulmonary embolism or bleeding is less than 1% in patients with treated DVT. The cost and effectiveness of clinical diagnosis are shown in Table 107-1.

The analysis is based on cost of the test, cost of hospitalization, and cost of treatment. The total cost of clinical diagnosis in 478 patients at $5513 per patient was $2,635,214. Thus the cost of clinical diagnosis for a yield of 201 patients with DVT correctly diagnosed and treated was $2,635,214, or $13,111 per patient.

The total cost of clinical diagnosis for a yield of 53 deaths from pulmonary embolism averted was $2,635,214; therefore, the cost for each death from pulmonary embolism averted was $49,721. Thus the cost effectiveness of a correct clinical diagnosis of DVT was $13,111 per patient treated and $49,721 for each pulmonary embolic death averted.

Venography

Venography is accepted as the diagnostic reference standard for identifying venous thrombosis against which non-invasive tests are measured. However, venography has disadvantages in that it is invasive and associated with patient morbidity and may not be readily available on an outpatient basis and so requires admission to the hospital. The cost will be considered on the basis of outpatient diagnosis and inpatient diagnosis.

Table 107-1. Cost effectiveness of clinical diagnosis alone

Cost		Effectiveness*
Intrinsic technical cost	$0	Correctly identified DVT in 201 patients
Cost of hospital room at $450/day for 10 days	$4500	Averted 53 deaths from pulmonary embolism by giving treatment to all 478 patients with a clinical diagnosis of DVT
Cost of therapy and laboratory testing and monitoring (inpatient and outpatient)	$1013	
Total cost per patient	$5513	
Total cost for 478 patients	$2,635,214	
COST EFFECTIVENESS OF DESIRED HEALTH EFFECT		
Cost for each correct diagnosis of DVT	$13,111	
Cost for each death from pulmonary embolism averted	$49,721	

*Desired health effect in 478 patients with clinical diagnosis of DVT.

Venography as an outpatient diagnostic approach. The cost and effectiveness of venography used as an outpatient diagnostic approach are shown in Table 107-2. Venography yielded negative results in 277 of 478 patients; thus the major cost incurred in this group was the cost of venography. The diagnosis of DVT was established in 201 patients (Fig. 107-1); thus the major costs incurred by these patients included not only the cost of venography but also of inpatient care and treatment. There were no deaths from pulmonary embolism (or bleeding).

As shown in Table 107-2, the total cost of this diagnostic approach in 478 patients was $1,484,777. Thus, the cost of using outpatient venography as a diagnostic approach for a yield of 201 patients with DVT correctly diagnosed and treated was $1,484,777. The cost for each patient with DVT correctly diagnosed and treated was therefore $7387.

The total cost of using outpatient venography as a diagnostic approach with a yield of 53 deaths from pulmonary embolism averted was $1,484,777. Therefore the total cost for each death from pulmonary embolism averted was $28,015.

Venography as an elective inpatient diagnostic approach. If immediate outpatient venography is not available, symptomatic patients may have to be admitted to the hospital for elective venography. Patients with clinically suspected DVT subsequently ruled out by elective venography had an average hospital stay of 3 days. If all 478 symptomatic patients were admitted to the hospital for elective venography, 277 patients (Fig. 107-1) would have been hospitalized unnecessarily, incurring the costs of anticoagulant therapy and hospitalization for 3 days. The cost and effectiveness of this diagnostic approach are shown in Table 107-3.

The total cost of this diagnostic approach in 478 patients was $1,952,353. Thus, the cost of using inpatient venography as a diagnostic approach for a yield of 201 patients with DVT correctly diagnosed and treated was $1,952,353, and the cost for each patient with DVT correctly diagnosed and treated was $9713.

The total cost of using inpatient venography as a diagnostic approach for a yield of 53 deaths from pulmonary embolism averted was $1,952,353; the cost for each death from pulmonary embolism averted was $36,837.

Table 107-2. Cost effectiveness of ascending venography as an outpatient diagnostic approach

Cost		Effectiveness*
Intrinsic cost of venography at $788/patient for 478 patients	$376,664	Correctly identified DVT in 201 patients
Cost of hospital room at $450/day for 10 days/patient for 201 patients with DVT	$904,500	Averted 53 deaths from pulmonary embolism by treating DVT in all 201 patients
Cost of therapy, laboratory tests, and monitoring at $1013/patient for 201 patients with DVT	$203,613	
Total cost for 478 patients	$1,484,777	
COST EFFECTIVENESS OF DESIRED HEALTH EFFECT		
Cost for each correct diagnosis of DVT	$7387	
Cost for each death from pulmonary embolism averted	$28,015	

*Desired health effect in 478 patients with clinical diagnosis of DVT.

Table 107-3. Cost effectiveness of ascending venography applied as an inpatient elective diagnostic approach

Cost		Effectiveness*
Intrinsic cost of venography at $788/patient for 478 patients	$376,664	Correctly identified DVT in 201 patients
Cost of hospital room at $450/day for 10 days/patient for 201 patients with DVT	$904,500	Averted 53 deaths from pulmonary embolism by treating DVT in all 201 patients
Cost of therapy, laboratory tests, and monitoring at $1013/patient for 201 patients with DVT	$203,613	
Cost of 3 days of in-hospital care and treatment with negative results at $1688/patient for 277 patients	$467,576	
Total cost for 478 patients	$1,952,353	
COST EFFECTIVENESS OF DESIRED HEALTH EFFECT		
Cost for each correct diagnosis of DVT	$9713	
Cost for each death from pulmonary embolism averted	$36,837	

*Desired health effect in 478 patients with clinical diagnosis of DVT.

Combined occlusive cuff impedance plethysmography–[125I]fibrinogen leg scanning: an alternative to venography

Combined IPG and [125I]fibrinogen leg scanning as an approach for diagnosing DVT is described in Chapter 104. The high sensitivity and specificity of combined IPG and leg scanning provide the clinician with a noninvasive alternative to venography that is versatile and can be performed at the patient's bedside or in the outpatient clinic or emergency room.[5,9]

The two tests combined detected DVT in 184 (92%) of 201 patients, proximal vein thrombosis in 138 of 139 (sensitivity, 99%), and calf vein thrombosis in 46 of 62 (sensitivity, 74%). The majority of calf thrombi not detected were in patients with long-standing symptoms, and their clinical significance is uncertain. Because they were inactive according to the [125I]fibrinogen uptake test, these thrombi were considered unlikely to extend proximally and to lead to clinically significant pulmonary embolism. Therefore these patients did not receive anticoagulant therapy, and none developed pulmonary embolism at early or long-term follow-up. Of the 31 patients with acute symptoms resulting from calf DVT, leg scanning detected calf DVT in 29 (sensitivity, 94%). These active calf thrombi are more likely to extend into the proximal veins if untreated, placing the patient at risk for massive pulmonary embolism. The combined approach yielded negative results in 256 of the 277 patients without venous thrombosis (specificity, 92%) and was falsely positive in 21 (8%) patients. All patients with proximal vein thrombosis or active calf vein thrombosis were given anticoagulant therapy. There were no deaths from pulmonary embolism or bleeding.[8] The cost and effectiveness of combined IPG and leg scanning are shown in Table 107-4.

The cost of this diagnostic approach in 478 patients was $1,296,987. Thus the cost of combined IPG and leg scanning as a diagnostic approach for a yield of 184 patients with DVT correctly diagnosed and treated was $1,296,987, and the cost for each patient with correctly diagnosed and treated DVT was $7049.

The total cost of combined IPG and leg scanning as a diagnostic approach for a total of 53 deaths from pulmonary embolism averted was $1,296,987. Therefore the cost for each death from pulmonary embolism averted was $24,471.

Serial occlusive cuff impedance plethysmography alone

IPG using the occlusive cuff technique is sensitive and specific for detecting proximal vein thrombosis but is insensitive for identifying calf thrombi. IPG is an objective diagnostic method that can be carried out in the outpatient clinic, ward, or emergency room.

IPG detected proximal vein thrombosis in 132 (95%) of 139 patients and calf DVT in 10 (16%) of 62. Thus a correct diagnosis was made in 142 (71%) of 201 patients with DVT. The IPG was falsely positive in 5 patients.

In a recently completed randomized clinical trial,[13] serial IPG alone was compared with a reference standard, combined IPG plus [125I]fibrinogen leg scanning, which is essentially as accurate as venography. IPG was performed serially to detect both proximal vein thrombosis and extending calf DVT. The important practical finding of this randomized trial was that it is safe to withhold anticoagulant therapy in patients with clinically suspected venous thrombosis if the results yielded by serial IPG remain negative.[13] On referral, IPG results were initially negative in 634 patients. Anticoagulant therapy was withheld in all 634 patients, who were then randomized to undergo noninvasive testing with serial IPG alone or with combined IPG and leg scanning. During the initial diagnostic assessment, none of these 634 patients died from pulmonary embolism. Of these, one suffered a submassive pulmonary embolism; this patient had been randomized to undergo combined testing with IPG plus leg scanning. Thus the frequency of pulmonary embolism in patients with negative IPG results at the time of referral in this study was 1 in 634 patients (0.16%; 95% confidence limits, 0.15% to 0.47%).

Anticoagulant therapy was withheld in all patients whose results of serial noninvasive testing remained negative and was commenced in any whose results became positive. All

Table 107-4. Cost effectiveness of combined IPG and [125I]fibrinogen leg scanning

Cost		Effectiveness*
Intrinsic cost of IPG at $79/patient for 478 patients	$37,762	Correctly identified DVT in 184 patients
Intrinsic cost of leg scanning at $270/patient for 478 patients	$129,060	Averted 53 deaths from pulmonary embolism by treating DVT in all 184 patients
Cost of hospital room at $450/day for 10 days/patient for 205 patients	$922,500	
Cost of therapy, laboratory tests, and monitoring at $1013/patient for 205 patients	$207,665	
Total cost for 478 patients	$1,296,987	
COST EFFECTIVENESS OF DESIRED HEALTH EFFECT		
Cost for each correct diagnosis of DVT	$7049	
Cost for each death from pulmonary embolism averted	$24,471	

*Desired health effect in 478 patients with clinical diagnosis of DVT.

patients were followed up at 3 months and 1 year. At 1 year, none of the 634 patients had died from pulmonary embolism. A total of 6 of 311 patients randomized to undergo noninvasive testing with serial IPG alone returned with an objectively documented venous thromboembolism, for a frequency of 1.9% (95% confidence limits, 0.4% to 3.4%); 7 of 323 patients randomized to receive combined IPG plus leg scanning returned with an objectively documented venous thromboembolism, for a frequency of 2.2% (95% confidence limits, 0.6% to 3.8%). Because the observed difference between the two diagnostic groups was 0.36%, which favors IPG alone, it is unlikely ($p < 0.05$) that a true difference in favor of serial IPG alone would be higher than 2.4% and the difference could be as much at 2.1% in favor of the combined approach. These findings indicate that IPG is as effective as the combined approach for the diagnosis of clinically suspected venous thrombosis when performed on the day of referral and, if negative, repeated the following day, again on day 5 to 7, day 10, and day 14.[13]

It has been shown that the combined approach of IPG plus leg scanning is essentially as accurate and safe as venography.[5,7,9] These observations, when taken together with the findings of the randomized trial, indicate that serial IPG alone is as effective as venography. The outcomes of long-term follow-up indicate that it is safe to withhold anticoagulant therapy in symptomatic patients when repeat evaluations with IPG yield consistently negative results. Thus the use of serial IPG alone is as effective as venography for the diagnosis of venous thrombosis and for averting death from pulmonary embolism in patients with clinically suspected DVT. The cost and effectiveness of serial occlusive cuff IPG used alone are shown in Table 107-5.

The total cost of this diagnostic approach in 478 patients was $848,173. Thus the cost of IPG used alone as a diagnostic approach for a yield of 142 patients with DVT correctly diagnosed and treated was $848,173, and the cost for each patient with DVT correctly identified and treated was $5973.

The total cost of using serial IPG alone as a diagnostic approach for a yield of 53 deaths from pulmonary embolism averted was $848,173. Therefore the cost for each death from pulmonary embolism averted was $16,003.

Comparison of diagnostic approaches by cost-effectiveness analysis

The cost effectiveness of each diagnostic approach is summarized in Table 107-6. The "worst" approach is clearly clinical diagnosis and the "best" approach is IPG alone performed serially.

COST EFFECTIVENESS OF DIAGNOSTIC APPROACHES FOR DVT IN PATIENTS WITH CO-MORBID CONDITIONS REQUIRING HOSPITAL ADMISSION

The assumption has been made in this economic analysis that the reason for admitting or keeping the patient in the hospital is the diagnosis of DVT. Clearly, a certain proportion of patients will have co-morbid conditions that may have been the primary reason for hospital admission or that may require continuing in-hospital care and treatment irrespective of the DVT. It is therefore inappropriate to charge the cost of the hospital room against the diagnostic approach in these patients.

Table 107-7 summarizes the cost effectiveness of the diagnostic approaches in these patients, excluding the cost of the hospital room. It is evident that the noninvasive tests are less expensive than venography. The most cost effective of the alternative approaches is serial IPG alone.

Relative cost effectiveness

The relative cost effectiveness of the diagnostic approaches in patients without co-morbid conditions requiring hospitalization is shown in Table 107-8. The net savings for each of the objective diagnostic approaches in comparison with clinical diagnosis is substantial. The greatest net savings is achieved with IPG alone, followed by the combination of IPG with leg scanning.

Similarly, the net savings from objective diagnosis can

Table 107-5. Cost effectiveness of serial IPG alone using the occlusive cuff technique

Cost		Effectiveness*
Intrinsic cost of IPG at $79/patient for 478 patients	$37,762	Correctly identified DVT in 142 patients
Cost of hospital room at $450/day for 10 days/patient for 147 patients with positive IPG results	$661,500	Averted 53 deaths from pulmonary embolism by treating DVT in all 142 patients†
Cost of therapy, laboratory tests, and monitoring at $1013/patient for 147 patients	$148,911	
Total cost for 478 patients	$848,173	

COST EFFECTIVENESS OF DESIRED HEALTH EFFECT		
Cost for each correct diagnosis of DVT	$5973	
Cost for each death from pulmonary embolism averted	$16,003	

*Desired health effect in 478 patients with clinical diagnosis of DVT.
†Calf DVT not detected in 52 patients and therefore not treated (see text).

Table 107-6. Cost effectiveness of diagnostic approaches for DVT

Diagnostic approach	Total cost for each patient with DVT correctly diagnosed ($)	Total cost for each death from pulmonary embolism averted ($)	Comment
Clinical diagnosis	13,111	49,721	All patients with clinically suspected DVT admitted to hospital and treated
Venography			
Outpatient	7387	28,015	Patients with findings positive for DVT admitted to hospital and treated
Inpatient	9713	36,837	All patients admitted to hospital and given treatment initially, but patients with findings negative for DVT subsequently discharged at a mean time of 72 hours
Combined IPG and leg scanning	7049	24,471	Patients with findings positive for DVT admitted to hospital and given treatment
IPG alone performed serially	5973	16,003	Patients with findings positive for DVT admitted to hospital and given treatment

Table 107-7. Cost effectiveness of diagnostic approaches for DVT excluding the cost of the hospital room in patients with other conditions requiring hospitalization

Diagnostic approach	Total cost for each patient with DVT correctly diagnosed ($)	Total cost for each death from pulmonary embolism averted ($)
Clinical diagnosis	2409	9136
Immediate venography	2887	10,949
Combined IPG and leg scanning	2035	7066
IPG alone	1315	3522

Table 107-8. Relative cost effectiveness of objective diagnostic approaches for DVT

Objective diagnostic approach and its cost for each correct diagnosis of DVT ($)		Net savings* for each correct diagnosis of DVT using objective diagnosis ($)
Venography		
Outpatient	7387	5724
Inpatient	9713	3398
Combined IPG and leg scanning	7049	6062
IPG alone	5973	7138

*Compared with clinical diagnosis at a cost of $13,111 for each correct diagnosis.

be calculated in patients with the clinical diagnosis of DVT who are in the hospital or admitted to the hospital for comorbid conditions. The least expensive approach is IPG alone, followed by IPG combined with leg scanning.

Future relevance of cost in this analysis

Although the actual cost of each component will be dictated by regional differences and will change in the future, the proportion each parameter contributes (to the total cost) will remain linked. Thus ranking of the diagnostic approaches from worst to best as determined by cost-effectiveness analysis should continue to be relevant. Inpatient diagnosis is likely to remain a major cost; therefore emphasis should be placed on outpatient diagnosis.[8]

CONCLUSION

The diagnostic approaches to DVT include clinical diagnosis, venography, and noninvasive approaches used alone or in combination. The clinical diagnosis of DVT is nonspecific and insensitive. In approximately 50% or more of

the patients with clinically diagnosed DVT, the results of objective testing are negative. Thus this approach is not cost effective because one of two patients with clinically diagnosed DVT is inappropriately admitted to the hospital and given anticoagulant therapy. Patients with DVT can be accurately identified by using venography or a combination of noninvasive tests.

At present, venography is the standard diagnostic reference test against which the noninvasive tests are evaluated. Among the disadvantages of venography, it is invasive, is associated with patient discomfort, and induces postvenography phlebitis in approximately 1% to 3% of patients.[4] In many centers, venography is not readily available on an outpatient basis; consequently, patients with clinically suspected DVT are admitted to the hospital, anticoagulant therapy is begun, and the diagnosis is confirmed or ruled out later by elective venography. This approach is not cost effective in patients subsequently found not to have DVT because they are admitted to the hospital unnecessarily and exposed to the hazards and added costs of anticoagulant therapy.[8]

In ranking the approaches discussed, it is evident that clinical diagnosis is the least cost effective. Serial IPG alone is the most cost effective and is as effective as the combined approach of IPG and leg scanning (and hence as effective as venography).[5,9,13] Serial IPG alone is less expensive than venography, is more versatile, and can be carried out in the outpatient clinic, ward, or emergency room. Noninvasive testing with serial IPG avoids the risk of unnecessary anticoagulant therapy in those patients who are subsequently shown by elective in-hospital venography not to have DVT, and its ease of access obviates the need to admit the patient to the hospital and the cost of an unnecessary hospital stay.

ACKNOWLEDGMENT

We thank Greg Stoddart, Ph.D., Health Economist, McMaster University, for assistance.

REFERENCES

1. Barrit DW, Jordan SL: Anticoagulant drugs in the treatment of pulmonary embolism: a controlled trial, *Lancet* 1:1309, 1960.
2. Basu D et al: A prospective study of the value of monitoring heparin treatment with the activated partial thromboplastin time, *N Engl J Med* 287:324, 1972.
3. Gallus AS, Hirsch J: Diagnosis of venous thromboembolism, *Semin Throm Hemost* 2:203, 1976.
4. Hull R, Hirsh J: Advances and controversies in the diagnosis, prevention and treatment of venous thromboembolism, *Prog Hematol* 12:73, 1981.
5. Hull R et al: Combined use of leg scanning and impedance plethysmography in suspected venous thrombosis: an alternative to venography, *N Engl J Med* 296:1497, 1977.
6. Hull R et al: Warfarin sodium versus low-dose heparin in the long-term treatment of venous thrombosis, *N Engl J Med* 301:855, 1979.
7. Hull R et al: Clinical validity of a negative venogram in patients with clinically suspected venous thrombosis, *Circulation* 64:622, 1981.
8. Hull R et al: Cost effectiveness of clinical diagnosis, venography, and noninvasive testing in patients with symptomatic deep-vein thrombosis, *N Engl J Med* 304:1561, 1981.
9. Hull R et al: Replacement of venography in suspected venous thrombosis by impedance plethysmography and ^{125}I-fibrinogen leg scanning: a less invasive approach, *Ann Intern Med* 94:12, 1981.
10. Hull R et al: Adjusted subcutaneous heparin versus warfarin sodium in the long-term treatment of venous thrombosis, *N Engl J Med* 306:189, 1982.
11. Hull R et al: Different intensities of oral anticoagulant therapy in the treatment of proximal-vein thrombosis, *N Engl J Med* 307:1676, 1982.
12. Hull R et al: The diagnosis of acute, recurrent, deep-vein thrombosis: a diagnostic challenge, *Circulation* 67:901, 1983.
13. Hull R et al: Diagnostic efficacy of impedance plethysmography for clinically suspected deep-vein thrombosis: a randomized trial, *Ann Intern Med* 102:21-28, 1985.
14. Kakkar VV et al: Natural history of post-operative deep-vein thrombosis, *Lancet* 2:230, 1969.
15. Mavor GE, Galloway JMD: The iliofemoral venous segment as a source of pulmonary embolism, *Lancet* 1:871, 1967.
16. Salzman EW, Deykin D, Shapiro RM: Management of heparin therapy, *N Engl J Med* 292:1046, 1975.
17. Weinstein MC, Stason WB: Foundations of cost-effectiveness analysis for health and medical practices, *N Engl J Med* 296:716, 1977.
18. White RH et al: Diagnosis of deep-vein thrombosis using duplex ultrasound, *Ann Intern Med* 111:297-304, 1989.
19. Zilliacus H: On specific treatment of thrombosis and pulmonary embolism with anticoagulants with particular reference to the post-thrombotic sequelae, *Acta Med Scand* [suppl] 171:1, 1946.

CHAPTER 108

Foot volumetry

OLAV THULESIUS

The number of noninvasive techniques for the diagnosis of chronic venous disease has been limited compared with the many such techniques available for the diagnosis of arterial disease,[4] and the numbers are disproportionate considering the high prevalence of chronic venous insufficiency. In a population study consisting of 4529 apparently healthy workers in Basel, Switzerland, 8% of those aged 25 to 54 years were found to have significant venous disease. If these findings are extrapolated to the whole Swiss population aged 25 to 74 years, the estimated prevalence of disease is 14%.[12]

Until recently, tests that assessed the function of the venous circulation consisted solely of those studying venous pressure changes during exercise. With the advent of slow-flow sensitivity software, color flow imaging has improved the quantitative evaluation of flow patterns in the deep venous system provided by duplex scanning, including that of perforator veins. This diagnostic modality is especially useful for the detection of persistent thrombotic changes and may aid in the quantitative evaluation of reflux in single vessels.

Volumetric techniques, however, can globally assess the two most important functional aspects of the venous circulation: (1) the venous pump and (2) venous reflux in both deep and superficial veins.

Volumetry is a truly noninvasive technique and is based on the concept that measurements of venous pressure and volume in the foot are governed by similar mechanisms.[11] During quiet standing, the hydrostatic pressure in the venous system of the lower extremity is a function of the vertical height of the blood column from the heart to the foot. In the presence of exercise and competent venous valves, standing venous pressure at the foot drops from 90 to 20 mm Hg.[9] This reduction in peripheral venous pressure is due to the central dislocation of blood that stems from the massaging action of the contracting calf muscles and the stretching forces of moving fascia acting on compressible vessels.

Competent valves disrupt the blood column on the venous side and thereby eliminate the hydrostatic pressure in the distal vessels; this leaves hydraulic pressure as the main component transmitted from the arterial side. This physiologic response of the peripheral venous pressure to exercise

in the foot has often been used for the quantitative evaluation of the calf muscle pump and the efficiency of venous valves. The variables assessed are the decrease in venous pressure and refilling time.[2]

Ambulatory venous pressure measurement, however, is an invasive technique that requires puncture of a foot vein, which may be uncomfortable and impractical when frequently repeated measurements are required. The noninvasive assessment of foot volume changes with exercise is much easier to perform, and the findings correlate well with pressure measurements.[3,6,7]

PRINCIPLE

The foot volumeter consists of an open, water-filled box designed to measure foot volume at rest and during exercise. The water level, which is initially 14 cm high, is sensed by a critically damped photoelectric float sensor; this operates an optical wedge whose output is monitored continuously on a strip-chart recorder. During exercise, blood is expelled from the foot vessels, causing the water to be displaced (reduced) in proportion to the volume of blood dislocated. During a series of knee bends, usually 15 to 20 performed in rapid succession, the blood volume gradually declines until it reaches a steady-state. After completion of the exercise, the blood volume takes varying lengths of time to return to its resting volume, depending on the rate of arterial inflow.

Normally, refilling flow is accomplished exclusively from the arterial side, but in cases of venous insufficiency, there is retrograde flow (reflux) from proximally located veins (Fig. 108-1). Usually two volumeters are used so that both feet can be measured simultaneously and volume is recorded on a two-channel recorder.

METHOD

The foot is placed in the volumeter, which is rapidly filled from a thermostated water line at a temperature of 32° C. Thereafter, calibration is performed with a water-filled syringe. Once a steady baseline is achieved with the patient standing, a standard exercise is performed, consisting of 20 knee bends in 40 seconds and paced by a metronome. To facilitate the exercise procedure, the patient grips handlebars

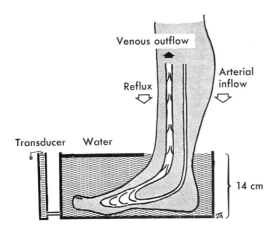

Fig. 108-1. Principle of volumetry: an open, water-filled box (plethysmograph) for continuous measurement of the water level.

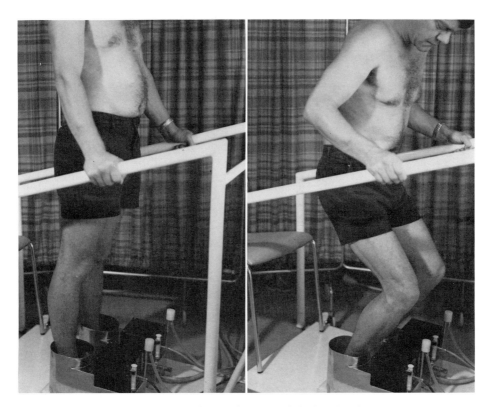

Fig. 108-2. Performance of foot volumetry with the knee-bending exercise.

with both hands (Figs. 108-2 and 108-3). After completing the exercise, the patient stands quietly until volume has been restored. To differentiate between superficial and deep venous insufficiency, measurements are also made after tourniquet compression of superficial veins at two levels: below the knee and at the ankle, just above the volumeter. After the exercise is completed, the water is sucked out of the volumeter and the total foot volume measured in a calibrated reservoir.

Fig. 108-4 shows a recording from a normal individual and one from a patient with varicose veins, together with

the different variables that can be determined from the curve. The most important variables are the expelled volume, characterizing the venous pump, and the refilling flow, reflecting the degree of reflux. The expelled volume is measured in absolute units (milliliters) or rendered in relation to the foot volume (per 100 ml) but becomes the relative expelled volume when expressed in this latter fashion.

Normally, refilling flow is equal to arterial inflow, but in patients with venous insufficiency, it also reflects retrograde flow through incompetent veins (reflux). Explanations and the abbreviations used to denote the different variables,

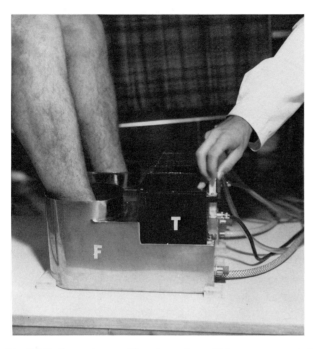

Fig. 108-3. Foot volumeter *(F)* and transducer *(T)* for measurement of the water level. Calibration with a syringe is shown.

Table 108-1. Volumetric variables with abbreviations and error of determination

Variable	Unit	Error (%)*
Foot volume (V)	ml	1.1
Expelled volume (EV)	ml	4.3
Expelled volume per 100 ml tissue (EVr)	ml/100 ml	(9.8)
Refilling flow (Q)	ml/100 ml·min	32.3
Time factor (Q/EVr)	1/min	—
Half refilling time (t/2)	sec	16.2 (25.7)
Refilling time (t₄)	sec	—

*Based on findings of Norgren et al[6] with those from Partsch[7] in parentheses.

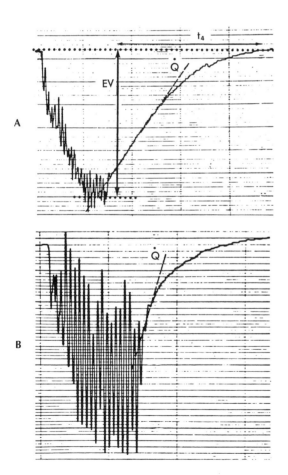

Fig. 108-4. Volumetric recordings from two patients. *A,* Normal individual. *B,* Patient with superficial venous insufficiency. *EV,* Expelled volume; *Q,* refilling flow; *t₄,* refilling time.

together with the percentage of error of the method, are given in Table 108-1. Table 108-2 lists the reference values from several investigators.

Another useful variable is the volume restitution time (*t* in seconds) or the more easily determined half-refilling time. The ratio of refilling flow and expelled volume constitute two of the most important measures of venous function.

CLINICAL APPLICATION

Foot volumetry evaluates the function of the peripheral venous system of the leg by assessing valvular function and the capacity of the calf-foot-pump. The most important variables are the expelled volume, refilling flow, and half-refilling time (Table 108-2).

To distinguish between superficial and deep vein insufficiency, measurements are repeated during tourniquet occlusion of superficial incompetent veins. Tourniquets can be applied at different levels to distinguish between insufficiency in the great and short saphenous vein. Furthermore, guided compression can eliminate reflux from incompetent perforator veins.

Foot volumetry can quantitate *the degree* of venous insufficiency and determine its location, as shown by several workers.[3,6,7] Volumetry is useful for the evaluation of therapeutic interventions and can be used in follow-up studies of patients after deep vein thrombosis to determine the incidence of postthrombotic valvular incompetence.[3,8]

DISCUSSION

Volumetry is a functional test of the venous circulation, and to obtain reliable information, it is necessary to adhere to a strict protocol. The water temperature must be kept between 30° C and 32° C; higher temperatures will increase arterial inflow to the foot and thus may obscure increments in flow due to reflux. Exercise must be standardized and should consist of 20 knee bends performed every other second with knee flexion of about 70°. The foot volume at rest may be a useful parameter if the effect of antiedematous therapy is being evaluated. Foot volume (V), in milliliters, can be predicted from an equation that incorporates the body surface area (BSA):

$$V = 617.3 \times BSA + 44.7$$

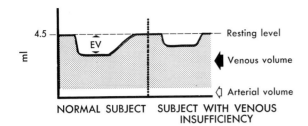

Fig. 108-5. The effect of exercise on expelled volume *(EV)*.

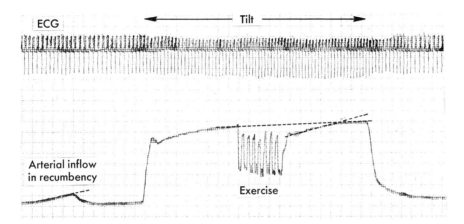

Fig. 108-6. Strain-gauge plethysmography on the foot using tilt table in a normal subject. Note that arterial inflow in recumbency is identical to the refilling flow after exercise.

Table 108-2. Normal values for volumetric parameters from three different studies*

Variable	Norgren et al[6]		Partsch[7]	Lawrence and Kakkar[3]
V = 617.3 × BSA + 44.7	—	—	1219.7 ± 163.9	—
EV	17.0 ± 7.5	8.8 ± 3.7	18.3 ± 6.8	21.2 ± 4.8
EVr	1.5 ± 0.5	0.8 ± 0.3	1.4 ± 0.4	1.9 ± 0.4
Q	2.3 ± 1.1	2.1 ± 0.7	2.2 ± 1.0	2.9
Q/EVr	1.6 ± 0.8	2.8 ± 1.2	1.5 ± 0.6	2.1 ± 0.9
t/2	25.9 ± 12.0	13.2 ± 5.0	26.4 ± 10.2	19.8 ± 8.3
t$_4$	101.2 ± 38.8	—	86.9 ± 34.3	—
n†	29	17	36	14
Age (yr)	31 (20 to 50)	68 (62 to 75)	35.4	Not stated

BSA, Body surface area.
*Abbreviations and units given in Table 108-1; mean values ± 1 standard deviation, range in parentheses.
†Number of observations.

As shown by Norgen et al[6] a useful criterion that discriminates normal individuals from patients with varicose veins and deep vein insufficiency is the ratio of refilling flow (Q) to the expelled volume (EVr):

$$Q/EVr$$

Exercise that activates the calf foot pump dislocates about 30% to 40% of the total blood volume contained in the vessels of the foot and mainly affects the volume of larger vessels; the remaining blood is stored in venules and capillaries. (This can be shown using a plethysmograph that tightly encloses the extremity and by the application of external pressure that squeezes out blood.[1])

Simultaneously measured intravenous pressure and volume curves show a marked similarity; both pressure and volume decrease during exercise and return slowly to resting levels, as shown in Fig. 108-5. From the combined application of volume and pressure changes, it is possible to calculate venous compliance.[1,5] A feature commonly seen after the completion of exercise is a more rapid return of the pressure curve to baseline. This may be due either to delayed compliance of the venous wall or to delayed filling with tissue fluid in the lymphatic system.

The advantages of foot volumetry are that it assesses the most distal parts of the leg, those most affected by hydrostatic pressure, and it closely depicts the status of venous pressure in a foot vein (Fig. 108-6). The method also reliably identifies the pathophysiologic changes associated with venous hypertension. This has recently been corroborated by Rosfors et al[10] who showed that the most distal assessment of venous function in the leg is the best way of determining the severity of venous disease and that clinically important deep vein insufficiency was especially prominent in patients with reflux in the distal posterior tibial veins.

REFERENCES

1. Christopoulos DC et al: Air-plethysmography and the effect of elastic compression on venous haemodynamics of the leg, *J Vasc Surg* 5:148, 1987.
2. Kriessmann A: Periphere Phlebodynamometrie, *Vasa* [suppl] 4:1, 1975.
3. Lawrence D, Kakkar VV: *Venous pressure measurement and foot volumetry in venous disease*. In Verstraete M, ed: *Techniques in angiology,* The Hague, 1979, Martinus Nijhoff.
4. Nicolaides AN, Christopoulos DC: Optimal methods to assess the deep venous system in the lower limb, *Acta Chir Scand* [suppl] 555:175-185, 1990.
5. Norgren L, Thulesius O: Pressure-volume characteristics of foot veins in normal cases and patients with venous insufficiency, *Blood Vessels* 12:1, 1975.
6. Norgren L et al: Foot volumetry and simultaneous venous pressure measurements for evaluation of venous insufficiency, *Vasa* 3:140, 1974.
7. Partsch H: *Simultane Venendruckmessung und Plethysmography am Fuss*. In May R, Kriessmann A, eds: *Periphere Venendruckmessung,* Stuttgart, 1978, Georg Thieme.
8. Partsch H: Funktionelle Indikation zur Krampfaderoperation, *Klin Wochenschr* 89:627, 1977.
9. Pollack AA, Wood EH: Venous pressure in saphenous vein at the ankle in man during exercise and changes in posture, *J Appl Physiol* 1:649, 1949.
10. Rosfors S et al: Severity and location of venous valvular insufficiency: the importance of distal valve function, *Acta Chir Scand* 156:689, 1990.
11. Thulesius O, Norgren L, Gjores JE: Foot volumetry: a new method for objective assessment of edema and venous function, *Vasa* 2:325, 1973.
12. Widmer L: *Peripheral venous disorders,* Berne, 1978, Hans Huber.

CHAPTER 109

Venous pressure measurements

NORMAN L. BROWSE

Although the pressure gradient between the left ventricle and the right atrium is sufficient to maintain continuous blood flow, the adoption by humans of the erect posture placed such a strain on the venous return from the lower limbs that a supplementary peripheral venous pump developed. Most chronic "venous" disease of the lower limb is caused by derangements of this peripheral pump.

Because the veins have functions other than simple blood conduction (e.g., thermoregulation), the peripheral venous system has become a complex two-chamber system. The superficial vessels, which are concerned with temperature control, form one chamber, which is connected to the vessels within the muscle pump, the second chamber, by small valved communicating (perforating) veins.

Any test that purports to measure the function of the peripheral venous pump should be able to measure all its properties, which constitutes the inflow to the pump, the pump ejection fraction, the competence of the valves between the chambers of the pump, the quantity of regurgitation through any set of incompetent valves, and the state of the outflow tract.

None of the current methods of investigation achieves this ideal, least of all the measurement of foot vein pressure. However, this is the oldest of the techniques available[3,4] and is customarily used as the standard for the comparative assessment of new methods.

When the calf pump is working normally, it ejects blood from within the muscles toward the heart along the deep axial veins. When the muscles relax, blood flows from the superficial veins into the intramuscular veins through the communicating veins. Consequently, the pressure in the superficial veins of the leg, which are on the upstream side of the pump, reflects calf pump efficiency in much the same way as central venous pressure reflects cardiac efficiency. However, it only indicates the overall effect of the pump and does not indicate the site or degree of any individual abnormality without the additional use of corrective tourniquets. When there are multiple pump defects, the measurement of foot vein pressure, even with the use of tourniquets, rarely gives anything more than a crude evaluation of total calf pump function.

METHODS

The vein

The foot is richly endowed with subcutaneous veins. Any one may be catheterized, but the most suitable is a vein running straight down the middle of the dorsum of the foot that can be entered 2 to 5 cm above an interdigital cleft so that the needle or catheter can lie comfortably inside the vein without impinging on the vein wall.

The catheter

Many workers use a short butterfly-type needle. This has two disadvantages. First, it is short and can slip out of the vein. To make the venipuncture simple and less painful, many clinicians are tempted to use a very fine needle. The second disadvantage is that fine needles damp the pressure-detecting system. Although the frequency of venous pressure changes is slow compared with the frequency of the arterial pressure wave, the best traces are obtained by using a catheter of a size that does not cause damping (e.g., a short, fine [0.5 mm, internal diameter] catheter inserted through a small stab wound in an anesthetized patch of skin).

Skin anesthesia

A small intradermal bleb of 2% lidocaine is sufficient to make the skin stab or venipuncture painless. The vein is marked with the patient standing, but the venipuncture is done with the patient lying down after producing venous congestion with an ankle tourniquet, since a number of patients faint if they feel pain while they are standing. It is not necessary to infiltrate deep beneath the skin. Anesthetic agents around the vein alter its tone.

Catheter, transducer, and recorder

It is important to use a transducer of sufficient sensitivity. The pressure may vary between 30 and 150 mm Hg, but the transducer must reliably detect changes of 2 to 5 mm Hg without excessive amplification. The frequency of the pressure waves depends on the type and rate of exercise, but the transducer should have a greater than 95% response to changes of at least 10 Hz. The center of the transducer diaphragm should be fixed level with the tip of the intravenous catheter. The connecting catheter should be as short as possible and not allowed to bounce about.

Any form of recorder may be used. The wider the paper and the tracing, the easier it is to measure gradients. Computerized systems are available that calculate the rate of change electronically and then present a number without displaying the tracing, but it is preferable to see the trace and decide that it is acceptable before making calculations from it.

System check

Transducer and pressure measurements have become so commonplace that many forget to check the system at regular intervals throughout a study. It is important to do the following:

1. Check that there are no air bubbles in any part of the catheter-transducer system.
2. Flush the catheter at regular intervals to prevent a blood clot from occluding its lumen. A continuous flushing system using heparinized saline solution prevents this complication.
3. Before each exercise test, put a very short high-pressure flush into the system and watch the trace. It should rise and fall vertically and return immediately to the baseline. Any tailing off of the rate of fall as it approaches its original resting level indicates damping caused by problems such as a clot in the catheter, bubbles in the system, too fine a catheter, the catheter tip resting on the vein wall, or an inadequate transducer. A "flush" should be seen in published recordings of pressure traces; it indicates that the operator knows the system and recognizes the problems.
4. Ask the patient to perform a Valsalva maneuver. Foot vein pressure should rise slightly if the system is working well.

Type of exercise

The venous pump must work with the patient standing, so foot vein pressures should be measured in this position. The most common form of exercise is to have the patient raise both heels off the ground as high as possible at a regular rate, usually one per second, in time to a metronome.

Many laboratories also assess calf pump function by foot volumetry[6]; the exercise for this test consists of repeated knee bending because the foot must remain still. It would seem sensible to use the same type of exercise for both methods, which means using knee bending for pressure studies.

The exercise should continue until a new stable pressure is reached. One of the objects of the test is to determine the maximum pressure fall obtainable. This is judged by watching the tracing. At least 2 and preferably 5 minutes' rest should be allowed between each period of exercise.

Tourniquets

The information gained from this test can be expanded by the application of tourniquets, which produce superficial vein obstruction. A tourniquet placed around the midthigh should prevent refilling down an incompetent long saphenous vein; one just below the knee should prevent refilling through both long and short saphenous veins; and one just above the ankle should stop refilling from all superficial to deep connections (i.e., the long and short saphenous veins and any incompetent communicating veins).

The problem is to find a tourniquet pressure that occludes the superficial but not the deep veins. In a leg with an average layer of fat, Nicolaides and Yao[5] have shown that a narrow (2.5-cm) cuff inflated to a pressure of 120 mm Hg at the ankle or 180 mm Hg at midthigh will occlude the superficial but not the deep veins. However, this does not hold in every case. The effect of the cuff will be affected by its width, the size of the leg, the depth of the fat layer, and the anatomy of the veins. There is no 100% reliable test to confirm superficial vein occlusion. The Doppler flow probe can be useful for detecting flow beneath the cuff and a helpful guide when adjusting the pressure in the tourniquet. An alternative technique is to inflate the tourniquet slowly until the respiratory fluctuations seen in the foot vein pressure disappear and then increase the tourniquet pressure by 10 mm Hg.

NORMAL FOOT VEIN PRESSURES
Resting pressure

The pressure in the veins of the feet when the patient is standing quietly is equal to the hydrostatic pressure produced by the column of blood between the head and the foot. It is usually 80 to 90 mm Hg, varies with the height of the patient, and shows small fluctuations corresponding to respiration.

Effect of exercise

Calf pump activity expels blood through the popliteal vein toward the heart. Between contractions, when the intramuscular vein pressure is zero, blood flows in from the subcutaneous veins through the communicating veins. The superficial vein pressure falls. Normally the pressure falls by 60% to 80%, that is, from 80 to 90 mm Hg down to 20 to 30 mm Hg. When the subject stops exercising, the pressure returns to the preexercise level. Three measurements can be made from the trace: the rate of fall, maximum fall, and rate of recovery.

Rate of fall. The rate of fall is affected by the power of the calf pump, obstruction or reflux in the pump outflow tract, and reflux back and forth between the superficial reservoir and the pump through the communicating veins, or the saphenopopliteal junction. The rate of fall is a measure of the rate of pump emptying and is difficult to measure accurately. It is also entirely dependent on the way the patient performs the exercise. It is not usually measured, since it is unusual to see the emptying time prolonged even in the presence of severe outflow obstruction.

Maximum fall. During the reduction of calf volume, the superficial venous pressure fluctuates in time to the heel raising. Once the maximum fall is reached, the fluctuations become smaller and it is easy to measure their upper and lower limits and calculate the mean. The mean lowest pressure is also visible for a brief moment after cessation of exercise. The percent fall in pressure is a good indicator of the overall efficiency of the calf muscle pump and the state of the inflow and outflow tracts. It is particularly affected by incompetent communicating veins and deep vein damage.[1,7]

Rate of recovery. The rate of recovery depends on the relative proportions of normal inflow from the arterial side of the circulation and retrograde flow down the deep and superficial veins. It is usually measured by drawing and extending the slope of the first few seconds of the pressure trace immediately after cessation of exercise and then calculating the time taken for the pressure to return to 50% or 90% of the resting level. All of these measurements should be repeated before and after the inflation of superficial vein−occluding tourniquets.

Normal values

Although the reduction of pressure is reproducible from laboratory to laboratory, the rates of emptying and refilling vary according to the nature of the exercise used. Each laboratory must establish its own normal values before attempting to assess patients with disordered calf pumps.

PRESSURE TRACES IN VENOUS DISEASE
Long saphenous vein incompetence

The most common abnormality of the venous system of the lower limb is simple long saphenous vein incompetence (LSI). The calf pump can usually cope with the extra load presented by reflux in this system of veins, and thus the rate and degree of foot vein pressure reduction during exercise may be normal or only just outside normal limits. The rate of refilling after exercise is increased and should be corrected by a midthigh superficial vein−occluding tourniquet. If LSI is the only abnormality, restoration of the pressure trace to normal by a midthigh cuff confirms the diagnosis and predicts a good response to long saphenous vein ligation. Pressure traces after the operation should show restoration to the normal range.

Short saphenous vein incompetence

The pressure profile of short saphenous vein incompetence (SSI) is similar to that of LSI and should be corrected by a below-knee superficial vein−occluding tourniquet. However LSI and SSI often occur simultaneously. In such cases, a midthigh tourniquet will prolong the refilling time but not restore it to normal, and the below-knee tourniquet will have a greater effect. If there is no communicating vein incompetence, a below-knee tourniquet should restore the pressure profile to normal in combined LSI and SSI as well as pure SSI and pure LSI.

Communicating vein incompetence

Incompetence of the communicating veins allows blood to flow into the superficial system at a variety of points between the knee and the ankle during calf muscle exercise. Consequently, the foot vein pressure fails to fall during exercise. If no other veins are incompetent, the refilling time is normal because there is not a large volume of blood available within the deep veins to flow outward into the superficial reservoir after exercise in the way that LSI allows, unless the whole of the deep system is also incompetent. A superficial vein−occluding tourniquet at the ankle may improve the pressure drop during exercise but rarely restores it to normal because (1) the communicating vein leak makes the whole pump inefficient, so it fails to empty the superficial veins of the foot, and (2) the tourniquet often fails to separate all the incompetent communicating veins from the foot because although most of them are above it, there is often a communicator below the tourniquet just behind and below the malleolus. Communicating vein incompetence is mainly diagnosed by exclusion, that is, when the above- and below-knee tourniquets fail to restore the refilling rate to normal and it is known by other means (usually ultrasonography or phlebography) that there is no deep axial vein obstruction or incompetence. The communicating vein leakage cannot be quantified by any of the superficial reservoir pressure- or volume-measuring techniques.

Deep axial vein obstruction

A major obstruction in the popliteal or femoral vein is expected to slow the rate of emptying during exercise and reduce the total expelled volume. Such changes are only apparent when the obstruction is extremely severe. In most cases there is sufficient power in the pump and the collateral vessels are big enough to allow normal emptying rates. Emptying also depends on the speed and strength of calf muscle contraction, a factor difficult to standardize. The absence of a detectable obstruction to outflow during laboratory exercise does not mean that one does not exist during the hyperemia of prolonged normal exercise.

If all of the collateral vessels bypassing a deep block are in the subcutaneous tissues, a superficial vein−occluding tourniquet may prolong the rate of emptying. This is a rare situation, and invariably there is edema and venous claudication.

The refilling rate should be normal in pure deep vein obstruction unless there are very inadequate collateral vessels. However, in most such limbs there is secondary incompetence of the superficial varicose veins, so the rate of refilling may be increased and the application of a midthigh cuff may prolong both emptying and refilling. Interpretation of such a pressure trace is extremely difficult.

Deep axial vein incompetence

Severe deep vein incompetence reduces pump efficiency and thus the expelled volume and the pressure fall of exercise and increases the rate of refilling. The rate of refilling will not be corrected by superficial vein−occluding cuffs regardless of where they are placed. However, because most of these patients have some degree of secondary superficial vein incompetence, there is usually some response to a midthigh tourniquet, which confuses the interpretation. Rapid refilling unaffected by a superficial vein–occluding cuff is one of the abnormalities best detected by foot vein pressure measurements.

ABSOLUTE VALUES

It can be seen from the preceding and from the singular lack of actual pressure measurements in this chapter that more is learned from a change in pressure profile in response to maneuvers such as the application of tourniquets than can be deduced from the absolute values of the pressures or their rate of change. Each laboratory must determine its own normal range, but most investigators quickly find that the normal range is so wide and the overlap between normal and abnormal so great that the interpretation of different values between individual patients is impossible. The only reliable and reproducible measurement is the 60% to 80% fall in foot vein pressure during exercise in normal individuals. Pressure falls of less than 60% signal an abnormality, but beyond this the investigator must rely on interpretation of the changes in pressure profile caused by the inflation of pneumatic cuffs at different positions on the leg. This is not a very scientific approach and emphasizes the fact that foot vein pressure measurements, although better than many other techniques, only indicate overall calf pump efficiency and the possible presence of superficial or deep reflux. Pressure measurements cannot determine individual abnormalities in the presence of multiple abnormalities—the usual clinical situation—and therefore cannot be used to assess treatment except when only one abnormality is corrected.[2]

CONCLUSION

Foot vein pressure measured during exercise, with and without the application of superficial vein–occluding tourniquets, gives a crude indication of calf pump function and may demonstrate the presence of superficial or deep vein reflux. The pressure changes do not give a precise measurement of any particular feature of calf pump function. In most cases, there is more than one abnormality of the pump, often undetected by the present forms of investigation and inadequately corrected by the current methods of treatment, so it is not surprising that pressure profiles are rarely restored to normal by surgery.

REFERENCES

1. Bjordal RI: Pressure patterns in the saphenous system in patients with venous leg ulcers, *Acta Chir Scand* 137:495, 1971.
2. Burnand KG et al: The relative importance of incompetent communicating veins in the production of varicose veins and venous ulcers, *Surgery* 82:9, 1977.
3. McPheeters HO, Merkel CE, Lundblad RA: The mechanics of the reverse flow of blood in varicose veins as proved by blood pressure readings, *Surg Gynecol Obstet* 55:298, 1932.
4. Moritz F, Tabora D: Uber eine Methode beim Menschen den Druck in oberflachlichen Venen exakt zu bestimmen, *Dtsche Arch Klin Med* 98:475, 1910.
5. Nicolaides A, Yao JST: *The investigation of vascular disorders,* Edinburgh, 1980, Churchill Livingstone.
6. Thulesuis O, Norgren L, Gjores JE: Foot volumetry: a new method for objective assessment of oedema and venous function, *Vasa* 2:325, 1973.
7. Warren R, White EA, Belcher CD: Venous pressure in the saphenous system in normal, varicose and postphlebitic extremities, *Surgery* 26:435, 1949.

CHAPTER 110

Preoperative mapping of the saphenous vein

ANN MARIE KUPINSKI, ROBERT P. LEATHER, BENJAMIN B. CHANG, and
DHIRAJ M. SHAH

Infrainguinal bypass procedures that use an autogenous saphenous vein can be aided greatly by a detailed preoperative venous assessment. Better information about the nature of the venous anatomy and any anatomic variations makes for improved use of veins[7] and more precise planning of the specific surgical approach for the bypass procedure.[4] It also can aid in the selection of the optimal vein, thus minimizing the dissection and reducing the frequency of wound complications.

Preoperative assessment of the saphenous veins can be achieved by clinical examination, venography, and real-time B-mode ultrasound scanning. In many patients, clinical examination by digital palpation or auscultation with a handheld Doppler stethoscope provides general knowlege about the venous anatomy below the knee but rarely furnishes adequate information about above-knee anatomy. Venography yields extensive details about the size, system configuration, cutaneous and deep branch points, valve locations, and any possible abnormalities. However, it is an invasive procedure and therefore carries a risk of causing local and systemic complications.

Duplex ultrasound scanning has become an established diagnostic tool in the vascular laboratory. Many investigators have used it to examine the deep femoral venous system for the presence of thrombi, valvular incompetence, recanalization, perforating veins, and other changes associated with acute or chronic deep vein thrombosis.[5,8] Other investigators have appraised its capability for assessing the adequacy of the superficial venous system for use as potential bypass graft material.[1,3,6] Duplex ultrasound scanning can be used routinely to preoperatively assess and map the saphenous vein system.

In a comparison of all three methods in more than 1900 distal arterial reconstructions for limb salvage, duplex scanning was found to be the most satisfactory technique for the preoperative assessment of saphenous veins for use as bypass conduits.

METHODS

During the past 6 years, duplex scanning has been used for the preoperative assessment of over 1500 saphenous venous systems, including 422 lesser saphenous systems. The majority of patients were male (65%). Initially, venous mapping was performed only on patients scheduled to undergo peripheral vascular procedures. During the past 2 years, its use has been extended to include those patients undergoing coronary artery bypass surgery. Of the total patient population undergoing preoperative venous mapping, 86% were scheduled for infrainguinal arterial reconstructions, and the remaining 14% were waiting to undergo coronary artery bypass grafting.

Both venography and duplex scanning were performed in the first 50 consecutive patients to compare the two techniques. In subsequent patients, venography was performed only when the ultrasound examination findings were considered inadequate.

More than 95% of the venous mapping procedures were performed using a 10-MHz mechanical sector probe equipped with a 4.5-MHz pulsed Doppler. To image deeper veins, a 7.5-MHz sector probe with a 4.0-MHz Doppler was occasionally used. The pulsed Doppler was used only to confirm venous patency. During the past year, color flow imaging was added to the laboratory protocol and is used in addition to gray-scale imaging to define those systems with questionable integrity.

To maximize venous pressure, the patient's limb is placed in a dependent position. If the patients' conditions allow, the examination is performed with them standing; if not, they sit upright on an examination table and dangle their legs over the side. Those who are unable to sit upright are placed in a 30° reverse Trendelenburg tilt, with their legs rotated externally and slightly flexed at the knee.

The examination begins at the knee. A transverse view is used to locate the greater saphenous vein because this allows easy visualization of the vein. The vein is lightly compressed to confirm patency. The greater saphenous vein is usually seen in apposition and deep to the superficial fascia. The vein is kept in the center of view and the probe is rotated into a sagittal scan to provide the best view of the vein's path. Care is taken to keep the probe perpendicular to the surface of the skin so that the vein is directly parallel to the ultrasound beam. When the vein is in full view, its

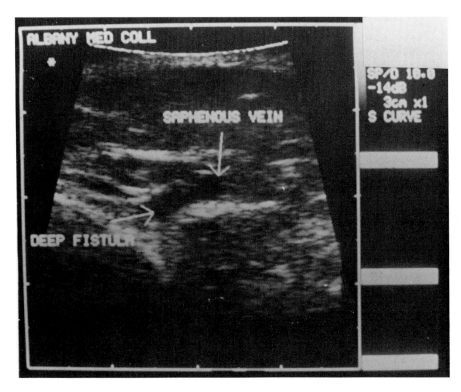

Fig. 110-1. A deep fistula originating laterally off the main trunk of the saphenous vein and penetrating the deep fascia of the limb to communicate to the deep venous system.

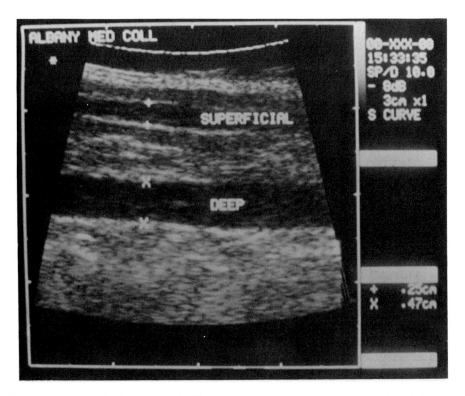

Fig. 110-2. A longitudinal scan of a double venous system found in the thigh portion of the greater saphenous vein.

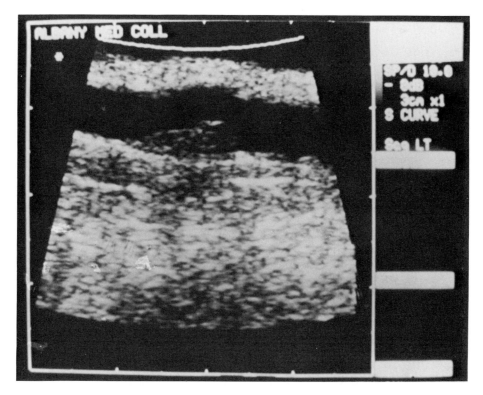

Fig. 110-3. A stenotic valve site with thrombus adherent behind the posterior leaflet.

position is marked with a small line by using a waterproof marker.* The vein is then traced, or "mapped," along its entire course. The acoustic coupling gel is used sparingly to keep the skin surface clear for marking.

Tributaries are more easily observed in the transverse scan. Anterior and posterior tributaries are marked *A* and *P*, respectively. Veins crossing the main system are marked with an *X* at the crossover point. Deep fistulas are marked *DF* (a deep fistula consists of communicating or perforating vein branches that directly connect the superficial saphenous venous system with the deep femoral venous system) (Fig. 110-1). Particular attention is paid to all tributaries in the thigh. They are followed to their completion to detect any possible double systems or closed circuits within the thigh. If a double system is found, the planar arrangement is recorded (Fig. 110-2). The internal vein diameter is measured and recorded for both the upper and lower parts of the thigh and calf. Optimally, this is done with the patient standing to maximize venous pressure. The diameters of any double systems are also measured to determine system dominance. Valves are easily seen; however, the positions are not marked unless they are stenotic or abnormal (Fig. 110-3).

When the venous assessment is complete, the acoustic-

coupling gel is wiped from the skin, and the preliminary map made with the waterproof marker is traced over using permanent marking ink. This creates an indelible surface map that lasts for 3 to 4 days and is resistant to preparation of the skin for surgery (Fig. 110-4).

The same technique is used to assess the lesser saphenous vein, which is examined with the patient standing, if possible. Otherwise, the examination is done with the patient prone. The termination of the lesser saphenous vein is easily located at the popliteal fossa where it branches off from the popliteal vein. It is followed distally and marked in the same manner as the greater saphenous vein. Branch points and internal vein diameters are also noted. Permanent marking ink is applied when the mapping is completed (Fig. 110-5).

RESULTS

In the original group of patients with peripheral vascular disease, preoperative mapping indicated vein unsuitability in 9.2% of the limbs because of discontinuity or absence of a segment due to thrombosis or disease. In an additional 9.7%, the adequacy of the vein was questionable because it either was thick walled or had an extremely small diameter despite being a continuous system from groin to ankle. Successful bypass was achieved using a continuous single vein in 97.8% of the limbs with a suitable vein, in 84.6% of the limbs with questionable veins (using in situ plus a transplanted free segment of vein), and in 80% of the limbs

---

*Liquid-Tip Felt Marker, #6173F or #1173F; Berol USA, Shelbyville, Tennessee.

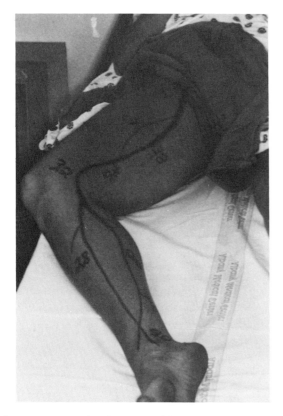

Fig. 110-4. A completed mapping of the greater saphenous vein.

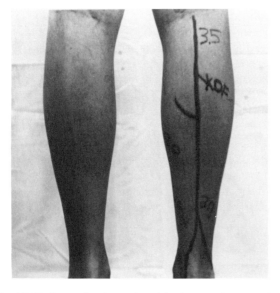

Fig. 110-5. A completed mapping of the lesser saphenous vein.

with unsuitable veins (using spliced and unspliced harvested vein grafts).

Of the patients with peripheral vascular disease who underwent mapping of the lesser saphenous vein, only seven had incomplete veins. Tributaries of the greater or lesser saphenous veins were used for spliced-vein grafting or for

lesser saphenous vein in situ bypass in those patients with incomplete greater saphenous systems. In this subgroup, 34% of the bypasses were made to the popliteal level and 66% were infrapopliteal.

The minimum follow-up period for all bypasses was 1 year, and the secondary patency rate during this time was 95%. The revision rate was 15.8%. An analysis of vein complexity (single versus double, triple, or branching systems) and revision rate showed no statistically significant difference ($p > 0.05$). The calf vein internal diameter, as measured by ultrasound at the time of mapping, was analyzed in terms of the revision rate and also showed no statistically significant difference (revised bypass calf vein internal diameter, 2.854 ± 0.713; nonrevised, 2.762 ± 0.21 [mean ± SD]).

In those patients undergoing coronary artery bypass surgery, 34% had clinically documented varicosities. In this subgroup of patients, 84% were found to have usable segments of saphenous vein. Many of the patients (62%) who were assessed before their coronary bypass surgery had undergone prior surgical procedures that involved the greater saphenous vein, and a suitable vein was found in 97%. In total, 98% of the patients who underwent mapping before their coronary bypass procedure proved to have a usable saphenous vein. In 94% of those patients who went on to surgery, the saphenous veins, either greater or lesser, were used as bypass conduits.

Mapping of the greater saphenous vein revealed various venous configurations. A standard saphenous vein consisting of a single medial dominant trunk in the thigh with an anterior dominant vein in the calf was observed in only 67% of the patients. Complete double venous systems were found in 8%, and branching double systems were found in 25%. The number of cutaneous tributaries varied greatly. Deep perforating veins were a fairly consistent finding; typically, one such vein was found at the level of the adductor hiatus and two or three were found at the calf.

With the exception of the first 50 patients studied, venography was performed in less than 5% of the patients who had vein mapping. In most instances, venography was carried out in patients who had complex saphenous systems or extremely small veins when more information was deemed necessary.

The time it takes to map a saphenous vein varies greatly. Simple, single systems of normal vein diameter can be mapped accurately in 20 to 30 minutes. Mapping complex systems with multiple crossing vein segments or saphenous systems with small diameters may take up to 60 minutes. Inexperienced technologists initially require up to 90 minutes to complete a mapping; but proficiency in mapping is usually achieved after 30 to 45 cases have been done.

DISCUSSION

The configuration of the saphenous venous system is seldom as simple as that depicted in most anatomy texts. The variations are comparable to those seen with venography.[7]

The internal diameter measurements obtained during the venous mapping procedure did not correlate with the rate of revision among the infrainguinal bypasses. Surgeons must bear in mind that these values represent internal diameter, not external diameter, and that they have been measured under normal venous pressure. Although the venous pressure is maximized by having the patient stand whenever possible, the pressure within the arterialized vein bypass is substantially greater. Thus the external diameter measured at the time of surgery can be at least 1 mm greater than the internal diameter noted at the time of venous mapping. The ultrasound-determined measurements of internal diameter should only be considered a rough estimation of vein size, and a final decision on the adequacy of conduit diameter should be made only upon surgical exposure.

Complete knowledge of saphenous venous anatomy is vital to achieving maximal use of veins in arterial bypass procedures. Clinical examination seldom provides sufficiently specific details of the venous anatomy. Venography, the previously established gold standard for venous assessment, provides the most extensive two-dimensional representation of venous anatomy.

Duplex ultrasound scanning provides a three-dimensional map plus information about tissue depth. This knowledge is extremely valuable when the surgeon is confronted with a double system in the thigh. Particularly relevant is whether the tributaries of a double system lie in the same anatomic plane. If the venous tributaries of a double system are superimposed on each other yet in different fascial planes, venography cannot discern which system is more superficial. The more superficial system is usually not the dominant system. When a Fogarty catheter is passed through the vein from the knee to the groin, the catheter will most likely travel up the vein within the same fascial plane.[2] A serious problem can arise if the diameter of the vein is not large enough to accommodate such instrumentation.

Duplex ultrasound vein mapping furnishes the surgeon with a detailed skin map of the course of the vein. These skin markings aid in the placement of surgical incisions and the selection of venous access points for instrumentation. Venous mapping also helps the surgeon avoid undermining and dissecting skin flaps while searching for a vein and determining unsuspected anatomic variations. In turn, the risk of wound complications can be minimized.

CONCLUSION

Duplex ultrasound vein mapping is a reliable noninvasive method of assessing the saphenous vein, and the resulting skin map is a useful guide for the surgeon. Venography provides excellent two-dimensional detail of saphenous venous anatomy but poses some risk to the patients. It is recommended that all patients undergo ultrasound saphenous vein mapping before distal arterial reconstruction. If the system is complex or the mapping ambiguous in any way, venography should then be performed. Duplex ultrasound vein mapping is the optimal technique for venous assessment in virtually all patients.

REFERENCES

1. Kupinski AM et al: Evaluation of saphenous veins for use as coronary artery bypass grafts, *J Vasc Tech* 16:124, 1992.
2. Leather RP, Karmody AM: In situ saphenous vein arterial bypass for the treatment of limb ischemia, *Adv Surg* 19:175, 1986.
3. Leather RP, Kupinski AM: Preoperative evaluation of the saphenous vein as a suitable graft, *Semin Vasc Surg* 1:51, 1988.
4. Leopold PW et al: Initial experience comparing B-mode imaging and venography of the saphenous vein before in situ bypass, *Am J Surg* 152:206, 1986.
5. Oliver MA: Duplex scanning in venous disease, *Bruit* 9:206, 1985.
6. Salles-Cunha SX et al: Pre-operative non-invasive assessment of arm vein to be used as bypass grafts in the lower extremities, *J Vasc Surg* 3:813, 1986.
7. Shah DM et al: The anatomy of the greater saphenous venous system, *J Vasc Surg* 3:273, 1986.
8. Sullivan ED, Peter DJ, Ganby JJ: Real time B-mode venous ultrasound, *J Vasc Surg* 1:465, 1984.

CHAPTER 111

Detection and quantification of venous reflux with duplex scanning

ANDREW N. NICOLAIDES, SPIROS N. VASDEKIS, and
DIMITRIS CHRISTOPOULOS

In recent years, duplex scanning has proved to be so accurate a method to detect deep vein thrombosis[2,16,18] that venography has become unnecessary in most cases. Its potential value in the assessment of chronic venous insufficiency has also been shown.[17] More recently, a team of researchers[11] has found that duplex scanning has the ability not only to detect the presence of reflux in individual veins but also to obtain quantitative measurements of such reflux. This ability, combined with the high-resolution images of the new-generation scanners that allow the visualization of venous valves (Fig. 111-1), has provided a powerful tool in the study of the venous system.[5,10-12] Finally, the introduction of color flow imaging has made the detection of reflux even simpler.

In the past, continuous wave Doppler ultrasound was used extensively to study the venous system.[1,8,9,14] However, one of its limitations is the inability to insonate an individual vein selectively because the technique detects signals from any other vessel lying in the path of the ultrasonic beam. In the groin, reflux can occur in a tributary of the long saphenous vein, the long saphenous vein itself, or the common femoral vein. Continuous wave Doppler ultrasound cannot distinguish reflux between these veins nor can it detect the presence of a double long saphenous vein. Although it can detect the presence of reflux in the popliteal fossa, it cannot detect the level of termination of the short saphenous vein.[3,19] Also, incompetence of the gastrocnemius or the Giacomini vein can be mistaken for reflux in the popliteal vein. These deficiencies have not been overcome by the introduction of duplex scanning into the study of venous disease.

The purpose of this chapter is to present the application and value of duplex scanning and color flow imaging in the assessment of chronic venous insufficiency.

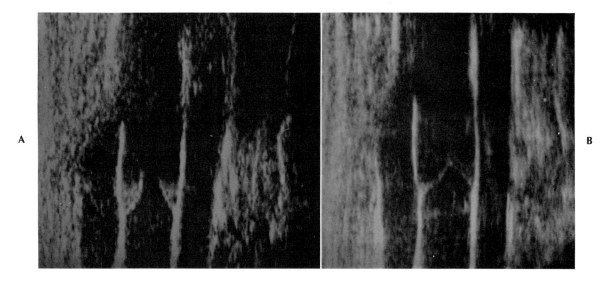

Fig. 111-1. High-resolution real-time B-mode image shows the popliteal artery, popliteal vein, and short saphenous vein. In **A** the popliteal valve is open, and in **B** it is closed (7.5-MHz linear array probe).

DETECTION OF REFLUX

A 10- or 7.5-MHz imaging probe with a 5- or 3-MHz pulsed Doppler ultrasound crystal is used. The saphenofemoral junction is examined first with the patient standing, facing the examiner, and holding onto a support, usually an orthopedic frame, to provide stability and eliminate unwanted contractions of the leg muscles. The weight of the patient is placed mainly on the opposite limb (Fig. 111-2). The probe is placed on the skin at the groin and pressed down lightly so that a longitudinal image of the common femoral

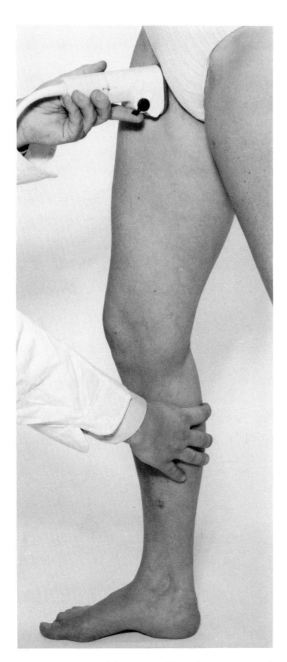

Fig. 111-2. Examination of the saphenofemoral junction is performed with the patient standing and with manual compression and sudden release of the calf.

vein, the long saphenous vein, and their junctions are obtained. Provided surgery has not been performed, the junction is always shown because of its constant anatomic position (Fig. 111-3). Two features of the area can be identified with real-time imaging: the movement of red cell aggregates, shown as echogenic intraluminar structures moving slowly cephalad,[15,20] and the movement of the venous valves during respiration, when no incompetence or thrombosis is present. The examination is performed with the patient standing because venous reflux is mainly the result of gravity and cannot be elicited as such with the patient lying down.

The sample volume is then positioned in the femoral vein 2 to 4 cm distal to the saphenofemoral junction with its beam at an angle of approximately 45° to the axis of the vessel. The calf muscles are compressed manually to show cephalad flow in the vein and are then released suddenly. In the presence of incompetence, sudden release of compression produces retrograde flow. This can be heard in the loudspeaker, and its gray-scale spectrum can be seen on the screen. They are both recorded on videotape. Absence of retrograde flow indicates competent valves (Fig. 111-4). The examination is repeated after the sample volume is positioned in the long saphenous vein 2 to 4 cm distal to the saphenofemoral junction. Retrograde flow (Fig. 111-5) indicates incompetent or absent valves.

The short saphenous and popliteal veins are examined in a similar way, with the patient standing and holding onto the frame but this time facing away from the examiner. The knee of the leg to be examined is flexed slightly, with the body weight placed mainly on the opposite leg, so that the skin over the popliteal fossa is relaxed (Fig. 111-6). The probe is placed on the skin and its position is adjusted so that three structures can be identified in a sagittal plane: the popliteal artery lying deepest, the popliteal vein lying more superficial and parallel to it, and the short saphenous vein most superficial (Fig. 111-1). Because of variations in the anatomy of the saphenopopliteal junction,[7,13] careful scanning above and below the popliteal fossa is necessary before the individual vein can be identified. The presence or absence of reflux is tested by compressing the calf manually and then suddenly releasing it after the sample volume is positioned in each individually identified vein. Other veins that should be identified and scanned for reflux are the veins of the gastrocnemius muscle. They drain into the popliteal or short saphenous vein[4] (Figs. 111-7 and 111-8).

The ability of duplex scanning to detect reflux in individual veins has shown for the first time that the diagnosis of gastrocnemius vein incompetence, which is often responsible for symptoms of swelling, heaviness, and a feeling of distention of the calf, can be made noninvasively (Fig. 111-9).

Identification of the saphenopopliteal junction

Reflux in the short saphenous vein is present in approximately 15% of all patients with varicose veins, and this is a common cause of recurrence of varices if unrecognized.

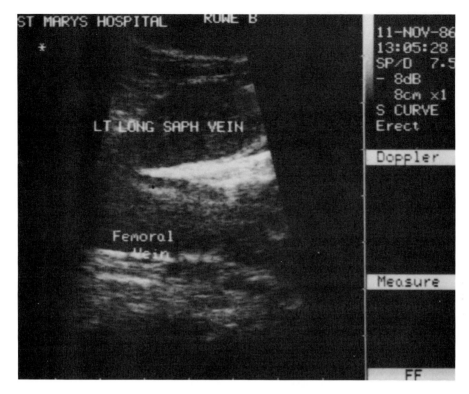

Fig. 111-3. B-mode real-time image of the saphenofemoral junction.

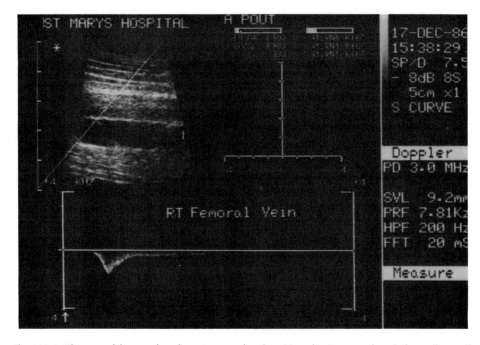

Fig. 111-4. The gate of the sample volume is opened and positioned to insonate the whole (wall to wall) lumen of the femoral vein. Flow is toward the heart on calf compression, and no evidence is seen of reflux on sudden release of the compression, indicating that the valves in the femoral vein are competent.

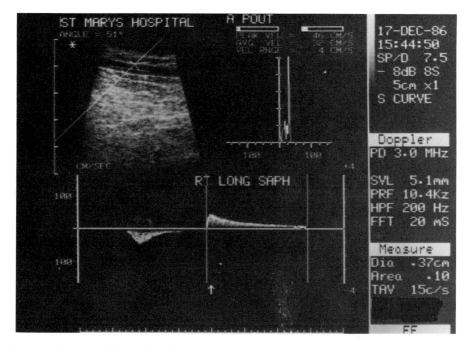

Fig. 111-5. The gate of the sample volume is opened and positioned to insonate the whole (wall to wall) lumen of the long saphenous vein. Flow is toward the heart on calf compression, and reflux is seen on sudden release of the compression, indicating that the long saphenous vein valves are incompetent.

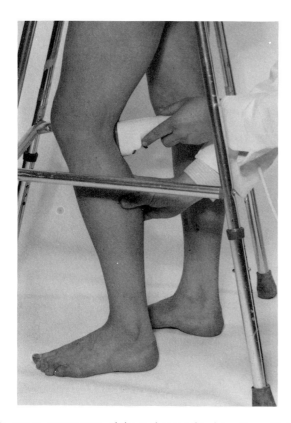

Fig. 111-6. Examination of the saphenopopliteal junction with the patient standing and holding onto an orthopedic frame. The patient's weight is mainly on the opposite leg.

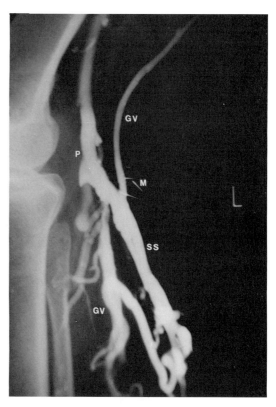

Fig. 111-7. Lateral view venogram obtained with contrast material injected into a varix of the short saphenous system shows the anatomy of the venous system at the popliteal fossa. *SS*, Short saphenous vein; *GV*, gastrocnemius vein; *P*, popliteal vein; *GT*, Giacomini vein; *M*, metal markers on the skin. (Courtesy JT Hobbs, London, England.)

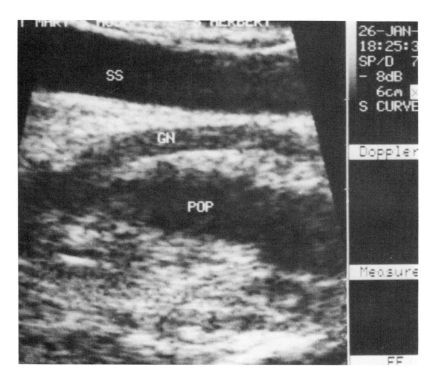

Fig. 111-8. Real-time B-mode image shows the gastrocnemius vein draining into the popliteal vein.

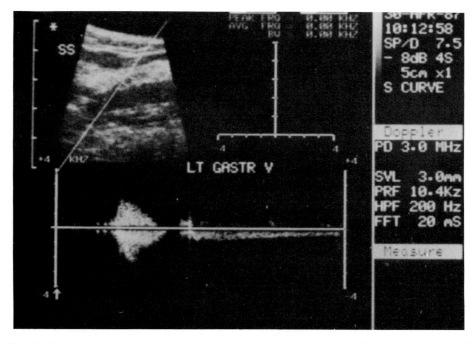

Fig. 111-9. Sample volume positioned in the gastrocnemius vein. Proximal flow occurs during calf compression and reflux on release of the compression. Simultaneous bidirectional flow indicates marked turbulence.

Because of the variable level of the saphenopopliteal junction and the need to ligate the incompetent short saphenous vein as close to the popliteal vein as possible to minimize the risk of recurrence, it was necessary in the past to do operative venography for correct placement of the skin incision. In a recent series[19] of more than 100 patients with varicose veins requiring ligation of the short saphenous vein as part of the operation because of reflux, duplex scanning was used before surgery to determine the level of the termination of this vein and this was marked on the skin. The skin mark was compared with the findings from operative venography and the junction found at surgery. Duplex scanning was 96% accurate. Consequently, operative venography may no longer be needed to identify the level of the saphenofemoral junction; the duplex scan can be used alone.

The value of duplex scanning

In an early study published in 1981[9] that used continuous wave Doppler ultrasound in patients with normal ambulatory venous pressures, the prevalence of false-positive reflux in the popliteal veins was 8%. Reflux had been assumed to exist in the popliteal vein because it could not be abolished by digital compression of the short saphenous vein. It is now possible to explain these false-positive results by showing with duplex scanning that such reflux is not in the popliteal but in the gastrocnemius veins.

A more recent study examined 96 limbs of 83 patients with chronic venous problems in whom preliminary screening with continuous wave pocket Doppler ultrasound had shown venous reflux in the popliteal fossa. Duplex scanning and venography were also performed in all. The gastrocnemius vein was incompetent in 26 (27%) limbs, and in 16, this was the only incompetent vein. The short saphenous vein was incompetent in 63 (65%) and the popliteal vein in 24 (25%) legs. Calf swelling was present in 24% of the limbs with reflux in the gastrocnemius vein but in only 16% of the whole group.[19]

Another vessel that may sometimes cause diagnostic problems is the Giacomini vein (Fig. 111-9). When present, it is the continuation of the short saphenous vein in the thigh and often terminates by joining the posteromedial tributary of the long saphenous or, rarely, the internal iliac vein. The irregular course of this vein and/or the presence of reflux in it can also make the diagnosis difficult. However, following the course of this vein with the imaging probe can solve this problem. When the anatomy of the area is unusual or not easily obvious, scanning transversely along the popliteal fossa can help show more accurately the anatomic relationship of the different vessels. Transverse scanning is particularly useful with color flow imaging because it provides an immediate indication of flow direction and thus identification of veins and arteries.

Perforating veins can be identified with real-time imaging by scanning transversely along the course of the long and short saphenous veins or the posterior arch of the long saphenous vein. For this part of the examination, the patient sits on a couch with the leg positioned vertically over the edge and the foot resting on a stool or low chair on which the examiner is sitting facing the patient. Perforating veins can be seen branching from the superficial veins toward the deep system. The probe is then rotated 90° so that the superficial and deep veins are visualized in a longitudinal plane with the perforating veins joining the two (Fig. 111-10). The sample volume is then positioned on the perforating veins, and distal compression is applied, followed by sudden release. The direction of flow from superficial to deep during the compression period can be identified, and the presence or absence of reflux on release of the compression determined. The Doppler spectrum of blood flow velocity detected in an incompetent perforating vein almost always shows simultaneous bidirectional flow, indicating turbulent flow (Fig. 111-11). Results of studies to correlate the finding of reflux in perforating veins with the findings of venography are not yet available.

QUANTIFICATION OF REFLUX

Duplex scanning has provided the ability to quantify reflux in individual veins. The method of examination is the same as the one previously described, but instead of manual compression of the calf, a Hokanson device and pneumatic cuff are used to ensure standard compression (70 mm Hg) and sudden release. The gate of the sample volume is adjusted so that insonation of the vein under examination is from wall to wall. The angle cursor is positioned along the axis of the vein (Fig. 111-12), and the Doppler spectrum is recorded on videotape during compression and release. The mean velocity at peak reflux in centimeters per second is determined. The diameter of the vein is also determined and is used to calculate the cross-sectional area (in square centimeters). Because the patient is standing and the vein is distended, it is considered to have a circular circumference. The flow (in milliliters per second) at peak reflux is obtained by multiplying the cross-sectional area by the mean velocity at peak reflux (Fig. 111-12).

The detection of reflux and the measurement of flow in milliliters per second at peak reflux in the axial veins (long saphenous, short saphenous, and femoropopliteal) were made in 47 limbs of patients who had chronic venous problems (varicose veins, skin changes, and/or ulceration). These measurements are shown in Figs. 111-13 and 111-14. They indicate that ulceration or skin changes do not occur when the sum of peak reflux in all the veins is less than 10 ml/sec. The prevalence of skin changes and/or ulceration is high when peak reflux exceeds 15 ml/sec, irrespective of whether such reflux is in the superficial or the deep veins.

The techniques described here are relatively tedious because most vessels visualized by B-mode real-time ultrasound have to be examined using gated Doppler ultrasound. Despite the help provided by the software of modern duplex scanning equipment for the calculation of mean velocity and diameter of the vessel at any instant, the rather long ex-

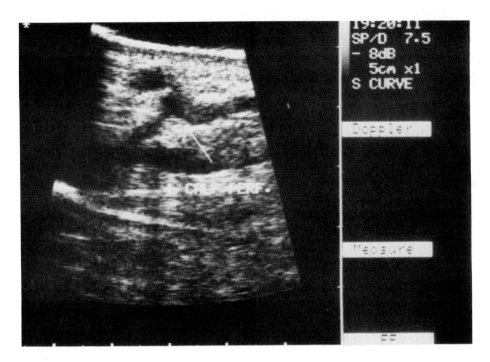

Fig. 111-10. B-mode image shows the calf perforating vein joining a superficial vein to a deep muscular vein.

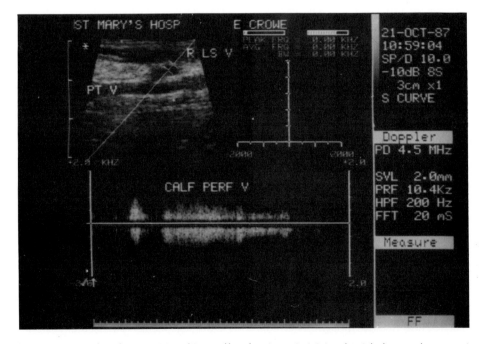

Fig. 111-11. Sample volume positioned in a calf perforating vein joining the right long saphenous vein *(RLSV)* with the posterior tibial vein *(PTV)*. Flow is bidirectional (turbulent) but mainly outward during calf compression and inward (superficial to deep) during release of the compression.

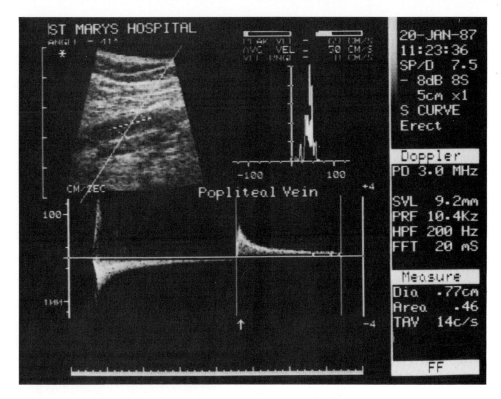

Fig. 111-12. Reflux in the popliteal vein. Average velocity at peak reflux (↑) is 30 cm/sec; diameter of popliteal vein *(Dia)* is 0.77 cm; cross-sectional area *(area)* is 0.46 cm². Flow at peak reflux = 30 × 0.46 = 13.8 ml/sec.

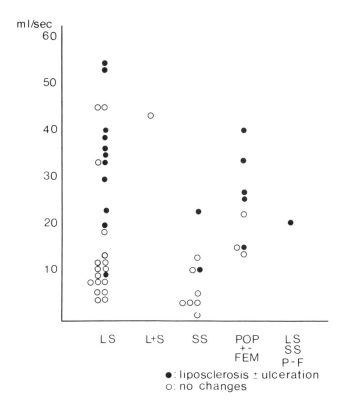

Fig. 111-13. Flow at peak reflux in the long saphenous *(LS)*, short saphenous *(SS)*, and femoropopliteal veins *(POP* and *FEM)* in 47 limbs of patients with venous insufficiency. Values of reflux present in more than one vein were added to obtain the value of overall reflux. The prevalence of liposclerosis and ulceration is high when flow at peak reflux is greater than 15 ml/sec irrespective of whether this reflux is in the superficial or deep venous system.

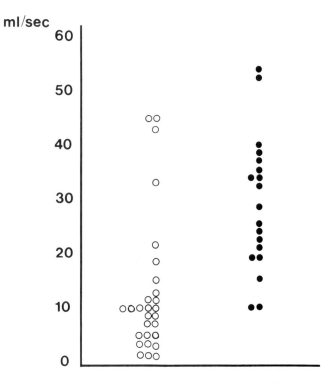

Fig. 111-14. The same data as in Fig. 111-13 but arranged in two groups according to the presence or absence of liposclerosis and/or ulceration.

amination period (half hour per limb) limits the number of patients that can be examined in a day. Thus the cost of duplex scanning is high compared with that of using a portable pocket Doppler probe. This is one reason duplex scanning should be used to supplement the Doppler examination done at the bedside or in the outpatient department when the diagnosis is difficult. In addition, training of the operator (examiner) is probably more difficult than that for carotid scanning. The variations of the venous anatomy and the lack of pulsatile flow make the identification of veins quite difficult. However, the advent of color flow imaging should overcome these problems.

COLOR FLOW IMAGING

Color flow imaging is a promising new technique. It provides instant visualization of blood flow and flow direction. These characteristics are important for venous assessment. The direction and magnitude of the Doppler frequency shift determine the hue and intensity, respectively, of the color. The color designation of the flow direction can be assigned by the operator. By convention, blue indicates flow toward the heart and red indicates flow away from the heart. The higher the velocity, the paler the color. Initial studies on arteries[6] have shown that flow can be quantified using color flow imaging and that flow patterns in specific areas, such as the carotid bulb, can be visualized with accuracy.

Examination of the venous system for reflux is performed using the same protocol as that for duplex scanning, with the patient standing. The veins are identified first by using the real-time monochrome B-mode. They appear as dark structures when the color is switched off. The gray-scale image is optimized by adjusting the attenuation curve for the tissues (Fig. 111-15, *A*), and the color is switched on. When the color is switched on, the pulsatile flow in the arteries becomes obvious (red). Distal compression results in augmentation of venous flow and increased Doppler shift frequency, which is assigned a color (blue) for flow toward the heart (Fig. 111-15, *B*). Sudden release of the distal compression will reveal reflux as a different color (red), indicating flow away from the heart (Fig. 111-15, *C*).

Use of this approach has made the detection of reflux at the saphenofemoral junction a simple matter. Use of a sample volume (as described with duplex scanning) is unnecessary, and thus the examination can be done quickly. Fig. 111-16 shows the findings in a patient with marked reflux in the long saphenous vein and no reflux in the common femoral vein distal to the saphenofemoral junction.

The measurement of reflux in milliliters per minute at any time during reflux using color flow imaging and the available software has also become a simple matter. Fig. 111-17 shows reflux in the long saphenous vein. The wide sample volume, the angle cursor in the axis of the vessel, and the colored pixels allow automatic calculation of flow and diameter at any instant.

Initial experience with color flow imaging and venography in a group consisting of 39 limbs showed that color

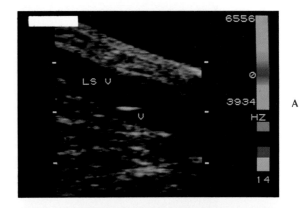

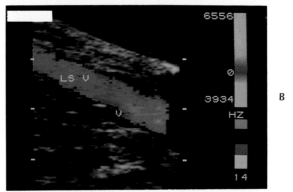

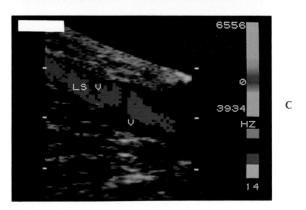

Fig. 111-15. *A,* B-mode gray-scale real-time image of long saphenous vein *(LSV)* in the thigh with remnant of a valve cusp *(V)*. *B,* Flow toward the heart (blue) during calf compression. *C,* Retrograde flow (red) immediately after release of the compression indicates the presence of incompetent valves.

flow imaging is as accurate as duplex scanning in detecting the anatomy of the popliteal fossa because the instrument used for color flow imaging also functions as a conventional duplex scanner.[19] The major advantage over duplex scanning is the potential to immediately identify the vessel with the retrograde flow, eliminating the need for multiple insonations with the sample volume at different sites. The average time required to scan the popliteal fossa with the duplex scanner is 10 minutes. With color flow imaging, this time has been reduced to 1 to 2 minutes. Fig. 111-18 is an example of reflux in only the short saphenous vein in a

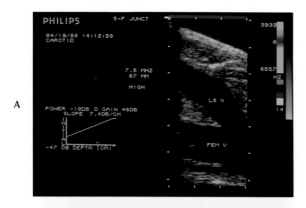

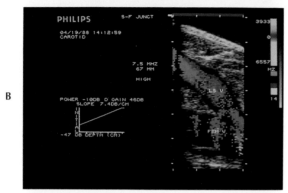

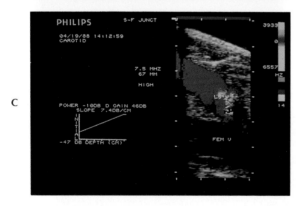

Fig. 111-16. *A,* B-mode gray-scale real-time image of the sapheno-femoral junction. *B,* Flow toward the heart (blue) during calf compression. *C,* Retrograde flow (red) in the long saphenous vein but not in the femoral vein distal to the saphenofemoral junction immediately after release of the compression.

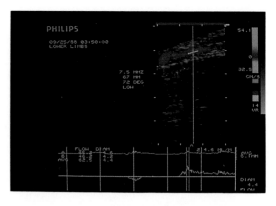

Fig. 111-17. Measurement of reflux in the long saphenous vein (red) on release of the calf compression. The area of blue indicates the turbulence produced by incompetent valve cusps. The sample-volume gate has been opened to provide wall-to-wall insonation, and the angle cursor has been positioned in the axis of the vessel. The diameter is measured automatically and depends on the number of colored pixels. Flow against time in milliliters per minute is recorded at the bottom of the screen. The first negative deflection indicates flow toward the heart during calf compression. The positive deflection indicates flow during reflux. Two cursors have been positioned at peak reflux when the flow was 62.5 ml/min.

patient with varicose veins. Fig. 111-19 is an example of reflux in the popliteal, gastrocnemius, and short saphenous veins in a patient with a postthrombotic limb. When more than one vein shows reflux, identification of individual veins is often made easy by scanning the popliteal fossa transversely but with the plane of the linear array probe at an angle of 20° to 30° to the horizontal plane (Fig. 111-20). Calf compression and sudden release are performed with the probe held in this position.

The direction of flow in perforating veins in the calf or thigh is shown without the need to also insonate each in-

dividual vessel with a sample volume. Tibial (Fig. 111-21), peroneal, and calf perforating veins are studied with the patient sitting at the end of a couch or table with the legs hanging vertically over the edge and the feet on a low stool. The examiner sits on this low stool facing the patient. Variations in flow during active muscle contractions (e.g., foot dorsiflexion) can be studied by color flow imaging. Initial observations have shown that the direction of flow through the perforating veins is more complicated than was originally thought. At the beginning of muscular contraction, the flow goes from the deep system through the incompetent perforating veins to the superficial veins. The perforating vein is subsequently partially or totally occluded during the muscular contraction, and this interrupts outward flow. During muscular relaxation, the flow is directed from the superficial to the deep veins (Fig. 111-22). This observation does not apply to enlarged perforating veins in which outward flow during muscle contraction is not interrupted. Care should be taken in interpreting the findings of color flow imaging because the color assignment depends on the Doppler frequency shift, which in turn depends on the angle of insonation. This is illustrated in Fig. 111-23. Flow in the posterior tibial vein is blue because it is away from the probe. Flow in the incompetent perforating vein and the long saphenous vein is red because it is toward the probe. Changes in the course of the perforating vein because of tortuosity may result in different color assignments, with each loop depending on the direction of flow relative to the probe (Fig. 111-24). In addition, when the course of the vessel parallels the transducer, no color is shown because there is no Doppler shift. This may be a potential source of error for the novice who may infer erroneously from this that the vein is not patent.

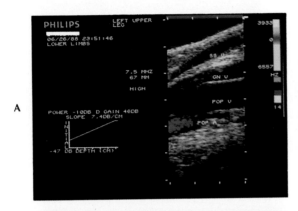

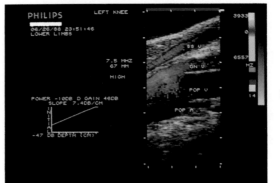

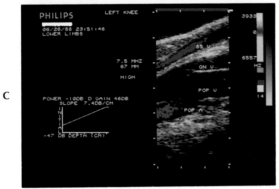

Fig. 111-18. *A,* B-mode real-time sagittal image of the popliteal fossa. Flow away from the heart (red) is seen in the popliteal artery *(POP A)* during systole. The lumens of the popliteal *(POP V),* gastrocnemius *(GN V),* and short saphenous veins *(SSV)* are black because of the very slow flow when the patient stands still. *B,* Flow toward the heart (blue) during calf compression. The popliteal artery is black during diastole because of slow flow. *C,* Retrograde flow (red) in the short saphenous vein immediately after release of the compression indicates incompetent valves in this vein. Absence of reflux in the gastrocnemius and popliteal veins indicates that the valves of these deep veins are competent.

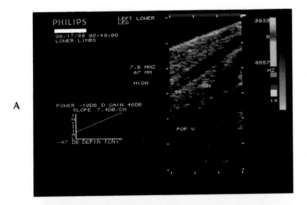

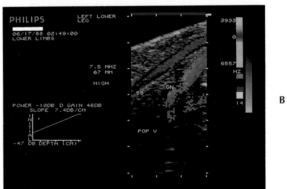

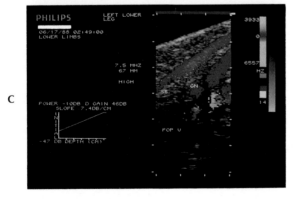

Fig. 111-19. *A,* B-mode real-time sagittal image of the popliteal fossa. *SS,* Short saphenous vein; *GN,* gastrocnemius vein; *POP-V,* popliteal vein. The popliteal artery is outside the plane of insonation, but the gastrocnemius artery (red) can be seen crossing the gastrocnemius vein. *B,* Flow toward the heart (blue) during calf compression in all three veins. *C,* Retrograde flow (red) indicates damaged incompetent valves in all three veins.

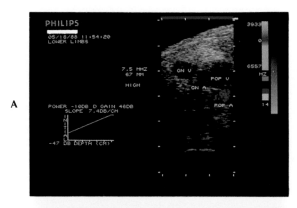

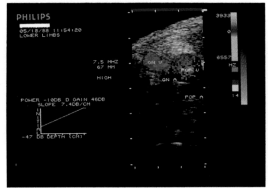

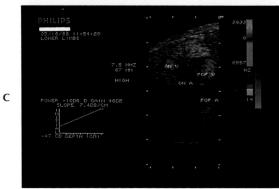

Fig. 111-20. A, B-mode real-time transverse image of the popliteal fossa. *GN V,* Gastrocnemius vein; *GN A,* gastrocnemius artery; *POP V,* popliteal vein; *POP A,* popliteal artery. The short saphenous vein is not seen because it is compressed by the probe. **B,** Flow toward the heart (blue) during calf compression in all gastrocnemius and popliteal veins. **C,** Retrograde flow (red) in both gastrocnemius and popliteal veins immediately after release of the compression.

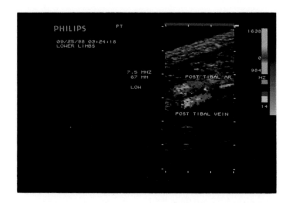

Fig. 111-21. Posterior tibial artery (red) and veins (blue) during calf compression.

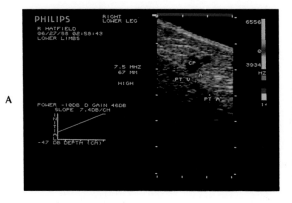

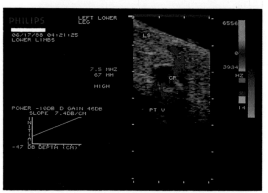

Fig. 111-22. A, B-mode real-time sagittal image of the posterior tibial vein *(PT V),* long saphenous vein *(LS),* and calf perforating vein *(CP).* Flow is toward the heart (blue) in the long saphenous and posterior tibial veins and outward (toward the probe) in the perforating vein during calf muscle contraction. **B,** Flow is reversed (red, i.e., from superficial to deep) during muscle relaxation. The outward flow during muscle contraction is characteristic of incompetent perforating veins.

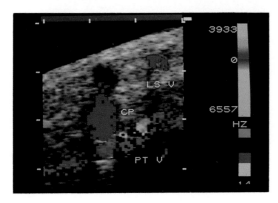

Fig. 111-23. Image during calf muscle contraction. Because of the angle of the probe, flow in the posterior tibial vein *(PT V)*, which is toward the heart but away from the probe, appears blue. Outward flow in the incompetent calf perforating veins *(CP)* and distal flow in the long saphenous vein *(LS V)* appears red because it is towards the probe.

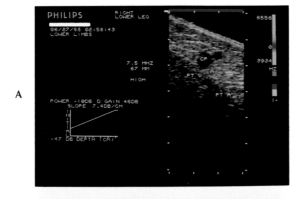

A

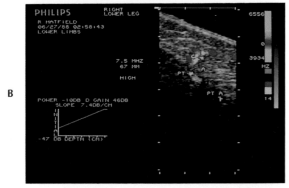

B

Fig. 111-24. *A,* B-mode real-time sagittal image of the posterior tibial artery *(PT A)*, posterior tibial vein *(PT V)*, and tortuous incompetent calf perforating vein. *B,* During calf compression, flow in the tibial veins is toward the heart and probe (blue). Outward flow in the perforating vein appears in both colors because of the tortuosity of the vein and turbulence of flow.

REFERENCES

1. Barnes RW et al: Noninvasive quantitation of venous reflux in the postphlebitic syndrome, *Surg Gynecol Obstet* 136:769, 1973.
2. Hannan LJ et al: Venous imaging of the extremities: our first twenty-five hundred cases, *Bruit* 10:29, 1986.
3. Hoare MC, Royle JP: Doppler ultrasound detection of saphenofemoral and saphenopopliteal incompetence and operative venography to ensure precise saphenopopliteal ligation, *Aust NZ J Surg* 54:49, 1984.
4. Hobbs JT: Errors in the differential diagnosis of incompetence of the popliteal vein and short saphenous vein by Doppler ultrasound, *J Cardiovasc Surg* 27:169, 1986.
5. Jaeger K, Bollinger A: *Evaluation of venous wall and valve motion.* In Negus D, Jantet G, eds: *Phlebology,* London, 1985, John Libby.
6. Keagy B et al: The use of angiodynography to quantify blood flow in the canine aorta, *J Vasc Surg* 6:269, 1987.
7. Kosinsky C: Observations on the superficial venous system of the lower extremities, *J Anat* 60:131, 1926.
8. Lewis JD et al: The use of venous pressure measurements and directional Doppler recordings in distinguishing between superficial and deep valvular incompetence in patients with deep venous insufficiency, *Br J Surg* 60:312, 1973.
9. Nicolaides AN et al: *Doppler ultrasound in the investigation of venous insufficiency,* In Nicolaides AN, Yao JST, eds: *Investigation of vascular disorders,* London, 1981, Churchill Livingston.
10. Rollins DL et al: *Characterisation of lower extremity chronic venous disease using real-time ultrasound imaging,* In Negus D, Jantet G, eds: *Phlebology,* London, 1985, John Libby.
11. Sandager G et al: Assessment of venous valve function by duplex scan, *Bruit* 10:238, 1986.
12. Semrow C et al: *Assessment of valve function using real-time B-mode ultrasound.* In Negus D, Jantet G, eds: *Phlebology,* London, 1985, John Libby.
13. Sheppard M: The incidence, diagnosis and management of saphenopopliteal incompetence, *Phlebology* 1:23, 1986.
14. Shull KC et al: Significance of popliteal reflux in relation to ambulatory-venous pressure and ulceration, *Arch Surg* 114:1304, 1979.
15. Sigel B et al: Comparison of clinical and Doppler ultrasound evaluation of confirmed lower extremity venous disease, *Surgery* 64:332, 1968.
16. Sullivan ED, David JP, Cranley JJ: Real-time B-mode venous ultrasound, *J Vasc Surg* 1:465, 1984
17. Szendro G et al: Duplex scanning in the assessment of deep venous incompetence, *J Vasc Surg* 4:237, 1986.
18. Talbot ST: Use of real time imaging in identifying deep venous obstruction: a preliminary report, *Bruit* 6:41, 1984.
19. Vasdekis SN et al: Comparison of clinical examination. Doppler ultrasound and duplex scanning with peroperative venography in the assessment of the short saphenous termination, *Br J Surg* 76:929, 1989.
20. Wolverson MK et al: The direct visualization of blood flow by real-time ultrasound: clinical observations and underlying mechanisms, *Radiology* 140:443, 1981.

CHAPTER 112

Quantification of venous reflux and outflow obstruction with air-plethysmography

ANDREW N. NICOLAIDES and DIMITRIS CHRISTOPOULOS

The symptoms of chronic venous insufficiency are produced by venous hypertension, which results from obstruction, reflux, or a combination of both (see Chapter 92). The traditional invasive methods of evaluating it—ascending and descending venography and ambulatory venous pressure (AVP) measurements—were accurate for detecting the problem and could somewhat quantify it but are now rarely used routinely because they have been superseded by duplex scanning and air-plethysmography (APG).[10] Before discussing APG, the respective contributions of these earlier tests is summarized.

ASCENDING VENOGRAPHY

Ascending venography can display the venous anatomy and can indicate the basic abnormality, but it cannot provide quantitative data. The main reasons for doing venograms are to confirm the presence and extent of outflow obstruction and to visualize the collateral circulation and potential sites of reflux.

Until recently, venography was considered the gold standard for anatomic visualization. However, the development of high-resolution real-time ultrasonic imaging equipment combined with Doppler ultrasound (duplex scanning) has produced a new noninvasive gold standard.[9,12,14,17,18] The availability of a number of noninvasive techniques that can quantify the severity of obstruction and reflux and complement duplex scanning now provides most of the answers, so venography tends to be performed in increasingly fewer patients (e.g., 3% to 4% of all patients with venous problems).

DESCENDING VENOGRAPHY

The aim of descending venography is to assess the extent of venous valve reflux and, by inference, the degree of valvular damage in the deep veins of the lower limb. The patient is placed in the 60°, semiupright position.[8] An 18-gauge end-hole venous catheter is positioned in the common femoral vein at the level of the pubic bone. Repeated boluses of isoosmolar contrast are injected. By determining the extent of distal reflux of the contrast material, this indicates the competence of the common femoral, superficial femoral, profunda femoris, and popliteal veins, as well as the saphenofemoral junction. Initially the examiner looks for spontaneous reflux, then asks the patient to do a Valsalva's maneuver, and next plantar flexes the foot gently but not against resistance as done for ascending functional venography.

Grades of reflux

Five grades of reflux (0 to 4) have been described (Table 112-1).[1,8] Although pathologic reflux through the popliteal vein is associated with symptoms, this association is not clear-cut. For example, in one study, reflux through the popliteal vein was noted in one of five limbs with skin changes or ulceration and in only 31% of postphlebitic limbs.[8] The poor association between popliteal reflux and symptoms may stem from two causes. Skin changes and ulceration can often occur when there is reflux in the superficial veins only, provided the retrograde flow at peak reflux exceeds 7 ml/sec.[4] The existence of competent popliteal valves does not exclude the possibility of postphlebitic changes that may be the result of reflux in the tibial veins and incompetent calf perforating veins.[11] Unfortunately, the

Table 112-1. Grades of reflux in the deep veins on descending venography

Grade no.	Description
Grade 0	No reflux below the confluence of the superficial and profunda femoris veins (i.e., the uppermost valve of the superficial femoral vein is competent)
Grade 1	Reflux beyond the uppermost valve of the superficial femoral vein but not below the middle of the thigh
Grade 2	Reflux into the superficial femoral vein to the level of the knee; popliteal valves competent
Grade 3	Reflux to a level just below the knee; incompetent popliteal valves but competent valves in the axial calf veins
Grade 4	Reflux through the axial veins (femoral, popliteal, and calf veins) to the level of the ankle

From Ackroyd JS, Lea Thomas M, Browse NL: Deep vein reflux: an assessment by descending venography, Br J Surg 73:31, 1986.

Table 112-2. The incidence of ulceration (active or healed) in relationship to ambulatory venous pressure in 251 limbs

No. of limbs	Pressure (mm Hg)	Incidence of ulceration (%)
34	<30	0
44	31-44	12
51	41-50	20
45	51-60	38
34	61-70	57
28	71-80	68
15	>80	73

From Christopoulos D, Nicolaides AN, Szendro: Venous reflux: quantification and correlation with the clinical severity of chronic venous disease, *Br J Surg* 75:352-356, 1988.

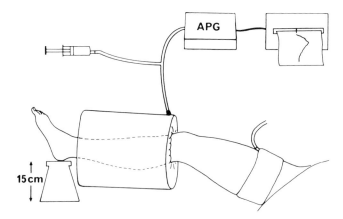

Fig. 112-1. An air-plethysmograph *(APG)* consists of a polyvinyl chloride *(PVC)* air chamber (5-L capacity) and a calibration syringe connected to a pressure transducer amplifier and recorder.

technique of descending venography as described here cannot demonstrate reflux in the tibial veins if the popliteal or more proximal valves are competent.

With the advent of duplex scanning ultrasonic equipment (see Chapter 111), a noninvasive method now exists for not only detecting but also quantitating reflux in individual veins so that descending venography is no longer necessary unless "floppy" valves are suspected, with a view toward performing valvuloplasty.

AMBULATORY VENOUS PRESSURE MEASUREMENTS

The original observation made in the 1940s of decreasing venous pressure in the foot during walking,[15] with gradual recovery to the resting value once walking stopped, formed the basis of the ambulatory venous pressure (AVP) measurements that were used to supplement the anatomic information provided by venography (see Chapter 109). In recent years, AVP measurements became the hemodynamic gold standard for the development of noninvasive methods of screening and diagnosis.[13] The correlation of AVP with the incidence of ulceration is shown in Table 112-2.

If there is severe outflow obstruction and deep venous reflux (including reflux in the popliteal vein), the AVP may actually increase during exercise because of the augmented blood flow resulting from exercise hyperemia. This is the group of patients who complain of "bursting" pain on walking (venous claudication), even though their popliteal valves are competent.

Because the measurement of ambulatory venous pressure is invasive, it cannot be repeated frequently or used as a screening test. Thus noninvasive screening tests, such as plethysmography, Doppler ultrasound, calf volume plethysmography, foot volumetry, and duplex scanning, have been developed for this purpose.

AIR-PLETHYSMOGRAPHY

APG was used in the early 1960s to study relative volume changes in the lower limb in response to postural alterations and muscular exercise.[2] Recent interest in reconstructive surgery of the deep veins has created a need for the non-

invasive quantitation of venous reflux and calf muscle pump ejection. Once it was possible to calibrate the APG, whole-leg volume changes as a result of exercise could be detected in both absolute (milliliters) and relative terms, thereby overcoming the limitations of segmental devices and water plethysmography (see Chapter 23).[3-7] Segmental volume changes measured with a strain gauge do not necessarily represent changes in the whole leg. In addition, because APG includes all the tissues between the knee and ankle, gravitationally induced tissue shifts in response to postural changes that interfere with segmental devices on the calf are less likely to occur.

The APG consists of a 35-cm-long, tubular, polyvinyl chloride air chamber (capacity, 5 liters) that encloses the whole leg from the knee to the ankle (Fig. 112-1). This device is inflated to 6 mm Hg and connected to a pressure transducer, amplifier, and recorder. (The pressure of 6 mm Hg is the lowest that can ensure good contact between the air chamber and the leg.) Calibration is performed by depressing the plunger of the syringe (Fig. 112-1), compressing the air in the system and reducing its volume by 100 ml, and then observing the corresponding pressure change. The plunger is then pulled back to its original position once the pressure in the air chamber returns to 6 mm Hg.

Initially, the patient is in the supine position with the leg elevated 45° to empty the veins and the heel resting on a support. After a stable baseline recording is obtained, the subject is asked to stand with the weight placed on the opposite leg while holding onto an orthopedic frame. Venous filling should produce an increase in the leg venous volume (Fig. 112-2), which is 100 to 150 ml in normal limbs and 100 to 350 ml in limbs with chronic venous insufficiency.

The venous filling index (VFI) is defined as the ratio of 90% of the venous volume (VV) divided by the time taken to achieve 90% of filling (VFT90), or VFI = 90% VV/VFT90. This is a measure of the average filling rate and is expressed in milliliters per second. The ranges of VFI in

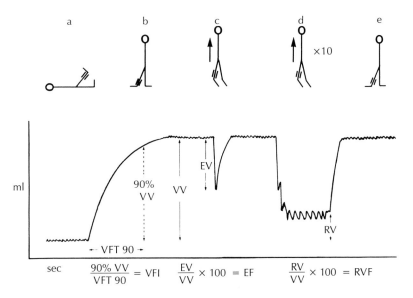

Fig. 112-2. Typical recording of volume changes during standard sequence of postural changes and exercise. Patient in supine position with leg elevated 45° *(a)*; patient standing with weight on nonexamined leg *(b)*; single tiptoe movement *(c)*; 10 tiptoe movements *(d)*; return to resting standing position as in *b* *(e)*. *VV*, Functional venous volume; *VFT*, venous filling time; *VFI*, venous filling index; *EV*, ejected volume; *RV*, residual volume; *EF*, ejection fraction; *RVF*, residual volume fraction. (From Christopoulos D et al: *J Vasc Surg* 5:148, 1987.)

normal limbs, limbs with superficial venous incompetence, and limbs with deep vein disease are shown in Fig. 112-3. A VFI of 2 ml/sec or less indicates absence of significant venous reflux and slow filling of the veins from the arterial circulation. A VFI greater than 7 ml/sec is associated with a high incidence of skin changes, chronic swelling, and ulceration irrespective of whether the reflux is in the superficial or deep venous system. The application of a narrow pneumatic tourniquet (2.5 cm wide) that occludes the superficial veins at the knee (long and short saphenous) can reduce the VFI to less than 5 ml/sec in limbs with primary varicose veins and competent popliteal valves but not those with incompetent popliteal valves identified on duplex scans.[8] In addition, measurements obtained before and after conventional surgery for superficial venous incompetence have shown that APG can effectively demonstrate the abolition of venous reflux.[8]

If the patient does one tiptoe movement with the weight on both legs and then returns to the initial position, the ejected volume (EV) (Fig. 112-2) and ejection fraction (EF) produced by the calf muscle contraction can be measured: EF = (EV/VV) × 100. The ranges of EF in normal limbs, limbs with primary varicose veins, and limbs with deep vein disease are shown in Fig. 112-4. If the patient does 10 tiptoe movements, the residual volume (RV) can be measured and the residual volume fraction (RVF) calculated as follows: RVF = (RV/VV) × 100 (Fig. 112-2). The ranges of RVF for different conditions in the limbs are shown in Fig. 112-5. There is a good linear correlation between RVF and ambulatory venous pressure (AVP) at the end of exercise (Fig. 112-6). This is not surprising because, at any time,

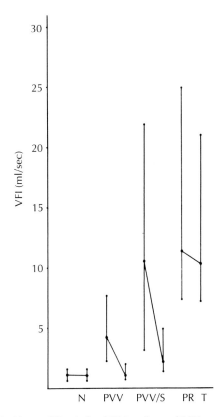

Fig. 112-3. Venous filling index *(VFI)* (median and 90% range) without and with a tourniquet *(T)* that occluded the superficial veins at the knee in normal *(N)* limbs, limbs with primary varicose veins without sequelae of chronic venous disease (liposclerosis and ulceration), primary varicose veins with sequelae of chronic venous disease *(PVV/S)*, and limbs with popliteal reflux *(PR)*. (from Christopoulos D et al: *J Cardiovasc Surg* 29:535, 1988.)

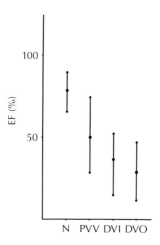

Fig. 112-4. Ejection fraction *(EF)* (median and 90% range) in normal *(N)* limbs, limbs with primary varicose veins *(PVV)*, deep venous incompetence *(DVI)*, and deep venous obstruction *(DVO)*.

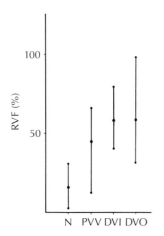

Fig. 112-5. Residual volume fraction *(RVF)* (mean and 90% range) in normal *(N)* limbs, limbs with primary varicose veins *(PVV)*, deep venous incompetence *(DVI)*, and deep venous obstruction *(DVO)*.

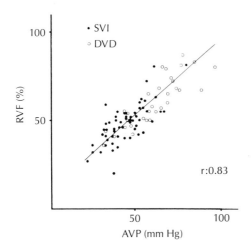

Fig. 112-6. Relationship between residual volume fraction *(RVF)* and ambulatory venous pressure *(AVP)* at the end of 10 tiptoe movements. ●, Limbs with superficial venous incompetence; O, limbs with deep venous disease. (From Christopoulos D et al: *J Vasc Surg* 5:148, 1987.)

Table 112-3. Incidence of ulceration in relationship to the RVF of the calf muscle pump in 175 limbs with venous disease

RVF (%)	No. of limbs	Incidence of ulceration
<30	20	0
31-40	24	8%
41-50	48	27%
51-60	43	42%
61-80	32	72%
80	8	87%

RVF, Residual volume fraction.

it is the amount of blood in the veins that determines the venous pressure. Table 112-3 shows how the incidence of ulceration increases in relation to the RVF.

These volume measurements have been used to study the efficacy of the calf muscle pump and to quantify the effect of therapeutic measures, such as compression and surgical intervention. They should be used not only to assess the effects of deep vein reconstruction but also to select likely candidates for such reconstruction.

OUTFLOW OBSTRUCTION

Outflow obstruction is suspected when swelling is the predominant symptom and the patient has a history of deep vein thrombosis plus there are prominent collateral venous channels in the groin above the pubis or the anterior abdominal wall. It should always be suspected in patients with postthrombotic limbs.

The resting venous pressure can be simply estimated by having the patient elevate the leg while supine then by observing the height (in centimeters) of the heel from the heart level when the prominent veins collapse.

Arm/foot pressure differential: the gold standard

The arm/foot pressure differential has been used by Raju[16] as another method of determining the severity of outflow obstruction. It consists of simultaneously measuring the pressure in the veins of the foot and hand with the patient in the supine position at rest. These pressures are measured again after reactive hyperemia is induced. In normal limbs, the arm/foot pressure differential is less than 5 mm Hg, which rises as much as 6 mm Hg during reactive hyperemia. Patients with venographic evidence of obstruction whose venous pressure at rest is less than 5 mm Hg but who show an increment of less than 6 mm Hg during reactive hyperemia are considered to be fully compensated (grade I). Using such measurements, Raju has classified four grades of limbs with outflow obstruction (Table 112-4).

Outflow fraction using APG

More recently, APG has been used to measure the 1-second venous outflow fraction (Fig. 112-7), and this has

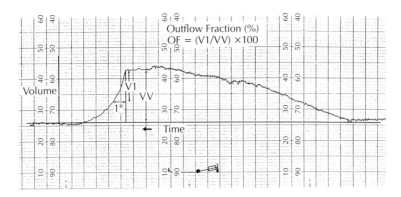

Fig. 112-7. Recording of outflow curve and calculation of outflow fraction *(OF)* using APG. *VV* represents the venous volume as a result of inflating a proximal thigh cuff to 80 mm Hg. V_1 is the decrease in the venous volume during the first second after the thigh cuff is deflated.

Table 112-4. Arm/foot pressure differential in limbs with outflow obstruction

Grade	ΔP at rest (mm Hg)	Pressure increment during hyperemia (mm Hg)
I. Fully compensated	<5	<6
II. Partially compensated	<5	>6
III. Partially decompensated	>5	>6 (often 10-15)
IV. Fully decompensated	>>>5 (often 15-20)	No further increase

ΔP, Arm/foot pressure differential.
From Raju S: New approaches to the diagnosis and treatment of venous obstruction, *J Vasc Surg* 4:42, 1986.

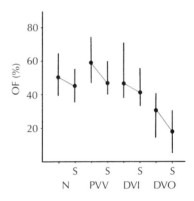

Fig. 112-8. Outflow fraction *(OF)* (median and 90% range) with and without *(s)* occlusion of the superficial veins in limbs of 50 normal volunteers *(N)*, 157 limbs with primary varicose veins *(PVV)*, 70 limbs with deep venous incompetence *(DVI)*, and 68 limbs with venographic deep venous occlusion *(DVO)*.

been found to represent more than 38% of the venous volume in normal limbs, 30% to 38% of the volume in limbs with mild to moderate obstruction, and less than 30% of the volume in limbs with severe obstruction. If the test is repeated with digital occlusion of the superficial veins that may be acting as collateral channels, this method can distinguish between limbs with and without obstruction, as confirmed venographically (Fig. 112-8).

The ability of the APG-determined 1-second outflow fraction to discriminate between limbs with an arm/foot pressure differential lower or higher than 5 mm Hg is shown in Fig. 112-9.

Venous outflow resistance

Venous outflow resistance can be calculated from the outflow curves of volume and pressure obtained simultaneously (Fig. 112-10). Pressure is measured by inserting a 21-gauge butterfly needle into a vein in the foot, and volume is determined by placing the air chamber of the APG around the leg. The foot itself is elevated 15 cm from the horizontal. A thigh cuff is inflated to 70 mm Hg for 2 minutes and then deflated suddenly (Fig. 112-11). The flow (Q) can be calculated at any point on the volume outflow curve from the

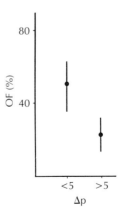

Fig. 112-9. Outflow fraction *(OF)* (median and 90% range) in 15 limbs with deep venous reflux but no obstruction (arm/foot pressure differential ΔP less than 5 mm Hg) and 8 limbs with venographic deep venous obstruction (ΔP greater than 5 mm Hg).

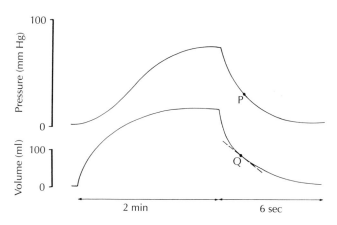

Fig. 112-10. Pressure and volume venous occlusion inflow and outflow curves. Pressure is recorded with a needle in a foot vein and volume with the APG (see Fig. 112-11).

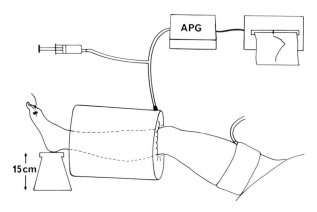

Fig. 112-11. Position of the leg and APG for recording the pressure and volume changes.

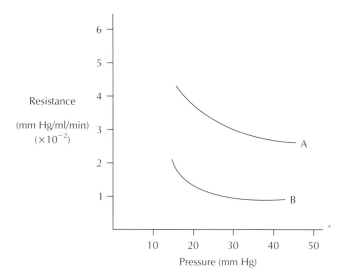

Fig. 112-12. Resistance plotted against pressure for a limb with outflow obstruction *(A)* and a normal limb *(B)*.

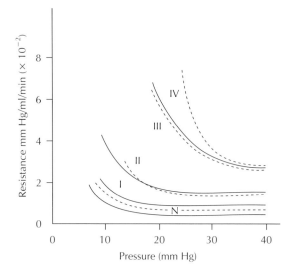

Fig. 112-13. Relationship between outflow resistance curves and Raju classification of grade I through IV outflow obstruction. *N*, Normal limbs.

tangent at that point (Fig. 112-10). The resistance (R) is calculated by dividing the corresponding pressure (P) from the pressure outflow curve by the flow: $R = P/Q$, and the value is expressed in mm Hg/ml/min. By calculating resistance at several points along the outflow curve and plotting it against pressure, this can demonstrate how the resistance changes with different pressures. Fig. 112-12 shows two such plots, one from a patient with outflow obstruction and the other from a normal limb. It can be seen that the relationship between resistance and pressure is not linear. At a high pressure, when the veins and collateral channels are distended, resistance is low. As the pressure decreases and the veins collapse, the resistance also decreases.

By measuring the outflow resistance in a large number of patients with and without various grades of obstruction (Raju test, Grades I to IV), a relationship between the two

methods has been found (Fig. 112-13). This resistance now serves as the gold standard to which noninvasive methods should be compared.

THE ROLE OF THE VARIOUS TESTS
The presence of obstruction and reflux

The evaluation of patients with chronic venous problems primarily consists of determining the presence or absence of outflow obstruction or reflux, or both, in the venous system. The history and clinical examination will identify the patient's problems and clinical picture. A continuous wave Doppler ultrasound evaluation in the clinic can confirm the presence of obstruction or reflux and indicate the site (obstruction, femoropopliteal or iliofemoral; reflux, saphenofemoral junction, saphenopopliteal, incompetent thigh perforating veins, or popliteal) in 90% of patients.

The remaining 10% will consist of complicated cases, and many of these patients will have had a previous operation on their veins or the results of their Doppler ultrasound examination are not clear. There is also a small group in whom incompetent calf perforating veins are suspected and need to be confirmed. In most of these patients, maximum venous outflow measurements (strain-gauge) and APG performed with a tourniquet placed at different levels can provide the necessary information.

Localization of obstruction and reflux

The accurate localization of venous obstruction in advance of surgery requires a venogram, although duplex scanning is proving equally helpful, particularly for lesions distal to the common femoral vein. Until recently, accurate localization of the sites of deep-to-superficial reflux (saphenofemoral, saphenopopliteal, incompetent thigh perforating veins, and calf perforating veins) and reflux in the deep veins (femoral, popliteal, and tibial) could only be achieved by venography. Duplex scanning is now proving to be a simpler and functionally more accurate test, so ascending functional or descending venography is now rarely performed. Duplex scanning is also the method of choice for localizing the site of incompetent perforating veins and the junction of the short saphenous with the popliteal vein.

These tests and the information they provide about the status of obstruction and reflux are adequate for the rational planning of management.

Quantitative measurements of obstruction and reflux

Quantitative measurements of outflow obstruction and reflux are needed for research purposes, particularly for studies of the natural history of different forms of chronic venous insufficiency and for the assessment of both established and new methods of treatment. These quantitative measurements have now opened up new avenues that have led to a better scientific basis for the management of patients. Until recently, the measurement of AVP was the only quantitative test. Although invasive, it could indicate the severity of venous hypertension by measuring the end result of both outflow obstruction and reflux. However, the new tests can discern the relative contribution of different abnormalities, such as venous obstruction and reflux in the superficial and deep veins. They can also show whether malfunction of the calf muscle pump is the result of intrinsic venous disease, a musculoskeletal problem, or both.

REFERENCES

1. Ackroyd JS, Lea Thomas M, Browse NL: Deep vein reflux: an assessment by descending venography, *Br J Surg* 73:31, 1986.
2. Allan JC: Volume changes in the lower limb in response to postural alterations and muscular exercise, *S Afr J Surg* 2:75-90, 1964.
3. Christopoulos D, Nicolaides AN: Noninvasive diagnosis and quantitation of popliteal reflux in the swollen and ulcerated leg, *J Cardiovasc Surg* 29:535-539, 1988.
4. Christopoulos D, Nicolaides AN, Szendro G: Venous reflux: quantification and correlation with the clinical severity of chronic venous disease, *Br J Surg* 75:352-356, 1988.
5. Christopoulos D et al: Objective noninvasive evaluation of venous surgical results, *J Vasc Surg* 8:683-687, 1988.
6. Christopoulos D et al: Air-plethysmography and the effect of elastic compression on venous haemodynamics of the leg, *J Vasc Surg* 5:148-159, 1987.
7. Christopoulos D et al: Pathogenesis of venous ulceration in relation to the calf muscle pump function, *Surgery* 106:829-835, 1989.
8. Herman RJ et al: Descending venography: a method of evaluating lower extremity valvular function, *Radiology* 137:63, 1980.
9. Hoare MC, Royle JP: Doppler ultrasound detection of sapheno-femoral and sapheno-popliteal incompetence and operative venography to ensure precise sapheno-popliteal ligation, *Aust NZ J Surg* 54:49, 1984.
10. Miller SS, Foote AV: The ultrasonic detection of incompetent perforating veins, *Br J Surg* 58:872, 1974.
11. Moore DJ, Himmel PD, Sumner DS: Distribution of venous valvular incompetence in patients with post-phlebitic syndrome, *J Vasc Surg* 3(1):49, 1986.
12. Nicolaides AN, Sumner DS, eds: *The investigation of patients with deep vein thrombosis and chronic venous insufficiency*, London, 1991, Med Orion.
13. Nicolaides AN, Zukowski AJ: The value of dynamic venous pressure measurements, *World J Surg* 10:9197, 1986.
14. O'Donnell J et al: Doppler examination vs clinical and phlebographic detection of the location of incompetent perforating veins, *Arch Surg* 112:31, 1977.
15. Pollack AA, Wood EH: Venous pressure in the saphenous vein in ankle in man during exercise and changes in posture, *J Appl Physiol* 1:649, 1949.
16. Raju S: New approaches to the diagnosis and treatment of venous obstruction, *J Vasc Surg* 4(1):42, 1986.
17. Szendro G et al: Duplex scanning in the assessment of deep venous incompetence, *J Vasc Surg* 4:237, 1986.
18. Vasdekis S: Quantification of venous reflux by means of duplex scanning, *J Vasc Surg* 10:670, 1989.

CHAPTER 113

Segmental evaluation of venous reflux

PAUL S. van BEMMELEN

Reflux in the venous system has been identified as one of the major causes of chronic venous insufficiency and stems either from congenital failure of competent venous valves to form or from thrombotic destruction of the valve cusps during and after an episode of phlebitis. Duplex scanning, which combines B-mode echo imaging with pulsed Doppler interrogation of the vessel under scrutiny, has permitted evaluation of the location and function of valves in the entire venous system of the lower extremity on a segmental basis. Real-time color flow imaging has made such examinations both easier and faster.

BASIS OF SEGMENTAL EXAMINATION

In the duplex method, a pulse of ultrasound is emitted, followed by a brief pause awaiting the reception of reflecting ultrasound from a certain depth. Because the velocity of ultrasound in tissue is known, the reflections of a circumscribed sample volume can be recorded. Further improvements in technology have made possible color flow imaging of veins.

The segmental evaluation of venous reflux consists of duplex interrogation at four vertical levels of the lower limb as compression of the segment distal to the scan head is released. The reflux-provoking test maneuver has been standardized by the use of pneumatic cuffs, which are automatically inflated to a level exceeding the hydrostatic pressure in the leg of a standing subject. The advantage of this maneuver is its applicability at all levels of the limb, whereas the effect of a Valsalva maneuver decreases with increasing distance from the abdomen. Although many examiners instinctively know that a Valsalva maneuver is not useful to test the competency of foot veins, the fact is this maneuver does not elicit reliable valve closure in a number of normal common femoral veins[12] because of the variable reflux velocity generated by the maneuver. A reflux velocity greater than 30 cm/sec is required for valves to close in supine patients. If this threshold is not exceeded, the Bernoulli effect is not sufficient to trigger closure. Low-velocity reflux is not prevented by an open valve. Manual compression is not reliable when performed proximal to the valve under study in a supine patient.[11] Manual compression distal to the valve under study is possible in a standing patient, but

it is usually necessary to use both hands to effectively empty a segment of the leg.

The following veins can usually be identified and tested for valve incompetence: common femoral, superficial femoral, profunda femoris (optional), popliteal, and posterior tibial at the level of the calf and ankle. The use of color flow imaging permits examination of the calf veins to also include the peroneal veins.

The anatomy of the superficial venous system is highly variable, particularly after previous surgery; therefore the examination must be tailored to the individual case. Because of the masking effect of obesity, especially in light of its high prevalence of 25% in the United States, and the large surface area of the entire leg (18% of the body surface), it is not practical to try to scan every square inch of the leg. The greater saphenous vein (GSV) and lesser (short) saphenous vein (LSV) are the most well known and consistent components of the superficial system. After surgical removal of a saphenous vein, the accessory branches become more important. Frequently noted are the anterolateral branch of the GSV in the thigh and the pretibial branches (usually of the GSV) on the ventral aspect of the lower leg. The accessory or second GSV is also usually noted after a stripping procedure. In practice, a lot of time is saved by integrating the examination of the superficial and deep systems and testing four vertical levels successively.

PROCEDURE FOR STANDING VENOUS SEGMENTAL DUPLEX SCANNING

The correct patient position for scanning is to have them stand on a platform and support their body weight on the contralateral leg while holding onto a frame (walker).[7] The muscles should be relaxed with the knee slightly bent. This position has been likened to that of a Greek statue.

A 24-cm-wide cuff is then placed around the thigh and connected to an air source with an automatic cuff inflator. The pressure is set at 80 mm Hg. The common femoral vein is located and the sample volume is positioned. The cuff is inflated for 3 seconds, and then reflux is measured during cuff deflation. The upper normal limit for maximum duration of reflux is 0.45 second.[10] The inflation-deflation maneuver is repeated with the sample volume in the superficial femoral vein and the proximal part of the GSV. The profunda femoris vein may be tested in the same way, but its clinical importance is uncertain.

Next, a 12-cm cuff is placed below the knee. The inflation pressure is set at 100 mm Hg and the popliteal vein is evaluated. If this vein is bifid, both veins must be tested. The LSV is tested in the same way; the exact site where the LSV enters the deep system is located. Well-known

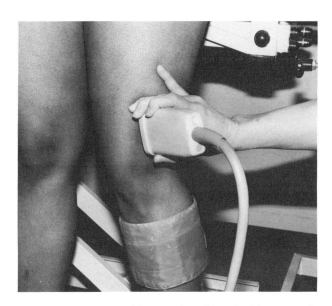

Fig. 113-1. Examination of the anterolateral branch of the GSV. Reflux is measured on deflation of the cuff, which is situated below the knee.

anatomic variations include a high entrance of the LSV at the dorsum of the thigh. On the medial side of the knee, the GSV is located and tested, and a possible second or accessory saphenous vein is sought. A transverse view is helpful for this purpose. The anterolateral branch of the GSV is usually immediately lateral to the patella and is also tested with the cuff below the knee (Fig. 113-1). Isolated incompetence of this vein occurs frequently and should certainly be expected if the origin of the GSV is incompetent but the vein is otherwise normal at the level of the knee.

The cuff is then moved to the ankle, and with the pressure set at 100 mm Hg, the deep calf veins are evaluated. Visualization of both the posterior tibial and peroneal veins is possible from the medial aspect of the leg using a 5-MHz transducer.[8] Fig. 113-2 is an example of the sort of incompetent calf veins seen during deflation of the cuff. At the midcalf level, the GSV often consists of two branches. One of these can swing dorsally toward the popliteal vein. This branch can be incompetent despite a competent main GSV at the knee. At the back of the calf, the small saphenous vein can be identified by its straight course and deep location near the muscle fascia (Fig. 113-3); it is tested at this level.

A 7-cm metatarsal cuff is placed around the foot and inflated to 120 mm Hg. The two posterior tibial veins are located on either side of the artery (Fig. 113-4). When a duplex scanner without color flow imaging is used, a small sample volume must be used and positioned accurately to eliminate possible confusion with the nearby superficial veins. Fig. 113-5 shows the short distance that can exist between incompetent superficial branches and normal posterior tibial veins at the ankle, which could easily create

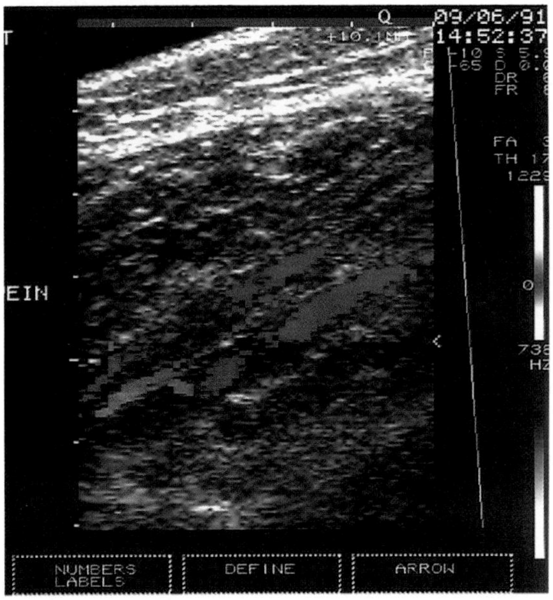

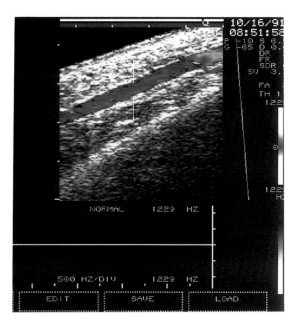

Fig. 113-2. Incompetence of deep calf veins in a patient with previous deep vein thrombosis. The flow direction to the feet is depicted in red. The head of the patient is to the left.

Fig. 113-3. Normal LSV. Note the straight course and deep location near the fascia. The antegrade flow during the augmentation phase (cuff inflation) is depicted in blue. The head of the patient is to the left.

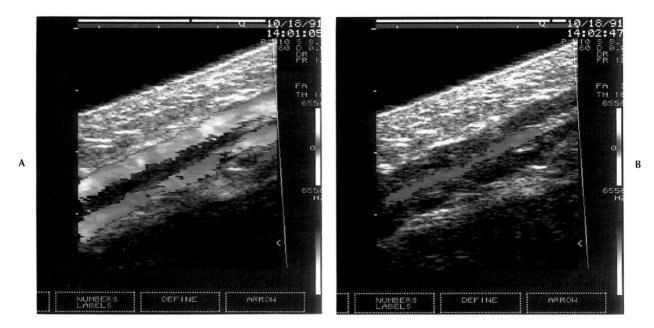

Fig. 113-4. **A,** Normal posterior tibial veins at the level of the ankle. Paired veins with antegrade flow during augmentation are shown. **B,** Normal posterior tibial veins. During cuff deflation, no reflux is noted in the veins, which are visible in black. The red vessel between the veins is the posterior tibial artery.

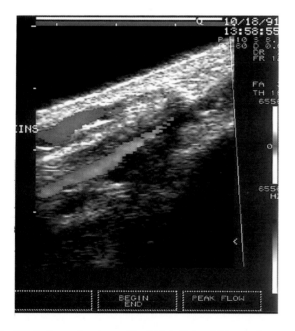

Fig. 113-5. Same situation as Fig. 113-4, *B.* In addition to the artery, an incompetent superficial vein is visible in red. The deep veins, which are normal, are in close proximity. This is difficult to appreciate with continuous wave Doppler only.

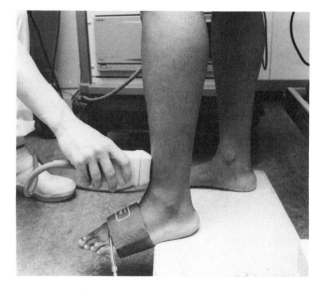

Fig. 113-6. Examination of the pretibial area. Care is taken not to exert any pressure on these veins, which would obliterate them.

confusion if these are assessed with continuous wave Doppler. At the ankle level, the GSV is tested near the medial malleolus. On the ventral aspect of the leg (Fig. 113-6), the pretibial branches are identified using a high-frequency probe and sufficient transmission gel to promote visualization of these very superficial branches (Fig. 113-7). The

gaiter area is further scanned to locate the posterior arch veins and any incompetent perforators.

If there is an unexplained transition of normal to incompetent superficial veins, this mandates a search for the site of incompetent perforators. These can be fairly large if located on the medial side of the thigh.

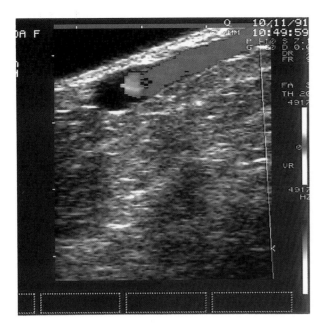

Fig. 113-7. Incompetent pretibial branches. Note the extremely superficial location immediately beneath the skin.

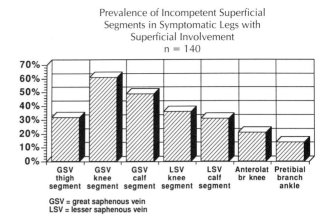

Fig. 113-8. Distribution of incompetent superficial segments in 140 legs, representing 93% of all legs referred for venous complaints.

CLINICAL EXPERIENCE
Ulceration

In a study of 25 legs with ulceration, 92% had involvement of the superficial veins.[13] There was also partial involvement of the deep veins in a majority of patients. The common femoral, superficial femoral, and popliteal veins were each incompetent in over 60% of the cases. The deep calf veins and deep ankle veins were each incompetent in 40% of the cases. Similar findings were subsequently reported by another group of investigators.[3]

Post deep vein thrombosis

In patients selected on the basis of a venographically confirmed history of deep vein thrombosis and normal ankle skin, isolated deep vein incompetence was noted frequently.[13] This incompetence included the popliteal vein and the superficial and common femoral veins but was relatively asymptomatic.

Stasis symptoms

A larger series consisting of 151 legs included patients with milder degrees of symptoms, such as fatigue upon standing and ankle swelling.[9] Most of these patients exhibited partial incompetence of their superficial veins, as summarized in Fig. 113-8. There was at least one segment of deep vein involvement in 42% of these patients.

Post saphenous vein stripping

Contrary to expectation, in the 30 legs that had undergone stripping of the entire long saphenous vein, superficial incompetence was usually found in the distribution of the

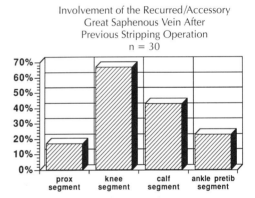

Fig. 113-9. Distribution of incompetent great saphenous segments in 30 legs that had undergone stripping of the entire (ankle to groin) GSV. Highest prevalence in knee and calf segments could be related to multiple saphenous veins in these areas.

removed GSV (Fig. 113-9). This could be due to incomplete removal of all saphenous branches near the entrance of the GSV in the femoral vein, as illustrated in Fig. 113-10, *B*. Fig. 113-10, *A* illustrates a typical case of incompetent proximal GSV, which has not been operated on. The recurrent GSV is more tortuous than the native GSV in this location. Another explanation for this incompetence could be the presence of a double saphenous vein or accessory saphenous vein that went undetected at the time of the original surgery. As shown in Fig. 113-9, a recurrent GSV is more common in the knee or calf than in the groin after a previous stripping operation. Fig. 113-11, *B* illustrates a recurrent calf GSV; this part of the vein is straight, with a diameter of 6 mm, and has no obvious features that distinguish it from an unoperated GSV in this location (Fig. 113-11, *A*).

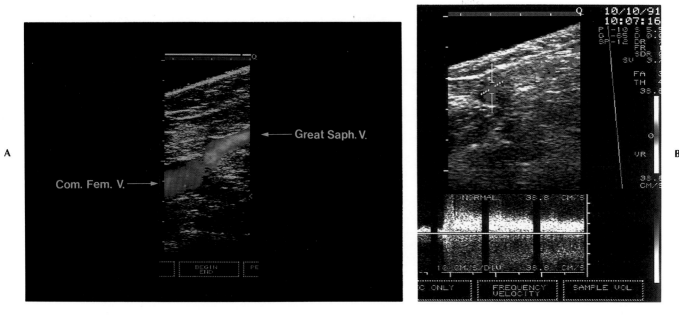

Fig. 113-10. **A,** Incompetent proximal GSV, with incompetent common femoral vein. The head of the patient is to the left. **B,** Incompetent recurrent vein in the groin after previous stripping. Note the irregular, tortuous vessel. Reflux is depicted in the spectrum (bottom) as a positive deflection.

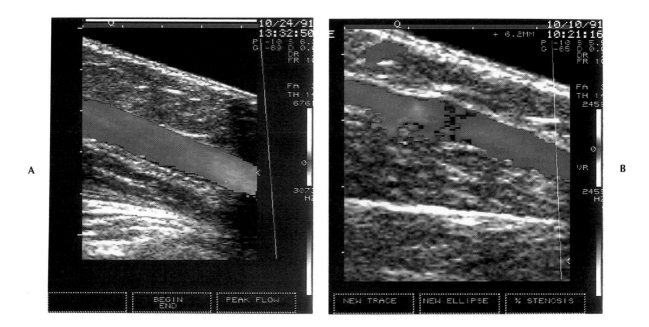

Fig. 113-11. **A,** Large diameter native GSV incompetence at the level of the calf. **B,** Recurrence after previous stripping operation. Often the diameter is smaller than that of the native GSV, with more irregularity and side branches.

CLASSIFICATION OF DEGREE OF SEGMENTAL INCOMPETENCE

Most veins were found to be only partially affected by valve incompetence. Although the involved segment is completely incompetent, the same vein can be normal at a more distal or proximal location. Of the 140 legs studied that had superficial incompetent segments (Fig. 113-8), the most fre-

quently involved segment (61%) was the GSV (or its recurrence after removal) at the knee. There was a 49% prevalence of GSV incompetence at the calf level. The proximal segment of the GSV at the thigh was incompetent in 32%, demonstrating the occurrence of distal GSV incompetence while the proximal part of the GSV was intact. The anterolateral branch of the GSV was incompetent in 21%, and

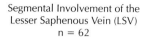
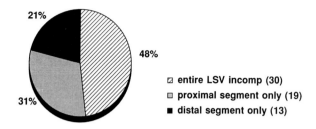

Segmental Involvement of the
Lesser Saphenous Vein (LSV)
n = 62

21%

48%

☑ entire LSV incomp (30)
☐ proximal segment only (19)
■ distal segment only (13)

31%

Fig. 113-12. Segmental involvement of the LSV. In the majority of cases, only part of this vein is incompetent.

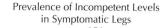
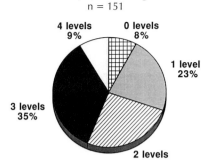

Prevalence of Incompetent Levels
in Symptomatic Legs
n = 151

4 levels   0 levels
9%   8%

1 level
23%

3 levels
35%

2 levels
26%

Fig. 113-13. Distribution of the number of incompetent levels in symptomatic legs. Of the total, 84% have one-, two-, or three-level involvement.

the pretibial branches of the GSV near the ankle were incompetent in 14%.

Lesser saphenous vein

Incompetence of the LSV is often segmental (Fig. 113-12); the proximal aspect was incompetent in 36%, and the calf aspect was incompetent in 31%. In more than half (52%) of the cases in which the LSV was affected, the incompetence was limited to one segment. If the distal half of the LSV remained normal, as seen in 26% of the cases, the reflux from the incompetent proximal part is diverted to superficial branches. When the proximal part of the LSV is normal, as noted in 21% of the cases, the reflux is often fed by a connecting branch from the GSV system (Giacomini vein).

Great saphenous vein

A GSV varicosity shows dilatation in the thigh and upper part of the lower leg, as discovered in previous studies.[1] Tortuosity is a feature of varicose tributaries, which can overlie the main trunk of the GSV. When 86 cases with GSV incompetence at the knee level were analyzed, the incompetence in less than half (n = 42) was contiguous from the origin of the GSV down to the knee. Of those with GSV incompetence at the knee but a normal proximal GSV, 34% had incompetent deep veins (superficial femoral vein–popliteal veins). In such cases, an incompetent deep-to-superficial perforating vein frequently was identified at the upper end of the incompetent GSV segment.

Classification. For the purpose of classification and stratification of patients, a system of anatomic levels[9] has been devised, and these levels consist of the thigh, knee, calf, and ankle. The maximum number of incompetent levels is four. Of 151 legs that underwent evaluation in the vascular laboratory (26% of the patients had undergone previous vein surgery), the numbers of incompetent levels were as follows (Fig. 113-13): Only 9% of the 151 legs with venous symptoms showed total incompetence that involved either four levels of the deep or superficial veins or a combination of both adding up to four-level involvement. A total of 35% had three-level disease; 26%, two-level disease; 23%, one-

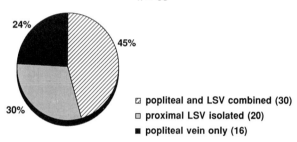

Association of Deep and Superficial
Incompetence at the Popliteal Fossa
n = 66

24%

45%

30%

☑ popliteal and LSV combined (30)
☐ proximal LSV isolated (20)
■ popliteal vein only (16)

Fig. 113-14. Distribution of isolated versus combined (deep and superficial) incompetence at the popliteal fossa. The majority of cases have isolated incompetence confined to either the popliteal or lesser saphenous system.

level disease; and no levels were involved in 8%. This normal finding is probably due to the fact that patients were selected on the basis of their complaints and not on the basis of physical findings or venograms.

RELATIONSHIP BETWEEN DEEP AND SUPERFICIAL INCOMPETENCE

The association of an incompetent deep segment with a contiguous superficial segment is a frequent but inconstant finding. The combined incompetence of the common femoral vein and the proximal GSV is probably a predisposing factor but not necessarily a result of previous thrombosis in the common femoral vein. Several observers have noted incompetent common femoral veins in approximately 70% of legs, together with primary varicose veins involving the proximal GSV.[2,13] Of 66 cases in which either the popliteal vein or the LSV, or both, were affected, the distribution was as follows (Fig. 113-14): 30 cases of combined incompetence (popliteal vein–LSV), 20 of isolated LSV incompetence (proximal segment) (Fig. 113-15), and 16 cases of isolated popliteal vein incompetence.

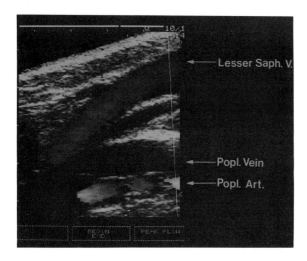

Fig. 113-15. Isolated incompetence of a large LSV in a patient with ulceration of the gaiter area. The LSV is shown in red during deflation of the cuff. The red vessel at the bottom is the popliteal artery. Immediately above the artery, a normal popliteal vein is visible in black. The head of the patient is to the left.

The diameters of the incompetent veins can vary: for the LSV, diameters ranged from 2 to 12 mm (mean, 6.2 ± 2.8 mm); for the GSV, diameters ranged between 2 and 19 mm (mean, 5.5 ± 2.7 mm), measured at the knee level. No normal values for GSV or LSV diameter are available for standing normal subjects, but considerable overlap is likely and would preclude attempts to predict competence based solely on the presence of a small diameter.

DISCUSSION AND CLINICAL IMPLICATIONS

There is some controversy regarding the importance of superficial vein incompetence to the pathogenesis of serious venous stasis problems, such as ulceration. The findings from classic studies that employed venous pressure measurements spawned the view that deep vein incompetence is responsible for ulceration, wheras superficial incompetence only leads to cosmetic and minor problems. The gold standard, venous pressure measurement, has recently been criticized because it makes use of tourniquets, which do not reliably occlude the superficial veins.[6] Failure to exclude the existence of superficial reflux will lead to a false-positive diagnosis of deep reflux, which could explain the systematic overestimation of the presence of deep incompetence noted in the past.

Recent studies using duplex imaging indicate that superficial incompetence does play a role in the pathogenesis of venous ulceration.[3,13] It was assumed that these incompetent superficial veins merely accompany a more severe deep incompetence that is not accessible to clinical diagnostic methods, but this has been disproved by duplex scans, which have shown no deep incompetence in a large percentage of patients with ulceration. Although continuous wave Doppler studies can successfully confirm reflux in suspected locations, scanning can exclude reflux in all areas.

Recognizing the clinical importance of incompetence of the LSV in chronic venous insufficiency is also a major step forward toward the development of correct treatment. LSV incompetence was noted in 41% of all legs that underwent venous evaluation. Previous literature regarding the anatomy

of the LSV[5] fostered the misconception that the LSV, due to its more muscular wall and greater number of valves, would be resistant to primary varicose degeneration. Ludbrook and Jamieson[4] suggested that LSV incompetence is only seen when the (deep) popliteal vein is incompetent; this is contradicted by the data presented in Fig. 113-14. Furthermore, even though the LSV is short, the data indicate that less than half of the incompetent LSVs are affected throughout. This means that less of the LSV may need to be removed at surgery, thus lowering the risk of damage to the adjacent cutaneous nerve.

The accurate localization and mapping of recurrent varicose veins after stripping of the GSV is important for treatment. Recurrent symptoms arising after surgical stripping are not necessarily due to deep reflux. More likely the recurrent superficial veins are in the knee and calf portions of the GSV, or the LSV incompetence was overlooked at the time of surgery. It is also important to keep in mind the frequent presence of incompetent accessory branches of the superficial system. Because the reflux in these treatable, superficial veins is probably adding to the reflux in the deep veins,[14] their eradication is probably also beneficial in the presence of deep incompetence, provided there is no obstruction to deep outflow.

CONCLUSION

Segmental duplex scanning for the detection of venous reflux is indicated in the following situations: varicose veins in obese patients, need for complete identification and treatment, recurrent varicose veins after previous surgery, ulceration in the gaiter area, and serious venous stasis complaints with or without subcutaneous induration. In these situations, segmental duplex examination can provide a systematic approach to the evaluation of the venous system, which can be affected by multiple combinations of incompetent parts.

ACKNOWLEDGMENT

The author wishes to thank Jeffrey L. Collins and Dianne L. Raymond for their preparation of the color flow illustrations.

REFERENCES

1. Cotton LT: Varicose veins, gross anatomy and development, *Br J Surg* 48:589-598, 1961.
2. Folse R: The influence of femoral vein dynamics on the development of varicose veins, *Surgery* 68:974-979, 1970.
3. Hanrahan LM et al: Distribution of valvular incompetence in patients with venous stasis ulceration, *J Vasc Surg* 13:805-812, 1991.
4. Ludbrook J, Jamieson GG: *Disorders of systemic veins.* In Sabiston DC, ed: *Davis Christopher textbook of surgery,* Philadelphia, 1977, Saunders.
5. Marinov G: Some differences between the long and short saphenous veins as regards the structure and vascularization of the wall and location of the valves, *Folia Morphol* 24:221-224, 1976.
6. McMullin GM, Coleridge Smith PD, Scurr JH: A study of tourniquets in the investigation of venous insufficiency, *Phlebology* 6:133-139, 1991.
7. Szendro G et al: Duplex scanning in the assessment of deep venous incompetence, *J Vasc Surg* 4:237-242, 1986.
8. van Bemmelen PS, Bedford G, Strandness DE: Visualization of calf veins by color flow imaging, *Ultrasound Med Biol* 16:15-17, 1990.
9. van Bemmelen PS, Van Ramshorst B, Eikelboom BC, Photoplethysmography re-examined: lack of correlation with duplex scanning, *Surgery* 112:544-548, 1992.
10. van Bemmelen PS et al: Quantitative segmental evaluation of venous valvular reflux with duplex ultrasound scanning, *J Vasc Surg* 10:425-431, 1989.
11. van Bemmelen PS et al: Evaluation of tests used to document venous valve incompetence, *J Vasc Tech* 14(2):87-90, 1990.
12. van Bemmelen PS et al: The mechanism of venous valve closure, *Arch Surg* 125:617-619, 1990.
13. van Bemmelen PS et al: Status of the valves in the superficial and deep venous system in chronic venous disease, *Surgery* 109:730-734, 1991.
14. Vasdekis SN, Clarke GH, Nicolaides AN: Quantification of venous reflux by means of duplex scanning, *J Vasc Surg* 10:670-677, 1989.

CHAPTER 114

Recent developments in venous photoplethysmography

ARNOST FRONEK

Impedance and strain-gauge plethysmographic methods are well accepted for the diagnosis of deep vein thrombosis (DVT) above the knee, but their ability to detect such obstructions below the knee is limited.[7,13,14,16] In addition, these plethysmographic methods, which are based essentially on the methodology originally developed by Wheeler et al,[20] are not useful for diagnosing venous valvular insufficiency.

Venous photoplethysmography (PPG) may be able to remedy some of the drawbacks of the other plethysmographic techniques because it can evaluate distal sites (ankle level) and because of its sensitive response to the presence of venous valvular insufficiency, indicated by the finding of a shortened refilling time.[1] This has been confirmed by other investigators using different probes.[12] These authors have also demonstrated an interesting relationship between the mean ambulatory venous pressure (AVP), measured immediately after the cessation of tiptoeing, and the refilling time (RT). The RT has been found to vary between 65 and 20 seconds when AVP is below 40 mm Hg, but an RT shorter than 15 seconds corresponds to an AVP higher than 40 mm Hg. No proportional correlation has been noted between RT and AVP when AVP was above 40 mm Hg, however. One of the most important variables influencing the reliability of the PPG system is the penetration of the light source. The light reflection rheograph (LRR), which was originally described by Blazek[2,3,4,21] and clinically evaluated by a number of authors,[15,17-19] proved to be a reliable system, primarily due to well-defined focusing and the standardized penetration of the light source (from 0.3 mm to 2.3 mm) that thus covered the subcutaneous venous plexus. The only disadvantage of this system was that it could not be calibrated. The response to dorsiflexion, which is the most widely used stress test to evaluate the efficacy of the venous pump, depends not only on the volume of blood displaced but also on a variety of optical conditions that influence the absorption and reflection of light, such as skin thickness, skin color, and initial local blood volume.

INSTRUMENTATION AND METHOD

A calibratable PPG system (C-PPG) has now been developed,[8] based on the principle of standardized change in light intensity, which thus produces a calibration signal to which all other changes are related. This is accomplished by inserting an adjustable resistance between the light-emitting diode (LED) and the power source (Fig. 114-1). The calibration signal can be obtained by short-circuiting the adjustable resistance, and the resulting change in current alters the voltage drop measured across an additional in-series small resistance. This change in the voltage drop is monitored and the resistance is adjusted to represent a predetermined change, usually 5%. By using an optical filter, the electrical change can also be correlated to a known optical density, thus recalling the original work by Hertzman.[9] For practical purposes, however, the percentage change of light intensity induced by a standardized current change fulfills the need to cancel the influence of skin thickness, skin color, and local blood volume. The increased light absorption caused by increased skin thickness, darker skin color, or increased local blood volume will reduce the calibration signal in the same proportion as the test-induced changes, such as dorsiflexion.

In a preliminary experimental study,[10] a linear correlation was found between the changes in blood volume and the optical density. Therefore changes in optical density, calibrated by the standardized reduction of light intensity, are expressed as a percentage change of the initial volume.

PRELIMINARY EVALUATION OF THE METHOD

A protocol similar to that used by Christopoulos et al[6] for air-plethysmography was used in a preliminary study in

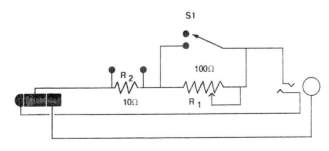

Fig. 114-1. The C-PPG calibration system. R_1, Resistance to be adjusted to produce a 5% voltage drop across resistance R_2; S_1, calibration switch (shortening the calibration resistance R_1).

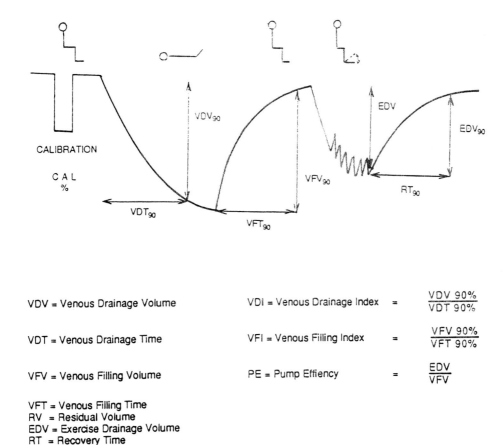

VDV = Venous Drainage Volume

VDT = Venous Drainage Time

VFV = Venous Filling Volume

VFT = Venous Filling Time
RV = Residual Volume
EDV = Exercise Drainage Volume
RT = Recovery Time

VDI = Venous Drainage Index $=\dfrac{VDV\ 90\%}{VDT\ 90\%}$

VFI = Venous Filling Index $=\dfrac{VFV\ 90\%}{VFT\ 90\%}$

PE = Pump Effiency $=\dfrac{EDV}{VFV}$

Fig. 114-2. Examination protocol: sitting, supine, sitting, and dorsiflexion.

which C-PPG was tested on normal control subjects and patients with venous disease.

The examination protocol was as follows (Fig. 114-2). After the calibration signal was recorded, the subject was moved from the sitting to the supine position. After a steady-state was reached, the subject sat up again. This was followed by the dorsiflexion exercise.

Fig. 114-3 summarizes the drainage or displaced volume that occurs under three conditions: normal, varicose veins, and venous ulcer, and Fig. 114-4 depicts the refilling time observed under these conditions. Combining the results obtained during the postural changes and dorsiflexion makes it possible to calculate the muscle pump efficiency, as described in Fig. 114-2.

Another direction was selected by the investigators at the Technical University in Aachen. Blazek et al[5] designed a computer-supported system that automatically controls the light intensity of the LED so that the input amplifier starts to operate only if a predetermined input voltage is reached. If the skin is dark, the light intensity is automatically in-

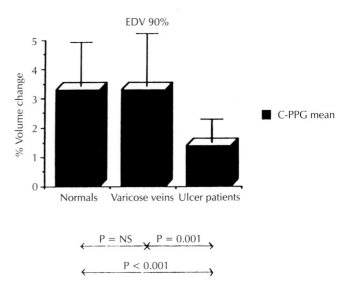

Fig. 114-3. Calibrated photoplethysmography (C-PPG). Changes in exercise drainage volume *(EDV)* in normal control subjects, patients with varicose veins, and patients with venous ulcers (mean and standard deviation).

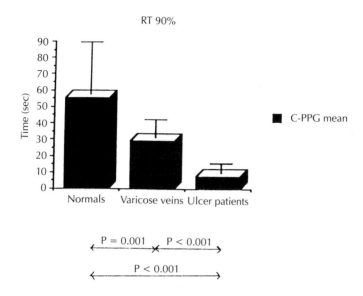

Fig. 114-4. Calibrated photoplethysmography (C-PPG). Recovery time *(RT)* in normal control subjects, patients with varicose veins, and patients with venous ulcers (mean and standard deviation).

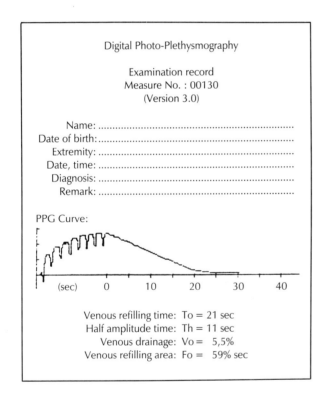

Fig. 114-5. Typical digital photoplethysmography (D-PPG) curve with the automatically evaluated parameters.

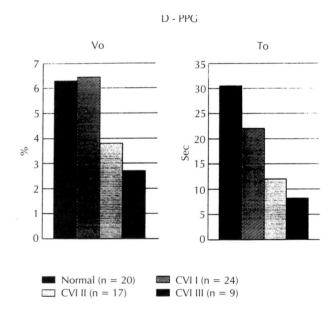

Fig. 114-6. Digital photoplethysmography (D-PPG): controls; *CVI*, Mild venous disease (Doppler positive but no trophic changes); *CVII*, moderate venous disease involving edema, white atrophy, induration, and hyperpigmentation; *CVIII*, severe venous disease including a healed or open ulcer.

creased, and vice versa if the skin is lighter or thinner. This system is called *digital-photoplethysmography* (D-PPG)* and includes both a measuring and a learning mode. The output is either printed immediately or the results of up to eight examinations can be stored and then printed. Fig. 114-5 represents a typical normal D-PPG tracing with the variables automatically evaluated.

The results of the automatic compensation (D-PPG) approach were compared with those yielded by a standard LRR instrument by recording the changes induced by dorsiflexion before and after covering the skin with dark paint (Lumicolor). Although the LRR-recorded changes were significantly reduced, the D-PPG–recorded changes remained essentially the same. Fig. 114-6 summarizes the results obtained from normal subjects and three groups of patients with increasingly severe venous disease.[11]

CONCLUSION

Quantitative PPG, either in the manual calibration (C-PPG) form or in the automatic computer-supported (D-PPG) form, represents a significant advance in the quantitative evaluation of venous hemodynamics, especially distal venous disorders and specifically venous valvular insufficiency and DVT below the knee.

Digital because of the digital circuitry used.

REFERENCES

1. Abramowitz HB et al: The use of photoplethysmography in the assessment of venous insufficiency: a comparison to venous pressure measurements, *Surgery* 86:434, 1979.
2. Blazek V: *Ein optoelektronisches Messverfahren zur farbvalenzmetrischen Bewertung der menschlichen Haut,* Aachen, Germany, 1979, Technische Hochschule (thesis).
3. Blazek V: *Medizinisch-Technische Grundlagen der Licht-Reflektions-Rheographie.* In May R, Stemmer R, eds: *Die Licht Reflektions-Rheographie,* Erlangen, 1984, Germany.
4. Blazek V, Wienert V: Funktionelle Diagnostik peripherer venoeser Abflussstoerungen, *Inform Arzt* 10:4-9, 1982.
5. Blazek V et al: Digitale Photoplethysmographie (D-PPG) für die Beinvenendiagnostik, *Phlebologie Proktologie* 18:91-97, 1989.
6. Christopoulos DG et al: Air-plethysmography and the effect of elastic compression on venous hemodynamics of the leg, *J Vasc Surg* 5:148-159, 1987.
7. Fronek A: *Noninvasive diagnostics in vascular disease,* New York, 1989, McGraw-Hill.
8. Fronek A, Bundens WP: Calibratable photoplethysmography (C-PPG), (submitted for publication).
9. Hertzman JB: The blood supply of various skin areas as estimated by the photoelectric plethysmograph, *Am J Physiol* 124:328-340, 1938.
10. Higgins JL Jr: *Photoplethysmography: theoretical and experimental considerations in the diagnosis of venous disease,* San Diego, 1988, University of California (thesis).
11. Kerner J, Schultz-Ehrenburg U, Blazek V: Digitale Photoplethysmograph (D-PPG), *Phlebologie Proktologie* 18:98-103, 1989.
12. Miles C, Nicolaides AN: *Photoplethysmography: principles and development.* In Nicolaides AN, Yao JST, eds: *Investigation of vascular disorders,* London, 1981, Churchill Livingstone.
13. Moore DJ, Himmel PD, Sumner D: Distribution of venous valvular incompetence in patients with the postphlebitic syndrome, *J Vasc Surg* 3:49-57, 1986.
14. Nicolaides AN, Christopoulos D, Vasdekis S: Progress in the investigation of chronic venous insufficiency, *Ann Vasc Surg* 3:278-292, 1989.
15. Nuzzaci G et al: Our experience on high reflection rheography (LRR): a new noninvasive method for lower limb venous examination, *Phlebology* 1:231-242, 1986.
16. Partsch H: Investigations on the pathogenesis of venous ulcers, *Acta Chir Scand* [suppl] 544:25-29, 1988.
17. Seycek J: Licht-Reflexions-Rheographie und blutige Venendruckmessung beim Arbeitstest im Stehen, *Vasa* 18:18-23, 1989.
18. Shepard AD, Mackey WC, O'Donnell TF: *Correlation of venous pressure measurements with LRR.* In May R, Stemmer R, eds: *Die Licht-Reflektions-Rheographie,* Erlangen, 1984, Germany.
19. Vanscheidt W et al: Malleoläre und plantare Licht reflexions rheographie, *Dermatol Monatsschr* 176:605-608, 1990.
20. Wheeler HB, O'Donnell JA, Anderson FA Jr: Occlusive impedance and pulmonary embolism, *Prog Cardiovasc Dis* 27:199, 1974.
21. Wienert V, Blazek V: Eine neue Methode zur unblutigen dynamischen Venendruckmessung, *Der Hautarzt* 33:498-499, 1982.

CHAPTER 115

Laser Doppler, oxygen, and CO_2 tension in venous hypertension

GIANNI BELCARO and ANDREW N. NICOLAIDES

Edema and capillary deposition of fibrin have been postulated to be the major factors responsible for the tissue damage, liposclerosis, and eventual leg ulceration in patients with postthrombotic limbs.[10,11,14] These pathologic changes are believed to stem from the effect of venous hypertension on the microcirculation. The chronic effect of venous hypertension on the skin of the perimalleolar region causes microcirculatory disturbances whose significance has only recently been understood.[13] It has now become possible to quantify these microcirculatory disturbances using noninvasive techniques such as laser Doppler flowmetry, transcutaneous Po_2 ($TcPo_2$) and Pco_2 ($TcPco_2$), strain-gauge plethysmography, and the vacuum suction chamber device. *Venous hypertensive microangiopathy* is the term used to refer to the anatomic and pathophysiologic changes that occur in the microcirculation as a result of venous hypertension and that are responsible for the characteristic clinical changes in the skin.

This chapter describes these microcirculatory changes and the methods available for their quantification, with special emphasis on laser Doppler, and elucidates their relative importance in the genesis of edema, lipodermatosclerosis, and ulceration. In addition, the beneficial effect on the microcirculation of various therapeutic measures known to heal leg ulcers is discussed.

SKIN BLOOD FLOW

Laser Doppler flowmetry has demonstrated that there is an increase in the skin red cell flux in limbs with venous hypertension, indicating increased skin blood flow at rest (resting flow [RF]) with a decrease or abolition of the normal vasomotor activity. These flux alterations are often associated with a decreased venoarteriolar response (VAR), which is the vasoconstrictor reflex induced by changes in posture when going from the supine to the standing position (Fig. 115-1).[6,16] This physiologic response minimizes the number of capillaries exposed to high pressure (and flow) in the standing position. An absent or reduced VAR therefore exposes a large number of capillaries to high pressure on standing and may be associated with increased capillary leakage and ankle edema.

The venoarteriolar response

In normal limbs, the precapillary resistance in the skin of the foot and the perimalleolar region increases on standing, thereby decreasing capillary blood flow.[15] This response limits the increase in capillary pressure determined by the vertical column of blood between the heart and foot.[18] This vasoconstrictive response may be mediated by a sympathetic axon reflex[16] and is made up of different components.

In a normal subject, lowering the leg and foot below the horizontal level elicits the VAR, producing a small decrease (10% to 20%) in skin red cell flux (Fig. 115-2). A greater decrease in this flux (40%) is observed on standing. A small decrease in flux is also observed when the subject is sitting while keeping the leg horizontal. Inflating a thigh cuff to 80 mm Hg to occlude the superficial venous system will also elicit a small decrease in flux but no further decrease when the leg is lowered below the horizontal level (Fig. 115-2).

Lowering one leg also sometimes produces a minimal decrease in the skin flow in the opposite limb, which is difficult to quantify. A sudden increase in venous pressure is an important stimulus for the VAR, which is mainly the result of a local reflex mechanism, with possibly a weak central component.

Normal skin blood flow

Only 5% to 10% of the total skin blood flow takes place through the nutrient capillaries that reach the outer layers of the dermis.[13] The number of nutrient capillary loops per unit area is related to the $TcPo_2$; the smaller the number of nutrient capillary loops per mm^2, the lower is the $TcPo_2$. Coherent light emitted by the laser Doppler probes penetrates only the superficial part of the dermis for 1 to 1.5 mm and thus measures red cell flux to a variable depth. It is therefore not surprising that $TcPo_2$ is not related to the red cell flux as measured by laser Doppler flowmetry. The thermoregulatory function and capacity of the skin causes great fluctuations in the total skin blood flow. Thus changes in flow, particularly in the deeper layers of the dermis, are not necessarily reflected by changes in laser Doppler measurements.

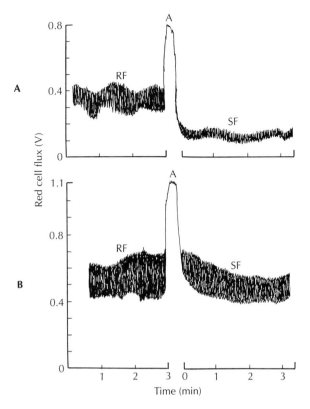

Fig. 115-1. Red cell flux in a normal limb **(A)** and in a limb with venous hypertension **(B).** (*RF,* Resting flow; *SF,* standing flow.) Note the presence of vasomotor waves at RF and the decreased red cell flux on standing *(SF)* as a result of the venoarteriolar response in the normal limb; also note the absence of vasomotor waves and high red cell flux both at rest and on standing, indicating the absence of the venoarteriolar response.

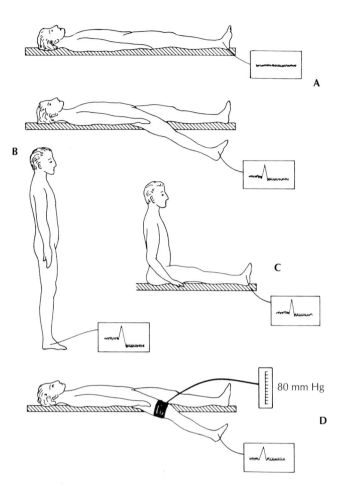

Fig. 115-2. The venoarteriolar response may be induced by foot dependency **(A),** standing **(B),** or sitting up **(C)** or by increasing the venous pressure by inflating a thigh tourniquet **(D).** In some patients with chronic venous insufficiency and severe venous hypertension, the venoarteriolar response is minimal.

The output signal from laser Doppler flowmeters is only directly proportional to the blood flow in the microcirculation and particularly in the superficial (less than 1 mm depth) skin vessels under certain specific but often not reproducible situations. The findings from comparative studies using television capillaroscopy indicate that laser Doppler flowmetry detects flow in subcapillary plexuses, superficial shunts, and capillary loops. Not surprisingly, the reflux responses yielded by the two techniques are broadly comparable.[20,24]

Laser Doppler probes record red cell flux, which is a function of the number of red cells, capillary loops, and velocity, in small areas of approximately 1 mm². One of the advantages of this approach is its ability to record vasomotor activity, which produces rhythmic fluctuations in blood flow. This is because vasoconstriction may be alternating with vasodilatation in one area while the opposite is occurring in an adjacent area. This vasomotor activity is associated with healthy skin and is a factor determining total skin blood flow. In pathologic situations such as inflammation, allergic reactions, and venous hypertensive microangiopathy, vasomotor activity appears to be altered or abol-

ished in conjunction with generalized vasodilatation causing a marked increase in local skin blood flow.

Skin blood flow and VAR in limbs with venous hypertension

In a recent study,[4,8] 20 patients with venous hypertension (postphlebitic limbs) and 25 normal controls matched for age and sex were studied. All subjects were studied with Doppler ultrasound and the presence of reflux in the popliteal vein confirmed in the patients and its absence confirmed in the control subjects. The ambulatory venous pressure (AVP) was measured in all patients by inserting a needle into a vein on the dorsum of the foot. The AVP was defined as the lowest pressure obtained during a 10-tiptoe exercise performed at the rate of one tiptoe per second.[17] Patients were selected to participate in the study if they had an AVP greater than 65 mm Hg (normal, less than 45 mm Hg) and small perimalleolar ulcers (area, 1.5 to 3 cm³).

The probe of the laser Doppler flowmeter* was attached

---

*Periflux; Perimed, Sweden.

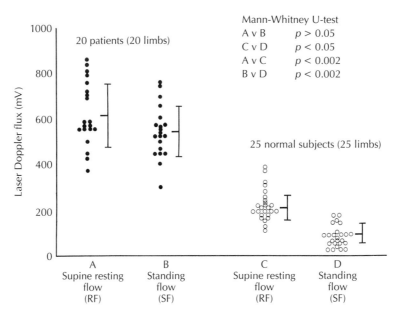

Fig. 115-3. The venoarteriolar response in 20 patients with chronic venous hypertension and in 25 normal subjects. Skin flux in normal subjects is lower and there is a significant decrease in flux on standing. The latter is almost abolished in patients.

to the skin of the perimalleolar region at least 1 cm proximal to the upper edge of the ulcer. After 30 minutes of acclimatization at a constant room temperature (21° C to 23° C), the baseline RF was recorded for 2 minutes. The subject was then asked to stand. The standing flux (SF) was recorded after a 4-minute interval for another 2 minutes. The RF and SF were measured in millivolts and expressed as the mean of the flux during the 2 minutes of measurement.

Fig. 115-3 shows the individual RF and SF readings obtained from the 20 postphlebitic and 25 normal limbs, along with the mean and standard deviation. The mean RF in the postthrombotic limbs was approximately three times greater than that in normal limbs. On standing, there was a small but insignificant decrease in the skin flux in the patients with postphlebitic limbs. In contrast, the decrease in flux in the normal limbs on standing was significant ($p < 0.01$). Thus the mean VAR (percentage decrease in flow on standing) was 14% in the postthrombotic limbs and 57% in the normal controls. The absolute decrease in the mean RF on standing was 86 perfusion units in the postthrombotic limbs and 108 perfusion units in the normal limbs.

The reduction or abolition of an effective precapillary vasoconstrictive response on standing will expose the capillary bed to a high hydrostatic load,[7,8,16] producing edema and thickening of the capillary basement membrane.[10,11] Prolonged venous hypertension with its consequential increased capillary fluid and protein loss will result in pericapillary fibrin deposition. This is probably enhanced by the low fibrinolytic activity often found in patients with postphlebitic limbs.[10,11] Findings from other studies on the microcirculation[8] are compatible with this theory.

The findings from laser Doppler studies suggest that in normal limbs when vasomotor activity is normal, only a portion of the capillaries, about 5 out of 10, are open at any one moment in horizontal positions. On standing, the VAR causes two or three additional capillaries to shut down so that only two or three capillary loops bear the high pressure when the venous system becomes full. Thus capillary flow is greatly reduced and capillary leakage is minimal (normal). In contrast, the skin blood flow in limbs with severe venous hypertension is, on average, increased threefold and vasomotor activity is minimal, indicating that most capillaries, perhaps 9 out of 10, are "open." This is similar to what happens in an inflammatory reaction. On standing, the VAR is minimal. Thus a large number of capillaries, about 8 out of 10, remain open, leading to increased capillary leakage that is proportional to the area of capillary endothelium exposed to the high flow and pressure.

This hypothesis has been tested in further studies in which the RF, SF, and VAR have been correlated with AVP, $TcPo_2$, $TcPco_2$, local skin temperature, capillary filtration, inhalation of CO_2, and the effect of various therapeutic measures (known to promote healing of leg ulcers) on the microcirculation. These findings are presented in the following sections.

CORRELATION OF RF, SF, AND VAR WITH AVP

AVP is linearly related to the incidence of ulceration.[19] The AVP and laser Doppler skin flux were measured in 15 healthy volunteers, 20 limbs with primary varicose veins and skin changes (no ulceration), and 30 limbs with deep vein disease and leg ulceration. The AVP in the limbs with primary varicose veins became normal when a below-knee or ankle pneumatic cuff (less than 45 mm Hg) that occluded

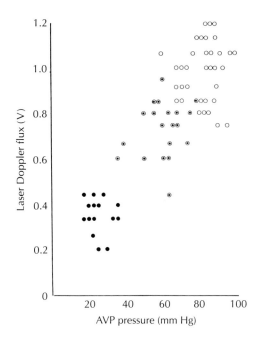

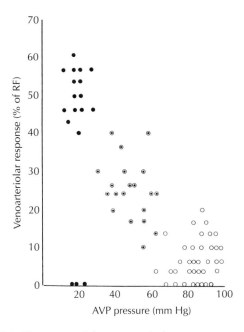

Fig. 115-4. The correlation between skin flux and ambulatory venous pressure measurements in normal subjects (●); patients with moderate venous incompetence due to superficial venous disease (◉); and patients with severe, chronic venous incompetence (○).

Fig. 115-5. The venoarteriolar response in the same groups as in Fig. 115-4.

the superficial veins was applied, but this did not take place in the limbs with deep vein disease.

Fig. 115-4 shows the correlation between AVP (without the application of tourniquets) and laser Doppler skin RF in normal subjects, patients with superficial vein incompetence, and those with deep vein incompetence. There is a linear relationship between the two ($r = 0.84$). Fig. 115-5 shows the relationship between the VAR and the AVP ($r = -0.79$) for the same three groups of subjects.

CORRELATION OF THE VAR, RF, AND SF WITH $TcPo_2$ AND $TcPco_2$

RF, SF, VAR, $TcPo_2$, $TcPco_2$, and AVP were measured from the perimalleolar region in 20 postthrombotic limbs (with popliteal vein reflux confirmed on duplex scanning) and 10 normal limbs. The instruments used for this study were the TSI Laserflo* and the Microgas.* The CombiSensor on the latter instrument allows the simultaneous measurement of Po_2 and Pco_2 at the same position on the skin (at a room temperature of $21°$ C $\pm 1°$ C).

The intercorrelation between all the parameters is shown in Fig. 115-6. The correlation of the $TcPo_2$ with all other measurements is poor ($r < 0.4$), whereas all other parameters are well intercorrelated ($r > 0.6$). There was a negative linear relationship between the Pco_2 and the VAR ($r = -0.72$), and it appears that a high Pco_2 is associated with a high resting skin blood flow and a poor VAR. It is not known whether the increased Pco_2 causes or results from

the vasodilatation, high skin blood flow, and abolition of vasomotor activity (vasoparalysis).

In an attempt to answer this question, CO_2 inhalation (5% for 15 minutes increasing to $TcPco_2$ by 20%) was administered in 10 normal volunteers. The resulting decrease in VAR is shown in Fig. 115-7, which demonstrates the powerful effect of Pco_2 on the microcirculation and indicates that the observed effects on venous hypertensive microangiopathy may stem from locally elevated Pco_2.

CORRELATION BETWEEN THE VAR AND THE INCREASE OF SKIN BLOOD FLOW INDUCED BY LOCAL TEMPERATURE ELEVATION

Skin blood flow increases when skin temperature is elevated (e.g., by a local thermostat applied to the skin around the probe). Fig. 115-8, upper chart shows the increase in skin flux in a normal subject when the skin temperature was raised from $26°$ C to $40°$ C over 15 minutes in a room at a constant temperature ($21°$ C $\pm 2°$ C). The probe was applied at the internal perimalleolar region.

Fig. 115-8, lower chart shows the increase in flux during local temperature elevation in a patient with venous hypertension, determined by popliteal vein incompetence (with skin ulceration). The tracing is obtained by a time averaging of 0.2 seconds. The baseline resting flux is higher in the lower chart and the flux increase is proportionally lower in the postphlebitic limb. The final flux level does not differ significantly between these two subjects, but the flux increased about 6.6 times in the normal subject and only 3.1 times in the patient.

*Kontron, United Kingdom.

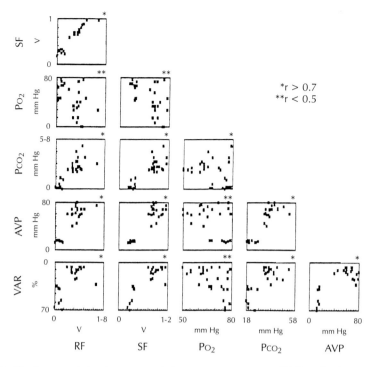

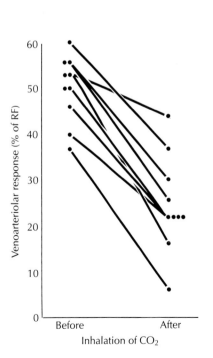

Fig. 115-6. The intercorrelation between ambulatory venous pressure *(AVP)* and microcirculatory parameters including transcutaneous Po_2 and Pco_2. The parameters with a good correlation ($r > 0.7$) are indicated with an asterisk. *(SD, Standing flux; RF, resting flux; VAR, venoarteriolar response.)*

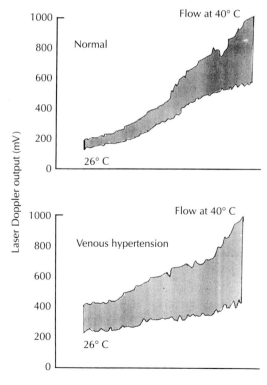

Fig. 115-7. The venoarteriolar response is reduced or abolished in normal subjects after inhalation of CO_2 (3%), indicating the effect of increased Pco_2 on the skin microcirculation.

Fig. 115-8. The increase in local skin flux after local temperature increase (from 26° C to 40° C) is lower in the skin of patients with venous hypertension.

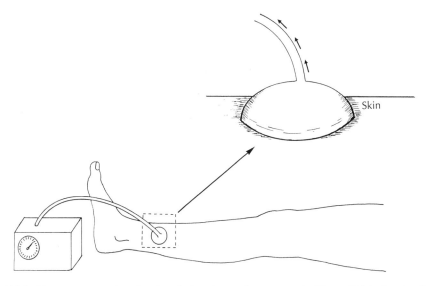

Fig. 115-9. The vacuum suction chamber device. A negative pressure (-30 mm Hg) in the chamber is maintained.

THE VAR AND CAPILLARY FILTRATION

In patients with diabetes and venous hypertension whose VAR is impaired, edema may occur as a result of high capillary pressure when subjects are in dependent positions. Thickening of the basement membranes, the histologic hallmark of microangiopathy in diabetics, is promoted by chronically raised capillary pressure.[24] Local capillary filtration and capillary permeability plus its variations may be evaluated in patients with venous hypertension using the vacuum suction chamber (VSC) (Fig. 115-9). In this method, a small plastic chamber is applied to the skin of the perimalleolar region and a negative pressure (-30 mm Hg) is exerted for 10 minutes.[3] The VSC produces a wheal, which is a round, flat-topped, pale red elevation in the skin that is evanescent and disappears within minutes or hours. Wheals are formed because of edema in the upper layer of the dermis and are due to increased capillary filtration arising from local capillary changes. Wheals produced by the VSC are recorded on serial photos taken every 5 minutes. In normal subjects, they disappear in less than 60 minutes.[3] The disappearance time of wheals in the perimalleolar region can be used to evaluate capillary filtration in pathologic conditions. The disappearance time of these wheals is then correlated with the VAR in the same area (Fig. 115-10).

Calibration of the technique has demonstrated a good correlation between the capillary filtration obtained by venous occlusion plethysmography and that revealed by the VSC.[3] However, evaluation of capillary permeability by venous occlusion plethysmography[21,23] is an expression of capillary filtration in the whole limb distal to the occlusion, in contrast to VSC, which evaluates local capillary permeability (i.e., in the perimalleolar region).

Strain-gauge plethysmography has also been used to evaluate the rate of ankle swelling. In this technique, the patient

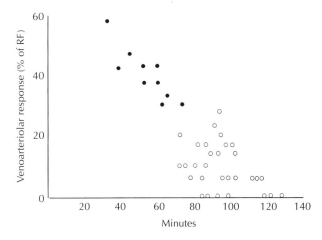

Fig. 115-10. The correlation between the venoarteriolar response and the time of disappearance of the wheal obtained with the VSC device. ●, Normal limbs; ○, venous hypertension (VH).

rests supine for 30 minutes at a constant room temperature and then stands holding onto a frame. The strain gauge is placed around the minimum circumference of the foot and records the increases in volume, which are considered proportional to the capillary filtration.[21,23] Fig. 115-11 shows the curve obtained in both a normal limb and a limb with venous hypertension caused by postphlebitic syndrome but not affected by lipodermatosclerosis or ulceration. The tangent to the curve between minute 7 and minute 10 is considered a measurement of capillary filtration.

This technique has revealed that there is a proportional increase in the rate of ankle swelling in patients with increased skin flux due to the postphlebitic syndrome.[4] It was also discovered that the increase in the rate of ankle swelling is proportional to the decrease in efficacy of the VAR.

Therefore it appears that there is a complex relationship between the increase in skin flux and PCO_2 and the decrease in VAR and the increase in capillary filtration, which then leads to edema and more progressively to extracapillary filtration of proteins and macromolecules, ultimately causing lipodermatosclerosis.

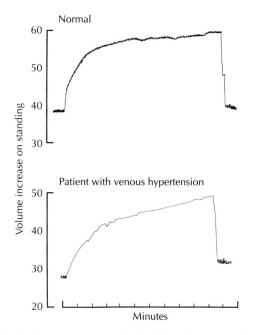

Fig. 115-11. The two curves obtained with strain-gauge plethysmography in normal volunteers and in subjects with venous hypertension. The tangent to the curve at 7 to 10 minutes is proportional to capillary filtration and indicates an increased filtration in the subject with venous hypertension.

THE EFFECT OF THERAPEUTIC MEASURES
The effect of elastic compression

In patients with chronic venous insufficiency, elastic compression has proved to be a beneficial measure through its action on the microcirculation.[1] Table 115-1 demonstrates the effect of 3 weeks of graduated elastic compression (25 mm at the ankle) in 32 patients with primary varicose veins, 31 patients with deep vein disease, and 15 normal volunteers who served as controls. There was a change in all variables toward normal. The RF decreased, the VAR improved, the $TcPO_2$ increased, and the $TcPCO_2$ decreased. In addition, these changes were associated with a decrease in the rate of ankle swelling, as measured by strain-gauge plethysmography.

The dramatic effects of elastic compression on skin flux are also shown in Fig. 115-12. In 76 postphlebitic limbs, the perimalleolar skin flux was recorded before and after 4 weeks of elastic compression using graduated below-knee stockings (ankle pressure, 25 mm Hg). The decrease in skin flux was significant after 4 weeks. (Normal values are shown for comparison.)

Effect of the sequential compression device

Intermittent pneumatic compression using the sequential compression device (SCD)* for 3 hours per day in addition to low-compression graduated elastic stockings accelerates the healing of leg venous ulcers approximately tenfold,[12,17] but until recently, little has been known about its effect on the microcirculation. The SCD consists of leggings containing multiple chambers that inflate sequentially from the foot and ankle toward the thigh. The pressure in any chamber is always lower than the pressure in the adjacent distal chamber. The compression cycle lasts for 11 seconds with a decompression period of 1 minute. The pressure is ad-

---

*Kendall, Cambridge, Mass.

Table 115-1. The effect of venous hypertension on the perimalleolar skin microcirculation and the effect of graduated elastic compression*

Variables	Normal	Primary VVs		DVD	
		Before GEC	After GEC	Before GEC	After GEC
No. of limbs	15	32	32	31	31
AVP range (mm Hg)	>30	39-57	39-57	43-79	43-79
Laser Doppler					
RF (red cell flux), mean (SD)	0.65 (0.6)	0.93 (0.11)	0.72 (0.1)	1.12 (0.8)	0.83 (0.9)
Percentage reduction of RF on standing due to VAR	37%	19%	26%	3%	16%
PO_2 (mm Hg), mean (SD)	74 (8)	65 (8)	69 (7)	52 (9)	66 (7)
PCO_2 (mm Hg), mean (SD)	28 (6)	33 (5)	30 (6)	38 (7)	32 (5)
Strain-gauge plethysmography					
Rate of ankle swelling (ml/100 ml/min), mean (SD)	1.01 (0.08)	1.54 (0.01)	1.34 (0.12)	1.95 (0.1)	1.44 (0.11)

VV, Varicose veins; *DVD*, deep vein disease; *GEC*, graduated elastic compression; *AVP*, ambulatory venous pressure; *RF*, resting flux; *VAR*, venoarteriolar response.
*Elastic compression consisted of 25 mm Hg at the ankle for 3 weeks.

justable, with a maximum attainable pressure of 65 mm Hg at the ankle.

A recent study has attempted to determine the effects of the SCD on the microcirculation of the skin in the gaiter area in patients with venous hypertension and skin changes or ulceration.[2] A total of 16 limbs in 11 patients with chronic hypertension and 12 limbs in 12 healthy volunteers were studied. The skin red cell flux was measured by laser Doppler flowmetry before, during, and after sequential compression. The probe was placed at least 2 cm distal to the edge of the ulcer outside the legging, and the mean RF was measured by taking the average flux obtained over a 5-minute period. The patient was then asked to stand, and flux was measured for the following 5 minutes; this SF is defined as the lowest mean flux during this period. The VAR was calculated from the equation: VAR = [(SF − RF)/RF] × 100. The occurrence of vasomotor waves was also observed.

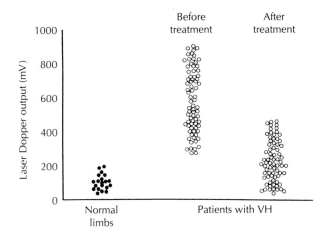

Fig. 115-12. Skin flux in normal limbs and in patients with venous hypertension before and after 4 weeks of treatment with elastic compression stockings.

Once these measurements were completed, the SCD was applied for 30 minutes while the patient rested supine. The compression period was set at 11 seconds, with a maximum pressure of 60 mm Hg and a deflation period of 60 seconds. Skin flux was continuously monitored by laser Doppler during the period of sequential compression. The time of onset of rhythmic vasomotor waves and the rate and amplitude of the waves were noted. At the end of the compression, the RF, SF, and VAR were measured again. The patient was then asked to lie down once more, and the skin flux was monitored by laser Doppler for 2 hours.

The mean skin blood flux (RF) in limbs with venous hypertension was 1.45 units. This was three times higher than that in controls ($p < 0.05$) (Table 115-2). The VAR, or the decrease in skin flux on standing, was lower (6.8%) than that in controls (35%) ($p < 0.05$). The vasomotor activity and amplitude of the vasomotor waves were both greatly reduced or missing compared with normal limbs (Table 115-3). There was a marked trend toward normal RFs; in addition, the vasomotor activity increased and vasomotor waves were observed. The vasomotor activity and amplitude of the vasomotor waves were both greatly reduced or absent compared with normal limbs. There was a marked trend toward normal RFs and vasomotor activity 10 and 30 minutes after the commencement of graduated intermittent sequential compression.

These improvements were still present 30 and 60 minutes after sequential compression had been stopped (Table 115-3). The mean VAR had also improved from 6.8% before compression to 23% ($p < 0.05$) 30 minutes after the end of compression. This improvement persisted at 60 minutes, although was reduced (14%, $p < 0.05$) (Table 115-3). In addition, vasomotion was clearly present 5 hours after the end of the sequential compression in all limbs treated.

The stimulation of the lower limb with intermittent sequential compression appears to induce vasomotor activity that produces decreased skin blood flow because some areas

Table 115-2. Skin red cell flux at rest and changes on standing before, during, and after sequential compression*

Timing	Resting flux (flux units, mean ± SD)		Venoarteriolar response (percentage flux decrease and range)		Vasomotion in patients
	Controls	Patients	Controls	Patients	
After 30 min rest	0.056 ± 0.03	1.45 ± 0.08†	35% (15-38)	6.8% (2-11)‡	Reduced or abolished
10 min after starting SCD	0.59 ± 0.03	1.10 ± 0.6‡§	—	—	Present, increased
30 min after starting SCD	0.67 ± 0.03	0.90 ± 0.5‡§	—	—	Present, increased
30 min after stopping SCD	0.47 ± 0.02	0.85 ± 0.5‡§	38% (15-36)	23% (9-29)‡‖	Present, increased
60 min after stopping SCD	0.44 ± 0.02	1.10 ± 0.6‡§	38% (14-38)	14% (7-27)‡§	Present, increased

SCD, Sequential decompression device.
*The study consisted of 11 patients with venous hypertension and 12 limbs in 12 normal controls.
†$P<0.025$ compared with controls.
‡$P<0.05$ compared with controls.
§$P<0.05$ compared with baseline.
‖$P<0.025$ compared with baseline.

Table 115-3. Measurements in the treatment group (mean ± SD)

Variables	Baseline measurements	Measurements after 6 weeks	Normal values* (95% confidence limits [mean ± 2 SD])
RF (mV)	372 ± 48	272 ± 63†	90-270
VAR (mV) ·	99 ± 24	148 ± 37†	40 ± 23
Increase in flow after warming (mV)	387 ± 8	537 ± 132‡	668 ± 110
P_{O_2} (mm Hg)	66 ± 4.4	75 ± 5.6‡	81 ± 7
P_{CO_2} (mm Hg)	31 ± 2.6	27 ± 2.4‡	25 ± 5
Leg volume (ml)	5088.7 ± 29	5029.6 ± 23	—

RF, Resting flow; *VAR*, venoarteriolar response.
*Normal values are based on findings from a previous study.[5,7]
†$P<0.05$.
‡$P<0.01$ (Mann-Whitney U-test).

vasoconstrict. A decrease in skin blood flow is itself a stimulus to further vasomotion and tends to perpetuate this phenomenon. It appears that elastic compression[7] and, as shown in this study, sequential compression induce this type of vasomotor activity, which persists well after the cessation of sequential compression. In other words, the application of intermittent graduated sequential compression initiates a normal phenomenon that possesses a self-perpetuating tendency.

The induction of vasomotor activity by graduated sequential pneumatic compression brings about normalization of local blood flow regulation. This response may stem from a direct stimulatory effect on vasomotor activity. However, another possible explanation for the microcirculatory response is that compression enhances the washout of metabolic or inflammatory mediators that cause the chronic vasodilatation seen in these patients.

The findings of this study may explain the accelerated healing of venous ulcers seen in patients with SCD. The persistence of vasomotor activity after the termination of compression is an important finding that needs additional investigation to determine the optimum compression (pressure and cycle), duration, and frequency of such treatment.

EFFECT OF FLAVONOIDS

Flavonoids have been used for many years to treat problems associated with varicose veins and deep vein insufficiency. Symptomatic relief has been reported to follow the administration of oral preparations.[5] Until recently, however, objective measurements for determining the effectiveness of this drug have been lacking.

In a recent study, 35 patients with venous hypertension who had ankle swelling and skin changes but no ulceration as a result of reflux in the popliteal vein were randomized into either a treatment or placebo group. All patients had an AVP greater than 55 mm Hg. Patients in the treatment group received an oral preparation of Venoruton (troxeruton), one sachet (1 gm) twice a day. The placebo group received the same dose (1 sachet) of lactose that was similar in appearance and taste to the active preparation. Elastic

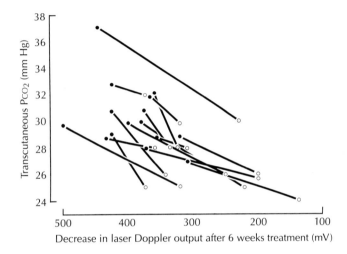

Fig. 115-13. The correlation between the transcutaneous P_{CO_2} and the decrease in laser Doppler output in patients treated with Venoruton for 6 weeks.

compression was not used during the study. RF, SF, VAR, the change in flux after warming, TcP_{O_2}, TcP_{CO_2}, and leg volume determined by water displacement were measured before and after 6 weeks of treatment.

At the beginning of the study, there was no significant difference between the mean values of all the measurements between the placebo and treatment group. There was also no significant change between the baseline measurements and the 6-week values in the placebo group. However, there were significant differences between the baseline measurements and those obtained at 6 weeks in the treatment group (Table 115-3). By plotting P_{CO_2} against RF before and after treatment, using all the readings, a linear relationship was found ($r = 0.78$) (Fig. 115-13).

CONCLUSION

The chronic effects of venous hypertension on the skin of the perimalleolar region cause microcirculatory disturbances (venous hypertensive microangiopathy) whose significance has only recently been understood. Quantitative noninvasive assessment of the microcirculatory disturbances has become possible with the advent of techniques such as laser Doppler flowmetry, $TcPO_2$ and $TcPCO_2$ measurements, strain-gauge plethysmography, and leg volumetry.

Both RF and SF are increased and the VAR is impaired in limbs with venous hypertension, and this exposes a large number of capillaries to high pressure on standing, which then provokes increased fluid leakage. This increased fluid loss is demonstrated by the increased rate of ankle swelling revealed by strain-gauge plethysmography. The increased skin blood flow and fluid leakage are associated with edema, eczema, and eventually ulceration. The increase in capillary filtration and the diffusion through capillaries is altered in the context of both diabetic microangiopathy and mild chronic venous incompetence.[9,22]

The induction of vasomotor activity, decrease in the resting flow, and improvement of the VAR brought about by elastic compression, intermittent sequential compression, and hydroxyethylrutosides such as Venoruton represent a normalization and are associated with a decrease in PCO_2, capillary filtration, and edema and an increase in PO_2.

For the first time, methods are now available that can document such changes and may be used in further research to establish the optimal regimen for both the mechanical and pharmacologic treatments.

REFERENCES

1. Belcaro G: The role of transcutaneous PCO_2 measurements in association with laser-Doppler flowmetry in venous hypertension, *Phlebology* 3:189, 1988.
2. Belcaro G, Nicolaides AN: *Acute effects of intermittent sequential compression in venous hypertension*, 5th Annual Venous Forum, Orlando, Fla, Feb 24-26, 1993.
3. Belcaro G, Rulo A: The study of capillary permeability in patients with venous hypertension by a new system: the vacuum suction chamber (VSC) device—a preliminary report, *Phlebology* 3:255, 1988.
4. Belcaro G, Christopoulos D, Nicolaides AN: Skin flow and swelling in postphlebitic limbs, *Vasa* 18:136, 1989.
5. Belcaro G, Rulo A, Candiani C: Evaluation of the microcirculatory effects of Venoruton (HR) in patients with chronic venous hypertension by laser-Doppler flowmetry, transcutaneous PO_2 and PCO_2 measurements, leg volumetry and ambulatory venous pressure measurements, *Phlebology* 41:847, 1988.
6. Belcaro G et al: Combined evaluation of postphlebitic limbs by laser-Doppler flowmetry and transcutaneous PO_2-PCO_2 measurements, *Vasa* 17:259, 1988.
7. Belcaro G et al: Evaluation of the effects of elastic compression in patients with post-phlebitic limb by laser Doppler flowmetry, *Phlebologie* 41:797, 1988.
8. Belcaro G et al: Blood flow in the perimalleolar skin in relation to posture in patients with venous hypertension, *Ann Vasc Surg* 1:5-7, 1989.
9. Bollinger A et al: Patterns of diffusion through skin capillaries in patients with long term diabetes, *N Engl J Med* 307:1305, 1982.
10. Browse NL, Burnand KG: The cause of venous ulceration, *Lancet* 2:243, 1982.
11. Burnand K et al: Venous lipodermatosclerosis: treatment by fibrinolytic enhancement and elastic compression, *Br Med J* 280:7, 1980.
12. Coleridge-Smith PD et al: Improved venous ulcer healing using intermittent pneumatic compression, *Phlebologie* 41:788-789, 1988.
13. Fagrell B: *Problems using laser-Doppler flowmetry on the skin in clinical practice*. In Belcaro G et al, eds: *Laser Doppler flowmetry: experimental and clinical applications*, London, 1993, Med Orion.
14. Gowland-Hopkins NF et al: Positron emission tomography in venous ulceration and liposclerosis: study of regional tissue function, *Br Med J* 286:333, 1983.
15. Hasselbach P et al: Microangiopathy in severe chronic venous insufficiency evaluated by fluorescence video-microscopy, *Phlebology* 1:159, 1986.
16. Hendriksen O: Local reflex in microcirculation in human subcutaneous tissue, *Acta Physiol Scand* 97:446, 1976.
17. Kolari PJ, Pekanmaki K: Effects of intermittent compression treatment on skin perfusion and oxygenation in lower limbs with venous ulcers, *Vasa* 16:312-317, 1987.
18. Levick JR, Michel CC: The effects of position and skin temperature on the capillary pressures in the fingers and toes, *J Physiol* (Lond) 274:97, 1978.
19. Nicolaides AN, Zukowski AJ: The value of dynamic venous pressure measurements, *World J Surg* 10:919, 1986.
20. Rayman G, Hassan A, Tooke JE: Blood flow in the skin of the foot related to posture in patients with diabetes mellitus, *Br Med J* 292:87, 1986.
21. Sigaard-Andersen J: Venous occlusion plethysmography on the calf, *Ugeskr Laeger* 17(suppl I), 1970.
22. Speiser DE, Bollinger A: Microangiopathy in mild chronic venous incompetence (CVI): morphological alterations and increased transcapillary diffusion detected by fluorescence videomicroscopy, *Int J Microcirc Clin Exp* 10:55, 1991.
23. Thulesius O: Capillary filtration under normal and pathological conditions, *Angiologia* 10:198, 1973.
24. Tooke JS, Ostergren J, Fagrell B: Synchronous assessment of human skin microcirculation by laser-Doppler flowmetry and dynamic capillaroscopy, *Int J Microcirc Clin Exp* 2:277, 1983.

CHAPTER 116

Upper extremity venous imaging with color flow Doppler

EDWARD G. GRANT

Color Doppler sonography is a promising technique for evaluating the venous system of the upper extremity and should be the primary screening method in patients with suspected thrombosis.[1,3] The prevalence of thrombosis in the upper extremity and thoracic inlet veins is growing with the expanded use of Hickman and other central venous catheters and pacemaker implants. In addition, the recent interest in physical fitness has spawned an increased number of young patients with spontaneous or effort-induced thrombosis. In the latter situation, there is no apparent predisposing factor and the patient is usually seen after engaging in recent vigorous exercise or weight lifting. In most of these cases, hypertrophy of the anterior scalene muscle or other thoracic outlet structures partially block the proximal subclavian vein, causing thoracic outlet syndrome and precipitating venous thrombosis. It is particularly important to diagnose effort-induced thrombosis early because a good outcome in an otherwise young, healthy individual can only be achieved by instituting prompt, effective treatment.

For some time, contrast-enhanced venography has been the standard method of assessing the upper extremity venous system and, in experienced hands, is relatively easy to perform. The procedure is carried out by injecting the contrast agent through intravenous lines inserted in both hands. The drawbacks associated with any such contrast evaluation remain, however, and include discomfort from extravasation at the injection site; a burning sensation in the arms, neck, and face; and the possible induction of thrombophlebitis in otherwise normal veins. Real-time and duplex Doppler sonography have been considered potential noninvasive screening procedures for some time. Unlike the veins of the legs, however, the subclavian vein is protected by the clavicle and therefore cannot be compressed, precluding the use of real-time ultrasound in cases of anechoic thrombus (Fig. 116-1). Duplex Doppler, on the other hand, although able to confirm the patency of individual vessels, is not an optimal method because veins may be difficult to locate and follow and peripheral venous spectral patterns may remain normal in spite of central occlusion when there is adequate collateral circulation (Fig. 116-2). The ability of color Doppler to provide anatomic images makes it an excellent method for evaluating the upper extremity veins. Normal vessels may be followed more easily and better differen-

tiated from collaterals, and compression is not needed. The accuracy of the color Doppler examination, however, depends on the location of the thrombus. A nonocclusive central clot may still be impossible to define and patients with chronic venous thrombosis may still need to undergo contrast-enhanced venography to distinguish the normal main vein from large collaterals.

SCANNING TECHNIQUE AND NORMAL ANATOMY

In preparation for scanning, the patient should be placed in the supine position and the arm to be examined extended comfortably so that it is at an approximate 90° to the chest (Fig. 116-3). Some clinicians scan while standing below the shoulder, although others advocate scanning from the head of the examining table.[3] By lightly placing the transducer over the proximal portion of the inner aspect of the upper arm in a transverse orientation, examiners should achieve adequate visualization of at least two major veins (the basilic and brachial venae comitantes) and the brachial artery. Because of the variable numbers of smaller veins and possible collaterals, the artery should be used as a landmark throughout the examination and confirms which of the veins is the main vessel. Turning longitudinally on the artery and adjacent basilic vein, the two vessels can be followed along the undersurface of the arm into the axilla, where the basilic and brachial venae comitantes join to form the axillary vein. An infraclavicular approach can be used to follow the axillary vein proximally beneath the pectoralis muscle and into the thoracic outlet, at which point it becomes the subclavian vein. The subclavian vein can usually be followed proximally for some distance by angling cephalad beneath the clavicle. Up to this point, scanning is best performed with a 5- or 7.5-MHz linear or curved array transducer (Fig. 116-4).

For examining the medial portion of the subclavian vein, its junction with the internal jugular vein, and the innominate vein, a supraclavicular or suprasternal approach is necessary. The examiner may begin by locating the jugular vein in the neck and following it to its junction with the subclavian vein. Although high-frequency linear probes are optimal for the jugular examination, the central veins (proximal jugular and subclavian as well as the innominate) are best evaluated using a lower-frequency (approximately 3.0

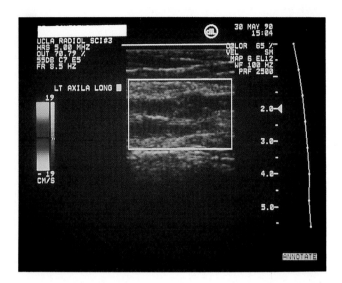

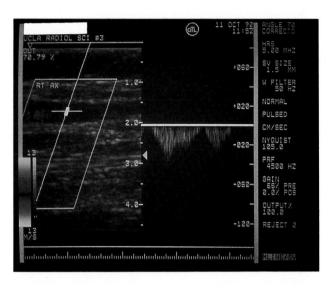

Fig. 116-1. Real-time imaging alone may successfully identify axillary or brachial vein thrombosis when the clot *(C)* is relatively echogenic. Unfortunately, the clot may be anechoic and impossible to identify with real-time imaging alone.

Fig. 116-2. Duplex sonography. When veins can be visualized with real-time imaging, duplex sonography can be used to evaluate the presence or absence of flow. Unfortunately, when veins are difficult to see with real-time imaging or in cases where collaterals may cause confusion, duplex scanning may not be adequate. A typical spectral pattern of upper extremity veins is illustrated. Note the two periods of forward flow (below baseline) with each cardiac cycle. Flow corresponds to the two phases of right atrial filling. Such pulsatile venous patterns should not be confused with arterial pulsations.

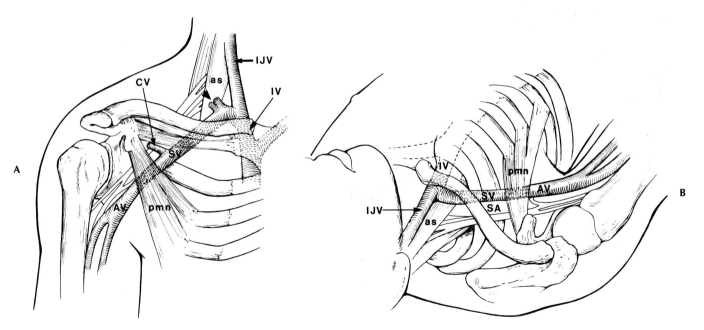

Fig. 116-3. Normal anatomy. *A,* The axillary vein *(AV)* lies behind the pectoralis minor muscle *(pmm)* and becomes the subclavian vein *(SV)* beyond the first rib. At least three constant branches join the subclavian vein: the cephalic vein *(CV)*, the external jugular, and the transverse cephalic vein *(arrowhead)*. All may serve as collaterals in patients with obstruction. Note the internal jugular vein *(IJN)* and innominate vein *(IV)*. *B,* An examiner's view shows vessels from another vantage point. The subclavian vein lies anterior to the anterior scalene muscle and is anterior and inferior to the subclavian artery.

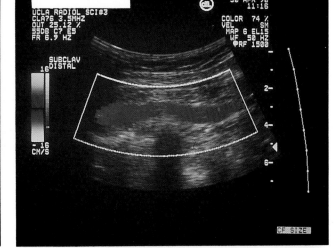

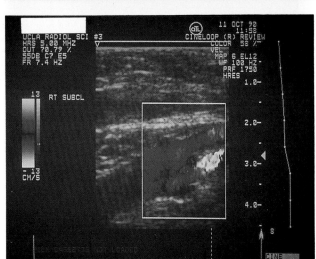

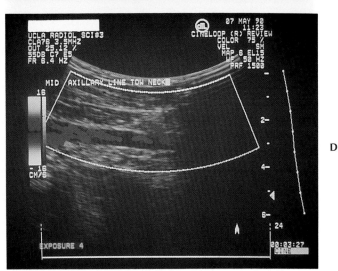

Fig. 116-4. Normal venous anatomy. **A,** The transverse image through the right upper arm reveals a normal brachial artery (red) and vein (blue). Note the presence of several smaller veins around the artery. These veins vary in size and position and represent the brachial venae comitantes. **B,** The longitudinal image of the distal subclavian vein shows the vessel to good advantage with the curved array transducer. Note the color assignment changes within the vessel as flow vectors change in relation to the transducer. The flow is initially toward the transducer and displayed in red and later is away from the transducer and displayed in blue. **C,** The right subclavian vein (S) is large and well defined in this patient. Note the cephalic vein (C) entering from above. **D,** The subclavian vein is followed proximally and eventually lost because of shadowing from the clavicle (arrows).

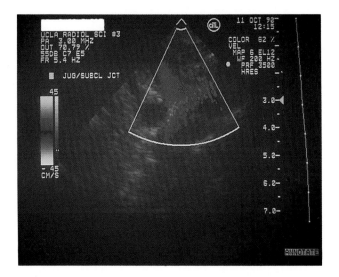

Fig. 116-5. The junction between the left jugular vein (J) and proximal subclavian vein (S) is delineated by using a sector-type transducer. The left innominate vein (I) can be followed beyond the venous junction.

MHz) sector-type transducer that achieves better imaging in areas with limited sonic access. In some patients, this type of transducer even allows imaging of the superior vena cava (Fig. 116-5).

THROMBOSIS OF UPPER EXTREMITY VEINS

Grassi and Polak[1] documented good results using color Doppler in the evaluation of acute effort-induced thrombosis of the subclavian and axillary veins. In the acute situation and when thrombus involves the veins in the arm or beyond the medial subclavian, the diagnosis is straightforward. Color Doppler visualizes the thrombosed vein as a tubular hypoechoic structure adjacent to the artery and flow is absent (Fig. 116-6). Spectral analysis may reveal monophasic flow because right atrial pulsatility is dampened by proximal

obstruction. This finding, however, is not invariably present and spectral patterns may be entirely normal. Collaterals are often visualized as venous structures in the soft tissues surrounding the thrombosed main vein, and their presence lends further support to the diagnosis. Spectral analysis may be used to confirm venous flow in suspected collaterals (Fig. 116-7). However, large collaterals should not be mistaken for the main vein. When the diagnosis is obvious (and it should be in most cases involving the arm or infraclavicular veins), no further imaging procedures are necessary.

Both acute and chronic thrombosis also often afflicts patients with central venous catheters, and the accuracy of diagnosis depends on the location and duration of the abnormality. When thrombosis involves the mid and distal subclavian, the axillary, or brachial veins, the diagnosis

A
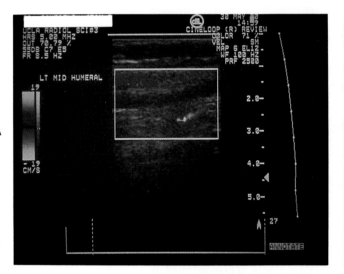
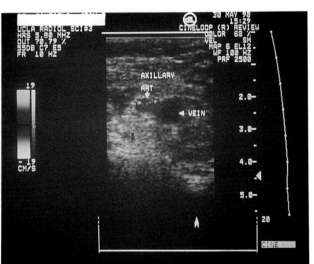
B

Fig. 116-6. Acute venous thrombosis. This 23-year-old weight lifter presented with an acutely swollen left arm. *A,* Longitudinal and *B,* transverse images in the left upper arm and axillary region reveal a prominent tubular hypoechoic thrombus occupying the left axillary vein. Note the adjacent axillary artery *(A)* and small venous collateral *(arrowheads).*

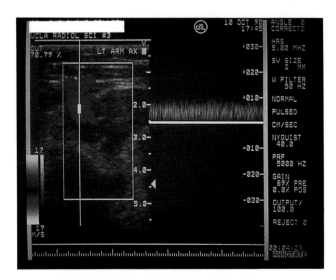

Fig. 116-7. Venous collaterals. The hypoechoic thrombus *(H)* fills the left axillary vein. The large collateral (shown in red) is identified adjacent to the main vessel. The structure is identified as a venous collateral by demonstrating monophasic flow with spectral analysis.

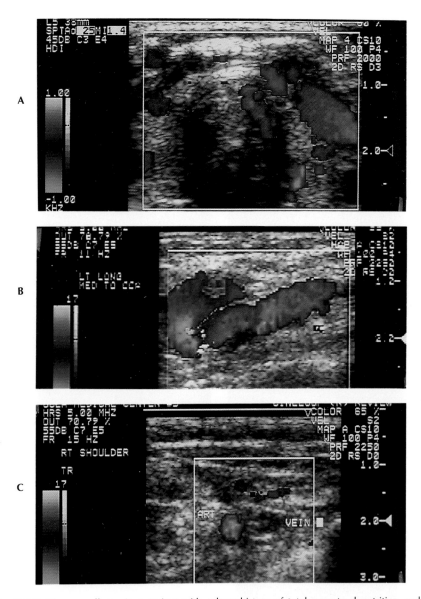

Fig. 116-8. Venous collapse in a patient with a long history of total parenteral nutrition and loss of multiple venous access sites. ***A,*** Color Doppler examination revealed numerous large collaterals in both sides of the neck. The thyroid *(T)* is filled with large collateral veins. ***B,*** A large venous structure *(V)* was initially thought to be the jugular vein but was medial to carotid and therefore a collateral. A normal jugular was absent on both sides. ***C,*** The scan through the distal right subclavian vessels shows a typical thrombus. Both femoral veins were also absent (or collapsed); the catheter was eventually inserted into the right hepatic vein under ultrasound guidance.

should be easy to make and the sonographic features should be similar to those of acute effort-induced thrombosis. Unfortunately, localized central thrombi may arise in these patients and be difficult or impossible to detect. The published experience thus far[1,3] indicates that sonographic accuracy is poor in these areas. However, these studies relied solely on linear array transducers and such instruments are extremely awkward when used in areas with limited acoustic windows. The use of sector-type transducers with small footprints remains to be evaluated.

In chronic thrombosis, significant collateral formation poses a major diagnostic challenge because collaterals are often large and may be easily mistaken for the main vein. Even the excellent anatomic detail provided by the color Doppler examination may be insufficient to allow differentiation between collaterals and normal veins. In patients with clinically suspected chronic thrombosis, the examination should begin in the upper arm for the purpose of orientation, and the normal main vein should be followed centrally. Any deviation from the expected normal anatomy or the identification of extra veins should be considered suspect and compared with the vessels of the opposite shoulder.

Patients with indwelling venous catheters may also have a venous obstruction without apparent intraluminal thrombus. In such patients, the veins may literally not be seen because the walls appear to collapse and fibrose together. It may be difficult to make a diagnosis in the subclavian vein where numerous collaterals may be present and easily confused with a normal main vein. This phenomenon frequently occurs in the jugular veins. In such patients, the normal jugular vein is not seen lateral to the carotid artery,

and numerous prominent venous collaterals are found in the surrounding soft tissues of the neck (Fig. 116-8).

In summary, color Doppler sonography is an excellent method for diagnosing acute venous thrombosis or for monitoring the course of patients undergoing treatment of a known clot. The method, however, does have limitations. Centrally located thrombi may be difficult to diagnose, and collaterals may be confused with normal vessels in patients with chronic phlebitis.

UPPER EXTREMITY ARTERIOVENOUS MALFORMATIONS

Arteriovenous malformations (AVMs) of the upper extremities are relatively unusual and may be either congenital or acquired. Patients with congenital AVMs may first be seen because of generalized enlargement of the affected limb or a soft tissue mass. When lesions are large, high-output congestive heart failure may exist as well. Acquired AVMs occur secondary to penetrating wounds or brachial arteriography, and most are asymptomatic. The findings yielded by color Doppler should be diagnostic in both varieties of AVMs, but the sonographic features of the two are quite different.

In congenital AVMs, the color examination will reveal an irregular knot of prominent vessels. Feeder vessels are often conspicuous and exhibit high-velocity, low-resistance flow; the draining veins may be arterialized. In patients who have undergone prior therapeutic embolization, vascular connections may be difficult to identify because main arteries have often been thrombosed. Color Doppler, however, is practical after therapeutic procedures and may be performed on a routine basis to determine if the lesion is recurring (Fig. 116-9). Color Doppler may also be useful at

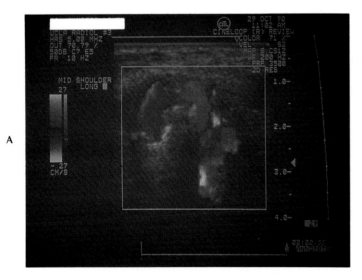
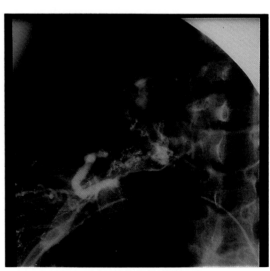

A

B

Fig. 116-9. Congenital AVM. *A,* The color Doppler sonogram of the right supraclavicular area reveals an unusual arcade of abnormal vessels. Extremely low-resistance spectral patterns were identified. The patient had undergone therapeutic embolization of congenital AVM immediately before the sonogram. *B,* An arteriogram performed after the embolization shows a dilated collection of veins *(arrows)* that correspond to the vessels seen on the color Doppler examination. This patient was followed at 6-month intervals; the lesion has remained stable over 2 years.

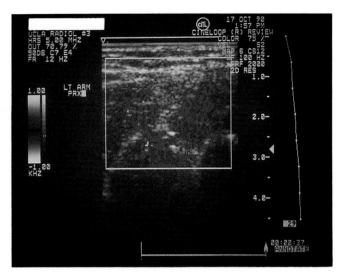

Fig. 116-10. Acquired AVM. Patient with oozing and a hematoma in the area of the puncture site after cardiac catheterization performed via the brachial route. *A,* A sonographic section taken somewhat below the puncture site reveals a well-defined artery (red) and vein (blue) and a small amount of extravascular color assignment in soft tissues. *B,* The area of AVM is defined by the presence of random color assignment in perivascular soft tissues. This so-called color Doppler bruit is diagnostic of an AVM. Color assignment beyond the vessels is secondary to tissue vibration around a jet of high-speed flow. In true AVMs, the color in soft tissues will not clear regardless of how low the gain settings are made.

the time of embolization to guide the initial percutaneous puncture of an optimal vessel for the local injection of embolic material.

Acquired AVMs are usually the result of a single direct communication between a main artery and the adjacent vein. These lesions tend to be relatively small (particularly those that occur after arteriography) and do not spawn the collection of dilated vessels typical of congenital AVMs. Only rarely does color Doppler actually define a jet of arterial flow in the vein.[2] Instead, a "color Doppler bruit"[4] is seen in the area of the communication, and this finding should be considered diagnostic (Fig. 116-10). Low-resistance flow in the artery and arterialization of the vein may be subtle or absent but, when present, may be used as confirmation of the existence of an AVM.

REFERENCES

1. Grassi CJ, Polak JF: Axillary and subclavian venous thrombosis: follow-up evaluation with color Doppler flow US and venography, *Radiology* 175:651-654, 1990.
2. Igidbashian VN et al: Iatrogenic femoral arteriovenous fistulae: diagnosis with color Doppler imaging, *Radiology* 170:749-753, 1989.
3. Knudson GJ et al: Color Doppler sonographic imaging in the assessment of upper-extremity deep venous thrombosis, *AJR* 154:399-403, 1990.
4. Middleton WD, Erickson S, Melson GL: Perivascular color artifact: pathologic significance and appearance on color Doppler US images, *Radiology* 171:647-652, 1989.

CHAPTER 117

Upper extremity venous imaging with duplex scanning

JOANN M. LOHR, THOMAS M. KERR, TREVOR M. VanWAGENEN, and JOHN J. CRANLEY

Duplex scanning has had a revolutionary impact on the vascular laboratory. It has become the standard noninvasive method for examining the carotid arteries,[1,2] the veins,[3,7,11,17,18] the arteries, and the soft tissues of the lower extremity[9] and is showing great promise for the examination of renal[13] and other visceral vessels of the abdomen.[16] In the upper extremity it is equally useful and easier to perform, plus it yields greater detail because of the decreased tissue mass involved.[10] The number of patients coming to the vascular laboratory for the evaluation of upper extremity problems is far less than the number coming for carotid or lower extremity testing. The study described in this chapter is a continuation of a previous review, such that the study period now extends from July 1984 to October 1991.[12] Duplex scanning was performed on 877 upper extremities. Table 117-1 lists the clinical indications for these scans. These scans represent 2.7% of all tests (n = 32,780), 4.7% of the duplex scans of the lower extremity (n = 18,736), and 7.1% of the scans done to evaluate carotid artery disease (n = 12,338) in this vascular laboratory.

MATERIAL AND METHODS

All scans were performed with a commercially available, high-resolution duplex instrument (Biosound 2000IIA, Biosound Phase II, or Acuson 128). The interpreter graded early scans for quality using the following system: poor, a portion of the scan was not interpretable; fair, the diagnosis could be made, but the entire scan was not well visualized; good, all structures were well visualized. Grading for quality was discontinued in 1989. The quality of a scan is reported as either acceptable or unacceptable. If unacceptable, repeat scanning or another modality was suggested.

All patient's hospital charts were reviewed and their medical history, hospital course, demographic information, treatment, and follow-up data obtained. The variables examined included symptoms and signs and their duration; the admitting diagnosis; possible hypercoagulable states; the presence, type, and extent of existing neoplasia; the presence and type of peripheral or central venous access; the type of venous catheter (single, triple-lumen, or Swan-Ganz); and its site of placement. Also analyzed was the composition of intravenous fluids administered. The diagnostic tests and location of the thrombi were reviewed, as well as the duration and type of anticoagulant or lytic therapy.

A standard laboratory protocol was followed for each duplex scanning session.[10] The upper extremity examination begins with a detailed assessment of signs and symptoms and past medical history plus risk-factor analysis. A very important aspect of the patient's history is whether intravenous catheters have been used and, if so, the location of insertion and the duration of use. The patient is then placed in the supine position and the examination begins with the radial vein, which is visualized from the wrist to the brachial vein. Next, the ulnar vein is followed from the wrist up to the antecubital fossa, where the ulnar and radial veins form the brachial vein. Then the brachial vein is followed into the upper arm. At the junction of the basilic and brachial veins, the axillary vein is formed. The axillary vein is followed under the shoulder in the direction of the clavicle. The junction of the cephalic and axillary veins forms the subclavian vein. The junction of the subclavian and jugular veins, including the innominate vein, is not routinely visualized because of its depth. Doppler signal analysis provides indirect information about the patency of these veins. The Doppler signal of the subclavian vein is assessed. Normally it is spontaneous and phasic with augmentation and shows no reflux. Next, the internal jugular vein is examined in a cephalad direction from the clavicle until it dives under the mandible. A Doppler signal is also obtained in the in-

Table 117-1. Indications for 877 consecutive upper extremity scans

Indication	No. (%)
Rule out thrombosis	430 (49)
Vein mapping	267 (31)
Graft surveillance	108 (12)
Rule out soft tissue abnormality	42 (5)
Arterial scans	30 (3)
TOTAL	877

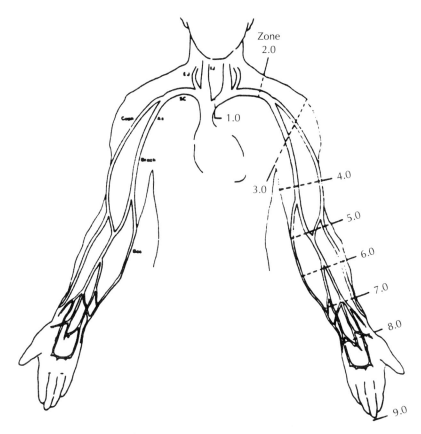

Fig. 117-1. Zones of reference for upper extremity venous scanning: suprasternal notch, 1.0; acromion, 3.0; antecubital fossa, 5.0; wrist, 8.0; and fingertips, 9.0.

ternal jugular vein, where spontaneous and phasic qualities are assessed.

Finally, the superficial veins are assessed by following the basilic vein along the ulna until it joins the brachial vein. The larger-diameter antecubital vein connects the basilic and cephalic systems at the antecubital fossa. The antecubital perforator is also seen connecting the cephalic and brachial veins. The cephalic vein is traced along the radius and upper arm and then joins with the axillary vein.

In this laboratory, the upper extremity is divided into zones for purposes of convenience in communicating the position of the probe and localizing abnormal findings discovered during the examination.[4] Each zone covers approximately 10 cm in length on the extremity. Zone 1 is located in the suprasternal notch, zone 3 is at the acromial clavicular process, zone 5 is at the antecubital fossa, and zone 8 is at the wrist (Fig. 117-1).

When a visible intraluminal thrombus is identified, several of its characteristics can be assessed to determine its relative age (Table 117-2). The clot may be either partially or totally occluding. If totally occluding, this indicates a more acute process. Free-floating thrombi are actually tethered distally but extend cephalad in the vein without a more proximal attachment to the vessel wall. These free-floating tails exhibit a side-to-side waving in the venous lumen that

can be induced by gently bouncing the probe on the skin or with respiration. Free-floating tails usually become attached to the venous wall within 1 to 2 weeks.

Clot retraction is defined as a concentric separation of the thrombus from the vein walls. There appears to be a very thin gap between the thrombus and the circumference of the venous wall. Retraction is thought to occur within a few hours of thrombus formation through clot contraction of the platelet, fibrin mesh formation, and extrusion of serum. This usually only lasts 1 to 2 weeks and then becomes adherent to the vein wall.

When the vein is dilated to a larger than normal diameter by a thrombus with a large cross section, this is referred to as *clot distention*. *Distention* in this context differs from the venous distention caused by obstruction or venous hypertension in the absence of an intraluminal thrombus. In the latter, it is possible to completely collapse the wall of the vein with the pressure of the probe and a Doppler signal is received. Veins exhibiting clot distention gradually shrink over several weeks to months.

An acutely thrombosed vein may be partially compressible, whereas a chronically thrombosed vein is not. Acute thrombi can be deformed by only light probe pressure. When viewed transversely, the round vein appears oblong. A thrombus remains soft for approximately 24 hours after for-

Table 117-2. Clot characteristics: relative value in clot aging

Characteristic	Acute value		Chronic value	
Degree of occlusion	Total	**	Partial	**
Free floating	Free	****	Stationary	**
Clot retraction	Retracted	***	Adherent	***
Clot distention	Distended	***	Contracted	**
Clot compressibility	Soft	****	Firm	*
Surface character	Smooth	**	Irregular	**
Echogenicity	Faint	*	Bright	*
Homogeneity	Homogeneous	**	Heterogeneous	**
Collaterals	Absent	*	Present	****
Recanalization	Absent	*	Present	****

From Karkow WS, Ruoff BA, Cranley JJ: *B-mode venous imaging.* In Kempczinski RF, Yao JST, eds: *Practical noninvasive vascular diagnosis,* Chicago, 1982, Mosby.
****, A diagnostic level; ***, good; **, fair; and *, poor (nondiagnostic). Each asterisk indicates the relative value assigned to each criterion in the interpretation of clot age; many criteria are only valuable when present, and the overall decision represents a weighted average.

mation. The clot surface may be smooth or irregular, and this is usually best assessed by a longitudinal view of the thrombus tip. Acute thrombi tend to have smooth rounded tips due to the continued surrounding flow.

Echogenicity is defined as an overall brightness of the clot compared with the surrounding tissues. Brightly echogenic thrombi tend to be more chronic, since they are more dense because of serum resorption. However, apparent changes in echogenicity may be influenced by alteration of the electrical gains of the instrument, the depth of the structure being accessed, and acoustic shadowing of the overlying tissues, making it a somewhat subjective finding. Homogeneity is also assessed. Acute thrombi tend to be more homogeneous, whereas chronic thrombi tend to be more heterogeneous.

The development of collateral venous channels is an absolute sign of chronic thrombosis. These channels are very small, lie parallel to the main trunk, and do not contain valves. Normal venous tributaries are larger, enter the main venous channel at an acute angle, and contain valves. Collateral venous channels are best visualized in a transverse view and may be visible as early as 1 to 2 weeks after the initial thrombosis but usually are not seen for a month or more after venous occlusion.

Recanalization is evidenced by an open, collapsible channel that runs through a thrombus. A recanalized channel is totally surrounded by clot. This tends to occur rather late.

Using the characteristics mentioned, thrombi can be classified as acute, chronic, or indeterminate. This classification must be based on the characteristics of the entire thrombus and not on an isolated segment because deep vein thrombosis is a continuing process. For this reason, a single thrombus may manifest various aging characteristics in differing regions. Repeat duplex scans are often necessary and frequently show the evolution of characteristics that were equivocal in the initial scans.

A total of 42 studies were performed to evaluate soft tissue abnormalities, but they can likewise be differentiated by their characteristics. The topic of pulsatile groin masses in patients with a history of femoral trauma was recently reviewed by Montefusco et al.[15] Features of pseudoaneurysms included visible intraluminal swirling and turbulent Doppler spectra. Frequently associated findings included a centrifugal thrombus with a superimposed arterial spectrum and a visible arterial laceration.

Abscesses, on the other hand, have hyperechoic contents, give off no Doppler signal, have inducible eddy motions, and frequently have an echo-dense capsule. Common associated findings include regional solidification.[15]

Hematomas exhibit a variable echo density, are noncompressible, have no fluid movement or clear margins, and give off no Doppler signal. If they are less than 12 hours old, there may be hypoechoic focal liquefaction. If they are more than 2 weeks old, dissection through the soft tissues is frequently seen.[15]

Edema fluid is radiolucent, follows tissue planes, and is not compressible. Lymph nodes are spherical and encapsulated with a mixed internal echogenicity and are noncompressible. Small lymph nodes may be invisible or difficult to see. Large lymph nodes, of course, are seen in the presence of infection, cellulitis, or tumor involvement. In fact, the duplex scan image of a large swollen lymph node shows an architecture strikingly similar to the cross section of a lymph node as depicted in pathology textbooks.

Cysts are best seen in a transverse view and stand out from the surrounding tissues. They are slightly echogenic and, in a transverse image, can be distinguished from the surrounding structures. They may be partially compressible. At times a cyst may compress an artery or vein, causing an increase in the peak velocity signal.

Duplex scanning is of special value for the evaluation of aneurysms and pseudoaneurysms and for graft surveillance. The past 5 years have witnessed the rapid expansion of the use of duplex imaging in the diagnosis and evaluation of upper extremity venous thrombosis and soft tissue abnormalities, and for arterial and graft evaluation. This area of clinical interest will likely continue to expand. Requests for examinations of the upper extremity have increased as more knowledge has been gained.

ACCURACY

In a multicenter collaborative study that assessed the accuracy of lower extremity duplex scanning, it was reported that the duplex scan was 97% sensitive in extremities with positive phlebograms.[4,5] The phlebogram was negative, however, in 191 extremities and was considered to be incorrect in 6 instances. Thus it was not a perfect standard when negative, and the duplex scan was slightly more accurate.

It has not been possible to generate similar data for the upper extremity because there is a blind area behind the clavicle. Thus a negative duplex scan does not absolutely

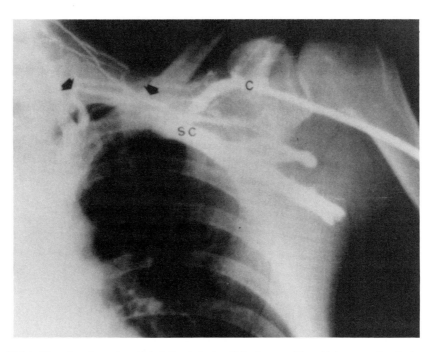

Fig. 117-2. Thrombus *(arrowheads)* in left subclavian *(SC)* diagnosed by phlebogram; the duplex scan was negative. In the mid and medial portion of the subclavian vein, the clavicle prevents visualization of clot and the cephalic vein (C) cannot be compressed. The Doppler signal may be unobtainable. (From Kerr TM et al: *Diagnosis of upper extremity venous thrombosis by duplex scanning.* In Bergan JJ, Yao JST, eds: *Venous disorders,* Philadelphia, 1991, Saunders.)

rule out thrombus in a subclavian vein. A phlebogram was requested whenever there was doubt, but only 8 were actually obtained. While all were confirmatory, it is possible that some subclavian vein thromboses were missed. In most cases, however, a negative scan and normal Doppler signals in the subclavian vein are accepted as evidence of a normal vein. Fig. 117-2 shows a thrombus in the left subclavian vein in a patient whose scan was negative. This patient was seen before this study was initiated. It is not known whether any patients with negative scans during this study were later found to have subclavian vein thromboses, but again, some may have been missed.

SIGNS AND SYMPTOMS

As in the lower extremity, the signs and symptoms of deep vein thrombosis of the upper extremity are not diagnostic. Of those scans done to rule out venous thrombosis, 63% (269 of 430) did not identify a clot. All these patients were referred to the vascular laboratory because they had symptoms, the most common ones being pain, tenderness, and swelling. Pain and tenderness were as common in the extremities that proved to have venous thrombosis as in those that did not. Swelling was more common in the extremities with confirmed thrombosis, but this was not a statistically significant finding.

SUPERFICIAL THROMBOPHLEBITIS

The diagnosis of superficial thrombophlebitis in both the upper and lower extremities has been considered to be made with certainty based solely on physical examination findings. However, duplex scanning has demonstrated that some of these thrombosed veins can extend far beyond the portion that is palpable in the superficial vein and can project into the deep system. In a recent review,[14] 31% of patients with superficial thrombophlebitis of the lower extremities were found to have at least one complication, in most cases consisting of extension into the deep system. In several instances, the same clinically unexpected extension was noted in the upper extremity, with the thrombus extending from a superficial vein in the forearm to the brachial vein.

VENOUS THROMBOSIS RESULTS

To assess the accuracy of duplex scanning in patients with suspected venous thrombosis, 877 consecutive upper extremity duplex scans were reviewed (Table 117-1). Of 430 scans performed, 161 (37%) were positive. A total of 284 thrombosed veins were identified, with two or more veins involved in many cases. A probable risk factor was identified in 99 extremities in which the thrombosis involved the subclavian or axillary vein, or both. An isolated internal jugular vein thrombosis was found in 11 extremities, and an isolated superficial vein thrombosis was detected in 51. Table 117-3 and Fig. 117-3 show a breakdown of the location of these thrombi.

Tables 117-4 and 117-5 show the associated risk factors. The most common was the insertion of a central or peripheral venous catheter, and this involved 64 of 99 (65%) patients with axillary-subclavian venous thrombosis. Table

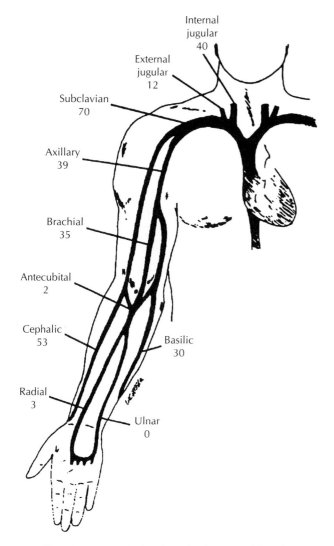

Fig. 117-3. Numerical and graphic location of thrombi.

117-4 also shows the risk factors when the indwelling catheter is excluded, and malignancy was then the most frequently identified risk factor. There were no identifiable risk factor in 101 patients with thromboses.

Table 117-6 lists the type of catheters used in those patients with confirmed thrombosis. Hyperalimentation formula had been infused in 27%.

Of 61 patients with axillary-subclavian vein thrombosis available for follow-up, 5 (8.2%) had a clinical diagnosis of pulmonary embolism and 2 died. The cause of death was believed to be a pulmonary embolism in both, although autopsies were not performed. Of these patients, 1 had had a negative lower extremity duplex scan and a negative venacavogram. Five upper extremity venograms and one phleborheogram had been obtained, all of which were positive. Two of the five emboli occurred in patients with axillary-subclavian thrombosis that developed while a catheter was in place, 2 patients did not have an indwelling catheter, and

Table 117-3. Veins involved by thrombosis in 161 upper extremities

Veins	No.
Subclavian	70
Cephalic	53
Internal jugular	40
Axillary	39
Brachial	35
Basilic	30
External jugular	12
Radial	3
Antecubital	02
Frequently encountered combinations	
Subclavian-axillary	36
Subclavian-axillary-brachial	29
Subclavian-axillary-brachial-internal jugular	16

Table 117-4. Axillary-subclavian thrombosis: associated risk factors in 99 patients

Risk factor	No.	%
Indwelling venous catheter	64	65
Excluding indwelling catheter (n = 35)		
Malignancy	14	40
Physical strain	7	20
Hypercoagulability	6	17
Obesity	4	11
Drug abuse	3	9
Pregnancy	1	3

Table 117-5. Isolated internal jugular vein thrombosis: associated risk factors in 11 patients

Risk factor	No.	%
Internal jugular venous line	8	73
Chronic renal failure	2	18
Neck abscess (drug abuse)	1	09

Table 117-6. Types of catheters associated with 119 cases of upper extremity venous thrombosis

Types of venous catheter	No.	%
Central catheter	84	71
Swan Ganz	22	26
Triple lumen	20	24
Unspecified	17	20
Porta-Cath	11	13
Dialysis	11	13
Pacemaker	3	4
Peripheral catheter (unspecified)	35	29

thrombosis arose at the site of a previous peripheral venous catheter in 1 patient.

Axillary-subclavian thrombosis that developed in 7 extremities was believed to have arisen from a peripheral intravenous site. In 5, the thrombi extended from the cephalic or basilic veins into the brachial and subclavian veins. When the thrombotic process extended into the jugular veins, it was included in the axillary-subclavian group. In addition, 11 cases of an isolated internal jugular vein thrombosis were diagnosed. In 8 it was related to an indwelling catheter. In 1 the thrombosis arose as the result of a neck abscess stemming from drug abuse, and 2 patients suffered from chronic renal failure. No pulmonary emboli or postthrombotic sequelae occurred in this group.

At 2 years, almost half of the patients with axillary-subclavian thrombosis were dead, indicating the high mortality in this group of patients. A total of 36% of the patients in this study complained of residual symptoms. It has been suggested that extending anticoagulation therapy beyond the acute event may decrease these sequelae.[6] However, this approach may be most effective in patients with catheter-associated thrombosis but not in those with other predisposing factors. It has also been reported[6,8] that there is less morbidity resulting from catheter-associated venous thrombosis than from primary venous thrombosis of the axillary-subclavian vein. This was also true in the review described here.

DISCUSSION

Major vein thrombosis of the upper extremities is becoming more common because of the frequent use of indwelling catheters, as indicated by the data shown in Tables 117-3 and 117-4. Excluding an indwelling catheter as a risk factor, malignancy was then the most common predisposing factor. All the cardiac patients with deep vein thrombosis had an indwelling catheter. This is probably related to the large catheters used in such patients. In 27% of the patients with a central catheter, hyperalimentation fluid was infused, adding to the risk. Quite unexpectedly, seven instances of a thrombus spreading from a superficial vein to the deep system were encountered.

CONCLUSION

Duplex scanning of the upper extremity is a practical method of diagnosing upper extremity venous thrombosis. The one blind area under the clavicle requires the use of phlebography in selected cases. The use of duplex imaging has expanded rapidly in recent years. The decreased mass of the upper extremity compared with the lower extremity makes duplex scanning easier and probably more accurate. The diagnosis of cysts, hemorrhage, aneurysms, and thrombosed grafts is also easily made and accurate. The use of duplex scanning to evaluate upper extremity abnormalities is expected to continue to expand.

REFERENCES

1. Barber FE et al: *Duplex scanner II for simultaneous imaging of artery tissues and flow,* IEEE publication 74, CHOop61SU, Ultrasonic Symposium Proceedings, New York, 1974, Institute for Electrical and Electronics Engineers.
2. Comerota AJ, Cranley JJ, Cook SE: Real time B-mode carotid imaging in diagnosis of cerebrovascular disease, *Surgery* 89:718-729, 1981.
3. Cranley JJ: Seeing is believing: a clot is a clot, on a duplex scan or a phlebogram, *Echocardiography* 4:423, 1987 (editorial).
4. Cranley JJ: *Diagnosis of deep venous thrombosis.* In Bernstein EF, ed: *Recent advances in noninvasive diagnostic techniques in vascular disease,* St Louis, 1990, Mosby.
5. Cranley JJ et al: Near parity in the final diagnosis of deep venous thrombosis by duplex scan and phlebography, *Phlebology* 4:71-74, 1989.
6. Donayre CE et al: Pathogenesis determines late morbidity of axillo-subclavian vein thrombosis, *Am J Surg* 152:179-184, 1986.
7. Flannagan LD, Sullivan ED, Cranley JJ: *Venous imaging of the extremities using real-time B-mode ultrasound.* In Bergan JJ, Yao JST, eds: *Surgery of the veins,* Orlando, Fla, 1984, Grune & Stratton.
8. Gloviczki P, Kazmier FJ, Hollier LH: Axillary-subclavian venous occlusion: the morbidity of a nonlethal disease, *J Vasc Surg* 4:333-337, 1986.
9. Johnston KW, Kassam M, Cobbold RSC: Relationship between Doppler pulsatility index and direct femoral pressure measurements in the diagnosis of aortoiliac occlusive disease, *Ultrasound Med Biol* 9:271-281, 1983.
10. Karkow WS, Ruoff BA, Cranley JJ: *B-mode venous imaging.* In Kempczinski RF, Yao JST, eds: *Practical noninvasive vascular diagnosis,* Chicago, 1987, Mosby.
11. Kerr TM et al: Analysis of 1084 consecutive lower extremities involved with acute venous thrombosis diagnosed by duplex scanning, *Surgery* 108:520-527, 1990.
12. Kerr TM et al: Upper extremity venous thromboses diagnosed by duplex scanning, *Am J Surg* 160:202-206, 1990.
13. Kohler TR et al: Noninvasive diagnosis of renal artery stenosis by ultrasonic duplex scanning, *J Vasc Surg* 4:450-456, 1986.
14. Lutter KS et al: Superficial thrombophlebitis diagnosed by duplex scanning, *Surgery* 110:42-46, 1991.
15. Montefusco C et al: The role of duplex ultrasonography in the differentiation of pseudoaneurysm, hematoma, and access, *J Vasc Tech* 14:11-17, 1990.
16. Nicholls SC et al: Use of hemodynamic parameters in the diagnosis of mesenteric insufficiency, *J Vasc Surg* 3:507-510, 1986.
17. Sullivan ED, Peter DJ, Cranley JJ: Real-time B-mode venous ultrasound, *J Vasc Surg* 1:465-471, 1984.
18. Talbot SR: Use of real-time imaging in identifying deep venous obstruction: a preliminary report, *Bruit* 6:41-42, 1982.

PART FOUR

NEW APPLICATIONS AND DIRECTIONS IN VASCULAR DIAGNOSIS

CHAPTER 118

Intravascular ultrasound imaging

RICHARD I. KITNEY

The current clinical interest in intravascular ultrasonic imaging arises primarily from a desire to image arterial plaque and also in response to the increasing use of angioplasty. To date, three techniques have been used for this purpose: contrast angiography, fiberoptic angiography, and intravascular ultrasonic imaging.

CONTRAST ANGIOGRAPHY

The most commonly used technique for imaging arterial disease has been contrast angiography. In this method, a small catheter is introduced into the arterial tree and radiopaque dye is injected. Several cardiac cycles are then recorded onto x-ray–sensitive cine film. However, this technique has a number of disadvantages in that it is difficult (1) to detect early or minimal atherosclerotic disease, (2) to determine the severity of the stenosis and vessel diameter, (3) to differentiate eccentric from concentric plaques, (4) to characterize the tissue composition of the plaque and distinquish between plaque and thrombus, and (5) to detect ulceration or dissection.[23]

FIBEROPTIC ANGIOGRAPHY

An alternative approach to contrast angiography is fiberoptic angiography. This technique, which is comparatively new, requires flushing of the blood from the region to be viewed—a somewhat cumberson procedure. Nevertheless, the method yields higher-resolution images than does contrast angiography and is capable of identifying such defects as luminal flaps and thrombi. One key disadvantage of the method is that direct viewing of the arterial wall will not divulge the presence of very early plaque and is incapable of any form of tissue characterization.

INTRAVASCULAR ULTRASONIC IMAGING

Intraluminal ultrasound techniques are a well-established part of the diagnostic methodology for evaluating other hollow viscera (e.g., rectal and vaginal ultrasound, transesophageal echocardiography). Endovascular transducers were first used more than 35 years ago, and a good review of early transducer technology has been published by Bom et al.[5] Nevertheless, the use of ultrasound to study the arterial wall from within the lumen—angioscopic ultrasound—is

in its clinical infancy. The past 10 years has seen growing interest in this technique, in parallel with the development of arterial angioplasty and related techniques.[28] This interest has led in turn to the allocation of significant resources into research and development in this area.[10]

The demand for better arterial imaging

Conventional contrast angiography that uses selective injection techniques provides the interventional cardiologist and radiologist with a "road map" that allows the identification and localization of atheromatous plaques throughout most of the arterial tree. These images also provide information about the arterial lumen. An abnormality of the arterial wall and the presence of atheromatous plaque must be inferred from changes in luminal caliber (Fig. 118-1). The method tends to underestimate the extent and severity of the atherosclerotic process, as borne out by pathologic findings obtained postmortem[3] and by findings yielded from intraoperative epicardial imaging using high-frequency ultrasonic transducers.[20] In addition, intraobserver and interobserver variability may be great.[30] Using fiberoptic angioscopy, the inner surface of the arterial wall can be visualized directly in real time, and this has contributed significantly to present understanding of acute ischemic syndromes.[29]

An alternative approach is to image with ultrasound from within the arterial lumen using a catheter-mounted transducer. This has several advantages over other types of imaging modalities. In particular, it enables the acquisition of real-time, high-resolution images without the need to obstruct blood flow. Furthermore, information about the full thickness of the arterial wall and not just the "visible" surface can be collected that may help in the differentiation between structures within the wall.

The demand for more detailed imaging of the arterial wall and for the ability to distinguish with greater certainty between different components within the wall has coincided with the advent of intraluminal treatment techniques that serve as alternatives to vascular surgery in patients with obstructive atherosclerotic arterial disease. In particular, second-generation therapeutic techniques, such as mechanical atherectomy and laser angioplasty, carry a significant

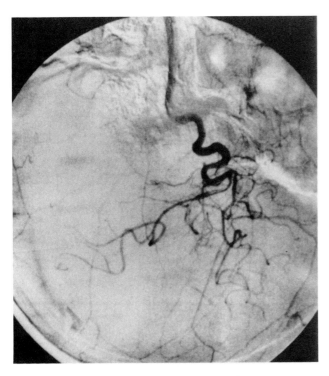

Fig. 118-1. An example of contrast angiography showing narrowing due to plaque. Note that the method gives low-resolution 3D images of the artery.

risk of major vessel-related complications. To minimize this risk, the operator needs an imaging technique that can characterize the whole arterial wall in real-time. Potentially, this need can be met by an intravascular, catheter-mounted ultrasonic imaging system—angioscopic ultrasound.[2,6]

Intravascular ultrasound is a logical extension of the use of balloon angioplasty and other intraarterial treatments. The method has a number of potential advantages: (1) it can produce high-resolution images of the arterial wall, (2) blood is effectively transparent to ultrasound, (3) it is possible to image plaque within the arterial wall in vivo, and (4) the method is minimally invasive. Although image-processing techniques have been applied to conventional angiograms to define sections of the arterial wall for the purposes of measurement, the inherent poor resolution of these images does not allow accurate definition of plaque. Similar techniques can be applied to two-dimensional (2D) monochrome intravascular images with far better results.[9]

THE DISEASE PROCESS

The arterial wall comprises an inner lining of endothelial cells and deep to that lie the intima, media, and adventitia. These different tissues have different acoustic impedances and can be identified using ultrasound. The earliest atherosclerotic lesions arise in the intimal region in the form of fatty streaks rich in lipid. These are thought to stem from an increased permeability to lipoprotein cholesterol in the arterial wall. The next stage in the process is for the fatty streak to broaden and incorporate increased amounts of free cholesterol, which become crystalline. This is believed to represent a predisease state and has therefore been called a *preatheroma*. This state can be considered to represent the transition between fatty streaks and atheromatous plaque.[7]

An atheromatous plaque is characterized by the presence of cholesterol monohydrate crystals. For an atheromatous plaque to form, fatty streaks must first appear, followed by thickening of the intima, foam cell formation, and finally cellular necrosis (Fig. 118-2). The intimal cells must enter a phase of positive cholesterol balance. Thus for the disease to occur, these cells must take up more cholesterol from lipoproteins or lipid particles than they are capable of metabolizing or secreting. From an imaging standpoint, the various stages of plaque development spawn different types of tissues possessing significantly different acoustic properties. Lipid pools acoustically resemble water and thus have a low acoustic signature. Conversely, necrotic structures are often highly calcified and have a high acoustic signature.

TRADITIONAL ULTRASONIC IMAGING METHODS

Much of the current clinical diagnosis of peripheral arterial disease relies on duplex ultrasonic scanners. Fig. 118-3 is a block diagram of a typical duplex scanner that can be divided into two sections, the B-mode image, which comprises a 2D monochrome arterial map, and a velocity estimate.

The B-mode image

The B-mode image is constructed from a series of A-scan lines. As displayed in Fig. 118-4, with the transducer in position for sector 1, the piezoelectric crystal on the scan head is energized and ultrasound is transmitted through the tissue. At every change in the histologic structure (acoustic interface), a partial reflection occurs, which is a function of the reflection coefficient of the medium. If the acoustic impedance of tissue sections a and b are defined as Z_a and Z_b, respectively, the reflection coefficient (R) can be defined as the following:

$$R = \frac{Z_b - Z_a}{Z_b + Z_a} \tag{1}$$

Equation 1 shows that when there is no change in acoustic impedance, $Z_a = Z_b$ and hence R is 0. Depending on the size of the acoustic impedance change at an interface, R will be large or small, in the range of 0 to 1. If A_i is the amplitude of the incident wave and A_r the amplitude of the reflected wave, then:

$$A_r = RA_i \tag{2}$$

The amplitude of the transmitted wave (A_t) is therefore $A_i - A_r$, and:

$$A_t = (1 - R) A_i \tag{3}$$

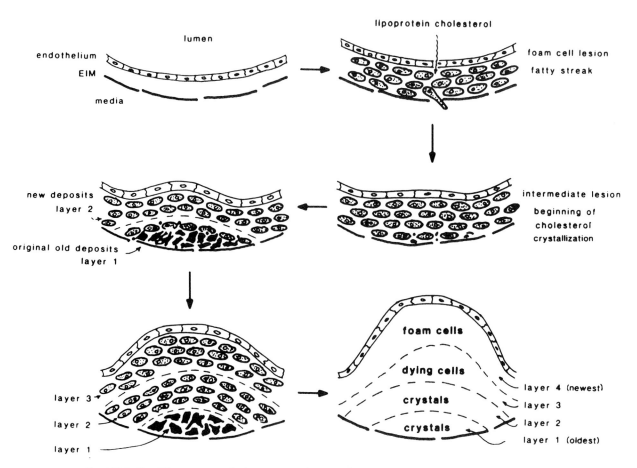

Fig. 118-2. Possible sequence of atherogenesis: the normal intima progresses through a series of stages to atheroma.

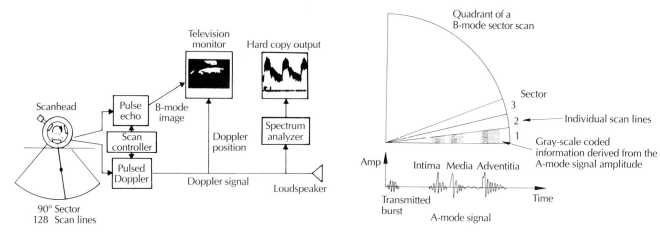

Fig. 118-3. A duplex scanner. The device can be split into two sections: the B-mode image with a 3D monochrome image of the arterial section and a velocity estimate calculated from the Doppler signal.

Fig. 118-4. Quadrant of a B-mode sector scan constructed from a series of individual A-mode scan lines.

When the ultrasonic transducer is operating in the receiving mode, a series of reflected waves will be received. The transmitted burst and the reflected signals from different acoustic interfaces are shown in the A-mode signal for sector 1 (Fig. 118-4). Two points should be noted from this:

1. The time axis on the received A-scan can be translated into distance by multiplying it by the velocity of sound.
2. The transmitted signal loses power at every acoustic interface; thus the reflected signal is often amplified according to the distance of its point of origin from the transducer.

Flow disturbance analysis and color flow mapping

The second approach to the study of arterial disease that is incorporated into a duplex scanner is the estimation of flow disturbance. In its simplest form, this comprises the determination of flow at a single point in the flow field, based on one sample volume or range cell. Flow is translated into velocity by the Doppler equation:

$$\Delta F = \frac{2F_0 \times V \times \cos\theta}{C} \tag{4}$$

where:

F_0 = The master oscillator frequency
C = The speed of sound
V = The speed of the particles
θ = The angle between the ultrasonic beam and the direction of motion.

The filtered signal, which is sometimes called the *audio Doppler signal,* is sampled at a particular depth at the pulse-repetition frequency (a typical value used for the study of peripheral disease is 20 kHz). A simplified mathematical expression of this signal is[27]:

$$y(t) = Re[\bar{s}(t) \times \exp(jw_D t)] \tag{5}$$

where:

w_D = The Doppler frequency shift and is frequently a function of time
$\bar{s}(t)$ = The complex envelope of the transmitted signal
c = A constant

The function $\bar{s}(t)$ introduces random-amplitude modulation in the frequency-modulated Doppler signal given by equation 5. The accurate estimation of Doppler frequency (w_D) in equation 5 is vital for the derivation of the pulsatile blood velocity waveform. Such a signal can carry important information concerning high-frequency flow structures.[18,25,26] These structures can be significant for the detection of arterial stenosis, as exemplified by the dog aorta model described in these papers.

The underlying assumption is that flow is disturbed by an arterial plaque, and thus there is a direct relationship between flow disturbance and the development of atherosclerotic plaque. This relationship is, however, complex.[15] The single-range cell approach to the tracking of blood flow has now been extended to multiple-range cells in which an entire section of the artery is imaged and blood velocity is color encoded. The color flow mapping technique results in a 2D scaler flow field. There are a number of problems with color flow mapping, although at present the method is generally considered to have definite clinical advantages over standard duplex scanning. Two of the principal problems of the approach are that (1) blood flow is really a three-dimensional (3D) vectorial flow field and (2) it is not possible to distinguish between the tortuosity of the vessel and a real change in velocity. Either of these phenomena can produce the same color flow map.

BASIC DESIGN OF INTRAVASCULAR IMAGING SYSTEMS

Intravascular imaging systems have largely evolved from standard duplex scanning technology. As previously described, the B-mode image produced by a duplex scanner is typically obtained from a series of A-mode scans, which are formed into a sector scan. A similar principle is applied in the case of intravascular ultrasound IVUS systems, except that the sector scan, which for example may be 90°, is replaced by a full 360° scan. Fig. 118-5 shows a typical A-mode scan obtained from the firing of a single crystal. This is then converted into a 360° B-mode scan, as illustrated in Fig. 118-6. In the case of analogue systems (which comprise the vast majority of the commercially available IVUS systems), the A-mode signals are continuously translated into the B-mode scan by converting the amplitude of the signal into a gray scale. The alternative is to digitize the radio-frequency A-mode signal and create a digital B-mode image. This method implies that the number of A-mode signals comprising the B-mode scan are predefined. However, with digital systems it is possible to employ sophisticated beam-forming techniques.[2]

A typical IVUS system has three main components: the ultrasonic catheter, the transceiver (which drives the ultra-

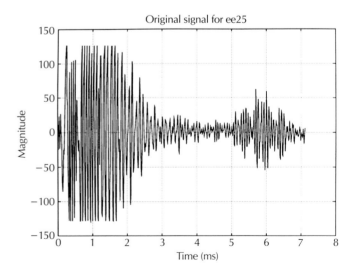

Fig. 118-5. An example of a typical A-mode scan line obtained from firing a single crystal. Note the echo from the arterial wall that begins to appear after 5 ms.

sonic crystals and receives the A-mode response), and the display system. The display system can include anything from simple analogue electronics, capable of producing a basic monochrome 360° raster scan, to highly sophisticated 3D visualization techniques based on the latest graphics work stations.[17] The next sections focus on the ultrasonic catheter and display technology. These are the two critical areas of IVUS technology that differentiate among the various systems under development. The design of transceiver technology will be considered only in relation to the processing of data and image formation.

INTRAVASCULAR CATHETER DESIGN

There are currently three basic types of intraarterial catheter designs: a single rotating crystal, a rotating mirror with a single fixed crystal, and a phased array. Only the last type has no moving parts.

Single rotating crystal catheters

A schematic of a single rotating crystal catheter is provided in Fig. 118-7. A key element in the design of an intraarterial catheter with a rotating mirror is the flexibility of the shaft, which must be consistent with the ability of the drive shaft to rotate the tip at a constant angular velocity, typically of the order of 4000 rpm. Even minor variations in speed can cause "image creep," as illustrated in Fig. 118-7. One potential advantage of this type of catheter is that because of the internal path of the ultrasound beam, the catheter can be placed very close to the arterial wall without the reflected signal interfering with the transmitted signal.

Rotating mirror catheters

The design of the rotating mirror catheter is similar to that of the single rotating crystal. Fig. 118-7 shows that the mirror is fixed to the drive shaft and reflects the ultrasonic beam. The advantage of this method over the rotating element catheter is that no electrical connections associated with the rotating parts are needed.

Phased array catheters

The third type of catheter, which is used in IVUS, is the phased array (Fig. 118-7). This differs in a number of important ways from the rotating element and rotating mirror types: (1) there are no moving parts, (2) the number of elements varies according to the lateral resolution required, (3) there is no internal dead zone path, and (4) there are multiple crystals, as opposed to single crystals, which are used in the other two types.

Table 118-1 lists the commercially available intravascular catheters. Only Endosonics manufactures phased array catheters. Because of the extreme difficulty in forming and machining solid ceramic material with an outer diameter of 1.8 mm for 5-French and 1.2 mm for 3.5-French catheters, they are believed to use PVDF (piezoelectric film). In the early 1970s, Bom, Lancee, and van Egmond[4] were able to produce a 32-element phased array catheter with an outer diameter of 3.2 mm mounted on a 9-French catheter and operating at 5.6 MHz.

A comparison of rotating and fixed element designs

Rotational catheters. Whether the rotational catheter has a fixed crystal, a rotating mirror, or vice versa, the advantages and disadvantages of this type of catheter are similar.

Advantages. The principal advantage of rotational catheters is that they represent a direct extension of existing

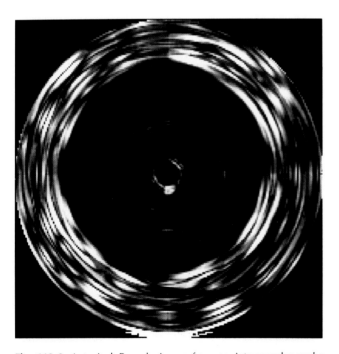

Fig. 118-6. A typical B-mode image from an intravascular probe placed in a section of a normal artery.

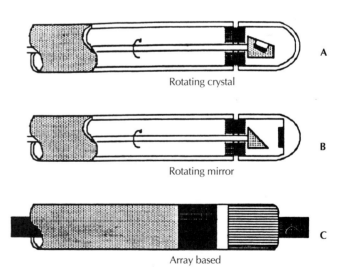

Fig. 118-7. Examples of different catheter designs. *A,* A single rotating crystal (rotation speed typically 3000 rpm). *B,* Rotating mirror design, with a fixed crystal shown in black at the tip. *C,* A phased array design comprising multiple crystals that are scanned electronically.

Table 118-1. Intravascular ultrasound catheter manufacturers*

Manufacturer	Available catheters	Transducer type	Frequency (MHz)
Endosonics	7.8F tip with 6.5F shaft	Stationary multielement dynamic aperature array, 64 elements	20
	5.5F tip with 4.5F shaft		20
Inter Therapy	4.9F tip with 5.9F shaft	Mechanically rotating transducer tip, rotating acoustic mirror and rotating piezoelectric crystal	20
Diasonics/Boston Scientific	6.6F	Mechanically rotating piezoelectric crystal, single element	20
	4.8F		20
Cardiovascular Imaging Systems (CVIS)	8F	Mechanically rotating acoustic mirror with fixed piezoelectric crystal	20
	5F		20

*The data represent the best estimates based on the available literature.

technology. This makes it possible to design relatively low-cost electronics to produce simple B-mode images that are largely based on modifications of existing ultrasonic technology used for external imaging. Another advantage is that there is a considerable internal ultrasonic path length that avoids a significant dead zone. (This is discussed in a later section.)

Disadvantages. There are a number of specific disadvantages of mechanically rotating catheters: (1) The configuration of such catheters consists of a central drive shaft with an outer cable, and thus it is not possible to put this type of catheter over a guide wire; (2) the rigid section of the tip is quite long, typically about 5 or 6 mm; (3) the mechanical drive can be unreliable, causing variations in speed that distort the images (image creep); (4) upsizing and downsizing of catheter designs using rotating crystals or mirrors is extremely difficult and usually requires a full redesign for each change in scaling; (5) to obtain accurate high-quality images, the tip of the rotating catheters must contain some form of stable coupling medium such as water; and (6) the cost of manufacturing such catheters in small sizes can be prohibitively expensive.

Phased array catheters. It is difficult to assess the full potential of phased array catheters because only one such device for intravascular imaging is currently on the market. The basic configuration typically comprises 32 or 64 elements placed on the tip of the catheter. These elements are energized by a number of wires inside the sheath and coupled to an electronic multiplexer tip at the transducer tip.

Advantages. A principal advantage of the phased array catheter is that it has no moving parts, so image creep can be eliminated. In addition, because the catheter comprises a phased array, it is possible to carry out image reconstruction using synthetic aperture techniques. Because of the design of the catheter, it is also possible to place it over a guide wire in the manner of more normal angioplasty procedures, and there is no problem with guide wire or strut artifacts.

Disadvantages. The principal disadvantage of phased array catheters is the low signal levels that can be obtained, stemming from the use of polyvinylidene (PVDF) instead of PZT. Phased array ultrasound systems consist of film-based transducers, as opposed to solid ceramic transducers. This typically results in an order of magnitude reduction in signal levels. To eliminate noise artifact, it is often necessary to ensemble average data. A second major disadvantage is that the technology is relatively new and requires the use of complex, and often slightly bulky, electronics, such as a multiplexer.

Specific design issues

Attenuation. Table 118-1 lists the different designs of catheters that are currently available. Apart from CVIS, all these catheters operate at 20 MHz. The choice of frequency is based on the fact that it is inversely proportional to the depth of penetration into the tissue because body tissues attenuate ultrasound signals at higher frequencies. The approximate relationship between attenuation and frequency is expressed as: attenuation = operating frequency × 1 dB/cm,[1] where the scaling factor is an average value calculated from soft tissue. Unlike external ultrasound systems, intravascular imaging systems can insonate tissue structures in the 20- to 40-MHz range. The frequency of the system is important for resolving the axial and lateral resolutions. From this simple analysis it would appear that operating at higher frequencies has distinct advantages. However, to obtain the appropriate range of a B-mode scan, it is customary to operate at 20 MHz, since this has been found to be an optimal frequency. The equation that is used to define the physical property of attenuation is frequency-dependent depth attenuation. The simple equation just given only works over the frequency range 20 to 30 MHz; at higher frequencies, the absorption is much greater and has a non-linear characteristic. A typical penetration depth for 20-MHz ultrasonic transducers is 1 to 2 cm.

Lateral and axial resolution

Axial resolution. Axial resolution is primarily a function of the frequency of the intravascular system and the type of tissue that is being insonated. For example, the speed of sound in water is 1480 m/sec, whereas in muscle it is 1580 m/sec. Thus for a particular imaging system with a burst length of 3 cycles operating at 20 MHz, the axial resolution will be *x* in water and *y* in muscle.

Lateral resolution. The lateral resolution of an ultrasound system is defined in terms of its ability to resolve individual reflecting targets that are perpendicular to the ultrasonic beam. The lateral resolution is best at points close to the catheter in the near field. For a circular transducer, the best lateral resolution is achieved at:

$$\frac{d^2}{4W}$$

where d is the diameter of the transducer and W is the wavelength. Thus, for a 20-MHz system, the wavelength is equal to 70 μm in water. If the diameter of the transducer is 1 mm, the best lateral resolution will be obtained at 3.6 mm from the transducer. This is the general range for intravascular imaging of the arterial wall.

Ringdown. Fig. 118-8 depicts the problem of ringdown in which an electronic excitation pulse causes the crystal on the catheter to ring. There are a number of ways in which ringdown can be minimized. One way is to damp the oscillation of the crystal. This can be achieved by the combination of appropriate backing materials with an appropriate matching layer over the crystal surface. Both work by optimizing the transfer of energy from the crystal to the medium to be imaged. Typically, backing layers consist of tungsten-loaded epoxy. An important criterion for the design of a backing layer is that the impedance of the backing and matching layer materials correspond as closely as possible to the impedance of the acoustic element. A second way to minimize ringdown is to use a greater path length between the ultrasonic crystal and the tissue that is being imaged. This can be achieved readily with rotating mechanical intravascular catheters, since either the crystal or the rotating mirror can be placed some distance from the tissue and produce a significant internal path length within the catheter.

Mechanical catheters are potentially better for minimizing ringdown because they can be placed against the artery wall.

Crystal response

Fig. 118-9 shows that the dimensions of the crystal consist of the width (W), the length (L), and the thickness (T). The two faces of the crystal are connected electrically and a voltage is applied. The applied voltage can take a number of forms, from a single pulse of known width to a sinusoidal burst consisting of a number of cycles. For the purposes of assessing the performance of the crystal, it is assumed that the lateral clamping of the crystal is effective. Therefore the resonance of the crystal is in the standard thickness mode in which the ratio of width to thickness is critical. A plot of the electromechanical coupling factor associated with the width-to-thickness mode is illustrated in Fig. 118-10. The figure shows that, for the piezoelectric crystal material considered here (PZT-5A), the maximum power transfer to the medium lies between 0.45 and 0.65 in the range. Although it is clear that the gain falls off outside this range, the quantity of the electric charge (Q) of the system is nevertheless low by comparison with many other resonance systems. Besides the loss of efficiency outside the preferred range, another problem is that the thickness mode is often subjected to interference from additional oscillations arising from resonances originating from the height and width modes.

In IVUS, the insonation frequency is typically around 20 MHz, and this corresponds to the following crystal dimensions: W, 40.8 μm; T, 74.2 μm; and L, more than 750 μm. The frequencies of the maximum (f_{max}) and minimum (f_{min}) impedances are related to the coupling coefficient (K_{eff}^2) as follows[12,13]:

$$K_{eff}^2 = \frac{\pi}{2}\left(\frac{f_{min}}{f_{max}}\right)\tan^{-1}\left(\frac{\pi f_{min}}{f_{max}}\right) \qquad (6)$$

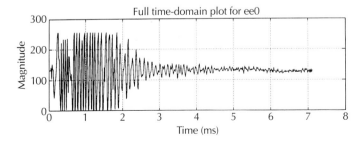

Fig. 118-8. The ringdown problem. The excitation burst occurs between 0.3 and 0.5 ms, followed 0.7 to 2.0 ms later by the ringdown, where the crystal continues to vibrate.

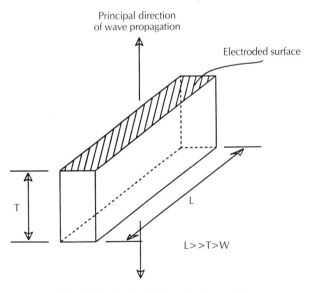

Fig. 118-9. A typical piezo-electric crystal.

Fig. 118-11 shows the operational impedances that can be obtained for different width-to-thickness ratios.

The backing layer. In medical applications, piezoelectric crystals are normally required to resonate into a low-impedance medium, such as water, or in the case of IVUS, into blood. As with other types of resonating systems, the object is for the pressure wave, which is generated by the vibration of the crystal, to be transmitted in a predefined direction

with a minimum reverberation within the transducer. This is normally achieved by using an appropriate backing layer or damping medium such that energy entering the backing layer is absorbed and as little as possible is reflected back into the crystal. It might appear that reflection of energy would strengthen the response of the transducer. However, this can actually result in multiple reflections and destructive interference. Using the transmission line analogue, the characteristic impedance of the backing layer Z_B is defined as:

$$Z_B = \sqrt{Z_t Z_W} \tag{7}$$

where Z_B, Z_T, and Z_L are the characteristic impedances of the backing layer, crystal, and the load (water or blood), respectively.

Fig. 118-12 illustrates the effects of different types of commonly used backing layers.

The matching layer. To achieve a maximal transfer of acoustic energy, it is also necessary to attach a matching layer to the front face of the crystal. This will typically improve the bandwidth and the transduction sensitivity. It is customary to use a quarter-wavelength matching layer, with the optimum acoustic impedance defined by:

$$Z_L = \sqrt{Z_T Z_W} \tag{8}$$

where Z_L, Z_T, and Z_W are again the characteristic impedances of the matching layer, crystal, and water, respectively.

Examples. For a typical PZT crystal operating in water, the matching layer will be optimized with a characteristic impedance of approximately 7 SI-MRayls. However, in practice up to a 20% variation can usually be tolerated. Two examples are given to illustrate the effect of the matching layer. In Fig. 118-13 no matching layer is present; *A* and

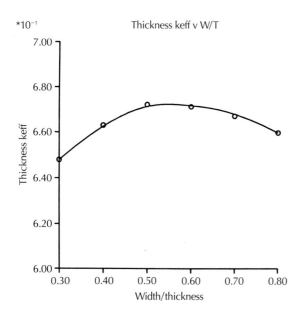

Fig. 118-10. Characteristic of power transfer as a function of the width thickness ratio of the piezo-electric crystal.

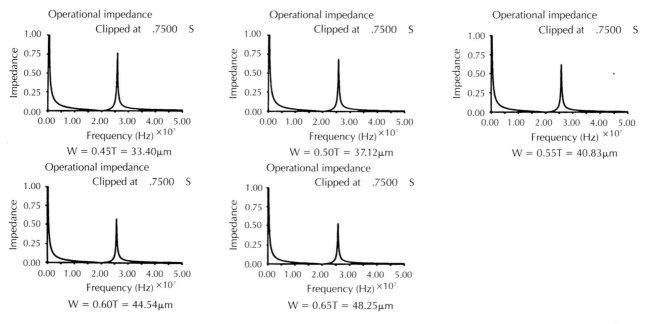

Fig. 118-11. Characteristics of operational impedances for a single crystal as a function of the width-to-thickness ratio.

B are the time and frequency plots, respectively. In the second case (Fig. 118-14), the matching layer is a single quarter-wavelength of tungsten-loaded epoxy (Z1, 7 SI-MRayls; T, 56.9 μm). These figures show that the matching layer produces an effective transfer of energy from the crystal to the medium.

Polyvinylidene transducers

There has been considerable interest in the use of piezopolymer materials such as PVDF as the ultrasonic trans-ducer on the catheter tip. Although it is relatively easy to etch the transducer elements using modified planar-printed circuit-board techniques, it is very difficult to obtain uniform backing and matching layers once the PVDF has been wrapped around the transducer tip.

The effect of different piezoelectric materials on pulse echo performance

Some advantage may be gained by using separate trans-ducer elements to perform the functions of transmission and

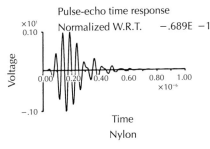

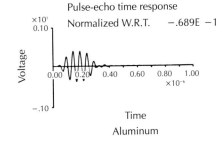

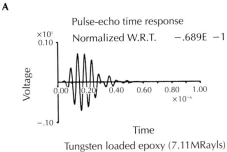

A

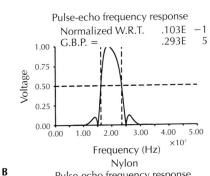

B

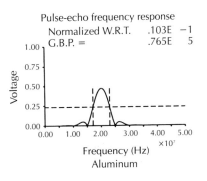

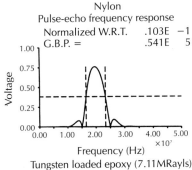

Fig. 118-12. *A,* Pulse echo time responses for different types of commonly used backing layer materials for a five-cycle tone burst with a cosine amplitude taper. *B,* The frequency spectra of the waveforms of *A.*

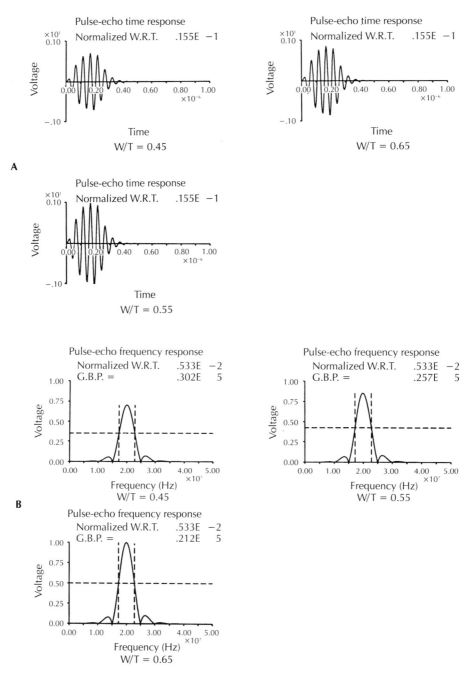

Fig. 118-13. A, Pulse echo responses for different width-to-thickness ratios with no matching layer. **B,** Frequency response spectra of the waveforms of **A.**

reception. Of particular interest for this purpose are flexible piezopolymer materials, such as PVDF, which provide good mechanical matching to water. Although relatively insensitive in transmission, such materials exhibit adequate reception performance when properly configured. Moreover, they are inherently lossy, resulting in low cross-talk properties. This is desirable for the fabrication of "monolithic" array structures, in which the array is defined solely by the electrode pattern. Such array structures, although less ef-

ficient than diced assemblies, possess considerable advantages in terms of consistent and repeatable manufacture.

For the present application (IVUS), one potential configuration involves a cylindrical piezoceramic transmitter, radiating in the radial direction directly through a separate PVDF array that is employed solely for reception beam forming and imaging. Because PVDF (characteristic impedance, 3.9 SI-MRayls) is well matched to the water load and if it is properly bonded to the ceramic, there should be no

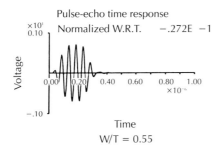

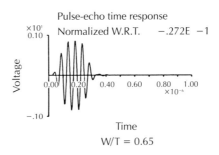

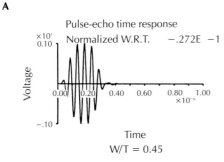

A

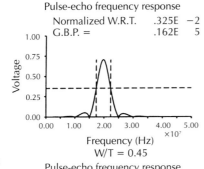

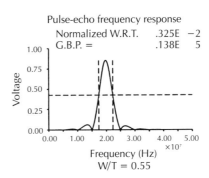

B

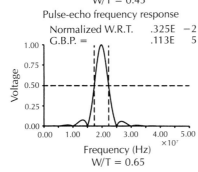

Fig. 118-14. **A,** The pulse-echo responses for different width-to-thickness ratios with a quarter wavelength tungsten-loaded epoxy matching layer. **B,** Frequency response spectra of the waveforms of **A.**

degradation in transmission, provided the piezopolymer layer is sufficiently thin.

To evaluate this concept, the following pulse-echo simulations were carried out:

- A PZT-5A transmitter, backed by tungsten-loaded epoxy of 15 SI-MRayls and operating at 20 MHz through a 40-μm layer of PVDF, which is matched to water via a quarter-wavelength layer (29 μm) of polystyrene
- A 40-μm (20-MHz) PVDF transducer, operating in pulse-

echo mode via a quarter-wavelength layer of polystyrene, backed by a lossy epoxy with a characteristic impedance of 2 SI-MRayls.

In both cases, the width of the transducer elements selected was 40.83 μm, corresponding to a ceramic aspect ratio of 0.55. The transmission conditions were the same as the ones described previously, using the 4-cycle tone burst. Two conditions of reception loading were evaluated, corresponding to 50 Ω and 1 MΩ connected directly across the PVDF receiver.[11]

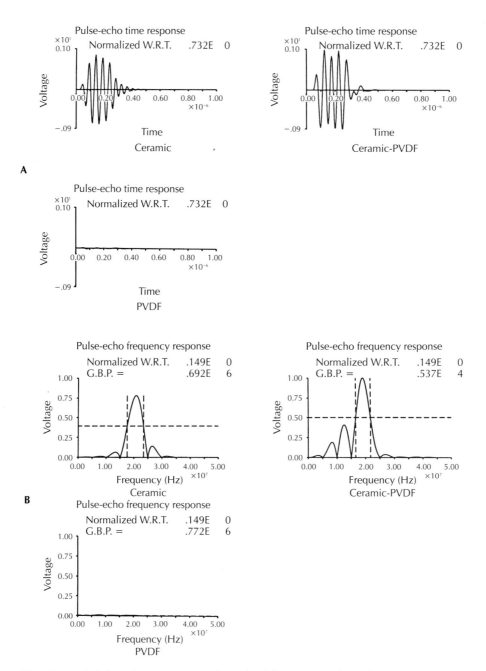

Fig. 118-15. *A,* Pulse echo response waveforms for different types of transducer materials: ceramic, ceramic-polyvinylidene film *(PVDF),* and PVDF for a 1 MΩ reception load. Note the very low amplitude response from PVDF. *B,* Frequency response spectra for the waveforms of *A.*

The results are shown in Figs. 118-15 and 118-16 for the 1-MΩ and 50-Ω reception loads, respectively. For completeness, the results for a PZT-5A device using a tungsten-loaded epoxy for backing (15 SI-MRayls) and quarter-wavelength matching (7 SI-MRayls) are shown on the same diagrams. From the simulations, the following observations can be made:

1. The PVDF-only structure is two orders of magnitude lower in sensitivity than either of the other pairs.

2. It is essential that a high-input resistance is connected across the PVDF in reception, thereby making sensitivity comparable with the ceramic element.

3. The frequency response is not unduly distorted by the presence of the PVDF layer, with the combination resonating close to 20 MHz. However, additional frequency components have been introduced in the stacked structure, as is evident from the distortion in the time-domain waveform of Fig. 118-15, *A.*

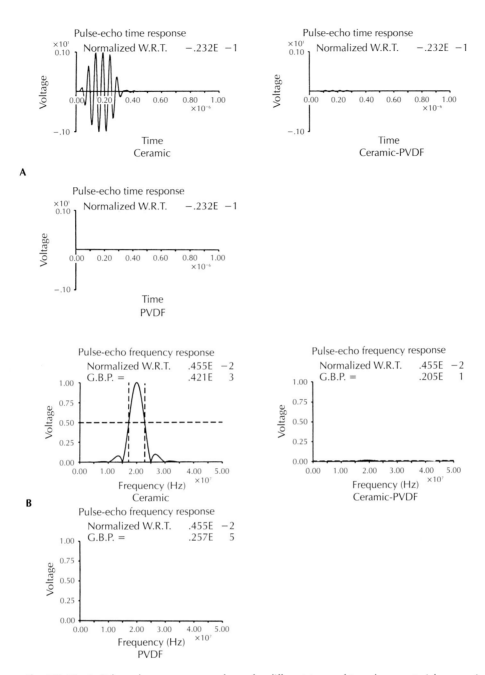

Fig. 118-16. A, Pulse echo response waveforms for different types of transducer materials: ceramic, ceramic-polyvinylidene film *(PVDF),* and PVDF for a 50 MΩ reception load. Note the very low amplitude response from PVDF. *B,* Frequency response spectra for the waveforms of *A.*

THREE-DIMENSIONAL SOLID MODELING IN THE STUDY OF ARTERIAL DISEASE

The use of ultrasound to study arterial disease is based on the assumption that plaque can be seen using B-mode imaging or detected from velocity disturbances caused by plaque. However, arterial structures and plaque are 3D structures. Hence, 3D imaging of such structures is seen as a worthwhile goal in its own right. More specifically, improved imaging techniques may reduce the risk that is associated with balloon and laser angioplasty, stemming from damage to the intimal surface of the vessel. Conventional contrast-enhanced radiographic techniques provide intermittent images with poor visualization of the intimal surface. Fiberoptic angioscopy improves resolution but requires flushing of blood with saline or complete obstruction to blood flow. Currently, it is impossible to obtain adequate information with real-time imaging about the effect of these procedures on the vessels being studied.

Over the past 15 years, interest in the use of computer graphics to represent and manipulate 3D objects has been increasing.[8,14] The main strategies that have been adopted are to represent the object in the form of either a wire or solid model. From a technical standpoint, the first option is far easier to implement, but it is relatively unrealistic for many applications. Therefore an increasing amount of work has been undertaken for the development of computer-based solid models of 3D objects. In such systems, objects are defined through their 3D coordinates or alternatively through the combination of a series of simple geometric shapes, called *primitives*. In general, it is possible to manipulate solid models constructed from geometric primitives and thus obtain cross-sections, perspective, and color-shaded images. A major problem arises when the object to be modeled does not conform to a combination of geometric primitive shapes (e.g., spheres, cylinders). As a result, for medical applications of 3D modeling, it is better to use a different approach.

3D space and object description. 3D modeling strategies are based on three approaches: constructive solid geometry (CGS), boundary representation (B-rep), and voxel space modeling. The first two techniques are discussed here.

Constructive solid geometry. CGS modeling is based on the fact that man-made objects can be built using simple geometric shapes. These primitives and objects are represented by sets of operators, for example, union and intersection, that are applied to primitives and positioned by means of translation and rotation. Fig. 118-17 shows a chess pawn that has been generated using this approach. The number of parameters required to define each primitive depends on its geometry. However, each primitive usually requires three coordinates for its center plus three angles of rotation.

A sphere requires an additional value, the radius; a cylinder requires two additional parameters, radius and length.

Because CGS objects are defined as conglomerates of primitives, any operation performed on an object must be performed on each of its constituent parts and the relative positions of each of the components maintained. This operation can be assisted by determining the intersection between a plane and the 3D model. In CGS modeling, this intersection is calculated by finding the intersection between every primitive and the given plane. CGS models must be computed each time they are used. Computing intersections and unions between primitives is very time consuming because the processing time increases not only as a function of the number of primitives but, more significantly, as a function of the number of interactions between primitives. Fig. 118-18 shows a CGS model of a carotid artery simulation using approximately 64 primitives organized in the form of rings. CGS modeling forms the basis of a large number of CAD/CAM packages in which synthetic objects can be modeled. However, CGS is not a good approach to the 3D modeling of anatomic or many biologic structures because of the large number of geometric primitives required.

Boundary representation. The B-rep approach to 3D modeling is a natural one because it is closely related to the methods used in 2D drawing. In the 2D case, a curve is represented by a sequence of x, y points connected in the simplest form by a straight line or lines. B-rep is a direct extension of this concept to the 3D case. In the 3D situation, volume is defined by surfaces that delimit it. The surfaces are described by sets of points (x, y, z), which are connected, again in the samples form, by straight lines. However, whereas in the 2D case the sequence of points gives the order of connection, in this instance such a simple connec-

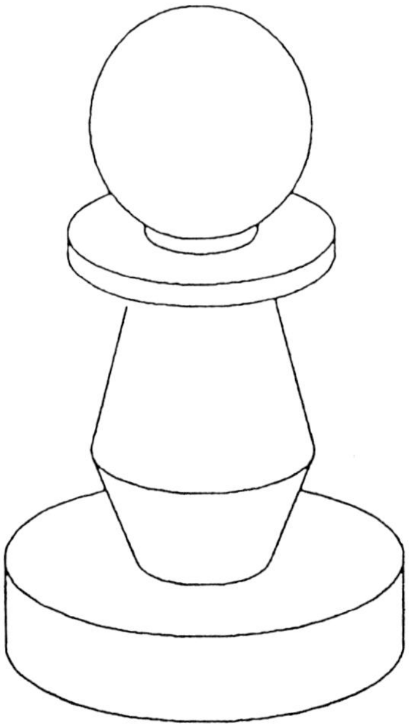

Fig. 118-17. Computer-based solid model of a chess pawn generated using the constructive solid geometry method.

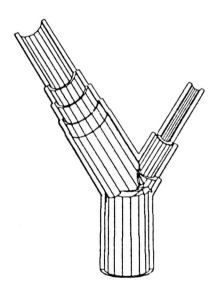

Fig. 118-18. A simple solid model of a carotid bifurcation generated using the boundary representative method from 64 rectangular elements of different sizes.

tion cannot be implemented because any point on the boundary surface is connected to more than one other point. Therefore the connection order must be precisely given using either explicit polygons or edges or by keeping a list of points and their connections. Usually the region within the polygons on the model surface is assumed to be planar (i.e., a facet); hence the method is referred to as *B-rep,* or faceted.

Data input to B-rep systems is usually performed either by defining a series of contours in different planes and then allowing the system to connect them or by defining primitives in a manner similar to that used in CGS. In the latter case, models are not stored as CGS models but as facets and vertices computed from the primitives as they are defined. B-rep is suitable when the structures to be modeled are smooth such that not too many facets are required to represent the volume adequately. Performing any operation on a B-rep model means processing all the facets individually. For B-rep models, finding the intersection between a given plane and the 3D model implies finding the intersection between the plane of each facet and the intersecting plane. If the intersection occurs within the facet, the intersection line must be computed; otherwise the facet is not intersected by the plane. For models with many facets, this operation is very time consuming. The strength of the B-rep method lies in the fact that it uses computer memory only as necessary, meaning that simple models are accurately represented by small amounts of memory. This leads to fast processing, which is one of the basic reasons why B-rep is so popular with 3D modeling packages designed for microcomputers. Because B-rep models are represented by their boundary surfaces, which in turn are made of facets, each facet must be oriented to convey the information both inside and outside the volume. This is usually done by keeping track of the direction of the vector normal to each facet, which is assumed to point outward from the model.[9]

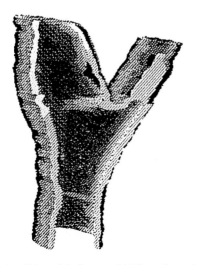

Fig. 118-19. A solid model of a carotid bifurcation using a parallel surface rendering and a large number of facets.

B-rep models are defined by a list of vertices of their connections and normal vector directions, and this list must be kept in strict order. If for any reason a single value in any of these lists is suppressed or even modified, the resulting model will bear little or no resemblance to the original model. By using B-rep, it is possible to define models that cannot be defined in the real world, such as the famous Escher objects.[22] Most of the CAD/CAM systems that are currently available make use of B-rep to define the solid model. Historically, B-rep models were the first to be implemented on computers, and consequently most of the theory and the computer techniques developed for the handling and viewing of 3D models were initially accomplished with B-rep objects. An example of a B-rep rendering from work on carotid bifurcations is shown in Fig. 118-19.

Computer system for 3D medical images

A typical image reconstruction system comprises two separate parts: object reconstruction and object handling and display (Fig. 118-20).

Object reconstruction. With object reconstruction software, a series of 2D tomographic slices are entered into the computer. These are then realigned in terms of distance and orientation to ensure that the most appropriate 3D model can be constructed. A typical method of reconstruction is to interpolate the 2D cross sections into 3D using spline functions techniques. Parallel 2D slices acquired from the artery under examination then comprise 2D images consisting of $M \times M$ picture elements or pixels. To transform 2D cross sections into 3D visualizations, the depth, or z dimension, needs to be added. This can be achieved by using a series of 2D pixel planes and lying *n* of them one behind the other. The 2D picture elements (pixels) then become volume elements (voxels), thereby informing the 3D image. A 3D object can thus be modeled in $M \times M \times N$ voxel space. The specific details of the strategies used in this form of contour definition and 3D interpolation are described elsewhere.[17]

Object handling and display. The requirements for image handling and display consist of a system that can rotate and slice in different orientations. Axial resolution is primarily a function of the frequency of the intravascular imaging and the type of tissue that is being investigated. For example, speed of sound in water is 1480 m/sec, and in muscle it is 1580 m/sec. Hence for a particular imaging system with a burst length of 3 cycles operating at 20 MHz, the axial resolution will be $\times F$ in water and y in muscle.

REVIEW OF DISPLAY TECHNIQUES
Ray tracing

Ray tracing from a point. As depicted in Fig. 118-21, in ray tracing from a point, the object is viewed as if seen by the eye. This means that points on surfaces, such as P_1 and P_2 in the figure, are observed through the view plane. P_1 and P_2 therefore reach the observer through the same pixel on the view plane. Unless otherwise constrained, the dis-

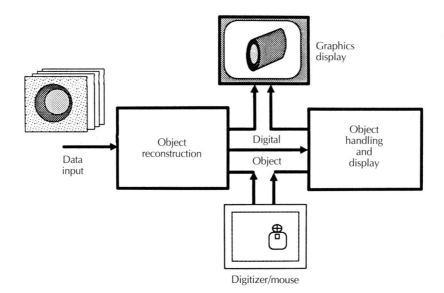

Fig. 118-20. A typical image reconstruction and manipulation system. The system consists of two parts: object reconstruction and object handling and display.

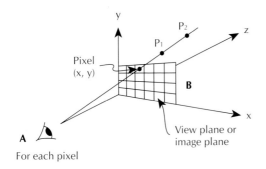

Fig. 118-21. *A,* Ray tracing from a point. *B,* Ray tracing from the image-plane.

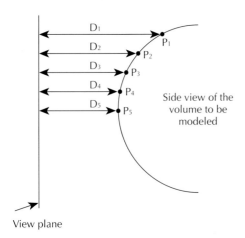

Fig. 118-22. The basis of z buffering. The distances from the viewplane to the points $P_1 \ldots P_n$ are stored in the Z-buffer matrix. Information pertaining to the nature of the point (e.g., gray level or pseudo color) is stored in a second matrix, the 0 matrix.

tance from the view plane to P_1 is noted. In this way, the surface of which P_1 is a part can be reproduced, but the surface of which P_2 is a part is lost. Alternatively, several surfaces can be stored in this way. Unless otherwise constrained, only the distance from the view plane to P_1 will be noted.

Ray tracing from the image plane. Ray tracing from the image plane is an alternative to ray tracing from a point. In this approach, points in the volume are mapped to single pixels on the image plane rather than back to a point (Fig. 118-21). However, the techniques for surface storage are similar to those used for ray tracing from a point. Again, only P_1 will be noted.

Z buffering

The distance information obtained from the ray tracing is stored in a 2D matrix in which P has N × M pixels. Therefore whether seen from a point or a plane, the distances from the view point or view plane are logged in P. Distance information relating to P_1, P_2, . . . P_n is stored in the P matrix. Fig. 118-22 shows that if in this case P_1, . . . P_n are all on the same surface of a volume, the information can be stored in the form of a column vector. In this way, using appropriate tissue characterization techniques, multilayered sections of anatomic structures can be preserved. Clearly, if a volume comprises only one or two layers, it may be appropriate to use B-rep techniques. However, for more complex structures, such as plaque in the arterial wall, voxel modeling is far more appropriate and can still be used in conjunction with the z buffer.

The O matrix. Information relating to the nature of the point, such as P_1, is stored in a second matrix, the O matrix. Where the O matrix is again normally N × M pixels, the z-buffer information comprises: (1) distance information—the P matrix and (2) point information—the O matrix.

Case 1: Simple surfaces. For simple models such as bone, this may consist of simple threshold information with a color assigned. Hence P_1, or $P(x_1, y_1) = D_1$ and $O(x_1, y_1) = O_1$. Similarly, $P(x_1, y_2) = D_2$ and $O(x_1, y_2) = O_2$, where $O_1 = O_2$. If every none-zero threshold value is assigned a single color, such as yellow, a single-colored solid object will be seen from the view plane. In this way, the entire surface can be represented by a single color.

Case 2: More complex surfaces. The use of P and O matrices can be particularly useful in their presentation of more complex anatomic structures. It is important to recognize that simple thresholding is often insufficient. Even the representation of histologic differences on the basis of amplitude variations in the A-mode signal is likely to be inadequate. More complex information concerning frequency and phase changes often needs to be incorporated. This can be effectively achieved by using a single P matrix coupled to a set of O matrices, each of which contains specific information about a particular voxel. For tissue type 1, P_1 and O_1 will be used. For tissue type 2, P_2 and O_2 will be used.

Basic reflection models

The reflection model is the basic factor in the appearance of a 3D shaded object. The choice of a particular reflection model can be important and the model used in given circumstances should be known. The basic equation is: light incident at a surface = reflected light + scattered light + absorbed light + transmitted light. The practical consequences of this model are shown in Fig. 118-23. It can be seen in this figure that the gradient shading in a simple model gives the specular component and the z-buffer image gives the diffuse component.

Specular reflection. As shown in Fig. 118-24, *A*, for simple specular reflection, the reflected component is a function of the cosine of the angle formed by the incident ray and a scan line constructed normal to the reflecting surface at the point of reflection.

Hence, in a simple specular reflection, the reflected component is related to $\cos\theta$.

Diffuse component. The diffuse component is obtained from the z-buffer information. Fig. 118-24, *B*, shows that if a perfect diffuser is assumed, light scatters equally in all directions. The intensity of the diffuse component (I_d) is defined by Lambert's law:

$$I_d = I_i k_d \cos\theta$$

or:

$$0 \leq \theta \leq 90°$$

A simple practical reflection model. The basic ideas relating to reflection models can therefore be incorporated into a simple practical reflection model as follows. This model comprises the sum of the specular and diffuse reflection components.

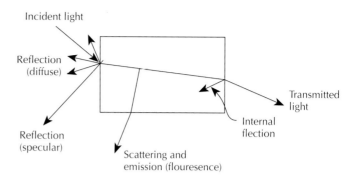

Fig. 118-23. The basis of reflection models that often consist of reflection, scattering, and transmitted components.

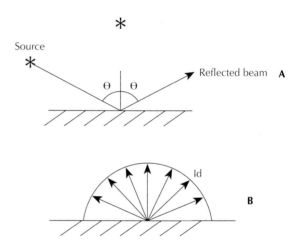

Fig. 118-24. A, Simple specular reflection. **B,** Diffuse component models.

The specular reflection component. Fig. 118-25 shows that the specular reflection component (I_s) as seen from the view plane can be presented as follows:

Path 1:

$$I_s = I_i$$

where:

$$I_i = \text{The incident component}$$

Path 2:

$$I_s = I_i \cos\theta$$

The diffuse component. This component is obtained from the z-buffer information.

The combined reflection model. As previously stated, for any point on the view plane, the combined reflection model comprises the sum of the specular and diffuse components. Referring to Fig. 118-25, it is clear that the total illumination (I_T) for the pixels P_1 and P_2 can be represented by the following:

$$I_T = I_s + I_z$$

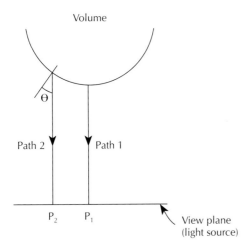

Fig. 118-25. A total illumination model.

$\partial y / \partial z$ is calculated in a similar way. The cosine between the normal to the surface and the observer is therefore given by:

$$\cos\theta = \frac{\left(\dfrac{\partial z}{\partial x}, \dfrac{\partial z}{\partial y}, -1\right) \cdot (0, 0, -1)}{\sqrt{\left(\dfrac{\partial z}{\partial x}\right)^2 + \left(\dfrac{\partial z}{\partial y}\right)^2 + 1}} \qquad (10)$$

Geometric transformations

Translation. If an object is displaced from its original position without rotation, this is called *translation*.

If the direction and displacement of the translation is described by a vector (v):

$$V = aI + bJ + cK$$

then the new coordinates of a translated point can be calculated by using the transformation:

$$T_v = \begin{bmatrix} x' = x + a \\ y' = y + b \\ z' = z + c \end{bmatrix}$$

which in the homogeneous matrix form becomes:

$$\begin{bmatrix} x' \\ y' \\ z' \\ 1' \end{bmatrix} = \begin{bmatrix} 1 & 0 & 0 & a \\ 0 & 1 & 0 & b \\ 0 & 0 & 1 & c \\ 0 & 0 & 0 & 1 \end{bmatrix} \begin{bmatrix} x \\ y \\ z \\ 1 \end{bmatrix}$$

Scaling. If the original object A (illustrated in Fig. 118-26) is defined by the identity:

$$\begin{bmatrix} 1 & 0 & 0 \\ 0 & 1 & 0 \\ 0 & 0 & 1 \\ 0 & 0 & 0 \end{bmatrix}$$

then, with a uniform scaling of 1.5 (Fig. 118-26), this becomes:

$$\begin{bmatrix} 1.5 & 0 & 0 \\ 0 & 1.5 & 0 \\ 0 & 0 & 1.5 \\ 0 & 0 & 0 \end{bmatrix}$$

Hence if s is the scaling factor, $s > 1$ is magnification and $s < 1$ is reduction.

If the origin remains fixed, scaling with respect to it is achieved by the transformation:

$$S_{sx,sy,sz} = \begin{bmatrix} x' = s_x \ x \\ y' = s_y \ y \\ z' = s_z \ z \end{bmatrix}$$

which in matrix form is:

$$S_{sx,sy,sz} = \begin{bmatrix} S_x & 0 & 0 \\ 0 & S_y & 0 \\ 0 & 0 & S_z \end{bmatrix}$$

Rotation. 3D rotation requires the definition of an angle of rotation and an axis of rotation.

The 2D example. Fig. 118-27 shows that the original position P is x_1, y_1 or, in complex form, $x_1 + jy$, or $re^{j\varnothing}$. Rotating to position p' gives the coordinates x_2, y_2, or

where:

$$I_z = \alpha P_z$$

i.e., a fraction of the z-buffer value (distance).

$$\therefore I_T = I_s + \alpha P_z,$$

which is the practical realization of a simple reflection model.

Image-based gradient shading

For image-based gradient shading, the z-buffer value is used to calculate the gradient. The normal vector N at any point on the visible surface, i.e., the surface of interest, can be computed as:

$$N = \frac{\partial z}{\partial x}, \frac{\partial z}{\partial y}, -1$$

where:

$$\frac{\partial z}{\partial x} \ and \ \frac{\partial z}{\partial y}$$

which are estimated from the digital data.

From the central difference approach[27]:

$$\frac{\partial z}{\partial x} = \frac{1}{2} [z(x + 1) - z(x - 1,y)] \qquad (9)$$

A simple method for overcoming discontinuities is for $\partial z / \partial x$ only to be accepted if $|\partial z / \partial x|$ is $< \epsilon$, where ϵ is a given threshold. Equation 9 then becomes:

$$\frac{\partial z}{\partial x} = \frac{1}{2} [z(x + 1y) - z(\partial - 1,y)] \ if \ \left|\frac{\partial z}{\partial x}\right| \le \epsilon$$

or:

$$\frac{\partial z}{\partial x} = \frac{1}{2} [z(x + i + 1,y) - z(x - i + 1,y)] \ if \ \left|\frac{\partial z}{\partial x}\right| > \epsilon$$

where i is such that:

$$\left|\frac{\partial z}{\partial x}\right| = MIN \left[\frac{1}{2} | z(x + i + 1,y) - z(x - i + 1,y) | \right]$$

$$for \ i = -1, 0, 1$$

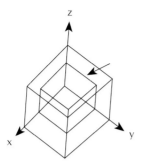

Fig. 118-26. Linear scaling change in three dimensions on a solid model, in this case by a factor of one and a half.

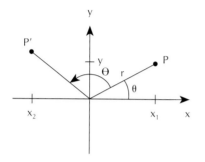

Fig. 118-27. 2D rotation of a single point (P to P').

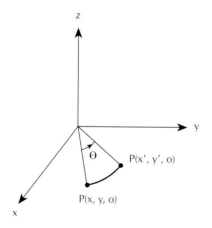

Fig. 118-28. 3D rotation of a single point (x,y,0) to x',y',0.

$re^{j(\emptyset + \theta)}$, which in contusion coordinates is: $r[\cos(\emptyset + \theta) + \sin(\emptyset + \theta)]$. Hence:

$$x_2 = r \cos(\emptyset + \theta)$$
$$= r(\cos\emptyset \cos\theta - \sin\emptyset \sin\theta)$$

But, $\cos\emptyset = r/x_1$ and $\sin\emptyset = r/y_1$:

$$\therefore x_2 = x_1 \cos\theta - y_1 \sin\theta$$

Similarly:

$$y_2 = r \sin(\emptyset + \theta)$$
$$= r(\sin\emptyset \cos\theta - \cos\emptyset \sin\theta)$$

which, as before, gives:

$$y_2 = y_1 \cos\theta + x_1 \sin\theta$$

The 3D example. Fig. 118-28 shows that for 3D space, rotation about the z axis can be defined as:

$$R_{\theta,k} = \begin{cases} x' = x\cos\theta - y\sin\theta \\ y' = x\sin\theta + y\cos\theta \\ z' = z \end{cases}$$

Similarly, rotation about the y axis can be defined as:

$$R_{\theta,j} = \begin{cases} x' = x\cos\theta - z\sin\theta \\ y' = y \\ z' = x\sin\theta + z\cos\theta \end{cases}$$

and rotation about the x axis is given by:

$$R_{\theta,I} = \begin{cases} x' = x \\ y' = y\cos\theta - z\sin\theta \\ z' = y\sin\theta + z\cos\theta \end{cases}$$

Matrix form. These transformations can be defined in matrix form as:

$$R_{\theta,k} = \begin{bmatrix} \cos\theta & \emptyset n\theta & 0 \\ \sin\theta & \cos\theta & 0 \\ 0 & 0 & 1 \end{bmatrix} \begin{bmatrix} x \\ y \\ z \end{bmatrix}$$

$$R_{\theta,j} = \begin{bmatrix} \cos\theta & 0 & \sin\theta \\ 0 & 1 & 0 \\ \sin\theta & 0 & \cos\theta \end{bmatrix}$$

$$R_{\theta,I} = \begin{bmatrix} 1 & 0 & 0 \\ 0 & \cos\theta & -\sin\theta \\ 0 & \sin\theta & \cos\theta \end{bmatrix}$$

VOXEL MODELING

A 2D image of an arterial cross section is composed of M × M picture elements, or pixels. This concept can be extended to the imaging of 3D objects. The depth, or z dimension, can be modeled by taking a series of 2D pixel planes and laying them one behind the other. The 2D picture elements (pixels) then become cubes. These cubes, which form the 3D image, are called *volume elements* or *voxels*. Thus a 3D object can be modeled in M × M × N voxel space. The current software, which produces full voxel space images, allows both 2D and 3D display and manipulation with the ability to transfer easily from one to the other. The design of the system also allows a wide range of operations to be performed on 3D solid models. These include rotation in all images by using a depth code, plane cuts so that any section of the model can be removed, and x-ray projection, in which a 3D structure can be made semi-transparent.

Application to arterial structures

By using voxel models, a series of 2D arterial slices can be used to produce a 3D image. This has been done and is described by Kitney, Moura, and Straughan.[17] An alternative approach is to visualize the artery under examination using a catheter-mounted sonographic probe. The morphologic information obtained is converted into a 3D solid model of the artery section under investigation. The probe can be used to generate data from arterial slices in parallel planes (Fig. 118-29). The time taken to acquire the data is small in comparison with the cardiac cycle; hence the slices can be aligned without significant movement error. If a single arterial slice is imaged in terms of n sets of polar coordinates, each contour can be described by:

$$R(i), \theta(i) \text{ for } i = 1 \ldots n$$

where $R(i)$ is the radius from the center of the image plane and $\theta(i)$ is the corresponding angular direction.

On the basis of this information, a contour can be drawn for a given slice that corresponds to a change in acoustic impedance. Multiple contours are similarly calculated. The information for a single slice is then contained in 2D pixel space. This process is repeated n times to generate the slices that form the 3D arterial volume. If the pixel space is composed of $M \times M$ pixels, the volume consists of $M \times M \times N$ voxels. This information is then used to construct a solid model of the arterial section. By using 3D voxel space, it is possible to produce x-ray–like transparent structures that allow close examination of the lumen.

One interpolation strategy is to assume that the radii vary linearly between the original slices. For example, three slices are separated in the digital science in such a way that they correspond to planes 10, 30, and 50. (The overall voxel space again is $M \times M \times N$.) It is then necessary to calculate the contours for planes 11 to 29 and for planes 31 to 49. To do this, it is assumed that any given radius will vary linearly between any two original consecutive slices, that is:

$$R(m,j) = \frac{(m - m_0)}{(m_1 - m_0) \times R(m_1,j) - R(m_0,j)} + R(m_0,j) \quad \textbf{(11)}$$

$$\text{for } m = m_0 + 1, m_1 - 1$$

when m is the mth slice to be calculated, m_0 is the position of the nearest "below" original slice, and m_1 the nearest "above" original slice. If equation 10 is applied to the linear interpolation problem previously defined, this yields:

$$R(m,j) = \frac{m - 30}{(50 - 30) \times [R(50,j) - R(30,j)]} + R(30,j) \quad \textbf{(12)}$$

Examples of results

Fig. 118-30, *A* shows a single histologic arterial cross section. Fig. 118-30, *C* shows the 3D reconstruction of a series of 30 arterial slices, one of which was shown in Fig. 118-30, *B*. This figure shows two important features of the 3D voxel modeling software. First, as can be seen in the cross section, various histologic segments of the arterial structures have been identified. With the current software, this can be achieved either manually by drawing contours on the screen with a mouse or automatically by using intelligent contouring software. (This identifies individual tissue regions and automatically color codes separate areas.) In this case (Fig. 118-30, *D*), two main areas have been identified. In fact, all the individual structures can be removed and replaced at will.

The importance of the technique is that arterial lesions

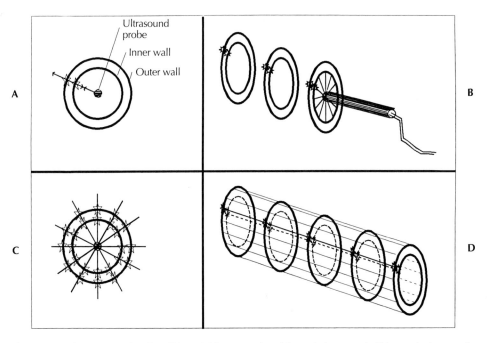

Fig. 118-29. Generation of a 3D solid model from a series of B-mode images. **A,** Firing a single crystal. **B,** Multiple crystal firing. **C,** Pull back to create a series of B-mode images. **D,** Creation of the solid model by 3D interpolation.

are essentially 3D structures and therefore can be rotated. One important feature of the voxel software is that multiple-orientation slicing can be carried out easily. This means that new 2D images can be constructed and further image processing undertaken. The 3D structure can be viewed as a

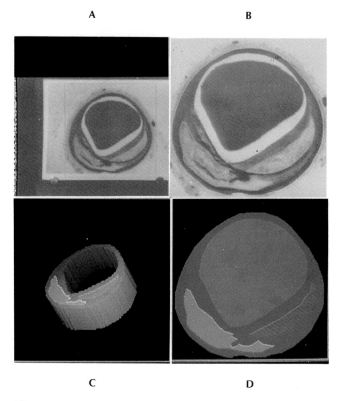

Fig. 118-30. Generation of a 3D solid model of an arterial specimen from a series of 3D histologic cross sections. **A,** a single 2D slice. **B,** The reconstructed 2D image. **C,** The 3D reconstruction of 30 arterial slices. **D,** Two areas of different types of plaque identified.

series of "microscope slides" as many times and from as many angles as considered appropriate. Fig. 118-31 shows a section of diseased aorta that has been imaged using an ultrasound probe. Fig. 118-31, *A* shows the artery viewed end-on. The plaque that has developed on the arterial wall between the 9- and 1-o'clock positions can be seen clearly. Fig. 118-31, *B* shows the 3D solid model of the artery rotated through 90° to give a side view. As shown in Fig. 118-31, *C* it is also possible to use the sonographically generated voxel data to produce an x-ray image. It can be seen from this figure that the vessel narrowing apparent in Fig. 118-31, *A* can now be studied over the entire length of the arterial segment. Like the full 3D shaded image (e.g., Fig. 118-31, *A* and *C*), the 3D x-ray model can also be rotated in any direction. Hence examination of the whole lumen can readily be achieved. Fig. 118-32 illustrates another aortic section. The upper panel is a photograph of the original pathologic specimen and the lower panel is the image reconstructed from the aortic specimen. The similarity of the two indicates the high-resolution imaging that is possible.

Tissue characterization by frequency tracking

Tissue characterization based on the A-mode signal of the ultrasound waveform typically comprises the detection of amplitude. Specifically, this approach involves the definition of the envelope, often in terms of the gray scale. Research has shown that this approach is inadequate because it yields considerable extra information in the spatial frequencies of the signal. To this end, advanced spectral estimators have been applied.[18,26] These papers focus on the use of linear estimators that use all-pole (AR) models incorporating Kalman filters. Theoretically such models have the advantage of requiring fewer terms than the AR type.

Frequency tracking is possible by maximizing the exact

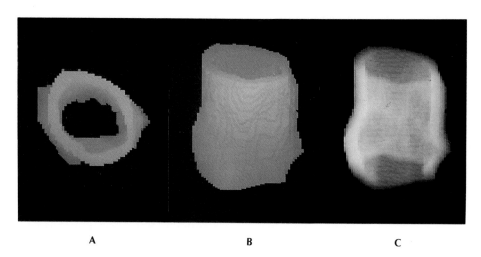

Fig. 118-31. Section of diseased aorta imaged by an IVUS probe. **A,** The artery viewed end-on. **B,** The 3D solid arterial model rotated through 90°. **C,** The x-ray version of the solid model generated with the system software.

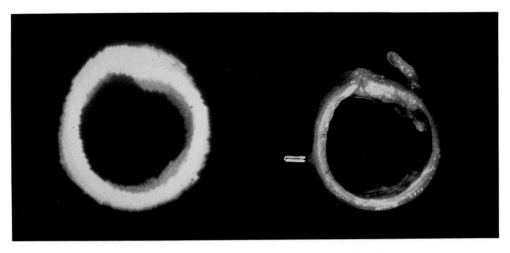

Fig. 118-32. A section of diseased aorta. The original pathologic specimen *(left)*. The image reconstructed from the aortic specimen *(right)*. The similarity of the two images is an indication of the type of high-resolution imaging that is possible using IVUS.

likelihood function of the autoregressive-moving average (ARMA) process of the form:

$$X_t = \sum_{k=1}^{p} a_k X_{t-k} + e_t + \sum_{k=1}^{q} b_k e_{t-k} \quad (13)$$

where $(a_1, a_2, \ldots, a_q)$ are the AR parameters, $(b_1, b_2, \ldots, b_q)$ are the MA parameters, and e_t is Gaussian noise. This method has been shown to provide good estimates of the ARMA coefficients over short records, especially when the poles or zeros happen to lie near or at the unit circle.[4] The spectrum is derived from the ARMA parameters as follows:

$$Y(f) = \sigma^2 f_s \left[\frac{\sum_{k=0}^{0} b_k \exp(j2\pi khf)}{1 - \sum_{k=1}^{p} a_k \exp(j2\pi khf)} \right] \quad (14)$$

where σ^2 is the variance of e_t, and f_s is the sampling frequency. The Kalman filter is applied sequentially to short sections of data to estimate the error of the ARMA process, whose likelihood is to be maximized. The mode of the spectrum in equation 2 is then taken to be the frequency estimate. Here a 6-pole, 5-zero ARMA model was applied to an A-mode signal. The results are consistent with previous work and show that it is possible to track spatial frequency changes accurately down to 1.5 cycles of the fundamental frequency. This results in a maximum spatial resolution of 0.075 mm. Fig. 118-33 illustrates an A-mode ultrasound signal obtained from an arterial wall. From left to right, the three main peaks correspond to the intima, media, and adventitia, respectively.

It is clear from Fig. 118-34 that the acoustic impedance changes relating to the intima, media, and adventitia have been detected in this case. The combination of envelope information and spatial frequency information yields a much more effective method for defining the histologic characteristics of the vessel acoustically.

The basis of this method is that the A-mode signal can be modeled by an all-pole filter driven from a white-noise source of zero mean and known variance. Hence, the nth output sample can be expressed as an autoregressive process:

$$y_n = a_1 y_{n-1} + y_{n-2} + \ldots + e_n \quad (15)$$

where $a_1 \ldots a_n$ are linear weighting coefficients and e_n is an error term. It can be shown that the linear spectral estimate is given by the equation:

$$S(f) = \frac{\sigma_n^2 T}{\left| 1 + \sum_{k=1}^{p} a_k \exp - j2\pi fkT \right|^2} \quad (16)$$

where T is the sampling interval and σ_n^2 the variance of the white-noise source.

The final stage in estimation of velocity from the Doppler signal is the application of a nonlinear filter. This filter is necessary because the estimate often contains a number of glitches that are unrepresentative of the surrounding estimates. Hence the filter is designed to automatically reduce such misrepresentation, if it occurs.

The effectiveness of the AR spectral estimator when applied to A-mode signals can be seen in Fig. 118-35, which shows the results of the analysis of the audio Doppler signal over one cardiac cycle. The signal was measured from a sample volume center line and 1.5 diameters downstream of an induced 50% stenosis in a dog aorta. Fig. 118-35 shows the result obtained using a 10-ms–window fast Fourier transform (FFT); Fig. 118-35 is the result obtained by using the described analysis protocol. When these results are compared with the hot film anemometer (HFA) measurement, the enhanced Doppler processing (based on linear estimation) shows a much better result than the FFT.

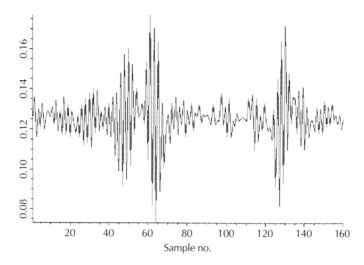

Fig. 118-33. An A-mode signal of the arterial wall obtained using IVUS. The three main peaks correspond to the intima, media, and adventitia.

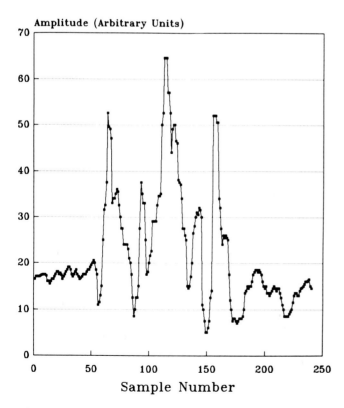

Fig. 118-34. A derived waveform representing the tissue of the arterial wall obtained from a combination of envelope information and spatial frequency information.

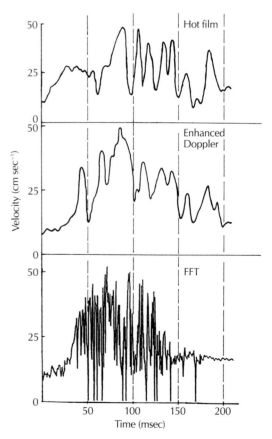

Fig. 118-35. The analysis of a single cardiac cycle velocity waveform calculated from a Doppler flow signal obtained one and a half diameters downstream of a 50% stenosis in a dog aorta. The velocity measured directly using a hot film anamometer, the velocity estimate obtained from an AR estimator ($p = 8$) with a 2 ms data window, and the velocity estimate obtained from an FFT estimator are shown.

The zoom Wigner transform. Although enhanced Doppler processing is a major improvement over the FFT, both methods suffer from the important drawback that the length of the time window determines the time resolution of the time-frequency plot representing the velocity waveform. Decreasing the interval length can lead to unstable spectral estimates and hence the introduction of artifacts. The Wigner transform, on the other hand, offers considerable potential advantages because it is a true time-frequency distribution. Investigators have developed a modified version of the Wigner transform that has the ability to zoom onto a frequency region of interest. In the case of a Doppler signal, this results in more accurate, higher-resolution tracking.

The method is based on the use of the chirp z-transform. If the n point sequence under consideration is defined as $x(n)$, then the z-transform of the sequence, $X(z)$, can be calculated at the points Z_m, where:

$$Z_m = AW^{-m}, m = 0, 1, \ldots M - 1 \qquad (17)$$
$$W = W_0 e^{-j\theta_0}, A = A_0 e^{j\theta_0}$$

$X(z)$ is calculated along a contour in the z-plane, which is in fact a spiral, and for A_0 and W_0, unity is an arc on the unit circle. The theoretical basis of the method is described by Kitney and Talhami.[16] Its primary advantage is that the operator is not forced to use the complete range of the upper unit semicircle. Any frequency range of interest, f_1 to f_2, can be specified. Hence it is possible to zoom onto the desired frequency region of the velocity waveform.

Fig. 118-36 shows a sample application of the zoom Wigner transform to a swept-frequency sine wave. In Fig. 118-36, *A*, the full frequency range is used (0 to 0.5 Hz) and the standard Wigner transform is applied. In the second case (Fig. 118-36, *B*), the range is restricted to 0 to 0.15 Hz and the zoom Wigner transform is used. From a comparison of the plots, it is clear that the zoom Wigner transform can resolve the frequency changes far more accurately.

Tissue characterization by edge detection. One of the aims of tissue characterization is to identify the boundaries of the structure of interest to isolate it from its surroundings. In many cases, when the structure of interest either stands out or can be described geometrically in a suitable way, this can be achieved more easily by means of edge detection techniques. These techniques are usually performed in three steps. The first, also called *early processing,* consists of applying local difference operators that measure discontinuity and can therefore detect edgy parts of an image. When using these operators, pixels within homogeneous regions produce low pixel values (black), whereas pixels placed at

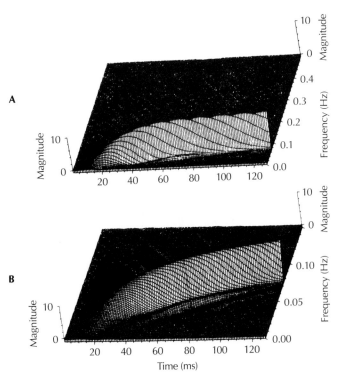

Fig. 118-36. Application of the zoom Wigner transform to a swept frequency sinewave. *A,* Over the full frequency range (0 to 0.5 Hz). *B,* With the range restricted to 0. to 0.15 Hz. Comparison of the plots shows that the zoom Wigner transform can resolve frequency changes far more accurately.

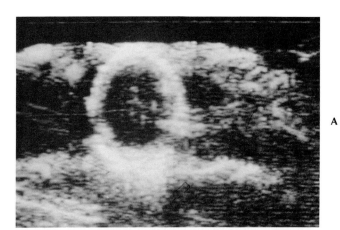

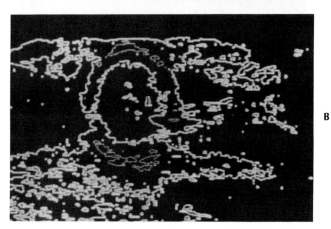

Fig. 118-37. A B-mode image of an arterial cross section. *A,* The image of the raw data. *B,* The same image after edge enhancement.

borders produce high intensities (white). The next step is to have the edge-enhanced image processed by some contour follower algorithm, which will furnish one-pixel-wide edge segments. Although in general these edge segments do not define clear regions and structures, they are used as the source of information for the next processing stage—contour detection. Fig. 118-37 shows a B-mode image of an arterial cross section. The upper panel illustrates the raw data and the lower panel shows the corresponding edge-enhanced image.

Contour detection involves defining both the basic geometric characteristics of the contours being sought and a series of rules for connecting the edge segments toward the formation of contours. Geometric coherence criteria are extremely dependent on the planned application and should be carefully chosen. Examples of coherence criteria are nonoverlapping pathways, roundish contours, and distance between segments less than a given threshold. Investigators have developed a method that has been successfully applied to the detection of coronary artery walls in cross-sectional slices for pathologic evaluation.[21] Besides making use of a great deal of *a priori* knowledge about the arterial wall contour geometry, the method uses a measure of roundness and heuristic search to detect roundish contours. Heuristic search is a technique that minimizes a cost function, which reflects how well the pathway being analyzed fits a description of the ideal contour sought. Because it is roundish contours that are being looked for, a cost function that leads to 0 when the contour is a perfect circle and to 1 when the surface area enclosed by the contour is null. Fig. 118-38 illustrates automatic wall contour detection, including the

digitized coronary artery cross-section *(A)*, the contour follower algorithm in progress *(B)*, the detected edge segments *(C)*, and the detected contour *(D)*. One of the main advantages of such a method is that it can fill in very wide gaps. It is a good example of how *a priori* knowledge of the structure's geometry can be used to increase an algorithm's reliability.

Tissue characterization by textural analysis. Another approach to the definition of tissue based on ultrasound is to compare textures.[19] In this approach, the comparison is done by identifying regions of interest. Typically, two regions of equal size are selected, the first, a region containing normal tissue, and the second, the area to be compared. The technique that has been developed for this purpose is based on Kolmogorov-Smirnov statistics. This method has two principal advantages: (1) it is a nonparametric approach and (2) it is a global technique in that it is insensitive to individual pixel values. After the selection of the two regions of interest, the cumulative frequency distribution for each region is determined and the maximum difference between the two characteristics is calculated. The maximum difference is a measure of similarity and is used to either reject or accept the hypothesis that the two regions pertain to the same structure.

Fig. 118-39 illustrates the use of this method in a B-mode image of the carotid artery. The square window in the ultrasound image is one of the two regions of interest to be compared. The right side of the figure shows their frequency-distribution characteristics. In this case, the method indicated that the two regions are not part of the same structure.

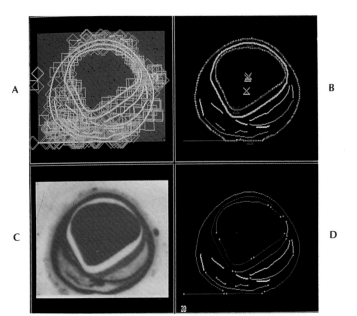

Fig. 118-38. Automatic wall contour detection. *A,* A digitized coronary cross section. *B,* The contour following algorithm in progress. *C,* The detected edge segments. *D,* The detected contours.

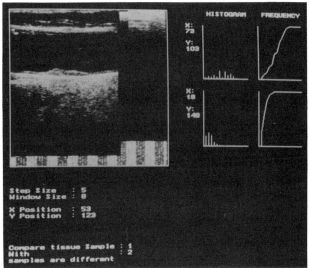

Fig. 118-39. Detection of differences in tissue characteristics by textural analysis and the use of Kolmogorov-Smirnov *(K-S)* statistics. The figure shows the original image together with the cumulative frequency histograms for two ROIs.

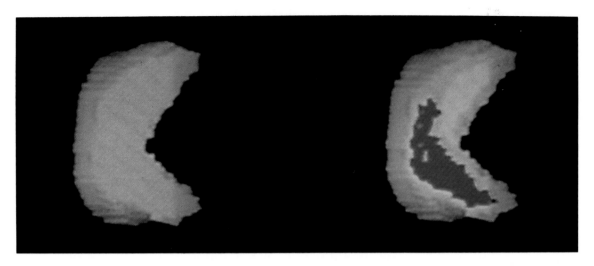

Fig. 118-40. A 3D solid model derived from IVUS data showing two areas of different plaque within the arterial wall. The result is important because it illustrates the ability of IVUS to image diseased tissue through the arterial wall at the stage before distortion of the lumen begins to affect flow.

CONCLUSION

Intravascular imaging is an important diagnostic tool, even when considering B-mode display only. The 3D imaging capability adds a new dimension to the intravascular study, allowing a much more detailed analysis of complex stenosis and arterial lesions. An example of the results of this procedure is illustrated in Fig. 118-40. Automatic procedures require sophisticated tissue characterization processing such as that using the methods discussed here. An important additional advantage of the method is that plaque within the arterial wall can be properly identified and visualized on the computer.

REFERENCES

1. Aerotech KB: Axial resolution, *Aero-Tech Rep* 1(1):1-3, 1978.
2. Metherell AF, eds: *Acoustical imaging,* New York, 1982, Plenum.
3. Arnett EN et al: Coronary arterial narrowing in coronary heart disease: comparison with cineangiographic and necropsy findings, *Ann Intern Med* 91:350-356, 1979.
4. Bom N, Lancee CTT, van Egmond FC: An ultrasonic intracardiac scanner, *Ultrasonics* 10:72-76, 1972.
5. Bom N et al: Early and recent intraluminal ultrasound devices, *Int J Card Imaging* 4:79-88, 1989.
6. Burrell CJ, Kitney RI, Rothman MT: Intravascular ultrasound imaging and three dimensional modeling of arteries, *Echocardiography* 7:475-484, 1990.
7. Davies MJ, Woolf N: *Atheroma—atherosclerosis in ischaemic heart disease. 1—The mechanisms,* Beijing, China, 1990, Science Press.
8. Farrell EJ: Visual interpretation of complex data, *IBM Sys J* 26:174-200, 1987.
9. Foley JD, van Dam A: *Fundamentals of computer graphics,* London, Amsterdam, 1984, Addison-Wesley.
10. Gussenhoven WJ, Bom N, Roelandt J, eds: *Intravascular ultrasound,* Dordrecht, Boston, London, 1991, Kluwer Academic.
11. Hayward G: Personal communication, 1991.
12. Hayward G, Gilles D: Five port lattice model for simulation of piezoelectric structures possessing twin, compressional modes of vibration, *Ultrasonics* 28:363-369, 1990.
13. Hayward G et al: A systems model of the thickness mode piezoelectric transducer, *J Acoust Soc Am* 72(2):369-375, 1984.
14. Herman GT, Liu HK: Three dimensional display of human organs from computer tomograms, *Comput Graph Image Processing* 9:1-21, 1979.
15. Khalifa MA, Giddens DP: Analysis of disorder in pulsatile flows with application to post-stenotic blood velocity measurements in dogs, *J Biomech* 11:129, 1987.
16. Kitney RI, Talhami HE: The zoom Wigner transform and its application to the analysis of blood velocity waveforms, *J Theor Biol* 129:395-409, 1987.
17. Kitney RI, Moura L, Straughan K: 3D visualisation of arterial structures using ultrasound and voxel modelling, *Int J Card Imaging* 4:135-143, 1989.
18. Kitney RI, Talhami HE, Giddens GP: The analysis of blood velocity measurements by autoregressive modeling, *J Theoret Biol* 120:419-442, 1986.
19. Kitney RI et al: 3D characterisation of the arterial wall using intravascular ultrasound, *Proc Comput Cardiol* pp 357-360, 1991.
20. McPherson DD et al: Delineation of the extent of coronary atherosclerosis by high frequency epicardial echocardiography, *N Engl J Med* 316:304-309, 1987.
21. Moura L, Kitney RI: A direct method for least-squares circle fitting, *Computer Physics Comm* 64:57-63, 1991.
22. Pipes A: Solid modellers: this year's style, *CAD/CAM Int* 9:20-23, 1985.
23. Sherman CT et al: Demonstration of thrombus and complex atheroma by in-vivo angioscopy in patients with unstable angina pectoris, *N Engl J Med* 315:913-919, 1986.
24. Smith GD: *Numerical solution of partial differential equations,* New York, London, 1965, Oxford University Press.
25. Talhami HE: Analysis and modelling of arterial blood velocity waveforms, London, 1985, University of London (thesis).
26. Talhami HE, Kitney RI: Maximum likelihood frequency tracking of the audio pulsed Doppler ultrasound signal using a Kalman filter, *Ultrasound Med Biol* 14:599-609, 1988.
27. Van Trees HL: *Detection, estimation and modulation theory, part III,* New York, 1971, John Wiley.
28. Yock PG, Linker D: Intravascular ultrasound: looking below the surface of vascular disease, *Circulation* 81:1715-1718, 1990.
29. Yock PG et al: *Intravascular ultrasound guidance during atherectomy.* In Tobis JM, Yock PG, ed: *Intravascular ultrasound imaging,* New York, London, 1992, Churchill Livingstone.
30. Zir LM et al: Inter-observer variability in coronary angiography, *Circulation* 53:627-632, 1976.

CHAPTER 119

Experimental applications of endovascular ultrasound

RODNEY A. WHITE, DOUGLAS M. CAVAYE, and GEORGE E. KOPCHOK

Intravascular ultrasound (IVUS) is developing rapidly both as a diagnostic imaging modality and as a method for guiding and evaluating therapeutic interventions. This chapter focuses on the experimental intravascular imaging investigations that preceded the widespread clinical evaluation and emphasizes its correlation with other imaging modalities.

INITIAL STUDIES
Morphologic evaluations

The findings from several studies have shown that IVUS can be used to accurately determine the dimensions of the luminal diameters and wall thickness of normal or minimally diseased arteries within 0.05 mm, both in vitro and in vivo, if the device is aligned properly in the vessel.* Delineation of the adventitial or outside diameter of the vessels may be less accurate and has shown a margin of error of as much as 0.5 mm in some cases. The precision of the measurements is affected by many variables that are discussed in detail in other sections of this book.

The images produced by IVUS catheters outline not only the luminal and adventitial surfaces of normal arterial segments but can also discriminate between normal and diseased vessel walls (Figs. 119-1 and 119-2). In muscular arteries, distinct wall layers may be visible, with the intima and adventitia more echogenic than the media (Fig. 119-1).[10] Smooth muscle in the media is hypoechoic, whereas collagen in the adventitia and elastin in the intima are hyperechoic. The exact thickness of the adventitia may be difficult to determine unless the vessel is surrounded by more or less echogenic tissues (e.g., fat). Small intimal lesions are quite well defined in muscular arteries because of their fibrous content (Fig. 119-1), but larger complex plaques may compress or shadow the medial detail. The three-layer vessel image seen in muscular arteries may be lost in smaller distal arteries and larger elastic arteries because the increased elastin content makes the media hyperechoic. In medium-sized distal vessels, such as the femoral artery, the media is visible but thinner than it is in more central vessels.

In soft tissue, the absorption coefficient for ultrasound energy is proportional to the frequency, whereas it is proportional to the square of the frequency in calcified tissue.[33] IVUS devices are thus quite sensitive for detecting calcified areas. Calcium shadows deeper structures such that the medial thickness may have to be estimated by comparing it to surrounding contours (Fig. 119-2). Gussenhoven et al[11] have described four basic types of plaque components in human atherosclerotic arteries that can be distinguished by in vitro IVUS imaging using a 40-MHz system. Hypoechoic images denote a significant deposit of lipid. Hypoechoic areas indicate fibromuscular tissue (intimal proliferation) as well as lesions composed of fibromuscular tissue and diffusely dispersed lipid. Bright echoes denote collagen-rich fibrous tissue, and bright echoes with shadowing behind the lesion represent calcium. With most IVUS devices, intraluminal thrombus can frequently be distinguished from the vessel wall. Recent thrombus may appear as a hyperechoic mass with some shadowing (loss of imaging) of tissue beyond it.

Comparison of IVUS to other imaging modalities

Several studies have compared the respective ability of IVUS and uniplanar angiography to determine the luminal dimensions of normal and moderately atherosclerotic human arteries.[22,29,30] Uniplanar angiography can be quite accurate for defining the luminal cross-sectional area if the vessel is circular, as it is in most normal and mildly diseased arteries. However, clinically significant atherosclerotic occlusive disease is usually eccentrically positioned in the lumen, which may be either circular or elliptical, although most are circular.[24,32,37] When the lumen is elliptical, biplanar angiograms are needed for the more accurate definition of luminal cross-sectional areas and calculation of the percentage area of stenosis.[27]

Investigations have also shown that luminal cross-sectional areas measured by IVUS correlate well with those calculated using angiography in normal and minimally diseased peripheral and coronary arteries.[29,33] In most studies in which the lumens have been only mildly elliptical, the cross-sectional areas seen on angiograms and measured using IVUS have been found to correlate significantly, but

---

*References 10, 13, 14, 17, 18, 19, 21, 22, 28, 36.

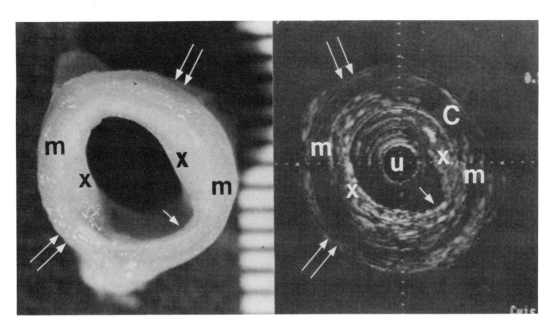

Fig. 119-1. Moderately diseased human atherosclerotic artery *(left)* and in vitro IVUS image of the specimen *(right)* demonstrating the luminal surface *(small arrow)*, fibrous plaque *(X)*, echolucent media *(m)*, and outside wall of the vessel *(double arrows)*. *(C)* denotes an area of shadowing beyond a mildly calcified lesion. *(u)*, Ultrasound probe. (Tabbara M et al: In vitro and in vivo evaluation of intraluminal ultrasound in normal and atherosclerotic arteries, *Am J Surg* 160:556-560, 1990.)

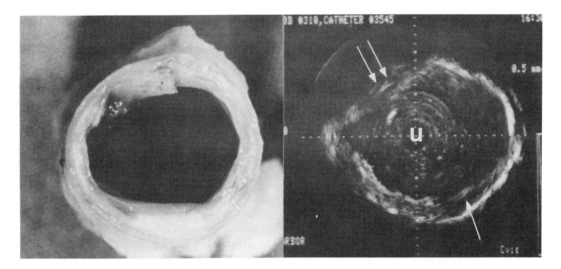

Fig. 119-2. Moderately diseased human iliac artery *(left)* and intraluminal ultrasound image *(right)* demonstrating the characteristic three-layer appearance of less diseased areas *(single arrows)* and shadowing and distortion of images in heavily calcified areas *(double arrows)*. u, Ultrasound probe. (Tabbara M et al: In vitro and in vivo evaluation of intraluminal ultrasound in normal and atherosclerotic arteries, *Am J Surg* 160:556-560, 1990.)

angiography has proved less accurate for calculating the luminal cross-sectional area in some severely diseased arteries with elliptical lesions. In elliptical lumens, the cross-sectional area calculated from angiograms is usually greater than that measured by IVUS.

IVUS has been shown to add other pertinent observations to those acquired by conventional imaging methods. Besides

angiography's limited ability to define the luminal dimensions and cross-sectional areas of elliptical and severely diseased vessels, it can provide no information about vessel wall morphology aside from the existence of calcification or aneurysms, which can be visualized on plain x-ray studies. Other imaging modalities, such as angioscopy, can clearly visualize the lumen of a blood vessel, but their ability

Table 119-1. Comparison of intraarterial imaging techniques

Imaging technique	Disease localization	Assessment of luminal dimensions and morphology	Characterization of plaque components	Vessel wall dimensions	Inspection of runoff vessels
Angiography	Gold standard	Yes, quantitative ($\pm 40\%$) in severely diseased arteries	Limited to calcification and ulceration	No	Yes
Angioscopy	Yes, limited to vessels large enough to accommodate catheter	Yes, qualitative	Only suggested by visual assessment	No	Limited to depth of field of angioscope
Intravascular ultrasound	Yes, limited to vessels large enough to accommodate catheter	Yes, best accuracy	Precise localization plus characterization (e.g., fibrous vs calcium vs thrombus)	Yes, limited by image quality	No

to define vessel wall morphology and the distribution of atherosclerotic lesions is limited. IVUS enhances the intraluminal perspective provided by angiography and angioscopy by defining luminal dimensions and vessel wall characteristics.[19,23,34]

The abilities of angiography, angioscopy, and IVUS to identify thrombus, residual stenosis, and vessel wall dissection after percutaneous coronary angioplasty have been compared, and angioscopy was found to be the most sensitive for visualizing thrombus.[20,23] Residual stenosis was underestimated by angiography, and IVUS proved to be the most accurate for this task. Angioscopy could not quantify stenosis but could only be used to estimate lesion size. Angioscopy was found to be the most sensitive method for determining dissection after dilatation. All three methods accurately identified atherosclerotic plaque. Angioscopy could depict surface features, such as pigmentation and thrombus, whereas IVUS was able to differentiate fibrous lesions from calcification in the arterial wall. This type of comparison emphasizes that angioscopy and IVUS each provide unique information not yielded by conventional angiography.

Validation of the data obtained from angioscopy and IVUS has also been achieved by comparing the sensitivity, specificity, and accuracy of both methods, separately and in combination, for determining the characteristics of normal and diseased arteries.[25] In normal vessels, the correlation of vessel wall dimensions was uniformly greater than or equal to 95%, but angioscopy showed an advantage because it could visually identify and inspect a thrombus. For specific evaluations, such as classifying atheroma as stable or disrupted, the sensitivities of both methods were slightly lower, although the specificity, accuracy, and predictive value for identifying lesions were each greater than 90%. The findings yielded by angioscopy and IVUS, either alone or in combination, demonstrated significant agreement with the histologic findings ($p < 0.001$). Table 119-1 compares the utility of angiography, angioscopy, and IVUS for char-

acterizing the morphology and distribution of vessel wall components.

Most investigators report that the currently available IVUS devices produce clear images of vessel anatomy under optimal conditions, but at times the instruments exhibit limited resolution in routine clinical situations. Careful positioning of catheter tips and appropriate probe-to-vessel size ratios are required to optimize visualization. Image quality is best when the catheter is parallel such that the ultrasound beam is perpendicular to the wall, and whereas minor angulations may affect the image. Eccentric positioning makes the near wall appear thicker and more echogenic. Calcium at the edge of a diverging beam may convey a misleading fibrotic appearance. Methods that can precisely identify the location and orientation of the probes are also needed. Some prototypes include the use of an image artifact that corresponds to an external mark on the catheter to define the orientation. With the further development of these instruments, the current limitations related to image resolution and position sensitivity should be overcome. The resolution of the images is improving rapidly as the clinical evaluation of these devices proceeds and the catheter-based technology progresses.

THREE-DIMENSIONAL ULTRASOUND IMAGING

Three-dimensional (3D) intravascular imaging of vessels is a recently available technique made possible by advances in personal computer hardware and innovative software.[5] 3D image reconstruction consists of three major computational steps: (1) segmentation and interpolation, (2) surface tracking, and (3) creation of rendered images. One approach* consists of a longitudinally aligned series of consecutive two-dimensional (2D) IVUS cross-sectional images that are stacked on top of each other (Fig. 119-3). After the stack of slices is obtained, a packed binary cubic voxel array is generated by combining segmentation, interpola-

---

*Image Comm Systems, Inc., Santa Clara, Calif.

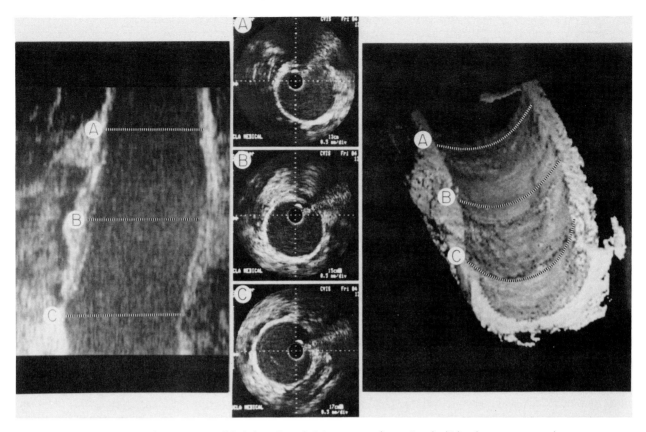

Fig. 119-3. The 2D images labeled *A, B,* and *C* (center panel) are "stacked" by the computer and correspond to the sites labeled with the same letter on the 3D image *(right)* and longitudinal section of the 3D image *(left)*. The longitudinal section of the 3D image is displayed on the computer monitor to allow optimal adjustments of the image density threshold and viewing orientation. (Cavaye DM et al: Three-dimensional vascular ultrasound imaging, *Am Surg* 57:751-755, 1991.)

tion, and efficient data packing. Because threshold-based segmentation is not perfect, objectlike structures and noise may clutter the binary information. The reconstructed image is therefore isolated from the clutter by tracking a specified connected surface of the image. This surface description is rendered to create a depiction of the surface on a computer screen.

Images may be acquired live or from videotape playback. The number of 2D images per 3D reconstruction is determined by the sampling rate and the total data acquisition time. Although image-sampling rates of between 32 and 256 are available in the software, 90 to 110 images per 5.0-cm segment is optimal. To obtain the images, the examiner positions the IVUS catheter at the proximal end of the segment to be reconstructed. The sampling gate is opened and the catheter is withdrawn manually through the organ segment at a rate of 1 cm/4 sec. A 5.0-cm-long segment is represented by 90 images acquired during the 20-second "pull through." A computer-processing time of approximately 10 seconds is required to complete the surface tracking and creation of a coronal 2D image. The organ segment is then viewed on a high-resolution gray-scale monitor in a longitudinal 2D view (Fig. 119-3). The image-density

threshold is adjusted to optimize the differentiation of structures. This is an important step, particularly when it is necessary to distinguish tissues with a similar echodensity (e.g., soft plaque versus thrombus). The 3D image is then displayed in multiple orientations as either a complete segment or in a longitudinal section, depending on the viewer's choice. The viewing angle is changed to allow inspection of the 3D image from all possible angles, both from within the lumen and from the adventitial surface. All data are stored on hard disk, making them available for review at a later time.

PRELIMINARY THERAPEUTIC APPLICATIONS

The therapeutic applications of IVUS are rapidly being developed. Several prototype instruments incorporate IVUS as the means for choosing the appropriate size and type of intraluminal device and for observing the immediate outcome of procedures. Results of recent studies have indicated that balloon size for use in percutaneous transluminal balloon angioplasty is often underestimated when selection is based on quantitative angiographic findings and that optimal balloon size is more accurately determined by IVUS.[2] Additional findings suggest that angiographic proof of the suc-

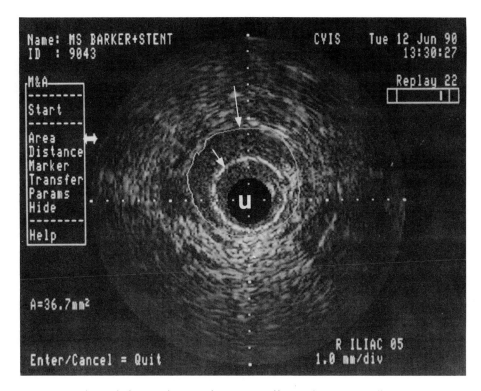

Fig. 119-4. Intraluminal ultrasound image of a 5.0 mm self-expanding stent *(small arrow)* in a 7.0 mm diameter canine iliac artery *(large arrow)*. Such an error in stent-vessel size matching results in the stent acting as a partial obstruction to blood flow. *u,* Ultrasound probe. (Cavaye DM et al: Intraluminal ultrasound assessment of vascular stent deployment, *Ann Vasc Surg* 5:241-246, 1991.)

cess of balloon angioplasty consists of disrupted calcified lesions (highly echoic components), with dissections extending into the media of the vessel; angiographically verified failure is implied when the lesions are nondisplaced or when circumferential dissections or intimal flaps form.[15] Angiographically confirmed success in the treatment of soft lesions (mildly echoic) is associated with superficial fissures or fractures of the luminal surface, but vessel recoil and luminal disruption or thrombosis at sites of plaque rupture lead to failure. Thus IVUS may provide information that can be used to select lesions for balloon therapy. Many studies have noted that IVUS can be used to document lesion characteristics, including eccentricity,[6,22] and to quantitate residual stenosis and dissections following dilatation.[6,9,22,31]

IVUS is also being investigated as a method for studying the mechanism of action and function of atherectomy devices, stents, and lasers.[3,4,12,26] For each type of device, the guidance and lesion assessment capabilities of IVUS in combination with the interventional components may delineate specific benefits for a particular approach. Figs. 119-4 and 119-5 highlight the potential for IVUS aiding in the deployment of intravascular stents and assessing the outcome of the procedure.

Additional studies have confirmed the utility of IVUS for identifying the important features of successfully performed endoluminal stenting of acute aortic dissections in

an experimental canine model.[4] 2D and 3D images can be used to delineate the proximal site and distal extent of the dissection, identify the relationship of the false lumen to major aortic branches, measure the aortic dimensions to allow selection of correct stent size, and confirm that the stent is being deployed in the true lumen to obliterate the false lumen. The ultrasound images also show whether the stents have been fully deployed and are more accurate than angiograms for evaluating this critical factor (Fig. 119-6).

An additional potential therapeutic application of IVUS, already investigated in preliminary studies, is to use it to guide laser angioplasty for the recanalization of small-diameter arterial occlusions.[1,35] The combination of IVUS and lasers is particularly appealing for the manufacture of cost-effective, miniaturized, precise ablation devices because the fiberoptic and microchip components used in these modalities can be integrated into low-profile catheter systems. Initial investigations have demonstrated the merits of IVUS-guided laser recanalization of experimental arterial occlusions, which is followed by concentric enlargement of the recanalization achieved by passing larger-diameter multifiber laser catheters over the initial concentrically placed laser fiber (Figs. 119-7 and 119-8). Although other interventional ablation devices such as atherectomy catheters may accomplish this same goal, so far only laser fiberoptics have best met the prerequisite of cost-effective miniaturization, since

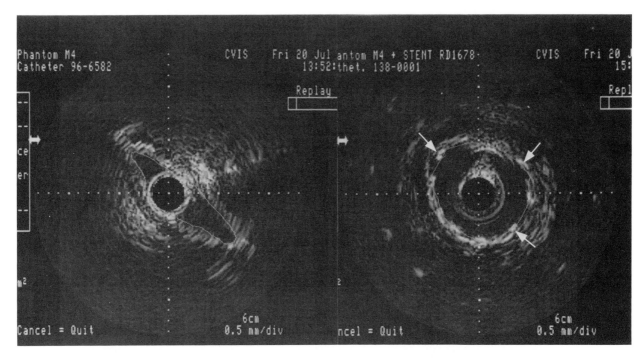

Fig. 119-5. Intraluminal ultrasound cross-sectional images *(left)* before and *(right)* after insertion of a 5.0 mm self-expanding stent into a formalin-preserved human superficial femoral artery. A dramatic change in the luminal shape is produced by the stent, resulting in an increase in cross-sectional area from 7.9 mm² to 16.7 mm² and an increase in the minimum/maximum diameter and ratio from 0.26 to 0.875. Arrows indicate stent struts. (Cavaye DM et al: Intraluminal ultrasound assessment of vascular stent deployment, *Ann Vasc Surg* 5:241-246, 1991.)

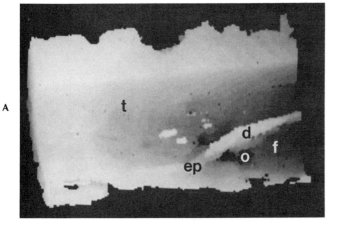 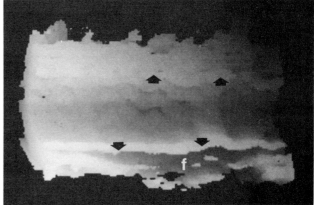

Fig. 119-6. *A,* Three-dimensional intravascular ultrasound image of aortic dissection before stent insertion showing the dissection flap and end point. *B,* After intravascular stent deployment, the dissection flap is forced against the aortic wall by the stent *(arrows),* leaving a residual false lumen filled with stagnant blood. *t,* True lumen; *f,* false lumen; *d,* dissection flap; *ep,* end point; *o,* lumbar artery orifice. (Cavaye DM et al: Usefulness of IVUS imaging for detecting experimentally induced aortic dissection and for determining the effectiveness of endoluminal stenting, *Am J Cardiol* 69:705, 1992.)

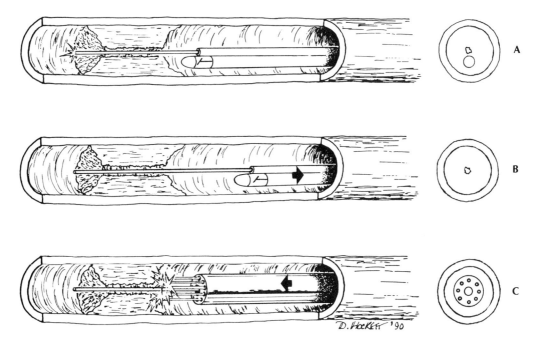

Fig. 119-7. The idealized ultrasound-guided laser recanalization of an experimental arterial occlusion. **A,** The laser fiberoptic is centered in the vessel lumen by coaxial alignment with the ultrasound catheters, followed by advancement of the fiber through the occlusion. **B,** Withdrawal of the ultrasound catheter leaving the laser fiberoptic positioned in the lesion. **C,** Passage of a multifiber laser catheter over the single fiberoptic to concentrically enlarge the vessel lumen. (White RA et al: IVUS-guided holmium:YAG laser recanalization of occluded arteries, *Lasers Surg Med* 12:239-249, 1992.)

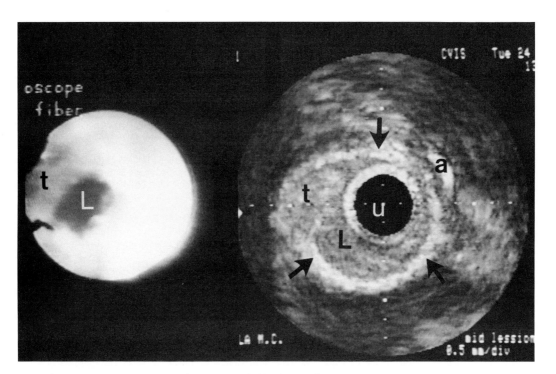

Fig. 119-8. Angioscopic view of an IVUS-guided laser recanalization after passage of a multifiber catheter over a concentrically positioned single fiber *(left)* and the IVUS image of the same site in the vessel *(right)*. *L,* Vessel lumen; *u,* position of the ultrasound probe on IVUS image; arrows outline the vessel wall on the IVUS image; *a,* artifact on the IVUS image to enable orientation of the probe and laser fiber. (White RA et al: IVUS-guided holmium:YAG laser recanalization of occluded arteries, *Lasers Surg Med* 12:239-249, 1992.)

the expense and technical difficulty of manufacturing many atherectomy devices increases with increased miniaturization.

3D real-time IVUS imaging of arterial lesions and recanalizations enhances the practicality of the guided ablation concept because it furnishes an easily interpretable reconstruction of the vessel and recanalization procedure. This ability to define the spatial arrangement of eccentrically positioned or variable-consistency plaque within a vessel makes 3D IVUS imaging a clinically applicable tool with unique diagnostic and therapeutic applications. Further refinements of this concept are represented by the forward-looking IVUS systems that are currently being developed and investigated. A particularly important contribution of IVUS to future endovascular device development is its ability to provide accurate control data that can be used to determine the efficacy of current devices and to define current failure mechanisms.

As can be inferred, conventional cineangiography does not supply adequately sensitive data regarding either the distribution and consistency of lesions or the outcome of current methods. Contemporary theories about recurrences (so-called restenosis) following interventional procedures are flawed by inaccurate control data regarding lesion morphology and distribution that has been measured or calculated from angiograms. In most cases, failures that are currently attributed to smooth muscle cell restenosis are actually due to inadequate removal of atherosclerotic lesions or to thrombosis and reorganization of residual intraluminal debris. The reportedly high recurrence rates associated with almost all interventional methods, particularly balloon angioplasty, stem primarily from inadequate removal of lesions and from trauma to the vessel wall that stimulates smooth muscle cell proliferation. The ability to accomplish long-term patency in most recanalized severely diseased human arteries using improved methods that debulk lesions in a less traumatic fashion has been demonstrated.[7] With the use of these improved methods, the 2-year patency documented by arteriography or duplex scanning approaches 70%. This degree of smooth muscle recurrence more closely approximates the known 10% to 15% luminal narrowing that occurs after surgical endarterectomy and negates the contemporary rapid restenosis concept. With refinement of the technique for IVUS-guided removal and debulking of lesions, the long-term patency may further improve and the complications from arterial wall dissection and perforation dramatically decrease.

FUTURE PERSPECTIVES

IVUS has important potential for both diagnostic and interventional applications. Future angioplasty guidance devices may combine the benefits of angioscopy and IVUS into a single, disposable delivery system suitable for incorporation into any mechanical or laser-based ablation device. Angioscopy would allow visual inspection of the lumen and ultrasound would define the vessel wall charac-

teristics and dimensions. Improved IVUS imaging will be achieved through both refinements in the 2D visualization of cross-sectional vessel wall anatomy and the 3D reconstruction of the vasculature from a sequence of ultrasound images.

IVUS devices are being evaluated clinically as a diagnostic aid for use during cardiac catheterizations in high-risk groups of patients for coronary artery disease, such as those with cardiac transplants. Future diagnostic capabilities may facilitate angioplasty device selection by identifying the tissue distribution in lesions. For example, the identification of highly calcified areas would indicate that pulsed-laser energy rather than balloon angioplasty be used. Quantitative analysis of ultrasound backscatter from the vessel wall may also increase the diagnostic sensitivity.[16] These devices may furnish information regarding the optimal amount of debulking necessary for successful angioplasty and enable studies to determine whether medial smooth muscle exposure leads to restenosis. The technology may also be used to identify the etiology of complications, such as intimal flaps that lead to restenosis or excessive lesion debulking that causes thinning of the vessel wall, precipitating aneurysm formation.

Additional possible applications for IVUS include many exciting vascular research areas such as determining blood vessel compliance,[8] identifying dynamic changes in the vascular wall caused by disease or pharmacologic intervention, and further elucidating the natural history of atherosclerosis and other arteriopathies. The combination of imaging technology with Doppler flow studies before and after interventions can assess both the hemodynamic effect of therapy and determine the presence or absence of any remaining disease.

REFERENCES

1. Aretz HT, Martinelli MA, LeDet EG: Intravascular ultrasound guidance of transverse laser coronary atherectomy, *Int J Card Imaging* 4:153-157, 1989.
2. Cacchione J, Nair R, Hodson J: Intracoronary ultrasound better than conventional methods for determining optimal PTCA balloon size, *J Am Coll Cardiol* 17:112A, 1991 (abstract).
3. Cavaye DM et al: Intravascular ultrasound assessment of vascular stent deployment, *Ann Vasc Surg* 5:241-246, 1991.
4. Cavaye DM et al: Usefulness of intravascular ultrasound imaging in detecting experimentally induced aortic dissection and for determining the effectiveness of endoluminal stenting, *Am J Cardiol* 69:705-707, 1992.
5. Cavaye DM et al: Three dimensional vascular ultrasound imaging, *Am Surg* 57:751-755, 1991.
6. Davidson CJ et al: Intracoronary ultrasound evaluation of interventional procedures, *Circulation* 82(suppl III):440, 1990 (abstract).
7. Graor RA et al: *Atherectomy of the superficial femoral and popliteal arteries: two year patency and factors influencing patency,* Presented at the meeting of the Society for Vascular Surgery, Los Angeles, Calif, June 1990.
8. Gordon M, Dick C, Jarvis G: Determination of regional arterial compliance by intravascular ultrasound, *Circulation* 84(suppl II):675, 1991 (abstract).
9. Gurley J et al: Comparison of intravascular ultrasound following percutaneous transluminal coronary angioplasty, *Circulation* 82:90, 1990 (abstract).
10. Gussenhoven WJ, Essed CE, Lancee CT: Arterial wall characteristics determined by intravascular ultrasound imaging: an in-vitro study, *J Am Coll Cardiol* 14:947-952, 1989.

11. Gussenhoven WJ et al: Intravascular echographic assessment of vessel wall characteristics: a correlation with histology, *Int J Card Imaging* 4:105-116, 1989.

12. Isner JM et al: Percutaneous intravascular US as adjunct to catheter-based interventions: preliminary experience in patients with peripheral vascular disease, *Radiology* 175:61-70, 1990.

13. Kopchok G, White R, White G: Intravascular ultrasound: a new potential modality for angioplasty guidance, *Angiology* 41:785-792, 1990.

14. Kopchok GE et al: Intraluminal vascular ultrasound: preliminary report of dimensional and morphologic accuracy, *Ann Vasc Surg* 4:291-296, 1990.

15. Leon M et al: Intravascular ultrasound assessment of plaque responses to PTCA helps to explain angiographic findings, *J Am Coll Cardiol* 17:47A, 1991 (abstract).

16. Linker DT et al: Analysis of back scattering ultrasound from normal and diseased arterial wall, *Int J Cardiol Imaging* 4:177-185, 1989.

17. Mallery JA et al: Assessment of normal and atherosclerotic arterial wall thickness with intravascular ultrasound imaging catheter, *Am Heart J* 119:1392-1400, 1990.

18. Meyer CR et al: Feasibility of high resolution intravascular ultrasonic imaging catheters, *Radiology* 168:113-116, 1988.

19. Neville RF et al: Validation and feasibility of in vivo intravascular ultrasound imaging with a new flexible catheter, *Surg Forum* 75:314-316, 1989.

20. Neville RF et al: Endovascular management of arterial intimal defects: an experimental comparison by arteriography, angioscopy, and intravascular ultrasonography, *J Vasc Surg* 13:496-502, 1991.

21. Nissen SE et al: Application of new phased-array ultrasound imaging catheter in the assessment of vascular dimensions, *Circulation* 81:660-666, 1990.

22. Nissen SE et al: Comparison of intravascular ultrasound and angiography in quantitation of coronary dimensions and stenoses in man: impact of lumen eccentricity, *Circulation* 82(suppl III):440, 1990 (abstract).

23. Ramee SR et al: Percutaneous coronary angioscopy versus intravascular ultrasound in patients undergoing coronary angioplasty, *J Am Coll Cardiol* 17:125A, 1991 (abstract).

24. Roberts RW: Coronary arteries in coronary heart disease: morphologic observations, *Pathobiol Annu* 5:249, 1975.

25. Siegel R, Ariani M, Fishbein M: Histopathologic validation of angioscopy and intravascular ultrasound, *Circulation* 84:109-117, 1991.

26. Smucker ML, Scherb DE, Howard PF: Intracoronary ultrasound: how much "angioplasty effect" in atherectomy? *Circulation* 82(suppl III):676, 1990 (abstract).

27. Sumner DS, Russell JB, Miles RD: *Pulsed Doppler arteriography and computer assisted imaging of carotid bifurcation.* In Bergan JJ, Yao JST, eds: *Cerebrovascular insufficiency,* New York, 1983, Grune & Stratton.

28. Tabbara M, Kopchok G, White R: In vitro and in vivo evaluation of intraluminal ultrasound in normal and atherosclerotic arteries, *Am J Surg* 160:556-560, 1990.

29. Tabbara MR et al: In-vivo human comparison of intravascular ultrasound and angiography, *J Vasc Surg* 14:496-504, 1991.

30. Tobis JM et al: The sensitivity of ultrasound imaging compared with angiography for diagnosing coronary atherosclerosis, *Circulation* 82(suppl III):439, 1990 (abstract).

31. Tobis J et al: Cross sectional morphology of balloon dilatation in vivo by intravascular ultrasound, *J Am Coll Cardiol* 17:157A, 1991 (abstract).

32. Waller BF: The eccentric coronary atherosclerotic plaque: morphologic observations and clinical relevance, *Clin Cardiol* 12:14-20, 1989.

33. West AL: *Endovascular ultrasound.* In Moore WS, Ahs SS, eds: *Endovascular surgery,* Philadelphia, 1989, Saunders.

34. White R: Indications for fiberoptic angioscopy and intraluminal ultrasound, *Compr Ther* 16:23-30, 1990.

35. White RA et al: Intravascular ultrasound guided holmium: YAG laser recanalization of occluded arteries, *Lasers Surg Med* 12:239-249, 1992.

36. Yock PG, Johnson EL, Linker DT: Intravascular ultrasound development and clinical potential, *Am J Card Imaging* 2:185-193, 1988.

37. Zarins C, Zatura MA, Glagov S: *Correlation of postmortem angiography with pathologic anatomy: quantitation of atherosclerotic lesions.* In Bond MG et al, eds: *Clinical diagnosis of atherosclerosis,* New York, 1983, Springer-Verlag.

CHAPTER 120

Clinical applications of intravascular ultrasound imaging

PAUL G. YOCK, PETER J. FITZGERALD, KRISHNANKUTTY SUDHIR, and THOMAS A. PORTS

The technology of intravascular ultrasound imaging is developing at a rapid pace. Although significant engineering efforts have been underway for only about 5 years, sophisticated, reliable catheters, approved by the Food and Drug Administration, are now available from four companies, and other developments are in progress.

New clinical knowledge about vascular disease has followed these technical developments closely. Scanning with ultrasound catheters provides a direct appreciation of the plaque burden present in clinically diseased arteries and a clinical means to view the natural history of the process. Also important is the opportunity to assess and monitor the results of different therapies for vascular disease, including surgery, catheter-based interventions, and pharmacotherapy. This chapter reviews some of the insights in these areas that have emerged from the early clinical studies with intravascular ultrasound.

DIRECT VISUALIZATION OF PLAQUE

Ultrasound is unique among the available and potential catheter-based imaging technologies in its ability to examine plaque and vessel walls beneath the luminal surface.[4,21,39] Fortunately, the media of muscular arteries such as the coronary and femoral systems is relatively hypoechoic compared with the intima and adventitia.[12,18,38] This provides a fairly distinct inner border from which accumulations of plaque can be discriminated (Fig. 120-1). The volume of plaque in a given segment of vessel can be determined by analyzing serial images.[8]

Several different components of plaque can be identified on the basis of their relative reflectivity of ultrasound. Fibrous tissue appears brighter than fibrofatty plaque on the images and is often seen in the form of a partial arc within the vessel wall.[13,17] Calcification is identified by even brighter reflectance accompanied by shadowing of tissue structures beyond the calcium deposits.[12] One problem associated with catheter ultrasound imaging is in discriminating between soft plaque and thrombus, which frequently have similar overall levels of reflectance. Advances in image processing, including so-called tissue characterization algorithms, may enhance the ability to make subtle tissue identifications that are difficult on the basis of the appearance of the images alone.[6] These methods involve computer-based analysis of either the texture of the video display or the spectral characteristics of the raw radiofrequency signal used to make the ultrasound images.[24]

Several studies have suggested that intravascular ultrasound is more accurate than angiography in measuring lumen cross-sectional area. This is particularly true in the postinterventional setting, in which the lumen contour may be complex as a result of dissection.[19,20,25,37] Although angioscopy is a better method for visualizing lumen surface details (and particularly for identifying thrombus), ultrasound is more readily quantitative. The ultrasound display screens have a calibration bar or grid that allows visual estimation of dimensions and includes software-based electronic calipers and area algorithms.

DIAGNOSTIC APPLICATIONS

The high resolution of intravascular ultrasound imaging and the ability to visualize plaque in depth have led investigators to identify several diagnostic areas of application for the technology. Clinically useful images have been obtained in aortic dissections in which the true and false lumens can be clearly located and the entry and exit sites specified.[36] Direct sizing of aortic aneurysms and identification of thrombus are also possible with the catheters, particularly at lower frequencies (10 to 20 MHz). In both dissections and aneurysms, the relative risk of passing the catheter must be weighed against the increased yield of information compared with computerized tomography or magnetic resonance imaging. If angiography is planned for the patient, catheter ultrasound imaging can add considerably to the detailed understanding of the process.

In the context of catheter-based vascular interventions, ultrasound can be used as a screening technique to help decide whether a particular lesion merits treatment. Again, it must be appreciated that catheter ultrasound is a relatively invasive imaging modality, which given the current generation of side-looking catheters, requires crossing of a lesion to obtain images. Recently, the feasibility of transvenous ultrasound imaging, which yields images of coronary arteries with the ultrasound transducer in an adjacent coronary vein, has been demonstrated.[31] It is worth empha-

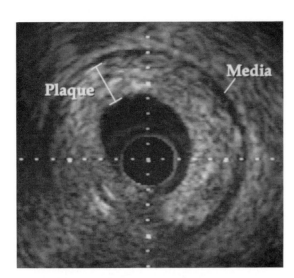

Fig. 120-1. Intravascular ultrasound scan from a coronary artery with a circumferential accumulation of soft plaque. The catheter is the dark circle in the center, positioned within an elliptical lumen (dark gray). The media is hypoechoic relative to the plaque. Calibration marks in the cross-hair are 0.5 mm.

sizing that the plaque burden revealed by intracoronary ultrasound is generally much greater than is evident from angiography and, for the present, decisions to intervene need to be based on clinical data and lumen caliber rather than on the amount of plaque present.

Catheter ultrasound has been advocated as a diagnostic tool in other arterial beds such as the pulmonary circulation. Pulmonary emboli have been detected in animal models, although the size of the catheters and the fact that a number of branches of the vessel may need to be scanned limit the practical applications of the technique in this setting.[23,28] Use of intravascular images to evaluate patients for pulmonary thrombectomy and endarterectomy has been described.[26]

GUIDANCE FOR BALLOON ANGIOPLASTY

Some of the mechanical factors that account for the success of balloon angioplasty also make it difficult to monitor the procedure accurately by angiography. In the majority of cases, successful dilatation of a diseased segment involves fracture of the plaque and/or tearing away from the normal wall components. This creates a complex and irregular lumen, which corresponds to a hazy or indistinct appearance on the angiogram. In these situations it is assumed that dissection or thrombus has been produced, but it is frequently not possible to have a complete understanding of the particular process involved with angiography.

Intravascular ultrasound has provided clinical confirmation of the mechanisms of angioplasty and has offered some new insights into the factors that control the response of the plaque to balloon inflation. Plaque tears and dissections are seen by ultrasound in a large proportion of balloon angioplasty cases (Fig. 120-2) in both peripheral and coronary vessels.[11,15,33] Investigators have speculated that the incidence of tears seen in coronary angioplasty (between 40% and 70%) may be an underestimation of the actual rate because of the tendency of the catheters to "prop up" torn portions of plaque against the vessel wall. Current coronary catheters are in the 3.5 to 4.3 Fr size range (1.1 to 1.4 mm in diameter), which is close to the lumen size in some cases. This issue is not as significant in the peripheral vessels, where the catheter-to-lumen ratio is typically somewhat smaller.

The clinical significance of the ability to detect plaque tears and dissections is unclear at this time. There is considerable evidence from both animal[27,30] and clinicopathologic studies[22,35] that true dissections, with tears extending into media or adventitia, stimulate a more aggressive proliferative response than tears remaining within the plaque substance. In the study by Nobuyoshi et al,[22] for example, the rate of myointimal proliferation was nearly double for subintimal tears compared with tears that did not extend into media. There is the prospect, therefore, that accurate imaging of postangioplasty tears could help identify a group of patients at high risk for restenosis.

Emerging data suggest that ultrasound may be able to not only identify dissections after balloon inflation but also identify plaques that are at a high risk of significant dissection in advance. Recent work from one laboratory has demonstrated that localized calcium deposits within plaque are a significant factor in promoting the formation of plaque tears.[5] Calcium deposits within lesions that are being treated by angioplasty are common; they occur in over 70% of coronary cases.[11] These localized deposits become sites of high shear stress during balloon inflation, since they are relatively hard compared with the surrounding plaque. Thus tears tend to occur more frequently in plaques with localized calcium deposits, to be located in association with the calcium, and to be larger when calcium is present. It is not clear, however, that localized calcium is associated with poor short- or long-term outcomes of balloon angioplasty. In fact, preliminary data from Tobis et al[34] suggest that concentric plaques without any calcium deposits may have a higher rate of restenosis (over 60%) than plaques with calcium. One explanation of this finding is that it may actually be favorable for some tearing of plaque to occur during the angioplasty process to release the constriction that the plaque creates at that segment of the vessel. If a segment stretches without tearing, rebound may be more likely to occur and negatively affect long-term patency. Myointimal hyperplasia may occur despite the lack of tearing, and the relatively small lumen may not be able to tolerate this tissue ingrowth.

Because of the potential for ultrasound to monitor and perhaps guide balloon angioplasty, several groups have undertaken development of combined balloon/ultrasound imaging catheters.[14,16] Hodgson et al[14] have pioneered the design and testing of a multielement combined catheter in

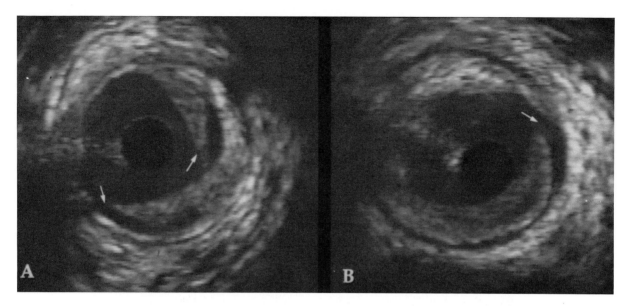

Fig. 120-2. Examples of dissection postballoon angioplasty in peripheral vessels. *A,* Two plaque tears *(arrows)* that remain within the plaque substance. The upper tear is associated with a localized calcium deposit (at 2 o'clock) that can be recognized both by the bright echo appearance and the shadowing beyond. *B,* Subintimal tear *(arrow)* extending into the media. The media is hypoechoic and is recognized as the thin dark band extending circumferentially under the plaque. (Courtesy Steven R. Bailey, San Antonio, Tex.)

which the transducer is placed behind the proximal shoulder of the balloon. This preserves the crossing profile of the balloon but allows for immediate inspection of the postprocedure result by sliding the deflated balloon forward. In initial clinical trials these investigators have documented that the operator's impression of the lumen is altered by the availability of the ultrasound images compared with angiography alone.[14] Isner et al[16] have tested a different catheter configuration in which a mechanical transducer is mounted centrally within the balloon. This allows direct visualization of the response of the plaque to balloon inflation. In preliminary clinical trials with this catheter, these investigators have documented that elastic recoil after balloon inflation is a common and significant factor in determining the result of the procedure.[16] They have also shown that plaque tears tend to occur at relatively low inflation pressures, typically in the range of 2 atm. Further trials with these devices are necessary to determine whether the information provided by ultrasound makes these combined catheters truly useful and cost effective.

PLAQUE REMOVAL METHODS: ATHERECTOMY AND LASER

Catheter-based plaque removal techniques such as atherectomy and laser provide a more direct example of the limitations of angiography as a guidance technique than does balloon angioplasty. Directional atherectomy, in which plaque specimens are removed from the side of the vessel wall, is the best studied of the second-generation catheter techniques and provides some interesting insights into the

problems of guidance. In the coronary atherectomy experience, 40% to 70% of cases have subintimal components— media or adventitia—present in the specimens retrieved from the artery.[9,29] Fortunately, the rates of frank perforation and pseudoaneurysm formation are very low. Original studies on restenosis suggested that recurrence rates were accelerated with subintimal sampling,[10] a finding that still appears to be true in peripheral cases.[2] A recent preliminary report of coronary atherectomy, however, suggests that medial sampling may be associated with a trend toward lower recurrence rates, perhaps because of the creation of a relatively large lumen that is able to tolerate some degree of intimal ingrowth.[40]

This deep tissue sampling, however, occurs in the context of incomplete plaque removal. In one preliminary study, the average percentage cross-sectional area still occupied by plaque at the end of a successful directional atherectomy procedure was 63%.[40] This result was despite a mean angiographic percent stenosis of 11% (Fig. 120-3). Thus when angiography alone is used as guidance, a considerable burden of plaque is left behind in the vessel, and inappropriately deep cuts are frequently made in some portion of the vessel wall. The main reasons for the large discrepancy between angiography and ultrasound are that (1) the "normal" reference site chosen for the angiographic percentage of stenosis calculations has an average plaque accumulation of 30% by ultrasound and (2) the atherectomy device dilates or "Dotters" the lumen as well as removes tissue, so the angiogram provides an optimistic assessment of the degree of plaque removal.

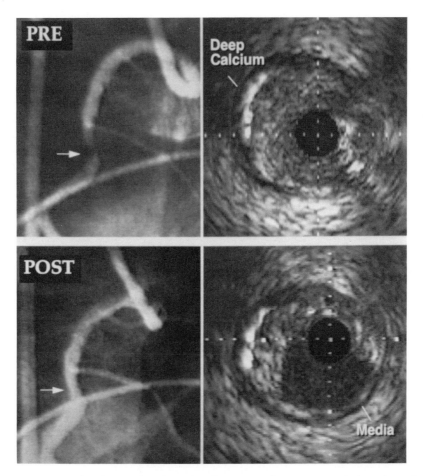

Fig. 120-3. Intravascular ultrasound guidance for atherectomy. The top two panels show the angiogram and ultrasound image preatherectomy. The ultrasound scan shows the catheter wedged in soft plaque, with a thin deposit of calcium at the luminal border between 9 and 11 o'clock. Post DCA (lower two panels). The angiographic result is excellent, but the ultrasound images show a large residual plaque. There is no evidence on the scan for medial encroachment.

Ultrasound also has demonstrated how calcium affects directional atherectomy. When calcium is deposited at the luminal surface, it is difficult for the current directional device to obtain samples from this portion of the plaque. Tissue retrieval in these cases is significantly diminished.[40] This phenomenon occurs despite the calcium not being apparent on fluoroscopy; it is the location of the calcium within the plaque and not the amount of calcium alone that appears to determine the success of tissue removal. Calcium buried deeper within the plaque substance is not an obstacle for the directional atherectomy device, which can remove the softer plaque down to the level of the calcification.

These findings suggest one way in which a triage strategy for device selection could be developed from specific information about plaque provided by ultrasound. If a significant layer of superficial calcification is detected on ultrasound scanning, it may be reasonable to use a calcium-avid device such as the Rotablator, which is a high-speed rotating burr capable of grinding through calcific deposits.

If a lesion is free of calcium or has a deposit deep at the medial border, directional atherectomy should be effective. If a laser catheter is selected, optimum energy and pulse parameters may be predictable on the basis of the amount of calcium to be encountered by the catheter.

Initial scanning of a vessel as a guide to the selection of therapy has some limitations because of the current state of the technology. With the present generation of side-looking catheters, it is necessary to cross the lesion before obtaining information about the type of plaque to be treated. With current 3.5 to 4.3 Fr catheters, many lesions are difficult to cross primarily. There is also theoretic concern about the effects of Dottering a lesion before delivering definitive therapy, although many of the current therapeutic devices have a significant Dottering effect. The industry is working to develop lower profile catheters and catheters with the ability to image forward from the catheter tip.

In addition to its ability to prescan a vessel to assist in the selection of an appropriate catheter, ultrasound may help direct plaque removal efforts to the appropriate portions of the vessel wall. Several research groups are currently using ultrasound with directional atherectomy to localize the portion of the vessel wall with the deepest plaque accumulation and to orient the directional atherectomy device accordingly. With the use of ultrasound guidance, some investigators have reduced subintimal sampling rates considerably without compromising the size of the lumen created. The long-term consequences of this targeted approach to atherectomy, however, are unclear.

Combining ultrasound imaging and atherectomy into a single catheter appears to be technically feasible[39] and has some obvious advantages. In preliminary in vitro and animal studies with a prototype device, real-time imaging guidance was highly useful in directing the cuts to areas of maximum plaque accumulation and in ensuring that cuts were not made into the subintimal space.[7]

A combined imaging catheter with a side-cutting laser has been developed by Aretz, Martinelli, and LeDet[1] and has also undergone preliminary animal testing. In this catheter a three-dimensional image of the vessel segment is built up by moving a single-element catheter within the

vessel. Firing of the laser is then directed according to this visitation map.

INTRAVASCULAR STENTING

Like balloon angioplasty, intravascular stenting is intrinsically a nondirectional procedure that is applied without attention to the exact orientation of the plaque within the wall or the plaque type. High-resolution imaging with intravascular ultrasound may still be useful in stenting, however, to assess the degree of apposition of the stent to the vessel wall. The struts of stents can be visualized relatively clearly with ultrasound, and the relationship of the struts to the vessel wall can be assessed (Fig. 120-4). It is possible that incomplete apposition of the stents with the resulting flow disturbance and increased exposure of metal may be a factor in promoting thrombosis.

Intravascular ultrasound is also contributing to the assessment of restenosis after stent placement. The struts of metallic stents can be identified within the substance of a restenosis lesion, which allows accurate measurements of restenosis to be performed. In a preliminary study by Bonner et al,[3] the major loss in lumen caliber after stent deployment

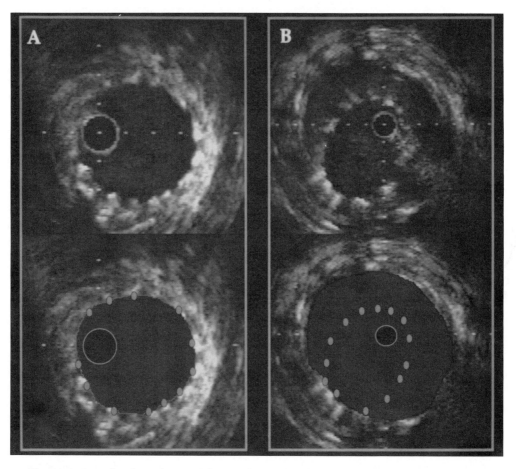

Fig. 120-4. Examples of complete (A) and incomplete (B) stent deployment in an iliac artery. The overlays in the bottom highlight the stent struts, which show up as bright reflections on the intravascular ultrasound scans.

could be attributed to narrowing of the stent scaffold itself over time, rather than ingrowth of hyperplastic tissue. The failure of the relatively rigid metallic stents to maintain sufficient radial forces raises the issue of whether different vessel segments have significantly different degrees of elasticity because of the composition of the plaque or other factors. These are issues that ultrasound imaging is well suited to explore.

ANTICIPATED TECHNICAL AND CLINICAL DEVELOPMENTS

In addition to the combined therapeutic/imaging catheters described, there are a number of technical developments that may enhance and expand the application of catheter ultrasound. Three-dimensional image reconstruction is a logical extension of cross-sectional vascular imaging (see Chapter 118). Current three-dimensional reconstructions are slightly limited in resolution and dynamic range, but early results from next-generation prototype systems (Fig. 120-5) suggest that three-dimensional images with full preservation of image quality are feasible. Combined two-dimensional and Doppler ultrasound imaging may provide more complete characterization of coronary structure and blood flow. It was recently demonstrated that one such system, comprising a two-dimensional imaging catheter over a Doppler guide wire, is a useful tool with which to assess coronary vascular reactivity in vivo.[32]

Tissue characterization techniques are methods of computer analysis of images or the raw ultrasound signal to extract more information about tissue types than is available from visual appearance alone. These techniques show considerable promise for helping to differentiate various plaque types (e.g., helping to discriminate a heavily lipid-laden plaque from a more fibrous lesion). Tissue characterization has already been applied to help overcome one of the significant limitations of intravascular ultrasound imaging, the inability to discriminate soft plaque from thrombus in some cases. Results from preliminary work suggest that analysis of the raw radiofrequency signal provides a statistically significant differentiation between these two tissue types (Fig. 120-6).

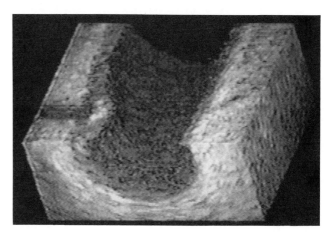

Fig. 120-5. Three-dimensional reconstruction of a clinical coronary artery study. One half of the vessel segment and surrounding tissue (a "hemisection"), approximately 1 cm long, is shown. On the left is a localized calcium deposit that shadows peripherally. The plaque is seen as a darker gray, fairly homogeneous concentric deposit compared with the somewhat brighter periadventitial tissue. A clear medial band is not seen in this image. The image was generated from a prototype system developed by Cardiovascular Imaging Systems, Inc. (Sunnyvale, Calif.) and Indec Systems (Capitola, Calif.)

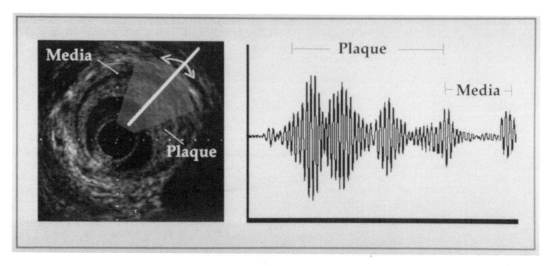

Fig. 120-6. Fundamentals of tissue characterization. The image on the left is constructed from raw radiofrequency information. One line of this information is shown on the right, with the corresponding tissue elements labeled. The image is created from the amplitude envelope of this signal. More information about specific tissue types, however, is available from computer analysis of the raw signal. The image and signal are from a prototype system (Cardiovascular Imaging Systems, Inc.) that provides combined imaging and tissue characterization.

CONCLUSION

The catheter and system technologies for intravascular ultrasound imaging are evolving rapidly. This new imaging modality shows strong promise for helping to delineate the specific features of atherosclerotic disease in the clinical setting and for helping to guide interventions such as balloon angioplasty and the newer, catheter-based methods. Early clinical studies suggest that a triage strategy for selection of devices may emerge from the information provided by the ultrasound scans. Ultrasound may also be useful in monitoring plaque removal treatments such as mechanical atherectomy and laser ablation. Major technical advances to be anticipated include the development of combined imaging/therapeutic devices and the evolution of sophisticated tissue characterization and three-dimensional image representation systems.

REFERENCES

1. Aretz HT, Martinelli MA, LeDet EG: Intraluminal ultrasound guidance of transverse laser coronary atherectomy, *Int J Cardiac Imaging* 4:153-157, 1989.
2. Backa D et al: Histologic comparison of atherectomy biopsies from coronary and peripheral arteries, *Circulation* 82(suppl III):III-34, 1990 (abstract).
3. Bonner RF et al: Acute and chronic compression of rigid slotted stents accounts for progressive lumen narrowing, *Circulation* 84:(suppl II):II-197, 1991 (abstract).
4. Coy KM, Maurer G, Siegel RJ: Intravascular ultrasound imaging: a current perspective, *J Am Coll Cardiol* 18:1811-1823, 1991.
5. Fitzgerald PJ, Ports TA, Yock PG: The contribution of localized calcium deposits to dissection post-angioplasty: an observational study using intravascular ultrasound, *Circulation* 1992 (in press).
6. Fitzgerald PJ et al: Distinction between soft plaque and thrombus by intravascular tissue characterization, *J Am Coll Cardiol* 17:111A, 1991 (abstract).
7. Fitzgerald PJ et al: Combined atherectomy/ultrasound imaging device reduces subintimal tissue injury, *J Am Coll Cardiol* 19:223A, 1992.
8. Galli FC et al: Direct measurement of plaque volume by three-dimensional ultrasound: potentials and pitfalls, *J Am Coll Cardiol* 19:115A, 1992 (abstract).
9. Garratt KN et al: Safety of percutaneous coronary atherectomy with deep arterial resection, *Am J Cardiol* 64:538-540, 1989.
10. Garratt KN et al: Restenosis after directional coronary atherectomy: differences between primary atheromatous and restenosis lesions and influence of subintimal tissue resection, *J Am Coll Cardiol* 16:1665-1671, 1990.
11. GUIDE Trial Investigators: Initial report of the "GUIDE" Trial for intravascular ultrasound imaging in coronary interventions, *J Am Coll Cardiol* 19:223A, 1992 (abstract).
12. Gussenhoven EJ et al: Intravascular echographic assessment of vessel wall characteristics: a correlation with histology, *Int J Cardiac Imaging* 4:105-116, 1989.
13. Gussenhoven EJ et al: Thinning of the media in atherosclerosis: an in vitro/in vivo intravascular echographic study, *Circulation* 82(suppl II):II-1817, 1990 (abstract).
14. Hodgson JM et al: Combined intracoronary ultrasound imaging and angioplasty catheter: initial in-vivo studies, *Circulation* 82(suppl III):III-676, 1990 (abstract).
15. Honye J et al: Morphological effects of coronary balloon angioplasty in vivo assessed by intravascular ultrasound imaging, *Circulation* 85:1012-1025, 1992.
16. Isner JM et al: How reliable are images obtained by intravascular ultrasound for making decisions during percutaneous interventions? Experience with intravascular ultrasound employed in lieu of contrast angiography to guide peripheral balloon angioplasty in 16 patients, *Circulation* 82(suppl III):III-440, 1990 (abstract).
17. Leon M et al: Intravascular ultrasound assessment of plaque responses to PTCA helps explain angiographic findings, *J Am Coll Cardiol* 17:47A, 1991 (abstract).
18. Meyer CR et al: Feasibility of high-resolution intravascular ultrasonic imaging catheters, *Radiology* 168:113-116, 1988.
19. Moriuchi M et al: The reproducibility of intravascular ultrasound imaging in-vitro, *J Am Soc Echocardiogr* 3:444-450, 1990.
20. Nissen SE et al: Comparison of intravascular ultrasound and angiography in quantitation of coronary dimensions and stenosis in man: impact of lumen eccentricity, *Circulation* 82(suppl III):III-440, 1990 (abstract).
21. Nissen SE et al: Intravascular ultrasound assessment of lumen size and wall morphology in normal subjects and patients with coronary artery disease, *Circulation* 84:1087-1099, 1991.
22. Nobuyoshi M et al: Restenosis after percutaneous transluminal coronary angioplasty: pathologic observations in 20 patients, *J Am Coll Cardiol* 17:433-439, 1991.
23. Pandian N et al: Intracardiac intravascular, two-dimensional, high-frequency ultrasound imaging of pulmonary artery and its branches in humans and animals, *Circulation* 81:2007-2012, 1990.
24. Picano E, Landini L, Lattanzi E: The use of frequency histograms of ultrasonic backscatter for detection of atherosclerosis in-vitro, *Circulation* 74:1093-1098, 1986.
25. Potkin BN et al: Coronary artery imaging with intravascular high-frequency ultrasound, *Circulation* 81:1575-1585, 1990.
26. Ricou F et al: Catheter-based intravascular ultrasound imaging of chronic thromboembolic pulmonary disease, *Am J Cardiol* 67:749-752, 1991.
27. Schwartz RS et al: Restenosis and the proportional neointimal response to coronary artery injury: results in a porcine model, *J Am Coll Cardiol* 267-274, 1992.
28. Schwartz S et al: Flow-directed, balloon-floation intravascular ultrasound catheter for percutaneous pulmonary artery imaging and intracardiac echocardiography, *J Am Coll Cardiol* 17:216A, 1991 (abstract).
29. Selmon MR et al: Retrieval of media and adventitia by directional coronary atherectomy by angiographic correlation, *Circulation* 82:III-624, 1990 (abstract).
30. Steele PM et al: Balloon angioplasty: natural history of the pathophysiological response to injury in pig model, *Circ Res* 57:105-112, 1985.
31. Sudhir K et al: Transvenous coronary ultrasound imaging: a novel approach to visualization of the coronary arteries, *Circulation* 84:1957-1961, 1991.
32. Sudhir K et al: Simultaneous intravascular two-dimensional and Doppler ultrasound: a new technique for in vivo assessment of coronary flow and vascular dynamics, *J Am Coll Cardiol* 19:140A, 1992 (abstract).
33. Tobis JM et al: Intravascular ultrasound cross-section imaging before and after balloon angioplasty in vitro, *Circulation* 80:873-882, 1989.
34. Tobis JM et al: Cross-sectional morphology of balloon dilatation in vivo by intravascular ultrasound, *J Am Coll Cardiol* 17:157A, 1991 (abstract).
35. Waller BF et al: Morphological observations late (>30 days) after clinically successful coronary balloon angioplasty, *Circulation* 1992 (in press).
36. Weintraub AR et al: Evaluation of acute aortic dissection by intravascular ultrasonography, *New Engl J Med* 323:1566-7, 1990.
37. White CW et al: Does visual interpretation of the coronary arteriogram predict the physiologic importance of coronary stenosis? *New Engl J Med* 310:819-824, 1987.
38. Yock PG, Linker DJ: Intravascular ultrasound: looking below the surface of vascular disease, *Circulation* 81:1715-1718, 1990.
39. Yock PG et al: Initial trials of a combined ultrasound imaging/mechanical atherectomy catheter, *J Am Coll Cardiol* 15:17A, 1990 (abstract).
40. Yock PG et al: Morphological features of successful coronary atherectomy determined by intravascular ultrasound imaging, *Circulation* 82(suppl III):III-676, 1990 (abstract).

CHAPTER 121

Ultrasound contrast agents

ROBERT F. MATTREY

The need for ultrasound contrast media has been recognized since the introduction of sonography to the clinical arena. Several factors have contributed to the slow progress: the pharmaceutical industry feared that intravenous injections would not be accepted because of practitioners' pride in the fact that sonography is painless and noninvasive, leaders in the field perceived a greater need for higher spatial resolution rather than contrast media, the mechanisms involved in ultrasound/tissue interaction have been difficult to master, and the combined clinical and pharmaceutical expertise required to develop such agents was scarce. The recent surge in interest and the significant investments being made by industry coincide with the wide acceptance of color Doppler imaging.

The color Doppler technique provides the sonographer with physiologic imaging of areas inaccessible to other methods. For the first time, it is widely apparent that sonography skirts the signal-to-noise limits. Vessels, although visible on gray scale, failed to fill with color when they were small, deep, or at suboptimal angles or when flow within their lumen was too slow to discriminate it from tissue motion. The need to boost the signal became much more apparent. Furthermore, the increased use of sonography as an intraoperative tool and as a guide to percutaneous intervention, coupled with the wide adoption of invasive sonography for endorectal, endovaginal, and endovascular imaging, has removed sonography from its noninvasive haven.

Because of the surprising acceptance of intravenous magnetic resonance contrast agents, combined with some significant research achievements, and the enormous market potential for ultrasonic agents that dwarf any other imaging modality, the pharmaceutical industry has geared up their research and development programs in this area. Ultrasound contrast agents have been upgraded from a mere curiosity to a high priority. The recent increase in publications describing various new agents and their potential applications provides a glimpse of the exciting new horizon for sonography, already the most versatile imaging modality. Imaging and quantification of flow, tissue perfusion including the myocardium, functional analysis of the left ventricle, and assessment of kidney function are some of the possibilities.

The ability to replace hysterosalpingography, cystography in the pediatric population, and voiding cystourethrography with nonionizing imaging is an added benefit. It may even be possible to improve abdominal imaging with orally administered ultrasound contrast agents.[14] With the increase in the number of investigators in the field and the increased capabilities made possible by the use of ultrasound contrast agents, progress is ensured.

Ultrasound contrast agents are presented here from a historical perspective without an exhaustive review of the field, which has been presented elsewhere.[1,12,21,28,29] Their potential applications in vascular and perfusion imaging are also described.

PHYSICAL BASIS OF CONTRAST MEDIA

The reflection of sound in tissues occurs when the sound beam strikes an interface that separates two regions with different acoustic impedance (Z). Z is equal to the product of mass density and acoustic velocity. The difference in Z between most tissues is on the order of 1% to 5%. The difference between fat and most tissues is approximately 15%.[27] Because the strength of the reflected signal is directly related to the normalized difference in Z [(Z1 − Z2)/ (Z1 + Z2), where *1* and *2* refer to tissue 1 and 2], it is not surprising that fat assumes the brightest signals on clinical ultrasound images. Contrast media typically take advantage of density and velocity to achieve greater reflectivity.

The size of the interface relative to the cross section of the sound beam is also important. When the reflective surface is smaller than the cross section of the beam, it scatters the sound wave in nearly all directions. Particles of ultrasound contrast media are considered scatterers because their diameter is much smaller than the beam width. Tissue texture depends on the number of scatterers present in the field and their spatial relationship. The image is the final result of interactions between the sound wave and the scatterers.[25] The interference occurs because the resolution of the sound wave is greater than that of the ultrasound beam. Although the effect of contrast media on the intensity of the backscattered signal can be predicted given the agent's sonographic properties, its effect on tissue echogenicity is more complex.

1001

Tissue echogenicity, or overall tissue brightness, is related to the number of dots and their brightness per square area (Fig. 121-1). The number of dots is related to the heterogeneity of the tissue or the number of discontinuities present per square area. The more heterogeneous the medium, the greater the number of dots generated. The brightness of the dot is related to the difference in the acoustic impedance of the two media on either side of the interface. Tissue contrast is generated when two tissues have differing heterogeneity (e.g., cystic versus solid, lymph node versus fat) or are made up of brighter reflectors produced by a greater difference in acoustic impedance between scatterers and background tissue, such as renal parenchyma and the peripelvic region.

Contrast materials can easily increase the number of reflectors in a region of interest by increasing the number of particles in the field (Fig. 121-1). This mechanism increases tissue echogenicity and the Doppler signal linearly with the concentration of the agent in the tissue or blood. The effect of contrast agents on the brightness of the dot is more complex and relates to their degree of reflectivity and spatial distribution. Reflectivity is related to the particle's scattering cross section, which is in turn related to particle size, the difference in the acoustic impedance of the agent and the surrounding medium, the particle elasticity, and the frequency of the interrogating sound wave.[21]

Particle size has a profound effect on reflectivity in that backscatter is related to the radius of the particle raised to the sixth power. However, particle size must be less than 5 μm to successfully traverse the capillary bed of the lung. The effect of the frequency used is also highly effective in that reflectivity is proportional to the inverse of the wavelength to the fourth power. Thus it is crucial in contrast development work to use the frequencies most commonly used in the clinical setting (3 to 7 MHz) to better predict the agent's clinical efficacy. Particle size, particle elasticity, and the bulk properties of the agent (acoustic impedance) greatly affect the scattering cross section of the particle. For instance, perfluorochemicals and air bubbles are 10 and 10^{10} times more reflective than a red blood cell, respectively. The elasticity of the particle, which is related to the compressibility of the agent and the stiffness of its outer shell, can dramatically affect reflectivity, allowing a particle with a small diameter (less than 5 μm) to increase its scattering cross section a few orders of magnitude to become effective at the clinical frequencies with a wavelength on the order of 200 to 500 μm.[21] Gas and to a much lesser degree fluorocarbons are compressible and can potentially exhibit this resonance phenomenon.

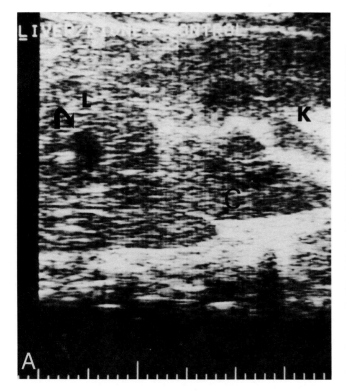
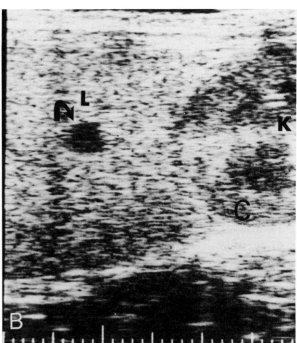

Fig. 121-1. Longitudinal scans taken at the level of the liver *(L)* and kidney *(K)* before *(A)* and 48 hours after *(B)* the infusion of a fluorocarbon emulsion show an increase in liver echogenicity relative to the renal cortex *(C)* because the liver accumulates fluorocarbon in the RE cells. The increase in brightness is related to an increase in the number of reflectors (note the improved definition of the intrahepatic vessel *[curved arrow]*) and an increase in the brightness of each reflector (compare liver to cortex reflector brightness). (From Mattrey RF et al: *J Ultrasound Med* 2:173, 1983.)

Attenuation, which is the loss of power of the sound beam as it travels through the medium (expressed as dB cm^{-1} MHz^{-1}), occurs when the energy of the sound wave is dissipated as it propagates through tissue by scattering, deflection, diffraction, and conversion to heat. Clinically, an attenuating tissue appears highly echogenic in the near field (because of increased scattering, including backscatter), with rapid loss of echogenicity and an inability to image the far field. Ultrasound contrast agents can produce significant attenuation. In fact, when the spacing between particles approaches a critical limit, the ultrasound beam is unable to penetrate the tissue, producing acoustic shadowing. The difference in attenuation between areas that collect the agent and those that do not can produce significant image contrast, a finding that has not been exploited to date.

The Doppler effect is produced when a detectable reflective surface is in motion relative to the transducer. If the reflected signal is above the noise level, a frequency shift can be calculated. Furthermore, because of the natural motion of tissues, a certain amount of shift occurs naturally and therefore small shifts are ignored. Signal processing techniques have been developed to discriminate among tissue motion, noise, and slow flow, decreasing the minimum detectable velocities to approximately 3 mm/sec under ideal conditions. It can be deduced that a small vessel would not carry enough reflectors to generate sufficient signal, or the small vessel may be deep enough that its signal is lost in the noise because of tissue attenuation, or the vessel may be imaged at a suboptimum angle (near perpendicular), offering very little frequency shift as if it had very slow flow. In addition, reflection from flowing blood decreases with

increasing shear, greatly affecting the smaller vessels where shear rates can be excessive.[15] Under these conditions, a stronger reflector within the vessel produces a greater signal-to-noise ratio, improving Doppler analysis (Figs. 121-2 and 121-3).

Doppler ultrasound is displayed as either a spectral pattern or a color display (Fig. 121-4). The horizontal direction on the spectral pattern represents time, the vertical direction represents frequency shift or velocity, and the brightness represents signal intensity (number of reflectors flowing at the same velocity). This display allows for quantitative analysis of velocities observed at one anatomic location over time. Color Doppler ultrasound, on the other hand, is qualitative. It provides the location of detectable motion within the entire region of interest at one time point. Red and blue are assigned to locations with motion that is either toward or away from the transducer. The brightness in the red or blue color reflects either peak or mean velocity detected at each location. Contrast media do not alter the envelope of the spectral pattern unless the signals emitted before contrast administration were near the detection limit. They merely increase the brightness and may actually fill the region within the envelope with a high contrast dose or gain setting (see Figs. 121-2 and 121-3). Similarly, contrast media should not alter the brightness of the red and blue on color images unless signals are near the detection limit. They do fill the image with more color by bringing into view additional regions of flow not detected before contrast administration (see Fig. 121-4); however, blooming around the vessels may occur depending on the contrast dose and the equipment used. There are several technical approaches used to produce color Doppler images, and most require the use

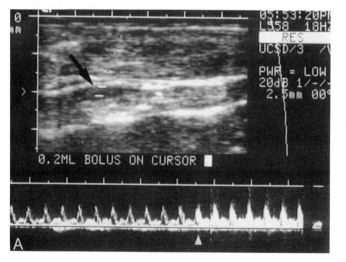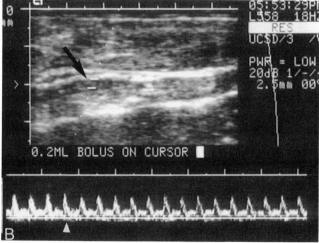

Fig. 121-2. Two frames taken approximately 10 sec apart from a continuous video recording showing the spectral Doppler waveform that was acquired from the aorta of a rabbit during the bolus administration of 0.2 ml of Albunex in the inferior vena cava. The spectral waveform displays time along the x-axis, frequency shift along the y-axis, and the reflected signal strength as brightness. Note the marked increase in brightness *(arrowhead)* when Albunex enters the sampling volume (arrow) *(A)* and then decreases to return to baseline within 10 to 12 seconds *(arrowhead)* *(B).* (From Hilpert PL et al: *AJR* 153:613, 1989.)

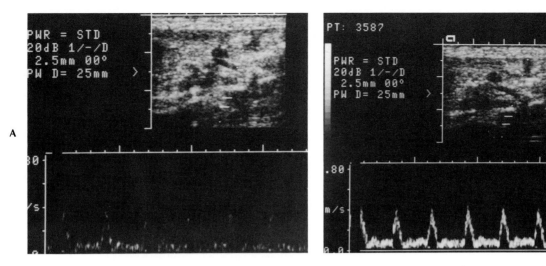

Fig. 121-3. Spectral Doppler waveform was acquired from the aorta of a rabbit before **(A)** and at the end of the infusion **(B)** of 3 ml/kg perflubron emulsion without altering any of the imaging parameters or transducer position. The gain setting at baseline was minimized to produce a faint spectral waveform to allow for the assessment of enhancement. Note the marked increase in brightness when perflubron was infused. This enhancement persisted for at least 1 hour. (From Satterfield R et al: *Invest Radiology* [in press].)

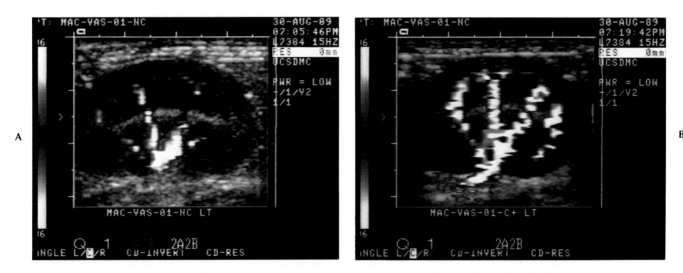

Fig. 121-4. The effect of perflubron emulsion on the visualization of intrarenal vessels is shown here before **(A)** and 15 minutes after **(B)** the infusion of 3 ml/kg. Note the overall increase in the color Doppler signal and the visualization of the arcuate ring at the corticomedullary junction not seen precontrast. (From Coley BD et al: *Kidney Int* 39:740, 1991.)

of larger voxels than those used in gray-scale imaging, which reduces spatial resolution. Large voxels are used to improve the signal-to-noise ratio and to decrease processing time so that near real-time frame rates are maintained. Although it is possible that the increase in the signal-to-noise ratio afforded by contrast agents would permit the use of smaller voxels to improve spatial resolution, no equipment manufacturer has yet optimized imaging to take advantage of this. Although all available color Doppler schemes will benefit from the use of contrast agents, some equipment will benefit more than others.

MILESTONES IN THE DEVELOPMENT OF CONTRAST AGENTS

Several classes of agents have been described to date. Only those that have been tested in vivo, have clinical potential, or have importance from a historical perspective are presented; omissions are not intentional.

One of the first reports of ultrasound contrast effect was from Gramiak and Shah[9] in the late 1960s. They reported the effect of intravenously administered saline solution on the cardiac chambers. Shortly thereafter, it was understood that this effect was caused by free air bubbles.[13] Although

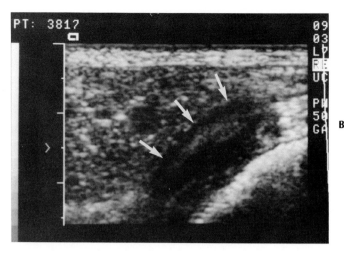

Fig. 121-5. Longitudinal scans taken over the inferior vena cava after the infusion of Fluosol ***(A)*** and perflubron emulsion ***(B)*** in two different rabbits. Note that the inferior vena cava, which is free of echoes, remains free of echoes after Fluosol ***(A)*** but fills with reflectors after perflubron *(arrows)* ***(B).*** When the image is frozen, the vessel that was quite apparent on real-time loses contrast with surrounding tissues. (From Satterfield R et al: *Invest Radiology* [in press].)

the free air bubbles are highly reflective, they have an extremely short half-life in blood because of the absence of a protective shell, exposing them to the collapsing forces of plasma. Should the bubbles survive long enough in the circulation, the bubble size prevents them from traversing the pulmonary capillaries to opacify the left ventricle. In the hope of increasing the stability and longevity of the bubble, Caroll et al[2] encapsulated gas within a gelatin protective shell. Among the types of encapsulated agents, the most advanced is the human albumin microsphere reported by Feinstein et al.[5] Clinical trials on this material, given the trade name Albunex,* have been completed for an echocardiographic application. SHU-454† and SHU-508† are galactose particles with the gas carried on the surface of the particle, an "inside-out" bubble.[6,7] These agents appear to be effective in opacifying the right ventricle. The SHU-508 formulation successfully crosses the lung to opacify the left ventricle.[7] Although gas-based contrast agents are extremely reflective and produce efficacious results at small dosages, they generally tend to be short lived in human plasma. In the case of the human albumin microspheres, echogenicity lasts several seconds and provides first-pass data (Fig. 121-2).[8,11] Many additional agents based on air bubbles are being proposed with different protective sleeves to increase their longevity in blood.

The first report that demonstrated successful and persistent tissue opacification from intravenous injections was in 1982 when a fluorocarbon emulsion (perfluorooctylbromide [PFOB]) was given to rabbits to produce liver and tumor image enhancement. The enhancement was observed for several days.[17] PFOB has since been given the generic name

perflubron by the USAN. It was also shown that tissue enhancement could also be observed with another fluorocarbon emulsion that at the time was an investigational drug, which was being tested in human beings for oxygen transport, called Fluosol* (Fig. 121-1).[18] The difference between these two agents is that perflubron emulsion is five times more concentrated than Fluosol, requiring one-fifth the volume to deliver an equal dose of fluorocarbon. The findings described in animals were later confirmed in human subjects.[19]

Further research and formulation changes in perflubron emulsions allowed the visualization of flow on gray scale (Fig. 121-5) and the enhancement of perfused tissues (Fig. 121-6) and Doppler signals (see Figs. 121-3 and 121-4).[16] It appears that the effect is dependent on the formulation, in that Fluosol failed to produce the vascular effects described for perflubron emulsion, neither the Doppler signal enhancement nor the visualization of flow on gray scale (Fig. 121-5). This occurred despite the fact that the perflubron emulsion was diluted to the same concentration as Fluosol and that both agents produced indistinguishable liver enhancement at 48 hours.[23] Although fluorocarbon emulsions are efficacious and produce a prolonged effect (in hours) on vascular and tissue enhancement, they are less effective than air and therefore require larger doses to produce a comparable echogenic effect.

In 1987, the use of solid particles, iodipamide ethyl ester, to opacify the liver was reported by Parker et al.[22] This formulation was recently improved by entrapping gas in the solid matrix, which increased reflectivity by a factor of 20.[26] Preliminary results with this new formulation show vascular

---

*Molecular Biosystems, San Diego, Calif.
†Echovist, Schering AG, Berlin, Germany.

*Alpha Therapeutic Corp., Los Angeles, Calif.

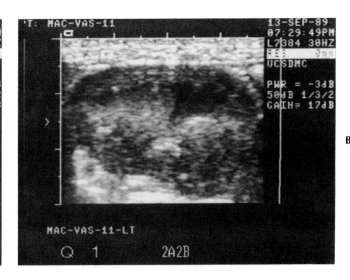

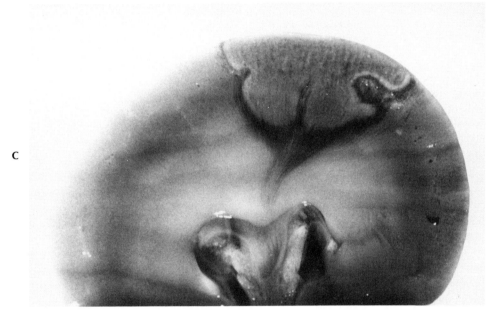

Fig. 121-6. Gray-scale visualization of partial renal infarction was not possible before contrast administration **(A).** The partial infarct, produced by embolizing a 1-mm bead into the renal artery, became apparent after the infusion of 3 ml/kg perflubron emulsion **(B)** and correlated precisely with the postmortem slice **(C).** Note that the medulla, which was hypoechoic relative to cortex precontrast **(A),** became more echogenic than cortex postcontrast **(B),** allowing the visualization of the extension of the infarct into the medulla. (From Coley BD et al: *Kidney Int* 39:740, 1991.)

and tissue enhancement from intravenous injections and suggest that the enhancement may persist for several minutes.

POTENTIAL USE OF CONTRAST AGENTS

Most of the work in ultrasound contrast agents has focused on their use as adjuncts to echocardiography to more clearly demarcate the endocardial surface or demonstrate valvular disease or intracardiac lesions. Although the ultimate goal is to demonstrate myocardial perfusion defects, this has only been possible with intraarterial injections. This discussion, however, is limited to the extra-cardiac applications, including vascular and organ imaging, which has been limited.

The major body of work in the nonechocardiographic application has been in liver, spleen, and tumor imaging. These are the regions in which contrast particles accumulate. Although liver and spleen image enhancement to visualize tumors would constitute a significant advance in sonography of the abdomen,[8,17-19] a sonographic contrast agent will have a greater and broader impact on clinical practice if it intensifies Doppler signals, visualizes vascular flow on gray scale, and enhances perfused tissues. The benefits of increasing Doppler signals are readily appreciated by practitioners in the field who are constantly attempting to probe deeper and smaller tumors and vessels. The benefit of visual-

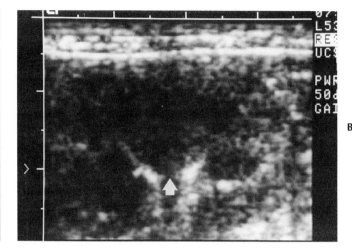

A   B

Fig. 121-7. The renal medulla is hypoechoic relative to the cortex in rabbits. It becomes more echogenic than the cortex after the infusion of perflubron emulsion *(arrow)* ***(A)*** because the contrast agent, which is limited to the vascular space, becomes more concentrated as it travels through the vasa recta. When the osmotic gradient is destroyed by furosemide administration, the echogenicity of the medulla is lost ***(B)***. (From Munzing D et al: *Kidney Int* 39:733, 1991.)

izing flow in vessels on gray scale is somewhat analogous to the addition of color Doppler imaging. However, it would not require sophisticated equipment, would not be susceptible to the artifacts of color Doppler imaging, and might provide greater spatial resolution. In cases in which the mere knowledge of whether flow is present or absent is needed (e.g., in testicular torsion,[10] venous obstruction[3]), visualization of flow on gray scale may suffice.

Gray-scale sonography without contrast enhancement has been limited to the assessment of tissue structure. The benefit achieved by enhancing perfused tissues could potentially bring to sonography a capability analogous to the accomplishments of intravenous contrast media for computerized tomography and magnetic resonance imaging. Such capability would allow the detection of renal function (Fig. 121-7),[20] and perfusion defects (see Fig. 121-6),[4] as well as alter the contrast between tumors and surrounding tissues,[16] and between the vascular and avascular regions in tumors and would markedly enhance imaging of hypervascular lesions.[24]

CONCLUSION

In the development of sonographic contrast media, the material properties of the agent significantly influence its efficacy. The important parameters are particle size, imaging frequency, density, compressibility, particle behavior (e.g., surface tension, internal pressure, bubble-like qualities), and biodistribution characteristics and tolerance. Particulate agents appear to be the most likely materials, and gas-filled particles are by far the most effective reflectors. However, further modification of the gas-based agents is required to lengthen their vascular longevity and increase their potential in nonechocardiographic applications, in which the fluorocarbon emulsions appear to be most promising. When the

field matures, sonography should reach new horizons and possibly achieve its maximum potential. Several agents may become available, each with unique properties and clinical utility, from which the practitioner may select the optimal system to answer the clinical question.

REFERENCES

1. Andre M, Nelson T, Mattrey R: Physical and acoustical properties of perfluorooctylbromide, an ultrasound contrast agent, *Invest Radiol* 25:983-987, 1990.
2. Caroll BA et al: Gelatin encapsulated nitrogen microbubbles as ultrasonic contrast agents, *Invest Radiol* 15:260-266, 1980.
3. Coley BD et al: Sonographic detection of deep venous thrombosis with PFOB "sonographic venography," [Abstract], *Radiology* 177 (suppl):215, 1990.
4. Coley BD et al: The potential role of PFOB enhanced sonography of the kidney. II. Detection of partial infarction, *Kidney Int* 39:740-745, 1991.
5. Feinstein SB et al: Safety and efficacy of a new transpulmonary ultrasound contrast agent: initial multicenter clinical results, *J Am Coll Cardiol* 16(2):316-324, 1990.
6. Fritzsch T, Schartl M, Siegert J: Preclinical and clinical results with an ultrasonic contrast agent, *Invest Radiol* 23 (suppl):S302-S305, 1988.
7. Fritzsch T et al: SHU 508, a transpulmonary echocontrast agent, *Invest Radiol* 25 (suppl):S160-S161, 1990.
8. Goldberg BB et al: Hepatic tumors: signal enhancement at Doppler US after intravenous injection of a contrast agent, *Radiology* 177:713-717, 1990.
9. Gramiak R, Shah PM: Echocardiography of the aortic root, *Invest Radiol* 3:356-366, 1968.
10. Heiberg E et al: Sonographic accuracy in testicular torsion: the utility of PFOB, a sonographic contrast agent [Abstract], *Radiology* 177 (suppl):177, 1990.
11. Hilpert PL et al: IV injection of air-filled human albumin microspheres to enhance arterial Doppler signal: a preliminary study in rabbits, *Am J Roentgenol* 153:613-616, 1989.
12. Hykes D, Hedrick W, Starchman D. *Ultrasound physics and instrumentation,* New York, 1985, Churchill Livingston.
13. Kremkau FW et al: Ultrasonic detection of cavitation at catheter tips, *Am J Roentgenol* 110:177-183, 1970.
14. Lund PJ et al: Cellulose as a gastrointestinal ultrasound contrast agent, *J Ultrasound Med* 10:S40, 1991.

15. Machi J et al: Relation of in vivo blood flow to ultrasound echogenicity, *J Clin Ultrasound* 11:3-10, 1983.

16. Mattrey RF: Perfluorooctylbromide: a new contrast agent for CT, sonography, and MR imaging, *Am J Roentgenol* 152:247-252, 1989.

17. Mattrey RF et al: Perfluorooctylbromide: a liver/spleen-specific and a tumor-imaging ultrasound contrast material, *Radiology* 145:759-762, 1982.

18. Mattrey RF et al: Perfluorochemicals as liver- and spleen-seeking ultrasound contrast agents, *J Ultrasound Med* 2:173-176, 1983.

19. Mattrey RF et al: Perfluorochemicals as US contrast agents for tumor imaging and hepatosplenography: preliminary clinical results, *Radiology* 163:339-343, 1987.

20. Munzing D et al: The potential role of PFOB enhanced sonography of the kidney. II. Detection of renal function and acute tubular necrosis, *Kidney Int* 39:733-739, 1991.

21. Ophir J, Parker KJ: Contrast agents in diagnostic ultrasound, *J Ultrasound Med Biol* 15:319-333, 1989.

22. Parker KJ et al: A particulate contrast agent with potential for ultrasonic imaging of liver, *Ultrasound Med Biol* 13(9):555-556, 1987.

23. Satterfield R et al: Comparison of perflubron emulsion and Fluosol-DA 20% as ultrasound contrast agents, *Invest Radiol* (in press).

24. Shiroma JT, Meyer CW, Mattrey RF: Improved detection of liver metastases in canine hemangiosarcoma using perfluorooctylbromide as an ultrasonic contrast agent: preliminary results. Presented at the meeting of the Veterinary Cancer Society, Auburn, Alabama, 1991.

25. Sommer FG, Sue JY: Image processing to reduce ultrasonic speckle, *J Ultrasound Med* 2:413-415, 1983.

26. Violante MR et al: Particle-stabilized bubbles for enhanced organ ultrasound imaging, *Invest Radiol* 26(suppl):S194-S197, 1991.

27. Wells PNT: *Physical principles of ultrasonic diagnosis*, London, 1969, Academic Press.

28. Wheatley M, Schrope B, Shen P: Contrast agents for diagnostic ultrasound: development and evaluation of polymer-coated microbubbles, *Biomaterials* 11:713-717, 1990.

29. Wood AB: *Textbook of sound*. London, 1964, G. Bell and Sons.

CHAPTER 122

Vector Doppler and complex blood flow

KIRK W. BEACH

Ultrasonic Doppler methods have been widely used for the diagnosis of arterial, venous, and cardiac diseases since Satamura first introduced the methods in 1957[21] and later were used for blood flow studies.[14,25] Doppler systems measure the velocity of blood or a component of that velocity. Accurate measurement of the velocity magnitude depends on the proper use of the Doppler equation[7]:

$$\Delta F = \frac{2F_0 \times V \times \cos\theta}{C}$$

where:

F = Frequency shift
2 = Round trip of the ultrasound
C/F_0 = Wavelength of ultrasound
$V \cos\theta$ = Closing speed between the erythrocytes and the Doppler transducer

To use the Doppler equation, the examiner must know the heading of the velocity vector (i.e., the direction in which it is moving). The Doppler equation is always tested in situations in which the heading of blood velocity is known. Often testing is done at the distal end of a long straight tube where the velocity vectors are known to be parallel to the axis of the tube. In other tests, moving strings or belts are used to calibrate Doppler instruments. Unfortunately, none of these tests is totally applicable to blood flow in human arteries, veins, and the heart. These anatomic channels frequently have short, curved sections with branches. Normal flow in these conduits is helical.[15,16,23,24,32]

HELICAL FLOW AND QUANTITATIVE LIMITATIONS

The presence of helical flow alters the simple relationship between blood velocity and volumetric flow rate,[8,11] as well as the simple relationship between velocity and Bernoulli pressure depression.[1,24,27,28] These are the two applications in which quantitative Doppler velocity measurements are compared with independent quantitative measurements. The volumetric flow rate is related to the velocity perpendicular to the area of a cross section of the blood vessel; the Ber-

noulli pressure drop is related to the kinetic energy of the blood, which in turn is related to the magnitude of the blood velocity.[1,12,13,24] The computation of volumetric flow rate closely agrees with independent measurements if a Doppler examination angle of 0° is used,[11] but the computations do not agree with independent measurements taken at other Doppler examination angles.[8] The computation of Bernoulli pressure drop agrees with independent measurements when a Doppler examination angle of 0° is used,[12] but the computations do not agree with independent measurements taken at other Doppler examination angles.[13] The source of the problem may be the often incorrect assumption that blood velocity vectors are parallel to the axis of the blood vessel.

When Doppler instruments are applied to helical flow (Fig. 122-1), widely different velocity measurements result from slight out-of-plane angulation of the Doppler transducer t. If the transducer $t1$ is positioned and angled so that the ultrasound beam $b1$ intersects the descending portion of the helix at a slightly obtuse angle, the directional Doppler frequency may be negative (Fig. 122-1, C). If the transducer

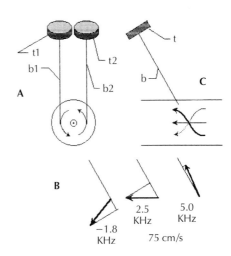

Fig. 122-1. During an arterial Doppler exam, the artery is viewed in longitudinal view to measure the Doppler examination angle. The transducer is adjusted to obtain the highest Doppler frequency holding the angle constant. This causes the examiner to tilt the scanhead to align with b2 and obtain a Doppler frequency of 5 kHz (**C**) rather than a lower value of 2.5 kHz from the centerstream or a reversal from b1.

This work is supported by NIH Specialized Center for Organized Research P50HL42270.

t2 is positioned and angled so that the ultrasound beam *b2* intersects the ascending portion of the helix at an acute angle to the ultrasound beam, the directional Doppler frequency will be positive and greater than expected from an independent measurement of the midstream velocity component parallel to the axis (Fig. 122-1, *C*). The pitch angle of normal helical blood flow varies during the cardiac cycle, sometimes reaching angles of 80° with the vessel axis.[15] To minimize variability in Doppler measurements, the examiner usually adjusts the angle of the scan plane to obtain the greatest possible Doppler frequency; this results in acquisition of the Doppler data from the portion of the helix that is most closely aligned with the ultrasound beam *b2* rather than velocity vectors that are parallel to the artery axis. Thus an inflated angle-adjusted velocity value is obtained.

In cardiac output measurements,[11] the ultrasound beam is aligned at an angle of 0° to the aortic axis; the cross-sectional area is perpendicular to that area. The computation does not require that the velocity magnitude be measured, only that the component perpendicular to the cross-sectional area be measured. Thus in this case, the measurement requirements and the measurement methods agree; correct measurements, compared with independent gold standards, are obtained. Helical flow cannot affect the results because the additional velocity components are not measured and the additional components do not contribute to volumetric flow, so the measurement limitations match the computational requirement at a Doppler examination angle of 0° to the axis of the cross-sectional area used in the computation.

In cardiac valvular pressure gradient measurements, the ultrasound beam is aligned with the stenotic jet by locating the window of view that results in the highest Doppler frequency. Therefore the Doppler examination angle between the blood velocity vector along the axis of the stenotic jet and the ultrasound beam is 0°, at least in the portion of the cardiac cycle during which the velocity is greatest.[12]

DETERMINATION OF COMPLETE VELOCITY DATA

In previous studies, investigators recognized that some problem existed in determining the true course of blood flowing through an artery and made attempts to measure the velocity magnitude and angle of blood flow through arteries.[2,4-6,9,10,18,22,29,31] None of these methods achieved commercial success because the implementation in an instrument was difficult, the application of such data in clinical measurement was cumbersome, and leadership to introduce the methods was lacking. One of the greatest difficulties of introducing such a method into medical practice is the display and application of the data.

TWO-DIMENSIONAL COLOR FLOW SYSTEMS

A two-dimensional color flow image shows flow away from the ultrasound transducer in one color and flow toward the transducer in another color (Fig. 122-2). If the axis of the blood vessel is tilted to the artery axis, the examiner often believes that the image shows the velocities or velocity

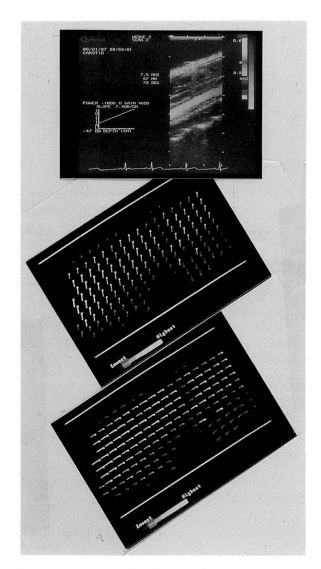

Fig. 122-2. A conventional two-dimensional color flow image *(top)* is formed by measuring the Doppler frequencies associated with the component of the velocity parallel to the ultrasound scan lines *(middle)*. When the image is viewed with the velocities assumed to be parallel to the artery axis, the colors are often assumed to represent velocities parallel to that axis *(bottom)*. (From Fitzgerald MP: *Two-dimensional vector Doppler imaging*, thesis, Seattle, 1987, University of Washington.)

components that are parallel to the artery axis (Fig. 122-2); however, this may not be the case.

VELOCITY VECTOR COORDINATE SYSTEMS

Complete data about the blood velocity require the acquisition of four values for each Doppler sample volume. Several combinations of four values are possible. One of the values is time in the cardiac cycle (or respiratory cycle for veins). The other three values indicate the magnitude and heading of the velocity. One combination of the three values, which is convenient to Doppler instrument design, is (1) the velocity vector component in the direction of the ultrasound transmit beam, (2) the velocity vector component perpendicular to the ultrasound beam but in the plane of the ultrasound image, and (3) the velocity vector component perpendicular to the plane of the ultrasound image. Conventional Doppler instruments display the time versus the first of these three numbers: the velocity magnitude in the direction of the ultrasound beam. Another combination of the three values is: (1) the velocity component in the cephalad direction, (2) the velocity component toward the patient's front, and (3) the velocity component toward the patient's left. These two are similar only if the ultrasound scan head is aligned with the axes of the patient's body. A more natural coordinate system for hemodynamic studies is (1) the velocity component parallel to the axis of the blood vessel, (2) the velocity component perpendicular to the vessel axis and in the plane of the nearest bifurcation, and (3) the velocity component perpendicular to that plane.

In all three of the preceding combinations, each component of the velocity can take on either positive or negative values. If the positive direction is cephalad, systolic arterial velocities in the neck are positive and systolic arterial velocities in the legs are negative. If the positive direction is away from the heart, all systolic arterial velocities are positive and all normal venous velocities are negative. The possibility of positive or negative velocity components is identified in most publications by the term *directional* or *bidirectional*. To avoid confusion with the former meaning of the word direction, in this chapter the word *heading* will be used to express the concept of the velocity vector along a line of any orientation with components along the axes as described. The term *heading* was taken from the concept of compass heading in navigation.

Although there are other combinations, one more method of describing the magnitude and heading of the velocity is (1) magnitude or speed, (2) angle between the velocity vector heading and the axis of the artery, and (3) angle between two planes: the plane including the velocity vector and the vessel axis and the plane of the nearest bifurcation. The angles used in this method can be visualized by imagining the sample volume at the center of the earth. The vector originates at the center of the earth and the length is indicated by the altitude of the tip (where altitude is measured from the earth center); thus the second angle in this combination is like latitude (angle from the equator) and the third angle is like longitude.

Any velocity vector can be represented by any of these methods. They are all equivalent, although one is often more useful than another. Some naturally arise from the measurement method: the cephalad-anterior-left velocity coordinate system is used in magnetic resonance flow measurement, the scan head–based coordinate system is used with ultrasound methods, and the artery-axis–based coordinate system is used with intravascular scan heads. A vector description in any coordinate system can be converted to an equivalent description in any other coordinate system.

Each possible Doppler sample volume in the plane of a

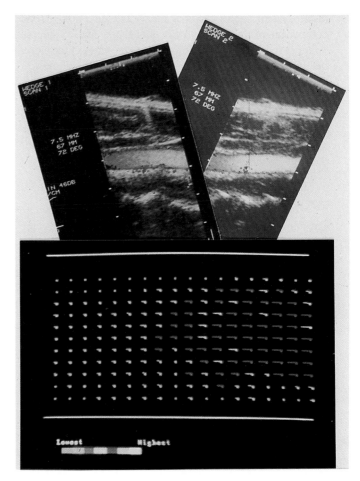

Fig. 122-3. In this case, most of the vectors are nearly parallel to the artery axis, but a few near the wall appear tilted. In the color scale left, red signifies flow toward the transducer array; in the right, red signifies flow away from the transducer array; and in the bottom, blue signifies low velocity and red signifies high velocity. These images were taken at the onset of systole. Because of the low sweep rate of the ultrasound scanner (54 cm/sec), the data on the left side of each image were acquired 55 ms earlier than the data on the right side. In this patient, the time for the velocity to change from presystolic velocities to 80% of peak systolic velocities is 23 ms. Thus the entire onset of systole occurs during the data acquisition for the middle half of this image. This accounts for the changes in velocity from the left portion of the image to the right portion. (From Fitzgerald MP: *Two-dimensional vector Doppler imaging,* thesis, Seattle, 1987, University of Washington.)

two-dimensional ultrasound image is described by the four values (time plus three for velocity). Comprehension of the display of these data is difficult. Conventional color flow images display data from each velocity sample volume in a plane, but the display of each sample volume is limited to one time in the cardiac cycle and one component of the velocity, with direction (positive or negative) and magnitude shown as color. This display can be extended to show the vector direction by the use of "flag" icons (Fig. 122-3). A spectral waveform shows data from one sample volume, time versus one component of the velocity vector with the additional information of strength of the signal and the presence of multiple frequencies in the signal. A velocity M-mode system shows the magnitude and direction of one component of velocity as color along one line of sample volumes indicated by position on the plane versus time along the horizontal axis.[20] With each kind of display, only a fraction of the data can be shown because the eyes and brain of the examiner cannot deal with more. Thus one problem with using the additional data about velocity heading and magnitude is selecting the portion of the data that will be most useful in reaching a correct (diagnostic) impression of the flow pattern.

ACQUISITION OF COMPLETE VELOCITY VECTOR INFORMATION

The two velocity components that describe a velocity vector in a plane taken from one Doppler sample volume at one moment in time can be measured by using a pulsed Doppler system with a single transmitter and two receivers. The method can be implemented with a conventional high-density linear array ultrasound scan head by using portions of the array for each function.

A two-dimensional vector Doppler system has been constructed[19] with a conventional pulsed Doppler transducer for transmitting and additional transducers for receiving. The transmitted pulse of ultrasound is scattered at all angles by clusters of erythrocytes in the sample volume (Figs. 122-

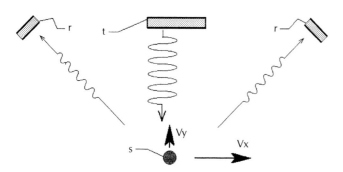

Fig. 122-4. An ultrasound pulse is transmitted into a patient's body by the central transducer *t*. Selected components of the ultrasound, scattered from clusters of erythrocytes in the sample volume *s*, headed toward the left and right transducers *(r)* are received and processed.

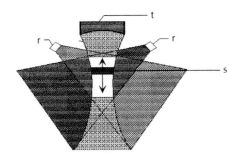

Fig. 122-5. The ultrasound transmitting transducer *t* is focused to ensure that the Doppler sample volume lies along a well-defined line. The receiving transducers *r* have wide beam patterns to ensure that they intersect the transmit beam pattern, even if the sample volume is adjusted over a range of depths.

4 and 122-5). Echoes can be received by a pair of separate receiving transducers, which are located on opposite sides of the transmitting transducer. The quadrature sum of the two Doppler-shifted frequencies received by the two receiving transducers is proportional to the velocity component (Vy) parallel to the transmitted ultrasound beam. This velocity vector component is the same velocity data obtained by a conventional pulsed Doppler system. The quadrature difference between the two received Doppler-shifted frequencies is proportional to the velocity component (Vx) perpendicular to Vy. The sum and difference of the received frequencies are obtained by a mixing process that is similar to radiofrequency Doppler demodulation (Fig. 122-6).

VECTOR DOPPLER DISPLAYS

Several means of displaying the multidimensional vector velocity data have been tried.[4,17,30] Time versus velocity in each of the two perpendicular headings can be shown as a pair of spectral waveforms (Fig. 122-7). This pair of tracings was simultaneously recorded from a sample volume in a human common carotid artery. The waveform of the blood velocity component perpendicular to the skin is shown (Fig. 122-7), with upward displacement of the tracing representing flow away from the ultrasound transducer. The waveform of the blood velocity component parallel to the skin is shown (Fig. 122-7, *B*), with upward displacement representing flow to the left. The systolic peak on the left of Fig. 122-7, *A* is aligned in time with a similar small peak on Fig. 122-7, *B*; this indicates that in systole, the blood velocity vector heading is tilted downward with respect to the skin.

The instantaneous velocity waveforms in Fig. 122-8 show velocity magnitude versus time and angle versus time from the common carotid artery. The waveforms are also derived from a time series of sequential velocity planes. The angle of the vector is nearly constant at 160°. As expected, the angle becomes uncertain when the velocity magnitude is near zero.

Fig. 122-9 shows an instantaneous polar plot with magnitude, angle, and confidence region (shown as a quadrilateral) at one point in time. The confidence region provides the examiner with an impression of the variance of the velocity. The angle variance and the magnitude variance are independent. Each contributes to an understanding of the disturbances in the flow. However, the diagnostic utility of these values is not yet clear.

Fig. 122-10 shows a trajectory of the vector termination with time in the cardiac cycle in the distal common carotid artery, just proximal to the carotid bifurcation. This display is a cumulative superposition of velocity data and is generated in real-time, providing a kinetic image. During the examination, the screen display is initiated; each 10 ms, a new point is added to the screen, representing a different 10 ms period during the cardiac cycle. All points are located to the left and below the central origin, showing that the velocity vectors representing each time period in the cardiac cycle are angled down and to the left. The trajectory of the

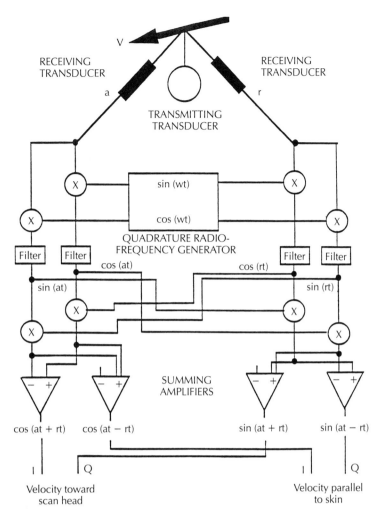

RECEIVING
TRANSDUCER

RECEIVING
TRANSDUCER

TRANSMITTING
TRANSDUCER

sin (wt)

cos (wt)

QUADRATURE RADIO-
FREQUENCY GENERATOR

Filter Filter

cos (at)

cos (rt)

Filter Filter

sin (at)

sin (rt)

SUMMING
AMPLIFIERS

cos (at + rt)   cos (at − rt)   sin (at + rt)   sin (at − rt)

I   Q   I   Q

Velocity toward
scan head

Velocity parallel
to skin

Fig. 122-6. A circuit schematic diagram for processing the echoes received by the receiving transducers shows conventional Doppler demodulation of each receiver above the low pass filters, followed by a quadrature multiplying and mixing network to obtain the sum of the Doppler frequencies from the pair of receiving transducers representing flow toward the transducers perpendicular to the skin and the difference of the Doppler frequencies from the pair of receiving transducers representing flow parallel to the skin.

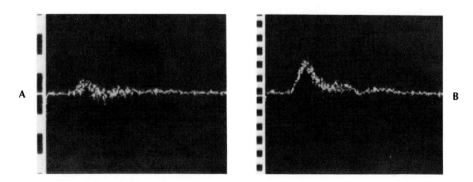

Fig. 122-7. The waveforms shows the velocity components perpendicular to the skin *(A)* and parallel to the skin *(B)*. The waveform was obtained by using the vector Doppler device shown in Figs. 122-5 and 122-6 on a human common carotid artery through the skin of the neck. (0 velocity can be determined from the scales on the left. Each black rectangle and each space represents 20 cm/sec, so the scale for *A* is magnified compared to the scale for *B*.) (From Overbeck JR, Beach KW, Strandness DE Jr: Vector Doppler: accurate measurement of blood velocity in two dimensions, *Ultrasound Med Biol* 18:19-31, 1992.)

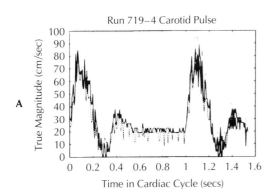

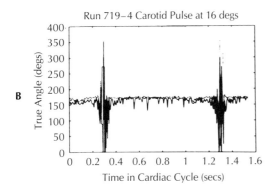

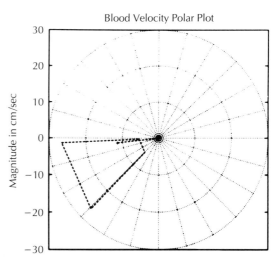

Velocity plotted at true angle and magnitude

Fig. 122-8. Velocity magnitude *(A)* and angle *(B).* The waveform was obtained by using the vector Doppler device shown in Figs. 122-5 and 122-6 on a human common carotid artery through the skin of the neck. Notice that as the velocity magnitude becomes small, the angle becomes undefined.

Fig. 122-9. The velocity vector magnitude and angle from an artery tilting slightly down and to the left is shown. The vector was determined from data acquired over 10 ms near peak systole. The quadrilateral around the vector termination shows the statistical confidence interval around the magnitude and angle. The waveform was obtained by using the vector Doppler device shown in Figs. 122-5 and 122-6 on a human common carotid artery through the skin of the neck. (From Overbeck JR, Beach KW, Strandness DE Jr: Vector Doppler: accurate measurement of blood velocity in two dimensions, *Ultrasound Med Biol* 18:19-31, 1992.)

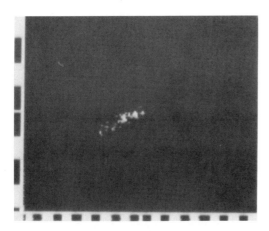

Fig. 122-10. The velocity vector magnitude and angle from an artery tilting slightly down and to the left is shown. Each vector was determined from data acquired over 10 ms. A total of 100 vector terminations are shown covering a period of 1 sec. The data were obtained by using the vector Doppler device shown in Figs. 122-5 and 122-6 on a human common carotid artery through the skin of the neck. 0 velocity in the vertical and horizontal directions can be determined from the scales on the bottom and left. Each black rectangle and each space represents 20 cm/sec so the vertical scale is magnified compared with the horizontal scale. (From Overbeck JR, Beach KW, Strandness DE Jr: Vector Doppler: accurate measurement of blood velocity in two dimensions, *Ultrasound Med Biol* 18:19, 1992.)

points demonstrates that in this volunteer patient, the systolic arterial flow is first directed from the common carotid artery into the external carotid artery; about 100 ms later, the flow is redirected into the internal carotid artery. This kind of detail on the changing direction of velocity vectors has never been possible with ultrasonic devices.

The time course of a blood velocity vector in two dimensions can be displayed in a projected view of a three-dimensional space that shows time along one coordinate and the vector direction along the other two coordinates (Fig. 122-11). A trajectory of the velocity vector is helpful in understanding the behavior of the vector (Fig. 122-11).

Velocity Vector with Time

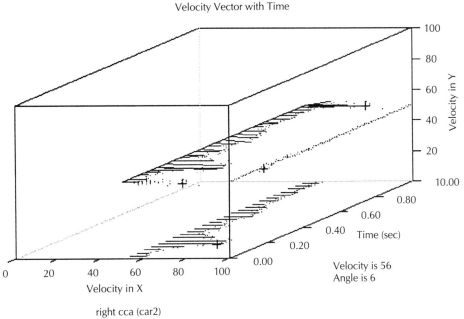

Velocity is 56
Angle is 6

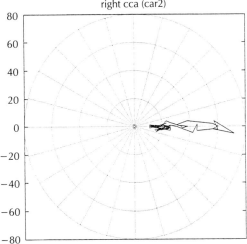

Fig. 122-11. The velocity vector magnitude and angle from a common carotid artery is shown. Each vector was determined from data acquired over 10 ms. A total of 100 vector terminations are shown covering a period of 1 sec. The data were obtained by using the vector Doppler device shown in Figs. 122-5 and 122-6 on a human common carotid artery through the skin of the neck. (Courtesy P.D. Waters.)

THREE-DIMENSIONAL VELOCITY INFORMATION

Three mutually perpendicular components of each velocity vector in the sample volume can be conveniently obtained by using a scan head with five ultrasound transducers on the skin as shown in Fig. 122-12. Four receiving transducers *ra*, *rb*, *rc*, and *rd* are located in a circle. Receiving transducers can be formed in pairs: *ra* and *rc*, *rb* and *rd*. Members of each pair are on diametrically opposite sides of the central transducer. Processing the echoes from the pair of transducers *ra* and *rc* to produce the quadrature difference frequency provides the blood velocity component with the X heading; processing the echoes from the other pair of transducers *rb* and *rd* to produce the quadrature difference frequency provides the blood velocity component in the Z heading.

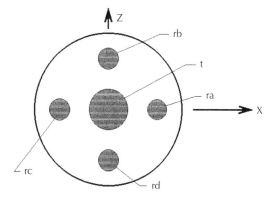

Fig. 122-12. By using a central transmitter *t* and a circle of receivers *r*, the examiner can determine the velocity components in the X and Z direction as well as in the Y direction. Velocity in the transverse X direction is obtained by taking the frequency difference between signals from *ra* and *rc*; velocity in the transverse Z direction is obtained by taking the frequency difference between signals from *rb* and *rd*.

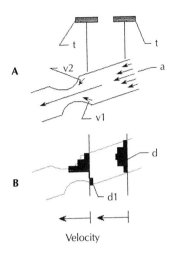

Fig. 122-13. When the blood velocity vectors converge at the entrance to a stenosis, a flow reversal with respect to the ultrasound lines appears at the deep wall. This does not represent retrograde flow in the artery. Flow magnitude and direction at each depth are shown as displacements from the zero velocity line. *A,* The velocity vectors. *B,* The resultant Doppler bidirectional frequency shifts at different depths.

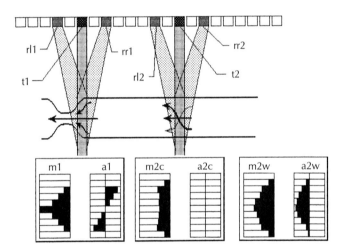

Fig. 122-14. By displaying the vector component parallel to the artery axis separate from the angle of the vector, details of both helical flow and a stenotic entrance are revealed. *m,* The velocity magnitude; *a,* the velocity heading angle. The *2c* data are taken from midstream in the artery, and *2w* data are taken from the wall of the artery where the helical velocity vector is ascending.

ENTRY INTO A STENOSIS

A conventional color Doppler system obtains only the velocity component perpendicular to the skin. At the entry to a stenosis, as the blood velocity vector on the deep side of the artery tilts toward the stenosis, it passes through a Doppler angle of 90° and thus creates a frequency increase in the ultrasound echo rather than a decrease like the rest of the velocity vectors. This area appears on the image as an anomalous flow reversal as shown in Fig. 122-13.

A two-dimensional vector Doppler system applied to the entry of a stenosis can prevent the appearance of this anomalous flow reversal (Fig. 122-14). With a vector Doppler system, the ultrasonic velocity signals from the region of the stenosis entry are received by the pair of receiving transducers (rr and r_1) and displayed as velocity magnitude versus depth m and heading angle versus depth a. The negative heading angle at the superficial side of the vessel, the high-velocity magnitude at the center, and the positive heading angle at the deep side of the vessel confirm the smooth laminar entry to a stenosis.

CONCLUSION

The history of ultrasound instrument development reveals that the introduction and initial testing of each development have preceded the wide clinical acceptance by nearly 10 years. Doppler ultrasonography,[21] introduced before 1960, became widely used after 1970; bidirectional Doppler ultrasonography,[26] introduced in 1969, became widely used in 1975; duplex scanning, first conceived in 1973, became widely used in 1980; color flow imaging,[3] first conceived in 1978, became widely used by 1985; phased linear arrays, conceived before 1976, came into common use by 1988 but are still under development.

The construction of the first vector Doppler instrument of the current design began in 1990; studies on earlier instruments and methods that addressed the same problem were published as early as 1974.[10] It is not possible to predict whether this technology will flourish beyond the novelty stage.

One thing is certain: there is still diagnostic information hidden in ultrasound echoes. Innovation will unlock the route to use that information for better diagnostic decisions. The final development of medical ultrasound diagnostic equipment is not here and will not be seen in this century.

ACKNOWLEDGMENT

Illustrations were prepared by Mary Patricia Fitzgerald, John R. Overbeck, and P. Dean Waters.

REFERENCES

1. Bernoulli D: *Hydrodynamica,* 1738.
2. Daigle RE et al: Nontraumatic aortic blood flow sensing by use of an ultrasonic esophageal probe, *J Appl Physiol* 38:1153-1160, 1975.
3. Eyer MK et al: Color digital echo/Doppler image presentation, *Ultrasound Med Biol* 7:21-31, 1981.
4. Fitzgerald MP: *Two-dimensional vector Doppler imaging,* thesis, Seattle, 1987, University of Washington.
5. Fox MD: *Crossed Beam Ultrasonic Flowmeter,* United States Patent No 4,062,237, issued Dec 13, 1977.
6. Fox MD: True volume flow measurement with multiple beam ultrasound Doppler, *Proceedings of the Thirteenth Annual Northeast Bioengineering Conference,* Institute of Electrical and Electronics Engineers Press, 2:357-60, 1987.
7. Franklin DL et al: A pulsed ultrasonic flowmeter, *Inst Radio Engineers: Trans Med Electronics* 6:204-206, 1959.
8. Gill RW: Measurement of blood flow by ultrasound: accuracy and sources of error, *Ultrasound Med Biol* 11:625-641, 1985.
9. Hansen PL: *Ultrasonic Transducer Devices,* United States Patent No 3,987,673, issued Oct 26, 1976.

10. Hansen PL, Cross G, Light H: *Beam-angle independent Doppler velocity measurement in superficial vessels.* In Woodcock JP, ed: *Clinical blood flow measurement,* London, 1974, Sector Publishing.
11. Hatle L, Angelsen B: *Cardiac output.* In *Doppler ultrasound in cardiology,* ed 2, Philadelphia, 1985, Lea & Febiger.
12. Hatle L, Angelsen B: *Pulsed and continuous wave Doppler in diagnosis and assessment of various heart lesions.* In *Doppler ultrasound in cardiology,* ed 2, Philadelphia, 1985, Lea & Febiger.
13. Kohler TR et al: Assessment of pressure gradient by Doppler ultrasound: experimental and clinical observations, *J Vasc Surg* 6:460-469, 1987.
14. Koneko Z et al: Studies on ultrasonic blood rheograph, *Brain Nerve* 72:921-935, 1960.
15. Ku DN et al: Hemodynamics of the normal human carotid bifurcation: in vitro and in vivo studies, *Ultrasound Med Biol* 11:13-26, 1985.
16. McConalogue DJ, Srivastava RS: Motion of a fluid in a curved tube, *Proc R Soc London* A307:37, 1968.
17. Napel S et al: Visualizing three-dimensional flow with simulated streamlines and three-dimensional phase-contrast MR imaging, *J Magnetic Resonance Imaging* 2:143-153, 1992.
18. Nealeigh RC, Miller CW, McLeod FD Jr: Venous ultrasound catheter-tip technique for evaluation of arterial hemodynamics, *J Appl Physiol* 41:946-952, 1976.
19. Overbeck JR, Beach KW, Strandness DE Jr: Vector Doppler: accurate measurement of blood velocity in two dimensions, *Ultrasound Med Biol* 18:19-31, 1992.
20. Reneman RS et al: Cardiovascular applications of multi-gate pulsed Doppler systems, *Ultrasound Med Biol* 12:357-370, 1986.
21. Satamura S: Ultrasonic Doppler method for the inspection of cardiac function, *J Acoust Soc Am* 29:1181-1185, 1957.
22. Schrank E et al: A triangulation method for the quantitative measurement of arterial blood velocity magnitude and direction in humans, *Ultrasound Med Biol* 16:499-509, 1990.
23. Stonebridge PA, Brophy CM: Spiral laminar flow in arteries? *Lancet* 338:1360-1361, 1991.
24. Strandness DE Jr, Sumner DS: The effects of geometry on arterial blood flow. In *Hemodynamics for surgeons,* New York, 1975, Grune & Stratton.
25. Strandness DE Jr, McCutcheon EP, Rushmer RF: Application of a transcutaneous Doppler flowmeter in evaluation of occlusive arterial disease, *Surg Gynecol Obstet* 122:1039, 1966.
26. Strandness DE Jr et al: Transcutaneous directional flow detection: a preliminary report, *Am Heart J* 78:65-74, 1969.
27. Texan M: A hemodynamic concept of atherosclerosis, with particular reference to coronary occlusion, *AMA Arch Intern Med* 99:418-427, 1957.
28. Texan M, Imparato AM, Lord JW Jr: The hemodynamic concept of atherosclerosis, *AMA Arch Surg* 80:47-53, 1960.
29. Uematsu S: Determination of volume of arterial blood flow by an ultrasonic device, *J Clin Ultrasound* 9:209-216, 1981.
30. Vera N et al: Visualization of complex flow fields, with applications to the interpretation of colour flow Doppler images, *Ultrasound Med Biol* 18:1-9, 1992.
31. Wei-qi W, Lin-xin Y: A double beam Doppler ultrasound method for quantitative blood flow velocity measurement, *Ultrasound Med Biol* 8:421-425, 1982.
32. Yearwood TL, Chanderin KB: Physiological pulsatile flow experiments in a model of the human aortic arch, *Biomech* 15:683-704, 1984.

CHAPTER 123

Magnetic resonance imaging and angiography

CHARLES B. HIGGINS

Magnetic resonance imaging (MRI) has several advantages that render it suitable for imaging the vascular system. These advantages include intrinsic contrast between the blood pool and vascular structures, negating the need for contrast media; multiple imaging planes, providing the ability to interrogate either parallel or perpendicular to the course of the vessel; a wide range of soft tissue contrast, permitting the depiction of perivascular as well as vascular structures; avoidance of ionizing radiation and contrast media, easing the concern for acquiring sequential investigations; and the ability to evaluate and quantify both structure and function of the vascular system.

The unique signal intensity of flowing blood obviates the need for contrast media to demarcate the blood pool. The appearance of flowing blood is nearly diametric on spin-echo (SE) compared with gradient echo (GRE) sequences. On standard SE images the blood pool is typically dark, whereas on GRE the flowing blood is bright. Whichever technique is used, the examination can usually be conducted without the use of contrast media.

The combination of imaging, either tomographic or projectional (magnetic resonance angiography [MRA]), and flow-sensitive techniques provides the capability for depicting structure and for quantifying blood flow volume and velocity during a single study. These velocity-encoded images can be acquired at multiple phases of the cardiac cycle to generate velocity (flow) versus time curves, which depict the flow characteristics of various vascular beds.

THORACIC AORTIC DISEASE

The complete evaluation of thoracic aortic disease requires information concerning luminal dimensions, velocity or rate of blood flow, status of the vessel wall, longitudinal extent of disease, relation and effect of disease to major aortic branches, and the effect of vascular disease on paraaortic structures. Some but not all of this information is obtained with angiography. Ultrasound also provides most of this information in the abdomen but has limited capability for evaluating thoracic vascular disease. Computerized tomography (CT) can acquire most of this information in both thorax and abdomen but requires contrast media for the purpose. MRI obtains all the critical information needed for

the diagnosis of vascular disease without the use of contrast media.

Considering the limitations and invasive features of other imaging modalities, MRI seems to be the procedure of choice for the evaluation of thoracic aortic disease. Furthermore, because it is completely noninvasive, it is the ideal technique for monitoring the progression of thoracic aortic abnormalities, such as thoracic aortic aneurysms and aortoannular ectasia.

The thoracic aorta is studied with both the SE and GRE techniques (Fig. 123-1). It is imaged in both the transverse and the sagittal or oblique sagittal planes. The sagittal or oblique sagittal planes are used to define the longitudinal extent of a lesion in relation to the origin of the aortic arch branches. The cine version of the GRE technique is used routinely for evaluating thoracic aortic disease. A four-level acquisition is done with placement of the levels equidistant from the sinus of Valsalva to the aortic arch.

Aortic dissection

MRI has been shown to be effective for the diagnosis of aortic dissection.* The definitive diagnosis of dissection requires the identification of the intimal flap. The intimal flap is readily discerned as a linear structure within the aorta (Figs. 123-1 and 123-2). When there is rapid flow in the true and false lumina, the intimal flap is observed between the flow void in both channels on SE images or as a low-intensity septum between the bright signal of the two channels on GRE images. In some instances, it may be possible to identify the entry point of the dissection. The dissection usually extends over a long segment of the aorta; however, focal dissection occurs infrequently.

Flow is sometimes slower in the false channel, causing partial or complete filling of this channel with a signal of variable intensity on SE images. The velocities of flow in the two channels can be measured by using a velocity-encoded cine MR sequence.[6,8] This observation enables differentiation between the true and false channels. MRI readily defines the presence of thrombosis of the false channel (Fig. 123-3). Even if the entire false channel is throm-

---

*References 2, 6, 8, 14, 15, 21, 27, 35, 36.

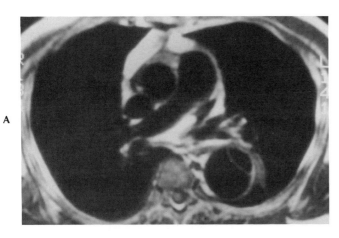

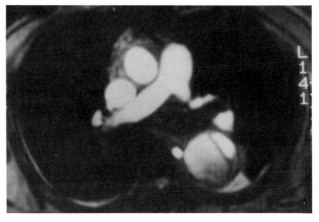

Fig. 123-1. ECG-gated *(A)* and GE *(B)* transaxial images at the descending thoracic aorta demonstrate an intimal flap in the descending aorta. This patient had previously undergone placement of a graft in the ascending aorta for treatment of type A aortic dissection. The intimal flap and patency of the false channel are evident after surgery.

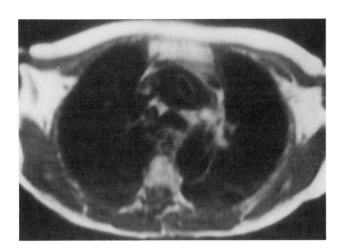

Fig. 123-2. ECG-gated transverse image of the thoracic aorta demonstrates a circumferential intimal flap in a patient with aortic dissection. This is a type A aortic dissection with involvement of the ascending aorta. In the ascending aorta, the intimal flap is recognized to be circumferential. High-velocity blood flow in the true and false channel outlines the intimal flap on the transverse image.

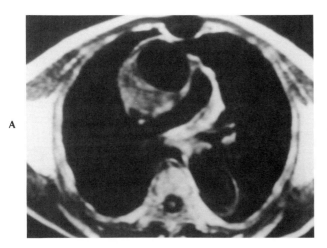

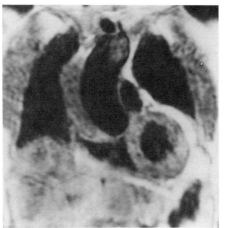

Fig. 123-3. ECG-gated transaxial *(A)* and coronal *(B)* images in a patient with type A aortic dissection. There is thrombosis of the false channel. The coronal image demonstrates a normal contour and diameter of the ascending aorta. The thrombosed false channel is readily recognized as extraluminal tissue on this image. Recognition of this extraluminal pathology might be difficult on a contrast angiogram.

bosed, MRI can still identify aortic dissection because it demonstrates intramural and intraluminal disease.

Signal within the false channel is caused by thrombus, slow flow, or a combination of the two. It is usually possible to differentiate between slow flow and thrombus. Because of the phenomenon of even-echo rephasing, there is both a relative (to other tissues) and absolute increase in MRI signal intensity on the second compared with the first echo image. Another method for differentiation is to obtain multiphase gated images. With this technique, images of the same anatomic level are acquired at five phases of the cardiac cycle. Because velocity of arterial flow varies during the cardiac cycle, the configuration and intensity of the intraluminal signal that is due to slow flow also varies. On the other hand, the signal of thrombus remains constant.

Phase images can also be used to distinguish thrombus from the signal of slowly moving blood.[28,29,31] Spins that move during the application of the gradient will appear different from stationary spins if phase images are examined. The intensity of voxels on such images is related to the phase variation of the spins flowing in a magnetic gradient. The phase variation is directly related to the velocity of motion.

MRI can identify the most precarious complication of dissection, which is leakage of blood from the aorta, resulting in hemorrhagic pericardial effusion, hemorrhagic pleural effusion, mediastinal hemorrhage, and periaortic hematoma. The signal intensity of blood within the first hours after hemorrhage may not be characteristically different from other fluid collections; however, hemorrhage usually has high intensity on T1-weighted spin-echo images. Furthermore, hemorrhage sometimes separates into two components: a medium-intensity clot component and a high-intensity (equal or higher than fat) serum component.

Because it is frequently possible to distinguish the true channel from the false one, MRI can sometimes determine whether aortic branches, such as the arch arteries and the celiac, superior mesenteric, and renal arteries, arise from the true or the false channel.[2] In addition, the presence of a flow void in the visceral vessels is indicative of patency of these arteries. Extension of the intimal flap into the aortic arch branches is also defined on MRI. Several reports that assess the capability of MRI for evaluating aortic dissection have appeared recently.[2,14,15,21,27] The diagnostic accuracy of MRI in aortic dissection was evaluated in a group of 54 consecutive patients with the use of receiver operating characteristic curves to confirm the diagnosis. The sensitivity at a specificity level of 90% was greater than 95% for two experienced reviewers.[21] MRI correctly distinguished between type A and type B dissections. The relationship of the dissection to the descending aorta, aortic arch, and descending aorta was indicated by multisectional transverse images. The transverse plane depicted the flap in all sections of the aorta; this was considered to be the essential imaging plane for identifying and determining the extent of the dissection.

The velocity-encoded cine MR technique has been used to demonstrate the flow pattern in the true and false lumina.[6,8] It can be used to distinguish between the signal caused by slow blood flow and thrombus in the false channel. Cine MRI can be used to demonstrate the motion of the intimal flap. Moreover, it may be the most effective imaging sequence to visualize a flap that is substantially mobile. Such a flap might be difficult to define with the SE technique because of its motion during the imaging sequence. Cine MRI can also be used to detect and assess the severity of aortic regurgitation caused by dissection. The aortic regurgitation is represented as a diastolic signal void in the left ventricle emanating from the aortic valve.[32] The volume of the signal void provides a means for estimation of the severity of regurgitation.[32]

Follow-up of aortic dissection. The type A dissection is treated by surgery, whereas the type B dissection is managed medically. With both forms of therapy, the aorta remains abnormal. After replacement of the ascending aorta with a graft, the false channel is frequently not obliterated and has been shown to be patent by follow-up CT[16] and MRI studies.[34] In both groups of patients, CT and MRI can be used to monitor the progression of disease and to detect such complications as aneurysm formation of the false channel and recurrent, progressive dissection at an early stage. MRI has demonstrated progressive, aneurysmal dilatation of the false channel in some type B dissections, false aneurysm at the anastomosis of a graft used to obliterate the false channel, persistent patency of the false channel after graft replacement of the descending aorta, and recurrent dissection of the abdominal aorta after surgical obliteration of type A dissection. Persistent patency of the false channel after surgery is observed in most patients.[34] Thrombosis of the false channel and remodeling of the thoracic aorta after treatment of type A dissection is observed in a minority of patients after operation. In some patients, thrombosis occurs in the false channel, but the true channel remains compressed.

CT and MRI can be used to trace the natural history of the false channel. A recent CT study[37] has shown a variable natural history with spontaneous obliteration or aneurysm formation of the channel in a minority of patients but persistent patency and no remarkable change in dimensions of the channel in the majority.

MRI is also an ideal method for sequential monitoring of the aorta in patients at a high risk for developing dissection. These are subjects with Marfan or Ehlers-Danlos syndrome and those with a familial history of aortic dissection.

Thoracic aortic aneurysm

MRI demonstrates concentric enlargement of the ascending or descending aorta in patients with thoracic aortic aneurysm[1,10,11,15] (Fig. 123-4). The outer diameter of the aneurysm and the size of the residual lumen have been readily visualized on transverse MRI. Because MRI shows the outer wall of the aneurysm, it can provide an accurate measure of the diameter of the aneurysm even when there

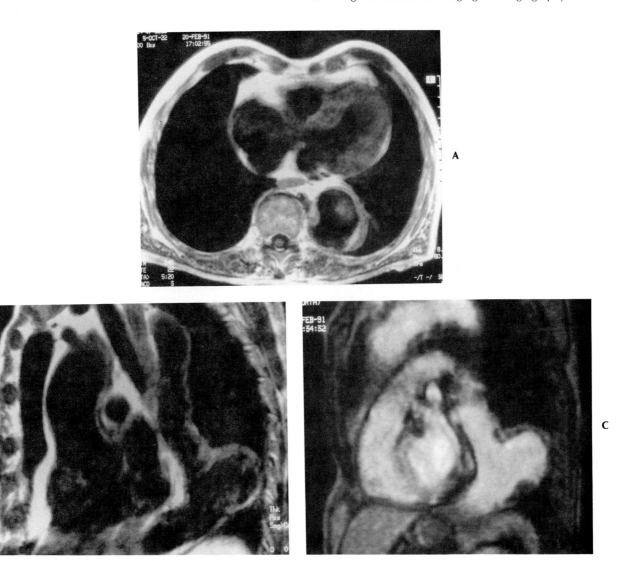

Fig. 123-4. ECG-gated SE transaxial *(A)* and sagittal images *(B)* and fast GRE sagittal image *(C)* in a patient with a large aneurysm of the descending thoracic aorta. The saccular aneurysm arises from the posterior aspect of the descending aorta. On one of the transaxial images, there is considerable signal within the aneurysm. This raised the possibility of thrombus within the aneurysm. The fast GRE image demonstrates bright signal intensity of the blood within the aneurysm and demonstrates that most of this signal on the SE image is caused by slow blood flow. A small mural thrombus is present. (Courtesy Charles Anderson, San Francisco, Calif.)

is wall thickening or mural thrombus (Figs. 123-4 and 123-5). On the other hand, angiography can only provide a definite measurement of the contrast-filled lumen. According to the experience of some investigators,[1,15] angiography in some patients underestimates the aneurysmal diameter in comparison with MRI. The longitudinal extent of the aneurysm can be discerned from sequential transverse tomograms and from sagittal (or left anterior oblique equivalent) tomograms. Huge aneurysms produce displacement and compression of cardiac chambers and other mediastinal structures.

Identification of different constituents of the aortic aneurysm is possible with MRI. Thrombus or atherosclerotic plaques are demonstrated as eccentric or concentric thickening of the aneurysmal wall (see Fig. 123-5). An old thrombus produces medium signal intensity on the first echo image and relatively lower signal on the second echo images. Conversely, a subacute thrombus has a substantially higher signal intensity on the first echo images and frequently shows a relatively higher signal intensity on the second echo image. In these cases, distinction between slow flow and fresh thrombus can be equivocal.

Detection of periaortic or mediastinal bleeding is a critical factor in the evaluation of symptomatic aneurysms. Hematoma produces a high signal intensity on T1-weighted images. This appearance is unlike most other fluids, which

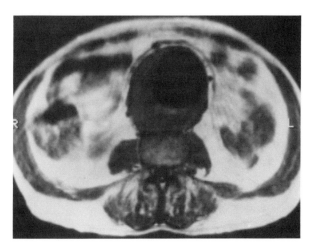

Fig. 123-5. Transverse SE image demonstrates a large aneurysm of the abdominal aorta. The aneurysm contains a substantial amount of mural thrombus. The inferior vena cava is compressed and essentially occluded by the aneurysm.

have low intensity on T1-weighted images; however, it should be noted that this characteristic appearance may not be present during the early hours after hemorrhage.

Dinsmore et al[10] reported the MRI features of 15 fusiform and 5 saccular aneurysms. An aneurysm was defined as a region of the aorta with a diameter greater than one and a half times normal. The structure and size of the aneurysm defined by MRI corresponded with the findings from other imaging modalities. Although there was aortic wall thickening in two patients and mural thrombus in others, the maximum diameter of the aneurysm as determined by MRI and angiography correlated closely. Presumably, the measurements were not made at the sites of wall thickening or thrombus, since angiography can accurately quantitate only the dimensions of the contrast-filled lumen. There was also agreement on the extent of the aneurysm as defined by MRI and angiography. The good correlation for the diameter of the aneurysm may reflect the large number of patients with Marfan syndrome in this study, since these patients tend to have thin-walled aneurysms of the sinuses of Valsalva and ascending aorta.

MRI seems to be a practical method for monitoring the progression of aneurysmal disease of the thoracic aorta. The noninvasive nature of the study makes it practical for periodic evaluation of patients with aortoanular ectasia, Marfan syndrome, and aneurysms. A diameter of the descending aorta in excess of 7.0 cm or a rapid increase in the aortic diameter may move the decision toward early operation. MRI can provide precise measurements of aortic dimensions. It is important to assess directly the actual aortic dimensions in patients in whom chest radiographs indicate an apparent impressive increase in the aortic shadow over a few years' duration. MRI has shown that such enlargement may be due to only a modestly dilated ascending aorta coupled with considerable elongation of the aorta (arteriomegaly).

Periaortic hematoma and mediastinal hemorrhage

MRI displays periaortic as well as intraluminal disease. Consequently, it demonstrates blood confined to a localized periaortic site or more extensive hemorrhage throughout the mediastinum in the extrapleural or pleural spaces. Thus MRI can be used for the definitive diagnosis of chest pain in a patient with a known or suspected thoracic aortic aneurysm. It can also demonstrate rupture of the false channel of an aortic dissection into the mediastinum or pericardium. The appearance of intracranial hemorrhage on T1- and T2-weighted images has been characterized clearly in relation to the age of the hematoma and the mechanisms responsible for the variable appearance. The appearance of hematoma in the thorax has not been as well characterized. A few cases in which mediastinal or pericardial blood caused a high signal on T1-weighted images have been encountered in patients in whom the onset of acute symptoms that were indicative of thoracic aortic hemorrhage occurred less than 24 hours before the MRI study.

The T1-weighted images are most useful in the diagnosis of aortic hemorrhage. The signal intensity of the blood is shown as being similar or only slightly less than fat as opposed to serous collections, which have low signal intensity similar to simple fluid such as urine. MRI can demonstrate the extent of the hemorrhage with confinement to the periaortic region, pleural space, subpleural space, pericardium, or generalized spread through the mediastinum.

Aortic thrombus

Aortic thrombus occurs frequently in the wall of aneurysms and sometimes at the site of atherosclerosis. Peripheral embolization is a complication of aortic thrombus. After peripheral embolization, the investigation for the source of the embolus is directed toward the left atrium, left ventricle, and aorta. The most frequent sources and clinical situations are the left atrium in patients with atrial fibrillation or the left ventricle in patients with recent myocardial infarction or dilated cardiomyopathy. Embolization from aortic thrombus is less frequent. There have been patients in whom the cause of peripheral embolization was thrombus in the aortic arch. These mural thrombi were disclosed by using electrocardiographic gated SE and cine MR images. Cine MR images are useful because they depict the motion of the clot within the aortic lumen. The SE images may be more difficult to interpret if slow flow produces an intraluminal signal. MRI can be used to provide a full investigation of the possible sources of peripheral embolization. This can be accomplished by imaging the entire thorax; thus evaluation of the left atrium, left ventricle, and aorta is accomplished by a single imaging study.

ABDOMINAL AORTIC DISEASE

Abdominal vascular anatomy and disease processes have been well defined by MRI.* These vessels are defined either with tomographic SE or GRE sequences or with MRA. Some

---

*References 3-5, 9, 13, 17-20, 24, 33.

vascular pathologic conditions, such as aneurysms, arterio-venous fistulas, and hemorrhage, can be adequately assessed in peripheral vessels. The most frequent disease process afflicting the peripheral vessels is obstructive atherosclerosis. Complete diagnosis, assessment of severity, and planning of therapy of obstructive peripheral vascular disease are most effectively accomplished by a projectional technique with high spatial resolution, such as angiography. MRA has evolved rapidly in the past few years, and it now constitutes an effective technique in specific circumstances for the evaluation of obstructive disease of the aorta, iliac, and lower limb arteries. Motion degradation in the abdomen and pelvis and limitation of imaging volume still hinder general acceptance of this technique for the evaluation of peripheral vascular disease. However, early reports suggest that it is or will be useful for specific indications such as the evaluation of renovascular hypertension,[22] assessment of superficial femoral and popliteal arteries before and after treatment such as angioplasty, and assessment of distal circulation for limb salvage operations.

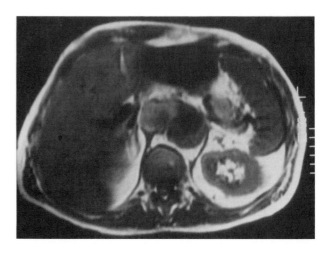

Fig. 123-6. Transaxial image of the abdomen in a patient with a suprarenal abdominal aortic aneursym. The aneurysm extends above the level of the celiac axis. Leakage of the aneurysm is demonstrated by the periaortic hematoma adjacent to the right side of the aorta and dissecting into the right crus of the diaphragm. There is thrombus in the aneurysm.

Abdominal aortic aneurysm

MRI can identify the presence, assess the diameter, and define the longitudinal extent of abdominal aortic aneurysms (AAAs).[3,13,24] It is accurate in defining the involvement of visceral arteries, including, most importantly, the renal arteries.[3] In the evaluation of AAAs, transverse MR images can determine the outer diameter of the aneurysm, dimension of the residual lumen, lamination of mural thrombus or atherosclerotic debris on the aneurysmal wall (Fig. 123-5), presence of periaortic hematoma (Fig. 123-6), and effect of the aneurysm on adjacent structures, especially the inferior vena cava. Sequential transverse images define the longitudinal extent and assess the possibility of extension to or above the level of the renal arteries. Neither angiography nor ultrasonography alone can provide all of these pieces of information. CT provides all of these observations but entails the use of contrast media and radiation exposure.

Several articles have now indicated the results of MRI for the evaluation of AAAs.[1,3,13,24] In one series of 27 patients with AAAs, the MRI findings were compared retrospectively with CT, ultrasonography, and angiography in 17 cases and prospectively with ultrasonography in 10 cases.[3] The measurement of the outer diameter of an AAA was similar for MRI, CT, and ultrasonography. MRI depicted the renal arteries in all 27 patients and identified extension to or above the renal arteries in the 8 patients in whom this was found during surgery (Fig. 123-6). Ultrasonography determined renal involvement in only 3 of these 8 patients; in 3 of the remaining 5 patients, ultrasonography could not definitely visualize the renal arteries. Extension of the aneurysm into the iliac arteries was demonstrated by MRI in all patients who had this condition. The extent of the aneurysm was best defined by the series of transverse images. Conversely, the entire length of the aneurysm could not be as closely defined by coronal images because of severe tortuosity of the aorta; however, coronal images occasionally clearly depicted the relationship of the AAA to the renal arteries.

MRI distinguished between mural thrombus filling much of the aneurysm and the central signal void representing the residual channel (see Figs. 123-5 and 123-6). Aneurysms with wide caliber sometimes had considerable signal from the moving blood, presumably because of lower velocity of flow in the expanded lumen. Slow flow within the residual lumen of the aneurysm was recognized as marked increase of intraluminal signal intensity on the second compared with the first SE image. Slowly flowing blood can usually be differentiated from mural thrombus within the aneurysm. The mural thrombus will usually demonstrate a decrease in signal on the second echo image rather than the marked increase in signal exhibited by slowly flowing blood (even echo rephasing of flowing blood); however, the signal intensity of some thrombi (presumably of more recent vintage) is fairly high and may even show some but not a marked increase of intensity on the second echo image. MRI can readily depict the narrowing and/or distortion of the inferior vena cava caused by an adjacent aneurysm (Fig. 123-5). MRI shows the low signal intensity of periaortic fibrosis occasionally associated with aneurysms. It also shows the high signal fluid collection that is indicative of periaortic hematoma (see Fig. 123-6).

The role of MRI in relation to ultrasound is considered secondary when used for the mere diagnosis of AAA and surveillance of its diameter. This notion is based on the finding that both methods provide equivalent estimates of the maximum diameter of the aneurysm. Because ultrasonography is less expensive and more widely available, it will likely be the initial diagnostic imaging modality. The unique role of MRI is for the preoperative definition of the longitudinal extent of the aneurysm, particularly for depicting involvement of the renal arteries. It should also be useful for evaluating the possibility of a leaking aneurysm with periaortic hematoma.

The advantages of MRI over angiography for the evaluation of AAA are its ability to provide a measure of the outer diameter of the aneurysm and the patent lumen, to depict the mural thrombus or atherosclerotic debris within the aneurysm, and to indicate the presence of periaortic hemorrhage.

Standard or fast GE (turbo) images are usually obtained as well as or in preference to SE images for the evaluation of AAA. These images are usually better for defining and separating the mural thrombus from slowly flowing blood in the dilated lumen. Turbo-GRE images acquired during the vascular phase of contrast enhancement produced by intravenously injected MR contrast media are effective for this purpose (see Fig. 123-4).

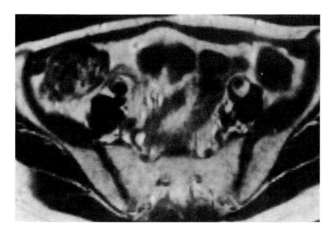

Fig. 123-7. Transverse SE images of the retroperitoneum by using a long TE (T2 weighted). The T2-weighted images show high signal fluid surrounding the two limbs of the graft. The perigraft fibrous capsule is also discernible.

Complications of aortoiliac and aortofemoral grafts

The major complications of grafts are perigraft hematoma, perigraft abscess, thrombus, and anastomotic pseudoaneurysm. Sequential CT and MR studies during the postoperative period indicate that hematoma, seroma, and other fluid collections can be observed in the perigraft region up to 3 months after surgery.[5,25] A hematoma older than 48 hours has high signal intensity on both T1- and T2-weighted images. A hematoma frequently separates into components with two distinct intensities. These are reasonably specific MR features of a hematoma. Sequential MR images in patients after surgery for the placement of aortoiliac or aortofemoral grafts indicate that fluid around the graft is a normal feature of healing and may be present for 2 to 3 months after surgery. Beyond this time, the graft is surrounded by fibrous tissue that causes a low signal intensity on T2-weighted images.

Perigraft abscesses show a somewhat variable signal intensity pattern; however, they usually have low intensity on T1-weighted images and high intensity on T2-weighted sequences (Figs. 123-7 and 123-8).[5] Since the perigraft region is usually free of fluid 2 to 3 months after surgery, the presence of a substantial perigraft fluid collection, in either the retroabdominal or retropelvic region, after this time is highly suggestive of a perigraft abscess. The inflammatory nature of the perigraft infection is usually reflected in the adjacent psoas muscle; there may be increased intensity of the psoas muscle. High intensity of the adjacent muscle has also been observed in patients with perigraft abscesses.

Transverse MR images at the level of the groin or lower pelvic region in perigraft abscess display the perigraft collection surrounding the graft and displacing the perigraft fibrous capsule away from the graft (Fig. 123-7). The fibrous capsule has low signal intensity. In such cases, transverse MR images of the pelvis and abdomen can be used to determine whether the infection extends into the retroperitoneum. A perigraft collection of high-intensity fluid

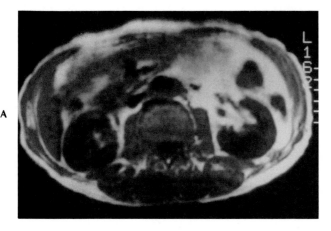
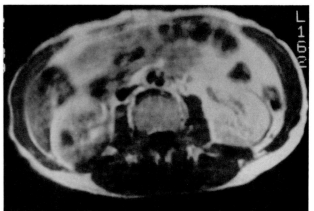

Fig. 123-8. T1-weighted images before *(A)* and after *(B)* the injection of MR contrast medium in a patient with an infected aortoiliac graft. The tissue surrounding the graft enhances in signal after administration of the contrast medium.

and alteration of intensity of the adjacent psoas muscle on T2-weighted images indicate this complication. After the injection of MR contrast media, the perigraft collection has shown enhancement (Fig. 123-8).

The pseudoaneurysm is recognized as either a disproportionate enlargement of the femoral or iliac artery at the expected anastomotic site or a vascular cavity projecting off the aorta, iliac, or femoral artery. The smaller saccular pseudoaneurysms usually have a flow void, and the connection with the parent vessel can be discerned. Conversely, some pseudoaneurysms may be enormous and show both regions of thrombus and slow flow within them.

MEASUREMENT OF BLOOD FLOW

Measurement of blood flow velocity with MRI has become practical in patients.[23,26,30] There are two methods for accomplishing this: time of flight method and phase change method.[23,26,30] The time of flight method is done by applying a preliminary radiofrequency pulse to a selected narrow slab of tissue that contains a blood vessel. The signal is removed from this slab of tissue so that when the blood vessel is imaged a short time later, the saturation tag is recognized downstream in the vessel. Since the time between presaturation and imaging acquisition is known and the distance between the site of presaturation of the slab of blood and its site on the image can be measured, the velocity can be simply calculated as $v = \Delta$ distance$/\Delta$ time. The second method—the phase change technique—is based on the phase shift of moving spins as they move along a magnetic field gradient. The extent of the phase shifts of moving spins is proportional to the velocity of motion along the velocity-encoded direction. Velocity encoding is performed by using bipolar gradient pulses. The direction of velocity encoding can be done in any orthogonal or oblique axis of the body. It can be done in one, two, or three dimensions.

Velocity encoding of blood flow in each voxel by the phase shift method provides two- or three-dimensional quantitative velocity mapping of the vascular system. The instantaneous flow in a vessel can be determined as the product of the cross-sectional area and mean velocity of blood flow in the vessel. The instantaneous flow in the ascending aorta can be determined by the product of the cross-sectional area and mean velocity of the blood within the aorta. The integration of the instantaneous flow at the base of the aorta through the cardiac cycle provides a measure of left ventricular stroke volume, and the same integration done at the proximal pulmonary artery is a measure of right ventricular stroke volume. The stroke volumes measured in this manner have correlated well with ventricular stroke volumes measured by planimetry of the adjacent cine MR images. Measurement of flow by velocity-encoded cine MRI should be accurate, provided that the flowing blood generates enough signal to calculate phase, the velocity phase–encoding gradients are accurately calibrated, and the correct range of velocity in the vessels being interrogated has been selected. The calculation of stroke volumes by the velocity-encoded

cine MRI technique has shown nearly equivalent values for the right and left ventricle in normal subjects. The technique is also capable of measuring blood flow volume separately in the right and left pulmonary arteries.[7] A distinctly different flow pattern in the pulmonary artery has been observed in patients with pulmonary hypertension compared with normal subjects when this technique was used.

MAGNETIC RESONANCE ANGIOGRAPHY

MRA has been effective for demonstrating disease in the extracranial and intracranial carotid circulation. The application of this technique in the chest, abdomen, and extremities is still undergoing development and is generally not universally available or reliable for clinical use. Some institutions have shown good results in the use of MRA for the detection of renovascular stenosis in patients with hypertension.[12,22] MRA has also been effective in displaying the arteries of the limbs (Fig. 123-9) and the aortoiliac circulation (Fig. 123-10). It is expected that with further development, the techniques will be important for the diagnosis of vascular disease in all regions of the body.

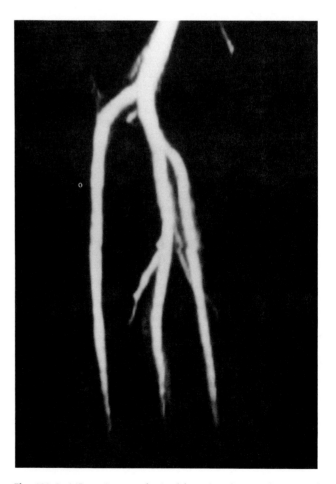

Fig. 123-9. MR angiogram obtained by using the two-dimensional time of flight technique shows the popliteal artery and trifurcation arteries in a normal subject.

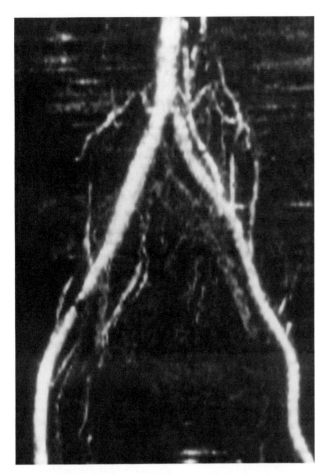

Fig. 123-10. MR angiogram obtained by using the two-dimensional time of flight technique shows a high-grade stenosis of the right external iliac artery.

REFERENCES

1. Amparo EG et al: Magnetic resonance imaging of aortic disease: preliminary results, *Am J Roentgenol* 143:1203, 1984.
2. Amparo EG et al: Aortic dissection: magnetic resonance imaging, *Radiology* 399-406, 1985.
3. Amparo EG et al: Comparison of magnetic resonance imaging and ultrasonography in the evaluation of abdominal aortic aneurysm, *Radiology* 154:451, 1985.
4. Auffermann W et al: MR imaging of complications of aortic surgery, *J Comput Assist Tomogr* 11:982-989, 1987.
5. Auffermann W et al: Incorporation versus infection of retroperitoneal aortic grafts: MR imaging features, *Radiology* 172:359-362, 1989.
6. Bogren HG et al: Magnetic resonance velocity mapping in aortic dissection, *Br J Radiol* 61:456-462, 1986.
7. Caputo GR et al: Right and left lung perfusion: in vitro and in vivo validation with oblique-angle, velocity-encoded cine MR imaging, *Radiology* 180:693-698, 1991.
8. Chang J-M et al: MR measurement of blood flow in the true and false channel in chronic aortic dissection, *J Comput Assist Tomogr* 15(3):418-423, 1991.
9. di Cesare E et al: Evaluation of hematoma by MRI in follow-up of aorto-femoral bypass, *Magn Reson Imaging* 9:247-253, 1991.
10. Dinsmore RE et al: Magnetic resonance imaging of thoracic aortic aneurysms: comparison of other imaging methods, *Am J Roentgenol* 146:309, 1986.
11. Dooms GC, Higgins CB: The potential of magnetic resonance imaging for thoracic aortic disease, *J Thorac Cardiovasc Surg* 92:1088-1095, 1986.
12. Edelman RR et al: Projection arteriography and venography: initial clinical results with MR, *Radiology* 172:351, 1989.
13. Evanocho AM, Oshbakken M, Weidner W: Comparison of NMR and angiography for preoperative evaluation of abdominal aortic aneurysm, *Magn Reson Imaging Med* 2:41, 1985.
14. Geisinger MA et al: Thoracic aortic dissection: magnetic resonance imaging, *Radiology* 155:407, 1985.
15. Glazer HS et al: The thoracic aorta studied by MR imaging, *Radiology* 157:149, 1985.
16. Guthaner DF et al: Fate of the false channel following surgical repair of aortic dissection: an angiographic study, *Radiology* 133:1-8, 1979.
17. Herfkens RJ et al: Nuclear magnetic resonance imaging of atherosclerotic disease, *Radiology* 148:161-166, 1983.
18. Hricak H, Higgins CB, William RD: NMR imaging in retroperitoneal fibrosis, *Am J Roentgenol* 141:35-38, 1983.
19. Hricak H et al: Abdominal venous system: assessment using MR, *Radiology* 156:415, 1985.
20. Justich E et al: Infected aortoileofemoral grafts: magnetic resonance imaging, *Radiology* 154:133-136, 1985.
21. Kersting-Sommerhoff B et al: Aortic dissection: sensitivity and specificity for MR imaging, *Radiology* 166:651-655, 1988.
22. Kim D et al: Abdominal aorta and renal artery stenosis: evaluation with MR angiography, *Radiology* 174:727, 1990.
23. Kondo C, Caputo GR, Higgins CB: Right and left ventricular stroke volume measurements with velocity encoded cine NMR imaging: in vitro and in vivo validation, *Am J Radiol* 157:9-16, 1991.
24. Lee JKT et al: Magnetic resonance imaging of abdominal aortic aneurysms, *Am J Roentgenol* 143:1197, 1984.
25. Marks AS et al: Natural history of abdominal aortic grafts by CT, *Radiology* 175(P):77, 1985.
26. Nayler GL, Fermin DN, Longmore DB: Blood flow imaging by cine MR, *J Comput Assist Tomogr* 10:715, 1986.
27. Pernes JM et al: MR evaluation of chronic aortic dissection, *J Comput Assist Tomogr* 11:975-981, 1987.
28. Rumancik WM et al: Cardiovascular disease: evaluation with MR phase-imaging, *Radiology* 166:63, 1988.
29. Tavares NJ et al: Detection of thrombus by using phase-image MR scans: ROC curve analysis, *Am J Roentgenol* 153:173-178, 1989.
30. Underwood SR et al: MR velocity mapping: clinical applications of a new technique, *Br Heart J* 57:404, 1987.
31. von Schultess GK, Augustiny N: Calculated T2 values versus phase-imaging for the dissection between flow and thrombus in MR imaging, *Radiology* 164:549, 1988.
32. Wagner S et al: Diagnostic accuracy and estimation of the severity of valvular regurgitation from the signal void on cine MR, *Am Heart J* 118:760-767, 1989.
33. Wesbey GE et al: Magnetic resonance applications in atherosclerotic vascular disease, *Cardiovasc Intervent Radiol* 8:342-350, 1986.
34. White R, Higgins CB: MR imaging of the aorta after surgery for aortic dissection, *Am J Radiol* 150:87-92, 1988.
35. White RD, Dooms GC, Higgins CB: State of the art in imaging: advances in imaging of thoracic aortic disease, *Invest Radiol* 21:761-778, 1986.
36. Yamada T, Tada S, Harada J: Aortic dissection without intimal rupture: diagnosis with MR imaging and CT, *Radiology* 168:347-352, 1988.
37. Yamaguchi T et al: False lumens in type III aortic dissections: progressive CT study, *Radiology* 156:757, 1985.

CHAPTER 124

Volume flow estimations

BRENDA K. ZIERLER and WILLIAM G. REISS

Hepatic blood flow (HBF) can be altered by pathologic, physiologic, and drug-induced mechanisms. Because HBF is a determinant of drug elimination for many drugs, it is important to accurately estimate HBF to predict how alterations in blood flow will ultimately affect systemic drug concentrations. With this knowledge, potential drug toxicity or interactions can be studied in a controlled environment and may ultimately be avoided in the clinical setting.

There are numerous methods for estimating HBF. Indirect methods include dye-clearance techniques based on Fick's principle and angiographic procedures.[4] Direct measurement techniques include electromagnetic flow meters, timed collection of hepatic vessel output, and Doppler sonography. Dye-clearance studies, specifically those with indocyanine green (ICG), have been the most common technique used in pharmacologic studies. This technique has been used to estimate HBF for over 30 years. ICG was believed to have a high extraction ratio (approximately 1), to be eliminated solely by the liver, to not distribute out of the vascular space, and to have pharmacokinetics that were constant over time. By measuring blood concentrations of ICG and calculating hepatic clearance, it was possible to estimate HBF. In more recent years, it has been shown that these basic assumptions about the behavior of ICG are not necessarily correct and that this method of estimating HBF may be inaccurate. Furthermore, hepatic clearance of ICG can range from -62% to 126% between days in the same individual.[1] This variance could obscure changes in liver blood flow caused by other drugs or disease states and has raised concern about the validity of using this technique for estimating HBF. The other available methods used for estimating HBF, except Doppler sonography, have the shortcoming of being invasive. The initial and subsequent liver duplex studies are described.

DUPLEX ESTIMATES OF VOLUME FLOW
Variability study

Because of the variability in ICG estimation of HBF, duplex ultrasound was used as a technique to noninvasively measure HBF estimates.[7] The initial liver research project began with a protocol that was devised to minimize variability of repeat HBF estimates, where HBF is expressed as:

$$\text{HBF} = \text{Time average velocity (TAV)} \times \text{Cross-sectional area} \quad (1)$$

In this protocol, measurement of total HBF was not performed, but flow in specific branches of the hepatic artery (HA), portal vein (PV), and hepatic vein (HV) was estimated on 2 separate days. This protocol was tested in 15 normal volunteers and revised and tested in an additional 15 volunteers to obtain the least variability in repeat HBF estimates.[16] Blood velocity and vessel diameter measurements were obtained five times over a period of 2 hours. No significant differences were seen in velocity or blood flow measurements within or between days. The interday coefficients of variation, which include intrasubject variability, were 10% to 15% and 14% to 20% for velocity and blood flow measurements, respectively.

Validation study

A validation study to examine the accuracy of duplex ultrasound measurements of volume flow was carried out in a baboon model.[17] A total of 14 anesthetized baboons were studied with a duplex scanner with a 7-MHz imaging transducer and 5-MHz pulsed Doppler ultrasound. B-mode ultrasound measurements of external iliac artery diameters were used for calculation of the cross-sectional area. Timed blood collections obtained via a cannula inserted into the common femoral artery and TAV measurements were simultaneously obtained over 6- to 15-second intervals. These measurements were repeated three to five times per animal, and different flow rates were obtained each time. There was no significant difference between the two methods of volume flow measurement. Linear regression analysis revealed a high degree of correlation ($r = 0.90$, slope $= 0.95$, $p = 0.0001$) between absolute and estimated blood flow. The absolute percentage error was $13\% \pm 8\%$. This study demonstrated that volume flow measured by duplex scanning correlates well with timed blood collections under the described conditions. The same protocol was used to measure changes in HBF before and after administration of drugs to perturb HBF.[2,3,12,13]

METHODS

Subjects

Subjects for the various liver research studies were normal, nonsmoking volunteers who ranged in age from 25 to 50 years, who were taking no medications, and who had a negative history for peripheral vascular or gastrointestinal disease. A large percentage of the subjects participated in all four of the research studies. All subjects were placed on a bland diet 1 day before the examination and fasted 12 hours before their scan to minimize bowel gas. Duplex scanning was performed in a quiet, darkened room after each subject rested in the recumbent position for approximately 30 to 60 minutes. Instruction on breathing and breath holding was given before the scanning began. Subjects were asked not to talk and to remain as still as possible for the duration of the examination. Subject cooperation was necessary for the successful completion of the study. Multiple measurements were made over a 2- to 6-hour period on two or three separate occasions per subject, depending on the particular research study.

Instrumentation

A duplex scanner* combining B-mode imaging and pulsed Doppler ultrasound was used to measure blood velocity parameters and vessel diameters. A 3.28-MHz sector scan head was used for both Doppler and B-mode measurements. The pulsed Doppler sample volume size was kept constant with a length of 1.5 mm. All data were recorded on videotape or on hard copy with a thermal printer. Hard copies of baseline B-mode images were obtained for each vessel in longitudinal and transverse sections. These were used as references during subsequent scans to aid in accurate placement of the sample volume to the same vessel site. Calibration of the duplex scanner was performed with a Doppler string target and a tissue phantom before the liver duplex research was done.[7]

Scanning technique

Velocity waveforms and B-mode images were obtained from branches of the HA, PV, and HV. From an anterior midline approach, the proper HA was located by following the common HA from its origin. Placement of the sample volume in the proper HA avoided branch angle effects from the celiac axis and provided a straight segment of the HA to obtain Doppler angles of less than 60° (Fig. 124-1). The characteristic waveform of the HA shows slightly turbulent forward flow in systole and high diastolic forward flow and is representative of blood flow that supplies an organ with low vascular impedance.[8] Peak systolic velocities are in the range of 50 to 100 cm/sec (Fig. 124-2).

The main PV is formed by the splenic and superior mesenteric veins, and it courses in the hepatoduodenal ligament to the porta hepatis. Within the liver, PV branches run parallel to HA branches. By using a transverse approach in

*Acuson 128, Acuson Corp., Mountainview, Calif.

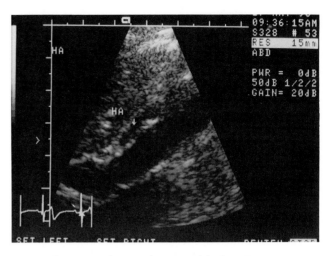

Fig. 124-1. The B-mode image of the hepatic artery.

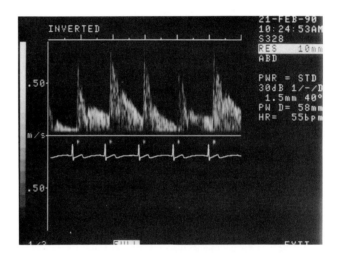

Fig. 124-2. The hepatic artery spectral waveform showing slightly turbulent forward flow in systole and high diastolic forward flow.

the right upper quadrant, the examiner followed the main PV to either a left or right PV branch (Fig. 124-3). Smaller, more favorable Doppler angles could be obtained in these branches. Because the walls of the PV are highly echogenic, they are easily distinguished from the HA and HVs. A normal PV waveform is characterized by continuous, mildly turbulent flow that varies with posture, exercise, dietary state, and respiration.[13] Mean and peak PV velocities range from 5 to 30 cm/sec (Fig. 124-4).

There are three major branches of the HV (right, middle, and left), which drain into the inferior vena cava. The HVs run between the hepatic segments. The hepatic veins were located by using a transverse approach in the right upper quadrant or by scanning between the ribs from a right lateral approach. The middle or right HVs were imaged and used for velocity and diameter measurements (Fig. 124-5). The

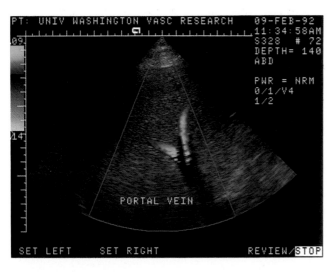

Fig. 124-3. The B-mode image of the main portal vein branching into the left and right portal veins.

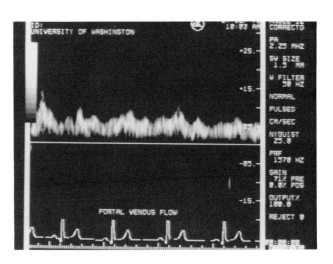

Fig. 124-4. A typical PV waveform characterized by slightly continuous, mildly turbulent flow.

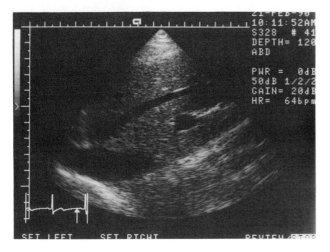

Fig. 124-5. The B-mode image of the middle hepatic vein.

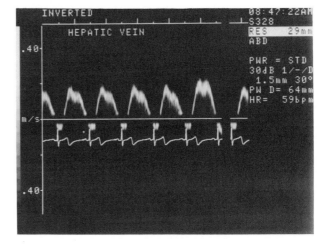

Fig. 124-6. An inverted hepatic vein waveform is obtained while the subject was breath holding at the end of expiration. This waveform is similar to the one of the vena cava and reflects the changes caused by the cardiac and respiratory cycles. A systolic reversal of flow in the waveform is due to the contraction of the right atrium.

characteristic HV flow pattern is similar to that of the vena cava and reflects the changes caused by the cardiac and respiratory cycles (Fig. 124-6). A systolic reversal of flow in the HV waveform is caused by the contraction of the right atrium. Peak systolic velocities range from 20 to 40 cm/sec depending on the angle of insonation.

Doppler angles and sample sites were held constant for each vessel for all study days. The Doppler sample volume was placed in the center of the flow stream to minimize branch angle effects associated with bifurcations and to avoid velocity gradients near the vessel walls.

An electrocardiogram with a cine loop function was used to obtain velocity and diameter measurements at specific times in the cardiac cycle. The sweep speed of the spectral display was reduced to 25 mm/sec, allowing for more cardiac cycles for the TAV measurements. This helped to reduce the beat-to-beat variability. Centering the zero baseline prevented skewing of the TAV, since the calculation of TAV incorporates the average value of weighted velocities on both sides of the baseline between the two calipers. The calculation of TAV is manufacturer specific, and the techniques described only pertain to a particular machine. The wall-filter setting was maintained at the lowest possible setting to prevent low frequencies from being eliminated.

All waveforms were obtained while the subject was holding a breath at the end of expiration. Pulsed Doppler spectral waveforms containing excessive noise caused by sample volume movement, wall motion, adjacent vessels, or an aliased signal were not used for analysis. Measurements obtained during rapid heart rates were also discarded.

Measurements

Peak systolic velocity (PSV), end-diastolic velocity (EDV), TAV, and vessel diameter measurements for the calculation of the area of an ellipse were obtained from the HA, PV, and HV. The PSV was determined by placing the caliper of the spectral display at the maximum velocity of a single representative cardiac cycle (Fig. 124-7). EDV was

determined by placing the caliper at the lowest velocity in diastole immediately before the systolic upstroke (Fig. 124-8). The TAV was obtained from the software within the duplex scanner. (It is the time average of the mean velocities of each of the velocity spectra that occur during an interval defined by the operator.) The intervals used began and ended with the same points in the cardiac cycle and typically included at least three to six cardiac cycles (Fig. 124-9).

For obtaining the cross-sectional vessel area, a static cross-sectional image of a specific vessel was captured on the screen for caliper placement. The first caliper was placed at the intima-lumen interface of the anterior wall, and the

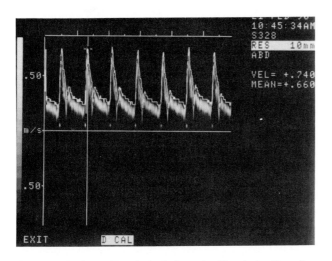

Fig. 124-7. Peak systolic velocity is determined by placing the caliper of the spectral display at the maximum velocity of a single representative cardiac cycle.

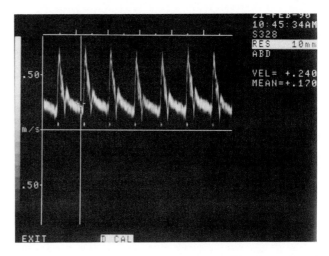

Fig. 124-8. End-diastolic velocity was determined by placing the caliper at the lowest velocity in diastole immediately before systolic upstroke.

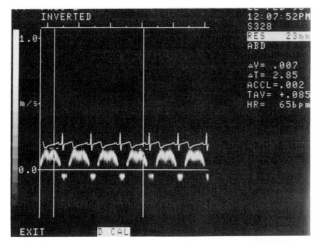

Fig. 124-9. The hepatic vein spectral waveform with a caliper placed at end-diastole of one cardiac cycle and a second caliper placed at end-diastole of the fourth subsequent cardiac cycle determining time average velocity (TAV). The TAV is a computer-derived value based on the time average of the mean velocities of each of the velocity spectra occurring during an interval defined by the operator.

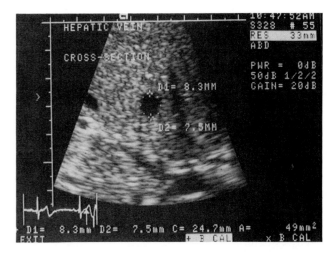

Fig. 124-10. The elliptical area of the hepatic vein. Diameter 1 (D1) is the distance between the anterior and posterior walls of the vessel cross section. Diameter 2 (D2) is then measured as the distance between the lateral walls at 90° to D1. Values for D1 and D2 are used to calculate the area of an ellipse (AE) as defined by the equation: AE = (D1 × D2 × 3.14/4).

second caliper was similarly placed at the posterior wall (Fig. 124-10). The distance between the anterior and posterior wall calipers was automatically measured and labeled as diameter 1 (D1). Diameter 2 (D2) is then measured as the distance between the lateral walls at 90° to D1.[7] The area of an ellipse was then calculated:

$$\text{Area of an ellipse} = (\text{D1} \times \text{D2} \times 3.14/4) \qquad (2)$$

Volume flow or HBF was then calculated with equation 1. End-diastolic ratio, which is the ratio of the EDV to the PSV, was also calculated. This ratio has been shown to reflect the degree of vascular resistance in the renal parenchyma.[8,10] Because increases in impedance of the liver are reflected in the waveform, the end-diastolic ratio was used to determine any changes in resistance after drug administration.

Sources of error

There are several potential sources of error in estimating blood flow with duplex ultrasound.[6,15,17] Volume flow measurements based on duplex ultrasound are calculated by using two values, the cross-sectional area of the vessel and the average rate of blood flow through the vessel over a specific period of time. Technical errors that contribute to the determination of blood flow include errors in the placement of calipers on the velocity waveforms and in the measurement of the vessel diameters, which is limited by the resolution of the B-mode image of the abdominal vessels.[15] Accurate repositioning of the Doppler sample volume during each repeat scan is necessary to provide measurement consistency.[6] There are several potential sources of error that can be introduced into the velocity measurements.[6,11,14] Errors in velocity determination are primarily caused by inaccuracy in measuring the angle of insonation of the Doppler beam. Because the cosine of this angle is used in the Doppler equation for calculating velocity from frequency shift, the extent of the error depends on the angle used. It increases as the angle approaches 90°.[11]

To appreciate the importance of HBF measurements, a brief review of the pharmacokinetics of drug metabolism and elimination is provided.

DRUG METABOLISM AND ELIMINATION

The liver is an important organ for the metabolism of many substrates. Drug molecules are one important class of substrates. Examples of drugs metabolized by the liver include theophylline, propranolol, warfarin, lidocaine, and carbamazepine. Under conditions that compromise the ability of the liver to metabolize (in effect, eliminate) drugs, the blood concentration of many drugs will be affected. Knowledge of the mechanism of hepatic drug metabolism is important to avoid potential drug toxicities.

HBF is an important determinant of drug elimination for many "high extraction ratio" drugs.[5] The extraction ratio actually quantifies the efficiency of the liver. A drug is considered to have a high extraction ratio if the liver is capable of extracting all or nearly all of the drug in one pass through the liver; that is, the extraction ratio is close to 1:

$$\text{ER} = \frac{C_A - C_V}{C_A} \qquad (3)$$

where ER is the extraction ratio and C_A and C_V denote drug concentrations in arterial and venous blood, respectively. It can be seen from this equation that when the liver is highly efficient at extracting a drug, the C_V approaches 0 and the ER approaches 1. Conversely, when the liver is inefficient at extracting a drug, the C_V is approximately equal to C_A, and the ER approaches 0. As a general rule, if the ER is greater than 0.8, the drug is considered to have a high extraction ratio. Examples of high extraction ratio drugs include propranolol, theophylline, and verapamil.

Hepatic drug clearance is a primary pharmacokinetic parameter that is related to the extraction ratio.[5] Clearance is actually a proportionality constant that relates rate of drug elimination to the blood concentration of the drug:

$$\text{Cl}_H = Q \times \text{ER} \qquad (4)$$

$$\text{Cl} = k \times V \qquad (5)$$

where Cl_H is hepatic drug clearance, Q denotes HBF, Cl is the overall systemic clearance of drug, k is the terminal elimination rate constant, and V is the apparent volume into which the drug distributes. In other words, clearance is the theoretical volume of blood from which all drug would appear to be removed on the basis of the apparent volume of drug distribution. Clearance is the pharmacokinetic parameter that actually determines the steady state concentration of a drug. As shown in equation 4, the elimination of high extraction ratio drugs is primarily dependent on HBF; therefore changes in the intrinsic ability to metabolize (the enzymatic quantity and/or quality of the liver) these drugs will have a minimal effect on systemic blood concentrations. That is, as ER approaches 1, Cl_H approximates HBF. For example, propranolol has an ER of approximately 0.8 and the average HBF is 1.5 L/min. If a patient is receiving a continuous intravenous infusion of 0.12 mg/min, the propranolol concentration after equilibration (C_{SS}, concentration at steady state) will be 0.1 mg/L (C_{SS} = rate of infusion divided by Cl_H). If HBF is increased to 3 L/min, the new C_{SS} will be 0.06 mg/L. This can be contrasted with a low ER drug such as theophylline. The ER of theophylline is approximately 0.06. With an infusion of 60 mg/hr and a QH of 1.5 L/min, the C_{SS} will be 10.7 mg/L. When the Q_H is changed to 3 L/min, C_{SS} only changes to 10.3 mg/L. This example reinforces the fact that changes in HBF have a much greater impact on steady-state drug concentrations of high extraction ratio drugs than on low extraction ratio drugs.

The difference between these types of drugs becomes even more dramatic when they are administered orally and systemic availability is effected. Presystemic elimination of the drug by the liver can be substantial when the drug has a high extraction ratio. This is because all drug administered orally must pass through the liver to reach the systemic circulation, and if the liver is efficient at extracting drug, much of the dose will be eliminated during the first pass. The systemic availability is the fraction of drug that reaches the systemic circulation after the first pass through the liver and is represented mathematically by:

$$F = 1 - ER \qquad (6)$$

where F is the fraction of the orally absorbed drug that reaches the systemic circulation. By changing the ER, the amount of drug systemically available will change. The extraction ratio can actually be affected by HBF.[5] That is, as blood flow increases, the ER actually decreases. This is believed to be due to the rate at which drug is being presented to the liver. If the rate is too fast, the liver's capacity to extract drug is surpassed, and drug simply passes through the liver without being extracted. This has been demonstrated in a clinical pharmacokinetic study in which hydralazine was administered concurrently with propranolol to transiently increase HBF.[9] The results of this study indicate that a greater concentration of propranolol was reached in the systemic circulation as the hydralazine dose was increased. The investigators concluded that this finding was probably due to a decreased removal of propranolol by the liver during initial transit from the gut to the systemic circulation. The authors postulate that one explanation for this is that the change in first-pass elimination is a transient change in splanchnic blood flow, altering the extraction ratio. On the basis of this information, if HBF is altered transiently during drug absorption and then returns to baseline thereafter, the elimination pharmacokinetics (after absorption) will be unaffected but the amount of drug that reaches the systemic circulation will change. This may have some significance in the clinical setting. That is, the amount of drug absorbed will increase, and this will result in an increase in the maximum drug concentration, which may have toxicologic or therapeutic implications.

RESULTS OF DUPLEX HBF MEASUREMENTS

Nifedipine is a calcium channel blocker that has been shown (with ICG methods) to increase HBF and was used as a probe in one study to determine whether duplex ultrasound can be used as a tool to estimate changes in HBF.[12] The effects of nifedipine on HBF were found to be more complex than a simple global increase in flow. The HA demonstrated a transient rise in blood flow soon after administration of

nifedipine, with a rapid return to baseline by 1 hour after dosing. Flow in the PV increased soon after drug administration, remained elevated for 3 hours, and then declined toward baseline. The flow changes in the HV paralleled those in the HA. The magnitude of the change in this vessel was greater than the changes in either the HA or HV.

Nitroglycerin has also been used as a probe, and the results indicate that the effects are highly complex, with blood flow decreasing in the HA and increasing in the HV.[13] The results of these two studies indicate that blood flow can be affected transiently and that this perturbation in flow may alter the disposition of co-administered drugs with a high extraction ratio as discussed earlier. Other drugs that have been studied with this technique are diclofenac and cimetidine.[2,3] Both of these drugs were found to have no effect on HBF. Knowledge of the effects of drugs on HBF is important because a drug may alter flow and ultimately affect the disposition of concurrently administered drugs.

REFERENCES

1. Bauer LA, Horn JR, Opheim KE: Variability of indocyanine green pharmacokinetics in healthy adults, *Clin Pharm* 8:54, 1989.
2. Bauer LA et al: Single and multiple doses of oral cimetidine do not change liver blood flow in humans, *Clin Pharmacol Ther* 48:195, 1990.
3. Bauer LA et al: Diclofenac does not change hepatic blood flow, *Clin Pharmacol Ther* 51:157, 1992 (abstract).
4. Bradley SE et al: The estimation of HBF in man, *J Clin Invest* 24:890, 1945.
5. Gibaldi M, Perrier D: *Pharmacokinetics*, ed 2, New York, 1980, Marcel Dekker.
6. Gill RW: Measurement of blood flow by ultrasound: accuracy and sources of error, *Ultrasound Med Biol* 11:625, 1985.
7. Horn JR et al: Estimation of hepatic blood flow in branches of hepatic vessels utilizing a noninvasive, duplex Doppler method, *J Clin Pharmacol* 30:922, 1990.
8. Kohler TR et al: Noninvasive diagnosis of renal artery stenosis by ultrasonic duplex scanning, *J Vasc Surg* 4:450, 1986.
9. McLean AJ et al: Interaction between oral propranolol and hydralazine, *Clin Pharmacol Ther* 27:726, 1980.
10. Norris CS et al: Noninvasive evaluation of renal artery stenosis and renovascular resistance, *J Vasc Surg* 1:192, 1984.
11. Phillips DJ et al: Should results of ultrasound Doppler studies be reported in units of frequency or velocity? *Ultrasound Med Biol* 15:205, 1989.
12. Reiss WG et al: The effects of oral nifedipine on HBF in humans, *Clin Pharmacol Ther* 50:379, 1991.
13. Reiss WG et al: The effects of sublingual nitroglycerin on HBF in volunteers, *Clin Pharmacol Ther* (submitted for publication).
14. Taylor DC et al: Duplex ultrasound scanning in the diagnosis of renal artery stenosis: a prospective evaluation, *J Vasc Surg* 7:363, 1988.
15. Taylor KJW et al: Blood flow in deep abdominal and pelvic vessels: ultrasound pulsed Doppler analysis, *Radiology* 154:487, 1985.
16. Zierler BK et al: Hepatic blood flow measurements by duplex ultrasound: how to minimize variability, *J Vasc Technol* 15:16, 1991.
17. Zierler BK et al: Accuracy of duplex scanning for measurement of arterial volume flow, *J Vasc Surg* 16:520, 1992.

INDEX